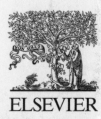
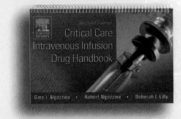
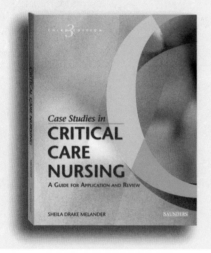
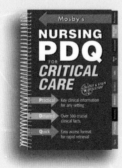
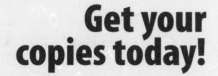

Thelan's

CRITICAL CARE NURSING

Diagnosis and Management

Thelan's
CRITICAL CARE NURSING

Diagnosis and Management

FIFTH EDITION

LINDA D. URDEN, DNSc, RN, CNA-BC, FAAN
Executive Director, Nursing Quality, Education & Research
Palomar Pomerado Health
Escondido, California;
Clinical Professor
Coordinator, Executive Nurse Leader Program
University of San Diego
San Diego, California

KATHLEEN M. STACY, MS, RN, CNS, CCRN
Nurse Manager/Critical Care Clinical Nurse Specialist
Intermediate Care Unit, Palomar Medical Center
Escondido, California;
Adjunct Faculty Member
School of Nursing, College of Health and Human Services
San Diego State University
San Diego, California

MARY E. LOUGH, MS, RN, CNS, CCRN, CNRN
Clinical Nurse Specialist, Medical/Surgical/Trauma ICU
Stanford University Hospital and Clinics
Stanford, California;
Associate Clinical Professor
Department of Physiological Nursing
University of California, San Francisco
San Francisco, California

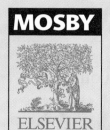
MOSBY
ELSEVIER

MOSBY
ELSEVIER

11830 Westline Industrial Drive
St. Louis, Missouri 63146

Notice

Nursing is an ever-changing field. Standard safety precautions must be followed, but as new
research and clinical experience broaden our knowledge, changes in treatment and drug therapy
may become necessary or appropriate. Readers are advised to check the most current product
information provided by the manufacturer of each drug to be administered to verify the
recommended dose, the method and duration of administration, and contraindications. It is the
responsibility of the licensed prescriber, relying on experience and knowledge of the patient, to
determine dosages and the best treatment for each individual patient. Neither the publisher nor the
author assumes any liability for any injury and/or damage to persons or property arising from this
publication.

The Publisher

ISBN-13   978-0-323-03248-3
ISBN-10   0-323-03248-6

Executive Publisher: Barbara Nelson Cullen
Senior Developmental Editor: Victoria Bruno
Publishing Services Manager: Deborah Vogel
Project Manager: Mary Drone
Designer: Jyotika Shroff

Printed in the United States of America

Last digit is print number: 9   8   7   6   5   4   3   2   1

About the Authors

Linda D. Urden, DNSc, RN, CNA-BC, FAAN

Linda Urden received her diploma in nursing from Barnes Hospital, St. Louis, Missouri; BSN from Pepperdine University, Malibu, California; MN, Cardiovascular Clinical Nurse Specialist, from UCLA; and DNSc from the University of San Diego. She is certified in Nursing Administration by the American Nurses Credentialing Center and is a Fellow in the American Academy of Nursing. Linda has held a variety of clinical and administrative positions, with accountabilities for quality, research, education, advanced practice, and outcomes management and measurement. In her various positions she has striven to create cultures that are sensitive to differentiated practice and to establish mechanisms that promote evidence-based practice and foster professional practice. She is the co-author of *Critical Care Nursing: Diagnosis and Management* and *Priorities in Critical Care Nursing*. Other publications are in the areas of heart failure, ethics, research, outcomes measurement, management and care delivery redesign, executive decision support databases, and collaborative practice models. In addition, she is a member of editorial boards and is a peer reviewer for several nursing journals. Her research is focused on clinical, fiscal, quality, and behavioral outcomes of care delivery and services.

Kathleen M. Stacy, MS, RN, CNS, CCRN

Kathleen Stacy has been a nurse for 27 years, the majority of which she has spent working in critical care. She graduated in 1978 with a BS in nursing from the State University of New York at Plattsburgh and in 1989 with an MS in critical care nursing from San Diego State University. She has held a variety of positions, including staff nurse, clinical educator, and outcomes manager. Currently Kathleen is the Nurse Manager and Clinical Nurse Specialist for the Intermediate Care Unit at Palo-mar Medical Center. As an advanced practitioner Kathleen collaborates with the health care team to facilitate the achievement of optimal outcomes for the critically ill patient. As a consultant she facilitates change to improve patient care. As an educator Kathleen develops and implements programs to assist the staff with acquisition of the skills and knowledge needed to care for the critically ill patient. As a researcher she facilitates, uses, and conducts nursing research. Kathleen also holds an adjunct faculty position at San Diego State University School of Nursing and has co-authored two critical care textbooks: *Critical Care Nursing: Diagnosis and Management* and *Priorities in Critical Care Nursing*.

Mary E. Lough, MS, RN, CNS, CCRN, CNRN

Mary Lough is a critical care nurse with more than 30 years of experience as a staff nurse, educator, and clinical nurse specialist. Mary received her BSN from the University of Manchester in England and her MS in cardiovascular nursing from the University of California, San Francisco (UCSF). She is the clinical nurse specialist for the medical/surgical/ trauma ICU at Stanford University Hospital and Clinics in Palo Alto, California. She is also an associate clinical professor in the Department of Physiological Nursing at her alma mater, UCSF. Mary has her own company called "Education PRN," through which she provides lectures and consulting.

Mary has been involved with all five editions of *Critical Care Nursing: Diagnosis and Management* as a writer or co-author and she also has published many other articles and research abstracts. As a clinician Mary appreciates the benefits of a clinically grounded textbook because when she began her career as a critical care nurse, so little information was available. Mary is married, has two children, and lives in San Carlos, California.

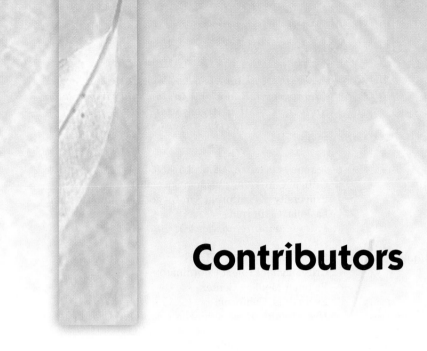

Contributors

Kara Adams, MS, RN, CCRN
Clinical Nurse Specialist
University Medical Center
Tucson, Arizona
Trauma

Deborah Barnes, MSN, RN, CCRN
AACN Practice Specialist
American Association of Critical-Care Nurses
Aliso Viejo, California
Perianesthesia Management

Patricia Gauntlett Beare, MSN, MED, PhD, RN
Louisiana State University Health Science School of Nursing
New Orleans, Louisiana
Gerontologic Alterations and Management

Jamie Blazek, BSN, MPH, FNP-C, CCTC, CNN
Liver Transplant Nurse Practitioner
Ochsner Clinic Foundation
Ochsner Multi-Organ Transplant Center
New Orleans, Louisiana
Organ Donation and Transplantation (Liver Transplantation)

Kim Blount, MSN, RN, CCRN
Cardiovascular Clinical Nurse Specialist
Carolinas Medical Center
Charlotte, North Carolina
Patient/Family Education

Mary Jo Burton, BSN, RN
Manager of Clinical Operations Organ Transplant Unit
Indiana University Hospital
Clarion Health Partners
Indianapolis, Indiana
Organ Donation and Transplantation (Kidney and Pancreas Transplantation)

Beverly Ann Carlson, MS, RN, CNS
Senior Research Consultant
Sharp Healthcare;
Lecturer, School of Nursing
San Diego State University
San Diego, California
Shock

Diana Clark, BS, MS, RN
President and Chief Operating Officer
LifeCenter Northwest Organ Donation Network
Bellevue, Washington
Organ Donation and Transplantation (Donor Management)

Karyn Denton, BSN
Senior Vice President and Chief Operating Officer
LifeCenter Northwest Organ Donation Agency
Bellevue, Washington
Organ Donation and Transplantation (Donor Management)

Joni L. Dirks, MS, RN, CCRN
Critical Care Educator
Sacred Heart Medical Center
Spokane, Washington
Cardiovascular Therapeutic Management

Lorraine Fitzsimmons, DNS, FNP, BC
Chair
Advanced Practice Nursing of Adults and Elderly;
Director
Adult and Geriatric Nurse Practitioner Program
San Diego State University School of Nursing
San Diego, California
Systemic Inflammatory Response Syndrome and Multiple Organ Dysfunction Syndrome

Celine Gelinas, PhD, BSc, MSc, RN
Postdoctoral Student
School of Nursing
McGill University
Montreal, Quebec
Canada
Pain and Pain Management

Major Pamela F. Godinez, BSN, MS, RN, CCRN
Clinical Nurse Specialist
Walter Reed Army Medical Center
Washington, D.C.
Gastrointestinal Disorders and Therapeutic Management

Christine Hartley, MS, RN, CNS
Heart and Lung Transplant Coordinator
Stanford Hospital and Clinics
Stanford, California
Organ Donation and Transplantation (Immune System, Transplant Drugs, Heart Transplantation, Heart and Heart-Lung Transplantation, Lung Transplantation)

Sara Horton-Deutsch, RN, DNSc, APN
Associate Professor
Indiana University School of Nursing
Indianapolis, Indiana
Psychosocial Issues

Karen Johnson, PhD, RN, CCRN
Associate Professor
University of Maryland School of Nursing
Baltimore, Maryland
Trauma

Karin T. Kirchhoff, MSN, MS, PhD
Rodefer Chair and Professor
School of Nursing
University of Wisconsin
Madison, Wisconsin
End of Life Issues

Julene B. Kruithof, MSN, RN, CCRN
Critical Care/Cardiovascular Educator
Spectrum Health
Grand Rapids, Michigan
High-Risk and Critical Care Obstetric Issues

Mary E. Lough, MS, RN, CNS, CCRN, CNRN
Clinical Nurse Specialist
Medical/Surgical/Trauma ICU
Stanford University Hospital and Clinics
Stanford, California;
Associate Clinical Professor
Department of Physiological Nursing
University of California, San Francisco
San Francisco, California
Agitation and Sedation Management; Cardiovascular Anatomy and Physiology; Cardiovascular Clinical Assessment; Cardiovascular Diagnostic Procedures; Cardiovascular Disorders; Renal Anatomy and Physiology; Renal Clinical Assessment and Diagnostic

Procedures; Renal Disorders and Therapeutic Management; Endocrine Anatomy and Physiology; Endocrine Clinical Assessment and Diagnostic Procedures; Endocrine Disorders and Therapeutic Management

Jeanne M. Maiden, MS, RN, CNS, CCRN
Critical Care Clinical Nurse Specialist
University of California San Diego/ Thornton Hospital
La Jolla, California
Pulmonary Diagnostic Procedures

Barbara Mayer, BSN, MS, RN
CNS/Magnet Project Coordinator
Palomar Medical Center
Escondida, California
Hematologic Disorders and Oncologic Emergencies

Kammie Monarch, MS, JD, RN
Chief Operating Officer
Sigma Theta Tau International Honor Society of Nursing
Indianapolis, Indiana
Legal Issues

Kerri J. Oates, MSN, MJ, CRNP
Pediatric Nurse Practitioner
Children's Hospital of Philadelphia
Philadelphia, Pennsylvania
The Pediatric Patient in the Adult Critical Care Unit

Colleen O'Leary-Kelley, PhD, RN, CCRN, CNS
Associate Professor
School of Nursing
San Jose State University
San Jose, California
Nutrition Alterations and Management

Laura Pagano, MS, ANP-GNP, CNS, CCRN, CDR
LCDR
US Navy Nurse Corps
Systemic Inflammatory Response Syndrome and Multiple Organ Dysfunction Syndrome

Beth Remsburg-Bell, MSN, RN
Clinical Operations Director
Duke Birthing Center
Duke University Health System
North Durham, North Carolina
High-Risk and Critical Care Obstetric Issues

Karen L. Rice, MSN, APRN, BC
Adult Nurse Practitioner/Clinical Specialist
Ochsner Clinic Foundation
New Orleans, Louisiana
Gerontologic Alterations and Management

Debra L. Ryan, BSN, RN, MN, CCRN
Clinical Nurse Specialist, Adult Critical Care
Spectrum Health
Grand Rapids, Michigan
High-Risk and Critical Care Obstetric Issues

Mary Schira, PhD, APRN, BC, ACNP
Associate Clinical Professor and Director
Acute Care and Emergency Nurse Practitioner Programs
The University of Texas at Arlington School of Nursing
Arlington, Texas
Renal Anatomy and Physiology; Renal Clinical
Assessment and Diagnostic Procedures

Carrie Sona, MSN, RN
Clinical Nurse Specialist, Surgical Services
Barnes Jewish Hospital
St. Louis, Missouri
Burns

Kathleen M. Stacy, MS, RN, CNS, CCRN
Nurse Manager/Critical Care Clinical Nurse Specialist
Intermediate Care Unit
Palomar Medical Center
Escondido, California;
Adjunct Faculty Member
School of Nursing, College of Health and Human Services
San Diego State University
San Diego, California
Pulmonary Anatomy and Physiology; Pulmonary Clinical
Assessment; Pulmonary Disorders; Pulmonary
Therapeutic Management; Neurologic Clinical
Assessment; Neurologic Disorders and Therapeutic

Management; Gastrointestinal Anatomy and Physiology;
Gastrointestinal Clinical Assessment and Diagnostic
Procedures; Nursing Management Plans

Sheila Cox Sullivan, MSN, PhD, RN, AS
Associate Professor and Associate Dean
Harding University College of Nursing
Searcy, Arkansas
Sleep Alterations and Management

Linda D. Urden, DNSc, RN, CNA-BC, FAAN
Executive Director
Nursing Quality, Education & Research
Palomar Pomerado Health
Escondido California;
Clinical Professor
Coordinator, Executive Nurse Leader Program
University of San Diego
San Diego California
Critical Care Nursing Practice; Ethical Issues

Anne W. Wojner, PhD, RN, CCRN, FAAN
President and Principle-Neuroscience Research
Health Outcomes Institute
The Woodlands, Texas
Neurologic Anatomy and Physiology

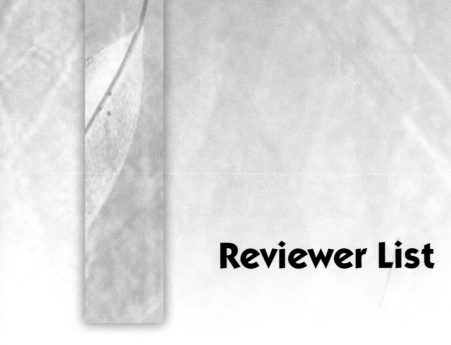

Reviewer List

Mike Aldridge, MSN, RN, CCRN
Nurse Educator
Pediatric Intensive Care Unit
Children's Hospital of Austin
Austin, Texas

Eugene F. Anderson, MSN, RN, CCRN
Clinical Educator
Good Shepherd Specialty Hospital
Allentown, Pennsylvania

Kathryn C. Anderson, RN, CEN, BA, ACLS
Vernon Urgent Care
Vernon, New Jersey

Marie K. Arnone, MA, RN, CCRN
Swedish Medical Center Providence Campus
Seattle, Washington

Karen K. Carlson, MN, RN, CCNS
Critical Care Clinical Specialist
Carlson Consulting Group
Bellevue, Washington

Elizabeth M. Carson EdD, RN
Saint Anthony College of Nursing
Rockford, Illinois

Mary Franklin, MS, RN, APRN, BC
Wayne State University College of Nursing
Detroit, Michigan

Cynthia A. Goodrich, MS, RN, CCRN
Airlift Northwest
Seattle, Washington

Allen Hanberg, MSN-RN
Weber State University
Ogden, Utah

Karen L. Harvey, RN
Spectrum Health Regional Burn Center
Grand Rapids, Michigan

Patricia A. Henry, MSN, RN, CNS, FNP, CCRN
Salinas Valley Memorial Healthcare System
Salinas, California

Melissa Lynn Hutchinson, RN, MN, CCRN, CWCN
VA Puget Sound Health Care System
Seattle, Washington

Marjorie Jannelle Justice, BSN, RN
St. Mary's Health System Inc.
Knoxville, Tennessee

Karen S. Kesten, MSN, RN, PCCN, CCRN
Washington Adventist Hospital
Takoma Park, Maryland;
Graduate Program
Georgetown University School of Nursing and Health Studies
Washington, D.C.

Dana Michelle Kyles, BSN, RN
Harborview Medical Center
Seattle, Washington

Janice G. Lanham, MSN, RN, FNP
Critical Care Clinical Nurse Specialist
Greenville Memorial Hospital
Greenville, South Carolina;
Faculty
University of Phoenix Online

Denise M. Lawrence, MS, ACNP
Hartford Hospital
Hartford, Connecticut

Rosanna LaMorte Marker-Faour, MSN, RN, CSN
Duquesne University
Pittsburgh, Pennsylvania

Abigail L. Plambeck, BSN, RN
Self-employed
Full time freelance writer for "The Wordsmith"
Milwaukee, Wisconsin

Teresita F. Proctor, MS, APRN, BC
Trinitas School of Nursing
Union County College
Elizabeth, New Jersey

Scott Thigpen, MSN, RN, CCRN, CEN
Assistant Professor of Nursing
South Georgia College
Division of Nursing
Douglas, Georgia

Susan C. Vaughn, MSN(c), BSN, RN
Home Care Specialist
Gentiva Health Services
Charlotte, North Carolina

Ron Whitten, MSN, RN, CEN, CCRN, ARNP
Kennewick General Hospital
Kennewick, Washington

Judith L. Williamson, MS, RN, AOCN
OSF Saint Anthony Medical Center
Rockford, Illinois

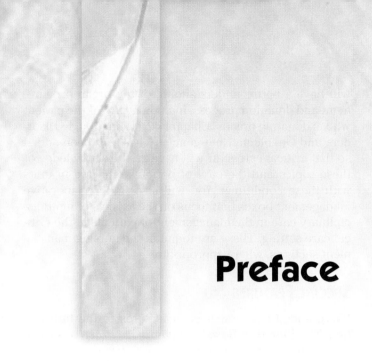

Preface

We are most grateful to the many students and nurses who made the previous editions of this book successful. The success has validated our commitment to proclaim the outstanding contributions of critical care nurses and to promote evidence-based nursing practice in the complex critical care environment. We actively solicited feedback from users of the previous editions and eagerly incorporated their comments and suggestions regarding format, content, and organization. And so, with this fifth edition, we again present to you a book that is thorough in all that is most pertinent to critical care nurses in a format that is organized for clarity and comprehension.

ORGANIZATION

The book's ten units are again organized around alterations in dimensions of human functioning that span biopsychosocial realms.

The content of Unit I, "Foundations of Critical Care Nursing," forms the basis of practice, regardless of the physiologic alterations of the critically ill patient. Although chapters in the book may be studied in any sequence, we recommend that Chapter 1, "Critical Care Nursing Practice," be studied first because it clarifies the major assumptions on which the entirety of the book is based. Chapter 2, "Ethical Issues," delineates ethical theories and strategies for dealing with the ethical dilemmas that arise on a daily basis in critical care. Chapter 3, "Legal Issues," provides a basis of information to help the critical care nurse be cognizant of practice issues that may have legal implications. Teaching and learning theory and strategies to best meet the learning needs of critical care patients are delineated in Chapter 4, "Patient/Family Education." Chapter 5, "Psychosocial Alterations," examines the theoretic basis and nursing process for alterations in self-concept and coping. Chapter 6, "Sleep Alterations and Management," examines a perennial problem in critical care. Chapter 7, "Nutritional Alterations and Management," examines the nutritional needs of the critically ill patient and provides specific recommendations for different disorders. The concepts of pain management in the critically ill are discussed in Chapter 8, "Pain and Pain Management." "Agitation and Sedation Management" are described in Chapter 9. Chapter 10, "End-of-Life Issues" delineates special needs for dealing with end of life and palliative care. Unit II, "Special Populations," addresses the needs of the critically ill pediatric, obstetric, and geriatric patient in the critical care unit, as well as the management of the recovery of the perianesthesia patient.

Unit III, "Cardiovascular Alterations" and Unit IV, "Pulmonary Alterations" are each structured with the following chapters:
- Anatomy and Physiology
- Clinical Assessment
- Diagnostic Procedures
- Disorders
- Therapeutic Management

This organization permits easy retrieval of information for students and clinicians and provides flexibility for the instructor to individualize teaching methods by assigning chapters that best suit student needs. Unit V, "Neurologic Alterations"; Unit VI, "Renal Alterations"; Unit VII, "Gastrointestinal Alterations"; and Unit VIII, "Endocrine Alterations," are organized similarly. However, in these units the assessment parameters such as clinical and diagnostic procedures are discussed in one chapter. In addition, disorders and therapeutic management are combined into one chapter.

Unit IX, "Multisystem Alterations," covers disorders that affect multiple body systems and necessitate discussion as a separate category. Unit IX consists of six chapters: Trauma, Shock, Systemic Inflammatory Response Syndrome and Multiple Organ Dysfunction Syndrome, Burns, Organ Donation and Transplantation, and Hematologic Disorders and Oncologic Emergencies.

Unit X, "Nursing Management Plans," contains management plans organized alphabetically by nursing diagnosis for easy access by students and practitioners.

Finally, the Appendix, "Physiologic Formulas for Critical Care," features commonly encountered hemodynamic, pulmonary, and other calculations and is presented in easily understood formulas. Recommendations for nutritional supplements also are included.

NURSING DIAGNOSIS AND MANAGEMENT

A dominant theme of the book continues to be nursing diagnosis and management, reflecting the strength of critical care nursing practice. Wherever possible, evidence-based critical care practice is incorporated into nursing interventions. To foster critical thinking and decision making, a boxed "menu" of nursing diagnoses complete with specific etiologic or related factors accompanies each medical disorder and major medical treatment discussions and directs the learner to Unit X, where appropriate nursing management is detailed. To facilitate student learning, the nursing management plans incorporate nursing diagnosis definition, etiologic or related factors, clinical manifestations, and interventions with rationale. The nursing management plans are liberally cross-referenced throughout the book for easy retrieval by the reader.

NEW TO THIS EDITION

We are very excited to provide you with a full-color text this edition. The full-color design and illustrations visually enhance the text, making it more appealing to the reader. Chapter 9, "Agitation and Sedation Management" has been added as a separate chapter due to the importance of these topics, related patient safety issues, and the increasing need for knowledge and competencies for nurses in these areas. Chapter 10, "End-of-Life Issues," has been added to this edition to enhance critical care nurse knowledge and understanding of the issues surrounding end of life, including palliative care and support for patients, families, and care providers. In Chapter 41, "Organ Donation and Transplantation," important information on the organ donation and procurement process has been added. It is believed that the learner

will have a better understanding of the organ procurement and donation process, including care of the patient who is donating organs. Chapter 42, "Hematologic Disorders and Oncologic Emergencies," has also been added so that critical care staff will have greater knowledge of these topics and the care of patients who are in units with these conditions. You will also find Collaborative Management boxes that focus on the aspects of multidisciplinary care in the management of patients in the critical care setting. These are found in the nursing management sections, where appropriate.

SPECIAL FEATURES

We've added two new special features to the fifth edition. The *Evidence-Based Collaborative Practice* special feature highlights important research-based articles on key topics in critical care nursing. The *Patient Safety Alert* feature highlights safety issues for the learner.

We've also retained many of the special features from the previous edition. *Clinical Applications* boxes are placed in most chapters or units. These cases promote student learning and critical thinking by illustrating the clinical course of a patient experiencing the history, clinical manifestations, treatment, and outcomes discussed in the related unit or chapter. Rationale for the clinical applications, continuations of the clinical applications discussed in the book, and additional clinical applications and questions are included on the Evolve website, which is available to all who purchase this text.

Nursing Interventions Classification (NIC) boxes are placed in the Therapeutic Management chapters. These boxes list the important nursing actions for a variety of nursing interventions that would be commonly incorporated in the management of a critically ill patient requiring a specific therapeutic treatment, such as mechanical ventilation. *Pharmacologic Management* tables are also found in the Therapeutic Management chapters. These boxes outline the common medications, along with any special considerations, used in treatment of the different disorders presented in the text. *Patient Education* boxes are placed in the Disorders chapters. These boxes list the special topics that should be taught to the patient and family to prepare them for discharge. Information that should be included as part of the patient's history has been incorporated into *Data Collection* boxes located in the Clinical Assessment chapters.

ANCILLARY PACKAGE

We are pleased to have a new, comprehensive student ancillary package for this edition: a new student CD-ROM bound into the text and the Evolve Learning Resources companion website for students and instructors.

STUDENT ANCILLARIES

This edition comes with a **new CD-ROM and companion Evolve Learning Resources** for students. The Evolve website is available at http://evolve.elsevier.com/Urden/criticalcare/

The new **Student CD-ROM** packaged with the text and the Evolve website both contain the following:

- Open Book Quizzes consisting of crossword puzzles, multiple-choice questions, fill-in-the-blank questions, and matching questions for each chapter.
- Monographs for the top 100 critical care drugs from **Mosby's Drug Consult.**
- A selection of assessment animations, audio/video clips, and images.
- Selected animations from **Pathophysiology Online,** including cardioembolic stroke and the six hallmarks of cancer.
- Fifteen procedures from the new edition of the **AACN Procedure Manual** linked to appropriate content in the corresponding chapter.
- A 200 question sample certification examination from **Dennison: Pass CCRN!, second edition.**
- Selected entries on Deep Vein Thrombosis and Pulmonary Embolism, and Acute Myocardial Infarction from **Schell: Critical Care Nursing Secrets.**
- PowerPoint presentation on sinus rhythm from **Aehlert: ECGs Made Easy, third edition** provides basic information and reinforces lectures on recognizing rhythms.
- Specific content accompanied by audio heart sounds and murmurs from **Erickson: Heart Sounds and Murmurs Across the Lifespan, fourth edition** provide better understanding of this complex concept for the student.
- **Discussions for the Clinical Applications** include the rationale for the clinical applications, continuations of the clinical application discussed in the book, and additional clinical applications and questions.
- Concept Map Creator allows users to create customized concept maps.
- WebLinks (Evolve only) are updated regularly and are organized by chapter, and gives the user the opportunity to explore additional content sources.

INSTRUCTOR ANCILLARIES

The Instructor's Resource, available both on the Evolve website and CD-ROM, provides a variety of aids to help enhance classroom instruction. Instructors also have access to the student resources listed above. The Instructor's Resource includes the following:

- **Instructor's Manual** complete with an overview, objectives, chapter outline, and teaching strategies for each chapter.
- **Test Bank** consists of approximately 1200 questions, including 200 in the alternate NCLEX format
- **PowerPoint** presentation by chapter consisting of a total of approximately 1500 lecture slides.
- **Image Collection** with approximately 400 images from the text and additional sources.
- **WebLinks** to various related websites that are keyed to the content of the book and constantly updated.

The **Evolve Learning System** is an interactive learning environment that works in coordination with *Thelan's Critical Care Nursing,* **fifth edition,** to provide Internet-based course management tools you can use to reinforce and expand concepts. You can use Evolve to:

- Publish your class syllabus, outline, and lecture notes.
- Set up "virtual office hours" and e-mail communication.
- Share important dates and information through the online class *Calendar.*
- Encourage student participation through *Chat Rooms* and *Discussion Boards.*

Thelan's Critical Care Nursing: Diagnosis and Management, fifth edition, represents our continued commitment to bringing you the best in all things a textbook can offer: the best and brightest in contributing and consulting authors, the latest in scientific research befitting the current state of health care and nursing, an organizational format that exercises diagnostic reasoning skills and is logical and consistent, and outstanding artwork and illustrations that enhance student learning. We pledge our continued commitment to excellence in critical care education.

Linda D. Urden
Kathleen M. Stacy
Mary E. Lough

Acknowledgments

A project of this book's magnitude is never merely the work of its authors. The concerted talent, hard work, and inspiration of a multitude of people have produced *Thelan's Critical Care Nursing: Diagnosis and Management*, fifth edition, and have helped to make it the state-of-the-science text we affirm it to be. A "tradition of publishing excellence" has been evident throughout our partnership with Elsevier. We deeply appreciate the assistance of Barbara Nelson Cullen, Executive Publisher, and Victoria Bruno, Senior Developmental Editor, who have helped us document and refine our ideas and transform our book into a reality. Their creativity, expertise, availability, and generosity of time and resources have been invaluable to us throughout this endeavor. We are also grateful to Mary Drone, Project Manager, for her scrupulous attention to detail.

Finally, we wish to thank those authors who contributed work to the first four editions of this book. Without the foundation they provided, a fifth edition would not have been born. We would like to acknowledge especially Lynne A. Thelan for her dedication to excellence and serving as the lead editor for three editions of *Critical Care Nursing: Diagnosis and Management*.

Linda D. Urden
Kathleen M. Stacy
Mary E. Lough

Contents

Detailed Contents

FOUNDATIONS OF CRITICAL CARE NURSING

CHAPTER 1

Critical Care Nursing Practice

OVERVIEW

Health care is undergoing dramatic change at a speed that makes it almost impossible to remain current and be proactive. The chaos and multiple challenges facing health care providers and consumers are evident in critical care, where new treatment modalities and technology interface with the continuing effort to strive for quality care and positive outcomes. Efficiency and cost-effectiveness in relation to health care services are frequently discussed and emphasized to all health care practitioners. To some, it appears that quality patient care has taken a back seat to the emphasis on cost containment and that quality and cost-effectiveness are not congruent. It is incumbent on all critical care health care providers to face these challenges both from their individual discipline's scope of practice and collectively from collaborative and interdisciplinary approaches.

The ever-changing health care environment creates multiple challenges for both providers and consumers of care. Sensitivity to the appropriate time to eliminate or modify practices and adopt innovations is key to maintaining quality, cost-effective care delivery. Willingness to step outside of traditional structures and roles is the first step in making necessary changes. Change is constant. Flexibility and adaptation to change are essential to maintaining personal and organizational balance and to surviving in today's health care environment.

The purpose of this chapter is to provide an overview of the evolution of critical care and to describe current issues and trends affecting the critical care nurse and interdisciplinary team. This chapter serves as the framework for the remainder of the book in the areas of professional nurse decision making, holistic care, and interdisciplinary collaboration.

HISTORY OF CRITICAL CARE

Critical care evolved from a recognition that the needs of patients with acute, life-threatening illness or injury could be better met if the patients were organized into distinct areas of the hospital. In the 1800s Florence Nightingale described the advantages of placing patients recovering from surgery in a separate area of the hospital. A three-bed postoperative neurosurgical intensive care unit was opened in the early 1900s at Johns Hopkins Hospital in Baltimore. This was soon followed by a premature infant unit in Chicago.[1]

Major societal issues also affected the development of intensive care as a specialty. During World War II, shock wards were established to care for those critically injured. The nursing shortage after the war forced the grouping of postoperative patients into designated recovery areas so that appropriate monitoring and care could be provided. The technologies and combat experiences of health care providers during the wars of the twentieth century also provided an impetus for specialized medical and nursing care in the civilian setting. The 1950s brought the new technology of mechanical ventilation and also the need to group patients receiving this new therapy into one location. By 1997 more than 5000 intensive care units were in operation in hospitals in the United States.[1]

CRITICAL CARE NURSING

Critical care nursing was organized into a specialty only less than 40 years ago; before that time critical care nursing was practiced wherever there were critically ill patients.[2] The development of new medical interventions and technology resulted in an increasing recognition that nursing was important in the monitoring and observation of critically ill patients. Physicians depended on nurses to watch for critical changes in the condition of patients in the physicians' absence and, sometimes, depended on the nurses to initiate emergency medical treatment.

As sophisticated technology began to support more elaborate medical interventions, hospitals began to organize separate units to make more efficient use of equipment and specially trained staff. Postoperative care, once provided by private duty nurses on general nursing wards throughout the hospital, was moved into recovery rooms where nurses with specialized knowledge regarding anesthesia recovery provided the patient care. Medical and surgical intensive care units served to segregate the most critically ill patients to locations where they could be cared for by nurses with specialized knowledge in those areas of care. By the 1960s nurses had begun to specialize their knowledge and practice into focused areas such as coronary care, nephrology, and intensive care. In the hospital units established for patients needing such specialized care, nurses assumed many functions and responsibilities formerly reserved for physicians and assumed a new authority by virtue of their knowledge and expertise.[3]

CONTEMPORARY CRITICAL CARE

Today critical care is provided to patients by a multidisciplinary team of health care professionals who have in-depth education in the specialty field of critical care. The team consists of physician intensivists, specialty physicians, nurses, advanced practice nurses and other specialty nurse clinicians, pharmacists, respiratory therapy practitioners, other specialized therapists and clinicians, social workers, and clergy. Critical care is provided in specialized units or departments, and importance is placed on the continuum of care, with an efficient transition of care from one setting to another.

Critical care patients are those who are at high risk for actual or potential; life-threatening health problems. Those who are more critically ill require more intensive and vigilant nursing care. There are over 400,000 nurses in the United States who care for critically ill patients. These nurses practice in a variety of settings: adult, pediatric, and neonatal intensive care units; step down, telemetry, progressive or transitional care units; cardiac catheterization labs; and postoperative recovery units.[4]

CRITICAL CARE NURSING ROLES

Nurses provide and contribute to the care of critically ill patients in a variety of roles. The most prevalent role for the professional registered nurse is that of direct care provider. The American Association of Critical-Care Nurses (AACN) has delineated role responsibilities important for the critical care nurse[4] (Box 1-1).

EXPANDED-ROLE NURSING POSITIONS

Expanded-role nursing positions interact with critical care patients, families, and the health care team. Nurse case managers work closely with the care providers to ensure appropriate, timely care and services and to promote continuity of care from one setting to another.

Other nurse clinicians such as patient educators, cardiac rehabilitation specialists, physician office nurses, and infection control specialists also contribute to the care. The specific types of expanded-role nursing positions are determined by patient needs and individual organizational resources.

ADVANCED PRACTICE NURSES

Advanced practice nurses (APNs) have met educational and clinical requirements beyond the basic nursing educational requirements for all nurses. The most commonly seen advanced practice nurses in the critical care areas are the clinical nurse specialist (CNS) and the nurse practitioner (NP) or acute care nurse practitioner (ACNP). APNs have a broad depth of knowledge and expertise in their specialty area and manage complex clinical and systems issues. The organizational system and existing resources of an institution determine what roles may be needed and how the roles function.

CNSs serve in specialty roles that use their clinical, teaching, research, leadership, and consultative abilities. They work in direct clinical roles and systems or administrative roles and in various other settings in the health care system. They may be organized by specialty, such as cardiovascular, or by function, such as cardiac rehabilitation. CNSs also may be designated as case managers for specific patient populations.

NPs and ACNPs manage direct clinical care of a group of patients and have various levels of prescriptive au-

---

Box 1-1

AACN CRITICAL CARE NURSE ROLE RESPONSIBILITIES

- Respect and support the right of the patient or patient's designated surrogate to autonomy and informed decision making.
- Intervene when the best interest of the patient is in question.
- Help the patient obtain necessary care.
- Respect the values, beliefs, and rights of the patient.
- Provide education and support help to the patient or patient's designated surrogate to make decisions.
- Represent the patient in accordance with the patient's choices.
- Support the decisions of the patient or patient's designated surrogate or transfer care to an equally qualified critical care nurse.
- Intercede for patients who cannot speak for themselves in situations that require immediate attention.
- Monitor and safeguard the quality of care that the patient receives.
- Act as liaison between the patient, the patient's family and other health care professionals.

From AACN Critical Care Nursing Fact Sheet, website: www.aacn.org, About Critical Care Nursing (Press Room).

thority, depending on the state and practice area in which they work. They also provide care consistency, interact with families, plan for patient discharge, and provide teaching to patients, families, and other members of the heath care team.[5]

CRITICAL CARE PROFESSIONAL ORGANIZATIONS

Professional organizations support critical care practitioners by providing numerous resources and networks. The Society of Critical Care Medicine (SCCM) is a multidisciplinary, multispecialty, international organization. Its mission is to secure the highest quality, cost-efficient care for all critically ill patients.[1] Numerous publications and educational opportunities provide cutting-edge critical care information to critical care practitioners.

The organization most closely associated with critical care nurses is the American Association of Critical-Care Nurses (AACN). It is the world's largest specialty nursing organization and was created in 1969. The purpose of AACN is "to promote the health and welfare of those experiencing critical illness or injury by advancing the art and science of critical care nursing and promoting environments that facilitate comprehensive professional nursing practice."[6] The top priority of the organization is education of the critical care nurse. AACN publishes numerous documents related to the specialty and is at the forefront of setting professional standards of care.

AACN serves its members through a national organization and many local chapters. The AACN Certification Corporation, a separate company, develops and administers a Critical Care Registered Nurse (CCRN) certification examination. The certification is valid for a 3-year period and is offered in adult, pediatric, neonatal, and progressive care specialties.

CRITICAL CARE NURSING STANDARDS

AACN has established nursing standards that provide a framework for critical care nurses. Nursing practice varies depending on the setting in which the nurse is employed and the patients cared for in that setting. The standards set forth by AACN describe the practice of the nurse who cares for an acutely or critically ill patient in the health care environment. The standards are authoritative statements that describe the level of care and performance by which the quality of nursing care can be judged. They serve as descriptions of the expected roles and responsibilities. Both the standards of care and the standards of professional practice are delineated.

The *Standards of Care for Acute and Critical Care Nursing* consists of six standards and are prescriptive of a competent level of nursing practice[7] (Box 1-2). The

Standards of Professional Practice for Acute and Critical Care Nursing include eight standards[7] (Box 1-3). Measurement criteria have also been formulated to evaluate the level of attainment of each standard.

EVIDENCE-BASED NURSING PRACTICE

Much of early medical and nursing practice was based on nonscientific traditions that resulted in variable and haphazard patient outcomes.[8] These traditions and rituals, which were based on folklore, gut instinct, trial and error, and personal preference, were often passed down from one generation of practitioner to another.[8-10] Examples of non–scientific-based critical care nursing practice include suctioning artificial airways every 2 hours; using iced saline injectable when measuring a cardiac output; always using lead II for cardiac monitoring; stripping chest tubes every 2 hours; and limiting visiting hours for all patients.[9]

The dramatic and multiple changes in health care and the ever-increasing presence of managed care in all geographic regions have placed greater emphasis on demonstrating the effectiveness of treatments and practices on outcomes.[11] In addition, emphasis is greater on efficiency, cost-effectiveness, quality of life, and patient sat-

---

Box 1-2

AACN STANDARDS OF CARE FOR ACUTE AND CRITICAL CARE NURSING

STANDARD OF CARE I: ASSESSMENT
The nurse caring for acute and critically ill patients collects relevant patient health care data.

STANDARD OF CARE II: DIAGNOSIS
The nurse caring for acute and critically ill patients analyzes the assessment data in determining diagnoses.

STANDARD OF CARE III: OUTCOME IDENTIFICATION
The nurse caring for acutely and critically ill patients identifies individualized, expected outcomes for the patient.

STANDARD OF CARE IV: PLANNING
The nurse caring for acutely and critically ill patients develops a plan of care that prescribes interventions to attain expected outcomes.

STANDARD OF CARE V: IMPLEMENTATION
The nurse caring for acutely and critically ill patients implements interventions identified in the plan of care.

STANDARD OF CARE VI
The nurse caring for acutely and critically ill patients evaluates the patient's progress toward attaining expected outcomes.

From *AACN Standards of Care for Acute and Critical Care Nursing*, Aliso Viejo, Calif, 1998, AACN.

Box 1-3

AACN STANDARDS OF PROFESSIONAL PRACTICE FOR ACUTE AND CRITICAL CARE NURSING

STANDARD OF PROFESSIONAL PRACTICE I: QUALITY OF CARE
The nurse caring for acute and critically ill patients systematically evaluates the quality and effectiveness of nursing practice.

STANDARD OF PROFESSIONAL PRACTICE II: INDIVIDUAL PRACTICE EVALUATION
The practice of the nurse caring for acutely and critically ill patients reflects knowledge of current professional practice standards, laws, and regulations.

STANDARD OF PROFESSIONAL PRACTICE III: EDUCATION
The nurse acquires and maintains current knowledge and competency in the care of acute and critically ill patients.

STANDARD OF PROFESSIONAL PRACTICE IV: COLLEGIALITY
The nurse caring for acute and critically ill patients interacts with and contributes to the professional development of peers and other health care providers as colleagues.

STANDARD OF PROFESSIONAL PRACTICE V: ETHICS
The nurse's decisions and actions on behalf of acutely and critically ill patients are determined in an ethical manner.

STANDARD OF PROFESSIONAL PRACTICE VI: COLLABORATION
The nurse caring for acute and critically ill patients collaborates with the team, consisting of patient, family, and health care providers, in providing patient care in a healing, humane, and caring environment.

STANDARD OF PROFESSIONAL PRACTICE VII: RESEARCH
The nurse caring for acute and critically ill patients uses clinical inquiry in practice.

STANDARD OF PROFESSIONAL PRACTICE VIII: RESOURCE UTILIZATION
The nurse caring for acute and critically ill patients considers factors related to safety, effectiveness, and cost in planning and delivering patient care.

From *AACN Standards of Care for Acute and Critical Care Nursing,* Aliso Viejo, Calif, 1998, AACN.

isfaction ratings.[12] It has become essential for nurses to use the best data available to make patient care decisions and carry out the appropriate nursing interventions.[12] By means of a scientific basis, with its ability to explain and predict, nurses are able to provide research-based interventions with consistent, positive outcomes. The content of this book is research-based, with the most current, cutting-edge research abstracted and placed throughout the chapters as appropriate to topical discussions.

The increasingly complex and changing health care system presents multiple challenges for creating an evidence-based practice. Not only must appropriate research studies be designed to answer clinical questions, but also research findings must be used to make necessary changes for implementation in practice. Multiple evidence-based practice and research utilization models exist to guide practitioners in the use of existing research findings. One such model is the *Iowa Model of Evidence-Based Practice to Promote Quality Care* that incorporates both evidence and research as the basis for practice.[13] Inquisitive practitioners who strive for best practices using valid and reliable data will demonstrate quality outcomes-driven care and practices.

HOLISTIC CRITICAL CARE NURSING

CARING

The high technology–driven critical care environment is fast paced and directed toward monitoring and treating life-threatening changes in patient conditions. For this reason, attention is often focused on the technology and treatments necessary for maintaining stability in the physiologic functioning of the patient. Great emphasis is placed on technical skills and professional competence and responsiveness to critical emergencies. Concern has been voiced about the lesser emphasis on the caring component of nursing in this fast-paced, highly technologic health care environment.[14,15] Nowhere is this more evident than in areas in which critical care nursing is practiced. It has been said that keeping the *care* in nursing care is one of our biggest challenges.[15] The critical care nurse must be able to deliver high quality care skillfully, using all appropriate technologies, while also incorporating psychosocial and other holistic approaches as appropriate to the time and condition of the patient.

The caring aspect between nurses and patients is most fundamental to the relationship and to the health care experience. The literature demonstrates that nurse clinicians focus on psychosocial aspects of caring, whereas patients place more emphasis on the technical skills and professional competence.[16] Physical and emotional absence, inhumane and belittling interactions, and lack of recognition of the patient's uniqueness indicate noncaring. Holistic care focuses on human integrity and stresses that the body, the mind, and the spirit are interdependent and inseparable. Thus, all aspects need to be considered in planning and delivering care.[17]

INDIVIDUALIZED CARE

The differences between nurses' and patients' perceptions of caring point to the importance of establishing individualized care that recognizes the uniqueness of each patient's preferences, condition, and both physiologic and psychosocial status. It is clearly understood by care providers that a patient's physical condition progresses at fairly predictable stages, depending on the presence or absence of comorbid conditions. What is not understood as distinctly is the effect of psychosocial issues on the healing process. For this reason, special consideration must be given to determining the unique interventions that will positively impact each individual patient and help the patient progress toward desired outcomes.

An important aspect in the care delivery to and recovery of critically ill patients is the personal support of family members and significant others. The value of both patient- and family-centered care should not be underestimated.[18,19] It is important for families to be included in care decisions and to be encouraged to participate in the care of the patient as appropriate to the patient's personal level of ability and needs.

CULTURAL CARE

Cultural diversity in health care is not a new topic but one that is gaining emphasis and importance as the world becomes more accessible to all as the result of increasing technologies and interfaces with places and peoples. Diversity includes not only ethnic sensitivity but also sensitivity and openness to differences in lifestyles, opinions, values, and beliefs. Over 28% of the U.S. population is made up of racial and ethnic minority groups.[20] The predominant minorities in the United States are Americans of African, Hispanic, Asian, Pacific Island, Native American, and Eskimo descent. Significant differences exist among their cultural beliefs and practices and the level of their acculturation into the mainstream American culture.[21]

Unless cultural differences are taken into account, optimal health care cannot be provided. More attention has been directed recently at determining the physiologic differences and those of disease development and progression among various ethnic groups. Death rates from cardiovascular disease are significantly higher for both black men and black women than for white men and white women. The prevalence of coronary heart disease is highest in black women, followed by that in Mexican American men.[22] An increased sensitivity to the health care needs and vulnerabilities of all groups must be developed by care providers.

Cultural competence is one way to ensure that individual differences related to culture are incorporated into the plan of care.[23,24] Nurses must possess knowledge about biocultural, psychosocial, and linguistic differences in diverse populations to make accurate assessments. Interventions must then be tailored to the uniqueness of each patient and family.

COMPLEMENTARY AND ALTERNATIVE THERAPIES

Recently consumer activism has increased; consumers are advocating for quality health care that is both cost-effective and humane. They are asking whether options other than traditional Western medical care exist for treating various disease conditions. The possibilities of using centuries-old practices that are considered alternative or complementary to current Western medicine have been in demand.[25] It is not uncommon now to see these various therapies in all health care settings, including the intensive care unit. These complementary therapies offer patients, families, and health care providers additional options to assist with healing and recovery.[26]

Two terms, *alternative* and *complementary*, have been in the mainstream for several years. *Alternative* denotes that a specific therapy is an option or alternative to what is considered conventional treatment of a condition or state. The term *complementary* was proposed to reflect that the therapies can be used as complementary or supportive to the conventional treatment.[26] The remainder of this section includes a brief discussion about nontraditional complementary therapies that have been used in critical care areas.

Spirituality and Prayer. As persons search for meaning and guidance in critical, emergent, and unexpected tragic circumstances, spirituality becomes more important.[27] Likewise, health care practitioners turn to their own spirituality to manage stress and find answers to the health care issues that they face on an intense, daily basis. Spiritual practices consist of meditation, prayer, and spiritual materials and are based on personal values and beliefs. Holt-Ashley[27] describes how to incorporate prayer into the critical care unit, concentrating on both patients and families and the nurse. The author also offers strategies for creating an environment that is conducive to spiritual well-being for both patients and staff.

Guided Imagery. One of the most well-studied complementary therapies is guided imagery, a mind-body strategy that is frequently used to decrease stress, pain, and anxiety.[28] Additional benefits of guided imagery have been shown to be (1) decreased side effects; (2) decreased length of stay; (3) reduced hospital costs; (4) enhanced sleep; and (5) increased patient satisfaction.[28] Guided imagery is a low-cost intervention that is relatively simple to implement. The patient's involvement in the process offers a sense of empowerment and accomplishment and motivates self-care.

Massage. Back massage as a once-practiced part of routine care of patients has been eliminated for various reasons, including time constraints, greater use of technology, and increasing complexity of care requirements. However, there is a scientific basis for concluding that massage offers positive effects on both physiologic and psychologic outcomes.

A comprehensive review of the literature revealed that the most common effect of massage was reduction in anxiety, with additional reports of significant decrease in tension. There was also a positive physiologic response to massage in the areas of decreased respiratory and heart rates and decreased pain. The effects on sleep were inconclusive. The authors concluded that massage is an effective complementary therapy for promoting relaxation and reducing pain and should be incorporated into nursing practice.[29]

Animal-Assisted Therapy. The use of animals has increased as an adjunct to healing in the care of patients of all ages in multiple settings. Pet visitation programs have been created in various health care delivery settings, including acute care, long-term care, and hospice. In the acute care area, animals are brought in to provide additional solace and comfort for patients who are critically or terminally ill. Fish aquariums are used also in both patient areas and family areas; they serve to humanize the surroundings. Scientific evidence indicates that animal-assisted therapy results in positive patient outcomes in the areas of attention, mobility, and orientation. Other reports have shown improved communication and mood in patients.[30]

NURSING'S UNIQUE ROLE IN HEALTH CARE

Today's health care environment necessitates a nursing framework that is flexible and responsive to the needs of the public that is served. The American Nurses Association has defined nursing as: "the protection, promotion, and optimization of health, and abilities, prevention of illness and injury, alleviation of suffering through the diagnosis and treatment of human response, and advocacy in the care of individuals, families, communities, and populations."[31] Although nursing has both independent and dependent nursing actions, it is essential that an interdependence with all health care professionals is actualized. It is through such collaborative efforts and exchanges of knowledge and ideas about care delivery that quality patient outcomes are made evident.[31,32]

CRITICAL CARE NURSING PRACTICE

Researchers have studied critical care nurses to better understand their clinical judgment and interventions and the link between the two.[33] They identified two major categories of thought and action and nine categories of practice that illustrate clinical judgment and the clinical knowledge development of critical care nurses. These major categories[33] are delineated in Box 1-4.

THE NURSING PROCESS

The nursing process is a method for making clinical decisions. It is a way of thinking and acting in relation to the clinical phenomena of concern to nurses. The nursing process is a systematic decision-making model that is cyclic, not linear. By virtue of its evaluation phase, the nursing process incorporates a feedback loop that maintains quality control of its decision-making outputs. The

---

Box 1-4

CATEGORIES OF CRITICAL CARE NURSING THOUGHT, ACTION, AND PRACTICE

THOUGHT AND ACTION
Clinical grasp and clinical inquiry: problem identification and clinical problem solving
Clinical forethought: anticipating and preventing potential problems

PRACTICE
Diagnosing and managing life-sustaining physiologic functions in unstable patients
Managing a crisis by using skilled know-how
Providing comfort measures for the critically ill
Caring for patients' families
Preventing hazards in a technologic environment
Facing death: end-of-life care and decision making
Communicating and negotiating multiple perspectives
Monitoring quality and managing breakdown
Exhibiting the skilled know-how of clinical leadership and the coaching and mentoring of others

---

nursing process is indeed a method for solving clinical problems, but it is not merely a problem-solving method. Similar to a problem-solving method, the nursing process offers an organized, systematic approach to clinical problems. Unlike a problem-solving method, the nursing process is continuous, not episodic. The six phases constitute a continuous cycle throughout the nurse's moment-to-moment data interpretation and management of patient care (Fig. 1-1).

Nursing Diagnosis. A dynamic thinking process that leads to a hypothesis for explaining clinical states is diagnostic reasoning.[34] By using this process that includes appropriate objective data, more accurate decisions can be made, with appropriate interventions to meet health care needs. Factors affecting diagnostic reasoning include patient factors such as acuity, altered mental status, multisystem disease, and rapidly changing physiologic status, and clinician factors such as clinical experience, knowledge, continuous stream of patient data, and uncertainty of data.[34]

The North American Nursing Diagnosis Association (NANDA) has supported the continued development and evolution of research-based nursing diagnoses.[35] With nursing diagnosis as a component of the decision-making method, there is a more systematic collection and interpretation of data. The most essential and distinguishing feature of any nursing diagnosis is that it describes a health condition *primarily resolved by nursing interventions or therapies.*

Nursing Interventions. Also known as *nursing orders* or *nursing prescriptions*, nursing interventions constitute the treatment approach to an identified health alteration. Interventions are selected to satisfy the outcome criteria and prevent or resolve the nursing diagnosis. It is important to link diagnostic labels with interventions and nurse-sensitive outcomes so that a consistent framework is available for evaluating nursing interventions and outcomes.

Intervention strategies that consist solely of monitoring, measuring, checking, obtaining physician orders, documenting, reporting, and notifying do not completely fulfill criteria for the treatment of a problem. Nursing interventions for nursing diagnoses designate therapeutic activity that assists the patient in moving from one state of health to another. Medically delegated actions, such as administering medications and initiating ventilator setting changes, are included in the interventions but with the emphasis placed squarely on the assessments and judgments the nurse makes in evaluating their effectiveness, patient tolerance, safety, dosage, titration, and discontinuance.

The Nursing Interventions Classification (NIC) framework contains 514 nursing interventions that are categorized into 30 classes and 7 domains.[36] Many nursing interventions are directly linked with NANDA nursing diagnoses. *Nurse-initiated treatments* are those interventions initiated by the nurse in response to a nursing diagnosis. The use of the NIC framework facilitates clinical decision making and provides a standardized language that describes the core of essential nursing interventions. An example of a NIC nursing intervention is presented in the following Nursing Interventions Classification feature on acid-base monitoring. In addition, the research base provides a method to link diagnoses with outcomes in the evaluation of care and services.[36]

Outcomes Evaluation. Evaluation of attainment of the expected patient outcomes occurs formally at intervals designated in the outcome criteria. Informal evaluation occurs continuously. The evaluation phase and the activities that take place within it are perhaps the most important dimensions of the nursing process (see Fig. 1-1). Evaluation of patient progress against a standard of nursing management incorporates accountability into the process—accountability to the standard of care. Lack of progress in outcome attainment or lack of progress in problem solving is readily identified and kept in check, and alternate solutions can then be proposed.

The Nursing Outcomes Classification (NOC) is a research-based model of 330 outcomes with definitions, indicators, and measurement scales for use with individual patients, families, and community and population levels.[37] NOC represents one way to standardize terminology for nurse-sensitive outcomes. The outcomes are not nursing assessments or diagnoses and are not prescriptive. The classification does not contain satisfaction outcomes. There are 17 measurement scales that use a five-point Likert-type scale. The model can be used to evaluate the totality of nursing interventions and track effectiveness of nursing on patient outcomes.

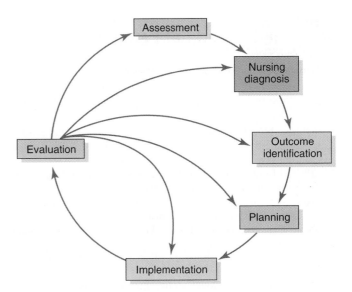

Fig. 1-1   Cyclic nature of the nursing process. Modified from Fortinash K, Holoday-Worret P: *Psychiatric nursing care plans,* ed 4, St Louis, 2004, Mosby.

INTERDISCIPLINARY PLANNING FOR CARE

The growing managed care environment has placed emphasis on examining methods of care delivery and processes of care by all health care professionals. Collaboration and partnerships have been shown to increase quality of care and services while containing or decreasing costs.[38,39] Early discharge planning and coordination of care in critical care units has been demonstrated to significantly influence patient outcomes.[40,41] It is now more important than ever to create and enhance partnerships, because the resulting interdependence and collaboration among disciplines is essential to achieving positive patient outcomes.

INTERDISCIPLINARY CARE MANAGEMENT MODELS

Several different models of care delivery and care management are used in health care. An overview of the various terms and models are presented in this chapter. The reader is encouraged to seek additional resources and consultation for a more in-depth explanation of the models.

Care Management. *Care management* is a system of integrated processes designed to enable, support, and coordinate patient care throughout the continuum of health care services. Care management takes place in many different settings; care is delivered by various professional health care team members and nonlicensed providers, as appropriate.

NIC   Acid-Base Monitoring

Definition: Collection and analysis of patient data to regulate acid-base balance

Activities

Obtain blood for determination of ABG levels, ensuring adequate circulation to the extremity before and after blood withdrawal.

Place blood samples for ABG determination on ice, as appropriate, and send to the lab.

Note patient's temperature and percent of oxygen administered at time blood was drawn.

Note if arterial pH level is on the alkaline or acidotic side of the mean (7.4).

Note if $Paco_2$ level shows respiratory acidosis, respiratory alkalosis, or normalcy.

Note if the HCO_3 level shows metabolic acidosis, metabolic alkalosis, or normalcy.

Examine the pH level in conjunction with the $Paco_2$ and HCO_3 levels to determine whether the acidosis/alkalosis is compensated or uncompensated.

Note the Pao_2, Sao_2, and hemoglobin levels to determine the adequacy of arterial oxygenation.

Monitor end-tidal CO_2 level, as appropriate.

Monitor for an increase in the anion gap (>14 mEq/L), signaling an increased production or decreased excretion of acid products.

Monitor for signs and symptoms of HCO_3 deficit and metabolic acidosis: Kussmaul respirations, weakness, disorientation, headache, anorexia, coma, urinary pH level <6, plasma HCO_3 level <22 mEq/L, plasma pH level <7.35, base excess ≤ 2 mEq/L, associated hyperkalemia, and possible CO_2 deficit.

Monitor for causes of possible HCO_3 deficit such as diarrhea, renal failure, tissue hypoxia, lactic acidosis, diabetic ketoacidosis, malnutrition, and salicylate overdose.

Administer oral or parenteral HCO_3 agents, if appropriate.

Administer prescribed insulin and potassium for treatment of diabetic ketoacidosis, as appropriate.

Monitor for signs and symptoms of HCO_3 excess and metabolic alkalosis: numbness and tingling of the extremities, muscular hypertonicity, shallow respirations with pause, bradycardia, tetany, urinary pH level >7, plasma HCO_3 level >26 mEq/L, plasma pH level >7.45, BE >2 mEq/L, associated hypokalemia, and possible CO_2 retention.

Monitor for possible causes of HCO_3 excess such as vomiting, gastric suction, hyperaldosteronism, diuretic

therapy, hypochloremia, and excessive ingestion of medications containing HCO_3.

Teach patient to avoid excessive use of medications containing HCO_3, as appropriate.

Administer pharmacologic agents to replace chloride, as appropriate.

Monitor for signs and symptoms of carbonic acid deficit and respiratory alkalosis: frequent sighing and yawning, tetany, paresthesia, muscle twitching, palpitations, tingling and numbness, dizziness, blurred vision, diaphoresis, dry mouth, convulsions, pH level >7.45, $Paco_2$ <35 mm Hg, associated hyperchloremia, and possible HCO_3 deficit.

Monitor for possible causes of carbonic acid deficits and associated hyperventilation such as pain, central nervous system (CNS) lesions, fever, and mechanical ventilation.

Sedate patient to reduce hyperventilation, if appropriate.

Administer pain medication, as appropriate.

Treat fever, as appropriate.

Administer parenteral chloride solutions to reduce HCO_3, while connecting the cause of respiratory alkalosis, as appropriate.

Monitor for signs and symptoms of carbonic acid excess and respiratory acidosis: hand tremor with extensions of arms, confusion, drowsiness progressing to coma, headache, slowed verbal response, nausea, vomiting, tachycardia, warm sweaty extremities, pH level <7.35, $Paco_2$ level >45 mm Hg, associated hypochloremia, and possible HCO_3 excess.

Monitor for possible causes of carbonic acid excess and respiratory acidosis such as airway obstruction, depressed ventilation, CNS depression, neurologic disease, chronic lung disease, musculoskeletal disease, chest trauma, infection, acute respiratory distress syndrome, cardiac failure, and use of respiratory depressant drugs.

Support ventilation and airway patency in the presence of respiratory acidosis and rising $Paco_2$ level, as appropriate.

Administer oxygen therapy, as appropriate.

Administer antimicrobial agents and bronchodilators, as appropriate.

Administer low-flow oxygen and monitor for CO_2 narcosis in cases of chronic hypercapnia.

From Dochterman JM, Bulechek GM: *Nursing interventions classification (NIC)*, ed 4, St Louis, 2004, Mosby.

Actual coordination of care and services may be done by health care staff or insurance/payor staff. Care management must be patient-focused, continuum-driven, results-oriented, and based on a team approach. Another term associated with this model of care is *disease state*

management, which connotes the process of managing a population's health over a lifetime. In disease state management, however, there is a focus on managing complex and chronic disease states, such as diabetes or heart failure, over the entire continuum.

Case Management. *Case management* is the process of overseeing the care of patients and organizing services in collaboration with the patient's physician or primary health care provider. The case manager may be a nurse, allied health care provider, or the patient's primary care provider. Case managers are usually assigned to a specific population group and facilitate effective coordination of care services as patients move in and out of different settings. Ideally, the case manager oversees the care of the patient across the continuum of care. Numerous reports have described the improved patient outcomes, decreased length of hospital stay, reduced readmission rates, and increased continuity of care associated with case management.[42-46]

Outcomes Management. *Outcomes management* refers to a model aimed at managing the outcomes of care by the use of various tools, quality improvement processes, and interdisciplinary team involvement and action. Specifically, emphasis is placed on consistent standards of care; measurement of disease-specific clinical outcomes, as well as patient functioning and well-being; and assessment of clinical and outcome data for the specific conditions.[47,48] Outcomes management also takes place in multiple settings across the continuum of care. Professional nurse outcomes managers ensure that variances from the plan of care are addressed in a timely manner, and they also examine aggregate information with the team for quality improvement in the interdisciplinary plan of care.

CARE MANAGEMENT TOOLS

Many quality improvement tools are available to providers for care management. The four tools addressed in this chapter are clinical pathway, algorithm, practice guideline, and protocol.

Clinical Pathway. The *clinical pathway* presents an overview of the entire multidisciplinary plan of care for routine patients. It focuses on the critical elements in the care of certain patient populations and may track variances from the pathway. Pathways are developed by a multidisciplinary team, based on a specific diagnosis or condition, and integrated with the latest research and best practices from the literature. Pathways are ideal for high-volume diagnosis groups that are amenable to standardization. Many pathways are incorporated into the medical record or are computerized, making them a permanent part of the clinical record.

Algorithm. An *algorithm* is a stepwise decision-making flowchart for a specific care process or processes. Algorithms are more focused than clinical pathways and guide the clinician through the "if, then" decision-making process, addressing patient responses to particular treatments. Well-known examples of algorithms are the advanced cardiac life support (ACLS) algorithms published by the American Heart Association.

Algorithms may be used with clinical pathways and are particularly helpful when patients develop variances from the pathway that are amenable to a concise decision-making guide. Whenever "bottlenecks" to a pathway occur, algorithms are considered an enhancement and serve to facilitate more timely clinical decision making. Weaning, medication selection, medication titration, individual practitioner variance, and appropriate patient placement algorithms have been developed to give practitioners additional standardized decision-making abilities.

Practice Guideline. A *practice guideline* is usually developed by a professional organization (e.g., American Association of Critical-Care Nurses, Society of Critical Care Medicine, American College of Cardiology, or government agencies such as the Agency for Health Care Research and Quality [AHRQ]). Practice guidelines are generally written in text prose style rather than in the flowchart format of pathways and algorithms. Practice guidelines are used as resources in formulating the pathway or algorithm.

Protocol. A *protocol* is a very common tool in research studies. Protocols are more directive and rigid than pathways or guidelines, and providers are not supposed to vary from a protocol. Patients are screened carefully for specific entry criteria before being started on a protocol. There are many national research protocols, such as those for cancer and chemotherapy studies. Protocols are helpful when built-in "alerts" signal the provider to potentially serious problems. Computerization of protocols assists providers in being more proactive regarding dangerous drug interactions, abnormal laboratory values, and other untoward effects that are preprogrammed into the computer.

Order Set. An *order set* consists of preprinted provider orders that are used to expedite the order process once a standard has been validated through analytical review of practice and research. Order sets complement and increase compliance with existing practice standards. They can also be used to represent the algorithm or protocol in order format.

MANAGING AND TRACKING VARIANCES

All variances must be addressed and managed in a timely manner by the health care team members.[49] All of the previously described care management tools provide methods to track variances. Whether variance coding is included on a pathway or is tracked by another quality improvement method, both individual and aggregate data must be assessed and analyzed. Except for protocols, which are more rigid and research-based, algorithms, pathways, and guidelines can be used according to the practitioner's discretion. Tracking variances from the expected standard is one method to determine the utility of the tools in particular settings and patient populations. There must be a link between the care management system and the quality improvement program so that changes, as appropriate, can be made to positively affect the outcomes of care and services.

REGULATORY ISSUES IN CRITICAL CARE

SAFETY

Patient safety has become a major focus of attention by health care consumers as well as providers of care and administrators of health care institutions. The Institute of Medicine publication *Crossing the Quality Chasm: A New Health System for the 21st Century* was released in 2001 and has been the impetus for debate and actions to improve the safety of health care environments. In this report, information and details were given indicating that health care harms patients too frequently and routinely fails to deliver its potential benefits.[50] Oftentimes, the definitions of medical errors and approaches to resolving patient safety issues differ among nurses, physicians, administrators, and other health care providers.[51]

Patient safety has been described as an ethical imperative, and one that is implied in health care professionals' actions and interpersonal processes.[52] Critical care units are prime examples of where errors may occur due to the hectic, complex environment where the margins of error are narrow and the demands for safety are crucial.[53] In this environment, patients are particularly vulnerable due to their compromised physiologic status, multiple technologic and pharmacologic interventions, and multiple care providers who frequently work at a fast pace. It is essential that care delivery processes that minimize the opportunity for errors are designed and that a "safety culture" rather than a "blame culture" is created.[54] When an injury or inappropriate care occurs, it is crucial that health care professionals promptly give an explanation of how the injury or mistake occurred and the short- or long-term effects to the patient and family. They should be informed that the factors involved in the injury will be investigated so that steps can be taken to reduce or avoid the likelihood of similar injury to other patients.

The Joint Commission on Accreditation of Healthcare Organizations (JCAHO) has approved 2005 National Patient Safety Goals (NPSGs)[55] that are to be implemented in healthcare organizations (Box 1-5).

The Safe Medical Device Act (SMDA) requires that hospitals report serious or potentially serious device-related injuries or illness of patients and/or employees to the manufacturer of the device, and if death is involved, to the Federal Drug Administration (FDA). In addition, implantable devices must be documented and tracked.[56] This reporting serves as an "early warning system" so that the FDA can obtain information on device problems. Failure to comply with the act is to result in civil action.

Box 1-5
2005 NATIONAL PATIENT SAFETY GOALS

- Improve the accuracy of patient identification
- Improve the effectiveness of communication among caregivers
- Improve the safety of using medications
- Eliminate wrong-site, wrong-patient, wrong-procedure surgery
- Improve the safety of infusion pumps
- Improve the effectiveness of clinical alarm systems
- Reduce the risk of health care–associated infections
- Accurately and completely reconcile medications across the continuum of care
- Reduce the risk of patient harm resulting from falls
- Reduce the risk of influenza and pneumococcal disease in institutionalized older adults
- Reduce the risk of surgical fires

PRIVACY AND CONFIDENTIALITY

In 1996 a landmark law was passed to provide consumers with greater access to health care insurance, promote more standardization and efficiency in the health care industry, and protect the privacy of health care data.[57] The Health Insurance Portability and Accountability Act of 1996 (HIPAA) has created additional challenges for health care organizations and providers due to the stringent requirements and additional resources needed in order to meet the requirements of the law. Most specific to critical care clinicians is the privacy and confidentiality related to protection of health care data. This has implications when interacting with family members as well as others, and the oftentimes very close work environment, tight working spaces, and emergent situations. Clinicians are referred to their organizational policies and procedures for specific procedures for their organizations.

REFERENCES

1. Society of Critical Care Medicine: www.sccm.org. Consumer information, *Brief History of Critical Care.*
2. Bengco A: The outlook is bright for critical care nurses, *Crit Care Nurse* 20(suppl 1):6, 2000.
3. Melosh B: Doctors, patients, and "big nurse": work and gender in the postwar hospital. In Lagemann E: *Nursing history: new perspectives, new possibilities*, New York, 1983, Teachers College Press.
4. American Association of Critical-Care Nurses: www.aacn.org. About Critical Care Nursing (Press Room).
5. Kleinpell R: Reports of role descriptions of acute care nurse practitioners, *AACN Clin Issues* 9(2):290-295, 1998.
6. American Association of Critical-Care Nurses: www.aacn.org. Fact sheet (Public Policy).
7. American Association of Critical-Care Nurses: www.aacn.org. *Practice resources.*

8. Omery A, Williams RP: An appraisal of research utilization across the United States, *J Nurs Adm* 29(12):50-56, 1999.
9. Wojner AW: Why do we do the things we do? Stop the carnage of nursing research, *AACN News* 17(4):2, 12, 2000.
10. Mick D: Folklore, personal preference, or research-based practice, *Am J Crit Care* 9(1):6-7, 2000.
11. Rosswurm MA, Larrabee JH: A model for change to evidence-based practice, *Image (IN)* 31(4):317-322, 1999.
12. McPheeters M, Lohr KN: Evidence-based practice and nursing: commentary, *Outcomes Manag Nurs Pract* 3(3): 99-101, 1999.
13. Titler MG et al: The Iowa model of evidence-based practice to promote quality care, *Crit Care Nurs Clin North Am* 13(4):497-509, 2001.
14. Panting K: Intensive care/intensive cure: the future of critical care? *Crit Care Nurse* 15(12):100, 1995.
15. Miller KL: Keeping the care in nursing care: our biggest challenge, *J Nurse Admin* 25(11):29-32, 1995.
16. Patistea E, Siamanta H: A literature review of patients' compared with nurses' perceptions of caring: implications for practice and research, *J Prof Nurs* 15(5):302-312, 1999.
17. Mariano C: Holistic ethics, *AJN* 101(1):24A-24C, 2001.
18. Warren NA: The phenomenon of nurses' caring behaviors as perceived by the critical care family, *Crit Care Nurs Q* 17(3):67-72, 1994.
19. Powers PH et al: The value of patient- and family-centered care, *Am J Nurs* 100(5):84-88, 2000.
20. Collins KS, Hall A: *US minority health: a chart book,* 1999, Commonwealth Fund.
21. Bushy A: Social and cultural factors affecting health care and nursing practice. In Lancaster J: *Nursing: issues in leading and managing change,* St Louis, 1999, Mosby.
22. Alspach G: Time for sensitivity training: cultural diversity in cardiovascular disease, *Crit Care Nurse* 20(3):14-24, 2000.
23. Gonzales R, Gooden M, Porter C: Eliminating racial and ethnic disparities in health care, *Am J Nurs* 100(3):56-58, 2000.
24. Leonard B, Plotnikoff GA: Awareness: the heart of cultural competence, *AACN Clin Issues* 11(1):51-59, 2000.
25. Lindquist R, Kirksey K: Preface, *AACN Clin Issues* 11(1): 1-3, 2000.
26. Kreitzer MJ, Jensen D: Healing practices: trends, challenges, and opportunities for nurses in critical care, *AACN Clin Issues* 11(1):7-16, 2000.
27. Holt-Ashley M: Nurses pray: use of prayer and spirituality as a complementary therapy in the intensive care setting, *AACN Clin Issues* 11(1):60-67, 2000.
28. Tusek DL, Cwynar RE: Strategies for implementing guided imagery program to enhance patient experience, *AACN Clin Issues* 11(1):68-76, 2000.
29. Richards KC, Gibson R, Overton-McCoy AL: Effects of massage in acute and critical care, *AACN Clin Issues* 11(1): 77-96, 2000.
30. Cole K, Fawlinski A: Animal-assisted therapy: the human-animal bond, *AACN Clin Issues* 11(1):139-149, 2000.
31. American Nurses Association: *Nursing's social policy statement,* ed 2, Washington, DC, 2003, The Association.
32. White KR, Begun JW: Profession building in the new health care system, *Nurs Adm Q* 20(3):79-85, 1996.
33. Benner P, Hooper-Kyriakidis P, Stannard D: *Clinical wisdom and interventions in critical care,* Philadelphia, 1999, Saunders.
34. Szaflarski NL: Diagnostic reasoning in acute and critical care, *AACN Clin Issues* 8(3):291-302, 1997.
35. North American Nursing Diagnosis Association: *Nursing diagnosis: definitions and classification,* Philadelphia, 2003, The Association.
36. Dochterman JM, Bulechek GM, editors: *Nursing interventions classifications (NIC),* ed 4, St Louis, 2004, Mosby.
37. Moorhead S, Johnson M, Maas M, editors: *Nursing outcomes classification (NOC),* ed 3, St Louis, 2004, Mosby.
38. Wheelan SA, Burchill CN, Tilin F: The link between teamwork and patients' outcomes in intensive care units, *Am J Crit Care* 12(6):527-534, 2003.
39. Boyle DK, Kochinda C: Enhancing collaborative communication of nurse and physician leadership in two intensive care units, *J Nurs Admin* 34(2):60-70, 2004.
40. Knaus W et al: An evaluation of outcome from intensive care in major medical centers, *Ann Intern Med* 104:410-418, 1986.
41. Kleinpell RM: Randomized trail of an intensive care unit-based early discharge planning intervention for critically ill elderly patients, *Am J Crit Care* 13(4):335-345, 2004.
42. Doerge JB: Creating an outcomes framework, *Outcomes Manag Nurs Pract* 4(1):28-38, 2000.
43. Flarey DL: Case management: a system for improving outcomes, *Nurs Leadersh Forum* 3(4):120, 143, 1998.
44. Kee CC, Borchers L: Reducing readmission rates through discharge interventions, *Clin Nurse Spec* 12(5):206-209, 1998.
45. Maljanian R, Effken J, Kaerhle P: Design and implementation of an outcomes management model, *Outcomes Manag Nurs Pract* 4(1):19-26, 2000.
46. Peters C, Cowley M, Standiford L: The process of outcomes management in an acute care facility, *Nurs Adm Q* 24(1): 75-89, 1999.
47. Wojner A: Outcomes management: an interdisciplinary search for best practice, *AACN Clin Issues* 7(1):133-145, 1996.
48. Wojner AW: Outcomes Management, St Louis Mo, Mosby, 2001.
49. Matea M, Newton C: Managing variances in case management, *Nurs Case Manag* 1(1):45-51, 1996.
50. Institute of Medicine: *Crossing the quality chasm: a new health system for the 21st century,* Washington, DC, 2001, National Academy Press.
51. Cook A et al: An error by any other name, *AJN* 104(6): 32-44, 2004.
52. White GB: Patient safety: an ethical imperative, *Nurs Economics* 20(4):195-197, 2002.
53. Benner P: Creating a culture of safety and improvement: a key to reducing medical error, *Am J Crit Care* 10(4):281-284, 2001.
54. Smith AP: In search of safety: an interview with Gina Pugliese, *Nurse Economics* 20(1):6-12, 2002.
55. Joint Commission for the Accreditation of HealthCare Organizations: www.jcaho.org. Facts about the 2005 National Patient Safety Goals.
56. Jensen JR: FDA's Safe Medical Device Act, *Risk Manag Rep* 1(2):1-4, 1997.
57. Center's for Medicare & Medicaid Services. www.cms.hhs.gov. Health Insurance Portability and Accountability Act (HIPAA)—Administrative Simplification.

CHAPTER 2

Ethical Issues

*I*t is essential that critical care nurses have an understanding of professional nursing ethics and ethical principles and that they are able to use a decision-making model to guide nursing actions. The purpose of this chapter is to provide an overview of principles and professional nursing ethics. An ethical decision-making model is described and illustrated. In addition, recommendations are given concerning methods to use when discussing ethical issues in the critical care setting.

DIFFERENCES BETWEEN MORALS AND ETHICS

Morals are the "shoulds," "should nots," "oughts," and "ought nots" of actions and behaviors and have been related closely to sexual mores and behaviors in Western society. Religious and cultural values and beliefs largely mold one's moral thoughts and actions. Morals form the basis for action and provide a framework for evaluation of behavior.

Ethics are concerned with the basis of the action rather than with whether the action is right or wrong, good or bad. Ethics implies that an evaluation is being made that is based on or derived from a set of standards.

MORAL DISTRESS

Moral distress has more recently been discussed in the literature as a serious problem for nurses. It occurs when one knows the ethically appropriate action to take, but cannot act upon it. It also presents when one acts in a manner contrary to personal and professional values. As a result, there can be significant emotional and physical stress that leads to feelings of loss of personal integrity and dissatisfaction with the work environment.[1] Relationships with both co-workers and patients are affected and can negatively impact the quality of care. There is also a great impact on personal relationships and family life. It is therefore important that nurses rec-

ognize moral distress and actively seek strategies to address the issue through institutional, personal, and professional organizational resources. Knowledge and application of ethical principles and guidelines will assist the nurse in daily practice when ethical dilemmas occur.

ETHICAL PRINCIPLES

Certain ethical principles were derived from classic ethical theories that are used in health care decision making. Principles are general guidelines that govern conduct, provide a basis for reasoning, and direct actions. The six ethical principles that are discussed in this chapter are autonomy, beneficence, nonmaleficence, veracity, fidelity, and justice (Box 2-1).

AUTONOMY

The concept of autonomy appears in all ancient writings and early Greek philosophy. In health care, autonomy can be viewed as the freedom to make decisions about one's own body without the coercion or interference of others. Autonomy is a freedom of choice or a self-determination that is a basic human right. It can be experienced in all human life events.

The critical care nurse is often "caught in the middle" in ethical situations, and promoting autonomous decision making is one of those situations. As the nurse works closely with patients and families to promote autonomous decision making, another crucial element becomes clear. Patients and families must have all of the information about a particular situation before they can make a decision that is best for them. They not only should be given all the pertinent information and facts but also must have a clear understanding of what was presented.[2] This is where the nurse is a most important member of the health care team—that is, as patient advocate, providing more information as needed, clarifying points, reinforcing information, and providing support

NIC Decision-Making Support

Definition: Providing information and support for a patient who is making a decision regarding health care

Activities

Determine whether there are differences between the patient's view of own condition and the view of health care providers.

Inform patient of alternative views or solutions.

Help patient identify the advantages and disadvantages of each alternative.

Establish communication with patient early in admission.

Facilitate patient's articulation of goals for care.

Obtain informed consent, when appropriate.

Facilitate collaborative decision making.

Be familiar with institution's policies and procedures.

Respect patient's right to receive or not to receive information.

Provide information requested by patient.

Help patient explain decision to others, as needed.

Serve as a liaison between patient and family.

Serve as a liaison between patient and other health care providers.

Refer to legal aid, as appropriate.

Refer to support groups, as appropriate.

From Dochterman JM, Bulechek GM: *Nursing interventions classification (NIC),* ed 4, St Louis, 2004, Mosby.

Box 2-1

ETHICAL PRINCIPLES IN CRITICAL CARE Comp: can double up.

Autonomy
- Beneficence
- Nonmaleficence
- Veracity
- Fidelity
  - Confidentiality
  - Privacy
- Justice/allocation of resources

---

during the decision-making process.[3] See the Nursing Interventions Classification (NIC) feature on nursing intervention activities that facilitate decision making.

BENEFICENCE

The concept of doing good and preventing harm to patients is a *sine qua non* for the nursing profession. However, the ethical principle of beneficence—which requires that one promote the well-being of patients—points to the importance of this duty for the health care professional. The principle of beneficence presupposes that harms and benefits are balanced, leading to positive or beneficial outcomes. In approaching issues related to beneficence, the instance of conflict with another principle, that of autonomy, is common. Paternalism exists when the nurse or physician makes a decision for the patient without consulting the patient.

Traditional health care has been based on a paternalistic approach to patients. Many patients are still more comfortable in deferring all decisions about care and treatment to their health care provider. Active involvement by various organizations, agencies, and consumer groups in regard to health care has demonstrated a trend toward the public's need and desire for more information about health care in general, as well as more about alternative treatments and providers. Paternalism, or maternalism in the case of female providers, may always be a possibility in the health care setting, but enlightened consumers are causing a change in this practice of health care professionals.

In the critical care setting, many instances of and possibilities for paternalistic actions by the nurse exist. Postoperative care, which is designed to assist the patient with achieving a quick recovery, is a good example of paternalistic action by the nurse. Encouraging the patient to turn, cough, and deep breathe and increasing activity in the form of dangling, sitting in a chair, and ambulating are all paternalistic actions when the patient is experiencing pain and sleep-deprivation and wanting to be left alone. However, at times the priorities of benefits and harms must be balanced. In these instances, the duty to do no harm—which is the next principle to be discussed—takes precedence over the need to avoid paternalistic actions. When ethical principles are in conflict, one must weigh all the benefits and choose the best principle to follow.

NONMALEFICENCE

The ethical principle of nonmaleficence, which dictates that one prevent harm and correct harmful situations, is a *prima facie* duty for the nurse. Thoughtfulness and care are necessary, as is balancing risks and benefits, which were discussed earlier with beneficence. Beneficence and nonmaleficence are on two ends of a continuum and are often adhered to differently, depending on the views of the practitioner.

A practitioner may consider long-term consequences and the good to society as a whole or the principle and its effect on the single individual in the situation. Such complex situations as quality of life versus sanctity of life are always difficult to analyze in the critical care setting, as well as in noncritical care settings.

VERACITY

Veracity, or truth-telling, is an important ethical principle that underlies the nurse-patient relationship. Veracity is important when soliciting informed consent because the patient needs to be aware of all potential risks of and benefits to be derived from specific treatments or their alternatives.[4,5] Once again the critical care nurse can be in the middle of a situation in which all of the facts and information about a particular treatment option are not disclosed. Sometimes information has been given accurately to the patient and family but has been delivered with bias or in a way that is misleading. Veracity must guide all areas of practice for the nurse, that is, in colleague relationships and employee relationships, as well as in the nurse-patient relationship.

FIDELITY

Another ethical principle that is closely related to autonomy and veracity is fidelity. Fidelity, or faithfulness and promise-keeping to patients, is also a *sine qua non* for nursing. It forms a bond between individuals and is the basis of all relationships, both professional and personal. Regardless of the amount of autonomy that patients have in the critical care areas, they still depend on the nurse for a multitude of types of physical care and emotional support. A trusting relationship that establishes and maintains an open atmosphere is one that is positive for all involved.[6]

As do all the other principles, fidelity extends to the family of the critical care patient. When a promise is made to family members that they will be called if an emergency arises or that they will be informed of any other special events concerning the patient, the nurse must make every effort to follow through on the promise. Fidelity will not only uphold the nurse-family relationship but will also reflect positively on the nursing profession as a whole and on the institution in which the nurse is employed.

Confidentiality is one element of fidelity that is based on traditional health care professional ethics. Confidentiality is described as a right whereby patient information can be shared only with those involved in the care of the patient. An exception to this guideline might be when the welfare of others will be put at risk by keeping patient information confidential. Again in this situation, the nurse must balance ethical principles and weigh risks with benefits. Special circumstances, such as the existence of mandatory reporting laws, will guide the nurse in certain situations.[7]

Privacy also has been described as being inherent in the principle of fidelity. It may be closely aligned with confidentiality of patient information and a patient's right to privacy of his or her person, such as maintaining privacy for the patient by pulling the curtains around the bed or making sure that he or she is adequately covered.

JUSTICE

The principle of justice is often used synonymously with the concept of allocation of scarce resources. Contrary to the belief of many people, health care is not a right guaranteed by the Constitution of the United States. Rather, it is the *access* to health care that should be provided to all people. With escalating health care costs, expanded technologies, an aging population with its own special health care needs, and (in some instances) a scarcity of health care personnel, the question of how to allocate health care becomes even more complex.

SCARCE RESOURCES IN CRITICAL CARE

Major factors influencing health care ethics are rapid health care cost inflation and the shrinking allocation of public funds to both primary and secondary care. As health care resources become increasingly scarce, allocation of resources to certain programs and rationing of resources within certain programs will become more evident.[8] Allocation of resources creates ethical challenges for health care practitioners facing the daily clinical realities.[9] Consulting ethicists and ending life support earlier in the management of some cases have been suggested as approaches to better manage costs.[10]

TECHNOLOGIES AND TREATMENTS

Limitations of resources force society and the critical care health professionals to reexamine the goals of critical care for patients. The application of new and/or experimental treatments and procedures needs to be carefully analyzed for each case, paying particular attention to the expected outcome.

Quality of life is an issue that should be considered carefully when examining the use of technologies. This issue is personal and value-laden; it is one that will be different for each individual involved and will depend on the various aspects of the case.[11,12] Quality of life has the dual dimensions of both objectivity and subjectivity. Objectivity examines the person's ability to function, whereas subjectivity analyzes his or her psychosocial state. Patients' treatment preferences reflect the value they place on different health outcomes.[13]

HEALTH CARE PERSONNEL

Critical care nurses are faced with rationing of critical care beds and nursing staff on a daily basis.[14] Strengths and weaknesses of the staff must be balanced with the needs of the patient. Orientation and other special circumstances—such as designation for charge nurse, trauma nurse, or code nurse—must be considered when scheduling staff and making assignments. Any inexperienced staff, float staff, or registry staff must be given appropriate orientation and backup during the shift.

Commonly a triage system for critical care units is called on when there are more admissions than available beds. The critical care nurse is instrumental in assisting the medical director to determine patient selection for transfer, if appropriate. Hospitals establish a set of standards, criteria, or guidelines for determining patient admission and transfer to and from critical care areas.

WITHHOLDING AND WITHDRAWING TREATMENT

The technologic support of life at all costs has recently been questioned by both health care professionals and health care consumers. Physicians and nurses who are closest to the issues have debated the moral and ethical implications and have looked to ethicists for guidance and legal opinions. Both medical and nursing associations have developed guidelines for their practitioners concerning withholding and withdrawing treatments. The decision to not employ aggressive measures or to discontinue treatments that have been in place is always difficult and stressful for all involved in the decision, particularly those who continue to care for the patient on a daily basis.[15]

There appears to be more reluctance to withdraw treatments, which is reflective of the ethical and moral conflicts within each of the practitioners. Withholding usually means that there is no hope for success from the onset, whereas withdrawing means surrendering hope. Also, difficult discussions must take place between the health care professionals and the family. Communication among care providers and with family is especially difficult when families are faced with choices about forgoing life-sustaining treatment. This is a time when families most need timely information, honesty, and care providers who are clear regarding treatment options. In addition, the care providers need to listen to the families and be informed about their loved one's wishes.[16]

MEDICAL FUTILITY

The concept of medical futility has resulted in various discussions and proposed criteria or formulas to predict outcomes of care.[17-19] Medical futility has both a qualitative and a quantitative basis and can be defined as "any effort to achieve a result that is possible but that reasoning or experience suggests is highly improbable and that cannot be systematically reproduced."[20]

Therapy or treatment that achieves its predictable outcome and desired effect is, by definition, effective. But effect must be distinguished from benefit. If that predictable and desired effect is of no benefit to the patient, it is nonetheless futile. It is suggested that when physicians conclude from either personal experiences or that of colleagues or from empiric data that a particular treatment has proved to be useless in the most recent 100 cases, the treatment should be considered futile.[20] It is incumbent on health care practitioners to make optimal use of health-related resources in a technically appropriate and effective manner.[21]

ETHICS AS A FOUNDATION FOR NURSING PRACTICE

Traditional theories of professions include a code of ethics upon which the practice of the profession is based. It is by adherence to a code of ethics that the professional fulfills an obligation to provide quality practice to society.

A professional ethic is based on three elements: (1) the professional code of ethics, (2) the purpose of the profession, and (3) the standards of practice of the professional. The code of ethics developed by the professionals is the delineation of its values and relationships with and among members of the profession and society. The need for the profession and its inherent promise to provide certain duties form a contract between nursing and society. The professional standards describe specifics of practice in a variety of settings and subspecialties. Each element is dynamic, and ongoing evaluations are necessary as societal expectations change, technologies increase, and the profession evolves.

NURSING CODE OF ETHICS

The American Nurses Association (ANA) *Code of Ethics for Nurses*[22] provides the major source of ethical guidance for the nursing profession. The nine statements of the code are found in Box 2-2.

The code was first adopted by the ANA in 1950 and has undergone revisions over the years. It provides a framework for the nurse to follow in ethical decision making and provides society with a set of expectations of the profession. When the requirements of the code are not in concert with the law, it is the nurse's obligation to uphold the code because of the societal commitment inherent in nursing.

Box 2-2

CODE OF ETHICS FOR NURSES

1. The nurse, in all professional relationships, practices with compassion and respect for the inherent dignity, worth, and uniqueness of every individual, unrestricted by considerations of social or economic status, personal attributes, or the nature of health problems.
2. The nurse's primary commitment is to the patient, whether an individual, family, group, or community.
3. The nurse promotes, advocates for, and strives to protect the health, safety, and rights of the patient.
4. The nurse is responsible and accountable for individual nursing practice and determines the appropriate delegation of tasks consistent with the nurse's obligation to provide optimum patient care.
5. The nurse owes the same duties to self as to others, including the responsibility to preserve integrity and safety, to maintain competence, and to continue personal and professional growth.
6. The nurse participates in establishing, maintaining, and improving health care environments and conditions of employment conducive to the provision of quality health care and consistent with the values of the profession through individual and collective action.
7. The nurse participates in the advancement of the profession through contributions to practice, education, administration, and knowledge development.
8. The nurse collaborates with other health professionals and the public in promoting community, national, and international efforts to meet health needs.
9. The profession of nursing, as represented by associations and other members, is responsible for articulating nursing values, for maintaining the integrity of the profession and its practice, and for shaping social policy.

Box 2-3

STEPS IN ETHICAL DECISION MAKING

1. Identify the health problem.
2. Define the ethical issue.
3. Gather additional information.
4. Delineate the decision maker.
5. Examine ethical and moral principles.
6. Explore alternative options.
7. Implement decisions.
8. Evaluate and modify actions.

listen, explain, and comfort can assist the nurse in determining unmet needs of patients.

As discussed earlier in this chapter, the critical care nurse encounters ethical issues on a daily basis. Because the nurse is on the "front line" with such issues as do-not-resuscitate (DNR) orders, response to treatments, and application of new technologies and new protocols, he or she may be the one person who best knows the patient's and/or family's wishes about treatment prolongation or cessation. Therefore it is important that the nurse be included as a member of the health care team that determines ethical dilemma resolution.

WHAT IS AN ETHICAL DILEMMA?

In general, ethical cases are not always clear-cut, or "black and white." The most common ethical dilemmas encountered in critical care are foregoing treatment and allocating the scarce resource of critical care. But how does one know that a true ethical dilemma exists?

Before the application of any decision model is made, it must be determined whether a true ethical dilemma exists. Criteria for defining moral and ethical dilemmas in clinical practice are threefold: (1) an awareness of the different options; (2) an issue that has different options; and (3) two or more options with true or "good" aspects, with the choice of one option compromising the option not chosen.

STEPS IN ETHICAL DECISION MAKING

To facilitate the ethical decision-making process, a model or framework must be used so that all involved will consistently and clearly examine the multiple ethical issues that arise in critical care. Steps in ethical decision making are listed in Box 2-3.

Step One. First, the major aspects of the medical and health problems must be identified. In other words, the scientific basis of the problem, potential sequelae, prognosis, and all data relevant to the health status must be examined.

ETHICAL DECISION MAKING IN CRITICAL CARE

THE NURSE'S ROLE

Benner described the concept of relational ethics of comfort, touch, and solace, and questioned whether it is an endangered art lost to times past. However, she and her colleagues did find that there are still many examples of such comforting in daily practice, despite the overwhelming use and emphasis on technologies in treating critically ill patients. Voice and touch are described as being central for the patient recovering from anesthesia. Critical decisions such as the conservative uses of restraints is another example related to comfort and ethical care of patients.[23] Acknowledging the importance of the nurse-patient relationship and establishing time to

NIC   Values Clarification

Definition: Assisting another to clarify her/his own values in order to facilitate effective decision making

Activities

Think through the ethical and legal aspects of free choice, given the particular situation before beginning the intervention.

Create an accepting, nonjudgmental atmosphere.

Use appropriate questions to assist the patient in reflecting on the situation and what is important personally.

Use a value sheet clarifying technique (written situation and questions), as appropriate.

Pose reflective, clarifying questions that give the patient something to think about.

Encourage patient to make a list of what is important and not important in life and the time spent on each.

Encourage patient to list values that guide behavior in various settings and types of situations.

Help patient define alternatives and their advantages and disadvantages.

Encourage consideration of the issues and consequences of behavior.

Help patient to evaluate how values are in agreement with or conflict with those of family members/significant others.

Support patient's decision, as appropriate.

Use multiple sessions, as directed by the specific situation.

Avoid use of the intervention with persons with serious emotional problems.

Avoid use of cross-examining questions.

From McCloskey JC, Bulechek GM: *Nursing interventions classification (NIC)*, ed 3, St Louis, 2000, Mosby.

Step Two. The ethical problem must be clearly distinguished from other types of problems. Systems problems (i.e., those resulting from failures and inadequacies in the organization and operation of the health care facility and the health care system as a whole) are often misinterpreted as being ethical issues. Occasionally, a social problem that stems from conditions existing in the community, state, or country as a whole is also confused with ethical issues. Social problems can lead to a systemic problem, which can constrain responses to ethical problems.

Step Three. Although categories of necessary additional information will vary, whatever is missing in the initial problem presentation should be obtained. If not already known, the health prognosis and potential sequelae should be clarified. Usual demographic data—such as age, ethnicity, religious preferences, and educational and economic status—may be considered in the decision-making process. The role of the family or extended family and other support systems must be examined. It is essential that any desires that the patient may have expressed about the treatment decision, either in writing or in conversation, are obtained.

Step Four. The patient is the primary decision maker and autonomously makes these decisions after receiving information about the alternatives and sequelae of treatments or lack of treatments. However, in many ethical dilemmas the patient is not competent to make a decision, as occurs when he or she is comatose or otherwise physically or mentally unable to make a decision. It is in these situations that surrogates are designated or court-appointed because the urgency of the situation requires a quick decision.

Others who are involved in the decision also need to be identified at this time, such as family, nurse, physician, social worker, clergy, and members of other disciplines having close contact with the patient. The role of the nurse must be examined. It may not be necessary for the nurse to make a decision at all; rather, the nurse's role may be simply to provide additional information and support to the decision maker.

Step Five. Personal values, beliefs, and moral convictions of all involved in the decision process need to be known. Whether actually achieved through a group meeting or through personal introspection, values clarification facilitates the decision process. See the Nursing Interventions Classification (NIC) feature on Values Clarification.

Professional ethical codes of the nurse and physician will serve as a foundation for future decisions. At this time, legal constraints or previous legal decisions regarding circumstances at hand will need to be assessed and acknowledged.

General ethical principles also have to be examined in regard to the case at hand. For instance, are veracity, informed consent, and autonomy being promoted? Beneficence and nonmaleficence will be analyzed as they relate to a patient's condition and desires. Close examination of these principles will reveal any compromise of ethical or moral principles for either the patient or the health care provider and will assist in decision making.

Step Six. After the identification of alternative options, the outcome of each action must be predicted. This analysis helps one to select the option with the best "fit" for the specific situation or problem. Both short-range and long-range consequences of each action must be examined, and new or creative actions must be encouraged. Consideration also must be given to the "no action" option, which is another choice.

Step Seven. When a decision has been reached, it is usually after much thought and consideration.

Step Eight. Evaluation of an ethical decision serves both to assess the decision at hand and to provide a basis for future ethical decisions. If outcomes are not as predicted, it may be possible to modify the plan or to use an alternative that was not originally chosen.

STRATEGIES FOR PROMOTION OF ETHICAL DECISION MAKING

The complexity of health care and frequent ethical dilemmas encountered in clinical practice demand the establishment of mechanisms used to address ethical issues found in hospitals and health care facilities. Four types of mechanisms are discussed briefly in this chapter: institutional ethics committees, inservice and education, nursing ethics committees, and ethics rounds and conferences.

INSTITUTIONAL ETHICS COMMITTEES

Although not required by law, many health care facilities have developed institutional ethics committees (IECs) as a way to review ethical cases that are problematic for the practitioner.[24-27] The three major functions of IECs are education, consultation, and recommendation to policy-making bodies. An IEC may function in a variety of ways. The committee may serve as consultants and make recommendations that are not binding. Another type may require that health care providers consult with the committee when there is an ethical problem, but recommendations are again not binding. The third approach requires that ethical dilemmas be presented to the committee, and that the recommendations made by the committee must be followed. Regardless of the type of IEC, ethics consultations can help to resolve conflicts that may otherwise prolong unwanted on nonbeneficial treatments.[28]

IECs very often comprise executive medical staff. Membership may include staff physicians, administrators, legal counsel, nurses, social workers, clergy, and community public volunteers. To fulfill its requirement for consultation, the committee must include members who not only have expertise but also are representative of various groups. Regardless of the type of committee model, consultation and support become available to the practitioners.

INSERVICE AND EDUCATION

Basic education about ethical principles and decision making is an important first step in facilitating ethical de-

cision making among nursing staff in the critical care area.[29] It is important for nurses to examine their own values, beliefs, and moral convictions. Nurses need to know and use the ANA *Code for Nurses* in their daily clinical practice. Treatment choices for patients and ethical issues involving patients, nurses, and medical colleagues must be explored and discussed in the classroom setting where no time constraints or extraneous distractions exist to interrupt the decision-making process.

NURSING ETHICS COMMITTEES

Nursing ethics committees provide a forum in which nurses can discuss ethical issues that are pertinent to nurses at the individual, the unit, or the department level.[30] Unlike the IEC, which involves treatment choices for patients, the nursing committee may or may not involve a patient situation. Depending on the specific goals of the committee, it can also serve as a resource to nursing staff, make recommendations to a policy-making body about a variety of professional issues, or actually formulate policies. It also may serve to educate the department on ethical and professional issues. Membership usually comprises representatives from all major clinical areas or divisions, educators, clinical nurse specialists, administrators, and other specialty staff. Some departments such as critical care may have their own unit or division committee.

ETHICS ROUNDS AND CONFERENCES

Ethics rounds at the unit level regarding patients in the unit can be done by nurses on a weekly or otherwise-established basis. Rounds educate the staff to problems and serve to be "preventive" when facilitated appropriately. During the discussion, potential problems may be identified early and actions can be taken to decrease or prevent the incidence of a problem. An individual patient ethics conference can be scheduled to include only the nursing staff or to include a multidisciplinary group to discuss unit issues. A patient ethics conference may function either as a liaison with the IEC or as an end in itself.

SUMMARY

The emergence of critical care as a specialty and the introduction of sophisticated technologic innovations into critical care units have had a great impact on health care professional practices. Ethical dilemmas are encountered daily in the practice of critical care. The critical nature of the situation and the speed that is required to make decisions often prevent practitioners from gaining insight into the desires, values, and feeling of patients.

The practitioner is often left with no clear ethical or legal guidelines, particularly in the fast-paced modern critical care unit. By assuming a solely technologic approach, practitioners will violate the rights of patients and their professional codes of ethics.

By using an ethical decision-making process, the rights of the patient will be protected and logical analysis of the case will lead to a decision that is made in the best interest of the patient. It is through moral reasoning and examining, weighing, justifying, and choosing ethical principles that patient rights and individuality will be upheld. The practice of nursing is built on a foundation of moral and ethical caring, and the critical care nurse is pivotal in identifying patient situations with an ethical component and can participate in the decision-making process.

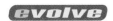 For a bonus clinical application on ethical issues, see the Evolve website.

REFERENCES

1. American Association of Critical Care Nurses: Position Statement: Moral Distress, Aliso Viejo, Calif, 7/8/04.
2. Correll N: Identifying patient's needs helps with ethical dilemmas, *AACN News* 17(6):4, 2000.
3. Singleton KA, Dever R: The challenge of autonomy: respecting the patient's wishes, *DCCN* 10(3):160, 1991.
4. Dennis BP: The origin and nature of informed consent: experiences among vulnerable groups, *J Prof Nurs* 15(5):285, 1999.
5. Crow KG, Matheson L, Steed A: Informed consent and truth telling: cultural direction of healthcare providers, *J Nurs Adm* 30(3):148, 2000.
6. Washington G: Trust: a critical element in critical care nursing, *Focus Crit Care* 17(5):418, 1990.
7. Pettrey L: Patient confidentiality: is it ever OK to tell? *AACN News* 17(4):5, 2000.
8. White J: Rationing health care resources, *Nurs Connect* 4(1):22, 1991.
9. Terry P, Rushton CH: Allocation of scarce resources: ethical challenges, clinical realities, *Am J Crit Care* 5(5):326, 1996.
10. Daly G: Ethics and economics, *Nurs Econ* 18(4):194, 2000.
11. Oleson M: Subjectively perceived quality of life, *Image J Nurs Sch* 22(3):187, 1990.
12. Kleinpell RM: Concept analysis of quality of life, *DCCN* 10(4):223, 1991.
13. Patrick DL et al: Validation of preferences for life-sustaining treatment: implications for advance care planning, *Ann Intern Med* 127(10):509, 1997.
14. Byers JF: Apply ethics to the allocation of healthcare resources, *AACN News* 17(2):2, 2000.
15. Dalinis P, Henkelman WJ: Withdrawal of treatment: ethical issues, *Nurs Manage* (Critical Care Edition) 27(9):32AA, 1996.
16. Norton SA et al: Life support withdrawal: communication and conflict, *A J Critical Care* 12(6): 548, 2003.
17. Noland LR: Medical futility: a bedside perspective, *AACN Clin Issues Crit Care Nurs* 5(3):366, 1994.
18. Montague J: A futile-care formula may ease end-of-life issues, *Hosp Health Netw* 8(4):176, 1994.
19. Taylor C: Medical futility and nursing, *Image J Nurs Sch* 27(4):301, 1995.
20. Schneiderman LJ, Jecker NS, Jonsen AR: Medical futility: its meaning and ethical implications, *Ann Intern Med* 112(12): 949, 1990.
21. Garman ME: Futile care: at what point have we done enough? *AACN News* 17(3):5, 2000.
22. American Nurses Association: *Code of ethics for nurses*, Washington, DC, 2001, The Association.
23. Benner P: Relational ethics of comfort, touch, and solace—endangered arts? *A J Crit Care* 13(4):346, 2004.
24. Bushy A, Raub JR: Implementing an ethics committee in rural institutions, *JONA* 21(12):18, 1991.
25. Bartels D, Youngner S, Levine J: Ethical committees: living up to your potential, *AACN Clin Issues Crit Care Nurs* 5(3):313, 1994.
26. Bosek MS: A comparison of ethical resources, *Medsurg Nursing* 2(4):332, 1993.
27. Feutz-Harter SA: Ethics committees: a resource for patient care decision-making, *JONA* 21(4):11, 1991.
28. Schneiderman LJ et al: Effect of ethics consultations on nonbeneficial life-sustaining treatments in the intensive care setting, *JAMA* 290(9):1166.
29. Corley MC, Selig P: Prevalence of principled thinking by critical care nurses, *DCCN* 13(2):96, 1994.
30. Buchanan S, Cook L: Nursing ethics committees: the time is now, *Nurs Manage* 23(8):40, 1992.

Legal Issues

OVERVIEW

Nursing is defined as the:
- Protection, promotion, and optimization of health and abilities;
- Prevention of illness and injury;
- Alleviation of suffering through the diagnosis and treatment of human responses; and
- Advocacy in the care of individuals, families, communities, and populations.[1]

Regardless of practice setting, the indicators of minimally competent nursing practice are broadly outlined in this definition, and further delineated in authoritative statements that are referred to as standards of practice and standards of professional performance. Standards of practice focus on care that is delivered throughout the nursing process to individuals, families, communities, and/or populations, while standards of professional performance articulate what is expected from nurses with regard to quality of care/practice, education, reflective practice, collegiality, ethics, research, resource utilization, and leadership. Standards of practice and standards for professional performance have recently been published by the American Nurses Association[1] and the American Association of Critical-Care Nurses,[3] and will be discussed later in more detail.

Nurses caring for acutely and critically ill patients alleged to have acted in a manner that is inconsistent with standards of care or standards of professional practice may find themselves involved in civil litigation that focuses in whole or in part on the alleged failure. For nurses caring for acutely and critically ill patients, the legal theories on which most civil cases against them are based include the following: negligence, negligence per se, malpractice, wrongful birth, wrongful death, defamation, assault and battery, loss of consortium, and emotional distress.

In this chapter these legal theories will be considered, as well as other issues that give rise to civil litigation in acute and critical care settings. These other issues include the respiratory management of acutely and critically ill patients and liability associated with blood transfusions, needle stick injuries, infection control, and informed consent.

NEGLIGENCE

Generally, negligence is failing to act as an ordinarily prudent person under similar circumstances. For a negligence-based cause of action to exist, there must have been a duty or obligation to conform to some standard, which was breached. The breach, in turn, must have caused some damage or injury. While negligence can occur whether or not an individual is acting in a personal or professional capacity, nurses commit negligence when they act in a manner that deviates from the standard of care and the deviation results in harm to patients for whom they care. When nurses are found to have acted negligently in their professional capacity, they are said to have committed malpractice. However, for liability to be imposed against a nurse, patient-plaintiffs must prove that the nurse had a duty to care for him or her and that the nurse breached that duty. In so doing, the breach must have caused damage that would not have occurred in the absence of negligence.

DUTY

Nurses assume a duty to provide care for patients that is consistent with the standard of care when a nurse-patient relationship is established. Providing care that is consistent with the standard of care requires nurses to protect patients from foreseeable injuries.

Cases from a number of states recognize the nurse-patient relationship as a separate and distinct relationship,[4] and as a prerequisite for determining whether or not a nurse owes the patient a duty to provide care in accordance with the requisite standard of care. If a nurse shows that he or she was not (1) assigned to that particular patient on the date that the negligence allegedly occurred, or (2) working the day or time the negligence allegedly occurred, no duty will be imposed on the nurse.

Because no duty will be imposed on the nurse, negligence allegations will fail.[5]

Although courts have been willing to construct parameters around a nurse's duty to his or her patient, when a patient establishes that a specific nurse rendered care, the nurse will have assumed a duty to provide reasonable care for the patient. A nurse's failure to provide reasonable care subjects the nurse to civil liability for negligence, where the patient proves that the failure caused damage or injury.

Lunsford v. Board of Nurse Examiners[6] illustrates this principle. In this case, Donald Wayne Floyd arrived at the emergency department of Willacy County Hospital in Raymondville, Texas, complaining of chest pain and pressure, as well as pressure that radiated down his left arm. Mr. Floyd arrived at the emergency department accompanied by Francis Farrell. Ms. Farrell attempted to have Mr. Floyd examined by a physician who was sitting at the nurses' station in the emergency department. The physician told Ms. Farrell that Mr. Floyd would need to first be seen by a nurse. Upon seeing nurse Lunsford, the physician instructed her to transfer Mr. Floyd to a neighboring hospital located 24 miles away in Harlingen, Texas because the equipment that would likely be needed to treat Mr. Floyd was already in use by another patient.

Lunsford interviewed Mr. Floyd and suspected cardiac involvement. Because of the transfer instruction that she received from the physician, she instructed Ms. Farrell to drive with her flashers on and to speed to get to the neighboring hospital. Reportedly, Lunsford also asked Ms. Farrell if she knew cardiopulmonary resuscitation (CPR), and suggested that she might need to perform CPR at some point on the way. Unfortunately, within approximately five miles of the Harlingen emergency department, Mr. Farrell died from cardiac arrest.

A complaint was subsequently filed with the Texas Board of Nurse Examiners alleging that Lunsford had acted negligently. After a hearing on the matter, the Texas Board of Nurse Examiners suspended the license of Lunsford for 1 year. Lunsford appealed the decision. The appellate court heard the appeal and determined that Lunsford as well as other nurses who are similarly situated have the duty to evaluate the status of persons who are ill and seeking professional help. In addition, the court determined that Lunsford as well as other nurses have a duty to implement care needed to stabilize a patient's condition and to prevent complications. According to this Texas Court of Appeals, Lunsford failed to act reasonably by breaching her duty to Mr. Floyd when she failed to do the following: assess him, inform the physician of the life and death nature of his condition, take appropriate action to stabilize him, and prevent his death. The court also pointed out that hospital policy or physician orders will not relieve a nurse of his or her duty to his or her patient.

Although the Texas Court of Appeals, as well as other courts throughout the United States, has determined that nurses have a duty to act reasonably when caring for patients, courts have limited the breadth of duties imposed on nurses in a number of specific instances. Nurses have been absolved of duties to assist patients who have no history of impaired mobility; and intervene when a physician exceeds the scope of consent (see *Kimball v. St. Paul Ins. Co.*,[7] *Daniel v. St. Francis Cabrini Hospital of Alexandria*,[8] and *Downey v. Mitchell*[9]).

What constitutes reasonable care has been the focus of many cases filed against health care professionals and the hospitals in which they practice. For nurses, there seems to be an emerging trend. Where the nurse reasonably executes every component of the nursing process by assessing, planning, implementing, and evaluating the care in accordance with the requisite standard of care, reasonable care will have been provided. Where, however, the nurse fails with regard to a single component of the nursing process, care provided to an acutely or critically ill patient will be deemed insufficient, unreasonable, and negligent.

A nurse's assessment-related failures include the failure to assess and analyze the level of care needed by the patient and to ascertain the patient's wishes with regard to self-determination. Planning-related failures include the failure of the nurse to diagnose appropriately. Implementation failures include the failure to communicate patient findings in a timely fashion; take appropriate action; document assessment findings, interventions, and the acutely or critically ill patient's responses to those interventions; and preserve patient privacy. Evaluation failures include the failure to act as a patient advocate.

ASSESSMENT FAILURES

FAILURE TO ASSESS AND ANALYZE THE LEVEL OF CARE NEEDED BY THE PATIENT

Nurses caring for acutely and critically ill patients have a duty to assess and analyze the level of care needed by the acutely or critically ill patient. Where a nurse allegedly fails to fulfill this responsibility, liability for negligence may be threatened. *Brandon HMA, Inc. D/B/A Rankin Medical Center v. Dawn Bradshaw*[10] demonstrates how courts handle failure to assess and analyze the level of care needed by acutely and critically ill patients.

In *Brandon*, Dawn Bradshaw contended that, while hospitalized at Rankin Medical Center (RMC) to be treated for bacterial pneumonia, she sustained permanent injuries because of negligence on the part of the nursing staff. The case was tried in front of a jury, and the jury agreed that Ms. Bradshaw sustained permanent, severe, oxygen deprivation–related brain damage because of the negligence of the nursing staff and awarded her $9,000,000 in damages.

The alleged failure occurred after a chest tube had been inserted; on the night shift a nurse allegedly failed to take vital signs between 11:00 PM and 3:30 AM until Dawn's condition had significantly worsened. At 3:30 AM Dawn was found to be nauseated, disoriented, sweating profusely, and unable to follow verbal commands. Approximately 10 minutes later, Dawn stopped breathing and had no pulse. A code was called, and CPR was administered. The code team arrived, and Dawn was revived. Subsequently, she was transferred to a rehabilitation facility specializing in treating brain injury patients and filed this negligence cause of action against RMC.

To withstand failure to assess and analyze allegations, it is not only important for nurses to assess and analyze the level of care needed by patients, but for nurses to document their assessment findings, as well as all actions taken to properly care for patients. Failure to assess and analyze, as well as failure to document the assessment findings, interventions, and the patient's response to those interventions, exposes a nurse and, in the case of *Brandon*, a hospital to liability for negligence.

FAILURE TO ASCERTAIN A PATIENT'S WISHES WITH REGARD TO SELF-DETERMINATION

Nurses caring for acutely and critically ill patients have a legal and ethical obligation to act in accordance with a patient's wishes with regard to self-determination. The standard was made explicit when the United States Supreme Court issued its opinion in *Cruzan v. Director, Missouri Department of Mental Health*.[11] In that case, the Supreme Court Justices ruled that competent adults have the right to decline any and all forms of medical intervention including life-saving or life-prolonging treatment. In the years following the issuance of this opinion, states have codified legislation that governs the creation, execution, and recognition of advanced directives. Nurses caring for the acutely and critically ill must know whether or not an advanced directive is in place for the patients for whom the nurse is caring. If one is in place, the terms of the directive must be known so that action consistent with those terms can be taken when and if the need arises.

Failure to abide by these wishes can lead to disciplinary action and civil liability. *Anderson v. St. Francis-St. George Hospital*[12] demonstrates how self-determination issues were dealt with in Ohio. In *Anderson*, Edward H. Winter was admitted to St. Francis-St. George Hospital because he was having chest pain and was fainting. After George E. Russo, Mr. Winter's treating physician, discussed treatment options with Mr. Winter, the physician entered a "no code" order in Mr. Winter's chart. Three days later, Mr. Winter began having ventricular tachycardia. A nurse defibrillated Mr. Winter and, when he re-

gained consciousness, he thanked the nurse for saving his life. When Russo was informed of Mr. Winter's condition he ordered that Lidocaine be administered. Two hours later Mr. Winter experienced another ventricular tachycardia episode, but it resolved spontaneously.

The next day, Russo ordered the discontinuation of Lidocaine and heart monitor. The day after that, Mr. Winter suffered a stroke that paralyzed his right side. Mr. Winter was eventually discharged, but his right side paralysis persisted until his death almost 2 years after his admission to St. Francis-St. George Hospital.

Before his death, Mr. Winter sued the hospital, alleging that it was negligent in failing to obey the "no code" order that had been issued. The Ohio Supreme Court eventually heard the case; the justices concluded that the interference in a person's right to die constituted a breach of the health care professional's duty to honor a patient's wishes. Despite that, the court ruled that Mr. Winter was not entitled to damages for the reasonably foreseeable damages associated with the unwanted resuscitation because he did not suffer harm as a result of the defibrillation.

PLANNING FAILURES

FAILURE TO APPROPRIATELY DIAGNOSE

Nurses caring for acutely and critically ill patients must plan effective courses of treatment. Such a course of treatment depends on a proper diagnosis. Historically, failure to diagnose cases have been filed against physicians, rather than nurses. However, nurses diagnosing patient conditions may find themselves the target of a failure-to-diagnose case, and need to be aware that liability may be imposed if the plan of care is based on an erroneous diagnosis.

IMPLEMENTATION FAILURES

FAILURE TO TIMELY COMMUNICATE PATIENT FINDINGS

Nurses spend more time with patients than any other health care professional. Nurses caring for acutely and critically ill patients spend even more time with their patients than do nurses in most other specialty settings. As a result, nurses caring for acutely and critically ill patients are in the best position to promptly detect changes in a patient's condition. Detection, however, is only the first step. Nurses caring for acutely and critically ill patients must promptly communicate troublesome patient findings. Failure to properly communicate patient findings can be devastating for patients, and can be the reason that patients file malpractice causes of action. *Gold v. United Health Service Inc.*[13] is a case involving failure to timely communicate patient findings, and illustrates the effects that these kinds of cases have on patients and on juries.

In *Gold*, Abraham Gold was born 10 weeks early at Charles S. Wilson Memorial Hospital in New York. Abraham is a spastic quadriplegic, and his parents alleged that his condition resulted from the negligence of the health care providers involved in his birth. The events giving rise to the lawsuit filed on Abraham's behalf occurred approximately 1 hour before Abraham was born. Abraham's mother, approximately 30 weeks pregnant, had been admitted for observation because she was having visual disturbances and headaches. Because of her pregnancy and neurologic condition, Kathryn Gold was being treated by her obstetrician, Donald Werner, and Jeffrey Ribner, a neurologist. At approximately 10:55 PM one evening, Kathryn Gold began having seizures. The nurse documented that grand mal seizures were occurring, but did not call the obstetrician or neurologist for 20 minutes. When she did call the neurologist, he testified that he ordered Dilantin to be administered. Dilantin was never administered by the nursing staff, because the nurse reportedly failed to inform the oncoming shift that the order had been given by the neurologist. Abraham was finally delivered via C-section, and was cared for in the neonatal intensive care unit. While a patient there, Abraham developed an *Escherichia coli* infection which caused him to go into septic shock.

The contention in this case was that the failure on the part of the nurse to timely communicate the seizure activity of Kathryn Gold caused damage to Abraham that had to be recognized via a monetary judgment. However, the defendant hospital and physicians alleged that Abraham's condition was a complication, rather than the result of any event surrounding his birth. The New York jury listened to the evidence presented by both sides and rendered a verdict in favor of Abraham for $103,127,355. In reaching their conclusion, the jury exonerated the physician defendants but held the hospital responsible for the negligence of the nurse.

Although *Gold* clearly conveys the obligation that nurses have to timely communicate patient findings, there are cases involving critical care patients that also make that point. *Denesia v. St. Elizabeth Community Health Center*[14] exemplifies how courts handle these kinds of failure to timely communicate cases.

In *Denesia* it was alleged that the death of Lucille Denesia was wrongful and the result of the nursing staff giving anticoagulation therapy and then failing to timely notify the physician of an alarmingly high partial thromboplastin time (PTT). Initially, Lucille Denesia was thought to be suffering a transient ischemic attack because of her history of atrial fibrillation. As a result, anticoagulation therapy was ordered. This therapy included an injection of heparin, followed by an intravenous (IV) infusion of that same drug, and the administration of oral Coumadin. After this treatment regime commenced,

a PTT test was ordered, and 1½ hour later, the laboratory called the results to the nurses' station reporting that Ms. Denesia's PTT was greater than 200 seconds. The nurse caring for Ms. Denesia called the primary treating physician to report the values, but the answering service the nurse called never contacted the physician. Approximately 1 hour and 10 minutes after the nurse called the answering service, Ms. Denesia started experiencing a headache; the electrocardiogram monitor showed 6 seconds of atrial beats with no corresponding ventricular response; and, when the nurse entered her room, Ms. Denesia was found to be vomiting but alert. Approximately 7 minutes after that, the nurse called Ms. Denesia's cardiologist. The nurse could not remember what she told the cardiologist, but stated that her practice was to report the patient's headaches, vomiting, and the results of the PTT test. The cardiologist contended that the nurse only reported that the PTT test had been done and that the nurse was waiting on the primary treating physician to return her call.

Approximately 1 hour and 15 minutes after the telephone conversation with the cardiologist, the nurse spoke with the primary treating physician. Again, she could not remember what she told him, but said that her practice was to report the PTT test result and the nausea and vomiting, as well as the headache Ms. Denesia was having. The primary treating physician testified that he was not informed of the PTT result, but that he ordered the IV infusion of heparin to be reduced. Twenty minutes after this conversation, Ms. Denesia vomited again. Antinausea medication was administered, but Ms. Denesia vomited again about 45 minutes later.

After these two vomiting episodes, Ms. Denesia rested comfortably for approximately 2 hours and 5 minutes. When she awoke, she vomited again, became lethargic, could not sit up, and her right hand grasp was found to be stronger than her left. The nurse called the primary treating physician again. The heparin infusion was discontinued. It was at this point that the primary treating physician testified that he learned of the abnormal PTT result. Twenty-five minutes later, Ms. Denesia was transferred to the intensive care unit because of continuing neurologic impairment. Two hours and 45 minutes later, her PTT was down to 27 seconds. However, Ms. Denesia lapsed into a coma and died from a massive cerebral hemorrhage.

While a jury initially rendered a decision against the estate of Ms. Denesia, the case was appealed to the Supreme Court of Nebraska, where the justices ordered that the case be retried because prejudicial jury instructions were given during the first trial. For nurses caring for acutely and critically ill patients, it is imperative that interactions with physicians be documented, whether in person or over the telephone, as well as the information conveyed during those interactions. Had the nurse taken the time to document what she told the cardiologist and the primary treating physician, this litigation may have been avoided.

FAILURE TO TAKE APPROPRIATE ACTION

Cases from across the country continue to affirm that it is the nurse's responsibility to take affirmative action when action is indicated. *Brookover v. Mary Hitchcock Memorial Hospital*[15] is one such case. In *Brookover*, Ronald Brookover had significant seizure activity that resulted in his need for a corpus callostomy, a surgical procedure performed in separate operations. Three days after the second surgery, Mr. Brookover got out of bed, fell, and broke his hip. The medical record indicated that Mr. Brookover was unrestrained and used his call light to indicate that he needed assistance. Based on this evidence, the hospital was found liable for Mr. Brookover's injury.

Another failure to take appropriate action case was tried in Colorado. That case was *Garcia v. United States.*[16] In *Garcia*, Candido Garcia was admitted to a Veteran's Administration Medical Center for the removal of a subdural hematoma. After surgery he began making snorting noises and emitting white bubbles at his mouth. Mr. Garcia's wife reported the occurrence to the nurse caring for him. The nurse, Margaret John, reportedly told the Mrs. Garcia that the extent of her responsibility was to ensure that the surgically inserted drainage tubes were kept clear. Doctors from a neighboring hospital were eventually called but were not informed of the emergency nature of the situation. The result was that Mr. Garcia did not receive proper medical assistance for a period of about 45 to 50 minutes. Following medical intervention, including a return trip to the operating room, Mr. Garcia was quadriplegic. At trial, the hospital was found to be negligent and liable for the damages sustained by Candido Garcia and awarded more than $2.3 million in damages, interest, and the cost of litigation to Mr. Garcia and his wife. In reaching its decision, the court found that the nursing staff should have recognized the emergency nature of the situation and taken proper steps to notify the attending physician.

Failure to take appropriate action in cases involving acutely and critically ill patients have not only included physician-notification issues, they have involved failure to follow physician orders,[17,18] failure to appropriately administer medication,[19-21] and failure to properly treat.[19] To avoid failure to take appropriate action allegations, nurses caring for acutely and critically ill patients need to recognize signs and symptoms of complications and patient compromise. Nurses must also ensure that those signs and symptoms are timely communicated to the physician, and take other affirmative action that is authorized and appropriate. In addition, patient findings, interventions and actions taken, and patient responses to those interventions must be documented.

FAILURE TO DOCUMENT

Not only are nurses caring for acutely and critically ill patients required to take appropriate action, but they are also required to accurately document their findings, interventions, and patients' response to those interventions. Failure to thoroughly and accurately document any aspect of care gives rise to negligence causes of actions. *Haney v. Alexander*, a case from North Carolina, demonstrates how courts and juries deal with a nurse's failure to properly document.

In *Haney* a nurse purportedly failed to take appropriate action and failed to properly document care rendered. Originally the trial court dismissed the hospital from the case. The physician-defendants later settled with the family. The family appealed the trial court's decision to dismiss the hospital, and citing the negligence of the nurse, the court of appeals agreed that the hospital should not have been dismissed and determined that a jury trial should be commenced.

In this case, a nurse caring for a patient experiencing atrial fibrillation failed to take, record, and communicate all of a patient's vital signs and failed to properly document the order and administration of Librium. Reportedly Librium had already been administered, but the on-call physician was told that Librium had not been administered, so the physician ordered again that Librium be given. The nurse gave the medication, and 45 minutes later the patient was found dead.

In reversing the trial court's previous decision to dismiss the hospital, the court of appeals concluded that the nurse was negligent in several respects. Specifically, the court of appeals observed that the events that led to the double administration of Librium could have prevented the patient from being able to communicate his worsening condition and receiving life-saving medical assistance.

Haney and *Denesia* are indicative of the need for nurses caring for acutely and critically ill patients to thoroughly document the care that is given, interventions and actions taken, and the response of the patient to those interventions and actions. Failure to thoroughly document opens the door for patient-plaintiffs to allege that the absence of documentation signals a breach of the standard of care.

FAILURE TO PRESERVE PATIENT PRIVACY

Nurses have a duty to preserve patient privacy. State and federal statutes and case law affirm this duty. *Doe v. Ohio State University Hospital and Clinics* explores the issue. In *Doe* a nurse taking care of a human immunodeficiency virus (HIV)–positive patient wrote his HIV status down on a laboratory requisition slip in the "other test" section of the form. This was done so that laboratory personnel could be alerted to the patient's HIV status. The patient was to have a complete blood count and potassium level drawn prior to having a lithotripsy performed to remove kidney stones. The laboratory staff interpreted the notation made by the nurse as an instruction to perform an HIV screen, and not a message regarding the patient's HIV status. The patient found out that the HIV screen had been done, and was outraged that the HIV testing had been done without his consent. This facility had a policy which prohibited HIV testing without informed consent being obtained by the physician.

The case was ultimately dismissed, but serves as a reminder to guard the privacy of every patient. Nurses can ensure that the privacy of acutely and critically ill patients is protected by following privacy-related regulations, policies, and procedures, and by refraining from having discussions about specific patients with anyone, except other health care professionals involved in the care of the patient. When discussing specific patients with other health care professionals, it is imperative that patient-specific discussions occur in non-public settings. Discussions about specific patients are never appropriate in public areas like elevators, cafeterias, gift shops, and parking lots.

EVALUATION FAILURES

FAILURE TO ACT AS A PATIENT ADVOCATE

From admission to discharge, nurses have a duty to act as a patient advocate. For nurses caring for acutely and critically ill patients, this duty imposes the responsibility to evaluate the care that is being given to patients. The landmark case failure to advocate case is *Darling v. Charleston Community Memorial Hospital*,[22] a case decided by the Illinois Supreme Court in 1965.

In *Darling*, Dorrence Darling II was an 18-year-old athlete who broke his leg playing football. He was taken to Charleston Community Memorial Hospital for treatment. Dorrence was placed in traction, and his broken leg was placed in a plaster cast. A heat cradle was used to dry the cast. Shortly after the cast had been applied, Dorrence began to complain of severe pain in the leg that had been broken. Dorrence's toes that protruded from the cast became swollen and dark in color and eventually became cold and insensitive to tactile stimulation.

The day after Dorrence had been admitted, his treating physician, John R. Alexander, notched the cast around Dorrence's toes. The next day, Alexander cut the cast approximately 3 inches from the foot toward Dorrence's knee. The day after that, Alexander used a Stryker saw to split the sides of the cast and cut both sides of Dorrence's broken leg. By this time, blood and other drainage was noted by the nursing staff. In addi-

tion, the room in which Dorrence was staying became filled with a noxious odor.

Fourteen days after his admission to Charleston Community Memorial Hospital, Dorrence was transferred to Barnes Hospital in St. Louis, Missouri. There he was cared for by surgeon Fred Reynolds. After multiple attempts to save the leg of Dorrence Darling, Reynolds finally had to amputate his lower leg approximately 8 inches below the knee.

Subsequently, Charleston Community Hospital and John R. Alexander were sued. The hospital, through the actions of the nursing staff and John R. Alexander, was alleged to have failed to treat Dorrence consistently with the requisite standard of care. With regard to the nursing staff, Darling alleged that they were negligent in assessing his deteriorating circulatory condition in accordance with hospital policy and procedure and that they failed to report the developments to the medical staff or hospital administration. A settlement was reached with the doctor, John R. Alexander, so the case against the hospital was presented to an Illinois jury. After listening to the evidence, the jury returned a verdict against the hospital for $150,000. The hospital appealed the decision, and the Supreme Court of Illinois eventually heard the appeal. In affirming the jury verdict, the Illinois Supreme Court justices determined that a jury could have reasonably concluded that the nurses involved in the care and treatment of Dorrence Darling were negligent in assessing his circulatory status. According to the court, if the nursing staff had promptly recognized that circulatory compromise was occurring, steps could have been taken to prevent the irreversible effects of prolonged inadequate circulation. Had they recognized the significance of the symptoms they were seeing, the nursing staff could have exercised their duty to inform hospital authorities so that appropriate action could be taken. Because they failed to act as patient advocate, Dorrence lost his leg, and the hospital was liable for their failure.

While *Darling* is a case that was decided in 1965, courts continue to hold that all nurses, including those caring for acutely and critically ill patients, have a nondelegable duty to act as patient advocate (see *NKC Hospital Inc. v. Anthony*[23] and *Reinen v. Northern Arizona Orthopedics*[24]). Failure to act as patient advocate exposes the nurse to substantial liability, but more importantly, exposes patients to life-altering and life-ending complications that could be avoided.

BREACH

Breach is the failure to act consistently with applicable standards of care. For a nurse to be found negligent, the patient must establish that the nurse had a duty to provide care and that the nurse failed to provide care consistent with those standards. Further, the nurse's failure, or breach, must have caused the damage(s) about which the patient seeks redress. An Idaho case exemplifies the courts' willingness to conclude that breach did not occur where the actions of nurses meet or exceed the standard of care.

In Idaho *Sparks v. St. Luke's Regional Medical Center*[25] was tried. In the case, the family of Thomas Sparks sued St. Luke's Regional Medical Center and treating physicians, alleging that their negligence resulted in Thomas Sparks sustaining brain damage after he was extubated and after he experienced cardiac arrest. The trial court granted the motion by St. Luke's to have judgment entered in its favor, and Sparks appealed the matter to the Idaho Supreme Court.

The Idaho Supreme Court reviewed the evidence presented by both parties and concluded that the nurses met the requisite standard of care. Therefore it found that no breach occurred. In fact, the court pointed out that Thomas Sparks presented evidence that recognized that the standard of care regarding the extubation and subsequent hospital care was met by the St. Luke's personnel. As a result, the ruling of the trial court was affirmed.

Sparks demonstrates that courts will consider whether or not something a nurse did or failed to provide the requisite standard of care. In so doing, applicable Nurse Practice Acts, professional practice standards, job descriptions, and policies/procedures/protocols/pathways, as well as other reference sources including case law, journal articles, textbooks, and other manuscripts determine the standard of care.

Nurse Practice Acts

Nurse Practice Acts (NPAs) provide statutory authority for the practice of nursing in every state within the United States. Nurses, as licensed and regulated health care professionals, are required to abide by the requirements of the applicable practice act. Failure to act consistently with NPA requirements exposes a nurse to civil liability in negligence or malpractice causes of action because the statutory standard was breached.

In NPAs the activities in which a registered nurse may engage are referred to as a nurse's scope of practice. Typically scope of practice activities for registered nurses include assessing the health status of individuals and groups; establishing a nursing diagnosis and goals to meet identified health care needs; creating and implementing a plan of care; prescribing and implementing interventions consistent with the plan of care; delegating nursing interventions to qualified others as the practice act permits; providing for the maintenance of safe and effective nursing care rendered directly or indirectly and evaluating patient responses to interventions; teaching the theory and practice of nursing; and collaborating with other health care professionals in the delivery of health care services.[26]

Professional Practice Standards

Actions which are consistent with professional practice standards will be evidence that the nurse did not breach his or her duty to patients. Therefore it is important to know what professional practice standards expect of nurses generally, as well as what is expected of nurses practicing in specialty settings. Standards of practice and standards of professional performance for nurses have been issued by the American Nurses Association as well as the American Association of Critical-Care Nurses. All nurses must practice in a manner that is consistent with the standards issued by the American Nurses Association. These standards promulgated by the American Nurses Association are listed at Box 3-1. Nurses caring for acutely and critically ill patients must also practice in accordance with the standards issued by the American Association of Critical-Care Nurses. These practice specialty standards are listed at Box 3-2.

Not only do these standards provide guidance for nurses, but they also provide definitive guidance in courtrooms. *Koeniger v. Eckrich*[27] is a case in which standards promulgated by the American Nurses Association were used in a case where the plaintiff alleged that standards of care were breached.

In *Koeniger* Winnfred Scoblic was admitted to Dakota Midland Hospital for surgical correction of incontinence. Two days later, J.A. Eckrich performed the surgery. After surgery, Ms. Scoblic had a temperature that fluctuated. On the day of discharge, Ms. Scoblic's temperature was 100.2° F. In spite of her temperature, Ms. Scoblic was discharged. Sixteen days after her original surgery, Ms. Scoblic was readmitted because of a fever and severe abdominal pain. She was diagnosed with septicemia. Two days later, Ms. Scoblic was transferred to the University of Minnesota Hospital. She died from multiple organ failure several weeks later.

On behalf of Ms. Scoblic, her daughter Patricia Koeniger filed a malpractice cause of action contending that the care rendered to her mother deviated from the standard of care. An expert retained by Koeniger used the standards published by the American Nurses Association and other general nursing treatises to conclude that the nursing staff failed to adhere to standards of care applicable to Ms. Scoblic as a postoperative urologic patient. At the trial court level, the case was dismissed. It was subsequently heard and reversed by the South Dakota Supreme Court. The South Dakota Supreme Court ordered that a trial occur so that jurors could have an opportunity to determine whether or not the actions on the part of the defendants caused the alleged wrongful death of Ms. Scoblic.

Job Descriptions/Contracts

Although standards of care are usually derived outside of any one specific institution, job descriptions and/or

Box 3-1

NURSING: SCOPE AND STANDARDS OF PRACTICE

The registered nurse does the following:

STANDARDS OF PRACTICE

Assessment
Collects comprehensive data pertinent to the patient's health or the situation

Diagnosis
Analyzes assessment data to determine the diagnoses or issues

Outcomes identification
Identifies expected outcomes for an individualized patient or situation plan

Planning
Develops a plan that prescribes strategies and alternatives to attain expected outcomes

Implementation
Implements the identified plan, including care coordination, health teaching and health promotion, consultation, prescriptive authority, and treatment and evaluation

Evaluation
Evaluates progress toward outcomes attainment

STANDARDS OF PROFESSIONAL PERFORMANCE

Quality of practice
Systematically enhances the quality and effectiveness of nursing practice

Education
Attains knowledge and competency that reflects current nursing practice

Professional practice evaluation
Evaluates one's own nursing practice in relation to professional practice standards and guidelines, relevant statutes, rules and regulations

Collegiality
Interacts with and contributes to the professional development of peers and colleagues

Collaboration
Collaborates with patient, family, and others in the conduct of nursing practice

Ethics
Integrates ethical principles in all areas of practice

Research
Integrates research findings into practice

Resource utilization
Considers factors related to safety, effectiveness, cost, and impact on practice in the planning and delivery of nursing services

Leadership
Provides leadership in the professional practice setting and the profession

From American Nurses Association: *Nursing: scope and standards of practice,* Washington, DC, 2004, The Association.

contracts delineating the terms of employment may be institution-specific. A nurse's job description and/or employment contract may contain provisions which require a nurse to act or refrain to act in a specific manner and within a specific period of time. Failure to adhere to those provisions could give rise to negligence causes of action where the patient-plaintiff asserts that the nurse failed to act in accordance with his or her job description or employment contract. Accordingly, job descriptions and employment contracts must be reflective of the standard of care, and expectations articulated in a manner which is reasonable.

POLICIES/PROCEDURES/PROTOCOLS/PATHWAYS

Nurses caring for acutely and critically ill patients are required to act in a manner that is consistent with organizational policies, procedures, protocols, and clinical pathways. Failure to act consistently with organizational policies, procedures, and protocols may result in liability where a patient is harmed because of the failure. Two cases are illustrative: *Teffeteller v. University of Minnesota,*[28] and *Ress v. Abbott Northwestern.*[29] In *Teffeteller*, a critically ill pediatric patient died from nar-

cotic toxicity because a nurse failed to follow the applicable protocol. In *Ress*, Randy Ress, an intensive care nurse contested being terminated. The hospital claimed that he was terminated because he failed to act in a manner consistent with past instruction, warning, and applicable protocols after he lavaged an endotracheal tube with iced, nonsterile saline and subsequently refused to promptly obtain a chest x-ray on a patient with gross hemoptysis. In upholding the termination decision, the Minnesota Supreme Court concluded that Randy Ress acted with willful disregard for the interests of Abbott Northwestern, and that he was disqualified from receiving unemployment benefits.

CAUSATION

In negligence causes of action focusing on care rendered by nurses, patients must prove that the nurse breached his or her duty to the patient and that the breach caused the patient to sustain injuries or damages for which he or she seeks monetary remuneration. Causation, as an element of negligence, is a pivotal element in civil cases filed against nurses. If causation is not proven by plaintiffs, there can be no recovery.

Box 3-2

STANDARDS FOR ACUTE AND CRITICAL CARE NURSING PRACTICE

The nurse caring for the acutely and critically ill patient observes the following:

STANDARDS OF CARE

Assessment
Collects relevant patient health data

Diagnosis
Analyzes the assessment data in determining diagnoses

Outcomes Identification
Identifies individualized, expected outcomes for patients

PLANNING
Develops a plan of care that prescribes interventions to attain expected outcomes

IMPLEMENTATION
Implements interventions identified in the plan of care

Evaluation
Evaluates the patient's progress toward attaining expected outcomes

STANDARDS OF PROFESSIONAL PERFORMANCE
Quality of care
Systematically evaluates the quality and effectiveness of nursing practice

Individual practice evaluation
Reflects knowledge of current professional standards, laws, and regulations

Education
Acquires and maintains current knowledge and competency in the care of acutely and critically ill patients

Collegiality
Interacts with and contributes to the professional development of peers and other health care providers as colleagues

Ethics
Makes decisions and takes actions on behalf of acutely and critically ill patients in an ethical manner

Collaboration
Collaborates with the team of patients, family, and health care providers in proving patient care in a healing, humane, and caring environment

Research
Uses clinical inquiry in practice

Resource utilization
Considers factors related to safety, effectiveness, and cost in planning and delivering patient care

From Medina J: *Standards for acute and critical care nursing practice,* ed 3, Aliso Viejo, Calif, 2000, American Association of Critical Care Nurses.

It should be no surprise, then, that nursing negligence cases focus on causation. If patients prove that the health care organization, or the nurse practicing in that setting, did or failed to do something which caused an injury, then they have met their burden of proof. If, on the other hand, patients fail to establish that some act or omission directly resulted in the injuries for which they are seeking compensation, or if health care organizations or nurses show that the complained-of injury was the result of something other than an action or omission which fell below the standard of care, then recovery will be denied. *McMullen v. Ohio State University Hospitals*[30] dealt with the causation issue, and was ultimately decided by the Ohio Supreme Court.

In *McMullen* a patient had been intubated and placed on a ventilator. Three days after she had been intubated, her oxygen saturation level suddenly dropped, as did her blood pressure, and she became cyanotic and dyspneic. The patient also developed a squeak, which the nurse thought was a cuff leak on the endotracheal tube. The nurse believed that the patient was dying and made a "stat" page so that on-call physicians would be notified. Prior to the arrival of the physicians, the nurse removed the patient's endotracheal tube. When the physicians ar-

rived, they attempted to reintubate the patient. It took more than 20 minutes for their reintubation attempts to be successful. The patient never resumed consciousness and died 7 days later.

The patient's estate brought a wrongful death cause of action against the Ohio State University Hospitals. The case went to trial, where damages were awarded to the patient's estate. Ohio State University Hospitals appealed the award to the Franklin County Court of Appeals. The Court of Appeals reversed the award to the patient's estate. The patient's estate then appealed the case to the Ohio Supreme Court. The Ohio Supreme Court, among other things, concluded that the decision of the Court of Appeals was erroneous and had be reversed, and that actions of the nurse directly caused the ultimate harm sustained by the patient. According to the Ohio Supreme Court, the nurse's removal of the patient's endotracheal tube was negligent and set into motion a chain of events that directly caused the patient to die.

DAMAGES

The fourth and final element of negligence is damages. Damages are derived from the harm or injury suffered by the acutely and critically ill patient, and are calculated as a dollar amount. In order for liability to be imposed against a nurse caring for an acutely and critically ill patient, that patient must prove that something the nurse did or failed to do was inconsistent with the standard of care, and that the inconsistency caused harm or injury for which the patient should be compensated.

In 1998, 36% of all medical malpractice cases filed resulted in jury verdicts in favor of patient-plaintiffs. In 2001 patient-plaintiffs won 27% of the medical malpractice cases tried in front of a jury, and 32% of those patient-plaintiff winners received $1,000,000 injury verdicts. Although the percentage of patient-plaintiff wins continues to decrease, jury awards are increasing. In 1997 the median jury award in medical malpractice cases was $515,738, whereas in 1998, the median jury award was up 46% to $755,530. Median jury awards were highest in childbirth cases at $2 million. Median awards in medication administration and misdiagnosis cases were more than $600,000, and median jury awards were $400,000, $300,000 and $230,000 in nonsurgical treatment cases, surgical matters, and health care professional-patient relationship cases, respectively.[31] In 2001 the median jury award in medical malpractice cases was $431,000.[32] This median award was almost 16 times higher than the median award of $27,000 in all other tort cases.

The number of nurses being named defendants in these cases is increasing. Some estimate that the number of nurses being named as individual defendants has increased 10% since 1995.[33] Accordingly, nurses caring for acutely and critically ill patients need to carefully consider whether or not to purchase professional liability insurance, and if so, the amount and type of coverage that is needed. Damage trends suggest that nurses caring for acutely and critically ill patients need to consider obtaining substantial insurance coverage.

NEGLIGENCE PER SE

Most courts have ruled that a statutory violation is negligence per se. Negligence per se allows patient-plaintiffs to conclusively establish a presumption of negligence and breach of a nurse's duty to the acutely and critically ill patient. However, a few courts hold that statutory violations give rise to a presumption with regard to the duty and breach components of a negligence cause of action, or that the statutory violation provides only threshold evidence of negligence. Regardless of the jurisdiction, however, statutory violations do assist patient-plaintiffs in proving that negligence occurred. This was the case in *Lama v. Borras.*[34] In that case, a patient acquired a postoperative infection, and the nurse failed to recognize the associated signs and symptoms. The court concluded that the nurse was negligent, and that the doctrine of negligence per se applied because the nurse's failure was a violation of Puerto Rico Health Regulations.

MALPRACTICE

Malpractice is professional misconduct or the failure to meet the requisite standard of care. While negligence may be committed by anyone, malpractice requires the alleged wrongdoer to have special standing as a professional. When an individual acts negligently in a personal rather than professional capacity, that individual would be subject to liability for negligence rather than malpractice. When a wrongdoer is a nurse caring for acutely and critically ill patients and is accused of acting or failing to act in a manner that is consistent with the standard of care, that nurse will be subject to liability for professional negligence or malpractice.

In civil cases alleging wrongdoing by health care professionals, the terms malpractice and negligence are used interchangeably, although there are courts which distinguish between the two causes of action. The malpractice-negligence distinction was addressed in *Candler General Hospital Inc. v. McNorrill.*[35] In that case, the court concluded that malpractice was merely a professional negligence act. According to the court, when acting in their professional capacity, nurses are subject to malpractice causes of action when patients assert that the nurse failed to meet the requisite standard of care.

In *Gould v. NY City Health and Hospital,*[36] the court looked at the elements that must be proven in a malpractice case and determined that there were three duties inherent in a malpractice cause of action. They were to (1) possess the requisite knowledge and skill possessed by an average member of the profession; (2) exercise reasonable and ordinary care in the application of professional knowledge and skill; and (3) use best judgment in the application of professional knowledge and skill. These duties are consistent with the duties nurses have in traditional negligence-based causes of action.

Griffin v. The Methodist Hospital[37] demonstrates that most courts treat malpractice cases like negligence cases. The only difference is that malpractice cases involve individuals with some special standing. In *Griffin,* Sharon Ann Griffin and her husband Dennis Griffin filed a malpractice cause of action against the Methodist Hospital and Sharon's treating physicians. They allege that Sharon sustained damages because of the negligent treatment of her treating physicians, and nursing staff while she was hospitalized at the Methodist Hospital. Specifically, Sharon alleged that her development of an Achilles tendon contraction was the result of negligence. The Methodist Hospital contended that despite Sharon's development of foot drop, the staff fully complied with applicable standards of care. As a result, the hospital asked the judge to dismiss the matter. The judge agreed. Sharon and her husband appealed the case to the Court of Appeals. After reviewing the case, the Court of Appeals determined that the case should not have been dismissed, and ordered that the matter be slated for trial.

Candler, Gould, and *Griffin* are similar and suggest that professional negligence and malpractice causes of action are treated similarly. Whether sued for professional negligence or malpractice, nurses will be required to defend their actions or alleged failures to act by showing how their actions or inactions were consistent with the standard of care.

WRONGFUL BIRTH

Wrongful birth claims are filed by parents who contend that they would have terminated their pregnancy had they known that their child was going to be born with severe birth defects. Typically, parents allege that the pregnancy would have been terminated had they been timely informed, through prenatal diagnostic tests, of the possibility of having a child with severe birth defects. Wrongful birth claims are distinguished from wrongful life and wrongful conception cases in that wrongful life cases are usually commenced by the child born with birth defects, rather than the child's parents. Wrongful birth claims, on the other hand, are designed to compensate parents, not the child. Alternatively, wrongful conception can be brought by a healthy child or that child's parents and usually allege the failure to perform a contraceptive procedure. *Smith v. Cote*[38] and *Duplan v. Harper*[39] are representative of the way that courts handle wrongful birth claims.

In *Smith,* Linda J. Smith, in her second trimester, underwent a rubella titer. Test results indicated that she had been exposed to rubella. Approximately 5 months later, Linda J. Smith gave birth to a full-term infant, Heather B. Smith. Heather was born with rubella syndrome, suffered from cataracts, multiple congenital heart defects, retardation, and significant hearing impairment. Heather was also legally blind. Approximately 4 years after Heather was born, Linda and Heather filed suit, alleging that Linda should have been tested for the disease in a timely manner and Linda should have been advised of the potential for delivering a baby with rubella-related birth defects.

The case was eventually heard by the New Hampshire Supreme Court, where the justices affirmed that wrongful birth actions would be recognized in New Hampshire and that damages could be recovered for extraordinary medical and educational costs associated with raising the impaired child, as well as extraordinary parental care and tangible losses attributable to the parents' emotional distress.

In *Duplan,* Roseann Duplan learned that she was pregnant after a pregnancy test was performed at the OB/GYN clinic at Tinker Air Force Base in Midwest City, Oklahoma. At that time, Roseann Duplan worked at a childcare center. Because she worked at a childcare center, Roseann Duplan knew that she was at an increased risk for contracting cytomegalovirus (CMV), a virus that is harmless for many people but which can cause serious birth defects if it is contracted during pregnancy. Consequently, she requested to be tested for CMV. She made multiple requests to have the test performed, but it was not performed until late in her pregnancy. When the test was finally performed, it indicated that Ms. Duplan had contracted a CMV infection in the first trimester of her pregnancy. A clinic nurse, Elizabeth Reed, reportedly informed Ms. Duplan that the CMV test was positive, and that the positive result meant that she was immune to CMV. Months later, Ms. Duplan delivered a severely mentally retarded baby boy.

Subsequently, this cause of action was filed. Ms. Duplan contended that her treating physician failed to discuss the CMV infection with her, failed to order the test in a timely manner, and did not follow the virus's impact on the unborn fetus. According to Ms. Duplan, the nurse failed to give accurate information about the meaning of the CMV test results.

At trial, the United States District Court found the treating physician and nurse negligent and awarded the Duplans $3,056,100 in damages. The case was appealed to the United States Court of Appeals. After reviewing the matter, the Court of Appeals affirmed the damage award.

Although wrongful birth claims do not typically emerge out of treatment rendered in acute or critical care settings, it is important for nurses caring for acutely and critically ill patients to know that this claim exists, and discuss fetal implications of treatment with that patient when caring for pregnant women.

WRONGFUL DEATH

Wrongful death causes of action are filed by the survivors of patients who allege that the patient died because of the negligence of health care organizations and/or health care professionals. *Reynolds v. Swigert*[40] *and Manning v. Twin Falls Clinic & Hospital*[41] provide insight into how courts handle wrongful death cases.

In *Reynolds,* a child had been seen three times as an outpatient. Despite these visits, the girl died from meningitis. Initially the child's mother took her to an ambulatory care clinic because she was listless and had a fever. Three days later, the mother took her daughter to an emergency department. There she was cared for by a nurse who wrote that the child had a fever, but failed to record any vital signs. The treating emergency room physician determined that the child had bronchopneumonia. He prescribed medications and discharged the child. The next day, the mother returned with the daughter to the emergency department, but was seen by a different physician. By that time, the girl was not eating and her neck was stiff. This time, the physician determined that the girl was suffering from meningitis. She was admitted to the hospital and died 4 days later.

After the child's death, the mother filed this wrongful death cause of action against the first emergency department physician and the hospital. The mother contended that the physician was negligent in failing to make the proper diagnosis while the child's illness was treatable, and in failing to perform an adequate physical examination. The mother also alleged that the emergency department nurse failed to perform an adequate physical examination. Specifically, the mother alleged that the nurse failed to take her daughter's vital signs. Expert testimony was used to establish that it was the responsibility of the emergency department nurse to take vital signs without being ordered to do so.

In *Manning*, the trial court determined that the nurse failed to exercise reasonable care, and was deemed negligent in the death of Daryl Manning, a 67-year-old man. Mr. Manning had been admitted to the hospital in the last stages of chronic obstructive pulmonary disease, hypoxemia, and increased carbon dioxide retention, and was on continuous supplemental oxygen via a nasal cannula. On his admission to the hospital, Mr. Manning was classified as a "no code." His condition steadily deteriorated, so Virginia L. Anderson, LPN, discontinued Mr. Manning's supplemental oxygen and began to transfer him to a private room. The family requested that oxygen be administered during the move, but the nurse declined to apply it, citing the proximity between the patient's current location and the private room. After the bed had been moved approximately 15 feet, Mr. Manning stopped breathing. Resuscitation was attempted, but when the physician who was aware of Mr. Manning's "no code" status arrived, resuscitative measures were discontinued. The family sued the hospital and two nurses. One nurse, Donna Gay Austin, RN, was relieved of all liability, but the jury determined that Virginia L. Anderson, LPN, was negligent in transferring Mr. Manning without using supplemental oxygen and awarded the Manning family compensatory, emotional distress, and punitive damages.

For families and health care professionals, wrongful death cases are among the most traumatic. It is in these cases that the life-and-death nature of the health care experience is exposed. In addition, it is in reviewing these kinds of cases that one learns that rarely at issue is the use, misuse, or malfunction of sophisticated, cutting-edge technology, or the miscalculation of a complex formula. On the contrary, a review of wrongful death cases suggests that the alleged failure at issue is typically much more basic and has more to do with paying attention. For instance, it is the failure to thoroughly assess patients, to take vital signs, to properly administer medication, and to administer portable oxygen to a respiratory-compromised patient that has been the focus of most of the wrongful death cases discussed in this chapter. To avoid wrongful death liability, it is imperative that nurses caring for acutely and critically ill patients pay attention, recognize the signs and symptoms of complications and compromise, and take authorized affirmative action to protect the patient.

DEFAMATION

Defamation causes of action can be filed against health care professionals where individuals believe that something the health care professional has said or written injures the patient's reputation. Any communication may be considered defamatory if it compromises a person's decency, respect for other, integrity, or reputation. If the defamatory communication is in writing, libel has been committed. If, on the other hand, the defamatory communication is verbal, slander has been committed.

To be successful, individuals alleging that they have been defamed must prove that the defamatory communication came from the defendant, and that the defamatory language pertained specifically to the plaintiff. In addition, the defamatory communication must have been published to a third person, and the plaintiff must have suffered damage to his or her reputation. Where defamation involves a public figure or a matter of public concern, the plaintiff must prove that the defamatory communication was false and was made with malice. *Meuser v. Rocky Mountain Hospital*[42] is a case in which a nurse-plaintiff alleged that a hospital administrator had defamed her.

In *Meuser*, Virginia T. Meuser alleged that the hospital administrator, Robert Pierce, defamed her in a letter which was published to other employees and in a statement to employees. In reviewing Meuser's defamation allegations, a Colorado Court of Appeals concluded that she failed to present clear and convincing evidence that the allegedly defamatory statements made by Pierce were false or that the defendant hospital or administrator entertained serious doubts about the truth of the statements. As a result, the trial court did not have jurisdiction to resolve the defamation claims.

ASSAULT AND BATTERY

Assault and battery are two separate torts that can be alleged by patients. Assault is any intentional act which creates reasonable apprehension of immediate harmful or offensive contact with the plaintiff. With assault, no actual contact is necessary. Battery, on the other hand, is any intentional act that brings about actual harmful or offensive contact with the plaintiff. In health care cases, assault occurs where a patient fears harmful or offensive touching. Harmful or offensive touching occurs where the patient has not consented to it. Battery occurs where the health care professional actually touches the patient in an unauthorized manner. Sexual misconduct, operating on an unauthorized body part, and removing the wrong limb constitute battery behaviors. In addition to battery, assault may also be alleged in these instances, if the patient is aware that he or she is going to be touched in a manner not authorized by informed consent.

Historically, assault and battery allegations have been treated differently than traditional negligence-based causes of actions. Because assault and battery are considered intentional acts, these offenses have not been routinely covered by professional liability insurers. However, two cases recently decided by the Alabama and South Dakota Supreme Courts have indicated that some assault and battery cases may be considered malpractice. In Alabama the case was *Mock v. Allen*,[43] whereas in South Dakota the case was *Martinmaas v. Engelmann*.[44]

LOSS OF CONSORTIUM

In addition to alleging negligence or malpractice, plaintiffs and their family members may also allege loss of consortium where their relationships with their spouses, children, or parents have suffered because of the professional negligence of the health care organization and/or nurse. Loss of consortium claims are based on the deprivation of an individual's right to enjoy the cooperation, company, affection, love, and aid of others, and are typically filed by family members of patients who have allegedly been treated negligently by health care professionals.

EMOTIONAL DISTRESS

Like loss of consortium claims, emotional distress claims can be added as causes of action in cases alleging that malpractice or negligence has occurred. Emotional distress claims may be classified as either intentional or negligent. Intentional emotional distress claims assert that the plaintiff acted in a way that intentionally caused emotional distress. Negligent emotional distress claims, however, do not contemplate an intentional act on the part of defendant-health care providers.

Regardless of the classification, emotional distress claims are alleged when an act is considered to be outrageous. Outrageous acts are those which are reckless and intolerable and have a tendency to shock the conscience. Because of the extreme nature of emotional distress claims, they are difficult for patients to prove.

OTHER ISSUES GIVING RISE TO CIVIL LITIGATION

While the issues discussed in this section could have been inserted and discussed as an example of negligence or malpractice, the nature of cases described in this section are such that special attention is warranted. These issues include the respiratory management of acutely and critically ill patients, liability associated with blood transfusions, needlestick injuries, infection control, and informed consent.

Respiratory Management. The management of an acutely or critically ill patient's respiratory status gives rise to more litigation than does the management of any other physiologic system. Between 1983 and 2004, eight published opinions regarding the alleged negligence associated with a critically ill patient's respiratory status were found at http://www.versuslaw.com. *Allman v. Holleman*,[45] published in 1983, was the oldest of the eight cases.

In *Allman*, Linda Allman was a 28-year-old patient who had been hospitalized because of a ruptured spleen. After surgery, Ms. Allman's endotracheal tube (ETT) became dislodged, she was reintubated. Subsequently the ETT became dislodged again, and efforts to revive her were unsuccessful. This case was filed, and a jury returned a verdict in favor of Ms. Allman.

Six years later, *Courteau v. Dodd*[46] was published. In *Courteau* the nasotracheal tube inserted into a nostril of a 20-year-old patient who sustained injury in a diving accident became dislodged. As a result, the patient suffered a myocardial infarction and massive brain damage. This case was filed, and then dismissed because of insufficient expert testimony.

In 1993 *Dixon v. Taylor*,[47] Willie L. Dixon was admitted to Watauga County Hospital for treatment for pneumonia. Later that day she was transferred to the intensive care unit because her condition began to deteriorate. In the early morning hours, just after being transferred to the intensive care unit, a Code Blue was called because Mrs. Dixon was in cardiac and respiratory arrest. During the code, she was intubated, but her physiologic condition stabilized. Approximately 17½ hours after being intubated, a critical care nurse and respiratory therapist extubated Mrs. Dixon. Nasal prongs were applied initially, but an oxygen mask was needed, so that respiratory therapist left the room to get the mask. When the respiratory therapist returned to her room, he realized that the patient was not breathing normally. The respiratory therapist examined her and found no air movement. Reintubation activities commenced.

However, bed rails had to be removed, the bed rolled down, and the restraints placed on Mrs. Dixon removed. In the process, Mrs. Dixon's heart stopped beating, and a Code Blue was called. During the second code, the nurse recording events on the Code Sheet noted that the respiratory therapist was unsuccessful at attempting to reintubate Mrs. Dixon. The issue was that the laryngoscope blade he was using was too small, and an appropriately sized blade could not be found in the crash cart. The crash cart had not been restocked after the first code, so the blade had to be obtained from the cardiac care unit across the hall.

When the appropriately-sized blade was found and taken to her room, Mrs. Dixon was quickly reintubated by a physician. She was placed on a ventilator and never regained consciousness. After the second code, Mrs.

Dixon was found to be brain-dead secondary to suffocation. She was eventually discharged from the hospital to a nursing home, where she died approximately 10 months later.

This cause of action was subsequently filed and tried before a jury. The jury returned a verdict in the amount of $900,000 to the estate of Mrs. Dixon, citing that the hospital, because of the actions of the respiratory therapist and nurse, was negligent in failing to adequately assess Mrs. Dixon as a candidate for extubation, failing to communicate concerns about her readiness for extubation to the physician prior to extubation, failing to stock the crash cart, and failing to properly position Mrs. Dixon after extubation for possible reintubation.

Four years later, *Moon v. St. Thomas*[48] was published. In this case, a portion of Mr. Moon's ETT had to be extricated from his airway after it had been transected by him biting through it. The family of Mr. Moon alleged that permitting him to bite on the ETT to the extent that it was transected was negligent, and that a bite block should have been inserted or the ETT repositioned to avoid the transection.

At the trial court level, the transection of this ETT was determined to be not reasonably foreseeable and dismissed the case. That decision was appealed, and one year later, the appellate court ordered the case to trial, concluding that a jury should determine whether inserting a bite block or repositioning the ETT was consistent with the standard of care.

Three years after the publication of the *Moon* decision, *Owensboro Mercy Health System v. Payne*[49] was decided. In this case, a jury awarded a man $2,270,000 in damages for the negligent transfer of Mr. Payne from the operating room to the critical care unit. Here, Mr. Payne was involved in a motor vehicle accident and because of extensive internal injuries, spent between 8 and 8½ hours in the operating room. At the conclusion of surgery, he was transferred to the critical care unit without supplemental oxygen being administered. This failure caused Mr. Payne to sustain a serious brain injury, causing him to be in a persistent vegetative state. Although this award was appealed, the appellate court affirmed the verdict at the trial court level.

A year after *Owensboro*, a defense verdict was rendered in *Martin v. St. Vincent Medical Center.*[50] In *Martin*, the family alleged that a certified registered nurse anesthetist (CRNA) punctured Mr. Martin's trachea while inserting an internal jugular line while he underwent a quadruple coronary artery bypass graft procedure. After surgery, Mr. Martin developed mediastinitis and died. His family filed this wrongful death cause of action, but the defense verdict was affirmed on appeal, citing in part the inability on the part of the Mr. Martin's family to affirmatively establish causation.

As in *Martin*, the patient-plaintiff in *Kent v. Baptist Memorial Hospital*[51] was denied a verdict in her favor.

The patient in *Kent* was a 16-year-old diabetic who experienced a diabetic seizure and went into septic shock. On her arrival to the hospital, she was unresponsive and had to be intubated. After she was intubated, she was transferred to another hospital. She was eventually extubated and filed this cause of action contending that she sustained vocal cord damage at intubation because the ETT was too large for her height and weight.

In *Miller v. Marymount Medical Center,*[52] a 31-year-old pregnant woman, Mrs. Miller, was admitted to Marymount Medical Center to give birth. Two days later, she gave birth via C-section to a healthy baby girl. Following the c-section, respiratory problems began. A chest x-ray taken the morning after the C-section revealed that Mrs. Miller had pneumonia. A blood gas taken that same morning indicated that her Po_2 was 64.4. Antibiotic therapy was started, and a nasal canula was applied to improve oxygenation. Mrs. Miller was also treated for pain and stress with Demerol and Vistaril injections. Throughout the day, respiratory distress continued.

At 9:45 PM that same night, her physician told the Miller family that a pulmonologist was going to be called. Five minutes later, the nurse administered Demerol and Vistaril injections. Ten minutes after the injections, Mrs. Miller's physician returned to her room to find Mrs. Miller unresponsive and in respiratory arrest. A code was called and 5 minutes later, Mrs. Miller was intubated, placed on an oxygen bag delivering 100% oxygen, and transferred to the intensive care unit. After she was intubated, another blood gas was taken and the Po_2 was 90. Twelve minutes after she was intubated and transferred to the intensive care unit, Mrs. Miller was breathing without assistance. However, she never regained consciousness, and was eventually transferred to a nursing home where she remains in a comatose state.

Her family filed this case. With regard to the nursing care rendered to Mrs. Miller, they alleged that the nursing staff failed to furnish treating physicians with up-to-date information about Mrs. Miller's symptoms and to obtain repeat blood gases as required by an order entered by Mrs. Miller's physician. They also contended that the administration of Demerol 10 minutes prior to her respiratory arrest was negligent as Demerol accelerates the progression of acute respiratory distress syndrome (ARDS). ARDS is the condition the experts retained by the family concluded that Mrs. Miller had the morning the chest x-ray was taken.

The trial lasted 7 days, and the jury returned a defense verdict because they were unable to definitively determine that negligence was the proximate cause of Mrs. Miller's injuries. This verdict was affirmed by the court of appeals, as well as the Kentucky Supreme Court.

Regardless of the verdict rendered, these cases serve as a stark reminder of the life-altering and life-ending implications associated with the management of the respiratory status of an acutely or critically ill patient. Consequently, nurses caring for respiratory compromised patients must diligently assess, plan, implement care, and evaluate these patients with laserlike precision. The life of the acutely or critically ill patient depends on it.

Blood Transfusions. *Tobin v. Providence Hospital*[53] serves as a reminder that blood transfusions carry with them considerable risks. In *Tobin*, Rollin Tobin underwent hip replacement surgery but died from sepsis and disseminated intravascular coagulation. The wife of Rollin Tobin asserted that he died because blood contaminated with *Yersinia* bacteria was administered to him during surgery.

Before surgery, Mr. Tobin donated three units of his own blood, and all three of those units were transfused in the operating room, as well as an additional, allogeneic unit. Following his death, the American Red Cross and the Centers for Disease Control and Prevention investigated the situation and determined that the fourth unit administered to Mr. Tobin was contaminated with *Yersinia* bacteria.

After his death, his family filed this wrongful death cause of action contending that failure to monitor or record his temperature before, during, and after that operation caused his death. This case went to trial, and the jury returned a verdict in the amount of $6,485,681.06 in favor of the estate of Mr. Tobin. Because there was an absence of testimony asserting the failure to monitor or record his temperature before, during, and after the operation, and other evidentiary errors, the Michigan Court of Appeals ordered a new trial.

Like managing a patient's respiratory status, the administration of blood and blood products, while routine in critical care settings, is a high-risk intervention that can prove to be deadly. *Tobin* is an example. To avoid liability associated with administering blood and blood products, carefully follow organizational procedures and/or protocols that govern the administration of blood and blood products. Then take the time to thoroughly document the care that was taken to protect the patient.

Infection Control. In *Carroll v. Sisters of St. Frances*,[54] Bessie Mae Carroll was visiting her sister, who was a patient in the critical care unit at St. Joseph Hospital when, after washing her hands, she attempted to remove a paper towel from the container located adjacent to the wash basin she was using. She thought the container was a paper towel dispenser, and inserted her right hand into the opening at the top of the container. When she did, three of her fingers were stuck by sharp objects. After telling a nurse that she hurt her fingers on the paper towel dispenser, the nurse told her that the container was not a paper towel dispenser, but a contaminated needle receptacle.

She developed a fear of contracting acquired immunodeficiency syndrome (AIDS) and filed this negligence-based cause of action, contending that the container had been placed too close to the wash basin and that their

should have been a warning placed on the container as to its purpose and contents.

At the trial court level the case was dismissed, but on appeal a trial was ordered so that the jury could determine whether or not her fear of acquiring AIDS was reasonable.

Piedmont Hospital v. Reddick,[55] like *Carroll*, arose out of an allegation that appropriate infection control standards were not followed. In *Piedmont*, James Davis died after contracting a fungal infection. His estate filed this cause of action contending that construction work performed in or near the intensive care unit where Mr. Davis was being treated caused the *Aspergillus* fungus to become airborne and transmitted to him.

The complaint asserted that construction work was performed without proper safeguards, and that in so doing, industry standards were breached. While there were a number of issues the Georgia Court of Appeals-Second Division addressed, the court ordered the case be tried as to the alleged negligence of the construction company and hospital.

Carroll and *Piedmont* demonstrate that infection control issues find their way to courtrooms across America. To minimize risks that are associated with these alleged infection control failures, sharps containers must be clearly labeled and positioned away from wash basins and paper towel dispensers. Before remodeling or other construction begins, the environment must be safeguarded from the airborne spread of deadly microorganisms.

Informed Consent. *Trombley v. Starr-Wood Cardiac Group, et al.*[56] is a case issued from the Alaska Supreme Court and arises out of a situation where a patient undergoing coronary artery bypass graft surgery told her surgeons that she did not want a vein to be harvested from her right leg because she had a history of phlebitis in that leg. The surgeons agreed to harvest a vein from her left leg, and never discussed with her the possibility of having to harvest a vein from her right leg. Despite this conversation and agreement, a vein was harvested from her right leg. After surgery the right leg incision was lapped over rather than stitched together and became infected, necessitating plastic surgery to remove dead tissue and stitch up the incision.

This malpractice case was subsequently filed, but was dismissed at the trial court level. Mrs. Trombley appealed that decision, and the Alaska Supreme Court determined that the decision of the trial court to dismiss her case was in error and ordered a trial. In reversing the decision of the trial court, the Alaska Supreme Court concluded that Mrs. Trombley had a right to insist that her right leg not be used as a harvest site. If, according to the court, her right leg was used without obtaining actual or implied consent, battery may have been committed. If battery occurred, the court observed that Mrs. Trombley would be entitled to damages for that cause of action as well.

CLINICAL APPLICATION

Legal Concepts

Assigned to your care is an aged patient who underwent a radical neck dissection over 1 year ago for laryngeal cancer. She has been returned to the intensive care unit for ventilatory management as she is being treated for pneumonia. The patient's stoma site has healed with some tracheal scar formation. Her intubation by the intensivist was difficult.

When the respiratory therapist asks your assistance in turning the patient, you agree to assist. As the patient is turned, the patient's endotracheal tube becomes completely dislodged. Efforts to reintubate the patient are unsuccessful, and the patient dies.

1. Was the care that was rendered substandard?
2. What is the duty that was owed and breached?
3. Are there challenges to causation?
4. How would the damages be valued?
5. Who may be held responsible for any alleged malpractice?

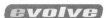 For the discussion of this Clinical Application and for an additional clinical application on legal concepts, see the Evolve website.

Box 3-3

SUMMARY OF ALLEGED FAILURES TO PROVIDE REASONABLE CARE TO ACUTELY AND CRITICALLY ILL PATIENTS

ASSESSMENT
Failure to assess and analyze the level of care needed by the patient; failure to ascertain the patient's wishes with regard to self-determination

PLANNING
Failure to diagnose appropriately

IMPLEMENTATION
Failure to timely communicate patient findings
Failure to take appropriate action
Failure to document assessment findings, interventions, and actions taken, as well as the patient's response to those interventions and actions
Failure to preserve patient privacy

EVALUATION
Failure to act as patient advocate

Although cases like *Trombley* have held physicians responsible for obtaining the consent of patients, nurses caring for acutely ill patients should consider obtaining informed consent before performing invasive procedures for which the nurse has been trained and is authorized to perform. Failure to obtain informed consent could lead to liability where a patient proves that damages occurred because of the negligence of the nurse in performing the invasive procedure.

SUMMARY

Protection, promotion, optimization, prevention, and alleviation are action words that convey the dynamic nature of the nurse's responsibility to take affirmative action when caring for acutely and critically ill patients. Standards of practice and standards of professional performance further delineate expectations of nurses generally, as well as those caring for acutely and critically ill patients. These standards have been promulgated by the American Nurses Association and the American Association of Critical-Care Nurses and have been discussed herein.

In addition, the legal theories on which civil litigation is based against nurses caring for acutely and critically ill patients have been considered; they include negligence, negligence per se, malpractice, wrongful birth, wrongful death, defamation, assault and battery, loss of consortium, and emotional distress. With regard to negligence, the alleged failures that give rise to civil liability have been summarized in Box 3-3.

Finally, the respiratory management of acutely and critically ill patients, as well as civil liability associated with blood transfusions, needlestick injuries, infection control, and informed consent has been outlined. Although these cases could have been discussed elsewhere, they highlighted situations in which nurses who care for acutely and critically ill patients need to be aware.

Regardless of the physiologic condition of the acutely and critically ill patient, nurses can minimize the risk of liability by daily coming to the practice setting focused on the care that must be given, and by paying attention to the signs and symptoms of complications and compromise. The risk of liability can be further diminished by taking affirmative action that is responsive to the patient's condition, and then thoroughly documenting what was done to protect the patient. Doing less may result in liability being imposed, but more importantly, could cost the acutely and critically ill patient his or her life. For further discussion, see the Clinical Application feature on Legal Concepts.

REFERENCES

1. American Nurses Association. *Nursing: Scope and Standards of Practice,* Washington, DC, 2004, American Nurses Association.
2. Deleted in proofs
3. American Association of Critical-Care Nurses, *Standards for Acute and Critical Care Nursing Practice,* Aliso Viejo, California, 2000, American Association of Critical-Care Nurses.
4. For example, **California**–Ybarra v. Spangard, 154 P.2d 687 (Cal. 1944); **Colorado**—Wood v. Rowland, 592 P.2d 1332 (Co. 1978); **Delaware**—Larrimore v. Homeopathic Hospital Association, 176 A.2d 362 (De. 1962); **Minnesota**—Plutshack v. University of Minnesota Hospital, 316 N.W. 2d 1 (Mn. 1982); **Montana**—Hunsaker v. Bozeman Deaconess Foundation, 588 P.2d 493 (Mt. 1978); **Pennsylvania**—Baur v. Mesta Machine Co., 176 A.2d 684 (Pa. 1962); **Texas**—Childs v. Greenville Hospital Authority, 479 S.W. 2d 399 (Tx. 1972).; and **Washington**—Stone v. Sisters of Charity of the House of Providence, 469 P.2d 229 (Wash. 1970).
5. Clough v. Lively, 387 S.E. 2d 573 (Ga. 1989).
6. 648 S.W. 391 (Tx.App. 1993).
7. 421 So. 2d 309 (La. 1982).
8. 415 So. 2d 586 (La. 1982).
9. 835 S.W. 2d 554 (Mo. 1992).
10. 809 So.2d 611 (Miss. 2001).
11. 497 U.S. 261 (1990).
12. 671 N.E. 2d 225 (Oh. 1996).
13. 98 LWUSA 51 (January 11, 1999).
14. 454 N.W. 2d 294 (Ne. 1990).
15. 893 F.2d 411 (1st Cir. 1990).
16. 697 F. Supp. 1570 (Co. 1988).
17. Keyser v. Garner, 922 P.2d 409 (Id. 1996).
18. Long v. Methodist Hospital of Indiana, 699 N.E. 2d 1164 (In. 1998).
19. Richardson v. James Miller, M.D., et al., 2000 TN. 0043340; www.versuslaw.com .
20. Ginsberg v. St. Michaels Hospital, 678 A. 2d 271 (N.J. 1996).
21. G.S. v. Department of Human Services, 723 A. 2d 612 (N.J. 1999).
22. Timblin v. Kent General Hospital, 1995 DE. 19001; www.versuslaw.coin.
23. Grayson v. The State of Oklahoma, et al., 838 P.2d 546 (Ok. 1992).
24. Taylor v. Cabell Huntington Hospital, 538 S.E. 2d 719 (W.V. 2000).
25. Scott v. Porter, 530 S.E. 2d 389 (S.C. 2000).
26. 323 S.E. 2d 430 (N.C. 1977).
27. 663 N.E. 2d 1369 (Oh. 1995).
28. 211 N.E. 2d 614 (11. 1974).
29. 849 S.W. 2d 564 (Ky. 1993).
30. 9 P.3d 314 (Az. 1998).
31. 768 P.2d 768 (Id. 1989).
32. NCSBN, p. 3 and 4.
33. 422 N.W. 2d 600 (S.D. 1988).
34. 645 N.W. 2d (Mn. 2002).
35. 448 N.W. 2d 519 (Mn. 1989).
36. 725 N.E. 2d 1117 (Oh. 2000).
37. Jury Verdict Research Report, April 12, 2000.
38. Cohen T: *Medical Malpractice Trials and Verdicts in Large Counties, 2001.* Bureau of Justice Statistics Civil Justice Data Brief, NCJ 203098, Department of Justice, Washington, D.C., April, 2004.
39. Stein T: On the Defensive, *Nurse Week/Health Week,* www.nurseweek.com/features/00-05/malpract.html May 15, 2000.
40. 16 F.3d 473 (1st Cir. 1994).
41. 354 S.E. 2d 872 (Ga. 1987).
42. 490 NYS 2d 87 (N.Y. 1985).
43. 948 S. W. 2d 72 (Tx. 1997).
44. 513 A.2d 341 (N.H.1986).
45. 188 F.3d 1195 (Ok. 1999).
46. 697 P. 2d 504 (N.M. 1979).
47. 830 P.2d 1185 (Id. 1992).
48. 685 P. 2d 776 (Co. 1984).
49. No. 1980985. June 30, 2000.
50. No. 2000. June 28, 2000.
51. 667 P.2d 296 (Ks. 1983).
52. 773 S.W. 2d 436 (Ark. 1989).
53. 431 S.E. 2d 778 (N.C. 1983).
54. 983 S.W. 2d 225 (Tn. 1998).
55. 2000.KY.0042192 www.versuslaw.com.
56. 755 N.E. 2d 926 (Oh. 2001).

CHAPTER 4

Patient/Family Education

CHALLENGES IN ACUTE CARE IN PATIENT/FAMILY EDUCATION

At no other point in history has the availability of information within the general population been so great. For example, televisions are practically in every home, computers with wireless access to the Internet are available for use anywhere at anytime, and cell phones are clipped to the waistbands of both the young and the old. It seems as if this century's population of adults cannot be without "knowing." The ease of access to the world's library of information meets a compulsive need to satisfy a desire for immediate gratification. Gathering information in bits and pieces from various sources allows people to collect information at their own pace and to gather as much or as little information as they desire. These "knowledge bites" are sorted and stored away in an individual's own cerebral "hard drive." The "file" is retrieved and "opened" whenever the situation warrants.

If alterations in health arise in daily life, people will use all available resources to discover information to help them cope and adapt to the new experience. This type of consumerism has developed a populace that is more educated in health matters than ever before. It is our duty as health professionals to assist patients and families with information gathering and self-care management skills so they can lead lives of the best quality possible. According to the Joint Commission on Accreditation of Healthcare Organizations (JCAHO), patients must receive "sufficient information to make decisions and to take responsibility for self-management activities related to their needs."[1] The goals, then, of patient/family education are to improve health outcomes by promoting healthy behavior and involvement in care and care decisions.[1]

Admission to an acute care unit is generally an unexpected event in anyone's life. The seriousness of the situation and unfamiliarity of the hospital/unit environment evokes a stress response in both patients and families. Nursing care is focused on improving the patient's physiologic stability and promoting end-organ tissue perfusion. Thus, promoting the most basic human physiologic survival need for cellular oxygenation is the priority. Al-

terations in normal functioning related to disease-process progression, sedation, assist devices, or mechanical ventilation contribute to the possibility of mental alterations in the patient. Sleep deprivation and sensory overload add to the complexity of the issues that affect the patient's ability to receive and understand medical information. Mental alterations may limit the effectiveness of the teaching-learning encounter. These physical and cognitive limitations prevent the patient from receiving or understanding information related to their care and impair their ability to make an informed decision.[2] At these times, critical life-or-death care decisions are transferred to a proxy, usually an immediate family member. The designated proxy will then have the responsibility to make informed treatment decisions for the patient. These types of situations present the nurse with special challenges in the education of both patients and families.

Acute illness will disrupt the "normalcy" of day-to-day life. Stress and crisis can develop within the family unit and stretch its members' coping resources.[3] These multiple emotional factors build barriers to the teaching-learning process and can become frustrating for both the learner and the nurse. So how, amidst the chaos, do bedside nurses effectively provide patient/family education that will optimize outcomes and deliver quality, cost-effective care? It is the nurse's responsibility to educate himself or herself on concepts that provide insight into the framework for patient/family education. Adult education concepts such as adult learning principles, types of educational needs, barriers to learning, stress and coping strategies, and evidence-based interventions must be used to develop an individualized education plan to meet the identified learning needs of the patient/family.

WHAT IS EDUCATION?

DEFINITION AND BENEFITS

Patient education is a process that includes the purposeful delivery of health-related information in order to promote changes in behavior that will optimize health practices and assist the individual in attaining new skills for living.[4,5] This concept can be overwhelming in today's fast-paced, technology-rich acute care environment. The bedside nurse must incorporate the abundant educational needs of the patient or family into the education plan as well as be aware of the requirements of regulatory agencies and the legalities of documenting the teaching-learning encounter.

Studies have documented that quality education shortens hospital length of stay, reduces readmission rates, and improves self-care management skills.[4-6] Complications associated with the physiologic stress response may be prevented if the patient or family perceives the educational encounter as positive. Positive encounters not only decrease the stress response, but also relieve anxiety, promote individual growth and development, and increase patient-family satisfaction.[4-6] The following are examples of positive outcomes associated with a structured teaching-learning process:[7,8]

- Clarification of patients' understanding and perceptions of their chronic illness and care decisions
- Improved health outcomes relative to self-management techniques such as symptom management
- Promotion of informed decision making and control over the situation
- Lessened emotional stress associated with an unfamiliar environment and unknown prognosis
- Improved adaptation to stressful situation
- Improved satisfaction with care received
- Improved relationship with health care team
- Promotion of self concept

THE PROCESS

The education process follows the same framework as the nursing process: assessment, diagnosis, goals or outcomes, interventions, and evaluation.[4] Box 4-1 lists the steps in this process. Although this chapter discusses these steps individually, in actual practice they may occur simultaneously and repetitively. The teaching-learning process is a dynamic, continuous activity that occurs throughout the entire hospitalization and may continue after the patient has been discharged. This process is often envisioned by the nurse as a time-consuming task that requires knowledge and skills to accomplish. Whereas knowledge and skills can be obtained, time in today's acute care unit is a diminishing commodity. Many nurses believe they cannot educate unless formal blocks of education time are planned during the shift. Although this type of education encounter is optimal, it is not realistic for contemporary nursing. The nurse must recognize that teaching occurs with every moment of a nurse-patient encounter.[9] Instructions for how to use to the call bell or explanations of events and sensations to expect during a bed bath could

---

Box 4-1

STEPS IN THE EDUCATION PROCESS

STEP 1: ASSESSMENT: INFORMATION GATHERING
Patient/family: culture, age-specific considerations
Actual and potential learning needs
Possible barriers to the teaching learning process

STEP 2: EDUCATION PLAN DEVELOPMENT
Identify needs and write expected outcomes
Design interventions: information to be taught, removal of barriers
Mobilize resources as needed to remove barriers and enhance communication of information

STEP 3: IMPLEMENTATION
Implement interventions for information sharing, learner participation in education process
Use written plan to structure the teaching encounter, cover essential information, and communicate outcomes between practitioners

STEP 4: EVALUATION
Evaluate learner response to the encounter, any need for follow-up teaching to attain goals
Evaluate learner comfort level with information: coping and adaptation

STEP 5: DOCUMENTATION
Document interventions used, resources used, information taught, and outcome of teaching encounter

---

be considered an education session. It is the nurse's role to recognize that education, no matter brief or extensive, affects the daily lives of each person with whom they come in contact. By following the nursing process both the physical assessment and education assessment can occur simultaneously.

STEP 1: ASSESSMENT

According to JCAHO, education provided should be appropriate to the patient's condition and should address the patient's identified learning needs.[1] The assessment is an important first step to providing need-targeted patient/family education. It begins on admission and continues until the patient is discharged. A formal, comprehensive, initial education assessment produces valuable information; however, it could take the nurse hours to complete. Therefore, the nurse must focus the initial and subsequent education assessments towards identifying gaps in knowledge related to the patient's current health-altering situation. Information must also be gathered on those factors that affect the education process and impair the ability of the patient or family to respond. These factors include the following: (1) cultural and religious views of illness or health; (2) emotional barriers; (3) desire and motivation; (4) physical or cognitive limitations; and 5) barriers to effective communication.[1]

EFFECTIVE QUESTIONING

Strategic questioning provides an avenue for the nurse to determine if the patient or family has any misconceptions about the environment, their illness, self-management skills, or the medication schedule. Health care providers use the term noncompliant to describe a patient or family who do not modify behaviors to the meet the demands of the prescribed treatment regimen, such as following the rules of a low-fat diet or medication dosing. However, the problem behind noncompliance may not be a conscious desire to defy the treatment plan, but an actual misunderstanding of the importance of the medication or how to take the medication. The technique of asking open-ended questions such as "can you tell me what you know about your medication?" will elicit more information about the patient's actual knowledge base than asking closed-ended questions such as "you know this is your water pill, right?" Open-ended questions provide the nurse an opportunity to assess actual knowledge gaps rather than assume knowledge by obtaining a yes-or-no response. These types of questions also assist the patient/family to tell their story of the illness and communicate their perceptions of the experience,[5] thus allowing the adult learner to feel respected and involved in the treatment process. Questions that elicit a "yes" or "no" response close off communication and do not provide for an interactive teaching-learning session. Box 4-2 contains sample questions the nurse can use in an assessment to obtain needed information. Generally, with practice and effort, it can be determined what educational information is needed in a brief period without a great deal of disruption in the routine care of the patient. It is important to note that patients and families are multidimensional. Even with good questioning skills the nurse cannot assess many aspects of the learner during initial contact or even during the hospital stay.

LEARNER IDENTIFICATION

Identifying learner characteristics benefits the nurse and results in optimal communication and the patient's understanding of information. As previously discussed, certain factors can affect the education process. Culture/ethnicity, age, and adult learning principles influence the manner in which information is presented and concepts are understood.[5,10]

Modern Family. A family can be defined as a group of individuals who are bonded by biologic, legal, and social relationships.[3] The modern family is diverse in ethnic backgrounds, sexual orientation, age, gender, work experience, physical or mental challenges, communica-

---

Box 4-2

OPEN-ENDED ASSESSMENT QUESTIONS

- Why have you come to the hospital today?
- What problem are you having:
- How can we help you today
- When did these problems start?
- Have you had these problems before?
- Have you been hospitalized for these problems before?
- Who is your doctor for this problem: Who is your family doctor?
- What medications are you taking?
- Can you tell me why you take each medication?
- How do you care for yourself at home? Do you have help?
- Are any family or friends with you today?
- Are these people your main support system?
- Are there any special needs, religious or otherwise, that we need to be aware of while you are in the hospital?
- What is your goal for coming to the hospital today?
- How can we help you reach this goal?
- Is there any information that I can give you right now that would help you understand more about why you are here or about your plan of care?
- What information have you received from other members of the health care team today?

---

tion skills, education backgrounds, work experience, geographic location, lived experiences, and religious beliefs.[11-13] If a picture of today's family were to be created, it would resemble that of a large patchwork quilt. Patches of different sizes, ethnicities, religions, cultures, attitudes, stages of development, and lived experiences would overlap and occupy their own individual spaces within the quilt framework. Bedside practitioners are expected to provide culturally competent care to each individual in the acute care setting. Culturally competent care is the delivery of sensitive, meaningful care to patients and families from diverse backgrounds.[13] This implies that the practitioner must value diversity and become knowledgeable concerning the cultural strengths and abilities of those for whom they care.[14] Communication and understanding impact the education process. Provision of language-appropriate literature and translation services, and recognition of cultural or religious differences in the perception of illness and treatment all influence the education encounter.[13]

Age-Specific Considerations. The acute care patient population differs not only in culture but also in age and stages of human development. Older adult patients may have more difficulty reading patient education material or the label on the bottle of prescription medication than younger adults. Printed materials with larger fonts may be needed for these patients. Older adults were not exposed to technology during their youth and may find it difficult to navigate the fragmented maze of today's health care. Because of advanced age, this population of adults may have prescriptions for multiple drug therapies. Education to prevent adverse drug reactions may be required because of the prevalence of multiple drug therapies.[15] Older adults may also be coping with end-of-life issues and are in need of information to make informed decisions. Young adults may struggle with the issue of how to incorporate intimacy into their lives without feeling isolated from the mainstream social scene. The need for privacy and peer support may be required to assist the young adult in coping with the current situation. The practitioner must recognize these age-specific issues and incorporate them into the education plan.[1]

Adult Learners. Adults learn, in large part, through lived experiences. The motivation to learn is internal and problem-oriented, focusing on life events. Malcolm Knowles described these principles of adult learning in a model known as *andragogy*. Adult learning theory stresses concepts of individualism, self-assessment, self-direction, motivation, experience, and autonomy. Adults tend to have a strong sense of self-concept, are goal-oriented learners, and like to make their own decisions.[16] They take responsibility and accountability for their own learning and want to be respected as individuals, as well as recognized for accomplished life experiences. Adults have individualized learning styles and often lack confidence in their ability to learn. Education is resisted when the information given is perceived to be in conflict with the individual's self-image.

The learning process generally involves altering some part of current behavior to produce changes in lifestyle, incorporating the new or chronic illness into day-to-day living. Coping mechanisms such as anger, disbelief, and denial affect the willingness of the patient or family to learn. The unwillingness to change behavior to manage health needs adds to the complexity of the acute care teaching-learning encounter. The nurse must provide need-to-know information in easy, understandable terms and in short bursts. Positive feedback and repetition of information may also be required before health education is incorporated into the patient's or family's bank of experiences.[16] Adults are sensitive about making mistakes and tend to view mistakes as failures. Learning situations that the patient/family interpret as belittling or embarrassing or that are perceived as not surmountable will be avoided or disregarded. The nurse should act more as a coach or facilitator of information instead of a didactic instructor.[10] It is important to remember that the teacher can only show the learner to the door; the learner must walk through that door on his or her own. Learning is an active process that occurs internally over time and cannot be forced. Bedside nurses are obliged to be proactive and to have a good understanding of adult learning theory, to incorporate its concepts into the as-

sessment of learning needs, development of an education plan, implementation of the plan, and evaluation of the outcomes of the education encounter.

EDUCATIONAL NEEDS

Learning needs can be defined as gaps between what the learner knows and what the learner needs to know; e.g., survival skills, coping skills, and/or ability to make a care decision. Identification of actual and perceived learning needs will direct the health care team to provide need-targeted education. Need-targeted or need-to-know education is directed at helping the learner to become familiar with the current situation. Patient/family educational needs can be placed into one or more of three categories: (1) information only (environment, visitation hours, get questions answered); (2) informed decision making (treatment plan, informed consent); and (3) self-management (recognition of problems and how to respond).[5,17] Patient education to be included in the education plan should address the plan of care, health practices and safety, safe and effective use of medications, nutrition interventions, safe and effective use of medical equipment or supplies, pain, and habilation or rehabilitation needs.[1]

Learning needs may change from day to day, shift to shift, or minute to minute. Educational needs are influenced by how the patient or the family perceive or interpret the acute illness.[18] Perceptions of experiences vary from person to person, even if two people are involved in the same event. This intense internal feeling affects one's desire to learn and understanding of the current situation. Satisfaction with the learning encounter is often judged to be positive if the nurse meets the patient's and family's expected learning needs. Congruency between nurse-identified needs and patient-identified needs brings about more positive learning experiences and encourages the learner to seek out further information. Therefore the nurse must actively listen, maintain eye contact, seek clarification, and pay attention to both verbal and nonverbal cues from the patient and the family in order to gather relevant information concerning perceived learning needs. The nurse should seek to first understand the learning need from the patient's point of view and then seek to be understood.

BARRIERS TO THE LEARNING PROCESS

Ability, Willingness, and Readiness. Assessing ability, willingness, and readiness to learn is an essential part of developing and implementing an education plan of care. The ability to learn is the capacity of the learner to understand, pay attention, and comprehend the material being taught. Willingness to learn describes the learner's openness to new ideas and concepts. Readiness to learn is the motivation to try out new concepts and behaviors.[5] Even if the amounts of inventive teaching methods, well thought-out education materials, and time are unlimited, learning will not take place if the patient or family is not ready, willing, and able to learn.[19] Several factors affect ability, willingness, and readiness to learn as well as the ability to cope and adapt to the current situation. These factors include physiologic, psychologic, sociocultural, financial, and environmental aspects.[5,10]

Physiologic Factors. The need for oxygen and thus survival predominates over any other human need. This need is described by a theory known as Maslow's hierarchy of human needs. It is a concept in which lower level, physiologic needs must be satisfied before an individual can move on to higher level, self-esteem–building issues. The motivation to meet the need to survive and to feel safe and secure predominates over the need to learn a lifestyle change such as smoking cessation. Only when lower-level needs are met can the patient be open to learning new concepts and skills. There is an instinctive need to decrease the effects of stressors and reestablish a normal daily routine. A physical assessment could supply the nurse with information concerning the patient's response to the stressors. Physiologic alterations in heart rate and blood pressure can be measured and taken into consideration during the teaching-learning encounter.[3] Sources of physiologic stress in the acutely ill include medications, pain, hypoxia, decreased cerebral and peripheral perfusion, hypotension, fluid and electrolyte imbalances, infection, sensory alterations, fever, and neurologic deficits.[10] Experiencing one or more of these stressors may completely consume all the patient's available energy and thoughts, thus affecting his or her ability to interact, comprehend, and respond to teaching.

Psychologic Factors. When confronted with life-altering situations such as admission to an acute care unit, both patients and families may well experience anxiety and emotional stress. Anxiety and fear disrupt the normalcy of day-to-day life. Sources of emotional stress include fear of death, uncertain prognosis, role change, self-image change, social isolation, disruption in daily routine, financial concerns, and unfamiliar critical care environment.[3,20] These intense emotions can lead to a crisis situation and alter the ability of the patient/family to cope.[21,22] During the acute illness, an individual's ability to process or retain information and ability to participate in the treatment plan could be altered.[2] If the disease process or physiologic stressors impair the patient's ability to make decisions, the burden of decision making will transfer to the family. Gender differences affect a patient's reaction to stress. For example, women who have experienced a myocardial infarction report higher anxiety levels than men at all points during the hospital stay.[23] Physiologic alterations caused by anxiety have been found to negatively impact both the recovery process and the long-term prognosis.[23] In acute situations the nurse may find it necessary to repeat information or limit teaching sessions to short bursts rather than one long encounter. Medical jargon should be limited and replaced by simple-to-understand terms. Provision of honest and accurate disease state information may decrease the effects of stressors and alleviate anxiety and fear.

Adaptation. A stressor can be described as any condition, situation, or perception that requires an individual to adapt.[20] All situations in an acute care facility may well be considered stressful. The capacity of an individual to adapt is paramount in breaking down emotional barriers that affect willingness and readiness for learning. Culture, beliefs, attitudes, and ability to mobilize resources affect one's ability to respond to a crisis situation.[24] General characteristics of the stages of adaptation to illness are outlined in Table 4-1, with corresponding applications for the teaching-learning process. Patients and families will move through these stages on an individual timeline and at a variable pace. A person may move back and forth between stages and may skip one all together. The patient and each member of the family could be experiencing different stages in the adaptation process at the same time. The education encounter may need to be modified to meet both the patient/family needs.

Coping. Coping refers to the way one manages stressful events that are straining or exceeding personal resources.[5,24] The stressful event is appraised according to the level of threat to the individual and is managed by focusing on either the problem at hand or the emotions felt at the moment.[25] Acute illness brings about disruption in the normalcy of day-to-day routines. Coping strategies are used by patient/family to help maintain control over the situation and encourage hope and stability in life. Disbelief and denial may be present anytime during the hospitalization. Phrases such as "why me" and "I can't believe this is happening" are common in the acute care setting. Other coping mechanisms, such as denial and anger, hamper the ability of the patient or the family to problem solve and cope with the situation. All are barriers to the ability of the patient to receive information and incorporate it into the self-concept. Adults must be ready and willing, both physically and emotionally, to learn. Therefore, teaching new skills or self-management techniques to the adult learner presents a special challenge to the nurse in acute care. For example, until the patient accepts the diagnosis of heart failure as part of who he or she is, he or she will not make appropriate changes in lifestyle to avoid an exacerbation of the disease.

Sociocultural Factors. Variables such as culture, ethnicity, values, beliefs, lifestyle, and family role influence the way an individual perceives illness, pain, and healing.[13] Culturally sensitive education strategies should be developed to communicate specific needs to other members of the health care team and achieve optimal learning outcomes.[1]

Table 4-1	Teaching-Learning Process in Adaptation to Illness	
Stage of Adaptation	Characteristic Patient Response	Implications for Teaching-Learning Process
Disbelief	Denial	Orient teaching to present. Teach during other nursing activities. Reassure patient about safety. Explain all procedures and activities clearly and concisely.
Developing awareness	Anger	Continue to orient teaching to present. Avoid long lists of facts. Continue to foster development of trust and rapport through good physical care.
Reorganization	Acceptance of sick role	Orient teaching to meet patient. Teach whatever patient wants to learn. Provide necessary self-care information; reinforce with written material.
Resolution	Identification with others with same problem; recognition of loss	Use group instruction. Use patient support groups and visits by recovered patients with same problem.
Identifying change	Definition of self as one who has undergone change and is now different	Answer patient's questions as they arise. Recognize that as basic needs are met, more mature needs will arise.

Financial Factors. Patients and families often worry about financial issues related to the hospitalization and the possibility of long-term disability. Examples of financial concerns are (1) fear of income loss related to time away from work or possible long-term disability; (2) how health care expenses will be paid; and (3) complex insurance coverage issues. Patients may be more concerned with the amount of out-of-pocket expenses they will have to pay for this illness rather than receiving information on symptom management strategies. It is important for the nurse to recognize these issues as patient concerns and mobilize resources to calm financial anxiety. Practitioners in other disciplines, especially social work, are available to assist patients and families obtain community resources to help cover expenses such as medication costs.

Environmental Factors. As discussed previously, the acute care environment can be considered a source of stress to the learner. Although sounds, people, and state-of-the-art equipment are familiar and mundane for the nurse, this environment may often appear foreign and intimidating to the patient/family. Prior exposure to an acute care unit is a double-edged sword. Depending on the outcome of the experience, whether positive or negative, it may either help alleviate or heighten anxiety. The nurse must pay attention to the patient-family perceptions of the environment and alter the teaching-learning encounter accordingly. Sleep cycle alterations caused by sleep deprivation, or sensory overload related to continuous noise from machines or people, will affect the patient's ability to concentrate and comprehend in-

formation. Allowing frequent uninterrupted rest periods, will assist the patient in obtaining structured sleep.[20]

For patients and families to value education, they must believe the information source is reliable. The bedside nurse is the most available source of information in the acute care unit. It is important for him or her to develop a rapport and establish a sense of trust within the nurse-patient relationship. These positive characteristics are recommended for a supportive learning environment. Assignment of multiple caregivers may negatively affect the ability of the patient/family to form a trusting relationship with the nursing staff. Arranging consistency in the assigned caregivers will help these promote rapport and trust, as well as decrease anxiety and enhance comfort level with the environment.[5,24]

STEP 2: EDUCATION PLAN OF CARE DEVELOPMENT

Education must be ongoing, interactive, and consistent with the patient's plan of care and education level.[1] The nurse must analyze information gathered from the assessment to prioritize both patient/family educational needs. The nursing diagnosis for deficient knowledge and accompanying interventions can be applied to any situation. The nurse must also consider the patient's physical and emotional status when setting education priorities. Ability, willingness, and readiness to learn are factors that impair acceptance of new information and add to the complexity of teaching-learning encounter. These factors should be recognized by the nurse prior to implementation of teaching. The written teaching plan should identify the learning need, goals or expected outcome of the teaching-learning encounter, interventions to meet that outcome, and appropriate teaching strategies.

Research and accepted national guidelines or standards can be used to assist the practitioner in developing an evidence-based plan for education. Examples of organizations that offer education standards are: American Association of Critical Care Nurses; American Heart Association Guidelines for Practice, Agency for Health Care Policy and Research, and the Society of Critical Care Medicine. A database for nursing interventions and outcomes has been developed out of research that began in the 1980s. This research is known as the IOWA Project. This body of research may be used in daily practice and can be found in two book publications: *Nursing Interventions Classifications* and *Nursing Outcomes Classifications*. These evidence-based interventions and outcomes assist the nurse in providing consistent outcomes and interventions from nurse to nurse, shift to shift, and discipline to discipline.

DETERMINING WHAT TO TEACH

It can be a difficult task to prioritize the multitude of learning needs that practitioners are required to address during a period in acute care. Learning needs in the intensive care unit (ICU), the progressive care, or the telemetry setting can be separated into four different categories to help set teaching priorities in each phase of the hospitalization (Table 4-2). Learning needs during the initial contact or first hours of hospitalization can be predicted. Education during this time frame should be directed toward the reduction of immediate stress, anxiety, and fear rather than future lifestyle alterations or rehabilitation needs. Interventions are targeted to promote comfort and familiarity with the environment and surroundings.[26] The plan should focus on survival skills, orientation to the environment and equipment, communication of prognosis, procedure explanations, and the immediate plan of care.

There are three learning domains to consider when developing an individualized education plan. The domains include knowledge, attitude, and skills. The knowledge domain is centered on the acquisition of information or facts about a given topic, such as listing the signs and symptoms of hypoglycemia and knowing what to do if you become symptomatic. A patient who has had diabetes for years will have different life experiences with his or her disease process than the newly diagnosed patient. Therefore, even though two patients have the same diagnosis, educational needs will differ. The attitude domain includes the incorporation of new values, beliefs, or attitudes into patients' behavior, such as believing smoking is bad for you and then exerting a con-

scious effort to stop. The skills domain is involved with the acquisition of skills that enable one to perform a new technique, such as endotracheal suctioning or dressing changes. The nurse may incorporate one or more of these domains into the education plan.

Both patients and families are attempting to cope with seriousness of the current situation and need information continually to adapt their behavior accordingly. Leske and Molter's hallmark research in the area of needs of the families of critically ill patients has provided nursing with a scientific body of knowledge for identification of actual learning needs in this population. Results of these studies found that families of critically ill patients needed to have their questions answered honestly and to have a feeling of hope.[27] The outcomes of this research can be used in developing interventions for the initial phase in the hospitalization process. Box 4-3 includes a sample listing of interventions that can be used to help meet the needs of the family. During this time of elevated stress, the nurse may have to refocus the patient/family to help concentrate efforts on coping with the present instead of dwelling on possibilities of the future. Not addressing these immediate concerns could result in further anxiety, affect ability to cope, and prevent open and honest communication.[3]

As the hospital length of stay increases, patients and families begin to adapt to the situation and learning needs change. The patient/family develop positive feelings of relief and happiness in the fact that survival has been achieved. Since lower-level, physiologic needs are

---

Box 4-3

INTERVENTIONS FOR IDENTIFIED PATIENT/FAMILY NEEDS

- Answer questions openly and honestly.
- Give as much or as little realistic information as the patient/family need to understand the situation or the patient's physiologic condition.
- Provide specific facts about the patient's daily or hourly progress.
- Provide information that is understandable and in simple terms.
- Use short sentences and incorporate only a couple of pieces of information at a time.
- Provide emotional comfort in order to reduce anxiety and facilitate the feeling of hope.
- Prepare the patient/family for their first visit to the unit.
- Explain possible patient appearance, purpose of equipment, family role in visitation, and unit environment.
- Keep the family informed and involved in the daily plan of care.
- Explain what procedures will be done, why they are being done, and what information is hoped to be gained from the procedure.

Table 4-2	Categories of Educational Needs in Acute Care
Phase	**Educational Needs**
Initial contact/first visit Focus on immediate needs	Preparation for the visit: patient representatives or nurses can prepare the family and patient for the first visit • What to expect in the environment • How long the visit will last • What the patient may look like (e.g., tubes, IVs) Orientation to unit/environment: call light, bed controls, waiting rooms, unit contact numbers Orientation to unit policies/hospital policies • HIPAA, advanced directives, visitation policies Equipment orientation: monitors, IV pumps, pulse oximetry, pacemakers, ventilators Medications: rationale, effects, side effects What to do during the visit: talk to the patient, hold patient's hand, length of visits (if applicable) Patient status: stable or unstable and what that terminology means What treatments and interventions are being done for the patient Upcoming procedures When the doctor visited or is expected to visit Disciplines involved in care and the services they provide Immediate plan of care (next 24 hours) Mobilization of resources for crisis intervention
Continuous care	Day-to-day routine: meals, lab visits, doctor visits, frequency of monitoring (VS), nursing assessments, daily weights, and shift routines Explanation of any procedures: expected sensations or discomforts (e.g., chest tube removal, arterial sheath removal) Plan of care: treatments, progress, patient accomplishments (e.g., extubation) Medications: name, why the patient is receiving them, side effects to report to the nurse or health care team Disease process: what it is and how it will affect life, symptoms to report to health care team How to mobilize resources to assist the patient/family in coping with stress and crisis: pastoral care, social workers, case managers, victim assistance, domestic violence Gifts: When a loved one is ill, it is traditional to send flowers, balloons, or cards. If your unit has any restrictions of gifts, make the family aware. Begin teaching self-management skills and discuss aftercare information.
Transfer to a different level of care	**SENDING UNIT** Acknowledge positive move out of critical care When the transfer will occur Why the transfer is occurring What to expect in the different unit Name of the new caregiver Availability of care provider Visiting hours Directions, how to get there; the new room number and phone number **RECEIVING UNIT** Orientation to environment, visitation policies, visitors Unit routine, meals shift changes, doctor visits Expectations about patient self care; ADLs Medication and diagnostic testing routine times
Planning for aftercare, discharge planning	Self-care management: symptom management, medication administration, diet, activity, durable medical equipment, tasks or procedures What to do for an emergency What constitutes an emergency or when to call the physician How to care for incisions or procedure sites
Completed throughout the hospital stay	Return appointment: name of physician practice, practice phone numbers and contacts Obtaining medications: prescriptions, pharmacy, special drug ordering information Required lifestyle changes: mobility and safety issues for the paraplegic or stroke victim, activities of daily living issues relative to medications or symptoms Potential risk modifications: smoking cessation, diet modifications, exercise Resources: cardiac rehabilitation, support groups, home care agencies
End-of-life care	End-of-life care: participation in care, services available, mobilizing resources Palliative care Hospice

ADLs, Activities of daily living; *VS,* vital signs.

met, the patient's efforts can be concentrated on modifying behavior to meet higher-level needs such as self-concept and self-actualization. Teaching during the continuous phase of nursing care is aimed at answering patient or family questions about the treatment plan or how the acute illness will impact their day-to-day lives. Education on lifestyle modification and self-management skills should be presented during this phase of nursing care. Discharge planning is also part of the education process and should start with admission to the hospital. Instructions for home care, also known as aftercare, should be accomplished prior to the day of discharge to avoid decreased retention of education that occurs with information overload.

WRITING GOALS OR OUTCOMES

An outcomes statement helps clarify to both the teacher and the learner what is to be taught, what is to be learned, what is to be evaluated, and what is to be documented. When goals or expected outcomes of the education encounter are clearly stated, both the teacher and the learner know the expectations and will do their best to achieve them. These statements differ from interventions in that they reflect what the learner is to accomplish, not what the nurse is to teach.[28] Identifying and writing outcomes may be the most difficult aspect in the development of the education plan of care. The written outcomes provide direction for the teaching-learning process and should be straightforward, attainable, and include one task or learning domain.[28]

There are essentially three components in the outcomes statement: (1) the individual who will meet the objective, (2) a measurable/observable verb, and (3) the content to be evaluated or learned. Examples of measurable verbs include define, list, identify, perform, prepare, and demonstrate, where as non-measurable, higher-level verbs include believe, value, and understand. Remember the KISS rule: Keep it Simple Simon. Outcomes should include behavioral lifestyle changes for self-management, psychomotor skill acquisition, and acquisition of knowledge. This is an example of a clearly stated outcome: the patient/family will list the signs and symptoms of postoperative infection.

DEVELOPING INTERVENTIONS

Interventions describe how a nurse will become involved in providing education to the patient or the family. Determining education interventions is part of clinical decision making.[29] Nurse-initiated interventions are based on clinical knowledge and judgment and have a direct impact on the outcome of the teaching encounter.[29] Although physiologic problems occupy most of the nursing plan of care, it is essential to incorporate teaching interventions into the daily plan in order to create positive patient outcomes. Nurses just entering the profession readily refer to education plans developed by experienced nurses to guide them in their new role of patient educator.[30] Carefully planned and developed interventions support nurses, patients, and families focused on achievable outcomes. Education interventions are targeted toward information to be taught, such as how to care and use oxygen or how to recognize signs and symptoms of an infection. The following is an example of a clearly stated research-based intervention: "instruct patient/family on proper name of prescribed diet."[29]

STANDARDIZED EDUCATION PLANS

Standardized education plans provide the health care team with consistent outcomes and interventions. Even though standardized plans are easy to implement, they must be individualized to meet the specific needs of the patient or family. Examples of standardized plans of care include patient pathways, traditional nursing care plans for Deficient Knowledge, and Nursing Interventions Classification (NIC) (see the NIC box). Examples of nursing management plans for Deficient Knowledge are included in Unit X.

STEP 3: IMPLEMENTATION

Once the assessment is completed and the education plan is developed, need-targeted education can commence. Beginning practitioners differ from experienced practitioners in their skills of implementing the EPOC. Experienced practitioners will use their intuition and knowledge base to anticipate learning needs and form a mental list of interventions and possible outcomes.[30] Those just starting in the profession need the concrete education plan that has been developed to guide the teaching-learning encounter.[30]

SETTING UP THE ENVIRONMENT

The optimal environment for learning is one that is nonthreatening, comfortable, open, and honest. As previously discussed, many factors concerning the acute care environment can be threatening or anxiety-producing. The practitioner must assess for these distractions and control them as much as possible. Providing the family with open visitation and access to the patient and health care providers can help decrease their anxiety level and improve satisfaction with care.[3] Current Health Insurance Portability and Accountability Act (HIPAA) requirements for patient confidentiality necessitate a need for privacy during the teaching-learning encounter. Bedside practitioner attention to this detail in open environments such as ICUs, waiting rooms, and emergency departments is important in creating an environment of trust and reassur-

NIC   Teaching: Disease Process

Definition: Assisting the patient to understand information related to a specific disease process

Activities

Appraise the patient's current level of knowledge related to specific disease process

Explain the pathophysiology of the disease and how it relates to the anatomy and physiology, as appropriate

Describe common signs and symptoms of the disease, as appropriate

Describe the disease process, as appropriate

Identify possible etiologies, as appropriate

Provide information to the patient about condition, as appropriate

Avoid empty reassurances

Provide the family/significant other(s) with information about the patient's progress, as appropriate

Provide information about available diagnostic measures, as appropriate

Discuss lifestyle changes that may be required to prevent future complications and/or control the disease process

Discuss therapy/treatment options

Describe rationale behind management/therapy/treatment recommendations

Encourage the patient to explore options/get a second opinion, as appropriate or indicated

Describe possible chronic complications, as appropriate

Instruct the patient on measures to prevent/minimize side effects of treatment for the disease, as appropriate

Instruct the patient on measures to control/minimize symptoms, as appropriate

Explore possible resources/support, as appropriate

Refer the patient to local community agencies/support groups, as appropriate

Instruct the patient on which signs and symptoms to report to health care provider, as appropriate

Provide the phone number to call if complications occur

Reinforce information provided by other health care team members, as appropriate

From Dochterman JM, Bulecheck GM: *Nursing interventions classification (NIC)*, ed 4, St Louis, 2004, Mosby.

ance. Supportive education promotes behaviors that facilitate motivation to learn and adherence to lifestyle changes.[31] The following is a list of strategies the practitioner can implement to facilitate learning.[31]

- Show empathy and concern. Actively listen to the learner and acknowledge lived experiences and ideas.
- Use language and nonverbal communication to enhance choice and promote problem solving.
- Reduce language that is controlling, criticizing, guilt provoking, judgmental, or punishing.
- Provide rationale for self-management behaviors: the importance of changing lifestyle to manage symptoms.

One example of the difference between supportive education and nonsupportive education is demonstrated by a patient diagnosed with chronic heart failure who is experiencing an exacerbation of symptoms related to dietary salt intake. Suppose the patient states that he or she is doing "OK" adhering to the low-salt diet but family members complain that he or she eats too many processed foods and too much take-out fast food. An example of a nonsupportive teaching phrase would be, "You know salt isn't good for you."[31] This phrase is judgmental, critical, and guilt provoking and makes an assumption of the patient's level of knowledge. By revising the wording in the phrase, the meaning of the information is changed. For example: "I know it is difficult not to eat all of your favorite foods. If you add salt, that is up to

you. Do you understand that salt will affect your heart condition?"[31] This supportive statement transfers accountability of performing the self-management skill from the nurse to the patient and motivates the patient to make the conscious decision to limit salt intake.

TEACHING STRATEGIES

It is important to remember that the nurse may be the first health care provider to initiate patient teaching. Bedside nurses are in a unique position to facilitate, mentor, and coach patients through the endless maze of information presented in the acute care arena. Information overload often occurs, and the information taught can easily be forgotten. Nurses may become frustrated when family members and patients ask the same questions repeatedly. Patience with repeated questioning is essential, since information taught may be lost within minutes after its presentation. Although health care providers would like patients and families to retain 100% of information given, in reality learning will not take place in one session or may not occur at all. An individual may be able to remember only two to three pieces of information in one education session.

Nurses are continuously interacting with patients and discussing their progress, updating them on treatment plans, and describing procedures. With that in mind, every patient contact can be thought of as a brief teaching-learning encounter. The nurse must use every teachable moment and take advantage of the patient's readiness and willingness to learn. When educating adults, a combination of teaching strategies should be used to facilitate both the giving and receiving of information. Each individual has a different learning style: visual, auditory, or tactile. Common strategies include discussion, demonstration, and use of media.

Discussion. Informal discussion can take place anywhere, at any time. This strategy allows for interaction between the teacher and the learner. Discussion occurs one-on-one or in groups. Education sessions need to be adapted quickly, as they are occurring, to meet the ever-evolving needs of the patient/family. Even though teaching through discussion is informal, the information given should promote the goals of the education plan. Focus on what the patient or family wants or *needs* to know at that moment, rather than on what might be *nice* to know. Obtaining and maintaining the learner's attention during discussion may be challenging. The nurse must utilize different teaching strategies and techniques and modify them frequently according to the situation and the patient or family response to the education.

Strategies used to maintain a positive teaching-learning encounter include:
- Addressing the patient/family by name.
- Clearly stating the purpose of the education encounter.
- Getting and keeping them involved in the learning process.
- Maintaining eye contact during the encounter.
- Keeping the encounter brief and to the point.
- Giving positive reinforcement.
- Communicating with other disciplines the patient/family progress and additional learning needs.[4,5]

Demonstration and Practice. Demonstration and practice are the best strategies for teaching technical skills. Adults learn best when they are able to participate in the learning process. Involving the learner, providing consistent step-by-step instructions, and presenting a visual demonstration of the skill being performed are all important strategies to achieve successful task acquisition. By allowing the patient or family to practice the skill in a simulated or real situation, the outcome of the teaching encounter can be evaluated. This strategy allows the nurse to offer positive reinforcement and constructive feedback during the learning encounter, thereby building learner confidence in performing the newly acquired skill. Many demonstration sessions and repetitive practice may be required for the patient or family to acquire and feel comfortable with the new skill.

Audio-Visual Media. The use of media in mainstream patient education is becoming more prevalent as a first-line teaching strategy. Media are an excellent tool to relay information to persons with any one of the three learning styles. Pamphlets, videos, and anatomical pictures or models are the most common types of audio-visual aids.

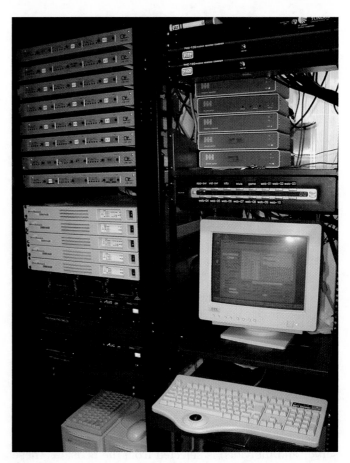

Fig. 4-1 This centrally located computer server contains over 350 videos for patient education purposes. The interactive television system permits the patient or family to access any education video at any time of day or any day of the week for learning purposes. (Courtesy Hospital Communication Systems, Pennsylvania.)

This teaching strategy supplies the learner with a large amount of information in a relatively short time period. Videos and written materials enable different nurses to distribute information that remains consistent from patient to patient/family to family. The use of media can assist practitioners to obtain informed consent as well as communicate current and future prescribed treatment plans. Media are used to educate patients on a variety of educational needs such as medications, disease process, procedures, symptom management, weight monitoring, lab tests, diet, surgery, and health maintenance issues. Patient education videos require the patient's attention for only a few minutes and supply the learner with "nice-to-know" as well as "need-to-know" information. Interactive video technology offers on-demand educational and health information video programs, which are delivered to the patient through the television. Patients and families are able to access education videos at anytime they desire during their hospital stay. The digital video system allows multiple TVs to show the same video at the same time. Fig. 4-1 shows the digital computer system. Fig. 4-2 shows

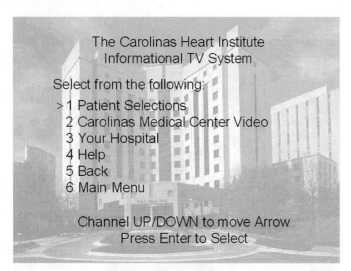

The Carolinas Heart Institute
Informational TV System

Select from the following:

> 1 Patient Selections
2 Carolinas Medical Center Video
3 Your Hospital
4 Help
5 Back
6 Main Menu

Channel UP/DOWN to move Arrow
Press Enter to Select

Fig. 4-2 This figure is an example of an initial television display screen. This screen may be customized according to the institution's specific needs. The menu may also be individualized to include categories of videos available at the institution. A system user guide is also noted on the screen. (Courtesy Hospital Communication Systems, Raleigh, NC, and Carolinas Heart Institute at Carolinas Medical Center, Charlotte, NC.)

the TV display of the education menu and the main screen. Bedside call systems are linked to the computer server and the video is selected from the bedside. These video systems can be customized to meet the needs of specialty patient populations (e.g., cardiac or obstetrics). Individual reports can be generated to list all educational films viewed during the patient's stay. Evaluation of learning can be achieved through the system by administration of a pretest or posttest available on the system.

Viewing a video does not ensure retention of information or knowledge acquisition. Patient education videos should not be used in place of patient/family interaction. After the patient watches the video the nurse must review the content and reiterate key points of information. This postvideo encounter is also used to evaluate the outcome of the teaching-learning encounter. If a nurse has never seen the video, it will be difficult to review the content with the patient or family. Therefore the nurse must also watch the video and choose key points to discuss with the learner in the postvideo discussion. Video presentation should be used to assist the learner in meeting identified educational needs.

Written Materials. Written media such as brochures, pamphlets, patient pathways, and booklets are commonplace in both outpatient and inpatient areas of health care. They are generally inexpensive and offer opportunities for a wide range of education: disease process education, risk factor modification information, procedure education, medication education, and use of medical equipment in the home setting. Written materials address multiple learning styles and offer learner-centered

teaching with concrete, basic information that can be placed at the learner's fingertips for immediate review, as well as future review anytime the learner desires. Multiple factors should be considered when choosing printed materials for patient education: target patient population, cultural considerations, age-specific considerations, and literacy.[6]

The practitioner must make sure that written materials are appropriate for the patient population as a whole and also for a particular individual patient or family. Literacy is the ability to use printed and written information to function in society, to achieve one's goals, and to develop one's knowledge and potential.[32] Persons with low literacy have trouble functioning in society. They may not be able to read a bus schedule, complete a simple form, or even follow the instructions on a bottle of aspirin. The term *health literacy* refers to the patient's ability to understand and communicate important medical and health information to members of the health care team.[33] Low literacy levels are considered a barrier to successful patient/family education and the teaching-learning process.[9]

If a person with a low literacy level cannot read the material or understand its meaning, he or she cannot perform self-management tasks to maintain health. This sets the patient and the family up for failure and being labeled noncompliant. Inadequate literacy is an independent risk factor for increasing hospital admissions among the elderly.[34] Nearly 20% of the U.S. adult population have low literacy skills and read at or below the fifth-grade reading level.[35] Typical patient education materials are written at or above the eighth- or ninth-grade reading level and may be out of reach for many readers.[5,36] A common misconception among health care providers is that reading levels are directly related to the level of education; the implication is that someone with a graduate-level education has a higher reading level than someone who only completed grade school. It is important to remember that this is not true; education levels do not necessarily correlate with the ability to read and comprehend health care information. Several tools are available to assist health care professionals to screen for low literary skills. The Rapid Estimate of Adult Literacy in Medicine (REALM) assesses the patient's ability to pronounce medical terms.[4] It takes only a few minutes to complete and is relevant to health care. Another literacy screening tool is the Test of Functional Health Literacy in Adults (TOFHLA). This tool assesses the ability of the individual to read and comprehend directions for taking medications, monitoring blood glucose, and keeping appointments.[37] The only drawback to this tool is it takes approximately 22 minutes to complete and may not be appropriate for the bedside practitioner to use.

Readability is another important factor in the consideration of printed educational materials. This term refers to the ease of how easy or hard the literature is to read.

Readability formulas are designed to make a quick, easy assessment of readability level in patient education materials. Formulas such as the Simplified Measure of Gobbledygook (SMOG), Suitability Assessment of Materials (SAM), and Fog and Fry assessment tools are available to assist practitioners in determining the readability of health education materials. Providing written education materials at the appropriate reading level is important, if the information is to be easily read and understood by the majority of patients and families. In order to assist the nurse in overcoming literacy-related barriers to health education, it is recommended that patient education materials be printed at or below the fifth-grade reading level.[35,38] Samples of health-related instructions at different reading levels are provided in Box 4-4.

Patients and families who cannot read and understand the written word provide a special challenge with regard to printed materials. Provision of educational materials with illustrations for those who cannot read or in Braille for the blind might be helpful. Also, it is important to note that a patient or a family's inability to read the English language does not mean they cannot understand directions and treatment regimens. Multilingual, written patient/family education materials are a necessity in any health care institution. There are many health education vendors that supply ready-made patient education materials. Examples are HERC publishing, Pritchett and Hall, and Krames. National associations such as the American Cancer Society, the American Lung Association, and the American Heart Association also publish patient education materials. Each of these companies has a website for easy viewing of sample patient education materials and pricing information. Prices for these materials can vary from pennies per pamphlet to several dollars; some pamphlets by national organizations are available free of charge to the consumer. When choosing standardized, printed education materials, there are several items to consider. Read the entire pamphlet or booklet to determine appropriateness of the material for the desired patient population. Ask the vendor to supply the reading level of the material and the method used to determine it. Also inquire about the frequency with which the printed material is updated to ensure that the patient or family have the most recent edition.

Thoroughly read the document for inconsistent information or information that is incongruent with a specific unit's treatment plan. For example, if the nurse educates the patient on a low-fat diet, but the pamphlet only teaches a low-salt diet, the patient may become confused and frustrated and not be able to determine which diet to follow at home. Another point to consider is whether the material contains information required by the institution and regulatory agencies such as JCAHO. Core measures outlined by JCAHO include certain items that must be included in discharge education and tracked by the institution. Certain materials may not properly fit

Box 4-4

SAMPLE OF DIFFERENT READING LEVELS

COLLEGE READING LEVEL
Consult your physician immediately with the onset of chest discomfort, shortness of breath, or increased perspiration.

TWELFTH-GRADE READING LEVEL
Call your physician immediately if you experience chest discomfort, shortness of breath, or increased sweatiness.

EIGHTH-GRADE READING LEVEL
Call your doctor immediately if you start having chest pain or shortness of breath or you feel sweaty.

FOURTH-GRADE READING LEVEL
Call your doctor right away if you start having chest pain, can't breathe, or feel sweaty.

with a unit's plan for education and therefore are not appropriate for that particular institution. Printed material should be an adjunct to patient-family education and match what is taught and practiced in a specific facility.

In those instances when predeveloped educational materials do not meet the need of the institution's patient population, the decision is made to develop internal patient education materials. Producing "home grown" educational materials can be time-consuming and difficult.[10] Time must be spent determining content, readability, and design. The practitioner must keep in mind that patients and families may receive a variety of educational materials during their hospital stay. Streamlining educational materials within an organization will decrease inconsistency of information, increase clarity of prescribed treatment, and help to avoid duplication of efforts between disciplines and shifts. Although providing written materials may seem like a quick and easy education method, the practitioner must still review the content with the patient or family to determine whether learning has occurred and whether there are any questions about the material.

Computer-Assisted Instruction. Computer-assisted instruction is a relatively new strategy to providing patient/family education. Even though personal computers are commonplace today, they may not be suitable for some individuals because comfort levels with the technical aspects of the computer vary from person to person. The learner should be able to pay attention to the material being presented and not be preoccupied with learning how to use the computer mouse. The costs of computers and new software development may prohibit institutions from considering them for their patient education programs. Software programs can be accessed via a single hard drive or through a server for multiple computer sites. The use of touch screen technology instead of the standard mouse opens up computer learning to many individuals who do not feel comfortable with technology. Touch screen technology is even available in local grocery stores for self-checkout. Computer screens may be placed in every patient room at the bedside for easy access to education videos or the Internet. Bedside computers provide the patient/family with an avenue to receive education on demand whenever they are ready, willing, and able. Computers offer self-directed learning. Since adults are self-directed individuals, they can go through the program at their own pace and spend as much or as little time as desired in one area of content. Computers stimulate all aspects of the adult learner, visual, auditory, and tactile.

Internet Websites. Patients and families often use Internet websites to research information regarding the illness or condition they are concerned with.[39] Information on the Internet is generally presented on an eighth-grade reading level.[9] Websites contain a wealth of information. However, the information is not regulated or controlled for reliability or validity.[39] Therefore not all information provided on every website is accurate. The nurse must advise the patient/family of this concern and ask them to print out and bring in such material so it can be discussed. Government websites, as well as those of professional organizations, reputable health care organizations, and consumer health groups, are some of sites available that offer trustworthy information for both the practioner and the lay public.[39]

Communication. Communicating information is essential to obtaining positive education outcomes. Interpreter services should be used if the patient or family is not fluent in the English language. Informational materials should be made available in other languages to facilitate the relaying of information and enhance self-care management skills after discharge.

All patients and families desire to be understood and have their concerns validated. This can be difficult for patients who are critically ill and whose ability to communicate to family and health care providers is impaired. Communication aids such as picture cards, picture boards, or word boards enhance the ability of the nurse to understand educational needs and communicate information. Augmentative and alternative communication (AAC) systems are available and may be considered for temporarily nonspeaking patients in the ICU. Technology which has generally been available in the outpatient setting to help persons who cannot speak is now becoming available for the intensive care environment. This technology is known as electronic voice output communication aids or VOCA. VOCA is a prerecorded, human or digitalized computer-generated voice message.[40] It can be beneficial for patients who awake, alert, but are unable to talk for reasons such as mechanical ventilation through an endotracheal tube or tracheostomy tube. Whole phrases, as opposed to pictures

or single words, are communicated to the health care team, for example, "I am having pain."[40] This technology can assist the patient to communicate comfort needs, anxiety, fears, and to ask questions concerning care or progress. Intubated patients describe the inability of families and caregivers to effectively understand their needs as an extremely stressful part of being in the ICU.[20] AACs can also assist the nurse to more effectively evaluate the outcome of education. Use of verbal, whole-sentence communication rather than traditional, nonverbal picture board communication has been found to decrease the guesswork in interpreting patient needs.[40]

CONSCIOUS AND UNCONSCIOUS PATIENTS

Patient education should not be reserved for the conscious and coherent patient only; it should be provided to the unconscious or sedated patient as well. Addressing the learning needs of this critically ill population of patients is challenging. These patients cannot communicate their educational needs, nor can they interact and participate in the learning process. Whereas it is truly not known what the unconscious or sedated patient hears or remembers, it is known that some sedated patients undergoing surgery remember discussions that took place among physicians and staff during the procedure. In addition, practitioners frequently tell family members to speak to the unconscious patient even though the patient cannot respond. Therefore, one should not ignore unconscious or sedated patients during the education process. These patients may not be able to respond or participate, and the effectiveness of the teaching process cannot be evaluated, but providing information regarding environment, procedures, sensations, and time of day is benevolent and may help to decrease immediate physiologic stress.

STEP 4: OUTCOME EVALUATION

Evaluation is the final component in the patient/family education process. The intent of evaluation is to determine the effectiveness of the educational interventions. The nurse must use his or her clinical judgment and knowledge of adult learning principles to determine how well the learner has met the expected outcomes and/or objectives. The evaluation process is continual and assesses the entire teaching-learning interaction, including the level of learner interest in the session, willingness to learn the content, and level of participation during the encounter. Evaluation should be completed at the end of each teaching-learning encounter. This allows the nurse to immediately present positive and constructive feedback to the patient/family, as well as revise the education plan to accommodate ongoing learning needs. It is also important to assess the response to teaching and determine whether follow-up education is required.

HOW TO EVALUATE

How does the nurse know if learning has occurred? Techniques such as verbalization of information, return demonstration, and physiologic measurement are common evaluation methods to determine the effectiveness of a teaching-learning encounter. Evaluation of knowledge retention can be completed by verbally questioning the learner. Questioning is an interactive process that assists the nurse in determining if the learner has retained the information taught. The nurse may ask the patient if he or she is able to list signs and symptoms of heart failure. Verbal questioning should not only occur immediately after the teaching event but also later, throughout the hospitalization, to assess knowledge retention. For example, the physician orders a new medication for the patient today, and the nurse educates that patient on the effects and side effects; tomorrow the nurse may assess retention by asking the patient if he or she remembers why he or she is taking the new medication. Common items that patients and families are asked to verbalize are reportable signs and symptoms, how to manage symptoms at home, when to take medication, how often the medication should be taken, and who to call for questions or concerns.

Changes in attitude, beliefs, or lifestyle are often difficult to evaluate, because learners could say they have changed their attitude when actually they have not. In this learning domain the nurse must use his or her detective skills to assess whether the individual has accepted the prescribed treatment plan and modified behavior accordingly. Sometimes the best way to evaluate a change in attitude is by observation and verbal questioning. An example might be a patient who has been asked to comply with a low-cholesterol diet; a food diary the patient has kept as requested provides some evidence as to what the patient has eaten. A wealth of information can also be obtained from the family concerning the patient's exhibited changes.

Physiologic evidence of the effectiveness of education can also be measured. Indicators such as blood cholesterol levels, blood pressure, heart rate, blood sugars, and weight can lead the practitioner to the conclusion that the patient/family may be having difficulties understanding or following through with the identified plan of care.[31] Adults generally want to comply with new expectations but often cannot for various reasons, for example, lack of money for medications or an inability to understand what is expected of them. Such barriers must be explored and included in the education plan.

Observation and return demonstration is the evaluation of choice for the skills learning domain. For the patient/family to be "checked off" on a particular skill, they should be able to perform it independently, using the nurse only as a resource for questions. Endotracheal suctioning, placing condom catheters, and performing dressing changes are examples of common tasks that patients and families may be asked to learn. Because of the increasingly complex care that patients now require at home after discharge, these skills may be the entire focus of teaching before discharge. It is important to remember that not every teaching moment is a success, and the nurse need not feel guilty or like a failure when the learner has not achieved the desired objective. Revisiting and revising the goals and objectives during the teaching-learning session may be necessary to meet the ever-changing needs of the patient or family.

STEP 5: DOCUMENTATION

Documentation of education is necessary to communicate education efforts to members of the health care team, patient/families, and regulatory agencies. The nurse should recognize that informal teaching at the bedside is education. It is important to document any information given to the patient on formal documents approved for use by each health care institution. In most institutions, formal education records are used to document education rendered by practitioners of any discipline involved in the care of a particular patient/family. These forms are communication tools used to indicate progress in the teaching-learning process from shift to shift, day to day, and discipline to discipline.[41] Documentation should include education from admission to discharge, on topics ranging from orientation to the environment to acquisition of self-management skills for home care.

WHAT SHOULD BE DOCUMENTED?

The complexity of information, demand by governing agencies, lawsuits, and the sheer volume of patients in and out of a unit are driving nurses to provide quality documentation of the education encounter.[41] Documentation of the teaching-learning process is multifaceted. The documentation form should "tell the story" of the education encounter from assessment to evaluation. Documentation of the education assessment should include learning preferences, factors that impair ability, readiness, and willingness to learn, and actual or perceived learning needs. Information should be noted on the interaction, material taught, supplemental materials distributed, response to the education, achievement of outcome, and any follow-up education or resources needed. The Nursing Outcomes Classification (NOC), clinical pathways, and patient education guides can provide a means of consistent documentation. Box 4-5 contains an example of a NOC evaluation for disease process.

Box 4-5

KNOWLEDGE: DISEASE PROCESS

Definition: Extent of understanding conveyed about a specific disease process

INDICATORS	NONE	LIMITED	MODERATE	SUBSTANTIAL	EXTENSIVE
Description of disease process	1	2	3	4	5
Description of cause or contributing factors	1	2	3	4	5
Description of risk factors	1	2	3	4	5
Description of effects of disease	1	2	3	4	5
Description of signs and symptoms	1	2	3	4	5
Description of usual disease course	1	2	3	4	5
Description of measures to minimize disease progression	1	2	3	4	5
Description of complications	1	2	3	4	5
Description of signs and symptoms of complications	1	2	3	4	5
Description of precautions to prevent complications	1	2	3	4	5

From Johnson M, Maas M, Morehead S: *Nursing outcomes classification (NOC),* ed 3, St Louis, 2004, Mosby.

Table 4-3	**Nursing Barriers to Education**	
Barrier	**Example**	**Solution**
Interruptions	Daily routines	Use all available teachable moments
Distractions	Tasks; medication administration	Turn TV off, minimize noise
	Phone calls	
	TV or other noise in patient's room	
Night shift	Patients are asleep	Plan education before bed
Sedation/pain medications	Narcotic analgesic	Teach before administering the medication
Nurse is unaware of what to teach	Diabetic education	Educate self

Adapted from London F: *No time to teach,* Philadelphia, 1999, Lippincott; Rankin S, Stallings K: *Patient education: principles and practice,* ed 4, Philadelphia, 2001, Lippincott.

FACTORS THAT AFFECT THE TEACHING-LEARNING PROCESS

Many factors can produce barriers to a successful teaching-learning process. Physiologic, psychologic, sociocultural, financial, and environmental factors previously discussed in the assessment portion of this chapter are known to affect the patient's and family's ability, willingness, and readiness to learn. Physical disabilities, impaired vision, and hearing loss will affect the learner's ability to read materials, listen to instructions, or perform a technical task.[42] If a technical task is required, ensure that the patient or family member has the physical ability or manual dexterity to perform the required skill. Provision of eyeglasses and hearing aids is essential to improving participation in learning. A number of other factors also have an impact on the teaching-learning process[5,10]:

- Lack of an accurate assessment
- Setting unrealistic goals
- Not involving the patient or the family in the process
- Overloading the learner with information

- Relying too heavily on resources
- Haphazard and non-directed teaching; lack of an education plan of care
- Time: teaching at the wrong time, hurried teaching, not paying attention to the learner
- Lack of trust and rapport between the teacher and learner
- Lack of communication among health care providers
- Language: communication barriers

Although this list may seem overwhelming, it is important to be proactive and to remove as many of these barriers as possible. It takes less time and fewer resources to start with a structured education plan than it does to start over after the teaching-learning process has begun.

Barriers to the teaching-learning process exist not only for the patient or family, but also for the bedside nurse. Time constraints, decreased length of stay, and daily routines interrupt or impair the nurse's ability to communicate information to the patient and the family. Table 4-3 includes common barriers to the education process experienced by nurses.

CLINICAL APPLICATION

Patient/Family Education Concepts

Anthony is an 18-year-old male who was involved in a motor vehicle collision 2 days ago. He and his girlfriend were on their way to a freshman party when a woman crossed the center line and hit them head-on. His girlfriend died at the scene. Anthony was airlifted to the trauma center. He arrived unconscious and in critical condition with multiple fractures, pulmonary contusions, pneumothoraces, a severe head injury, and internal injuries. Since admission he has received multiple fluid boluses and blood products and has had surgery for a splenectomy and to externally fixate left leg fractures. He has a ventriculostomy, a pulmonary artery catheter, an arterial line, a Foley catheter, and chest tubes and is intubated and on the ventilator. Anthony remains in critical condition. His current plan of care involves maintaining stable hemodynamics with vasopressor therapy, sedation to decrease oxygen consumption and intracranial pressure (ICP), and other supportive care. He is 12 kg over his admission weight, and his facial features are distorted as a result of the fluid.

His mother and father have been at the hospital, living in the ICU waiting room, since the accident. They have never been in an ICU before and are frightened by all the tubes and machines connected to their son. Anthony's mother brings in a pad of paper with questions on it for each visit. She has asked several questions repeatedly and still hesitates to touch her son during visits. She states, "I don't ever know where to touch him with all those IVs and tubes." Anthony's parents have been emotional during visits, but they talk to him and tell him who has visited and that they are praying for him. Anthony has responded to them only once, by squeezing their hand. They are concerned about the way he looks, when he will wake up and talk to them, and whether he will be able to return to college and when. They have elected not to tell him about the death of his girlfriend at this time. His father is also concerned about the finances of this hospitalization because he is self-employed and has limited insurance.

1. What are the five steps in the teaching-learning process?
2. What immediate and long-term learning needs do you assess that Anthony and his parents have?
3. What are the top three needs of Anthony's family. Explain why you chose those three.
4. What would you determine to be the expected outcome(s) for their education plan of care?
5. In which domain(s) of learning will you focus your education for Anthony's parents?
6. Are any factors present that will affect Anthony's and his parent's ability, willingness, and readiness to learn? Explain why they will have an effect.
7. What teaching strategies would be best for this situation?
8. What techniques would you use to evaluate the teaching-learning process in this situation?

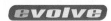 For the discussion of this Clinical Application and an additional clinical application on patient/family education concepts, see the Evolve website.

PREPARING THE PATIENT/FAMILY FOR TRANSFER

Transferring a patient from the one acute care area to another is no small event. It can produce anxiety and create stress. Patients and families have learned and adapted to their current situation. They have grown to know the staff, the environment, and expected routine of care (see the Clinical Application feature on Patient/Family Education Concepts).

In the critical care environment they will have become dependent on the monitors, equipment, constant nursing attention, and abundant information received while in the critical care unit. The patient will have become secure knowing that his or her immediate physiologic and emotional needs are being met. A strong bond develops between the staff and the family. Many patients and families are reluctant to give up that bond and feel their needs will not be met as well on an unfamiliar unit with unfamiliar people and routines. To avoid anxiety and provide the patient/family with some control over the event, practitioners need to prepare them for the transfer process.

Preparation for transfer should start after the patient has been stabilized and the life-threatening event that resulted in hospitalization has subsided. The stressor at this point is not the now-familiar critical care environment, but the unfamiliar step-down environment. Explanations as to where the patient will be transferred, the reason for transfer, and the name of the nurse who will be providing care should be provided as soon as known. Before transfer, information about how care will change, what self-care will be expected, and visiting hours should be provided to the patient/family. Family members should also be contacted concerning exactly when the patient will be transferred so either they can be present during the transfer or they can be made aware of the patient's new location.

The education plan of care and tips learned by the critical care staff about that particular patient/family should be communicated to the step-down unit staff. Most of the patient transfers made from the critical care unit to a step-down unit are planned events. At times, however, unplanned or unexpected transfers do occur. This usually happens when the critical care unit requires a bed space for a more seriously ill patient. This situation arises during the day or often during the night, and the transfer occurs quickly. Families may be present in the hospital or may have gone home for the evening. This sudden need to transfer the patient can produce as much anxiety as the initial event, primarily because they may not feel ready for the transfer or they may feel they have lost control of the situation. Providing the patient/family with concrete evidence of improvement, such as more favorable vital signs or the need for fewer medications or tubes, can reassure them of improvement in the patient's condition before unplanned transfers occur.

SUMMARY

In the current health care arena, a collaborative, well organized, need-targeted education plan of care is essential to improving health outcomes and decreasing lengths of stay. Incorporating adult learning principles, performing an accurate assessment, developing a learner-oriented teaching plan, using effective teaching skills, and evaluating progress are prime components of a successful teaching-learning interaction. With time and education, practitioners will develop these skills and become advocates in empowering patients and families to take charge of their own health-related behaviors.

REFERENCES

1. Joint Commission on Accreditation of Healthcare Organizations (JCAHO): 2004 *Comprehensive accreditation manual for hospitals*, Oakbrook Terrace, Ill, 2004, The Commission.
2. Davis N et al: Improving the process of informed consent in the critically ill, *JAMA* 289(15):1963-1968, 2003.
3. Leske J: Comparison of family stresses, strengths, and outcomes after trauma surgery, *AACN Clin Issues Crit Care* 14(1):33-41, 2003.
4. Redman BK: *The practice of patient education*, ed 9, St Louis, 2004, Mosby.
5. Rankin S, Stallings K: *Patient education: principles and practice*, ed 4, Philadelphia, 2001, Lippincott.
6. Wei H, Camargo C: Patient education in the emergency department, *Acad Emerg Med* 7(6):710-717, 2000.
7. Briggs L et al: Patient-centered advance care planning in special patient populations: a pilot study, *J Prof Nurs* 20(1):47-58, 2004.
8. Moorhead S, Johnson M, Maas M: *Nursing outcomes classification (NOC)*, ed 3, St Louis, 2004, Mosby.
9. Burkhead V et al: Enter: a care guide for successfully educating patients, *J Nurses Staff Dev* 19(3):143-146, 2003.
10. Phillips LD: Patient education: understanding the process to maximize time and outcomes, *J Intraven Nurs* (22)1:19-35, 1999.
11. Glittenburg J: A transdisciplinary, transcultural model for health care, *J Trans Nurs* 15(1):6-10, 2004.
12. Walsh S: Formulation of a plan of care for culturally diverse patients, *Int J Nurs Terminol Classif* 15(1):17-26, 1999.
13. Leininger M, McFarland M: *Transcultural nursing*, ed 3, New York, 2002, McGraw Hill.
14. Suh EE: The model of cultural competence through an evolutional concept analysis, *J Transcultural Nurs* 15(2):93-102, 2004.
15. Blount KA, Moore LA: Medications and the elderly, *Crit Care Nurs Clin North Am* 14(1):111-119, 2002.
16. Knowles MS: *The modern practice of adult education: from pedagogy to andragogy*, New York, 1976, Cambridge Books.
17. London F: *No time to teach*, Philadelphia, 1999, Lippincott.
18. Gentz C: Perceived learning needs of the patient undergoing coronary angioplasty: an integrative review of the literature, *Heart Lung* 29(3):161-172, 2000.
19. Ruzicki D: Realistically meeting the educational needs of hospitalized acute and short stay patients, *Nurs Clin North Am* 24(3):629-637, 1989.
20. Thomas L: Clinical management of stressors perceived by patients on mechanical ventilation, *AACN Clin Issues Crit Care* 14(1):73-81, 2003.
21. Leske JS: Protocols for practice: applying research at the bedside, *Crit Care Nurs* 18(4):92-95, 1998.
22. VanHorn E, Fleury J, Moore S: Family interventions during the trajectory of recovery from cardiac event: an integrative literature review, *Heart Lung* 31(3):186-198, 2002.
23. An K et al: A cross-sectional examination of changes in anxiety early after acute myocardial infarction, *Heart Lung* 33(2):75-82, 2004.
24. Leske JS: Family stresses, strengths, and outcomes after critical injury, *Crit Care Nurs Clin North Am* 12(2):237-244, 2000.
25. Lazarus RS, Folkman S: *Stress, appraisal, and coping*, New York, 1984, Springer.
26. Laubach E: How to communicate with seriously ill patients, *Nurs Manage* 31(4):24H-24J, 2000.
27. Leske J: Overview of family needs after critical illness: from assessment to intervention, *AACN Clin Issues Crit Care* 2(2):220-26, 1991.
28. Saunders R: Constructing a lesson plan, *J Nurses Staff Dev* 19(2):70-78, 2003.
29. Dochterman JM, Bulechek GM: *Nursing interventions classification (NIC)*, ed 4, St. Louis, 2004, Mosby.
30. Benner C, Tanner C, Chelsa C: *From beginner to expert: excellence and power in clinical nurse practice*, Menlo Park, 1984, Addison-Wesley.
31. Clark P, Dunbar S: Family partnership intervention: a guide for family approach to care of patients with heart failure, *AACN Clinical Issues* 14(4):467-476, 2003.
32. Kaestle C et al: *Adult literacy and education in America*, Washington, DC, 2001, U.S. Dept of Education.
33. Wilson J: The crucial link between literacy and health, *Ann Intern Med* 139(10):875-878, 2003.
34. Baker DW et al: Functional health literacy and the risk of hospital admission among Medicare managed care enrollees, *Am J Pub Health* 92(8):1278-1283, 2002.
35. Doak C et al: Improving comprehension for cancer patients with low literacy skills: strategies for clinicians, *CA Cancer J Clin* 38(3):151-162, 1998.
36. Doak C, Doak L, Root J: *Teaching patients with low literacy skills*, ed 2, Philadelphia, 1996, Lippincott.
37. Quirk P: Screening for literacy and readability: implications for the advanced practice nurse, *Clin Nurse Spec* 14(1):26-32, 2000.

38. Kingbeil C, Speece M, Schubiner H: Readability of pediatric patient education materials, *Clin Pediatr* 34(2):96-102, 1995.

39. Jones J: Patient education and the use of the Internet, *Clin Nurs Spec* 17(6):281-283, 2003.

40. Happ MB, Roesch TK, Garrett K: Electronic voice-output communication aids for temporarily non-speaking patients in a medical intensive care unit: a feasibility study, *Heart Lung* 33(2):92-101, 2004.

41. Russell C, Freiburghaus M: Heart transplant patient teaching documentation, *Clin Nurs Spec* 17(5):249-257, 2004.

42. Bruccoliere T: How to make patient teaching stick, *RN* 63(2):34-38, 2000.

Psychosocial Alterations

PSYCHOSOCIAL ALTERATIONS, COPING MECHANISMS, AND MANAGEMENT

Patients requiring critical care must cope with a variety of stressors. A patient's response to these stressors depends on individual differences, such as age, gender, social support, cultural background, medical diagnosis, current hospital course, and prognosis. A person's perceptions of self and relationships with others, of spiritual values, and of self-competency in social roles also play a major role in how he or she will respond to stress and illness. The purpose of this chapter is to provide a theoretic basis for understanding these various issues and to provide the nurse with additional insight into implementing holistic nursing care.

The human self-concept is a major concern for nurses because nursing interventions that do not consider the individual in his or her wholeness—including the self-concept—will probably not be effective. The self-concept comprises attitudes about oneself; perceptions of personal abilities, body image, and identity; and a general sense of worth. The stressors imposed by physical illness, trauma, and surgical procedures can cause disturbances in the self-concept. A person's response to these stressors depends on a variety of individual differences, as just mentioned.

The following discussions address the nursing diagnoses related to self-concept disturbances imposed by critical stages of illness (i.e., Disturbed Body Image, Situational Low Self-Esteem, Ineffective Role Performance, Ineffective Coping, Compromised Family Coping) as developed by the North American Nursing Diagnosis Association (NANDA).[1] The four subcomponents of the human self-concept are depicted in Fig. 5-1. Evaluation of each subcomponent as a way of understanding and intervening with an individual patient will be discussed. Stuart's stress adaptation conceptual model[2] is presented as a means to address coping mechanisms and holistic methods of care. Some of the various stressors experienced in the critical care setting are depicted in Box 5-1.

The selected diagnoses presented relate to the major concerns and problems common to the critical care setting. Customary responses to stress, such as anxiety and depression, are described, as well as the risks for spiritual distress, powerlessness, hopelessness, and self-directed violence (suicide). Delirium, or acute confusion, frequently experienced by the critical care patient, is also discussed, as are the psychosocial needs of specific populations including the elderly, chronically ill persons with acute exacerbations, persons with suppressed immune systems, and transplant recipients. Ways to enhance patient coping mechanisms and support family and friends with an attitude of care, openness, and warmth are presented. These interpersonal skills lead to effective interventions. A Clinical Application is presented at the conclusion of this chapter to illustrate the potential psychosocial alterations and coping measures that can be used and to stimulate critical decision making.

HOLISTIC NURSING PRACTICE

Holistic nursing care requires consideration of all factors, individual and environmental, that affect the patient's or client's well-being and the ability to cope with crises such as an acute or chronic illness. The nurse must have a sound knowledge base of anatomy and physiology, disease processes, remedial measures, and human responses. The critical care nurse should not only be able to work with technology but also needs to "know the patient" in order to humanize and individualize the care. The value of "presence," being attuned to the patient's needs, represents the caring aspect of nursing and can assist in early identification of patient problems.[3,4] Decisions to implement interventions are then based on an understanding of the patient's experiences, cultural beliefs, behavior patterns, feelings, and preferences (Table 5-1).[5-9]

Research conducted by Jenny and Logan[10] asked patients to provide examples of nurse caring behaviors. Positive comments included alleviating discomfort, car-

Box 5-1

STRESSORS IN THE CRITICAL CARE SETTING

Patients' experience of critical illness and care vary. However, each patient must cope with at least some of the following stressors:
- Threat of death
- Threat of survival, with significant residual problems related to the illness/injury
- Pain or discomfort
- Lack of sleep
- Loss of autonomy over most aspects of life and daily functioning
- Loss of control over environment, such as loss of privacy and exposure to light, noise, and general activity of the critical care unit, including the care of other patients
- Daily hassles or common frustrations
- Loss of usual role and, with that, the arena in which usual coping mechanisms serve the patient
- Separation from family and friends
- Loss of dignity
- Boredom broken only by brief visits, threatening stimuli, and frightening thoughts
- Loss of ability to express self verbally when intubated

Effects and response to the stressors depend on the individual's perception of the intensity of the stress and the following factors:
- Acute/chronic duration of stressors
- Cumulative effect of simultaneous stressors
- Sequence of stressors
- Individual's previous experience with stressors and coping effectiveness
- Amount of social support

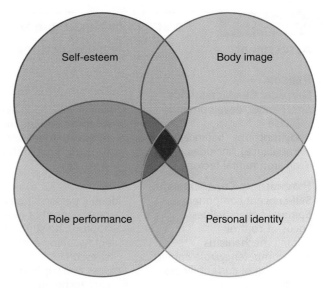

Fig. 5-1 Four subcomponents of the human self-concept.

ing attitudes and behaviors, advocacy, encouragement, and respect for the individual. Comments regarding noncaring behaviors were related to task-oriented behaviors and impersonal communication. The art of caring requires skills in communication and interpersonal relationships, a personal commitment, and the ability to create a sense of trust.

EFFECTS OF STRESS ON MIND/BODY INTERACTIONS

Stress of any type—whether positive or negative, biologic, psychologic, or social—elicits the same physical responses.[11] Extensive literature exists describing the relationship between the mind/body interactions and the immune response to stress. All personal resources can be depleted by exposure to severe or prolonged stress. Several studies have shown the effects of different life events such as an acute illness that is perceived to be a threat to personal integrity.[12-14] When an illness requires

hospitalization, the effect of this event can be further compounded when admission to an intensive care unit (ICU) becomes necessary.

The ICU environment can be frightening. Technologic equipment can control one's breathing and prevent speaking. Invasive procedures, abrupt or continual noises, loss of privacy, sleep interruptions, pain, medications, isolation, and minimal contact with significant support persons all create feelings of powerlessness and loss of control. Disorientation, which is common for patients in the ICU, is influenced by several factors, including the severity of the physical problem, chemical imbalances, sensory overload or deprivation, and previous experiences with the health care system. In addition to these factors are personal variables (i.e., biologic factors, social roles, and the person's emotional responses of anxiety, confusion, or depression).[5,13] However, for some individuals the ICU is perceived as a safe environment where life-saving procedures are immediately at hand and administered by highly competent caregivers.

Three of the principal stress theories proposed by scientists describe stress in terms of a stimulus, a response, and a transaction.[11,15-17] Hans Selye's pioneer work[11] portrayed the body responses to the stress stimulus as the general adaptation syndrome (GAS). Stimulation of the sympathetic nervous division of the autonomic nervous system (ANS) and the release of neurotransmitters and endocrine hormones occur in the initial stage, which is commonly referred to as the "fight or flight" response. Elevations in blood pressure, tachycardia, increased muscle tone, increased alertness, and "free floating" anxiety are some of the responses. A stage of exhaustion occurs when all reserves have been depleted, leading to further complications and/or death. Reversal of these processes can be accomplished through restoring re-

Table 5-1	Paradigm of Nursing in the Implementation of Holistic Patient-Centered Care	
Assessment	**Nursing Actions**	**Expected Outcomes**
PERSON		
BIOLOGIC CHARACTERISTICS		
Age, gender, developmental phase	Focus all actions toward total strengths/ needs of patient, including aspects related to environment and health status; use theoretic knowledge base for comparison purposes	Continuity of care will be provided
Body functions (balance/ imbalance) (includes internal environmental factors)		
PSYCHOLOGIC CHARACTERISTICS		
Self-concept components	Identify person's perception of current ill- ness, control of events, and availability of appropriate support system	Patient will have realistic expectations of outcomes from current illness and its impact on physical and mental health
Spiritual beliefs/values		
Locus of control		
Coping mechanisms	Identify coping mechanisms with previous stressors	Patient will use effective coping mechanisms in response to illness- related stressors
Role competency/role conflict		
Perception of current illness	Assess and support ability to learn new self- care techniques	Patient will participate in self-care, learn new psychomotor skills to achieve confidence in skill perform- ance
Intellect		
SOCIAL ASPECTS		
Interrelationships	Provide positive, honest feedback	Patient will place trust in caregivers and verbalize satisfaction with care or express need for changes
Availability of support system	Establish trust	
ENVIRONMENT		
Cultural/ethnic/societal influ- ences	Identify influencing factors in external environment that facilitate/inhibit pa- tient's coping with current health problem	Inhibiting factors will be minimized; facilitative factors will be enhanced
Area of residence, condition of living quarters/workplace	Collaborate with health care team members in providing holistic care	Collaborative team efforts will pro- mote holistic approach to decision making; family will be included in decisions
Access to available community resources—transportation, food, sanitation, support services	Provide safe, comfortable environment that is as stress-free as possible during hospi- talization	Hospital environment will be modi- fied to provide safe, secure atmo- sphere
Access to recreation facilities	Encourage positive interactions with signifi- cant others	Significant others will have central role in providing social support; pa- tient will not be isolated
Membership/attendance at religious/social functions		
Availability of significant others in social support system		
HEALTH		
Current and past mental/ spiritual/physical health status	Encourage positive interactions with signifi- cant others	Patient and family will have knowl- edge about illness and prognosis and can plan realistically for future
Life-style practices	Instruct person and family on self-care activities	Patient can implement a balanced plan of care for self
Type of coping mechanisms	Involve family in patient-centered activities as early as possible; support family members	Family caregivers will recognize own limits and seek help
Attitude toward life		

serves with the use of medications, nutrition, stress re- duction measures, and psychotherapy. Selye's work con- tinues to be the primary framework for stress and coping theories.

Nuerberger[15] was the first to propose that a person's emotional response to stress (or a perceived threat), de- scribed as "shutting down," is the result of overstimula- tion of the parasympathetic nervous system. He labeled this survival tactic as the general inhibition syndrome (GIS), or the "possum response." The use of defense mechanisms such as withdrawal, avoidance, and detach- ment are typical behaviors of this type of response.[2,17] Both ANS responses are protective measures. Imbal- ances of either system can be detrimental.

The extensive work of Lazarus and others[16,17] provides the framework for transactional theories on stress that suggest that the way that people cope with stress may be more important to overall morale, social function, and health/illness states than the frequency and severity of stress episodes. The person confronted by stress first makes a *cognitive appraisal* of its intensity. Response to the stressor depends on the perceived degree of threat imposed. A *secondary appraisal* determines what the response will be or what coping method to use to minimize the threat.

Coping, or adaptation, is an ongoing process involving both cognitive and physiologic neural-chemical and endocrine processes. The individual's sensitivity and vulnerability to the stressor are the determining factors of emotional and behavioral responses.[17,18] Therefore what may be an acutely stressful event to one person is not necessarily perceived as stressful by another. A person may employ different coping mechanisms to various stressors or to the same stressor at different times. A mechanism that is ineffective in one situation may be appropriate in another. Each person comes to an illness with a history and knowledge of the particular situation and its impact on life. Interpretation of the event and the responses depend on this history. The history changes with each new encounter.[2,11,12,17]

The Stuart stress adaptation model[2] addresses nursing interventions for persons whether they are sick or well. Concepts depicting biologic and psychologic responses to stress parallel those of the stress theories presented. Precipitating stressors may arise from the individual's internal or external environment; adaptation may depend on the number of stressors and the timing of their occurrence, as well as the degree of change that is represented. The accumulation of daily hassles can often influence a person's response to a major stressor. Personal characteristics that facilitate constructive adaptation to stress include hardiness, resilience, hope, a positive self-concept and internal locus of control, a sense of belonging, and the presence of social support.[19-21] Use of maladaptive, or destructive, measures may temporarily minimize anxiety but do not resolve the personal conflicts. There are four stages of nursing activities: (1) stabilization of the patient in a time of crisis; (2) providing symptom relief and assessment of the person's coping responses; (3) reinforcement of adaptive behaviors and improved patient functioning; and (4) implementing strategies for health promotion and accomplishing optimal quality of life.

ANXIETY AS A RESPONSE TO STRESS

Anxiety is a normal subjective human response to a perceived or actual threat to self-integrity, which can range from a vague, generalized feeling of discomfort to a state of panic and loss of control. Anxiety is the most common of all mental illnesses.[22] Symptoms of anxiety closely parallel the biologic stress responses described earlier. The initial emotional responses of excitement and heightened awareness diminish as anxiety levels increase, the individual's perceptual field narrows, and problem-solving and coping skills are lost. Prolonged stress can exhaust available resources.

An acute or chronic illness, facing a real or anticipated loss, being hospitalized, and any other event that is perceived as stressful can be triggers for anxiety. The nature of the stressor and the bio-psycho-social conditioning of the person being stressed can be the determining factors of a response.[7,17,23,24] Individuals who possess an anxiety trait may have poorer coping mechanisms and respond quite differently to an anxiety-producing situation than do individuals who do not possess this trait (See Unit X).

Anxiety elicits changes in the neurohumoral release patterns involving the neurotransmitters, including acetylcholine, norepinephrine, dopamine, serotonin, and their corresponding receptors. The complex and elusive integration of these responses within the central nervous system relies on communication between the cerebral cortex, the limbic system, the thalamus, the hypothalamus, the pituitary gland, and the reticular activating system. The cortex is involved with cognition, attention, and alertness, whereas emotional responses to stress are located in the limbic system. The corticotropin-releasing factor (CRF) controls the endocrine response and the norepinephrine pathway that is active in regulating the sympathetic branch of the ANS. It is suggested that a positive feedback system between the CRF and the ANS occurs when the increased activation in one system influences an increased activation in the other system. It is also proposed that large amounts of circulating CRF can accelerate behavioral responses, that is, anxiety and hypersensitivity, to stressful stimuli.[25,26]

ANXIETY AND PAIN

A cyclic relationship exists between levels of anxiety and perceptions and tolerance of pain. This relationship varies according to whether pain is produced by disease processes or invasive procedures, is acute or chronic, or is anticipatory. Pain affects the whole person. It has been defined as "an unpleasant sensory and emotional experience associated with actual and potential damage, or described in terms of such damage."[25] Pain also is multidimensional in nature, necessitating comprehensive assessment and management. In high acuity areas, pain can be caused by a variety of sources such as injured tissues, imposed immobility, intubation, lighting, noise, and interrupted sleep.

When an illness or pain is severe enough, the person experiencing it is forced to conserve all energies and focus inward to gain control of anxiety feelings. The person may startle easily, become irritable, display anger and rage, be vigilant and wary of caregivers, or be demanding. The person has a tendency to blame others, to be confused, and to be indecisive. The person may withdraw from interpersonal contact and indicate that the situation is overwhelming.[2,22] It is crucial for the nurse to identify the cause of the patient's pain, validate observations with the patient, and identify a plan for pain management. (For detailed information on pain management, see Chapter 8.)

Once pain management has been addressed, the nurse evaluates for ongoing anxiety. Again the nurse needs to identify the cause of a patient's anxiety and to validate observations with the patient. Medications frequently administered in the ICU can contribute to anxiety feelings; they include theophylline, anticholinergics, dopamine, levodopa, salicylates, and steroids.[22,25,26] Whether the causes of anxiety are biochemically induced or genetic factors or are secondary to a threat imposed in an emergency or a crisis situation, for interventions to be effective, one must take all factors into consideration. Panic attacks (outcomes of severe anxiety), which are frequent occurrences in the ICU, can also produce physiologic symptoms such as tachycardia, hyperventilation, and dyspnea.[2]

SELF-CONCEPT

THEORETIC BASIS

The terms *self-concept* and *self-esteem* have often been used synonymously. No clear-cut distinctions have been made. However, theoretic models used in the development of measurements refer to the self-concept as the "self-schema," or knowledge, of abilities, beliefs, and values that influence behavior during interactions with others in the social and cultural environments, whereas self-esteem is most closely linked to one's sense of self-worth.[2,27,28] Although the self-concept is relatively stable, it can be modified by the developmental phases and social roles a person experiences over a lifetime.[2,29] The nursing discipline has chosen the multidimensional construct of self-concept because it is useful for understanding individuals in regard to regulating health and illness behaviors and for distinguishing the importance of the environment on these behaviors (see Fig. 5-1).[29]

GENERAL DISTURBANCES IN SELF-CONCEPT

Any event with unpredictable body changes and functions requires adjustments in the self-concept, as well as a realistic readjustment to the role limitations that are imposed. These adjustment stages are complex and highly individualized.

A person faced with an intolerable situation may panic, may display behavior that distorts reality, and may exhibit excessive demands or be suspicious of motives and methods of the caregivers. Depression and anxiety are common reactions as the person experiences a loss of control and worries over outcomes.[30] The illness experience may have different meanings for individuals from different cultures and ethnic groups. Assessment of their needs can be elicited through use of tools that include questions that are sensitive to cultural values.[9] Patients in critical care units usually do not have time to adjust to the illness conditions and may exhibit signs of shock, numbness, and avoidance of reality and be unable to clearly understand the implications of the situation.[2,11,31-34] The patient is usually transferred to an intermediate unit before a true acknowledgment phase occurs. However, establishing rapport, repeating information as needed, and assuring the patient of their immediate safety are appropriate interventions. As patients begin to deal with what has happened to them, active listening, conveyance of validation, empathy, warmth, and reassurance help patients understand that they are being heard by a caring professional.

DISTURBED BODY IMAGE

Body image is the mental picture an individual has of his or her body and its physical functioning at any given time. It includes attitudes and feelings about one's body in reference to appearance, build, health, performance ability, and gender-related concepts.[2,14,34-36] The body image develops over time from internal-sensation postural changes, contact with people and objects in the environment, emotional experiences, and fantasies.[22,35] Stein[27] suggests that the ability to project possible images of one's self in the future that are highly desirable or feared can play a powerful role in motivating and regulating goal-directed behavior.

Disturbances in body image arise when the person fails to perceive or adapt to the changes that are imposed by age, disease, trauma, or surgery. In some instances, the person may feel betrayed by the body, which no longer seems "normal." Body image may also be altered by the need to incorporate a prosthetic device or a donated body part.[37-40] The disease or problem may be corrected by surgery and treatments; however, whenever the result is visible to the patient and others, the change in body image can arouse intense feelings of anger, frustration, depression, and powerlessness.[14,38] The critical care nurse often begins the process of helping the patient live with this permanent alteration. Interventions by the nurse and others on the health team focus on helping the person manage the physical changes and the psychosocial alterations.

DISTURBANCES IN SELF-ESTEEM

Self-esteem, or self-measurement of one's worth, develops as a part of self-concept through the perceived appraisals of significant others.[41] The need for self-esteem is a part of the hierarchy of human needs postulated by Maslow.[42] Having high self-esteem helps one deal with the environment and face the maturational and situational crises of life more easily. Persons with well-developed self-esteem are at less risk for disturbances of self-esteem than those with poorly developed self-esteem.[20,35]

Self-esteem has been studied often in a variety of contexts and is an important concept for nurses, who have a significant impact on ill patients, to understand.[6,28,43] Illness can rob the person of perspective and shrinks both the familiar world and the one of possibility, often leading to low self-esteem and feelings of powerlessness, helplessness, and depression.[44,45] A low self-regard impairs one's ability to adapt. The person may refuse to participate in self-care, exhibit self-destructive behavior, or be too compliant—asking no questions and permitting others to make all decisions.[23,41,45] For the critical care nurse who values a holistic approach to treatment, requesting psychologic and/or psychiatric consultation and ongoing treatment is essential when patients jeopardize their own safety or the safety of others. Ideally this type of comprehensive approach to recovery includes the provision of ongoing supportive and adjustment psychotherapy.

DISTURBANCES IN PERSONAL IDENTITY, OR SELF-IDENTITY

"Self-identity is different from self-concept in that it refers to a feeling of distinctness from others."[27,33] It represents a whole picture of the self, or "who I am," through a combination of conscious and unconscious perceptions. When behaviors are in accordance with the self-concept, the self-identity is confirmed, or reinforced. Ego-identity is developed throughout the life span and is influenced by sociocultural norms, gender roles, and interpersonal relationships.

Personal identity disturbance is the inability to differentiate the self as a unique and separate human being from others within a social environment, and this sense of depersonalization engenders a high level of anxiety.[41] This problematic aspect of the self-concept is most often seen during maturational or situational crises and in mental illnesses including anxiety disorders. Additional causes of personal identity disturbance are use of psychoactive drugs; biochemical imbalances in the brain; organic brain disorders of dementia, amnesia, or delirium; or any traumatic insult to the brain. A careful nursing assessment and appropriate interventions, such as psychiatric referral, are needed because of the varied causes of identity disturbances.

INEFFECTIVE ROLE PERFORMANCE

Roles are sets of socially expected behavior patterns that individuals fulfill throughout the life span.[2,29] In-

teractions with others that create and modify these roles are an important part of the self-concept. Primary roles are those associated with gender, age, and developmental stage. Secondary roles include membership in a family, and tertiary roles are those assumed by choice, such as an occupation. Illness, when it occurs, disrupts secondary and tertiary roles, and responses can be affected by primary role characteristics. The rapid and potentially drastic changes that accompany critical illness may seriously interfere with role relationships, expectations, or abilities in role performance. Role performance alterations often are referred to as *role strain*, *role stress*, or *role insufficiency*. In helping patients with disruption of roles it is important to explore their feelings, generate and explore alternatives, and identify resources available that would allow them to resume a relatively normal life as soon as possible.

POWERLESSNESS

Powerlessness, as a nursing diagnosis, is defined as the perception of the individual that his or her own action will not significantly affect an outcome.[41] Unrelieved powerlessness may result in hopelessness, which is discussed in the next section.

The causes of powerlessness include factors in the health care environment, interpersonal interactions, one's culture and religious beliefs, illness-related regimen, and a lifestyle of helplessness. The range in levels of powerlessness varies and depends on the person's perceived sense of control, the amount of loss experienced, and the availability of social support. Powerlessness can be manifested by delayed decision making or refusal to make decisions, and expressions of self-doubt in role performance. Frustration, anger, and resentment over being dependent on others often occur and are exhibited as verbal expressions regarding dissatisfaction with care.[44]

Individuals vary in the amount of control they prefer.[45] The critical care unit routines may oppose or preclude any control by the patient. The person for whom control is important should be helped to continue to control as many areas of his or her life as possible. On the other hand, a patient must be given the opportunity to choose not to control.

Rotter's early research[46] on human behavior and perception of control has been particularly helpful in explaining the variability of responses people have in similar situations. He proposed the two major concepts of internal vs. external locus of control. Individuals who have internal locus of control perceive themselves to be responsible for the outcome of events. Individuals with external locus of control believe their actions will have no effect on outcomes of a situation. The scale to measure internal/external locus of control developed by Rotter is useful in assessing this personality trait. However, later situation-specific measures are better predictors than the original global scale.

Another aspect of powerlessness is *learned helplessness*, or *excessive dependence*.[45] A person who repeatedly experiences uncontrollable situations loses the motivation for making decisions about life events. Some people assume a martyr role and accept the illness state as their fate, thus doing nothing to improve their status. Others may find the sick role a gratifying means for gaining control over others by using their symptoms to gain attention.[47] Setting limits on these behaviors, encouraging independence and participation in self-care, counseling, and involving family members in establishing realistic goals are helpful strategies to assist the person to diminish this manipulative behavior. However, for persons who have a premorbid mental health history of excessive dependence, limit-setting may aggravate an already difficult situation. Persons may become very angry and/or withdrawn. These patients require a comprehensive mental health assessment, a carefully considered treatment plan, and ongoing psychotherapy. Therapy begins with the development of trust, open dialogue, and a discussion of realistic expectations that encourages small measurable improvements in self-care over time. It is essential that the critical care nurse work in concert with the mental health professionals to ensure continuity of care. Working together with the patient will set a nonthreatening tone and aid in beginning to diminish these dependent behaviors.

Critically ill patients generally have experienced a rapid onset of illness without time to acquire the illness role. If control is defined as the ability to determine the use of time, space, and resources, admission to a critical care unit strips away control of this power. On admission, persons lose their independent status. They become patients. Choice of clothing and use of other personal belongings are usually restricted in a critical care unit. Patients cannot decide who enters the room, who provides personal care, or who intrudes with painful treatments. Hospital rules are usually not open to modification. Patients may feel anxious because they are separated from a familiar environment and have restrictions on who may visit them.

Poor interactions with the health care providers may make the situation worse. Patients may react aggressively, may try bargaining, or may refuse to comply with diagnostic and treatment regimens. They may resent the close scrutiny of the nurses and physicians and the invasion of their privacy. By virtue of their experiences with critical illness and care, people may lose sight of areas of influence they still do retain over themselves because so much control has been taken from them. Nurses can emphasize the patient's influence on control and thus help to preserve it.[3,44]

HOPELESSNESS

Hopelessness is a subjective state in which an individual sees limited or no alternatives or personal choices available and is unable to mobilize energy on his or her own behalf.[41] Boling[48] has proposed a new nursing diagnosis entitled Defect in Hope. To help clarify hopelessness, the following definition of hope is included: a feeling that provides comfort while enduring life threats and personal challenges; a feeling that what is wanted will happen; a desire that is accompanied by anticipation or expectation. Most people agree that an element of hope must be maintained, no matter how hopeless things appear. Hope is a force that helps one survive.[18,49] An interdisciplinary concept analysis of hope and hopelessness in the literature from theology, medicine, nursing, and psychology revealed that absolute hopelessness is viewed as incompatible with life. Hope often arises in the presence of crisis and instills vigorous resistance to giving up. The help of others in the situation supports the patient's belief.[3,19] Hope wards off despair, mental anguish, disorganization, and helplessness.[49]

When people expect something to happen, they usually act in ways that increase the likelihood that the expectations will be met.[27] The expectation, whether positive or negative, becomes stronger the more times the "reinforcing circle" occurs. This process is defined as a *self-fulfilling prophecy*.

The critically ill patient is a multiproblem patient. Nurses and physicians are tempted to focus on the crisis and the use of technical equipment and to overlook the patient in his or her totality. The health care team may stereotype patients and underestimate their individual strengths.[4,34] The very nature of the critical care unit is frightening and increases the patient's sense of vulnerability and the fear of death. Therefore, it is important to foster a realistic sense of hope in the patient.[41,50] The critical care nurse can project an attitude of hope and identify some aspect of the situation in which hope is warranted, no matter how grave the situation, and attempt to channel feelings toward some positive outcome.

When the situation moves from hopeful to hopeless in the critical care unit, deciding to write a "do-not-resuscitate" order must be carefully considered.[51,52] Of special importance is the need to recognize that members of the health care team and the family may reach this decision at varying times.[9,53] However, it is important to not avoid difficult conversations and to keep patients and families informed. Careful medical and nursing assessments and the use of family and team conferences to foster communication, as well as enlisting the assistance of a spiritual counselor, can make these situations less frustrating for all concerned.

Families also need hope. Nursing strategies for supporting the family include clarifying any distorted thinking, providing opportunities for the family to be with the

---

Box 5-2

STRATEGIES TO INSPIRE HOPE IN FAMILIES OF CRITICALLY ILL PATIENTS

RESPONDING TO FAMILY CONCERNS
- Explore own feelings about interacting with families of critically ill patients and end-of-life issues
- Use active listening, therapeutic communication skills, and touch (when appropriate); allow family to share concerns; avoid giving messages that convey false hope
- Establish mutually trusting relationship with patient and family
- Provide comfort and pain relief care to patient; demonstrate caring attitude
- Provide adequate/appropriate information regarding patient's condition/progress; clarify misinformation
- Express empathy; consider impact of patient's illness on roles within the family; respect membership in nontraditional family structures
- Assess ability to cope; recognize that family members may use defense mechanisms to cope with anxiety and/or crisis situation; accept individual responses to stress (which usually are not characteristic of usual behavior)
- Be sensitive to reactions to adverse changes in patient's condition; observe for expressions of anticipatory grief, helplessness, hopelessness, and depression
- Address spiritual needs through facilitating contacts with chaplain/spiritual counselor; notify family about areas available for privacy/meditation

- Support processes that are meaningful to family and congruent with their cultural beliefs/values

RESPONDING TO FAMILY'S PHYSICAL NEEDS
- Encourage members to attend to own health and physical needs—nutrition, rest, and sleep
- Provide information about available community resources for personal needs

FAMILY PARTICIPATION
- Prepare family regarding the patient's condition and behaviors; instruct them about ICU environment before first visit; monitor interactions with patient; discourage confrontations between them; remove overemotional person from unit; provide support until she/he can gain control of emotions
- Involve family in decision making and in participation in basic patient care activities (they can be a patient's major support system)
- When possible, have family select one person to serve as liaison at interdisciplinary team planning sessions and to be the contact for scheduling visits and receiving updates of information to decrease uncertainties the family may have
- Use expertise of interdisciplinary team to provide social support, to explore the meaning of the crisis, to expand the coping repertoire, and to help maintain caring relationships between family members

Data from Wheeler RW: Helping families cope with death and dying, *Nursing* 98(7):25-30, 1996; Czerwiec M: When a loved one is dying: families talk about nursing care, *Am J Nurs* 96(5):32-36, 1996; Durhan E: How patients die, *Am J Nurs* 97(12):41-46, 1997; Powers P et al: The value of patient- and family-centered care, *Am J Nurs* 100(5):84-88, 2000; and Barry P: *Psychosocial nursing: assessment and intervention in care of the physically ill,* ed 3, Philadelphia, 1996, Lippincott.

---

patient, presenting realistic patient outcome expectations, and expanding the coping repertoire of the family.[9,51,52,54] See Box 5-2 for additional strategies.

SPIRITUAL DISTRESS

Spiritual distress has been defined as the disruption in the life principle that pervades a person's entire being and that integrates and transcends one's biologic and psychosocial nature.[41] Adherence to a particular philosophic, psychologic, sociologic, or political belief may bring a sense of one's value and of life's meaning. Threats imposed by any physiologic or psychologic illness and prolonged pain and suffering can challenge a person's spirituality.[33] Life-threatening illness causes a person to face his or her own mortality. The provision of holistic nursing care is not limited to meeting a person's religious needs; it also encompasses all that provides meaning to life.

A person in spiritual distress may question the meaning of suffering and death in relation to a personal belief system. Anger toward God or a supreme being, feelings

of self-blame, or regret over inability to practice belief rituals may be expressed. Individuals may even question the necessity for the therapeutic regimen. Spiritual care, then, has been described as health-promoting interventions to relieve responses to stress that affect spiritual perspectives of individuals or groups.[41] Creating an environment of compassion where patients feel their emotional and spiritual needs are met is at the heart of holistic care.[55] Listening to the patients' concerns, offering support, and/or enlisting the support of a spiritual counselor can promote the healing process.

MENTAL STATUS CHANGES REQUIRING EVALUATION

Two medical diagnoses are associated with mental status changes that should be distinguished from the nursing diagnosis of Ineffective Coping. These clinical states, delirium and major depression, call for a medical and/or nurse specialist psychiatric evaluation and medical intervention.

ACUTE CONFUSION/DELIRIUM

Acute confusion, which encompasses global cognitive impairment, has not been clearly or consistently defined.[57,58] Synonyms include delirium (the medical term), intensive care unit (ICU) psychosis, postcardiotomy delirium, and acute brain failure.[2] Additional terms are acute mental status change, acute organic reaction, metabolic encephalopathy, and reversible cognitive dysfunction. Orientation to person, time, or place and the ability to reason, follow directions, process incoming stimuli, or maintain concentration are lost. Confused persons may be aware of these disturbances and fear that they are "losing their minds." The confused state is a secondary response to organic causes, that is, hypoxia, drugs, or fluid and electrolyte imbalances, or to inorganic causes such as stress and sleep deprivation. Onset is abrupt, and duration can be shortened if early diagnosis and treatment are initiated. It is estimated that confusion develops in 50% of hospitalized elderly patients; however, it is often misdiagnosed because of inaccurate assessment and assumptions that a mental deterioration is the result of the effects of aging.[59,60] More than 80% of reports of confused status in the elderly are attributed to organic causes; dehydration and recent falls, hip fractures, and polypharmacy are additional risk factors for confusion. Behavioral symptoms may be subtle and varied. Prodromal symptoms include insomnia, distractibility, drowsiness, anxiety, and nightmares. Symptoms of acute confusion resemble those of dementia, which makes differentiation between the two conditions more difficult. However, dementia, which cannot be reversed, has a gradual onset and is of long duration.

Approximately 10% to 15% of all hospitalized medical-surgical patients experience symptoms of delirium. This percentage is increased by 30% to 40% in the critical care setting. Hospital stays are prolonged for this population.[57] An increased level of confusion may be the first indicator of a biologic problem or may be the result of environmental stressors. The nurse must continually assess cognitive function. Several tools for assessing this are available. The Mini-Mental State Examination (MMSE), developed by Folstein, Folstein and McHugh,[61] is the most popular and easy to administer. Items included on the examination relate to orientation, comprehension, recall, and following commands. (Further comments about the full MMSE are discussed in Assessment.) The Delirium Rating Scale (DRS/DRS-98) can also help confirm diagnosis.[62]

ETIOLOGY

Understanding the causes and symptoms of delirium, knowing the people who are at risk for developing delirium, and using appropriate measures to minimize causal factors are primary aspects of the critical care nurse role. The majority of the time, the exact etiology is unknown.

Three predisposing contributors to the development of delirium are (1) age 60 years or over, (2) presence of brain damage, and (3) presence of a chronic brain disorder, such as Alzheimer's disease. Cognitive dysfunctions are believed to occur when "there is a widespread reduction of cerebral oxidative metabolism and an imbalance of neuro-transmission."[25,57,58] (Box 5-3)

Drugs that are commonly used in the ICU contribute to delirium. Some of these are digitalis, antibiotics, steroids, beta-blockers, and respiratory stimulants. Additional causes of delirium include sleep deprivation, sensory deprivation or overload, and immobilization, all of which are events commonly encountered in the ICU.[22]

The patient in the ICU is deprived of the restorative benefits of deep sleep and the rapid eye movement (REM) phase of sleep because of frequent interruptions by equipment noises, voices, and procedures. Constant, bright overhead lights, the absence of day-night cycles, immobility, pain, and medications contribute to the patient's disorientation to time and place. Daytime napping, complaints of fatigue, slurred speech, as well as depression, cognitive impairment, and hallucinations can result. Delayed recovery, increased length of hospital stay, and the seriousness of sleep deprivation are closely related.

To improve the ICU environment, a number of hospitals across the nation have introduced physical changes in the ICU to reduce noise levels (e.g., installation of acoustic tiles, carpets, and private rooms). Team members also have suggested several corrective measures, such as keeping noise levels to a minimum, scheduling procedures as much as possible so as to avoid waking the patient, lowering the lighting intensity at intervals, and holding conversations and verbal shift reports at a distance outside of the patient's hearing range.[58] Distraction measures such as soft music in the ICU also orient individuals to their surroundings and provide both a stimulus and a calming effect.[63]

The literature reports more than 30 terms for describing the confusion syndrome.[57-60] Many of the terms are misleading, are narrow in scope, and give cause for overlooking some of the possible reasons for the behaviors. The classification of mental disorders in the *Diagnostic and Statistical Manual (DSM-IV-TR)*[64] uses the term *delirium* as the only official designation for this syndrome and has established specific criteria to be used for making this diagnosis.[29]

ASSESSMENT

Three forms of delirium have been identified—hyperactive, hypoactive, and a mixture of both forms.[2,57,58] The patient with the hyperactive form may become violent; remove intravenous lines, dressings, and catheters; be extremely restless and try to get out of bed; pick at things in the air; and call out to persons who are not

Box 5-3

DEFINING CHARACTERISTICS OF DELIRIUM/ACUTE CONFUSION AND ETIOLOGIC FACTORS

DEFINING CHARACTERISTICS
Displays at least two of the following:

Early Signs/Symptoms
- Sudden onset of global cognitive function impairment (from hours to days)
- Restlessness, agitation, combative behavior
- Drowsiness—can lead to loss of consciousness
- Slurred speech, inappropriate statements, or "word salad," and mumbling
- Inappropriate gestures, short attention span—needs questions repeated; inability to learn new material
- Disordered awake-sleep cycle
- Disorientation to person, time, place, situation
- Difficulty in separating dreams from reality—may experience bizarre dreams/nightmares
- Anger at staff for continued questions about his or her orientation

Later Signs/Symptoms
- Symptoms tend to fluctuate throughout the day and night
- Early symptoms continue—may be more frequent and of longer duration
- Illusions
- Hallucinations
- Extreme agitation—attempts to climb out of bed, pull out catheters, rip off dressings
- Calling out in loud voice; may swear; attempt to bite or hit people who approach person

Etiologic Factors
- Fluid and electrolyte imbalances
- Potential for organ dysfunction (hepatic, renal, gastrointestinal, cardiac, respiratory) because of oxygenation
- Delay in metabolism and excretion of drugs, thus prolonging half-life and increasing drug's effect or interaction with other drugs
- Immune-suppressant drugs' side effects
- Narcotic analgesics
- Hypersensitivity to drugs
- Surgical time (or on by-pass equipment) more than 4 hours
- Stressors in ICU (also refer to Box 5-1)
- Physical and mental status of patient before surgery—preexisting medical conditions (e.g., diabetes, epilepsy, neoplasm)
- Withdrawal symptoms (e.g., alcohol, drugs, amphetamines)
- Minimal accessibility to social-spiritual/family support

Data from Geary S: Intensive care unit psychosis revisited: understanding and managing delirium in the critical care setting, *Crit Care Nurs Q* 17(1):51-63, 1994; Hall G, Wakefield B: Acute confusion in the elderly: what to do when the clouds roll in, *Nursing CE Handbook* (on-line), March 1998, Springhouse; and American Psychiatric Association: *Diagnostic and statistical manual of mental disorders-DSM-IV-TR,* ed 4, Washington, DC, 2000, The Association.

there. Sympathetic nervous system responses of tachycardia, dilation of pupils, diaphoresis, and facial flushing are evident. In the hypoactive form, persons complain of extreme fatigue, are slow to respond, and have hypersomnolence that can progress to loss of consciousness. At times these individuals are absorbed in a dreamlike state, mumble to themselves, experience vivid hallucinations, and make inappropriate gestures. The third form is a mixture of agitation and hypoactive behaviors that can vary throughout the day. Symptoms and hallucinations seem to worsen during the night—often referred to as *sundowner's syndrome*—with more lucid intervals occurring during the day.

THE MENTAL STATUS EXAMINATION

The mental status examination (MSE) is a full, criteria-based assessment of the patient's cognitive function and thought processes. Although the examination is rarely conducted in its entirety in the critical care setting, knowledge of its main components will enhance the nurse's effectiveness in collecting data, will improve the nurse's use of accepted terminology in documentation of

findings, and will help the nurse identify issues that require further assessment. This tool can be useful in evaluating the nursing diagnoses of Deficient Knowledge, Disturbed Sensory Perception, and Disturbed Thought Processes.

Components of the Mental Status Examination. Categories of the MSE include: (1) general description of appearance, speech, motor activity, and behaviors noted during the interview process; (2) emotional state covering mood and affect; (3) perceptions of experiences; (4) thought content and process; (5) level of consciousness; and (6) cognitive abilities (i.e., memory, level of concentration and calculation ability, judgment, and insight). Refer to Box 5-4 for categories of measurement, which are organized around theoretic concepts.[2,29,64a]

Several shorter instruments to assess mental function have been developed. The MMSE,[61] mentioned earlier, is particularly useful in evaluating the elderly. Each item is tied to a score that when totaled will provide an estimate of function depending on age, education, and language origin. Another rapid assessment tool by Pfeiffer[65] registers the person's orientation, memory, thought processes, and attention span.

Box 5-4

COMPONENTS OF THE MENTAL STATUS EXAMINATION

Documentation of the assessment of mental status is indicative of the person's mental status at the specific time of the interview and/or observation.

ASSESSMENT CRITERIA

- *Orientation and level of awareness:* A common measurement for evidence of confusion is asking patients if they know who they are and where they are, as well as asking them to state the day of the week, the month, or the year.
- *Appearance and behavior:* General observations include the patient's appearance and behaviors in terms of their consistency with a normal range in age, station in life, general health, and nutritional status.
- *Speech and communication:* Speech may be garbled, slurred, distinct, rapid or slow, and volume may be loud or soft. Person may remain mute. Nonverbal communication such as eye contact, gestures, and posture are indicators of the patient's mood, thought formation, and content. It is important to evaluate the match between verbal and nonverbal communication patterns.
- *Mood/affect:* Communication with caregivers and family may be normal, or there may be wide mood swings in emotions. Anxiety, fear, or apathy; lethargic or agitated behaviors; and unusual gestures may be demonstrated.
- *Thinking process:* Illogical statements, rapid speaking with quick shifts from one idea to another (flight of ideas), disconnected mixture of unrelated words (word salad), delusions, hallucinations, or obsessive behavior may be present at various times. Memory impairment may be masked by the patient's attempt at "filling in the gaps" with false statements.
- *Memory:* Recent memory is the first to be impaired and is most often seen in persons with chronic organic mental disorder (which is irreversible), with acute organic mental disorders, or with depression.

Recent memory refers to recall of events that have occurred within the recent past. This is assessed by asking orientation to person, time, and place. Long-term memory is assessed by asking person to describe childhood events. Questions can be asked conversationally without causing person to feel being "cross-examined."

- *Perception:* Perception of self, environment, and interpersonal relationships is derived through the senses of vision, hearing, touch, and smell. Defense mechanisms used during times of stress or illness can distort perception of reality. Visual, auditory, or tactile hallucinations are frequently experienced by patients in ICU. Hypnagogic hallucinations are false sensory perceptions that occur during the twilight period between wakefulness and sleep. (This can be a common occurrence for well persons, especially during times of severe stress or fatigue.)
- *Abstract thinking and judgment:* Differences between concrete and abstract thinking include logical reasoning in problem solving and providing a solution to a hypothetical problem.

PSYCHOSOCIAL CRITERIA

- *Stressors:* Internal (mental or physical illness, perceived loss); external (actual loss of something significant to person)
- *Coping skills:* Methods used in adaptation to stressors
- *Relationships:* Type of interrelationships congruent with developmental stage (includes sexual relationship)
- *Cultural:* Ability to adapt as appropriate to norms for an identified group
- *Spiritual:* Values/beliefs that are considered to be satisfying, worthwhile, and comforting
- *Occupational:* Involvement in useful, rewarding activity (work, school, recreation) that is congruent with developmental stage

Data from Stuart G: A stress adaptation model of psychiatric nursing care. In Stuart GW, Laraia MT, editors: *Principles and practices of psychiatric nursing,* ed 6, St Louis, 2005, Mosby; Hollinger-Smith L: The elderly. In Fortinash K, Holoday-Worret P, editors: *Psychiatric mental health nursing,* ed 3, St Louis, 2004, Mosby.

MEDICAL AND NURSING MANAGEMENT OF MENTAL STATUS CHANGES

The American Psychiatric Association has developed a practice guideline for the treatment of patients with delirium.[66] Psychiatric consultation and management are preferred, with communication among the primary treatment team, the critical care nurse, and the family. The treatment of choice is to diagnose and treat the underlying medical condition that is causing the delirium. Once this is done it is important to treat the ongoing symptoms that are distressing the patient. Sedation is

prescribed for patients with hyperactive delirium. A neuroleptic drug such as haloperidol, commonly used for neurotic and personality disorders, is useful in the treatment of delirium. Currently, haloperidol is considered to be the drug of choice, and a regular dosing schedule is preferred rather than waiting until symptoms recur before giving another dose. A typical regimen is as follows: *mild agitation,* 1 to 3 mg; *moderate agitation,* 5 to 7 mg; and *severe agitation,* 10 mg or more.[67] However, some patients may have a paradoxical effect to haloperidol, worsening the delirium. If continued dosing increases agitation, administration should be discontinued. A combination of haloperidol and lorazepam, a benzodiazepine drug that produces sedative effects, allows lower doses of each drug to be given, is very effective, and produces fewer side effects. Benzodiazepine monotherapy should be avoided unless the delirium is attributable to sedative or alcohol withdrawal.

The newer atypical antipsychotics appear to provide similar efficacy and are better tolerated; however, few randomized and controlled trials have been reported. Risperidone, Olanzapine, Quetiapine, and Ziprasidone have been shown to be effective for the treatment of delirium in retrospective case reports.

When delirium is considered to be secondary to pain, narcotics can be administered. However, the paradoxical effects of depressed respirations and cardiac output can exacerbate the delirium. The elderly patient, particularly, benefits from smaller doses given on a regular basis.[58] The use of barbiturates is no longer recommended as routine treatment, but they are used in the treatment of barbiturate withdrawal–induced delirium.

Finally, neuromuscular blocking agents are sometimes used for severely agitated patients who are on mechanical ventilation to affect a decrease in oxygen consumption, to promote synchrony with the ventilator, and to increase tissue oxygenation. These complex drugs can be dangerous but do not affect consciousness, cognition, or pain levels; thus sedatives or analgesics should be added as appropriate.[57,58]

MAJOR DEPRESSIVE EPISODE

A major depressive episode is a mood disorder of at least 2 weeks' duration, characterized by depressed mood, diminished interest or pleasure in usual activities, insomnia, poor appetite, psychomotor retardation or agitation, and loss of energy. Patients with this disorder also may report feelings of hopelessness, worthlessness, and guilt. Recurrent thoughts of death, loss of interest in life, and recurrent suicidal ideation may be present.[68] Major depression may complicate the patient's underlying physical illnesses; for example, asthma, headaches, ulcers, arthritis, and coronary heart disease may be exacerbated to the point of a life-threatening situation.[2,68] Depression deepens, and suicide ideation frequently resurfaces after surgery if a life-threatening diagnosis is confirmed.

The nurse who suspects that the patient is severely depressed can assess thought content by using the MSE. The nurse can listen empathetically and convey to the patient that recovery from the depression is expected, while understanding that the patient's depression cannot be overcome by cheerfulness or reassurance. If the patient is on suicide precautions, the nurse safeguards the patient according to department policy and procedure and alerts all on the health care team and the family. The nurse also informs the patient that precaution measures are being taken as a safeguard until his or her mood improves. Requesting a comprehensive mental health assessment provided by a mental health professional would provide the means for giving proper attention to the patient's mind-body experience.

SUICIDE

Depression is mentioned as a causal factor in 30% to 70% of suicide attempts by the high-risk groups of youth, ages 15 to 24; the elderly population over 65; and individuals with psychiatric disorders. Suicide rates for persons with acquired immunodeficiency syndrome (AIDS) have been reported to be 66 times greater than that of the general population.[34] Suicide has been described as a self-destructive response to a stimulus resulting from an undesirable, unacceptable, or overwhelming event; as a response to overcome high anxiety feelings about abandonment by God or significant others; as a hostility toward self; and as the only solution for ending a helpless or hopeless situation. Suicide is the eighth-leading cause of death in the United States, statistically represented by 30,000 deaths annually that result from more than one million reported suicide attempts, although the actual number may be underreported.[2,69]

Etiologic factors in the suicide risk profile include both bio-psychologic and sociologic circumstances. Biopsychologic events may involve living within the limits of a chronic disease or facing an acute, life-threatening illness and pain such as that produced by cancer and end-stage renal failure.[34] Depression is associated with irregularities in the levels of serotonin, dopamine, norepinephrine, and gamma-aminobutyric acid (GABA), the neurotransmitters in the brain that regulate mood. Genetic predisposition toward suicidal and antisocial behavior also may play a role. Frontal lobe dysfunction has been associated with the feelings of hopelessness and worthlessness that contribute to depression. Other psychologic factors are negative thinking patterns and reduction of positive reinforcement. Comorbidity with a psychiatric disorder is the highest indicator in the risk profile. "The common emotions of suicide are helplessness and hopelessness. The common consistency in suicide is lifelong patterns of failure, stress, duress, and threats to self-esteem."[69]

Nurses in high acuity and emergency settings will be challenged by patients who have attempted suicide or are at risk for doing so. Persons with cognitive impairment resulting from delirium effects of medications, fluid and electrolyte imbalances, anoxia, surgery, or trauma are at greatest risk for attempting suicide. Hallucinations may compel their self-destructive behavior.[70]

A primary focus for care of the person with self-destructive behavior is protection from harm.[2,70,71] Nurses also must consider their own responses to patients' self-destructive behaviors, which can enhance or inhibit their interactions with patients. Interventions may include removal of harmful objects; consistent supervision; active listening; contracting with the individual to cease harmful activities; promoting the person's self-esteem and self-control in regulating emotions and behaviors, which frequently includes administration of anxiolytic medications as well as mobilizing social support systems; and providing mental health education.

When a person commits suicide, nurses also can be involved with providing care for the survivors, who may be at increased risk for similar actions. Feelings of guilt or anger over why the suicide occurred need to be expressed by the survivors, and they need to learn how to deal with the stigma that is frequently associated with the suicide event.[2,69-71]

Clark's suicide risk factor inventory[72] provides a useful assessment tool. Each of the six dimensions contains items related to high-risk behaviors. The presence of an illness, pain, or a crisis situation of a developmental or situational nature; the person's age; the type of coping skills used; daily activities; level of self-concept; expressions of hopelessness and suicidal intent; and history of recent trauma are some of the areas that are covered. Identified risk factors can be used to design appropriate interventions.

COPING

Patients requiring critical care must cope with a variety of stressors (see Box 5-1). As mentioned earlier, each patient's response to these stressors is unique and depends on a variety of environmental factors and individual differences. The nurse's knowledge of assessment, diagnosis, and effective coping strategies also will affect how well the patient copes. The uncomfortable effects of a situation, such as anxiety or grief and loss of control, can lessen the effectiveness of coping mechanisms when people are faced with serious problems that they cannot overcome using familiar behaviors.

Coping is defined as a dynamic process involving cognitive and behavioral efforts to manage specific internal and/or external demands that are perceived to be exceeding the person's resources.[16,17] Aquilera[73] states that coping activities encompass all the diverse behaviors that people use to meet actual or potential demands. The available coping mechanisms are those behaviors that a person draws on that have been found to be effective in the past. The key to effective coping is using the best strategy or mix of strategies in a given situation.

NANDA[1] defines *Ineffective Coping* as "the impairment of adaptive behaviors and problem-solving abilities of a person meeting life's demands and roles." The defining characteristics of Ineffective Coping usually associated with critical illness include the following: verbalization of an inability to cope or to ask for help, and being unable to meet personal basic needs. The person exhibits inappropriate use of defense mechanisms and cannot problem solve. The person may display destructive behavior toward self and others.

COPING MECHANISMS

When a patient copes effectively, what he or she is doing to cope often goes unnoticed. Emotionally the patient seems relatively comfortable, is a cooperative recipient of care, and exhibits nonproblematic behavior. The patient may be using multiple appropriate coping mechanisms that help to manage a problem or a stressful situation. The following discussion covers several coping mechanisms that may or may not be effective, depending on the degree to which they are used. Some authors differentiate between coping mechanisms that relate to adjusting, adapting, and successfully meeting a challenge and defense mechanisms that are automatic self-protective measures that develop in response to an internal or external stressor.[12,34,74] Examples of the latter include denial, acting-out behavior, avoidance, hypochondriasis, passive-aggressive behavior, and projection.

REGRESSION

Regression is an unconscious defense mechanism that involves a retreat, in the face of stress, to behavior characteristic of an earlier developmental level.[75] Regression allows the patient to give up his or her usual role, autonomy, and privacy to become the passive recipient of medical and nursing care. In fact, the patient who does not regress jeopardizes his or her own care. However, the patient who becomes too regressed presents another problem. Regression is a normal reaction to severe burns. The person may become childlike in interactions with staff. Behaviors such as whining, clinging to staff, and attempting to keep the nurse at the bedside constantly are not uncommon. In both cases the patient must know the limits set on behavior if he or she is to receive essential care. The patient is best served when limits are set in a supportive manner.

Although the behavior of these patients can provoke confrontations or reprimands, this should be avoided. Such responses from staff may only worsen a situation in which a patient is already struggling with issues of dependence and autonomy.

SUPPRESSION

Suppression is a conscious, intentional process in which patients push ideas, problems, or desires out of their conscious thoughts.[74] Patients often use suppression when their problems are overwhelming and they are in no position to resolve them. For example, before becoming ill an individual may have been struggling to meet financial obligations, but now uses suppression to postpone dealing with this concern until further along in the recovery phase.

DENIAL

According to NANDA, denial includes both conscious and unconscious attempts to disavow knowledge or the meaning of an event.[1] In this text the psychoanalytic definition of denial—"an unconscious defense mechanism that reduces anxiety by eliminating or reducing the seriousness of the perceived threat"—will be used to allow for the distinction between denial and suppression. When used by a critically ill patient, denial reduces the anxiety and the perceived threat level of the illness.[75] The degree to which denial is used varies among patients and may vary in the same patient at different times.

Patients also may deny different aspects of the illness. Some deny the probable medical significance of symptoms, as in the case of the 55-year-old cardiologist who interprets severe substernal chest pain as indigestion or the case of the quadriplegic who cheerfully insists he will be back on his feet in no time. Other patients cannot recognize signs of illness that are obvious to others, as in the case of the patient who cannot "see" the gangrenous foot requiring amputation.[75]

Other people cannot readily influence the beliefs of a patient using denial. For example, the patient who is denying a myocardial infarction is not convinced of its occurrence by being shown the cardiogram interpretation or laboratory reports. The patient is best served by the nurse who recognizes his need to deny at the present time but who watches for cues from the patient that indicate readiness to accept the reality of the medical diagnosis. A patient with a tracheostomy may refuse to look at her body, avoid mirrors, and fear rejection by others because of her appearance. Forcing her to look at herself before she is ready can be extremely detrimental.

TRUST

Trust manifests itself in the critical care patient as the belief that the staff will get him or her through the illness, managing any untoward event that might occur. Trust is an unconscious process in which the patient transfers the trust learned in early significant relationships onto caregivers in the present.[2,47] For example, a patient with severe burns must learn to trust her caregivers. Intense fear of pain or of falling when being moved from a stretcher to the Hubbard tank can affect other coping skills as well.

HOPE

Although hope has long been recognized as a significant factor in patient recovery and survival, the phenomenon receives little attention until the patient comes to feel hopeless. Hope is the expectation that a desire will be fulfilled. It can exist even in the face of a realistic appraisal of a grim situation.[52] Hope supports the patient and helps him or her endure the physical and psychologic insults that are a part of the daily experience. Hope is central to resilience and spiritual strength.[30]

HARDINESS AND RESILIENCE

Hardiness and resilience are multidimensional concepts that depict an individual's capacity for mastering stressful situations and viewing adverse circumstances as challenges and are attributed to persons who have an internal locus of control. Individuals who are resilient view themselves as "overcomers" rather than just "survivors"; they feel stronger for persevering. A "self-healing personality" is often ascribed to a person of resilience. Resilience has been associated with the strength of the human spirit and the will to survive.[20,33,76-78]

SPIRITUAL BELIEFS AND PRACTICES

Spiritual beliefs and practices may provide the patient with some measure of acceptance of an illness, a sense of mastery and control, a source of hope and trust beyond the limits the staff can provide, and the strength to endure the current stress. A patient may discuss personal beliefs and concerns openly or view the subject as a private and personal matter.[6,79-84]

USE OF FAMILY SUPPORT

The patient can use the presence of a supportive family to cope with critical illness. The patient with a supportive family knows that family members share a past and hope for a future with the patient. They love the patient as a person and a member of the family. The patient also realizes that family members know him or her in ways the staff cannot. With them, the patient may know that his or her experience is truly understood, even when little is said. Family members also can be involved in the patient's personal care and can attend to the practical problems the patient cannot, such as managing finances.[85] Family members can help the nurse to understand and know the patient especially when patients are unable to communicate themselves.

SHARING CONCERNS

Sharing concerns with a caring and understanding listener can relieve some of the patient's spiritual and emotional distress. The patient is consoled knowing that he or she is not alone and that someone knows and cares about what is being experienced (as mentioned earlier in the discussion of suicidal ideation).[4,34,69] The patient may share concerns with family members. However, the patient may be reluctant to upset loved ones further or may have a family in which such communication is not the norm. A patient who relies on this coping mechanism will benefit from a nurse who recognizes when a patient needs to talk and who knows how to listen.

COPING ASSESSMENT

Ineffective coping may be suggested in patient behaviors. Overt hostility, severe regression, or noncompliance with treatment may suggest ineffective coping. The patient may also report such problems as severe anxiety, despondence, or despair. The nurse who suspects that coping is ineffective should consider a number of factors before questioning the patient directly.[34]

It is not always clear whether the patient's coping is truly ineffective and intervention by the nurse is indicated. Witnessing problematic behavior can be very uncomfortable, especially when that behavior is directed at the caregiver(s). Careful evaluation of one's reaction to the behavior is needed to discover whether patient care can continue to be provided objectively by the nurse alone or consultation with others on the team is needed to alleviate the problem.[4,44]

ENHANCING THE COPING PROCESS

SUPPORTING THE PATIENT

Attention to the total patient is an ultimate goal of nursing care. Nightingale believed that it was "unthinkable to consider sick humans as mere bodies who could be treated in isolation from their minds and spirits."[82] Essential techniques for effective interventions include an attitude of caring; openness and warmth; and withholding judgment until you "know" the patient (have an understanding of the individual's perception about self), the current illness or problem, and the type of social support available. Assessment skills are essential, as is a willingness to become involved when the potential or actual use of ineffective coping mechanisms exists.

Teaching the patient new coping skills may be impossible, since individuals have a repertoire of defense and coping mechanisms—conscious and unconscious—that are automatically brought into play when facing stressful situations. A person who is experiencing extreme psychologic stress cannot learn new methods to manage these defense mechanisms. However, the nurse may help to reduce the level of anxiety by employing active listening, by encouraging support from family members and other caregivers, and by introducing changes in the environment as appropriate. In doing so, the nurse can facilitate the changes the patient must make. It is extremely

important that the patient express an interest in learning and recognize a personal need for help.[2,84]

A patient's trust in the nurse's competence in the physical and technical aspects of care aids in the patient's participation. Hope is instilled when the nurse and other caregivers display a sense of realistic optimism regarding the patient's progress. It is essential that patients receive honest feedback, for patients are keen observers of their caregivers and read them well. Trust and hope are easily lessened when inappropriate information is given.

SUPPORTING FAMILY MEMBERS

Patient-centered care is also family-centered care. Consideration of nonbiologic or nonlegal partners of the patient as members of the patient's support system is also necessary in providing holistic care. The nurse's support of family members at the bedside can enhance the value of the visits for the patient. Patients often look to the family for love, understanding, and support and for care of matters to which they cannot attend themselves. Although the nurse cannot perform full family assessment and give ongoing support to all family members, the critical care nurse can observe the quality of the patient-family interaction and formulate interventions that will aid the family in supporting the patient.[4,37,43]

An illness of a family member can be a hardship on the total family. The illness (or death) of a patient can affect the health of other family members—particularly an elderly spouse.[51,85] Reactions to the stress are similar to the emotions experienced by the patient. The extended waiting time between visits with the patient, lack of information or misinterpretation of information, disruption in family roles and routines, being in an unfamiliar and challenging environment, and worrying over outcomes, finances, and additional responsibilities can be overwhelming. Disorganization and emotional turmoil may result. Sleep deprivation is a frequent experience leading to confusion and inability to make decisions.

Family members also may react to the crisis with expressions of anger and hostility toward the patient or staff or may be immobilized.[6,52] The family member may be at a loss for what to say or do during visits with the patient. The nurse might find some words to put the family member at ease and offer a suggestion for what to say to his or her loved one.

If the family member is so upset that he or she completely loses composure, a brief attempt at supporting this family member away from the bedside may be an adequate intervention. In doing so, the nurse may determine that the family member needs the assistance of a consistent outside source of support and therefore may consult with another member of the health care team such as the psychiatric nurse consultant, the pastor/chaplain, or a social worker.

Family members need understanding, respect, and emotional support. A study of patients' perspectives on health care revealed that their definition of patient-centered care included early involvement of their families in their care and decision making; support, accommodation, and respect for their family and friends; and accurate, updated information.[38,52]

Families often must deal with the impending death of a loved one when the patient's condition deteriorates in spite of all efforts. Anticipatory grief is a process that is filled with emotional upheaval that can be as intense as when the loved one actually dies.[51,53,86] At such time, they are particularly sensitive to the nurse's words and actions and may misinterpret them as signs of indifference. This may be particularly true for the nontraditional family members. It is essential that the health care team convey understanding and acceptance of the patient and his or her family. Some of the interventions that are meaningful to the family are reassurance that the patient is receiving adequate pain medication, telling them what to expect as the dying process progresses, and helping them to comfort the patient with their presence. After the death, allow the family members to spend some time alone with the patient; be supportive of them as they work through their grief. Recognition of cultural and religious factors and incorporating them into the plan of care are also beneficial to the family.[9,52]

A study by Powers et al[54] revealed that nurses did discuss care plans with patients and their families; however, they did not inquire whether the plans were acceptable. The majority of the respondents wanted to be more involved. A pilot program in patient and family-centered care was initiated that included the families in ongoing planning sessions. The program received very positive responses from everyone. Because of the success of this program, hospital-wide planning sessions were implemented. The nurse-patient relationship was strengthened, patients and families reported that anxieties were decreased, and they expressed satisfaction with the increased participation in the plan of care.

SUPPORTING SPIRITUAL CARE

Spiritual need assessment is often inadequate when patients are asked only about their religious affiliation. If no affiliation is mentioned, no further questions are asked of the patient regarding spiritual matters. The right to receive care that respects individual spiritual values was added to the Joint Commission standards in 1998.[79] Spirituality is a basic human phenomenon that helps create meaning in the world and can be experienced before any awareness of religious beliefs.[30,87] Separation from philosophical and religious rituals and ties, together with intense suffering, can induce spiritual distress for patients and their families. Probing questions such as "How can a caring God let this happen?," "Why

me?," or "Am I being punished for some wrong that I have done?" are common indicators of spiritual distress. Some individuals may question their very existence and may even display anger toward religious representatives. Others may accept their illness as fate or just punishment and resist help, give up, and wait to die.[88]

Philosophical belief practices can directly affect caregiving practices such as diet and hygiene and rituals surrounding birth, death, and medical interventions. The nurse should have a basic understanding of the various religious tenets of Eastern and Western philosophies and how they may affect a patient's plan of care.[2,81,82]

Patients easily succumb to feelings of helplessness and powerlessness in the technologic, impersonalized environment of the ICU. Including a pastor or chaplain on the health care team is also an important aspect of holistic care. The chaplain may be the best person to assess spiritual needs and to assist patients and their families with coping with the crisis. Providing access to religious rituals, prayer, and scriptures and readings are meaningful strategies in alleviating stress. The patient, with the help of the agency chaplain, pastor, or counselor, can identify inner resources of strength, meaning, and purpose to help cope with the crisis event. The spiritual leader is also valuable in ethical decisions such as termination of life support and can be of great assistance to the health care team as their own personal resources are drained as a result of the sustained or cumulative assistance they have provided to others in crisis.[82]

Spiritual health has been found to be associated with hardiness, a composite measure composed of commitment, challenge, a sense of control, and a mark of psychologic health.[9,82,87] Spiritual well-being also can refer to one's valuing of goodness, love, and relatedness to others or a general feeling of having a purposeful and fulfilled life.

SUPPORTING COMPLEMENTARY THERAPIES

The field of complementary therapies is evolving. The purpose of these therapies and practices is to help maintain wellness, and when necessary, facilitate the body's own healing responses to restore balance and harmony. Integrative health care implies blending conventional health care with complementary therapies, accompanied by open communications among practitioners and conscious recognition of the possible synergy. Integrative health care, like nursing, holds a holistic philosophy.

Interest in complementary therapies has increased dramatically in the past decade, and the national demand for these services has reached unprecedented levels. The most recent utilization study, in 2001, studied time trends and found that almost 70% of adults in the United States had used at least one complementary therapy in their lifetime.[89] The number of hospitals providing complementary therapies is also growing. Nursing, in turn, is returning to those holistic roots with an increased awareness and integration of complementary therapies. Today, nursing combines biomedical understanding of disease and treatment with the caring behaviors and treatments that have been part of holistic nursing practice throughout history.[90]

The importance of complementary therapies in modern health care has been recognized at the national level. In 1998 Congress established the National Center for Complementary and Alternative Medicine to facilitate the evaluation of alternative medical treatment modalities and to provide a public information clearinghouse and a research-training program. Music therapy, relaxation, guided imagery, art therapy, therapeutic massage, and mindfulness meditation are a few of the complementary therapies currently being evaluated by nurses. Smith and colleagues examined the effects of therapeutic massage on pain, sleep, symptom distress, and anxiety in hospitalized cancer patients.[91] Significant decreases in pain and symptom distress were attributed to therapeutic massage. Bauer-Wu and colleagues recently completed a study examining the feasibility of mindfulness meditation in patients undergoing bone marrow transplantation. At the completion of the intervention, patients reported improved psychologic functioning, decreased symptom distress, and subjective benefits of improved coping and quality of life.[92] Although more research is needed to support the value of complementary therapies on selected outcomes related to the symptoms of critically ill hospitalized patients, early studies are supporting the potential for complementary therapies as a therapeutic nursing intervention.

CARE OF SPECIFIC POPULATIONS

CHRONICALLY ILL PERSONS IN THE ICU

Chronic illnesses have a direct effect on a successful outcome of a critical illness incident. The typical length of stay in the ICU is 2 to 4 days; however, this time may be extended for a week or more for a chronically ill patient who becomes acutely ill.[93] Usually this type of patient is older; has multiple system problems such as cardiac, respiratory, and renal disturbances; has nutritional deficits; and has diminished reserves resulting from the prolonged stress of coping with the primary problem. These individuals are at high risk for developing episodes of mental confusion or delirium. They often have difficulty adjusting to the ICU environment, the isolation from family, and their reactions to medications. Sensory deficits in hearing and vision also may complicate their course of recovery. When possible, the patients should be allowed to wear their hearing aids and glasses.

Care of chronically ill patients can be very costly, and fewer than 50% live to be discharged. Two similar longitudinal studies[94,95] compared the effects of care provided for the critical condition of chronically ill patients in traditional ICUs and in low-technology special care units (SCUs). Outcomes of complications, length of stay, costs, recovery and survival rates, and patient/family satisfaction were examined. Patients were carefully selected for placement in the two groups. The average age of the participants was 64 years, and respiratory and cardiac illnesses were the common chronic problems. The average hospital stay was 32.2 days.

In the study by Douglas et al,[94] SCUs were designed with private rooms to ensure privacy and to promote sleep, and a nursing care management model, including experienced staff, was used. The family-oriented units allowed unlimited visiting hours and arrangements for overnight stays by family members, if desired. Care in the ICUs followed the traditional protocols, limited visits with family, and used a primary care model under the supervision of physicians. Few significant outcome differences were found in either the Douglas or the Fisher and Hegge study.[94,95] However, costs were drastically lower in the SCUs, primarily because of the reduction in diagnostic costs and the minimal use of high-technology equipment other than mechanical ventilators.

According to Rudy et al,[93] chronically ill patients survive one complication only to succumb to another. When complications do occur, the patient and family must make difficult decisions regarding whether to extend further aggressive treatment or to restrict treatment, for example, making "do-not-resuscitate" decisions. The frequent and close contact with the health care team and the friendlier environment of the SCU would facilitate making those decisions.

Both studies demonstrated the efficacy of care in the SCU was equal to the care provided in the ICU. Satisfaction with care was implied. These studies contribute to the early body of knowledge that carefully selected, highly vulnerable patients can be appropriately cared for outside the ICU. These studies also support the social support theories by including the patients and their families in making treatment choices.

Nurses caring for these patients should be especially aware of the particular needs, watch for early signs of disorders, and act promptly to avoid major complications. Patience, excellent therapeutic communication skills, and a solid foundation in geriatric nursing are valuable attributes.[30]

CARE OF ELDERLY TRAUMA PATIENTS

By the year 2010 it is estimated that there will be more than 39 million senior adults (over 65 years of age), the fastest growing portion of the population in the United States. By 2020 this number is expected to soar to 69 million.[96] As this population increases, the number of trauma injuries for these individuals also will increase.

Trauma injuries caused by falls, burns, and motor vehicle accidents combined are the fifth-leading cause of death for elderly persons. The mortality rate resulting from such injuries is significantly higher for this population than for younger persons.[95,97] Contributing factors to these injuries include polypharmacy, chronic illnesses, sensory deficits (diminished vision, hearing, and sense of touch and slowing of psychomotor and cognitive responses), and osteoporosis. Because of osteoporosis, these individuals are more susceptible to fractures of extremities (especially the hip) and to spinal cord injuries.

Often the elderly receive less analgesic medication than do younger patients; however, it is not known whether this is because of differences in their perception and tolerance of pain or whether pain relief measures are adequate. Zalon's phenomenologic study of the pain experience of frail elderly women after surgery[97] concluded that these elders tended to endure pain as a part of life and trusted nurses to recognize signs of pain and to attend to pain-relief measures as needed. The women did not ask for pain relief until they could no longer cope. Lying still was one of the means they used to control the pain; using distractive measures and asking for pain relief at bedtime also were mentioned. Some women feared addiction and loss of control, which resulted in their greater endurance of pain. Managing postoperative pain was easier for the women than dealing with the presurgery pain that was associated with fear and anxiety.

The ICU and perioperative nurses must carefully evaluate the geriatric trauma patient for fluid and electrolyte imbalances; signs of impaired renal, respiratory, and circulatory function; and pain. All of these factors can contribute to psychosocial alterations. Because of the potential delay in elimination of medications, these patients may have mental status changes related to the many drug and narcotic side effects.[30,32,93]

CARE OF PATIENTS WHO REQUIRE TRANSPLANTS

Advances in technology have contributed to the belief that any organ can be replaced. People often have unrealistic expectations about what can or cannot be done to help them.[7,98] Statistics reported by the scientific registry of the United Network for Organ Sharing (UNOS)[99] revealed that more than 85,000 persons are on the national waiting list for donor organs. (This number includes those who are waiting for more than one organ.)

Waiting for a donor organ can be an emotional drain on the recipient. The recipient may experience guilt, knowing that a sacrifice is being requested from a living donor or that someone else must die so that the recipient can live. At the same time, the recipient realizes that his or her own death may come before an organ is available. These patients and their families experience a gamut of emotions. Concerns include worry over the financial burden, stress on the family, anxiety over the possible rejection of the transplanted organ, and the consequences of taking immune-suppressant drugs for the remainder of one's life. The fear of infections is ever present because becoming ill may delay or deny a recipient's eligibility for the surgery.[100]

Persons receiving bone marrow transplants experience a complex process involving repeated hospital stays of various lengths. Coping with prolonged isolation and the side effects of immune-suppressant drugs and body radiation can be very taxing. The fear of rejection is a major concern. The donor, who often is a family member, may experience guilt feelings if the graft fails. The nurse's role is critical in maintaining hope during these periods. Demonstrating patience and empathy with the patient's and the family's array of emotions is very important.[99]

The number of persons with end-stage renal disease who require dialysis has increased to more than 275,000, and more than 60,000 are awaiting kidney transplant procedures.[99,101] However, the availability of donor organs is much less than the demand. Nearly half (43%) of the transplant organs are now supplied by living donors. Success rates of the surgery range between 91% and 97%, and costs have decreased to one third the cost of dialysis. Most individuals awaiting kidney transplants must endure dialysis several times a week for many months or years, which is extremely costly, time-consuming, and stress-producing.

Psychologic evaluation is an essential component of the preoperative work-up to determine the patient's ability to cope with the necessary life-long medical regimen and the ability to accept the donated organ as a part of the body. Postsurgical quality-of-life perceptions may be affected by internal and external environmental factors, gender differences regarding self-image and self-esteem and functioning ability, as well as social support and cultural and religious values.[37] Emotions also can be exacerbated by the presence of steroid medications.[102]

Living donors also are evaluated psychologically. A donor must offer the kidney freely, without coercion, and must fully understand the possible risks and benefits of the procedure. Most kidney transplant patients will experience at least one episode of rejection. The threat of rejection can cause much anxiety. Although a second kidney transplant may be possible if a suitable organ can be found, progression of the disease process may preclude the patient's chances of survival during the waiting period. Psychosocial nursing care for these patients is challenging, because they face the wide-ranging emotions of hope or hopelessness, anxiety, despair, grief, helplessness, and depression.[40,98]

Annually, the national statistics have reported more than 4000 individuals awaiting heart transplants; however, only one half of the needed hearts have been avail-

CLINICAL APPLICATION

Psychosocial Concepts

Nancy Donovan, a 32-year-old single mother of two boys, ages 5 and 8 years, was admitted to the intensive care burn unit with partial-thickness and full-thickness burns over 40% of her body—affecting portions of her face, anterior chest, arms, and legs. She had been using cleaning fluid near a gas water heater in the garage. She appears highly anxious and in intense pain and has symptoms of shock. As a result of potential airway problems, she has been intubated and placed on a ventilator. Fluid requirements have been calculated, and an IV started; an indwelling catheter has been inserted. Her prognosis is guarded. A neighbor activated the 911 emergency response system and alerted Nancy's parents, who live in a town 20 miles away. The children, who were in school at the time of the accident, are staying with the neighbor until the grandparents arrive. Although initial treatment is directed toward physical stabilization, Nancy's psychologic responses to this crisis also must receive

prompt attention. Severe burn injuries pose a major coping challenge to any person, even though the individual is considered to be "psychologically healthy."

Early Posttrauma Phase

1. Because Nancy cannot verbally communicate with you, what behaviors/symptoms would you assess to support the nursing diagnosis of Anxiety Related to Pain?
2. What measures would you take to establish a trusting relationship between you and Nancy?
3. How would you prepare Nancy's parents for their first visit to the burn unit?
4. What would be your response when they asked about the seriousness of her burn injuries?
   What additional information would you like to have from Nancy's parents to assist you in planning and providing psychologic care for her?

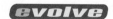 For the discussion of the questions and a continuation of this Clinical Application and for an additional clinical application on managing a patient with delirium/acute confusion, see the Evolve website.

able. During that same annual period, approximately 222 people have needed heart-lung transplants, and less than one third of these double-transplant surgeries can be performed. Roark[103] indicated that the average waiting period for donor organs is 1 to 2 years. Stressors are greater than ever as the number of potential recipients increases, and 24% to 30% of these individuals die before a heart becomes available.[102]

Patients and families have much information to process concerning the uncertain future of a transplant recipient and the prediction of an average survival rate of 1 year. Average costs are $250,000 during the first year and $20,000 for annual follow-up.[99] Many ethical issues surround the people involved in the process of procuring donor organs. A multidisciplinary health care team consisting of the nurse, the chaplain, psychiatric consult, social services, the patient, and the family is extremely helpful in resolving these issues and in making decisions.[38,102] New regulations initiated in 1998 require the education of a "designated requestor," one who would approach the family of a potential organ donor. These changes offer new opportunities for nurses to educate families regarding their options as well as informing individuals regarding their own decision to be a donor. It is estimated that the donor supply would be increased by 20% through such education.[103] The patient and family experience a variety of emotional responses after surgery; these range from the initial euphoria that comes from receiving a second chance at life to the anguish felt over the death of the donor. They also must deal with ac-

ceptance of another person's heart, dependence on immune suppressants, and the ever-present fear of organ rejection. The nurse can be a valuable resource for individuals learning to cope with these emotions.

It is predicted that hospitals will become more specialized and organ transplants will become more common. Rejection of human and animal transplants will most likely be conquered. By 2020 most hospitalized patients will be older, will experience multisystem failures, and will have major trauma injuries and/or complex surgeries. A major challenge then will be addressing the many moral and ethical issues regarding the balance of the rights of individuals and the rights of society.[104] Advanced knowledge, decision making, and expertise in technologic skills will be required; however, caring attitudes and interpersonal and therapeutic communication skills will still be essential components of the nursing role.

SUMMARY

Several authors have emphasized the caring aspect of nursing. Although the ICU environment is not always conducive to nurses doing more than just managing the physiologic needs of critically ill patients, it is paramount, as demonstrated by the discussion in this chapter, that nurses consider the mind-body links in providing holistic nursing care and promoting patient recovery. One aspect of critical care nursing is knowing what emotional and behavioral responses should be expected in a given patient care situation and recognizing atypical responses. The placement of these responses within a theoretical context is an important tool in assessment and in providing appropriate interventions.

As health care teams have gained prominence during the past few years, some emphasis has been placed on the need for interdisciplinary collaboration in providing high quality care. Major psychosocial nursing diagnoses related to self-concept, self-esteem, and self-image were discussed in this chapter, as well as those of delirium (acute confusion), depression, violence toward self (actual and potential), spiritual distress, and ineffective individual and family coping (see Unit X for the nursing management plans for specific psychosocial alterations).

REFERENCES

1. North American Nursing Diagnosis Association: *Nursing diagnosis: definitions and classifications,* St Louis, 2003-2004, The Association.
2. Stuart G: A stress adaptation model of psychiatric nursing care. In Stuart GW, editor: *Principles and practices of psychiatric nursing,* ed 6, St Louis, 2004, Mosby.
3. Radwin LE, Alster K: Individualized nursing care: an empirically generated definition, *Int Nurs Rev* 49(1):54-63, 2002.
4. Snyder M, Brandt C, Tseng Y: Use of presence in the critical care unit, *AACN Clin Issues* 11(1):27-33, 2000.
5. Benner P, Tanner C, Chesla C: *Expertise in nursing practice,* New York, 1998, Springer.
6. Phillips S, Benner P, editors: *The crisis of care: affirming and restoring caring practices in helping professions,* Washington, DC, 1994, Georgetown University.
7. Gordon S, Benner P, Noddings N, editors: *Caregiving: readings in knowledge, practice, ethics, and politics,* Philadelphia, 1996, University of Pennsylvania.
8. Down J: Therapeutic nursing and technology: Clinical supervision and reflective practice in a critical care setting. In Freshwater D, editor: *Therapeutic nursing: improving patient care through self awareness and reflection,* London, 2002, Sage.
9. Spector R: *Cultural diversity in health and illness,* ed 6, Upper Saddle River, NJ, 2003, Prentice-Hall Health.
10. Jenny J, Logan J: Caring and comfort metaphors used by patients in critical care, *Image J Nurs Sch* 28(4):349-352, 1996.
11. Selye H: *Stress in health and disease,* Boston, 1976, Butterworth.
12. Bauer S: *Psychological and immunological correlates of surviving breast cancer,* dissertation, Chicago, 1997, Rush University.
13. Motzer SA et al: Natural killer cell function and psychological distress in women with and without irritable bowel syndrome, *Biol Res Nurs* 4(1):31-42, 2002.
14. Dropkin MJ: Anxiety, coping strategies, and coping behaviors in patients undergoing head and neck cancer surgery, *Cancer Nurs* 24(2):143-148, 2001.
15. Neurberger P: *Freedom from stress: a holistic approach,* Honesdale, Pa, 1981, The Himalayan International Institute of Yoga Science and Philosophy.
16. Lazarus R, Folkman S: *Stress, appraisal, and coping,* New York, 1984, Springer.
17. Lazarus R, Lazarus B: *Passion and reason: making sense of emotions,* New York, 1994, Oxford University.
18. Morse J: Responding to threats to integrity of self, *Adv Nurs Sci* 19(4):21-36, 1999.
19. Morse J, Penrod J: Linking concepts of enduring, uncertainty, suffering, and hope, *Image J Nurs Sch* 31(2):145-150, 1999.
20. Tusaie K, Dyer J: Resilience: a historical review of the construct, *Holistic Nursing Practice* 18(1):3-8, 2004.
21. Wagnild G, Young H: Development of psychometric evaluation of the resilience scale, *J Nurs Meas* 1(2):165-178, 1993.
22. Doenges ME, Moorhouse MF: *Nurse's pocket guide: diagnoses, interventions, and rationales,* ed 7, Philadelphia, 2004, FA Davis.
23. McCloskey J, Bulechek GM: *Nursing interventions classification (NIC),* ed 3, St Louis, 2000, Mosby.
24. Marcus PE: Anxiety and related disorders. In Fortinash K, Holoday-Worret P, editors: *Psychiatric mental health nursing,* St Louis, 2004, Mosby.
25. Porth C: *Pathophysiology: concepts of altered health states,* ed 5, Philadelphia, 1998, Lippincott.
26. O'Leary A et al: Stress and immune function. In Miller T, editor: *Clinical disorders and stressful life events,* Madison, Conn, 1997, International Universities.
27. Stein K: Schema model of the self-concept, *Image J Nurs Sch* 27(3):187-192, 1995.
28. Coopersmith S: *The antecedents of self-esteem,* San Francisco, 1967, WH Freeman.
29. Fortinash KM: The nursing process. In Fortinash KM, Holoday-Worret PA, editors: *Psychiatric mental health nursing,* ed 3, St Louis, 2004, Mosby.
30. O'Neill D, Kenny E: Spirituality and chronic illness, *Image J Nurs Sch* 30(3):275-280, 1998.
31. Giarelli E: Spiraling out of control: one case of pathologic anxiety as a response to a genetic risk of cancer, *Cancer Nurs* 22(5):327-339, 1999.
32. Keough V, Letizia M: Perioperative care of elderly trauma patients, *AORN J* 63(5):932-937, 1996.
33. Pettie D, Triolo A: Illness as evolution: the search for identity and meaning in the recovery process, *Psych Rehab J* 22(3):255-262, 1999.
34. Minarik P: Psychosocial intervention with ineffective coping responses to physical illness: depression-related. In Barry P, editor: *Psychosocial nursing,* ed 3, Philadelphia, 1996, Lippincott.
35. Byrne B: *Measuring self-concept across the life span,* Washington, DC, 1996, American Psychiatric Association.
36. Price B: A model for body-image care, *J Adv Nurs* 15:585, 1995.
37. Johnson C et al: Racial and gender differences in quality of life following kidney transplantation, *Image J Nurs Sch* 30(2):125-129, 1998.
38. DePalma J, Townsend R: Ethical issues in organ donation and transplantation: are we helping a few at the expense of many? *Crit Care Nurs Q* 19(1):1-9, 1996.
39. Hunter A, Chandler G: Adolescent resilience, *Image J Nurs Sch* 31(3):243-247, 1999.
40. Juneau B: Psychologic and psychosocial aspects of renal transplantation, *Crit Care Nurs Q* 7(4):62-66, 1995.
41. McFarland G, McFarland E: *Nursing diagnosis and interventions,* ed 3, St Louis, 1997, Mosby.
42. Maslow H: *Motivation and personality,* New York, 1954, Harper & Row.

43. Edmisson K: Psychosocial dimensions of medical-surgical nursing. In Hawks J, Keene AM, Black JM, editors: *Medical-surgical nursing*, ed 6, Philadelphia, 2000, Saunders.

44. Nield-Anderson L et al: Responding to difficult patients, *Am J Nurs* 99(12):27-33, 1999.

45. Hollinger-Smith L: Growth and development across the life span. In Fortinash K, Holoday-Worret P, editors: *Psychiatric mental health nursing*, ed 3, St Louis, 2004, Mosby.

46. Rotter JB: Generalized expectancies for internal versus external control of reinforcement, *Psychol Monogr* 80(1): 1-28, 1966.

47. Beyea S: Collaboration in health practice. In Blais K et al: *Professional nursing practice: concepts and perspectives*, ed 4, Menlo Park, Calif, 2001, Addison Wesley.

48. Boling A: *Defect in hope*, Presentation at Joint Southern California STTI Chapters Research Conference, October 10-12, 1996.

49. Herth K: Abbreviated instrument to measure hope: development and psychometric evaluation, *J Adv Nurs Res* 17: 1251-1259,1992.

50. Morse J, Doberneck B: Delineating the concept of hope, *West J Nurs Res* 27(4):277-278, 1995.

51. Wheeler RW: Helping families cope with death and dying, *Nursing* 98(7):25-30, 1996.

52. Czerwiec M: When a loved one is dying: families talk about nursing care, *Am J Nurs* 96(5):32-36, 1996.

53. Durhan E: How patients die, *Am J Nurs* 97(12):41-46, 1997.

54. Powers P et al: The value of patient and family-centered care, *Am J Nurs* 100(5):84-88, 2000.

55. Nussbaum GB: Spirituality in critical care: patient comfort and satisfaction, *Crit Care Nurs Q* 26(3):214-220, 2003.

56. Reference deleted in proofs.

57. Geary S: Intensive care unit psychosis revisited: understanding and managing delirium in the critical care setting, *Crit Care Nurs Q* 17(1):51-63, 1994.

58. Hall G, Wakefield B: Acute confusion in the elderly: what to do when the clouds roll in, *Nursing CE Handbook* (online), March 1998, Springhouse.

59. Mentes J et al: Acute confusion indicators: risk factors and prevalence using MDS data, *Res Nurs Health* 22:95-105, 1999.

60. Burke MM, Laramie J: *Primary care of the older adult*, St Louis, 2004, Mosby.

61. Folstein MF, Folstein SE, McHugh PR: "Mini-mental state": a practical method for grading the cognitive state of patients for the clinician, *J Psychiatr Res* 12(3):189-198, 1975.

62. Trzepacz PT et al: Validation of the delirium rating scale-revised-98: comparison with the delirium rating scale and the cognitive test for delirium. *J Neurospychiatr Clin Neurosci* 13:229-242, 2001.

63. Johnston K, Rohaly-Davis J: An introduction to music therapy: helping oncology patients in the ICU, *Crit Care Nurs Q* 18(4):54-60, 1996.

64. American Psychiatric Association: *Diagnostic and statistical manual of mental disorders DSM-IV-TR*, ed 4, Washington, DC, 2000, The Association.

64a. Barry P: *Psychosocial nursing: assessment and intervention in care of the physically ill*, ed 3, Philadelphia, 1996, Lippincott.

65. Pfeiffer E: A short portable mental status questionnaire for the assessment of organic brain deficit in elderly patients, *J Am Geriatr Soc* 23(10):433-441, 1975.

66. American Psychiatric Association: Practice guidelines for the treatment of patients with delirium. *Am J Psychiatry* 156(5 Suppl):1-20, 1999.

67. Barber JM. Pharmacologic management of integrative brain failure, *Crit Care Nurs Q* 26(3):192-207, 2003.

68. Hagerty B, Patusky KL: Mood disorders: depression and mania. In Fortinash K, Holloday-Worret P, editors: *Psychiatric mental health nursing*, ed 3, St Louis, 2004, Mosby.

69. Marcus P: Suicide. In Fortinash K, Holoday-Worret P, editors: *Psychiatric mental health nursing*, ed 3, St Louis, 2004, Mosby.

70. Badger J: Reaching out to the suicidal patient, *Am J Nurs* 95(3):24-31, 1995.

71. Rabie D et al: Suicide prevention control, *Am J Nurs* 99(12):53-57, 1999.

72. Clark MJ: *Community health nursing handbook*, Stamford, Conn, 1999, Appleton & Lange.

73. Aquilera DC: *Crisis intervention: theory and methodology*, ed 7, St Louis, Mosby, 1998.

74. Holoday-Worret P: Foundations of psychiatric mental health nursing. In Fortinash K, Holoday-Worret P, editors: *Psychiatric mental health nursing*, ed 3, St Louis, 2004, Mosby.

75. Beyers M: The new reality, *JONA* 20(6):5-6, 1996.

76. Coward D: Facilitation of self-transcendence in a breast cancer support group. II, *Oncol Nurs Forum* 30(2):291-300, 2003.

77. Mynatt S: Increasing resiliency to substance abuse in recovering women with comorbid depression, *J Psychosoc Nurs Ment Health Serv* 36(1):28-36, 1998.

78. Tolsma AN: *Evaluation of theoretical model of resilience and salient predictors of resiliency in a sample of community based elderly*, dissertation, Ann Arbor, Mich, 1995, University of Michigan.

79. Sumner C: Recognizing and responding to spiritual distress, *Am J Nurs* 98(1):26-30, 1998.

80. Armentrout D: Heart cry: a biblical model of depression, *J Psychol Christianity* 14(2):101-111, 1995.

81. Dossey B, Dossey L: Holistic modalities and healing moments, *Am J Nurs* 98(6):44-47, 1998.

82. Gillman J: Religious perspectives on organ donation, *Crit Care Nurs Q* 22(3):19-29, 1999.

83. Holt-Ashley M: Nurses pray: use of prayer and spirituality as complementary therapy in the intensive care setting, *AACN Clin Issues* 11(1):60-67, 2000.

84. Lougren G, Astrom G, Engstrom B: A care policy and its implementation, *Int J Nurs Practice* 7(2):92-103, 2001.

85. Johnson S et al: Perceived changes in adult family members' roles and responsibilities during critical illness, *Image J Nurs Res* 27(3):238-243, 1995.

86. Buchanan H, Geubtner M, Snyder C: Trauma bereavement program: review of development and implementation, *Clin Care Nurs Q* 19(1):35-44, 1996.

87. Frankl V: *Man's search for meaning*, New York, 1959, Washington Square Press.

88. Shelly J: *Spiritual care: a guide for caregivers*, Downers Grove, Ill, 2000, Intervarsity Press.

89. Kessler R et al: Long-term trends in the use of complementary and alternative medical therapies in the United States, *Ann Intern Med* 135(4):262-268, 2001.

90. Libster M: Demonstrating care: the art of integrative nursing, Independence, Ky, 2001, Thompson Delmar Learning.

91. Smith M, Kemp J, Hemphill L, Vojir C: Outcomes of therapeutic massage for hospitalized cancer patients, *J Nurs Scholarship* 34(3):257-262, 2002.

92. Bauer-Wu S: Facing the challenges of stem cell/bone marrow transplantation with mindfulness mediation, 2004, Dana Farber/Harvard Cancer Center, unpublished manuscript.

93. Rudy E et al: Patient outcomes for the chronically critically ill: special care unit versus intensive care unit, *Nurs Res* 44(6):324-331, 1996.

94. Douglas S et al: Survival experience of chronically critically ill patients, *Nurs Res* 45(2):73-77, 1996.

95. Fisher C, Hegge M: The elderly women at risk, *Am J Nurs* 100(6):54-59, 2000.

96. Aging in the 21st Century. Administration on Aging. National Aging Information Center. This report was prepared by Jacob Siegel with the administration, U.S. Department of Health and Human Services. Retrieved from the Internet at www.aoa.gov.STATS/aging21/demography.htm, June 10, 2004.

97. Zalon M: Pain in frail, elderly women after surgery, *Image J Nurs Sch* 29(1):21-26, 1997.

98. Decker W: Psychosocial considerations for bone marrow transplant recipients, *Crit Care Nurs Q* 17(4):67-73, 1995.

99. United Network for Organ Sharing, National patient waiting list. Retrieved from the Internet at www.unos.org/newsroom/criticaldata_main.htm on June 10, 2004.

100. Bartucci MR: Kidney transplantation: state of the art, *AACN Clin Issues* 10(2):153-163, 1999.

101. U.S. Renal Data System 2002. Annual Report www.usrd.org. Located through the National Kidney Foundation on the Internet at www.kidney.org.

102. AACN Cardiopulmonary Update. Part III. Wyeth-Ayerst Nursing Fellows program Supplement to *AJN* 99(5): 2000. Also available at www.nursingcenter.com/ce/test/article.

103. Roark D: Overhauling the organ donation system, *Am J Nurs* 100(6):45-48, 2000.

104. Hupfeld S: Through the looking glass: tomorrow's hospital, *RN* 63(6):52-59, 2000.

Sleep Alterations and Management

Sleep is the only medication that gives ease.— Sophocles

Nurses who have an appreciation of the importance of sleep place a higher priority on protection of patients' sleep.[1] Health care providers interrupt patients' sleep for assessment, treatments, or interventions, and environmental noise, pain, and/or anxiety also disturb it.[2] Although prioritizing care is essential, the consequence of sleep interruptions by the nurse is not merely sleep-deprived patients; alterations in sleep patterns can delay physical and mental healing.[1] To facilitate both sleep and healing, critical care nurses need to understand the essentials of sleep and chronobiology, the effect of pharmacologic therapy on sleep, and the consequences of disrupted sleep. The purpose of this chapter is to acquaint nurses with the characteristics of normal human sleep and chronobiology, changes in sleep associated with aging and pharmacology, and abnormal sleep patterns that may affect critically ill patients. Finally, research-based nursing care for critically ill patients with sleep disturbances is discussed.

NORMAL HUMAN SLEEP

SLEEP PHYSIOLOGY

Humans spend about one third of their lives engaged in a process known as *sleep*. Although little is now known about the physiologic process or the depths to which it affects us, researchers are learning more about sleep every day. The behavioral definition of sleep is a reversible behavioral state of perceptual disengagement from and unresponsiveness to the environment.[3] Sleep is a basic human need, just as food and water are. For patients to regain and maintain their optimal physical and emotional health, they must be able to get adequate amounts of quality sleep. To help patients obtain their optimal amount of sleep, a nurse must first understand what constitutes normal sleep and how the nursing diagnosis and intervention plan can contribute to accomplishing this goal.

Polysomnography is the collection of multiple channels of physiologic data to assess sleep and its disorders using various electrodes.[4] Electroencephalography (EEG) electrodes are attached to the patient's scalp to measure brain waves. Changes in the EEG frequency (number of waveforms) and amplitude (height of waveform) over the course of the study allow the sleep to be scored into stages. Sleep stages are distinguished primarily by the EEG waveforms they produce. Sleep is scored by each 30-second epoch or segment of the tracing. The criteria for scoring sleep in infants differ from those used for adults.

Electrooculography (EOG) measures eye movement activity. The study can help to determine when the patient is in rapid eye movement (REM) sleep; it also can establish when sleep onset occurs as reflected by slow, rolling eye movements. Electromyography (EMG) involves leads placed over various muscle groups. When placed over the chin, the leads can help detect muscle atonia associated with REM sleep. Intercostal leads detect respiratory effort, whereas leads over the anterior tibialis detect leg movements that may be causing the patient to arouse. The electrocardiogram (ECG) shows any cardiac abnormalities, oximetry monitors the oxygen saturation levels, and piezo elastic bands around the chest and abdomen detect respiratory disorders such as apnea. Thermocouples are used to monitor airflow through the nose and mouth.

SLEEP STAGES

NREM Sleep. Humans experience three states of being. They are either awake (Fig. 6-1), in rapid eye movement (REM) sleep, or in nonrapid eye movement (NREM) sleep, which can be further divided into stages 1 through 4, with each stage being a progressively deeper sleep state. Adults usually enter sleep through NREM stage 1 sleep (Fig. 6-2), which is a transitional, lighter sleep state from which the patient can be easily aroused by light touch or softly calling his or her name.

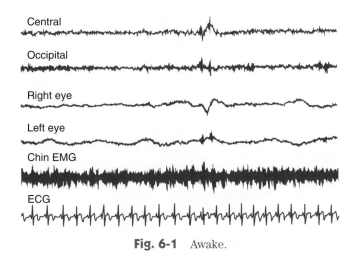

Fig. 6-1 Awake.

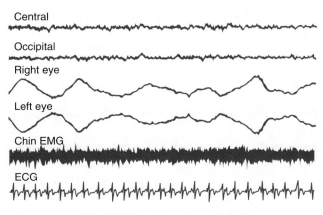

Fig. 6-3 NREM stage 2 sleep.

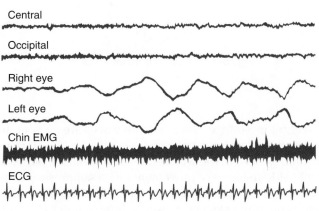

Fig. 6-2 NREM stage 1 sleep.

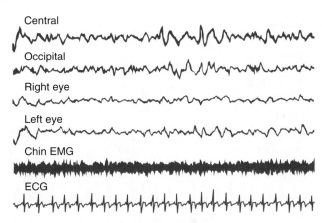

Fig. 6-4 Delta sleep NREM stage 3.

Stage 1 comprises 2% to 5% of a night's sleep and is demonstrated by an EEG pattern of low-voltage, mixed-frequency waveforms with vertex sharp waves. The EOG during stage 1 may demonstrate slow, side-to-side eye movement. A patient with severely disrupted sleep may experience an increase in the amount of stage 1 sleep throughout the sleep cycle. As a patient makes the transition from awake to asleep, a brief memory impairment may result.[5] This may mean that the patient may not remember educational or care instructions given by the nurse during the transition between sleep and wake states. Patients sometimes may experience muscle jerks and recall vivid images upon awakening. These are called *hypnic myoclonia;* although not pathologic, they can cause the patient to awaken feeling frightened.

Stage 2 NREM sleep (Fig. 6-3) occupies about 45% to 55% of the night, with sleep deepening and a higher arousal threshold being required to awaken the patient. Changes seen in the EEG pattern include sleep spindles and K complexes. As stage 2 continues, high-voltage, slow-wave activity begins to appear. When these slow waves represent 20% of the EEG activity per page, they

will meet the criteria for stage 3 sleep, which constitutes 3% to 8% of the cycle. In stage 3 NREM (Fig. 6-4) sleep, slow waves continue to develop until 50% of the EEG waveforms are slow wave, which meets the criteria for stage 4 sleep. Stage 4 (Fig. 6-5) comprises 10% to 15% of the cycle. Stages 3 and 4 often are combined and referred to as *slow-wave sleep,* or *delta sleep.* Delta sleep has the highest arousal threshold. NREM sleep usually occupies 70% to 75% of the sleep cycle, with REM sleep comprising 20% to 25%.

NREM sleep is dominated by the parasympathetic nervous system. The body tries to maintain a homeostatic regulation, and this causes a decreased level of energy expenditure. Blood pressure, heart and respiratory rates, and metabolic rate return to basal levels. EMG levels are lower in NREM as opposed to wake states but not as low as those seen in REM sleep. Sweating or shivering that a patient may experience with temperature extremes occurs in NREM sleep but ceases during REM sleep.[3]

During slow-wave sleep, 80% of the total daily growth-stimulating hormone is released, which works to stimu-

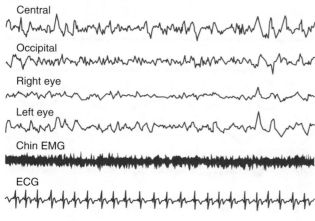

Fig. 6-5 Delta sleep NREM stage 4.

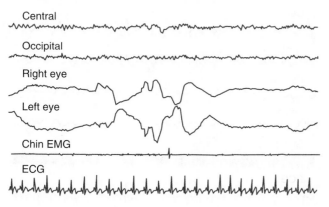

Fig. 6-6 REM sleep.

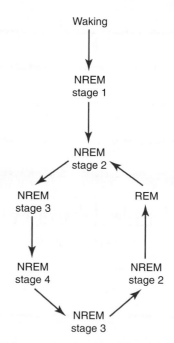

Fig. 6-7 The cyclic nature of sleep.

late protein synthesis while sparing catabolic breakdown. The release of other hormones, such as prolactin and testosterone, suggests that anabolism is occurring during slow-wave sleep. Cortisol release peaks during early morning hours, whereas melatonin is released only during darkness and thyroid-stimulating hormone is inhibited during sleep. Thus activities associated with stage 4 NREM (see Fig. 6-5) include protein synthesis and tissue repair, such as the repair of epithelial and specialized cells of the brain, skin, bone marrow, and gastric mucosa.[6] Some propose the theory that NREM sleep is a restorative period that relieves the stresses of waking activities, whereas REM sleep serves to refuel creative brain stores.

REM Sleep. REM sleep occupies about 20% to 25% of the night in healthy young adults and is sometimes known as the *dream stage*. However, dreaming is not the exclusive property of any one stage. REM can be viewed as a highly active brain in a paralyzed body and is frequently referred to as a *paradoxic sleep*. The paradox is that some areas of the brain remain very active, whereas others are suppressed. EEG waveforms (Fig. 6-6) are rel-

atively slow voltage, and sawtooth waves are present. Increased cortical activity occurs, with the EEG pattern resembling those of the wake state. Synchronized bursts of rapid side-to-side eye movements with suppressed EMG activity, or muscle atonia, are seen indicating functional paralysis of the skeletal muscles. Infants enter sleep onset through REM and spend about 50% of their night in REM sleep.

The sympathetic nervous system predominates during REM sleep.[6] Oxygen consumption increases, and blood pressure, cardiac output, and respiratory and heart rates become variable. The body's response to decreased oxygen levels and increased carbon dioxide levels is lowest during REM sleep. Cardiac efferent vagus nerve tone is generally suppressed during REM sleep, and irregular breathing patterns can lead to oxygen reduction, particularly in patients with pulmonary and cardiac disease. An increase in premature ventricular contractions and tachydysrhythmias may be associated with respiratory pauses during REM sleep.[6] Arterial pressure surges and increases in heart rate, coronary arterial tone, and blood viscosity may cause the combination of plaque rupture and hypercoagulability in persons with cardiac disease.[7]

SLEEP CYCLES

NREM and REM sleep cycles alternate (Fig. 6-7) throughout the night. Sleep onset usually occurs in stage 1 sleep, progressing through stages 2 to 4 and then going back to stage 2, at which time the person usually enters

REM. This first cycle usually takes about 70 to 100 minutes, with later cycles lasting 90 to 120 minutes. Four to five cycles are completed during normal adult sleep. NREM sleep predominates during the first third of the night, whereas REM is more prominent during the last third. Brief episodes of wakefulness (usually less than 5%) tend to intrude later into the night and are usually not remembered the next morning.

The amount of sleep required is uncertain. No set number of hours has been established, and sleep length may be determined by many factors, including genetic predisposition. A sufficient amount of sleep has been achieved when one awakens without the alarm and gets through the day without feeling sleepy.

SLEEP CHANGES IN AGING

Important changes in sleep occur with aging, and critical care nurses must consider these changes when planning care for elderly clients. Assessment for sleep disturbances in the elderly is particularly essential since lack of sleep can compromise daytime function, thereby lowering quality of life.[8]

Elders most commonly complain about either excessive sleepiness or insomnia, and current research offers justification for both of these complaints.[9] Sleep pattern changes in older adults include fewer episodes of stages 3 and 4 NREM and REM sleep.[10] Elders also report that they do not sleep as soundly or feel as rested after awakening.[11] One reason for this may be that elders do not consolidate their sleep into one session. They may go to bed, awake 4 hours later, stay awake for an extended period, and then go back to sleep, resulting in fragmented sleep patterns.[8] Many of the diseases associated with aging may contribute to these nocturnal arousals, including diabetes, nocturia, cardiovascular symptoms, chronic pain, and depression.[8,12,13] In addition, sleep-related respiratory disorders and increased incidence of periodic leg movements in elders may further disrupt their sleep.[14] Increasing age brings many physical and social changes with which the elder must cope. Assessment of elder clients must always include sleep history as an indicator of mental health because depression is a common struggle for the elderly.[15]

One common misconception is that elders require less sleep than younger adults do. Because their sleep is not as consolidated as that of younger adults, elders often take daytime naps to satisfy their sleep needs. In a study involving 45 healthy subjects at least 78 years of age and 33 healthy adults ages 20 to 30 years, Buysse et al[11] found that these elders napped an average of 3.4 times in 14 days as opposed to 1.1 times for young controls (n = 33). In addition, the elders went to bed earlier, slept less time, and did not sleep through the night as well as the control group. These findings are consistent with those of other investigators reviewed by Bliwise.[12]

Ancoli-Israel[10] believes that elders lose the ability to sustain a sleep state because of alterations in their circadian rhythms. Their internal clocks reset, causing them to become sleepy during the early evening and awaken during the early morning. Combined with fragmented sleep, this change in the internal clock leads to increased daytime sleepiness and napping. Elders who are constantly battling fatigue are less involved socially and mentally, resulting in decreased quality of life, and may be at risk for higher mortality.[16]

In critical care areas, nurses need to identify these altered sleep patterns as well as other impediments to adequate rest and methods to minimize acute disruption of sleep while accommodating age-related changes in sleep patterns. Authorities on sleep[17] recommend the use of nonpharmacologic means to promote sleep such as control of environmental noise and light, use of white noise, music, massage, and/or allowing specified blocks of time for sleep. It is also important for nurses to educate patients about the changes in sleep that result from aging and teach sleep hygiene practices such as adhering to regular bedtimes and rising times and avoiding napping.

CHRONOBIOLOGY

Sleep is not merely a response to fatigue. A complex group of interacting systems determines the timing and depth of sleep. The following section reviews circadian and homeostatic processes and theories of sleep regulation.

CIRCADIAN SYSTEM

Many body systems cycle within approximately a 24-hour period, hence the name *circadian rhythm* (circa = about, dia = day).[18] Among these systems is the sleep-wake rhythm.[18] A bundle of cells in the anterior hypothalamus, known as the *suprachiasmatic nucleus*, functions as the pacemaker for these rhythms.[18] The circadian system facilitates cycling of the prescribed functions within a predictable period, but the functions are also influenced by other conditions, such as social activity, posture, and physical environment.[18] Rhythms can be seasonal or ultradian (less than a day). One example of an ultradian rhythm is the pattern of sleep during one night's sleep, in which the sleeper cycles between stages.

Under normal conditions, a person's rhythms interact and influence one another. For example, when body temperature is lowering, a person is more likely to sleep, and as the body temperature rises in early morning hours, people awaken.[19] Another example is the melatonin cycle, which tends to run in synchrony with the sleep-wake cycle.[20,21]

External influences such as posture, exercise, and light also influence the sleep circadian rhythm.[22] These external influences, known as *zeitgebers*, can shift the rhythm, causing it to peak at different times, or fragment it. Light is the most influential zeitgeber for sleep;[23,24] therefore critical care nurses need to limit the light in the environment during nocturnal hours to facilitate sleep and circadian continuity in their patients.

HOMEOSTATIC MECHANISM

The recent history of the sleep obtained by an individual also influences timing and depth of sleep. Known as the *homeostatic process of sleep regulation*, this determinant of sleep is linked to how much sleep the individual has had previously. Essentially, someone who is sleep-deprived will sleep more readily, regardless of circadian phase, whereas someone who is well rested will not fall asleep readily.[25] The amount of slow-wave sleep (stages 3 and 4 NREM sleep) reflects sleep intensity,[24,25] and individuals recovering from sleep deprivation have increased amounts of slow-wave sleep.

CIRCADIAN AND HOMEOSTATIC INTERACTION

Circadian and homeostatic processes function together to ensure optimal sleep for an individual. However, researchers can study each process separately using desynchrony protocols. These protocols isolate the circadian process from the homeostatic process by imposing a set sleep-wake routine that is not 24 hours in length. This allows the subject's intrinsic circadian rhythm to emerge, which is usually slightly longer than 24 hours long.[26] In essence, these studies have shown that homeostatic processes primarily regulate slow-wave activity, and the ratio of REM to NREM sleep is primarily regulated by the interaction of circadian and homeostatic processes.[25]

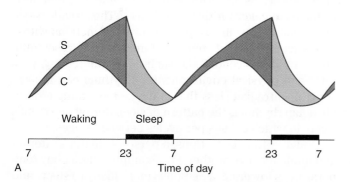

Fig. 6-8 Two-process model of sleep regulation. *A,* Time course of homeostatic process *S* and circadian process *C*. *S* rises during waking and declines during sleep. The intersection of *S* and *C* defines time of wake-up. (Modified from Borbely AA: A two-process model of sleep regulation, *Hum Neurobiol* 1:195, 1982.)

MODELS OF SLEEP REGULATION

A variety of models for sleep regulation exist, and research to determine the adequacy of these explanations is ongoing. The two-process model suggests that sleep in humans is controlled by an interaction of the circadian process (C) and the homeostatic process (S). The interplay of these two processes sets the timing for sleep and wake.[25,26] As the sleep circadian rhythm wanes, it intersects the homeostatic rhythm and the sleeper awakens (Fig. 6-8).

A second model is the two-oscillator model.[27] This theory suggests the existence of two separate circadian modulators, x and y. X is a strong oscillator that controls body temperature, REM sleep, and cortisol levels, whereas the weaker y oscillator controls sleep. A variant of this model considers temperature as factor x and deems the thermoregulatory mechanism to be the most important factor in sleep regulation.[28] This model does not acknowledge the role of homeostasis in sleep regulation.

SUMMARY OF CHRONOBIOLOGY

In the critical care environment, light is often needed to facilitate assessment or nursing actions. Frequent interruptions to sleep that are associated with bright light and social interaction may cause circadian disruption and result in sleep loss and slowed healing. Interventions that assist in maintaining patient orientation such as use of natural light, putting clocks and updated calendars where patients can see them, and facilitating the patient's normal schedule and sleep rituals are important methods of supporting circadian processes.

PHARMACOLOGY

It is essential that nurses understand the relationship between various medications and the sleep of patients in the critical care unit. Pathophysiology and age may profoundly affect not only medication absorption and elimination but also how patients cope with their illness and their ability to maintain health.

Hypnotics are considered the drugs of choice to treat insomnia. Insomnia is a patient complaint of inability to initiate or maintain sleep. Acute stress such as admission to a critical care unit may cause some patients to experience acute sleep-onset insomnia. Hypnotics tend to promote lighter sleep stages and have a higher lipophilicity, which can cause the elderly to experience an increased drug half-life.[29,30] Care should be used in the administration and dosage of hypnotics in the elderly. This age-group may experience night terrors, nightmares, and increased agitation. Their metabolism of hypnotics can be inhibited by the use of steroids or can be accelerated in those who smoke. Hypnotics may also produce anterograde amnesia, which is a memory failure of information processed after the drug is consumed. Patients with normal ventilation should not be affected by the mild respiratory depression caused by hypnotics, although patients with chronic obstructive pulmonary disease (COPD) and sleep-disordered breathing may be affected.

Stimulants produce increased arousal, behavioral activation, and alertness. They can be divided into three classes: direct-acting sympathomimetics such as phenylephrine; indirect-acting sympathomimetics (methylphenidate, amphetamine, and mazindol); and stimulants that are not sympathomimetics such as caffeine. Side effects can include irritability, talkativeness, sweating, anorexia, gastrointestinal complaints, dyskinesias, insomnia, and palpatations.[31] Stimulants can be used for patients who experience disabling symptoms of sleepiness resulting from narcolepsy, idiopathic central nervous system hypersomnia, or sleep deprivation. Stimulants should be used only when sustained alertness is required for the individual or public safety.

Stimulants possess a high abuse potential. A sequence of euphoria, dysphoria, paranoia, and psychosis can occur after a single exposure, and sustained use can lead to cognitive and behavioral disorders. Proper dosing and a structured management plan are recommended for stimulant use. This includes patient education with treatment goals, beginning with low doses, emphasizing good sleep hygiene such as naps, and adjusting the dosage according to clinical information.[32] Stimulants should be included as part of a treatment plan only to decrease excessive somnolence. Sustained use of high-dose stimulants can lead to cognitive and behavioral disorders.[32] Effective sleep hygiene and attention to other substances or medications that may affect sleep may be beneficial for patients who want to avoid the abuse potential.

Many people use alcohol to assist them in falling asleep. Alcohol is a central nervous system sedative and will cause suppression of REM sleep. More than two alcoholic drinks may cause an increase in NREM stages 1 and 2 and decrease the onset of slow-wave sleep. Alcohol also may cause shallow, fragmented sleep and may precipitate or aggravate an existing obstructive sleep apnea condition. In a Gallup survey of the general population, people with insomnia tend to self-medicate with alcohol.[33] Of those polled, 40% used either alcohol or over-the-counter medications (OTCs), 28% used alcohol, and 23% used only OTCs.

Recently many people have turned to alternative medicine in the form of herbs to treat their sleep problems. Because these are not considered prescription drugs, patients do not always inform their caregivers that they are using them. Some herbs are considered effective hypnotics, whereas others may be used as stimulants. It is the responsibility of the nurse to inquire about all medications used, whether they are prescription or over-the-counter.

Healthy patients may respond differently to medications than do patients with illness. Patients may come to the critical care unit with impaired sleep or poor cognitive function. Beta-blockers are known to produce nightmares and have disruptive effects on sleep quality in some individuals.[34] The effects of various drug combinations are not well known.

In patients requiring continuous sedation, propofol (Diprivan) is a common choice. It is unclear whether sedation is an adequate replacement for natural sleep; however, investigators have shown that rats injected with higher doses of propofol experienced decreased sleep latency as well as increases in NREM and total sleep time.[35] The adequacy of this sleep in humans remains an area of concern.

The critical care nurse will need to assess the patient's need for sedative and analgesic medications. The nurse has a responsibility to administer these medications in the most efficient manner to promote sleep and to monitor effectiveness. This can be achieved through assessment, including a drug history, diagnostic test results, and review of the patient's medical history. Information from that assessment will assist the nurse to formulate a nursing diagnosis with outcome criteria and interventions. Evaluation of the patient will ensure that the desired outcomes are achieved. Drugs that disrupt sleep and wakefulness are discussed in the Pharmacologic Management table.

ABNORMAL SLEEP

SLEEP PATTERN DISTURBANCE IN CRITICALLY ILL PATIENTS

Definition. Sleep disturbance in critically ill patients is defined as insufficient duration or stages of sleep that results in discomfort and interferes with quality of life. When ill, most individuals need more sleep than usual, and sleep seems to promote recovery. Studies have demonstrated that the nocturnal sleep of patients in critical care units is severely disturbed, even though many receive medications to promote sleep.[36,37] Few studies have examined the effectiveness or the side effects of sedative-hypnotics in vulnerable populations such as the elderly and critically ill. Studies in younger, healthy populations show that some sedative-hypnotics may produce disturbances in sleep architecture, diminished daytime performance, residual daytime fatigue, dependence, tolerance, and REM suppression and rebound.[30]

Etiology and Pathophysiology. Normal sleep is a period of decreased physiologic workload for the cardiovascular system. Insufficient sleep in acutely and critically ill patients has been associated with physiologic and psychologic exhaustion and may delay recovery

Pharmacologic Management: Drugs That Affect Sleep and Wakefulness

MEDICATION CLASS	DRUG	EFFECT	COMMENTS
Hypnotics[29]	Benzodiazepines	↓ SWS, ↑ TST, ↓ WASO, ↓ stage 1 sleep, mild REM suppression	↑Apnea, ↑ daytime residual sedation, mild respiratory depression, ↓ psychomotor function
Immediate-acting	Quazepam	Half-life 20-120 hr	
	Temazepam	Half-life 8-20 hr	
Long-acting	Flurazepam, HCl	Half-life 40-250 hr	
Rapid-acting	Triazolam	Half-life 2-6 hr	Rebound insomnia
	Estazolam	Half-life 8-24 hr	
	Nonbenzodiazepines	No effect on REM or SWS	
Rapid-acting	Zolpidem	Half-life 1 hr	
	Zaleplon	Half-life 1 hour	No cognitive or performance impairment; ↓ abuse potential; can be taken in middle of night
Stimulants[32]	Nicotine	↑ SL, ↓ TST, ↓ REM	
	Amphetamines	↓ REM, ↓ SWS, ↓ TST, ↑ WASO	Less daytime fatigue
Nonsympathomimetics	Xanthine derivatives: coffee, chocolate, tea; scopolamine; strychnine; pentylenetetrazol; modafinil	↓ TST, ↓ REM, ↓ SWS, ↑ SL, ↑ WASO	
Direct sympathomimetics	Isoproterenol, epinephrine, norepinephrine, phenylephrine, phenylpropanolamine, apomorphine	↑ Wake, ↑ REM onset, ↓ fatigue, ↓ sleepiness	↑ Blood pressure, ↓ heart rate
Indirect sympathomimetics	Amphetamine, methamphetamine, cocaine, piperacillin (Pipradol), methylphenidate, tyramine	↑ WASO, ↑ daytime SL, ↓ sleepiness	Narcolepsy treatment, ↑ cognitive tasks
	Pemoline		Possible liver damage
Antihypertensives[34]			
Beta antagonists	Propranolol, metoprolol	↑ Wake, TWT, SL, ↓ REM	Insomnia, nightmares
Alpha$_2$ agonists	Atenolol, clonidine	↓ REM, ↓ TST in hypertensives, ↑ TST in normal subjects	Nightmares, sedation, ↓ concentration, mental slowing
	Methyldopa	↑ REM, ↑ TST	Sedation, insomnia, nightmares
Diuretics	Hydrochlorothiazide, chlorthalidone, indapamide	No data	CNS effects unlikely
Vasodilators	Hydralazine	No data	Depression, insomnia, anxiety
Catecholamine depletors	Reserpine	↑ REM and stage shifts	
Calcium antagonists	Verapamil, nifedipine, diltiazem, amlodipine, felodipine, nisoldipine	No data	Insomnia, nightmares, depression, sedation, difficulty concentrating
Antihistamines[34]	H$_1$ antihistamines (chem. class: selective histamine H$_1$-receptor antagonist) (e.g., diphenhydramine, hydroxyzine, triprolidine)	↑ Drowsiness, ↓ SL	Impaired daytime performance

REM, Rapid eye movement; *SEM*, slow eye movement; *SL*, sleep latency; *SWS*, slow-wave sleep; *TST*, total sleep time; *TWT*, total wake time; *WASO*, wake after sleep onset.

Pharmacologic Management: Drugs That Affect Sleep and Wakefulness—cont'd

MEDICATION CLASS	DRUG	EFFECT	COMMENTS
Antihistamines —cont'd	H$_1$ antihistamines (*chem. class:* ethanolamine derivative H$_1$-receptor antagonist) (e.g., loratadine, terfenadine)	No sedation effects	
	Histamine$_2$ antagonists (e.g., cimetidine, ranitidine)	May cause insomnia or somnolence	Drowsiness in patients; renal impairment
Antidepressants[34]			
Tricyclic antidepressants	Amitriptyline, doxepin, imipramine (Trimipramine), clomipramine, desipramine, nortriptyline, protriptyline	↑ TST, ↓ wake	↓ Psychomotor and cognitive performance and daytime drowsiness
Selective serotonin reuptake inhibitors	Fluoxetine	↑ TST, ↑ wake, ↑ stage 1, ↑ SEM	Mild ↑ in psychomotor performance
	Paroxetine	↑ Wake, ↓ TST, ↑ stage 1, ↑ SL	
	Sertraline	No data	Insomnia 7%-16%
	Fluvoxamine	↓ TST, ↑ wake, ↑ stage 1, ↑ SL	
	Citalopram	No change	Insomnia, no impairment in performance
	Trazodone	Variable, may ↑ TST, ↓ SL	↓ Cognitive performance in elderly
Monoamine oxidase inhibitors	Phenelzine, tranylcypromine, moclobermide, brofaromine	↑ Daytime sleepiness because of ↓ TST, ↑ wake	Some improved psychomotor performance

from illness. These effects include mental status change, also known as *ICU (intensive care unit) psychosis.*[7] In another study, sleep debt was found to produce the following effects: decreased glucose tolerance, decreased thyrotropin concentrations, increased evening cortisol production, and increased nervous system activity.[38] A general consensus among sleep experts and researchers is that sleep deprivation results in psychologic alterations such as changes in mood and performance, fatigue, increased irritability, and feelings of persecution.

The intensification of pain related to sleep disturbance is a significant problem in acutely and critically ill patients. Sunshine et al[39] relate that a potential theory for pain alleviation from massage therapy is linked to quiet or restorative sleep. During deep sleep, somatostatin is normally released. Without this substance, pain is experienced. Substance P is released when an individual is deprived of deep sleep, and substance P is noted for causing pain. Thus when people are deprived of deep sleep, they may have less somatostatin and increased substance P, which results in greater pain, and more sleep disruption.

Sleep disturbance in critically ill patients may stem from psychologic stress associated with critical illness and the critical care environment, surgical stress, noise, interruptions for care, painful procedures or physiologic processes, excessive bright light, and muscular and joint discomfort that result from bed rest. Of 84 patients' recollections about sleep-disturbing factors in the critical care unit, the most frequently mentioned factors included an inability to get comfortable or lie comfortably (recalled by 70% of patients), inability to perform one's usual routine before going to sleep (57% of patients), anxiety (55% of patients), and pain (54% of patients).[40] The stressful nature of the critical care environment and uncertainty and worry regarding the outcomes of a critical illness may explain why some patients have such difficulty sleeping while hospitalized. These concerns are not culturally isolated. A Swedish study identified pain, anxiety, and environmental noise among factors that interfered with sleep.[41]

Another source of sleep disturbance in critically ill patients is surgical stress. A general inflammatory response caused by the heart-lung machine or the incisions, altered endocrine neuro-metabolism control, and the effects of medications such as benzodiazepines, barbiturates, scopolamine, and systemic opioids may disturb sleep.[42]

Bright nocturnal light, excessive noise, and frequent interruptions for care procedures also may disturb sleep in critically ill patients. In a study of light and sound levels and interruptions to sleep in medical and respiratory critical care units, light levels maintained a day-night rhythm, with peak levels dependent on window orientation. Peak sound levels were extremely high in all areas and exceeded recommendations of the Environmental Protection Agency as acceptable for a hospital. Patient interruptions for care procedures tended to be erratic, leaving little time for condensed sleep.[43] However, one group determined that noise and nursing interventions explained fewer than 30% of sleep interruptions.[44] Identifying additional factors that create these sleep disruptions remains an area of potential research.

In a study of the sleep of 38 male patients before and after coronary artery bypass grafting, the investigators found that there was a decrease in sleep at night, and an increase in daytime sleep in the immediate postoperative period.[45] Nocturnal sleep was reduced to a mean of 253.6 minutes, and the minutes of stages 3 and 4 NREM sleep also were decreased. However, daytime sleep increased. The total sleep time during the 24-hour period before surgery, the first 24-hour period after surgery, and the second 24-hour period after surgery was 421.1, 483.2, and 433.2 minutes, respectively. This study supports the need for daytime napping immediately after coronary artery bypass graft surgery.

Not surprisingly, mechanical ventilation, and the required care associated with it, contributes to sleep disturbances. Cooper et al[46] studied 20 subjects on mechanical ventilation classified as critically ill; based on polysomnography (PSG)-accepted criteria, none of these patients had normal sleep. Twelve did not experience sleep at all, and the remaining eight demonstrated PSG findings consistent with severely disrupted sleep. The magnitude of sleep disruption found in the latter group was similar to the excessive daytime sleepiness and cognitive impairment of patients with untreated obstructive sleep apnea. Unfortunately, additional evidence suggests that sleep disturbances associated with prolonged mechanical ventilation do not resolve with extubation and discharge.[47,48] These findings emphasize the nursing responsibility to promote and protect the sleep of patients in the critical care environment.

Assessment and Diagnosis. Assessment of the patient on admission to the critical care unit includes a description of multiple sleep-related factors: the normal sleep pattern, including awakenings, naps, normal bedtime, and waking time; customary habits that enhance sleep (e.g., number of pillows, extra blankets, bedtime rituals, and medications); any recent changes in the patient's normal sleep pattern resulting from the acute illness; recent history of difficulty falling asleep or staying asleep, snoring, gasping for breath at night, stopping breathing at night, or excessive daytime sleepiness; frequency and duration of daytime naps; and the severity, duration, and history of chronic illnesses and disturbances that may disrupt sleep, such as COPD, arthritis, nocturnal angina, reflux esophagitis, and nocturia.

The patient's psychologic response to admission to the critical care unit needs to be assessed, along with the noise level in the patient's immediate environment. The critical care nurse needs to elicit any history of snoring because of its relationship to sleep apnea and sleep disturbances. One effective way to assess the quality of the patient's sleep is for the nurse to ask the patient how his or her sleep in the hospital compares with sleep at home. Because individuals differ in their sleep behaviors and requirements, a flexible, individualized plan of care must be formulated to promote rest and sleep.

Compiling a sleep record of a patient's sleep for 48 to 72 hours may assist in assessing actual quantity of sleep in addition to assessing necessary and unnecessary awakenings. The sleep record includes the date and time, whether the patient was awake or asleep, and any procedures that necessitated waking the patient. A 24-hour flow sheet such as is common in critical care units could include an area for documentation of sleep.

Just as nurses document other data relevant to the patient's recovery, sleep periods of more than 90 minutes in duration, number and length of awakenings, and total possible sleep time should be recorded and evaluated.

Medical Management. Medical management of sleep pattern disturbance in critically ill patients consists of sedative-hypnotics. Nonbenzodiazepine short-acting hypnotics, zolpidem and zaleplon, have few side effects and little effect on sleep architecture. Because of their short half-life, they may be repeated once during the night. Although hypnotics may assist the patient to fall asleep, it is a nursing responsibility to provide an environment and care procedures that promote sleep and allow patients to stay asleep.

Nursing Management. If one of the primary causes of the sleep pattern disturbance for a patient hospitalized in the critical care unit is a state of heightened anxiety and discomfort, nursing interventions such as massage that promote relaxation and comfort may be effective. In a review of 22 articles investigating the effects of massage on relaxation, comfort, and sleep, massage consistently reduced anxiety and pain.[49] Another research-based intervention is audiotapes of ocean sounds or other relaxing auditory sounds. Williamson[50] found that an audiotape of the ocean or the rain significantly increased sleep quality in patients in a progressive care unit. Providing a relaxed, caring environment that encourages confidence in care providers may also assist the patient to relax. In addition, allowing close family members to sit quietly at the bedside while the patient rests may comfort both the family and the patient and allow the patient to rest better.

Nurses can limit interruptions for care procedures and coordinate the care among other disciplines to allow patients time for consolidated nocturnal sleep time and a daytime nap. Draperies or blinds should be opened during the day to allow patients to receive bright natural light and to help orient them to time of day, with lights dimmed at night. Noise from staff, squeaky carts, alarms, televisions, slamming doors, and ringing phones should be minimized. Offering the patient ear plugs may help decrease noise and promote sleep. Outcomes of these nursing interventions can be assessed and documented on the 24-hour flow sheet. One group reported that an enforced afternoon quiet time resulted in benefits for patients as well as the multidisciplinary team.[51]

Also, it is important for nurses to instruct patients who have had coronary artery bypass graft surgery about sleep disturbance, which commonly persists up to 1 year after the operation. In a study of the sleep patterns of 22 women over a 6-month period using a wrist-worn actigraph, sleep gradually became less fragmented and more consolidated over time.[42]

Often nurses have influence on the design of critical care units. Critical care units should be designed with private rooms and acoustical features that limit noise.

SLEEP APNEA SYNDROME

Definition, Etiology, and Pathophysiology. Sleep apnea syndrome, sometimes called *sleep-disordered breathing*, occurs when airflow is absent or reduced. Apneas during sleep can be divided into three types: (1) obstructive, (2) central, and (3) mixed. In obstructive apnea the absence of airflow is caused by an obstruction in the upper airway. Complete obstruction lasting 10 seconds or longer is referred to as an *obstructive apnea*, whereas a partial obstruction is known as a *hypopnea*. In central apnea, airflow is absent because of lack of ventilatory muscle effort. The third type of sleep apnea syndrome, mixed, occurs when a combination of both obstructive and central patterns occurs in one apneic event. An apnea-hypopnea index (the number of apneas and hypopneas per hour divided by the hours of sleep) of five or greater is diagnostic of sleep apnea syndrome.[52]

All types of sleep apnea syndrome are accompanied by arterial desaturation and potentially by hypoxemia, which may cause pulmonary vasoconstriction and an increased systemic vascular resistance. However, desaturation and hypoxemia are most severe in the obstructive type. Although the pathophysiology of obstructive sleep apnea (OSA) is unclear, hypotheses suggest that the various types of sleep apnea are all actually part of a disease continuum. Failure of the central respiratory rhythm control center to generate a stable rhythm is thought to be the basic defect responsible for sleep apnea syndrome. Cyclic oscillations occur with greater frequency at night and are further exacerbated by mouth breathing.[53]

OBSTRUCTIVE SLEEP APNEA

Definition, Etiology, and Pathophysiology. OSA syndrome occurs when at least five apnea or hypopnea events occur per hour of sleep caused by an obstruction in the upper airway. Studies show that among employed people 30 to 60 years old, at least 2% of women and 4% of men have severe OSA.[54] The incidence of OSA is believed to increase with age. Consequences include chronic hypoventilation syndrome, arousals that fragment sleep, cardiovascular changes such as hypertension, stroke, ischemic heart disease, insulin resistance, ventricular hypertrophy, and nocturnal angina.[55] Because of the cardiovascular complications and accidents caused by sleepiness, OSA is a significant condition that should be effectively evaluated.

The cause of OSA is not entirely understood; however, upper airway structure, hormonal balance, and neural control are implicated. Factors that contribute to OSA are (1) anatomic narrowing of the upper airway, (2) increased compliance of the upper airway tissue, (3) reflexes affecting upper airway caliber, and (4) pharyngeal inspiratory muscle function.[53] Computerized tomographies of awake subjects have shown that patients with OSA have narrower airways than normal subjects. The narrower the airway, the more easily it becomes obstructed.

Upper airway patency is also affected by upper airway function, which is under the control of the respiratory motor neurons. During sleep, this control varies and causes decreased neural activity, thereby narrowing the airway. This effect is especially prevalent during REM sleep when the motor neurons are hypotonic. Unstable control of the respiratory nerves of the diaphragmatic, intercostal, and upper airway muscles can cause sleep apneas.[53] Hypothyroidism can alter respiratory controls and therefore contribute to OSA. Other contributing disorders are exogenous obesity, kyphoscoliosis, and autonomic dysfunction.

The patient with OSA develops cycles of hypoxemia, hypercapnia, and acidosis with each episode of apnea until he or she is aroused and airflow resumes. Alveolar hypoventilation accompanies each episode of apnea and results in hypercapnia. Between episodes, alveolar ventilation improves so that overall there is no retention of CO_2.

With obstruction, inspiratory subatmospheric intrathoracic pressures are abnormally elevated. This leads to a tendency for airways to collapse, resulting in both hemodynamic and electrocardiographic changes. The extremely elevated pressures that occur in individuals with OSA who have apneic episodes in both REM and NREM stages cause systemic and pulmonary hypertension. Systemic pressures of 200/120 mm Hg (awake control: 130/80 mm Hg) and pulmonary artery pressures of 80/54 mm Hg (awake control: 30/20 mm Hg) have been reported.[55] Cardiac dysrhythmias associated with obstructive apnea include bradycardias, sinus arrest, and occasionally, second-degree heart blocks. After resumption of airflow, tachycardias commonly occur. Thus bradycardia-tachycardia syndrome is associated with OSA.[55]

Assessment and Diagnosis. Careful monitoring of oxygen saturation and breathing patterns can help the critical care nurse identify this syndrome and assist in its diagnosis and treatment. Patients at risk for OSA may have the following: snoring, obesity, short, thick neck circumference, cardiovascular disease, systemic hypertension, pulmonary hypertension, sleep fragmentation, gastroesophageal reflux, and an impaired quality of life. Apneas may occur in people whose throats are abnormally small or collapsible. Muscles that would normally hold the throat open relax while the patient is asleep. Snoring is caused when those soft tissues in the throat vibrate. Snoring often precedes the complaint of daytime sleepiness, and the intensity increases with weight gain and alcohol ingestion.[53]

Males with a collar size of 17 and females with a size 16 are thought to have an increased incidence of apnea. Friedman and others have shown a clinical correlation between modified Mallampiti grade (MMP), tonsil size, body mass index, and the severity of apnea. These assessments are used by anesthesiologists to determine intubation difficulty.[56]

OSAs frequently end in brief EEG arousals. Patients may experience hundreds of arousals and not even realize they awaken hundreds of times during the night. These arousals cause the patient to experience sleep fragmentation and daytime sleepiness, which can lead to irritability, poor job performance, troubled relationships, depression, and impaired quality of life.

Diagnosis of OSA syndrome is made with polysomnography, an overnight sleep study. Polysomnography is used to determine the number and length of apnea episodes and sleep stages, number of arousals, airflow, respiratory effort, and oxygen desaturation.

Medical Management. For patients with mild OSA (apnea-hypopnea index of 5 to 10), weight loss, sleeping on the side if apneas are associated with sleeping on the back, avoidance of sedative medications and alcohol before bedtime, and the avoidance of sleep deprivation may be all that is necessary. Moderate to severe levels of apnea may be treated with mechanical, surgical, or pharmacologic therapy. Treatment can vary depending on the type and severity of illness.

Continuous positive airway pressure (CPAP) via nasal mask is the treatment of choice. CPAP machines are simply pressure generators with the effective pressure being determined during the titration part of the polysomnography. This holds the airway open and prevents collapse. The patient wears a small, triangle-shaped mask over the nose. CPAP will treat not only the obstruction but also the snoring, choking, and gasping that accompanies it, as well as provide cardiovascular benefits. CPAP, although the treatment of choice, is effective only if the patient is compliant with therapy. Regular attendance at CPAP clinics can improve patient compliance.[57] When a patient cannot tolerate the continuous pressure of CPAP, bi-modal positive airway pressure (BiPAP), which provides separate pressures for inspiration and expiration, may be tried.

Dental appliances or bite blocks can be used to pull the jaw forward and open the airway. These devices must be fitted by a dentist and are not always as effective as CPAP. Various surgical treatments are available for treatment of apnea and snoring. Patients with mild OSA or snoring alone may undergo an outpatient procedure called *laser uvulopalatopharyngoplasty (LAUP)*, which uses lasers to remove excess tissue at the soft palate level. For patients who snore but do not have apnea, somnoplasty may provide relief. Somnoplasty involves inserting a small electrode into the soft palate and heating the tissue, causing the area to shrink and tighten.[58]

Uvulopalatopharyngoplasty (UPPP) was one of the earlier surgeries used to treat OSA. Essentially, a large tonsillectomy is performed and all redundant tissue is removed. Only about 50% of patients experience sleep apnea improvement.[58] Complications include speech impairment, inability to eat, hemorrhage, and infection. Although tracheostomy was the original surgery procedure used to treat OSA, it is now used only in the most severe cases of apnea that do not respond to other treatments.

Treatment of OSA with medication is usually a last resort and has proved to be very disappointing. Protriptyline has been shown to decrease apnea and reduce excessive daytime sleepiness by decreasing REM sleep apnea frequency that increases during REM sleep. Oxygen may be used to lower hypoxemia and nocturnal desaturations.

Nursing Management. The nurses' role in the management of sleep apnea includes educating the patient and family about the syndrome and the consequences of noncompliance of treatment regimens. This education may also include preoperative teaching for any surgery procedures such as UPPP. Monitoring of patients with OSA while in critical care should include assessment of the breathing patterns, hours of sleep, and pulse oximetry.

Nasal CPAP is most effective when patients are properly fitted with the nasal mask and have clear instructions regarding use. Several types and sizes of masks are available, including one type called a *nasal pillow*, which does not cover the nose but instead fits into the nostrils. If patients are admitted to the critical care unit with a history of OSA, they need to use their home CPAP mask and equipment as part of their regular sleep routine. Compliance with the CPAP system can be enhanced by the nurse. Nursing care includes ensuring proper fit of the CPAP mask, no air blowing into the patient's eyes, correct airway pressure, no pressure sores from the mask, and no gastric insufflation.

Postoperative monitoring after UPPP includes risk of aspiration, pain management, anxiety relief, patient education, and monitoring for respiratory complications, hemorrhage, infection, impaired speech, nutritional concerns, and sleep disturbance (see the Nursing Diagnoses box).

CENTRAL SLEEP APNEA

Definition, Etiology, and Pathophysiology. Central sleep apnea can be seen on polysomnography as an absence of airflow and respiratory effort for at least 10 seconds. A complete loss of electromyographic activity by the respiratory muscles would be expected since central sleep apnea is defined as a pause in respiration without ventilatory effort.[59]

A chemoreceptor sensitive to the levels of carbon dioxide resides within the brain. When these levels rise too high, ventilatory efforts are increased to blow off the excess carbon dioxide. This negative feedback loop exists to provide a homeostatic balance in the carbon dioxide and oxygen levels of the body. Whereas OSA results from an obstructed or collapsed airway, patients with central sleep apnea suffer from a lack of ventilatory effort. This can be seen in patients who suffer from cardiopulmonary disease such as COPD or heart failure, because their chemoreceptors have become adjusted to an increased carbon dioxide level. Javaheri[60] found in his study of patients with congestive heart failure that as many as 40% suffer from central sleep apnea. Central sleep apnea is therefore not a single disease, but rather a group of disorders in which breathing ceases momentarily during sleep because of the transient withdrawal of central nervous system drive to the muscles of respiration.[61] It is not uncommon for a patient who experiences central sleep apnea to also have some obstructive events.

Central sleep apnea may result from many physiologic or pathophysiologic events.[59] Possible causes of nonhypercapnic central sleep apnea include periodic breathing at high altitude, renal/metabolic disturbances, Cheyne-Stokes breathing, and idiopathic central apnea seen at sea level. Hypercapnic central sleep apnea can occur in many neuromuscular conditions such as spinal cord or brain injury, encephalitis, brain stem neoplasm or infarcts, muscular dystrophy, myasthenia gravis, bulbar poliomyelitis, and postpolio syndrome.

Assessment and Diagnosis. Clinical characteristics of hypercapnic central sleep apnea include respiratory failure, cor pulmonale, peripheral edema, polycythemia, daytime sleepiness, and snoring. Patients with nonhypercapnic central sleep apnea have clinical features very similar to those of OSA. Nonhypercapnic central sleep apnea characteristics include daytime sleepiness, insomnia or poor sleep, mild or intermittent snoring, and awakenings accompanied by choking or feeling short of breath, and frequently the patients are of normal body weight. Diagnosis is made by overnight polysomnography or sleep study, which will determine the respiratory and sleep patterns of the patient.

Medical Management. Because there are two types of central sleep apnea, there are two therapeutic approaches depending on the cause of the apnea. The hypercapnic patient who has worsening hypoventilation during sleep is best served by nocturnal ventilation. Most such patients experience some respiratory muscle failure. One treatment for the nonhypercapnic or heart failure patients is nasal CPAP, which also may provide a beneficial cardiovascular effect. Nocturnal oxygen supplementation may be effective as well. If CPAP is not tolerated, pharmacologic management may be tried. Medroxyprogesterone, a respiratory stimulant, may improve ventilation in selected patients.[59] Acetazolamide, a carbonic anhydrase inhibitor that can result in metabolic acidosis, also may decrease frequency of apneas. Several studies have reported the development of obstructive apnea in patients successfully treated for central apnea.[60]

Nursing Management. For the nurse caring for a patient with central sleep apnea, patient and family education about the patient's condition and treatment regimen can help to ensure patient compliance. The nurse needs to address any fear or anxiety about going to sleep. Nurses also need to caution patients to avoid alcohol or sedative medications. Weight loss is recommended if the patient is obese. The nurse needs to carefully monitor and assess the respiratory status of the patient. For more information, see the Clinical Application on Sleep Alterations discussed in the text and the bonus feature on the website.

NURSING DIAGNOSES

Status Post-Uvulopalatopharyngoplasty

- Risk for Aspiration risk factors: impaired laryngeal sensation or reflex; impaired laryngeal closure or elevation; decreased lower esophageal sphincter pressure
- Acute Pain related to transmission and perception of cutaneous, visceral, muscular, or ischemic impulses
- Disturbed Sleep Pattern related to fragmented sleep
- Anxiety related to threat to biologic, psychologic, and/or social integrity
- Deficient Knowledge related to lack of previous exposure to information

CLINICAL APPLICATION

Sleep Alterations

DR is a 43-year-old severely obese, self-employed man. His medical history includes excessive daytime sleepiness, hypertension, and sinus brady-tachy dysrhythmia. He received a diagnosis of obstructive sleep apnea (OSA) 2 years ago, and his health care provider prescribed nasal continuous positive airway pressure (CPAP) for use at night. However, DR has been, for the most part, noncompliant because of reported discomfort and interference with his sex life.

DR's hypertension has required increasing medication, and he has begun to develop cardiomegaly. His business suffers from his inability to stay awake and focus. His wife and he started sleeping in separate rooms because of his snoring. These circumstances have prompted DR's physician to recommend surgical correction of DR's airway. He refused to consider a tracheostomy but agreed to uvulopalatopharyngoplasty despite the 50% chance of success. He presents to critical care after surgery with an oral endotracheal tube connected to supplemental oxygen with spontaneous respiration.

1. What risk factors for OSA does DR have?
2. What factors caused the physician to recommend surgical correction for DR's OSA?
3. Does DR's history of sleep-disordered breathing affect the type of pain relief medication he should be given after surgery? Why or why not?

    DR has an uncomplicated recovery until extubation. At that time, his voice is greatly changed beyond normal intubation changes.
4. Is this an expected complication of uvulopalatopharyngoplasty? Why or why not? What are common complications of this surgery?
5. What nursing interventions are needed for DR at this time?

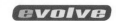 For the discussion of this Clinical Application and for an additional clinical application on sleep, see the Evolve website.

REFERENCES

1. Evans JC, French DG: Sleep and healing in intensive care settings, *DCCN* 14(4):189-199, 1995.
2. Richards KC: Effect of a back massage and relaxation intervention on sleep in critically ill patients, *Am J Crit Care* 7(4):288-299, 1998.
3. Carskadon MA, Dement WC: Normal human sleep: an overview. In Kryger MH, Roth T, Dement WC, editors: *Principles and practice of sleep medicine,* ed 3, Philadelphia, 2000, Saunders.
4. Rechtschaffen A, Kales A: *A manual of standardized terminology, techniques, and scoring system for sleep stages of human subjects,* Bethesda, Md, 1968, U.S. Department of Health, Education, and Welfare.
5. Douglas NJ: Respiratory physiology: control of ventilation. In Kryger MH, Roth T, Dement WC, editors: *Principles and practice of sleep medicine,* ed 3, Philadelphia, 2000, Saunders.
6. Davidhizar RE, Poole VL, Giger JN: What nurses need to know about sleep, *J Nurs Sci* 1:61-67, 1995.
7. Krachman SL, D'Alonzo GE, Criner GJ: Sleep in the intensive care unit, *Chest* 107(6):1713-1720, 1995.
8. Vitiello MV: Normal versus pathologic sleep changes in aging humans. In Kuna ST, editor: *Sleep and respiration in aging,* St Louis, 1991, Mosby.
9. Ancoli-Israel S et al: Identification and treatment of sleep problems in the elderly, *Sleep Med Reviews* 1:3-17, 1997.
10. Ancoli-Israel S: Sleep problems in older adults: putting myths to bed, *Geriatrics* 52(1):20-30, 1997.
11. Buysse DJ et al: Napping and 24-hour sleep/wake patterns in healthy elderly and young adults, *J Am Geriatr Soc* 40(8):779-786, 1992.
12. Bliwise DL: Normal aging. In Kryger MH, Roth T, Dement WC, editors: *Principles and practice of sleep medicine,* ed 3, Philadelphia, 2000, Saunders.
13. Bliwise DL, King AC, Harris RB: Habitual sleep durations and health in a 50-65 year old population, *J Clin Epidemiol* 47(1):35-41, 1994.
14. Sloan E, Flint A: Circadian rhythms and psychiatric disorders in the elderly, *J Geriatr Psychiatry Neurol* 9(4):164-170, 1996.
15. Zarit S, Zarit J: *Mental disorders in older adults,* New York, 1998, Guilford Press.
16. Foley DJ et al: Sleep complaints among elderly persons: an epidemiologic study of three communities, *Sleep* 18(6):425-432, 1995.
17. Richards KC: Sleep promotion, *Crit Care Nurs Clin North Am* 8(1):39-52, 1996.
18. Schwartz W: A clinician's primer on the circadian clock: its localization, function, and resetting, *Adv Intern Med* 38:81-106, 1993.
19. Carrier J et al: Amplitude reduction of the circadian temperature and sleep rhythms in the elderly, *Chronobiol Int* 13(5):373-386, 1996.
20. Haimov I, Lavie P: Potential of melatonin replacement therapy in older patients with sleep disorders, *Drugs Aging* 7(2):75-78, 1995.
21. Czeisler CA, Cajochen C: Melatonin in the regulation of sleep and circadian rhythms. In Kryger M, Roth T, Dement WC, editors: *Principles and practice of sleep medicine,* ed 3, Philadelphia, 2000, Saunders.
22. Czeisler CA, Khalsa S: The human circadian timing system and sleep-wake regulation. In Kryger M, Roth T, Dement WC, editors: *Principles and practice of sleep medicine,* ed 3, Philadelphia, 2000, Saunders.
23. Hauri P: *Sleep disorders,* Kalamazoo, Mich, 1992, Upjohn.
24. Dijk DJ, Czeisler CA: Contribution of the circadian pacemaker and the sleep homeostat to sleep propensity, sleep structure, electroencephalographic slow waves, and sleep spindle activity in humans, *J Neurosci* 15(5 Pt 1):3526-3538, 1995.

25. Borbely AA: *Sleep* homeostasis and models of sleep regulation. In Kryger M, Roth T, Dement WC, editors: *Principles and practice of sleep medicine,* ed 3, Philadelphia, 2000, Saunders.

26. Borbely AA, Achermann P: Sleep homeostasis and models of sleep regulation, *J Biol Rhythms* 14(6):557-568, 1999.

27. Kronauer RE et al: Mathematical model of the human circadian system with two interacting oscillators, *Am J Physiol* 242(1):R3-R17, 1982.

28. Nakao M et al: Dynamical features of thermoregulatory model of sleep control, *Jpn J Physiol* 45(2):311-326, 1995.

29. Henderson WB: Hypnotics: basic mechanisms and pharmacology. In Kryger M, Roth T, Dement WC, editors: *Principles and practice of sleep medicine,* ed 3, Philadelphia, 2000, Saunders.

30. Roehrs T, Roth T: Hypnotics: efficacy and adverse effects. In Kryger M, Roth T, Dement WC, editors: *Principles and practice of sleep medicine,* ed 3, Philadelphia, 2000, Saunders.

31. Koob GF: Stimulants: basic mechanisms and pharmacology. In Kryger M, Roth T, Dement WC, editors: *Principles and practice of sleep medicine,* ed 3, Philadelphia, 2000, Saunders.

32. Mitler MM: Stimulants: efficacy and adverse effects. In Kryger M, Roth T, Dement WC, editors: *Principles and practice of sleep medicine,* ed 3, Philadelphia, 2000, Saunders.

33. Ancoli-Israel S, Roth T: Characteristics of insomnia in the United States: results of the 1991 National Sleep Foundation Survey. I, *Sleep* 22(suppl 2):S347-S353, 1999.

34. Schweitzer PK: Drugs that disturb sleep and wakefulness. In Kryger M, Roth T, Dement WC, editors: *Principles and practice of sleep medicine,* ed 3, Philadelphia, 2000, Saunders.

35. Tung, A, Bluhm, B, Mendelson, WB: The hypnotic effect of propofol in the medial preoptic area of the rat, *Life Sciences* 69:855-862, 2001.

36. Edell-Gustafsson U et al: Nurses' notes on sleep patterns in patients undergoing coronary artery bypass surgery: a retrospective evaluation of patient records, *J Adv Nurs* 20(2):331-336, 1994.

37. Gabor, JY, Cooper,AB, Hanly, PJ: Sleep disruption in the intensive care unit, *Curr Opin Crit Care* 7:21-27, 2001.

38. Spiegel K, Leproult R, Van Cauter E: Impact of sleep debt on metabolic and endocrine function, *Lancet* 354:1435-1439, 1999.

39. Sunshine W et al: Massage therapy and transcutaneous electrical stimulation effects on fibromyalgia, *J Clin Rheumatol* 2:18-22, 1997.

40. Simpson T, Lee ER, Cameron C: Patients' perceptions of environmental factors that disturb sleep after cardiac surgery, *Am J Crit Care* 5(3):173-181, 1996.

41. Frisk, U, Nordstrom, G: Patients sleep in an intensive care unit—patients' and nurses' perception, *Intens Crit Care Nurs* 19:342-349, 2003.

42. Redeker NS et al: Sleep patterns in women after coronary artery bypass surgery, *Appl Nurs Res* 9(3):115-122, 1996.

43. Meyer TJ et al: Adverse environmental conditions in the respiratory and medical ICU settings, *Chest* 105(4):1211-1216, 1994.

44. Gabor, JY et al: Contribution of the intensive care unit environment to sleep disruption in mechanically ventilated patients and health subjects, *Am J Respir Crit Care Med* 167:708-715, 2003.

45. Edell-Gustafsson UM, Hetta JE: Anxiety, depression, and sleep in male patients undergoing coronary artery bypass surgery, *Scand J Caring Sci* 13(2):137-143, 1999.

46. Cooper, AB, Thornley, KS, Young, GB, et al: Sleep in critically ill patients requiring mechanical ventilation, *Chest,* 117:809-818, 2000.

47. Combes, A et al: Morbidity, mortality, and quality-of-life outcomes of patients requiring >14 days of mechanical ventilation, *Crit Care Med,* 31(5):1373-1381, 2003.

48. Chisti, A et al: Sleep-related breathing disorders following discharge from intensive care, *Int Care Med,* 26:426-433, 2000.

49. Richards KC, Gibson R, Overton-McCoy AL: Effects of massage in acute and critical care, *AACN Clin Issues* 11(1):77-96, 2000.

50. Williamson JW: The effects of ocean sounds on sleep after coronary artery bypass graft surgery, *Am J Crit Care* 1(1):91-97, 1992.

51. Lower, J, Bonsack, C, Gulon, J: High-tech high-touch: Mission possible? *Dimens Crit Care Nurs,* 21(5):201-205, 2002.

52. Kryger MH: Management of obstructive sleep apnea-hypopnea syndrome: overview. In Kryger MH, Roth T, Dement WC, editors: *Principles and practice of sleep medicine,* ed 3, Philadelphia, 2000, Saunders.

53. Hudgel DW: Mechanisms of obstructive sleep apnea, *Chest* 101(2):541-549, 1992.

54. Young T et al: The occurrence of sleep-disordered breathing among middle-age adults, *N Engl J Med* 328(17):1230-1235, 1993.

55. Weiss JW, Launois SH, Anand A: Cardiorespiratory changes in sleep-disordered breathing. In Kryger MH, Roth T, Dement WC, editors: *Principles and practice of sleep medicine,* ed 3, Philadelphia, 2000, Saunders.

56. Friedman M, Landsberg R, Caldarelli D: Clinical predicators of obstructive sleep apnea, *Sleep* 23:A268, 2000.

57. Neumeyer et al: Compliance of CPAP in patients with obstructive sleep apnea who are enrolled in a CPAP clinic, *Sleep* 23:A257, 2000.

58. Krug P: Snoring and obstructive sleep apnea, *AORN J* 69:792-797, 1999.

59. White DP: Central sleep apnea. In Kryger M, Roth T, Dement W, editors: *Principles and practice of sleep medicine,* ed 3, Philadelphia, 2000, Saunders.

60. Javaheri S: A mechanism of central sleep apnea in patients with heart failure, *N Engl J Med* 341(13):949-954, 1999.

61. Bradley T, Phillipson E: Central sleep apnea, *Clin Chest Med* 13(3):493-505, 1992.

CHAPTER 7

Nutrition Alterations and Management

NUTRIENT METABOLISM

ENERGY-YIELDING NUTRIENTS

The energy-yielding nutrients are carbohydrates, proteins, and fats. They are composed mostly of carbon, hydrogen, and oxygen. For proper metabolic functioning, adequate amounts of vitamins, electrolytes, minerals, and trace elements also must be supplied to the human body. The process by which nutrients are used at the cellular level is known as *metabolism*. The major purposes of metabolism of the energy-yielding nutrients are the production of energy and the formation and preservation of lean body mass.

Carbohydrates. Through the process of digestion, carbohydrates are broken down into glucose, fructose, and galactose. After absorption from the intestinal tract, fructose and galactose are converted to glucose, the primary form of carbohydrate used by the cells. Glucose provides the energy needed to maintain cellular functions, including transport across cell membranes, secretion of specific hormones, muscle contraction, and synthesis of new substances. Most of the energy produced from carbohydrate metabolism is used to form adenosine triphosphate (ATP), the principal form of immediately available energy within all body cells. One gram of carbohydrate provides approximately 4 kcal of energy.

One form of carbohydrate that is poorly digested by the majority of the world's adults is lactose, or milk sugar. In lactose intolerance, the individual lacks lactase, the intestinal enzyme required for digestion of lactose. Consumption of lactose causes abdominal cramping, bloating, and diarrhea. The individual with lactose intolerance may tolerate cheeses, yogurt, acidophilus milk, and buttermilk, since these products contain less lactose than unmodified milk. In addition, lactase enzyme supplements are available to be taken orally, and many markets now sell milk that has been treated with lactase.

Inside the cell, glucose is stored either as glycogen (the storage form of carbohydrate) or lipid (fat) or it is metabolized for the release of energy. Liver and muscle cells have the largest glycogen reserves. In addition to glucose obtained from glycogen, glucose can be formed from lactate,

amino acids, and glycerol. This process of manufacturing glucose from nonglucose precursors is called *gluconeogenesis*. Gluconeogenesis is carried out at all times, but it becomes especially important in maintaining a source of glucose in times of increased physiologic need and limited supply. Only the liver and, to a lesser extent, the kidney are capable of producing significant amounts of glucose for release into the blood for use by other tissues.

Proteins. Proteins are made up of chains of amino acids. Each amino acid consists of carbon, hydrogen, and oxygen, and nitrogen in the form of one or more amine groups ($-NH_2$). Amino acids are the protein components that can be used by cells.

Proteins have important structural and functional duties within the body. Proteins provide the structural basis of all lean body mass, such as the vital organs and skeletal muscle. Proteins are important for visceral (cellular) functions such as initiation of chemical reactions (hormones and enzymes), transportation of other substances (e.g., apoproteins and albumin), preservation of immune function (e.g., antibodies), and maintenance of osmotic pressure (albumin) and blood neutrality (buffers). Some amino acids are used for energy, providing approximately 4 kcal/g.

Proteins are synthesized constantly, broken down into amino acids, and then resynthesized into new protein. This three-step process is called *protein turnover*. The rate of turnover is fastest (often only a few hours) in enzymes and hormones involved in metabolic activities. In very active tissues—such as those of the liver, kidney, and gastrointestinal mucosa—protein turnover occurs every few days. If necessary, 90% of the amino acids released by tissue breakdown can be reused, with the diet providing the remaining 10% of the amino acids needed for protein synthesis. In the injured or undernourished individual, many of the amino acids released by tissue breakdown may be used for gluconeogenesis. To preserve lean body mass, adequate energy must be supplied by the diet so that most of the amino acids from the diet and from tissue breakdown can be used for tissue synthesis, rather than gluconeogenesis.

Proteins, which often consist of hundreds or even thousands of amino acids, are too large to be absorbed intact under normal circumstances. Through digestion the proteins are broken down into amino acids and dipeptides or tripeptides (composed of two or three amino acids, respectively) that can be absorbed across the intestinal wall. Certain amino acids are essential; that is, they cannot be produced by the body and must be supplied through the diet. Essential amino acids include valine, leucine, isoleucine, lysine, phenylalanine, tryptophan, threonine, and methionine, as well as histidine and arginine in infants. Other amino acids are nonessential and can be manufactured by the body under normal circumstances if the essential amino acids are in adequate supply. Some amino acids that may be nonessential in healthy adults become essential during illness. For example, histidine is an essential amino acid for adults with renal failure, and glutamine may be essential for individuals with trauma, sepsis, or other physiologic types of stress.

The amine group is essential for protein synthesis, but it is the nonamine portion of the molecule (the "keto-acid") that is used in gluconeogenesis. If a ketoacid is used for gluconeogenesis, the amine group can be excreted in the urine as ammonia or urea. Therefore if the rate of gluconeogenesis rises, urinary nitrogen excretion also rises. In assessing protein nutrition, it is common to measure nitrogen balance, or the amount of nitrogen excreted compared with that consumed. Normally most of the body's nitrogen losses are in the urine, so in determining nitrogen balance, urinary nitrogen excretion is measured (preferably over a 24-hour period). Nitrogen (protein) intake is recorded over the same time period, and losses of nitrogen from feces and other routes (e.g., sloughing of skin cells) are usually estimated.

Most healthy adults are in "nitrogen equilibrium," meaning that they excrete the same amount of nitrogen that they consume. Individuals who excrete less nitrogen than they consume are said to be in *positive nitrogen balance;* this occurs during growth, pregnancy, and healing. Individuals who excrete more nitrogen than they consume are in *negative nitrogen balance.* Negative nitrogen balance is common in the early period after trauma or surgery. When the rate of gluconeogenesis is high (as may occur in the trauma patient who is initially too unstable to be fed), extensive loss of body proteins can occur. These losses include both structural (e.g., muscle) and visceral proteins. Visceral proteins, including immunoglobulins, albumin, and complement, are critical for survival. Preservation of body protein is therefore a key goal of nutritional support of critically ill patients.

Fat (Lipids). Lipids include fatty acids, triglycerides (three fatty acids bound to a glycerol backbone), phospholipids (lipids containing phosphate groups), cholesterol, and cholesterol esters. Aside from their involvement in such functions as the maintenance of cell membranes and the manufacture of prostaglandins, lipids—primarily in the form of triglycerides—provide a stored source of energy. They are calorically dense mole-cules, providing more than twice the amount of energy per gram (9 kcal) as protein and carbohydrates.

Most dietary lipids—consisting primarily of triglycerides—are too large to be absorbed intact and are partially broken down (hydrolyzed) in the intestine to form monoglycerides and diglycerides, which contain one or two fatty acids, respectively, bound to glycerol.

Bile salts produced in the liver are detergents, and they promote the formation of micelles (emulsions of fatty acids, monoglycerides, and bile salts). Long-chain fatty acids, which contain more than 12 carbon atoms, are very insoluble in water; they are found mainly in the interior of the micelle. The external portion of the micelle (which includes the glycerol part of the triglycerides) is more water soluble than the interior portion. This allows the micelle to cross the unstirred water layer that coats the intestinal absorptive surface.

Once inside the intestinal cells, monoglycerides and long-chain fatty acids rejoin to form triglycerides, and they are surrounded by specific proteins to form chylomicrons. These chylomicrons are transported out of the intestine through the lymphatic system, finally entering the blood circulation through the thoracic duct. Some of the chylomicrons are taken up by the liver, but the majority are directly transported to other tissues. Short-chain fatty acids (less than 8 carbon atoms long) and medium-chain fatty acids (8 to 12 carbon atoms long) are more water soluble than longer fatty acids; triglycerides containing these fatty acids can be absorbed without hydrolysis and are soluble enough to be transported to the liver via the portal vein, without chylomicron formation. Short- and medium-chain fatty acids have advantages in nutritional care of patients who have insufficient bile salt formation or inadequate intestinal surface area for absorption of long-chain fatty acids.

With the aid of the enzyme lipoprotein lipase, triglyceride-containing chylomicrons are broken down outside the cell and enter the cell as fatty acids and glycerol. (Heparin stimulates lipoprotein lipase, and low doses of heparin are sometimes given to patients receiving intravenous lipid emulsions to improve lipid use.) Insulin also stimulates the cellular uptake of triglycerides. Once inside the cell, the fatty acids are either oxidized (metabolized for energy) or reformed into triglycerides for storage. During an overnight fast, prolonged starvation, or metabolic stress when the carbohydrate supply is limited, the blood glucose level declines, and consequently, insulin levels decrease. In response, a process called *lipolysis* causes the breakdown of intracellular triglycerides, which provides fatty acids for energy production and glycerol for gluconeogenesis.

The fatty acids released from adipose tissue can be used by the liver, heart, or other tissues. In the liver, fatty acids are broken down to ketones (betahydroxybutyrate, acetoacetate, and acetone). In the absence of glucose, fatty acid breakdown and ketone production are increased. Ketones can be directly oxidized by skeletal muscle and used for energy. During prolonged starvation, the brain—which normally uses glucose—converts to using ketones as its primary energy source. This is a body defense mechanism to ensure a supply of energy when carbohydrate intake is low.

Protein-Calorie Malnutrition. Malnutrition results from the lack of intake of necessary nutrients or improper absorption and distribution of them, as well as from excessive intake of some nutrients. Malnutrition can be related to any essential nutrient or nutrients, but a serious type of malnutrition found frequently among hospitalized patients is protein-calorie malnutrition (PCM). Poor intake or impaired absorption of protein and energy from carbohydrate and fat worsens the debilitation that may occur in response to critical illness. In PCM the body proteins are broken down for gluconeogenesis, reducing the supply of amino acids needed for maintenance of body proteins and healing. Malnutrition can be caused by simple starvation—the inadequate intake of nutrients (e.g., in the patient with anorexia related to cancer). It also can be the result of an injury that increases the metabolic rate beyond the supply of nutrients (hypermetabolism). In the seriously ill patient, if malnutrition occurs, usually it is the result of the combined effects of starvation and hypermetabolism.

Metabolic Response to Starvation and Stress. To understand the development of malnutrition in the hospitalized patient, the nurse must understand the metabolic response to starvation and physiologic stress. Changes in endocrine status and metabolism work together to determine the onset and extent of malnutrition. Nutritional imbalance occurs when the demand for nutrients is greater than the exogenous nutrient supply. The major difference between one who is starved and one who is starved and injured is that the latter has an increased reliance on tissue protein breakdown to provide precursors for glucose production to meet increased energy demands. Therefore, although carbohydrate and fat metabolism are also affected, the main concern is with protein metabolism and homeostasis.

During an acute, nonstressed fast, blood levels of glucose and insulin fall and glucagon levels rise. Glucagon stimulates the liver to release glucose from its glycogen reserves, which become exhausted within a few hours. Glucagon also stimulates gluconeogenesis, and skeletal muscle provides a large amount of the substrates required for gluconeogenesis. As fasting progresses, fat becomes the primary source of fuel, and consequently the blood ketone levels begin to increase. Once the circulating ketone level rises, the brain is able to use ketones for 70% of its energy, thereby decreasing the total body's reliance on glucose as an energy source. As gluconeogenesis from protein precursors decreases, protein breakdown and nitrogen excretion also slow. Some tissues—such as red blood cells, the renal medulla, and 30% of brain cells—are obligatory glucose users, and these continue to require a small amount of amino acids for gluconeogenesis. However, endogenous protein stores are "spared" from use for gluconeogenesis to a major extent, and protein homeostasis is partially restored.

Critically ill patients are at risk for a combination of starvation and the physiologic stress resulting from injury, trauma, major surgery, and/or sepsis. Starvation occurs because the person must have nothing by mouth (NPO) for surgical procedures, is unable to eat because of disease-related factors, and/or is hemodynamically too unstable to be fed. The physiologic stress causes an increased metabolic rate (hypermetabolism) that results in a rise in oxygen consumption and energy expenditure.

The hypermetabolic process results from increased catabolic hormone changes caused by the stressful event. The sympathetic nervous system is stimulated, causing the adrenal medulla to release catecholamines (epinephrine and norepinephrine). Other hormones released in response to stress include glucagon, adrenocorticotropic hormone (ACTH), and antidiuretic hormone (ADH), as well as glucocorticoids and mineralocorticoids (e.g., cortisol and aldosterone). Cytokines are peptide messengers secreted by macrophages as part of the inflammatory response and serve as hormonal regulators of the immune system. Cytokine levels increase in response to sepsis and trauma. Important cytokines include tumor necrosis factor (TNF), cachectin, interleukin-1 (IL-1), and interleukin-6 (IL-6). All of these hormonal changes cause nutrient substrates, primarily amino acids, to move from peripheral tissues (e.g., skeletal muscle) to the liver for gluconeogenesis.

Unfortunately this mobilization of substrates occurs at the expense of body tissue and function at a time when the needs for protein synthesis (e.g., for wound healing and acute phase proteins) also are high. Hyperglycemia results from the effects of increased catecholamines, glucocorticoids, and glucagon. Again, the body relies on its protein stores to provide substrates for gluconeogenesis, because glucose now becomes the major fuel source. Loss of protein results in a negative nitrogen balance and weight loss. Catabolism may be unresponsive to nutrient intake.

IMPLICATIONS OF UNDERNUTRITION FOR THE SICK OR STRESSED PATIENT

As many as 12% to 50% of hospitalized patients are at risk for malnutrition.[1-5] Although illness or injury is the major factor contributing to development of malnutrition, other possible contributing factors are lack of communication among the nurses, physicians, and dietitians responsible for the care of these patients; frequent diagnostic testing and procedures, which lead to interruption in feeding; medications and other therapies that cause anorexia, nausea, or vomiting and thus interfere with food intake; insufficient monitoring of nutrient intake;

and inadequate use of supplements, tube feedings, or total parenteral nutrition (TPN) to maintain the nutritional status of these patients.

Nutritional status tends to deteriorate during hospitalization unless appropriate nutrition support is started early and continually reassessed. Malnutrition in hospitalized patients is associated with a wide variety of adverse outcomes. Wound dehiscence, pressure ulcers, sepsis, infections, respiratory failure requiring ventilation, longer hospital stays, and death are more common among malnourished patients.[6-8] Decline in nutritional status during hospitalization is associated with higher incidences of complications, mortality, and increased length of stay and higher hospital costs.

ASSESSING NUTRITIONAL STATUS

A nutrition screening should be conducted on every patient. A brief questionnaire to be completed by the patient or significant other, the nursing admission form, or the physician's admission note usually provides enough information to determine whether the patient is at nutritional risk (Box 7-1). Any patient judged to be nutritionally at risk needs a more thorough nutrition assessment.

Nutrition assessment involves collection of four types of information: (1) anthropometric measurements, (2) biochemical (laboratory) data, (3) clinical signs (physical examination), and (4) diet and pertinent health history. This information provides a basis for (1) identifying patients who are malnourished or at risk of malnutrition, (2) determining the nutritional needs of individual patients, and (3) selecting the most appropriate methods of nutrition support for patients with or at risk of developing nutritional deficits. Nutrition support is the provision of specially formulated or delivered oral, enteral, or parenteral nutrients to maintain or restore optimal nutrition status.[9] The nutrition assessment can be performed by or under the supervision of a registered dietitian or by a nutrition care specialist (e.g., a nurse with specialized expertise in nutrition). See Fig. 7-1 to assess the route of administration of specialized nutrition support.

ANTHROPOMETRIC MEASUREMENTS

Height and current weight are essential anthropometric measurements, and they should be measured rather than obtained through patient or family report. The most important reason for obtaining anthropometric measurements is to be able to detect changes in the measurements

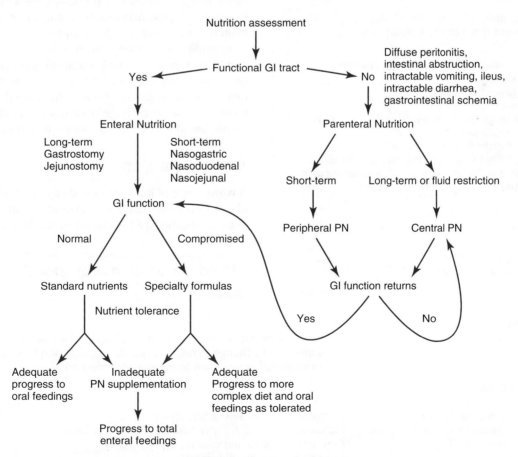

Fig. 7-1 Route of administration of specialized nutrition support. (From ASPEN, Board of Directors, and the Clinical Guidelines Task Force: Guidelines for the use of parenteral and enteral nutrition in adult and pediatric patients, *JPEN J Parenter Enter Nutr* 26[suppl 1]:8SA, 2002.)

over time (e.g., response to nutritional therapy). They are also used as an indicator of underweight or overweight. The patient's measurements may be compared with standard tables of weight-for-height or standard growth charts for infants and children. Another simple and reliable tool for interpreting appropriateness of weight for height for adults and older adolescents is the body mass index (BMI).

$$BMI = weight \div height^2$$

Weight is measured in kilograms and height in meters. A chart is available for estimating BMI and classifying it without performing any calculations (Fig. 7-2). BMI can be classified as follows: (1) underweight, less than 18.5; (2) desirable, 18.5 to 24.9; (3) overweight, 25 to 29.9; and (4) obese, 30 or greater.[10]

It may be impossible to measure the height of some patients accurately. Total height can be estimated from knee height.[11] To measure knee height, bend the knee 90 degrees and measure from the base of the heel to the anterior surface of the thigh.

For men:

$$height (cm) = 6419.0 - (0.04 \times age\ in\ years) + (2.02 \times knee\ height\ [cm])$$

For women:

$$height (cm) = 84.88 - (0.24 \times age\ in\ years) + (1.83 \times knee\ height\ [cm])$$

During critical illness, changes in anthropometric measures such as weight are more likely reflective of changes in body water and its distribution. Therefore good judgment must be used in interpreting anthropometric data. As an example, edema may mask significant weight loss or underweight. Despite these limitations, weight remains an important measure of nutritional status. Moreover, any history of recent weight change must be evaluated. A woman who was obese 4 months ago and has lost 15 kg (33 lb) since then may be at nutritional risk even if her current weight is appropriate for her height.

In addition to height and weight data, other measurements such as arm muscle circumference, skinfold thickness, and body composition (proportion of fat and lean tissue, determined by bioelectric impedance or other methods) are sometimes performed, but these measurements are of limited use in critically ill patients.[12]

BIOCHEMICAL DATA

A wide range of laboratory tests can provide information about nutritional status. Those most often used in the clinical setting are described in Table 7-1. As the table

---

Box 7-1

PATIENTS WHO ARE AT RISK FOR MALNUTRITION

ADULTS WHO EXHIBIT ANY OF THE FOLLOWING:
- Involuntary loss or gain of a significant amount of weight (>10% of usual body weight in 6 months, >5% in 1 month), even if the weight achieved by loss or gain is appropriate for height
- Weight 20% more or less than ideal body weight, or body mass index <18.5 or >25
- Chronic disease
- Chronic use of a modified diet
- Increased metabolic requirements
- Illness or surgery that may interfere with nutritional intake
- Inadequate nutrient intake for >7 days
- Regular use of three or more medications
- Poverty

INFANTS AND CHILDREN WHO EXHIBIT ANY OF THE FOLLOWING:
- Low birth weight
- Small for gestational age
- Weight loss of 10% or more
- Weight-for-length or weight-for-height <5th percentile or >95th percentile
- Increased metabolic requirements
- Impaired ability to ingest or tolerate oral feedings
- Inadequate weight gain or a significant decrease in an individual's usual growth percentile
- Poverty

Table 7-1   Common Blood and Urine Tests Used in Nutrition Assessment

Test	Comments/Limitations
SERUM PROTEINS	
Albumin or prealbumin	Levels decrease with protein deficiency but also in liver failure; albumin levels are slow to change in response to malnutrition and repletion; prealbumin levels fall in response to trauma and infection
HEMATOLOGIC VALUES	
Anemia	
Normocytic (normal MCV, MCHC)	Common with protein deficiency
Microcytic (decreased MCV, MCH, MCHC)	Indicative of iron deficiency (can be from blood loss)
Macrocytic (increased MCV)	Common in folate and vitamin B_{12} deficiency
Lymphocytopenia	Common in protein deficiency

MCH, Mean corpuscular hemoglobin; *MCHC,* mean corpuscular hemoglobin concentration; *MCV,* mean corpuscular volume.

emphasizes, no diagnostic tests for evaluation of nutrition are perfect, and care must be taken in interpreting the results of the tests.[13]

CLINICAL OR PHYSICAL MANIFESTATIONS

A thorough physical examination is an essential part of nutrition assessment. Box 7-2 lists some of the more common findings that may indicate an altered nutritional state. It is especially important for the nurse to check for signs of muscle wasting, loss of subcutaneous fat, skin or hair changes, and impairment of wound healing.

DIET AND HEALTH HISTORY

Information about dietary intake and significant variations in weight is a vital part of the history. Dietary intake can be evaluated in several ways, including a diet record, a 24-hour recall, and a diet history. The diet record, a listing of the type and amount of all foods and beverages consumed for some period (usually 3 days), is useful for evaluating the patient's intake in the critical care setting if the adequacy of intake is questionable. However, such a record reveals little about the patient's habitual intake before the illness or injury. The 24-hour

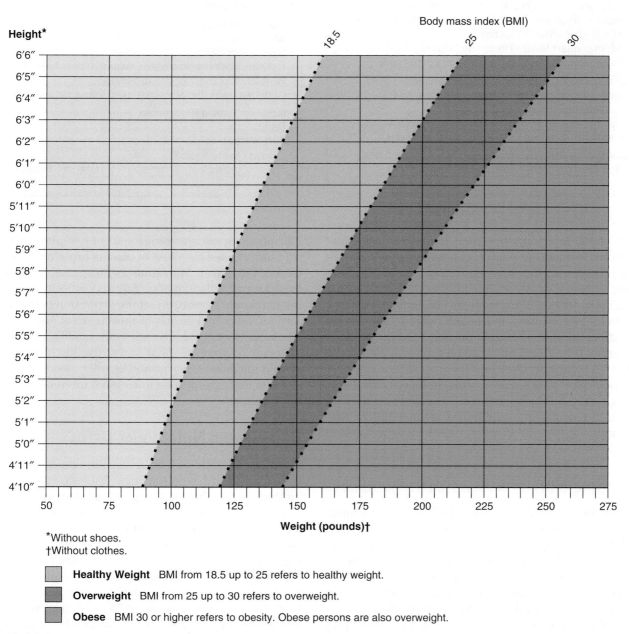

*Without shoes.
†Without clothes.

Healthy Weight BMI from 18.5 up to 25 refers to healthy weight.

Overweight BMI from 25 up to 30 refers to overweight.

Obese BMI 30 or higher refers to obesity. Obese persons are also overweight.

Fig. 7-2 Chart for estimating and categorizing body mass index (BMI). To use, find the point where body weight and height intersect. (Modified from Report of the Dietary Guidelines Advisory Committee on the dietary guidelines for Americans, Washington, DC, 2000, USDA and DHHS.)

Box 7-2

CLINICAL MANIFESTATIONS OF NUTRITIONAL ALTERATIONS

MANIFESTATIONS THAT MAY INDICATE PROTEIN-CALORIE MALNUTRITION
- Hair loss; dull, dry, brittle hair; loss of hair pigment
- Loss of subcutaneous tissue; muscle wasting
- Poor wound healing; decubitus ulcer
- Hepatomegaly
- Edema

MANIFESTATIONS OFTEN PRESENT IN VITAMIN DEFICIENCIES
- Conjunctival and corneal dryness (vitamin A)
- Dry, scaly skin; follicular hyperkeratosis, in which the skin appears to have gooseflesh continually (vitamin A)
- Gingivitis; poor wound healing (vitamin C)
- Petechiae; ecchymoses (vitamin C or K)
- Inflamed tongue, cracking at the corners of the mouth (riboflavin [vitamin B_2], niacin, folic acid, vitamin B_{12}, or other B vitamins)
- Edema; heart failure (thiamine [vitamin B_1])
- Confusion; confabulation (thiamine [vitamin B_1])

MANIFESTATIONS OFTEN PRESENT IN MINERAL DEFICIENCIES
- Blue sclerae; pale mucous membranes; spoon-shaped nails (iron)
- Hypogeusia, or poor sense of taste; dysgeusia, or bad taste; eczema; poor wound healing (zinc)

MANIFESTATIONS OFTEN OBSERVED WITH EXCESSIVE VITAMIN INTAKE
- Hair loss; dry skin; hepatomegaly (vitamin A)

Box 7-3

NUTRITION HISTORY INFORMATION

INADEQUATE INTAKE OF NUTRIENTS
Alcohol abuse
Anorexia, severe or prolonged nausea or vomiting
Confusion, coma
Poor dentition
Poverty

INADEQUATE DIGESTION OR ABSORPTION OF NUTRIENTS
Previous gastrointestinal surgeries, especially gastrectomy, jejunoileal bypass, and ileal resection
Certain medications, especially antacids and histamine H_2-receptor antagonists (reduce upper small bowel acidity), cholestyramine (binds fat-soluble nutrients), and anticonvulsants

INCREASED NUTRIENT LOSSES
Blood loss
Severe diarrhea
Fistulae, draining abscesses, wounds, decubitus ulcers
Peritoneal dialysis or hemodialysis
Corticosteroid therapy (increased tissue catabolism)

INCREASED NUTRIENT REQUIREMENTS
Fever
Surgery, trauma, burns, infection
Cancer (some types)
Physiologic demands (pregnancy, lactation, growth)

recall of all food and beverage intake is easily and quickly performed, but it too may not reflect the patient's usual intake and thus has limited usefulness. The diet history consists of a detailed interview about the patient's usual intake, along with social, familial, cultural, economic, educational, and health-related factors that may affect intake. Although the diet history is time-consuming to perform and may be too stressful for the acutely ill patient, it does provide a wealth of information about food habits over a prolonged period and also provides a basis for planning individualized nutrition education, if changes in eating habits are desirable. Other information to include in a nutrition history is listed in Box 7-3.

EVALUATING NUTRITION ASSESSMENT FINDINGS

It is rare for a patient to exhibit a lack of only one nutrient. Usually nutritional deficiencies are combined, with the patient lacking adequate amounts of protein, calories, and possibly vitamins and minerals. A common form of combined nutritional deficit among hospitalized patients is protein-caloric malnutrition (PCM). Two types of PCM are kwashiorkor and marasmus.

Kwashiorkor results in low levels of the serum proteins *albumin, transferrin,* and *prealbumin;* low total lymphocyte count; impaired immunity; loss of hair or hair pigment; edema resulting from low plasma oncotic pressure caused by a loss of plasma proteins; and an enlarged, fatty liver. Marasmus is recognizable by weight loss, loss of subcutaneous fat, and muscle wasting. In the marasmic person, creatinine excretion in the urine is low, an indication of loss of muscle mass. Because PCM weakens muscles, increases vulnerability to infection, and can prolong hospital stays, the health care team should diagnose this serious disorder as quickly as possible so that appropriate nutritional intervention can be implemented.

DETERMINING NUTRITIONAL NEEDS

A variety of methods can be used in clinical practice to estimate caloric requirements. Indirect calorimetry, a method by which energy expenditure is calculated from oxygen consumption (Vo_2) and carbon dioxide production (Vco_2), is the most accurate method for determining caloric needs.[14] Indirect calorimetry is useful in those patients suspected to have a high metabolic rate. This test can also analyze substrate use, which can be extrapolated from Vo_2 and Vco_2 during a steady state of respiration. The respiratory quotient (RQ) is equal to the Vco_2 divided by the Vo_2. Fat, protein, and carbohydrates each have a unique RQ (0.7, 0.8, and 1.0, respectively). The RQ identifies which substrate is being preferentially metabo-

Table 7-2	Estimating Energy Needs		
Category	**Description**	**Calories/kg**	**Calories/lb**
Obese	More than 40% over ideal body weight, or BMI >30	21	9.5
Sedentary	Relatively inactive individual without regular aerobic exercise; hospitalized patient without severe injury or sepsis	25-30	11-13.5
Moderate activity or injury	Individual obtaining regular aerobic exercise plus routine activities; patient with trauma or sepsis	30-35	13.5-16
Very active or severe injury	Manual laborer or athlete in very active training; patient with major burns or trauma	40	18

lized and may provide target goals for calorie replacement.[14] The test can be performed on spontaneously breathing patients as well as those who require mechanical ventilation. Some ventilators are constructed so that they can perform indirect calorimetry. However, for most patients, indirect calorimetry requires the use of a metabolic cart, which is not available in all institutions. To maintain accuracy and reliability of measurement, several testing criteria must be met.[15] In addition, information received from the metabolic cart is limited—measurements are conducted over a relatively brief period (often only 20 to 30 minutes) and may not be representative of energy expenditure over the whole day.

Calorie and protein needs of patients are often estimated using formulas that provide allowances for increased nutrient usage associated with injury and healing. Although indirect calorimetry is considered the most accurate method to determine energy expenditure, estimates using formulas have demonstrated reasonable accuracy.[16,17] Commonly used formulas can be found in the Appendix. Some "rules of thumb" are also available to provide a rough estimate of caloric needs so that nurses and other caregivers can quickly determine if patients are being seriously overfed or underfed (Table 7-2).

The goal of nutrition assessment is to obtain the most accurate estimate of nutritional requirements. Both underfeeding and overfeeding must be avoided during critical illness. Overfeeding results in excessive production of carbon dioxide, which can be a burden in the person with pulmonary compromise. In addition, overfeeding increases fat stores, which can contribute to insulin resistance and hyperglycemia. Hyperglycemia increases the risk of postoperative infections in both diabetic and nondiabetic individuals.[18-20] Therefore hyperglycemia is a complication to be avoided if at all possible.

NUTRITION AND CARDIOVASCULAR ALTERATIONS

Diet and cardiovascular disease may interact in a variety of ways. On the one hand, excessive nutrient intake—manifested by overweight or obesity and a diet rich in

Box 7-4

COMMON FINDINGS IN NUTRITION ASSESSMENT OF THE PATIENT WITH CARDIOVASCULAR DISEASE

ANTHROPOMETRIC MEASUREMENTS
Overweight or obesity; underweight (cardiac cachexia)
Abdominal fat: increased risk of cardiovascular disease with waist measurement >102 cm (>40 in) for men and >88 cm (>35 in) for women

BIOCHEMICAL (LABORATORY) DATA
Elevated total serum cholesterol, LDL cholesterol, and/or triglycerides

CLINICAL FINDINGS
Wasting of muscle and subcutaneous fat (cardiac cachexia)

DIET OR HEALTH HISTORY
Sedentary lifestyle
Excessive intake of saturated fat, cholesterol, salt, and/or alcohol
Angina, respiratory difficulty, or fatigue during eating
Medications that impair appetite (e.g., digitalis preparations, quinidine)

LDL, Low-density lipoprotein.

cholesterol and saturated fat—is a risk factor for development of arteriosclerotic heart disease. On the other hand, the consequences of chronic myocardial insufficiency can include malnutrition.

NUTRITION ASSESSMENT IN CARDIOVASCULAR ALTERATIONS

A nutrition assessment provides the nurse and other members of the health care team the information necessary to plan the patient's nutrition care and education. Common findings in the nutrition assessment of the cardiovascular patient are summarized in Box 7-4. The major nutritional concerns relate to appropriateness of body weight and the levels of serum lipids and blood pressure. Guidelines for more extensive nutrition assessment are provided on p. 100.

NUTRITION INTERVENTION AND EDUCATION IN CARDIOVASCULAR ALTERATIONS

Myocardial Infarction

Short-Term Interventions. In the early period after a myocardial infarction (MI), nutrition interventions and education are designed to reduce angina, cardiac workload, and risk of dysrhythmia. Meal size, caffeine intake, and food temperatures are some of the dietary factors that are of concern. Small, frequent snacks are preferable to larger meals for patients with severe myocardial compromise or postprandial angina.

If caffeine is included in the diet, its effects should be monitored. Because caffeine is a stimulant, it might be expected to increase heart rate and myocardial oxygen demand. In the United States and in most industrial nations, coffee is the richest source of caffeine in the diet, with about 150 mg of caffeine per 180 ml (6 fluid oz) of coffee. In comparison, the caffeine content of the same volume of tea or cola is approximately 50 mg or 20 mg, respectively. Very hot or very cold foods should be avoided as they can potentially trigger vagal or other neural input and cause cardiac dysrhythmias.

Long-Term Changes. The focus of nutritional and lifestyle interventions for the person who has had one MI or is at increased risk for heart disease are directed at primary and secondary prevention strategies. These strategies include weight reduction, if the person is overweight, and control of cholesterol, fat, and saturated fat intake. Most of the education regarding these changes will take place in the rehabilitation period. However, during the acute phase of recovery, the patient and family may have an interest in learning more about risk reduction.

For the individual who is overweight or obese, gradual loss of weight (0.45 to 0.9 kg [1 to 2 lb] per week) is the goal.[10] Weight loss can be achieved through moderate exercise (with the physician's approval) and reduction of dietary intake by 500 to 1000 kcal/day. A balanced low-fat, low-calorie diet is recommended. There is insufficient evidence to support the efficacy and safety of low-carbohydrate diets for weight loss.[21] The most recent guidelines for the National Cholesterol Education Program (NCEP) Adult Treatment Panel III (ATP III) support lipid-lowering therapy through adoption of a low saturated–fat and low-cholesterol diet, maintenance of a healthy weight, and regular physical activity.[22] New features include recommendations of low-density lipoprotein (LDL) cholesterol levels of 100 mg/dl as optimal, and increased focus on the metabolic syndrome.[23,24]

Metabolic syndrome, or insulin resistance syndrome, is associated with increased risk for cardiovascular disease and has been recognized as a secondary target of lipid-lowering therapy after LDL cholesterol reduction and recommended use of weight reduction and increased physical activity.[25]

Elevated plasma levels of homocysteine, derived from the essential amino acid *methionine*, are a risk factor for heart disease. Homocysteine can damage the endothelium of the blood vessels, cause proliferation of smooth muscle in the vessel walls, and activate platelets and the coagulation cascade, contributing to thrombus formation. Adequate amounts of folic acid (400 mcg/day or more), along with vitamins B_{12} and B_6, can reduce homocysteine levels.[26] Folic acid (also known as *folate*) is found in green, leafy vegetables and many fruits, and in fortified flour and cereals.

For hypertensive cardiac disease, sodium chloride restriction is recommended. Some individuals have been shown to be more salt-sensitive than others, and this salt sensitivity contributes to hypertension. Adoption of a healthy lifestyle is critical for the prevention of high blood pressure (BP) and is an indispensable part of the management of those with hypertension.[27] Weight loss of as little as 10 pounds reduces BP. BP is also benefited by adoption of the Dietary Approaches to Stop Hypertension (DASH)[28] eating plan, which comprises a diet rich in fruits, vegetables, and lowfat dairy products with a reduced content of dietary cholesterol as well as saturated and total fat. It is rich in potassium and calcium content. Dietary sodium should be reduced to no more than 100 mmol per day (2.4 g of sodium). Alcohol intake should be limited to no more than 1 oz (30 ml) of ethanol per day in men and no more than 0.5 oz of ethanol in women.

Heart Failure. Nutrition intervention in heart failure (HF) is designed to reduce fluid retained within the body and thus reduce the preload. Because fluid accompanies sodium, limitation of sodium is necessary to reduce fluid retention. Specific interventions include limiting salt intake, usually to 5 g a day or less, and limiting fluid intake as appropriate. If fluid is restricted, the daily fluid allowance is usually 1.5 to 2 L per day, to include both fluids in the diet and those given with medications and for other purposes (see Heart Failure in Chapter 18).

Cardiac Cachexia. Malnutrition is common in patients with HF. The term cachexia is derived from the Greek words *kakos*, meaning "bad," and *hexis*, meaning "condition." It is characterized by weight loss, anorexia, weakness, early satiety, and edema.[29] Cachexia is seen in a variety of disorders, including cancer and cardiac failure. It is well recognized as an independent predictor of higher mortality in patients with HF.[30] Sodium and fluid restriction are appropriate interventions. It is important to concentrate nutrients into as small a volume as possible and to serve small amounts frequently, rather than three large meals daily, which may overwhelm the patient. The individual should be encouraged to consume calorie-dense foods and supplements.

Because the patient is likely to tire quickly and to suffer from anorexia, enteral tube feeding may be necessary. Most commonly used tube feeding formulas provide 1 calorie per milliliter, but more concentrated products are available to provide adequate nutrients in a smaller volume. The nurse must monitor the fluid status of these patients carefully when they are receiving nutrition support. Assessing breath sounds and observing for presence and severity of peripheral edema and changes in body weight are performed daily or more frequently. A consistent weight gain of more than 0.11 to 0.22 kg (0.25 to 0.5 lb) per day usually indicates fluid retention rather than gain of fat and muscle mass.

NUTRITION AND PULMONARY ALTERATIONS

Malnutrition has extremely adverse effects on respiratory function, decreasing surfactant production, diaphragmatic mass, vital capacity, and immunocompetence. Patients with acute respiratory disorders find it difficult to consume adequate oral nutrients and can rapidly become malnourished. Individuals who have an acute illness superimposed on chronic respiratory problems are also at high risk. Nearly three fourths of patients with chronic obstructive pulmonary disease (COPD) have had weight loss.[31] Patients with undernutrition and end-stage COPD, however, often cannot tolerate the increase in metabolic demand that occurs during refeeding. In addition, they are at significant risk for development of cor pulmonale and may fail to tolerate the fluid required for delivery of enteral or parenteral nutrition support. Prevention of severe nutritional deficits, rather than correction of deficits once they have occurred, is important in nutritional management of these patients (see "Acute Respiratory Failure" and "Long-term Mechanical Ventilator Dependence" in Chapter 23).

NUTRITION ASSESSMENT IN PULMONARY ALTERATIONS

Common findings in nutrition assessment related to pulmonary alterations are summarized in Box 7-5. Guidelines for more extensive nutrition assessment are provided on p. 100. The patient with respiratory compromise is especially vulnerable to the effects of fluid volume excess and must be assessed continually for this complication, particularly during enteral and parenteral feeding.

NUTRITION INTERVENTION AND EDUCATION IN PULMONARY ALTERATIONS

Prevent or Correct Undernutrition and Underweight. The nurse and dietitian work together to encourage oral intake in the undernourished or potentially undernourished patient who is capable of eating. Small, frequent feedings are especially important, because a very full stomach can interfere with diaphragmatic movement. Mouth care should be provided before meals

and snacks to clear the palate of the taste of sputum and medications. Administering bronchodilators with food can help to reduce the gastric irritation caused by these medications.

Because of anorexia, dyspnea, debilitation, or need for ventilatory support, however, many patients will require enteral tube feeding or total parenteral nutrition (TPN). It is especially important for the nurse to be alert to the risk of pulmonary aspiration in the patient with an artificial airway. To reduce the risk of pulmonary aspiration during enteral tube feeding, keep the patient's head elevated at least 45 degrees during feedings, unless contraindicated; keep the cuff of the artificial airway inflated during feeding, if possible; monitor the patient for increasing abdominal distention; and check tube placement before each feeding (if intermittent) or at least every 4 to 8 hours if feedings are continuous.

Avoid Overfeeding. Overfeeding of total calories or of carbohydrate or lipid alone can impair pulmonary function. The production of carbon dioxide (Vco_2) increases when carbohydrate is relied on as the primary energy source. This is unlikely to be significant in the patient who is eating foods. Instead, it is an iatrogenic complication of TPN, in which glucose is often the predominant calorie source, or occasionally of tube feeding in a patient with a very high carbohydrate formula. Excessive calorie intake can raise $Paco_2$ sufficiently to make it difficult to wean a patient from the ventilator. A balanced regimen with both lipids and carbohydrates providing the nonprotein calories is optimal for the patient with respiratory compromise, and the patient needs to be reassessed continually to ensure that caloric intake is not excessive.[9]

Excessive lipid intake can impair capillary gas exchange in the lungs, although this is not usually sufficient to produce an increase in $Paco_2$ or decrease in Pao_2.[32] However, the patient with severe respiratory al-

---

BOX 7-5

COMMON FINDINGS IN NUTRITION ASSESSMENT OF THE PATIENT WITH PULMONARY DISEASE

ANTHROPOMETRIC MEASUREMENTS
Underweight

BIOCHEMICAL (LABORATORY) DATA
Elevated Pco_2 related to overfeeding

CLINICAL FINDINGS
Edema, dyspnea, signs of pulmonary edema related to fluid volume excess

DIET OR HEALTH HISTORY
Poor food intake related to dyspnea, unpleasant taste in the mouth from sputum production or bronchodilator therapy; endotracheal intubation preventing oral intake

teration may be further compromised by lipid overdose. If lipid intake is maintained at no more than 2 g/kg/day, lipid excess is rarely a problem. Serum triglyceride levels greater than 400 mg/dl may indicate inadequate lipid clearance and a need to decrease the lipid dosage.

Prevent Fluid Volume Excess. Pulmonary edema and failure of the right side of the heart, which may be precipitated by fluid volume excess, further worsen the status of the patient with respiratory compromise. Maintaining careful intake and output records allows for accurate assessment of fluid balance. Usually the patient requires no more than 35 to 40 ml/kg/day of fluid. For the patient receiving nutrition support, fluid intake can be reduced by using 20% lipid emulsions as a source of calories, by using tube feeding formulas that provide at least 2 calories/ml (the dietitian can recommend appropriate formulas), and by choosing oral supplements that are low in fluid. Some examples are cottonseed oil (Lipomul [Upjohn]), an oral lipid supplement providing 6 calories/ml, and powdered glucose polymers, which increase caloric intake without increasing volume. The nurse plays a valuable role in continually reassessing the patient's state of hydration and alerting other team members to changes that may indicate the need for an increase or decrease in fluid intake.

NUTRITION AND NEUROLOGIC ALTERATIONS

Because neurologic disorders such as stroke and closed head injury tend to be long-term problems, they necessitate good nutritional care to prevent nutritional deficits and promote well-being.

NUTRITION ASSESSMENT IN NEUROLOGIC ALTERATIONS

Nutrition-related assessment findings vary widely in the patient with neurologic alterations, depending on the type of disorder present. Some common assessment findings are listed in Box 7-6. Guidelines for more extensive nutrition assessment are provided on p. 100.

NUTRITION INTERVENTION AND EDUCATION IN NEUROLOGIC ALTERATIONS

Prevention or Correction of Nutritional Deficits

Oral Feedings. Patients with dysphagia or weakness of the swallowing musculature often experience the greatest difficulty in swallowing foods that are dry or thin liquids, such as water, that are difficult to control. For these patients, the nurse, the dietitian and the speech therapist can work together to plan suitable meals and evaluate patient acceptance and tolerance (see "Stroke" in Chapter 27).

Box 7-6

COMMON FINDINGS IN NUTRITION ASSESSMENT OF THE PATIENT WITH NEUROLOGIC ALTERATIONS

BIOCHEMICAL (LABORATORY) DATA
Hyperglycemia (with corticosteroid use)

CLINICAL FINDINGS
Wasting of muscle and subcutaneous fat related to disuse or to poor food intake

DIET OR HEALTH HISTORY
Poor food intake related to altered state of consciousness, dysphagia or other chewing or swallowing difficulties, ileus resulting from spinal cord injury or use of pentobarbital
Hypermetabolism resulting from head injury
Pressure ulcers

Soft, moist foods are usually easier to swallow than dry ones. An upright sitting position is preferable during meals, if possible, to allow gravity to facilitate effective swallowing. Water and other thin liquids may be especially difficult for the person with swallowing dysfunction to manage. Beverages may be thickened with commercial thickening products, with infant cereal, or with yogurt if the patient has difficulty swallowing thin fluids. Fruit nectars may be better tolerated than thinner juices.

The patient should not be rushed while eating because this may increase the risk of pulmonary aspiration. Providing small amounts of food at frequent intervals rather than larger amounts only at mealtimes may help the patient feel less need to hurry. Suction equipment should be kept available in case aspiration does occur. Dysphagia is frustrating and frightening for the patient and requires much understanding and patience by the family and caregivers.

Tube Feedings or TPN. Patients who are unconscious or unable to eat because of severe dysphagia, weakness, ileus, or other reasons require tube feedings or TPN. Prompt initiation of nutrition support must be a priority in the patient with neurologic impairments. Needs for protein and calories are increased by infection and fever, as may occur in the patient with encephalitis or meningitis. Needs for protein, calories, zinc, and vitamin C are increased during wound healing, as occurs in the trauma patient and the patient with pressure ulcers.

Patients with neurologic deficits have an increased risk of certain complications (particularly pulmonary aspiration) during tube feeding and therefore require especially careful nursing management. Patients of most concern are (1) those with an impaired gag reflex, such as some patients with cerebral vascular accident; (2) those with delayed gastric emptying, such as patients in the early period after spinal cord injury and patients with head injury treated with barbiturate coma; and (3) patients likely to experience seizures. To help prevent pulmonary aspiration, the patient's head is kept elevated, if not contraindicated; when elevation of the head is not possible, administering feedings with the patient in the prone or lateral position will allow free drainage of emesis from the mouth and decrease the risk of aspiration (see "Aspiration Lung Disorder" in Chapter 23).

Administering phenytoin with enteral formulas decreases the absorption of the drug and the peak serum level achieved. A problem arises when a patient is receiving continuous enteral feedings and also requires anticonvulsant therapy. One way to deal with the problem is stop the feeding for 1 to 2 hours before and after phenytoin administration.[33] Even when this practice is followed, the patient may require a higher phenytoin dosage than normal to maintain therapeutic serum concentrations. When continuous feedings are discontinued and the patient resumes eating meals or receives intermittent enteral feedings, the phenytoin dosage must be adjusted appropriately. Phenytoin levels should be monitored carefully in patients receiving enteral feedings. The infusion rate may need to be increased to account for the time that the enteral feeding is held for phenytoin administration.

Hyperglycemia is a common complication in patients receiving corticosteroids. Regular monitoring of blood glucose is an important part of care of such patients. They may require insulin to control the hyperglycemia.

Prompt use of nutrition support is especially important for patients with head injuries because head injury causes marked catabolism, even in patients who receive barbiturates, which should decrease metabolic demands. Head-injured patients rapidly exhaust glycogen stores and begin to use body proteins to meet energy needs, a process that can quickly lead to PCM. The catabolic response is partly a result of corticosteroid therapy in head-injured patients. However, the hypermetabolism and hypercatabolism are also caused by dramatic hormonal responses to this type of injury.[34] Levels of cortisol, epinephrine, and norepinephrine increase as much as 7 times normal. These hormones increase the metabolic rate and caloric demands, causing mobilization of body fat and proteins to meet the increased energy needs. Furthermore, head-injured patients undergo an inflammatory response and may be febrile, creating increased needs for protein and calories. Improvement in outcome and reduction in complications have been observed in head-injured patients who receive adequate nutrition support early in the hospital course.[34,35] (see "Traumatic Brain Injuries" in Chapter 37).

Prevention of Overweight and Obesity. Many stable patients with neurologic disorders are less active than their healthy counterparts and require fewer calories. Thus they may become overweight or obese if given normal amounts of calories for their age and gender. Within 1 or 2 months after spinal cord injury, substantial amounts of muscle atrophy and loss of body mass begin to occur as a result of denervation and disuse. Consequently, body weight and caloric needs decline. Ideal body weights for paraplegics and quadriplegics are less than those for healthy adults of the same height.[36] Stable, rehabilitating paraplegics need approximately 27.9 calories/kg/day, and quadriplegics need approximately 22.7 calories/kg/day.[36,37] Patients with dysphagia or extreme swallowing musculature weakness may rely on very soft, easy-to-chew foods that are usually more dense in calories than are bulky, high-fiber foods. Thus they also may gain unneeded weight that will hamper their care and impede mobility. For these reasons, nutrition teaching of the patient and family coping with a spinal cord injury should include instruction about prevention of undesirable weight gain. Decreased use of high-fat foods—such as shakes, ice cream, butter, margarine, and pastries—will help to reduce calorie intake. Fruits and vegetables without added fat or sauces are good choices because they are generally low in fat and supply fiber needed to help maintain regular bowel habits.

NUTRITION AND RENAL ALTERATIONS

Providing adequate nutrition care for the patient with renal disease can be extremely challenging. Although renal disturbances and their treatments can markedly increase needs for nutrients, necessary restrictions in intake of fluid, protein, phosphorus, and potassium make delivery of adequate calories, vitamins, and minerals difficult. Thorough nutrition assessment provides the basis for successful nutrition management in patients with renal disease.

NUTRITION ASSESSMENT IN RENAL ALTERATIONS

Some common assessment findings in individuals with renal disease are listed in Box 7-7. Guidelines for more extensive nutrition assessment are provided on p. 100.

NUTRITION INTERVENTION AND EDUCATION IN RENAL ALTERATIONS

Nutritional needs of patients with renal disease are complex. The goal of nutrition intervention is to balance adequate calories, protein, vitamins, and minerals, while avoiding excesses of protein, fluid, electrolytes, and other nutrients with potential toxicity.

Protein. The kidney is responsible for excreting nitrogen from amino acids or proteins in the form of urea. Thus, when urinary excretion of urea is impaired in renal failure, blood levels of urea rise. Excessive protein intake may worsen uremia. However, the patient with renal failure often has other physiologic stresses that actually increase protein/amino acid needs: losses because of dialysis, wounds, and fistulae; use of corticosteroid drugs that exert a catabolic effect; increased endogenous secretion of catecholamines, corticosteroids, and glucagon, all of which can cause or aggravate catabolism; metabolic acidosis, which stimulates protein breakdown; and catabolic conditions, such as trauma, surgery, and sepsis.[38] Therefore patients with acute renal failure need adequate amounts of protein to avoid catabolism of body tissues. Patients with acute renal failure who are malnourished should receive approximately 1.5 to 1.8 g protein/kg/day to limit catabolism.[9]

Patients with stable acute renal failure without evidence of fluid overload or electrolyte or acid-base disturbances can often be managed conservatively without dialysis. However, when renal function worsens, some form of renal replacement therapy (RRT) is required to maintain homeostasis and prevent metabolic complications. Types of RRT include peritoneal dialysis, intermittent hemodialysis, and continuous arteriovenous (A-V) hemofiltration.[38] During hemodialysis, amino acids are freely filtered and lost but proteins such as albumin and immunoglobulin are not. Both proteins and amino acids are removed during peritoneal dialysis, creating a greater nutritional requirement for protein.[39,40] Protein needs are estimated at approximately 1.1 to 1.4 g/kg/day for stable patients receiving hemodialysis or hemofiltration, and 1.2 to 1.5 g/kg/day for those receiving peritoneal dialysis.[41] Protein needs may be higher depending on the level of stress.[42]

Fluid. The patient with renal insufficiency usually does not require a fluid restriction until urine output begins to diminish. Patients receiving hemodialysis are limited to a fluid intake resulting in a gain of no more than

0.45 kg (1 lb) per day on the days between dialysis. This generally means a daily intake of 500 to 750 ml plus the volume lost in urine. With the use of continuous peritoneal dialysis, hemofiltration, or hemodialysis, the fluid intake can be liberalized.[41] This more liberal fluid allowance permits more adequate nutrient delivery, whether by oral, tube, or parenteral feedings. Enteral formulas containing 1.5 to 2 calories/ml or more provide a concentrated source of calories for tube-fed patients who require fluid restriction. Intravenous lipids, particularly 20% emulsions, can be used to supply concentrated calories for the TPN patient. Intradialytic TPN can be given during hemodialysis sessions to some malnourished patients; it supplies an additional source of nutrients at a time when the fluid can be rapidly removed in dialysis.[39]

Energy (Calories). Energy needs are not increased by renal failure, but adequate calories must be provided to avoid catabolism.[38,41] It is essential that the renal patient receive an adequate number of calories to prevent catabolism of body tissues to meet energy needs. Catabolism not only reduces the mass of muscle and other functional body tissues but also releases nitrogen that must be excreted by the kidney. Adults with renal insufficiency need about 30 to 35 calories/kg/day to prevent catabolism and ensure that all protein consumed is used for anabolism rather than to meet energy needs.[41] After renal transplantation, when the patient usually receives large doses of corticosteroids, it is especially important to ensure that caloric intake is adequate (usually 25 to 35 calories/kg/day) to prevent undue catabolism.

Glucose in the peritoneal dialysate may be a significant calorie source and a contributing factor in hypertriglyceridemia. Approximately 70% of the glucose instilled during peritoneal dialysis to serve as an osmotic agent may be absorbed, and this must be considered part of the patient's carbohydrate intake. The glucose monohydrate used in intravenous and dialysate solutions supplies 3.4 calories/g. Thus if the patient receives 4.25% glucose (4.25 g glucose/100 ml solution) in the dialysate, he or she receives the following:

$$42.5 \text{ g/L} \times 70\% \times 3.4 \text{ calories/g} = 101 \text{ calories/L of dialysate}$$

To help control hypertriglyceridemia, only about 30% to 35% of the patient's calories should come from carbohydrates, including glucose from the dialysate, with the major portion of dietary carbohydrate coming from complex carbohydrates.

Consuming at least 20 to 25 g of fiber daily can help to control triglyceride levels. Sources of dietary fiber include cooked dried beans and peas (5 to 7 g fiber/0.5 cup); cereals containing whole grains (not 100% bran); berries, apples, oranges, pears, corn, and peas (3 to 5 g/serving); whole grain breads and most fruits and vegetables other than those listed above (1 to 2 g/serving). Wheat bran is a good source of fiber (5 to 10 g/oz), but it is also a good source of phosphorus and therefore may cause renal failure to progress more rapidly. For the tube-fed patient, a formula containing dietary fiber can be chosen. To help control hypertriglyceridemia and to provide concentrated calories in minimal fluid, fat may need to supply as much as 40% of the patient's calories.

Hypercholesterolemia is commonly found in patients with renal failure, so unsaturated fats and oils (corn, soybean, sunflower, safflower, cottonseed, canola, and olive) are preferred over saturated fats (primarily from meats and dairy products), which tend to raise cholesterol levels. The necessary restriction of meat, milk, and other protein foods in the diet will help lower cholesterol and saturated fat intake. Intravenous lipids and the long-chain fats found in most commercial enteral formulas are primarily polyunsaturated. Avoiding alcohol or limiting alcohol intake to occasional small servings also helps to reduce hypertriglyceridemia.

Other Nutrients. Certain nutrients such as potassium and phosphorus are restricted because they are excreted by the kidney. The patient has no specific requirement for the fat-soluble vitamins A, E, and K, because they are not removed in appreciable amounts by dialysis and restriction generally prevents development of toxicity. Patients with ESRD may have decreased clearance of vitamin A and levels should be monitored.[9] On the other hand, needs for several water-soluble vitamins and trace minerals are increased in the dialysis patient because they are small enough to pass freely through the dialysis filter. Vitamin and minerals should be supplemented as necessary.[41]

NUTRITION AND GASTROINTESTINAL ALTERATIONS

Because the gastrointestinal (GI) tract is so inherently related to nutrition, it is not surprising that impairment of the GI tract and its accessory organs has a major impact on nutrition. Two of the most serious GI-related illnesses seen among critical care patients are hepatic failure and pancreatitis. Therefore this discussion focuses on these disorders.

NUTRITION ASSESSMENT IN GASTROINTESTINAL ALTERATIONS

Some common assessment findings in individuals with GI disease are listed in Box 7-8. Guidelines for more extensive nutrition assessment are provided on p. 100.

NUTRITION INTERVENTION AND EDUCATION IN GASTROINTESTINAL ALTERATIONS

Hepatic Failure. The liver is the most important metabolic organ and is responsible for carbohydrate, fat and protein metabolism, vitamin storage and activation, and detoxification of waste products. Hepatic failure is

---

Box 7-8

COMMON FINDINGS IN NUTRITION ASSESSMENT OF THE PATIENT WITH GASTROINTESTINAL DISEASE

ANTHROPOMETRIC MEASUREMENTS
Underweight related to malabsorption (from inadequate production of bile salts and/or pancreatic enzymes), anorexia, or poor intake (because of pain caused by eating)

BIOCHEMICAL (LABORATORY) DATA
Hypoalbuminemia (may be the result primarily of liver damage and not malnutrition)
Hypocalcemia related to steatorrhea
Hypomagnesemia related to alcohol abuse
Anemia related to blood loss from bleeding varices

CLINICAL FINDINGS
Wasting of muscle and subcutaneous fat
Confusion, confabulation, nystagmus, and/or peripheral neuropathy related to thiamine deficiency caused by alcohol abuse (Wernicke-Korsakoff syndrome)

DIET OR HEALTH HISTORY
Steatorrhea

---

associated with a wide spectrum of metabolic alterations. Because the diseased liver has impaired ability to deactivate hormones, levels of circulating glucagon, epinephrine, and cortisol are elevated. These hormones promote catabolism of body tissues and cause glycogen stores to be exhausted. Release of lipids from their storage depots is accelerated, but the liver has decreased ability to metabolize them for energy. Furthermore, inadequate production of bile salts by the liver results in malabsorption of fat from the diet. Therefore body proteins are used for energy sources, producing tissue wasting. The branched-chain amino acids (BCAAs)—leucine, isoleucine, and valine—are especially well used for energy, and their levels in the blood decline. Conversely, levels of the aromatic amino acids (AAAs)—phenylalanine, tyrosine, and tryptophan—rise as a result of tissue catabolism and impaired ability of the liver to clear them from the blood. BCAAs are not as dependent on liver metabolism as the AAAs are.[43] The AAAs are precursors for neurotransmitters within the central nervous system (serotonin and dopamine). Rising levels of AAAs cause encephalopathy by promoting synthesis of false neurotransmitters that compete with endogenous neurotransmitters. In addition, the damaged liver cannot clear ammonia from the circulation adequately, and ammonia accumulates in the brain. The ammonia may contribute to the encephalopathic symptoms and also to brain edema.[9,43]

Monitoring Fluid and Electrolyte Status. Ascites and edema occur because of a combination of factors. There is decreased colloid osmotic pressure in the plasma, because of the reduction of production of albumin and other plasma proteins by the diseased liver, increased portal pressure caused by obstruction, and renal sodium retention from secondary hyperaldosteronism. To control the fluid retention, restriction of sodium (usually 2000 mg) and fluid (1500 ml or less daily) is generally necessary, in conjunction with administration of diuretics. Patients are weighed daily to evaluate the success of treatment. Physical status and laboratory data must be closely monitored for deficiencies of potassium, phosphorus, and vitamins A, D, E, and K, and zinc.[9]

Provision of a Nutritious Diet and Evaluation of Response to Dietary Protein. PCM and nutritional deficiencies are common in hepatic failure. The causes of malnutrition are complex and usually related to decreased intake, malabsorption, maldigestion, and abnormal nutrient metabolism. Nutrition intervention is individualized and based on these metabolic changes. A diet with adequate protein helps to suppress catabolism and promote liver regeneration. Stable patients with cirrhosis usually tolerate 0.8 to 1 g protein/kg/day. Patients with severe stress or nutritional deficits have increased needs—as much as 1.2 to 2 g/kg/day.[43] Aggressive treatment with medications including lactulose, neomycin, or metronidazole is considered first-line therapy in the management of acute hepatic encephalopathy. In a minority of patients, pharmacotherapy may not be effective, and protein restriction to as little as 0.5 g/kg/day or less may be necessary for brief periods. Chronic protein restriction is not recommended as a long-term management strategy for patients with liver disease.[9,43]

Anorexia may interfere with oral intake, and the nurse may need to provide much encouragement to the patient to ensure intake of an adequate diet. Prospective calorie counts may need to be instituted to provide objective evidence of oral intake. Small, frequent feedings are usually better tolerated by the anorexic patient than are three large meals daily. Soft foods are preferred because the patient may have esophageal varices that might be irritated by high-fiber foods. If patients are unable to meet their caloric needs, they may require oral supplements or enteral feeding. Small-bore nasoenteric feeding tubes can be used safely without increasing risk of variceal bleeding.[43] TPN should be reserved only for patients who are absolutely unable to tolerate enteral feeding.[9] Diarrhea from concurrent administration of lactulose should not be confused with feeding intolerance.

A diet adequate in calories (at least 30 calories/kg daily) is provided to help prevent catabolism and to prevent the use of dietary protein for energy needs.[44] In cases of malabsorption, medium-chain triglycerides (MCTs) may be used to meet caloric needs. Pancreatic enzymes may also be considered for malabsorption problems.

BCAA-enriched products have been developed for enteral and parenteral nutrition of patients with hepatic disease. These products may be used in patients with acute hepatic encephalopathy who do not tolerate standard diets or enteral formulas, or who are unresponsive to lactulose. However, no substantial evidence exists showing BCAAs are superior to standard formulas in regards to nitrogen balance or as treatment for encephalopathy.[9,43] The patient who undergoes successful liver transplantation is usually able to tolerate a regular diet with few restrictions. Intake during the postoperative period must be adequate to support nutritional repletion and healing; 1 to 1.2 g protein/kg/day and approximately 30 calories/kg/day are usually sufficient. Immunosuppressant therapy (corticosteroids and cyclosporine or tacrolimus) contributes to glucose intolerance. Dietary measures to control glucose intolerance include (1) obtaining approximately 30% of dietary calories from fat; (2) emphasizing complex sources of carbohydrates; and (3) eating several small meals daily. Moderate exercise often helps to improve glucose tolerance.

Pancreatitis. The pancreas is an exocrine and endocrine gland required for normal digestion and metabolism of proteins, carbohydrates, and fats. Acute pancreatitis is an inflammatory process that occurs as a result of auto-digestion of the pancreas by enzymes normally secreted by that organ. Food intake stimulates pancreatic secretion and thus increases the damage to the pancreas and the pain associated with the disorder. Patients usually present with abdominal pain and tenderness and elevations of pancreatic enzymes. A mild form of acute pancreatitis occurs in 80% of patients requiring hospitalization, and severe acute pancreatitis occurs in the other 20%.[45] Patients with the mild form of acute pancreatitis do not require nutrition support and generally resume oral feeding within 7 days. Chronic pancreatitis may develop and is characterized by fibrosis of pancreatic cells. This results in loss of exocrine and endocrine function because of the destruction of acinar and islet cells. The loss of exocrine function leads to malabsorption and steatorrhea. In chronic pancreatitis, the loss of endocrine function results in impaired glucose intolerance.[45]

Prevention of Further Damage to the Pancreas and Preventing Nutritional Deficits. Effective nutritional management is a key treatment for patients with acute pancreatitis or exacerbations of chronic pancreatitis. The concern that feeding may stimulate the production of digestive enzymes and perpetuate tissue damage has led to the widespread use of TPN and bowel rest. Recent data suggest that enteral nutrition infused into the distal jejunum bypasses the stimulatory effect of feeding on pancreatic secretion and is associated with fewer infectious and metabolic complications compared to TPN.[46,47]

The results of randomized studies comparing TPN with total enteral nutrition (TEN, or enteral tube feeding) indicate that TEN is preferable to TPN in patients with severe acute pancreatitis, reducing costs and the risk of sepsis and improving clinical outcome.[46-48] Patients unable to tolerate TEN should receive TPN, and some patients may require a combination of TEN and TPN to meet nutritional requirements.[49,50] Low-fat enteral formulas and those with fat provided by MCTs are more readily absorbed than formulas that are high in long-chain triglycerides (e.g., corn or sunflower oil).

When oral intake is possible, small frequent feedings of low-fat foods are least likely to cause discomfort.[47] Alcohol intake should be avoided because it worsens the tissue damage and the pain associated with pancreatitis. Guidelines for treatment of diabetes (see following sections) are appropriate for the care of the person with glucose intolerance or diabetes related to pancreatitis.

NUTRITION AND ENDOCRINE ALTERATIONS

Endocrine alterations have far-reaching effects on all body systems, and thus they affect nutritional status in a variety of ways. One of the most common endocrine problems, both in the general population and among critically ill patients, is diabetes mellitus.

NUTRITION ASSESSMENT IN ENDOCRINE ALTERATIONS

The nutrition assessment process is summarized on p. 100. Because of the prevalence of patients with non–insulin-dependent diabetes mellitus (type 2) among the hospitalized population and the association of type 2 diabetes with overweight, the nutritional problems most commonly noted in patients with endocrine alterations are overweight and obesity. Hyperglycemia and hyperlipidemia are other common findings in the individual with diabetes.

NUTRITION INTERVENTION IN ENDOCRINE ALTERATIONS

Nutrition Support and Blood Glucose Control. Patients with insulin-dependent diabetes mellitus (type 1 diabetes) or endocrine dysfunction caused by pancreatitis often have weight loss and malnutrition as a result of tissue catabolism because they cannot use dietary carbohydrates to meet energy needs. Although patients with type 2 diabetes are more likely to be overweight than underweight, they too may become malnourished as a result of chronic or acute infections, trauma, major surgery, or other illnesses.[51] Nutrition support should not be neglected simply because a patient is obese, because PCM develops even among such patients. When a patient is not expected to be able to eat for at least 5 to 7 days or inadequate intake persists for that period, initiation of tube feedings or TPN is indicated. No disease process benefits from starvation, and development or progression of nutritional deficits may contribute to complications (e.g., pressure ulcers, pulmonary or urinary tract infections, and sepsis, which prolong hospitalization, increase the costs of care, and may even result in death).

Blood glucose control is especially important in the care of surgical patients. Poorly controlled diabetes reduces immune function by impairing granulocyte adherence, chemotaxis, and phagocytosis.[18,19] In surveys of critically ill patients undergoing a variety of elective surgeries and coronary artery surgery,[18] glucose levels of 206 to 220 mg/dl or higher during the first 24 to 36 postoperative hours were associated with higher rates of nosocomial infection than lower glucose levels.[18,52] To maintain tight control of blood glucose, glucose levels are monitored regularly, usually several times a day, until the patient is stable. Patients unable to tolerate oral diets or enteral feeding may require TPN to meet nutritional requirements during acute illness.[53] Regular insulin added to the solution is a common method of managing hyperglycemia in the patient receiving TPN. The dosage required may be larger than the patient's usual dose because some of the insulin adheres to glass bottles and plastic bags or administration sets. Multiple injections or, preferably, a continuous infusion of regular insulin may be used to maintain tight control of blood glucose in the enterally-fed patient.[54] Although further study is needed, the following glucose goals are recommended: 80 mg/dL to 120 mg/dL in critically ill patients in ICU; and 100 mg/dL to 150 mg/dL for stable patients on the wards.[53]

In patients receiving enteral tube feedings, the postpyloric route (via nasoduodenal, nasojejunal, or jejunostomy tube) may be the most effective, since gastroparesis may limit tolerance of intragastric tube feedings.[55] Postpyloric feedings are given continuously because dumping syndrome and poor absorption may occur if feedings are given rapidly into the small bowel. Continuous enteral infusions are associated with improved control of blood glucose. Fiber-enriched formulas may slow the absorption of the carbohydrate, producing a more delayed and sustained glycemic response. Most standard formulas contain balanced proportions of carbohydrate, protein and fats appropriate for diabetic patients. Specialized diabetic formulas have not shown improved outcomes compared to standard formulas.[54]

Severe Vomiting or Diarrhea in the Patient With Type 1 Diabetes Mellitus. When insulin-dependent patients experience vomiting and diarrhea severe enough to interfere significantly with oral intake or result in excessive fluid and electrolyte losses, adequate carbohydrates and fluids must be supplied. Nausea and vomiting should be treated with antiemetic medication.[55] Delayed gastric emptying is common in diabetes and may improve with administration of prokinetic agents.[55] Small amounts of food or liquids taken every 15 to 20 minutes are generally the best tolerated by the patient with nausea and vomiting. Foods and beverages containing approximately 15 g of carbohydrate include ½ cup regular gelatin, ½ cup custard, ¾ cup regular ginger ale, ½ cup regular soft drink, and ½ cup orange or apple juice. Blood glucose levels should be monitored at least every 2 to 4 hours.

NUTRITION EDUCATION IN DIABETES

Optimal control of blood glucose in both type 1 and type 2 diabetes is associated with a decreased risk of development of retinopathy, neuropathy, and other long-term complications.[51] Self-monitoring of blood glucose is essential in maintaining diabetic control, and nutrition is considered the most critical component of diabetes care in achieving blood glucose goals.[56] Meals are based on heart-healthy diet principles according to which saturated fat and cholesterol are limited and protein covers 15% to 20% of total calories. Instead of focusing on the type of carbohydrate, the emphasis is on the total amount of carbohydrate in each meal. The majority of carbohydrate foods should be whole grains, fruits, vegetables and low-fat milk; some sucrose-containing foods can be included as part of the total carbohydrate allowance.[57] Evidence-based medical nutrition therapy supports a consistent carbohydrate meal plan for diabetic patients.[20] The meal plan is based on the amount of carbohydrate that is consistent from meal to meal each day. Although exact calorie levels are not specified, a typical daily menu provides approximately 1500 to 2000 calories with a range of three to five carbohydrate foods at each meal, each containing 15 g of carbohydrate.[57]

Careful monitoring of dietary intake and blood glucose levels are essential during critical illness so nutritional needs are met and glucose control is maintained. Avoidance of overfeeding will limit hyperglycemia and associated complications. Insulin can be adjusted to maintain blood glucose control based on frequent monitoring. Intensive insulin therapy has been shown to reduce mortality in critically ill surgical patients.[18] However, it is not known whether the reduction in mortality is a result of lower blood glucose, the administration of insulin, or a combination of both. It is vital for the dietitian to work closely with the interdisciplinary team to determine feeding methods, appropriate enteral formulas, and the amounts of protein, lipid, and carbohydrate supplied in parenteral nutrition.[20]

ADMINISTERING NUTRITION SUPPORT

NURSING MANAGEMENT OF NUTRITION SUPPORT

Nutrition support is an important aspect of the care of critically ill patients. Maintenance of optimal nutritional status may prevent or reduce the complications associated with critical illness and promote positive clinical outcomes.[58] Critical care nurses play a key role in the delivery of nutrition support and must work closely with dietitians and physicians in promoting the best possible outcomes for their patients.

Nutrition support is the provision of oral, enteral, or parenteral nutrients. It is an essential adjunct in the prevention and management of malnutrition in critically ill patients.[9] The goal of nutrition support therapy is to provide enough support for body requirements, to minimize complications, and to promote rapid recovery. Critical care nurses must have a broad understanding of nutrition support—the indications as well as the prevention and management of associated complications.

Whenever possible, the enteral route is the preferred method of feeding. The proposed advantages of enteral nutrition over TPN include lower cost, better maintenance of gut integrity, and decreased infection and hospital length of stay.[9] A recent review of the literature comparing TEN and TPN indicates that enteral nutrition is indeed less expensive than TPN and is associated with lower risk of infection.[59] However, other research in a variety of patient populations found no difference in risk of infection between TEN and TPN.[60-62] The GI tract plays an important role in maintaining immunologic defenses, which is why nutrition by the enteral route is believed to be more physiologically beneficial than TPN. Some of the barriers to infection in the GI tract include neutrophils; the normal acidic gastric pH; motility, which limits GI tract colonization by pathogenic bacteria; the normal gut microflora, which inhibit growth of or destroy some pathogenic organisms; rapid desquamation and regeneration of intestinal epithelial cells; the layer of mucus secreted by GI tract cells; and bile, which detoxifies endotoxin in the intestine and also delivers immunoglobulin A (IgA) to the intestine. A second line of defense against invasion of intestinal bacteria is the gut-associated lymphoid tissue (GALT).[63] The systemic immune defenses in the GI tract are stimulated by the presence of food within the GI tract. In animal models, resting the GI tract by providing TPN contributes to "bacterial translocation," whereby bacteria normally found in the GI tract cross the intestinal barrier, are found in the regional mesenteric lymph nodes, and give rise to generalized sepsis. However, there is insufficient evidence in humans that TPN causes atrophy of the intestinal mucosa or that enteral nutrition prevents bacterial translocation.[64,65]

Oral Supplementation. Oral supplementation may be necessary for patients who can eat and have normal digestion and absorption but simply cannot consume enough regular foods to meet caloric and protein needs. Patients with mild to moderate anorexia, burns, or trauma sometimes fall into this category. To improve intake and tolerance of supplements, there are several steps for the critical care nurse to take:

1. Collaborate with the dietitian to choose appropriate products and allow the patient to participate in the selection process, if possible. Milk shakes and instant breakfast preparations are often more

palatable and economical than are commercial supplements. However, intolerance of lactose is common among adults. Furthermore, many disease processes (e.g., Crohn's disease, radiation enteritis, human immunodeficiency virus [HIV] infection, severe gastroenteritis) can cause lactose intolerance. Individuals with this problem require commercial lactose-free supplements or milk treated with lactase enzyme.

2. Serve commercial supplements well-chilled or on ice, because this improves flavor.
3. Advise patients to sip formulas slowly, consuming no more than 240 ml over 30 to 45 minutes. These products contain easily digestible carbohydrates. If formulas are consumed too quickly, rapid hydrolysis of the carbohydrate in the duodenum can contribute to dumping syndrome, characterized by abdominal cramping, weakness, tachycardia, and diarrhea.
4. Record all supplement intake separately on the intake-and-output sheet so that it can be differentiated from intake of water and other liquids.

Enteral Nutrition. Enteral nutrition or tube feedings are used for patients who have at least some digestive and absorptive capability but are unwilling or unable to consume enough by mouth. Patients with profound anorexia and those experiencing severe stress that greatly increases their nutritional needs (e.g., those with major surgery, burns, or trauma) often benefit from tube feedings. Individuals who require elemental formulas because of impaired digestion or absorption or the specialized formulas for altered metabolic conditions (Table 7-3) usually require tube feeding because the unpleasant flavors of the free amino acids, peptides, or protein hydrolysates used in these formulas are very difficult to mask.

Immune-enhancing formulas (IEFs) have emerged as a means to protect and stimulate the immune system. Some of the enterally delivered nutrients that may benefit critically ill patients include fiber, the amino acids glutamine and arginine, the omega-3 fatty acids, and the nucleotide ribonucleic acid (RNA).[66] Fiber is not digested by humans but can be metabolized by gut bacteria to yield short-chain fatty acids, the primary fuel of the colon cells. Glutamine is the major fuel of the small intestinal cells. It is considered a nonessential amino acid, but becomes "conditionally essential" in illness. It has been shown to improve mortality and infectious morbidity in critically ill patients.[67-69] Arginine is involved in protein synthesis and also is a precursor of nitric oxide, a molecule that stimulates vasodilation in the GI tract and heart and mediates hepatic protein synthesis during sepsis.[66] The omega-3, or n-3, fatty acids, derived primarily from fish oils, are involved in synthesis of eicosanoids (molecules with hormone-like activity)—prostaglandins, prostacyclin, and leukotrienes—and thus may modulate the inflammatory response.

There are a variety of commercial enteral feeding products, some of which are designed to meet the specialized needs of the critically ill. Products designed for the stressed patient with trauma or sepsis are usually rich in glutamine, arginine, branched amino acids (a major fuel source, especially for muscle), and antioxidant nutrients, such as vitamins C, E, and A and selenium.[70] The antioxidants help to reduce oxidative injury to the tissues (e.g., from reperfusion injury). Despite the fact that IEFs may reduce the incidence of infectious complications, the efficacy and safety of these formulas in critically ill patients has not yet been clearly demonstrated.[71-74]

Early enteral nutrition, administered with the first 24 to 48 hours of critical illness, has been advocated as a way to reduce septic complications and improve feeding tolerance in critically ill patients. Although studies[75] have shown a lower risk of infection and decreased length of stay with early enteral nutrition, the actual benefit of early enteral nutrition compared with enteral nutrition delayed a few days remains controversial.[9,76] Current guidelines support the initiation of nutrition support in critically ill patients who will be unable to meet their nutrient needs orally for a period of 5 to 10 days.[9] To avoid complications associated with intestinal ischemia and infarction, enteral nutrition must be initiated only after fluid resuscitation and adequate perfusion have been achieved.[77,78]

Critically ill patients may not tolerate early enteral feeding because of impaired gastric motility, ileus, or medications administered in the early phase of illness. This is particularly true for patients receiving gastric enteral feeding.[79] The assessment of enteral feeding tolerance is an important aspect of nursing care. Monitoring of gastric residual volume is a method used to assess enteral feeding tolerance. However, evidence suggests that gastric residuals are insensitive and unreliable markers of tolerance to tube feeding.[58,80] There is little evidence to support a correlation between gastric residual volumes and tolerance to feedings, gastric emptying, and potential aspiration. Except in selected high-risk patients, there is little evidence to support holding tube feedings in patients with gastric residual volumes less than 400 ml.[80] Gastric residual volume should be evaluated within the context of other gastrointestinal symptoms. Prokinetic agents, including metoclopromide and erythromycin, have been used to improve gastric motility and promote early enteral nutrition in critically ill patients.[81-83]

Enteral Feeding Access. Achievement of enteral access is the cornerstone of enteral nutrition therapy. Several techniques can be used to facilitate enteral access. These include surgical methods, bedside methods, fluoroscopy, endoscopy, air insufflation, and prokinetic agents.[9] Placement of feeding tubes beyond the stomach (postpyloric) eliminates some of the problems associated with gastric feeding intolerance. However, placement of postpyloric feeding tubes is time-consuming and may be costly. Tubes with weights on the proximal end are avail-

Table 7-3	Enteral Formulas		
Formula Type	**Nutritional Uses**	**Clinical Examples**	**Examples of Commercial Products (Manufacturer)**
FORMULAS USED WHEN GI TRACT IS FULLY FUNCTIONAL			
Polymeric (standard): Contains whole proteins (10%-15% of calories), long-chain triglycerides (25%-40% of calories), and glucose polymers or oligosaccharides (50%-60% of calories); most provide 1 calorie/ml	Inability to ingest food Inability to consume enough to meet needs	Oral or esophageal cancer Coma, stroke Anorexia resulting from chronic illness Burns or trauma	Ensure (Ross) NuBasics (Nestlé) IsoSource (Novartis) Pediasure (Ross), for children ages 1-10 Boost (Mead Johnson)
High-nitrogen: Same as polymeric except protein provides >15% of calories	Same as polymeric, plus mild catabolism and protein deficits	Trauma or burns Sepsis	IsoSource HN (Novartis) Osmolite HN (Ross) Ultracal (Mead Johnson)
Concentrated: Same as polymeric except concentrated to 2 calorie/ml	Same as polymeric, but fluid restriction needed	Heart failure Neurosurgery COPD Liver disease	Deliver 2.0 (Mead Johnson) TwoCal HN (Ross) Nutren 2.0 (Nestlé)
FORMULAS USED WHEN GI FUNCTION IS IMPAIRED			
Elemental or predigested: Contains hydrolyzed (partially digested) protein, peptides (short chains of amino acids), and/or amino acids, little fat (<10% of calories) or high MCT, and glucose polymers or oligosaccharides; most provide 1 calorie/ml	Impaired digestion and/or absorption	Short bowel syndrome Radiation enteritis Inflammatory bowel disease	Criticare HN (Mead Johnson) Vital High Nitrogen (Ross) Reabilan HN (Nestlé)
DIETS FOR SPECIFIC DISEASE STATES*			
Renal failure: Concentrated in calories; low sodium, potassium, magnesium, phosphorus, and vitamins A and D; low protein for renal insufficiency; higher protein formulas for dialyzed patients	Renal insufficiency Dialysis	Predialysis Hemodialysis or peritoneal dialysis	Suplena (Ross) Renalcal (Nestlé) Nepro (Ross) Magnacal Renal (Mead Johnson)
Hepatic failure: Enriched in BCAA; low sodium	Protein intolerance	Hepatic encephalopathy	NutriHep (Nestlé) Hepatic-Aid II (B Braun+ McGaw)
Pulmonary dysfunction: Low carbohydrate, high fat, concentrated in calories	Respiratory insufficiency	Ventilator dependence	NutriVent (Nestlé) Pulmocare (Ross)
Glucose intolerance: High fat, low carbohydrate (most contain fiber and fructose)	Glucose intolerance	Individuals with diabetes mellitus whose blood sugar is poorly controlled with standard formulas	Glucerna (Ross) Choice dm (Mead Johnson) Diabeti Source (Novartis) Glytrol (Nestlé)
Critical care, wound healing: High protein; most contain MCT to improve fat absorption; some have increased zinc and vitamin C for wound healing; some are high in antioxidants (vitamin E, β-carotene); some are enriched with arginine, glutamine, and/or omega-3 fatty acids	Critical illness	Severe trauma or burns Sepsis	Immun-Aid (B Braun+ McGaw) Impact (Novartis) Perative (Ross) Crucial (Nestlé) TraumaCal (Mead Johnson)

*These diets may be beneficial for selected patients; costs and benefits must be considered.
BCAA, Branched chain-enriched amino acid; *COPD,* chronic obstructive pulmonary disease; *GI,* gastrointestinal; *MCT,* medium-chain triglyceride.

able; these were originally designed for postpyloric feeding in the belief that that they would be more likely than unweighted tubes to pass spontaneously through the pyloric sphincter. However, randomized trials with the two types of tubes have shown that unweighted tubes are more likely to migrate through the pylorus than weighted tubes.[83a] In addition, the weights sometimes cause discomfort while being inserted through the nares. Therefore unweighted tubes may be preferable.

Once the tube is placed, correct location must be confirmed before feedings are started and regularly throughout the course of enteral feedings. Radiographs are the most accurate way of assessing tube placement, but repeated radiographs are costly and can expose the patient to excessive radiation. Once correct placement has been confirmed, marking the exit site of the tube to check for movement is helpful. Alternative methods for confirming tube placement have been researched that attempt to verify placement in the stomach or small intestine. An inexpensive and relatively accurate alternative method involves assessing the pH of fluid removed from the feeding tube; some tubes are equipped with pH monitoring systems. Assessing both the pH and the bilirubin concentration of fluid aspirated from the feeding tube is a new method for confirming tube placement.[84]

Location and Type of Feeding Tube. Decisions regarding enteral access should be determined based on gastrointestinal anatomy, gastric emptying, and aspiration risk.[9] Nasal intubation is the simplest and most commonly used route for enteral access. This method allows access to the stomach, duodenum, or jejunum. Tube enterostomy—a gastrostomy or jejunostomy—is used primarily for long-term feedings (6 to 12 weeks or more) and when obstruction makes the nasoenteral route inaccessible. Tube enterostomies may also be used for the patient who is at risk for tube dislodgment because of severe agitation or confusion. A conventional gastrostomy or jejunostomy is often performed at the time of other abdominal surgery. The percutaneous endoscopic gastrostomy (PEG) tube has become extremely popular because it can be inserted at the bedside without the use of general anesthetics. Percutaneous endoscopic jejunostomy (PEJ) tubes are also used.

Postpyloric feedings via nasoduodenal, nasojejunal, or jejunostomy tubes are commonly used when there is a high risk of pulmonary aspiration, because theoretically the pyloric sphincter provides a barrier that lessens the risk of regurgitation and aspiration.[85] However, some studies have demonstrated that gastric feeding is safe and not associated with an increased risk of aspiration.[86-88] Postpyloric feedings have an advantage over intragastric feedings for patients with delayed gastric emptying, such as those with head injury, gastroparesis associated with uremia or diabetes, or postoperative ileus. Delivery of enteral nutrition into the small bowel is associated with improved tolerance,[89] higher calorie and protein intake,[90]

and fewer gastrointestinal complications.[79] Small bowel motility returns more quickly than gastric motility after surgery, and thus it is often possible to deliver transpyloric feedings within a few hours of injury or surgery.[85] See Fig. 7-3 for location of tube feeding sites.

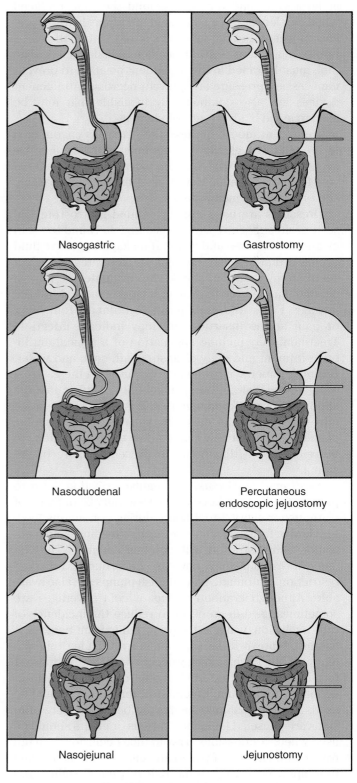

Nasogastric

Gastrostomy

Nasoduodenal

Percutaneous endoscopic jejuostomy

Nasojejunal

Jejunostomy

Fig. 7-3   Tube feeding sites.

Assessment and Prevention of Feeding Tube Complications. Nursing care of patients receiving enteral nutrition involves prevention and management of complications associated with this form of therapy. Nursing management of these problems is summarized in Table 7-4. The skin around the feeding tube should be cleaned at least daily and the tape around the tube replaced whenever loosened or soiled. Secure taping helps to prevent movement of the tube, which may irritate the nares or oral mucosa or result in accidental dislodgment. The tube must be taped in the dependent position to prevent unnecessary pressure and prevent necrosis. Attachment devices are also commercially available that may be used to avoid inadvertent dislodgment.

To prevent mouth dryness, the patient is encouraged to breathe through the nose as much as possible. Frequent mouth care will clear the palate of unpleasant flavors from the formula, as well as clean the teeth, tongue, and oral mucous membranes.

Dressings are used initially around gastrostomy insertion sites. The dressing is changed daily and the skin cleansed with soap and water. If leakage of gastric fluid occurs around a gastrostomy tube, the integrity of the gastrostomy balloon should be evaluated.[91] Karaya powder can be used to protect the peristomal skin from leakage. Fever, redness, purulent drainage, foul odor, or pain at the insertion site may indicate infection. Treatment may include application of a topical antibiotic ointment and daily cleansing with soap and water. Buried bumper syndrome may occur when the gastrostomy device disk, or bumper, is pulled tight against the abdominal wall. To prevent this, it is necessary to minimize tension on the disk. The tube may also become dislodged. If it is a new gastrostomy tube, it will need to be reinserted within hours to prevent closure of the stoma.

Feeding Tube Occlusion. Regular irrigation helps to prevent feeding tube occlusion. Generally 20 to 30 ml of warm water every 3 to 4 hours during continuous feedings and before and after intermittent feedings and medication administration will maintain patency.[9] The volume of irrigant may have to be reduced for fluid restriction. Automatic enteral flush pumps are also available. Although cranberry juice or cola beverages are sometimes used in an effort to reduce the incidence of tube occlusion, water is the preferred irrigant because it has been shown to be superior in maintaining tube patency.[92] Tube occlusion may occur as a result of stagnant formula, inadequately crushed pills, or medication interactions with formula. Enteral infusion pumps should be used, and tubes should be flushed before feeding infusions are paused. Liquid medications or elixirs should be used whenever possible to avoid tube occlusion with pill fragments. The use of pancreatic enzymes in the feeding tube appears to reduce the risk of tube clogging, and

may also be successful in removing a clog once it has formed.[92,93]

Aspiration. Pulmonary aspiration of enteral formulas and subsequent pneumonia is a serious complication of enteral feeding in critically ill patients. Risk factors for aspiration of enteral feeding include decreased level of consciousness, supine position, and swallowing disorders.[94] See Fig. 7-4 for aspiration risk factors. To reduce the risk of pulmonary aspiration of formula during enteral feeding, the nurse must keep the head of the bed elevated unless contraindicated; temporarily stop feedings when the patient must be supine for prolonged periods; position the patient in the right lateral decubitus position whenever possible to encourage gastric emptying; use postpyloric feeding methods; keep the cuff of the endotracheal tube inflated as much as possible during enteral feeding, if applicable; and be alert to any increase in abdominal distention.

Two bedside methods have been used to detect pulmonary aspiration of enteral feeding. One is the addition of blue dye to the enteral formula and observation of the patient for any dye-tinged tracheal secretions, and the other is glucose testing of tracheal secretions to detect the presence of the glucose-containing enteral formula. The glucose oxidase method may cause false-positive reactions if blood is present. It also has a low sensitivity when low-glucose formulas are used, and it also has questionable specificity.[95] There is no established protocol for blue dye testing. Although it has been used routinely in clinical practice for several years, there is no evidence to support its efficacy or safety. It lacks sensitivity and specificity in ruling out aspiration. Numerous clinical reports of systemic absorption of blue dye and adverse outcomes have been described.[96,97] Glucose oxidase testing and blue food coloring are not recommended as appropriate methods for detecting aspiration of enteral feedings.[96,98]

Gastrointestinal Complications. Diarrhea is common in patients receiving enteral nutrition, with incidence ranging from 2% to 70%.[99] It is generally defined as 3 or more liquid stools per day or at least 250 ml liquid stool collected in a rectal bag.[100] Diarrhea in enterally-fed critically ill patients has many factors. Common causes include medications, malabsorption, formula contamination, or low-fiber formulas. While the cause of diarrhea is being determined, nurses must provide adequate fluid and electrolyte replacement, maintain skin integrity, and administer antidiarrheal agents. To prevent complications, stool must be checked for infection, especially *Clostridium difficile*, before antidiarrheal drugs can be administered.[101] Constipation is a complication of enteral feeding that may result from dehydration, bedrest, opioid administration, or lack of adequate fiber in enteral formulas. Pasty stools are normal in enterally-fed patients. Bowel move-

Table 7-4	Nursing Management of Enteral Tube Feeding Complications	
Complication	**Contributing Factor(s)**	**Prevention/Correction**
Pulmonary aspiration	Feeding tube positioned in esophagus or respiratory tract	Check tube placement before intermittent feeding and every 4-6 hr during continuous feedings by checking the pH of fluid aspirated from the tube (usually gastric juice pH is <3.5).
	Regurgitation of formula	Elevate head to 45 degrees during feedings unless contraindicated; if head cannot be raised, position patient in lateral (especially right lateral, which facilitates gastric emptying) or prone position to improve drainage of vomitus from the mouth. Keep cuff of endotracheal or tracheostomy tube inflated during feedings, if possible.
		Metoclopramide may improve gastric emptying and decrease the risk of regurtation.
		Evaluate feeding tolerance every 2 hr initially, then less frequently as condition becomes stable; intolerance may be manifested by bloating, abdominal distention and pain, lack of stool and flatus, diminished or absent bowel sounds, tense abdomen, increased tympany, nausea and vomiting, residual volume >200 ml aspirated from an NG tube or >100 ml aspirated from a gastrostomy tube (but a high residual volume in the absence of other abnormal findings may not be grounds for stopping feedings); (measuring residual volumes is a controversial practice; see the section on tube occlusion that follows); if intolerance is suspected, abdominal radiographs may be done to check for distended gastric bubble, distended loops of bowel, or air/fluid levels.
Diarrhea	Medications with GI side effects (antibiotics, digitalis, laxatives, magnesium-containing antacids, quinidine, caffeine, and many others)	Evaluate the patient's medications to determine their potential for causing diarrhea, consulting the pharmacist if necessary.
	Hypertonic formula or medications (e.g., oral suspensions of antibiotics, potassium, or other electrolytes), which cause dumping syndrome	Evaluate formula administration procedures to be sure that feedings are not being given by bolus infusion; administer the formula continuously or by slow intermittent infusion.
		Dilute enteral medications well.
	Bacterial contamination of the formula	Use scrupulously clean technique in administering tube feedings; prepare formula with sterile water if there are any concerns about the safety of the water supply or if the patient is seriously immunocompromised; keep opened containers of formula refrigerated, and discard them within 24 hr; discard enteral feeding containers and administration sets every 24 hr; hang formula no more than 4-8 hr unless it comes prepackaged in sterile administration sets.
	Fecal impaction with seepage of liquid stool around the impaction	Perform a digital rectal examination to rule out impaction; see guidelines for prevention of constipation that follow.
Constipation	Low-residue formula, creating little fecal bulk	Consult with the physician regarding the possibility of using a fiber-containing formula.
Tube occlusion	Medications administered via tube (which either physically plug the tube or coagulate the formula, causing it to clog the tube)	If medications must be given by tube, avoid use of crushed tablets; consult with the pharmacist to determine whether medications can be dispensed as elixirs or suspensions; irrigate tube with water before and after administering any medication; never add any medication to the formula unless the two are known to be compatible.
	Sedimentation of formula	Irrigate tube every 4 hr during continuous feedings and after every intermittent feeding.

GI, Gastrointestinal; *NG,* nasogastric.

Continued

Table 7-4	Nursing Management of Enteral Tube Feeding Complications—cont'd	
Complication	**Contributing Factor(s)**	**Prevention/Correction**
Tube occlusion —cont'd	Aspirating gastric contents to measure residual volumes (acidified protein from the formula clots in the tube)	It has been suggested that aspiration of gastric residuals be avoided with small-bore feeding tubes (8 Fr) and that patient tolerance be assessed by physical examination; if residuals are measured, flush the tube thoroughly after returning the formula to the stomach.
Gastric retention	Delayed gastric emptying related to head trauma, sepsis, diabetic or uremic gastroparesis, electrolyte balance, or other illness	The cause must be corrected if possible; consult with the physician about use of postpyloric feedings or metoclopramide to stimulate gastric emptying; encourage patient to lie in right lateral position frequently, unless contraindicated.

Modified from Moore MC: *Pocket guide to nutritional care,* ed 4, St Louis, 2000, Mosby.

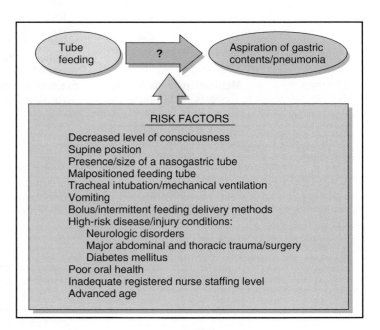

Fig. 7-4 Factors that influence aspiration. (From Proceedings from N.A. Summit on Aspiration, *JPEN* 26(6):S27, 2002.)

ments should be assessed daily. The nurse must ensure adequate fluid and fiber intake, promote optimal mobility, and administer laxatives and stool softeners as necessary.[102]

Formula Delivery. Careful attention to administration of tube feedings can prevent many complications. Very clean or aseptic technique in the handling and administration of the formula can help prevent bacterial contamination and a resultant infection. When using cans of formula transferred to a feeding container, wash hands and tops of cans before opening, hang enough formula for just 8 hours of infusion, and do not add new formula to formula already hanging. Closed systems that use a prefilled sterile container that can be spiked with the enteral tube are also available.

Tube feedings may be administered intermittently or continuously. Bolus feedings, which are intermittent feedings delivered rapidly into the stomach or small bowel, are likely to cause distention, vomiting, and dumping syndrome with diarrhea. Instead of using bolus feedings, nurses can gradually drip intermittent feedings, with each feeding lasting 20 to 30 minutes or longer, to promote optimal assimilation. The question of which feeding schedule—continuous or intermittent—is superior in critically ill patients remains unanswered.

Adequacy of Enteral Nutrition. Critically ill patients have so many needs for care that it is easy to overlook the importance of nutrition. A growing number of critical care studies have shown that critically ill patients receive considerably less enteral nutrition than required.[103-106] This is a complication unique to enteral nutrition not observed with TPN. The discrepancy in nutritional intake is due to a variety of causes including patient factors (e.g., high residual volumes, emesis, abdominal distention), tube-related factors (e.g., occlusion, malposition) and treatment-related factors (e.g., interruptions caused by procedures, airway management, and medications).[104] Inadequate enteral nutrition delivery is also related to physician-prescribing practices in the intensive care unit (ICU).[106] The enteral delivery practices in ICU and clinician concerns about aspiration may lead to inappropriate and prolonged interruptions in enteral feeding. Chest physiotherapy, suspicion of formula in the tracheobronchial secretions, and excessive gastric retention of formula are examples of appropriate reasons for stopping feedings. Enteral nutrition delivery practices that are evidence-based are necessary for optimal nutritional outcomes in critically ill patients.

Total Parenteral Nutrition. Total parenteral nutrition (TPN) refers to the delivery of all nutrients by the intravenous route. It is used when the GI tract is not functional or when nutritional needs cannot be met solely via the GI tract. Likely candidates for TPN include patients who have a severely impaired absorption (as in short bowel syndrome, collagen-vascular diseases, or radiation enteritis), intestinal obstruction, peritonitis, or prolonged ileus. In addition, some postoperative, trauma, or burn patients may need TPN to supplement the nutrient intake that they are able to tolerate via the enteral route.

Types of Parenteral Nutrition. TPN involves administration of highly concentrated dextrose that ranges from 25% to 70%, providing a rich source of calories. Such highly concentrated dextrose solutions are hyperosmolar, as much as 1800 mOsm/L, and therefore must be delivered through a central vein.[107] Peripheral parenteral nutrition (PPN) has a glucose concentration of 5% to10% and may be delivered safely through a peripheral vein. PPN solution delivers nutrition support in a large volume that cannot be tolerated by patients who require fluid restriction. It provides short-term nutrition support for a few days to less than 2 weeks.

Regardless of the route of administration, both PPN and TPN provide glucose, fat, protein, electrolytes, vitamins, and trace elements. Although dextrose–amino acid solutions are commonly thought of as good growth media for microorganisms, they actually suppress the growth of most organisms usually associated with catheter-related sepsis, except yeasts. However, because the many manipulations required to prepare solutions increase the possibility of contamination, TPN solutions are best used with caution. They should be prepared under laminar flow conditions in the pharmacy, with avoidance of additions on the nursing unit. Solution containers need to be inspected for cracks or leaks before hanging, and solutions must be discarded within 24 hours of hanging. An in-line 0.22 μm filter, which eliminates all microorganisms but not endotoxins, may be used in administration of solutions. Use of the filter, however, cannot be substituted for good aseptic technique.

Nursing Management of Potential Complications. Nursing management of the patient receiving TPN includes catheter care, administration of solutions, prevention or correction of complications, and evaluation of patient responses to intravenous (IV) feedings. Refer to Table 7-5 for nursing management of TPN complications. Evaluation of patient response is discussed later in this chapter.

Because TPN requires an indwelling catheter in a central vein, it carries an increased risk of sepsis as well as potential insertion-related complications such as pneumothorax and hemothorax. Air embolism is also more likely with central vein TPN. Patients requiring multiple IV therapies and frequent blood sampling usually have multilumen central venous catheters, and TPN is often infused via these catheters.

Some clinical studies have reported that catheter-related sepsis is higher with multilumen catheters; others have found no difference compared with single-lumen catheters.[108] Clearly patients requiring multilumen catheters are likely to be very ill and immunocompromised, and scrupulous aseptic technique is essential in maintaining multilumen catheters. The manipulation involved in frequent changes of IV fluid and obtaining blood specimens through these catheters increases the risk of catheter contamination. Peripherally inserted central catheters (PICCs) allow central venous access through long catheters inserted in peripheral sites. This reduces the risk of complications associated with percutaneous cannulation of the subclavian vein and provides an alternative to PPN.[109]

The indwelling central venous catheter provides an excellent nidus for infection. Catheter-related infections arise from endogenous skin flora, contamination of the catheter hub, seeding of the catheter by organisms carried in the bloodstream from another site, or contamination of the infusate. Good hand washing and scrupulous aseptic technique in all aspects of catheter care and TPN delivery are the primary steps for prevention of catheter-related infections. Other measures to reduce the incidence of catheter-related infections include using maximal barrier precautions (i.e., cap, mask, sterile gloves, sterile drape) at the time of insertion, tunneling the catheter underneath the skin, use of a 2% chlorhexidine

Table 7-5	Nursing Management of TPN Complications	
Complication	**Clinical Manifestations**	**Prevention/Correction**
Catheter-related sepsis	Fever, chills, glucose intolerance, positive blood culture	Use aseptic technique when handling catheter, IV tubing, and TPN solutions; hang a bottle of TPN no longer than 24 hr, lipid emulsion no longer than 12-24 hr; use an in-line 0.22 μm filter with TPN to remove microorganisms; avoid drawing blood, infusing blood or blood products, piggybacking other IV solutions into TPN IV tubing, or attaching manometers or transducers via the TPN infusion line, if at all possible. If catheter-related sepsis is suspected, remove catheter or assist in changing the catheter over a guidewire and administer antibiotics as ordered.
Air embolism	Dyspnea, cyanosis, apnea, tachycardia, hypotension, "millwheel" heart murmur; mortality estimated at 50% (depends on quantity of air entering)	Use Luer-Lok connections; use an in-line air-eliminating filter; have patient perform Valsalva maneuver during tubing changes; if the patient is on a ventilator, change tubing quickly at end expiration; maintain occlusive dressing over catheter site for at least 24 hr after removing catheter to prevent air entry through catheter tract. If air embolism is suspected, place patient in left lateral decubitus and Trendelenburg positions (to trap air in the apex of the right ventricle, away from the outflow tract) and administer oxygen and CPR as needed; immediately notify physician, who may attempt to aspirate air from the heart.
Pneumothorax	Chest pain, dyspnea, hypoxemia, hypotension, radiographic evidence, needle aspiration of air from pleural space	Thoroughly explain catheter insertion procedure to patient, because when a patient moves or breathes erratically he or she is more likely to sustain pleural damage; perform x-ray examination after insertion or insertion attempt. If pneumothorax is suspected, assist with needle aspiration or chest tube insertion, if necessary.
Central venous thrombosis	Edema of neck, shoulder, and arm on same side as catheter; development of collateral circulation on chest; pain in insertion site; drainage of TPN from the insertion site; positive findings on venogram	Follow measures to prevent sepsis; repeated or traumatic catheterizations are most likely to result in thrombosis. If thrombosis is confirmed, remove catheter and administer anticoagulants and antibiotics as ordered.
Catheter occlusion or semiocclusion	No flow or a sluggish flow through the catheter	If infusion is stopped temporarily, flush catheter with saline or heparinized saline. If catheter appears to be occluded, attempt to aspirate the clot; if this is ineffective, physician may order thrombolytic agent such as streptokinase, alteplase (t-PA) instilled in the catheter.
Hypoglycemia	Diaphoresis, shakiness, confusion, loss of consciousness	Infuse TPN within 10% of ordered rate; monitor blood glucose until stable after discontinuance of TPN. If hypoglycemia is present, administer oral carbohydrate; if the patient is unconscious or oral intake is contraindicated, the physician may order a bolus of IV dextrose.
Hyperglycemia	Thirst, headache, lethargy, increased urinary output	Administer TPN within 10% of ordered rate; monitor blood glucose level at least daily until stable; the patient may require insulin added to the TPN if hyperglycemia is persistent; sudden appearance of hyperglycemia in a patient who was previously tolerating the same glucose load may indicate onset of sepsis.

Modified from Moore MC: *Pocket guide to nutritional care,* ed 4, St Louis, 2000, Mosby.
CPR, Cardiopulmonary resuscitation; *IV,* intravenous; *TPN,* Total parenteral nutrition.

preparation for skin cleansing; no routine replacement of the central venous catheter for prevention of infection; and use of antiseptic/antibiotic-impregnated central venous catheters.[110]

Metabolic complications associated with parenteral nutrition include glucose intolerance and electrolyte imbalance. Slow advancement of the rate of TPN (25 ml/hr) to goal rate will allow pancreatic adjustment to the dextrose load. Capillary blood glucose should be monitored every 4 to 6 hours. Insulin can be added to the TPN solution or can be infused as a separate drip to control glucose levels. Rapid cessation of TPN may not lead to hypoglycemia; however, tapering the infusion over 2 to 4 hours is recommended.[111]

Serum electrolytes are obtained upon starting TPN. During critical illness, levels should be monitored and corrected daily, and then weekly or twice weekly once the patient is more stable. The refeeding syndrome is a potentially lethal condition characterized by generalized fluid and electrolyte imbalance. It occurs as a potential complication after initiation of oral, enteral, or parenteral nutrition in malnourished patients. During chronic starvation, several compensatory metabolic changes occur. The reintroduction of carbohydrates and amino acids leads to increased insulin production. This creates an anabolic environment that increases intracellular demand for phosphorus, potassium, magnesium, vitamins, and minerals.[112] These metabolic demands result in severe shifts from the extracellular compartment. Increased insulin levels also result in fluid retention. Severe hypophosphatemia, hypokalemia, and hypomagnesemia result in altered cardiac, gastrointestinal, and neurologic function. In particular, hypophosphatemia causes a decrease in 2,3-diphosphosoglycerate (2,3 DPG) and also limits the many reactions that require ATP. As a result, hypophosphatemia and other electrolyte deficiencies may lead to respiratory failure, congestive heart failure, and dysrythmias.

It is important to anticipate refeeding syndrome in patients who may be at risk. Patients with chronic malnutrition or underfeeding, chronic alcoholism, or anorexia nervosa or those maintained NPO for several days with evidence of stress are at risk for refeeding syndrome.[113] In high-risk patients, nutrition support should be started cautiously at 25% to 50% of required calories and slowly advanced over 3 to 4 days as tolerated. Close monitoring of serum electrolytes before and during feeding is essential. Normal values do not always reflect total body stores. Correction of preexisting electrolyte imbalances are necessary prior to initiation of feeding. Continued monitoring as well as supplementation with electrolytes and vitamins is necessary throughout the first week of nutrition support.[113]

Lipid Emulsion. Lipids or fat emulsions provide calories for energy and prevent essential fatty acid depletion. In contrast to dextrose–amino acid solutions, IV lipid emulsions provide a rich environment for the growth of bacteria and fungi including *Candida albicans*. Furthermore, lipid emulsions cannot be filtered through an in-line 0.22 μm filter, because some particles in the emulsions have larger diameters than this. Lipids may be infused into the TPN line downstream from the filter. No other drugs should be infused into a line containing lipids or TPN. Lipid emulsions are handled with strict asepsis, and they must be discarded within 12 to 24 hours of hanging. There is a trend toward mixing lipid emulsions with dextrose–amino acid TPN solutions; these are called 3-in-1 solutions or total nutrient admixtures (TNA). Consolidating the nutrients in one container is more economical and saves nursing time, although TNA solutions may be less stable.[107]

EVALUATING RESPONSE TO NUTRITION SUPPORT

A multidisciplinary approach is required in evaluating the effects of nutrition support on clinical outcomes. Assessment of response to nutrition support is an ongoing process that involves anthropometric measurements, physical examination, and biochemical evaluation. Daily monitoring of nutritional intake is an important aspect of critical care and is a key element in preventing problems associated with underfeeding and overfeeding. Daily weights and the maintenance of accurate intake-and-output records are crucial for evaluating nutritional progress and the state of hydration in the patient receiving nutrition support. Serum levels of electrolytes, calcium, phosphorus, and magnesium serve as a guide to the amount of these nutrients that has to be supplied; blood urea nitrogen and creatinine levels reflect the adequacy of renal function to handle nutrition support; blood glucose is an indicator of the patient's tolerance of the carbohydrate; prealbumin is an indicator of the adequacy of nutrition support; and serum triglyceride concentrations (in patients receiving intravenous lipid emulsions) reflect the ability of the tissues to metabolize the lipids. It is within the scope of practice for critical care nurses to calculate caloric requirements and analyze daily caloric delivery, advocate for early nutrition support, and minimize feeding interruptions through careful patient assessment and interruption analysis. In addition to monitoring changes in weight and laboratory values, the nurse is the health care team member who has the most constant contact with the patient; therefore he or she is uniquely qualified to evaluate feeding tolerance and adequacy of delivery. For additional information, see the Clinical Application feature on Nutrition Concepts in the text and the bonus feature on the website.

CLINICAL APPLICATION

Nutrition Concepts

Bill R. is a 28-year-old man brought to the emergency department after an accident in which his motorcycle hit a road sign. On arrival, Bill is alert and communicative, but his skin is cool and clammy. Bruising is evident over the upper abdomen, and Bill complains of pain in the left upper quadrant. Admission vital signs are the following: blood pressure 80/52, heart rate 132, respiratory rate 28, and temperature 95° F. Laboratory values are remarkable for hematocrit 32% and hemoglobin 10 g/dl. The patient's height is 5'7" (170 cm), and weight is 156 lb (71 kg). X-ray films reveal fractures of the mandible, three ribs, and the pelvis.

Bill remains hypotensive after administration of 3 L of IV fluids and 3 units of whole blood. He is taken to the operating room where he undergoes a partial splenectomy, repair of the remaining spleen, repair of hepatic lacerations, and stabilization of the mandible. A jejunostomy tube is inserted intraoperatively, and Bill is begun on prophylactic antibiotic therapy. On postoperative day one his vital signs are stable, and his hematocrit is 30%. Bowel sounds are active.

1. Why are no feedings begun via the jejunostomy tube?
2. What metabolic and nutritional changes are likely to be occurring at this time?

Bill becomes increasingly agitated and tremulous on postoperative day one and begins having hallucinations. He denies alcohol abuse, but a family member indicates that Bill consumes a six-pack of beer "most days." Bill is begun on lorazepam IV for delirium tremens. The physician orders thiamine hydrochloride 100 mg IM daily for 3 days. Jejunostomy feedings are initiated on postoperative day three.

3. In view of Bill's history of heavy alcohol use, he is at risk for deficiency of what nutrients?
4. Why was such a large dose of thiamine hydrochloride ordered? (The recommended daily allowance [RDA] for thiamine for a man of Bill's age is 1.2 mg/day.)
5. What nutrients are of special concern in the postoperative period?

6. What type of tube feeding product is most appropriate for Bill?
7. Give an estimate of Bill's caloric needs.
8. On what schedule should the feedings be administered?

Bill tolerates jejunostomy feedings well, and his IVs are discontinued on the fourth postoperative day. The antibiotics and lorazepam are given in oral liquid formulations via the jejunostomy tube.

9. What precautions should be followed in administering the medications?

Bill begins having four to five loose stools a day. The jejunostomy feedings are reduced, but the diarrhea continues.

10. What likely causes of diarrhea should be explored?

Bill's temperature increases to 103.3° F, and he complains of severe pain over the left upper quadrant of the abdomen. The abdominal wound is reddened, with gaping between sutures and purulent drainage at one site. IV antibiotics are resumed, with the enteral dosages discontinued.

11. Because diarrhea limits the amount of enteral feeding that Bill can tolerate, what alternative(s) is (are) appropriate for him?

The lorazepam dosage is tapered and then discontinued as Bill's symptoms of delirium tremens improve. At the same time, the diarrhea decreases markedly. Wound healing continues to be poor.

12. What changes in his nutritional regimen should be considered?
13. What parameters should be examined in updating Bill's nutrition assessment data?

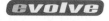 For the discussion of this Clinical Application and for an additional clinical application on nutritional alterations and management, see the Evolve website.

REFERENCES

1. Huang YC et al: Nutritional status of mechanically ventilated critically ill patients: comparison of different types of nutrition, *Clin Nutr* 19(2):101-107, 2000.
2. Kelly IE et al: Still hungry in hospital: identifying malnutrition in acute hospital admissions, *Q J Med* 93:93, 2000.
3. Waitzberg DL, Caiaffa WT, Correia MI: Hospital malnutrition: the Brazilian national survey (IBRANUTRI): a study of 4000 patients, *Nutrition* 17(7):573-580, 2001.
4. Pirlich M et al: Prevalence of malnutrition in hospitalized medical patients: impact of underlying disease, *Dig Dis* 21(3):245-251, 2003.
5. Kyle UG et al: Prevalence of malnutrition in 1760 patients at hospital admission: a controlled population study of body composition, *Clin Nutr* 22(5):473-481, 2003.
6. Braunschweig C, Gomez S, Sheehan PM: Impact of declines in nutritional status on outcomes in adult patients hospitalized for more than 7 days, *J Am Diet Assoc* 100:1316-1322, 2000.
7. Mathus-Vliegen EMH: Nutritional status, nutrition and pressure ulcers, *Nutr Clin Pract* 16: 286-291, 2001.
8. Rubinson L et al: Low caloric intake is associated with nosocomial bloodstream infections in patients in the medical intensive care unit, *Crit Care Med* 32:350-357, 2004.

9. August D et al: Guidelines for the use of parenteral and enteral nutrition in adult and pediatric patients, *JPEN J Parenter Enteral Nutr* 26:18SA-19SA, 33SA-41SA, 65SA-70SA, 78SA-81SA, 90SA-91SA, 2002.

10. National Heart, Lung, and Blood Institute: *Clinical guidelines on the identification, evaluation, and treatment of overweight and obesity in adults*, Washington, DC, 1998, NIH.

11. Gianino S, St. John RE: Nutritional assessment of the patient in the intensive care unit, *Crit Care Nurs Clin North Am* 5:1-16, 1993.

12. Ravasco P et al: A critical approach to nutritional assessment in critically ill patients, *Clin Nutr* 21(1):73-77, 2002.

13. Raguso C, Dupertuis YM, Pichard C: The role of visceral proteins in the nutritional assessment of intensive care unit patients, *Curr Opin Nutr Metabol Care* 6:211-216, 2003.

14. Fung EB: Estimating energy expenditure in critically ill adults and children, *AACN Clin Issues* 11(4):480-497, 2000.

15. McCarthy MS: Use of indirect calorimetry to optimize nutrition support and assess physiologic dead space in the mechanically ventilated ICU patient: a case study approach, *AACN Clin Issues* 11(4):619-630, 2000.

16. Cheng CH et al: Measured versus estimated energy expenditure in mechanically ventilated critically ill patients, *Clin Nutr* 21(2):165-172, 2002.

17. Alberda CL et al: Energy requirements in critically ill patients: how close are our estimates? *Nutr Clin Pract* 17(1):38-42, 2002.

18. Van den Berghe, G et al: Intensive insulin therapy in critically ill patients, *N Engl J Med* 345:1359-1367, 2001.

19. Rassias AJ et al: Insulin increases neutrophil count and phagocytic capacity after cardiac surgery, *Anesth Analg* 94:1113-1119, 2002.

20. Clement S et al: Management of diabetes and hyperglycemia in hospitals, *Diabetes Care* 27:553-591, 2004.

21. Bravata DM et al: Efficacy and safety of low-carbohydrate diets: a systematic review, *JAMA* 289:1837-1850, 2003.

22. Executive summary on the third report of the national cholesterol education program (NCEP) expert panel on detection, evaluation, and treatment of high blood cholesterol in adults (Adult Treatment Panel III), *JAMA* 285:2486-2497, 2001.

23. Lipsy RJ: The National Cholesterol Education Program Adult Treatment Panel III guidelines, *J Managed Care Pharm* 9(1 suppl):2-5, 2003.

24. Brewer HB: New features of the National Cholesterol Education Program Adult Treatment Panel III lipid-lowering guidelines, *Clin Cardiol* 26:19-24, 2003.

25. Ginsberg HN: Treatment for patients with the metabolic syndrome, *Am J Cardiol* 91(7):29-39, 2003.

26. Warren CJ: What is homocysteine? *Am J Nurs* 99:39, 1999.

27. Chobanian AV et al: Seventh report of the Joint National Committee on Prevention, Detection, Evaluation, and Treatment of High Blood Pressure, *Hypertension* 42(6):1206-1252, 2003.

28. Sacks FM et al: Effects of blood pressure of reduced dietary sodium and the dietary approaches to stop hypertension (DASH) diet, *N Engl J Med* 344(1):3-10, 2001.

29. Barber MD: The pathophysiology and treatment of cancer cachexia, *Nutr Clin Pract* 17:203-209, 2002.

30. Gerasimos S et al: Leptin levels in cachetic heart failure patients, *Int J Cardiol* 76:117-122, 2000.

31. Cochrane WU, Afolabi OA: Investigation into the nutritional status, dietary intake and smoking habits of patients with chronic obstructive pulmonary disease, *J Hum Nutr Diet* 17(1):3-11, 2004.

32. Driscoll DF: Intravenous lipid emulsions: 2001, *Nutr Clin Pract* 16:215-218, 2001.

33. Dickerson RN, Tidwell AC, Brown RO: Adverse effects from inappropriate medication administration via a jejunostomy feeding tube, *Nutr Clin Pract* 18:402-405, 2003.

34. Donaldson J, Borzotta MA, Matossian D: Nutrition strategies in neurotrauma, *Crit Care Nurs Clin North Am* 12(4):465-475, 2000.

35. Taylor SJ et al: Prospective, randomized, controlled trial to determine the effect of early enhanced enteral nutrition on clinical outcome in mechanically ventilated patients suffering head injury, *Crit Care Med* 27(11):2525-2531, 1999.

36. Cox SA et al: Energy expenditure after spinal cord injury: an evaluation of stable rehabilitating patients, *J Trauma* 25:419, 1985.

37. Aquilani R et al: Energy expenditure and nutritional adequacy of rehabilitation paraplegics with asymptomatic bacteriuria and pressure sores, *Spinal Cord* 39:437-441, 2001.

38. Kapadi FN et al: Special issues in the patient with renal failure, *Crit Care Clin* 19:233-251, 2003.

39. Charney P, Charney D: Nutrition support in renal failure, *Nutr Clin Pract* 17:226-236, 2002.

40. Case KO, Cuddy PG, McGurk EP: Nutrition support in the critically ill patient, *Crit Care Nurs Q* 22(4):75-89, 2000.

41. Wiggins KL, Harvey KS: A review of guidelines for nutrition care of renal patients, *J Renal Nutr* 12(3):190-196, 2002.

42. Scheinkestel CD et al: Prospective randomized trial to assess caloric and protein needs of critically ill, anuric, ventilated patients requiring continuous renal replacement therapy, *Nutrition* 19:909-916, 2003.

43. Patton KM, Aranda-Michel J: Nutritional aspects in liver disease and liver transplantation, *Nutr Clin Pract* 17:332-340, 2002.

44. Florez DA, Aranda-Michel J: Nutritional management of acute and chronic liver disease, *Sem Gastrointest Dis* 13(3):169-178, 2002.

45. Khokhar AS, Seidner DL: The pathophysiology of pancreatitis, *Nutr Clin Pract* 19:5-15, 2004.

46. Avgerinos C et al: Nutritional support in acute pancreatitis, *Dig Dis* 21(3):214-219, 2003.

47. Russell MK: Acute pancreatitis: a review of pathophysiology and nutrition management, *Nutr Clin Pract* 19:16-24, 2004.

48. Al-Omran M, Groof A, Wilke D: Enteral versus parenteral nutrition for acute pancreatitis, *Cochrane Database of Systematic Reviews* 1:1-19, 2003.

49. Dejong CH, Greve JW, Soeters PB: Nutrition in patients with acute pancreatitis, *Curr Opin Crit Care* 7(4):251-256, 2001.

50. Abou-Assi S, O'Keefe SJ: Nutrition support during acute pancreatitis, *Nutrition* 18:938-943, 2002.

51. Woolf SH et al: Controlling blood glucose levels in patients with type 2 diabetes mellitus: an evidence-based policy statement by the American Academy of Family Physicians and American Diabetes Association, *J Fam Pract* 49(5):453-460, 2000.

52. Umpierrez GE et al: Hyperglycemia: an independent marker of in-hospital mortality in patients with undiagnosed diabetes, *J Clin Endocrinol Metabol* 87:978-982, 2002.

53. McMahon MM: Management of parenteral nutrition in acutely ill patients with hyperglycemia, *Nutr Clin Pract* 19:120-128, 2004.

54. Charney P, Hertzler SR: Management of blood glucose and diabetes in the critically ill patient receiving enteral feeding, *Nutr Clin Pract* 19:129-136, 2004.

55. Jones MP: Management of diabetic gastroparesis, *Nutr Clin Pract* 19:145-153, 2004.

56. Paul E: New interventions in diabetes with medical nutrition therapy, *Case Manager* 13(2):78-81, 2002.

57. American Diabetes Association: Evidence-based nutrition principles and recommendations for the treatment and prevention of diabetes and related complications (Position Statement), *Diabetes Care* 26(suppl 1):S51-S61, 2003.

58. Swanson RW, Winkelman C: Special feature: exploring the benefits and myths of enteral feeding in the critically ill, *Crit Care Nurs Q* 24(4):67-74, 2002.

59. Braunschweig CL et al: Enteral compared with parenteral nutrition: a meta-analysis, *Am J Clin Nutr* 74(4):534-542, 2001.

60. Bozzetti F et al: Perioperative total parenteral nutrition in malnourished, gastrointestinal cancer patients: a randomized, clinical trial, JPEN *J Parenter Enteral Nutr* 24:7-14, 2000.

61. Braga ML et al: Early postoperative enteral nutrition improves oxygenation and reduces costs compared with parenteral nutrition, *Crit Care Med* 29(2):242-248, 2001.

62. Woodcock NP et al: Enteral versus parenteral nutrition: a pragmatic study, *Nutrition* 17(1):1-12, 2001.

63. Langkamp-Henken B: If the gut works, use it: but what if you can't? *Nutr Clin Pract* 18:449-450, 2003.

64. Jeejeebhoy KN: Total parenteral nutrition: potion or poison? *Am J Clin Nutr* 74(2):160-163, 2001.

65. Alpers DH: Enteral feeding and gut atrophy, *Curr Opin Nutr Metabol Care* 5:679-683, 2002.

66. Schloerb PR: Immune-enhancing diets: products, components, and their rationales, *JPEN J Parenter Enteral Nutr* 25(2):S3-S7, 2001.

67. Kelly D, Wischmeyer PE: Role of L-glutamine in critical illness: new insights, *Curr Opin Nutr Metabol Care* 6:217-222, 2003.

68. Wernerman J: Glutamine and acute illness, *Curr Opin Crit Care* 9:279-285, 2003.

69. Boelens PG et al: Glutamine alimentation in catabolic state, *J Nutr* 131:2569S-2577S, 2001.

70. Preiser J-C et al: Enteral feeding with a solution enriched with antioxidant vitamins A, C, and E enhances the resistance to oxidative stress, *Crit Care Med* 28(12):3828-3832, 2000.

71. Heyland DK et al: Should immunonutrition become routine in critically ill patients? A systematic review of the evidence, *JAMA* 286(8):944-953, 2001.

72. Heyland DK: Immunonutrition in the critically ill patient: putting the cart before the horse? *Nutr Clin Pract* 17:267-272, 2002.

73. Montejo JC et al: Immunonutrition in the intensive care unit: a systematic review and consensus statement, *Clin Nutr* 22(3):221-233, 2003.

74. Stechmiller JK, Childress B, Porter T: Arginine immunonutrition in critically ill patients: a clinical dilemma, *Am J Crit Care Nurs* 13(1):17-23, 2004.

75. Marik PE, Zaloga GP: Early enteral nutrition in acutely ill patients: a systematic review, *Crit Care Med* 29(12):2264-2270, 2001.

76. Jeejeebhoy KN: Enteral feeding, *Curr Opin Clin Nutr Metabol Care* 5:695-698, 2002.

77. Zaloga GP, Roberts PR, Marik PE: Feeding the hemodynamically unstable patient: a critical evaluation of the evidence, *Nutr Clin Pract* 18:285-293, 2003.

78. Moore FA, Weisbrodt NW: Gut dysfunction and intolerance to enteral nutrition in critically ill patients, *Nestle Nutrition Workshop Series & Clinical Performance Programme* 8:149-170, 2003.

79. Montejo JC et al: Multicenter, prospective, randomized, single-blind study comparing the efficacy and gastrointestinal complications of early jejunal feeding with early gastric feeding in critically ill patients, *Crit Care Med* 30(4):796-800, 2002.

80. McClave SA, Snider HL: Clinical use of gastric residual volumes as a monitor for patients on enteral tube feeding, *JPEN J Parenter Enteral Nutr* 26(suppl 6):S43-S50, 2002.

81. Berne JD et al: Erythromycin reduces delayed gastric emptying in critically ill trauma patients: a randomized, controlled trial, *J Trauma* 53(3):422-425, 2002.

82. Booth CM et al: Gastrointestinal promotility drugs in the critical care setting: a systematic review of the evidence, *Crit Care Med* 30(7):1429-1435, 2002.

83. Doherty WL, Winter B: Prokinetic agents in critical care, *Crit Care* 7(3):206-208, 2003.

83a. Lord LM et al: Comparison of weighted vs. unweighted enteral feeding tubes for efficacy of transpyloric intubation, *JPEN J Parenter Enteral Nutr* 17(3):271-273, 1993.

84. Metheny NA et al: pH and concentration of bilirubin in feeding tube aspirates as predictors of tube placement, *Nurs Res* 48:189, 1999.

85. Heyland DK et al: Effect of postpyloric feeding on gastroesophageal regurgitation and pulmonary microaspiration: results of a randomized controlled trial, *Crit Care Med* 29(8):1495-1501, 2001.

86. Esparza J et al: Equal aspiration rates in gastrically and transpylorically fed critically ill patients, *Intensive Care Med* 27:660-664, 2001.

87. Neumann DA, DeLegge MH: Gastric versus small-bowel tube feeding in the intensive care unit: a prospective comparison of efficacy, *Crit Care Med* 30(7):1436-1438, 2002.

88. Marik PE, Zaloga GR: Gastric versus post-pyloric feeding: a systematic review, *Crit Care* 7(3):R46-R51, 2003.

89. Davies AR et al: Randomized comparison of nasojejunal and nasogastric feeding in critically ill patients, *Crit Care Med* 30(3):586-590, 2002.

90. Kearns PJ et al: The incidence of ventilator-associated pneumonia and success in nutrient delivery with gastric versus small intestine feeding: a randomized clinical trial, *Crit Care Med* 28(6):1742-1746, 2000.

91. Grant MJC, Martin S: Delivery of enteral nutrition, *AACN Clin Issues* 11(4):507-516, 2000.

92. Lord LM: Restoring and maintaining patency of enteral feeding tubes, *Nutr Clin Pract* 18:422-426, 2003.

93. Bourgault AM et al: Prophylactic pancreatic enzymes to reduce feeding tube occlusions, *Nutr Clin Pract* 18:398-401, 2003.

94. Metheny NA: Risk factors for aspiration, *JPEN J Parenter Enteral Nutr* 26(6):S26-S33, 2002.

95. Metheny NA, Aud MA, Wunderlich RJ: A survey of bedside methods used to detect pulmonary aspiration of enteral formula in intubated tube-fed patients, *Am J Crit Care* 8:160-169, 1999.

96. Maloney JP, Ryan TA: Detection of aspiration in enterally fed patients: a requiem for bedside monitors of aspiration, *JPEN J Parenter Enteral Nutr* 26(6):S34-S41, 2002.

97. Lucarelli MR et al: Toxicity of food drug and cosmetic blue no. 1 dye in critically ill patients, *Chest* 125(2):793-795, 2004.

98. McClave SA et al: North American summit on aspiration in the critically ill patient: consensus statement, *JPEN J Parenter Enteral Nutr* 26(6):S80-S85, 2002.

99. Ringel AF, Jameson GL, Foster ES: Diarrhea in the intensive care patient, *Crit Care Clin North Am* 11:465-477, 1995.

100. Bliss DZ, Guenter PA, Settle RG: Defining and reporting diarrhea in tube-fed patients: what a mess! *Am J Clin Nutr* 55:753-759, 1992.

101. Bliss DZ et al: Fecal incontinence in hospitalized patients who are acutely ill, *Nurs Res* 49(2):101-108, 2000.

102. Mostafa SM et al: Constipation and its implications in the critically ill patient, *Br J Anaesth* 91(6):815-819, 2003.

103. Elpern EH et al: Outcomes associated with enteral tube feedings in a medical intensive care unit, *Am J Crit Care* 13:221-227, 2004.

104. Engel JM et al: Enteral nutrition practice in a surgical intensive care unit: what proportion of energy expenditure is delivered enterally? *Clin Nutr* 22(2):187-192, 2003.

105. Krishnan JA et al: Caloric intake in medical ICU patients: consistency of care with guidelines and relationship to clinical outcomes, *Chest* 124:297-305, 2003.

106. DeJonghe B et al: A prospective survey of nutritional support practices in intensive care unit patients: What is prescribed? What is delivered? *Crit Care Med* 29(1):8-12, 2001.

107. Worthington P, Gilbert KA, Wagner BA: Parenteral nutrition for the acutely ill, *AACN Clin Issues* 11(4):559-579, 2000.

108. Dobbins BM et al: Each lumen is a potential source of central venous catheter-related bloodstream infection, *Crit Care Med* 31(6):1688-1690, 2003.

109. Orr ME: The peripherally inserted central catheter: what are the current indications for its use? *Nutr Clin Pract* 17:99-104, 2002.

110. O'Grady NP et al: Guidelines for the prevention of intravascular catheter-related infections, *Infect Control Hosp Epidemiol* 23(12):759-769, 2002.

111. Speerhas R et al: Maintaining normal blood glucose concentrations with total parenteral nutrition: is it necessary to taper total parenteral nutrition? *Nutr Clin Pract* 18: 414-416, 2003.

112. Crook MA, Hally V, Panteli JV: The importance of the refeeding syndrome, *Nutrition* 17:632-637, 2001.

113. Hearing SD: Refeeding syndrome, *BMJ* 328(7445):908-909, 2004.

CHAPTER 8

Pain and Pain Management

Pain is an important stressor for patients in critical care settings.[1-7] Many sources of pain have been identified such as acute illness, surgery, trauma, invasive equipment, nursing and medical interventions, and immobility.[8-10] Moderate to severe pain is experienced by patients in critical care, which reinforces the importance of providing attention to pain.[4,5,11-18]

IMPORTANCE OF PAIN ASSESSMENT

Because pain is an important problem in critical care, its detection is a priority. To detect pain, it has to be adequately assessed. The Agency for Health Care Policy and Research (AHCPR)[19] proposed guidelines and recommendations for the assessment of acute pain. They reinforce McCaffery's[20] suggestion that the patient's self-report of pain be obtained as often as possible because it represents the most valid measure of pain. Unfortunately in critical care, many factors affect verbal communication with patients: the administration of sedative agents, mechanical ventilation, and the patient's change in level of consciousness.[8,21-22] These obstacles make pain assessment more complex. Nevertheless, except for being unable to speak, many intubated patients can communicate that they have pain by using facial expressions or hand motions, or by seeking attention with other movements.[4] Pain scales have also been used with intubated patients, who point on them to communicate about their pain.[5,13-14] When the patient is unable to express himself in any way, observable indicators, clustered as behavioral and physiologic ones, become unique indices for pain assessment.[4,8,9,21,23-26] In this situation, the AHCPR[19] strongly recommends that these indicators become part of pain assessment.

Moreover, pain assessment is an important part of the quality of care provided to critically ill patients and an essential part of nursing practice.[27] Because nurses are at the patient's bedside on a continuous basis, they play a major role in pain assessment and management.[28] Despite the growing body of research conducted in the field of pain in acute and critical care, pain is still undertreated.[5,11,12,14,16-18,29-37] Lack of education regarding pain, as well as underestimation of patients' pain, and incomplete and difficult pain assessment have been identified as significant barriers to adequate pain management.[12,17,18,25,27,30,31,36-42]

Undetected and untreated pain can lead to many complications involving the cardiovascular, pulmonary, and neurologic systems.[13,21,25,43-45] Conversely, an adequate pain assessment can lead to better treatment and a decrease in the risks of complications in critically ill patients.[23,46]

Because of the significance of pain in the critically ill patient, guidelines and standards of care for pain assessment and management were developed in the United States (AHCPR[19] and JACHO[47]) and in Canada (CCHSA).[48] In addition, the American Association of Critical-Care Nurses (AACN) identified pain as a priority area for nursing research, and many nursing professional organizations have developed pain management position statements.[49-50] Many health care agencies have increased their vigilance regarding the patient's pain and its management, including designating pain assessment as the fifth vital sign.[51] With the frequency of the diagnosis of pain and the professional responsibility to manage pain, the critical care nurse must understand the mechanisms, assessment process, and appropriate therapeutic measures for managing pain.

This chapter provides nurses with a better understanding of the physiology of pain. It will also demonstrate indicators that can be used for pain assessment and pain management in critically ill patients.

A DEFINITION AND DESCRIPTION OF PAIN

Pain is an unpleasant sensory and emotional experience associated with actual or potential tissue damage.[52] Pain is recognized as a subjective and multidimensional experience.[25,53-55] Its subjective characteristic implies that pain is whatever the experiencing person says it is and exists whenever he or she says it does.[20] Its multidimensional characteristics include many components including physiologic, sensory, affective, cognitive, and behavioral ones.[25,56-58] The physiologic component refers to nociception and the stress response. The sensory component is the perception of many characteristics of pain such as intensity, location, and quality. The affective component includes negative emotions such as anxiety and fear that may be associated with the experience of pain. The cognitive component refers to the interpretation of pain by the person who experiences it. Finally, the behavioral component includes the strategies used by the person to express, avoid, or control pain.

The major types of pain are acute and chronic. Acute pain is short-lasting, usually less than 6 months in duration, and implies tissue damage that is usually from an identifiable cause.[21,58-60] Acute nociceptive pain is associated with the inflammatory process[61] caused by trauma, surgery, or an acute illness.[8,59,62,63] If undertreated, acute pain can become chronic pain.[64]

Chronic pain persists over time, following the process of healing from the original injury, and may or may not be associated with an illness.[60] Chronic pain develops when the healing process is incomplete or when there is permanent damage to the nervous system. It has also been associated with a prolonged stress response.[57]

Both acute and chronic pain can be divided into somatic, visceral, or neuropathic origin. Somatic pain involves superficial tissues such as the skin, muscles, joints, and bones. Its location is well defined. Visceral pain involves organs such as the heart, stomach, and liver. Its location is diffuse and can be referred. Finally, neuropathic or deafferentation pain is described as an abnormal sensory process caused by changes in the excitability of nerve cells. These changes are associated with the acute inflammatory process or with nociceptive nerve damage that can be caused by surgery or an illness process.[65-67] The origin of the pain may be peripheral or central. Neuralgia and phantom pain are peripheral deafferentation pains. Cerebrovascular accidents can cause central deafferentation pain.[34] Neuropathic pain can be difficult to manage and frequently requires a multimodal approach.[68]

Pain in critical care is a subjective and multidimensional experience. Its components are physiologic, sensory, affective, cognitive, and behavioral. Pain experienced by critical care patients is mostly acute and has multiple origins. An understanding of the physiology of pain provides a foundation for assessment and treatment.

PHYSIOLOGY OF PAIN

NOCICEPTION

Nociception is the term used to describe how pain becomes conscious.[68] Four processes are involved in nociception:[3,46,66,68-70]

1. Transduction.
2. Transmission.
3. Perception.
4. Modulation.

Illustrations of the four processes are provided in Figs. 8-1 and 8-2.

Transduction. Transduction refers to mechanical (e.g., surgical incision), thermal (e.g., burn), or chemical (e.g., toxic substance) stimuli that damage tissues. In critical care, many nociceptive stimuli exist including the patient's acute illness condition, technology used for patients, and multiple interventions that have to be done for them. These stimuli, also called stressors, stimulate the liberation of many chemical substances such as prostaglandins, bradykinin, serotonin, histamine, glutamate, and substance P.[43] These neurotransmitters stimulate peripheral nociceptive receptors and thus serve to initiate nociceptive transmission.

Transmission. As a result of transduction, an action potential is produced and is transmitted by nociceptive nerve fibers in the spinal cord that reach higher centers of the brain. This is called transmission and represents the second process of nociception. The principal nociceptive fibers are the A-delta and C fibers. Small diameter, myelinated Aδ fibers transmit well-localized, sharp pain. Small diameter, unmyelinated C fibers transmit diffuse, dull, and aching pain. These fibers transmit the noxious sensation from the periphery to the dorsal route of the spinal cord. With the liberation of substance P, these fibers then synapse with ascending spinothalamic fibers to the central nervous system (CNS). These spinothalamic fibers are clustered into two specific pathways: neospinothalamic (NS) and paleospinothalamic (PS). Generally, the A-delta fibers transmit the pain sensation to the brain within the NS pathway, whereas the C fibers use the PS pathway.[69]

Through synapsing of nociceptive fibers with motor fibers in the spinal cord, muscular rigidity can appear because of a reflex activity.[43] Muscular rigidity can be a behavioral indicator associated with pain. It can contribute to immobility and decrease diaphragmatic excursion. This can lead to hypoventilation and hypoxemia.[43,46] Hypoxemia can be detected by monitoring pulse oximetry (SpO_2) and oxygen arterial pressure (PaO_2). In intubated patients, the alarms of the ventilator could also indicate the presence of pain.[23]

Perception. The pain message is transmitted by the spinothalamic pathways to centers in the brain where it is perceived. Pain sensation transmitted by the NS pathway reaches the thalamus, while the pain sensation transmitted by the PS pathway reaches brain stem, hypothalamus, and thalamus.[69] These parts of the CNS contribute to the initial perception of pain. Projections to the limbic system allow for the expression of the affective component of pain.[55,71] From these lower parts of the CNS, many projections reach higher parts of the

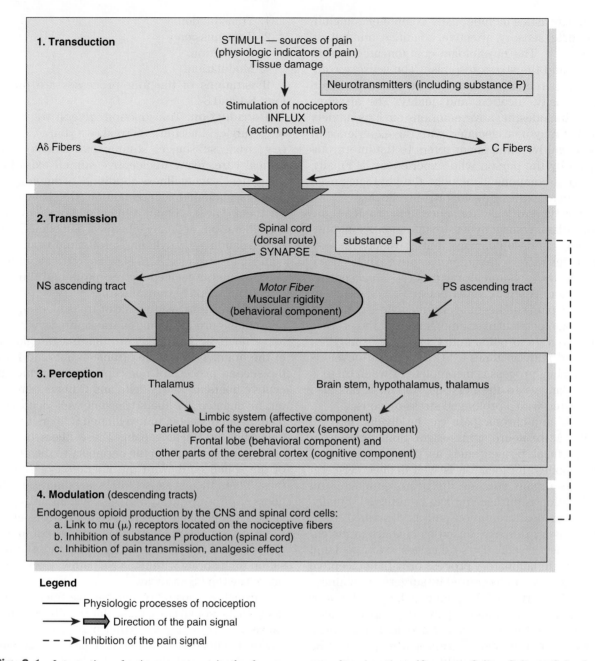

1. Transduction

STIMULI — sources of pain
(physiologic indicators of pain)
Tissue damage

Neurotransmitters (including substance P)

Stimulation of nociceptors
INFLUX
(action potential)

Aδ Fibers   C Fibers

2. Transmission

Spinal cord
(dorsal route)
SYNAPSE

substance P

NS ascending tract   PS ascending tract

Motor Fiber
Muscular rigidity
(behavioral component)

3. Perception

Thalamus   Brain stem, hypothalamus, thalamus

Limbic system (affective component)
Parietal lobe of the cerebral cortex (sensory component)
Frontal lobe (behavioral component) and
other parts of the cerebral cortex (cognitive component)

4. Modulation (descending tracts)

Endogenous opioid production by the CNS and spinal cord cells:
  a. Link to mu (μ) receptors located on the nociceptive fibers
  b. Inhibition of substance P production (spinal cord)
  c. Inhibition of pain transmission, analgesic effect

Legend

——— Physiologic processes of nociception

⟶ ▭▷ Direction of the pain signal

– – –▷ Inhibition of the pain signal

Fig. 8-1 Integration of pain assessment in the four processes of nociception. (Courtesy Celine Gelinas, School of Nursing, McGill University, Canada.)

CNS. More specifically, projections to the sensory cortex located in the parietal lobe allow the patient to describe the sensory characteristics of his or her pain, such as location, intensity, and quality.[55,69,72-74] The cognitive component of pain involves many parts of the cerebral cortex and is complex. These three components (affective, sensory, and cognitive) represent the subjective interpretation of pain. Parallel to this subjective process, certain facial expressions and body movements are behavioral indicators of pain occurring as a result of pain fiber projections to the motor cortex located in the frontal lobe.[54,75]

Modulation. Modulation is the liberation of endogenous opioids by the CNS such as beta-endorphins, enkephalins, and dynorphins. Endogenous opioids inhibit through the descending pathways the transmission of pain sensation in the spinal cord and produce analgesia. These substances link to mu receptors located on nociceptive fibers, inhibiting the liberation of substance P and blocking the transmission of the pain sensation.[54,69]

In summary, nociception is an important physiologic mechanism of pain that can integrate many components of pain for its assessment. In transduction, stimuli are sources of pain that can be considered as physiologic in-

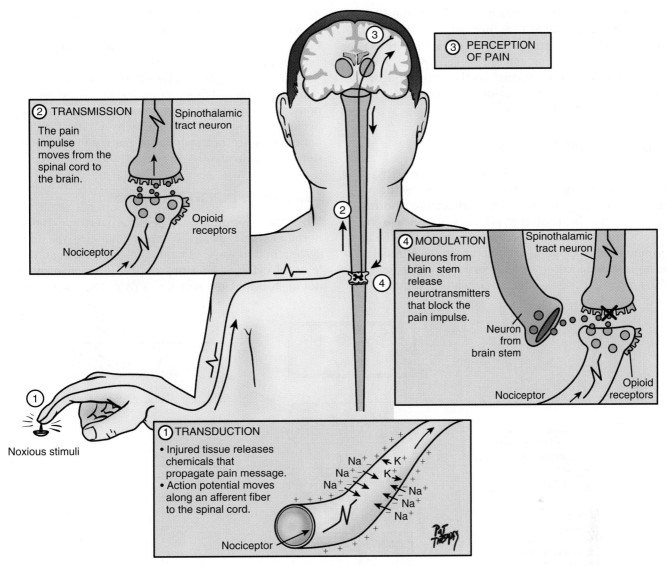

Fig. 8-2   Illustration of the four processes of nociception. (From Jarvis C: *Physical examination and health assessment,* ed 4, Philadelphia, 2004, Saunders, p 209.)

dicators for pain assessment. In transmission, muscular rigidity is a reflex activity and can be observed as a behavioral indicator associated with pain. In perception, the patient's self-report of affective, sensory, and cognitive information can be obtained.

BIOLOGIC STRESS RESPONSE

A biologic stress response is activated by pain, an obvious stressor.[25,43,45] This stress response involves the nervous, endocrine, and immune systems in the hypothalamo-pituitary-adrenal axis (HPA).[76,77] The biologic stress response includes a short-term direct response, a mid-term indirect response, and a long-term indirect response. A depiction of stress mechanisms is presented in Fig. 8-3.

SHORT-TERM DIRECT RESPONSE

In the presence of pain, the hypothalamus releases corticotropin-releasing factor (CRF), which activates the sympathetic nervous system (SNS). Then, norepinephrine is released from the terminals of sympathetic nerves, and epinephrine is released from the adrenal cortex. This mechanism constitutes the short-term direct stress response. The effects of these stress hormones allow for the observation of physiologic responses associated with the activation of SNS. For instance, increased blood pressure (BP) and increased heart rate (HR) are common signs of acute pain.[78-79] Moreover, increased respiratory rate (RR), perspiration, and pupil dilation can be observed.[25]

If pain persists over time or if injuries are located in the bladder or the intestines, the parasympathetic nervous system (PNS) may be dominant. Thus, the BP and HR may decrease rather than increase.[8] In addition, different responses to stressors involving PNS or SNS patterns have been documented.[80] Thus, the absence of pain-related indicators related to the activation of the sympathetic nervous system does not necessarily imply an absence of pain sensation.[79]

MID-TERM INDIRECT RESPONSE

Following the short-term direct response, the CRF is released from the hypothalamus and stimulates the anterior pituitary to release adrenocorticotropic hormone (ACTH), and the posterior pituitary to release vasopressin, the antidiuretic hormone. This is called the midterm indirect response. ACTH activates the adrenal cortex to release aldosterone and cortisol. Vasopressin and aldosterone increase sodium and water retention. This

increases intravascular volume and decreases diuresis, increases blood pressure and cardiac preload. In addition, cortisol may contribute to multisystemic responses such as infection and hyperglycemia.[77]

At mid-term pain could be associated with decreased diuresis, increased blood pressure, increased central venous pressure (CVP), and increased pulmonary artery occlusion pressure (PAOP). However, changes in these parameters are not specific to pain, and their correlations with pain are not supported by empirical data.

LONG-TERM INDIRECT RESPONSE

When the stress response persists over time, the stress hormones, specifically cortisol, influence the immune system in two ways: (1) immunosuppression and (2) release of cytokines.[81] However, these mechanisms have not been associated with acute pain. Their potential role

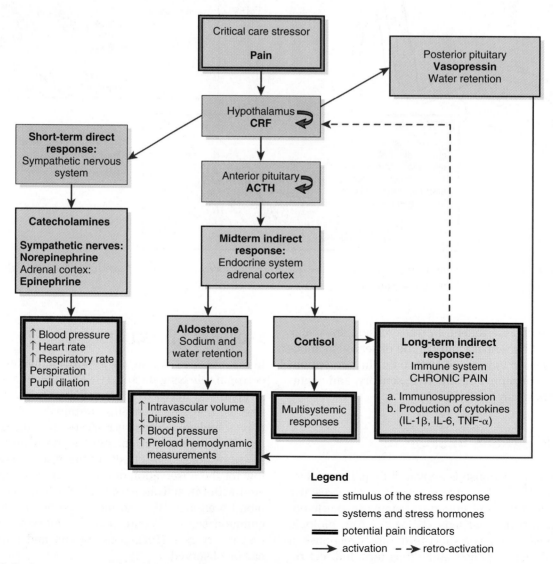

Fig. 8-3 Integration of potential physiologic pain indicators in the biologic stress response. (Courtesy Celine Gelinas, School of Nursing, McGill University, Canada.)

in the chronic pain process is currently under investigation. Cytokines could prolong by retroactivation the release of cortisol, which may exacerbate tissue damage contributing to the chronic pain process.[57,82] Therefore the long-term indirect response of stress does not seem to be relevant to acute pain.

In summary, the biologic stress response activated by pain allows for the observation of relevant physiologic signs that could be associated with pain. The signs related to the short-term direct response are the result of SNS activation. Other signs such as decreased diuresis and increased CVP, with increased PAOP pressure, relate to the mid-term indirect stress response. Finally, the immune system is involved in the long-term indirect response of stress. No acute pain indicators have yet been associated with this process. All the indicators identified within the biologic stress response are nonspecific to pain. Most of them have not been studied empirically

within the context of pain in critically ill patients. However, because of their theoretic association with pain, they may be used as a guide in pain assessment.

A FRAMEWORK FOR PAIN ASSESSMENT

As a framework, Melzack[56,57] developed a multidimensional theory that provides a relevant operational definition of pain and an appropriate model for pain assessment. This theory integrates the physiologic mechanism of pain (nociception) with the stress response. It also includes components of pain relevant for its assessment.

The model for pain assessment proposed by Melzack can be adapted for clinical use (Fig. 8-4). Pain indicators can be clustered into nonobservable/subjective and observable/objective categories. Nonobservable indicators constitute subjective information (i.e., the patients' self-

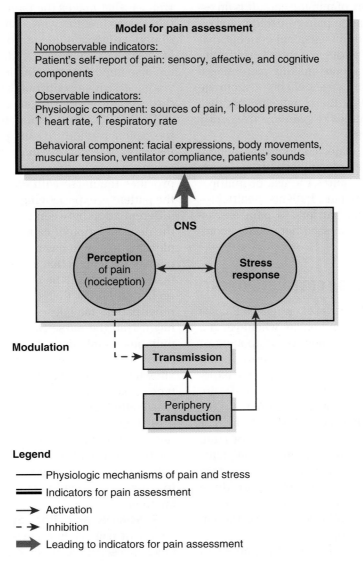

Fig. 8-4 Adaptation of the Multidimensional Theory of Melzack. (From Melzack R: Pain and stress: a new perspective. In Gatchel RJ, Turk DC, editors: *Psychological factors in pain,* New York, 1999, Guilford Press, p 98)

report of pain, including the sensory, affective, and cognitive components of pain). Observable indicators include physiologic and behavioral indicators. That can be detected by health professionals to document pain assessment. Physiologic indicators can be easily documented in critical care settings because of their continuous monitoring. Some measurable components are blood pressure, heart rate, respiratory rate, and oxygen saturation. These physiologic indicators are common to every critical care setting. Behavioral indicators include facial expression, body movements, and rigid posture that can be documented by nurses through observation. By using a model such as the one presented here, nurses can conduct a systematic assessment of pain in critically ill patients.

PAIN ASSESSMENT

Pain assessment is a vital part of nursing care. It is an essential prerequisite for adequate pain control and/or relief. Pain is a subjective, multidimensional concept that is complex to assess. Many factors may alter verbal communication in critically ill patients, making pain assessment more difficult. This situation should not discourage nurses from assessing pain in these patients, because acute pain is a stressor. Sources of pain are frequently present in critically ill patients.

Pain assessment has two major components: nonobservable/subjective and observable/objective. The complexity of pain assessment requires the use of multiple strategies by critical care clinicians. Patients, health professionals, and organizational barriers to pain assessment and management are addressed here, and recommendations proposed.

PAIN ASSESSMENT: THE SUBJECTIVE COMPONENT

Pain is recognized as a subjective experience. Pain is whatever the patient says it is and exists whenever the patient says it does.[20] Thus the subjective component of pain assessment refers to the patient's self-report of pain about his or her sensorial, affective, and cognitive experience of pain. Since it is the most valid measure of pain, the patient's self-report must be obtained as often as possible.[9,19,83] Mechanical ventilation should not prevent nurses from documenting patients' self-reports of pain. Many intubated patients can communicate having pain[25] or can use pain scales by pointing on them.[5,13-14] Before concluding that a patient is unable to self-report, three attempts to ask the patient about pain are recommended.[9] Sufficient time should be allowed for the patient to respond with each attempt.

If sedation and cognition levels allow the patient to give more information about pain, a multidimensional assessment can be documented. Multidimensional pain assessment tools, including the sensorial, affective, and cognitive components, are available (e.g., Brief Pain Inventory,[84] Initial Pain Assessment Tool,[68] and the short-form McGill Pain Questionnaire[85]). Because intubated patients receive sedative and analgesic agents, a tool must be shrot enough to be completed. For instance, the short form McGill Pain Questionnaire takes 2 to 3 minutes to complete[85] and has been used with intubated patients.[5,13,14]

The patient's self-report of pain can also be obtained by questioning the patient using the mnemonic PQRSTU[86]:

P: provocative or palliative/aggravating factors
Q: quality
R: region or location, radiation
S: severity and other symptoms
T: timing
U: understanding.

P: Provocative or Palliative/Aggravating Factors. The *P* indicates what provokes or causes the patient's pain and what he was doing when the pain appeared, as well as what makes the pain better or worse. The example of deep breathing intensifying the chest pain because of pericarditis is an illustration of an aggravating factor. Moderating factors that reduce the pain or discomfort are also important to establish. A knowledge of any alleviating activities contributes to the patient's plan of care throughout the continuum of care.

Q: Quality. The *Q* refers to the quality of the pain, or the pain sensation that the patient is experiencing. For instance, the patient may describe the pain as dull, aching, sharp, burning, or stabbing. This information provides the nurse with data regarding the type of pain the patient is experiencing (i.e., somatic or visceral). The differentiation between types of pain may contribute to the determination of cause and management. For example, a patient who has had open-heart surgery may complain of chest pain that is shooting or burning. This information would lead the nurse to investigate for cutaneous or bone injuries that can result from sternotomy. Another patient may describe a sharp thoracic pain, which might lead the nurse to consider a visceral pain due to pulmonary embolism. A verbal description of pain is important also because it provides a baseline description, allowing the critical care nurse to monitor changes in the type of pain, which could indicate a change in the underlying pathology.

R: Region, Radiation. *R* is normally easy for the patient to identify, although visceral pain is more difficult for the patient to localize.[25,68,87] If the patient has difficulty naming the location or is intubated, ask the patient to point to the location on him- or herself or on a simple anatomic drawing.[25]

S: Severity and Other Symptoms. The severity or intensity of pain, *S*, is a measurement that has undergone much investigation. Multiple visual analog scales are available, as well as the descriptive and numeric pain intensity scales that are often used in the critical care environment (Fig. 8-5). In addition, visual analog scales and numeric and

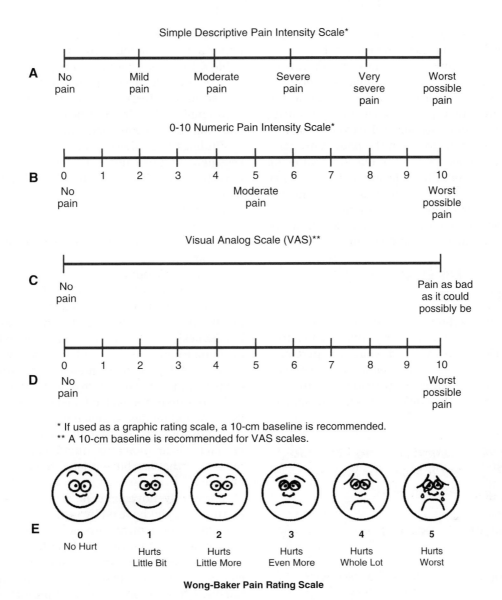

Fig. 8-5   Pain intensity scales. **A,** Simple descriptive pain intensity scale; **B,** numeric pain intensity scale; **C,** visual analog scale; **D,** simple descriptive pain intensity scale; **E,** Wong-Baker FACES pain rating scale. (**E** From Wong DL: *Whaley & Wong's essentials of pediatric nursing,* ed 6, St Louis, 2001, Mosby.)

descriptive pain intensity scales have been used in critically ill patients, intubated or not.[5,13,14,79,88,89] The Faces Pain Rating Scale has been identified as the easiest pain intensity scale by adults in acute and critical care settings.[90,91]

Many critical care units use a specific pain intensity scale. The use of a single tool provides consistency of assessment and documentation. The employment of a pain intensity scale is useful in the critical care environment.[58] Asking the patient to grade the pain on a scale of 0 to 10 is a consistent method and aids the nurse in objectifying the subjective nature of the patient's pain. However, the patient's tool preference should be considered.

S also refers to other symptoms accompanying the patient's pain experience such as shortness of breath, nausea, and fatigue. Anxiety and fear are common emotions associated with pain.

T: Timing. The *T* is also used to document the onset, duration, and frequency of pain. This information can help to determine if the origin of the pain is acute or chronic. Duration of pain can indicate the severity of the problem. For instance, a cardiac patient with pain duration of less than 5 minutes may experience angina, but pain that persists for longer than this may indicate a myocardial infarction.

U: Understanding. The *U* is the patient's perception of the problem or his cognitive experience of pain. Patients with known cardiac problems can tell the nurse if their pain is the same as they had during myocardial infarction.

Patients with a cerebral hemorrhage often describe experiencing the worst headache they have ever had.

Because of the patient's change in communication, lack of concentration secondary to sedation therapies, and the life-or-death immediacy of most actions in the critical care environment, pain assessment is often reduced to one dimension: sensorial. Kwekkeboom and Herr[9] recommend starting to ask if the patient has pain or not by using a simple "yes or no" question, allowing the patient to answer verbally, by head nodding, or other signs. This way is easier for intubated patients, who cannot express themselves verbally, to communicate with clinicians. In addition, pain intensity and location are necessary for the initial assessment of pain.[92,93]

PAIN ASSESSMENT: THE OBSERVABLE/ OBJECTIVE COMPONENT

Besides the patients' self-report of pain, nurses can rely on observation of behavioral and physiologic indicators which may manifest with pain and which are part of a complete pain assessment.[19] These should not be substituted for a self-report as long as the patient is able to communicate in any way. On the other hand, when the patient is unable to express him- or herself, these indicators give important information for pain assessment.[4,8,9,21,23-26] Table 8-1 lists behavioral and physiologic indicators that may be associated with pain. These indicators are highlighted in the literature, and some have been supported with empiric data from critical care or post–anesthesia care unit (PACU) adult patients.[4,78,79,88,89,94]

Findings from these studies can be used in pain assessment of the critically ill. Facial expressions of pain have been widely studied in adults. There are four primary facial movements:

1. Brow lowering.
2. Orbit tightening.
3. Levator contraction (deepening of the nasolabial furrow).
4. Eyelid closing.[95]

The presence of the first three facial movements may suggest moderate pain, whereas the presence of all four facial movements may suggest severe pain.[95] Payen and colleagues[78] used this gradation of intensity of facial expression for pain assessment in critically ill unconscious patients. A higher pain intensity was related to an increase number of facial movements. Physicians and critical care nurses recognize facial expression (e.g., frowning, eye tightening, grimacing, tears) as an important indicator for pain assessment.[92] The facial expression of grimacing is an indicator often recorded by critical care nurses[79,96] that has been related to patient-reported pain intensity.[88,97]

Many body movements have been described in the literature that can be used by critically ill patients to communicate their pain to nurses.[4] Being immobile, moving slowly or with caution, touching the pain site or tubes, moving arms or legs, and restlessness are relevant indicators of pain identified by physicians and critical care nurses.[92] Nurses' observation of protection movements, like trying to reach or touching the pain site or the tubes while being positioned, are associated with critically ill patients' self-report of pain.[97] Restlessness is often identified as a body movement associated with pain.[79,88,89,96] However, the absence of movement was often recorded by nurses as a pain behavior in postoperative critical care patients.[79] Some patients are unable to communicate pain with behaviors because of exhaustion. This could be one explanation for the absence of movement; patients may also have learned that movement increased pain. Interestingly, in the study of Gelinas and colleagues,[92] some physicians and nurses made a distinction about body movements, based on the patient's level of consciousness. They noted that unconscious patients may be more agitated, while conscious patients tend to remain immobile in order to protect themselves from having pain.

Muscular tension is another potential behavioral pain indicator. It has been related to patient-reported pain intensity[88,89,97] and identified as a pain behavior in critically ill patients.[79,96] When a patient is tense, rigid, spas-

Table 8-1	Behavioral and Physiologic Indicators for Pain Assessment	
Indicator for Pain Assessment	**Description**	
BEHAVIORAL		
Facial expression	Grimacing, frowning, wincing, eyes squeezed closed, teeth clenched, wrinkled brow, teary/crying	
Body movements	Immobile, slow/cautious movements, touching the pain site or tubes, seeking attention through movements, restlessness	
Muscular tension	Rigid, tense, stiff, splinting	
Compliance with the ventilator	Coughing, turning the alarms on, fighting the ventilator	
Sounds or vocalizations	Groaning, moaning, sighing, sobbing, grunting	
PHYSIOLOGIC		
Heart rate	Increase or decrease	
Blood pressure	Increase or decrease	
Respiratory status	Increase or decrease rate, decrease depth	
Spo_2	Decrease	
End-tidal CO_2	Increase or decrease	
Perspiration	General	
Pallor	Skin	
Pupil	Dilation	

tic, and resistive to being turned, critical care nurses have noted this as an indicator of pain.[92]

An intubated patient's noncompliance with the ventilator was first studied as an indicator of pain by Payen and colleagues.[78] Although this behavioral indicator has been widely studied for sedation assessment,[98-100] noncompliance with the ventilator deserves to be documented empirically in intubated patients. It has been identified by physicians and critical care nurses as a potential indicator of pain in intubated patients and has been documented to be associated with patients' self-report of pain.[92,97] In other words, patients experiencing pain were coughing into their endotracheal tubes and triggering ventilator alarms or blocking ventilation.

Patients' sounds or vocalizations may be used for pain assessment in critically ill extubated patients.[79,88,89] Pain-related vocalizations include sighing, groaning, moaning, crying, or sobbing.[88,89] These types of vocalizations were found to be related to patient-reported pain intensity.[88-89,97] Patient vocalization was the third-most recorded pain indicator by critical care nurses in their pain assessments.[79]

Research concerning physiologic indicators has shown that increased mean arterial pressure (MAP) and increased HR are associated with acute pain caused by a nociceptive procedure in critically ill unconscious patients.[78] Gelinas and others[97] documented an increase in MAP, HR, RR, SpO_2, and end-tidal CO_2 in response to a nociceptive procedure (positioning) in critically ill pa-

tients. Only increased HR was associated with the patients' self-report of pain. These indicators are frequently reported by critical care nurses for pain assessment.[79,92] These physiologic indicators occur when the sympathetic nervous system is activated during a biologic stress response. The vital signs are commonly monitored in critical care settings, which make them useful for pain assessment. However, the use of physiologic indicators for pain assessment must be used with caution.

Some of these observable indicators were included in tools developed and validated for clinical use in critical care: PACU Behavioral Pain Rating Scale (PACU BPRS),[88] Pain Assessment and Intervention Notation (PAIN),[79] Behavioral Pain Scale (BPS),[78] and Critical-Care Pain Observation Tool (CPOT)[94,101] (Table 8-2). Although these tools have limitations, they may help support pain assessment in critical care especially in uncommunicative patients. Research is still needed to improve the use of observable indicators for pain assessment in critically ill patients. It is also important to remember that absence of observable indicators (behavioral and physiologic) does not mean absence of pain.[94] This is what makes its assessment so complex. Many factors may explain the lack of a physiologic response. Some therapies employed in the critical care area are designed to block the SNS response to stress. Critical care nurses must also be aware that behavioral and physiologic indicators are not specific to pain. They can indicate other problems (e.g., anxiety, delir-

Table 8-2   Description of the Critical-Care Pain Observation Tool (CPOT)

Indicator	Description	Measurement Scale	
Facial expression	No muscular tension observed	Relaxed, neutral	0
	Presence of frowning, brow lowering, orbit tightening, and levator contraction	Tense	1
	All previous facial movements plus eyelid tightly closed	Grimacing	2
Body movements	Does not move at all (doesn't necessarily mean absence of pain)	Absence of movements	0
	Slow, cautious movements, touching or rubbing the pain site, seeking attention through movements	Protection	1
	Pulling tube, attempting to sit up, moving limbs/thrashing, not following commands, striking at staff, trying to climb out of bed	Restlessness	2
Muscular tension	No resistance to passive movements	Relaxed	0
Evaluation by passive flexion and extension of upper limbs	Resistance to passive movements	Tense, rigid	1
	Strong resistance to passive movements, incapacity to complete them	Very tense or rigid	2
Compliance with the ventilator (intubated patients)	Alarms not activated, easy ventilation	Tolerating movements	0
	Alarms stop spontaneously	Coughing but tolerating	1
	Asynchrony: blocking ventilation, alarms frequently activated	Fighting ventilator	2
or			
Vocalization (extubated patients)	Talking in normal tone or no sound	Talking in normal tone or no sound	0
	Sighing, moaning	Sighing, moaning	1
	Crying out, sobbing	Crying out, sobbing	2

Courtesy Celine Gelinas, School of Nursing, McGill University, Canada.

Table 8-3	Components to Include for Complete Pain Assessment Documentation		
Pain Documentation	**Description**		
Sources of pain	Admission diagnosis (acute illness, trauma, surgery) Invasive equipment (e.g., endotracheal tube, venous lines, chest tube) Nursing interventions (e.g., positioning, endotracheal suctioning) Medical interventions Immobility		
Patient's self-report	**SENSORY** 1. Intensity (pain scale)* 2. Location 3. Quality 4. Aggravating/alleviating factors 5. Onset/time * The first pain information to focus on in the patient's self-report.	**AFFECTIVE** 1. Emotions	**COGNITIVE** 1. Meaning of pain 2. Impact of pain
Observable indicators	**PHYSIOLOGIC** 1. Blood pressure (BP) 2. Heart rate (HR) 3. Respiratory rate (RR)	**BEHAVIORAL** 1. Facial expressions 2. Body movements 3. Muscular tension, rigidity (posture) 4. Compliance with the ventilator (intubated patients) 5. Vocalizations (extubated patients)	
Intervention for pain	Always conduct pain assessment before and after an intervention for pain (pharmacologic and nonpharmacologic) is undertaken as an on-going assessment.		

Courtesy Celine Gelinas, School of Nursing, McGill University, Canada.

ium) or can be influenced by different pharmacologic therapies.

Pain is considered the fifth vital sign,[102,103] and including pain assessment with other routinely documented vital signs may help ensure that pain is assessed and controlled for all patients on a regular basis.[103] This would ensure that pain is detected and treatment implemented before the patient develops complications associated with unrelieved pain. This is accomplished by nurses' remaining aware of sources of pain in their critically ill patients.

Use of a pain flow sheet in critical care settings allows for on-going pain assessment before and after an intervention for pain.[30,104,105] This could facilitate and reinforce the assessment process. Recommendations of information to include in complete pain assessment documentation are proposed in Table 8-3.

PATIENT BARRIERS TO PAIN ASSESSMENT AND MANAGEMENT

DIFFICULTY IN COMMUNICATING

The most obvious patient barrier to the assessment of pain in the critical care population is an alteration in the ability to communicate. The patient who is intubated cannot verbalize a description of the pain. If the patient can communicate in any way, such as by head nodding or pointing, then he or she may report the pain in that manner. The patient who can write a description may be able to thoroughly describe the pain in writing. It is with nonverbal patients that the nurse relies on behavioral and physiologic clues to assess the presence and intensity of pain. Because the nurse cannot be sure of the predictability of the indicators that she or he observes, other sources of assessment must be addressed. The patient's family can contribute significantly in the assessment of pain. The family is intimately familiar with the patient's normal responses to pain and can assist the nurse in identifying such clues. If there is absolutely no observable evidence to support a diagnosis of pain, the clinician needs to use the concept that if the trauma, disease, injury, or procedure is painful for most patients, it is painful for this patient, too.[68]

ALTERED LEVEL OF CONSCIOUSNESS

The patient in a coma presents a dilemma for the critical care nurse. Since pain recognition depends on cortical response, there is the mistaken belief that the patient without higher cortical function has no perception of pain.[87,106] Conversely, the inability to interpret the nociceptive transmission does not negate the transmission. Interviews by Lawrence[107] with 100 patients who experienced being unconscious revealed that they could hear, understand, and respond emotionally to what was being said while they were unconscious. An oncology nurse shared her experience caring for a patient who became comatose and still felt pain while unconscious.[108] Experts recommend assuming that unconscious patients have pain and that they should be treated the same way as conscious patients when they are exposed to sources of pain.[109,110] Payen and others[78] demonstrated that behavioral and physiologic indicators of pain can be observed in reaction to a painful procedure in critically ill unconscious patients. These indicators of pain have been observed during a painful procedure in critically ill patients no matter what their level of consciousness.[97] Knowing this, the critical care nurse can initiate a discussion with the other members of the health care team to formulate a plan of care for the coma patient's comfort.

THE ELDERLY

Many elderly patients do not complain much about pain. Some misconceptions such as believing that pain is a normal consequence of aging, or being afraid to disturb the health care team, are barriers to pain expression for the elderly.[111,112] Delirium, dementia, or cognitive deficits present additional barriers to pain assessment. In elderly patients with cognitive deficits, 20% are unable to communicate pain verbally.[27,113] Observation of behaviors becomes the only way to determine the presence of pain in this population. Some tools have been developed and validated for members of this specific population, who often experience chronic pain (e.g., Checklist for Nonverbal Pain Indicators [CNPI],[114] Discomfort Scale–Dementia Alzheimer Type [DS-DAT],[115] and Pain Assessment Checklist for Seniors With Limited Ability to Communicate [PACSLAC][116]). Otherwise, most elderly patients with or without cognitive deficits are able to give a self-report of pain. Vertical pain intensity scales are easily understood by this group of patients and their use is recommended (see Fig. 8-5).[117]

NEONATES AND INFANTS

At these stages of development, verbal communication is impossible; this is an important barrier to pain assessment. The misconception that preterm neonates are incapable of pain sensation has persisted for a long time. Recent evidence has supported the idea that both term and preterm neonates have the anatomic and functional capacity for pain sensation at birth.[118] The Premature Infant Pain Profile (PIPP) is a valid tool for pain assessment of this population and has been implemented in many clinical settings.[119] Many tools have been developed and validated for clinical use for term neonates and preverbal infants (e.g., COMFORT scale,[120] *C*rying—*R*equires O_2 for saturation >95—*I*ncreased vital signs—*E*xpression—*S*leepless [CRIES],[121] Nursing Assessment of Pain Intensity [NAPI],[122] Neonatal Infant Pain Scale [NIPS],[123] and Scale for Use in Newborns [SUN][124]). It is important to note that these tools include behaviors specific to infants, such as crying, and that physiologic indicators (e.g., heart rate and pulse oximetry) are more sensitive for pain in this population when compared to adults.

CULTURAL INFLUENCES

Another barrier to accurate pain assessment are cultural influences on pain and pain reporting.[125,126] These cultural influences may be compounded if the patient speaks a language other than that of the health team members. In order to facilitate communication, the use of a pain intensity scale in the patient's language is relevant. The 0 to 10 numeric pain scale and the Wong-Baker FACES Scale have been translated into many different languages.[68]

Although this chapter does not address specific cultural groups and their typical responses to pain, a few generalizations can be made. First, when assessing a patient from a cultural group different from your own, avoid the assumption that the patient will have a specific response to pain or exhibit a particular behavior because of his culture. Patients are individual in their responses to pain. The health care practitioner might unjustly assign or expect behaviors that a patient will not exhibit. A second consideration that is commonly overlooked is the role of pain in the life of the patient. The nurse must communicate with the patient or the family to ascertain what that role is.

Some cultures believe that God's test or punishment takes the form of pain. Persons of such cultures would not necessarily believe that the pain should be relieved. Other cultures perceive pain as being associated with an imbalance in life. Persons of these cultures believe they need to manipulate the environment to restore balance to control pain.[126]

The complexities and intricacies of cultural beliefs require much greater discussion than is possible here. It is important for the nurse to support, whenever possible, the special beliefs and needs of the patient and his family to provide the most therapeutic environment for healing to occur.

LACK OF KNOWLEDGE

A relatively overlooked patient barrier to accurate pain assessment is the public knowledge deficit regarding pain and pain management. Many patients and their families are frightened by the risk of addiction to pain medication. They fear that addiction will occur if the patient is medicated frequently or with amounts of opiates necessary to relieve the pain. This concern is so powerful for some that they will deny or deliberately underreport the frequency or intensity of pain. Another misconception held by some patients is the expectation that unrelieved pain is simply part of a critical illness or procedure.[127] Many patients have no memory of receiving an explanation of their pain management plan.[30] With that in mind, it is important that the critical care nurse teach both the family and the patient about the importance of pain control and the use of opioids in treating the critically ill patient.

HEALTH PROFESSIONAL BARRIERS TO PAIN ASSESSMENT AND MANAGEMENT

The health professional's beliefs and attitudes about pain and pain management are frequently a barrier to accurate and adequate pain assessment. This can lead to poor management practices.[68,128,129] It is well documented that the study of pain assessment and management is lacking in most nursing schools and in nursing textbooks.[105,127,128] Multiple studies conducted by pain experts McCaffery and Pasero have documented nurses' misconceptions or lack of knowledge regarding addiction, physiologic dependence, drug tolerance, and respiratory depression.[68] The problematic misconception on the part of nurses is that the patient must have a physiologic and behavioral response to pain that matches the nurse's concept of what a patient in pain looks like (i.e., the patient must have a marked change in vital signs and be moaning, writhing, and crying to truly be in pain). This hampers appropriate management of the patient's pain. The critical care nurse must remember that pain is what the patient states it is and that no additional finding is necessary to treat the patient's pain.[68]

Nursing concerns with addiction can contribute to misinterpretation of signs during the pain assessment process. Addiction rates for patients in acute pain who receive opioid analgesics are less than 1%.[68] Some of the false beliefs that surround addiction result from a lack of knowledge about the terms *addiction* and *tolerance*. Addiction is defined by a pattern of compulsive drug use that is characterized by an incessant longing for an opioid and the need to use it for effects other than pain relief. Tolerance is defined as a diminution of opioid effects over time. Physical dependence and tolerance to opioids may develop if the drug is given over a long period. Physical dependence is manifested by withdrawal symptoms when the opioid is abruptly stopped.[68] If this is an anticipated problem, withdrawal may be avoided by simply weaning the patient from the opioid slowly to allow the brain to reestablish neurochemical balance in the absence of the opioid.[25]

Another concern of the health care professional is the fear that aggressive management of pain with opioids will cause critical respiratory depression. Opioids can cause respiratory depression, but in the critically ill this is a rare phenomenon. The incidence of respiratory depression is less than 1%.[130] Respiratory depression from the administration of opioids can be managed with diligent assessment practices that are discussed later.

ORGANIZATIONAL BARRIERS TO PAIN ASSESSMENT AND MANAGEMENT

The organizational system influences pain and pain management practices as well as associated outcomes. Failure to make pain management a priority is the initial barrier. Failure to adopt standard pain assessment tools or to provide staff with sufficient time to assess and document pain, and a lack of accountability for pain management practices are observed in some organizations.[47] Evidence continues to demonstrate the lack of documentation of pain assessment and the undertreatment of pain in critical care settings.[18,33-35,37-39,96] The lack of collaboration between physicians and nurses is still identified as a barrier to effective pain management.[94,131]

Since unrelieved pain is harmful to patients and increases the cost of care, it needs to be a priority of care for the health organization. Every organization must analyze its pain management issues and practices and provide education to staff about pain and pain management. Now that pain is considered as the fifth vital sign, pain assessment must be included in documentation systems as a standard.[102,103] Pain has to be assessed in all critically ill patients, regardless of their clinical condition or their level of consciousness.[97,103] The implementation of pain assessment tools is essential so that the health care team can establish a common language of communication. This facilitates interprofessional collaboration. There must be increased commitment to clinical practice guidelines and standards for pain assessment and management (e.g., JCAHO[47]) in healthcare institutions. In addition, strategies to enhance collaboration among health professionals may include interdisciplinary care rounds or case reviews. Patients have the right to be consulted about their pain care plan, and they should be involved in making decisions.[103] The organization must continually evaluate outcomes and work to improve the quality of pain management.

PAIN MANAGEMENT

The management of pain in the critically ill patient is as multidimensional as the assessment. It is a multidisciplinary task. The control of pain can be pharmacologic, nonpharmacologic, or a combination of the two therapies. Pharmacologic pain management is predominantly used in critical care.

PHARMACOLOGIC CONTROL OF PAIN

The pharmacologic management of pain has infinite variety in the critical care unit. Although this chapter is not an in-depth discussion of pharmacology, some commonly administered agents are discussed. Pain pharmacology is divided into three categories of action: opioid agonists (morphine, fentanyl, hydromorphone, meperidine, codeine, and methadone); nonopioids (acetaminophen, nonsteroidal antiinflammatory drugs [NSAIDs]); and adjuvants (anticonvulsants, antidepressants, local anesthetics). How pain is approached and managed is a progression or combination of the available agents, the type of pain, and the patient response to the therapy. Fig. 8-6 illustrates the analgesic action sites in relation to nociception.

OPIOID ANALGESICS

The opioids most commonly used and recommended as first-line analgesics are the agonists. These opioids bind to mu- (μ-) receptors (transmission process, Fig. 8-6), which appear to be responsible for pain relief. Additional pharmacologic information is presented in the Pharmacologic Management Table. As a clinical practice guideline, scheduled opioid doses or a continuous infusion is preferred over an "as needed" regimen to ensure consistent analgesia in critically ill patients.[132]

Morphine. Morphine is the most commonly prescribed opioid in the critical care unit.[25] Because of its water-solubility, morphine has a slower onset of action and a longer duration compared with the lipid-soluble opioids (such as fentanyl). This puts it and hydromorphone among the preferred opioids for intermittent therapy.[132] Morphine has two main metabolites, morphine-3-glucuronide (M3G, inactive) and morphine-6-glucuronide (M6G, active). M6G is responsible for the analgesic effect but may accumulate and cause excessive sedation in patients with renal failure or hepatic dysfunction.[133,134] Morphine is available in a variety of delivery methods. It is the standard by which all other opioids are measured. It is also the agent that most closely mimics the endogenous opioids in the human pain modification system.

Morphine is indicated for severe pain. It has additional actions that are helpful for managing other symptoms. Morphine dilates peripheral veins and arteries, making it useful in reducing myocardial workload. Morphine is also viewed as an antianxiety agent because of the calming effect it produces.[135]

Many side effects have been reported with morphine (see Pharmacologic Management Table on Pain). The hypotensive effect can be particularly problematic in the hypovolemic patient. The vasodilation effect is potentiated in the volume-depleted patient; therefore, hemodynamic status must be carefully monitored.[136] Volume resuscitation restores blood pressure in the event of a prolonged hypotensive response.

A more serious side effect requiring diligent monitoring is the respiratory depressant effect. Opioids may cause this complication because they reduce the responsiveness of carbon dioxide chemoreceptors in the respiratory center located in the medulla.[130] Although infrequent, this effect can have significant sequelae for the critically ill patient. A subset of patients is at greater risk of respiratory depression after morphine administration. This subset includes newborns (younger than 6 months) and the elderly patient with chronic obstructive pulmonary disease or known obstructive sleep apnea syndrome, as well as patients who are opiate-naïve (receiving opiates for less than a week), and patients with renal failure.[133,134] The critical care nurse must monitor the patient intensively in order to prevent such a complication. Monitoring of patients receiving opioid analgesics is discussed in more detail in a later section of this chapter. In addition to side effects common to all opioids, morphine may stimulate histamine release from mast cells, resulting in cardiac instability and allergic reactions.[138]

Fentanyl. Fentanyl is a synthetic opioid preferred for critically ill patients with hemodynamic instability or morphine allergy. It is a lipid-soluble agent which has a more rapid onset than morphine and a shorter duration.[133,134] The metabolites of fentanyl are largely inactive and nontoxic, which makes it an effective and safe opioid. The use of fentanyl in the critical care unit is growing in popularity, and it is the preferred agent for acutely distressed patients. Fentanyl or hydromorphone is also recommended in hemodynamically unstable or renally impaired patients.[132] It is available in a variety of forms: intravenous (IV), intraspinal, and transdermal. The transdermal form is commonly referred to as the *Duragesic patch* or the *72-hour patch.*

Because the side effects of fentanyl are similar to those of morphine, the nurse must monitor carefully the hemodynamic and respiratory response. When fentanyl is given by rapid administration and at higher doses, it has been associated with the additional hazard of bradycardia and rigidity in the chest wall muscles.[132,133] The use of transdermal fentanyl is rarely indicated in the critically ill patient. The customary use of this form is for those experiencing chronic pain or cancer pain, and in critical care it is used for the patient who requires extended pain control. Transdermal delivery requires 12 to 16 hours for onset of action and has a duration of 72 hours.[68] If this delivery method is used, the patient will require other opioid management until the transdermal fentanyl takes effect.[106]

Hydromorphone. Hydromorphone is a semisynthetic opioid that has an onset of action and a duration similar to morphine.[133,134] It is an effective opioid with multiple routes of delivery. It is more potent than morphine. Hydromorphone should be used with caution in patients with renal or hepatic failure because its metabolite, hydromorphone-3-glucuronide, accumulates and can cause central nervous system toxicity. Studies have shown that some side effects (e.g., pruritus, sedation, nausea and vomiting) may occur less with hydromorphone than morphine.[139]

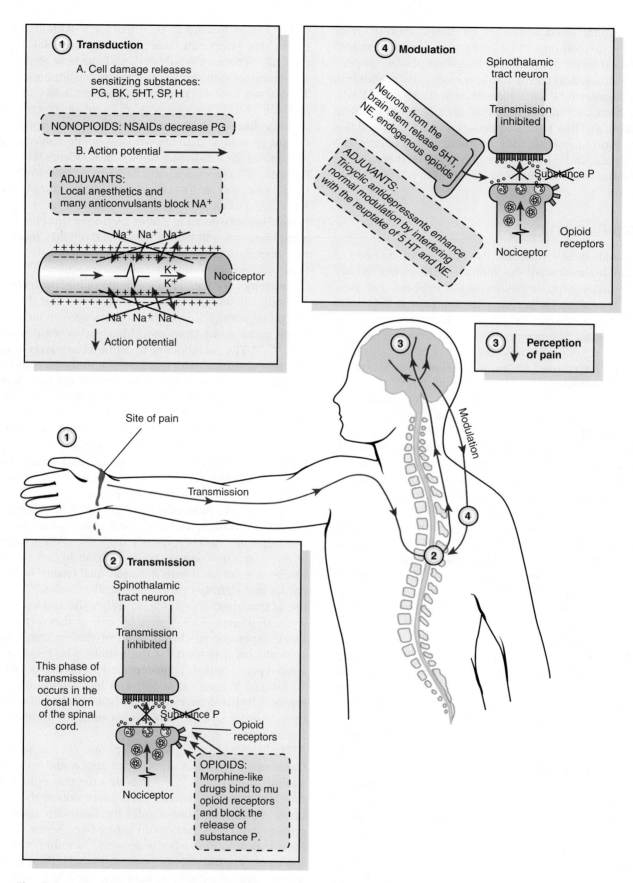

Fig. 8-6　Nociception and analgesic action sites. (From McCaffery M, Pasero C: *Pain: clinical manual for nursing practice*, ed 2, St Louis, 1999, Mosby, p 107.)

Pharmacologic Management: Pain

Drug	Dosage	Onset (min)	Duration (h)	Available Routes	Properties	Side Effects and Comments
Morphine	1-4 mg IV bolus 1-10 mg IV infusion	5-10	3-4	PO, SL, R, IV, IM, SC, EA, IA	Analgesia Antianxiety	Standard for comparison Side effects: sedation, respiratory depression, euphoria/dysphoria, hypotension, nausea, vomiting, pruritus, constipation, urinary retention M6G can accumulate in renal failure or hepatic dysfunction patients
Fentanyl	25-100 mcg IV bolus 25-200 mcg IV infusion	1-5	0.5-4	OTFC, IV, IM, TD, EA, IA	Analgesia Antianxiety	Same side effects as morphine Rigidity with high doses
Hydromorphone (Dilaudid)	0.2-1 mg IV bolus 0.2-2 mg IV infusion	5	3-4	PO, R, IV, IM, SC. EA, IA	Analgesia Antianxiety	Same side effects as morphine
Meperidine (Demerol)	75-100 mg IM	5-10	2-4	PO, IV, IM, SC, EA, IA	Analgesia	Seem to cause less constipation, urinary retention, pruritus, sedation and nausea than morphine Neurotoxicity (normeperidine) High doses may cause agitation, muscle jerking, seizures or hypotension Use with care in patients with renal failure, convulsive disorders, and dysrhythmias
Codeine	15-30 mg IM, SC	10-20	3-4	PO, IM, SC	Analgesia (mild-to-moderate pain)	Lacks potency (unpredictable absorption, and not all patients convert it to an active form to achieve analgesia) Most common side effects: lightheadedness, dizziness, shortness of breath, sedation, nausea, and vomiting
Methadone (Dolophine)	5-10 mg IV	10	4-8	PO, SL, R, IV, SC, IM, EA, IA	Analgesia	Usually less sedating than morphine but repeated doses can result in accumulation and can cause serious sedation (2-5 days)
Acetaminophen	650 mg Maximum 4g/day	20-30	4-6	PO, R	Analgesia Antipyretic	Rare side effects Hepatotoxicity
Ketorolac (Toradol)	15-30 mg IV	<10	6-8	PO, IM, IV	Analgesia Minimum antiinflammatory effect	Short-term (<5 days) Side effects: gastric ulceration, bleeding, exacerbation of renal insufficiency Use with care in elderly, and renal failure patients

EA, Epidural analgesia; *IA*, intrathecal analgesia; *IM*, intramuscular; *IV*, intravenous; *M6G*, morphine-6-glucuronide; *OTFC*, oral transmucosal fentanyl citrate; *PO*, oral; *R*, rectal; *SC*, subcutaneous; *SL*, sublingual; *TD*, transdermal.

Meperidine. Meperidine (Demerol) is a less potent opioid with agonist effects similar to morphine. It is considered the weakest of the opioids and must be administered in large doses to be equivalent in action to morphine.[140] The duration of action is short, so dosing is frequent. A major concern with this drug is the metabolite *normeperidine*. Normeperidine is a CNS-neurotoxic agent. At high doses in the renal- or hepatic-compromised patient or in the elderly patient, it may induce a CNS toxicity including irritability, muscle spasticity, tremors, agitation, and seizures.[134,141] Research has also shown that meperidine can cause postoperative delirium in patients of all ages.[142] Although meperidine is useful in short-term specific conditions (e.g., treating postoperative shivering); it should be avoided in patients who require longer periods of analgesia. Any patient receiving meperidine for pain control must be carefully monitored for signs of toxicity. The AHCPR guidelines suggest its use be limited to those patients with a documented sensitivity or allergic response to other μ-agonists.[19]

Codeine. Codeine has limited use in the management of severe pain. It is rarely used in the critical care unit. It provides analgesia for mild to moderate pain. It is usually compounded with a nonopioid (e.g., acetaminophen). To be active, codeine has to be metabolized in the liver to morphine.[143] Codeine is only available through oral, intramuscular (IM), and subcutaneous (SC) routes; therefore its absorption can be reduced in the critical care patient by altered gastrointestinal motility and decreased tissue perfusion.[144]

Methadone. Methadone is a synthetic opioid with morphinelike properties but provides less sedation. It is longer acting than morphine with a long half-life. This makes it difficult to titrate in the critical care patient. Methadone lacks active metabolites, and 60% of it is eliminated by nonrenal routes, so it doesn't accumulate in patients with renal failure.[145] Methadone is recommended to be used as a second-line opioid analgesic.[146] It is a good alternative for the patient who has a long recovery ahead with an anticipated prolonged ventilatory wean.[133]

PREVENTING AND TREATING RESPIRATORY DEPRESSION

Respiratory depression is the most life-threatening opioid side-effect. The risk of respiratory depression increases when other drugs with CNS-depressant effects (e.g., benzodiazepines, antiemetics, neuroleptics, and antihistamines) are concomitantly administered.[68,147,148] Respiratory depression is defined as a decrease in the rate or depth of respirations, not necessarily a specific number of respirations per minute. This means that a patient breathing deeply but less than 10 times per minute may not have respiratory depression. A change in the patient's level of consciousness or an increase in sedation normally precedes respiratory depression.

Monitoring patients before and after opioid administration for the following parameters, every 1 to 2 hours for the first 24 hours and every 2 to 4 hours afterwards, depending on the patient's clinical condition, is the best way to prevent respiratory depression:
- Pain intensity (using a valid pain scale)
- Respiratory rate and depth
- Blood pressure and heart rate
- Sedation level (using a valid sedation scale, see Chapter 9)
- Oxygen saturation using pulse oximeter (SpO_2)
- Loud snoring

Loud snoring doesn't necessarily indicate that the patient has a comfortable status. Loud snoring is frequently a sign of respiratory depression associated with airway obstruction by the tongue, leading to hypoxemia and then possibly cardio-respiratory arrest. Monitoring pulse oximetry (SpO_2) is highly recommended to detect any deterioration in the patient's respiratory condition.[137] A patient snoring after the administration of an opioid requires the critical care nurse to observe closely.

Critical respiratory depression can be readily reversed with the administration of the opiate antagonist *naloxone*. The usual dose is 0.4 mg, which is mixed with 10 ml of normal saline (for a concentration of 0.04 mg/ml). Naloxone is normally given intravenously, very slowly, while the patient is carefully monitored for reversal of the respiratory signs. Because the duration of naloxone is shorter than most opioids, another dose of naloxone may be needed as early as 30 minutes after the first dose. Naloxone administration can be discontinued as soon as the patient is responsive to physical stimulation and able to take deep breaths. The nurse must monitor sedation and respiratory status and remind the patient to deep breathe every 1 to 2 minutes until he or she becomes more alert. The benefits of reversing respiratory depression with naloxone must be carefully weighed against the risk of a sudden onset of pain and the difficulty achieving pain relief. In order to prevent this from occurring, it is important to provide a nonopioid medication for pain management.[68]

NONOPIOID ANALGESICS

The use of nonopioids in combination with an opioid is now recommended in selected critical care patients.[132] They may reduce opioid requirement and provide greater analgesic effect, through their action at the peripheral and central levels.[47,149] Pharmacologic information is presented in the Pharmacologic Management Table.

Acetaminophen. Acetaminophen is an analgesic used to treat mild to moderate pain. It inhibits the synthesis of neurotransmitter prostaglandins in the CNS and this is why it has no antiinflammatory properties.[150] Acetaminophen is metabolized by two pathways: major (nontoxic metabolite) and minor (toxic metabolite which is rapidly converted into a nontoxic form by glutathione). In an acetaminophen overdose a larger amount is processed by the minor pathway, resulting in a larger quantity of toxic metabolites. This may cause damage to the liver. Side effects are rare at therapeutic doses (total daily dose should not exceed 4000 mg).[68] Nonopioids are rarely used alone in critical care patients. When calculating the total daily dose of acetaminophen the nurse must consider the other products containing acetaminophen (e.g., Empracet) that the patient may receive. Special care must be taken of patients with hepatic dysfunction or malnutrition (alcohol consumption).[132]

Nonsteroidal Antiinflammatory Drugs. The use of nonsteroidal antiinflammatory drugs (NSAIDs) in combination with opioids is indicated in the patient with acute musculoskeletal and soft tissue inflammation.[68,151] The mechanism of action of NSAIDs is to block the action of cyclooxygenase (COX, which has two forms: COX-1 and COX-2), the enzyme that converts arachidonic acid into prostaglandins. This inhibits the production of prostaglandins (transduction process, see Fig. 8-6). This action occurs in the PNS and the CNS components of pain. NSAIDs can be grouped in two categories: (1) first-generation (COX-1 and COX-2 inhibitors; e.g., aspirin, ibuprofen, naproxen, ketorolac), and (2) second-generation (COX-2 inhibitors, e.g., celecoxib, rofecoxib). The inhibition of COX-1 is thought to be responsible for many of the side effects such as gastric ulceration, bleeding due to platelet inhibition, and acute renal failure. In contrast, the inhibition of COX-2 is responsible for the suppression of pain and inflammation.[150] Second-generation NSAIDs are associated with minimal risk of serious adverse effects, but their role in the critically ill remains unknown.[132]

Ketorolac is the most appropriate NSAID for use in the critical care setting. Research has shown that it is a safe and effective agent for postoperative pain.[63] Patients who received ketorolac in conjunction with an opioid had better pain relief and fewer side effects than patients who received just an opioid.[152] Not all critically ill patients are candidates for ketorolac therapy because of its side effects. Caution is advised in the elderly or patients with renal impairment because of slower clearance rates in these individuals. Because ketorolac is an NSAID, monitoring for clumping of platelets is of primary importance. Laboratory data should be evaluated for an increase in bleeding time, and the patient should be assessed for any signs of abnormal bleeding. Of particular concern is any evidence of gastrointestinal (GI) bleeding.[153] Moreover, a prolonged use of ketorolac of more than 5 days has been associated with an increase in renal failure and bleeding.[154,155] It is important to consider the concurrent use of opioids and NSAIDs to affect pain modification at both areas of transmission and transduction. This combination of agents often significantly reduces the amount of opioids required for effective pain management.

Other pharmacologic agents, in addition to those discussed, are used in the critical care unit. The most important factor to be considered in the management of pain with any pharmacologic agent is the careful assessment and reassessment of the patient's pain status during the administration of the drug. The need to adjust the dosage, increase the frequency, or change the agent will be based on assessment findings. The use of a pain flow sheet allows an on-going pain assessment and a complete documentation of pain and pain management in the critical care setting.[30,105]

Adjuvants. Even if not widely mentioned in the critical care literature, adjuvants can be helpful for pain relief in patients with complex pain syndromes such as neuropathic pain or for other specific purposes (e.g., procedural pain). Anticonvulsants (e.g., carbamazepine, phenytoin, gabapentin) are first-line analgesics for lancinating neuropathic pain. Although the specific mechanism for pain relief is not known, analgesia probably results from the suppression of Na+ discharges, reducing the neuronal hyperexcitability (action potential) in the transduction process (see Fig. 8-6).[68] Antidepressants (e.g., amitriptyline, imipramine, desipramine) are also considered as analgesics in a variety of chronic pain syndromes such as headache, arthritis, low back pain, neuropathy, central pain, and cancer pain. The analgesic dose is often lower than that required to treat depression. The mechanism of analgesia most widely accepted is the ability of antidepressants to block the reuptake of neurotransmitters serotonin and norepinephrine in the CNS. This increases the activity of the modulation process (see Fig. 8-6).[68]

Anesthetics may also be used in the critical care setting. Ketamine is a dissociative anesthetic agent that has analgesic properties. It was traditionally used via IV route for procedural pain in burn patients. It is also available in enteral routes. Compared to opioids, ketamine has the benefit of sparing the respiratory drive. It has many side effects related to the release of catecholamines and the emergence of delirium. For this reason, ketamine is not recommended for routine therapy in critically ill patients.[63,133] Before administering ketamine to a patient, the dissociative state should be explained to him or her. Dissociative state refers to the feelings of separateness from the environment, loss of control, hallucinations, and vivid dreams. The use of benzodiazepines (midazolam) can reduce the incidence of this unpleasant effect.[68] Lidocaine is another anesthetic that can be used for procedural and acute pain or for some patients with chronic neuropathic pain.[68] When used locally, anesthetics act through the transduction process (see Fig. 8-6).

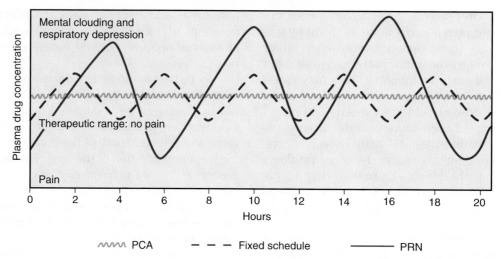

Fig. 8-7   Fluctuations in opioid blood levels seen with three dosing procedures. (From Lehne RA: *Pharmacology for nursing care,* ed 5, Philadelphia, 2004, Saunders, p 243.)

DELIVERY METHODS

The most common route for drug administration is the intravenous route—via continuous infusion, bolus administration, or patient-controlled analgesia (PCA). Traditionally the choice has been IV bolus administration. The benefits of this method are the rapid onset of action and the ease of titration. The major disadvantage is the rise and fall of the serum level of the opioid, leading to periods of pain control with periods of breakthrough pain (Fig. 8-7).[150,156]

Continuous infusion of opioids via an infusion pump provides constant blood levels of the ordered opioid. This promotes a consistent level of comfort. It is a particularly helpful method of administration during sleep because the patient awakens with an adequate level of pain relief.[157] It is important that the patient be given the loading dose that relieves the pain and also raises the circulating dose of the drug. After the basal rate is established, the patient maintains a steady state of pain control unless there is additional pain from a procedure, an activity, or a change in the patient's condition. Orders for additional boluses of opioid must be available.

PATIENT-CONTROLLED ANALGESIA

Patient-controlled analgesia (PCA) is a method of delivery, via the IV route and an infusion pump, that allows the patient to self-administer small doses of analgesics. Different opioids can be used, but the most extensively used is morphine.[150] This method of medication delivery allows the patient to control the level of pain and sedation and to avoid the peaks and valleys of intermittent dosing by the health care professional (see Fig. 8-7). The patient can self-administer a bolus of medication the moment the pain begins, thus acting preemptively. Nursing management of the patient using a PCA pump is de-

scribed in the Nursing Interventions Classification (NIC) feature.

Certain patients are not candidates for PCA. Alterations in the level of consciousness or mentation preclude the patient understanding the use of the equipment. The very elderly or patients with renal or hepatic insufficiency may require careful screening for PCA.

Allowing the patient to self-administer opioid doses does not diminish the role of the critical care nurse in pain management. The nurse advises for necessary changes to the prescription and continues to monitor the effects of the medication and doses. The patient is closely monitored during the first 2 hours of therapy and after every change in the prescription. If the patient's pain does not respond within the first 2 hours of therapy a total reassessment of the pain state is essential. The nurse monitors the number of boluses the patient delivers. If he or she is bolusing more often than the prescription, the dose may be insufficient to maintain pain control. Naloxone must be readily available to reverse adverse opiate respiratory effects. Ideally the patient undergoing an elective procedure requiring opioid analgesia postoperatively is instructed in the use of PCA during preoperative teaching. This allows the patient to become comfortable with the concept of self-medication before use.

INTRASPINAL PAIN CONTROL

Intraspinal anesthesia uses the concept that the spinal cord is the primary link in nociceptive transmission. The goal is to mimic the body's endogenous opioid pain modification system by interfering with the transmission of pain and providing an opiate-receptor binding agent directly into the spinal cord. The benefits of the intraspinal route include good to excellent pain control with typically lower doses of opioids, increased patient mobility, minimal sedation, and increased patient satisfaction.[158]

NIC	Patient-Controlled Analgesia Assistance

Definition: Facilitating patient control of analgesic administration and regulation

Activities

Collaborate with physicians, patient, and family members in selecting the type of narcotic to be used

Recommend administration of aspirin and nonsteroidal antiinflammatory drugs in conjunction with narcotics, as appropriate

Avoid use of meperidine (Demerol)

Ensure that patient is not allergic to analgesic to be administered

Teach patient and family to monitor pain intensity, quality, and duration

Teach patient and family to monitor respiratory rate and blood pressure

Establish nasogastric, venous, subcutaneous, or spinal access, as appropriate

Modify that the patient can use a patient-controlled analgesia (PCA) device: is able to communicate, comprehend explanations, and follow directions

Collaborate with patient and family to select appropriate type of patient-controlled infusion device

Teach patient and family members how to use the PCA device

Assist patient and family to calculate appropriate concentration of drug to fluid, considering the amount of fluid delivered per hour via the PCA device

Assist patient or family member to administer an appropriate bolus loading dose of analgesic

Teach patient and family to set an appropriate basal infusion rate on the PCA device

Assist patient and family to set the appropriate lockout interval on the PCA device

Assist patient and family in setting appropriate demand doses on the PCA device

Consult with patient, family members, and physician to adjust lockout interval, basal rate, and demand dosage, according to patient responsiveness

Teach patient how to titrate doses up or down, depending on respiratory rate, pain intensity, and pain quality

Teach patient and family members the action and side effects of pain-relieving agents

Document patient's pain, amount and frequency of drug dosing, and response to pain treatment in a pain flow sheet

Recommend a bowel regimen to avoid constipation

Consult with clinical pain experts for a patient who is having difficulty achieving pain control

From Dochterman JM, Bulechek GM: *Nursing intervention classification (NIC)*, ed 4, St Louis, 2004, Mosby.

Also, the hemodynamic status of the patient changes very little.

Intraspinal anesthesia is particularly appropriate for pain in the thorax, upper abdomen, and lower extremities. The two intraspinal routes are intrathecal and epidural (Fig. 8-8). Regardless of the route the effects of the opioid agonist used will be the same; so assessment parameters are the same as those used for other routes. Nursing management of the patient receiving intraspinal analgesia is described in the Nursing Interventions Classification (NIC) feature.

INTRATHECAL ANALGESIA

Intrathecal (subarachnoid) opioids are placed directly into the cerebral spinal fluid and attach to spinal cord receptor sites. Opioids introduced at this site act quickly at the dorsal horn. The dural sheath is punctured, eliminating the barrier for pathogens between the environment and the cerebral spinal fluid. This creates the risk of serious infections. The intrathecal route is usually reserved for intraoperative use. Single-bolus dosing provides short-term relief for pain that is short-lived (e.g., the pain

of labor and delivery is well managed using this regimen).[153] Side effects of intrathecal pain control include postdural puncture headache and infection.

EPIDURAL ANALGESIA

Epidural analgesia is commonly used in the critical care unit after major abdominal surgery, nephrectomy, thoracotomy, and major orthopedic procedures.[5] Certain conditions preclude the use of this pain control method: systemic infection, anticoagulation, and increased intracranial pressure. Epidural delivery of opiates provides longer-lasting pain relief with lower doses of opiates. When delivered into the epidural space, 5 mg of morphine may be effective for 6 to 24 hours, compared with 3 to 4 hours when delivered intravenously. Opioids infused in the epidural space are more unpredictable than those administered intrathecally. The epidural space is filled with fatty tissue and is external to the dura mater. The fatty tissue interferes with uptake and the dura acts as a barrier to diffusion, making diffusion rate difficult to predict.

The rapidity of the diffusion of the drug is determined by the type of drug used. The drugs are either hy-

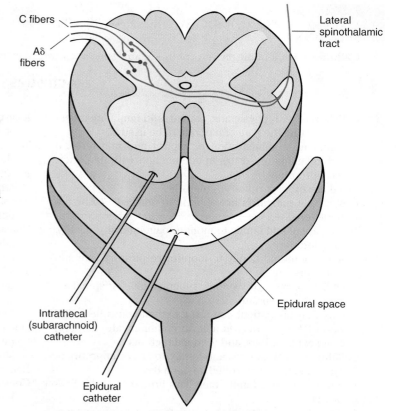

Fig. 8-8 Intraspinal catheter placement in spinal cord cross section. (See p. 125 for description of C and Aδ fibers.)

NIC　Analgesic Administration: Intraspinal

Definition: Administration of pharmacologic agents into the epidural or intrathecal space to reduce or eliminate pain

Activities

Check patency and function of catheter, port, and/or pump

Ensure that IV access is in place at all times during therapy

Label the catheter and secure it appropriately

Ensure that the proper formulation of the drug is used (e.g., correct concentration and preservation-free)

Ensure narcotic antagonist availability for emergency administration, and administer per physician order, as necessary

Start continuous infusion of analgesic agent after correct catheter placement has been verified, and monitor rate to ensure delivery of prescribed dosage of medication

Monitor temperature, blood pressure, respirations, pulse, and level of consciousness at appropriate intervals, and record on flow sheet

Monitor level of sensory blockade at appropriate intervals and record on flow sheet

Monitor catheter site and dressings to check for a loose catheter or wet dressing, and notify appropriate personnel per agency protocol

Administer catheter site care according to agency protocol

Secure needle in place with tape, and apply appropriate dressing according to agency protocol

Monitor for adverse reactions, including respiratory depression, urinary retention, undue somnolence, itching, seizures, nausea, and vomiting

Monitor orthostatic blood pressure and pulse before the first attempt at ambulation

Instruct patient to report side effects, alterations in pain relief, numbness of extremities, and need for assistance with ambulation if weak

Follow institutional policies for injection of intermittent analgesic agents into the injection port

Provide adjunct medications as appropriate (e.g., antidepressants, anticonvulsants, and nonsteroidal antiinflammatory agents)

Increase intraspinal dose, based on a pain intensity score

Instruct and guide patient through nonpharmacologic measures (e.g., simple relaxation therapy, simple guided imagery, and biofeedback) to enhance pharmacologic effectiveness

Instruct patient about proper home care for external or implanted delivery systems, as appropriate

Remove or assist with removal at catheter according to agency protocol

---

From Dochterman JM, Bulecheck GM: *Nursing interventions classification (NIC)*, ed 4, St Louis, 2004, Mosby.

drophilic or lipophilic. Hydrophilic drugs are water soluble and penetrate the dura slowly, giving them a longer onset and duration of action. Morphine is hydrophilic. Lipophilic drugs are lipid soluble; they penetrate the dura rapidly and therefore have a rapid onset of action and a shorter duration of action.[5] Fentanyl is lipophilic.

The dura acts as a physical barrier and causes delay in diffusion of the drug. When compared with the intrathecal route, it allows more drug to be absorbed in the systemic circulation, requiring greater doses for pain relief.[158] Drugs delivered epidurally may be bolused or continuously infused. Epidural analgesia is being used more often in the critical care environment and requires careful monitoring.

The nurse must assess the patient for respiratory depression. This phenomenon may occur early in the therapy or as late as 24 hours after initiation. The epidural catheter also puts the patient at risk for infection. The efficiency of this pain control method and the increased mobility of the patient does not diminish the nurse's responsibility to monitor and evaluate the outcomes of the pain management protocol in use.

EQUIANALGESIA

At some point in the patient's recovery, strong opioids are replaced by more moderate agents. In doing any conversion the goal is to provide equal analgesic effects with the new agents. This concept is referred to as *equianalgesia*. The critical care nurse is the practitioner most likely to convert the patient from parenteral medication to oral medication in preparation for a change in the level of care or for discharge. There is the misconception that when a patient is able to take oral medication the pain is less severe. The change to oral medications does not indicate a need for less medication.

The nurse needs to practice equianalgesia when converting the patient. Because of the variety of agents and routes, the professional pain organizations have developed equianalgesia charts for use by the health care professional. All critical care units need to have a chart posted for easy referral. Table 8-4 provides the equianalgesia dose for different drugs used in clinical practice.

NONPHARMACOLOGIC METHODS OF PAIN MANAGEMENT

Numerous methods of pain management other than drugs appear in the critical care literature.[159,160] In most instances these therapies augment and enhance the pharmacologic management of the patient's pain. Stimulating other non–pain-sensory fibers (alpha-beta) present in the periphery modifies pain transmission.[54] These fibers are stimulated by thermal changes, as in the application of heat or cold, and by simple massage. The use of massage has been a mainstay in the nursing management of the patient in pain. It is an appropriate pain management technique for most critically ill patients.

TRANSCUTANEOUS ELECTRICAL NERVE STIMULATOR

The nonpain-sensory fibers (alpha-beta) in the periphery are stimulated by the action of the transcutaneous electrical nerve stimulator (TENS). The use of TENS has contraindications in the critical care unit. Since the device is controlled by the patient, mentation must be intact. TENS is also contraindicated in patients with pacemakers or automatic implantable defibrillators, because these devices may recognize and erroneously interpret the TENS electrical signal. TENS therapy is efficient, patient-controlled pain management for orthopedic, obstetric, and some postoperative pain states.

COGNITIVE TECHNIQUES

Using the cortical interpretation of pain as the foundation, a number of interventions are known to reduce the patient's pain report. These modalities include cognitive techniques: patient teaching, relaxation, distraction, guided imagery, and music therapy.[68,159,160] Teaching may help the patient decrease distress and improve pain control. Other techniques are discussed in the following paragraphs.

Relaxation. Relaxation is a well-documented method for reducing the distress associated with pain. Although not a substitute for pharmacology, relaxation is an excellent adjunct for controlling pain.[161] Relaxation decreases oxygen consumption and muscle tone and can decrease heart rate and blood pressure. Relaxation gives the patient a sense of control over the pain and reduces muscle tension and anxiety. Not all patients are interested in relaxation therapy. For those patients, deep-breathing exercises may be helpful and frequently lead to relaxation. Excellent references for thorough techniques in relaxation therapy are available.[68]

Distraction. The patient and family may provide information about other sources of distraction for the patient. Determining what distraction therapies the patient normally uses may provide a clue to which might work during the illness. Some persons are distracted by television; however, for others television is a source of increased anxiety. Do not assume that the patient does or does not want to watch television until you determine whether it will be beneficial or harmful to the patient.

The key to success with any of these therapies is understanding their mechanism of action so that the therapy matches the needs of the patient. All of the previously mentioned interventions require the patient's cooperation. There must be some commitment to the treatment on the part of the patient. When handled effec-

Table 8-4	Equianalgesic Chart: Approximate Equivalent Doses of Opioids for Moderate-to-Severe Pain		
Analgesic	**Parenteral (IM, SC, IV) Route [1,2] (mg)**	**PO Route[1] (mg)**	**Comments**
MU OPIOID AGONISTS			
MORPHINE	10	30	Standard for comparison; multiple routes of administration; available in immediate-release and controlled-release formulations; active metabolite M6G can accumulate with repeated dosing in renal failure
CODEINE	130	200 NR	IM has unpredictable absorption and high side effect profile; used PO for mild-to-moderate pain; usually compounded with nonopioid (e.g., Tylenol No. 3)
FENTANYL	100 mcg/h parenterally and transdermally ≅ 4 mg/h morphine parenterally; 1 mcg/h transdermally ≅ 2 mg/24h morphine PO	—	Short half-life, but at steady state, slow elimination from tissues can lead to a prolonged half-life (up to 12 h); start opioid-naïve patients on no more than 25 mcg/h transdermally; transdermal fentanyl NR for acute pain management; available by oral transmucosal route
HYDROMORPHONE (Dilaudid)	1.5	7.5	Useful alternative to morphine; no evidence that metabolites are clinically relevant; shorter duration than morphine; available in high-potency parenteral formulation (10 mg/ml) useful for SC infusion; 3 mg rectal ≅ 650 mg aspirin PO; with repeated dosing (e.g., PCA), it is more likely than 2-3 mg parenteral hydromorphone = 10 mg parenteral morphine

-- fold here --

LEVORPHANOL (Levo-Dromoran)	2	4	Longer-acting than morphine when given repeatedly; long half-life can lead to accumulation within 2-3 days of repeated dosing.
MEPERIDINE	75	300 NR	No longer preferred as a first-line opioid for the management of acute or chronic pain due to potential toxicity from accumulation of metabolite, normeperidine; normeperidine has 15-20 h half-life and is not reversed by naloxone; NR in elderly or patients with impaired renal functions; NR by continuous IV infusion
METHADONE (Dolophine)	10	20	Longer-acting than morphine when given repeatedly; long half-life can lead to delayed toxicity from accumulation within 3-5 days; start PO dosing on PRN schedule; in opioid-tolerant patients converted to methadone, start with 10%-25% of equianalgesic dose
OXYCODONE	—	20	Used for moderate pain when combined with a nonopioid (e.g., Percocet, Tylox); available as single entity in immediate-release and controlled-release formulations (e.g., OxyContin); can be used like PO morphine for severe pain
OXYMORPHONE (Numorphan)	1	10 rectal	Used for moderate-to-severe pain; no PO formulation

[1] Duration of analgesia is dose dependent; the higher the dose, usually the longer the duration.

[2] IV boluses may be used to produce analgesia that lasts approximately as long as IM or SC doses. However, of all routes of administration, IV produces the highest peak concentration of the drug, and the peak concentration is associated with the highest level of toxicity, e.g., sedation. To decrease the peak effect and lower the level of toxicity, IV boluses may be administered more slowly, e.g., 10 mg of morphine over a 15 minute period, or smaller doses may be administered more often, e.g., 5 mg of morphine every 1-1.5 hours.

FDA, Food and Drug Administration; *NR*, not recommended; ≅, roughly equal to.

IM, Intramuscular; *IV*, intravenous; *M6G*, morphine-6-glucuronide; *NR*, not recommended; *PCA*, patient-controlled analgesia; *PO*, by mouth; *PRN, pro re nata* (as needed); *SC*, subcutaneous.

tively, nonpharmacologic tools can assist in pain management. An increasing number of therapies are appearing in critical care research. It is important for practitioners to be aware of the current literature on this topic so they can provide the most effective and current interventions to manage the patient's pain.

Guided Imagery. Guided imagery is a technique that uses the imagination to provide control over pain. It can be used to distract or relax. Guiding a patient to a place in his or her imagination that is pain free and relaxing takes a considerable time commitment on the part of the nurse. Although this may be difficult in the critical care environment, it may be beneficial.[160]

Music Therapy. Music therapy is a commonly used intervention for relaxation. Music that is pleasing to the patient may have soothing effects.[162,163] Ideally the music should be supplied by a small set of headphones. This method also serves to minimize the distracting and anxiety-producing noises of a critical care unit.[164] It is important to educate the patient and family regarding the role of music in relaxation and pain control and also to provide music of the patient's choice.

Table 8-4	Equianalgesic Chart: Approximate Equivalent Doses of Opioids for Moderate-to-Severe Pain—cont'd		
Analgesic	**Parenteral (IM, SC, IV) Route [1,2] (mg)**	**PO Route[1] (mg)**	**Comments**
AGONIST-ANTAGONIST OPIOIDS: Not recommended for severe, escalating pain. If used in combination with mu agonists, may reverse analgesia and precipitate withdrawal in opioid-dependent patients.			
BUPRENORPHINE (Buprenex)	0.4	—	Not readily reversed by naloxone; NR for laboring patients
BUTORPHANOL (Stadol)	2	—	Available in nasal spray
DEZOCINE (Dalgan)	10	—	
NALBUPHINE (Nubain)	10	—	
PENTAZOCINE (Talwin)	60	180	

Selected References For more complete information and additional references, see Pasero C, Portenoy RK, McCaffery M: Opioid analgesics, pp. 161-299. In McCaffery M, Pasero C: *Pain: clinical manual*, St Louis, 1999, Mosby, pp 241-243.
American Pain Society (APS): *Principles of analgesic use in the treatment of acute and cancer pain*, ed 3, Glenview, Ill, 1992, APS.
Lawlor P, Turner K, Hanson J, et al: Dose ratio between morphine and hydromorphone in patients with cancer pain: a retrospective study, *Pain* 72(1,2):79-85, 1997.
Manfredi PL, Borsook D, Chandler SW, et al: Intravenous methadone for cancer pain unrelieved by morphine and hydromorphone: clinical observations, *Pain* 70:99-101, 1997.
Portenoy RK: Opioid analgesics. In Portenoy RK, Kanner RM, editors: *Pain management: theory and practice*, Philadelphia, 1996, FA Davis Company, pp. 249-276.

Equianalgesic Chart
Approximate equivalent doses of PO nonopioids and opioids for mild-to-moderate pain

ANALGESIC	PO DOSAGE (mg)
Nonopioids	
Acetaminophen	650
Aspirin (ASA)	650
Opioids*	
Codeine	32-60
Hydrocodone†	5
Meperidine (Demerol)	50
Oxycodone††	3-5
Propoxyphene (Darvon)	65-100

* Often combined with acetaminophen; avoid exceeding maximum total daily dose of acetaminophen (4000 mg/day).

† Combined with acetaminophen, e.g., Vicodin, Lortab.

†† Combined with acetaminophen, e.g., Percocet, Tylox. Also available alone as controlled-release OxyContin and immediate-release formulations.

A Guide to Using Equianalgesic Charts

- Equianalgesic means approximately the same pain relief.
- The equianalgesic chart is a guideline. Doses and intervals between doses are titrated according to individual's response.
- The equianalgesic chart is helpful when switching from one drug to another, or switching from one route of administration to another.
- Dosages in the equianalgesic chart for moderate-to-severe pain are not necessarily starting doses. The doses suggest a ratio for comparing the analgesia of one drug to another.
- For elderly patients, initially reduce the recommended adult opioid dose for moderate to severe pain by 25% to 50%.
- The longer the patient has been receiving opioids, the more conservative the starting dose of a *new* opioid.

Selected References: For more complete information and additional references, see McCaffery M, Portenoy RK: Nonopioids: acetaminophen and nonsteroidal antiinflammatory drugs, pp. 241-243. In McCaffery M, Pasero C: *Pain: clinical manual*, St Louis, 1999, Mosby, p. 133.
American Pain Society (APS): *Principles of analgesic use in the treatment of acute pain and cancer pain*, ed. 3, Glenview, IL, APS, 1992.
Kaiko R et al: Analgesic efficacy of controlled-release (CR) oxycodone and CR morphine, *Clin Pharmacol Ther* 59:130, 1996.
■ From McCaffery M, Pasero C: *Pain: clinical manual*, St Louis, 1999, Mosby.

SUMMARY

Today's health care environment mandates that patients experience positive outcomes as rapidly as possible. Because pain is a major barrier to early mobility and rapid return to a pre-illness state; pain management is of paramount importance to the critical care nurse. Since the critically ill patient is the most difficult to assess and manage, the critical care nurse must develop the skill and intervention techniques necessary to manage complex pain states. As patient advocate the nurse assumes the responsibility for establishing pain control as a priority for the health care team.[165] The nurse's role and responsibility become more important as the regulating agencies and professional bodies focus more attention on the area of patient pain. The nurse's knowledge and understanding of pain and its implications for patients are the foundations for meeting patients' pain needs safely and efficiently.

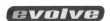 For bonus Clinical Applications on pain and pain management, see the Evolve website.

REFERENCES

1. Cochran J, Ganong LH: A comparison of nurses' and patients' perceptions of intensive care unit stressors, *J Adv Nurs* 14:1038, 1989.
2. Hallenberg B, Bergbom-Engberg I, Haljamäe H: Patients' experiences of postoperative respirator treatment—influence of anaesthetic and pain treatment regimens, *Acta Anaesthesiol Scand* 34:557, 1990.
3. Puntillo KA: The phenomenon of pain and critical care nursing, *Heart Lung* 17:262, 1988.
4. Puntillo KA: Pain experience of intensive care unit patients, *Heart Lung* 19:526, 1990.
5. Puntillo KA: Dimensions of procedural pain and its analgesic management in critically ill surgical patients, *Am J Crit Care* 3:116, 1994.
6. Turner JS et al: Patients' recollection of intensive care unit experience, *Crit Care Med* 18:966, 1990.
7. Wilson VS: Identification of stressors related to patients' psychologic responses to the surgical intensive care unit, *Heart Lung* 16:267, 1987.
8. Christoph SB: Pain assessment: the problem of pain in the critically ill patient, *Crit Care Nurs Clin North Am* 3:11, 1991.
9. Kwekkeboom KL, Herr K: Assessment of pain in the critically ill, *Crit Care Nurs Clin North Am* 13:181, 2001.
10. Murray MJ: Pain problems in the ICU, *Crit Care Clin* 6:235, 1990.
11. Desbiens NA et al: Pain and satisfaction with pain control in seriously ill hospitalized adults: findings from the SUPPORT research investigations, *Crit Care Med* 24:1953, 1996.
12. Ferguson J, Gilroy D, Puntillo K: Dimensions of pain and analgesic administration associated with coronary artery bypass grafting in an Australian intensive care unit, *J Adv Nurs* 26:1065, 1997.
13. Puntillo KA, Weiss SJ: Pain: its mediators and associated morbidity in critically ill cardiovascular surgical patients, *Nurs Res* 43:31, 1994.
14. Puntillo KA et al: Patients' perceptions and responses to procedural pain: Results from Thunder Project II, *Am J Crit Care* 10:238, 2001.
15. Stanik-Hutt J et al: Pain experiences of traumatically injured patients in a critical care setting, *Am J Crit Care* 10:252, 2001.
16. Valdix SW, Puntillo KA: Pain, pain relief and accuracy of their recall after cardiac surgery, *Prog Cardiovasc Nurs* 10:3, 1995.
17. Watt-Watson J et al: Relationship between nurses' pain knowledge and pain management outcomes for their postoperative cardiac patients, *J Adv Nurs* 36:535, 2001.
18. Whipple JK et al: Analysis of pain management in critically ill patients, *Pharmacotherapy* 15:592, 1995.
19. Agency for Health Care Policy and Research (AHCPR): Acute pain management: operative or medical procedures and trauma, part 1, *Clinical Pharmacy* 11:309, 1992.
20. McCaffery M: *Nursing management of the patient with pain*, ed 2, Philadelphia, 1979, Lippincott.
21. Hamill-Ruth RJ, Marohn L: Evaluation of pain in the critically ill patient, *Crit Care Clin* 15:35, 1999.
22. Shannon K, Bucknall T: Pain assessment in critical care: what have we learned from research, *Intensive Crit Care Nurs* 19:154, 2003.
23. Kaiser KS: Assessment and management of pain in the critically ill trauma patient, *Crit Care Nurs Q* 15:14, 1992.
24. Mlynczak B: Assessment and management of the trauma patient in pain, *Crit Care Nurs Clin North Am* 1:55, 1989.
25. Puntillo KA: *Pain in the critically ill: assessment and management*, Gaithersburg, Md, 1991, Aspen.
26. Solomon P: The clinical utility of pain behavior measures, *Phys Rehab Med* 12:193, 2000.
27. Ferrell B, Wheden M, Rollins B: Pain and quality assessment/improvement, *J Nurs Care Qual* 9:69, 1995.
28. Bellinger K et al: The impact of nursing on pain management. In Weiner R, editor: *Pain management: a practical guide for clinicians*, Sonora, Calif, 1998, CRC Press.
29. Carr ECJ, Thomas VJ: Anticipating and experiencing postoperative pain: the patient's perspective, *J Clin Nurs* 6:191, 1997.
30. Carroll KC et al: Pain assessment and management in critically ill postoperative and trauma patients: a multisite study, *Am J Crit Care* 8:105, 1999.
31. Celia B: Age and gender differences in pain management following coronary artery bypass surgery, *J Gerontol Nurs* 26(5), 2000.
32. Choiniere M et al: Comparisons between patients and nurses assessment of pain and medication efficacy in severe burn injuries, *Pain* 40:143, 1990.
33. Lay TD et al: Analgesics prescribed and administered to intensive care cardiac surgery patients: does patient age make a difference? *Prog Cardiovasc Nurs* 11:17, 1996.
34. Maxam-Moore VA, Wilkie DJ, Woods SL: Analgesics for cardiac surgery patients in critical care: describing current practice, *Am J Crit Care* 3:31, 1994.
35. Puntillo KA et al: Practices and predictors of analgesic interventions for adults undergoing painful procedures, *Am J Crit Care* 11:415, 2002.
36. Stannard D et al: Clinical judgment and management of postoperative pain in critical care patients, *Am J Crit Care* 5:433, 1996.
37. Tittle M, McMillan SC: Pain and pain-related side effects in an ICU and on a surgical unit: nurses' management, *Am J Crit Care* 3:25, 1994.
38. Camp LD, O'Sullivan PS: Comparison of medical, surgical and oncology patients' descriptions of pain and nurses' documentation of pain assessments, *J Adv Nurs* 12:593, 1987.
39. Idvall E, Ehrenberg A: Nursing documentation of postoperative pain management, *J Clin Nurs* 11:734, 2002.
40. Manias E, Botti M, Bucknall T: Observation of pain assessment and management—the complexities of clinical practice, *J Clin Nurs* 11:724, 2002.
41. Paice JA, Mahon SM, Faut-Callahan M: Factors associated with adequate pain control in hospitalized postsurgical patients diagnosed with cancer, *Cancer Nurs* 14:298, 1991.
42. Sullivan LM: Factors influencing pain management: a nursing perspective, *J Post Anesth Nurs* 9:83, 1994.
43. Carr DB, Goudas LC: Acute pain, *Lancet* 353:2051, 1999.
44. O'Gara PT: The hemodynamic consequences of pain and its management, *J Intensive Care Med* 3:3, 1988.
45. Wild L: Transition from pain to comfort: managing the haemodynamic risks, *Crit Care Nurs Q* 15:46, 1992.
46. Cheever KH: Reducing the effects of acute pain in critically ill patients, *Dimensions Crit Care Nurs* 18:14, 1999.
47. Joint Commission on Accreditation of Healthcare Organizations (JCAHO): *Pain: current understanding of assessment, management, and treatments*, Oakbrook Terrace, Ill, 2001, JCAHO.
48. Canadian Council on Health Services Accreditation (CCHSA), *Inclusion of pain management in the achieving improved measurement*, www.cchsa.ca, 2003.
49. American Nurses Association: *Position statement: promotion of comfort and relief in the dying patient*, Washington, DC, 1992, The Association.

50. Lindquist R, Banasik J, Barnsteiner J: Determining AACN's research priorities for the 90s, *Am J Crit Care* 2:110, 1993.
51. Joint Commission on Accreditation of Healthcare Organizations: *Joint Commission on Accreditation of Healthcare Organizations comprehensive accreditation manual for hospitals,* Oakbrook Terrace, Ill, 2000, JCAHO.
52. International Association for the Study of Pain (IASP), Subcommittee on Taxonomy: Pain terms: a list with definitions and notes on usage, *Pain* 6:249, 1979.
53. Loeser JD, Cousins MJ: Contemporary pain management, *Med J Aust* 153:208, 1990.
54. Melzack R, Wall PD: Pain mechanisms: a new theory. *Science* 150:971, 1965.
55. Melzack R, Casey KL: Sensory, motivational, and central control determinants of pain: a new conceptual model. In Kenshalo D, editor: *The skin senses,* Springfield, 1968, Charles C Thomas.
56. Melzack R: From the gate to the neuromatrix, *Pain* (suppl 6):S121-S126, 1999.
57. Melzack R: Pain and stress: a new perspective. In Gatchel RJ, Turk DC, editors: *Psychological factors in pain,* New York, 1999, Guilford Press.
58. McGuire D: Comprehensive and multidimensional assessment and measurement of pain, *J Pain Symptom Manage* 7:312, 1992.
59. Cousins M: Acute and postoperative pain. In Wall PD, Melzack R, editors: *Textbook of pain,* New York, 1994, Churchill Livingstone.
60. McGuire DB: Measuring pain. In Frank-Stromberg M, Olsen SJ, Pender NJ, editors: *Instruments for clinical health-care research,* ed 2, Massachusetts, 1997, Jones and Bartlett.
61. Levine J, Taiwo Y: Inflammatory pain. In Wall PD, Melzack R, editors: *Textbook of pain,* New York, 1994, Churchill Livingstone.
62. Loeser JD, Melzack R: Pain: an overview, *Lancet,* 353:1607, 1999.
63. Summer GJ, Puntillo KA: Management of surgical and procedural pain in a critical care setting, *Crit Care Nurs Clin North Am* 13:233, 2001.
64. Katz J et al: Acute pain after thoracic surgery predicts long-term post-thoracotomy pain, *Clin J Pain* 12:50, 1996.
65. Hayes C, Molloy AR: Neuropathic pain in the perioperative period, *Int Anesthesiol Clin* 35:67, 1997.
66. Siddall PJ, Cousins MJ: Neurobiology of pain, *Int Anesthesiol Clin* 35:1, 1997.
67. Woolf CJ, Mannion RJ: Neuropathic pain: aetiology, symptoms, mechanisms, and management, *Lancet* 353:1959, 1999.
68. McCaffery M, Pasero C: *Pain: clinical manual for nursing practice,* ed 2, St Louis, 1999, Mosby.
69. Melzack R, Wall PD: *The challenge of pain,* ed 2, London, 1996, Penguin.
70. Wallace KG: The pathophysiology of pain, *Crit Care Nurs Q* 15:1, 1992.
71. McKenna JE, Melzack R: Analgesia produced by lidocaine microinjection into the dentate gyrus, *Pain* 49:105, 1992.
72. Bromm B: Consciousness, pain, and cortical activity. In Bromm B, Desmedt JE, editors: *Pain and the brain: from nociception to cognition,* New York, 1995, Raven Press.
73. Tasker RAR et al: Analgesia produced by injection of lidocaine into the lateral hypothalamus, *Pain* 31:237, 1987.
74. Vaccarino AL, Melzack R: Temporal processes of formalin pain: differential role of the cingulum bundle, fornix pathway and medial bulboreticular formation, *Pain* 49:257, 1992.
75. Behbehani MM: Physiology and mechanisms of pain. In Parker MM, Shapiro MJ, Porembka DT, editors: *Critical care: state of the art,* California, 1995, Society of Critical Care Medicine.
76. Selye H: *Stress without distress,* Philadelphia, 1974, JB Lippincott.
77. McCance KL, Huether SE: *Pathophysiology : the biologic basis for disease in adults and children,* ed 3, St Louis, 1998, Mosby.
78. Payen JF et al: Assessing pain in the critically ill sedated patients by using a behavioral pain scale, *Crit Care Med* 29:2258, 2001.
79. Puntillo KA et al: Relationship between behavioral and physiological indicators of pain, critical care self-reports of pain, and opioid administration, *Crit Care Med* 25:1159, 1997.
80. Hurwitz BE et al: Differential patterns of dynamic cardiovascular regulation as a function of task, *Biol Psychol* 36:75, 1993.
81. Rabin BS et al: Bidirectional interaction between the central nervous system and the immune system, *Crit Rev Immunol* 9:279, 1989.
82. Sapolsky RM: Stress, glucocorticoids, and damage to the nervous system: the current state of confusion, *Stress* 1:1, 1996.
83. Ste-Marie B: *American Society of Pain Management Nurses: Core curriculum for pain management nursing,* Philadelphia, 2002, Saunders.
84. Daut RL, Cleeland CS: The prevalence and severity of pain in cancer, *Cancer* 50:1913, 1982.
85. Melzack R: The short form McGill Pain Questionnaire, *Pain* 30:191, 1987.
86. Jarvis, C: *Physical examination and health assessment,* ed 4, Philadelphia, 2004, Saunders.
87. Caillet R: *Pain: mechanisms and management,* Philadelphia, 1993, Davis.
88. Mateo OM, Krenzischek DA: A pilot study to assess the relationship between behavioral manifestations and self-report of pain in postanesthesia care unit patients, *J Post Anesth Nurs* 7:15, 1992.
89. Webb MR, Kennedy MG: Behavioral responses and self-reported pain in postoperative patients, *J Post Anesth Nurs* 9:91, 1994.
90. Carey SJ et al: Improving pain management in an acute care setting: the Crawford Long Hospital of Emory University Experience, *Orthopaed Nurs* 16:29, 1997.
91. Stuppy DJ: The Faces Pain Scale: Reliability and validity with mature adults, *Appl Nurs Res* 11:84, 1998.
92. Gelinas C et al: Les indicateurs de la douleur en soins critiques (Pain indicators in critical care), *Perspective Infirmière* 2(4):12-22, 2004.
93. Puntillo KA: Pain management. In Schell HM, Puntillo KA, editors: *Critical care nursing secrets,* Philadelphia, 2001, Hanley & Belfus.
94. Gelinas C: *Développement et validation d'une grille d'observation de douleur auprès d'une clientèle adulte de soins critiques présentant ou non une altération du niveau de conscience* (Development and validation of the Critical-Care Pain Observation Tool [CPOT] among critically ill adult patients with or without an alteration of the level of consciousness), Doctoral Thesis, Faculty of Nursing, Laval University, Quebec City, Canada, 2004.
95. Prkachin KM: The consistency of facial expressions of pain: a comparison across modalities, *Pain* 51:297, 1992.

96. Gelinas C et al: Pain assessment and management in critically ill intubated patients: a retrospective study, *Am J Crit Care* 13:126, 2004.

97. Gelinas C et al: *Observable indicators of pain in cardiac surgery ICU patients,* National Teaching Institute (NTI), American Association of Critical-Care Nurses (AACN), Annual Congress, Orlando (Florida), Oral presentation, May 15-20, 2004. Retrieved from the Internet at http://www.aacn.org/AACN/NTIPoster.nsf/vwdoc/2004RESCGelinas?opendocument.

98. Harris CE et al: Use of propofol by infusion for sedation of patients undergoing haemofiltration—assessment of the effect of haemofiltration on the level of sedation and on blood propofol concentration, *J Drug Devel* 4 (suppl 3): 37, 1991.

99. Devlin JW et al: Motor Activity Assessment Scale: a valid and reliable sedation scale for use with mechanically ventilated patients in an adult surgical intensive care unit, *Crit Care Med* 27:1271, 1999.

100. Riker RR, Graser GL, Cox PM: Continuous infusion of haloperidol controls agitation in critically ill patients, *Crit Care Med* 22:433, 1994.

101. Gelinas C et al: Validation of the Critical-Care Pain Observation Tool (CPOT) in adult patients, *Am J Crit Care,* submitted 2005.

102. Lynch M: Pain as the fifth vital sign, *J Intravenous Nurs* 24:85, 2001.

103. Wild LR: Pain management: an organizational perspective, *Crit Care Nurs Clin North Am* 13:297, 2001.

104. Faries JE et al: Systematic pain records and their impact on pain control, *Cancer Nurs* 14:306, 1991.

105. Voigt L, Paice JA, Pouliot J: Standardized pain flowsheet: impact on patient-reported pain experiences after cardiovascular surgery, *Am J Crit Care* 4:308, 1995.

106. Halloran T, Pohlman A: Managing sedation in the critically ill patient, *Crit Care Nurse* 5(suppl 4):1, 1995.

107. Lawrence M: The unconscious experience, *Am J Crit Care* 4:227, 1995.

108. Stephens ST: A promise to Billie, *Nursing* April:96, 1994.

109. Bushnell MC: Perception of pain in the persistent vegetative state? (Commentaries), *Eur J Pain* 1:167, 1997.

110. Klein M: Perception of pain in the persistent vegetative state? (Letter to the Editor), *Eur J Pain* 1:165, 1997.

111. Forrest J: Assessment of acute and chronic pain in older adults, *J Gerontol Nurs* October:15, 1995.

112. Gibson MC: Improving pain control for the elderly patient with dementia, *Am J Alzheimers Dis Other Demen* January/February:10, 1998.

113. Miller J et al: The assessment of discomfort in elderly confused patients: a preliminary study, *J Neurosci Nurs* 28:175, 1996.

114. Feldt KS: The Checklist of Nonverbal Pain Indicators (CNPI), *Pain Manag Nurs* 1:13, 2000.

115. Hurley AC et al: Assessment of discomfort in advanced Alzheimer patients, *Res Nurs Health* 15:369, 1992.

116. Fuchs-Labelle S, Hadjistavropoulos T: Development and preliminary validation of the Pain Assessment Checklist for Seniors with Limited Ability to Communicate (PACSLAC), *Pain Manag Nurs* 5:37, 2004.

117. Herr KA, Mobily PR: Comparison of selected pain assessment tools for use with the elderly, *Appl Nurs Res* 6:39, 1993.

118. Anand KJS: The applied physiology of pain. In Anand KJS, McGrath PJ, editors: *Pain in neonates,* Amsterdam, 1993, Elsevier.

119. Stevens B et al: Premature Infant Pain Profile: development and initial validation, *Clin J Pain* 12:13, 1996.

120. Ambuel B et al: Assessing distress in pediatric intensive care environments: the COMFORT scale, *J Pediatr Psychol* 17:95, 1992.

121. Krechel SW, Bildner J: CRIES: a new neonatal postoperative pain measurement score. Initial testing of validity and reliability, *Paediatr Anaesth* 5:53, 1995.

122. Stevens B: Development and testing of a pediatric pain management sheet, *Pediatr Nurs* 16:543, 1990.

123. Lawrence J et al: The development of a tool to assess neonatal pain, *Neonatal Network* 12:59, 1993.

124. Blaner T, Gerstmann D: A simultaneous comparison of three neonatal pain scales during common NICU procedures, *Clin J Pain* 14:39, 1998.

125. Jurf J, Nirschl A: Acute postoperative pain review and update, *Crit Care Nurs* Q 16:8, 1993.

126. Bozeman M: Cultural aspects of pain management. In Salerno E, Willens J, editors: *Pain management handbook: an interdisciplinary approach,* St Louis, 1996, Mosby.

127. Ulmer J: Identifying and preventing pain mismanagement. In Salerno E, Willens J, editors: *Pain management handbook: an interdisciplinary approach,* St Louis, 1996, Mosby.

128. Alpen M, Titler M: Pain management in the critically ill: what do we know and how can we improve? *AACN Clin Issues Crit Care Nurs* 5:159, 1994.

129. Sun X, Weissman C: The use of analgesics and sedatives in the critically ill patient: physician's order versus medication administered, *Heart Lung* 23:169, 1994.

130. Pasero CL, McCaffery M: Avoiding opioid-induced respiratory depression, *Amer J Nurs* April:25-31, 1994.

131. Kirkchhoff LT, Beckstrand RL: Critical care nurses perceptions of obstacles and helpful behaviors in providing end-of-life care to dying patients, *Am J Crit Care* 9:96, 2000.

132. Jacobi J et al: Clinical practice guidelines for the sustained use of sedatives and analgesics in the critically ill adult, *Crit Care Med* 30:119, 2002.

133. Liu LL, Gropper MA: Postoperative analgesia and sedation in the adult intensive care unit: a guide to drug selection, *Drugs* 63:755, 2003.

134. Volles DF, McGory R: Pharmacokinetic considerations, *Crit Care Clin* 15:55, 1999.

135. Salerno E: Pharmacologic approaches to pain. In Salerno E, Willens J, editors: *Pain management handbook: an interdisciplinary approach,* St Louis, 1996, Mosby.

136. Paice J: Pharmacologic management. In Watt-Watson J, Donovan M, editors: *Pain management: nursing perspective,* St Louis, 1992, Mosby.

137. Yantis MA: Obstructive sleep apnea syndrome, *Am J Nurs* 102:83, 2002.

138. Barke KE, Hough LD: Opiates, mast cells and histamine release, *Life Sci* 53:1391, 1993.

139. Sarhill N, Walsh D, Nelson KA: Hydromorphone: pharmacology and clinical applications in cancer patients, *Support Care Cancer* 9:84, 2001.

140. Wild L: Intravenous methods of analgesia for pain in the critically ill. In Puntillo K, editor: *Pain in the critically ill: assessment and management,* Gaithersburg, Md, 1991, Aspen.

141. Jacox A et al: *Management of cancer pain: clinical practice guideline,* No. 9, AHCPR Publication No. 94-0592, Rockville, Md, U.S. Public Health Service, March 1994, AHCPR.

142. Marcantonio ER et al: The relationship of post-operative delirium with psychoactive medications, *JAMA* 272:1518, 1994.

143. Reisine T, Pasternak G: Opioid analgesics and antagonists. In Hardman JG, Limbird LM, editors: *Goodman &*

Gilman's the pharmacological basis of therapeutics, ed 9, New-York, 1996, McGraw-Hill.

144. McGory R: Pharmacokinetic and pharmacodynamic concerns in the critically ill. In Hamill RJ, Rowlingson RC, editors: *Handbook of critical care pain management,* New York, 1994, McGraw-Hill.

145. Davis MP, Walsh D: Methadone for relief of cancer pain: a review of pharmacokinetics, pharmacodynamics, drug interactions and protocols of administration, *Support Care Cancer* 9:73, 2001.

146. World Health Organization (WHO): *Cancer pain relief,* Geneva, 1986, WHO.

147. Levine RL: Pharmacology of intravenous sedatives and opioids in critically ill patients, *Crit Care Clin* 10:709, 1994.

148. Murray MJ, Deruyter ML, Harrison BA: Opioids and benzodiazepines, *Crit Care Clin* 11:849, 1995.

149. Petuda VA, Ballabio M, Stefanini S: Efficacy of propacetamol in the treatment of postoperative pain. Morphine sparing effect in orthopedic surgery, Italian Collaborative Group on Propacetamol, *Acta Anaesthesiol Scand* 42:293, 1998.

150. Lehne RA: *Pharmacology for nursing care,* ed 5, Philadelphia, 2004, Saunders.

151. Spross J, Singer M: Patients with cancer. In Watt-Watson J, Donovan M, editors: *Pain management: nursing perspective,* St Louis, 1992, Mosby.

152. Ready LB et al: Evaluation of intravenous ketorolac administered by bolus of infusion for treatment of postoperative pain, *Anesthesiology* 80:1277, 1994.

153. American Society of Hospital Pharmacists: *American hospital formulary service drug information* 99, Bethesda, Md, 1999, The Association.

154. Feldman HI et al: Parenteral ketorolac: the risk for acute renal failure, *Ann Intern Med* 126:193, 1997.

155. Strom BL et al: Parenteral ketorolac and risk of gastrointestinal and operative site bleeding, *JAMA* 275:376, 1996.

156. McKenry L, Salerno E: *Mosby's pharmacology in nursing,* ed 20, St Louis, 1998, Mosby.

157. Collins P, Spunt A, Huml M: Symptom management. In Salerno E, Willens J, editors: *Pain management handbook: an interdisciplinary approach,* St Louis, 1996, Mosby.

158. Dyble K: Epidural and intrathecal methods of analgesia in the critically ill. In Puntillo K, editor: *Pain in the critically ill: assessment and management,* Gaithersburg, Md, 1991, Aspen.

159. Rietman L: Pain management. In Chulay M, Guzzetta C, Dossey B, editors: *AACN Handbook of critical care nursing,* Stamford, Conn, 1997, Appleton & Lange.

160. Gujol M: A survey of pain assessment and management practices among critical care nurses, *Am J Crit Care* 3:123, 1994.

161. Miller KM, Perry PA: Relaxation technique and postoperative pain in patients undergoing cardiac surgery, *Heart Lung* 19:136, 1990.

162. Broscious SK: Music: An intervention for pain during chest tube removal after open heart surgery, *Am J Crit Care* 8:410, 1999.

163. Courts N: Nonpharmacologic approaches to pain. In Salerno E, Willens J, editors: *Pain management handbook: an interdisciplinary approach,* St Louis, 1996, Mosby.

164. Edgar L, Smith-Hanrahan C: Nonpharmacologic pain management. In Watt-Watson J, Donovan M, editors: *Pain management: nursing perspective,* St Louis, 1992, Mosby.

165. Meehan D et al: Analgesic administration, pain intensity, and patient satisfaction in cardiac surgical patients, *Am J Crit Care* 4:435, 1995.

CHAPTER 9

Agitation and Sedation Management

O ne of the unique challenges facing all critical care nurses is the need to deliver nursing care, while assuring that the critically ill patient does not suffer physical pain or psychologic stress. This chapter complements the discussion on pain management in the previous chapter. The known strategies and very real challenges of providing sedation management are explained and explored.

PATIENT AGITATION AND NEED FOR SEDATION/ANALGESIA

One of the challenges facing clinicians is how to provide a therapeutic environment for patients in the alarm-filled, emergency-focused critical care unit. Rest and relaxation can be difficult to find. As many as 74% of critical care patients demonstrate some degree of agitation during their critical care hospitalization.[1] Many patients report upsetting dreams, hallucinations, nightmares, and flashbacks once they are recovered. The many causes of this agitation include painful procedures, invasive tubes, sleep deprivation, fear, anxiety, and the stress associated with critical illness. Some patients experience a post-traumatic stress disorder (PTSD) syndrome after prolonged hospitalizations.[1]

The goal of recent clinical practice guidelines is to increase the awareness of these issues within the medical and nursing community.[2] When the sedation assessment, as with the pain assessment, is recognized as a *fifth vital sign*, nurses may be able to decrease the incidence of agitation and delirium in critically ill patients.

The need for analgesics and sedatives to maintain patient safety and comfort is important, but it is increasingly recognized that excessive sedation can prolong the duration of mechanical ventilation, create physical and psychologic dependence, and increase the length of the hospital stay.[3] The goal is to find a balance between providing compassionate patient care and avoiding oversedation.

ASSESSING LEVEL OF SEDATION

SEDATION SCALES

The use of scoring systems to assess and record levels of sedation and agitation is now strongly recommended.[2] Four frequently used scales are the Ramsey Scale, the Riker Sedation-Agitation Scale (SAS), the Motor Activity Assessment Scale (MAAS), and the Richmond Agitation-Assessment Scale (RAAS) (Table 9-1).[3,4] Frequent assessment of the patient's motor activity and sedation level is helpful to titrate continuous infusions of sedatives such as propofol or lorazepam. Collaboratively, the critical care team must decide which level of sedation is most appropriate for an individual patient.[2,3]

Sedative levels are standardized using the descriptors "light," "moderate," and "deep" to describe the level of sedation (Box 9-1).[2,3] *Light sedation*, or "minimal" sedation, is used when the goal of sedative therapy is to relieve anxiety and ensure patient comfort while allowing the patient to remain responsive to the environment. A recent research survey of critical care nurses found most believe that treating patient's anxiety is both beneficial and important.[5] *Moderate sedation*, also called "conscious" or "procedural" sedation, is used in conjunction with analgesia to ensure patient comfort during a painful or invasive procedure (e.g., bronchoscopy). *Deep sedation* is used when the patient must be unresponsive so that care may be delivered safely. For example in the management of acute respiratory distress syndrome (ARDS), deep sedation and analgesia may be required to achieve ventilator synchrony.[3] By contrast, when a patient is weaning from the ventilator, only light sedation may be necessary. During ventilator-weaning trials, it is more reasonable to limit sedation so that the patient is comfortable and arousable to voice while avoiding the twin perils of agitation and oversedation.

The first step in assessing the agitated patient is to rule out any sensations of pain.[3] Clinical assessment is more challenging when the patient is obtunded or has an

Table 9-1	Sedation Scales	
Score*	Description	Definition

RIKER SEDATION-AGITATION SCALE (SAS)[1]

7	Dangerous agitation	Pulls at endotracheal tube (ETT), tries to remove catheters, climbs over bedrail, strikes at staff, thrashes side to side
6	Very agitated	Does not calm despite frequent verbal reminding of limits, requires physical restraints, bites ETT
5	Agitated	Anxious or mildly agitated, attempts to sit up, calms down to verbal instructions
4	Calm and cooperative	Calm, awakens easily, follows commands
3	Sedated	Difficult to arouse, awakens to verbal stimuli or gentle shaking but drifts off again, follows simple commands
2	Very sedated	Arouses to physical stimuli, but does not communicate or follow commands, may move spontaneously
1	Unarousable	Minimal or no response to noxious stimuli, does not communicate or follow commands

MOTOR ACTIVITY ASSESSMENT SCALE (MAAS)[2]

6	Dangerously agitated	No external stimulus required to elicit movement; is uncooperative, pulls at tubes/catheters, thrashes side to side, strikes at staff, tries to climb out of bed, does not calm down when asked
5	Agitated	No external stimulus required to elicit movement; attempts to sit up or move limbs out of bed, does not consistently follow commands (e.g., will lie down when asked, but soon reverts back to attempts)
4	Restless and cooperative	No external stimulus required to elicit movement; picks at sheets/tubes or uncovers self, follows commands
3	Calm and cooperative	No external stimulus required to elicit movement; adjusts sheets/clothes purposefully, follows commands
2	Responsive to touch or name	Opens eyes, raises eyebrows, or turns head toward stimulus; or moves limbs when touched or when name loudly spoken
1	Responsive only to noxious stimulus	Opens eyes, raises eyebrows, or turns head toward stimulus; or moves limbs with noxious stimulus
0	Unresponsive	Does not move with noxious stimulus

RAMSEY SCALE[3]

1	Awake	Anxious and agitated or restless, or both
2		Cooperative, oriented, and tranquil
3		Responds only to commands
4	Asleep	Brisk response to light glabellar tap or loud auditory stimulus
5		Sluggish response to light glabellar tap or loud auditory stimulus
6		No response to light glabellar tap or loud auditory stimulus

RICHMOND AGITATION-SEDATION SCALE (RASS)[4,5]

−5	Unresponsive	No response to voice or physical stimulation
−4	Deep sedation	No response to voice, but any movement to physical stimulation
−3	Moderate sedation	Any movement, but no eye contact to voice
−2	Light sedation	Briefly, less than 10 seconds, awakening with eye contact to voice
−1	Drowsy	Not fully alert, but has sustained—more than 10 sec—awakening with eye contact to voice
0	Alert and calm	
1	Restless	Anxious or apprehensive but movements not aggressive or vigorous
2	Agitated	Frequent nonpurposeful movement or patient-ventilator dyssynchrony
3	Very agitated	Pulls on or removes tubes or catheters or has aggressive behavior toward staff
4	Combative	Overly combative or violent, immediate danger to staff

References

1. Riker RR, Picard JT, Fraser GL: Prospective evaluation of the Sedation-Agitation Scale for adult critically ill patients, *Crit Care Med* 27(7):1325-1329, 1999.
2. Devlin JW et al: Motor Activity Assessment Scale: a valid and reliable sedation scale for use with mechanically ventilated patients in an adult surgical intensive care unit, *Crit Care Med* 27(7):1271-1275, 1999.
3. Ramsey MA et al: Controlled sedation with alphaxalone-alphadolone, *Br Med J* 2:656-659, 1974.
4. Sessler CN et al: The Richmond Agitation-Sedation Scale: validity and reliability in adult intensive care unit patients, *Am J Respir Crit Care Med* 166(10):1338-1344, 2002.
5. Ely EW et al: Monitoring sedation status over time in ICU patients: reliability and validity of the Richmond Agitation-Sedation Scale (RASS), *JAMA* 289(22):2983-2991, 2003.

Box 9-1

LEVELS OF SEDATION

LIGHT SEDATION (MINIMAL SEDATION, ANXIOLYSIS)
Drug-induced state during which patients respond normally to verbal commands. Although cognitive function and coordination may be impaired, ventilatory and cardiovascular functions are unaffected.

MODERATE SEDATION WITH ANALGESIA (CONSCIOUS SEDATION, PROCEDURAL SEDATION)
Drug-induced depression of consciousness during which patients respond purposefully to verbal commands, either alone or accompanied by light tactile stimulation. No interventions are required to maintain a patent airway, and spontaneous ventilation is adequate. Cardiovascular function is usually maintained.

DEEP SEDATION AND ANALGESIA
Drug-induced depression of consciousness during which patients cannot be easily aroused but respond purposefully after repeated or painful stimulation. The ability to maintain ventilatory function independently is impaired. Patients require assistance in maintaining a patent airway, and spontaneous ventilation may be inadequate. Cardiovascular function is usually maintained.

GENERAL ANESTHESIA
Drug-induced loss of consciousness during which patients are not arousable, even by painful stimulation. The ability to maintain ventilatory function independently is impaired, and assistance to maintain a patent airway is required. Positive-pressure ventilation may be required because of depressed spontaneous ventilation or drug-induced depression of neuromuscular function. Cardiovascular function may be impaired.

Data from Joint Commission on Accreditation of Healthcare Organizations: *Comprehensive accreditation manual for hospitals,* Oakbrook Terrace, Ill, 2000, The JCAHO; and Jacobi J et al: *Crit Care Med* 30(1):119-141, 2002.

artificial airway in place. If the patient can communicate, the 0 to 10 verbal pain scale is very useful. If the patient is intubated and cannot vocalize, assessing pain becomes considerably more complex. Once medication for pain has been provided, the next step is to determine the minimum level of sedation required. If deep or moderate sedation is being applied, it is essential that all members of the health care team are qualified and have appropriate credentials to manage sedative medications and any potential patient complications that arise.[2,3]

CONTINUOUS NERVOUS SYSTEM MONITORING

One of the challenges with deep sedation is recognizing whether a patient is effectively sedated and pain free. Two clinicians evaluating the same patient may not agree about whether the level of applied sedation and

analgesia is appropriate; one may describe the patient as "oversedated," and the other may describe the patient as "inadequately sedated."[2] Clinical parameters such as heart rate and blood pressure are not always reliable, because these can be changed by other conditions.

In an attempt to clarify clinical assessment of depth of consciousness some hospitals use continuous monitoring of the electroencephalogram (EEG) for sedated, mechanically ventilated patients. The United States Food and Drug Administration (FDA) has approved two modified continuous EEG monitoring systems. The first, and most widely used, system in critical care units is the bispectral index (BIS).[6,7] The BIS system uses sensor electrodes on a single band placed on the patient's forehead. The other continuous EEG monitoring system monitors a "Patient State Index" (PSI) via an electrode array that is also placed on the forehead.[8] Both systems analyze the patient's EEG signals to detect the effect of sedatives and anesthetics on the brain. These technologies have been successfully used in the operating room when the patient is under general anesthesia and are increasingly used in the critical care unit for ventilated patients who are deeply sedated or are sedated and pharmacologically paralyzed. Both systems calculate a number on a scale from 0 to 99 or 100. A value greater than 95 indicates wakefulness, and a value less than 50-60 indicates the patient is unconsciousness or deeply sedated with a low probability of mental recall of events. A value below 20 denotes an extremely deep level of sedation sufficient to cause brain-wave suppression. Unless the goal is to achieve a level of sedation equivalent to a barbiturate coma, brain wave suppression is not desirable. Both systems incorporate an electromyogram (EMG) sensor to filter out erroneous muscle movement that may distort the numerical sedation value.[6-8]

Continuous nervous system monitoring via EEG definitely has a role for the most critically ill patients who are deeply sedated, are receiving opiate analgesia, and are pharmacologically paralyzed, although research outside the operating room is limited at this time.[9]

It is recommended that all critically ill, intubated, mechanically ventilated patients have a stated goal for analgesia and sedation (Fig. 9-1).[3] Once the sedation goal is articulated and documented, the ongoing use of a validated assessment scale is recommended to facilitate consistency between the various health care practitioners (see Table 9-1).

COMPLICATIONS OF SEDATION

Oversedation is recognized as a state of unintended patient unresponsiveness in which the patient resides in a state of suspended animation that resembles general anesthesia.[10] Prolonged deep sedation is associated with significant complications of immobility, including pressure ulcers, thromboemboli, gastric ileus, nosocomial pneumonia, and delayed weaning from mechanical ventilation.

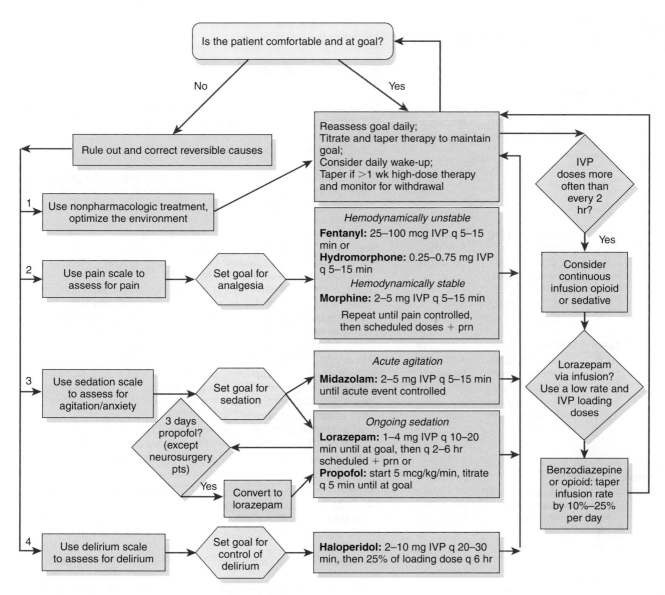

Fig. 9-1   General guidelines for sedation and analgesia management of mechanically ventilated critical care patients. Doses are approximate for a 70-kg (154-pound) adult. *IVP,* Intravenous push; *q,* every; *prn,* as needed. (From Jacobi J et al: *Crit Care Med* 30(1):119-141, 2002.)

Too little sedation is equally hazardous. Most nurses have experienced the challenge of caring for a patient who unexpectedly removes the endotracheal or nasogastric tube. Unplanned extubation in restless, anxious, agitated patients occurs in 8% to 10% of intubated patients after an average of 3.5 days in the critical care unit. Of self-extubations, 6% cause significant complications including aspiration, dysrhythmias, bronchospasm, and bradycardia.[10]

SELECTING MEDICATIONS FOR SEDATION

Several categories of sedatives are commercially available. None of these medications has any analgesic prop-erties. Therefore, if the patient is experiencing pain, analgesia must be administered in addition to any seda-tive agents. Sedative agents include the benzodi-azepines, anesthetic agents such as propofol, and the central alpha agonists (see the Pharmacologic Manage-ment Table on Sedation).[3]

BENZODIAZEPINES

Benzodiazepines are sedative-hypnotics with powerful amnesic properties that inhibit reception of new sensory information.[3,10] Benzodiazepines do not have analgesic properties. The most frequently used critical care benzo-diazepines are *diazepam* (Valium), *midazolam* (Versed), and *lorazepam* (Ativan). Midazolam is recommended for control of acute short-term agitation because of an intra-

Pharmacologic Management: Sedation

DRUGS	DOSAGE	ACTIONS	SPECIAL CONSIDERATIONS
Benzodiazepines			
Diazepam	0.03-0.1 mg/kg every 0.5-6 hr (slow IV intermittent doses)	Anxiolysis Amnesia Sedation	*Onset:* 2-5 minutes following IV administration. *Side effects:* hypotension, respiratory depression. *Half-life of parent compound:* long, from 20-120 hours. Contains active sedative metabolites that also contribute to prolonged sedative effect. *Drug tolerance:* physical tolerance develops with prolonged use, and more drug is required to achieve same effect over time. Slow wean required from diazepam after continuous prolonged use. Phlebitis in peripheral IV.
Lorazepam	0.02-0.06 mg/kg every 2-6 hr (slow IV intermittent doses) 0.01-0.1 mg/kg/ hr (continuous infusion)	Anxiolysis Amnesia Sedation	*Onset:* 5-20 minutes following IV administration. *Side effects:* hypotension, respiratory depression. *Half-life of parent compound:* relatively long, ranges from 8-15 hours. Sedative effect is also prolonged. *Drug tolerance:* physical tolerance develops with use, and higher drug dosage is required to achieve same effect over time. Slow wean required from Lorazepam after continuous prolonged use. Solvent-related acidosis/renal failure at high doses.
Midazolam	0.02-0.08 mg/kg every 0.5-2 hr (slow IV intermittent doses) 0.04-0.2 mg/kg/ hr (continuous infusion)	Anxiolysis Amnesia Sedation	*Onset:* 2-5 minutes following IV administration. *Side effects:* hypotension, respiratory depression. *Half-life of parent compound:* ranges from 3-11 hours. Sedative effect prolonged when midazolam infusion has continued for many days. This is due to presence of active sedative metabolites. Sedative effect also prolonged in renal failure. *Drug tolerance:* physical tolerance develops with prolonged use, and higher drug dosage is required to achieve same effect over time. Slow wean required from midazolam after prolonged use.
Anesthetic Agents			
Propofol	5-80 mcg/kg/min (continuous infusion)	Anxiolysis Amnesia Sedation	*Onset:* 1-2 minutes, very rapid onset following IV administration. *Side effects:* hypotension, respiratory depression (patient must be intubated and mechanically ventilated to eliminate this complication). *Half-life of parent compound:* 2-8 minutes when used as a short-term agent. *Sedative effect:* can range from 26-32 hours with prolonged continuous IV infusion. Effective short-term anesthetic agent, useful for rapid "wake-up" of patients for assessment. If continuous infusion is used for many days, emergence from sedation can take hours or days. Sedative effect is dependent upon dose of drug administered, depth of sedation, and length of time sedated. Change IV infusion tubing every 12 hours. Requires a dedicated IV catheter and tubing (do not mix with other drugs). Monitor serum triglyceride levels.
Neuroleptic Agents			
Haloperidol	0.03-0.15 mg/kg every 0.5-6 hr (IV intermittent doses) 0.04-0.15 mg/kg/ hr (continuous infusion)	Antipsychotic Antidelirium	*Onset:* 3–20 minutes following IV administration. *Half-life of parent compound:* 18-54 hours. Used in management of delirium. Sedation is an unintended side effect. Measure QT interval at baseline and periodically during haloperidol infusion. Active metabolites may cause extrapyramidal symptoms (EPS). Anticholenergic agent may be administered if EPS occur.

IV, Intravenous; *min,* minute; *EPS,* extrapyramidal symptoms.

Pharmacologic Management: Sedation—cont'd

Drugs	Dosage	Actions	Special Considerations
Alpha-Adrenergic Receptor Agonists			
Dexmedeto-midine	1 mcg/kg initial loading dose over 20 minutes. 0.2-0.7 mcg/kg/hr (continuous infusion)	Anxiolysis Analgesia Sedation	*Half-life:* approximately 2 hours. Duration of infusion up to 24 hours only. Bolus dosing is not recommended. Maintenance infusion is adjusted to achieve desired level of sedation.

venous (IV) onset of action of under 3 minutes.[3,10] However, when midazolam is administered for longer than 24 hours as a continuous infusion, the sedative effect is prolonged by active metabolites.[3]

When long-term sedation is required, converting to a continuous infusion of lorazepam is recommended (see Fig. 9-1). One advantage of lorazepam for long-term sedation is that it does not have active metabolites that contribute to the overall sedative effect. Lorazepam has a slow onset, which makes it unsuitable for the treatment of acute agitation. As would be expected, the recovery time from a sedated state takes longer when infusing lorazepam (Ativan) compared with midalozam (Versed); the higher the dose infused, the longer the recovery time for both drugs.[11] Mechanically ventilated patients who were sedated with a continuous infusion of lorazepam for 72 hours emerged from light sedation in 11.9 hours, whereas recovery from deep sedation took 31.1 hours. By contrast, in the same research study, patients who were sedated with a continuous midazolam infusion emerged from light sedation in 3.6 hours and from deep sedation in 14.9 hours.[11] Clearly, even within the class of benzodiazepines it is important to select the sedative agent carefully, anticipating how long the patient will be sedated and how long it will take to recover from the sedative state.

The major unwanted side effects associated with the benzodiazepines are dose-related respiratory depression and hypotension.[10] If needed, *flumazenil* (Romazicon) is the antidote used to reverse benzodiazepine overdose in symptomatic patients.[10] Flumazenil should be avoided in patients with benzodiazepine dependence because rapid withdrawal can induce seizures.[10]

ANESTHETIC AGENTS

Propofol (Diprivan) is an IV-delivered general anesthetic agent.[3,12,13] At high doses (greater than 100 to 200 mcg/kg/minute), propofol is intended to produce a state of general anesthesia in the operating room.[13] In the critical care unit, propofol is prescribed at lower doses to induce a state of deep sedation (5 to 50 mcg/kg/min).[13] The clinical advantage of propofol is its very short half-life and rapid elimination from the body. It does not have active metabolites.[12,13] This drug is especially suitable for management of the agitated neurologic patient with brain injury. Propofol quickly crosses the blood brain barrier, slows cerebral metabolism, and decreases elevated intracranial pressure (ICP).[13]

With short-term administration the drug infusion can be turned off, and the patient can be fully alert within 30 minutes. The half-life is 2 to 4 minutes with short-term use.[13] If propofol is infused for several days, the wake-up time is also prolonged.[12,14] If propofol is infused for over 10 days the half-life extends to 1 to 3 days.[13] Propofol is not a reliable amnesic, and patients sedated with only propofol can have vivid recollections of their experiences. It is therefore important to add an opiate such as *fentanyl* to ensure adequate amnesia.[12]

Significant disadvantages of propofol are mainly related to the high lipid content. It comes packaged in a glass container and has the appearance of milk. Propofol is emulsified in a soybean intralipid emulsion that delivers 1.1 kcal/ml as fat. These calories must be taken into account when assessing nutritional intake.[13] Propofol can elevate serum triglyceride levels and has been associated with pancreatitis. The lipid emulsion can also act as a potential medium for bacterial growth. Administration requires a dedicated IV line, and all IV solution and tubing must be changed every 12 hours.[13] Propofol shares with other sedatives the propensity for hypotension when delivered rapidly.[12,13]

Propofol Infusion Syndrome (PIS) is a rare complication of prolonged, high-dose propofol administration. It occurs more commonly in children than in adult critically ill patients. The syndrome includes cardiac arrest, myocardial failure, metabolic acidosis, rhabdomyolysis, and hyperkalemia that occur on day 4 or 5 following very high-dose propofol infusion.[15,16] Clinicians are advised not to administer dosages above 5 mg/kg/hour for longer than 48 hours. Propofol is prescribed only for intubated patients.

CENTRAL ALPHA AGONISTS

Two central alpha-adrenergic agonists are available for sedation: clonidine (often prescribed as a Catapres patch) and dexmedetomidine (Precedex as a continuous infusion). *Clonidine* is prescribed for patients experiencing withdrawal syndromes. *Dexmedetomidine* is a newer alpha-2 agonist recently approved for use as a short-term sedative (less than 24 hours) for the mechanically ventilated patient. It is prescribed in some hospitals to wean patients from short-term ventilation after cardiac surgery.[17,18] At this time there is not enough information to determine whether dexmedetomidine will have a wider role in sedation therapy lasting more than 24 hours.[3]

The choice of sedative is very patient- and situation-specific. If the need is for *short-term* sedation (less than 24 hours) the most frequently used sedatives are midazolam or propofol.[3,10-14] Both these drugs may be combined with a short-acting opioid analgesic (e.g., fentanyl). If the need is for *intermediate-term* sedation (1 to 3 days), the most frequently prescribed drugs again are propofol and midazolam, plus an opiate. If the need is for *long-term* sedation, the recommended agent is lorazepam.[3] Research using continuous EEG monitoring has shown that patients who receive continuous sedative infusions are more deeply sedated than patients who are given sedatives as an IV bolus; patients receiving continuous infusions are also more likely to be oversedated.[19]

MANAGING DRUG DEPENDENCE AND WITHDRAWAL

The question of which drugs to use for prolonged sedation is complex. Long-term patients are frequently mechanically ventilated and often seriously ill for weeks or months. To tolerate the ventilator and other procedures, patients must receive sedation and analgesia. When it is time to decrease the sedation, many patients have become physically and psychologically dependent, and as the drug dosage is reduced, they become highly agitated.

Physical symptoms of agitation can include increased heart rate, blood pressure, and respiratory rate. Other notable symptoms include lack of self-awareness, unawareness of surroundings, very short-term memory for information, irritability, anxiety, confusion, delirium, and even seizures.[3] Patients may pull at the tubes and attempt to climb out of bed, and can represent a danger to themselves, the nurse, and family visitors. The temptation to resedate is powerful, because it is painful to watch a patient experience the stages of withdrawal. During this period the patient does not sleep well, even when sedation provides the appearance of sleep.

One innovative strategy to avoid pitfalls of sedative dependence and withdrawal is a planned "daily drug holiday." This means that all sedative and analgesic agents are turned off once a day and the patient is allowed to awaken.[20,21] The patient is carefully monitored, and when consciousness and awareness are attained, an assessment of level of consciousness and neurologic function is performed. When using protocols that incorporate daily interruption of sedative infusions, it is imperative that accurate assessment be performed and documented during the wake-up period. Also, if the patient becomes agitated, it is essential that a protocol be in place to the nurse to restart the sedatives, plus opiates if applicable.[20,21] One protocol scheduled the daily interruption of sedatives in the morning and, after a full assessment, recommended restarting the sedative and opiate infusions at 50% of the previous morning dose and adjusting upward until the patient was comfortable.[20,21] Initially it was believed that patients would be highly agitated during each interruption. However, because the patients had less sedative and opiate medication accumulated, they were less restless in the wake-up period. The intubated patients who were woken up daily by turning off the sedative infusions (either propofol or midalozam) experienced a lower rate of medical complications and lower levels of posttraumatic stress disorder (PSTD).[21-22]

An important nursing responsibility is to prevent the patient from coming to harm during drug withdrawal (Table 9-2). Some movement in bed is expected, but extreme restlessness increases myocardial oxygen consumption and work of breathing and activates the sympathetic nervous system. If the patient is seriously agitated, it is vital to consult with the physician and pharmacist to establish an effective treatment plan that will allow weaning from these agents without harm. The approach to avoidance of drug dependence and withdrawal symptoms is not yet fully delineated but clearly requires a multidisciplinary effort with ongoing evaluation using an established assessment scale (see Table 9-1).

ASSESSING FOR DELIRIUM

Delirium is described as a reversible global impairment of cognitive processes, usually of sudden onset, coupled with disorientation, impaired short-term memory, altered sensory perceptions (hallucinations), abnormal thought processes, and inappropriate behavior. Delirium is probably more prevalent than generally recognized and is difficult to diagnose in the critically ill patient. The incidence ranges from 30% to 70% in medical-surgical critical care patients (Box 9-2).[3,23] Delirium increases both hospital stay and mortality in patients who are mechanically ventilated.[24] The increase in mortality remains true even after controlling for associated variables such as coma, sedatives, and analgesic administration.[24]

Table 9-2	Signs and Symptoms of Sedative/Analgesic Drug Withdrawal*	
System	**Opiate Withdrawal**	**Benzodiazepine Withdrawal†**
Neurologic	Delirium, tremors, seizures	Agitation, anxiety, delirium, tremors, myoclonus, headache, seizures, fatigue, paresthesias, sleep disturbances
Hemodynamic	Tachycardia, hypertension (SNS stimulation)	Tachycardia, hypertension (SNS stimulation)
Sensory	Dilation of pupils, teary eyes, irritability, increased sensitivity to pain, sweating, yawning	Increased sensitivity to light/sound, sweating
Musculoskeletal	Cramps, muscle aches	Muscle cramps
Gastrointestinal	Vomiting, diarrhea	Nausea, diarrhea
Respiratory	Tachypnea	Tachypnea

*Data on propofol is limited, but withdrawal symptoms after prolonged use similar to those of the benzodiazepines. (Jacobi 2002)
†Not all symptoms are seen in all patients (Jacobi 2002; Szokol 2001).
SNS, Sympathetic nervous system.

Box 9-2

CAUSES OF DELIRIUM IN CRITICALLY ILL PATIENTS

METABOLIC
Acid-base disturbance
Electrolyte imbalance
Hypoglycemia

INTRACRANIAL
Epidural/subdural hematoma
Intracranial hemorrhage
Meningitis
Encephalitis
Cerebral abscess
Tumor

ENDOCRINE
Hyperthyroidism/
   hypothyroidism

Addison's disease
Hyperparathyroidism
Cushing's syndrome

ORGAN FAILURE
Liver encephalopathy
Uremic encephalopathy
Septic shock

RESPIRATORY
Hypoxemia
Hypercarbia

DRUG RELATED
Alcohol withdrawal
Drug-induced
Heavy metal poisoning

Adapted from Szokol JW, Vender JS: *Crit Care Clin* 17(4):821-842, 2001.

When patients are agitated, restless, and pulling at tube and lines, they are often identified as delirious. In this scenario, delirium may be described as *ICU psychosis* or *Sundowner syndrome.* However, the delirious patient is not always agitated, and it is much more difficult to detect delirium when the patient is apparently calm.[3,23,25] The major categories to assess include (1) acute onset of mental status changes or fluctuating course, (2) inattention, (3) disorganized thinking, and (4) altered level of consciousness, which can include any level of consciousness other than "alert" (vigilant, lethargic, stupor, coma). Routine assessment for the presence of delirium is recommended in critical care patients.

Specific scoring scales are available to assess for delirium, and an experienced psychiatric consultant can be helpful.[25]

SELECTING MEDICATIONS FOR MANAGING DELIRIUM

Unfortunately the medications typically prescribed for sedation and analgesia may exacerbate the symptoms of delirium. Sedatives make delirious patients confused, less responsive, and more obtunded,[23] thus creating a situation that can also lead to a paradoxical increase in agitation. The neuroleptic drug haloperidol (Haldol) is frequently prescribed. This antipsychotic agent stabilizes cerebral function by blocking dopamine-mediated neurotransmission at the cerebral synapses and in the basil ganglia. Delirium is reduced, but the patient tends to have a flat affect and diminished interest in surroundings, and with higher doses becomes sedated. Electrocardiographic (ECG) monitoring is recommended because neuroleptic agents produce dose-dependent QT interval prolongation, with an increased incidence of ventricular dysrhythmias.[10]

PREVENTING AGITATION AND DELIRIUM

Agitation and delirium are common in critically ill patients.[3,23,25] Causes of delirium are multifactorial, but *sleep deprivation* is a universal experience that may contribute.[26] Even when patients are apparently "sleeping," if the sleep is induced by sedatives, opiates, neuromuscular blockade, or neuroleptics, it is unlikely that this represents true rapid eye movement (REM) sleep. Similar to pain assessment, self-report of sleep deprivation is considered the most accurate measure.

EVIDENCE-BASED COLLABORATIVE PRACTICE

Sedation in the Critically Ill

The key recommendations from the clinical practice guideline for the sustained use of sedatives and analgesia in the critically ill adult, based upon research and expert panel opinion, are as follows:

Assessment, Communication, and Documentation

1. Frequent assessment of critically ill patients is mandated to determine if sedation and analgesia are required and appropriate as part of the plan of care.
2. A sedation goal or endpoint should be established for each patient at the beginning of therapy; for example, "a calm patient that can be easily aroused with maintenance of the normal sleep-wake cycle." Some patients may require deep sedation to facilitate synchrony with mechanical ventilation.
3. Need for sedation should be reevaluated on a frequent basis as the clinical condition of the patient changes.
4. Sedation regimens should be written with the flexibility to allow titration to the desired endpoint, anticipating fluctuations in sedation requirements throughout the day.
5. Use of a validated sedation assessment scale to standardize assessment among clinicians, document the patient's level of sedation and response to sedatives is recommended. Vital signs such as blood pressure or heart rate are not sufficiently specific or sensitive to serve as indicators of sedation effectiveness.
6. Sedation and analgesia goals must be communicated to all caregivers and to the patient and family.
7. Due to insufficient research, using sedation monitors that interpret EEG data are not endorsed for monitoring critical care patients.

Agitation

8. Sedation of agitated critically ill patients should be started only after providing adequate analgesia and providing treatment for reversible physiologic causes of agitation.
9. Cautious use of sedatives is warranted for patients not yet intubated because of the risk of respiratory depression.

Drug Therapy

10. Midazolam or diazepam should be used for rapid sedation of acutely agitated patients.
11. Propofol is the preferred sedative when rapid awakening for rapid neurologic assessment or extubation is important.
12. Midazolam is recommended for short-term use only, as it provokes unpredictable awakening and time to extubation when infusions continue longer than 48-72 hours.
13. Lorazepam is the recommended sedative when prolonged mechanical ventilation is required, via intermittent IV administration or continuous infusion.

Avoidance of Complications

14. The titration of the sedative dose to a defined endpoint is recommended with systemic tapering of the dose, or daily interruption with retitration to minimize prolonged sedative effects.
15. Triglyceride concentrations should be monitored after 2 days of propofol infusion, and total caloric intake from lipids should be included in the nutrition support prescription.
16. The potential for opioid, benzodiazepine, and propofol withdrawal should be considered after high doses of more than approximately 7 days of continuous therapy. Doses should be tapered systematically to prevent withdrawal symptoms.

Delirium

17. Routine assessment for the presence of delirium is recommended. The CAM-ICU is noted as a promising assessment tool for delirium.
18. Haloperidol is the preferred agent for the treatment of delirium in critically ill patients.
19. ECG monitoring for detection of potential QT interval prolongation and dysrhythmias is recommended when haloperidol is administered.

Sleep

20. Sleep promotion should include optimization of the environment and non-pharmacologic methods to promote relaxation with adjunctive use of hypnotics.

Data from Jacobi J et al: Clinical practice guidelines for the sustained use of sedatives and analgesics in the critically ill adult, *Crit Care Med 30*(1):119-141, 2002.
CAM-ICU, Confusion Assessment Method—ICU instrument; *EEG*, electroencephalogram; *ECG*, electrocardiogram; *IV*, intravenous.

The *nonpharmacologic* strategies used to prevent agitation and delirium are similar to those used to control pain. These methods include back massage, music therapy, noise reduction in the environment, decreasing lights at night to promote sleep, clustering nursing care to provide some uninterrupted rest periods, and speaking in a calm, quiet, and gentle voice.[2,3,9,10,12,13,25,26]

COLLABORATIVE MANAGEMENT

Collaborative management of anxiety, agitation, and sedation is a responsibility shared by all members of the health care team (see the Evidence-Based Collaborative Practice feature on Sedation in the Critically Ill). Recognition of the problem is the first step toward a solution to establish a more effective standard of patient care in sedation/analgesia management. It is important to involve families and significant companions in the plan of care for effective management of both pain and sedation.

SUMMARY

The goal of making the critical care unit a therapeutic healing environment is shared by patients, families, and health care practitioners alike.[1] Critical care nurses remain challenged by limitations in the medications and monitoring tools currently available.[6] Sedatives for short-term use are fairly well delineated, but no ideal agent is available for long-term sedation.[27] New clinical practice guidelines have resulted in a renewed emphasis on finding appropriate levels of sedation, both to provide comfort and to avoid oversedation.[3] The critical care nurse is in a pivotal position to act as a patient advocate so that all aspects of patient comfort are assessed as the "fifth vital sign."

REFERENCES

1. Fraser GL, RR Riker: Monitoring sedation, agitation, analgesia, and delirium in critically ill adult patients, *Crit Care Clin* 17(4):967-987, 2001.
2. Joint Commission on Accreditation of HealthCare Organizations (JCAHO): Standards and intents for sedation and analgesia care in the revisions to anesthesia care standards. In *Comprehensive accreditation manual for hospitals,* Oakbrook Terrace, Ill, 2000, JCAHO.
3. Jacobi J et al: Clinical practice guidelines for the sustained use of sedatives and analgesics in the critically ill adult, *Crit Care Med* 30(1):119-141, 2002.
4. Consensus conference on sedation assessment: a collaborative venture by Abbott Laboratories, American Association of Critical-Care Nurses, and Saint Thomas Health System, *Crit Care Nurse* 24(2):33-41, 2004.
5. Frazier SK et al: Critical care nurses' beliefs about and reported management of anxiety, *Am J Crit Care* 12(1):19-27, 2003.
6. Arbour R: Continuous nervous system monitoring, EEG, the bispectral index, and neuromuscular transmission, *AACN Clin Issues* 14(2):185-207, 2003.
7. Arbour R: Using bispectral index monitoring to detect potential breakthrough awareness and limit duration of neuromuscular blockade, *Am J Crit Care* 13(1):66-73, 2004.
8. Drover DR et al: Patient State Index: titration of delivery and recovery from propofol, alfentanil, and nitrous oxide anesthesia, *Anesthesiology* 97(1):82-89, 2002.
9. McGaffigan PA: Advancing sedation assessment to promote patient comfort, *Crit Care Nurse* 22(suppl):29-36, 2002.
10. Young CC, Prielipp RC: Benzodiazepines in the intensive care unit, *Crit Care Clin* 17(4):843-862, 2001.
11. Barr J et al: A double-blind, randomized comparison of IV lorazepam versus midazolam for sedation of ICU patients via a pharmacologic model, *Anesthesiology* 95(2):286-298, 2001.
12. Angelini G, Ketzler JT, Coursin DB: Use of propofol and other nonbenzodiazepine sedatives in the intensive care unit, *Crit Care Clin* 17(4):863-880, 2001.
13. Whitcomb JJ, Huddleston MC, McAndrews KL: The use of propofol in the mechanically ventilated medical/surgical intensive care patient: is it the right choice? *Dimens Crit Care Nurs* 22(2):60-63, 2003.
14. Barr J et al: Propofol dosing regimens for ICU sedation based upon an integrated pharmacokinetic-pharmacodynamic model, *Anesthesiology* 95(2):324-333, 2001.
15. Cremer OL et al: Long-term propofol infusion and cardiac failure in adult head-injured patients, *Lancet* 357(9250):117-118, 2001.
16. Kang TM: Propofol infusion syndrome in critically ill patients, *Ann Pharmacother* 36(9):1453-1456, 2002.
17. Coursin DB, Maccioli GA: Dexmedetomidine, *Curr Opin Crit Care* 7(4):221-226, 2001.
18. Herr DL, Sum-Ping ST, England M: ICU sedation after coronary artery bypass graft surgery: dexmedetomidine-based versus propofol-based sedation regimens, *J Cardiothorac Vasc Anesth* 17(5):576-584, 2003.
19. de Wit M, Epstein SK: Administration of sedatives and level of sedation: comparative evaluation via the Sedation-Agitation Scale and the Bispectral Index, *Am J Crit Care* 12(4):343-348, 2003.
20. Kress JP et al: Daily interruption of sedative infusions in critically ill patients undergoing mechanical ventilation, *N Engl J Med* 342(20):1471-1477, 2000.
21. Schweickert WD et al: Daily interruption of sedative infusions and complications of critical illness in mechanically ventilated patients, *Crit Care Med* 32(6):1272-1276, 2004.
22. Kress JP et al: The long-term psychological effects of daily sedative interruption on critically ill patients, *Am J Respir Crit Care Med* 168(12):1457-1461, 2003.
23. Szokol JW, Vender JS: Anxiety, delirium, and pain in the intensive care unit, *Crit Care Clin* 17(4):821-842, 2001.
24. Ely EW et al: Delirium as a predictor of mortality in mechanically ventilated patients in the intensive care unit, *JAMA* 291(14):1753-1762, 2004.
25. Marshall MC, Soucy MD: Delirium in the intensive care unit, *Crit Care Nurs Q* 26(3):172-178, 2003.
26. Honkus VL: Sleep deprivation in critical care units, *Crit Care Nurs Q* 26(3):179-189, 2003.
27. Arbour RB, Ponzillo JJ: *Appropriate utilization of intravenous sedatives and analgesics used in the care of the critically ill patient,* monograph, Bloomsbury, NJ, 2002, Medical Education Resources MED-DOC.

CHAPTER 10

End-of-Life Issues

End of life has not been thought of as an important clinical topic in critical care. Since the primary purpose of admission of patients to a critical care unit is for aggressive, life-saving care, the death of a patient is generally regarded as a failure. Because the culture is that of saving lives, the language around end of life is stated in negative terms such as forgoing life-sustaining treatments, do not resuscitate (DNR), and withdrawal of life support. At times the phrase *withdrawal of care* is used—imagine the impact of that phrase on families. This lack of end-of-life language has hampered literature-searching until recently, the low yield leading those looking for information to think nothing has been done on end of life in the critical care unit. In fact the medical subject headings (MeSH) term for withdrawal of life support is "passive euthanasia." Content on end of life in critical care textbooks, both medical[1] and nursing,[2] is minimal; further, the first textbook on end of life in critical care was only published in 1998[3] and the second in 2001.[4]

More attention is being given to the quality of the end-of-life experience of the critically ill with recognition of the numbers of patients who die in critical care units. The focus of the content in this chapter will be on the evidence we have for the care we are rendering to the dying critical care patient and his or her family, and care that is recommended by evidence, research reports, and summaries of research and guidelines.

END-OF-LIFE EXPERIENCE IN CRITICAL CARE

This attention to end of life in hospitalized patients has increased since the publication of the Study to Understand Prognoses and Preferences for Outcomes and Risks of Treatments (SUPPORT).[5] In this major report, more than 9000 seriously ill patients in five medical centers were studied. Despite an intervention to improve communication, shortcomings were found, aggressive treatment was frequent, only one half of physicians knew their patients' preferences to avoid cardiopulmonary resuscitation (CPR), more than one third of patients who died spent at least 10 days in a critical care unit, and for 50% of conscious patients, family members reported moderate to severe pain at least half of the time.

Following closely after the publication of the SUPPORT study, the Institute of Medicine (IOM) released a report, *Approaching death: improving care at the end of life.*[6] The group detailed deficiencies in care and gave seven recommendations to improve care:

1. Patients with fatal illnesses and their family should receive reliable, skillful, and supportive care.
2. Health professionals should improve care for the dying.
3. Policymakers and consumers should work with health professionals to improve quality and financing of care.
4. Health profession education should include end-of-life content.
5. Palliative care should be developed, possibly as a medical specialty.
6. Research on end of life should be funded.
7. The public should communicate more about the experience of dying and options available.

In SUPPORT and in the IOM report, critical care patients were included with other hospitalized patients. In order to describe the number of deaths in critical care units, Angus and colleagues reviewed hospital discharge data from six states and the National Death Index. Of the more than 500,000 deaths studied, 38.3% were in hospitals, and 22% (59% of all hospital deaths) occurred after admission to the critical care unit. Terminal admissions associated with critical care accounted for 80% of all terminal hospitalization costs.[7] The likelihood of dying in hospital increased from age 25 to 74, and the likelihood of dying after critical care unit admission remained 25% of all deaths for each age category. Although 90% of people would prefer to die in their own homes,[6] more than 20% of those who died in this review received high-tech aggressive care before they died.

ADVANCE DIRECTIVES

Although advance directives, also known as a *living will* or a *health care power of attorney*, were encouraged to ensure patients received the care they desired, the enactment has been less than desired. Like other preventive measures, it is underused, even though it is inexpensive and potentially effective.[8] Prevalence rates of advance directives were 30% or less in a group 65 years or older, but only 15% had discussed their wishes with their primary physician, which is a bigger issue.[9] Even when advance directives are present, the question arises as to whether they are applicable; in other words, "Is this a terminal illness?"

ADVANCE CARE PLANNING

Cultural influences in the United States discourage discussion of death. To actually plan for decisions to be made when one is incompetent is difficult, however help-ful they would be for those families members left to make those decisions. Advance care planning for those with chronic illness would be advantageous for all involved, especially where there are repeated critical care unit admissions involved. Communication of the patient's wishes between primary care providers and intensivists is critical. If patients have stated desires, those should be communicated when patients are transferred. If the patient has not specified his or her preferences, that too is important and should be communicated to new health care providers; if patients desire aggressive care, it should be offered as appropriate. If aggressive care is not how the patient wishes to be managed, then patients, families, and care providers could be so informed and families would not be left in emergency situations trying to decide what to do. Emotional support for the patient and the family as they discuss advance care planning in the critical care setting is described in the Nursing Interventions Classification (NIC) feature on Family Support.

NIC   Family Support

Definitions: Promotion of family values, interests, and goals

Activities

Assure family that best care possible is being given to patient

Appraise family's emotional reaction to patient's condition

Determine the psychological burden of prognosis for family

Foster realistic hope

Listen to family concerns, feelings, and questions

Facilitate communication of concerns/feelings between patient and family or between family members

Promote trusting relationship with family

Accept the family's values in a nonjudgmental manner

Answer all questions of family members or assist them to get answers

Orient family to the health care setting, such as hospital unit or clinic

Provide assistance in meeting basic needs of family, such as shelter, food, and clothing

Identify nature of spiritual support for family

Identify congruence between patient, family, and health professional expectations

Reduce discrepancies in patient, family, and health professional expectations through use of communication skills

Assist family members in identifying and resolving any conflict in values

Respect and support adaptive coping mechanisms used by family

Provide feedback for family regarding their coping

Counsel family members on additional effective coping skills for their own use

Provide spiritual resources for family, as appropriate

Provide family with information about patient's progress frequently, according to patient preference

Teach the medical and nursing plans of care to family

Provide necessary knowledge of options to family that will assist them to make decisions about patient care

Include family members with patient in decision making about care, when appropriate

Encourage family decision making in planning long-term patient care affecting family structure and finances

Acknowledge understanding of family decision about post-discharge care

Assist family to acquire necessary knowledge, skills, and equipment to sustain their decision about patient care

Advocate for family, as appropriate

Foster family assertiveness in information-seeking, as appropriate

Provide opportunities for visitation by extended family members, as appropriate

Introduce family to other families undergoing similar experiences, as appropriate

Give care to patient in lieu of family to relieve then and/or when family is unable to give care

Arrange for ongoing respite care, when indicated and desired

Provide opportunities for peer group support

Refer for family therapy, as appropriate

Tell family members how to reach the nurse

Assist family members through the death and grief processes, as appropriate

From Dochterman JM, Bulechek GM: *Nursing interventions classification (NIC)*, ed 4, St Louis, 2004, Mosby.

ETHICAL/LEGAL ISSUES

Legal and ethical principles guide many of our decisions in caring for the dying patient and the family. The patient is respected as autonomous and able to make his or her own decisions. When the patient is unable to make decisions, the same respect should be accorded to surrogates. These wishes may have been put in writing by the patient as an advance directive. The Patient Self-Determination Act supports the patient's right to control future treatment in the event the individual cannot speak for him or herself.

Two of the basic principles underlying the provision of health care are beneficence and nonmaleficence. Beneficence is the principle of intending to benefit the other through one's actions. Nonmaleficence means to do no harm. Sometimes, at end of life, these are seen in conflict, such as when resuscitation is attempted under beneficence but does cause harm.

COMFORT CARE

The decision to withdraw life-sustaining treatments and switch to comfort care at end of life should be made with as much involvement of the patient as possible, including physical presence of the patient in decision making or procuring paper documents if the patient is not able to be present. If neither is available, the patient's intent as understood from discussions or knowledge of the patient should guide the decision whether or not to withdraw treatment. Withholding and withdrawing are considered to be morally and legally equivalent.[10] However, families have more stress in withdrawing treatments than in withholding them,[11] so treatments should not be started that the patient would not want or that would not benefit him or her.

The goal of withdrawal of life-sustaining treatments is to remove treatments that are not beneficial and may be uncomfortable. Any treatment in this circumstance may be withheld or withdrawn. Once the goal of comfort has been chosen, each procedure should be evaluated to see if it is necessary, or if it causes discomfort. If discomfort is caused, those treatments do not need to be continued. Forgoing life-sustaining treatments is not the same as active euthanasia or assisted suicide. Killing is an action causing another's death, whereas allowing dying is avoiding any intervention that interferes with a natural death following illness or trauma.[3]

IMPACT OF DNR ORDERS

A do-not-resuscitate (DNR) order should prevent the initiation of CPR. In a review of 25 years since the DNR was established, Burns[12] found that those with a DNR order sometimes received less care, and some treatments were withheld[13] without those changes being specified in the DNR order. DNR is sometimes thought to mean Do Not Care, but that is not the intent. DNR orders should be written before withdrawal of life support; this will prevent any unfortunate errors in unwanted resuscitation during the time period between initiation of withdrawal and the actual death.

PROGNOSTICATION

Why patients who will die soon would have received life-prolonging therapy shortly before their death can be partially explained by a series of studies. Physicians' ability to prognosticate has been found to be limited[14,15]; in general, time to death is overestimated. Patients' wishes are usually not known, or when known, are vague[16] or change over the course of an illness.[17] Care is often not in accord with patient wishes, and this is more prevalent when comfort care is desired over aggressive care.[18] Skills in communication and end-of-life care are not emphasized in medical curricula.[19,20] The very skills that would enable assessment of patient wishes are not well developed.

CARDIOPULMONARY RESUSCITATION

One decision to be made as death approaches, the do-not-resuscitate order, is frequently delayed.[21] However, the benefits of resuscitation may be overestimated both for survival and for the more relevant outcome of functional status. In a metaanalysis of 51 studies, Ebell and colleagues found that the overall survival to discharge after in-hospital CPR was 13.4%. A decreased rate of immediate survival was found for patients with acquired immune deficiency syndrome, those with a hematocrit above 35%, and those who were male. Decreased survival to discharge was related to sepsis on the day before resuscitation, cancer with or without metastasis, dementia, elevated serum creatinine level, African-American race, and dependent status. CPR was originally developed for those with coronary artery disease, and they are the most likely to survive resuscitation to discharge, as well as those who suffer cardiac arrest in the critical care unit.[22] Brindley found the same overall survival to hospital discharge (13.4%) in a retrospective study of hospital charts. The patients in the study were all inpatients who had gone through resuscitation. FitzGerald and others[23] found that functional status among almost one half of the survivors of in-hospital CPR had deteriorated compared with their condition 2 months before the event. After 6 months, 30% of those patients had died, and two thirds continued to lose function. Despite these dismal statistics, CPR is offered as an option without fully informing patients or families of the low possibility of survival, the pain and suffering involved during and after the procedure, and the potential for decline in functional status.

PROGNOSTIC TOOLS

There are two common tools for estimating critical care unit mortality: Acute Physiology and Chronic Health Evaluation (APACHE) and multiple organ dysfunction score (MODS).[24] However, when these were compared to physician estimates of intensive care unit survival less than 10%, the physician estimate was associated with subsequent life-support limitation. Physician estimate was more powerful in predicting mortality than illness severity, organ dysfunction, and use of inotropes or vasopressors.[25]

Despite this information and these tools, uncertainty remains a major issue in decision making, not only for physicians but for patients and families[17] as well. Because one is never sure and because few patients who were never thought likely to survive actually return to visit a critical care unit, professionals are not confident about issues of survivability. In addition, many families cling to small hopes of survival and recovery.

COMMUNICATION AND DECISION MAKING

Communication with the patient and family is critically important.

PATIENT COMMUNICATION

Patients' capacity for decision making is limited by illness severity; they are too sick or are hampered by the therapies or medications used to treat them.[26] As decision making is required, the patient is the first person to be approached. Information that can assist the clinical team to facilitate and support health-related decision making is provided in the Decision-Making Support Nursing Interventions Classification (NIC) feature in Chapter 2. When the patient is not able to safely make health care decisions, because of disease progression or the therapy used for treatment, written documents such as a living will or a health care power of attorney should be obtained when possible. See more on power of attorney for health care in the earlier section in this chapter on advance care planning. Without those documents, wishes of the patient should be ascertained from those closest to the patient. Some states have a legal order of priority for surrogates.

FAMILY COMMUNICATION

How questions are asked of surrogates is extremely important. The question is not: "What do you want to do about (patient's name)?" but rather, "What would (patient's name) want if he knew he were in this situation?" The consequences of the questions for the family are vastly different. The former has a greater likelihood of engendering guilt over "pulling the plug." The latter question gives more the sense of fulfilling what the patient wanted. Sometimes this discussion is held in the family meeting where a general sense of goals can be discussed. As families make decisions, they appreciate support of those decisions, and that support can reduce the burden they experience.

Family members have reported dissatisfaction with communication and decision making.[27] Increasing the frequency of communication and sharing concerns early in the hospitalization will make subsequent discussions easier for both the patient and family and the health professional. Having the entire critical care unit team present for morning rounds is one method of improving communication.[28]

CULTURE AND RELIGIOUS INFLUENCES

Cultural and religious influences on attitudes and beliefs about death and dying differ dramatically. Those cultures of the predominant religions commonly seen in the surrounding community should be familiar to the local health care team. These differences may affect how the health care team is viewed, how decisions are made, whether aggressive treatment is preferred, how death is met, and how grieving will occur.[29,30] One's own attitude toward the specific practices of a culture should be that of assessment[31] and respect. Interpreters are necessary when the patient or the family do not speak English.

HOSPICE

Although hospice care has been available, patients and families frequently view that method of support the last months of a patient in end-stage illness as "giving up." Health professionals can assist patients and families by providing information about the hospice benefit. Some hospices are offering to partner with critical care units in the provision of end-of-life care and in the process of withdrawal of ventilatory support.

WITHDRAWAL OR WITHHOLDING OF TREATMENT

Discussions about the potential for impending death are never held early enough. Usually the first discussion is around the discontinuation of life support. The late timing of that first discussion is an issue, since sometimes families have arrived at the notion of withdrawal before physicians.[26,32] Physicians could give families time to adjust by providing discussions early on about prognosis, goals of therapy, and patient's wishes.[33]

PROACTIVE APPROACH

Once a poor prognosis is established, a length of time can elapse before end-of-life treatment goals are established. Campbell and Guzman[34] recommended a proactive case-finding approach by palliative care personnel to decrease hospital length of stay for patients with multiorgan system failure and global cerebral ischemia. They shortened the time between identifying the poor prognosis and establishing comfort care goals, decreased length of critical care unit stay for patients with multisystem organ dysfunction, and reduced the cost of care.

DISAGREEMENT AND DISTRESS FOR CAREGIVERS

Nurses and doctors frequently disagree about the futility of interventions. Sometimes nurses consider withdrawal before physicians and patients and feel like the care they are giving is unnecessary and possibly harmful. Nurses in one study were found to be more pessimistic but more often correct than physicians in the prognosis of dying patients, but the nurses proposed treatment withdrawal in some very sick patients who survived.[35] This issue is a serious one for critical care nurses, since the score on the emotional exhaustion subscale of the Maslach Burnout Inventory and the score on the frequency subscale on the Moral Distress Scale were found to correlate in a group of 60 critical care nurses.[36]

BARRIERS TO DYING

Ellershaw identified a number of barriers to diagnosing dying: hope for the patient to improve, unclear diagnosis, pursuance of futile interventions, disagreement about the patient's condition, failure to recognize key signs and symptoms, poor ability to communicate, fears about foreshortening life, concerns about withdrawal and withholding, and medico-legal issues.[37] Further, the usefulness of prognostic models is to predict mortality rates for groups of critical care patients, rather than to guide specific decisions to forego treatment.[38]

STEPS TOWARD COMFORT CARE

If a series of interventions is to be withdrawn, usually dialysis is discontinued first along with diagnostic workups and vasopressors. Next, intravenous fluids, monitoring, laboratory tests, and antibiotics are stopped.[38] Withdrawal of specific treatments may have effects necessitating symptom management. Withdrawal of dialysis may cause dyspnea from volume overload, which may necessitate the use of opioids or benzodiazepines. Efforts to discontinue artificial feeding may be met with concern from the family, since offering food has high social significance.

PALLIATIVE CARE

Those patients who are identified as being near the end of life require aggressive care for their symptom management, provided by a team of health professionals. The most relevant clinical goal should be to palliate these unpleasant situations by assessing for them and implementing appropriate interventions.[3] Palliative care guidelines have been released by a consortium of organizations concerned with palliative care and end-of-life care, and these may provide guidance when the usual first-line treatments do not promote comfort for critically ill patients who are near death.[39] Palliative care has been thought of as desirable only when the patient nears death or when several interventions have been tried for management of symptoms without success. However, recent publications such as these guidelines and the IOM report *Improving Palliative Care for Cancer*[40] stated that palliative care ideally begins at the time of diagnosis of a life-threatening illness and continues through cure, or until death and into the family's bereavement period.

PAIN MANAGEMENT

Since many critical care patients are not conscious, assessment of pain and other symptoms becomes more difficult.[41] Gelinas and colleagues[42] recommended using signs of body movements, neuromuscular signs, facial expressions, or response to physical examination for pain assessment in patients with altered consciousness (see Chapter 8). Foley,[43] while acknowledging the usual three-step approach of the World Health Organization, admitted that in critical care units, step 3 is frequently used because of the intensity of the pain. Nonopioid drugs are the first-line approach, followed by adding an opioid for additional analgesia when relief is not obtained. Since opioids provide sedation and anxiolysis as well as analgesia, they are particularly beneficial in the ventilated patient. Morphine is the drug of choice, and there is no upper limit in dosing.[3] In nonventilated patients, sedation may cause respiratory depression,[43] and nonopioids or specific anesthetic agents may be more appropriate. Jacobi and others have published a guideline for the sustained use of sedatives and analgesia[44] (see Chapter 9); it is also available on the Society of Critical Care Medicine's website (www.sccm.org).

SYMPTOM MANAGEMENT

Campbell,[3] in her chapter on "Usual care requirements for the patient who is near death," listed the following symptoms as necessary parts of the assessment: dyspnea, nausea and vomiting, edema and pulmonary edema, anxiety and delirium, metabolic derangements, skin integrity, and anemia and hemorrhage.

DYSPNEA

Campbell recently published a review of terminal dyspnea and respiratory distress.[45] Dyspnea is best managed with close evaluation of the patient and the use of opioids, sedatives, and nonpharmacologic interventions (oxygen, positioning, and increased ambient air flow). Morphine reduces anxiety and muscle tension and increases pulmonary vasodilation. Benzodiazepines may be used in patients who are not able to take opioids, or for whom the respiratory effects are minimal. Benzodiazepines and opioids should be titrated to effect.

NAUSEA AND VOMITING

Nausea and vomiting are common and should be treated with antiemetics. The cause of nausea and vomiting may be intestinal obstruction. Treatment for decompression may be uncomfortable in dying patients, so its use should be weighed using a benefit/burden ratio.

FEVER AND INFECTION

Fever and infection will necessitate assessment of the benefits of continuing antibiotics so as not to prolong the dying process.[3] Management of the fever with antipyretics may be appropriate for patient comfort, but other methods such as ice or hypothermia blankets should be balanced against the amount of distress the patient would experience.

EDEMA

Edema may cause discomfort, and diuretics may be effective if kidney function is intact. Certainly dialysis would not be warranted at end of life. The use of fluids may contribute to the edema when kidney function is impaired and the body is slowing its functions. In a Database of Abstracts of Reviews of Effectiveness (DARE) report,[46] little relationship was found between thirst and fluid therapy or fluid status.

ANXIETY

Anxiety should be assessed verbally, if possible, or by changes in vital signs or restlessness. Benzodiazepines, especially midazolam with its rapid onset and short half-life, are frequently used.

DELIRIUM

Delirium is commonly observed in the critically ill and in those approaching death. Haloperidol is recommended as useful, and restraints should be avoided. Kehl[47] has published a review of available literature. She concluded that despite the recommendations of most authors to use neuroleptic medications as a treatment for restlessness, a number of studies demonstrated the effectiveness of other medications such as benzodiazepines (notably midazolam and lorazepam), or phenothiazines, either alone or in combination.

METABOLIC DERANGEMENT

Treatments for metabolic derangements, skin problems, anemia, and hemorrhage should be tempered with concerns for patient comfort. Only those interventions promoting comfort should be performed. Patients do not necessarily feel better "when the lab values are right," if they had to have invasive treatments to get there.

PROVIDING COMFORT

The nursing interventions at end of life should focus on the provision of comfort care as an active, desirable, and important service. Unnecessary checks of vital signs, laboratory work, and any treatment that does not promote comfort should be avoided. Positioning the patient who is actively dying has as its purpose only comfort, not the schedule to promote skin integrity. Coordinating this care with the many members of the critical care team is important to ensure consistency across disciplines and across shifts. When symptom management is not successful in ensuring comfort, the services of the Pain Team or the Palliative Care Service may be required.

NEAR DEATH AWARENESS

Two hospice nurses[48] have described a phenomenon of near death awareness. The same behaviors may be seen in conscious critical care patients near death. Having an awareness of the phenomenon will allow for more careful assessment of behaviors that could be interpreted as delirium, acid-base imbalance, or other metabolic derangements. These behaviors include communicating with someone who is not alive, preparing for travel, describing a place they can see, or even knowing when death will occur.[49]

WITHDRAWAL OF MECHANICAL VENTILATION

During the family meeting where a decision to withdraw life support is made, a time to initiate withdrawal is usually established. For example, a distant family member may need to arrive, and then the procedure will occur. Where possible, the patient should be moved to a separate or special room. It is helpful if noninvolved staff are alerted to the fact that a withdrawal is occurring. A neutral sign hung on the door or use of a special room may caution staff to avoid loud conversations and laughter, which is quite upsetting to families present.

Pacemakers or implantable cardioverter-defibrillators should be turned off to prevent patient distress from their firing[50] and to avoid interfering with the pronouncement of death.[38] Neuromuscular blocking agents should be discontinued, since paralysis precludes the assessment of patient discomfort and the means of the patient to communicate with loved ones. Time for clearance of the medication should be included in the schedule.[38]

The removal of monitors is usually recommended.[10] However, physicians may use the monitor to assess the distress of the patient during the withdrawal process to adjust the amount of medication needed. Families may glance at the monitor to verify that electrical activity has ceased since the appearance of death may be too subtle to detect. If not needed, monitors should be removed to make the room appear as normal as possible.

OPIOIDS AND SEDATIVES

Opioids and benzodiazepines are the most commonly administered medications, since dyspnea and anxiety are the usual symptoms related to ventilator withdrawal. Campbell[3] stated that brain-dead patients do not require sedation and patients with brainstem activity only may not show signs of distress or need sedation. Von Gunten and Weissman[51] recommended sedating all patients, even those who are comatose. They recommend a bolus dose of morphine, 2 to10 mg IV, and a continuous morphine infusion at 50% of the bolus dose per hour. Midazolam, 1 to 2 mg IV, is given, followed by an infusion at 1 mg/hour. The intent is to provide good symptom control so that doses accelerate until patient comfort is achieved. Additional medication should be available at the bedside for immediate administration when patient discomfort is observed.

VENTILATOR SETTINGS

After patient comfort is achieved, reduction of ventilator settings occurs. An experienced physician, a respiratory therapist, and a nurse should be present during this time. Ventilator alarms should be turned off. Which method of withdrawal is adopted is usually up to clinician preference. The choice of terminal wean as opposed to extubation is made based on considerations of access for suctioning, appearance of the patient for the family, how long the patient will survive off the ventilator, and whether the patient has the ability to communicate with loved ones at the bedside.

If terminal wean is used, first positive end-expiratory pressure (PEEP) is reduced to normal, then the mode is set to patient control. Next the Fio_2 is reduced to 0.21 (21%). All of these steps are taken slowly while observ-

ing the patient for distress or anxiety. If extubation is used immediately, rather then at the end of the terminal wean, the family should be prepared for airway compromise and the appearance of the patient.

All patients do not require the same ventilator weaning or extubation protocols. For example, Campbell[3] recommends turning off the ventilator and extubating patients who are brain-dead; placing patients who have brainstem-only injuries on a T-piece; and using terminal weaning for those with altered consciousness or those who are conscious. The terminal wean offers the most control over secretions, respiratory noises, and gasping.

PROFESSIONAL ISSUES/HEALTH CARE SETTINGS

Professional issues surround the provision of palliative care within traditional acute and clinical settings. In critical care units, care may be managed by an intensivist or by a "committee" of specialists, seldom by the family physician who knows the patient. The use of consultants may be limited. Palliative care specialists might be advisable at times, but they are considered to be "outsiders" and are infrequently invited. How the consultation is arranged may vary by institution. "Turf" issues should not be the reason patients do not get the care they need.

EMOTIONAL SUPPORT FOR THE NURSE

Nurses who care for the dying patient need to have that work as valued as are the "high tech" functions in the critical care unit. At times, critical care units have several nurses who seem to be the ones who are relied upon to give end-of-life care or to assist with withdrawal of life support. When there are several deaths together in time, those nurses may be called on frequently. Some consideration in assignment should be given when a nurse has more than one death in a shift or a week. Taking a new admission is also difficult immediately following a death, sometimes before the family has left the unit. Nurse administrators can provide some additional resources, debriefing, or time off when the burden has been high. Critical care nurses have reported that colleagues' comments of support are also helpful.[52]

ORGAN DONATION

The Social Security Act Section 1138[53] requires that hospitals have written protocols for the identification of potential organ donors. The Joint Commission on the Accreditation of HealthCare Organizations (JCAHO) has a standard on organ donation, LD.3.110.[54] Although an impending death marks a difficult time for family members, the nurse must notify the organ procurement official to approach the family with a donation request. Those individuals have training to make a supportive request and are the ones to decide if a family should not be approached based on the patient's disease. Although organ donation may not be appropriate in some cases, tissue donation remains a consideration. More information is available in Chapter 41.

BRAIN DEATH

Death may be pronounced when the patient meets a list of neurologic criteria. However, there are differences among hospital policies for certification of brain death, which may permit differences among the circumstances under which patients are pronounced dead in different U.S. hospitals.[55] Families do not understand the meaning of brain death, and they are less likely to donate organs when they believe the patient will not be dead until the ventilator is turned off and the heart stops.[56] How these conversations are held will determine families' understanding and positively affect donation. Campbell[3] recommended not suggesting that the organs are alive while the brain is dead, but rather that the organs are functioning as a result of the machines used. Chapter 26 contains more information on the specifics of brain death.

FAMILY CARE

In this chapter, the term *family* means whatever the patient states is the family. An integral part of the patient-family dyad, families expect a "cure" for any condition the patient may have; they do not expect to receive "bad news." They look for the good news in any message received from caregivers and are surprised when told that death is the only outcome possible.[52] Families need assistance in forming their expectations about outcomes. It is preferable to have ongoing communication about patient progress, rather than waiting until the patient is near death and then communicating with the family.

COMMUNICATION NEEDS

Families have complained about infrequent physician communication,[57] unmet communication needs in the shift from aggressive to end-of-life care,[58] and lacking or inadequate communication.[59] Sometimes families are not ready to receive the prognosis and engage in decision making.[60] Communication seems to be the most common source of complaint in families across studies and should be at the center of efforts to improve end-of-life care.

The health care team can reinforce to the family the legitimacy of expressing feelings of disappointment, sadness, and loss. It is important that the family is made aware that the patient was more than simply a clinical disease and that he or she was recognized as an individual while in the critical care unit. Ways to address the cultural, social, and emotional issues surrounding the expression of grief are listed in the Nursing Interventions Classification (NIC) feature on Grief Work Facilitation.

NIC   Grief Work Facilitation

Definition: Assistance with the resolution of a significant loss

Activities

Identify the loss
Assist the patient to identify the nature of the attachment to the lost object or person
Assist the patient to identify the initial reaction to the loss
Encourage expression of feelings about the loss
Listen to expression of grief
Encourage discussion of previous loss experiences
Encourage the patient to verbalize memories of the loss, both past and current
Make empathetic statements about grief
Encourage identification of greatest fears concerning the loss
Instruct the phases of the grieving process, as appropriate
Support progression through personal grieving stages
Include significant others in discussions and decisions, as appropriate

Assist patient to identify personal coping strategies
Encourage patient to implement cultural, religious, and social customs associated with the loss
Communicate acceptance of discussing loss
Answer children's questions associated with the loss
Use clear words, such as *dead* or *died*, rather than euphemisms
Encourage children to discuss feelings
Encourage expression of feelings in ways comfortable to the child, such as writing, drawing, or playing
Assist the child to clarify misconceptions
Identify sources of community support
Support efforts to resolve previous conflict, as appropriate
Reinforce progress made in the grieving process
Assist the identifying modifications needed in lifestyle

From Dochterman JM, Bulechek GM: *Nursing interventions classification (NIC)*, ed 4, St Louis, 2004, Mosby.

WAITING FOR "GOOD NEWS"

Patients and families do not come to the critical care unit with the expectation of death. Even those who have had previous admissions expect to be "saved." They tend to listen to imparted information looking for good news; even when "bad news" is given, they may initially deny it or have great difficulty taking it in.[59] Having this in mind while talking to families may assist professionals in interpreting families' responses.

Preparing families for changes in the patient as the health condition deteriorates helps them make plans. They need to know if other family members should be called, if someone should spend the night, or if financial arrangements should be changed before an impending death (e.g., to enable the widow to have access to funds). Anticipated changes can be described to prepare families.

Families may refuse to forgo life-supporting treatments and want "everything done" because of mistrust of health professionals, poor communication, survivor guilt, or religious/cultural reasons.[26] Effective communication throughout the hospitalization, as well as providing information throughout the stay, predisposes the family to better acceptance of "news" as the patient deteriorates.

FAMILY MEETINGS

Families may experience a sense of crisis as emergencies occur, or as the patient deteriorates or dies. There will be various responses to the news of the death. They could show anger or quiet, emotions or stoicism. Culture or religious beliefs may affect their response to news. It is helpful to ask if they would like to see a chaplain or a social worker. Quiet and calm, some privacy, and support are always appreciated.

Family meetings in the presence of the critical care team have been one method used to arrive at a common understanding of the patient's prognosis and goals for future care.[61,62] An analysis of the amount of opportunity families had to speak in these meetings revealed that when families had greater opportunity to talk, their satisfaction with physician communication increased and their ratings of conflict with the physician decreased. Abbott and colleagues[63] discussed families' descriptions, 1 year after decisions about withdrawal of life support, of conflict centering on communication and the behavior of the staff. After the patient's death, greater family satisfaction with withdrawal of life support was associated with the following measures:

- The process of withdrawal of life support being well explained
- Withdrawal of life support proceeding as expected
- Patient appearing comfortable
- Family/friends prepared

- Appropriate person initiating discussion
- Adequate privacy during withdrawal of life support
- A chance to voice concerns[64]

FAMILY PRESENCE DURING CPR

To be helpful, family presence during procedures or resuscitative attempts[65] should be coupled with staff support. Critical care nurses and emergency nurses have taken family members to the bedside for resuscitation or invasive procedures, but most did not have written policies for family presence.[66] At times these experiences provide opportunities for the family to be supportive of the patient. At other times the family may become more aware of what is involved in decisions they have made on behalf of the patient. Seeing the steps of resuscitation may make clearer the impact of decisions made or delayed.

VISITING HOURS

Providing the visiting time to help family members say good-bye is an important function. Family members may have difficulty in seeing the person they knew among all the tubes. Coaching can be provided about how to approach the patient and that the patient may still be able to hear despite appearing to be nonresponsive. Visitors should be permitted to the extent possible, not interfering with other patients' privacy or rest. Children, unless they represent a significant source of infection, should be able to say good-bye as well, but they may need adult assistance in understanding the situation. Families may have religious or cultural ceremonies that are important for them to perform before the patient dies or experiences withdrawal of life support. These should be encouraged and facilitated as much as possible.

Continuity of care by the same nurse is important. As the patient nears death, nurses have sometimes stayed with the family after the end of a shift when death was imminent, so that they would not need to adjust to another person at this difficult time.[52]

FOLLOWING DEATH

Following the death, the family may wish to spend time at the bedside. The families' time with the body should be unhurried, and private. They need adequate room to sit and spend time. They can be asked if they need assistance or resources, and whether they wish to be alone or have someone nearby. Frequently the bed is needed for another patient and juggling is required to ensure that the family has sufficient time even as another patient needs to be admitted. Supporting families after a death involves immediate bereavement support, information on what to do about the death, bereavement support for the future, contact with the family after death, and as-

EVIDENCE-BASED COLLABORATIVE PRACTICE

End-of-Life Care

The key recommendations of the guidelines for *end-of-life care in the intensive care unit*, based on research and expert panel review, are as follows:

The management of patients at the end of life can be divided into two phases:

1. The first phase concerns the pursuit of shared decision making that leads from the pursuit of cure or recovery to the pursuit of comfort and freedom from pain.
2. The second phase concerns the actions that are taken once this shift in goals has been made and focuses on both the humanistic and technical skills that must be enlisted to ensure that the needs of the patient and family are met.

This guideline focuses predominantly on the second phase.

Needs of the Patient, Family, and Clinical Team

1. **Needs of the patient**

Many patients have lost consciousness before the decision is made to move to palliative care. The following are five patient-centered domains of good end-of-life care:
   - Receiving adequate pain and symptom management
   - Avoiding inappropriate prolongation of dying
   - Achieving a sense of control
   - Relieving burden
   - Strengthening relationships with loved ones

2. **Needs of the family**

The 10 most important needs of families of critically ill dying patients are the following:
   - To be with the dying person
   - To be helpful to the dying person
   - To be informed of the dying person's changing condition
   - To understand what is being done to the patient and why
   - To be assured of the patient's comfort

   - To ventilate emotions
   - To be assured that their decisions were right
   - To find meaning in the dying of their loved one
   - To be fed, hydrated, and rested

3. **Needs of the clinical team**
   - Multidisciplinary teamwork
   - Administrative support that values intensive palliative care
   - Opportunity for bereavement and debriefing

Comfort and Freedom From Pain

4. **Clinical assessments and interventions**
   - Assessment of pain
   - Assessment of suffering
   - Use of medications to relieve pain and suffering
   - Alleviation of symptoms such as dyspnea, nausea and vomiting, thirst, skin irritation, anxiety, and delirium
   - Avoid use of restraints

5. **Terminal weaning vs. extubation**
   - Terminal wean
   - Extubation

Decisions about how to discontinue ventilatory support depend on the patient's clinical condition, the patient's wishes, if known, family concerns, and the prior experiences of the clinical team.

Sensitivity After the Death

6. **Procedures**
   - Cultural or religious requests
   - Organ donation
   - Autopsy

Sometimes families may have specific requests related to religion or culture. Also, there are several procedures that may occur following the death of a patient, and the family must be approached with sensitivity and a consciousness that they are grieving the loss of a loved one.

Data from Truog RD et al: Recommendations for end-of-life care in the intensive care unit: the Ethics Committee of the Society of Critical Care Medicine, *Crit Care Med* 29(12):2332-2348, 2001.

---

sessment of the quality of care the patient experienced.[67] Having material already prepared with the necessary after-death information is quite helpful at this time. Nurses need to be aware of their own judgment on what is an appropriate response, since individuals respond differently to the same news, even within the same family.

COLLABORATIVE CARE

The ability to provide collaborative, compassionate end of life care is the responsibility of all clinicians who

work with the critically ill (see the Evidence-Based Collaborative Practice feature on End-of-Life Care). In 2001 the Society of Critical Care Medicine published "Recommendations for end-of-life care in the intensive care unit" to provide guidance for end-of-life care.[68] The Robert Wood Johnson Foundation (RWJF) Critical Care End-of-Life Peer Workgroup identified seven end-of-life care domains for use in the intensive care unit:

1. Patient- and family-centered decision making
2. Communication
3. Continuity of care
4. Emotional and practical support

5. Symptom management and comfort care
6. Spiritual support
7. Emotional and organizational support for intensive care unit clinicians[69]

SUMMARY

Recently, individuals[70] and groups[71] have developed Websites of online tools to improve end-of-life care. Critical care unit staff will be able to assess the quality of their end-of-life care by assessing perceptions of families and staff, auditing documentation,[72] or making observations of care. We need to put the same attention into improving our end-of-life care that we do into our skills of ECG interpretation or hemodynamic monitoring.

REFERENCES

1. Rabow MW et al: End-of-life care content in 50 textbooks from multiple specialties, *JAMA* 283(6):771-778, 2000.
2. Kirchhoff KT et al: Analysis of end-of-life content in critical care nursing textbooks, *J Professional Nurs* 19(6):372-381, 2003.
3. Campbell ML: *Forgoing life-sustaining therapy: How to care for the patient who is near death,* Aliso Viejo, Calif, 1998, AACN.
4. Curtis JR, Rubenfeld GD, editors: *Managing death in the intensive care unit: the transition from cure to comfort,* Oxford, 2001, Oxford University Press.
5. The SUPPORT Principal Investigators: a controlled trial to improve care for seriously ill hospitalized patients. The study to understand prognoses and preferences for outcomes and risks of treatments (SUPPORT), *JAMA* 274(20):1591-1598, 1995.
6. Field MJ, Cassell CK, editors: *Approaching death: improving care at the end of life,* Washington, DC, 1997, National Academy Press.
7. Angus DC et al.: Use of intensive care at the end of life in the United States: an epidemiologic study, *Crit Care Med* 32(3):638-643, 2004.
8. Gillick MR: Advance care planning, *N Engl J Med* 350(1):7-8, 2004.
9. Gordon NP, Shade SB: Advance directives are more likely among seniors asked about end-of-life care preferences, *Arch Intern Med* 159(7):701-704, 1999.
10. Rubenfeld GD, Crawford SW: Withdrawal of life-sustaining treatment. In Curtis JR, Rubenfeld, GD, editors: *Managing death in the intensive care unit: The transition from cure to comfort,* Oxford, 2001, Oxford University Press.
11. Tilden V et al: Family decision-making to withdraw life-sustaining treatments from hospitalized patients, *Nurs Res* 50(2):105-115, 2001.
12. Burns JP et al: Do-not-resuscitate order after 25 years, *Crit Care Med* 31(5):1543-1550, 2003.
13. Keenan CH, Kish SK: The influence of do-not-resuscitate orders on care provided for patients in the surgical intensive care unit of a cancer center, *Crit Care Nurs Clin North Am* 12(3):385-390, 2000.
14. Christakis NA, Lamont EB: Extent and determinants of error in doctors' prognoses in terminally ill patients: prospective cohort study, *BMJ* 320(7233):469-472, 2000.
15. Lynn J et al.: Prognoses of seriously ill hospitalized patients on the days before death: implications for patient care and public policy, *New Horiz* 5(1):56-61, 1997.
16. McDonald DD et al: Communicating end-of-life preferences, *West J Nurs Res* 25(6):652-666, discussion 667-675, 2003.
17. Fried TR, Bradley EH: What matters to seriously ill older persons making end-of-life treatment decisions? A qualitative study, *J Palliat Med* 6(2):237-244, 2003.
18. Teno JM et al: Medical care inconsistent with patients' treatment goals: association with 1-year Medicare resource use and survival, *J Am Geriatr Soc* 50(3):496-500, 2002.
19. Mularski RA et al: Educational agendas for interdisciplinary end-of-life curricula, *Crit Care Med* 29(2 Suppl):N16-23, 2001.
20. Wood EB et al: Enhancing palliative care education in medical school curricula: implementation of the palliative education assessment tool, *Acad Med* 77(4):285-291, 2002.
21. Covinsky KE et al: Communication and decision-making in seriously ill patients: Findings of the SUPPORT project. The study to understand prognoses and preferences for outcomes and risks of treatments, *J Am Geriatr Soc* 48(5 Suppl):S187-193, 2000.
22. Ebell MH et al: Survival after in-hospital cardiopulmonary resuscitation. A meta-analysis, *J Gen Intern Med* 13(12):805-816, 1998.
23. FitzGerald JD et al: Functional status among survivors of in-hospital cardiopulmonary resuscitation. SUPPORT investigators study to understand progress and preferences for outcomes and risks of treatment, *Arch Intern Med* 157(1):72-76, 1997.
24. Marshall JC et al: Multiple organ dysfunction score: a reliable descriptor of a complex clinical outcome, *Crit Care Med* 23(10):1638-1652, 1995.
25. Rocker G et al: Clinician predictions of intensive care unit mortality, *Crit Care Med* 32(5):1149-1154, 2004.
26. Prendergast TJ, Puntillo KA: Withdrawal of life support: intensive caring at the end of life, *JAMA* 288(21):2732-2740, 2002.
27. Baker R et al: Family satisfaction with end-of-life care in seriously ill hospitalized adults, *J Am Geriatr Soc* 48(5 Suppl):S61-69, 2000.
28. Curtis JR: Communicating about end-of-life care with patients and families in the intensive care unit, *Crit Care Clin* 20(3):363-380, viii, 2004.
29. Lipson JG et al: *Culture & nursing care : a pocket guide,* San Francisco, 1996, UCSF Nursing Press, v 303.
30. Degenholtz HB et al: Race and the intensive care unit: disparities and preferences for end-of-life care, *Crit Care Med* 31(5 Suppl):S373-378, 2003.
31. Crawley LM et al: Strategies for culturally effective end-of-life care, *Ann Intern Med* 136(9):673-679, 2002.
32. Breen CM et al: Conflict associated with decisions to limit life-sustaining treatment in intensive care units, *J Gen Intern Med* 16(5):283-289, 2001.
33. Curtis JR, Patrick DL: How to discuss dying and death in the ICU. In Curtis JR, Rubenfeld GD, editors: *Managing death in the intensive care unit: the transition from cure to comfort,* Oxford, 2001, Oxford University Press.
34. Campbell ML, Guzman JA: Impact of a proactive approach to improve end-of-life care in a medical ICU, *Chest* 123(1):266-271, 2003.
35. Frick S et al: Medical futility: predicting outcome of intensive care unit patients by nurses and doctors—a prospective comparative study, *Crit Care Med* 31(2):456-461, 2003.
36. Meltzer LS, Huckabay LM: Critical care nurses' perceptions of futile care and its effect on burnout, *Am J Crit Care* 13(3):202-208, 2004.

37. Ellershaw J, Ward C: Care of the dying patient: the last hours or days of life, *BMJ* 326(7379):30-34, 2003.

38. Faber-Langendoen K, Lanken PN: Dying patients in the intensive care unit: forgoing treatment, maintaining care, *Ann Intern Med* 133(11):886-893, 2000.

39. National Consensus Project for Quality Palliative Care: *Clinical Practice Guidelines for Quality Palliative Care*, 2004, website: http://www.nationalconsensusproject.org/index.html.

40. Foley KM, Gelband H, editors: *Improving palliative care for cancer*, Washington, DC, 2001, National Academy Press.

41. Mularski RA: Pain management in the intensive care unit, *Crit Care Clin* 20(3):381-401, viii, 2004.

42. Gelinas C et al: Pain assessment and management in critically ill intubated patients: a retrospective study, *Am J Crit Care* 13(2):126-135, 2004.

43. Foley KM: Pain and symptom control in the dying ICU patient. In Curtis JR, Rubenfeld GD, editors: *Managing death in the intensive care unit: the transition from cure to comfort*, Oxford, 2001, Oxford University Press.

44. Jacobi J et al: Clinical practice guidelines for the sustained use of sedatives and analgesics in the critically ill adult. [Erratum appears in *Crit Care Med* 30(3):726, 2002], *Crit Care Med* 30(1):119-141, 2002.

45. Campbell ML: Terminal dyspnea and respiratory distress, *Crit Care Clin* 20(3):403-417, viii-ix, 2004.

46. N. H. S. Centre for Reviews & Dissemination: The effects of fluid status and fluid therapy on the dying, *Database of Abstracts of Reviews of Effectiveness*, 3:2003.

47. Kehl KA: Treatment of terminal restlessness: a review of the evidence, *J Pain Palliat Care Pharmacother* 18(1):5-30, 2004.

48. Callanan M, Kelley P: *Final gifts: understanding the special awareness, needs, and communications of the dying*, New York, 1997, Bantam.

49. Marchand L: Fast fact and concepts #118: near death awareness, 2004, End of life physician education resource center (EPERC), website: www.eperc.mcw.edu/.

50. Mueller PS et al: Ethical analysis of withdrawal of pacemaker or implantable cardioverter-defibrillator support at the end of life, *Mayo Clin Proc* 78(8):959-963, 2003.

51. von Gunten C, Weissman DE: Fast facts and concepts #34: symptom control for ventilator withdrawal in the dying patient (Part II), 2001, End of life physician education resource center (EPERC), website: www.eperc.mcw.edu/.

52. Kirchhoff KT et al: Intensive care nurses' experiences with end-of-life care, *Am J Crit Care* 9(1):36-42, 2000.

53. Social Security Administration: Hospital protocols for organ procurement and standards for organ procurement agencies, website: http://www.ssa.gov/OP_Home/ssact/title11/1138.htm.

54. Joint Commission on the Accreditation of Healthcare Organizations: Hospital standard on organ donation and procurement, 2004 comprehensive accreditation manual for hospitals leadership chapter: standard LD.3.110, Chicago, 2004, JCAHO.

55. Powner DJ et al: Variability among hospital policies for determining brain death in adults, *Crit Care Med* 32(6):1284-1288, 2004.

56. Siminoff LA et al: Families' understanding of brain death, *Prog Transplant* 13(3):218-224, 2003.

57. Heyland DK et al: Family satisfaction with care in the intensive care unit: results of a multiple center study, *Crit Care Med* 30(7):1413-1418, 2002.

58. Norton SA et al: Life support withdrawal: communication and conflict, *Am J Crit Care* 12(6):548-555, 2003.

59. Kirchhoff KT et al: The vortex: families' experiences with death in the intensive care unit, *Am J Crit Care* 11(3):200-209, 2002.

60. Murphy PA et al: Under the radar: contributions of the SUPPORT nurses, *Nurs Outlook* 49(5):238-242, 2001.

61. Ambuel B, Weissman D: Fast fact and concept No. 16; conducting a family conference, 2001, End of Life Physician Education Resource Center (EPERC), website: www.eperc.mcw.edu/.

62. Curtis JR et al: The family conference as a focus to improve communication about end-of-life care in the intensive care unit: opportunities for improvement, *Crit Care Med* 29(2 Suppl):N26-33, 2001.

63. Abbott KH et al: Families looking back: one year after discussion of withdrawal or withholding of life-sustaining support, *Crit Care Med* 29(1):197-201, 2001.

64. Keenan SP et al: Withdrawal of life support: how the family feels, and why, *J Palliat Care* 16(Suppl):S40-44, 2000.

65. Emergency Nurses' Association: *Family presence at the bedside during invasive procedures and resuscitation*, Des Plaines, Ill, 2001, The Association.

66. MacLean SL et al: Family presence during cardiopulmonary resuscitation and invasive procedures: practices of critical care and emergency nurses, *Am J Crit Care* 12(3):246-257, 2003.

67. Shannon SE: Helping families cope with death in the ICU. In Curtis JR, Rubenfeld GD, editors: *Managing death in the intensive care unit: the transition from cure to comfort*, Oxford, 2001, Oxford University Press.

68. Truog RD et al: Recommendations for end-of-life care in the intensive care unit: the Ethics Committee of the Society of Critical Care Medicine, *Crit Care Med* 29(12):2332-2348, 2001.

69. Clarke EB et al: Quality indicators for end-of-life care in the intensive care unit, *Crit Care Med* 31(9):2255-2262, 2003.

70. Curtis JR: End-of-life care research program, 2004, website: http://depts.washington.edu/eolcare/currentprojects/.

71. Promoting Excellence in End-of-Life Care, Promoting Excellence Tools. 2004, website: http://www.promotingexcellence.org/.

72. Kirchhoff KT et al: Assessment of documentation on withdrawal of life support in adult ICU patients, *Am J Crit Care* 13(4):328-334, 2004.

SPECIAL POPULATIONS

CHAPTER
11

The Pediatric Patient in the Adult Critical Care Unit

*T*his chapter covers some of the developmental and physiologic differences between adults and children older than 1 month. Although children may experience similar medical conditions to adults, they are assessed and managed differently. During periods of stress, children can maintain physiologic stability for a period, but then they can decompensate quickly. Children are not "small adults." Many of the laboratory values, medications, blood product dosages and methods of administration, and other therapeutic modalities differ from those used with adults.

Most children admitted to critical care units are younger than 5 years and therefore are less able to understand their circumstances and less able to verbalize their needs. Parents are the major sources of comfort for their children. They may also recognize subtle changes in their child's condition because they know their child better than anyone. Because of this, parental concerns must be addressed and parents must be present at the bedside as much as possible.

Even though some critically ill children can be managed in adult critical care units, there are certain situations in which children need the services of various pediatric subspecialties and/or pediatric intensivists and must be transferred to tertiary care pediatric critical care units. Some examples are children requiring high-frequency ventilation, extracorporeal membrane oxygenation (ECMO), cardiac surgery, and treatment for some neurologic conditions that require intracranial pressure (ICP) monitoring. In addition, transfer is considered for children who do not respond to treatment.

RESPIRATORY SYSTEM

ANATOMY AND PHYSIOLOGY

Upper Airway. The upper airway of the infant and child is different from that of the adult. The epiglottis of the newborn is located at the level of cervical spine 1 (C1) and the older infant's is located at C3, as opposed to an adult's, which is located at C4 to C5.

The infant's epiglottis is large and floppy, and because of its high placement, it can press against the pharyngeal soft palate on inspiration. The infant's tongue is also large, relative to head size, and fills the oral cavity. Because of this anatomy, the infant is generally an obligate nose breather until between 4 and 6 months of age, after which the larynx descends with growth.[1] Oral breathing is a very complex process for an infant, and it never occurs alone. Oronasal breathing is possible, but only up to 30% to 40% of ventilation can be provided orally. During sleep, oronasal breathing can occur spontaneously and last for about 20 seconds.

The larynx of the infant and young child, unlike that of the adult, is funnel-shaped, with the narrowest portion at the cricoid ring.[1] It also is pliable because of cartilage that is less developed, making it easier to collapse on inspiration or expiration. With changes in intrathoracic pressure, collapse can occur even with crying.[2] By 8 to 10 years of age the larynx has grown cylindric; has assumed the narrowest portion at the glottic opening; and has increased in length, width, and internal diameter. By 12 years of age the diameter has grown to 1.8 cm.[3]

The submucosal layer of the larynx is also more loose in the infant and young child, so fluid can accumulate more easily in that space.[4] With the airway's relatively rigid confines, any accumulation of fluid encroaches into the airway space. Along with a shorter and narrower airway, any decrease in airway radius leads to a greater exponential increase in airflow resistance, which increases the work of breathing. Turbulent airflow, such as occurs with crying, doubles the already increased airflow resistance.[5] Fig. 11-1 illustrates the changes in airway diameter and airflow resistance with obstruction from edema in an adult and in an infant. The infant or child with an abnormally small jaw and low-set ears must be considered as having a potentially difficult airway to manage and must have a consult with an anesthesiologist if airway management is required. Congenital malformations of the airway occur in utero at the same time these types of facial malformations occur.[1]

Lower Airway. Alveolar collapse is more likely in the infant and young child because of the smaller alveolar

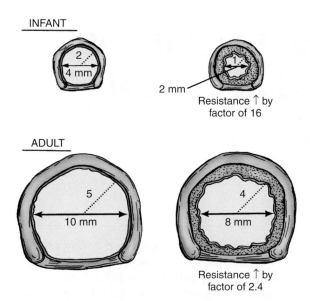

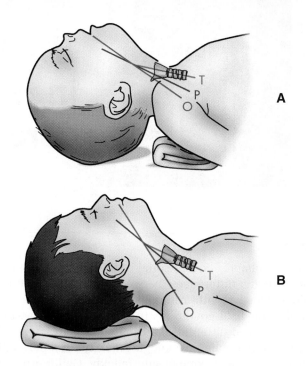

Fig. 11-1 Effects of edema on airway resistance. Proportional increases in airflow resistance with 1 mm of circumferential edema in the infant versus the adult. (From Zander J, Hazinski MF: Pulmonary disorders. In Hazinski MF, editor: *Nursing care of the critically ill child,* ed 2, St Louis, 1992, Mosby.)

Fig. 11-2 Correct airway positioning for ventilation of **A,** an infant, and **B,** a child. Better airflow is provided with a straight alignment of the oropharynx *(O),* pharynx *(P),* and trachea *(T).*

size. The infant and young child are at greater risk for ventilation-perfusion mismatch and atelectasis without this collateral ventilation.

The infant and child have a higher metabolic rate than does the adult; therefore oxygen consumption per kilogram is higher. Therefore hypoxemia develops more rapidly in the context of respiratory compromise for the child than for the adult.[3]

Chest Mechanics. The infant's and young child's respiratory mechanics are very different from the older child's or adult's.[3,6] In the infant and young child the chest wall is more compliant because the bones are smaller and more cartilaginous. The ribs are more horizontally placed, providing less of a bellowing action on inspiration. Accessory muscles are less developed, so the external intercostals do not contribute to pulling the ribs up on inspiration. The diaphragm is more horizontal in the chest and tends to pull the lower ribs inward on inspiration. Because of these mechanics, the infant and toddler depend almost totally on diaphragm contraction for lung expansion. Anything that impedes diaphragmatic contractions can result in respiratory compromise. With any decrease in lung compliance, as with lung disease, diaphragmatic contractions, which cause decreased intrathoracic pressure, will produce intercostal and substernal retractions.[6] The greater the chest wall retractions, the more the diaphragm must contract to offset the changes in intrathoracic pressure and to generate an adequate tidal volume.

In the normal infant, apnea can occur as an indirect result of paradoxic chest movement (diaphragm contractions pushing the abdomen out with the chest wall sinking in). This produces decreased lung volumes, leading to hypoxemia.

ASSESSMENT AND OXYGEN DEVICES

The infant or child usually experiences respiratory failure more often than primary cardiac failure. Unlike the older adult who may have underlying cardiovascular disease, the infant and child tend to demonstrate bradycardia and apnea in cardiopulmonary failure and not ventricular dysrythmias.[7] For the infant or child who is conscious and needs supplemental oxygen, the device of comfort must be selected.[3] Minimizing anxiety and fear in the child is paramount to decrease the work of breathing. Table 11-1 outlines the assessment areas for the infant or child at risk for respiratory failure.[3]

Airway Positioning. Knowledge of childhood anatomy is necessary to establish a patent airway. The infant or toddler younger than 2 years, because of the large occiput, needs to have a small roll or towel placed under the upper shoulders, with the jaw slightly extended into a "sniffing" position.[3] This displaces the tongue and lines up the posterior pharynx and tracheal opening for a clear airway. For the infant younger than 6 months, correct head positioning still may not prevent the large tongue from falling back into the posterior pharynx. Oral airways must not be used unless the infant is unconscious because the airway tip can stimulate laryngospasm as a result of the higher placement of the larynx. Try side-lying placement, with the neck in a neutral position.[3] The older child needs to have a folded towel placed under the head, with the neck in an extended position to maintain a patent airway.[5] Fig. 11-2 illustrates proper head positioning in the infant and child. The con-

Table 11-1	Significant Findings of the Infant or Child at Risk for Respiratory Failure	
Assessment Area	**Physical Findings**	**Discussion Points**
Respiratory rate	• Infant: >60/min • Child: >40/min • Slow or irregular	Tachypnea usually first sign of distress in an infant; fatigue is a common contributing factor in respiratory failure
Mechanics	• Retractions (intercostal, supraclavicular, substernal) • Paradoxic movements (chest in and abdomen out) • Grunting • Stridor • Wheezing	 Closing of the glottis to create "auto-PEEP" to keep alveoli open at end-expiration Sign of upper airway obstruction Sign of lower airway obstruction
Air entry	• Changes in pitch rather than volume of breath sounds	Chest expansion can sometimes be barely perceptible in a normal, spontaneously breathing infant; the small, thin chest wall causes breath sounds from any area of the lungs to be easily referred throughout the chest, even over fluid or atelectasis; listen for bilateral breath sounds high in the axillae, because these are the two most separated points
Color/temperature	• Central coolness, pallor, or cyanosis	Peripheral changes may be normal in the infant or child
Heart rate	• <5 years: <60 or >180 beats/min • 5-10 years: <60 or >160 beats/min • >10 years: <50 or >140 beats/min	The infant and child have limited ability to increase stroke volume; therefore with hypoxemia the heart rate increases to improve cardiac output. If bradycardia occurs with cardiorespiratory distress, arrest may be imminent.
Neurologic	• Infant: hypotonia • Child: irritability • Decreased level of consciousness	Sign of hypoxia for infants An early sign of hypoxia, often manifested as a decreased responsiveness to parents or to pain

PEEP, positive end-expiratory pressure.

scious child must be allowed to assume a position of choice for airway maintenance.

Supplemental Oxygen Devices. Many of the oxygen devices used for adults are used also for children. Some additions include oxygen hoods, for infants up to 1 year of age, which are clear plastic boxes that envelop the head and allow full vision of the head and access to the body; oxygen tents, which are used less often; and oxygen "blow-by," which uses oxygen tubing or a hose to blow oxygen toward the child's face without touching him or her. Oxygen masks can aggravate and upset the child and often are repeatedly pushed off. In contrast, the child or parent can hold the blow-by tubing himself or herself, ensuring greater compliance and resulting in oxygen saturations higher than those from oxygen masks.

An adult-size, self-inflating resuscitation bag can be carefully used on an infant, providing only the force needed to cause appropriate chest expansion.[3] An appropriately-sized bag minimizes the potential for overinflating the lungs. Bag sizes, along with other supplemental oxygen devices and oxygen administration, are outlined in Table 11-2. There must be no leaf-flap outlet valves when a self-inflating bag is used to assist spontaneous ventilation in an infant, because the infant cannot generate enough negative inspiratory pressure to open the valve.[3] Bags equipped with spring-loaded positive end-expiratory pressure (PEEP) valves to provide constant positive airway pressure (CPAP) must not be used with the spontaneously breathing child for the same reason previously discussed.[3] Anesthesia ventilation bags have no flow valves that require opening on inspiration and therefore can be used to provide supplemental oxygen, PEEP, or CPAP to the spontaneously breathing infant or child.[3] Pressure manometers can be attached to the ventilation bags to measure peak inspiratory pressure. Ventilatory masks are measured in the child as in the adult—from the bridge of the nose to before the end of the chin.

ENDOTRACHEAL INTUBATION

Procedure. Endotracheal tube (ETT) placement and management for the infant and the young child differ from those for the adult. Preoxygenation is especially important for the infant, who has higher resting oxygen demands.[8] The infant also has a smaller lung volume, resulting in smaller oxygen reserves. Intubation attempts, therefore, need to be shorter in duration (less than 30 seconds) with the infant than with the older child or adult.[3] Box 11-1 provides formulas for ETT measurements in the child. For the child younger than 2 years, there is no formula. ETT size is matched to the infant's age (Table 11-3).[3,8] When placed, the tip of the ETT should be 1 to 2 cm above the carina, about level with T2.[1] This level, confirmed on a chest radiograph, is just below where the clavicles connect to the spine, or at the third rib. Table 11-3 outlines approximate sizes for various pieces of intubation equipment for infants and children. After the equipment is placed, bilateral breath sounds in the infant should be assessed high in the axillae and over the abdomen.[3,8] The easy transmission of sounds in the chest of the child can be mistaken for breath sounds if there is accidental esophageal intubation.

ETT dislodgment can occur very easily in the infant or young child. The tip of the ETT is pulled upward with neck extension or when the head is turned completely to the side. Conversely, the ETT moves downward with neck flexion. With the existing short trachea of the young child, an ETT placed higher or lower can become dislodged or intubate the bronchus. ETT obstruction can occur also with high placement, neck flexion, or head rotation, which can cause the bevel of the ETT to press against the tracheal wall, occluding the lumen. Secretions and mucus plugs may more easily occlude the lumen of a small-diameter ETT.

Securing Endotracheal/Nasotracheal Tubes. The small infant or child has less facial area for tape adherence for securing the tubes. A method with a low inci-

---

Box 11-1

ENDOTRACHEAL TUBE MEASUREMENT

ENDOTRACHEAL TUBE (ETT) SIZE
- Formula >2 years old: **(age in years + 16) ÷ 4**
- Infant/toddler sizes based on age
- For any age: can compare circumference of child's little finger with external diameter size of ETT
- Cuffed tube: external diameter one-half size smaller than appropriate-size uncuffed tube

ETT DEPTH OF INSERTION
- Formula (from teeth to midtrachea): **internal diameter ETT × 3**

ETT CUFF PRESSURE
- Allow for a barely sealed air leak

Table 11-2	Supplemental Oxygen Devices and Oxygen Administration in Infants and Children	
Device	**Administration**	**Discussion Points**

Nasal cannula	• Young infant[26-27]
	  0.5 L/min = 28% O_2
	  1.0 L/min = 32% O_2
	  2.0 L/min = 35% O_2
	• Child
	  Same as adult settings*
		Minute volume, inspiratory/expiratory times, and amount of mouth breathing affects infant Fio_2 via a nasal cannula differently than for an adult given the same gas flow and O_2 percent[26-29]

Oxygen hood[1]	• 10-15 L/min = nearly 100% O_2	Use with infants <1 year old
Oxygen blow-by	• 10-15 L/min = nearly 100% O_2	Better tolerated than oxygen masks Allows child or parent to hold tubing

Self-inflating resuscitation bag[24]	• Infant
	  <3 months old: ¼-L bag
	  3 months-4 years old: ½-L bag
	• Child
	  5-10 years old: 1 L bag
	  >10 years old: 1.5 L bag
		Do not use bags with leaf-flap outlet valves or with spring-loaded PEEP valves[1]

Anesthesia bag[1,4]	• Spontaneously breathing
	  Flow rate 3 times minute ventilation
	• Non–spontaneously breathing
	  <10 kg: 2 L/min flow rate
	  0-15 kg: 3.5-4 L/min flow rate
	  >50 kg: 6 L/min flow rate	

PIP[25]	• ≤20-30 cm H_2O	
Ventilatory mask size[3]	• <6 months old: 0 • 6 months-3 years old: 1 • 3-6 years old: 2 • >6 years old: 3	Fit and placement on face same as for adult

*See Table 24-1 for adult settings.
PIP, Peak inspiratory pressure.

dence of accidental extubation uses two pieces of cloth tape, split halfway down the middle, creating a Y shape. Fig. 11-3 illustrates this technique. The skin of the child is more fragile than that of an adult. Cloth tape can be irritating. Duoderm can be applied to the cheeks, with the securing tape attached on top of the Duoderm, or a zinc oxide–based "pink tape" can be used.

Mechanical Ventilation. Numerous types of unconventional mechanical ventilation are used in the infant or child, such as inverse inspiratory:expiratory (I:E) ratio, high-frequency flow interruption, high-frequency positive pressure, high-frequency jet, high-frequency oscillation, and airway pressure release. For most infants and children, standard means of positive-pressure ventilatory support, using volume- or pressure-controlled ventilators, are used. The type of ventilation chosen depends on the child's size, minute ventilation requirements, and lung compliance. Several positive-pressure ventilators are available for the infant or small child, and adult ventilators can be made functional for the older child. A continuous-flow, time-limited ventilator in intermittent mandatory ventilation (IMV) mode is commonly used with an infant or toddler. Continuous flow offsets the infant's inability to generate enough negative pressure to open an inspiratory demand valve.[9]

For the older child, noncontinuous-flow, volume-limited ventilation in synchronized intermittent mandatory ventilation (SIMV) mode is used most often. Pressure support ventilation is also used in the child as the sole ventilatory mode if respiratory mechanics and work of breathing are stable, or to assist with spontaneous breathing, especially during the weaning process.[9] Table 11-4 outlines ventilator settings for initiating positive-pressure ventilation for the infant and child.[9]

Ventilator-patient asynchrony can arise from several causes. The Hering-Breuer reflex is a vagal reflex in which the child's sensing of positive lung inflation sets off immediate expiration, and lung deflation stimulates inspiration. Apnea, or active expiration during the ventilator's inspiratory cycle, also can cause asynchrony. The

Table 11-3	Approximate Sizes of Intubation Equipment and Tracheostomy Tubes for Infants and Children							
Age	3 mo	6 mo	1 yr	3 yr	6 yr	8 yr	12 yr	16 yr
Weight	6 kg	8 kg	10 kg	15 kg	20 kg	25 kg	40 kg	60 kg
ETT size (mm)*	3.0-3.5	3.5-4.0	4.0-4.5	4.5-5.0	5.0-5.5	6.0 c/u	7.0 c	7.0-8.0 c
Blade †	0-1 s	0-1 s	1 s	2 s	2 s	2 s/c	3 s/c	3 s/c
Stylet F	6	6	6	6	14	14	14	14
Suction catheter F (fr)‡	6-8	8	8	8-10	10	10-12	12-14	12-14
SHILEY TRACHEOSTOMY								
Shiley size (mm)	0	1	1-12	4	4	4	6	6
Internal diameter (mm ID)	3.4	3.7	3.7-4.1	5	5	5	7	7
Length (cm)	4	4.1	4.1-4.2	4.6	4.6	4.6	6.7	6.7

*Cuffed/uncuffed (c/u).
†Straight or curved (s/c).
‡Catheter size twice the internal diameter size of any tracheal tube.
F *(fr)*, French; *ID*, internal diameter.

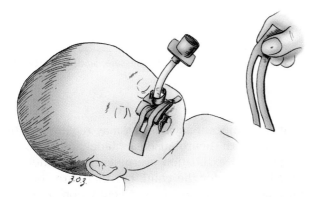
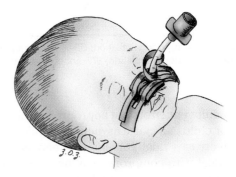

Fig. 11-3   Securing of endotracheal tube with split taping. (Modified from Zander J, Hazinski MF: Pulmonary disorders. In Hazinski MF, editor: *Nursing care of the critically ill child*, ed 2, St Louis, 1992, Mosby.)

Table 11-4	Initiating Positive-Pressure Ventilation in the Infant or Child	
Parameter	**Setting**	**Discussion Points**
Rate of Fio_2	Age-based to maintain Pao_2 >70 mm Hg	
Tidal volume	10-15 ml/kg	Includes compressibility of ventilator circuit tubing and dead space
I:E	Age-specific, usually 1:2	Increase expiratory time with obstruction disease
Inspiratory time	0.4-0.5 seconds	
PEEP or CPAP	Starts at 3 cm H_2O and increases by 2-3 cm increments	Maintain Pao_2 >70 mm Hg with nontoxic O_2 (0.40-0.50) without causing circulatory depression; PEEP >15 cm warrants a pulmonary artery catheter to measure circulatory status; volutrauma must be addressed with pneumothorax suspicions

I:E, Inspiratory: expiratory: *PEEP,* positive end-expiratory pressure; *CPAP,* constant positive airway pressure.

Table 11-5	Guidelines for Discontinuing Positive-Pressure Ventilation in the Infant or Child	
Weaning Ventilatory Mode	**Ventilatory Parameter**	**Discussion Points**

Non-PSV	• Rate: decrease by 2-5 breaths/min (may be 1 breath/min in chronic conditions)
	  Infant: down to minimum of 4 breaths/min
	  Child: possibly down to spontaneous breathing with CPAP trials
	• PEEP/CPAP: decrease by 2-3 cm H_2O
	  Infant: down to 2-3 cm H_2O
	  Child: down to <5 cm H_2O
		Rapidity of each change can be variable, from hourly to every couple of weeks; for infants, rates must not go fewer than 4 breaths/min just before extubation, since ETT creates airway resistance and the work of breathing may be increased too much with total spontaneous breathing[45,46]

PSV	• Fio_2: decrease by 5%-10%, to <0.40-5.0 • With SIMV: decrease rate first, down to CPAP • Pressure: to achieve tidal volume of 10-15 ml/kg; then decrease to 5 cm H_2O	To maintain Pao_2 >70 mm Hg or Sao_2 >93% See previous guidelines for rate and pressure changes

Extubation	• Vital capacity:
	  Infant/toddler: >15 ml/kg when crying[37]
	  Older child: >10-15 ml/kg
	• Negative inspiratory pressure:
	  Infant/toddler: >45 cm H_2O when crying[37]
	  Older child: >20-30 cm H_2O
	• Minute ventilation doubled
	• Pao_2 >60-70 mm Hg at an Fio_2 >0.4
	• $Paco_2$ 35-45 mm Hg
		Positive gag/cough reflex
		Can tolerate own secretions

PSV, Pressure support ventilation; *CPAP,* constant positive airway pressure; *PEEP,* positive end-expiratory pressure; *SIMV,* synchronized intermittent mandatory ventilation; *ETT,* endotracheal tube.

use of adult ventilators not appropriately adapted for the infant or child can cause asynchrony.[9] Because the small child decreases tidal volume and increases respiratory rate to deal with compromise, adult ventilators may not sense rapidly enough, if at all, these spontaneous respiratory efforts, which then lead to increased work of breathing.

Asynchrony can lead to poor oxygenation or volu-trauma. Significant asynchrony may require sedation or sedation with neuromuscular blockade. Criteria for weaning and extubation are much more extensive for the adult than for the child, but there are some guidelines. IMV or pressure support ventilation (PSV) is used to wean from positive-pressure ventilation. PSV allows the child to have greater control over breathing, and asynchrony is not a problem.[9] Table 11-5 outlines guidelines for weaning and extubation.[9] Supplemental oxygen must be supplied after extubation via nasal cannula, ventilation mask, or oxygen hood. Nasal or facial CPAP also can be given, but if the child fights this, it is best to remove it to minimize oxygen demands and prevent postextubation complications.

Extubation Complications. A postextubation croup can occur in the small child. Manifestations arising from airway edema include hoarseness, stridor, or a crowing cough that begins immediately or up to 3 hours after extubation. Initial treatment consists of keeping the child calm. Procedures must be withheld if possible and crying averted to avoid increasing airway resistance. Hold supplemental humidified oxygen at the child's mouth immediately after extubation, and continue to provide cool mist. More severe symptoms can be treated with racemic epinephrine and/or intravenous IV or inhaled steroid therapy. Intubation equipment and personnel qualified to intubate should be available for 4 hours after extubation.

TRACHEOSTOMIES

Several types of tracheostomy tubes are available for the child, with the plastic, single-cannula type the most popular for in-hospital care because they have few complications. Silastic tubes have been recommended for the infant and child because they are pliable and bend with tracheal movement. Uncuffed tubes are generally used for the infant and small child, allowing for a larger airway lumen. A snug fit is necessary with a tube size of 0.5 mm larger than an appropriately-sized ETT, because placement is below the cricoid ring. Cuffed tubes can be used with the older child. See Table 11-3 for tracheostomy tube sizes for the infant and child.

If accidental decannulation occurs in a new tracheostomy, pulling on the stay sutures allows for tube replacement in most instances. In the child who has had a long-term tracheostomy, usually for tracheal stenosis, reinserting a tracheal tube after accidental decannulation can be very difficult. Tracheomalacia with cricoid cartilage collapse can develop, resulting in upper airway obstruction once the tube is no longer in place. In some cases, an airway can be reestablished only surgically. In others, an ETT that is a size smaller can be inserted into the stoma; otherwise the child may have to be orally/nasally intubated.

VIRAL RESPIRATORY INFECTIONS

Viral respiratory infections are characterized with respect to time, person, and place. Many of the common viral respiratory infections exhibit predictable seasonality.[10] For example, influenza and respiratory syncytial virus (RSV) occur prominently in winter, whereas rhinoviruses are prominent in autumn and spring.[10] Many viruses are responsible for both mild and severe respiratory infections. Influenza produces the most severe illnesses in most age groups. RSV produces severe disease in the very young.

Pathophysiology. Viral respiratory infections often lead to bronchiolitis, an acute inflammatory disease of the lower small airways that may lead to obstruction.[11] It occurs in children younger than 2 years, most often in infants younger than 1 year, and is most severe in infants younger than 6 months. Many different viruses can cause bronchiolitis, but RSV is the major cause.[10] RSV occurs primarily from late fall to early spring. It is highly contagious and spread by direct close contact through droplets. The virus is shed for 3 to 8 days, but in young infants virus shedding can occur for up to 4 weeks.[12] The virus can exist on environmental surfaces for many hours and on the hands for at least 30 minutes, resulting in a high rate of nosocomial spread by hospital staff.[11] Reinfections occur frequently but are generally milder after infancy.

RSV has an overall low mortality, but infants with congenital heart disease have a mortality rate of 37%. Those with cystic fibrosis or bronchopulmonary dysplasia or who are immunocompromised are also at greater risk for more serious disease and for occurrence beyond 1 year of age. The chance of recovery from RSV can be excellent, but reactive airway disease is common for several years after infection.[13] RSV involves inflammation of respiratory epithelium, leading to necrosis. The epithelium is replaced with nonciliated tissue. Submucosal edema forms with lymphocytic infiltrates and other alveolar debris. Obstruction occurs from mucus secretions and debris not being cleared because of the lack of ciliated epithelium. Pathologic pulmonary dynamics involve lung hyperinflation almost two times normal. Obstruction occurs in a patchy distribution with complete obstruction, leading to atelectasis and partial obstruction, which results in hyperinflation. Inspiratory resistance and expiratory resistance are present, along with ventilation/perfusion mismatch, which lead to hypoxemia. Minute ventilation is increased significantly so that a normal $Paco_2$ can be maintained. Respiratory failure ensues with a rising $Paco_2$ (greater than 65 mm Hg).[14]

Clinical Assessment. The first symptoms to appear are those of an upper respiratory tract infection—sneezing and rhinorrhea. In many cases a family member has had a respiratory illness. After 2 to 3 days respiratory distress ensues, with increased respirations, coughing, nasal flaring, chest retractions, wheezing, irritability, and possible feeding difficulties. Fever and lung rhonchi may or may not occur. Once bronchiolar obstruction is evident, the illness is at its peak. Improvement is gradual, and by 2 weeks the infant usually has recovered.[14]

Treatment. The overall treatment goal in RSV is supportive. Because of the highly contagious nature of RSV, place the infant in contact isolation. Other infants with RSV, as well as staff caring for them, must be grouped together to prevent nosocomial spread of the infection.[13]

Oxygen continues to be the primary therapy[15] to decrease work of breathing and oxygen demands. Depending on the severity of illness, the infant can receive supplemental humidified oxygen via mask, tent, nasal CPAP (despite lung hyperinflation), or mechanical ventilation.[15] Inhaled β_2-agonists may be tried because of the expiratory resistance, but the beneficial effects can be variable.[16] Euvolemia must be maintained through careful use of diuretics and fluid restriction[15] because pulmonary edema can occur from greater negative intrapulmonary pressures or from fluid leaks with epithelial necrosis. Administration of an antiviral agent, ribavirin, is controversial.[17] It possibly has greater effect in the mechanically ventilated infant.[18] It is a broad-spectrum, aerosolized agent that can be administered over a 6-hour period.[19] When given to the mechanically ventilated infant, ribavirin crystallizes in ventilator and endotracheal tubes, necessitating meticulous attention to frequent ventilator tubing changes and ETT assessments for obstruction.

In addition, the teratogenicity of ribavirin in humans has been questioned, although no effects have been reported in humans after 7 years of usage. The drug can be absorbed through the respiratory tract from the environment, as it is released from respirator equipment, or from the infant's secretions. The infant needs to be in contact isolation only because of the RSV, not because of the exposure to ribavirin. Standard surgical masks, gloves, or gowns provide no protection from the ribavirin. Caution must still be exercised, and pregnant staff must not provide care. Because ribavirin causes crystallization of particles, contact lenses can be damaged; however, close-fitting goggles can be worn. All staff and visitors need to be warned of the possible hazards of ribavirin. The infant can be placed with other infants receiving ribavirin; placement must be in a well-ventilated room with at least six air changes/hour.[11]

Currently, there are two methods of preventing RSV infection in children that are high risk for developing severe infections. RSV-IGIV (Respigam) was approved by the FDA for prevention of severe RSV in children less than 24 months of age with chronic lung disease or premature birth (35 weeks gestation). RSV-IGIV consists of mostly immunoglobulin G and trace amounts of immunoglobulin A and M.[10] Palivizumab (Synagis 7) is a monoclonal antibody that is used to prevent serious lower respiratory tract disease caused by RSV in high-risk pediatric patients. High-risk patients are those who are premature or who have chronic lung disease or congenital heart disease.[20] Researchers have found that in infants less than 35 weeks' gestation, only 2.3% required hospitalization and only 0.5% required intensive care unit (ICU) admission. Palivizumab is administered monthly during the RSV season, with an average of five to six doses.[20]

STATUS ASTHMATICUS

Pathophysiology. Asthma is a state of diffuse, reversible airflow obstruction that results from inflammation and edema, bronchoconstriction, and increased mucus secretion. Status asthmaticus is moderate to severe airflow obstruction that is refractory to intensive treatment with bronchodilators.[21] Clinical findings in status asthmaticus demonstrate lung hyperinflation and air trapping, increased minute ventilation and ventilation/perfusion mismatch with hypoxemia and hypercapnia, metabolic and respiratory acidosis, right and left ventricular strain from increased pulmonary vascular resistance, and increased cardiac workload to maintain an elevated cardiac output in the face of increased afterload.[15,21,22] Risk factors for a life-threatening event include wide fluctuations in peak expiratory flow rate (PEFR), an increase $\leq 10\%$ in PEFR or forced expiratory volume over 1 second (FEV_1) over emergency room measurement, a PEFR or FEV_1 of $\leq 25\%$ of predicted value for age, a $Paco_2$ ≥ 40 mm Hg, and an age of 1 year or younger.[23]

Clinical Assessment. Assessing severe asthma in the infant is different as compared to the older child because of the anatomic and physiologic differences between them. Physiologic changes can progress rapidly to respiratory failure in the infant. Table 11-6 outlines guidelines for assessing severe asthma in infants and children.[22]

Treatment. Optimal treatment is based on three components: environmental control, pharmacologic therapy, and patient education. There is a strong relationship between allergy and asthma; therefore, steps are taken to reduce exposure to allergens. Some examples of environmental triggers are tobacco smoke, dust mites, animal dander, and indoor mold.

Pharmacologic therapy is based on the concept that asthma is chronic inflammation. A short acting bronchodilator should always be available. The first-line controller for children of all ages is an inhaled corticosteroid. For children with moderate persistent asthma, a long-acting bronchodilator and an inhaled corticosteroid are used. Children with severe persistent asthma are placed on a long-acting bronchodilator and a high-dose corticosteroid. Intensive care management of the child with status asthmaticus involves humidified oxygen to maintain an oxygen saturation of more than 95%, continuously nebulized selective β_2-agonists, IV methylprednisolone, IV aminophylline, and possibly IV terbutaline.[23] If $Paco_2$ is more than 55 mm Hg or increasing more than 5 to 10 mm Hg/hour, if pulsus paradoxus is more than 30 mm Hg, or if acidosis or continual hypoxemia occurs, mechanical ventilation must be considered. Chest percussion and vibration are contraindicated in status asthmaticus and are not useful for the patient recovering from severe asthma.[23,24] Minimizing the child's anxiety is crucial. Sedating medications must be used very cau-

Table 11-6	Guidelines for Assessing Severe Asthma in Infants and Children		
Assessment Area	Physical Findings		Discussion Points
	Infant	Child	
Respiratory rate	Increase of >50% above normal	Can range from normal to >95 percentile for age	Sleeping rates in infants and resting rates in children are good measures of obstruction; awake or activity rates are too variable
Level of consciousness	Decreased	May be decreased	Assess response to parents and pain
Accessory muscle use	Retractions in less-than-severe states	Severe intercostal, tracheosternal, and sternocleidomastoid retractions and nasal flaring	In infants, compliant chest wall produces retractions earlier in course
			In children, retractions and flaring correlate well with degree of obstruction and with PEFR of <50% of predicted for age
Color	Pallor, grayness, or cyanosis	Possible cyanosis	
Dyspnea		Can speak only single words or short phrases; cannot count to 10 in one breath	
Quality of cry	Softer and shorter as FEV_1 decreases		
O_2 saturation	<90% in less-than-severe states	<90% on room air	Infants have greater ventilation-perfusion mismatch
			In children, hypoxemia correlates well with degree of obstruction
Breath sounds	Wheezing; then becoming inaudible because of decreased air movement	Same as in infant	Presence and volume of wheezing is the least-sensitive predictor of obstruction
$Paco_2$	If >50 mm Hg or if rising 5-10 mm Hg/hr, consider mechanical ventilation	Can range from <40 mm Hg with respiratory distress to >40 mm Hg as air movement significantly decreases	$Paco_2$ is best measure of ventilation in infants.
			A continually rising $Paco_2$ of >40 mm Hg in a child occurs when PEFR is <20% of predicted for age
PEFR		<50% of predicted for age or personal best	Best objective measure of obstruction; used in children >5 years of age; requires cooperation
Feeding/sucking ability	Decreased or absent		

PEFR, Peak respiratory flow rate; *FEV₁,* formed expiratory volume over 1 second.

tiously in the nonintubated child. Environmental measures to promote comfort, decrease noxious stimuli, and enhance personal security (e.g., presence of parents) must be used (see "The Ill Child's Experience of Critical Illness," p. 201).

APNEA

Pathophysiology. Apnea occurs most often in the preterm infant and is a function of immaturity, but it can occur in older infants as well. Pathologic apnea in the full-term infant is defined as ineffective or absent respirations for more than 16 seconds, with or without hypotonia, cyanosis, or bradycardia.[25] This is to be differentiated from periodic or disorganized breathing. These conditions have shorter periods of apnea, interspersed with rapid or irregular breathing. Some periodic breathing can be normal at any age.[25] Three types of apnea exist: central, obstructive, and mixed.[26]

Central apnea involves failure of the respiratory centers in the brain to stimulate ventilation. Obstructive apnea involves a blocked airway; however, respiratory efforts can still be made but they do not generate adequate gas exchange. Mixed apnea has both central and obstructive components and accounts for about 50% of cases.[26]

Aside from congenital etiologies, apnea may be a symptom of many reversible disorders.[26] Central apnea can occur with sepsis, electrolyte disorders, hypoglycemia, and hypothermia; cardiorespiratory disease involving hypoxemia or respiratory muscle fatigue; or central nervous system (CNS) infections, seizures, hydrocephalus, or conditions related to increased ICP. Obstructive apnea can occur with tonsil and adenoid hypertrophy, abnormally large tongues, abnormally small mandibles, and vascular rings; after surgical correction for cleft palate; and with other forms of airway obstruction.[26]

Apnea may appear as an apparent life-threatening event (ALTE), which used to be referred to as *near-miss SIDS* (sudden infant death syndrome). ALTE is defined as an event that was frightening to the observer, coupled with an assumption that death would have occurred without intensive intervention. For instance, the child displayed some combination of apnea, color change, marked change in muscle tone, and/or choking or gagging.[23]

Monitoring. An episode of secondary central apnea can result from hospital procedures such as suctioning or stimulating the larynx, passage of a nasogastric (NG) tube, after lung hyperinflation, or with feedings. Obstructive apnea can be brought on with neck flexion, pressure beneath the chin or on the lower rim of an applied face mask, or with supine positioning. A ventilation bag and a mask should be at the bedside. Because ineffective respiratory efforts may be sensed as normal respirations, cardiac and/or pulse oximetry monitoring should be in place.

Treatment. Episodes of apnea must first be treated with gentle shaking of the infant or tapping the bottoms of the infant's feet while observing for return of effective respirations. Slight extension of the neck to reopen the airway can be attempted. If recovery does not occur, manual ventilation with bag and mask at the infant's normal respiratory rate for age should be performed at the fractional inspired oxygen concentration (FiO_2) level the infant was previously receiving. This manual ventilation should continue until normal respiratory pattern and heart rate return. For frequent episodes (more than two to three per hour) or for those who require prolonged manual ventilation, other treatments include prone positioning, rocker beds, recurrent cutaneous stimulation, nasal CPAP (for mixed or obstructive apneas only), or a switch to continuous gavage feedings. Surgery may be necessary for obstructive apnea, or CNS respiratory stimulants may be used when no other correctable cause of apnea exists. Ultimately, mechanical ventilation may be needed. If there is no correctable cause, home monitoring may be necessary until the infant matures.

CARDIOVASCULAR SYSTEM

ANATOMY AND PHYSIOLOGY

The differences in cardiovascular function between children and adults are related to early physical development and the presence or absence of congenital cardiac disease. Congenital heart defects (CHDs) occur during the embryologic development of the heart, whereas acquired defects occur after birth. Some cases of CHDs are caused by single gene or chromosomal abnormalities, and others are the result of exposure to teratogens such as the rubella virus, but in most cases the cause is unknown.[27] The heart develops from the third to eighth week of gestation, so development is complete before the woman may definitely know that she is pregnant.

The design of fetal circulation allows prenatal needs to be met as well as permits the modifications at birth that support the postnatal circulation.[27] Before the child is born, the lungs are essentially nonfunctional, the liver is partially functional, and the brain requires the highest oxygen concentration. The structures that support fetal circulation and bypass the lungs and liver are the foramen ovale, ductus arteriosus, ductus venosus, the umbilical arteries, and the umbilical vein (Fig. 11-4). After the child is born, the lungs and liver begin normal function, so the structures of fetal circulation are no longer needed. The foramen ovale closes, and the ductus arteriosus, the ductus venosus, and the umbilical vessels become ligaments (Fig.11-5). During fetal life, the patency of the ductus arteriosus is controlled by the low oxygen content and exogenous prostaglandins.[27] Thus postnatally, hypoxia maintains patency of the ductus arteriosus. Before repair of some congenital defects, it is essential that the ductus arteriosus remain open so that the newborn receives a pulmonary vasculature vasodilator, such as prostaglandin E_1 (PGE_1) continuous IV drip. At birth, pulmonary resistance is high but quickly falls to adult levels in the first few weeks of life. In newborns, hypoxia, acidosis, and hypothermia may result in pulmonary vasoconstriction. This can lead to right-to-left (pulmonary-to-systemic) shunting of blood through the ductus arteriosus and foramen ovale. Treatment includes oxygenation, mechanical ventilation with hyperventilation to produce alkalosis, sedation, and keeping the newborn warm.

ASSESSMENT

Assessment of the cardiovascular (CV) system in the child includes the complete health history, including birth history and physical assessment. As the pediatric data base is completed for the child with cardiac disease, the parents may report any of the following: poor feeding with fatigue noted during feeding, diaphoresis with feeding, weight loss or inability to gain weight, respiratory problems such as dyspnea or tachypnea, frequent respiratory infections, cyanosis, and fatigue during play. Heart rate and blood pressure (BP) should be within normal range for age (Tables 11-7 and 11-8). Auscultate the heart for extra heart sounds and murmurs. Physiologic splitting of the second heart sound (S_2) is usually more pronounced in the pediatric patient. A widely fixed split S_2 is heard in children who have a secundum atrial septal defect. Sinus dysrhythmia is normal

in the child, particularly during rest or sleep. To monitor perfusion, pedal pulses and capillary refill are evaluated hourly. Urine output must be at least 1 ml/kg/hr.

HEMODYNAMIC MONITORING

Hemodynamic monitoring may be indicated in the critically ill pediatric patient. Issues in monitoring are related to the smaller size of the pediatric patient; fluid

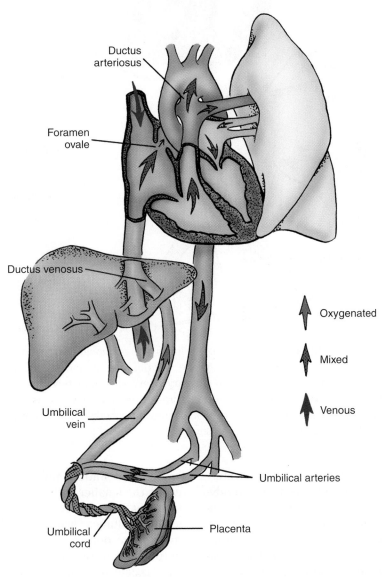

Fig. 11-4   Fetal circulation. Fetal blood is oxygenated in the placenta (which is a less-efficient oxygenator than the lungs). The oxygenated blood enters the fetus through the umbilical vein and enters the ductus venosus, bypassing the hepatic circulation and flowing into the inferior vena cava. When this blood reaches the right atrium, it is diverted by the crista dividens toward the atrial septum and flows through the foramen ovale into the left atrium. The blood then passes through the left ventricle and ascending aorta to perfuse the head and upper extremities. This pathway allows the best-oxygenated blood from the placenta to perfuse the fetal brain. Venous blood from the head and upper extremities returns to the fetal heart through the superior vena cava, enters the right atrium and ventricle, and flows into the pulmonary artery. Because pulmonary vascular resistance is high, this blood is diverted through the ductus arteriosus into the descending aorta. Ultimately, much of this blood will return to the placenta through the umbilical arteries. (Modified from Hazinski MF: *Nursing care of the critically ill child,* ed 2, St Louis, 1992, Mosby.)

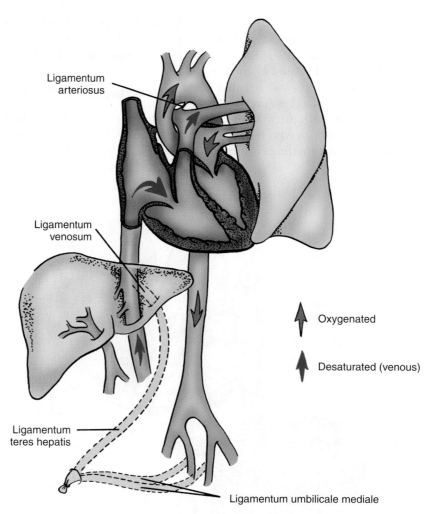

Ligamentum
arteriosus

Ligamentum
venosum

Ligamentum
teres hepatis

Ligamentum umbilicale mediale

Oxygenated

Desaturated (venous)

Fig. 11-5   Postnatal circulation. Blood is oxygenated in the lungs, and pulmonary vascular resistance is low. Systemic venous (desaturated) blood returns to the heart through the superior and inferior vena cavae. This blood then flows through the right atrium and right ventricle, into the pulmonary artery, and ultimately into the pulmonary circulation. Oxygenated blood from the lungs returns to the left atrium through the pulmonary veins. This blood passes into the left ventricle and flows into the aorta and systemic arteries to perfuse the body. (Modified from Hazinski MF: *Nursing care of the critically ill child,* ed 2, St Louis, 1992, Mosby.)

overload and blood loss are concerns. To accurately monitor intake, all fluid used for intravascular hemodynamic monitoring lines must be given by volume infusion pumps. Heparinized fluid is given in each line and only small volumes of blood are drawn for laboratory tests. Each medical facility that cares for pediatric patients has policies for how much blood to draw for each test. All flush volumes are recorded as intake, an accurate record is kept of the amount of blood lost, and periodically the child receives replacement. See Table 11-9 for pediatric blood volumes.

When continuously monitoring the blood pressure in the child, the arterial reading is considered more accurate than the cuff pressure. Korotkoff sounds are more difficult to hear when the BP is low. A size 4 or 5 French (Fr) pulmonary artery catheter is used for the child. The child's vessel must be large enough to accept the 4 Fr

catheter to initiate pulmonary artery monitoring. Because the smaller catheters have smaller balloons, refer to the catheter for balloon volume. To limit fluid intake, smaller volumes (usually 3 or 5 ml) of injectant are used for cardiac output studies. See Table 11-10 for cardiac output and stroke volume values. Left atrial pressure (LAP), central venous pressure (CVP), and pulmonary artery pressure (PAP) in the child are comparable with adult values. Hemodynamic parameters are related to the body surface area of the child. The normal cardiac index for children is 3.5 to 5.5 L/min/m^2, which is higher than that of adults. The right ventricular stroke work index of 5 to 7 g/m^2 is slightly less than the adult value.[28] When evaluating hemodynamic parameters, always relate the numbers to the clinical condition of the child. If the numbers do not correlate, revaluate calibration and zeroing of the monitoring equipment.

Table 11-7	Normal Heart Rates in Children	
Age	Awake Heart Rate (per minute)	Sleeping Heart Rate (per minute)
Neonate	100-180	80-160
Infant (6 mo)	100-160	75-160
Toddler	80-110	60-90
Preschooler	70-110	60-90
School-age child	65-110	60-90
Adolescent	60-90	50-90

From Hazinski MF: *Nursing care of the critically ill child,* ed 2, St Louis, 1992, Mosby.

Table 11-8	Normal Blood Pressures in Children*	
Age	Systolic Pressure (mm Hg)	Diastolic Pressure (mm Hg)
Birth (12 hr, <1000 g)	39-59	16-36
Birth (12 hours, 3 kg)	50-70	25-45
Neonate (96 hr)	60-90	20-60
Infant (6 mo)	87-105	53-66
Toddler (2 yr)	95-105	53-66
School age (7 yr)	97-112	57-71
Adolescent (15 yr)	112-128	66-80

From Hazinski MF: *Nursing care of the critically ill child,* ed 2, St Louis, 1992, Mosby.
*Blood pressure ranges taken from the following sources: **Neonate:** Versmold H et al: Aortic blood pressure during the first 12 hours of life in infants with birth weight 610-4220 g, *Pediatrics* 67:107, 1981. Tenth-ninetieth percentile ranges used. **Others:** Horan MJ, chairman: Task Force on Blood Pressure Control in Children, report of the Second Task Force on Blood Pressure in Children, *Pediatrics* 79:1, 1987. Fiftieth-ninetieth percentile ranges indicated.

CONGENITAL HEART DEFECTS

Some CHDs can be diagnosed by ultrasound before birth, and some parents decide to deliver these babies at a tertiary center affiliated with a pediatric cardiac surgery program. Other newborns with cardiac anomalies are diagnosed after birth and transferred to tertiary care centers for further evaluation and, often, immediate surgery. Certain defects are completely repaired in the first few days of life, other defects are repaired in stages, and some are repaired once the child is older. Infants with CHDs may develop complications after discharge after a surgical procedure or while waiting for surgery, and may be admitted to an adult critical care unit. Examples of

Table 11-9	Calculation of Circulating Blood Volume
Age	Blood Volume (ml/kg)
Neonates	85-90
Infants	75-80
Children	70-75
Adults	65-70

From Hazinski MF: *Nursing care of the critically ill child,* ed 2, St Louis, 1992, Mosby.

Table 11-10	Normal Pediatric Cardiac Output and Stroke Volume		
Age	Cardiac Output (L/min)	Heart Rate	Normal Stroke Volume
Newborn	0.8-1.0	145	5 ml
6 mo	1.0-1.3	120	10 ml
1 yr	1.3-1.5	115	13 ml
2 yr	1.5-2.0	115	18 ml
4 yr	2.3-2.75	105	27 ml
5 yr	2.5-3.0	95	31 ml
8 yr	3.4-3.6	83	42 ml
10 yr	3.8-4.0	75	50 ml
15 yr	6.0	70	85 ml

From Hazinski MF: *Nursing care of the critically ill child,* ed 2, St Louis, 1992, Mosby.

postoperative surgical complications in the pediatric cardiac patient are wound infection, pericardial effusion, pleural effusion, and dysrhythmia.

In the past, congenital heart defects were classified as cyanotic or acyanotic defects. In reality, though, children with acyanotic defects may develop cyanosis. Distinguishing the anomalies by hemodynamic pathophysiology is a more accurate method of classification. There are four defining pathophysiologic characteristics[29] (Fig. 11-6):

1. Increased pulmonary blood flow.
2. Decreased pulmonary blood flow.
3. Mixed blood flow.
4. Obstruction of flow of blood out of the heart.

At birth, pulmonary vascular resistance is high but decreases after the first few weeks of life. If a left-to-right (systemic-to-pulmonary) shunt is present, pulmonary blood flow increases and the child may develop congestive heart failure (CHF). Decreased pulmonary flow occurs when blood flow is obstructed from the right side of the heart to the pulmonary circulation or in the presence of a right-to-left (pulmonary-to-systemic) shunt. Mixed

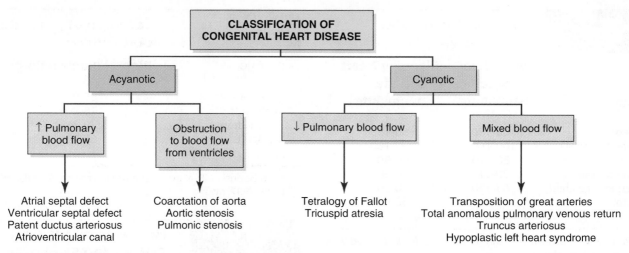

Fig. 11-6 Comparison of acyanotic-cyanotic and hemodynamic classification systems of congenital heart disease. (From Wong D et al: *Whaley and Wong's nursing care of infants and children*, ed 6, St Louis, 1999, Mosby.)

blood flow results from the mixing of oxygenated and deoxygenated blood. Obstruction of blood flow to the ventricles occurs with stenotic semilunar valves or a narrowed aorta. When caring for a child with surgical repair of cardiac defects, the nurse must know the actual circulation of blood (e.g., has a palliative procedure been done, has total correction been done, or will this patient require additional stages of repair in the future). Complications of CHD include CHF, hypoxemia, dysrhythmias, endocarditis, shock, and cardiac arrest. Any of these complications may result in the admission of the child to the critical care unit.

Heart Failure

Heart failure (HF) may occur in children with CHD, after surgical repair of congenital defects, and in severe anemia.[30-31] Classifications and pathophysiology of HF are similar to those of the adult patient. Symptoms of HF are related to the pathophysiologic processes of left and right ventricular failure and high and low output failure (see Chapter 18). Children usually exhibit manifestations of both right- and left-sided failure rather than one or the other.[28] The infant exhibits a change in responsiveness and may be lethargic or irritable. Respiratory distress is present with dyspnea; tachypnea; intercostal, substernal, sternal, or supraclavicular retractions; nasal flaring; or grunting. Grunting occurs during expiration when the infant breathes against a closed glottis to maintain positive end-expiratory pressure. Crackles may be auscultated in the infant.[28] During abdominal assessment, the liver may be palpated and is usually full and low in the infant with HF. In children younger than 5 years, the liver is normally palpated at the costal margin to 1 cm below. With decreased cardiac output and perfusion, the infant's extremities are cool, pedal pulses are weak, capillary refill is slow, skin is mottled, and blood

pressure is decreased. The infant is easily fatigued, feeds poorly, and may become dehydrated. Infants usually do not have fluid or sodium restrictions.

Digoxin is the inotropic drug of choice for HF.[31] The dosage is ordered in micrograms and is double-checked for accuracy. When the child is receiving digoxin, observe for signs of digitalis toxicity and periodically monitor the child's digoxin level. Cardiac dysrhythmias may indicate toxicity. Bradycardia is most common, but any dysrhythmia may be noted.[28,31] Inotropic agents, vasodilators, and/or diuretics may be ordered. Serum potassium levels are closely monitored with diuretic therapy.

Hypoxemia

Cyanosis is present in children with certain congenital heart defects. Cyanosis is visible when there is 5 g of reduced hemoglobin per 100 ml of blood[28,32] and the arterial oxygen saturation is at or less than 75% to 85%.[28] Hypoxemia may be caused by respiratory or cardiac disease. Cyanosis that decreases with crying is thought to be respiratory in origin, whereas cyanosis that increases with crying is usually cardiac in origin.[28] Some children with CHD manifest hypercyanotic spells. This is most common in children with tetralogy of Fallot, and these episodes often are called "Tet spells." During these episodes the child becomes very cyanotic, hypoxic, and tachypneic and may lose consciousness or develop seizures. These spells are dangerous because the child may develop severe hypoxemia and possible cerebral hypoxia; cerebral vascular accidents or death may occur during these episodes.[32] Treatment of hypercyanotic spells includes soothing the child while placing him or her in a knee-chest position and administering oxygen and physician-ordered morphine and fluid boluses. This child may need intubation, mechanical ventilation, and treatment of metabolic acidosis.

DYSRHYTHMIAS

Electrophysiology and electrocardiography principles are similar in the adult and pediatric patients (see Chapters 15 and 17). Differences include a faster heart rate in children and the variances in the PR and QT intervals related to the rapid heart rate. See Table 11-7 for normal pediatric heart rates. At birth the right ventricle is thicker than the left ventricle. Right ventricular dominance of the newborn period is replaced by left ventricular dominance in childhood and in adulthood. Anatomic changes are most rapid in the first month, and by 6 months of age the left ventricle is dominant. With increasing age the heart rate decreases and the PR interval, QRS duration, and QT interval increase.[33]

In the pediatric patient, monitoring of respiratory rate and oxygen saturation is done concurrently with cardiac monitoring. It is important to recognize the manifestations of impending respiratory failure in the pediatric patient, since respiratory failure precedes cardiac failure and potential cardiac arrest. Electrocardiogram (ECG) monitoring electrodes are placed along the nipple line on the chest to facilitate monitoring the cardiac rate and rhythm and the respiratory rate. Refer to the instructions for pediatric monitoring provided with the monitoring equipment.

Dysrhythmias are common in the child with underlying rhythm abnormalities and CHD and may occur in children with metabolic disorders. Other conditions that may cause dysrhythmias are abnormal potassium or calcium levels, hypoxia, acidosis, and hypothermia. A decrease in heart rate is an ominous sign in the pediatric patient. Asystole is the most common cardiac arrest rhythm, and bradycardia is the second most common cardiac arrest–associated rhythm.[3] Ventricular fibrillation and pulseless ventricular tachycardia are uncommon pediatric rhythms.[3]

Supraventricular Tachycardia. The most common symptomatic tachydysrhythmia in children is supraventricular tachycardia (SVT). P waves may or may not be seen, and the rate often exceeds 220 beats/min. Wide QRS supraventricular tachycardia is relatively rare in children, so any wide QRS tachycardia must be treated as ventricular in origin until proved otherwise.[1] If the child in SVT is unstable and shows signs of decreased cardiac output, direct current (DC) cardioversion is indicated.[34] The initial energy dose is 0.5 joules (J)/kg, and if the tachydysrhythmia persists, the dose is doubled.[3] In the stable child, procedures may include eliciting the diving reflex and other vagal maneuvers, pharmacologic therapy, and overdrive pacing. The drug of choice is adenosine.[35] The dose is 0.1 mg/kg rapid IV push and may be increased by 0.05 mg/kg increments every 2 minutes to a maximum of 0.25 mg/kg up to 12 mg or until termination of SVT.[35] Rapid IV push is essential because of the drug's half-life of 10 seconds.[9] IV verapamil is not recommended for young children because it has been associated with severe hypotension and cardiac arrest in infants younger than 1 year.[28,35]

Bradycardias. Bradycardias are the most common dysrhythmias in the pediatric patient and can result from hypoxia, acidosis, and/or hypothermia. Bradycardia is defined as a cardiac rate less than the low limit for age. Bradydysrhythmias include sinus node dysfunction, heart block, and effects from pharmacologic therapy. Treatment includes adequate oxygenation, epinephrine, atropine, transthoracic pacing, and chest compressions.[3] To initiate transthoracic pacing, adult electrodes are used if the child weighs more than 15 kg; if the child weighs less than 15 kg, use the small or medium pediatric electrodes. The child may require sedation, intubation, and mechanical ventilation for successful transcutaneous pacing. The procedure results in mild to moderate discomfort, and it is seldom possible in the unsedated child. The pacing pads cover a large area of the child's chest as compared with the adult's. Pad placement is the same as with the adult unless the child has dextrocardia. The condition of the skin is closely monitored.

BACTERIAL ENDOCARDITIS

Bacterial endocarditis may occur in children with CHD but, as in adults, may also occur in children with no history of cardiac disease. The most common causative organisms are *Streptococcus* and *Staphylococcus*; rarely is the organism fungal. Manifestations in children are myalgias, arthralgias, headache, general malaise, fever, or the occurrence of an embolic event.[36] Most patients have a positive blood culture. It is essential to recognize bacterial endocarditis in children, since the risk of death is great if antibiotics are not started early in the infective process. Antibiotic treatment usually lasts at least 6 weeks, and children usually stay in the hospital for treatment.

SHOCK IN INFANTS AND CHILDREN

Shock is classified as hypovolemic, cardiogenic, or distributive. Septic shock is the classification of distributive shock most common in children.

Hypovolemic Shock. Hypovolemic shock may occur from severe vomiting or diarrhea and the resultant fluid loss, or from blood loss caused by trauma or other bleeding problems. Treatment of hypovolemic shock is volume replacement. Albumin or other colloids may be given at 10 to 20 ml/kg.[31] Packed red cells are given for blood loss, starting with 10 ml/kg. Isotonic crystalloids (normal saline/Ringer's lactate) may be given initially in doses of 10 to 20 ml/kg rapidly by IV route. Crystalloids rapidly diffuse into the interstitial space, so only minimal volume is available in the intravascular space to increase circulating volume. The child must be closely monitored for tissue perfusion.

Cardiogenic Shock. Cardiogenic shock results from pump failure in congenital cardiac disease. The child develops tachycardia as a mechanism to increase cardiac output. Children have small stroke volumes, so increasing the heart rate increases cardiac output. The child will have decreased urine output (less than 0.5 to 1 ml/kg/hr), gain weight, and retain fluid. Crackles may be heard on lung auscultation, and frothy sputum may be present. Intubation and mechanical ventilation may be required. IV fluids may be given to optimize left ventricular end-diastolic pressure unless CVP or pulmonary artery occlusion pressure (PAOP) is elevated. If fluid overload is present, inotropic support is provided. Vasodilators may also be required. These vasoactive medications are usually prepared using the rule of sixes (Box 11-2) and are infused in mcg/kg/min in the pediatric patient. It is recommended that these drugs be infused through a central line.[3] A multilumen CVP catheter is often inserted to administer vasopressors, fluids, and other medications.

Sepsis/Septic Shock. "Rule out sepsis" may be an admitting diagnosis for the pediatric patient. Infants and very young children are at particular risk for developing sepsis or septic shock. This risk is increased when the patient has invasive monitoring lines, undergoes diagnostic testing, or has surgery. The child exhibits manifestations of systemic inflammatory response syndrome (SIRS) or severe sepsis or septic shock. Instead of temperature elevation, the infant or child may have a low temperature or temperature instability. Level of consciousness changes, and the child may be irritable, restless, or lethargic. Urine output is decreased, the skin may be warm or mottled, and peripheral pulses may be strong and bounding. The child does not feed well, and decreased fluid intake may precipitate dehydration. Blood pressure is maintained within normal limits from activation of the body's compensatory mechanisms. Parents may remark that the child "does not seem right" or "something is different" with the child. Always listen to the parents' assessment of the child's status.

Treatment of SIRS includes administration of oxygen, fluids, and antibiotics, but the most effective treatment of SIRS is prevention. Hand washing before and after patient contact is essential. Sterile technique is maintained during suctioning, while managing invasive lines, and during dressing changes and wound care.

Severe sepsis or septic shock is diagnosed when perfusion decreases and the child becomes hypotensive. If the child is receiving inotropics, the BP may be normal but there is a change in perfusion. The patient exhibits metabolic acidosis and hypoxemia, requiring intubation, mechanical ventilation, sedation, fluids, and vasopressor medications. Complications of septic shock include acute respiratory distress syndrome, acute renal failure, disseminated intravascular coagulation, and multiple organ dysfunction syndrome (MODS).

CARDIOPULMONARY ARREST

The pediatric patient must be assessed for manifestations of respiratory failure and sepsis because failure to recognize these problems may result in the development of cardiopulmonary failure and respiratory or cardiac arrest. In the pediatric patient, respiratory arrest usually precedes cardiac arrest. In an arrest situation, oxygen is administered and an airway established and maintained (see "Assessment and Oxygen Devices," p. 178). For a cardiac arrest, compressions are started and an IV or intraosseous (IO) line established. Intraosseous placement is recommended as an alternative means to deliver intravenous fluids and medications in children under 6 years of age when vascular access is not obtained within 90 seconds or three attempts. The preferred site is the broad, flat portion of the anteromedial surface of the tibia approximately 1 to 2 cm below the tibial tuberosity. Other interventions are based on the cardiac rhythm and cause of the arrest.

Pulseless arrest includes asystole, ventricular fibrillation, pulseless ventricular tachycardia, and electromechanical dissociation (EMD).[3] Treatment of asystole includes cardiopulmonary resuscitation (CPR), airway maintenance with oxygenation, and an IV or IO access. Epinephrine is the drug of choice. The first dose of epinephrine is 0.01 mg/kg (1:10,000, 0.1 ml/kg) given IV or IO; or, if given endotracheally (ET), the dose is 0.1 mg/kg (1:1,000, 0.1 ml/kg). The second dose, given IV, IO, or ET, is 0.1 mg/kg (1:1,000, 0.1 ml/kg). Subsequent doses may be given IV or IO in a dose up to 0.2 mg/kg. It is important

---

Box 11-2

RULE OF SIXES FOR PREPARING VARIABLE CONCENTRATIONS OF VASOACTIVE DRUGS

I. For drugs infused in doses of mcg/kg/min (or multiples):
  A. Multiply weight (in kilograms) by 6; place this number of milligrams of drug in solution *totaling* 100 ml
  B. Then 1 ml/hr delivers 1 mcg/kg/min
II. For drugs infused in doses of 0.1 mcg/kg/min (or multiples):
  A. Multiply weight (in kilograms) by 0.6; place this number of milligrams of drug in solution *totaling* 100 ml
  B. Then 1 ml/hr delivers 0.1 mcg/kg/min
III. For any concentration of a drug:

$$\text{Rate (ml/hr)} = \frac{\text{weight (kg)} \times \text{dose (mcg/kg/min)} \times 60 \text{ min/hr}}{\text{concentration (mcg/ml)}}$$

Modified from Hazinski, MF: *Nursing care of the critically ill child,* ed 2, St Louis, 1992, Mosby.

to note that the volume of epinephrine administered is 0.1 ml/kg whether conventional or high-dose epinephrine is given. The dose of epinephrine is determined by the concentration of the drug (1:10,000 vs. 1:1,000).[3]

Acidosis during resuscitation is corrected by effective ventilation and systemic perfusion. Sodium bicarbonate is considered only for documented severe acidosis associated with prolonged cardiac arrest, unstable hemodynamic state, hyperkalemia, or tricyclic antidepressant overdose. It is uncertain whether atropine is useful in the treatment of asystole; clinical studies have failed to document its efficacy. A vagolytic dose (0.2 mg/kg and a minimum dose of 0.1 mg/kg) may be given. A dose smaller than the minimum dose may produce paradoxic bradycardia.[3] Defibrillation is not indicated for the treatment of asystole in the child. If EMD results in pulseless electrical activity, the cause should be determined; the treatment is the same as for asystole.

For ventricular fibrillation or pulseless ventricular tachycardia, electrical defibrillation (2 J/kg) is the treatment of choice. Defibrillate up to three times if needed (2 J/kg, 4 J/kg, 4 J/kg). If defibrillation is unsuccessful, epinephrine is given, and lidocaine (1 mg/kg) is helpful in preventing the recurrence of ventricular fibrillation.[3] Bretylium may also be used.

Bradydysrhythmias including sinus bradycardia, sinus node arrest with a slow junctional or ventricular escape rhythm, and various degrees of atrioventricular (AV) blocks are the most common terminal rhythms in children.[3] Hypoxemia, hypotension, and acidosis interfere with sinus node function and conduction of the cardiac impulse. CPR is required in the child if the heart rate is less than 60 bpm and is associated with poor systemic perfusion. Vascular access is started, either IV or IO. Epinephrine is given, as it is for pulseless arrest. Atropine may be given, and cardiac pacing may be indicated.

After arrest, the goals are to restore adequate blood pressure and effective perfusion and to correct hypoxia and acidosis. The inotropic agents *dopamine, dobutamine,* and *epinephrine* are used, but in the pediatric patient, epinephrine is the drug of choice.[3]

One other product that may be useful in pediatric arrest is the Broselow Pediatric Resuscitation Tape. This tape is color coded for each pediatric age-group and provides resuscitation information based on the length and estimated weight of the child.[37]

NERVOUS SYSTEM

ANATOMY

The nervous system grows rapidly before birth, and growth continues during infancy and childhood. In comparison with the adult, the infant/toddler's head size is proportionally larger than the rest of the body. The skull is more flexible because the skull bones are not fused

and are separated by spaces called *fontanelles.* The anterior fontanelle is the junction of the coronal, sagittal, and frontal sutures, whereas the posterior fontanelle is the junction of the parietal and occipital bones. By 3 months of age, the posterior fontanelle is usually closed, and the anterior fontanelle is closed by 20 months of age.

PHYSIOLOGY

Both cerebral blood flow and oxygen consumption are increased in childhood in relation to increased metabolic needs. Hyperemia, tissue hypoxia, and acidosis result in cerebral arterial dilation and increased cerebral blood flow. Hyperventilation decreases cerebral blood flow, but severe hypercarbia may result in decreased oxygen consumption and use. The normal cerebral perfusion pressure (CPP) values in children are unknown. It is thought that CPP should be in the range of 40-60 mm Hg, but this figure may vary since perfusion is determined by blood flow and not blood pressure.[28] CPP must be maintained at a level to maintain blood flow.

THERMOREGULATION

Monitoring and maintaining the infant's temperature is a priority of pediatric nursing care. With a proportionally larger body surface and an increased metabolic rate, infants are predisposed to heat loss. The presence of minimal subcutaneous fat in the newborn results in increased heat loss in cold environments. Older children shiver to increase temperature, but the infant cannot shiver effectively. In the newborn, heat is produced by a process called *chemical (nonshivering) thermogenesis.* Cold stress must be avoided because hypoxia, metabolic acidosis, or hypoglycemia may occur. Sudden infant temperature changes may also lead to apneic spells, especially during rapid rewarming. Nursing interventions to decrease heat loss include maintaining the infant in flexed position and avoiding heat transfer by radiation, convection, conduction, or evaporation. Infants may be placed in incubators or under radiant warmers.

ASSESSMENT

Cognitive function cannot be evaluated until the preschool and early childhood years, but level of consciousness (LOC), movement, and pupils can be evaluated in the pediatric patient. The Glasgow Coma Scale (GCS) is used for older children and has been modified for use in infants and younger children (Table 11-11). Evaluation of reflexes in children is comparable to that of adults, with a couple of exceptions. Although a positive Babinski reflex is an abnormal response in an adult, this response is normal in the child until ages 1½ to 2½ years.[34] In the first few months of life, grasp is reflexive in the infant. With severe neurologic disease or injury, grasp may re-

Table 11-11	Modified Glasgow Coma Scale for Infants and Children		
	Child	**Infant**	**Score**
Eye opening	Spontaneous	Spontaneous	4
	To verbal stimuli	To verbal stimuli	3
	To pain only	To pain only	2
	No response	No response	1
Verbal response	Oriented, appropriate	Coos and babbles	5
	Confused	Irritable cries	4
	Inappropriate words	Cries to pain	3
	Incomprehensible words or non-specific sounds	Moans to pain	2
	No response	No response	1
Motor response	Obeys command	Moves spontaneously and purposefully	6
	Localizes painful stimulus	Withdraws to touch	5
	Withdraws in response to pain	Withdraws in response to pain	4
	Flexion in response to pain	Decorticate posturing (abnormal flexion) in response to pain	3
	Extension in response to pain	Decerebrate posturing (abnormal extension) in response to pain	2
	No response	No response	1

Modified from Davis RJ et al: Head and spinal cord injury. In Rogers MC, editors: *Textbook of pediatric intensive care,* Baltimore, 1987, Williams & Wilkins; James H, Anas N, Perkin RM: *Brain insults in infants and children,* New York, 1985, Grune & Stratton; and Morray JP et al: *Crit Care Med* 12:1018,1984.

vert back to a reflex as opposed to a purposeful response, so the grasp response may not indicate improvement of the child's neurologic status.

A situation referred to as the "talk and die phenomenon" may occur in both adults and children.[28] In this situation, the child with a closed head injury is awake and alert on admission to the hospital, but suddenly the child's condition deteriorates and brain stem herniation and death result. Several hours after admission to the hospital, LOC changes and the pupils dilate. The severity of the head injury is not initially recognized, but severe brain damage has occurred and the child does not respond to treatment. The causes of death are cerebral herniation and ischemia. The pediatric patient with head injury requires careful assessment and ongoing, frequent monitoring.

SEIZURES

Seizures are brief manifestations of the brain's electrical system that result from cortical neuronal discharge. Seizures are the most commonly observed neurologic deficit in children and can occur with a variety of CNS conditions (Box 11-3). Seizures are more common during the first 2 years of life. Brain injuries are the most common cause in the first few months of life, whereas infections are a common cause in older infants and toddlers. In preschoolers and older children, epilepsy is the most common cause. As children enter adolescence, hormonal and metabolic changes may alter the seizure threshold. The child who is in an unconscious state must

Box 11-3

ETIOLOGY OF SEIZURES IN CHILDREN

NONRECURRENT (ACUTE)	RECURRENT (CHRONIC)
Febrile episodes	Idiopathic epilepsy
Intracranial infection	Epilepsy secondary to:
Intracranial hemorrhage	Trauma
Space-occupying lesions (cyst, tumor)	Hemorrhage
Acute cerebral edema	Anoxia
Anoxia	Infections
Toxins	Toxins
Drugs	Degenerative phenomena
Tetanus	Congenital defects
Lead encephalopathy	Parasitic brain disease
Shigella, Salmonella	Hypoglycemia injury
Metabolic alterations	Epilepsy—sensory stimulus
Hypocalcemia	Epilepsy-stimulating states
Hypoglycemia	Narcolepsy and catalepsy
Hyponatremia or hypernatremia	Psychogenic
Hypomagnesemia	Tetany from hypocalcemia, alkalosis
Alkalosis	Hypoglycemic states
Disorders of amino acid metabolism	Hyperinsulinism
Deficiency states	Hypopituitarism
Hyperbilirubinemia	Adrenocortical insufficiency
	Hepatic disorders
	Uremia
	Allergy
	Cardiovascular dysfunction or syncopal episodes
	Migraine

From Hockenberry MJ: *Wong's nursing care of infants and children,* ed 7, St Louis, 2003, Mosby.

be evaluated for a history of seizures, since unconsciousness may be the result of a postictal state. Clinical manifestations of seizures may be more subtle in the infant because of immaturity of the CNS. Some common behaviors seen with subtle seizures include (1) tonic horizontal deviations of the eyes with or without nystagmoid jerking; (2) repetitive blinking or fluttering of the eyelashes; (3) drooling, sucking, and/or tongue thrusting; and (4) swimming or rowing movements of the arms with occasional bicycling movements of the legs. Apnea may also occur, so respiratory status must be closely monitored. Seizures must be differentiated from jitteriness in infants. With jitteriness, the predominant type of movements is tremors characterized by alternating rhythmic movements of equal rate and magnitude. Both jitteriness and seizures may be observed in the infant with asphyxia, hypoglycemia, or hypocalcemia. Laboratory studies help determine the metabolic status of the infant.

Nursing management of seizures includes monitoring respiratory status and perfusion, assessing for the cause of the seizure, determining methods to prevent additional seizures, providing a safe environment for the child, and documenting the seizure activity. Children admitted to the critical care unit may require intubation for respiratory complications of seizures, for the sedative effects of anticonvulsants, or for status epilepticus. Anticonvulsant therapy may be indicated for prolonged or recurrent seizures. Phenobarbital, phenytoin (Dilantin), and benzodiazepines (lorazepam, diazepam) may be ordered for the child.

STATUS EPILEPTICUS

Status epilepticus is a medical emergency and is characterized by prolonged or repeated seizure activity.[38] Causes are high fever, meningitis, encephalitis, metabolic disorders, and abrupt stoppage of anticonvulsant drugs. There is an increase in cerebral blood flow, metabolic requirements, and oxygen needs. Cerebral edema may occur. An electroencephalogram (EEG) may be required to confirm status epilepticus in patients in deep coma or with pharmacologic paralysis. Treatment includes short-term administration of anticonvulsants, such as diazepam, lorazepam, and midazolam; airway maintenance, including intubation and oxygenation; barbiturate coma; or general anesthesia.[38] Nursing management includes monitoring the airway, perfusion, BP, heart rate, and neurologic status.

BACTERIAL MENINGITIS

Meningitis, an inflammation of the meninges and cerebrospinal fluid (CSF), is more common in children than in adults. Children younger than 5 years are affected more often, but school-age children and adolescents are also at risk. The causes of meningitis are septic (bacter-

ial or fungal) or aseptic (viral), but the information in this section pertains to bacterial meningitis. Common causative organisms are *Haemophilus influenzae*, type B, *Streptococcus pneumoniae*, and *Neisseria meningitidis;* other causative organisms are β-hemolytic streptococcus, *Staphylococcus aureus*, *Escherichia coli*, *Pseudomonas*, and *Listeria monocytogenes*. Invasion of microorganisms triggers the inflammatory response, and a purulent exudate is produced. Cerebral blood flow is decreased in meningitis, and aggressive hyperventilation may reduce cerebral blood flow below ischemic levels in children.[39]

Clinical manifestations include fever, chills, headache, vomiting, irritability or lethargy, photophobia, nuchal rigidity, and positive Kernig's or Brudzinski's sign. In meningococcemia, petechiae and purpura may be observed.[39] Lumbar puncture is the diagnostic test for meningitis. CSF studies show elevated white blood cell count, increased protein, and decreased glucose. The CSF/blood-glucose ratio is usually less than 0.40.[39] The child with meningitis is isolated during initial antibiotic treatment and for 24 hours after appropriate antibacterial therapy is started. Health care providers must use appropriate precautions because they are also at risk. Broad-spectrum antibiotics may be administered until the specific organism is identified, and then the appropriate drug is given. Antibiotics for meningitis are given in high doses and must be given at the scheduled times to maintain adequate blood levels. Acetaminophen may be given for elevated temperature; aspirin must not be used. Adequate hydration is maintained. Complications of bacterial meningitis include seizures; increased ICP; septic shock; cerebral ischemia, causing neurologic compromise; and possible loss of digits or distal parts of extremities in the case of meningococcemia.

Nursing management includes maintaining universal and isolation precautions; providing a quiet environment; monitoring neurologic, respiratory, and cardiovascular status; measuring and documenting head circumference in the child younger than 2 years; administering antibiotics and pain medications; and providing family education and support. The child may develop sequelae of meningitis, which include hearing loss, mental retardation, hydrocephalus, and death. There is now a vaccine for *H. influenzae*, type B (HIB), and the first dose is given when an infant is 2 months of age. Also, just available is a vaccine for *S. pneumoniae*, Prevnar-7 conjugate vaccine. It is given at 2, 4, 6, and 12 to 15 months of age.

HEAD TRAUMA

Trauma is the leading cause of death in the child older than 1 year, with head trauma a major determinant of pediatric mortality. Head trauma is more common in males—results of motor vehicle accidents (MVAs), falls, violence, or abuse.[40] The child in a motor vehicle accident may be an occupant of a vehicle or be a bicyclist or pedestrian. Falls are a common cause of head injuries in children younger than 2 years because the child's head size is proportionally larger in relationship to total body size. Child abuse is the most common cause of head injury in the first year of life.[40]

Definitions and descriptions of the various types of head injuries are similar to those for the adult. Though the pathophysiology of head injury is similar in adults and children, there are variations in the nursing assessment and management for the pediatric patient. During infancy, the most common causes of head injury are child abuse and falls.[40] The abused infant may be admitted to the critical care unit in serious condition with a severe head injury. One form of abuse in which there are no external signs of head injury is shaken baby syndrome. The patient exhibits changes in neurologic status that result from violent shaking. Diagnostic evaluations reveal subdural hematoma and retinal hemorrhage.[41] When completing the admission assessment, the nurse may find inconsistency in information provided about the injury or a history of injury that does not fit the described circumstances. There may be a history of emergency department visits and may be previous hospital admissions for evaluation of neurologic deficits. If child abuse is suspected, health care personnel have a legal obligation to report concerns to the appropriate child protection agency.

Falls occur in infants and children as they become more mobile. Infants can roll off beds, sofas, and changing tables. As the toddler begins to walk and climb, falls can result from an unsteady gait or a normal curiosity. Because the child's head is larger in proportion to the rest of the body, the child often lands head first in a fall. MVAs are the leading cause of death in the child older than 1 year.[41] Prevention is the best treatment for MVAs. Correct use of infant seats, seat belts, and helmets and caution when walking, playing near the street, or driving will decrease the incidence of head injury. The nurse is an advocate for child safety, providing information to parents on maintaining a safe environment to prevent injuries.

Firearms are the lethal weapons used in most homicides in older children and in most completed teenage suicides.[40] The child with a gunshot wound to the head is stabilized, a computed tomography (CT) scan may be obtained, and the child is taken to surgery for débridement of the wound. Children who are victims of gunshot wounds to the head usually do not survive.

Complications of head injuries include hemorrhage, infections, cerebral bleeding, cerebral edema, seizures, and brain herniation. Treatment is based on the complication manifested by the patient. Both epidural and subdural hematomas occur in children, but epidural hematoma occurs less frequently in the infant or toddler.[42] Treatment for epidural hematoma is surgical intervention. Subdural hematoma is more common in children

and may result from falls and abuse, including violent shaking.[41] Treatment of subdural hematoma may be frequent subdural taps or surgical intervention.

Children, especially infants, are at risk for infection after head injury. The child admitted to the critical care unit with a head injury must be constantly monitored for cerebral edema and signs of increased ICP. Two other potential complications of head injury—diabetes insipidus and syndrome of inappropriate antidiuretic hormone (SIADH)—are discussed in Chapter 36.

Nursing interventions include precise neurologic assessment, including using the GCS and monitoring for signs of increased ICP. The frequency of assessment is related to the severity of the injury. Observe behaviors in relationship to the developmental level and usual behavior of the child. Maintain IV fluid restriction and monitor respiratory status, ventilation parameters, and arterial blood gases. Provide pharmacologic paralysis or barbiturate coma if needed per the medical management plan. Administer diuretics, osmotic agents, antibiotics, pain medications, sedatives, and antipyretics. Children who survive severe head injury often require extended rehabilitation services. Involve the pediatric rehabilitation team in the care of the child while the child is in the critical care unit.

Working with the family of the child with a head injury is challenging. Information given to the parents must be accurate and consistent. The parents may be guilt-ridden, especially if they feel they might have been able to prevent the injury. Parents are encouraged to interact with the child soothingly and gently, even if the child cannot respond. Reading books, making a tape of home activities, and bringing in familiar toys or stuffed animals are ways to involve the family in the care of the child.

If the child is not expected to survive, the parents are informed. The child may be evaluated for brain death. Before the tests begin, the parents are offered the opportunity to spend time with the child. If brain death has occurred, the parents are told the test results. Parents may be asked to participate in the decision of when, but not if, to discontinue support. Special circumstances such as the impending arrival of a grandparent may influence the timing of the decision. Parents must be allowed to spend as much time as they desire with the child.

GASTROINTESTINAL SYSTEM/FLUIDS/NUTRITION

ANATOMY AND PHYSIOLOGY

Coordination of sucking, swallowing, esophageal peristalsis, and breathing is established just after birth. Infant sucking, which is also a reflex, can be nutritive or nonnutritive. Nonnutritive sucking involves no swallowing; occurs at a rapid rate; has self-soothing capacities, which can also be used with the intubated infant; and affects the postprandial process. Nutritive sucking involves moving food from the mouth through the small intestines. It involves bursts of about 10 to 30 sucks, interspersed with one to four swallows.[47] The quality of nutritive sucking is one of several indicators of illness in the infant. The sucking involves a considerable amount of motor activity, and when changes in oxygen demand and consumption occur during illness, the infant will fatigue more readily and sucking will be weaker or even abate.

After birth, growth and maintenance of the small intestine require not only nutritional components but also the stimulation that comes from having food present in the gut lumen. The infant's and young child's intestinal tracts are larger per body weight than the adult's. Sodium and water conservation in the large intestine is immature in the infant, which accounts for the increased number of stools produced each day.[43] For the first 2 years of life, gut immunity is lower[43] and there is greater mucosal binding for bacterial toxins. With these differences of immunity, sensitivity, and greater potential for fluid loss, the infant and toddler have a greater morbidity and mortality with enteric infections than does the adult.[44]

ASSESSMENT AND TREATMENT

The child's fluid requirements involve not only replacing output and insensible losses but also extra fluid for the production of new intracellular and extracellular fluid during growth. Fluid maintenance for the child with normal renal and cardiac status can be calculated using several formulas, but these account only for basal metabolic needs and growth.[45] Table 11-12 provides formulas for normal fluid and electrolyte maintenance for the infant and child. Box 11-4 provides adjustments to fluid maintenance based on level of activity or increased metabolic rate from disease.[45]

One of the common ways a pediatric patient will present with fluid volume deficit is with vomiting and diarrhea. When considering fluid requirements, the bedside nurse can assess the pediatric patient for signs and symptoms of dehydration. The degree of dehydration can be classified as *mild*, *moderate*, or *severe*:

- Mild dehydration: the child is restless, thirsty, and alert; normal pulse rate and strength; normal blood pressure, respiratory rate, and fontanelle; skin readily retracts when pinched; moist mucous membranes; normal urine output. Approximately 4% to 5% body weight loss.
- Moderate dehydration: the child is thirsty, restless, lethargic, irritable; rapid/weak pulse; respirations may be deep, and rate may be rapid; sunken fontanelle; normal or low blood pressure; skin retracts slowly when pinched; dry mucous membranes; urine is dark and amount reduced. Approximately 6% to 9% body weight loss.

Box 11-4

ADJUSTMENTS TO FLUID MAINTENANCE

Fever/hypothermia: Increases/decreases 12% for each degree greater/less than 37.8° C rectal
Tachypnea: Increases 25%-30%
Humidified mechanical ventilation: Decreases 12%
Activity: Non–critically ill resting child: increases 10%
  Restless/active child: increases 30%
Diaphoresis: Increases 10%-25%
High humidity environment: Decreases 25%-40%

Table 11-12	Normal Fluid and Electrolyte Maintenance for Infants and Children	
	Infant/Child Weight	**Total Amount**
Fluids	1-10 kg	(100 ml/kg/day)
	11-20 kg	(1000 ml + 50 ml/each kg over 10 days)
	>20 kg	(1500 ml + 20 ml/each kg over 20 days)
		or
		100 ml/100 kcal/day can be used for children of any weight
		or
		1500 ml/m²/day can be used for children >10 g
Sodium		2-4 mEq/kg/day
Potassium		2-3 mEq/kg/day
Hourly fluid maintenance	1-10 kg	4 ml/kg/hr
	11-20 kg	40 ml + 2 ml/kg over 10 kg
	>20 kg	60 ml + 1 ml/kg over 20 kg

Modified from Roberts KE: Fluid and electrolyte regulation. In Curley M, Smith J, Moloney-Harmon P: *Critical care nursing of infants and children*, ed 2, Philadelphia, 2001, Saunders.

Table 11-13	TPN Administration for Term Infants and Children*	
	10-30 kg Child	**<10 kg Child**
DEXTROSE (need to calculate dextrose from all IV lines)		
Amount/rate	Initiate at 4-8 mg/kg/min	Same
	Maximum 10-17 mg/kg/min	Same
	Increase rate by 1.5-4 mg/kg/min	0.3-0.8 mg/kg/min
	or	or
	2.5%-5% dextrose/day	0.5%-1% dextrose/day
IV limits		
Peripheral	12.5% maximum	Same
Central	35% maximum	Same
LIPIDS		
Amount	1-4 g/kg/day	1-3 g/kg/day
(Minimum of 2%-4% of kcal/day of fat to prevent essential fatty acid deficiency)		
Rate	<0.25 g/kg/hr	Same
(Administer concomitantly with PN solution over 24 hours)		
AMINO ACIDS		
Amount/rate	Initiate at 1 g/kg/day	Same
	Maximum 1-2.5 g/kg/day	Same
	Increase rate by 0.5-1 g/kg/day	Same
MAXIMUM FLUID VOLUMES[47]		
	4000 ml/m²/day	200 ml/kg/day

*>30 kg, use adult recommendations.
TPN, Total parenteral nutrition; *IV,* intravenous; *PN,* parenteral nutrition.

- Severe dehydration: the child is drowsy, limp, cold, and sweaty, and extremities may be cyanotic; rapid/feeble pulse, sometimes difficult to palpate; respirations are deep, and rate is rapid; fontanelle is very sunken; no urine for several hours; no tears; eyes are very sunken. Approximately >10% body weight loss.[28]

Fluid and electrolyte requirements are based on the history, degree of dehydration, and presenting symptoms. The infant and child also need more calories per body weight than the adult for energy expenditure, because of growth. The first fluid formula listed in Table 11-12 can also be used for determining calories in the infant and child (substituting kcal for ml). This formula already provides for a 30% increase in calories, exceeding the basal metabolic rate needed for average hospital activity. Approximate daily weight gain in the growing child or adolescent is the following: 0 to 3 months of age—30 g/day; 3 to 12 months—15 g/day; 1 to 10 years—7 g/day; young adolescent—225 g/day; and older adolescent—300 g/day.[46,47] This should be considered when evaluating for fluid overload in the child.

Total Parenteral Nutrition. Providing needed calories in the face of fluid restrictions is a significant problem with the critically ill infant and child. Table 11-13 outlines daily dextrose, lipid, and amino acid amounts;

administration rates; and intravenous line concentration limits for the infant and child receiving total parenteral nutrition (TPN).[46]

Dextrose solutions initially are titrated up over several days to reach desired caloric levels to prevent hyperglycemia and to allow endogenous insulin secretions to adjust.[46,47] The seriously ill infant or child does better with lipids administered concomitantly with dextrose/amino acids over 24 hours, not only to decrease the solution's osmolarity and increase longevity of cannulated vessels but also to minimize fat intolerance. If TPN is to be cycled, the titration for a child weighing less than 30 kg occurs over 2 hours, with the rate increased or decreased by half each hour. If TPN is to be discontinued, the rate can be tapered over 24 hours without hypoglycemia occurring, as long as enteral nutrition is tolerated. Enteral caloric intake generally increases milliliter-for-milliliter with TPN decreases. When the child can tolerate 75% of desired caloric hourly volume, TPN can be discontinued.[46,47]

Gavage Feeding. Many different formulas are available for the infant and child based on age, host factors, and nutritional requirements. Amounts for formula feeds are based on needed kcal/kg/day and tolerance.[46] For the full-term infant younger than 1 year, cow's milk (Enfamil, Similac) or soy-based formulas (Isomil, ProSobee) are

Table 11-14	Guidelines for Gavage Feeding in Infants and Children				

Age	3 mo	6 mo	2 yr	5 yr	10 yr
Tube size	6 Fr	8 Fr	10 Fr	12 Fr	14 Fr

Method	Initial Volume/Rate	Advancement Volume/Rate
Bolus	2-5 ml/kg every 3-4 hr over 20 min	2-5 ml/kg every other feeding
Continuous	1-2 ml/kg/hr; initial volume not to exceed 55 ml/hr regardless of child's weight	1-2 ml/kg every 8-12 hr

Fr, French.

most commonly given. Human breast milk is highly recommended.[46] PediaSure is designed specifically for the 1- to 6-year-old age-group. Adult formulas can be given to the child older than 6 years. Osmolite and Isocal are preferred for their isotonicity and caloric and protein content.[48] It is not necessary to routinely dilute feedings. Full-strength formulas can be given safely to the ill child.[46] Continuous gavage feedings have advantages over bolus feedings. The risk for aspiration is less, particularly for the infant with reflux. Increased GI absorption and increased growth can occur. Diarrhea can also be managed with continuous feedings.[46]

Feeding tubes can be placed orally or nasally in the infant, but indwelling tubes are usually placed nasally. Determining the insertion length of a nasogastric tube in the child has traditionally been the same as that in the adult—naris to ear to xyphoid process. However, it is possible that this measurement does not always allow for all the side holes of a feeding tube to be in the stomach. Measuring to a point between the xyphoid and the umbilicus is a safer method. Table 11-14 provides guidelines for gavage feeding tube sizes and feeding rates in infants and children.[46]

Gavage feeding in the infant occurs with nonnutritive sucking during some portion of the feeding time, if possible. The emotional and GI benefits of nonnutritive sucking were discussed earlier in this chapter. In addition, to minimize aspiration, the head of the bed or crib should be elevated for all infants receiving enteral formulas.

PAIN MANAGEMENT

The past 20 years of research has witnessed remarkable growth in pediatric pain management. Research has proven that infants and children do feel pain; when they are not treated, there is an increased morbidity and mortality and hyperalgesia, and there can be a negative impact on development.[49] Pain is "an unpleasant sensory and emotional experience associated with actual or potential tissue damage."

PHYSIOLOGY AND PHARMACOKINETICS

Neurotransmitters and peripheral and central neural pathways for pain transmission are developed and are functional before birth. The cardiorespiratory, hormonal, and metabolic responses to pain are the same in the child as in the adult.[50] The infant younger than 1 to 2 months may have a more immature blood-brain barrier, allowing greater permeability of water-soluble opioids, such as morphine. The infant also has less protein-binding with morphine.[51] By the time the child is 2 months of age, the elimination half-life and plasma drug clearance for morphine and its derivatives are equal to those of an adult.

The physiologic effects of untreated pain in the child can result in the following[53]:
- Hyperglycemia from decreased insulin secretion with breakdown of carbohydrate and fat stores
- Metabolic acidosis from increased use of fat
- Increased corticosteroids, growth hormone, and catecholamines
- Increased pulmonary vascular resistance
- Hypoxemia

ASSESSMENT

Pain assessment is the key to good pain management. Many of the factors that influence an adult's pain also influence a child's. One of the differences, though, is the influence of parental anxiety and behavior regarding their child's overall experience of pain. Although most of the pain research has involved procedural pain, it is important to be cognizant of the acute and chronic pain and distress associated with the critical care unit and its repetitive procedures.

The child may not spontaneously express his or her need for pain treatment. Staff need to be vigilant and actively explore a child's level of pain whenever the potential for pain exists. Self-report scales have been found to be the most accurate measurement of pain,[54] but these cannot be used with the preverbal child, the child who cannot comprehend the request to symbolically identify pain, or the child who has a significantly altered LOC. For the child up to 3 years old, behavioral scales are used as the primary source for pain assessment, with physiologic parameters secondary.[55] Crying, motor activity, and facial expression are the components that generally comprise behavioral scales.[55]

For the child at least 6 years old, self-reports are the primary assessment tool, with behavioral scales secondary. For the child 3 to 6 years old, self-reports can be used but with a caveat. Many self-report scales have been tested as effective with this age-group, but the young child 3 to 4 years old may have difficulty using them.[55] Cognitive ability may not be advanced enough yet, or the child may have regressed in cognitive ability because of the illness. The child's rating may indicate a mood state and not pain. With this age-group, self-reports and behavioral scales may need to be used in tandem.[56]

If obtaining a self-report of pain is not possible, numeric rating scales or behavioral assessments can be done by parents or staff.[57] Parental ratings of their child's pain depend on the parent-child relationship, the parents' beliefs about pain, and their own emotional state.[57] Using behavioral scales to measure pain intensity may not always give a true reflection of a child's pain. Severe pain can be felt without any manifestation of expectable behaviors.[58] See Fig. 8-5 for pain rating scales.

TREATMENT OF PAIN

There are general principles that are applied to management of pain in children:

- *Prevention of pain.* If pain can be anticipated, pain should be treated prophylactically.
- *Adequate assessment.* Developmentally appropriate assessment tools
- *Multimodal approach.* Analgesics, physical strategies such as massage, acupuncture, hot/cold therapies, behavioral/cognitive/psychologic
- *Parental involvement.* Parents are the best source of information about their child. They can be taught different strategies to help their child with their pain.
- *Nonnoxious routes.* Route of administration of analgesia should be as painless as possible.
- *Pain control during procedures.* Inadequate pain control during procedures can create an atmosphere of anxiety and increased pain during subsequent procedures.[49]

NONSTEROIDAL ANTIINFLAMMATORY DRUGS

Nonsteroidal antiinflammatory drugs (NSAIDs) are very effective for the management of mild to moderate pain and can be used in combination with opioids. The drawback to NSAIDs is that there is a ceiling effect and that they affect the gastric mucosa and platelet aggregation.[49]

OPIOID ANALGESICS

The most commonly used narcotics for the child are morphine and fentanyl.[59] Methadone is used for weaning from iatrogenic narcotic dependency.[60] Meperidine is not a drug of choice because it causes depressed cardiac output and tachycardia and its metabolite lowers seizure threshold and causes hyperexcitability with multiple dosing.[59] Opioids are given by IV push (IVP) continuous infusion, or in epidurals and caudals. Because some believe that the older infant continues to be overly sensitive to the respiratory depressant effects of opioids beyond the neonatal period, some health care providers are hesitant to administer these drugs.[59] Respiratory depression is not a common side effect, and hesitancy in administering these drugs to an infant 2 months or older is unwarranted. When opioids are given in age-appropriate dosages, no differences in incidence of respiratory depression have been reported.[61] The standard dose of morphine for a child is 0.1 mg/kg. The Acute Pain Management Guideline Panel still suggests caution when administering morphine to a nonintubated infant younger than 6 months and recommends one third of the regular child's dose (0.03 mg/kg). Table 11-15 outlines dosages of morphine and fentanyl for the infant and child.[59]

Topical Anesthetics. Immunizations, intravenous lines, and venipuncture produce pain and anxiety. EMLA Cream, a combination of lidocaine and prilocaine, was introduced in the 1990s. It takes at least 1 hour to produce acceptable anesthesia. ElaMax is a topical formulation of 4% lidocaine that is encapsulated by liposomes, which create lipid solubility and allow transdermal drug delivery. ElaMax provides anesthesia in about 30 minutes.[49] Lidocaine iontophoresis allows for the active transdermal delivery of lidocaine under the influence of a low level electric current. It is currently available under the name Numby Stuff. Numby provides topical anesthesia in as little as 10 minutes.[49]

PSYCHOSOCIAL ISSUES OF THE CHILD AND FAMILY

Admissions to a critical care unit include children with illnesses, injuries, and imminent deaths that are often unanticipated by the family. In a crisis situation, the parents can be overwhelmed and be focused solely on the physiologic well-being of their child. If the child is conscious, he or she desperately needs the continual physical presence and emotional support of the parents; yet, this is a time when it can be very difficult for the parents to help their child emotionally. Critical care staff need to be knowledgeable about childhood cognitive and emotional development and family dynamics to assist the

Table 11-15	Opioid Dosages for Infants and Children	
Agent	**Age**	**Dosage**
MORPHINE		
ROUTE		
IVP	<6 months	0.03-0.05 mg/kg/dose
	>6 months	0.1 mg/kg/dose
Continuous infusion	<6 months	0.01-0.015 mg/kg/hr + IVP loading dose
	>6 months	0.02-0.03 mg/kg/hr + IVP loading dose
PCA		20 mcg/kg/bolus; 6 boluses/hr; 8-10 min lockout
		or
		0.02-0.03 mg/kg/hr continuous + boluses
Epidural		0.03–0.1 mg/kg bolus q 6-12 hr
FENTANYL		
ROUTE		
IV (short procedure)		2-3 mcg/kg/dose (if sedation used: 1-2 mcg/kg/dose)
Continuous infusion (intubated)		10 mcg/kg loading dose + 2.5 mcg/kg/hr
Epidural		0.2 – 2 mcg/kg/hr, possibly with bupivacaine

IVP, Intravenous push, *PCA,* patient-controlled analgesia; *IV,* intravenous.

family through this kind of crisis. This section can only introduce common issues.

THE ILL CHILD'S EXPERIENCE OF CRITICAL ILLNESS

The emotional reactions of the child to hospitalization depend on the type and quantity of stress produced by the illness itself, the hospitalization experience, and the notions that the child has about the situation. The final outcome is influenced, in part, by the child's age, level of development, adaptive capacity to control (within reason) the fears and anxieties that are provoked, the kinds of hospital procedures done, the attitude and reactions of parents and staff, and the environmental conditions of the hospital. A child in the critical care unit experiences significant stress, and the important question is whether the child's capacity to cope in an age-appropriate fashion, either physically or emotionally, is exceeded. See the Clinical Application feature at the end of this chapter for a discussion on "Pediatric Concepts."

The critically ill child needs, foremost, the physical presence of the parents (or primary caretaker) at the bedside. Unrestricted visitation (i.e., 24 hours/day) for parents is imperative. They are the most reassuring persons in the child's eyes and are needed psychologically by the child to believe that he or she will not be abandoned, left to be unsafe, or left in pain and distress. The child, even more so than the adult patient, also needs to be protected from staff who would discuss the child's case at the bedside. Anxiety and fear are easily heightened when the child recognizes scary words or fills in ambiguities heard with his or her own distorted interpretations. For the child who is very ill and prostrate,

anxieties may fester within the child, unbeknown to staff.

In the critically ill child it may be difficult to differentiate withdrawal from fatigue. Parental touch and verbalizations are extremely important to provide reassurance that the child is not alone. These are also needed for the child who is heavily sedated or unconscious, since some level of awareness may still exist. Other age-appropriate sensory stimuli, such as soft objects for rubbing on the face, favorite snuggle toys from home, special objects that may have a feel or smell that the child can identify, audio cassettes of the mother's and/or family members' voices speaking to the child or reading a book, or a cassette with favorite music, can be used as soothing measures for a child of any age. For the school-age child, repeated orientation to time, day, and place also can be reassuring, whereas the younger child's primary concern is whether the parents are present.

Noxious procedures must be preceded by gently bringing the infant or child to a state of arousal. Even in depressed states of consciousness, gently speaking or stroking the child is done first. For the infant and toddler, someone (ideally the parent) needs to provide comfort and distraction during and after the procedure. A child of this age does not understand procedural explanations and apologies for performing them. An overall emotional tone of calmness and quiet soothing in body language and voice volume can be helpful in minimizing anxiety.

The child 3 to 7 years old also needs this same emotional tone from staff and parents to assist him or her in tempering anxiety. A child this age also needs a brief explanation of what will be done. The purpose of the ex-

CLINICAL APPLICATIONS

Pediatric Concepts

A 2-month-old infant is admitted directly to the intensive care unit with a history of vomiting and diarrhea over the past 24 hours. The mother reports that the infant was irritable yesterday but today is more lethargic; she has had three wet diapers over the past 24 hours; and the urine appears dark. She continues not to tolerate formula or Pedialyte. Physical assessment reveals the following—weight: 6.84 kg (weight 1 week prior: 7.6 kg), which represents a 10% loss; temperature: 38.5° C; pulse: 180; respiratory rate: 46-50; BP: 80/43; pulse oximetry: 97%. The infant's lips and mucous membranes are dry and tacky. Her fontanelle is sunken. Extremities are cool and mottled, nail beds are dusky, and capillary refill is 3 seconds. Pulses are rapid and weak. The infant is lethargic.

1. As the bedside nurse, what is the priority in caring for this infant?

2. What category of shock applies to this situation?
3. Describe the pathophysiology of hypovolemic shock in the pediatric patient.
4. What are the two goals of therapy?
5. What level of dehydration does this infant appear to suffer?
6. Determine the estimated fluid deficit (ml/kg).
7. Calculate the daily fluid requirement for a 6.84-kg infant.
8. What is the fluid of choice to treat the volume deficit?
9. What is the initial therapy for volume resuscitation? After the infant has received the initial volume replacement, she is arousable; vital signs are the following— pulse: 160; BP: 84/40; CVP: 1-2 mm Hg.
10. What is the next step in the treatment of her fluid deficit?

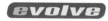 For the discussion of this Clinical Application and for an additional clinical application on supraventricular tachycardia, see the Evolve website.

planation is not to impart educational information but rather to mute the sense of bodily assault by removing some of the surprise and by providing a working language for the child. The form of the explanation should be brief—only one or two sentences. Also, because of the underdeveloped sense of time, procedures are spoken about only just before they are to be done. By the same token, the child must not overhear talk from staff about procedures to be done in the future.

For the child 8 to 10 years old, the process is much the same, except that the older child can usually understand a fuller explanation of the procedure. Depending on how ill the child is, he or she may desire more rationale as a way of coping by using intellectual means. The child of this age feels he or she has more self-control over some aspects of illness or injury. Acknowledgments of possible feelings after the procedure must also occur. Because of the child's greater ability to remember and to comprehend time, statements can now include reference to feelings about the repetition of procedures, the dread of future ones, the lack of control over them, or the child's wish to be able to make someone else the recipient of the procedures.

The older school-age child, although having a better understanding of his or her body and illness, still does not fully grasp what role the health care professionals play in recovery. The child younger than 11 years cannot fully understand how treatment goals are accomplished because of the limits in logical reasoning.

However, the bond between the health care professional and the child-patient can occur by helping to verbalize the child's feelings without belittling or condemning him or her.

In the adolescent, any type of behavioral regression that is seen in the younger child can occur, but the emphasis is different on the issues of privacy, boundaries, immobility, body image, and abandonment from family, peers, and pets. The young adolescent has a greater concern about separation from mother. Despite the ability for abstract reasoning, anxiety can bring on a cause-and-effect type of thinking. The adolescent, as does the younger child, fears pain and is very threatened by invasive procedures. With adolescents' cognitive grasp of the finality of death, when they are surrounded by others who might or actually do die, they can worry deeply about their own mortality. Adolescents may also fear recovery if hospitalization is believed to be a respite from intense family conflicts.

THE PARENTS' EXPERIENCE OF A CHILD'S CRITICAL ILLNESS

Parents of the critically ill child experience a great deal of stress and anxiety, regardless of the severity of the child's illness or length of stay in the critical care unit.

Parents experience common issues when their child is admitted to the critical care unit. With a sudden illness or injury, denial often is present. Parents may question the diagnosis or want to prove the physician wrong. The situation can feel unreal—as if it were not happening to them. It may be difficult to grasp the totality of what has happened to their child. They can feel immobile and not know what they should do next. The parents may find it difficult to remember and process explanations given to them about what is happening with their child. This is usually a defense against pain. This forgetting can result in some parents feeling that staff do not explain very much to them. Other parents may feel that this is a sign of their own inadequacy. Out of embarrassment, they may be reluctant to ask for explanations to be repeated, especially more than once. They may then query others who may not be qualified to answer to their specific situation. Some parents may appear outwardly as competent and composed during the height of the crisis, but this should not be interpreted as them actually being less stressed or anxious.

Parents need to be reunited with their child, if this is their wish, as soon as they have been prepared about what to expect. Having them wait until all assessments are done and the room is cleaned up is unnecessary. But parents may be afraid to see their child. Changes in the child's appearance and in the child's emotional reactions can be very upsetting to parents. If the child is conscious and relatively alert, the parents need to be informed that their child may show some form of regressive behavior, such as withdrawal or anger, which is expectable given the stress of the situation and the degree of illness or injury. Parents also can feel frightened about touching or talking to their child, believing this may harm the child. They must be told that it is okay to do this and that if there are any concerns, staff will be present in the room.

Intense anxiety is another emotion that can make parents question whether their reactions are normal. They wonder how other parents feel or behave. They can be extremely frightened by the intensity of their feelings and may wonder whether they will have a breakdown. These feelings are common in a crisis, and parents need to hear that their feelings are understandable. Some parents may behave with hostility toward staff or family members. On the other hand, some may behave quite rigidly—visiting only briefly or not asking questions in an attempt to maintain composure.

Guilt is another emotion that can torment parents. They may feel responsible for their child's condition. Alternatively, now that the child is ill or injured, parents may feel troubled by previously held negative feelings toward the child. These feelings may revolve around the normal exasperation of rearing a child, or the parents may have had ambivalence about having the child at all.

Anger is an emotion that usually takes its toll after the crisis period, usually with longer critical care unit stays. Destructive anger occurs when parents seek justification for their anger by blaming others for their child's condition. They are unreasonably critical of staff and feel be-littled by them. A common occurrence is alienation between spouses. Either different coping styles or one parent blaming the other prevents them from supporting each other.

Another situation that can occur with prolonged hospitalization of a child is the mother becoming totally devoted to the ill child. She lives at the hospital and is very involved in her child's care but abandons interest in any other children at home or other family members. This is often a consequence of and begets further blame, anger, and alienation between the spouses. This situation requires intensive social work intervention and can result in a breakdown of the marriage.

REFERENCES

1. Backofen JE, Rogers MC: Upper airway disease. In Rogers MC, editor: *Textbook of pediatric intensive care*, ed 2, vol 1, Baltimore, 1992, Williams & Wilkins.
2. Williams PL, editor: *Gray's anatomy: the anatomical basis of medicine and surgery*, ed 38, New York, 1995, Churchill Livingstone.
3. Chameides L, Hazinski MF: *Textbook of pediatric advanced life support*, Dallas, 1994, American Heart Association.
4. Roberts KB: Upper airway obstruction. In Roberts KB, editor: *Manual of clinical problems in pediatrics*, ed 4, Boston, 1995, Little, Brown.
5. Cote CJ, Todres ID: The pediatric airway. In Cote CJ et al, editors: *A practice of anesthesia for infants and children*, ed 2, Philadelphia, 1993, Saunders.
6. Papastamelos C et al: Developmental changes in chest wall compliance in infancy and early childhood, *J Appl Physiol* 78:179, 1995.
7. Manno M: Cardiopulmonary arrest and resuscitation. In Roberts KB, editor: *Manual of clinical problems in pediatrics*, ed 4, Boston, 1995, Little, Brown.
8. Backofen JE, Rogers MC: Emergency management of the airway. In Rogers MC, editor: *Textbook of pediatric intensive care*, ed 2, vol 1, Baltimore, 1992, Williams & Wilkins.
9. Martin LD et al: Principles of respiratory support and mechanical ventilation. In Rogers MC, editor: *Textbook of pediatric intensive care*, ed 2, vol 1, Baltimore, 1992, Williams & Wilkins.
10. Monto A: Occurrence of respiratory virus: time, place and person, *Pediatr Infec Dis J* 23:S58-64, 2004.
11. Welch JA et al: Staff nurses' experience as co-investigators in a clinical research project, *Pediatr Nurs* 16:364, 1990.
12. American Academy of Pediatrics Committee of Infectious Disease: Use of ribavirin in the treatment of respiratory syncytial virus infection, *Pediatrics* 92:501, 1993.
13. American Academy of Pediatrics: Summary of infectious diseases. In Peter G, editor: *Red book: report of the committee on infectious diseases*, ed 23, Elk Grove Village, Ill, 1994, American Academy of Pediatrics.
14. Roberts KB: Bronchiolitis. In Roberts KB, editor: *Manual of clinical problems in pediatrics*, ed 4, Boston, 1995, Little, Brown.
15. Helfaer MA et al: Lower airway disease: bronchiolitis and asthma. In Rogers MC, editor: *Textbook of pediatric intensive care*, ed 2, vol 1, Baltimore, 1992, Williams & Wilkins.

16. Alario A et al: The efficacy of nebulized metaproterenol in wheezing infants and young children, *Am J Dis Child* 146: 412, 1992.
17. Groothius JR et al: Early ribavirin treatment of respiratory syncytial viral infection in high-risk children, *J Pediatr* 117: 792, 1990.
18. Smith DW et al: A controlled trial of aerosolized ribavirin in infants receiving mechanical ventilation for severe respiratory syncytial virus infection, *N Engl J Med* 325:24, 1991.
19. Englund JA et al: High-dose, short-duration ribavirin aerosol therapy compared with standard ribavirin therapy in children with suspected respiratory syncytial virus infection, *J Pediatr* 125:635, 1994.
20. Kiernan M: Contemporary Forum: Nursing of the Hospitalized Child. *"What's new in asthma and bronchiolitis,"* New Orleans, May 2000.
21. Lasley M: New treatments for asthma, *Pediatr Rev* 24:7, July 2003.
22. Stokes DC: Respiratory failure and status asthmaticus. In Roberts KB, editor: *Manual of clinical problems in pediatrics,* Boston, 1995, Little, Brown.
23. Malfino N et al: Respiratory arrest in near-fatal asthma, *N Engl J Med* 324:285, 1991.
24. Scarfone R., Friedlaender, E. Corticosteroids in acute asthma: past, present, and future. *Pediatr Emerg Care* 19:5, 2003.
25. Ruggins N: Pathophysiology of apnea in preterm infants, *Arch Dis Child* 66:70, 1991.
26. Finer N et al: Obstructive, mixed, and central apnea in the neonate: physiological correlates, *J Pediatr* 121:943, 1992.
27. Moore KL, Persaud TVN: *The developing human, clinically oriented embryology,* ed 5, Philadelphia, 1993, Saunders.
28. Hazinski MF: *Nursing care of the critically ill child,* ed 2, St Louis, 1992, Mosby.
29. Gaedke-Norris MK, Roland JA: Perioperative management of pulmonary circulation in children with congenital cardiac defects, *AACN Clin Issues Crit Care Nurs* 5:255, 1994.
30. Burton DA, Cabalka AK: Cardiac evaluation of infants, *Pediatr Clin North Am* 41:991, 1994.
31. Emmanouilides GC et al, editors: *Moss and Adams heart disease in infants, children and adolescents including the fetus and young adults,* ed 5, Baltimore, 1995, Williams & Wilkins.
32. O'Brien P, Smith PA: Chronic hypoxia in children with cyanotic heart disease, *Crit Care Nurs Clin North Am* 6:215, 1994.
33. Park MK, Guntheroth WG: *How to read pediatric ECGs,* ed 3, St Louis, 1992, Mosby.
34. Chang A et al: *Pediatric cardiac intensive care,* Baltimore, 1998, Williams & Wilkins.
35. The Johns Hopkins Hospital Department of Pediatrics, Barone M, editor: *The Harriet Lane handbook,* ed 14, St Louis, 1996, Mosby.
36. Hockenberry MJ: Pediatric variations of nursing interventions. In Hockenberry MJ: *Wong's nursing care of infants and children,* ed 7, St Louis, 2003, Mosby.
37. Luden RC et al: Length-based endotracheal tube and emergency equipment in pediatrics, *Ann Emerg Med* 8:900, 1992.
38. Lacroix J et al: Admissions to a pediatric intensive care unit for status epilepticus: a ten-year experience, *Crit Care Med* 22:827, 1994.
39. Carno M: Meningococcemia: recognizing and reducing complications in pediatric patients, *AACN Clin Issues Crit Care Nurs* 5:278, 1994.
40. Moloney-Harmon PA, Czerwinski SJ: Caught in the crossfire: children, guns, and trauma, *Crit Care Nurs Clin North Am* 6:525, 1994.
41. Wong DL, editor: *Whaley and Wong's nursing care of infants and children,* ed 5, St Louis, 1995, Mosby.
42. Curley MAQ, Smith JB, Moloney-Harmon PA, editors: *Critical care nursing of infants and children,* Philadelphia, 1996, Saunders.
43. Weaver LT: Anatomy and embryology. In Walker WA et al, editors: *Pediatric gastrointestinal disease: pathophysiology, diagnosis, management,* ed 2, vol 1, St Louis, 1996, Mosby.
44. Udall JN, Watson RR: Development of immune function. In Walker WA et al, editors: *Pediatric gastrointestinal disease: pathophysiology, diagnosis, management,* ed 2, vol 1, St Louis, 1996, Mosby.
45. Adelman RD, Solhung MJ: Fluid therapy. In Behrman RE, Kliegman RM, Arvin AM, editors: *Nelson textbook of pediatrics,* ed 15, Philadelphia, 1996, Saunders.
46. Kovacevich DS, editor: *Parenteral and enteral nutrition manual,* ed 7, Ann Arbor, Mich, 1994, University of Michigan Medical Center.
47. Kerner JA: Parenteral nutrition. In Walker WA et al, editors: *Pediatric gastrointestinal disease: pathophysiology, diagnosis, management,* ed 2, vol 2, St Louis, 1996, Mosby.
48. Sinden AA, Dillard VL, Sutphen JL: Enteral nutrition. In Walker WA et al, editors: *Pediatric gastrointestinal disease: pathophysiology, diagnosis, management,* ed 2, vol 2, St Louis, 1996, Mosby.
49. Zempsky W, Schechter N: What's new in the management of pain in children, *Pediatr Rev* 24:10, 2003.
50. Anand KJS, Hickey PR: Pain and its effects in the human neonate and fetus, *N Engl J Med* 317:1321, 1987.
51. Bhat R et al: Pharmacokinetics of a single dose of morphine in preterm infants during the first week of life, *J Pediatr* 117:477, 1990.
52. Reference deleted in proofs.
53. Anand KJS, Carr DB: The neuroanatomy, neurophysiology, and neurochemistry of pain, stress, and analgesia in newborns and children, *Pediatr Clin North Am* 36:795, 1989.
54. Acute Pain Management Guideline Panel: *Acute pain management: operative or medical procedures and trauma.* Clinical practice guideline, AHCPR Pub No 92-0032, Rockville, Md, 1992, Agency for Health Care Policy and Research, Public Health Service, US Department of Health and Human Services.
55. Stein PR: Indices of pain intensity: construct validity among preschoolers, *Pediatr Nurs* 21:119, 1995.
56. McGrath PA: Pain in the pediatric patient: practical aspects of assessment, *Pediatr Ann* 24:126, 1995.
57. Finley GA et al: Parents' management of children's pain following "minor" surgery, *Pain* 64:83, 1996.
58. Hammers JPH et al: The influence of children's vocal expression, age, medical diagnosis, and information obtained from parents on nurses' pain assessment and decisions regarding intervention, *Pain* 65:53, 1996.
59. Yaster M et al: Pain, sedation, and post-operative anesthetic management in the pediatric intensive care unit. In Rogers MC, editor: *Textbook of pediatric intensive care,* ed 2, vol 2, Baltimore, 1992, Williams & Wilkins.
60. Anand KJS, Arnold JA: Opioid tolerance and dependence in infants and children, *Crit Care Med* 22:334, 1994.
61. Lynn AM et al: Respiratory effects of intravenous morphine infusions in neonates, infants, and children after cardiac surgery, *Anesth Analg* 77:695, 1993.

CHAPTER 12

High-Risk and Critical Care Obstetric Issues

*D*uring the past few years the worlds of critical care and obstetrics have seen a new emphasis on collaboration and integration. Traditionally the two specialties have been separated, in part because of the typical normalcy and health-oriented approach of obstetrics and the crisis and illness orientation of critical care. Pregnancy alters the function of virtually every organ system and therefore the baseline state and patient response to physiologic changes are very different in the pregnant patient. Fetal considerations are often very important in designing and leading the clinical approach to the critically ill woman. There are many common conditions in pregnancy that require special medical care. Each of these conditions has associated complications that have the potential for serious morbidity and mortality.

It is important to recognize that critical care obstetrics encompasses two distinct populations: women with preexisting disease who become pregnant and women with normal pregnancies who become compromised by critical illness or injury. The two priorities for the pregnant critically ill woman are supporting fetal growth and development and optimizing the maternal and family experience.

It is impossible to discuss every aspect of management of the critically ill obstetric patient in one chapter. Instead, the focus and goal of this chapter is twofold: first, to provide a synopsis of the more commonly seen conditions or concerns in the realm of critical care obstetrics; and second, to emphasize the collaborative nature of this emerging field, recognizing that the manifestations and management of critical illness are typically identical in pregnant and nonpregnant patients, although the data value changes associated with pregnancy must be considered. Nursing management, unless unique to the critically ill obstetric patient, is not detailed here.

RISKS TO FETAL DEVELOPMENT

Factors that influence embryonic and fetal development may be intrinsic or extrinsic in nature. Intrinsic factors such as chromosomal abnormalities and congenital anomalies account for 25% to 28% of all birth defects.[1] Extrinsic factors such as radiation exposure, bacterial, fungal, and viral infections, medication exposure, and "unknown" causes account for those remaining.[1] Exposure to ionizing radiation is usually not of concern until more than 5 to 15 rads (cGy) have been exceeded. Table 12-1 lists radiation exposure of common radiologic studies.[2-5]

Medication use in critically ill obstetric patients requires analysis of the risk:benefit ratio. Often the benefit may outweigh the potential fetal risk when all factors are considered. It is important to remember the influence that drug exposure can have on the developing fetus. See Box 12-1 for Food and Drug Administration (FDA) labels regarding a drug's risk to a fetus.[6,7]

Technologic advances, improvements in maternal-fetal diagnostics, and aggressive neonatal interventions have improved the survival of extremely low–birth weight infants. Current research places minimal viability parameters between 23 and 26 weeks' gestation and fetal weight between 500 and 1000 g (0.5 and 1 kg). Critical care clinicians may encounter situations in which extrauterine viability, fetal outcomes, and maternal stability are uncertain. Clinical decisions must be made in light of the maternal-fetal risk:benefit ratio. Personal, cultural, spiritual, and social beliefs regarding viability may affect the clinical decision-making process. Parental and family beliefs and desires may conflict with those of the health care team. When confronting the dilemma of viability, the parameters of gestational age, fetal weight, parental desires, and maternal-fetal mortality must be considered.

PHYSIOLOGIC ALTERATIONS IN PREGNANCY

During pregnancy the woman's body undergoes profound physiologic changes. These changes are necessary to maintain the pregnancy and to allow for fetal growth and development. So dramatic are the changes that they

Table 12-1	Radiation Dose from Radiologic Studies
Radiologic Study	**Estimated Fetal Dose (rads [cGy]) (1×10^{-5} Gy)**
Chest x-ray	8
Skull x-ray	4
Cervical spine x-ray	2
Thoracic spine x-ray	402
Lumbar spine x-ray	275
Abdominal x-ray	185
IV/Retrograde pyelography	585
Upper GI x-ray	330
Lower GI x-ray	465
Pelvimetry	750
Hip x-ray	100
Lower extremity x-ray	1

Gy, Gray: *IV,* intravenous; *GI,* gastrointestinal.

Box 12-1

FDA CATEGORIES OF LABELING FOR DRUG USE IN PREGNANCY

- Category A—Controlled studies in women fail to demonstrate risk to the fetus in the first 12 weeks. Possibility of fetal harm is remote.
- Category B—Animal studies do not indicate a risk to the fetus. Well-controlled studies with pregnant mothers fail to demonstrate a risk to the fetus.
- Category C—Studies have shown teratogenic effects in animal studies. There are no controlled studies in women.
- Category D—Evidence of fetal risk exists, but benefits in life-threatening or serious disease may make it acceptable despite risks.
- Category X—Studies demonstrate fetal abnormalities, or there is evidence of risk from human experience. The risk clearly outweighs the benefit.

Data from Briggs G, Freeman R, Yaffe S: *Drugs in pregnancy and lactation,* ed 5, Baltimore, 1998, Williams & Wilkins; Riordan J, Auerbach K: *Breastfeeding and human lactation,* ed 2, Boston, 1999, Jones & Bartlett.

Box 12-2

PRIMARY FUNCTIONS AND IMPLICATIONS OF ESTROGEN AND PROGESTERONE

FUNCTIONS/EFFECTS OF ESTROGEN
Promote growth and function of the uterus
Cause uterine musculature hypertrophy and hyperplasia
Increase blood supply to uteroplacental unit
Promote breast (ductal, alveolar, nipple) development
Increase pliability of connective tissue
- Relax pelvic joints and ligaments
- Allow for cervical softening
Promote sodium and water retention
Produce psychologic changes leading to emotional lability
Decrease gastric secretion of hydrochloric acid and pepsin
Increase sensitivity to carbon dioxide (CO_2) levels in the blood
Produce integumentary changes
- Hyperpigmentation
- Striae gravida
Affect blood component concentrations
- Increase fibrinogen (factor 1) concentration
- Decrease plasma protein concentration
- Cause leukocytosis

FUNCTIONS/EFFECTS OF PROGESTERONE
Decrease maternal smooth muscle contractility
- Uterus: prevent contractility
- Gastrointestinal tract: contribute to nausea, heartburn, and constipation
- Renal: contribute to urinary dilation leading to urinary stasis
- Vascular: dilate vessels and contribute to peripheral edema
Produce metabolic effects
- Reset hypothalamus up approximately 0.2° C (0.5° F)
- Promote fat storage
Stimulate respiratory center to decrease CO_2 retention
Stimulate secretion of sodium in the urine, thereby stimulating aldosterone production
Promote breast development and inhibit the action of prolactin

would probably be considered pathologic in the non-pregnant woman. Adaptations occur in nearly every organ system, beginning during the first week of gestation and continuing until up to 6 weeks after delivery. The only system where there are no documented characteristic changes is the nervous system. Understanding the physiologic adaptations is important to the management of the critically ill pregnant woman. In the limited space of this text there is not room for an exhaustive descrip-

tion of each adaptation. Physiologic changes are summarized, with special attention given to those areas that affect or are affected by critical illness or injury. The authors refer the reader to a comprehensive obstetric text for expanded detail.

ENDOCRINE SYSTEM

Hormonal changes are critically important to the initiation and maintenance of pregnancy. Maintenance of adequate estrogen and progesterone levels is essential (Box 12-2). During pregnancy, estrogen production increases approximately 1000-fold.[8] Progesterone is essential for maintenance of pregnancy and is first produced by the corpus luteum and then by the placental unit. Human placental lactogen (HPL) promotes maternal breakdown of lipids, causing increased levels and use of free fatty acids, and has an anti-insulin effect, contributing to hyperglycemia. HPL also contributes to breast growth and development, preparing the breasts for lactation. Thyroid enlargement and stimulation occur during pregnancy, causing an increase of approximately 25% in the maternal basal metabolic rate.

REPRODUCTIVE SYSTEM

Reproductive organs undergo remarkable changes during pregnancy. The uterus increases in weight 20 times and alters its capacity from 10 mL to 4.5 to 5 L. The uterus grows out of the pelvic cavity, displacing intestines laterally and superiorly. When the pregnant woman assumes a supine position, the gravid uterus may compress the inferior vena cava and aorta, decreasing venous return to the heart.

Uterine blood flow increases dramatically as pregnancy progresses—from 50 ml/min at 10 weeks to 500 ml/min at 40 weeks.[9,10] Major expansion of the uterine vascular bed contributes to the development of decreased systemic vascular resistance.

CARDIOVASCULAR SYSTEM

Pregnancy is characterized as a hyperdynamic (high-flow), low-resistance state. This is facilitated through adaptations in blood volume, cardiac structure, cardiac output, vascular resistance, and heart rate.[11]

Blood volume changes are as follows:
- Total blood volume increases approximately 30% to 40%, or 1 to 1.5 L.
- Blood volume maximizes between the twenty-sixth and thirty-fourth week.
- Red blood cell volume increases approximately 20%.
- Plasma volume increases 45% to 50%.
- Total body water increases by approximately 6 to 8 L.
- Colloid oncotic pressure (COP) decreases.

Cardiac structural changes are as follows:
- Heart is displaced to the left and upward and rotates slightly anteriorly.
- There are no characteristic electrocardiographic changes.
- Left axis deviation may occur because of mechanical displacement.
- Cardiac volume increases slightly because of increased volume and hypertrophy.

Cardiac auscultatory changes areas follows:
- There is a physiologic S_1 (first heart sound) split.

Table 12-2	Positional Cardiac Output Changes in Pregnancy
Maternal Position	**Cardiac Output (L/min)**
Knee-chest	6.9 ($\pm$2.1)
Right lateral	6.8 ($\pm$1.3)
Left lateral	6.6 ($\pm$1.4)
Sitting	6.2 ($\pm$2.0)
Supine	6.0 ($\pm$1.4)
Standing	5.4 ($\pm$2.0)

- S_3 (third heart sound) development is considered normal.
- Systolic murmurs develop in 90% of all pregnant women.
- Diastolic murmurs develop in 20% of all pregnant women.
- Murmurs are generally physiologic in nature and disappear after delivery.

Blood pressure variations may occur during pregnancy. Blood pressure may decrease slightly during the first trimester, reach a low point in the second trimester, and then return to normal for the duration of the pregnancy. Postural hypotension may occur with sudden position changes or supine positioning.

Cardiac output (CO) changes begin early in the first trimester, peak at the end of the second trimester, and remain elevated until term. CO increases 30% to 50% during pregnancy, with normal levels usually 6 to 7 L/min.[9] Changes are attributed to increased blood volume, increased heart rate, and decreases in systemic vascular resistance. Heart rate increases 10 to 15 beats/minute during the second trimester and usually returns to normal 6 weeks postpartum. CO varies markedly depending on maternal position[11] (Table 12-2). The American College of Obstetricians and Gynecologists (ACOG) has defined indications for hemodynamic monitoring in pregnancy[12] (Box 12-3). Table 12-3 summarizes hemodynamic value changes associated with pregnancy, and are most reflected in the third trimester.[11,13]

PULMONARY SYSTEM

Pulmonary physiologic changes are essential to provide adequate oxygenation for the mother's increased metabolic demands, as well as for the dependent fetus. As the uterus grows, it causes diaphragmatic elevation of approximately 4 cm, decreasing lung length. Compensatory and hormonal changes cause lower rib flaring and thoracic cage enlargement of 5 to 7 cm.[10,11]

Oxygen consumption increases approximately 15% to 25% throughout pregnancy. To meet these needs for addi-

Table 12-3	Hemodynamic Changes Associated With Term Pregnancy	
Parameter	**Pregnancy Normal Value**	**Change**
Mean arterial pressure (mm Hg)	90 ± 6	No significant change
Central venous pressure (mm Hg)	8 ± 2	No significant change
Pulmonary artery wedge pressure (mm Hg)	4 ± 3	No significant change
Heart rate (beats per minute)	83 ± 10	Increase 17%
Cardiac output (L/min)	6.2 ± 1.0	Increase 43%
Systemic vascular resistance (dynes/sec/cm^{-5})	1210 ± 266	Decrease 21%
Pulmonary vascular resistance (dynes/sec/cm^{-5})	78 ± 22	Decrease 34%
Serum colloid oncotic pressure (mm Hg)	18 ± 1.5	Decrease 14%
Left ventricular stroke work index (g-m/m^2)	48 ± 6	No significant change

Box 12-3

INDICATIONS FOR HEMODYNAMIC MONITORING IN PREGNANCY

- Severe pregnancy-induced hypertension with persistent oliguria or pulmonary edema
- Massive hemorrhage or volume replacement needs
- Adult respiratory distress syndrome
- Shock of unknown etiology
- Sepsis with oliguria or refractory hypotension
- Cardiovascular decompression during intrapartum or intraoperative periods
- Chronic disease during labor or intraoperatively (New York Heart Association Classification III or IV cardiac disease)
- Pulmonary edema, oliguria, or heart failure refractory to treatment or of unknown etiology

Table 12-4	Physiologic Adaptation of the GI System During Pregnancy
GI Function Change	**Presumed Cause**
Heartburn	Progesterone and estrogen; size of gravid uterus impeding gastroesophageal junction
Bleeding gums	Hyperemia
Constipation	Progesterone, causing decreased motility and intestinal secretion, enhanced water absorption
Hemorrhoids	Hyperemia, pelvic congestion, obstruction of venous return
"Morning sickness" or nausea	Increased levels of estrogen and human chorionic gonadotropin (HCG)
Risk for aspiration	Displacement of lower esophageal sphincter and reduced gastric motility
Gallstones	Decreased gallbladder activity, impaired emptying

tional oxygen, ventilatory changes (Fig. 12-1) must occur. Vital capacity remains unchanged during pregnancy; however, there is an increase in tidal volume and slight increase in respiratory rate. Together these account for an increase in minute ventilation by approximately 50% at term.

Hyperventilation is normal and is mediated primarily by the effects of progesterone on the respiratory center. Hyperventilation causes a normal decrease in Paco$_2$ levels to approximately 28 to 32 mm Hg.[10,11] The resulting alkalosis is compensated by increased renal excretion of bicarbonate. Normal maternal Pao$_2$ is 101 to 108 mm Hg.[10,11] The maternal oxyhemoglobin dissociation curve shifts to the right, facilitating the exchange of carbon dioxide from the fetus to the mother and the exchange of oxygen from the mother to the fetus.

GASTROINTESTINAL AND GENITOURINARY SYSTEMS

Both functional and structural gastrointestinal (GI) and genitourinary (GU) system changes occur in pregnancy. Physiologic adaptations of the GI system are summa-

rized in Table 12-4. Genitourinary structural changes include slight enlargement of the kidneys; dilation of pelvic, caliceal, and ureteral structures; bladder displacement forward and upward; and impaired blood and lymph drainage after the second trimester. Increases in blood volume and cardiac output, lowered systemic vascular resistance, and hormonal effects contribute to the primary physiologic functional changes summarized in Table 12-5.[8-10,14] The greater increase in glomerular filtration rate over renal plasma flow increases the proportion of filtered plasma. This lowers serum plasma protein concentration and colloid oncotic pressure. The increase in filtration also enhances the renal clearance of many substances, causing decreased plasma levels. Urea and creatinine are excreted more efficiently, and there-

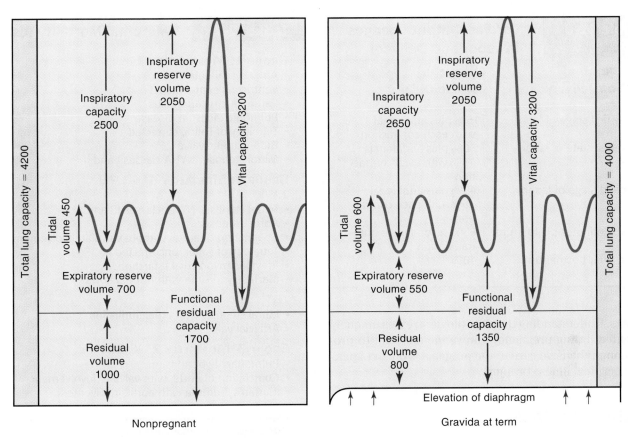

Fig. 12-1 Pulmonary volumes and capacities (in milliliters) during pregnancy, labor, and the postpartum period. (From Bonica JJ: *Principles and practice of obstetric analgesia and anesthesia,* Philadelphia, 1967, FA Davis.)

Table 12-5	Renal Physiologic Changes in Pregnancy	
Parameter	**Percent Change**	**Normal in Pregnancy**
Renal blood flow	Increase 25%-50%	1250-1500 ml/min
Glomerular filtration rate	Increase 50%	140-170 ml/min
Renal plasma flow	Increase 35%	700-900 ml/min

fore normal adult values signify decreased renal function in the pregnant patient. Normal pregnant serum creatinine levels are 0.46 mg/dl, and blood urea nitrogen (BUN) levels are 8.2 mg/dl.[9,14]

Glycosuria and mild proteinuria are common in pregnancy but may be indicative of underlying pathology. While glomerular filtration is increased, tubular reabsorption of glucose and protein cannot increase proportionately, resulting in glycosuria and proteinuria. Both occurrences warrant further investigation in pregnancy.

PHYSIOLOGIC CHANGES DURING LABOR AND DELIVERY

Labor and delivery bring additional stresses to the maternal system, especially as a result of the pain and anxiety associated with labor. The most dramatic requirements are in the cardiopulmonary systems. During labor, uterine contractions produce cyclic autotransfusions of approximately 300 to 500 ml. Delivery of the fetus produces a final autotransfusion of approximately 1000 ml into the maternal vascular system.[10] This occurs because of the contracted uterus shunting its blood, sudden removal of fetal supply demands, and resolution of vena caval compression. Table 12-6 summarizes the cardiac output changes in labor and delivery.[11,15]

Normal blood loss from a vaginal birth is more than 600 ml[11,14]; blood loss from cesarean births usually is 1000 ml.[8] The cardiopulmonary changes occurring during labor and delivery are of significant concern, since they occur over a short time and maternal decompensation may occur.

In summary, maternal physiology is profoundly and rapidly affected by pregnancy. Adaptations begin early in the pregnancy and continue through the postpartum period, gradually returning to prepregnant states over

Table 12-6	Cardiac Output Changes in Labor and Delivery
Stage of Labor/Delivery	**Change in Cardiac Output**
Early first stage of labor	↑15% plus additional 15% with each contraction
Last first state of labor	↑ 30% plus additional 15% with each contraction
Second stage of labor	↑ 45% plus additional 15% with each contraction
First 5 minutes postpartum	↑ 65% secondary to auto-transfusion
First hour postpartum	↑ 40%

Table 12-7	Maternal Mortality Risks

GROUP 1: MORTALITY <1%
- Atrial septal defect
- Ventricular septal defect
- Patent ductus arteriosus
- Pulmonic tricuspid disease
- Tetralogy of Fallot, corrected
- Bioprosthetic valve
- Mitral stenosis, NYHA classes I and II

GROUP 2: MORTALITY 5%-15%
2A
- Mitral stenosis, NYHA classes III and IV
- Aortic stenosis
- Coarctation of aorta, without valvular involvement
- Tetralogy of Fallot, uncorrected
- Previous myocardial infarction
- Marfan syndrome with normal aorta

2B
- Mitral stenosis with atrial fibrillation
- Artificial valve

GROUP 3-MORTALITY 25%-50%
- Pulmonary hypertension
- Coarctation of aorta, with valvular involvement
- Marfan syndrome with aortic involvement

NYHA, New York Heart Association.

6 weeks. Understanding the physiologic stresses uniquely presented during pregnancy allows the clinician to provide comprehensive care to the pregnant woman experiencing critical illness or injury.

CARDIAC DISEASE

There are several general considerations in the care of the pregnant woman with cardiac disease. Cardiac disease during pregnancy may be a result of preexisting conditions, such as congenital diseases, or may be a result of primary cardiac disease arising during pregnancy. Prepregnancy counseling is highly recommended for women with known cardiac disease. Counseling includes determining the New York Heart Association (NYHA)[16] functional class (see Chapter 18) of the woman, as well as determining the maternal and fetal risks associated with the pregnancy[17] (Table 12-7). Major fetal risks include fetal development of congenital heart disease, prematurity, intrauterine growth restriction (IUGR), and intrauterine fetal demise (IUFD). During the prenatal period, anticoagulant therapy is frequently recommended secondary to the already hypercoagulable state of pregnancy or preexisting conditions. Anticoagulant therapy using heparin is recommended because of the teratogenic effects of oral agents.[6] Special consideration must be given to physical assessment during the antepartum period. Normal physiologic changes, such as murmur development or shortness of breath, may mask symptoms of cardiac disease or make diagnosis more challenging. Method and timing of delivery are decided primarily by obstetric considerations, taking into account the woman's ability to tolerate the labor process and associated physiologic changes. Selection of anesthesia techniques involves weighing risks and benefits of the procedures. As a general rule, most patients tolerate

epidural anesthesia more favorably than general anesthesia (see Chapter 14).

PREGNANCY WITH PREEXISTING HEART DISEASE

Much progress has been made during the past two decades in managing preexisting cardiac disease in the pregnant woman. Women in NYHA class I or II generally have a favorable prognosis in pregnancy; however, the dramatic physiologic changes present a significant confounding variable.

Atrial Septal Defect. Atrial septal defect (ASD) is the most common congenital anomaly seen during pregnancy, and the majority of women with ASD tolerate pregnancy, labor, and delivery without complications. The decrease in systemic vascular resistance (SVR) lessens the degree of left-to-right shunt, whereas the hypervolemic state may slightly worsen the shunt and increase right ventricular workload. The most common complications seen with ASD are dysrhythmias, heart failure, and thromboembolism.

Ventricular Septal Defect. The outcome for the pregnant woman with ventricular septal defect (VSD) and resultant left-to-right shunt depends on the size of the defect, with larger defects producing a less favorable prognosis. In the absence of significant symptoms and pulmonary hypertension, pregnancy is typically well tolerated. Therapy is aimed at early recognition and treatment of signs of cardiac failure. Common complications include tachycardias, heart failure, and pulmonary hypertension.

Patent Ductus Arteriosus. In general, patent ductus arteriosus (PDA) is well tolerated during pregnancy, labor, and delivery. Precautions against the risks of infective endocarditis and thromboembolism may be taken. Severe PDA can produce large left-to-right shunts, producing pulmonary hypertension that is associated with significant maternal mortality.

Pulmonic/Tricuspid Disease. Isolated pulmonic or tricuspid valvular disease is uncommon but may be seen during the peripartum period. Because of the right-sided nature of the lesions, pregnancy, labor, and delivery are generally well tolerated in spite of the hypervolemic state. The mainstay of treatment focuses on cautious fluid administration and balance.

Valve Prosthesis. Management of the pregnant woman with a prosthetic valve focuses on maintenance of adequate anticoagulation to prevent thromboembolism and on infective endocarditis prophylaxis. Pregnant women with biologic valves usually do not require anticoagulation during pregnancy unless evidence of thromboembolic disease or atrial fibrillation is present. Biologic valves are associated with slightly lower mortality risks, since anticoagulation is normally not required with their use.

Mitral Stenosis. The presence of a stenotic mitral valve is the most common rheumatic valve disease. The primary concern with mitral stenosis during pregnancy is the impedance to ventricular filling, which produces a relatively fixed cardiac output. Additional risks include thromboembolism and dysrhythmias, especially atrial fibrillation. Cardiac output in the face of mitral stenosis is determined by two primary factors: length of diastolic filling and left ventricular preload. The length of diastolic filling may be negatively affected because of the normal hypervolemic state of pregnancy. In addition, discomfort or anxiety associated with labor may produce tachycardia, which can drastically impede ventricular filling, producing an even lower cardiac output with resultant cardiac failure and pulmonary edema. Tachycardia is commonly managed with beta-blockade therapy.

Maintenance and management of left ventricular preload is the second important consideration in mitral stenosis. Patients may require high normal or slightly elevated left ventricular filling pressures to maintain adequate flow across the stenotic mitral valve. Caution must be used when employing therapies that decrease preload, such as diuresis or epidural anesthesia. Invasive hemodynamic monitoring may be indicated to carefully tailor therapy (refer to "Bedside Hemodynamic Monitoring," p. 355).

In the immediate postpartum period, careful monitoring is essential because of the massive fluid shifts and large increases in cardiac output. Authorities recommend that optimal predelivery pulmonary artery occlusion pressures be maintained at 14 mm Hg or less to accommodate the increase in occlusion pressure of up to 16 mm Hg that can be associated in the immediate postpartum period.[11]

Aortic Stenosis. Aortic stenosis (AS) is often accompanied by other valvular disease, especially disease affecting the mitral valve. The hallmark of AS is decreased left ventricular ejection. Mild AS is usually well tolerated during pregnancy because of the natural hypervolemic state. Significant AS can produce left ventricular hypertrophy and dilation. Thromboembolic prophylaxis is advised. Critical to successful management is maintenance of cardiac output through prevention of hypovolemia, especially at the time of delivery. Any factor that diminishes venous return or produces hypotension worsens the effects of AS and significantly reduces cardiac output. The overall reported range for mortality is 17%.[11]

Tetralogy of Fallot. The four primary lesions associated with tetralogy of Fallot include VSD, overriding aorta, right ventricular hypertrophy, and pulmonary stenosis. Women with corrected tetralogy of Fallot generally can tolerate pregnancy well. Although rare, if the congenital anomalies are not corrected, maternal mortality and fetal complications increase significantly. Cardiopulmonary function must be maximized by measures including the treatment of dysrhythmias and the use of prophylaxis for endocarditis. Considerations during labor and delivery include maintenance of adequate preload and blood pressure.

Previous Myocardial Infarction. The outcome of the pregnant woman with previous myocardial damage depends on many factors. The length of time between the myocardial event and delivery is especially important. Increased myocardial oxygen demands during pregnancy must be considered, and therapy is usually supportive in nature. Careful attention to preload is essential to prevent burdening the heart and producing congestive failure (see "Heart Failure," p. 414).

Marfan Syndrome. Marfan syndrome is characterized by connective tissue weakness that can lead to aortic root and wall weakness. Mitral valve prolapse is commonly seen. Prognosis is based on aortic root diameter, with most authorities citing 4.0 cm as maximal, after which significant increases in mortality occur.[18-19] Prevention of tachydysrhythmias and hypertension is recommended, along with endocarditis prophylaxis. Beta-blockade therapy may be initiated for cardiac rate control and to decrease pressure on the weakened aortic wall. Goals of management include maintenance of cardiac output to meet physiologic needs without producing undue stress on the aortic wall. Careful blood pressure maintenance is essential. Differential diagnosis of chest and back pain is essential, along with recognition of other signs of aortic dissection (see "Aortic Dissection," p. 426).

Pulmonary Hypertension and Eisenmenger Syndrome. Pulmonary hypertension during pregnancy may be primary or idiopathic. Eisenmenger syndrome develops when, in the presence of a congenital left-to-right shunt (a result of ASD, VSD, or PDA), progressive pulmonary hypertension leads to shunt reversal or bidirectional shunting.[11] Regardless of the cause, the risk of sudden death because of pulmonary hypertension in pregnancy is 50%, and deaths have been reported up to 4 to 6 weeks postpartum.[18,20] Avoidance or termination of pregnancy is commonly recommended. If pregnancy is continued, therapeutic management is directed at avoidance of pulmonary vasoconstrictors, thromboembolism, and hypotension; maintenance of adequate preload and oxygenation; fetal surveillance; and reduction of stress at the time of delivery.

Coarctation of the Aorta. Coarctation of the aorta may occur in isolation or, most often, in combination with valvular or septal anomalies. Patients with uncomplicated coarctation of the aorta who are relatively asymptomatic (NYHA Class I or II) have demonstrated good prognosis and minimal risk of complications or death.[11] Intrapartal management focuses on the prevention of hypertension to avoid aortic wall stress. Careful management of fluid balance and left ventricular function must occur to prevent congestive heart failure and to promote adequate perfusion.

CARDIAC DISEASE ARISING DURING PREGNANCY

Peripartum Cardiomyopathy. Women who have no evidence of previous cardiac disease but have cardiac failure during the last month of pregnancy or within the first 6 months postpartum are considered to have peripartum cardiomyopathy. To confirm the diagnosis, other causes of cardiac failure must be ruled out. Peripartum cardiomyopathy accounts for less than 1% of all cardiac problems associated with pregnancy[23] and carries mortality ranging from 25% to 50%.[11] Controversy continues regarding exact etiologies of peripartum cardiomyopathy, with viral and immune etiologies the leading suspected causes.

Symptomatology is identical to classic cardiac failure, as is the treatment of rest, sodium and fluid restriction, inotropes, diuretics, and afterload reduction. Anticoagulation is commonly employed to prevent thromboembolism. Treatments specific to the suspected cause, such as immunosuppressive therapy, may be used as well.

Acute Myocardial Infarction. Although acute myocardial infarction (AMI) is rare during pregnancy, mortality ranges from 35% to 45%, depending on the timing of the myocardial event, with increased mortality if delivery occurs within 2 weeks of infarction.[22] The dramatic physiologic demands throughout pregnancy challenge the woman's cardiovascular system and can cause ischemia, leading to infarction. Clinical diagnostics are similar to those for standard AMI detection, although diagnosis must be made with consideration of the normal physiologic cardiovascular changes. Treatment of AMI during pregnancy is focused on balancing myocardial oxygen supply and demand. Management may include nitrate and/or beta-blockade therapy, cardiac monitoring, oxygen therapy, management of pain and anxiety, and afterload reduction. Special consideration is given to the maternal physiologic demands required during the labor and delivery processes. Operative delivery interventions, such as forceps or cesarean section, may be necessary (see "Myocardial Infarction," p. 439).

Shock. Shock is best defined as tissue hypoxia that is a result of decreased perfusion. Because pregnancy is a hyperdynamic, low-resistance state with increased oxygen delivery and consumption requirements, the management of shock in the pregnant patient necessitates a different approach than for the nonpregnant patient. Normal physiologic adaptations that occur during pregnancy alter ranges in vital signs and laboratory values. Frequently the clinician may be obtaining data from and managing two patients, both mother and fetus. Finally, there are causes for shock in pregnancy and immediately postpartum that must be considered in addition to routine causes (see "Shock," p. 1009.)

Hemorrhagic, septic, and cardiogenic shock are most commonly seen in pregnancy; neurogenic shock is an infrequent occurrence. Causes of hemorrhagic shock unique to pregnancy include abruptio placentae, ectopic pregnancy, placenta previa, and postpartum hemorrhage.[11] Postpartum hemorrhage can be attributed to uterine atony, genital tract lacerations, hematoma formation, retained placenta, and uterine prolapse.[11] Unique causes of septic shock in the pregnant patient include chorioamnionitis, septic abortion, and postpartum pyelonephritis.[11] Cardiogenic shock is most frequently a result of the presence of severe valve disease. Regardless of the cause, whether specific to pregnancy or not, the occurrence of shock requires aggressive intervention with treatment of the underlying cause.

Management of shock in pregnancy focuses on optimizing maternal stability in an effort to provide the most stable *in utero* environment. Clinical judgments include assessment of the risks and benefits of therapeutic interventions and fetal viability. Consideration must be given to the potential vasoconstrictive nature of some pharmacotherapeutics and the potential for uteroplacental insufficiency.

Resuscitation. The occurrence of cardiopulmonary arrest during pregnancy is relatively rare. Successful management of the pregnant patient requires integration of physiologic changes present during pregnancy and adaptations for those from standard resuscitative guidelines. Fetal outcomes are directly related to the mother's condition and well-being. The interrelationship between fetal and maternal well-being may present unique ethical dilemmas for health care providers and family members. Etiologies, predisposing factors, and accompanying rationale for cardiopulmonary arrest during pregnancy are summarized in Table 12-8.

Basic Cardiac Life Support. American Heart Association recommendations[23] include only minor deviations from usual procedure. Critically important is the facilitation of venous return. This is accomplished through lateral displacement of the uterus, either through manual manipulation or through use of a wedge under the woman's hip. Airway management includes early intubation, if possible, because of the increased physiologic demands for oxygen delivery and the increased risk of aspiration. Because of the hyperemic nature of pregnancy and the risk for bleeding, nasal intubation must be avoided. No differences are required in compression ratio or depth. Physiologic adaptations in pregnancy place the woman at greater risk for complications from cardiopulmonary resuscitation, such as fractured ribs and sternum, hemothorax, hemopericardium, and internal organ damage. Specific organs of concern include the uterus, the spleen, and the liver.

Evaluation of fetal tolerance of the mother's condition is essential during cardiopulmonary arrest. Fetal hypoxia may develop because of decreased uteroplacental perfusion. Fetal gestational age is a prime consideration when determining course of action. Before the twenty-fourth week of gestation, resuscitative efforts are focused primarily on maternal outcome. After the twenty-fourth week of gestation, evaluation includes both maternal and fetal response to resuscitative efforts. Emergent cesarean section may be undertaken for fetal distress or to improve maternal status, although consideration also must be given to the stress that cesarean section produces. In late pregnancy, maternal and fetal outcomes are enhanced if delivery is accomplished within 15 minutes of cardiac arrest.[24]

Advanced Cardiac Life Support. There are no specific alterations of advanced life support guidelines for resuscitation during pregnancy. Pharmacologic and electrical therapeutic interventions are carried out as usual, although there are minor considerations in the case of pregnancy. Epinephrine may decrease uteroplacental perfusion because of its vasoconstrictive nature; however, the benefits outweigh the risks of administration. Lidocaine crosses the placenta but in therapeutic levels does not have adverse fetal or uteroplacental effects. If maternal toxicity occurs, fetal cardiac and central nervous system depression may occur. Fetal bradycardia is associated with bretylium administration; therefore careful fetal monitoring is recommended. There are no contraindications for use of atropine in pregnancy. Administration of sodium bicarbonate is to be undertaken cautiously. Maternal acidosis increases uteroplacental adrenergic reactivity and must be avoided, although maternal alkalosis may impair oxygen exchange to the fetus. Electrical therapies such as defibrillation, cardioversion, and pacing are not contraindicated in pregnancy.

HYPERTENSIVE DISEASE

Hypertensive disease is a potentially life-threatening complication of pregnancy affecting 6% to 8% of all pregnancies,[25] is the second leading cause of death in childbearing women, and contributes to high rates of newborn morbidity and mortality.[11,26-28] Maternal complications include pathologic compromise of the cardiovascular, pulmonary, renal, neurologic, and hepatic systems[29-31] (Table 12-9). Current understanding of hypertensive disease in pregnancy is based on (1) a classification according to manifestations and time of onset in relation to gestation; (2) the fact that pregnancy can induce hypertension in women without a history of high blood pres-

Table 12-8	Etiology of Cardiopulmonary Arrest in Pregnancy
Cause	**Discussion**
Preexisting cardiac disease	Dramatic volume changes and cardiac output requirements may be greater than diseased heart's ability to tolerate
Acute cardiac disease	May occur during pregnancy in relation to increased myocardial demands
Pregnancy-induced hypertension	May induce multisystem dysfunction
Anaphylaxis/laryngeal edema	May occur as reaction to medications used to treat urinary infections
Preexisting asthma	Stress induced by pregnancy may compromise maternal ability to maintain adequate oxygenation
Aspiration pneumonia	May occur as a result of gastrointestinal sphincter incompetence
Pulmonary embolism	Hypercoagulable nature of pregnancy, venous stasis
Hypermagnesemia	Therapeutically used for seizure prevention, increased levels depress reflexes and may cause respiratory depression and subsequent arrest
Anesthesia	Complications from local, spinal, epidural, or general anesthesia used to facilitate delivery
Other causes	Sepsis, trauma, amniotic fluid embolism, drug overdose

Table 12-9	Complications of Hypertensive Disease in Pregnancy
Body System	**Complication**
Cardiovascular	Dysrhythmias, congestive heart failure, severe hypertension
Pulmonary	Pulmonary edema, acute airway obstruction
Renal	Oliguria, renal failure, acute tubular necrosis (ATN)
Neurologic	Cerebral edema, eclampsia, cerebral hemorrhage, coma
Hepatic	Necrosis, rupture, periportal and subcapsular hemorrhage
Hematologic	Disseminated intravascular coagulation (DIC), hemolysis thrombocytopenia

sure; and (3) the fact that elevated blood pressure in pregnancy can occur without the presence of generalized edema or proteinuria (transient hypertension). Proper diagnosis of hypertensive complications is critical and requires in-depth knowledge of disease pathophysiology to prevent or decrease the risk of maternal/fetal compromise.

CLASSIFICATION OF HYPERTENSION

The National Institutes of Health Working Group on High Blood Pressure has endorsed the classification and terminology of ACOG for hypertensive disease in pregnancy.[25,28,31] These definitions have proven useful in establishing consistent guidelines for pregnancy management[32]:

  I. Chronic hypertension: Hypertension before conception, or diagnosed before 20 weeks gestation
  II. Preeclampsia-eclampsia: Systemic syndrome of hypertensive disease with proteinuria diagnosed after 20 weeks' gestation. Eclampsia indicates the additional presence of convulsions.
  III. Preeclamsia superimposed on chronic hypertension: May be before 20 weeks or have sudden onset.
  IV. Gestational hypertension: Hypertension without proteinuria

PREECLAMPSIA

Preeclampsia is characterized by widespread physiologic changes including vasospasms in the arterial systems that result in endothelial damage, platelet aggregation, and decreased vascular volume. Current research suggests two stages of disease progression: alterations to placental perfusion (stage 1) and maternal syndrome

(stage 2).[33] The widespread arteriolar vasospasms result from abnormal sensitivity to vasoconstrictor substances of vascular smooth muscle, leading to injury of the endothelial lining. These generalized cyclic vasospasms lead to tissue ischemia and eventually end-organ dysfunction[30] (Fig. 12-2).

Patients with preeclampsia or chronic hypertension may have a significant decrease in circulating plasma volume as a result of damage done by vasospasms.[29] These vasospasms are the result of an imbalance of sensitivity to vasoconstrictive substances such as angiotensin II, prostacyclin, and thromboxane A_2.[34] It is theorized that patients with hypertensive disease have a higher cardiac output and lower systemic vascular resistance in early pregnancy, which precedes an elevation in blood pressure and the classic manifestations of preeclampsia. This theory suggests that patients progress from a high–cardiac output, low-resistance state to a low–cardiac output, high-resistance state, leading to multisystem organ dysfunction. Approximately 50% of all patients are intravascularly volume depleted, 30% demonstrate normal hemodynamic functioning, and the remaining 20% have intravascular volume overload.

Current research and a lack of randomized large trials show there may be no clear benefit of antihypertensive treatment for pregnant women with mild to moderate hypertension. Antihypertensive therapy is used to reduce arterial vasospasms and decrease blood pressure, reducing left ventricular workload and enhancing placental and renal perfusion. Hypertensive control also decreases the potential for maternal cerebral vascular accidents. The goal of antihypertensive therapy is to maintain diastolic pressures less than 90 mm Hg.[11,29] Methyldopa is the drug of choice for treating chronic hypertension during pregnancy. Vasodilators, such as Hydralazine, are the most common first-line medications used for management of hypertensive crisis. Betablockers, such as labetalol, are common second-line drugs when hypertension remains refractory to first-line management. Sodium nitroprusside is rarely used antepartally or intrapartally, but it may be administered to the severe preeclamptic-eclamptic patient when first-line drugs have failed. It's use is considered only when delivery is imminent or during the postpartum period, since thiocyanate is the metabolite. Nifedipine is a calcium channel blocker that must be used cautiously when given concurrently with magnesium sulfate ($MgSO_4$), because exaggerated hypotension may occur.

HEMOLYSIS, ELEVATED LIVER ENZYMES, LOW PLATELET SYNDROME

Hemolysis, elevated liver enzymes, low platelet (HELLP) syndrome is an associated syndrome that affects 4% to 12% of patients with severe preeclampsia-eclampsia.[11,35]

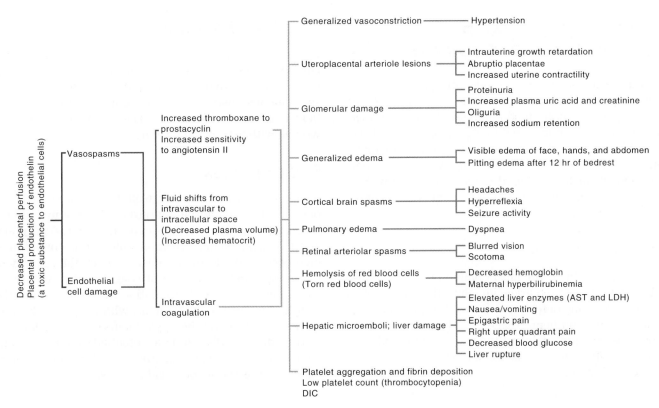

Fig. 12-2 Pathophysiologic changes of pregnancy-induced hypertension. *AST,* Aspartate aminotransferase (SGOT); *LDH,* lactic dehydrogenase; *DIC,* disseminated intravascular coagulation. (From Gilbert E, Harmon J: *Manual of high risk pregnancy and delivery,* ed 3, St Louis, 2003, Mosby.)

Patients are critically ill and may require invasive hemodynamic monitoring. Maternal mortality ranges from 3.5% to 24%, whereas perinatal mortality ranges from 10% to 60%[36-38] and is related to damage done by cyclic arterial vasospasms. Approximately 10% to 20% of pregnant patients with HELLP syndrome will not have elevated blood pressure diagnostic of hypertensive disease.[29] The clinical manifestations of HELLP syndrome may suggest a multitude of other clinical diagnoses. Misdiagnosis is common and may result in a delay of correct treatment. Therefore any pregnant woman demonstrating clinical manifestations must be diagnosed with HELLP syndrome. Complications of HELLP syndrome include abruptio placentae, liver hematoma, disseminated intravascular coagulation (DIC), pulmonary edema, liver rupture, and acute renal failure.[11]

The treatment goals of severe preeclampsia are to prevent seizures, decrease arterial spasms, and effect prompt delivery of the fetus. $MgSO_4$ is the standard treatment for prevention and control of seizure activity in preeclampsia-eclampsia. Typical anticonvulsant therapies such as phenytoin, phenobarbital, or diazepam are not used, because they address primarily neurologic dysfunction rather than vasospastic disease. Serum magnesium levels of 4 to 7 mEq/L are thought to be therapeutic for prevention of seizure activity. A loading dose of 4 to 6 g is given via infusion pump over 15 to 20 minutes, followed by a maintenance infusion of 2 to 3 g/hour.

Control of eclamptic seizures is accomplished through administration of 4 to 6 g of intravenous $MgSO_4$ over 5 to 10 minutes. This bolus is followed by a continuous infusion of 2 to 3 g/hour. If a patient has a recurrent seizure, another 2 to 4 g bolus can be given over 3 to 5 minutes. Occasionally, a patient will have continuing seizure activity in spite of magnesium therapy, necessitating intubation, ventilatory support, and consideration of delivery.[36,39]

Collaborative management for patients with severe preeclampsia-eclampsia or HELLP syndrome is key to the stabilization of mother and fetus. Continuous assessment of the cardiovascular, renal, central nervous, and pulmonary systems provides early indications of worsening maternal condition. Fetal surveillance may include continuous fetal monitoring, biophysical profile, and fetal lung maturity testing. Delivery of the fetus may be indicated because of maternal condition or presence of fetal compromise. The goal of the health care team is to accurately monitor ongoing organ system dysfunction and prevent further damage leading to end-organ failure and maternal-fetal mortality.

OBSTETRIC DISSEMINATED INTRAVASCULAR COAGULATION

Obstetric causes of DIC include abruptio placentae, preeclampsia-eclampsia, dead fetus syndrome, septic abortion, and amniotic fluid embolus. Pathophysiologic mechanisms are summarized in Fig. 12-3. Primary treatment goals include identification of the underlying disorder, removal of the trigger or initiating event, and volume replacement, including blood component therapy. Secondary treatment may include anticoagulation therapy (see Chapter 39).

ABRUPTIO PLACENTAE

Abruptio placentae is the most common obstetric cause of DIC. Of mothers experiencing abruption, 20% have a significant clotting defect, with 25% of this group experiencing postpartum hemorrhage.[29,40] The basic elements of treatment include delivery, the removal of blood clots from the uterus, blood component therapy, and fluid volume resuscitation.

DEAD FETUS SYNDROME

Dead fetus syndrome is consistent with a true chronic DIC condition. The onset is gradual over 2 to 4 weeks. Of women who experience fetal demise, 80% will have spontaneous onset of labor. Treatment of the stable patient is delivery of the fetus. Heparin may be used for women with associated coagulopathy.

SEPTIC ABORTION

Septic abortion is another well-documented cause of obstetric DIC. Bacterial endotoxins are the most likely initiating mechanism. The clinical findings of gram-negative septic shock are applicable to this condition. A high correlation seems to exist between the severity of the disease and the degree of coagulopathy. Aggressive antibiotic therapy and evacuation of the uterus are the frontline therapies for patients who are hemodynamically stable. Heparin therapy remains controversial.

Hypertensive disease is a potentially life-threatening complication of pregnancy, affecting 6% to 8% of all pregnancies[41]; it is the second leading cause of death in child-

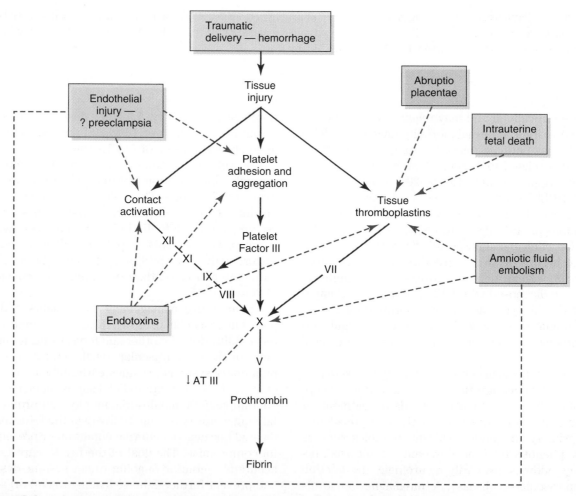

Fig. 12-3 Pathophysiologic mechanisms in obstetric disseminated intravascular coagulation (DIC). *AT,* Antithrombin. (From Clark S et al: *Handbook of critical care obstetrics,* Boston, 1994, Blackwell Scientific.)

bearing women and contributes to high rates of newborn morbidity and mortality.[11,26-28] Maternal complications include pathologic compromise of the cardiovascular, pulmonary, renal, neurologic, and hepatic systems[29,31] (Table 12-9). Current understanding of hypertensive disease in pregnancy is based on (1) a classification according to manifestations and time of onset in relation to gestation; (2) the fact that pregnancy can induce hypertension in women without a history of high blood pressure; and (3) the fact that elevated blood pressure in pregnancy can occur without the presence of generalized edema or proteinuria (transient hypertension). Proper diagnosis of hypertensive complications is critical and requires in-depth knowledge of disease pathophysiology to prevent or decrease the risk of maternal/fetal compromise.

PULMONARY DYSFUNCTION

Pulmonary dysfunction carries clinical significance because of the normally slightly hyperoxygenated condition associated with the physiologic changes in pregnancy. Compromise of respiratory function places both the mother and fetus at risk for harm. Maternal hypoxia can be the end result of several conditions, including pneumonia, asthma, trauma, acute respiratory distress syndrome (ARDS), and pulmonary embolism. Contributing factors (e.g., smoking, drug use, preexisting disease states), manifestations, and management differ very little from that which is seen in the nonpregnant individual. Common to these respiratory disorders is the issue of maternal-fetal hypoxia. Maternal hypoxia is defined by a PaO_2 less than 100 mm Hg, an SpO_2 less than 95%, a $PaCO_2$ greater than 35 mm Hg, a pH less than 7.40, and an SvO_2 less than 60%. Hyperventilation, shortness of breath, and dyspnea are commonly seen in pregnancy and must be differentiated from the usual maternal complaints.

ASTHMA

Although asthma often can be easily managed, it has previously been associated with an increased incidence of hyperemesis gravidarum, preeclampsia, chronic hypertension, preterm labor, perinatal mortality, spontaneous abortion, complicated labor, and low birth weight.[42,43] Ongoing studies indicate maternal and fetal outcomes are related to the severity of the disease and the degree of control achieved with medical management.[44] It is estimated that approximately one third of patients will experience no change in asthma symptoms, one third will see improvement, and one third will have worsening of symptoms. The peak incidence of asthma exacerbation is at 24 to 36 weeks' gestation and during labor, with relative improvement in the last month.[42] The lessening of asthma symptoms during pregnancy is the result of smooth muscle relaxation secondary to progesterone. Decreased

cell-mediated immunity and an increased level of corticosteroids may assist in diminishing the inflammatory response. Increased cyclic adenosine monophosphate (AMP) levels are also present and aid in maintaining an ongoing energy supply to cells. At the same time, other factors may contribute to worsening of symptoms. Nasal congestion, decreased functional residual volume, anxiety, noncompliance with medical regimens, stress, exercise, exposure to allergens, environmental irritants, respiratory infections, and smoking can contribute to exacerbation of asthma symptoms.[42,45] The decrease in cell-mediated immunity may predispose the mother to viral infections. Pregnancy in itself does not generally change peak flow rate.[42] Management recommendations include use of a peak flow meter twice a day to assist in objectively measuring maternal pulmonary function. If peak flow rates fall to 50% to 80% of the patient's norm, symptoms are reviewed and the management plan is reevaluated. Flow rates less than 50% of the patient's norm signal the need for rapid assessment and intervention.[44]

PNEUMONIA

Pneumonia can result from a variety of factors and is often associated with asthma. Exacerbations are more common in the second and third trimesters and are often associated with other maternal disease processes.[46] Prior respiratory disease, concurrent illness, tobacco use, and anemia have all been linked with an increased maternal risk of pneumonia. Physiologic changes of pregnancy decrease the mother's ability to clear secretions and place her at increased risk for gastric aspiration. The severity of aspiration correlates directly to aspirate amount, particulate content, and pH. Typically the pneumonia is of a bacterial origin; however, a variety of organisms can be seen. Some of the most common pathogens identified are *Streptococcus pneumoniae* (represents over 50% of bacterial pneumonias), *Staphylococcus aureus*, *Haemophilus influenzae*, *Mycoplasma*, *Chlamydia*, and influenza viruses.[42,43,46] Pregnant women experiencing a varicella infection have a 45% to 50% chance of developing varicella pneumonia, which carries a 35% to 40% mortality rate. *Pneumocystis carinii* pneumonia and resistant strains of tuberculosis are a growing concern, given that the majority of women who are human immunodeficiency virus–positive (HIV–positive) or have acquired immunodeficiency syndrome (AIDS) are in their reproductive years.

ACUTE RESPIRATORY DISTRESS SYNDROME

ARDS in pregnancy is often the result of a variety of conditions, including tocolytic administration (agents used to stop labor) leading to pulmonary edema, preeclampsia-eclampsia, abruptio placentae, postpartum hemorrhage, and amniotic fluid embolism (AFE). Some of the most common causes of ARDS in the perinatal patient are sepsis resulting from pyelonephritis, chorioamnionitis, IUFD, septic abortion, and postpartum endometritis. Women at risk for development of ARDS need to be assessed for early signs of worsening or changing dyspnea and tachypnea. As ARDS evolves, pulmonary function rapidly deteriorates over a 24-hour period. Symptoms, including diffuse or basilar rales, bilateral opacities on the chest x-ray, and a deteriorating PaO_2 with increasing FiO_2 demands, need to be excluded from other etiologies, such as fluid overload and cardiac failure that can sometimes be seen in the last trimester (see "Acute Lung Injury," p. 622).

Management of Respiratory Failure. Management of maternal hypoxia includes restoration and maintenance of the hypervolemic state without inducing fluid overload and further compromising cardiopulmonary function. Because colloidal osmotic pressure is decreased, great care must be taken to prevent the development of pulmonary edema when providing fluid replacement therapy. Oxygen is administered at a high flow rate via mask to achieve an optimal PaO_2 greater than 100 mm Hg and an SpO_2 greater than 95%. Noninvasive mechanical ventilation should be avoided or used with caution due to the risk of gastric aspiration.[42] If intubation is required, placement of an orotracheal tube is more desirable than a nasotracheal tube because of hyperemic nasal passageways. If nasotracheal intubation is required, the smallest tube possible that will still allow adequate ventilation is used. Gastric decompression is instituted with a small-bore nasogastric or orogastric tube. When initiating mechanical ventilation, the normal tachypnea, increased tidal volume (6 to 8 ml/kg lean body weight[43]), and decreased functional residual volume occurring in pregnancy should be considered when selecting settings. Caution must be taken to maintain the maternal $PaCO_2$ of 30 to 32 mm Hg, since respiratory alkalosis can lead to decreased uterine blood flow. Pulmonary compliance should be routinely assessed to evaluate the effectiveness of interventions. Pulmonary compliance may decrease from the normal average of 75 ml/cm H_2O to 20 ml/cm H_2O in severe ARDS.[11] Pharmacologic therapies must consider maternal-fetal risk and benefits. The Pharmacologic Management table summarizes obstetric concerns of common drugs used in pulmonary dysfunction.[42,43,45,46]

Pharmacologic Management: Pulmonary Dysfunction During Pregnancy

DRUG	CONSIDERATIONS
Antibiotics	Cephalosporins, erythromycin are generally well tolerated
	Sulfites should be avoided
	Vancomycin, aminoglycosides, tetracycline can lead to fetal toxicity
	Acyclovir improves maternal morbidity and appears to improve fetal outcomes
Inhaled corticosteroids	Beclomethasone generally considered safe
Systemic corticosteroids	Documentation of decreased birth weights and increase in small-for-date babies
	Majority of drug is metabolized by placental enzymes before entering fetal circulation
	Small amount of steroid may cross into breast milk, yet it is still considered safe to breastfeed
Nonsteroidal antiinflammatory drugs (NSAIDs)	Cromolyn and nedocromil are generally considered safe
	Not associated with increased risks to fetus
Adrenergic agonists	Epinephrine and isoproterenol may contribute to maternal-fetal tachycardia
	Albuterol and terbutaline have fewer side effects and may have the additional benefit of tocolytic actions
Leukotriene receptor antagonist	Appears to be safe for management of chronic mild to moderate asthma
Theophylline	Not commonly used because of maternal side effects
	Recommended that serum levels be maintained between 5 and 12 mg/ml to prevent complications of toxicity
Analgesics	Morphine and meperidine should be avoided in active labor since they can worsen bronchospasm
	Will cross the placenta and should be considered when completing a fetal assessment
	Fentanyl may be a better agent to use
	Epidural analgesia is considered safe
Beta-mimetic tocolytics	Contraindicated since can worsen maternal lung damage
Labor induction	Oxytocin is the drug of choice
	Prostaglandin F_2 should be avoided since it is a bronchoconstrictor
Neuromuscular blockade	Can be administered safely as long as peripheral nerve testing is conducted to monitor drug dosages
	Will cross the placenta, and this should be considered when assessing fetal activity

PULMONARY EMBOLISM

Thromboembolic disorders including pulmonary embolism (PE) occur secondary to a variety of reasons, many of which are related to the physiologic changes in pregnancy. Also of consideration is the increasing frequency of long term bedrest for high-order multiple pregnancies, premature labor, and other high-risk conditions. The greatest risk for developing PE is in the immediate postpartum period, especially if a C-section was performed. Two thirds of the patients who die from PE expire within 30 minutes of the initial event. Assessment, management, and complications associated with PE are essentially no different from those of the nonpregnant woman; however, differential diagnosis of anaphylactoid syndrome of pregnancy must be considered. Heparin is administered initially intravenously and then subcutaneously for the remainder of the pregnancy, since warfarin sodium derivatives are known fetal teratogens that readily cross the placenta. Unfractionated heparin does not cross the placenta or become excreted in breast milk, and low–molecular weight heparin does not cross the placenta.[47,48] Heparin induced thrombocytopenia (HIT) is a serious complication and has been estimated to occur in 1% to 30% of patients receiving heparin.[47] A vena caval filter may be implanted, but a suprarenal position is selected to prevent restriction of venous blood coming from the left ovary and draining into the left renal vein (see "Pulmonary Embolism," p. 635).

ANAPHYLACTOID SYNDROME OF PREGNANCY

Anaphylactoid syndrome of pregnancy was previously known as amniotic fluid embolism (AFE). The National Amniotic Fluid Embolus Registry data suggests the process is more comparable to anaphylaxis than embolism. ASP/AFE is rare, yet it is associated with mortality rates of 60% to 70% and is the leading maternal cause of death.[49-51] The most common precipitating factors associated with the syndrome are a large fetus, multiparity, premature separation of the placenta, IUFD, tumultuous labor, and small tears in the endocervical veins that may occur during normal labor.[52,53] Placental abruption is seen in almost half the cases, with fetal death having occurred before the event.[53]

Sudden onset of symptoms during or immediately after delivery can lead to the suspicion of ASP/AFE. Acute respiratory distress, shock out of proportion to blood loss, chills, fever, shivering, sweating, and cardiovascular collapse are observed. In a small percentage of patients a grand mal seizure may be the initial symptom. Pulmonary edema is present and is followed by acute cardiovascular collapse. Chest pain and bronchospasm are uncommon. More then 50% of patients die within the first hour, and 40% of survivors develop DIC.[49,53]

Diagnosis is confirmed by the presence of fetal squamous cells, lanugo, vernix caseosa, meconium, and mucin in blood aspirated from the pulmonary artery. Chest x-rays may show pulmonary edema, effusions, and cardiac enlargement. Management consists of maintaining oxygenation and supporting cardiac function. Inotropic support is provided, fluids are replaced, and blood components are administered. Other therapies such as low-dose heparin, bronchodilators, and steroids may also be used.

TRAUMA

Trauma in the pregnant woman is the leading cause of nonobstetric death; it has been estimated to be around 6% to 7%, although a precise number is difficult to obtain since injuries can range from minor to life threatening.[50,54,55] The primary cause of trauma is motor vehicle accidents. Domestic violence should also be considered when blunt trauma is seen, especially to younger patients, or injuries involving the face, head, abdomen or breasts.[56,57] It may be difficult to differentiate between damage occurring as a result of an accidental fall and that of having been pushed or struck; therefore the patient should be carefully interviewed. Reports of violence were more likely to be associated with alcohol consumption, smoking, inadequate prenatal care (contributing to low birth weight), as well as a history of a fetal death and previous induced and/or spontaneous abortion.[57] Burn injuries are uncommon. The severity of maternal total body surface area (TBSA) of thermal injury correlates with fetal outcomes.[55] Approximately 10% of injuries occur in the first trimester, 40% occur in the second trimester, and 50% occur in the third trimester.[59] As women continue to work late into their pregnancies and become involved in higher-risk activities, the type and severity of injuries may begin to increase. Mechanisms that produce injuries in pregnant patients are no different from those that injure nonpregnant women.

Management of trauma during pregnancy and in the first 6 weeks postpartum is essentially, with a few exceptions, no different from the management of trauma for any other patient (see Chapter 37). Normal physiologic changes associated with pregnancy may mask assessment findings and therefore affect decisions about interventions that are provided (Table 12-10). It is recommended that any pregnant woman beyond 22 to 24 weeks' gestation who experiences trauma should receive at least 4 hours of fetal monitoring. A critical point to remember is that the first priority is to provide whatever interventions would normally be provided to the nonpregnant woman, with the goal being to keep the mother alive. Keeping the mother alive is the best thing that can be done for the fetus, even though some of the

Table 12-10	Initial Assessment and Management of Obstetric Trauma
Assessment	**Management/Rationale**

PRIMARY SURVEY

AIRWAY

Signs of obstruction

Same as for nonpregnant patient	Remove visible debris with caution because of ↑ hyperemia of nasal/oral area
	Decrease risk of aspiration (because of enlarged uterus and effects of progesterone) by lateral tile or by inserting NG/OG tube
	Emergency cricoid thyrotomy/tracheotomy, if performed, is done above usual site because of upward displacement of thoracic structures

BREATHING

Signs of ineffective respiration

Same as for nonpregnant patient with exception of the following: ABGs: Spo$_2$ <95 Pao$_2$ <100 mm Hg Pco$_2$ >30 mm Hg pH <7.40 Tidal volume <800 ml Labored respirations RR <20 beats/min or >24 beats/min	100% oxygen by mask since passages tend to be hyperemic and there is tendency for breathing through mouth
	Elevate HOB if possible to decrease pressure on thoracic structures caused by elevated diaphragm
	Oral intubation using smaller size (5.5-7.0 Fr) endotracheal tubes to ↓ risk of bleeding caused by ↑ vascularity of area
	Gastric decompression with OGT (or small NGT if pt. does not tolerate OGT placement) since prone to ileus and gastric reflux
	Physiologic monitoring (RR, Spo2, Etco$_2$)
	Obtain ABGs, CXR
	Emergent needle decompression/chest tube insertion for hemopneumothorax. May need to reassess entry point because of upward/outward displacement of thorax

CIRCULATION

Signs of ineffective circulation

Same as for nonpregnant patient with exception of the following: SBP <100 mm Hg MAP <60 mm Hg CVP <4 mm Hg Pale, moist, cool skin	DPL can be performed; open technique is usually preferred
	Assess for possible placental abruption
	Normally hypervolemic, skin is warm and slightly moist because of progesterone and may mask signs of hypoperfusion
	CVC or large-bone IV access upper extremity sites because of potential for impeded venous return from lower extremities
	Fluid resuscitation
	LR—recommended since has potential to metabolize into bicarbonate via intrinsic body pathways; cannot administer blood products through same IV line
	0.9 NS—can administer blood products through line; may decrease risk of developing maternal alkalosis (as compared with LR)
	O-negative blood—can be given until type/cross done
	Replace 3 ml per 1 ml of blood lost to compensate for hypervolemia associated with pregnancy
	Use caution because of ↑ risk of pulmonary edema caused by ↓ colloidal osmotic pressure
	May apply MAST but DO NOT inflate abdominal compartment
	Tilt to side, even if on back board, to maximize venous return

SECONDARY SURVEY

FOCUSED OB HISTORY

Gestational age	Keep mother alive
Single vs. multiple pregnancy	Keep baby where it is
Number of pregnancies, live births, abortions	Vaginal examination to determine fetal presentation, status of amniotic membrane, presence of fetal parts or umbilical cord in vagina
Name of obstetrician	Avoid manipulating cord → spasms
Rh factor	Emergent delivery vaginal vs. cesarean; live vs. perimortem
Prenatal complications	

ABGs, Arterial blood gases; *bpm,* breaths per minute; *BUN,* blood urea nitrogen; *CBC,* complete blood count; *CVC,* central venous catheter; *CVP,* central venous pressure; *CXR,* chest x-ray; *DPL,* diagnostic peritoneal lavage; *ECG,* electrocardiogram; *Etco$_2$,* end tidal CO; *FHR,* fetal heart rate; *Hct,* hematocrit; *Hg,* hemoglobin; *HOB,* head of bed; *IV,* intravenous; *LR,* lactated Ringer's; *MAP,* mean arterial pressure; *MAST,* military antishock trousers; *Na+,* sodium; *NG,* nasogastric; *NGT,* nasogastric tube; *NS,* normal saline; *OB,* Obstetric; *OG,* orogastric; *OGT,* orogastric tube; *RBC,* red blood cell; *RR,* respiration rate; *SBP,* systolic blood pressure; *WBC,* white blood cell.

Table 12-10	Initial Assessment and Management of Obstetric Trauma—cont'd
Assessment	Management/Rationale

SECONDARY SURVEY—CONT'D
FOCUSED OB HISTORY—CONT'D
Past vaginal drainage, bleeding, clots
Past abdominal pain/uterine contractions

MATERNAL STUDIES
Unexpected diagnostic study results

CBC	Insert urinary Foley catheter with caution—risk of bleeding because of ↑ pelvic vascularity; consider using a smaller size catheter
WBC >18,000/mm³	
RBC <6,500,000/mm³	Consider significance of positive toxicity results—is the fetus at risk for issues such as drug withdrawal or fetal alcohol syndrome?
Hg <12 g/dl	
Hct <32%	Hct/Hg values that are below those identified may put both the mother and fetus at risk for hypoxia
Platelets <200,000/mm³	
Fibrinogen >400 mg/dl	Use caution when performing rectal examination to assist in determining fetal position/traumatic damage—pelvic vascular congestion contributes to development of hemorrhoids and predisposes mother to bleeding from this site
Chemistries:	
BUN <9 mg/dl	
Creatinine >0.5 mg/dl	Obtain radiologic studies as needed; however, implement measures to decrease risk to fetus
Na⁺ slight ↑	
Glucose slight ↓	May see left axis deviation on 12-lead ECG as a normal variant

FETAL STUDIES
Signs of fetal distress

FHR <100-110	Ultrasound to elevate fetus
Nonreassuring patterns on fetal monitor	Assess fundal height, firmness, contractions, q30min
Fundal height not appropriate for gestational age	Fetal monitoring (with pocket Doppler, ultrasound, or fetal monitor) as allowed based on interventions provided to mother
Vaginal drainage, bleeding, clots present	Differentiate uterine pain/contractions from other sources of abdominal pain
Abdominal pain/uterine firmness/contractions present	Administer tocolytics as needed
Amniocentesis:	L/S ratio and presence of PG to determine fetal lung maturity
Presence of RBCs	Kleihauer-Betke: indicates a break in the integrity of placental circulation if fetal cells are present
Lecithin/sphingomyelin (L/S) ratio and presence of phosphatidylgycerol (PG)	
Kleihauer-Betke test to detect presence of fetal blood in maternal bloodstream	

TERTIARY SURVEY

ASPECT OF CARE	PURPOSE
Administer "follow up meds"	Prophylactic measures:
	Antibiotics—choose broad-spectrum, nonteratogenic agents
	Tetanus toxoid—does not cross placenta
	Rh-negative mothers:
	Can become Rh immunized within 72 hrs
	Administer Rh₀ (D) immune globulin (RhoGAM) (300 mcg/15 ml fetal blood) if:
	Possibility of mother having received Rh-positive blood
	Breach in integrity of the placenta of an Rh-positive fetus as evidenced by positive Kleihauer-Betke test

interventions may produce transient alterations in fetal blood flow. Hesitation in providing necessary interventions increases the risk of harming both the mother and fetus. An exception to this situation may occur after the fetus has reached the state of viability and the mother is at risk for immediate demise. In this situation it may be decided to perform an emergent cesarean section to save the infant. To achieve the most optimal fetal outcome, a perimortem C-section should be performed within 4 to 5 minutes in a patient who is unresponsive to cardiopulmonary resuscitation (CPR).[11,55,59,60] Removal of the fetus may also increase the potential survival of the mother by relieving fetal compression of the aorta and vena cava thereby improving venous return and cardiac output, increasing in intravascular volume secondary to uterine autotransfusion, enhancing more effective chest compressions and improving the functional residual capacity.[60]

TYPES OF INJURIES

Types of injuries can vary with the stage of pregnancy. In the first trimester, common injuries are associated with falls resulting from fainting from fatigue, hypoglycemia, and normal physiologic changes. The fetus is usually well protected from external trauma, since the uterus is located within the pelvis and is protected by bony structures. In the second trimester, as the enlarging uterus expands up out of the pelvis, maternal abdominal organs are displaced upward and laterally. Some protection is provided to the maternal abdominal organs, since the uterus/fetus now occupies much of the abdominal cavity; however, the growing fetus becomes more vulnerable to injury. By the third trimester the fetus has begun to settle into the pelvis in preparation for birth. Hyperventilation and fainting are common as the fetus grows and places greater metabolic demands on the mother. As relaxin secretion increases, the end effect of relaxed pelvis ligaments can lead to lordosis and pelvic tilt. This produces a change in gait and in the center of gravity/balance, which can increase the risk of falls.

SPECIFIC BODY SYSTEM INJURIES

Cardiovascular. Manifestations related to cardiovascular injury may be masked because of normal physiologic changes in pregnancy. The hypervolemic, low systemic–resistance state that occurs during pregnancy can mask shock, since significant blood volume can be lost before the classical manifestations are seen.[11,61] Lower extremity wounds may bleed more vigorously than might be expected because of venous congestion of the lower extremities.

Pulmonary. The most commonly fractured ribs are the middle ribs (5 through 9). The upper ribs (1 through 4) are associated with potential damage to the great vessels and the spine. The lower ribs (10 through 12) are as-

sociated with diaphragmatic, liver, and spleen damages. It should be taken into consideration that as pregnancy progresses, the anteroposterior diameter of the chest increases, the length decreases, and abdominal organs shift.

Neurologic. Spinal cord injury (SCI) in pregnancy may be either acute (as the result of recent trauma) or may be chronic (due to preexisting damage). Initial management of acute SCI is the same as for nonpregnant patients, including the administration of steroids. Adequate uterine perfusion can be evaluated by observing for a reassuring fetal heart rate tracing and lack of uterine contractions.[62] SCI patients, as are pregnant women, are at high risk for development of deep vein thrombosis, which necessitates the provision of prophylactic anticoagulation. Vaginal delivery is possible; however, patients with injuries above T6 are more likely to develop autonomic dysreflexia (ADR) and therefore may require assisted vaginal delivery or a C-section.[62,63] Disruption of autonomic nervous system activity is not associated with labor dysfunction. Uterine sensory nerves enter the spinal cord at T11 to L1; therefore women with SCI above T10 are unable to feel uterine contractions. They must rely on uterine palpation and symptoms such as shortness or breath and abdominal/leg spasms. Epidural anesthesia in early labor may be provided, since uterine contractions are associated with ADR. If severe irreversible brain damage or maternal brain death occurs, it is possible that the fetus may remain viable and continue to develop in utero. The issue of pregnancy maintenance in an irreversibly brain-damaged or brain-dead mother remains a controversial ethical issue.

Abdomen/Pelvis. Failure to wear or improper use of seat belts can lead to blunt abdominal injury. Penetrating abdominal injuries are also seen, with gunshot and stab wounds being the most common causes of abdominal injury. The engorgement of pelvic vasculature increases the risk of retroperitoneal hemorrhage after lower abdominal trauma. Because the uterus displaces maternal abdominal structures, the traditional assessment findings and sites of referred pain may be altered. Diagnostic peritoneal lavage (DPL) may be performed; however, a supraumbilical site (if uterus is palpable above the pubis) using the open technique using direct visualization is preferred. The use of ultrasound to detect intraperitoneal fluid/hematoma can be used in place of DPL. Peritoneal signs such as tenderness, rigidity, and rebound tenderness are unreliable indicators because of stretching of the abdominal wall. Bowel sounds may be absent, since pregnant women are prone to ileus. All of these factors can contribute to delayed detection of abdominal injuries. Pelvic fractures can potentially injure the reproductive and urinary structures, although pelvic injury is not an absolute contraindication to vaginal delivery. Additional studies must be obtained before a final decision is made.

Reproductive System. Until 12 weeks' gestation the uterus is a pelvic organ. As the uterus enlarges, it can assist in protecting other organs but it becomes more vulnerable to injury. Direct trauma to the uterus/placenta reverses protective hemostasis by releasing an increased concentration of placental thromboplastin, a plasminogen activator, from the myometrium. The uteroplacental bed functions as a dilated, passive, low-resistance system that lacks autoregulation and therefore has few, if any, compensatory mechanisms. The body perceives the uterus as a peripheral or nonvital organ. Because the uteroplacental system receives 20% to 30% of maternal cardiac output, maintenance of adequate circulating blood volume is essential to ensure adequate blood flow. The abdomen must be palpated to assess uterine position, size, and firmness; the presence of contractions; and the fetal position. Abruptio placentae, commonly seen with pelvic fractures, may occur immediately, within 48 hours, or up to 5 days after injury. Uterine damage/rupture is rare, but if it occurs, it is commonly at the fundus or the site of a previous cesarean section and almost always results in fetal death. Even if there was no identifiable damage to the reproductive system, there may be an increased risk for premature rupture of membranes (PROM), premature labor, fetal/maternal hemorrhage, or fetal damage or demise. It is generally recommended that pregnant patients with trauma be admitted to the hospital for 24 to 48 hours of fetal monitoring, since there may be latent injuries or the need for tocolytics.

Fetal Injuries. The fetus is usually well cushioned by amniotic fluid, the gravid uterus, and the abdominal wall, which all serve to distribute the force of injury. The most common cause of fetal death is maternal death. Placental abruption and fetal skull fracture, secondary to engagement of the fetal head into the pelvis, and intracranial hemorrhage have been identified as leading causes of fetal death. Potential predictors of fetal demise vary, depending on the study. Increased injury severity score (ISS), decreased hemoglobin level, need for blood replacement, presence of DIC, and abruptio placentae have been associated with increased fetal mortality.

NEUROLOGIC DYSFUNCTION

No known neurologic changes are associated with pregnancy, yet women may have preexisting neurologic conditions. There are a large variety of neurologic conditions (see Chapter 27), but only those conditions associated with the potential to place the mother and fetus at risk are discussed in this chapter.

EPILEPSY

Some of the most common maternal neurologic disorders are seizures, although seizures do not appear to increase the risk of pregnancy-induced hypertension (PIH), premature delivery, or other common complications. The frequency of seizures during pregnancy, with preexisting epilepsy, has been known to increase by 30% to 50%.[64-66] This is thought to be a result of reduced plasma concentrations and altered pharmacokinetics secondary to impaired absorption. Failure to adjust drug doses to compensate for increased maternal vascular volume, electrolyte changes, increased renal clearance, hormonal changes that alter hepatic enzyme systems responsible for drug metabolism, respiratory alkalosis, sleep deprivation, which lowers the seizure threshold, and noncompliance with medical regimen because of nausea, vomiting, or fear of harming the fetus have all been identified as increasing the risk of seizure activity.[64,66,67] Efforts must be made to differentiate neurologic etiologies (i.e., epileptic) from nonneurologic etiologies (e.g., PIH), since management is significantly different. The major goals in managing the epileptic patient are to keep the mother seizure-free and to minimize the risk of fetal teratogenic effects from anticonvulsant medications. Discontinuing anticonvulsant drugs should be considered if the electroencephalogram (EEG) shows lack of ectopic activity and if the patient has been seizure-free on long-term, low-dose drugs. Discontinuing medications must be carefully balanced against the potential development of seizures, since fetal damage resulting from hypoxia during seizures can occur.

Management focuses on identifying the minimal drug dose required to prevent seizures and drugs that pose the least risk for fetal harm. Although most anticonvulsant drugs have been associated with fetal abnormalities, studies have shown that 95% of fetuses are unaffected.[64] Because anticonvulsants interfere with folic acid metabolism, which can lead to maternal macrocytic anemia and fetal neural tube defects, folic acid supplements should be given. Polypharmacotherapy with multiple anticonvulsant agents must be avoided since this practice is associated with an increased risk of fetal damage. During the last month of pregnancy, supplemental vitamin K may be administered to protect the newborn against bleeding caused by vitamin K depletion.[64,65] As maternal physiology gradually returns to the nonpregnant state, drug doses may need to be reduced in the first 2 to 3 weeks postpartum.[64]

INTRACRANIAL HEMORRHAGE

The most common cause of intracranial hemorrhage (ICH) in pregnancy is subarachnoid hemorrhage secondary to a ruptured cerebral aneurysm or arteriovenous malformation.[11] Mortality rates for pregnant patients with ICH are estimated to be 30% to 40%.[11,65] Patients with PIH and associated ICH may account for as many as 60% of deaths associated with eclampsia.[29] Although it has been theorized that physiologic changes of pregnancy place increased strain on previously weakened cerebral vessels, clinical data have not supported this. Management of ICH is only slightly different in the pregnant patient. Hypotensive agents such as sodium nitro-

CLINICAL APPLICATION

Critical Care Obstetric Concepts

Mrs. B is a 35-year-old G8, P5, AB2 woman at 35 weeks' gestation admitted to rule out a deep vein thrombosis in her right lower extremity. Significant medical history includes eye surgery at age 15 for detached retina, legally blind, and Marfan syndrome. Current medications include metoprolol (Lopressor), ferrous sulfate, prenatal vitamins, and eyedrops. Peripheral Doppler studies were negative. Cardiac ultrasound documented mild aortic insufficiency and mitral regurgitation and an aortic root diameter of 4.8 cm without evidence of dissection. A non–stress test (NST) revealed fetal heart tone (FHT) of 140s to 150s with good variability.

1. What are the priorities in the care of Mrs. B?
2. What referrals would be necessary to manage Mrs. B's care?

   An amniocentesis completed 11 days after admission revealed fetal maturity. A 6 lb, 9 oz baby girl was delivered by cesarean section with Apgar scores of 8 and 9 at 1 and 5 minutes. Epidural anesthesia was used, and Mrs. B experienced an uneventful postoperative recovery. At 24 hours after surgery, Mrs. B experienced severe chest pain.
3. What differential diagnoses should be considered?

   Mrs. B underwent emergent aortic repair, aortic valve replacement, and reimplantation of coronary arteries and was transferred to the critical care unit postoperatively.

Her assessment in the immediate postoperative period included the following: temp = 34.6° C; HR = 118; RR = 8; BP = 103/66; SaO_2 = 98%; CO = 3.2 L/minute; SVR = 1582 dynes/sec/cm^{-5}; SvO_2 = 43%; PAP = 28/16 mm Hg; and PAWP = 14 mm Hg. Arterial blood gas values were the following: pH = 7.40; PCO_2 = 40 mm Hg; PO_2 = 122 mm Hg; bicarbonate = 24 mEq/L; and O_2 saturation = 98%. Mrs. B.'s mechanical ventilator settings are FiO_2 = 50%; TV = 800; AC = 8; and PEEP = +5.

4. Evaluate Mrs. B's immediate postoperative status. What are the initial priorities?
5. Normal values for vital signs and laboratory values change with pregnancy. How long after delivery should the values associated with pregnancy be used rather than the usual normal values?

   Mrs. B was started on dopamine and dobutamine drips to support cardiac output. Arrangements were made for Mrs. B's baby girl to visit her. Mrs. B had previously expressed the desire to breastfeed her infant.
6. What nursing measures are necessary to support Mrs. B's maternal experience?

   Two days after surgery, Mrs. B was weaned from the ventilator, extubated, and placed on 6 L of nasal oxygen. She was still requiring dobutamine and dopamine drips for cardiac support.
7. What are the next priorities in Mrs. B's care?

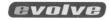 For the discussion of this Clinical Application and for an additional clinical application on critical care obstetric concepts, see the Evolve website.

---

prusside are commonly used to maintain the blood pressure within a desired range but must be used with great caution if the patient has not yet delivered. Hypotension and toxic effects of nitroprusside can pose significant risk to the fetus.

MYASTHENIA GRAVIS

The few studies that have been conducted on patients with myasthenia gravis (MG) suggest that two thirds of patients will experience either no change or an improvement in their condition during pregnancy.[67-70] MG may first manifest itself during pregnancy or in the postpartum period.[71] Postpartum exacerbations are relatively common; therefore routine physician follow-up every 2 weeks for the first 6 weeks is recommended. Management during pregnancy should be the same as when the patient is not pregnant, although interventions may be required in the second stage of labor when the abdominal muscles are required for pushing. Past studies have shown that the presence of MG is associated with higher occurrence of delivery complications necessitating the interventions such as forceps, vacuum-assisted delivery,

and C-section if the mother cannot effectively push with contractions.[72] There is increased maternal sensitivity to medications such as narcotics, central nervous system (CNS) depressants, neuromuscular blockers, some anesthetics, and tocolytic agents. A myasthenic crisis may occur if magnesium sulfate is administered. Epidural medications may be safely used to decrease pain and fatigue during labor. Critical respiratory muscle fatigue is best assessed by measurement of the forced vital capacity.[71] Maternal antibodies to neurotransmitters may cross the placenta and cause the fetus to have transient symptoms of MG, manifested by respiratory depression, poor tone, weak cry, and poor sucking; however, these symptoms spontaneously subside in 2 to 4 weeks.[70,72,73]

SUMMARY

Caring for the critically ill obstetric patient presents multiple challenges. Obstetric patients may be critically ill secondary to preexisting disease or the advent of critical illness or injury during pregnancy (see the Clinical Application feature). Central to optimal care is the persistent application of physiologic changes of pregnancy to normal adult values. It must be remembered that symptomatology may be altered because of the pregnant state. Understanding the intricate maternal-fetal relationship provides practitioners with a focus of maintaining maternal stability to enhance uteroplacental perfusion and an optimal *in utero* environment. All potential therapeutic interventions must be weighed in light of the risk:benefit ratio to maternal-fetal status. Critical situations may bring personal, cultural, social, spiritual, and/or ethical values into conflict. Decision making must be done in collaboration with family and health care team members, and all options should be considered. Finally, determining an appropriate environment for care can be a challenge. Some institutions have created dedicated obstetric intensive care units, whereas others provide care in either the obstetric care unit or critical care unit. Regardless of the location, the key factor is collaboration among specialties to optimize maternal-fetal outcomes and facilitate the family experience.

REFERENCES

1. Niebyl J: Teratology and drugs in pregnancy. In Scott JR et al, editors: *Danforth's obstetrics and gynecology*, ed 9, Philadelphia, 2003, Lippincott.
2. DiSaia PJ: Radiation therapy in gynecology. In Scott JR et al, editors: *Danforth's obstetrics and gynecology*, ed 9, Philadelphia, 2003, Lippincott.
3. Harrison BP, Crytal CS: Imaging modalities in obstetrics and gynecology, *Emerg Med Clin North Am* 21:711-735, 2003.
4. Goodsitt MM, Christodoulou EG: Imaging safety in the fetus. In Pearlman MD, Tintinalli JE, editors: *Emergency care of the woman*, New York, 1998, McGraw Hill.
5. VanHook JW: Trauma in pregnancy, *Clin Obstet Gynecol* 45(2):414-424, 2002.
6. Briggs G, Freeman R, Yaffe S: *Drugs in pregnancy and lactation*, ed 5, Baltimore, 1998, Williams & Wilkins.
7. Riordan J, Auerbach K: *Breastfeeding and human lactation*, ed 2, Boston, 1999, Jones & Bartlett.
8. May K, Mahlmeister L: *Maternal and neonatal nursing: family-centered care*, ed 3, Philadelphia, 1994, Lippincott.
9. Cunningham FG et al: *Williams' obstetrics*, ed 20, Norwalk, Conn, 1997, Appleton & Lange.
10. Harvey MG: Physiologic changes of pregnancy. In Harvey CJ: *Critical care obstetrical nursing*, Gaithersburg, Md, 1991, Aspen.
11. Dildy G et al, editors: *Critical care obstetrics*, ed 4, Malden, Mass, 2004, Blackwell.
12. American College of Obstetricians and Gynecologists: *Invasive hemodynamic monitoring in obstetrics and gynecology*, Technical Bulletin 121, 1988.
13. Clark S et al: Central hemodynamic observations in normal third trimester pregnancy, *Am J Obstet Gynecol* 161:1439-1442, 1989.
14. Monga M, Creasy R: Cardiovascular and renal adaptation to pregnancy. In Creasy R, Resnik R, editors: *Maternal-fetal medicine*, ed 4, Philadelphia, 1999, Saunders.
15. Troiano NH: Cardiac diseases in pregnancy. In Mandeville LK, Troiano NH, editors: *High-risk intrapartum nursing*, Philadelphia, 1999, Lippincott.
16. Criteria Committee of the New York Heart Association: *Nomenclature and criteria for diagnosis of disease of the heart and great vessels*, ed 6, Boston, 1964, Little, Brown.
17. American College of Obstetricians and Gynecologists: *Cardiac disease in pregnancy*, Technical Bulletin 168, 1992.
18. Jelsema R, Cotton D: Cardiac disease. In James DK et al, editors: *High risk pregnancy: management options*, ed 2, Philadelphia, 1999, Saunders.
19. Rutherford JD, Hands M: Pregnancy with preexisting heart disease. In Douglas PS, editor: *Cardiovascular health and disease in women*, Philadelphia, 1993, Saunders.
20. Shabetai R: Cardiac disease. In Creasy R, Resnik R, editors: *Maternal-fetal medicine*, ed 4, Philadelphia, 1999, Saunders.
21. Reference deleted in proofs.
22. Clark SL: Cardiac disease in pregnancy, *Am J Obstet Gynecol* 19:237-253, 1987.
23. American Heart Association: *Textbook of advanced cardiac life support*, Dallas, 1994, The Association.
24. Luppi CJ: Cardiopulmonary resuscitation in pregnancy. In Mandeville LK, Troiano NH, editors: *High-risk intrapartum nursing*, Philadelphia, 1999, Lippincott.
25. National High Blood Pressure in Pregnancy Education Program Working Group: *Working group report on high blood pressure in pregnancy*, 2000, (NHBPEP) Publication.
26. Berg CJ et al: Pregnancy-related mortality in the United States, 1987-1990, *Obstet Gynecol* 88:161-167, 1996.
27. Grimes DA: The morbidity and mortality of pregnancy: still risky business, *Am J Obstet Gynecol* May 170(5pt2):1489-1494, 1994.
28. American College of Obstetricians and Gynecologists: *Invasive hemodynamic monitoring in obstetrics and gynecology*, Technical Bulletin 219, 1996.
29. Clark S et al: *Handbook of critical care obstetrics*, Boston, 1994, Blackwell Scientific.
30. Gilbert E, Harmon J: *Manual of high risk pregnancy and delivery*, ed 3, St Louis, 2003, Mosby.
31. Peters RM, Flack JM: Hypertensive disorders of pregnancy, *J Obstet Gynecol Neonatal Nurs* 33(2):209-214, 2004.
32. American College of Obstetricians and Gynecologists: *Hypertension in pregnancy.* (ACOG Practice Bulletin No 29). Washington, DC, 2001, The College.
33. Roberts JM et al: Summary of the NHLBI Working Group on research on hypertension in pregnancy, *Hypertension* 41: 437-445, 2003.
34. Walsh S: Preeclampsia: an imbalance in placental prostacyclin and thromboxane production, *Am J Obstet Gynecol* 152:335-340, 1985.
35. Leicht TG, Harvey CJ: Hypertensive disorders in pregnancy. In Mandeville LK, Troiano NH, editors: *High-risk intrapartum nursing*, Philadelphia, 1999, Lippincott.
36. Sibai B, Mabie C: Hemodynamics of preeclampsia, *Clin Perinatol* 18(4):727-747, 1991.
37. Sibai BM: Treatment of hypertension in pregnant women, *N Engl J Med* 335:257-264, 1996.
38. Wolf JL: Liver disease in pregnancy. *Med Clin North Am* 80:1167-1187, 1996.
39. Villar M, Sibai B: Eclampsia, *Obstet Gynecol Clin North Am* 15(2):355-377, 1988.
40. Clark S: Critical care obstetrics. In Scott JR et al, editors: *Danforth's obstetrics and gynecology*, ed 8, Philadelphia, 1999, Lippincott.
41. Report of the National High Blood Pressure Education Working Group on High Blood Pressure in Pregnancy, *Am J Obstet Gynecol* 183(1):s1-22, 2000.
42. Graves CR: Acute pulmonary complications during pregnancy, *Clin Obstet Gynecol* 45(2):369-376, 2002.

43. Wendel PJ: Asthma in pregnancy, *Obstet Gynecol Clin North Am* 28(3):537-551, 2001.
44. Lavery P: Asthma. In Queenan J, editor: *Management of high-risk pregnancies,* ed 4, Cambridge, Mass, 1996, Blackwell Science.
45. Kochenour N: Asthma. In Queenan J, Hobbins J, editors: *Protocols for high-risk pregnancies,* ed 3, Cambridge, Mass, 1996, Blackwell Science.
46. Ramsey PS, Ramin KD: Pneumonia in pregnancy, *Obstet Gynecol Clin North Am* 28(3):553-569, 2001.
47. Andres RL, Miles, A: Venous thromboembolism and pregnancy, *Obstet Gynecol Clin North Am* 28(3):613-630, 2001.
48. Dizon-Townson D: Pregnancy-related venous thromboembolism, *Clin Obstet Gynecol* 45(2):363-368, 2002.
49. Clark SL et al: Amniotic fluid embolism: analysis of a national registry, *Am J Obstet Gynecol* 172:1158-1169, 1995.
50. Naylor DF, Olson MM: Critical care obstetrics and gynecology, *Crit Care Clin* 19(1):127-149, 2003.
51. Davies S: Amniotic fluid embolus: a review of the literature, *Can J Anaesth* 48:88-98, 2001.
52. DeJong, MJ, Fausett MB: Anaphylactoid syndrome of pregnancy: a devastating complication requiring intensive care, *Crit Care Nurse* 23(6):42-48,2003.
53. Dildy GA, Clark SL: Anaphylactoid syndrome of pregnancy (amniotic fluid embolism). In Dildy, GA editor: *Critical care obstetrics,* ed 4, Malden, Mass, 2003, Blackwell Scientific.
54. Stone I: Trauma in the obstetric patient, *Obstet Gynecol Clin North Am* 3:459-785, 1999.
55. American College of Obstetricians and Gynecologists: *Obstetric aspects of trauma management,* Educational Bulletin 251, September 1998.
56. American College of Obstetricians and Gynecologists: *Domestic violence,* Educational Bulletin 257, December 1999.
57. Lipsky S, et al: Impact of police reported intimate partner violence during pregnancy on birth outcomes, *Obstet Gynecol* 102(3):557-564, 2003.
58. Reference deleted in proofs.
59. Stallard TC, Burns B: Emergency delivery and perimortem C-section, *Emerg Med Clin N Am* 21:679-693, 2003.
60. Whitty JE: Maternal cardiac arrest in pregnancy, *Clin Obstet Gynecol* 45(2):377-392, 2002.
61. Colburn V: Trauma in pregnancy, *J Perinat Neonat Nurs* 3:21-32, 1999.
62. Pereira L: Obstetric management of the patient with spinal cord injuries, *Obstet Gynec Survey* 58(10):678-686, 2003.
63. American College of Obstetricians and Gynecologists: *Obstetric management of patients with spinal cord injuries,* Committee Opinion 275, 2002.
64. Kochenour NK: Epilepsy. In Queenan JT, Hobbins JC, editors: *Protocols for high risk pregnancies,* ed 3, Cambridge, Mass, 1996, Blackwell Science.
65. Samuals P: Neurologic disorders. In Gabbe S, Niebyl J, Simpson J, editors: *Obstetrics: normal and problem pregnancies,* ed 3, New York, 1999, Churchill Livingstone.
66. Pschirrer ER, Monga M: Seizure disorders in pregnancy, *Obstet Gynecol Clin North Am* 28(3):601-611, 2001.
67. Plauche WC: Myasthenia gravis in mothers and their newborns, *Clin Obstet Gynecol* 34(1):82-99, 1991.
68. Batocchi A et al: Course and treatment of myasthenia gravis during pregnancy, *Neurology* 52(3):447-452, 1999.
69. Aminoff M: Neurologic disorders. In Creasy R, Resnik R, editors: *Maternal-fetal medicine,* ed 4, Philadelphia, 1999, Saunders.
70. Donaldson J: Neurologic complications. In Burrow G, Duffy T, editors: *Medical complications during pregnancy,* ed 5, Philadelphia, 1999, Saunders.
71. Vincent A et al: Myasthenia gravis, *Lancet* 357:2122-2128, 2001.
72. Hoff JM et al: Myasthenia gravis: consequences for pregnancy, delivery, and the newborn, *Neurology* 61:1362-1366, 2003.
73. Donaldson J: Neurologic disorders of pregnancy. In Reece E, Hobbins J, editors: *Medicine of the fetus and mother,* ed 2, Philadelphia, 1999, Lippincott-Raven.

CHAPTER 13

Gerontologic Alterations and Management

*P*atients in critical care units include an increasing number of older adults. As of 2002 the United States population older than 65 years reached 35.6 million, accounting for 12.3% of the overall population. Those in the 65- to 74-year age-group numbered 18.3 million; 75 to 84 year olds accounted for 12.7 million; and those in the 85-year or older age group numbered 6 million. This latter group is expected to reach 9.6 million by 2030.[1] In 2001 a 65-year-old woman had a life expectancy of 19.4 more years, whereas men could expect to live another 16.4 years.[1]

Statistics for 2003 showed that 38.6% of older persons described their health as excellent or very good. The most frequently occurring chronic disorders include hypertension (49.2%), arthritis (36.1%), heart disease (31.1%), cancer (20%), and diabetes (15%).[2] More than half of this population reported severe disability. In addition, older adults accounted for 39.1% of all hospital stays and more than half of all healthcare days.[2] Hospital admissions for older adults increased 8% since 1990, with a 1-day decline in the average length of stay (most recently, 5.8 days).[1] Older adults average $3586 per year out-of-pocket medical expenses (a 45% increase since 1992), which is 12.8% of their total income (three times as much as younger adults).[1]

The process of senescence (growing old) is characterized by tissue and organ changes. This, in combination with the prevalence of chronic conditions in the older adult, contributes to increased morbidity and mortality in the critical care unit. Aging is accompanied by physiologic changes in the cardiovascular, respiratory, renal, gastrointestinal, hepatic, integumentary, immune, and central nervous systems. With advancing age the incidence of disease increases, with cardiovascular and neoplastic diseases being the most common causes of death.[3] However, although physiologic decline and disease processes influence each other, physiologic decline occurs independently of disease and is responsible for the development of symptoms at an earlier stage of disease in older adults than in their younger counterparts.[3] Therefore changes in physiologic function are important

to consider when caring for the older adult patient. The purpose of this chapter is to acquaint the critical care nurse with literature and research on the age-associated changes in physiologic function in healthy older adults and to describe implications for this population in critical care.

CARDIOVASCULAR SYSTEM

Advancing age has many effects on the cardiovascular system. With advancing age both the myocardium and the vascular system undergo a multitude of anatomic and cellular changes that alter the function of both the myocardium and peripheral vascular system.[4] These changes in cardiovascular function significantly impact critical illness in the older adult because of the age related effects on cardiovascular structure and function. In addition, since age is a major risk factor for cardiovascular disease in the older adult, this high-risk population will encounter more cardiovascular events when admitted for noncardiac problems to the critical care unit.[5]

AGE-RELATED CHANGES IN MYOCARDIAL STRUCTURE AND FUNCTION

Myocardial collagen content increases with age.[6,7] Collagen is the principal noncontractile protein occupying the cardiac interstitium.[8] Increased myocardial collagen content renders the myocardium less compliant; therefore, a decrease in myocardial compliance can adversely affect diastolic filling (through decreased distensibility and dilation) and myocardial relaxation. Consequently, the left ventricle must develop a higher filling pressure for a given increase in ventricular volume. Decreased left ventricular compliance may be evident in the older adult by the presence of an S_4 heart sound.[9]

The functional consequence of these changes could be an increase in myocardial oxygen consumption. Under normal physiologic conditions, an increase in myocardial oxygen demand is met with a corresponding increase in coronary artery blood flow. However, in the presence of coronary artery disease, coronary artery blood flow can be limited because of atherosclerotic-mediated narrowing of the coronary arteries. Hence the older patient is at risk for developing myocardial ischemia and/or infarction. Clinical manifestations of myocardial ischemia include electrocardiographic (ECG) changes and chest pain. However, the sensation of chest pain may be altered in the older adult. Nadelmann et al[10] found that complaints of chest pain were absent in 50% of older adult patients (older than 74 years) who sustained a myocardial infarction. Others[11] have also reported that chest pain in the older adult is less intense and of shorter duration and originates in other areas of the chest besides the substernal region. Atypical symptoms, such as dyspnea, confusion, and failure to thrive are frequently the only symptoms associated with myocardial infarction in this high-risk population.[12] The aging heart also undergoes a modest degree of hypertrophy that is similar to pressure overload–induced hypertrophy. Such hypertrophy entails a thickening of the left ventricular wall without appreciable changes in left ventricular cavity size.[13] However, increases in left ventricular cavity size associated with aging occur only in men.[12] The increase in left ventricular wall thickness is a result primarily of an increase in muscle cell size. In older individuals the myocardial hypertrophy may be caused by corresponding increases in aortic impedance and systemic vascular resistance.[14]

Myocardial contractility depends on numerous factors. However, the most important determinants of myocardial contraction are the intracellular level of free calcium and the sensitivity of the contractile proteins for calcium.[14,15] Because peak contractile force in the senescent myocardium is unaltered, this suggests that neither the amount of intracellular free calcium during systole nor the sensitivity of the contractile proteins for calcium is altered. The prolonged duration of contraction (systole) is caused in part by a slowed or delayed rate of myocardial relaxation, which may be an adaptive mechanism to preserve contractile function compromised by age-related increases in afterload.[4,15]

AGE-ASSOCIATED CHANGES IN HEMODYNAMICS AND THE ELECTROCARDIOGRAM

Resting (supine) heart rate decreases with age.[16,17] Cinelli et al[16] reported a decrease in the resting heart rate from 78.8 beats/min in young adults to 62.3 beats/min in older adults. Heart rate is an important determinant of cardiac output (CO), and the normal resting heart beats approximately 70 times a minute. At rest or with minimal activity, the older adult probably will not experience any untoward cardiovascular effect (i.e., a decrease in CO) with a heart rate of 62 beats/min. However, if the heart rate response is attenuated during exercise, the older person's capacity for exercise may be lim-

ited. In addition, intrinsic heart rate also decreases with aging.[17] The intrinsic heart rate is the heart rate in the absence of parasympathetic and sympathetic influences. In healthy, resting individuals, parasympathetic (cholinergic) influences predominate, causing a heart rate of approximately 70 beats/min.[11] In the absence of both parasympathetic and sympathetic influences, the heart rate of young adults averages about 100 beats/min (intrinsic heart rate). Jose[18] found that the intrinsic heart rate (in the presence of both sympathetic and parasympathetic blockers) in a 20-year-old person was 100 beats/minute, as compared with a heart rate of 74 beats/min in an 80-year-old man. This decrease in intrinsic heart rate may in part explain the decrease in the resting (supine) heart rate that occurs with aging.

Resting CO and stroke volume are not changed with advancing age. Rodeheffer et al[19] studied subjects without coronary artery disease or other types of illnesses over a 30- to 80-year period and found no changes in the resting CO or the cardiac index in participants.[19] At rest, left ventricular end-diastolic volume (preload), end-systolic volume, and the ejection fraction are not affected by age.[20] In the elderly human myocardium, the early diastolic filling period and isovolumic phase of myocardial relaxation are prolonged.[20-22] However, these changes, although suggestive of diastolic dysfunction, do not translate into decreases in end-diastolic volume or stroke volume.[21,22] Finally, aging is associated with a moderate increase in pulmonary artery pressure.[23]

Advancing age produces changes in the ECG. R wave and S wave amplitude significantly decrease in persons older than 49 years, whereas QT duration increases[24] (Table 13-1). The increase in the duration of the QT interval is reflective of the prolonged rate of relaxation.[24] The frontal plane axis shifts downward from 48.93 to 38.83 degrees between the ages of 30 and 49 years, which is suggestive of a modest degree of cardiac enlargement or hypertrophy.[24] The incidence of asymptomatic cardiac dysrhythmias increases in elderly patients.[25] The most common dysrhythmia occurring in older individuals is the premature ventricular contraction (PVC). Carom et al.[26] and Fleg and Kennedy[27] report that 70% to 80% of all patients older than 60 years experience PVCs. In a healthy geriatric population (60 to 85 years old), 24-hour ambulatory ECG recordings revealed that 78 of the 98 subjects studied experienced asymptomatic ventricular ectopic beats. Other common types of dysrhythmias are sinus node dysfunction (atrial fibrillation, atrial flutter, or paroxysmal supraventricular tachycardia) and atrioventricular conduction disturbances.[20,24,25] Because the majority of patients are asymptomatic, the use of antidysrhythmics is generally not recommended. The side effects and toxic effects of antidysrhythmics impose more of a risk, as compared with the risk of mortality or morbidity related to the dysrhythmia.[25,28] In contrast, for patients who are symptomatic and have malignant ven-

Table 13-1	Age-Related Changes in Electrocardiographic Variables			
	Age (in years)			
ECG Variable	**Younger Than 30**	**30-39**	**40-49**	**Older Than 49**
R wave amplitude (mm)	10.43	10.53	9.01	9.25
S wave amplitude (mm)	15.21	14.21	12.22	12.42
Frontal plane axis (degrees)	48.93	48.13	36.50	38.83
PR duration (ms)	15.89	16.23	16.04	16.25
QRS duration (ms)	7.64	7.51	7.36	8.00
QT duration (ms)	37.83	37.50	37.99	39.58
T wave amplitude (ms)	5.21	4.57	4.31	4.42

Data from Bachman S, Sparrow D, Smith LK: Effect of aging on the electrocardiogram, *Am J Cardiol* 48:513, 1981.

tricular dysrhythmias (sustained ventricular tachycardia and/or fibrillation), pharmacologic therapy is warranted.[25,28] More recent studies support the addition of cardiac-resynchronization therapy rather then pharmacologic therapy alone in those patients with advanced heart failure as a mechanism to further reduce mortality associated with dysrhthymias.[29]

AGE-RELATED CHANGES IN BARORECEPTOR FUNCTION

Baroreceptor-reflex function is altered with aging.[30] Baroreceptors are mechanoreceptors that respond to stretch and other changes in the blood vessel wall and are located at the bifurcation of the common carotid artery and aortic arch.[14] Impulses arising in the baroreceptor region project to the vasomotor center (nucleus of tractus solitarius) in the medulla. Abrupt changes in blood pressure caused by increases in peripheral resistance, CO, or blood volume are sensed by the baroreceptors, resulting in an increase in the impulse frequency to the vasomotor center within the medulla. This increase inhibits vasoconstrictor impulses arising from the vasoconstrictor region within the medulla.[14] The result is a decrease in heart rate and peripheral vasodilation; both of these effects return the blood pressure to within normal limits. The baroreflex can be tested by measuring the heart rate response (i.e., increase or decrease in heart rate) after the administration of either a pressor or depressor agent and by changing a person's position from lying to standing. Yin et al[31] and Elliott et al[32] found an attenuated increase in heart rate response in elderly subjects after the infusion of phenylephrine, an alpha$_1$-adrenoreceptor agonist that produces vasoconstriction and increases the blood pressure. Likewise, the baroreflex-mediated tachycardia response to depressor agents is also attenuated in older adults.[31] There are several reports of an attenuation in the heart rate response of older adults after changes in position (supine to standing).[33,34]

When an individual changes his or her position from supine to standing, the distribution of blood volume changes. This can result in a reduction in CO and hence blood pressure.[14] However, when a person changes position, there are simultaneous baroreceptor-mediated increases in the heart rate that maintain blood pressure by increasing CO. The baroreceptor-reflex response also mediates changes in the peripheral resistance and force of myocardial contraction, which likewise serve to offset the drop in blood pressure. It was once thought that postural hypotension occurred more frequently in older adults and was an age-related phenomenon. However, the prevalence of postural hypotension is actually quite low in older adults.[35,36] The prevalence of orthostatic hypotension is greater in institutionalized geriatric patients who are receiving antihypertensive medications.[34]

LEFT VENTRICULAR FUNCTION DURING EXERCISE IN THE OLDER ADULT

In most individuals, aging is associated with a decline in exercise performance. Exercise performance depends on a multitude of physiologic variables. Cardiac performance and the ability of the heart to increase and maintain CO are critical for increasing oxygen delivery to the peripheral tissues. During exercise, CO is increased by several mechanisms; however, the most important mechanisms include an increased heart rate, an increased inotropic state of the myocardium, and a decreased aortic impedance.[19] Some reports suggest that changes in exercise performance are related to a decrease in the maximal cardiac output achieved with exercise. However, Rodeheffer et al[19] reported that the older adult's diminished ability to exercise is not due to a decrease in the maximal CO that can be achieved during exercise. These investigators found no difference in CO response to different levels of exercise in subjects from the Baltimore Longitudinal Study of Aging.[19] With advancing age, the maximal heart rate achieved during exercise is attenuated; however, the decreased heart rate response is accompanied by an increase in left ventricular end-diastolic volume (LVEDV) and stroke volume (SV). This augmentation in LVEDV and SV offsets the attenuated heart rate response and maintains CO in exercise. Changes in aortic impedance have not been studied in older individuals; however, in animal models, blood pressure and systemic vascular resistance are increased during exercise in senescent, but not young adult, animals.[37] In summary, in healthy older individuals there is no age-associated decline in cardiac output during exercise; however, other factors such as neural functioning, skeletal and joint functioning, as well as pulmonary function, may limit an older individual's ability to exercise.

The Peripheral Vascular System

The effects of aging on the peripheral vascular system are reflected in the gradual but linear rise in systolic blood pressure up until age 80, when values tend to plateau.[20,38,39] Diastolic blood pressure is less affected by age and generally remains the same or decreases.[38,39] Important determinants of systolic blood pressure include the compliance of the vasculature and the blood volume within the vascular system. Similar to the heart, the compliance of the vasculature is determined by its cell type and tissue composition. With advancing age, the intimal layer thickens, principally because of an increase in smooth muscle cells (that have migrated from the medial layer), and the amount of connective tissue (collagen and elastic tissue) increases.[38] These changes occur in the intima of the large and distal arteries. This gradual decrease in arterial compliance or "stiffening of the arteries" is sometimes referred to as arteriosclerosis. Arteriosclerotic changes are also accompanied by changes caused by atherosclerosis, which is the accumulation within a vessel of lipoproteins and fibrinous products such as platelets, macrophages, and leukocytes.[40] The consequences of arteriosclerotic and atherosclerotic processes are that the arteries become progressively less distensible and the vascular pressure-volume relationship is altered. These changes are clinically significant, because small changes in intravascular volume are accompanied by disproportionate increases in systolic blood pressure.[41] The decrease in arterial compliance and disproportionate increase in systolic blood pressure may lead to an increase in afterload and the development of concentric (pressure-induced) ventricular hypertrophy in the older adult.[41]

It is well recognized that increased serum lipoprotein levels are risk factors in the development and progression of atherosclerosis.[40] Lipoprotein levels increase with advancing age. However, innumerable factors can influence serum lipoprotein levels, making it very difficult to determine whether such changes contribute to the aging of the peripheral vascular system.[42,43] Serum lipoproteins are particles that contain varying amounts of cholesterol, triglycerides, phospholipids, and apoproteins.[40] The five principal serum lipoproteins are chylomicrons, low-density lipoproteins (LDLs), very–low-density lipoproteins (VLDLs), intermediate-density lipoproteins (IDLs), and high-density lipoproteins (HDLs). The lipoprotein classification is based on the lipoprotein's size and relative concentration of cholesterol, triglycerides, and apoproteins.[40] In men, the serum total cholesterol level (all of the lipoproteins combined) increases progressively from 150 to 200 mg/dl between the ages of 20 and 50 years and remains relatively unchanged until the age of 70 years.[43] As would be predicted, the age-related changes in serum LDL levels parallel the changes in the total serum cholesterol level. All lipoprotein fractions transport cholesterol; however, in healthy people, three fourths of the total cholesterol is transported within the LDL.[40] There are relatively few age-related changes in VLDL and HDL levels in men. In men, serum triglyceride levels peak at approximately age 40 and then decrease.[42,43]

In women, serum total cholesterol levels are low between the ages of 20 and 50 years.[42,43] However, between the ages of 55 and 60 years, serum total cholesterol levels progressively increase, usually simultaneously with changes in the hormonal production of estrogen.[43] The increase in total serum cholesterol levels is primarily the result of an increase in the LDL fraction and, to a lesser extent, the VLDL and HDL fractions, which do not change appreciably with age in women. In women, serum triglyceride levels progressively increase with age.[43]

Arterial pressure is also governed by the amount of blood volume, which in turn is regulated by plasma levels of sodium and water and the activity of the renin-angiotensin system (RAS).[44] Plasma renin activity declines with age, and aging per se has no appreciable effect on sodium and water homeostasis.[45,46] However, as noted, there are age-related changes in tubular function, as well as a decrease in the glomerular filtration rate (GFR), both of which can affect overall sodium and water homeostasis. Circulating levels of sodium-regulating hormones, such as natriuretic hormone, aldosterone, and antidiuretic hormone (ADH), are not appreciably altered by advancing age.[46,47] However, a delayed natriuretic response after sodium loading and plasma volume expansion and diminished renal response to ADH secretion have been reported in older adults.[47]

Cardiovascular System Summary

- Aorta and other arteries become stiff and less pliable, leading to increased workload on the heart to perfuse tissue
- Systolic and diastolic pressures increase, along with an increase in systemic vascular resistance and a decrease in cardiac output
- There is a loss of capacity in the myocardium and arterial system and decreased ability to respond and re-

Table 13-2	Age-Related Changes in Commonly Performed Pulmonary Function Tests		
Pulmonary Function Test	Description	Standard Lung Volume and Capacity (ml)	Age-Related Change (ml)
Total lung capacity	Vital capacity plus residual volume	6000	No change
Vital capacity	Amount of air exhaled after a maximal inspiration	5000	3750
Tidal volume (V_T)	Amount of air inhaled or exhaled with each breath	500	No change
Residual volume (RV)	Amount of air left in lungs after forced exhalation	1200	↓ 1800
Inspiratory reserve volume (IRV)	Amount of air that can be forcefully inhaled after inspiring a normal V_T	3100	↓ 2800
Expiratory reserve volume (ERV)	Amount of air that can be forcefully exhaled after expiring a normal V_T	1200	↓ 1000
Forced expiratory volume in 1 sec (FEV_1)	Volume exhaled in the first second of a single forced expiratory volume; expressed as a percent of the forced vital capacity	80%	↓ 75%

cover from periods of physiologic and psychologic stress
- A decreased myocardial efficiency results in less relaxation during diastole
- The alteration in baroreceptor function leads to changes in compensatory responses

PULMONARY SYSTEM

Many of the changes in the pulmonary system that occur with aging are reflected in tests of pulmonary function and include changes in thoracic wall expansion and respiratory muscle strength, morphology of alveolar parenchyma, and decreases in arterial oxygen tension (Pao_2)[48,49] (Tables 13-2 and 13-3). These changes occur progressively as age advances and should not alter the elderly person's ability to breathe effortlessly. However, factors such as repeated exposure to environmental pollutants, cigarette smoking, and frequent pulmonary infections can accelerate age-related changes, thereby making it difficult to identify the age-associated changes in pulmonary function.[50] Interestingly, Thurlbeck[51] did not find age-related morphologic changes in the lung tissue of aging mice raised in a pollution- and infection-free environment, suggesting the immense effect of environmental variables on pulmonary function.

THORACIC WALL AND RESPIRATORY MUSCLES

With advancing age, the chest wall (thoracic skeleton) and vertebrae undergo a small degree of osteoporosis, and at the same time the costal cartilages that connect the rib cage become calcified and stiff. These changes may produce kyphosis and reduce chest wall compliance, respectively (Fig. 13-1).[48,49,52,53] The functional effect is a decrease in thoracic wall excursion. Other

Table 13-3	Progressive Changes in Arterial Oxygen Tension (Pao_2) and Carbon Dioxide Tension ($Paco_2$)	
Age-Group (years)	Pao_2 (mm Hg)	$Paco_2$ (mm Hg)
<30	94	39
31-40	87	38
41-50	84	40
51-60	81	39
>60	74	40

Modified from Sorbini CA et al: Arterial oxygen tension in relation to age in healthy subjects, *Respiration* 25:3, 1968.

factors, such as an increase in abdominal girth and change in posture, also decrease thoracic excursion. These anatomic changes are reflected by an increase in residual volume and decrease in vital capacity (see Table 13-2).

The strength of the respiratory muscles gradually decreases: the diaphragm and both the external and internal intercostal muscles. The diaphragm is the most important inspiratory muscle because its movement accounts for 75% of the change in intrathoracic volume during quiet respiration.[54] The respiratory muscles are composed of skeletal muscle fibers.[55] During aging, skeletal muscle progressively atrophies and its energy metabolism decreases, which may partially explain the declining strength of the respiratory muscles.[55,56] In addition, there is an age-associated decrease in the effectiveness of the cough reflex, which is possibly caused by a decrease in ciliary responsiveness and motion.[49,57] These changes underscore the importance of deep

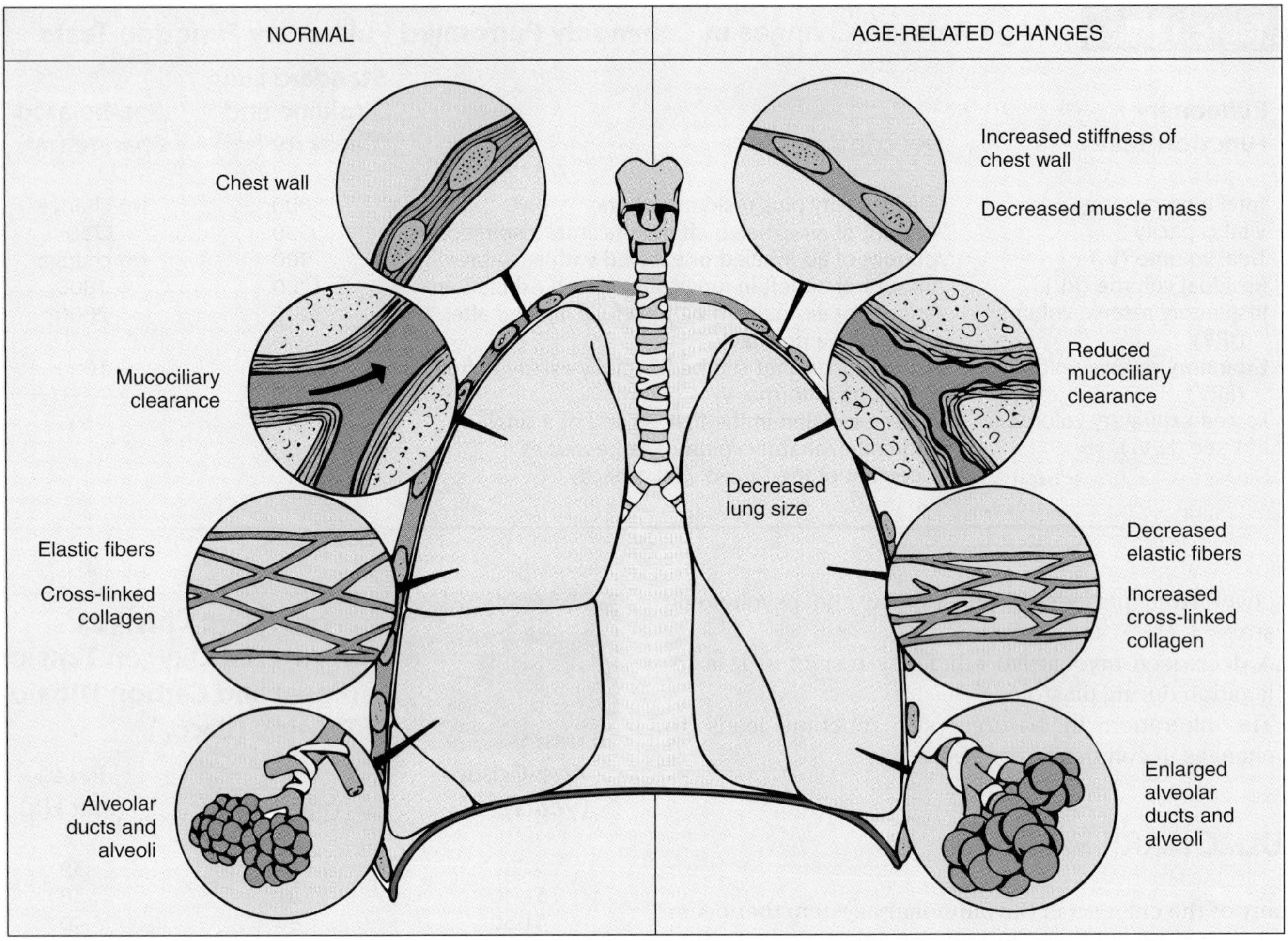

Fig. 13-1 Age-related changes in the respiratory system. With advancing age, the compliance of the chest wall and lung tissue changes. There is also a reduced clearance of mucus by the cilia that line the pulmonary tree and an enlargement of the alveolar ducts and alveoli. More age-related changes in respiratory function are described in the text.

breathing and coughing for the bedridden older patient in the critical care unit.

As noted, the age-associated changes in pulmonary function do not alter the older adult's ability to breathe effortlessly. However, the decrease in respiratory muscle strength may be a limiting factor during exercise because the respiratory muscles—specifically the accessory inspiratory muscles (sternocleidomastoid, scalene, and trapezius)—facilitate inspiration during exercise. However, this theory is not supported by the findings of Belman and Gaesser,[58] who reported that although ventilatory muscle strength improved after elderly men and women received ventilatory muscle training, neither submaximal nor maximal exercise tolerance improved.

ALVEOLAR PARENCHYMA

With advancing age a diminished recoil (or increased compliance) of the lung occurs.[59] The reduced recoil results from the increase in the ratio of elastin to collagen

content that occurs with advancing age.[60] Collagen, elastin, and reticulin are the primary connective tissue proteins of the lung tissue.[61,62] They are responsible for the elasticity and performance of the airways of the lung. Whereas total lung collagen remains unaltered, the amount of elastin increases with age in the interlobular septa and pleura and possibly within the bronchi and their vessels.[61,62] These anatomic changes are reflected by an increase in residual volume and a decrease in forced expiratory volume. An additional anatomic structural change includes an increase in the size of the alveolar ducts, which occurs after 40 years of age.[48] The bronchial enlargement displaces inhaled air volume away from the alveoli that line the alveolar ducts (see Fig. 13-1).[48] Ventilation and the process of oxygen and carbon dioxide exchange (diffusion) depend on numerous factors, one of which is the surface area available for diffusion. A displacement of inhaled air volume away from the alveoli limits the surface area available for gas exchange. This may in part explain the progressive and linear decrease in the pulmonary diffusion capacity, which depends on both the surface area and capillary blood volume. There are reports that capillary blood volume and surface area decrease with advancing age.[63]

PULMONARY GAS EXCHANGE

The arterial oxygen tension (PaO_2) decreases with age, such that the median PaO_2 for healthy persons older than 60 years is 74.3 mm Hg, as compared with 94 mm Hg for younger adults.[64] In contrast, arterial carbon dioxide ($PaCO_2$) does not change with advancing age (see Table 13-3).[64] The decrease in PaO_2 may be the result of an increase in the closing volume in the dependent lung zones during resting tidal breathing in older subjects.[65,66] Consequently, dependent lung zones may be ventilated intermittently, leading to regional differences in ventilation. It is possible that alterations in blood volume and vascular resistance within the pulmonary circulation may also contribute to ventilation/perfusion (V/Q) mismatching. Other factors, such as smoking and pulmonary disease, also have an impact on the level of arterial oxygenation.

LUNG VOLUMES AND CAPACITIES

With advancing age, total lung capacity and tidal volume do not change[52] (see Table 13-2). Residual volume (RV) increases with age, paralleling the decrease in chest wall compliance and reduced strength of the respiratory muscles (see Table 13-2).[48] The increase in RV may also add to the diminished strength of the inspiratory muscles by stretching the diaphragm and altering the tension-length relationship. Results from studies are conflicting with regard to age-related changes in functional residual capacity (FRC), which is the volume of air in the lungs at the normal resting end-expiratory position. There are reports of both no change[67] and decreases[52] in FRC in elderly persons. The balance of two opposing forces, the elastic recoil of the lung and the outward recoil of the chest wall, determine the FRC.[54] These factors change in opposite directions with age: the elastic recoil of the lung decreases, thereby increasing compliance; and the outward recoil of the chest wall decreases, thus decreasing the compliance of the chest wall. One would predict that because these factors change in opposite directions, FRC would remain unaltered. In fact, Knudson et al.[67] found no change in FRC in older adults, supporting this prediction.

Other lung volumes that decrease with age include the inspiratory reserve volume (IRV) and the expiratory reserve volume (ERV).[50,52] The decrease in the ERV is the result of an increase in the RV. The decrease in IRV, however, has been found only in studies reporting a corresponding increase in FRC. See Table 13-2 and Fig. 13-1 for a summary of age-related changes in pulmonary function.

The following dynamic measurements of lung volume are decreased in aging: maximal expiratory flow rate, maximal midexpiratory flow rate, forced expiratory volume in 1 second (FEV_1), and the ratio of FEV_1 to forced vital capacity.[68,69] Dynamic measurements of lung volume reflect changes in airflow rate; airflow rate depends on the resistance of airways and chest wall compliance. Hence the age-related decrease in the dynamic lung volume is probably caused by decreased chest wall compliance, increased likelihood of small airways closing during forced expiratory efforts (increasing airway resistance), and decreased strength of expiratory muscles.[70]

PULMONARY SYSTEM SUMMARY

- Lung tissue stiffens
- Diffusion of gases is impaired by 8% per year after age 65
- There is a decrease in vital capacity and maximal breathing capacity
- Increased weakness of diaphragm and abdominal and accessory muscles leads to decreased ability to inhale and exhale

RENAL SYSTEM

Aging produces changes in renal structure and function, many of which begin at approximately 30 to 40 years of age.[71,72] One of the prominent changes is a decrease in the number and size of the nephrons, which begins in the cortical regions and progresses toward the medullary portions of the kidney.[73] The decrease in the number of nephrons corresponds to a 20% decrease in the weight of the kidney between 40 and 80 years of age.[73] Initially this loss of nephrons does not appreciably alter renal function because of the large renal reserve: the kidney contains approximately 2 million to 3 million nephrons, all of which are not needed to maintain adequate fluid and acid-base homeostasis. However, with time the geriatric patient also loses this renal reserve.[73] Nephron loss is caused by a gradual reduction in blood flow to the glomerular capillary tuft.[74] Total renal blood flow declines after the fourth decade of life[71] because of hyaline arteriosclerosis.[74,75] The etiology of this vascular lesion within the glomerular tuft is unknown. By the eighth decade of life, 50% of the glomeruli are lost as a result of this arteriolar hyalinization.[73]

FLUID FILTRATION

The glomerular filtration rate decreases with advancing age.[71-73] The GFR is the volume of fluid traversing the glomerular membrane in a given period and is an important regulator of water and solute excretion. GFR depends on the permeability of the glomerular capillary and the surface area available for filtration, as well as the balance of pressure gradients between the glomerular capillary and Bowman space.[44] In older adults the decrease in GFR is most likely caused by the decrease in nephron number as well as the decrease in renal blood flow.[71,72] Even though the remaining nephrons adapt to the loss of nephrons by glomerular hyperfiltration and increased solute load per nephron, the reduced GFR predisposes the older adult to adverse drug reactions and drug-induced renal failure. Some drugs are excreted unchanged in the urine, whereas other drugs have active or nephrotoxic metabolites that are excreted in the urine. In addition, the senescent kidney is more susceptible to injury by hypotensive episodes because of the age-related decrease in renal blood flow and reduced pressure gradient across the afferent arteriole.[72,76]

Age-related changes also occur in tubular function. The functions that are primarily carried out in the renal tubules are sodium and water concentration and conservation, and acidification of the urine.[44,72] These functions are governed by the amount of sodium and water delivered to the tubules and overall acid-base balance. The age-related changes in tubular function become apparent when extreme changes occur in the body fluid composition or acid-base balance. For example, with systemic acidosis the rate and amount of total acid excretion (bicarbonate, titratable acid, and ammonium) are reduced.[71,72,76] This predisposes the older adult patient to metabolic acidosis, volume depletion, and hyperchloremia. However, at a normal pH level, the kidney of an older adult can maintain acid-base homeostasis.

There is a diminished ability of the senescent kidney to excrete a free water load, conserve water during periods of dehydration, and conserve sodium during periods of low salt intake.[71] Age-related changes also occur in extrarenal mechanisms, such as the decreased activity and responsiveness of the senescent kidney to the sympathetic nervous system and renin-angiotensin-aldosterone system, which are important in integrating overall fluid homeostasis and maintaining blood pressure in response to changes in body position.[45,72]

RENAL SYSTEM SUMMARY

- A decreased renal blood flow leads to a decrease in glomerular filtration and decreased renal tubule function
- There is decreased elimination of physiologic substances (blood urea nitrogen, or BUN, and creatinine)

GASTROINTESTINAL SYSTEM

AGE-RELATED CHANGE

Age-related gastrointestinal changes occur in the processes of swallowing, motility, and absorption.[77,78] Swallowing may be difficult for the older adult because of incomplete mastication of food within the oral cavity.[78]

The result of deteriorating dentition, diminished lubrication (secondary to salivary dysfunction), and ill-fitting dentures, incomplete mastication can put the older adult patient at risk for aspiration.[77,78] In addition, the number and velocity of the peristaltic contractions of the older adult's esophagus decreases and the number of nonperistaltic contractions increases.[78]

These changes in esophageal motility are referred to as *presbyesophagus*. These changes may predispose the patient to erosion of the esophageal wall (recurrent esophagitis), because food remains in the esophagus longer. In addition, bed rest and reclining in a supine position for a prolonged period can cause esophageal reflux, which also can lead to esophagitis.

The aging process produces thinning of the smooth muscle within the gastric mucosa.[78,79] The epithelial layer of the gastric mucosa, which contains the chief and parietal cells, undergoes a modest degree of atrophy, resulting in the hyposecretion of pepsin and acid, respectively.[78,80] However, with aging, gastritis-induced achlorhydria (decreased acid secretion) is prevalent. Therefore it remains unknown whether the changes in gastric acid secretion are a result of age-related changes or a disease process such as gastritis.

Mucin secretion from the mucus cells decreases, thereby altering the protective function of the gastric mucosal (bicarbonate) barrier. Because of this, the stomach wall is more susceptible to acid injury, thus increasing the incidence of gastric ulcerations.[78,81] Aging does not appreciably alter gastric emptying of solid foods. However, Moore et al[82] found a delay in the emptying of liquids from the stomach in older adults. No changes in small intestinal peristalsis or segmental movements with aging have been reported.[83] Alterations within the small intestine include a decrease in intestinal weight after the age of 50 and a flattening and shortening of jejunal villi.[83] Age produces no change in the small intestine's absorption of fats and proteins; however, decreased carbohydrate absorption has been reported.[84,85] A gradual decline in albumin is also evidenced with increased age; however, serum levels generally remain within normal limits in healthy older adults.[85] Although most vitamins and minerals are normally absorbed, absorption of fat-soluble vitamin A is increased and there is the potential for impaired absorption of vitamin D.[85] In those patients who are not hypochlorhydric, iron is normally absorbed. However, the absorption of both zinc and calcium decreases with advancing age.[78,85] In summary, age-associated changes in gastrointestinal function occur; however, these changes are not of sufficient magnitude to produce malnutrition in healthy individuals.

LIVER

With advancing age both hepatocyte number and liver weight decrease.[86] Also, total liver blood flow decreases significantly, such that between 25 and 65 years of age, total liver blood flow decreases by 50%.[86-88] The liver has many complex functions, including carbohydrate storage, ketone body formation, reduction and conjugation of adrenal and gonadal steroid hormones, synthesis of plasma proteins, deamination of amino acids, synthesis and storage of cholesterol, urea formation, and detoxification of toxins and drugs. Age-related changes in hepatic function include a reduction in synthesis of cholesterol, total bile acid pool, and bile acid from cholesterol.[88] There is also a reduced capacity of the liver for regeneration in response to injury when compared to a younger population. However, despite these age-related changes, liver function is not appreciably altered.[88] Several tests of liver function, such as serum bilirubin, alkaline phosphatase, and aspartate aminotransferase (AST) levels, are not altered with advancing age. However, because of the decrease in total liver blood flow, first-pass clearance of drugs is somewhat reduced. The most important age-related change in liver function is the decrease in the liver's capacity to metabolize drugs.[89,90] Although clinical tests of liver function do not reflect this change in metabolism, it is well recognized that drug side effects and toxic effects occur more frequently in older adults than in young adults.[90] This reduced drug-metabolizing capacity is caused by a reduction in the activity of the drug-metabolizing enzyme system, microsomal ethanol oxidizing system, and decrease in total liver blood flow.[87,91] Those drugs that are dependent on the cytochrome P-450 group of liver enzymes are the most affected because of age-associated changes causing as much as a 50% decline in enzymatic function.[88]

GASTROINTESTINAL SYSTEM SUMMARY

- Gastric emptying, splenic blood flow, and GI motility are decreased; GI pH and thinning or reduction of absorptive surface of the gut are increased
- Absorption rates are decreased
- Bacterial colonization of duodenum is increased
- There is a decline in drug metabolism by hepatic enzymes

CENTRAL NERVOUS SYSTEM

COGNITIVE FUNCTIONING AND AGING

Cognitive functioning involves the process of transforming, synthesizing, storing, and retrieving sensory input. Additional components include perception, attention, thinking, memory, and problem solving. For the aging individual, cognition is altered by the speed at which information is processed and retrieved.[92] Performance on timed tests declines slowly past the age of 20 years. Intelligence remains fairly stable past the age of 30 years until one reaches the mid-80s. Although the rate at which

complex tasks are completed may be diminished, these age-related changes are not synonymous with cognitive impairment. Marked deterioration of any component of cognitive functioning is not a normal expectation of the aging process.[93] Although some type of cognitive change, such as mild memory dysfunction, is generally apparent with increasing age, this decline may represent a change in individual need rather than a change in function. However, cognitive impairment in older adults more commonly results from acute and chronic etiologies. Acute problems such as infection, fluid, electrolyte, and metabolic imbalances, or medication-induced events are generally reversible once identified. Long-term chronic impairment develops from more organic causations such as those associated with neurodegenerative dementias (i.e., Alzheimer's type, Lewy body disease) or nonneurodegenerative types (i.e., multiinfarct dementia, traumatic brain injury).

Although dementia is pathology-based and not necessarily an expected outcome of aging, there is an increased incidence associated with advanced age, particularly in those over age 85.[93] Alzheimer's disease is identified by amyloid-containing neuritic plaques and intraneuronal neurofibrillary tangles in various areas of the cortex.[94] Alzheimer's disease is characterized initially by progressive short-term memory loss, which progresses to long-term memory loss. Marked decline in memory ultimately leaves the individual functionally impaired and physically dependent. In contrast, nonneurodegenerative dementias, such as multiinfarct types, present as fixed deficits associated with the area of brain injury. Unlike with the Alzheimer's type, cognitive impairment may be associated with significant impairment following stroke rather than over time.[95]

CHANGES IN STRUCTURE AND MORPHOLOGY

The brain decreases approximately 20% in size between 25 and 95 years of age (Fig. 13-2).[93,96] The reduced brain weight may be related in part to the overall decrease in the number of neurons that occurs with advancing age. Neurons are lost from the hippocampus, the amygdala, and the cerebellum and from areas of the brain stem such as the locus ceruleus, the dorsal motor nucleus of the vagus, and the substantia nigra.[92] This is in contrast to areas such as the hypothalamus, where very few neurons disappear with advancing age.[96] In addition, portions of the cerebral cortex atrophy, principally the frontal and temporal cortical association areas (the superior frontal gyrus and superior temporal gyrus, respectively).[97]

The cerebral ventricles enlarge and develop an asymmetric appearance.[98] Cerebrospinal fluid (CSF) also accumulates in the ventricles; however, total brain CSF is not increased.[98] Accompanying the loss of neurons are changes in the ultrastructure and intracellular

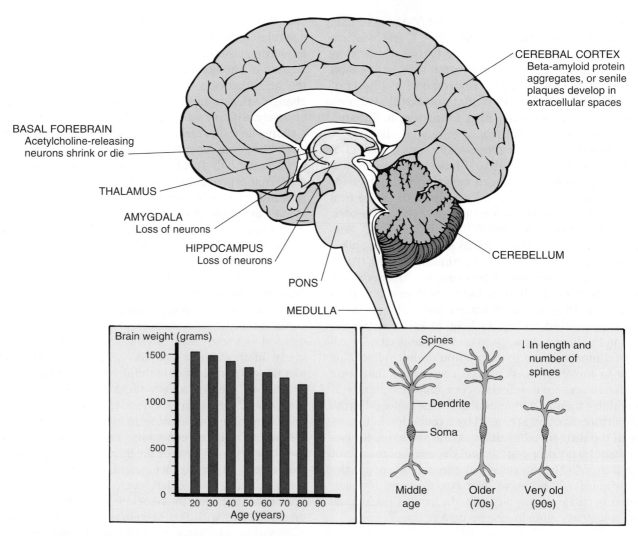

Fig. 13-2   Summary of age-related changes in the brain. (From Soelkoe DJ: *Sci Am* 267:135, 1992.)

structures of the neuron.[99] The neuron is composed of a cell body, a dendrite, and an axon. Dendrites are long, spiny processes extending out from the cell body. One of the most ubiquitous changes in the aging brain is a decrease in the number of dendrite spines. Interestingly, between middle and late old age the length of the dendritic spines increases, but then it decreases after late old age (older than 90 years).[93,96] Also, large neuron shrinking and degenerative changes occurring in the cell bodies and axons of certain acetylcholine-secreting neurons have been reported. These changes may explain alterations in the processing and receiving of information.[93]

With advancing age, lipofuscins, neuritic plaques, and neurofibrillary bodies appear within the cytoplasm of the neuron.[96] Lipofuscins, or age pigment, are granules containing a dark, fluorescent pigment. They are derived from lipid-rich membranes that have been partially disintegrated and oxidized. It is still not clear whether lipofuscin accumulation is harmful to the brain.[96] Neuritic, or senile, plaques are aggregates of the beta-amyloid pro-

tein, and they also accumulate in the brain of normal senescent persons. Neuritic plaques are found in the hippocampus, the cerebral cortex, and other brain regions.[95,96] Neurofibrillary tangles, which are bundles of helically-shaped wound protein filaments, occur in the hippocampus with advancing age in healthy persons.[97] However, they are present in larger numbers in persons with neuropathologic disorders such as Alzheimer's disease. It has been suggested that neurofibrillary tangles could interfere with neuronal signaling.[93,96]

In the senescent brain, synaptogenesis (synaptic regeneration) still occurs after partial nerve degeneration.[99] After a nerve fiber is damaged, neighboring undamaged neurons often sprout new fibers and form new connections. However, synaptogenesis occurs at a slower rate in the older brain.[99]

NEUROTRANSMITTER SYNTHESIS

Advancing age is associated with changes in neurotransmitter function. Altered neurotransmitter function can result from changes in the available precursors for neurotransmitter synthesis, changes in the neurotransmitter receptor, and changes in the activity of the enzymes that synthesize and degrade the neurotransmitter. Different methods are used to examine changes in neurotransmitter function, and these methods include measuring neurotransmitter levels, neurotransmitter turnover, and receptor number and binding. Changes in neurotransmitter systems in the aging brain are equivocal, more than likely a result of the different methods used to study neurotransmitter systems.[100] For example, in some studies, neurotransmitters have been quantified by measuring (1) the concentration of the neurotransmitters, (2) the breakdown or activation products, and (3) the activity of the enzyme responsible for the synthesis or breakdown of the neurotransmitters. Gottstein and Held[101] suggested that age-related changes in neurotransmitter levels may cause a "desynchronization" in neurotransmission, thereby affecting many neurologic functions. Acetylcholine (ACh), dopamine (DA), serotonin (5-HT), glutamate, and γ- (gamma-) aminobutyric acid (GABA) all decrease with increasing age. In addition to age-related neurotransmitter dysfunction, certain disorders frequently encountered in the older adult, such as Alzheimer's disease, Parkinson's disease, multiple sclerosis, depression, and delirium, may further contribute to neurologic dysfunction associated with neurotransmitters.[102] Similarly, many medications (i.e., histamine blockers, benzodiazepines, anticholinergics, antiarrhythmics, antimicrobials, antiemetics) administered in critical care directly affect neurotransmitter function and contribute to the incidence of delirium.[103,104]

CEREBRAL METABOLISM AND BLOOD FLOW

Cerebral blood flow (CBF) decreases with advancing age. This decrease parallels the decrease in brain weight and is most likely caused by the reduction in neuron number and metabolic needs of the cerebral tissue.[92,101] Cerebral blood flow is also influenced by age-related changes in blood pressure, barometric response to positional change, and the severity of cerebrovascular disease.[105]

CENTRAL NERVOUS SYSTEM SUMMARY

- There are changes in gyral function, formation of neurofibrillary tangles, and a decrease in brain volume
- Senile plaque formation increases
- The dilation of the ventricle results in a decrease in number of Purkinje cells and loss of cells in the vestibular system
- There are changes in neurotransmitter synthesis and function, and there is degeneration of the blood-brain barrier

IMMUNE SYSTEM

Several changes in immune function render the older adult more susceptible to infections.[106-111] Infections in the geriatric population are associated with higher rates of mortality.[111] Common infections in the older adult include bacterial pneumonia, urinary tract infection, intraabdominal infections, gram-negative bacteremia, and decubitus ulcers.[111] The reasons for the increased susceptibility are multifactorial and include changes in cell- and humoral-mediated immunity; breakdown in physical barriers, such as the skin and oral mucosa; and changes in nutrition.

CELL-MEDIATED AND HUMORAL-MEDIATED IMMUNITY

Immune system function depends on many cell types with distinct functions. T cells are the primary effector of cell-mediated immunity, whereas bone marrow–derived B cells produce antibodies that are the effector cells of humoral-mediated immunity.[106,108,110] With aging, cell-mediated immunity declines. Even though the total number of T cells remains unchanged with advancing age, T-cell function decreases.[108,110] For example there is a decrease in T-cell production of interleukin-2 (IL-2) and in differentiation of T cells into effector cells. IL-2 is essential for activating B cells, which eventually differentiate into antibody-secreting cells. Subsets of T cells mature into cytotoxic cells, whereas other T cells activate B cells and stimulate B-cell proliferation. Changes in B-lymphocyte function are not as well understood, even though with age the ability of B cells to produce antibodies into new antigens declines.[106,108] Although there is no evidence that age-associated changes directly affect phagocytosis and chemotaxis or the bactericidal action of neutrophils, compromised immune-mediated responses have been identified in areas with reduced blood supply such as the skin.[106]

ADDITIONAL RISK FACTORS

Multiple concurrent chronic illnesses produce systemic stressors that ultimately diminish immune functioning. The critical care nurse must be aware that an exacerbation of preexisting illness such as diabetes or emphysema may present itself before infection is suspected. Introducing bacteria through invasive devices such as central lines or chest tubes may threaten an already suppressed immune system. One must also consider nutritional deficiencies, particularly protein malnutrition, which are a common problem among the elderly. Inadequate protein intake can develop from prolonged anorexia and cognitive impairment. Protein malnutrition is associated with a shrinkage of lymphoid tissue, which then diminishes T-cell functioning and cell-mediated immunity.[109]

Furthermore, inadequate emptying of urine secondary to bed rest, obstruction, or side effects from anticholinergic medications can result in stagnation of urine and recurrent urinary tract infections. Long-term placement of urinary catheters is a significant source of bacteriuria. However, treatment with antibiotic therapy is not indicated unless the patient becomes symptomatic with anorexia or cognitive impairment or has a history of a chronic illness such as diabetes or chronic obstructive pulmonary disease.[106,111,112]

IMMUNE SYSTEM SUMMARY

- The number of gamma and helper T cells increases; suppressor/cytotoxic T lymphocytes decrease; germinal centers of lymph nodes decrease; and plasma cells and lymphocytes in the bone marrow increase
- Cell surface characteristics of lymphocytes change
- There are impaired humoral immune and antibody responses

CHANGES IN PHARMACOKINETICS AND PHARMACODYNAMICS

The many benefits of modern advancements in pharmacologic therapy are frequently counterbalanced by adverse drug effects, medication interactions, and therapeutic failure.[107] Adverse drug effects and medication interactions are related to pharmacokinetics and pharmacodynamics. There are many age-related changes in drug pharmacokinetics, which is the manner in which the body absorbs, distributes, metabolizes, and excretes a drug.[90,91,107] The aging process is associated with changes in gastric acid secretion, which can alter the ionization or solubility of a drug and hence its absorption[90,91] (Table 13-4).

Drug distribution depends on body composition, as well as the physiochemical properties of the drug. With advancing age, fat content increases, lean body mass decreases, and total body water decreases, which can alter the drug disposition.[91] For example, because of the increase in the ratio of body fat content to body weight, lipophilic drugs have a greater volume of distribution per body weight in older adults as compared with younger adults. Other age-related factors[90,113] affecting drug disposition are listed in Table 13-4.

As noted, the senescent liver and kidneys are less able to metabolize and excrete drugs, which also affects clinical outcomes. For example, the rate of absorption, time to peak plasma concentration, and clearance of loop diuretics is reduced in older adults, which may necessitate high dosing regimens in order to facilitate diuresis.[114,115] This poses an increased risk of metabolic acidosis, since the higher diuretic dose increases competition for the organic acid transport pathway at the proximal tubule. Using the example of diuretics, bioavailability between

Table 13-4	Age-Related Changes in Pharmacokinetics	
Pharmacokinetic Parameter	**Definition**	**Age-Related Changes**
Absorption	Receptor-coupled or diffusional uptake of drug into tissue	Decreased absorptive surface area of small intestine Decreased splanchnic blood flow Increased gastric acid pH Decreased gastrointestinal motility
Distribution	Theoretic space (tissue) or body compartment into which free form of drug distributes	Decreased lean body mass and total body water Increased total body fat Decreased serum albumin level Increased alpha$_1$-acid glycoprotein
Metabolism	Chemical change in drug that renders it active or inactive	Decreased liver mass Decreased activity of microsomal drug-metabolizing enzyme system Decreased total liver blood flow
Excretion	Removal of drug through an eliminating organ, which is often the kidney; some drugs are excreted in the bile or feces, in the saliva, or via the lungs	Decreased renal blood flow and glomerular filtration rate Decreased distal renal tubular secretory function

Data from Gilman AG et al, editors: *Goodman and Gilman's the pharmacological basis of therapeutics,* ed 8, London, 1990, Pergamon Press; Vestal RE, Cusack BJ: Pharmacology and aging. In Schneider EL, Rowe JW, editors: *Handbook of the biology of aging,* San Diego, 1990, Academic Press.

agents may also be variable. For instance, bumetanide has a fairly consistent bioavailability in advanced age, whereas that of furosemide varies from 20% to 80%.[115]

Similarly, other drugs associated with management of common disorders seen in critically ill patients—such as digoxin, angiotensin II-converting enzyme (ACE) inhibitors and angiotensin II receptor blockers (ARBs)[115,116]—have delayed excretion, increased serum concentration, and more prolonged duration of action because their excretion parallels GFR (which decreases with age).[110] See Table 13-4 for age-related changes in drug pharmacokinetics and the Pharmacologic Management table[76,114-122] for the potential side effects, nursing interventions, and/or special considerations for frequently used pharmacologic agents in the elderly patient in the critical care unit.

Age-related changes in pharmacodynamics have also been reported. Pharmacodynamics refers to the pharmacologic or physiologic response to a drug that occurs after the drug interacts with its receptor on the plasma membrane. The chronotropic and inotropic effects of (beta-adrenergic agonists reportedly decrease in elderly patients.[123,124] There also are reports that age produces no change in heparin-stimulated increases in partial thromboplastin time, whereas the effects of warfarin (Coumadin) are very susceptible to medication interactions.

The use of multiple medications in the presence of multiple comorbidities has been associated with an increase in adverse drug reactions. Although this is not always avoidable, it is important to avoid choosing an agent for its side effect profile (e.g., diphenhydramine for sedative effects) and monitor the effects of the chosen agent. A major cause of therapeutic failure is the underuse or inappropriate use of drug therapy that is indicated for the treatment of a particular problem. It is not uncommon for delirium not associated with a withdrawal syndrome to be treated with benzodiazepines in critical care. However, this frequently makes agitation worse, once the sedative effects are gone, in comparison to a low dose antipsychotic agent.[103,104,125]

PHYSICAL EXAMINATION AND DIAGNOSTIC PROCEDURES

The various physiologic changes that occur with aging warrant special physical examination techniques.[126] The clinician must distinguish between changes in health caused by physiologic as opposed to pathologic processes; therefore the nurse must ensure that the physical examination is conducted under optimal conditions. When beginning a physical examination, the clinician should consider the ability of the gerontologic patient to cooperate and hear, as well as his or her activity level. In addition, the patient's comfort and energy levels must be considered. Before beginning an examination, the nurse

must ensure that the room's noise level and temperature and the patient's position in the bed are optimal and comfortable.[127]

HEAD AND NECK

Normal funduscopic findings include a diminished pupillary response to penlight, a decrease in near and peripheral vision, and a loss of visual acuity to dim light. These changes result from an increase in opacity of the lens and a decrease in ciliary movement.[128,129] It is not uncommon to find irises that are pale blue or light gray, which stems from a decrease in melanocyte production.[128,129] Around the periphery of the iris, fat deposits may also be found, which are referred to as arcus senilis. The eyes also may appear sunken or recessed because of a loss of subcutaneous tissue. These clinical manifestations may also be signs of dehydration; however, in older adults, these are normal findings. The pupils may appear small, which can be unrelated to changes in neurologic status or medication administration. The pupil at age 60 is one third the size of a pupil at age 20.[129] Patients may complain of dry, itching eyes, which result from a decrease in lacrimal activity.[129]

Although healthy older adults generally do not have any remarkable deficit in taste, smell is significantly diminished.[130] However, taste is likely to be markedly affected in the patient with metabolic imbalance who is receiving multiple medications.

Loss of dentition is not a normal process of aging. It indicates poor nutrition and/or poor oral hygiene. Older adults commonly experience gradual hearing loss.[131] On physical examination, the older adult may have a reduced ability to distinguish low- and high-pitched sounds and may have difficulty in understanding high-pitched and rushed speech. The hearing loss is related to atrophy of the auditory nerve and the organ of Corti.[131]

INTEGUMENTARY AND MUSCULOSKELETAL SYSTEMS

As noted, the loss of elastic and connective tissue causes the skin to wrinkle; both skin wrinkles and sagging may be found over many areas of the body. The appearance and number of skin wrinkles also depend greatly on environmental agents and exposure to ultraviolet rays.[132] The nurse will also find that underlying structures such as the veins and muscles are more visible because of the transparency of the skin. Because of the loss of skin turgor, especially in the hands, the nurse assesses for dehydration by pinching the skin tissue over the sternum or forehead (see Table 13-5 for age-related changes in the skin and their related nursing interventions).

The nurse may also find multiple ecchymotic areas because of decreased protective subcutaneous tissue

Pharmacologic Management: Gerontologic Patients[38,105,116]

PHARMACOLOGIC AGENT	DRUG ACTIONS	ADVERSE DRUG EFFECTS*	NURSING INTERVENTIONS AND/OR SPECIAL CONSIDERATIONS
ACE Inhibitors Captopril Enalapril	Inhibits the conversion of angiotensin I to angiotensin II	Hypotension, especially in patients taking diuretics Hypokalemia	Monitor HR and BP Monitor serum creatinine level Monitor serum K^+ level Excreted by the kidney so the dosage is reduced if the GPR is reduced
Diuretics Bumex Lasix	Inhibits Na^+ and Cl^- absorption from the proximal tubule and loop of Henle	Hypokalemia Volume depletion	Reduced rate of clearance and magnitude of the diuretic response
Cardiac Glycosides Digoxin Dopamine Dobutamine	Inhibits the sarcolemmal Na^+-K^+-ATPase α_1-adrenergic agonist, dopaminergic agonist Sympathomimetic, beta$_1$-adrenergic agonist	Digitalis toxicity Ectopic beats, hypotension	Monitor HR and serum K^+ and serum digoxin levels Verapamil, quinidine, and amiodarone increase serum digoxin levels
Antidysrhythmics Procainamide Lidocaine	Decreases myocardial conduction velocity and excitability and prolongs myocardial refractoriness Decreases automaticity (especially in Purkinje fibers) and prolongs conduction and refractoriness	Procainamide toxicity Dizziness, paresthesia, and drowsiness at lower plasma concentrations	Procainamide is converted to its active metabolite, N-acetylprocainamide (NAPA), in the liver; NAPA may accumulate and cause side effects, even though the procainamide plasma level is within therapeutic range Can be administered only parenterally
Calcium Channel Blockers Verapamil Nifedipine Diltiazem	Blocks the entry of Ca^{++} through voltage-dependent Ca^{++} channels and decreases SA automaticity and AV conduction	Constipation May alter liver function Headaches, tachycardia, palpitations, flushing, and ankle edema Constipation	Monitor liver function tests Contraindicated in heart failure, sick sinus syndrome, or first-degree AV block Calcium channel blockers have a negative inotropic effect, but nifedipine produces less of a negative inotropic effect as compared with verapamil Monitor liver function tests Contraindicated in heart failure, sick sinus syndrome, or first-degree AV block

Data modified from Creasy WA et al: *J Clin Pharmacol* 26:264, 1986; Gilman AG et al, editors: *Goodman and Gilman's the continued pharmacologic basis of therapeutics*, London, 1990, Pergamon Press; Hockings N, Ajayi AA, Reid JL: *Br J Pharmacol* 21:341, 1986; Lynch RA, Horowitz LN: *Geriatrics* 46:41, 1991; Pederson KE: *Acta Med Scan* 697(suppl 1);1, 1985; Vidt GD, Borazanian RA: *Geriatrics* 46:28, 1991; Wall RT: *Clin Geriatr Med* 6:345, 1990; Watters JM, McClaran JC: The elderly surgical patient. In Wilmore DW et al, editors: vol vii, *Special problems*, New York, 1990, Scientific American.

HR, Heart rate; *BP*, blood pressure; *K*$^+$, potassium; *Ca*$^{++}$, calcium; *GFR*, glomerular filtration rate; *Na*$^+$, sodium; *Cl*$^-$, chloride; *SA*, sinoatrial; *AV*, atrioventricular; *CNS*, central nervous system.
*Not all side effects are listed for each drug.

Pharmacologic Management: Gerontologic Patients—cont'd

PHARMACOLOGIC AGENT	DRUG ACTIONS	ADVERSE DRUG EFFECTS	NURSING INTERVENTIONS AND/OR SPECIAL CONSIDERATIONS
Narcotic Analgesics			
Meperidine	Blocks the transmission of pain and inhibits the release of substance P; site of action is within the CNS	Respiratory depression and oversedation Tremors and muscle twitches related to effects of the metabolite normeperidine	Accumulation of normeperidine can produce CNS hyperexcitability
Morphine	Synthetic analgesic; mechanism similar to meperidine	Respiratory depression and oversedation	The volume of distribution for morphine is small; hence plasma and tissue levels are greater at a specific plasma concentration

Table 13-5	Age-Related Changes in the Integumentary System	
Skin Problem	**Underlying Mechanisms**	**Nursing Interventions**
Delayed wound healing	↓ Vascular supply to dermis ↓ Connective tissue layer ↓ SQ tissue layer Impaired inflammatory response ↓ New connective tissue proliferation	Use nonrestrictive dressings Weigh patient daily Support nutritional needs
Thermoregulation	↓ SQ tissue layer ↓ Number of capillary arterioles supply skin ↓ Number of eccrine (sweat glands)	Monitor room temperature
Pressure ulcers	↓ Flattening of capillary bed ↓ Thinning of epidermis	Reposition patient every 2 hours Use pressure-relieving devices
IV infiltrations	↓ Connective tissue layer Vascular fragility	Monitor peripheral IV site hourly Discontinue IV at first sign of infiltration
Diminished skin turgor	↓ Connective tissue layer ↓ Eccrine and sebaceous gland activity	Bathe with tepid water Avoid use of deodorant soap

IV, Infiltration; *SQ,* subcutaneous.

layers, increased capillary fragility, and flattening of the capillary bed, which predispose older adults to developing ecchymoses.[133-135] In conjunction with frequent aspirin use, these physiologic factors result in increased bleeding tendencies and the appearance of ecchymotic areas. However, areas of ecchymosis may also indicate elder abuse.

Changes that occur in the musculoskeletal system are a decrease in lean body mass; a compression of the spinal column, which results from the thinning of cartilage between vertebrae; and a decrease in the mobility of skeletal joints.[136,137] Despite the ubiquitous finding of reduced joint mobility, no exact physiologic process gives rise to the altered mobility. It is possible that the reduced synovial fluid production that occurs with aging causes changes in function. This may produce some changes in range of motion.

Bone demineralization afflicts both men and women as they age; however, it occurs four times more often in women than in men. Bone demineralization refers to an increase in osteoplast and osteoclast activity, which decreases calcium absorption into the bone.[137] Mineral loss (calcium and phosphorus), along with a decrease in bone mass, is referred to as *osteoporosis.*[137] Osteoporosis produces bones that are more "porous" or fragile. With extensive bone demineralization, an elderly patient may sustain multiple fractures. There is an accelerated incidence of osteoporosis in women, which occurs after the onset of menopause. A decrease in estrogen is implicated in this process, because estrogen replacement may arrest the osteoporosis process (although it will not reverse the process). The exact mechanism whereby estrogen affects bone mass is unknown. Evidence indicates that estrogen stimulates intestinal absorption of calcium, and the loss of estrogen action after menopause may in part be related to postmenopausal osteoporosis.[137] Decreased intake of dietary calcium, immobility, excess glucocorticoid secretion, and smoking all contribute to the development of osteoporosis. The nurse should be alert for physical signs of deformities associated with osteoporosis, such as kyphosis or scoliosis, which may place limitations on physical mobility and/or lead to gait instability.

RESPIRATORY AND CARDIOVASCULAR SYSTEMS

Many of the physiologic changes that occur with aging and the mechanisms underlying them have been addressed previously. The physical correlates to these changes are only noted in this section. On inspection of the aging thorax, the nurse will find a greater anterior-posterior diameter and some degree of kyphosis. On initial auscultation, bibasilar crackles may be heard; however, with several deep breaths and coughing, they should be cleared. Bibasilar crackles that do not clear with deep inspirations are suggestive of pathology. The cough reflex also is diminished, which predisposes the elderly patient

to aspiration. No changes are noted with palpation, but the nurse needs to assess for areas of tenderness, which could be the result of old fractures. Increased resonance is noted with percussion. Changes in tests of pulmonary function are noted in Tables 13-2 and 13-3.

There are relatively few modifications in the assessment of cardiovascular function and age-related physical findings in the older adult. As noted, resting heart rate decreases and systolic blood pressure increases with age. Manifestations of left ventricular hypertrophy and aortic sclerosis may include a prominent cardiac apex impulse, a prominent S_4 (fourth heart sound) at the cardiac apex, a single S_2 (second heart sound) (with expiration), and a short, early-peaking systolic murmur.[136]

GASTROINTESTINAL AND RENAL SYSTEMS

On physical examination of the nonobese older adult, the abdominal organs are more easily palpated because of a decrease in subcutaneous tissue. Despite a change in gastrointestinal (GI) motility, bowel sounds are normoactive. There are no remarkable physical assessment considerations with the hepatic-biliary and renal systems and no age-related change in liver function tests. BUN and serum creatinine levels can be normal or decreased in older adults (Box 13-1). As noted, the GFR decreases with age. In the hospital the GFR is estimated by the creatinine clearance. Endogenous creatinine is a metabolic by-product of muscle metabolism that is excreted by the kidney and is not reabsorbed. Usually the creatinine clearance is estimated by collecting a 24-hour urine sample to measure creatinine excretion. With advancing age, muscle mass decreases, thereby reducing the renal load of serum concentration of creatinine. Therefore in the geriatric patient, neither the creatinine excreted nor the plasma creatinine level may reflect the change in GFR. In older adults the Cockroft-Gault equation often is used to assess creatinine clearance (CrCl) and GFR (ml/min) because it incorporates serum creatinine levels, body weight, age, and gender as variables.[73] The Cockroft-Gault equation follows:

Males:

$$CrCl \text{ (ml/min)} = \frac{(140 - age)}{72 \times serum\ creatinine} \times weight\ (kg)$$

Females:

$$CrCl = 0.85 \times male\ CrCl$$

Box 13-1 lists the effects of aging on other laboratory tests that may or may not have clinical significance.[107,138]

CENTRAL NERVOUS SYSTEM

Physical examination of the central nervous system begins with a review of the older patient's mental status. The nurse assesses the patient's level of consciousness,

---

Box 13-1

EFFECTS OF AGING ON VARIOUS LABORATORY VALUES

VALUES THAT DO NOT CHANGE WITH AGE
Hemoglobin/hematocrit
Platelet count
White blood cell count with differential
Serum electrolytes
Coagulation profile
Liver function tests
Thyroid function tests
↔ or ↓ Blood urea nitrogen
↔ or ↓ Creatinine

VALUES THAT CHANGE WITH AGE BUT HAVE LITTLE CLINICAL SIGNIFICANCE
↓ Calcium
↑ Uric acid

VALUES THAT CHANGE WITH AGE AND HAVE CLINICAL SIGNIFICANCE
↓ Erythrocyte sedimentation rate
↓ Arterial oxygen pressure
↑ Blood glucose
↓ or ↑ Serum lipid profile
↓ Albumin

From Duthie EH Abbasi AA: *Geriatrics* 46:41, 1991.
↔, No change; ↓, decreased; ↑ increased.

Table 13-6	Summary of Age-Related Physiologic Changes and Related Clinical Considerations
Age-Related Effect	**Clinical Considerations**

CARDIOVASCULAR SYSTEM

↓ Inotropic and chronotropic response of myocardium to catecholamine stimulation ↑ Myocardial collagen content ↓ Baroreceptor sensitivity Prolonged rate of relaxation ↓ Compliance of blood vessels	The increase in CO achieved during stress or exercise is achieved by an increase in diastolic filling (increased dependence on Starling's law of the heart) Leads to a decrease in the compliance of the ventricle (higher filling pressures are needed to maintain stroke volume) ↑ Tendency for orthostatic hypotension after prolonged bed rest or if patient is taking antihypertensive medication or has systolic hypertension May predispose the elderly patient to hemodynamic derangements in the presence of tachydysrhythmias, hypertension, or ischemic heart disease ↑ Peripheral vascular resistance and blood pressure

RESPIRATORY SYSTEM

↓ Strength of the respiratory muscles, recoil of lungs, chest wall compliance, and efficiency and number of cilia in airways ↓ Pao_2 level	↑ Susceptibility to aspiration, atelectasis, and pulmonary infection Patient may require more frequent deep breathing, coughing, and position change ↓ Ventilatory response to hypoxia and hypercapnia ↑ Sensitivity to narcotics

RENAL SYSTEM

↓ GFR ↓ Ability to concentrate and conserve water ↓ Ability to excrete salt and water loads, as well as urea, ammonia, and drugs ↓ Response to an acid load	Careful observation of patient when administering aminoglycosides, antibiotics, and contrast dyes May predispose patient to development of dehydration and hypernatremia, especially if patient is fluid-restricted and insensible losses are high (e.g., during mechanical ventilation or fever) Observe for clinical manifestations of fluid overload and drug reactions After an acid load (i.e., metabolic acidosis) the elderly patient may be in a state of uncompensated metabolic acidosis for a longer period

LIVER

↓ Total liver blood flow	Adverse drug reactions, especially with polypharmacy

GASTROINTESTINAL SYSTEM

Diminished ability to swallow Impaired esophageal motility Delayed emptying of liquids ↓ Stool weight and transit time	May predispose elderly patient to aspiration pneumonia Assess for proper fit of dentures and ability to chew Flex head forward 45 degrees Develop awareness for complaints of food or medications "sticking in throat" Assess for complaints of heartburn or epigastric discomfort Avoid prolonged supine position Examine abdomen for distention Investigate complaints of anorexia Obtain thorough bowel history and note routine use of laxatives Increase intake of dietary fiber and assess for fecal incontinence and impaction

NEUROLOGIC SYSTEM

↑ Cranial dead space ↓ Number of neurons and dendrites and length of dendrite spines Delay in the rate of synaptogensis Changes in neurotransmitter turnover	Elderly persons may sustain a significant amount of hemorrhage before symptoms are apparent Delayed or impaired processing of sensory and motor information May cause desynchronization of neurotransmission

Modified from Rebenson-Piano M: *Crit Care Q* 12:1, 1989.
CO, Cardiac output; *GFR,* glomerular filtration rate.

ability to communicate and follow commands, and short- and long-term memory. In the critical care unit, parameters may be altered by hypoxia, electrolyte imbalances, or various medications. The practitioner may observe that the patient occasionally forgets minor details. The slow, gradual decline in some cognitive functions as evidenced by forgetfulness is considered normal.[139,140] However, forgetting important information such as name, address, and marital status is not part of the normal aging process. Although some older adults may have problems with short-term memory, long-term memory is intact. Older adults are commonly labeled "demented" or "confused." These cognitive syndromes have different etiologies and are not a normal part of aging. See Foreman, Gillies, and Wagner[141] for further review of impaired cognition in the older adult patient. It is important to remember that hearing dysfunction associated with aging affects spoken communication. Therefore careful attention should be taken in assessing cognition to assure that responses to questions are in response to the question actually posed. The neurologic examination for the geriatric patient always includes an assessment of muscle strength, reflexes, sensation, and cranial nerves.[142] There may be some changes in fine and gross motor skills. Handgrip strength declines with age and may correlate with a decreased ability to perform fine motor activity (e.g., tying a shoelace). Age diminishes the geriatric patient's vibratory sense, primarily in the lower extremities. Reflexes are slowed, which is caused by neuronal loss.[142] Neurologic deficits may ultimately alter the patient's ability to perform self-care. In addition, changes in older adults' cognitive function may al-

ter their ability to follow instructions and interpret patient-teaching instructions regarding their care in the critical care unit. Also, the critical care nurse evaluates the patient's gait if the patient is ambulatory.

IMMUNE SYSTEM

Infections in the older adult initially appear as an acute onset of mental status changes, anorexia, urinary incontinence, falls, or generalized weakness.[111,143] However, these may be signs of a urinary tract infection or pneumonia, two common infections in older adults. As noted, the response of the immune system is attenuated; therefore signs such as fever and chills initially may be absent.

SUMMARY

The older adult requires more intense observation and consideration in the critical care unit because his or her system has become less adaptable to stress and illness. (For further discussion, see the Clinical Application feature.) Table 13-6 summarizes the major changes in the various systems, along with clinical considerations.[144] As shown in Fig. 13-3, many physiologic changes occur with advancing age, and each change may render a particular system less adaptable to stress. In addition, the change in one system may affect another system in the presence of disease. The inability to adapt poses a significant risk for functional decline after discharge. Older adults at the greatest risk include those with poor nutritional status or cognitive dysfunction, and those who re-

---

CLINICAL APPLICATION

Gerontologic Concepts

Mr. S, a 72-year-old retired construction worker, was admitted through the emergency room with an acute exacerbation of chronic bronchitis. Since admission, his respiratory distress has increased, his oxygenation status has worsened, and his work of breathing is rapidly leading to fatigue.

1. What evidence of Mr. S's respiratory status would the nurse assess for on inspection?
2. What changes might the nurse expect to see related to Mr. S's age?
3. What respiratory physiologic changes are expected because of Mr. S's age, and how would they impact his risk of chronic obstructive pulmonary disease (COPD) exacerbation?
4. Analyze the following diagnostic data, describing the effects aging may have on the results:

a. Chart data:
   - Vital signs: HR, 154 (irregular); RR, 28 (labored, shallow); BP, 104/62; T, 99.5° F (oral)
   - Laboratory data: ABGs—pH, 7.21; PaO_2, 45 mm Hg; $PaCO_2$, 65 mm Hg; HCO_3, 28 mEq/L; O_2 saturation, 78%; CBC—WBC, 12,000/mm³; RBC, 6.5 million/mm³; Hct, 65%
   - ECG: Atrial fibrillation with a rapid ventricular response
b. Physical data: Extreme shortness of breath, unable to talk, currently receiving O_2 via Venturi face mask at 40% FIO_2, minimally productive weak cough, lethargic, unable to follow simple commands.
5. In planning Mr. S's care, what alterations will you make because of his age?

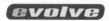 For the discussion of the Clinical Application and for an additional clinical application on gerontologic alterations, see the Evolve website.

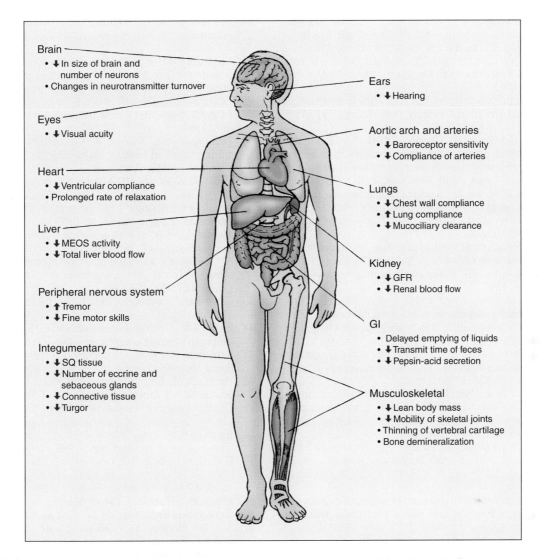

Fig. 13-3 Summary of the physiologic changes that occur in all systems and that the critical care nurse must consider in caring for the elderly patient in the critical care unit. *MEOS,* Microsomal enzyme oxidative system; *GFR,* glomerular filtration rate; *GI,* gastrointestinal; *SQ,* subcutaneous.

quired assistance with at least two activities of daily living before admission.[145]

The critical care nurse must also be aware of socioeconomic factors that confront older adult patients, as well as lifestyle adjustments such as the death of a spouse or friend. Changes in Medicare payment for hospitalization and medication have also placed a financial burden on such patients. To provide the best care and prevent iatrogenic complications, the critical care nurse must consider all physiologic and psychologic factors that affect the older adult patient.

REFERENCES

1. *Profile of Older Americans:* 2003, Administration on Aging, US Department of Health and Human Services; www.aoa.dhhs.gov/aoa/stats/profile/default.html.

2. Hall MJ, Owings MF: 2000 National hospital discharge survey, *Advance Data* 329:1-20. DHHS Publication No. 2002-1250.

3. Resnick NM: Geriatric Medicine. In Braunwald E et al, editors: *Harrison's principles of internal medicine,* ed 15, New York, 2001, McGraw Hill.

4. Levine BS, Craven RF: Physiologic adaptations with aging. In Woods SL et al, editors: *Cardiac nursing,* ed 5, Philadelphia, 2005, Lippincott Williams & Wilkins.

5. Polanczyk C et al: Impact of age on perioperative complications and length of stay in patients undergoing noncardiac surgery, *Ann Intern Med* 134:637, 2001.

6. Eghbali M et al: Collagen accumulation in heart ventricles as a function of growth and aging, *Cardiovasc Res* 23:723, 1989.

7. Wegelius O, von Knorring J: The hydroxyproline and hexosamine content in human myocardium at different ages, *Acta Med Scand Suppl* 412:233, 1964.

8. Katz AM: Heart failure. In Fozzard HA et al, editors: *The heart and cardiovascular system,* New York, 1991, Raven.

9. Eaton L: Cardiovascular function. In Lueckenotte AG, editor: *Gerontologic nursing*, ed 2, St Louis, 2000, Mosby.

10. Nadelmann J et al: Prevalence, incidence and prognosis of recognized and unrecognized myocardial infarction in persons aged 75 years or older: The Bronx aging study, *Am J Cardiol* 66:533, 1990.

11. Mukerji V, Holman AJ, Alpert MA: The clinical description of angina pectoris in the elderly, *Am Heart J* 117:705, 1989.

12. Lakatta EG, Schulman SP, Gerstenblith G: Cardiovascular aging in health and therapeutic considerations in older patients with cardiovascular diseases. In Fuster V, et al, editors: *Hurst's the heart*, ed 10, New York, 2001, McGraw-Hill.

13. Gerstenblith G et al: Echocardiographic assessment of normal adult aging population, *Circulation* 56:273, 1977.

14. Opie LH: *The physiology of the heart and metabolism*, New York, 1991, Raven.

15. Lakatta EG et al: Prolonged contraction duration in the aged myocardium, *J Clin Invest* 55:61, 1975.

16. Cinelli P et al: Effects of age on mean heart rate variability, *Aging* 10:146, 1987.

17. Ribera JM et al: Cardiac rate and hyperkinetic rhythm disorders in healthy elderly subjects: evaluation by ambulatory electrocardiographic monitoring, *Gerontology* 35:158, 1989.

18. Jose AD: Effect of combined sympathetic and parasympathetic blockage on heart rate and cardiac function in man, *Am J Cardiol* 18:476, 1966.

19. Rodeheffer RJ et al: Exercise cardiac output is maintained with advancing age in human subjects: cardiac dilation and increased stroke volume compensate for a diminished heart rate, *Circulation* 69:203, 1984.

20. Aronow WS: Effects of aging on the heart. In Tallis RC, Fillit HM, editors: *Brocklehurst's textbook of geriatric medicine and gerontology*, ed 6, London, 2003, Churchill Livingstone.

21. Bonow RO et al: Effects of aging on asynchronous left ventricular regional function and global ventricular filling in normal human subjects, *J Am Coll Cardiol* 11:50, 1988.

22. Miller TR et al: Left ventricular diastolic filling and its association with age, *Am J Cardiol* 58:531, 1986.

23. Davidson WR, Fee WC: Influence of aging on pulmonary hemodynamics in a population free of coronary artery disease, *Am J Cardiol* 65:1454, 1990.

24. Bachman S, Sparrow D, Smith LK: Effect of aging on the electrocardiogram, *Am J Cardiol* 48:513, 1981.

25. Horwitz LN, Lynch RA: Managing geriatric arrhythmias. I. General considerations, *Geriatrics* 46:31, 1991.

26. Carom AJ et al: The rhythm of the heart in active elderly subjects, *Am Heart J* 99:598, 1980.

27. Fleg JL, Kennedy HL: Cardiac arrhythmias in 9 healthy elderly population: detection by a 24-hour ambulatory electrocardiography, *Chest* 81:638, 1982.

28. Aronow WS: Cardia arrhythmias. In Tallis RC, Fillit HM, editors: *Brocklehurst's textbook of geriatric medicine and gerontology*, ed 6, London, 2003, Churchill Livingstone.

29. Bristow MR et al: Cardiac-resynchronization therapy with or without an implantable defibrillator in advanced chronic heart failure, *N Engl J Med* 350:2140, 2004.

30. Docherty JR: Cardiovascular responses in aging: a review, *Pharmacol* Rev 42:103, 1990.

31. Yin FCP et al: Age-associated decrease in ventricular response to haemodynamic stress during beta-adrenergic blockade, *Br Heart J* 40:1349, 1978.

32. Elliott HL et al: Effects of age in the responsiveness of vascular alpha-adrenoreceptors in man, *J Cardiovasc Pharmacol* 4:388, 1982.

33. Strogatz DS et al: Correlates of postural hypotension in a community sample of elderly blacks and whites, *JAGS* 39:562, 1991.

34. Applegate WB et al: Prevalence of postural hypotension at baseline in the systolic hypertension in the elderly program (SHEP) cohort, *J Am Geriatr Soc* 39:1057, 1991.

35. Smith JJ et al: The effect of age on hemodynamic response to graded postural stress in normal men, *J Gerontol* 42:406, 1987.

36. Dambrink JHA, Wieling W: Circulatory response to postural change in healthy male subjects in relation to age, *Clin Sci* 72:335, 1987.

37. Yin FCP, Weisfeldt ML, Milnor WR: Role of aortic input impedance in the decreased cardiovascular response to exercise in aging dogs, *J Clin Invest* 68:28, 1981.

38. Potter JF: Hypertension. In Tallis RC, Fillit HM, editors: *Brocklehurst's textbook of geriatric medicine and gerontology*, ed 6, London, 2003, Churchill Livingstone.

39. Schoenberger JA: Epidemiology of systolic and diastolic systemic blood pressure elevation in the elderly, *Am J Cardiol* 57:45c, 1986.

40. Lawn RM: Lipoprotein(a) in heart disease, *Sci Am* 266:54, 1992.

41. Rowe JW: Clinical consequences of age-related impairments in vascular compliance, *Am J Cardiol* 60:68G, 1987.

42. Kreisberg RA, Kasim S: Cholesterol metabolism and aging, *Am J Med* 82:54, 1987.

43. Davis CE et al: Lipoprotein-cholesterol distributions in selected North American populations: The Lipid Research Clinics Program Prevalence Study, *Circulation* 2:302, 1980.

44. Rose BD: *Clinical physiology of acid-base and electrolyte disorders*, New York, 1989, McGraw-Hill.

45. Hall JE, Coleman TG, Guyton AC: The renin-angiotensin system: normal physiology and changes in older hypertensives, *J Am Geriatr Soc* 37:801, 1989.

46. Crane MG, Harris JJ: Effect of aging on renin activity and aldosterone excretion, *J Lab Clin Med* 87:947, 1976.

47. Sica DA, Harford A: Sodium and water disorders in the elderly. In Zawada ET, Sica DA, editors: *Geriatric nephrology and urology*, Littleton, Mass, 1985, PSG Publishing.

48. Webster JR, Kadah H: Unique aspects of respiratory disease in the aged, *Geriatrics* 46:31, 1991.

49. Connolly MJ: Age-related changes in the respiratory system. In Tallis RC, Fillit HM, editors: *Brocklehurst's textbook of geriatric medicine and gerontology*, ed 6, London, 2003, Churchill Livingstone.

50. Connolly MJ: Asthma and chronic obstructive pulmonary disease. In Tallis RC, Fillit HM, editors: *Brocklehurst's textbook of geriatric medicine and gerontology*, ed 6, London, 2003, Churchill Livingstone.

51. Thurlbeck WM: Growth, aging and adaptation. In Murray JF, Nadel JA, editors: *Textbook of respiratory medicine*, Philadelphia, 1988, Saunders.

52. Levitzky MG: Effects of aging on the respiratory system, *Physiologist* 27:102, 1984.

53. Mittman C et al: Relationship between chest wall and pulmonary compliance and age, *J Appl Physiol* 20:1211, 1965.

54. West JB: *Respiratory physiology*, ed 5, Baltimore, 1995, Williams & Wilkins.

55. Rizzato G, Marazzine L: Thoracoabdominal mechanisms in elderly men, *J Appl Physiol* 28:457, 1970.

56. Gutmann E, Hanzlikova V: Fast and slow motor units in aging, *Gerontology* 22:280, 1976.

57. Pontoppidan HH, Beecher HK: Progressive loss of protective reflexes in the airway with advance of age, *JAMA* 1974:2209, 1960.

58. Belman MJ, Gaesser GA: Ventilatory muscle training in the elderly, *J Appl Physiol* 64:899, 1988.

59. Knudson RJ et al: Changes in the normal maximal expiratory flow-volume curve with growth and aging, *Am Rev Respir Dis* 127:725, 1983.

60. Turner JM, Mead J, Wohl ME: Elasticity of human lungs in relation to age, *J Appl Physiol* 25:664, 1968.

61. Pierce JA, Hocott JB: Studies on the collagen and elastin content of the human lung, *J Clin Invest* 39:8, 1960.

62. Pierce JA, Ebert RV: Fibrous network of the lung and its change with age, *Thorax* 20:469, 1965.

63. Semmens M: The pulmonary artery in the normal aged lung, *Br J Dis Chest* 64:65, 1970.

64. Sorbini CA et al: Arterial oxygen tension in relation to age in healthy subjects, *Respiration* 25:3, 1968.

65. LeBlanc P, Ruff F, Milic-Emili J: Effects of age and body position on "airway closure" in man, *J Appl Physiol* 28:448, 1970.

66. Holland J et al: Regional distribution of pulmonary ventilation and perfusion in elderly subjects, *J Clin Invest* 47:81, 1968.

67. Knudson RJ et al: Effect of aging alone on mechanical properties of the normal adult human lung, *J Appl Physiol* 43:1054, 1977.

68. Knudson RJ et al: The maximal expiratory flow-volume curve: normal standards, variability, and effects of age, *Am Rev Respir Dis* 113:587, 1976.

69. Gold WM: Pulmonary function testing. In Murray JF et al, editors: *Textbook of respiratory medicine*, ed 3, Philadelphia, 2000, Saunders.

70. Wahba WH: Influence of aging on lung function: clinical significance of changes from age twenty, *Anesth Analg* 62:764, 1983.

71. Weder AB: The renally compromised older hypertensive: therapeutic considerations, *Geriatrics* 46:36, 1991.

72. Maddox DA, Alavi FK, Zawada ET: The kidney and aging. In Massry SG, Glassock RJ, editors: *Textbook of nephrology*, ed 4, Philadelphia, 2001, Lippincott Williams & Wilkins.

73. Gilbert BR, Vaughan ED: Pathophysiology of the aging kidney, *Clin Geriatric Med* 6(1):12, 1990.

74. Kasiske BL: Relationship between vascular disease and age-associated changes in the human kidney, *Kidney Int* 31:1153, 1987.

75. Anderson S, Brenner BM: Effects of aging on the renal glomerulus, *Am J Med* 80:435, 1986.

76. Watters JM, McClaran JC: The elderly surgical patient. In Wilmore DW et al, editors: *Care of the surgical patient*, (vol VII, *Special Problems*), New York, 1990, Scientific American.

77. Tepper RE, Katz S: Geriatric gastroenterology: overview. In Tallis RC, Fillit HM, editors: *Brocklehurst's textbook of geriatric medicine and gerontology*, ed 6, London, 2003, Churchill Livingstone.

78. Greenwald DA, Brandt LJ: The upper gastrointestinal tract. In Tallis RC, Fillit HM, editors: *Brocklehurst's textbook of geriatric medicine and gerontology*, ed 6, London, 2003, Churchill Livingstone.

79. Altman DF: Changes in gastrointestinal, pancreatic, biliary and hepatic function in aging, *Gastroenterol Clin North Am* 19:227, 1990.

80. Thomson AB, Keelan M: The aging gut, *Can J Physiol Pharmacol* 64:30, 1986.

81. Bansal SK et al: Upper gastrointestinal hemorrhage in the elderly: a record of 92 patients in a joint geriatric/surgical unit, *Age Aging* 16:279, 1987.

82. Moore JG et al: Effect of age on gastric emptying of liquid-solid meals in man, *Dig Dis Sci* 28(4):340, 1983.

83. Schuster MM: Disorders of the aging GI system, *Hosp Prac* 11:95, 1976.

84. Curran J: Overview of geriatric nutrition, *Dysphagia* 5:72, 1990.

85. Tepper RE, Katz S: Geriatric gastroenterology: overview. In Tallis RC, Fillit HM, editors: *Brocklehurst's textbook of geriatric medicine and gerontology*, ed 6, London, 2003, Churchill Livingstone.

86. Sato TG, Miwa T, Tauchi H: Age changes in the human liver of the different races, *Gerontology* 16:368, 1970.

87. Bach B et al: Disposition of antipyrine and phenytoin correlated with age and liver volume in man, *Clin Pharmacokinet* 6:389, 1981.

88. James OFW: The liver. In Tallis RC, Fillit HM, editors: *Brocklehurst's textbook of geriatric medicine and gerontology* ed 6, London, 2003, Churchill Livingstone.

89. Schmucker DL, Wang RK: Age-related changes in liver drug metabolism: structure versus function, *Proc Soc Exp Biol Med* 165:178, 1980.

90. Guay DRP et al: The pharmacology of aging. In Tallis RC, Fillit HM, editors: *Brocklehurst's textbook of geriatric medicine and gerontology*, ed 6, London, 2003, Churchill Livingstone.

91. Yuen GJ: Altered pharmacokinetics in the elderly, *Clin Geriatric Med* 6:257, 1990.

92. Stuart-Hamilton IA: Normal cognitive aging. In Tallis RC, Fillit HM, editors: *Brocklehurst's textbook of geriatric medicine and gerontology*, ed 6, London, 2003, Churchill Livingstone.

93. Quinn J, Kaye J: The neurology of aging, *Neurologist* 7:98, 2001.

94. Wilcock GK: Alzheimer's disease. In Tallis RC, Fillit HM, editors: *Brocklehurst's textbook of geriatric medicine and gerontology*, ed 6, London, 2003, Churchill Livingstone.

95. Rockwood K, Erkinjuntti T: Vascular dementia. In Tallis RC, Fillit HM, editors: *Brocklehurst's textbook of geriatric medicine and gerontology*, ed 6, London, 2003, Churchill Livingstone.

96. Arriagada P et al: Neurofibrillary tangles but not senile plaques parallel duration and severity of Alzheimer's disease, *Neurology* 42:631, 1992.

97. Selkoe DJ: Aging brain, aging mind, *Sci Amer* 267:134, 1992.

98. Morris JC, McManus DQ: The neurology of aging: normal versus pathologic change, *Geriatrics* 46:47, 1991.

99. Lytle LD, Altar A: Diet, central nervous system, and aging, *Fed Proc* 38:2017, 1979.

100. Cotman CW: Synaptic plasticity, neurotropic factors and transplantation in the aged brain. In Schneider EL, Rowe JW, editors: *Handbook of the biology of aging*, San Diego, 1990, Academic Press.

101. Gottstein U, Held K: Effects of aging on cerebral circulation and metabolism in man, *Acta Neurol Scand Suppl* 72:54-55, 1979.

102. Meara J: Parkinsonism and other movement disorders. In Tallis RC, Fillit HM, editors: *Brocklehurst's textbook of geriatric medicine and gerontology*, ed 6, London, 2003, Churchill Livingstone.

103. Pompei P: Delirium. In Tallis RC, Fillit HM, editors: *Brocklehurst's textbook of geriatric medicine and gerontology*, ed 6, London, 2003, Churchill Livingstone.

104. Litton KA: Delirium in the critical care patient: what the professional staff needs to know, *Crit Care Nurs Q* 26:208, 2003.

105. Potter JF: Hypertension. In Tallis RC, Fillit HM, editors: *Brocklehurst's textbook of geriatric medicine and gerontology*, ed 6, London, 2003, Churchill Livingstone.

106. Gravenstein S, Fillit HM, Ershler WB: Clinical immunology of aging. In Tallis RC, Fillit HM, editors: *Brocklehurst's textbook of geriatric medicine and gerontology*, ed 6, London, 2003, Churchill Livingstone.

107. Hanlon JT, Lindblad C, Maher RL, Schmader K: Geriatric pharmacotherapy. In Tallis RC, Fillit HM, editors: *Brocklehurst's textbook of geriatric medicine and gerontology*, ed 6, London, 2003, Churchill Livingstone.

108. Miller RA: Immune system. In Masoro EJ, editor: *Handbook of physiology: aging*, New York, 1995, Oxford University Press.

109. Terpenning MS, Bradley SF: Why aging leads to increased susceptibility to infection, *Geriatrics* 46:77, 1991.

110. Miller RA: The aging immune system: primer and prospectus, *Science* 273:70, 1996.

111. Rajagopalan S, Moran D: Infectious disease emergencies in older adults, *Clin Geriatr* 9:1, 2001; website: http://www.mmhc.com/engine.pl?station=mmhc&template=cgfull.html&id=1003.

112. President's Commission for the Study of Ethical Problems in Medicine and Biomedical and Behavioral Research: *Deciding to forgo life-sustaining treatment: a report on the ethical, medical and legal issues on treatment decisions*, 1993, Washington, DC, US Government County Office.

113. Schwertz DW, Bushmann MT: Pharmacogeriatics, *Crit Care Q* 12:26, 1989.

114. Gilman AG et al, editors: *Goodman and Gilman's the pharmacological basis of therapeutics*, ed 8, London, 1990, Pergamon.

115. Gillespie ND, Struthers AD: Chronic cardiac failure. In Tallis RC, Fillit HM, editors: *Brocklehurst's textbook of geriatric medicine and gerontology*, ed 6, London, 2003, Churchill Livingstone.

116. The SCOPE Study Group: The study on cognition and prognosis in the elderly (SCOPE): principal results of a randomized double-blind intervention trial, *J Hypertension* 21:875, 2003.

117. Mooradian AD: An update of the clinical pharmacokinetics, therapeutic monitoring techniques and treatment recommendations, *Clin Pharmacokinet* 18:165, 1988.

118. Creasy WA et al: Pharmacokinetics of captopril in elderly healthy male volunteers, *J Clin Pharmacol* 26:264, 1986.

119. Hockings N, Ajayi AA, Reid JL: Age and the pharmacodynamics of angiotensin converting enzyme inhibitors, enalapril and enalaprilat, *Br J Pharmacol* 21:341, 1986.

120. Pederson KE: Digoxin interactions: the influence of quinidine and verapamil on the pharmacokinetics and receptor binding of digitalis glycosides, *Acta Med Scand* 697 (suppl 1):1, 1985.

121. Lynch RA, Horowitz LN: Managing geriatric arrhythmias. II. Drug selection and use, *Geriatrics* 46:41, 1991.

122. Vidt GD, Borazanian RA: Calcium channel blockers in geriatric hypertension, *Geriatrics* 46:28, 1991.

123. Bertel O et al: Decreased beta-adrenoreceptor responsiveness as related to age, blood pressure and plasma catecholamines in patients with essential hypertension, *Hypertension* 2:130, 1980.

124. Kendall MJ et al: Responsiveness to beta-adrenergic receptor stimulation: the effects of age are cardioselective, *Br J Clin Pharmacol* 14:821, 1982.

125. Balas MC, Gale M, Kagan SH: Delirium doulas: an innovative approach to enhance care for critically ill older adults, *Crit Care Nurse* 24:36, 2004.

126. Fields SD: History-taking in the elderly: obtaining useful information, *Geriatrics* 46(8):26, 1991.

127. Geokas MC: The aging process, *Ann Intern Med* 113:455, 1990.

128. Mobbs CV: Neurobiology of aging. In Tallis RC, Fillit HM, editors: *Brocklehurst's textbook of geriatric medicine and gerontology*, ed 6, London, 2003, Churchill Livingstone.

129. Brodie SE: Aging and disorders of the eye. In Tallis RC, Fillit HM, editors: *Brocklehurst's textbook of geriatric medicine and gerontology*, ed 6, London, 2003, Churchill Livingstone.

130. Blandford G: Eating disorders. In Tallis RC, Fillit HM, editors: *Brocklehurst's textbook of geriatric medicine and gerontology*, ed 6, London, 2003, Churchill Livingstone.

131. Weinstein BE: Disorders of hearing. In Tallis RC, Fillit HM, editors: *Brocklehurst's textbook of geriatric medicine and gerontology*, ed 6, London, 2003, Churchill Livingstone.

132. Brooke RC, Griffiths CE: Aging of the skin. In Tallis RC, Fillit HM, editors: *Brocklehurst's textbook of geriatric medicine and gerontology*, ed 6, London, 2003, Churchill Livingstone.

133. Jones PL, Millman A: Wound healing and the aged patient, *Nurs Clin North Am* 25(1):263, 1990.

134. Kelly L, Mobily PR: Iatrogenesis in the elderly, *J Geron Nurs* 17(9):24, 1991.

135. Shenefelt PD, Fenske NA: Aging and the skin: recognizing and managing common disorders, *Geriatrics* 45(10):57, 1990.

136. Francis RM: Metabolic bone disease. In Tallis RC, Fillit HM, editors: *Brocklehurst's textbook of geriatric medicine and gerontology*, ed 6, London, 2003, Churchill Livingstone.

137. Tobias JH, Sharif M: Bone and joint aging. In Tallis RC, Fillit HM, editors: *Brocklehurst's textbook of geriatric medicine and gerontology*, ed 6, London, 2003, Churchill Livingstone.

138. Duthie EH, Abbasi AA: Laboratory testing: current recommendations for older adults, *Geriatrics* 46:10, 1991.

139. Quinn J, Kaye J: The neurology of aging, *The Neurologist* 7:98, 2001.

140. Howieson DB et al: Natural history of cognitive decline in the old, *Neurology* 60:1489, 2003.

141. Foreman MD, Gillies DA, Wagner D: Impaired cognition in the critically ill elderly patient: clinical implications, *Crit Care Q* 12:61, 1989.

142. Boss BJ: Normal aging in the nervous system: implications for SCI nurses, *SCI* 8(2): 42, 1991.

143. Henshke PJ: Infections in the elderly, *Med J Aust* 158:830, 1993.

144. Piano MR: The physiologic changes that occur with aging, *Crit Care Q* 12:1, 1989.

145. Covinsky KE et al: Loss of independence in activities of daily living in older adults hospitalized with medical illnesses: increased vulnerability with age, *J Am Geriatr Soc* 51:451, 2003.

CHAPTER 14

Perianesthesia Management

Many advances in anesthetic agents and monitoring have resulted in more precise and safer delivery of anesthetic agents. However, caring for the critically ill patient who is emerging from anesthesia requires diligent monitoring of the patient's physical and psychologic status to prevent potential complications that may occur as a result of the anesthetic agents or techniques. To provide safe and competent patient care, the critical care nurse needs to be aware of anesthetic agents and techniques and the physiologic and psychologic responses of patients who are subjected to anesthesia.[1,2]

SELECTION OF ANESTHESIA

The complex structure of the anesthetic agents, combined with potential drug interactions and the patient's physical condition, can make it difficult to predict exactly how the patient will respond when emerging from anesthesia. An understanding of general principles prepares the nurse for the most commonly expected outcomes.[2,3] The American Society of Anesthesiologists (ASA) physical status classification is a widely accepted method of preoperative patient evaluation. It serves as a guide to communicate clinical conditions and predict risks for anesthesia (Box 14-1).[4]

The type of anesthesia used for surgery may be local, regional, or general. Local and regional anesthetics eliminate the sensation of pain to a specific part of the body without loss of protective reflexes or consciousness. In addition many patients will also receive intravenous sedation with benzodiazepines to relieve anxiety, provide amnesia, and promote relaxation. Local anesthesia with sedation is commonly referred to as conscious or procedural sedation. Depending on the amount of sedation given and the patient' response, the level of consciousness can range from light to deep. For further discussion on sedation see Chapter 8. Regional anesthesia is achieved through the use of nerve blocks or spinal or epidural catheters. Spinal anesthesia involves injecting

the lumbar subarachnoid space with local anesthetics. Epidural anesthesia involves injecting the epidural space with local anesthetics and/or narcotics. Both spinal and epidural anesthesia cause sensory and motor anesthesia. The advantages of epidural over spinal anesthesia are decreased incidence of spinal headache and increased ability to provide postoperative pain management. General anesthesia is a controlled state of unconsciousness, the patient is not arousable, there is partial or complete loss of protective reflexes, and the airway needs to be continuously monitored and maintained. The preferred method of maintaining the patient's airway during general anesthesia is with an endotracheal tube.[3-5]

Several factors influence the choice of anesthetic agent and the mode of delivery. They include the age and physical status of the patient, the type of surgery, the skills of the anesthesiologist and surgeon, and the patient's wishes.

GENERAL ANESTHESIA

The objectives of general anesthesia are analgesia, amnesia/hypnosis, blocking of reflexes, and skeletal muscle relaxation. There are four distinct phases or stages of anesthesia.

Stage I, commonly called the stage of analgesia, begins with the initiation of an anesthetic agent and ends with the loss of consciousness. This stage has been described as the lightest level of anesthesia and represents mild sensory and mental depression. Patients can open their eyes on command, breathe normally, and maintain protective reflexes. The patient's pain threshold is not appreciably lowered during this stage.[2,3,5]Stage II, also called the stage of delirium, begins with the loss of consciousness and ends with the onset of a regular pattern of breathing and the disappearance of the eyelid reflex. It is characterized by excitement, which can include uncontrolled movement and potentially dangerous responses to noxious stimuli. Other responses include vomiting, laryngospasm, tachycardia, and even cardiac

Box 14-1

ASA CATEGORIES

Category 1—Normal, healthy patient
Category 2—Patient with mild systemic disease
Category 3—Patient with severe systemic disease
  (hypertension, diabetes)
Category 4—Patient with severe systemic disease that is
  a threat to life
Category 5—Patient with high morbidity
Category 6—Brain death

ASA, American Society of Anesthesiologists.

Box 14-2

IDEAL CHARACTERISTICS OF ANESTHETIC AGENTS/ADJUNCTS

Rapid onset of action
Controllable duration of action
Identifiable levels of depths
Technically easy to administer
No untoward effects on vital signs
No toxic metabolites
Predictable elimination
High specificity of action
High margin of safety
Useful with all ages
Cost-effective
Rapid emergence

arrest. If vomiting occurs, the patient is at risk for aspiration because of the loss of protective reflexes that is associated with this stage of anesthesia. With the use of newer and faster-acting anesthetic agents this stage is passed through rapidly, decreasing the risk of complications. In addition, the use of short-acting barbiturates during the induction of anesthesia facilitates rapid transition through stage II.[2,3,5]

Stage III is the stage of surgical anesthesia. It is defined as lasting from the onset of regular pattern of breathing to cessation of breathing. This is the goal for anesthesia, since the response to surgical incision is absent. Patients experience a depression in all elements of nervous system function (i.e., sensory depression, loss of recall, reflex depression, some skeletal muscle relaxation). Each anesthetic agent affects the patient's clinical signs differently; therefore monitoring the effects of anesthesia depends on the specific properties of each agent.[2,3,5]

Stage IV is considered the stage of overdose and occurs when the patient receives too much anesthesia. In this stage the patient will show signs of circulatory failure, and full cardiovascular and pulmonary support must be provided.[2,3,5]

During general anesthesia the goal is to keep the patient in Stage III. If the patient is not given enough anesthesia the patient may experience recall or awareness during surgery. If the patient is given too much anesthesia, stress on the patient and recovery time increase. The level of anesthesia is monitored by subjective and objective methods. Subjective methods include hemodynamic changes, pupil dilation, sweating, and lacrimation. Objective monitoring techniques include spontaneous surface electromyogram, lower esophageal contractility, heart rate variability, and evoked potentials. Bispectral index (BIS) is the newest technique for monitoring levels of anesthesia. Studies show that the BIS values correlate with the stages of anesthesia. The BIS monitoring system is currently being studied in the operating room and in critical care units to monitor depth of anesthesia and level of sedation.[6-9]

ANESTHETIC AGENTS

Usually two or more anesthetic agents are used in combination to achieve the desired level of anesthesia. In order to anticipate the patient's response, it is important for the nurse to have knowledge of the anesthetic agents that are used and the usual physiologic effects.

The ideal characteristics of anesthetic agents and adjuncts are listed in Box 14-2.[2]

INHALATION AGENTS

Inhalation agents are be used for induction and maintenance of anesthesia or in combination with other anesthetic agents to maintain Stage III anesthesia. Their exact mechanism of action is unknown, but all cause central nervous system depression and a state of unconsciousness that is deep enough to allow surgery. The Pharmacologic Management table on Inhalation Anesthetics lists the inhalation anesthetics presently used and their chief characteristics, effects, and nursing implications.[10]

INTRAVENOUS ANESTHETICS

Because inhalation anesthetics can produce adverse effects such as vasodilation, hypotension, dysrhythmias, and myocardial depression, other medications and methods of delivery were sought to provide general anesthesia. Intravenous (IV) anesthetics are now commonly used in the perioperative period. IV anesthetics are grouped by their primary pharmacologic action as nonopioid or opioid intravenous agents. The nonopioid agents are further divided into the barbiturates, nonbarbiturates, and tranquilizers. These drugs can be administered by intermittent IV push dosing to induce anesthesia or be administered by continuous IV drip to maintain anesthesia.[2,11]

Pharmacologic Management: Inhalation Anesthetics

DRUG	CHARACTERISTICS	EFFECTS	CONSIDERATIONS
Nitrous oxide	Light anesthetic; carrier for other inhalation agents; always given with oxygen	Anesthetic and analgesic; little pulmonary, cardiac, or CNS effects; increases intracranial pressure; amnesia	Eliminated via ventilation; nausea and vomiting; diffusion hypoxia; mild myocardial depression
Halothane (Fluothane)	Nonpungent, nonirritating odor; less likely to cause laryngospasms; pediatric agent	Bronchodilator; decreases mucociliary function and pharyngeal reflex	Myocardial depression; decreases SVR, contractility, and cardiac output; hepatotoxicity; "halothane shakes"; may trigger malignant hypothermia
Enflurane (Ethrane)	Used for deliberate hypotension cases	Vasodilator; marked cardiovascular stability; good operative analgesic; pleasant induction and emergence	Decreases SVR and seizure threshold; less nausea and vomiting
Isoflurane (Forane)	Pungent ether-like odor; low potential for toxicity; successful ambulatory agent	Higher cardiovascular stability; potentiates muscle relaxants	Mild depression of spontaneous ventilation; postoperative shivering; fewer dysrhythmias noted
Desflurane (Suprane)	Strong, pungent odor; rapid onset; requires warmed vaporizer for administration	Minimal metabolism; respiratory depression; cardiovascular depression; no lingering analgesia	Observe for breath holding; coughing and laryngospasm; needs immediate analgesia
Sevoflurane (Ultane)	Little pungency; pediatric anesthetic	Minimal airway irritation; rapid elimination; great precision and control over anesthetic depth	May trigger malignant hypothermia; observe for breath holding

CNS, Central nervous system; *SVR*, systemic vascular resistance.

NONOPIOID INTRAVENOUS ANESTHETICS

The nonopioid drugs appear to interact with γ- (gamma) aminobutyric acid (GABA) in the brain. GABA is an inhibitory neurotransmitter. Activation of the GABA receptors inhibits the postsynaptic neuron and results in a loss of consciousness. Barbiturates bind to GABA postsynaptic receptors, inhibiting neuronal activity and causing a loss of consciousness. Tranquilizers such as benzodiazepines potentiate the action of GABA, leading to inhibition of neuronal activity. Nonbarbituate induction agents, such as etomidate, antagonize the muscarinic receptors in the central nervous system (CNS) and work as opioid agonists, resulting in a hypnotic state and loss of consciousness.[2,11] The Pharmacologic Management table on Nonopiod Intravenous Anesthetics presents the nonopioid intravenous anesthetics and their effects and nursing considerations.

Benzodiazepine Antagonists. Flumazenil (Romazicon) antagonizes or reverses the sedative, amnesic, anxiolytic, and muscle-relaxant effects of benzodiazepines. However, flumazenil does not reverse benzodiazepine-induced respiratory or cardiac depression. Flumazenil is specific for the benzodiazepine receptors, and thus it also does not reverse the effects of barbiturates or opiates. It should be used with great caution in patients who

have a history of seizures or chronic benzodiazepine usage, as it can precipitate seizures. The incidence of postoperative nausea and vomiting is also increased with its use. Because flumazenil has a shorter duration of action than most of the benzodiazepines, the risk of resedation can occur after the initial dose starts to wear off, especially when high doses of benzodiazepines are administered. Therefore the patient must be monitored for resedation and other residual effects. If the patient develops signs of resedation, flumazenil is repeated at 20-minute intervals. Flumazenil has proven to be a valuable asset in the care of the patient who has received an excessive dose of a benzodiazepine such as midazolam or lorazepam. Consequently, flumazenil is very useful intraoperatively, postoperatively, and in the intensive care unit.[2,11,12]

Physostigmine (Antilirium), an anticholinesterase drug that inhibits the enzyme acetylcholinesterase, is a nonspecific reversal agent for benzodiazepines, scopolamine, and ketamine. It results in an increase in the availability of acetylcholine at the receptor sites, which counteracts the negative effects of GABA, reversing the CNS side effects. Because this drug is a nonspecific agent, it can cause a number of vagally mediated cholinergic side effects, including nausea, vomiting, salivation, bradycardia, bronchospasm, and seizures. Because of its

Pharmacologic Management: Nonopioid Intravenous Anesthetics

CATEGORY	DRUG	CHARACTERISTICS	EFFECTS	CONSIDERATIONS
Barbiturates	Thiopental (Pentothal)	Good patient acceptance; quick onset; very brief duration; no analgesia	CNS depression; spontaneous ventilation arrested; loss of laryngeal reflexes; causes histamine release (vasodilation, hypotension, and flushing)	IV administration painful; may cause myoclonus and hiccoughs; increased risk of aspiration
	Methohexital (Brevital)	Similar to thiopental but twice as potent; used in pediatric patients; no analgesia; hepatic metabolism	Similar to thiopental; lowers seizure threshold (epileptiform)	Similar to thiopental; burns when given IV
Nonbarbiturates	Etomidate (Amidate)	Agent of choice in patient with cardiovascular disease	Heart rate and cardiac output remain constant; minimal negative inotropic effects; suppression of adrenal function	May cause nausea and vomiting; burns when given IV; may cause myoclonus and hiccoughs
	Propofol (Diprivan)	No analgesic effect; avoid in patients with coronary stenosis, ischemia, and hypovolemia; antiemetic properties; hepatic metabolism	Patient wakes up clearly and quickly, myocardial depressant; may decrease blood pressure 20% to 25%	Rapid emergence may hasten pain awareness; low incidence of postoperative side effects; burns when given in small veins
Dissociative anesthetic	Ketamine (Ketalar)	Profound analgesia and anesthesia; provides amnesia; may be used alone, may be given IV or IM	Produces cardiovascular and respiratory stimulation; may increase blood pressure and heart rate 10% to 50%; increases intracranial pressure	Monitor for and prevent emergent reactions; titrate pain medications
Butyrophenones	Haloperidol (Haldol)	Limited use in anesthesia because of long duration; antipsychotic; antiemetic		High incidence of extrapyramidal reactions
	Droperidol (Inapsine)	Major tranquilizer; works with CNS as dopamine antagonist; hepatic metabolism	Prevents and treats nausea and vomiting; neuroleptic, causing amnesia or indifference to surroundings; adrenergic blocker, causing extrapyramidal muscle movements, hypotension, and peripheral vasodilation	Postanesthetic dysphoria (internalized overwhelming fear); effects last longer than narcotics
Benzodiazepines	Diazepam (Valium)	Rapid onset; long half-life; potent amnesic; effective anxiolysis; renal excretion		Titrate pain medications; monitor vital signs for respiratory depression
	Midazolam (Versed)	Rapid onset; short duration; potent amnesic; effective anxiolysis; hepatic metabolism		Lower dose in elderly, debilitated, COPD, and liver disease patients; titrate pain medications; monitor vital signs
	Lorazepam (Ativan)	Slow onset of action; long duration; anticonvulsant action; renal excretion	Pronounced sedation; minimal cardiovascular effects	Poor IV compatibility; titrate pain medications; monitor vital signs and for respiratory depression; which for orthostatic hypotension

CNS, Central nervous system; *IV*, intravenous; *IM*, intramuscular; *COPD*, chronic obstructive pulmonary disease.

nonspecific properties, physostigmine is rarely used for the reversal of benzodiazepines.[2]

OPIOID INTRAVENOUS ANESTHETICS

Opioid IV anesthetics play an important role in clinical anesthesia. These drugs enhance the effectiveness of inhalation agents by providing the analgesic portion of the anesthetic process. In addition, the use of opioids allows for reduction in the concentration of the inhalation agent to be administered, resulting in a safer process. When opioids are administered, they bind to specific receptors and produce a morphinelike or opioid agonist effect. Opioids are used to manage acute and chronic pain and are administered for general anesthesia, sedation, and pain relief during regional anesthesia; thus they are important in all phases of the perioperative experience.[2,11] The Pharmacologic Management table on Opioid Adjunctive Agents presents a summary of clinical uses and nursing implications for the most frequently used opioids.

Opioid Antagonists. Opioid antagonists are used to reverse the effects of opioids, particularly respiratory depression. The drug of choice in perianesthesia care is naloxone (Narcan). Naloxone competes with and displaces the opioid on the receptor site, and therefore it reverses both the respiratory depressant and analgesic effects of opioids. Naloxone is titrated to the patient's response. The onset of action is 1 to 2 minutes, and if after 3 to 5 minutes adequate reversal has not been achieved, naloxone administration is repeated until reversal is complete. If the patient shows no sign of reversal, assessment of the pharmacologic agents administered is indicated. The effects of drugs such as halothane, barbiturates, and muscle relaxants are not reversed by naloxone.[12,13]

The duration of action of naloxone is 1 to 4 hours. If long-acting opioids are used, the patient must be monitored for respiratory insufficiency because the depressant effects of the opioids may return. Often a low-dose, continuous IV drip of naloxone proves effective. One adverse effect to watch for when excessive doses of naloxone are given is an increase in blood pressure, which may be in response to pain. Too-rapid reversal may induce nausea, vomiting, diaphoresis, or tachycardia. During the reversal procedure, vital signs are monitored closely. Naloxone must be used with caution in patients with cardiac irritability.[12,13]

Naloxone does not produce respiratory depression as do other narcotic antagonists, nor does it produce any significant side effects or pupillary constriction. Naloxone reverses natural or synthetic opioids, propoxyphene (Darvon), and the opioid antagonist and analgesic pentazocine (Talwin). It must be administered with great caution in patients who are physically dependent on opioids, because reversal may precipitate an acute withdrawal syndrome.[12,13]

NEUROMUSCULAR BLOCKING AGENTS

Neuromuscular blocking agents (NMBAs), or muscle relaxants, interrupt the transmission of impulses from the nerve to the muscle, causing a decrease in muscle activity. Decreasing muscle activity allows the surgeon to operate in a quiet field and decreases the need for deep anesthesia. They have contributed greatly to clinical anesthesia. However, the use of NMBAs is not limited to the operating room; they are used to facilitate endotracheal intubation, terminate laryngospasm, eliminate chest wall rigidity that may occur after the rapid injection of potent opioids, and to facilitate mechanical ventilation by producing total paralysis of the respiratory muscles. NMBAs cause paralysis of the respiratory muscles, and the patient receiving these agents will require support of ventilation with either a hand-held bag-valve-mask or a mechanical ventilator. It is important to

Pharmacologic Management: Opioid Adjunctive Agents

AGENTS	
Meperidine (Demerol)	Butorphanol (Stadol)
Morphine	Nalbuphine (Nubain)
Fentanyl (Sublimaze)	Dezocine (Dalgan)
Sufentanil (Sufenta)	Buprenorphine (Buprenex)
Alfentanil (Alfenta)	Ketorolac (Toradol)
Pentazocine (Talwin)	

CLINICAL USES	IMPLICATIONS	CONSIDERATIONS
Preoperative sedation	Monitor for hypotension	Keep Narcan available
Induction of anesthesia	Monitor for bradycardia	Keep resuscitation equipment available
Maintenance of anesthesia	Monitor for respiratory depression	Respiratory depressant effect may outlast
Postoperative pain management	May cause nausea and vomiting	analgesia

Pharmacologic Management: Neuromuscular Blocking Agents

	AGENTS	
LONG ACTING	**INTERMEDIATE ACTING**	**SHORT ACTING**
Pancuronium (Pavulon) Gallamine (Flaxedil) Metocurine (Metubine) Doxacurium (Nuromax) Pipecuronium (Arduran)	Atracurium (Tracrium) Vecuronium (Norcuron)	Mivacurium (Mivacron) Alcuronium (Alloferin) Rocuronium (Zemuron) Succinylcholine (Anectine)—depolarizing agent
CHARACTERISTICS	**IMPLICATIONS**	
Compete with acetylcholine at the myoneural junction Shorter acting; most appropriate for anesthesia Provide surgical relaxation Facilitate intubation Assist in ventilatory support	**Depolarizing** Reversible only with time Use cautiously in patients with neuromuscular disease, such as myasthenia gravis or muscular dystrophy Adverse effects include bradycardia, tachycardia, ventricular dysrhythmias, asystole, hypertension, hyperkalemia Increases intraocular, intracranial, and intragastric pressure Precipitates muscle fasciculations and pain Prolongs respiratory depression Histamine release causes hypotension Use cautiously in patients with head injury, cerebral edema, trauma, burns, electrolyte imbalances, and renal or hepatic disease Be alert for manifestations of malignant hyperthermia	**Nondepolarizing** Reversible with time and anticholinesterase Use cautiously in patients with hepatic or renal disease, obesity, asthma, or COPD Adverse effects include tachycardia, hypertension, hypotension, bronchospasms, and flushing

COPD, Chronic obstructive pulmonary disease.

remember that NMBAs do not have analgesic, amnesic, anxiolytic, or sedative effects. The paralyzed patient is not able to communicate his or her needs; NMBAs must be used in combination with other medications to prevent pain and provide sedation.[3,14,15]

Skeletal muscle contraction occurs when acetylcholine is released from the motor neuron and binds to receptor sites on the muscle fiber (neuromuscular junction), resulting in depolarization. Skeletal muscle relaxation occurs when the release of acetylcholine ceases and any residual acetylcholine is destroyed by the enzyme acetylcholinesterase, resulting in repolarization. Neuromuscular blocking agents interfere with the relationship between acetylcholine and the receptor. There are two general categories of skeletal muscle relaxant: nondepolarizing and depolarizing.[14-16]

Depolarizing agents compete with acetylcholine at the neuromuscular junction causing the muscle to depolarize and inhibiting repolarization. The muscle stays in a prolonged depolarized state and movement is inhibited. The principal depolarizing skeletal muscle agent is succinylcholine (Anectine). Once the succinylcholine attaches to the receptor, a brief period of depolarization occurs, which is manifested by transient muscular fasciculations.

Succinylcholine has a rapid onset, 30-60 seconds, and a short duration of action, 5 to10 minutes. It is frequently used to facilitate intubation. The actions of succinylcholine cannot be pharmacologically reversed.[2,5,14,17] Nondepolarizing NMBAs are generally longer-acting than depolarizing agents. Nondepolarizing agents do not cause muscle contraction or depolarization. They compete with and block the uptake of acetylcholine at the muscle receptor site and prevent repolarization. Sustained muscle relaxation occurs, and voluntary control of skeletal muscle contraction is weakened or lost.[2,5,14,16]

The Pharmacologic Management table on Neuromuscular Blocking Agents presents a pharmacologic overview of the commonly used skeletal muscle relaxants. A number of factors can potentiate the effects of nondepolarizing NMBAs, as well as antagonize them; these factors are listed in Box 14-3.[15,16]

Neuromuscular Blocking Agent Antagonists. The pharmacologic actions of nondepolarizing NMBAs can be reversed by anticholinesterase drugs such as neostigmine (Prostigmin). These drugs increase the amount of acetylcholine available at the receptor sites by preventing its destruction by acetylcholinesterase. This promotes more effective competition of acetylcholine with

Box 14-3

FACTORS INFLUENCING NEUROMUSCULAR BLOCKADE

POTENTIATE

Hypocalcemia
Hypokalemia
Hyponatremia
Hypermagnesemia
Acidosis
Hypothermia
Antibiotics (gentamicin;
   tobramycin; amikacin;
   kanamycin; neomycin;
   polymyxin A, B, and E;
   clindamycin; tetracyclines;
   piperacillin; streptomycin)
Antidysrhythmics
   (procainamide, lidocaine,
   quinidine)
β-adrenergic blockers
Calcium channel blockers
Diuretics (furosemide,
   thiazides)

Droperidol
Inhalation agents
Cyclosporine
Lithium
Dantrolene
Etomidate
Hepatic failure
Renal failure
Neuromuscular diseases

ANTAGONIZE

Phenytoin
Carbamazepine
Aminophylline
Theophylline
Sympathomimetic
   agents
Corticosteroids
Azatioprine

the nondepolarizing skeletal muscle relaxant that is occupying the receptor sites. Because of the increased availability and mobilization of the acetylcholine, the concentration gradient favors acetylcholine and the removal of the nondepolarizing agent from the receptors, resulting in the return of normal skeletal muscle depolarization and contraction.[15] These drugs also produce undesired side effects by increasing the level of acetylcholine at receptor sites in the heart, the lungs, the eyes, and the gastrointestinal tract, which can lead to bradycardia, bronchospasm, miosis, and increased peristalsis and secretion. To prevent or minimize these effects, anticholinergic agents such as atropine or glycopyrrolate (Robinul) are given with the reversal agent.[2,4,5,10] The Pharmacologic Management table on NMBA Reversal Agents outlines the common NMBA reversal agents used in anesthesia and their nursing implications.

PERIANESTHESIA ASSESSMENT AND CARE

The goal of patient management in the immediate postoperative period is the recognition and immediate treatment of any problems in order to eliminate or lessen complications that may occur. This requires the collaborative effort of the nurse, the anesthesiologist, and the surgeon. Physical assessment of the postanesthesia patient begins immediately on admission to the unit. The nurse admitting the patient receives a report from the anesthesiologist. The nurse should get information re-

lated to the patient's general condition, the operation performed, the type of anesthesia administered, estimated blood loss, total intake and output during surgery, and any problems or complications encountered in the operating room.[2]

Assessment of the cardiopulmonary system is the immediate priority. The patient's airway is assessed to ensure it is patent, and the patient's breathing pattern is evaluated to ensure that it is unlabored. The patient's blood pressure, pulse, rate of respiration, and oxygen saturation level are checked and recorded. All dressings and drains are quickly inspected for gross bleeding.[19] Once these initial observations are made, it is essential to systematically assess the patient's total condition.[2]

RESPIRATORY FUNCTION

Because patients have experienced some interference with their respiratory system, postanesthesia maintenance of adequate gas exchange is a crucial aspect of care in the immediate postoperative period. It is for this reason that most experts suggest routine oxygen administration in the immediate postoperative phase. Any change in respiratory function must be detected early so that appropriate measures can be taken to ensure adequate oxygenation and ventilation. Respiratory function is evaluated using physical assessment skills: inspection, palpation, percussion, and auscultation. Several preexisting conditions can increase the probability that ventilatory support will be needed in the postoperative period. These include preexisting lung disease, thoracic or upper abdominal surgery, history of smoking, recent opioid administration, and/or low oxygen saturation before surgery.[2]

Pulse oximetry, a noninvasive technique, measures oxygen saturation of functional hemoglobin. Pulse oximetry can be used to identify hypoxemia and it should be used on all postoperative patients. In addition, if the patient is intubated and being mechanically ventilated, capnography can be used to assess the adequacy of ventilation. Arterial blood gas measurements can be used to definitively confirm abnormal pulse oximetry or capnography values. Normal pulse oximetry values are 97% to 99%; however, preanesthetic baseline values must be noted. Some patients may normally have lower saturation values on room air for a variety of reasons, and attempting to maintain higher oxygen saturation levels may result in prolonged oxygen therapy.[20]

Routine oxygen administration in the postanesthesia recovery period can be accomplished with nasal cannula (prongs) or face mask. Surgery and anesthesia often interrupt the normal functioning of the nose, so humidification or nebulization with oxygen delivery may be needed. Humidifiers convert water from the liquid to the gaseous state, whereas nebulizers produce tiny water particles. This is especially helpful at higher flow rates.[21]

Pharmacologic Management: NMBA Reversal Agents

DRUG	CHARACTERISTICS	EFFECTS	CONSIDERATIONS
Neostigmine (Prostigmin)	Binds with cholinesterase and inactivates it Preserves endogenous anticholinesterase	Antidote for nondepolarizing neuromuscular blockers Prevents postoperative distention and urinary retention Muscarinic effects cause bradycardia, bronchoconstriction, peripheral vasodilation, and coronary vasoconstriction	Does not cross blood-brain barrier Lasts 30-90 min May be given with atropine and glycopyrrolate to decrease muscarinic effects Use cautiously in patients with asthma or coronary disease
Pyridostigmine (Regonol)	Analog of neostigmine, with fewer adverse effects Only 20% as potent as neostigmine Rapid onset of action (5-15 min)	Antidote for nondepolarizing neuromuscular blocking agents Muscarinic effects less severe than those of neostigmine	Longer half-life Lasts 120 min May be given with atropine and glycopyrrolate Use cautiously in patients with asthma, peptic ulcer, epilepsy, or pregnancy
Edrophonium (Tensilon)	Cholinergic Short-acting anticholinesterase	Parasympathetic effects: GI: salivation, dysphasia, nausea, vomiting, increased peristalsis CV: bradycardia, cardiac dysrhythmias, hypotension Respiratory: increased pharyngeal and tracheobronchial secretions EENT: Lacrimation, miosis, diplopia	Must be given with atropine Very rapid onset, but brief duration of action Use cautiously in presence of asthma, peptic ulcer, or bradycardia
Atropine	Anticholinergic Antimuscarinic Chronotropic stimulator in event of bradycardia	Preanesthetic medication to prevent or reduce respiratory tract secretions Restoration of cardiac rate during anesthesia Antidote for cholinesterase inhibitors Causes decreased sweating and predisposition to heat prostration	Crosses blood-brain barrier Ensures adequate hydration Provides temperature control to prevent hyperpyrexia
Glycopyrrolate (Robinul)	Similar to atropine Longer duration	Less incidence of dysrhythmias Slow increase in heart rate Protection against peripheral muscarinic effects of neostigmine and pyridostigmine	Does not cross blood-brain barrier Contraindicated in presence of glaucoma, peptic ulcer, or COPD

GI, Gastrointestinal; *CV*, cardiovascular; *EENT*, eye(s), ear(s), nose, throat; *COPD*, chronic obstructive pulmonary disease.

Some patients recovering from anesthesia may require mechanical ventilation. Various modes, such as positive end-expiratory pressure (PEEP), continuous positive airway pressure (CPAP), and synchronized intermittent mandatory ventilation (SIMV), are used to improve the respiratory status of the patient.[21]

STIR-UP REGIMEN

The stir-up regimen is probably the most important aspect of perianesthesia nursing management. The basics of the regimen are aimed at the prevention of complications, primarily atelectasis and venous stasis. Five major activities—deep-breathing exercises, coughing, position-ing, mobilization, and pain management—constitute the stir-up regimen.[22]

Deep-Breathing Exercises. The major factor contributing to postoperative pulmonary complications is low lung volumes resulting from a shallow, monotonous, sighless breathing pattern caused by general anesthesia, pain, and opioids. Therefore the patient must be stimulated to take three or four deep breaths every 5 to 10 minutes. Full lung expansion is important, and every effort must be made to enhance the patient's ability to accomplish it.

The sustained maximal inspiration (SMI) maneuver is a method to enhance the lung volumes of postoperative patients. The SMI maneuver consists of having the patient inhale as close to lung capacity as possible and, at the peak of inspiration, having the patient hold that volume for 3 to 5 seconds before exhaling it. This maneuver is more effective than simple deep breathing in preventing reduced lung volumes in the immediate postanesthesia periods. If the patient's vital capacity is inadequate or because anesthesia respiratory depression is prolonged, deep breathing and the SMI maneuver may be augmented with a manual resuscitation bag connected to an oxygen source or with an intermittent positive-pressure breathing apparatus.

Incentive spirometry (IS) has become increasingly popular and is used to assist with preventing and treating atelectasis, promoting normal lung expansion, and improving oxygenation. IS devices allow patients visual feedback and observation of inspiratory volume. Instruction and practice before surgery provides patients with the opportunity to master the device and establish their baseline before anesthetic and surgical interventions.[22]

Coughing. The patient must be instructed to cough, as well as perform SMI maneuvers. The best way to clear the air passages of obstructive secretions is with a purposeful cough. For the patient recovering from anesthesia, the cascade cough is the most effective coughing maneuver. Instruct the patient to take a rapid, deep inhalation. This will increase the volume of air in the lungs and dilate the airways, allowing air to pass behind the retained secretions. On exhalation, have the patient perform multiple coughs. With each cough the length of the airways increases, enhancing the effectiveness of the cough. Coughing should only be done in the patient with secretions, since it can promote atelectasis.[22]

Coughing is most effective with the patient sitting upright. Splinting of incisions and adequate analgesia facilitate coughing. If the patient is unable to sit upright, place the patient in a side-lying position with hips and knees flexed, or in a semi-Fowler's position with the head and arms supported with pillows and the knees flexed. This will decrease abdominal tension and allow maximal movement of the diaphragm, improving the effectiveness of the cough.

Between cascade cough maneuvers, the patient is encouraged to inhale and close the glottis. This dilates the airways, increases intrathoracic pressure, and compresses the smaller airways, pushing the secretions toward the larger airways where they can be expectorated in succeeding cough maneuvers.

When a large amount of secretions accumulates in the patient's lungs that cannot be handled effectively by coughing, suctioning must be instituted. Suctioning is not without complications and should be done only when necessary and not routinely.[22]

Positioning. Patients recovering from anesthesia are maintained in a semiprone, side-lying position when possible. The semiprone position promotes maintenance of a patent airway, prevents aspiration, and permits optimal ventilation of the lower lung lobes. Frequent repositioning of patients (at least every hour) from side to side is essential for the prevention of atelectasis and venous stasis. Patients are encouraged to turn and change positions as soon as possible.

Mobilization. To prevent venous stasis, patients must be encouraged to move their legs and arms rhythmically, flexing and extending their extremities. Mobilization and flexion of the muscles aids venous return, improves cardiac output (CO), and prevents venous stasis and the formation of deep vein thrombosis.[22]

Pain Management. Adequate pain control is a major consideration in the recovering patient (Box 14-4). Without it, it is difficult to implement the first four stir-up regimen's interventions. Poorly controlled pain may have serious consequences in terms of hemodynamic responses to catecholamines and of physical limitations on respiratory function. On the other hand, the medications used to control pain may in themselves have deleterious effects on hemodynamic and respiratory function. Opioids depress the cough reflex, ciliary activity, and the respiratory center in the brain and should not be used indiscriminately. However, if the patient refuses to deep breathe, cough, or move because of pain, he or she is at risk for postoperative respiratory and/or embolic complications.

Pain accelerates the cardiovascular system by activating the sympathetic nervous system and the adrenal system. Normally this will cause an increase in heart rate and blood pressure. However, anesthesia and some cardiac medications can blunt the sympathetic response; thus asking the patient his or her pain level is the most valid method of assessing pain levels (see Chapter 8 for more in-depth discussion). It has been suggested that pain, especially at upper abdominal and thoracic sites, decreases or eliminates the normal sighing (yawning) mechanism. The absence of an appropriate sigh leads to reduced lung volumes and, ultimately, to atelectasis and pneumonia. Appropriate pain relief in these patients will reduce the postoperative incidence of atelectasis and pneumonia.[23]

Once the assessment has been made and it has been determined that the patient is indeed experiencing acute postoperative pain, certain interventions are suggested. If the patient has received an inhalation anesthetic, such as isoflurane, enflurane, or halothane, and demonstrates manifestations of acute pain, relief is instituted early in the postanesthetic period. Similarly, patients receiving a nitrous oxide–opioid technique are medicated early in the immediate postoperative period, particularly if the intraoperative opioids were of short duration. If medications such as sufentanil, meperidine (Demerol), and morphine are used intraoperatively, opioids must be administered with caution to avoid respiratory depression as a result of the synergistic action of the intraoperative and postoperative opioid agonists. Finally, if the patient received droperidol intraoperatively or preoperatively, great caution must be used, because opioid agonists as well as barbiturates are significantly potentiated by this

Box 14-4

ASPAN POSITION STATEMENT ON PAIN MANAGEMENT

ASPAN has the responsibility for defining the practice of perianesthesia nursing. An integral part of this responsibility involves identifying the educational requirements and competencies essential to perianesthesia nursing practice and the educational needs of the patients and family regarding pain assessment and management.

ASPAN sets forth this position statement to promote the optimal level of practice and to present a consistent standard of care that documents sound clinical judgment in the management of postoperative pain.

BACKGROUND

ASPAN has defined a standard for pain management (Standard XI) with the intent of providing guidelines, which represent what is believed to be an optimal level of practice. To assist members in achieving this standard, ASPAN published pain management competency material in the Competency Based Orientation and Credentialing Program. In response to continued concerns from perianesthesia nurses, ASPAN's Standards and Guidelines Committee conducted a review of literature to identify current issues related to pain assessment and management. The following issues were identified:

1. As many as 50% of postoperative patients in both hospitals and outpatient surgical centers are undermedicated and suffer unrelieved pain.[1-4]
2. The practice of undermedicating for pain occurs regardless of the patient's age.[5,6]
3. Frequently the patient's self-report of pain is not taken into consideration when choosing the dosage of medication to give for pain relief.[7,8]
4. Inadequate pain management affects postoperative recovery and behaviors associated with that recovery.[5,6,9]
5. A prevalent cause of ineffective pain management is the professional's lack of knowledge related to pain physiology, medications, and protocols.[4,10]
6. There is still an overriding concern that the use of opioids in the treatment of acute postoperative pain control will contribute to psychologic dependence.[11]
7. Patient and family education addressing postsurgical pain management remains inconsistent.[12]
8. Pain management should begin preoperatively with patient and family education addressing use of a pain scale as well as methods of postoperative pain control.
9. The Agency for Health Care Policy and Research (AHCPR) suggests that practitioners are too rigid when managing acute postoperative pain and should set goals to reduce its incidence and severity. Guidelines have been published by this agency for acute pain management.[13]

POSITION

It is therefore the position of ASPAN that a collaborative plan should be developed between the anesthesia department and the perianesthesia nurses to address pain management within the perianesthesia setting. The following points of action should be addressed:

1. The goal should be to relieve as much pain as possible to allow for activity, relaxation, prevention of complications, and promotion of optimal health and healing.

2. Areas of education in pain management for health care professionals should include the following:
   a. Physiology of pain management.
   b. Assessment techniques
   c. Methods of intervention (pharmacologic and non-pharmacologic)
   d. Management of side effects and complications related to each intervention
   e. Evaluation of successful management
   f. Ethical considerations
   g. Age and cultural considerations
   h. Patient and family education issues
3. Whenever possible, the patient's plan of care for pain management should begin during the preoperative interview.
4. The patient's self-report of pain is the best measurement tool to use when assessing pain.
5. The use of reliable and valid pain scales should be a standard part of the pain assessment.
6. Measurement of outcomes should reflect timely, appropriate interventions and achievement of desired effects.

EXPECTED OUTCOMES

Perianesthesia nurses need to familiarize themselves with this position statement and inform and educate peers, nurse managers, hospital administrators, and physicians.

Anesthesiologists and perianesthesia nurses need to collaborate in the development of a multidisciplinary plan of care (protocol, critical pathway, care map, etc.) to provide safe, appropriate, and effective pain management.

ASPAN, as the voice of perianesthesia nursing practice, must externalize this information by sharing this position statement with regulatory agencies and professional organizations that interface with perianesthesia nursing areas.

APPROVAL OF STATEMENT

This statement was recommended by a vote of the ASPAN Board of Directors on April 16, 1999, and approved by a vote of the ASPAN Representative Assembly on April 18, 1999, in Honolulu, Hawaii.

REFERENCES

1. Anonymous: Most patients face pain, often unrelieved, after surgery, *Am J Nurs* 96(3):68, 1996.
2. Campese C: Development and implementation of a pain management program, *AORN J* 64:931-940, 1996.
3. Bormann D, Hansen K: Improving pain management through staff education, *Nurs Manage* 28(7):55-57, 1997.
4. Thornborough J: Developing a pain management protocol in the PACU, *Surg Nurse* 20(5):23-27, 1998.
5. Fortin J, Schwartz-Barcott D, Rossi S: The postoperative pain experience: a description based on the McGill Pain Questionnaire, *Clin Nurs Res* 1(3)292-304, 1992.
6. Pasero C, McCaffrey M: Managing postoperative pain in the elderly, *Am J Nurs* 96(!0):38-46, 1996.
7. Reid D et al: Postoperative pain, *Can Nurse* 88(7):55, 1992.

By the American Society of PeriAnesthesia Nurses, 10 Melrose Avenue, Suite 110, Cherry Hill, NJ 080037-3696; toll-free (877)737-9696, fax: (856) 616-9601. E-mail: aspan@aspan.org. Copyright 1997-2001, American Society of PeriAnesthesia Nurses.

Box 14-4

ASPAN POSITION STATEMENT ON PAIN MANAGEMENT—cont'd

8. Malek C, Olivieri R: Pain management: documenting the decision-making process, *Nurs Case Manage* 1(2):64-76, 1996.
9. Getker-Black S et al: Preoperative self-efficacy and post-operative behaviors, *Appl Nurs Res* 5(3):134-139, 1992.
10. Carr E: Overcoming barriers of effective pain control, *Prof Nurse* 12:412-416, 1997.
11. Aiher J et al: Children win with improved pain management, *Can Nurse* 88(1)19-21, 1992.
12. Jones S, Villalobos J: Incorporating clinical research findings into practice, *J Nurs Staff Dev* 12(1):46, 1996.
13. Agency for Health Care Policy and Research: *Acute pain management in infants, children, and adolescents: operative and medical procedures,* Rockville, Md, 1992, Department of Health and Human Services.

BIBLIOGRAPHY

ANA: *Code for nurses with interpretative statements,* Washington, DC, 1995, American Nurses Association.

Anonymous: Surgical patient's no. 1 fear: pain, *Today's Surgical Nurse* 18:7, 1996.

ASPAN: *Competency-based orientation and credentialing program,* Cherry Hill, NJ, 1997, American Society of PeriAnesthesia Nurses.

Bishop A, Scudder J: *Nursing ethics: therapeutic caring presence,* Boston, 1996, Jones and Bartlett Publishers.

Heiser R et al: The use of music during the immediate postoperative recovery period, *AORN J* 65:777-778, 781-785, 1997.

Miaskowski C et al: Interdisciplinary guidelines for the management of acute pain: Implications for quality improvement, *J Nursing Care Qual* (Education of) 7:1-6, 1992.

Schwartz-Barcott C, Fortin J, Kim-Hesook S: Client-nurse interaction: testing for its impact in preoperative instruction, *Int J Nurs Stud* 31:23-35, 1994.

Wong D: Video Presentation. Pain Assessment in Children and Infants.

butyrophenone tranquilizer. Because of the synergistic effects of the medications, it may be necessary to decrease the amount of opioids administered in the first 24 hours following administration of anesthesia, but this must always be based on the patient's report of pain and clinical status.[10,24,25]

CARDIOVASCULAR FUNCTION

Evaluation of the cardiovascular system involves assessment of the heart, circulating blood, and the arteriovenous system. These three basic components control CO. Tissue perfusion depends on a satisfactory CO; therefore most of the assessment is aimed at evaluating this component.[27]

In most patients the nurse will utilize physical assessment skills to evaluate the patient's cardiovascular function. The patient's overall condition is observed, especially skin color and turgor. Peripheral cyanosis, edema, jugular venous distention, shortness of breath, and many other findings may be indicative of cardiovascular problems. In addition to checking all operative sites for blood loss, the amount of blood lost during surgery and the patient's most recent hemoglobin level are noted.[18]

The patient's blood pressure (BP) must be assessed and correlated to the preoperative assessment, intraoperative course, and anesthetic course. The major component of systolic pressure is stroke volume, and the major component of diastolic pressure is systemic vascular resistance (SVR). Changes in the patient's systolic or diastolic pressure and/or narrowing of the pulse pressure may indicate cardiovascular comprominse.[18] Peripheral pulses are as-

sessed bilaterally. The rate, character, and any irregularities are documented and reported to the physician if clinically indicated.[18] Electrocardiographic (ECG) monitoring is also essential in the immediate postoperative recovery period. Dysrhythmias of any type may occur at any time and in any patient during the postoperative period.[18]

Two components of CO are heart rate and stroke volume. If CO is compromised, one of the first compensatory responses is an increase in heart rate, followed by peripheral vasoconstriction. However medications such as β-blockers and angiotensin-converting enzyme inhibitors, as well as anesthetic agents, can impair the patient's ability to initiate that response. It is important for the nurse to be aware of the patient's preoperative medications and the impact they may have in the initial phase of recovery. Hemodynamic monitoring is commonly used with higher acuity patients in the postanesthesia recovery period. Hemodynamic monitoring is usually accomplished via a pulmonary artery catheter and intraarterial blood pressure monitoring.

CENTRAL NERVOUS SYSTEM FUNCTION

Assessment of the CNS in the immediate postanesthesia period generally involves only gross evaluation of behavior, level of consciousness, intellectual performance, and emotional status. Anesthetic agents are usually reversed before the patient leaves the operating room, so the nurse should anticipate that the patient will be responsive. However, even if anesthesia is not reversed, most patients will respond within 90 minutes from time of admission to the unit. A more detailed assessment of the

CNS is necessary for patients who have undergone CNS surgery.[2]

Occasionally a patient becomes agitated and thrashes about; this behavior is referred to as emergence delirium. It occurs more often in adolescents and young adults than in patients of other age-groups. Emergence delirium also tends to occur more commonly in patients who have undergone intraabdominal and intrathoracic procedures.[2,28]

THERMAL BALANCE

The measurement of the patient's body temperature in the immediate postanesthesia recovery period is particularly important. Factors influencing the body temperature include type of anesthesia, preoperative medication, age of patient, site and temperature of intravenous fluids, body surface exposure, temperature of irrigation solutions, temperature of the ambient air, and vasoconstriction (secondary to blood loss or anesthetic agents). Both hypothermia (temperature below 36° C) and hyperthermia (temperature above 38° C) are associated with physiologic alterations that may interfere with recovery.[29]

The body maintains its temperature between a narrow range of 36° and 38° C. This is accomplished by a balance of heat production and heat loss that is controlled by the thermoregulation mechanisms in the CNS. These mechanisms receive input from various thermoreceptors located in the skin, nose, oral cavity, thoracic viscera, and spinal cord. These thermoreceptors then send sensory information in hierarchic order to the spinal cord, reticular formation, and the primary control center in the hypothalamic region of the brain.[29]

The central temperature controls maintain body temperature via physiologic and behavioral responses. The physiologic thermoregulatory responses consist of sweating, shivering, and alterations in peripheral vasomotor tone. These responses fine-control the regulatory process of body temperature; consequently, heat is conserved via vasoconstriction and lost via vasodilation and sweating. The physiologic responses also can lower the metabolic rate to decrease heat production, and increase muscle tone and shivering to increase heat production. Behavioral thermoregulation is accomplished by subjective feelings of discomfort or comfort. For example, in a hot environment a person seeks air conditioning and in a cold environment a person seeks heat. Behavioral thermoregulation is a stronger response mechanism, but it cannot fine-tune body temperature as can the physiologic responses.[29]

The accuracy of axillary, rectal, or oral measurements is frequently debated. Shell (skin) temperatures can be measured at the axilla or forehead with temperature strips. Invasive techniques that use the pulmonary artery, tympanic membrane, or bladder as a site for monitoring are more accurate. Whatever method, trending is essential in the immediate postanesthesia recovery period.[29]

FLUID AND ELECTROLYTE BALANCE

Evaluation of a patient's fluid and electrolyte status involves total body assessment. Imbalances readily occur in the postoperative patient because of a number of factors, including the restriction of food and fluids preoperatively, fluid loss during surgery, and stress. The normal body response to stress, surgery, trauma, and anesthesia is to release the antidiuretic responsible for the retention of water and sodium. In addition, postanesthesia patients often have abnormal avenues of fluid loss after surgery.

Each patient must be evaluated to determine his or her baseline requirements and the fluid needed to replace abnormal loss. Most patients in the immediate postanesthesia recovery period receive IV fluids. It is important to know what fluids, if any, are to follow and whether the infusion is to be discontinued. All IV sites are checked regularly for signs of extravasation, phlebitis, and infection.

Oral intake is prohibited after anesthesia until the patient regains laryngeal and pharyngeal reflexes. These reflexes are demonstrated by the patient's ability to gag and swallow effectively. In addition, the management of postoperative nausea and vomiting remains critical.

Normal output in the average adult results from urinary output and insensible losses, including evaporation of water from the skin and exhalation during respiration. A lower-than-normal urinary output can be expected in the immediate postanesthesia recovery period as a result of the body's normal reaction to stress. Specific gravity determines whether to suspect dehydration as opposed to renal insufficiency. External losses from vomiting, nasogastric tubes, T-tubes, and wound drainage are assessed and monitored. Accurate measurement and recording of all intake and output is vital in the assessment of the patient's fluid and electrolyte status.[30]

In the surgical patient, intravenous access to the circulatory system is necessary for the administration of anesthesia, resuscitation drugs, blood and blood products, and fluid and electrolyte solutions. Postoperative parenteral fluid requirements vary with the patient's preoperative status and with the surgical procedure. Disease processes, tissue injuries, and operative procedures greatly influence the physiology of fluids and electrolytes in the body.

In deciding the type of fluid to use in the postanesthesia recovery period, one can differentiate between crystalloids and colloids, maintenance and replacement fluids, or fluids of differing tonicity. Because of the large variety of fluid solutions, some general guidelines are recommended in clinical practice. Crystalloids are generally used as maintenance fluids to compensate for insensible fluid losses and as replacement fluids to correct body fluid deficits (i.e., treatment of specific fluid and electrolyte disturbances). Maintenance fluid requirements are calculated according to body weight and are used to replace insensible losses from the lungs, skin, urine, and feces. Adults typically require 1.5 to 2 ml/kg/hr. When used to replace blood loss the replacement factor is 5 ml of crystalloid for each 1 ml of blood loss. Isotonic solutions, 0.9% normal saline (NS), or lactated Ringer's (LR) are usually administered in the immediate postoperative period. Colloids generally are used for fluid replacement associated with severe hypotension or shock resuscitation. They generally do not leave the intravascular space and therefore require lower infusion volumes to achieve volume replacement.[30]

The goal of fluid therapy in the immediate postanesthesia recovery period is the restoration of blood volume and tissue perfusion. Recovery after surgery is a dynamic process, and fluid reassessment is conducted periodically. Fluid challenges may be necessary in the hypovolemic patient or in the patient with clinical manifestations of hypoperfusion. The decision of whether to use crystalloids or colloids for fluid resuscitation is complex, controversial, and often determined by physician preference. Either meets the replacement needs of the patient and achieves the desired outcome when administered appropriately. As with any therapeutic intervention, complications can occur with fluid administration and the patient should be monitored closely.

Blood and blood components are reserved for specific patient situations. Red blood cells are indicated to increase oxygen-carrying capacity in patients with anemia. Platelets are used to treat bleeding associated with deficiencies in platelet number or function. Fresh-frozen plasma is transfused to increase clotting factor levels in patients with demonstrated deficiencies. A good understanding of fluid types available, of a systematic approach to evaluating fluid depletion, and of the indication for blood component therapy allows the nurse to make appropriate decisions when implementing fluid therapy in the immediate postanesthesia period.[2]

PSYCHOSOCIAL STATUS

Assessment of the patient's psychosocial and emotional well-being is an important component of perianesthesia care. As with any other assessment, this must be made in the context of the whole patient. Almost all patients experience a degree of anxiety about anesthesia and the surgical procedure and a fear of postoperative pain. The physical manifestations include increased HR and BP; pale, cool skin; increased respiratory rate; increased muscle tone; restlessness; agitation; and dilated pupils.[31]

In 2003 the American Society of Perianesthesia Nurses published a position statement on visitation (Box 14-5). This statement recognizes that research shows that visitation during the postanesthesia period benefits both the patient and the family.

OTHER POSTANESTHESIA CARE UNIT NURSING CONSIDERATIONS

Assessment and nursing care are based on the complexity and acuity of the patient in the postanesthesia care unit (PACU). Patient classification systems capture data that are used to predict patient acuity and forecast nursing workload.[32]

Concerns are growing regarding the use of PACU as an overflow unit for critically ill patients. Issues surrounding these concerns are competencies of staff; adequacy of equipment, medications, supplies, and technology; and appropriate nurse staffing.[33] Refer to Box 14-6 for guidelines for the overflow of critical care patients into the PACU.[34]

GENERAL COMFORT MANAGEMENT

General comfort and safety measures are important parts of postanesthesia care. For safety, at least two nurses (one of whom is a registered nurse) must always be present whenever patients are recovering. An unconscious patient must never be left alone, and side rails must be raised on the bed whenever direct care is not being provided. The wheels of the bed must be locked to prevent sliding when care is being rendered.

General physical measures such as cleanliness must not be overlooked in the postanesthesia recovery period. Comfort measures, important to the total well-being of postanesthesia patients, are often forgotten in the hustle of caring for them. As soon as the patient is settled into the unit and has been assessed, all excess skin preparations and electrodes are removed; in addition to providing comfort, washing off excess skin preparations gives the nurse an excellent opportunity to further assess the patient's general condition. A back rub at this time may prevent later complaints of discomfort from positioning for long periods in the operating room. This is also a good time to change the patient's position, assist with range of motion exercises, and encourage deep breathing. Frequent position changes help prevent atelectasis, promote circulation, and prevent pressure sores from developing on the skin surfaces.

Mouth care is comforting to the patient who not only has had nothing by mouth but has been medicated with an anticholinergic or glycopyrrolate to reduce secretions. When patients are fully conscious and their laryngeal reflexes have returned, they can rinse their mouth with mouthwash and water. Ice chips and small sips of water or juice may be offered to patients who can tolerate fluids. A non–petroleum-based ointment is applied to the lips after mouth care to prevent drying and consequent cracking.

Patients often complain of being cold when returning from the operating suite. This is a result of the effects of anesthesia and premedications and the cool atmosphere

Box 14-5

A Position Statement on Visitation in Phase I Level of Care

ASPAN HAS THE responsibility for defining the practice of perianesthesia nursing. An integral part of this responsibility is to promote comfort and satisfaction among patients and families. The specialty of perianesthesia nursing encompasses the care of the patient as well as the family and significant other along the perianesthesia continuum of care. ASPAN sets forth this position statement to support the needs of both patients and families as it relates to family visitation in the phase I level of care.

Background
Historically, PACUs have been closed units. A patient's family waited anxiously while the patient recovered in the PACU. In recent years, there have been rapid advances in anesthesia management with shorter-acting anesthetic agents and increased use of regional anesthetic techniques. There is a growing body of nursing research in support of family visitation and presence at the bedside. ASPAN supports the reevaluation of the needs of both patients and families while striving to maintain quality services across the continuum of patient care. In response to the concerns of many perianesthesia nurses from around the country, the Standards and Guidelines Committee conducted a review of literature and gathered information from various institutions to identify issues related to visitation in phase I level of care.

A review of current nursing practice revealed a wide range of family visitation practices across the country, ranging from no visitation, visitation for ICU/overnight patients, visitation for pediatric patients only, to an open family visitation policy. Perianesthesia nurses also vary in their concerns regarding family visitation as it relates to the following:
1. Issues of patient confidentiality
2. Pain and comfort management
3. Procedures done in Phase I level of care
4. Potential for emergency situations
5. Unclear family expectations regarding visitation guidelines

A growing body of research supports both patients' and families' needs for increased visitation in the ICUs. In addition, research directly related to the PACU setting reveals that family visitation in Phase I level of care benefits both patients and families. The concept of family visitation has gained increased acceptance by nurses when a well-developed visitation program is established.

Position
Therefore, it is the position of ASPAN that visitation in the Phase I level of care is supported and that perianesthesia nurses develop guidelines within their own settings to incorporate this into their practice. Guidelines should include the following:
1. Appropriate education for patients and families regarding family visitation to maintain a safe and beneficial experience.
2. The confidentiality of all patients shall be maintained.
3. The visit will take place at an appropriate time for the patient, visitor, and clinical staff.
4. Perianesthesia nurses should work together with hospital administration to establish a well-organized family visitation program supported by appropriate personnel to meet the needs of families in this unique setting.

Expected Outcomes
Perianesthesia nurses need to familiarize themselves with this position statement, current literature, and research in support of family visitation. Perianesthesia nurses should work together with hospital administration to develop organized methods of increasing communication with families throughout the perianesthesia experience and providing appropriate support personnel to establish a visitation program in the Phase I level of care that meets the needs of patients, families, and clinical staff. ASPAN, as the voice of perianesthesia nursing practice, must externalize this information by sharing this position statement with all disciplines that interface with the practice of perianesthesia patients and families.

©2003 by American Society PeriAnesthesia Nurses.

of the operating suite. The normothermic patient may shiver or complain of feeling cold, so warm blankets may provide psychologic comfort. Blankets of any type must not, however, obscure the intravenous lines, arterial lines, or other monitoring apparatuses from the direct view of the attending nurse. The patient's temperature must be monitored closely to avoid overheating.

In addition to the physical comfort measures, remember to provide psychologic comfort. Reorientation, especially to time and place, is important to the postanesthesia patient, as is constant reassurance that the surgery is completed and that all went well. The nurse's presence at the bedside or gentle touch may also be comforting to the patient.[22]

MANAGEMENT OF POSTANESTHESIA PROBLEMS AND EMERGENCIES

In the immediate postoperative period significant physiologic changes occur as the patient emerges from the effects of anesthesia. Factors that influence the development of problems are listed in Box 14-7.[35]

RESPIRATORY PROBLEMS AND EMERGENCIES

Respiratory problems occur with some regularity in the postanesthesia period. Remember that all general anesthetic agents and opioid analgesic drugs have respiratory depressant effects. Acute pain also impairs the ability to

Box 14-6

A JOINT POSITION STATEMENT ON ICU OVERFLOW PATIENTS*

ISSUE

A phase 1 postanesthesia care unit (PACU) is a critical care area providing postanesthesia nursing care for patients immediately after operative and invasive procedures prior to discharge to the phase II ambulatory setting, the inpatient surgical unit and the intensive care unit.

Perianesthesia nurses have identified concerns regarding the increasing use of the phase 1 postanesthesia care unit (PACU) for the care of the surgical and nonsurgical intensive care unit (ICU) patients when ICU beds are not available in the facility.

PURPOSE

As professional societies involved in the provision of care for operative and invasive procedures and critically ill patients, the American Society of PeriAnesthesia Nurses (ASPAN), the American Association of Critical-Care Nurses (AACN), and the American Society of Anesthesiologists (ASA) collaborated to develop criteria for the purposes of maintaining quality care in the PACU, ensuring quality care for the intensive care unit patient, and promoting the safe practice of perianesthesia nursing and critical care nursing.

ASPAN exists to promote quality and cost-effective care for patients, their families and the community through public and professional education, research and standards of practice. ASPAN has the responsibility for defining the practice of perianesthesia nursing. An integral part of this responsibility involves identifying the educational requirements and competencies essential to perianesthesia practice as well as recommending acceptable staffing requirements for the perianesthesia environment.

AACN was established to provide the highest quality resources to maximize nurses' contributions to care for critically ill patients and their families. AACN provides and inspires leadership to develop standards and guidelines that establish work and care environments that are respectful, healing, and humane.

ASA was established to raise and maintain the standard of the medical practice of anesthesiology and improve the care of the patient during anesthesia and recovery, and is involved in the provision of critical care medicine in the intensive care unit.

BACKGROUND

In response to concerns expressed by perianesthesia nurses around the country, the ASPAN Standards and Guidelines Committee conducted a review of current literature and perianesthesia nursing practice to identify issues related to the care of critically ill surgical and nonsurgical patients in phase 1 PACUs during times when all other ICU beds are full. The review identified the following trends:

1. Staffing requirements identified for phase 1 PACUs may be exceeded during times when PACUs are being utilized for ICU overflow patients.[1]

2. The phase 1 PACU nurse may be required to provide care to a surgical or nonsurgical ICU patient he/she has not been properly trained to care for or for which he/she has not had the required care competencies validated.[1]

3. Phase 1 PACUs may be unable to receive patients normally admitted from the operating room when staff is being utilized to care for ICU overflow patients.[1]

4. Because the need to send ICU overflow patients to the phase 1 PACU does not occur regularly, both the PACU and hospital management may not be properly prepared to deal with the admission and discharge of phase 1 PACU and ICU patients.[1]

STATEMENT

Therefore when it is necessary to admit ICU overflow patients, or prolong the stay of the surgical ICU patient in the phase 1 PACU, ASPAN, AACN, and ASA recommend that the following criteria be met:

1. It must be recognized that the primary responsibility for phase 1 PACU is to provide the optimal standard of care to the postanesthesia patient and to effectively maintain the flow of the surgery schedule.

2. Appropriate staffing requirements should be met to maintain safe, competent nursing care of the postanesthesia patient as well as the ICU patient.[2] Staffing criteria for the ICU patient should be consistent with ICU guidelines and based on individual patient acuity and needs.[3]

3. Phase 1 PACUs are by their nature critical care units and, as such, staff should meet the competencies required for the care of the critically ill patient. These competencies should include, but are not limited to, ventilator management, hemodynamic monitoring, and medication administration, as appropriate to their patient population.

4. Management should develop and implement a comprehensive resource utilization plan with ongoing assessment that supports the staffing needs for both the PACU and ICU patients when the need for overflow admission arises.[3]

5. Management should have a multidisciplinary plan to address appropriate utilization of ICU beds. Admission and discharge criteria should be utilized to evaluate the necessity for critical care and to determine the priority for admissions.[3]

EXPECTED ACTIONS

ASPAN, AACN and the ASA committees (Anesthesia Care Team, Critical Care Medicine and Trauma Medicine) recognize the complexity of caring for patients in a dynamic healthcare environment where reduced availability of resources and expanding roles for the registered nurse have an impact on patient care. Thus we encourage all members to actively pursue the education and development of competencies required for the care of the critically ill patient in the perianesthesia environment. We also encourage members to actively identify strategies for collaboration and problem solving to address complex staffing issues.

*Developed by the American Society of PeriAnesthesia Nurses: American Association of Critical-Care Nurses; American Society of Anesthesiologists: Anesthesia Care Team Committee; Committee on Critical Care Medicine and Trauma Medicine; June 2000.

Box 14-6

A JOINT POSITION STATEMENT ON ICU OVERFLOW PATIENTS—cont'd

This information and position is to be shared with all individuals, organizations, and institutions involved in the care of the critically ill patient in the perianesthesia environment.

REFERENCES

1. Johannes MS: A new dimension of the PACU: the dilemma of the ICU overflow patient, *J Peri Anesth Nurs* 9:297-300, 1994.

2. ASPAN: Resource 3: *Patient classification/recommended staffing guidelines in the standards of perianesthesia nursing practice,* 27-28, Thorofare, NJ, 1998, American Society of PeriAnesthesia Nurses.
3. Medina J: *Staffing blueprint: constructing your staffing solutions,* Alisa Viejo, Calif, 1999, AACN.

Box 14-7

FACTORS INFLUENCING THE DEVELOPMENT OF POSTOPERATIVE PROBLEMS

Intraoperative complications
Type of anesthetic technique
Preoperative condition of patient
Length and type of surgery
Urgency of surgery
Poorly controlled pain
Other drugs administered intraoperatively
Changes in fluid status and elderly balance
Alterations in body temperature

breathe deeply. Most respiratory problems are related to upper airway obstruction, though other problems can occur, including acute respiratory failure, aspiration, pulmonary edema, and respiratory arrest.[36]

Airway Obstruction. Slack nasal or oropharyngeal muscles, rigid neck muscles, or secretions in the upper respiratory tract can cause obstruction of the airway. Soft tissue obstruction occurs when the pharynx is blocked and air cannot flow in and out. The most common cause of soft tissue obstruction is the tongue. Clinical manifestations of an airway obstruction include snoring, stridor, flaring of the nostrils, retractions at the intercostal spaces and the suprasternal notch, abnormal use of accessory muscles, asynchronous movements of the chest and abdomen, increased pulse rate, decreased oxygen saturation level, and decreased breath sounds.

Management of an airway obstruction begins with immediate recognition. Stimulation may be all that is necessary to relieve the obstruction and obtain a patent airway. With the nonreactive patient, the head tilt–chin lift maneuver or elevation of the mandible at its angles (jaw thrust) will displace the tongue and open the airway. If patency of the airway cannot be achieved by either of these methods, an oropharyngeal or nasopharyngeal airway is inserted. A nasopharyngeal airway is usually better tolerated, although it can occasionally cause nasal bleeding. Oropha-

ryngeal airways should only be used in an unconscious patient because they can cause gagging, vomiting, and laryngospasm in the awake patient. The patient can also be turned on his or her side to a lateral position, which will facilitate the displacement of the tongue and drainage of secretions. If the obstruction is still unrelieved, positive-pressure mask ventilation, intubation, tracheotomy, or cricothyrotomy may be required.[3,4,35,38]

Laryngeal Edema. Laryngeal edema is defined as swelling of the laryngeal tissue. This edema can cause varying degrees of airway obstruction. Manifestations include stridor, retraction, hoarseness, and a crouplike cough. Apprehension and restlessness may be present in the awake patient.

Management consists of placing the patient in the upright position; using cool, humidified oxygen; and administering nebulized racemic epinephrine. If the laryngeal edema is a result of an allergic reaction, the reaction must be managed with epinephrine, bronchodilators, and antihistamines. Reintubation is performed only if the patient's symptoms cannot be controlled with an inhalation treatment within 30 minutes, hypercarbia persists, or the patient appears to be in respiratory distress. If reintubation is done, the endotracheal tube must be at least one size smaller than the previous tube used and an air leak must be present around the cuff.[37,38]

Laryngospasm. Laryngospasm is caused by reflex contractions of the pharyngeal muscles, resulting in spasms of the vocal cords and the inability of the patient to take a breath. The spasms may result in either a partial or complete airway obstruction. Involvement of the intrinsic laryngeal muscles causes a reflex closure of the glottis, which results in an incomplete obstruction. Involvement of the extrinsic muscles causes a reflex closure of the larynx, which results in a complete airway obstruction. Signs and symptoms of laryngospasm include dyspnea, hypoxia, hypoventilation, absence of breath sounds, and hypercarbia. Crowing sounds may be heard if the spasm is incomplete. The chest does not expand normally, and a rocking motion of the chest wall that stimulates abdominal breathing may be present. The patient panics if awake.

Several factors can help identify the patient at risk for a laryngospasm. Preoperatively, risks include a history of asthma, chronic obstructive pulmonary disease (COPD), or smoking. Intraoperatively, risks include the use of an endotracheal tube (ETT), anesthetic agents, "light" anesthesia, multiple attempts at intubation, or surgical airway manipulation. After surgery, risks include coughing, "bucking" on the ETT, repeated suctioning, or excessive secretions in the nasopharyngeal area. Laryngospasm may also be precipitated by irritants and foreign bodies.

Laryngospasm is an emergency that requires an immediate response; otherwise, the patient may rapidly deteriorate. Management is initiated by removing the stimulus, along with any irritants such as secretions, blood, or an artificial airway that is too long. The patient's head must be hyperextended and positive-pressure mask ventilation instituted on 100% oxygen. The anesthesiologist is notified immediately. If complete obstruction is unrelieved by positive-pressure ventilations, a small dose of succinylcholine (10 to 20 mg) may be needed to relax the vocal cords to allow for ventilation. Positive-pressure mask ventilation is continued until full muscle function has resumed. Endotracheal intubation is required if the laryngospasm persists or if refractory hypoxemia develops, though it may cause further irritation of the airways. Medications that may be used in the treatment of laryngospasm include lidocaine, steroids, and atropine.

After the spasm, the patient continues to receive supplemental oxygen until stable. It is also important at that time for the nurse to reassure the patient that the spasm has resolved. The patient's feelings of being unable to breathe during laryngospasm are intense, and emotional support from the nurse is imperative.[5,37,39]

Bronchospasm. Bronchospasm is a lower airway obstruction that is characterized by spasmodic contractions of the bronchial tubes. Bronchial airway constriction is a result of an increase in smooth muscle tone in the airways, and bronchospasms develop when the smooth muscles constrict and obstruct the airway. Inflammation has also been recognized as a fundamental component of bronchospasms.

Bronchiolar constriction may be centrally generated, as in asthma, or it may be a local response to airway irritation. Manifestations include wheezing; noisy, shallow respirations; chest retractions; and use of accessory muscles. The patient can exhibit shortness of breath, coughing, and a prolonged expiratory phase of respiration. In addition, hypertension and tachycardia may be present. The patient's level of consciousness may range from lethargy to extreme anxiety.

Patients who smoke and those with chronic bronchitis have essentially irritable airways that react to stimulation. A preoperative history of asthma, a recent upper respiratory infection, severe emphysema, pulmonary fibrosis, or radiation pneumonitis are indicators of a greater risk of bronchospasm. Stimuli that produce a bronchospasm postoperatively include secretions, vomitus, and blood. Patients who have had laryngoscopy, bronchoscopy, or other surgical stimulation are also at increased risk of bronchospasm. Some drugs are also thought to predispose the patient to developing bronchoconstriction resulting from cholinomimetic stimulation; these drugs include physostigmine, neostigmine, edrophonium, and barbiturates. Other histamine-releasing drugs such as tubocurarine, morphine, metocurine, and atracurium may potentially foster bronchospasm.

Bronchospasm is treated initially by removing any possible irritants or drugs. The first line of therapy consists of inhaled bronchodilators. These inhalants cause fewer cardiovascular side effects than systemically administered drugs. Common inhalant medications used are isoetharine, metaproterenol, albuterol, and beclomethasone. Systemic bronchodilators and antiinflammatory agents may also be required at times. Epinephrine or isoproterenol is occasionally needed as a continuous infusion. Methylprednisolone given intravenously manages the inflammatory aspect of bronchospasm. Cholinergics have been given by nebulizer to decrease secretions.[37,39]

Noncardiogenic Pulmonary Edema. Pulmonary edema may be defined simply as increased total lung water. Fluid can accumulate in the interstitial spaces or in the alveoli as the result of cardiogenic or pulmonary capillary etiology. Noncardiogenic pulmonary edema in the postanesthesia recovery period can result from pulmonary aspiration, blood transfusion reaction, allergic drug reaction, upper airway obstruction, or sepsis. The most common causative factor seems to be an upper airway obstruction, usually laryngospasm. Often a short episode of airway obstruction in the operating room had occurred. Noncardiogenic pulmonary edema has also occurred after the administration of naloxone to patients who have received general anesthesia. The reversal of the analgesics causes a rise in the level of adrenal catecholamines, which can lead to pulmonary hypertension and probably increased pulmonary vascular permeability.

During laryngospasm, the patient is inhaling against a closed glottis. This generates an increase in negative intrathoracic pressure. A tremendous subatmospheric transpulmonary pressure gradient is created that causes transudation, or leaking of fluid, from the pulmonary capillaries into the interstitium.

Management of the patient consists of maintenance of an unobstructed airway and supplemented oxygen to correct hypoxemia. Those patients who cannot maintain adequate oxygenation with a mask may require the use of CPAP or even mechanical ventilation with PEEP. The use of PEEP or CPAP improves hypoxemia by restoring the functional residual capacity. Vigorous pulmonary toilet may be required, as well as the use of hemodynamic monitoring if the patient's blood pressure is labile and fluid balance is difficult to maintain.

Diuretics and fluid restriction are usually a part of the treatment regimen. Morphine can be titrated to relieve anxiety. Corticosteroid therapy can be used to decrease laryngeal edema and stabilize the pulmonary membrane. Noncardiogenic pulmonary edema occurs rapidly and requires early assessment and immediate intervention.[40,41]

Aspiration. Aspiration can be defined as the passage of regurgitated gastric contents or other foreign materials into the trachea and down to the smaller air units. It can occur during the period of reduced protective airway reflexes. The most common and severest form of aspiration is the aspiration of gastric contents. The gastric acid in gastric contents damages the alveolar and capillary endothelial cells. Fluid rich with protein leaks into the interstitium and alveoli. This results in atelectasis and consolidation. Pulmonary compliance and functional residual capacity are decreased, and airway resistance and intrapulmonary shunting are increased, with hypoxemia resulting.

If aspiration is suspected, management begins with lowering the patient's head, if possible. The patient is positioned to the side or the head is turned to the side to permit gravity to pull secretions from the trachea. Management centers on promoting tissue oxygenation by maintaining arterial oxygenation via CPAP and supplemental oxygen. Positive-pressure ventilation via mask can be applied if the patient is awake and can protect his or her airway or via an ETT if the patient cannot tolerate the mask or requires higher levels of airway pressure.[37,39]

Hypoxemia. Administration of oxygen by face mask to recovering patients is routine because of the many factors that can lead to hypoxemia in the postoperative patient. Respiratory depressant effects of residual agents may result in a shallow breathing pattern with increased dead space–to–tidal volume ratio. This is even more evident in patients after upper abdominal surgery, and the reduction in the effective ventilation can have serious effects on oxygenation.[35]

The most common cause of hypoxemia is ventilation-perfusion mismatching. Atelectasis often occurs as a result of bronchial obstruction by secretions or blood. Reduction in functional residual capacity (FRC) is caused by the effects of anesthesia and, in the case of upper abdominal surgery, by the surgical procedure. When FRC falls below closing capacity, dependent alveoli occlude, leading to increased mismatching. Impairment of hypoxic pulmonary vasoconstriction by inhalation agents and some vasoactive drugs potentiates this effect.[37]

Hypoventilation. Central respiratory depression is caused by all anesthetic agents. This may lead to significant hypoventilation and hypercarbia. Impaired respiratory muscle function, particularly after upper abdominal surgery, may contribute to the problem of carbon dioxide elimination. Incomplete reversal of neuromuscular blockade must also be considered. Other contributory factors may include tight dressings and body casts, obesity, and gastric dilation. In addition, increased carbon dioxide production may occur as a result of shivering or sepsis. This leads to hypercarbia in patients unable to increase ventilation enough to compensate.

Hypercarbia resulting from postoperative hypoventilation may cause hypertension and tachycardia, increasing the risk of myocardial ischemia in susceptible individuals. Hypoventilation, by itself or in combination with the other factors previously discussed, can cause hypoxemia. Very high levels of carbon dioxide may have sedative effects. Evaluation of suspected hypoventilation requires measurement of arterial blood gases.

Careful titration of opioid antagonists, such as naloxone, may be effective in improving ventilation without compromising pain relief. Planning ahead to provide adequate postoperative pain relief is essential for maintaining adequate postoperative ventilation, particularly in patients undergoing abdominal or thoracic procedures. Placing obese patients in a head-up position and relieving the effects of tight dressings and casts can also be important. Hypoventilation that cannot be improved sufficiently by noninvasive means requires intubation and mechanical ventilation until the patient can maintain adequate ventilation.[35,39]

CARDIOVASCULAR PROBLEMS AND EMERGENCIES

In the immediate postoperative period, cardiovascular complications causing an alteration in CO can occur. These include anesthetic effects on cardiac function, myocardial dysfunction, dysrhythmias, hypertension, and hypotension. These conditions may occur individually or in combination.[42]

Effects of Anesthesia on Cardiac Function. In the immediate postoperative period the residual effects of anesthetic agents and their adjuncts must be considered in the evaluation of a patient who has cardiac dysfunction. Volatile anesthetic agents such as halothane, enflurane, and isoflurane can cause a dose-related reduction in myocardial function. Halothane causes a drop in blood pressure primarily because of a reduction in heart rate and myocardial contractility. It produces only a slight reduction in SVR. Enflurane not only decreases contractility but also reduces SVR. Isoflurane has the most significant hypotension action and the least negative inotropic effects of the three agents. The actions of these agents may be noted for several hours after the conclusion of surgery.[2,4] Nitrous oxide is an inhalation agent that demonstrates insignificant cardiac depression. However, the combined action of opioids given during emergence from nitrous oxide can result in marked cardiovascular depression.[2]

Therapy directed toward mitigating the myocardial depressant effects of inhalation anesthetic agents is primarily that of increasing preload. Elevation of the legs and a crystalloid fluid bolus are commonly sufficient treatment, but ephedrine or other positive inotropic agents may be needed.[10]

Individually most opioids and benzodiazepines only moderately depress cardiac function. Opioids reduce the sympathetic response and enhance vagal and parasympathetic tone. This results in vasodilation and a decreased in SVR. Benzodiazepines also cause vasodilation and a decrease in the SVR. Used in combination, these medications can have a significant effect on the cardiovascular system. Specifically, the overall reaction may include a lowered SVR, heart rate, ventricular contractility, catecholamine level, baroreceptor reflex, CO, and blood pressure. Aggressive administration of crystalloid solutions may be required to counteract these effects. High-dose opioids combined with vecuronium produce a negative inotropic and chronotropic effect. Patients may require short-term vascular support until these medications dissipate.[13]

In contrast to most opioids, meperidine has a greater effect in diminishing myocardial contractility. Meperidine can cause histamine release, which can lower SVR and blood pressure. Sufentanil also has myocardial depressant effects but with less hemodynamic instability than meperidine. Barbiturates depress the activity of the vasomotor center, causing peripheral vasodilation and hypotension. These actions are dose-related and more marked in the presence of underlying cardiovascular disease. Ketamine has a direct myocardial depressant effect that is usually counterbalanced by its indirect effect on the autonomic nervous system to increase heart rate and blood pressure. In patients who are unable to mount a sympathetic response to stress, ketamine causes a net decrease in CO. Propofol causes a dose-dependent decrease in blood pressure primarily because of a decrease in SVR. This must be considered when caring for patients who are hypovolemic or have minimal cardiac reserves.[39,43]

Local anesthetic agents may cause cardiovascular toxicity if inadvertently injected into the systemic circulation or if excessive dosage of the agent is used. A decrease in myocardial contractility, reduction in SVR, and diminished CO have been observed secondary to these agents. The extent of cardiovascular compromise appears to occur in a dose-related fashion. Management of the cardiovascular complications associated with local anesthetic agents includes measures to increase preload, namely elevation of legs and fluid administration. In refractory cases, ephedrine may also be needed.[2,4]

Myocardial Dysfunction. During the immediate postoperative period, the causes of myocardial depression include pathologic processes and aberrant physiologic states, in addition to anesthetic side effects. These processes may occur alone or in combination and may be particularly hazardous in the presence of underlying cardiac disease.

Myocardial ischemia results from an imbalance of oxygen supply and demand. Commonly, ischemia is a result of a decrease in myocardial blood flow that is usually secondary to atherosclerosis, vasospasm, or hypotension. In the postoperative period, the stress of surgery and the action of certain anesthetic agents can increase myocardial ischemia.[42]

Dysrhythmias. In the immediate postanesthetic period, patients are predisposed to a variety of cardiac dysrhythmias. The most common dysrhythmias are sinus tachycardia, sinus bradycardia, premature ventricular contractions, supraventricular tachydysrhythmias, and ventricular tachycardia. If any of these are present, a thorough investigation of the disturbance must be undertaken, not just a reflex treatment.

Accurate interpretation and identification of the dysrhythmia are essential, because therapeutic intervention is based on diagnosis. Appropriate skin preparation and lead placement are extremely important to ensure a clear, readable tracing, free from artifact. Additional 12-lead electrocardiographic capabilities should be used if an interpretation cannot be made from bedside monitoring tracings.

The hemodynamic effects of the dysrhythmia also should be thoroughly assessed. The clinical presentation of the dysrhythmia determines the severity of underlying cardiac disease and the type of treatment. Tachydysrhythmias shorten diastolic filling time and interfere with coronary artery perfusion. These two effects, coupled with an increase in myocardial oxygen consumption, may produce cardiac decompensation. Bradycardia can produce a clinically significant decrease in CO if stroke volume is limited by underlying cardiac disease or if the venous return is reduced. Finally, the cause of the rhythm disturbance should be considered.[43]

The causes of postoperative dysrhythmias are variable. Circulatory instability; preexisting heart disease; an increase in vagal tone; drugs; pain; electrolytic disturbances; and alterations in acid-base balance, oxygenation, and ventilation are most common.

General anesthesia lowers the dysrhythmia threshold of the myocardium. Inhalation agents such as halothane, enflurane, and isoflurane sensitize the myocardium to catecholamines and depress sinoatrial (SA) and atrioventricular (AV) nodal function. Junctional rhythms and premature ventricular contractions are the most commonly seen dysrhythmias. Ketamine produces sympathetic stimulation, resulting in tachycardia and hypertension. Succinylcholine stimulates the cholinergic receptors, enhancing vagal tone, and it can produce sinus bradycardia or junctional escape rhythms. Opioids may cause bradycardia because of direct stimulation of the vagus nerve.

In addition, endogenous catecholamine levels in postoperative patients are elevated because of the pain and stress of surgery. Increased catecholamine levels increase sinus and AV node rates, as well as atrial and ventricular irritability. The direct result is tachydysrhythmias and atrial or ventricular premature contractions.[42,43]

Postoperative Hypertension. Hypertension is not an unusual occurrence in the immediate postoperative period. The diagnosis of hypertension must be considered in the context of an elevated blood pressure in relation to the patient's preoperative and intraoperative blood pressure range. Most commonly, postoperative hypertension is related to fluid overload, heightened sympathetic nervous system activity, or preexisting hypertension. Postoperative hypertension, even as a transient episode, may have significant cardiovascular and intracranial consequences, and therefore aggressive diagnosis and treatment are indicated.

Increased sympathetic tone in the immediate postoperative period may be secondary to the stress of surgery; postoperative pain; anxiety or restlessness during emergence from anesthesia; bladder or bowel distention; or hypothermia. Stimulation of the autonomic nervous system can occur because of hypoxia or hypercarbia. These factors can occur alone or in combination.

Pain is one of the most common sources of increased sympathetic tone. Administering adequate amounts of analgesics, repositioning the patient for comfort, providing reassurance, and limiting environmental stimuli can contribute to alleviating postoperative pain and to lowering blood pressure. Hypothermia and shivering also contribute to postoperative hypertension and are easily treated with warm blankets, warming devices, warm intravenous fluids, and heated humidified oxygen. Bladder distention contributes to postoperative hypertension and must be alleviated. Placement of a urinary catheter may be needed. Hypoxia and hypercarbia must also be treated.

Pharmacologic treatment of postoperative hypertension includes the use of vasodilators, adrenergic inhibitors, and calcium channel blockers. The use of these agents is necessary when hypertension persists despite conservative measures previously mentioned.[36,42]

Postoperative Hypotension. Maintenance of blood pressure depends on adequate preload, myocardial contractility, and afterload. The most common cause of hypotension is intravascular volume depletion caused by inadequate replacement of blood loss, third space fluid loss, insensible loss, and urinary output. Pulmonary embolism may also reduce preload by blocking flow of blood to the left side of the heart. Reduced myocardial contractility may be a result of the effects of anesthetic drugs, myocardial ischemia, or dysrhythmias. Reduced afterload in the form of low SVR may occur as a result of sepsis, hyperthermia, sympathectomy, or large arteriovenous shunts, as seen in chronic liver failure.

Prolonged hypotension can lead to serious ischemic organ damage. Prompt treatment is essential. If the underlying cause is not immediately apparent, the first treatment is an attempt to increase preload by elevating the patient's legs and infusing fluids. Examination of the ECG monitor for dysrhythmias or evidence of ischemia may help guide therapy. Also, the lungs are examined for evidence of pulmonary edema or tension pneumothorax. Vasopressors may be administered to maintain perfusion while additional monitoring modalities are evaluated and established. Insertion of a central venous catheter allows measurement of right ventricular filling pressure and may be used to guide fluid administration in patients with normal myocardial function. In the presence of left ventricular dysfunction or when the etiology remains unclear, a pulmonary artery catheter may be inserted to guide therapy through evaluation of left-sided filling pressure, CO, and SVR. The use of additional fluids, inotropic agents, or vasoconstrictor or vasodilator drugs is determined by these measurements.[36,37]

THERMOREGULATORY PROBLEMS AND EMERGENCIES

Patients recovering from anesthesia usually experience some form of thermoregulatory imbalance (i.e., a core body temperature that is outside the normothermic range of 36° to 38° C). Both hypothermia and hyperthermia can occur in the postoperative patient. Management of these alterations is important because they are associated with other physiologic alterations that may interfere with recovery.

Hypothermia. Hypothermia is a common occurrence both intraoperatively and postoperatively because the conditions associated with surgery and anesthesia typically inhibit the body's heat-generating mechanisms and favor its heat-loss mechanisms.[44] It occurs when systemic heat loss lowers core body temperature below 36° C. Causes of hypothermia include wound and skin exposure, respiratory gas exchange, fluid and blood administration, use of mechanical warming/cooling devices, chemical reactions, alterations in body temperature regulation, and disease states. Clinical manifestations of hypothermia include bluish tint to the skin (peripheral cyanosis); shivering and an increase in metabolic rate (early sign); dysrhythmias; and a decrease in metabolic rate (late sign), oxygen consumption, muscle tone, heart rate, and level of consciousness.[29]

Hypothermia has several adverse effects, including discomfort, vasoconstriction, and shivering. It depresses the myocardium and increases susceptibility to ventricular dysrhythmias. Significant hypothermia slows metabolic processes, leading to reduced drug biotransformation and impaired renal transport. This may prolong drug effects and delay emergence.[44]

Shivering. Shivering may be a result of either the compensatory response to hypothermia or the effects of anesthetic agents, and it can produce a 500% increase in the metabolic rate. Under these conditions, increased oxygen consumption and greater carbon dioxide production can increase the ventilatory requirements. If these requirements are not met, the $PaCO_2$ increases and the PaO_2 can decrease, especially if any significant intrapulmonary shunting coexists. The demand for blood flow by the diaphragm can increase sharply, requiring CO and myocardial workload to increase, resulting in an increase in myocardial oxygen consumption. This can result in myocardial ischemia, particularly in elderly patients or in patients with coronary artery disease.[44]

Vasoconstriction, a particularly deleterious consequence of postoperative hypothermia, may be responsible for unexplained hypertension in the recovery room. Because vasoconstriction can increase systemic vascular resistance and myocardial workload, the potential for myocardial ischemia exists. In addition, vasoconstriction can mask hypovolemia, and sudden reductions in blood pressure can occur as the patient warms and vasodilates.[45] Delayed drug clearance as a consequence of hypothermia is particularly significant in elderly patients who may already have impaired drug-clearing mechanisms and a decreased metabolic rate. For example, the maximal rate of renal excretion of a drug can decline by 10% for every 0.6° C drop in body temperature. In addition, elderly hypothermic patients are more likely to have residual paralysis because of muscle relaxants that are difficult to reverse pharmacologically.[46]

Management of the hypothermic patient is directed toward the restoration of normothermia. Rewarming prevents the thermoregulatory responses to cold, such as shivering. Management depends on the degree of temperature loss. If the patient's body temperature is between 36° and 37° C, the patient can simply be covered with warmed blankets, and heat lamps can be used to keep the patient adequately warm. If the patient's body temperature is less than 36° C, rapid rewarming is required to decrease the possible complications of hypothermia and the postanesthesia recovery time. Convective warming devices provide a safe and effective means of rewarming the patient. In patients with a normal metabolic rate, a setting of "low" or "medium" increases the mean body temperature at about 1° C per hour. A "high" setting increases the mean body temperature about 1.5° C per hour.[2,4] Other methods of rewarming are thermal mattresses, fluid and blood warming, and environmental warming. Supplemental oxygen must be administered to meet the increased metabolic demand in shivering patients. Patients who are shivering may respond to a small dose of meperidine (Demerol).[45]

Hyperthermia. By definition, hyperthermia occurs at any core body temperature above normal. Severe, clinically significant hyperthermia results when core temperature exceeds 40° C. Though not as common perioperatively as hypothermia, hyperthermia is nevertheless a serious complication of surgery. Postoperative temperature elevations may be caused by accidental overwarming of the patient during surgery, infection, sepsis, and transfusion reactions. As an elevated temperature increases oxygen demand and subsequently ventilatory and cardiac workload, a hyperthermia patient with poor cardiac reserve suffers serious consequences.[47]

Postoperative fever must be distinguished from other hyperthermic syndromes. A fundamental difference exists between fever and specific hyperthermic states. In nonfever-related hyperthermic states, body temperature rises above normal despite the body's heat-dissipating mechanisms (e.g., vasodilation, sweating). Therefore excessive heat gain, secondary to either internal or external factors, exceeds the body's cooling capabilities with a consequent rise in body temperature.[2,4]

In contrast, fever results from a resetting to a higher temperature from the normal set point. Until the body reaches its new set point temperature, heat-generating mechanisms (i.e., vasoconstriction and shivering) are activated. Once the new set point temperature is reached, there is an equilibrium between heat generation and heat loss. Unlike hyperthermia, with fever there is no physiologic activity to bring body temperature back to normal. Factors that can contribute to raising core body temperature and fever during the perioperative period are listed in Box 14-8.[2,44]

Primary therapy for hyperthermia includes cooling and decreasing thermogenesis. Cooling by either evaporative or direct external methods has proved effective. This includes ice packs, a cool environment, and cooling blankets. Gastric and bladder lavage have also proved effective. Although physical cooling is an appropriate therapy for other hyperthermias, attempts to cool a febrile patient may be resisted by the thermoregulatory system. Consequently, the first course of action is to restore normothermia with the use of antipyretic drugs. Antipyretics are useful because they have the ability to prevent prostaglandin synthesis in the hypothalamus. Measures to manage the febrile patient include using antipyretics (as indicated), providing a sponge bath with tepid water, keeping the environment cool, using a cooling blanket for sustained fever, and monitoring fluid and electrolyte balance as fluid needs increase during fever. The possibility of malignant hyperthermia (MH) must always be considered.[47]

Malignant Hyperthermia. Malignant hyperthermia is a genetically determined condition. MH is precipitated by certain general inhalation anesthetics, depolarizing skeletal muscle relaxants, local anesthetics, and stress. The incidence of MH ranges from 1 in 15,000 in children to 1 in 50,000 in adults. The onset of MH usually occurs during induction of anesthesia. However, there have been reports of it occurring up to 72 hours after

Box 14-8

FACTORS INFLUENCING TEMPERATURE AND FEVER

CAUSES OF ELEVATED CORE TEMPERATURE
Blood transfusion
Drug-induced fever
Overuse of techniques to prevent hypothermia
Hypothalamic injury
Malignant hyperthermia
Warm environment
Use of anticholinergics
Endocrine disorders
Neurogenic hyperthermia

CAUSES OF POSTOPERATIVE FEVER
Atelectasis
Wound infection
Abscess formation
Fat emboli after bone trauma
Drug reactions
Malignancy
Silent aspiration
Dehydration
Blood transfusion reaction
Central nervous system damage
Urinary tract infections
Phlebitis/deep vein thrombosis
Pulmonary emboli

Box 14-9

SIGNS AND SYMPTOMS OF MALIGNANT HYPERTHERMIA

Hypoxemia
Metabolic acidosis
Respiratory acidosis
Hyperkalemia
Myoglobinuria
Elevated creatine phosphokinase
Tachycardia
Tachypnea
Ventricular dysrhythmias
Cyanosis
Skin mottling
Fever—hot, flushed skin
Rigidity
Profuse sweating
Unstable blood pressure

Modified from Drain CB, editor: *Perianesthesia nursing: a critical care approach,* ed 4, Philadelphia, 2003, Saunders.

the triggering agent is introduced. Because successful management of MH depends on early assessment and prompt intervention, the nurse must be knowledgeable in the pathophysiology and treatment of this syndrome.[47]

Identification before anesthesia of patients who may be susceptible to MH is of major therapeutic importance. On history and physical examination, MH-susceptible patients usually demonstrate some subclinical weakness or abnormality, such as deficient fine motor control. Many complain of muscle cramps that occur spontaneously, during an infectious illness, or during or after exercise. Patient history or genealogy going back two generations may be positive. Physical examination may reveal myopathies such as cryptorchidism, pectus carinatum, kyphosis, lordosis, ptosis, or hypoplastic mandible. Electromyographic changes are seen in fewer than half of MH-susceptible patients. Measurement of blood creatine phosphokinase (CPK) is usually about 70% reliable in determining susceptibility to MH.[2,4]

The most definitive test for detecting MH susceptibility is a biopsy of skeletal muscle. Samples are obtained from the quadriceps muscles and are subjected to isometric contractor testing. The skeletal muscle of the MH-susceptible patient has an increased isometric tension when exposed to caffeine or halothane.[48]

When a susceptible patient is exposed to a triggering agent for MH, such as halothane, the clinical features are produced by an excess of calcium ions in the myoplasm. With an elevated calcium ion concentration in the myoplasm, skeletal muscle contraction is intense and prolonged, leading to a hypermetabolic state of acid and heat production. More specifically, heat is produced by the accelerated and continued synthesis and use of adenosine triphosphate (ATP) during glycolysis. The metabolic by-product of glycolysis, lactic acid, is transported to the liver and then back to the metabolically active muscle, where the cycle repeats. Respiratory and metabolic acidosis develop because of this hypermetabolic state, and symptoms such as tachycardia, tachypnea, ventricular dysrhythmias, and unstable blood pressure appear. Because of intense vasoconstriction the skin is mottled and cyanotic.[48] Box 14-9 lists the clinical manifestation of MH.

Elevated body temperature can actually be a late sign of MH. For this reason, the nurse must not prolong the assessment of the patient on the assumption that the patient's temperature must be significantly elevated before intervention is attempted. Once the patient's temperature begins to rise, it may increase at a rate of 0.5° C every 15 minutes and may approach levels as high as 46° C.[2]

Muscle rigidity occurs in about 75% of the patients who experience MH. This is especially true in MH-susceptible patients after the administration of succinylcholine. In fact, muscle rigidity may be so severe that the nurse cannot open the patient's mouth to insert an airway. The onset of skeletal muscle rigidity after the administration of succinylcholine could be a sign of impending development of MH.[47]

Various environmental stimuli and pharmacologic agents can stimulate an acute episode of MH (Box

Box 14-10

ENVIRONMENTAL AND PHARMACOLOGIC TRIGGERS OF MALIGNANT HYPERTHERMIA

ENVIRONMENTAL STIMULI
Extensive skeletal muscle injury
Emotional crisis
Very hot and humid weather
Strenuous and prolonged exercise

PHARMACOLOGIC AGENTS
Halothane
Enflurane
Isoflurane (?)
Succinylcholine
d-Tubocurarine
Gallamine (?)
Amide local anesthetics—lidocaine, mepivacaine, bupivacaine, etidocaine
Caffeine

From Drain CB, editor: *Perianesthesia nursing: a critical care approach*, ed 4, Philadelphia, 2003. Saunders

14-10). Fatigue, emotional upset, or very hot and humid weather can trigger a waking febrile episode. The anesthetic agents that may trigger MH seem to affect the sarcoplasmic reticulum. Because of their widespread use, halothane and succinylcholine are the most common triggering agents. Local anesthetics, such as lidocaine, are also triggering agents. It has been demonstrated that lidocaine causes the release of calcium ions into the mycoplasma in vitro. In MH-susceptible patients or in patients who have had an episode of MH in the operating room, all possible triggering agents must be stringently avoided. As another precaution, because emotional upsets trigger MH, nurses must provide a stress-free environment for the MH-susceptible patient.[46,47]

The cornerstone of the successful management of MH is early detection. If the patient develops acute MH, all inhalation anesthetics are stopped, the patient is hyperventilated with 100% oxygen, sodium bicarbonate (1 to 2 mg/kg) is administered, and dantrolene is given. It is important to know how to administer dantrolene. It must be diluted with sterile water. Cooling measures, such as administering cold IV fluids, packing the patient in ice, and irrigating body cavities (e.g., stomach, bladder) with cold fluids, are initiated. Accurate intake and output records are essential because large amounts of fluids and diuretics are given. Laboratory tests, such as complete blood counts (CBC) and coagulation studies, are closely scrutinized for signs of bleeding or the onset of disseminated intravascular clotting. Ongoing ECG and temperature monitoring are also essential. It is recommended that all emergency drugs be available on a special cart, either in the operating room or in the postanesthesia care unit.[46,47]

NEUROLOGIC PROBLEMS AND EMERGENCIES

Almost all patients exhibit some level of arousal within 90 minutes after anesthesia is completed. Although many factors are known to prolong anesthetic effects, most reports of delayed arousal and emergence delirium are anecdotal.

Delayed Arousal. Delayed awakening after general anesthesia is a common and often easily explained problem. The etiology can usually be attributed to prolonged action of anesthetic drugs, metabolic causes, or neurologic injury. In most cases the prolonged sedation is the result of residual general anesthetic. Hypoventilation resulting from high concentration of inhaled anesthetic limits the exhalation of the agent and prolongs its retention. Opioids used as adjunct therapy may contribute to hypercarbia and sedation as well. Hypothermia, advanced age, hepatic dysfunction, and renal disease may contribute to prolonged recovery from anesthetics by heightening sensitivity, delaying elimination, or both. The use of premedication may also prolong recovery, especially if narcotics or benzodiazepines, particularly diazepam, are used.[49]

In addition to experiencing a slowing elimination of potent inhalation anesthetic, the hypoventilating patient may develop hypoxia and hypercapnia. The ensuing hypercapnia may cause significant narcosis, as well as potentiate the depressive effects of the anesthetics. In the diabetic patient, the administration of chlorpropamide or excessive insulin preoperatively may cause postoperative hypoglycemia, unconsciousness, or even coma.[50]

Severe electrolyte disturbances are most commonly seen after excessive water absorption during transurethral prostate surgery. The subsequent dilution hyponatremia may manifest as sedation, coma, or hemiparesis. Dilution hyponatremia may also be seen after the inappropriate release of antidiuretic hormone. Hypocalcemia after parathyroid surgery may result in delayed awakening. High magnesium levels after the prolonged administration of magnesium sulfate to the eclamptic or preeclamptic patient may also result in prolonged postoperative sedation, as well as muscle weakness after general anesthetic cesarean section.[30]

Neurologic injury and subsequent unconsciousness may be the result of an unsuspected cerebral vascular accident. Intracranial hemorrhage may result from hypertensive responses to anesthetic or surgical manipulations, especially in the patient receiving anticoagulant therapy. Paradoxical air emboli may cross a patent foramen ovale in the presence of a right-to-left shunt. Direct emboli from cardiac valves, intracardiac thrombi, and atherosclerotic vessels may also be a threat. Fat emboli can occur after massive long-bone or tissue damage and may not appear until during or after surgical manipulation or reduction of the fracture. Deliberate, induced hypotension in normal patients is not usually associated with neurologic damage. However, uncontrolled intraoperative hypotension may result in ischemia, especially in the patient with hypertension or carotid occlusive disease.[49]

The successful management of delayed arousal depends on careful consideration of the differential diagnosis. A thorough review of the patient's preoperative medical condition and the intraoperative course, both surgical and anesthetic, usually points to an etiology. If the cause of the sedation is not immediately obvious, the first consideration must be assessing the patient's oxygenation and ensuring adequate gas exchange. Pulse oximetry, end-tidal carbon dioxide measurement, and arterial blood gas values can give an estimate of any ventilatory depression and rule out ongoing hypoxia and hypercarbia factors.[49,51]

If the cause is thought to be residual inhalation anesthetic, maintaining adequate ventilation should be sufficient treatment. If available, mass spectrophotometry can provide an estimate of exhaled anesthetic concentrations and confirm the diagnosis. Residual opioids can be reversed by naloxone, and anticholinergic CNS depression can be reversed by physostigmine. Physostigmine has been reported to reverse sedation from other hypnotics and general anesthetics as well. The benzodiazepine antagonist flumazenil has been shown to directly antagonize the CNS sedative and amnesic effects of the benzodiazepines.[2]

Body temperature is determined and warming instituted if hypothermia exists. Serum electrolytes and magnesium and calcium levels are checked if ion disturbance is suspected. Blood for a serum glucose assay may also be drawn, but the simple fingerstick glucose determination is faster and accurate enough to exclude hypoglycemia from consideration if normal. Other laboratory tests may be useful, as well, if hepatic or renal disease is being considered. Unless perioperative events point specifically to it, neurologic injury is usually a diagnosis of exclusion. If other causes of prolonged arousal have been excluded, a thorough neurologic consultation is obtained.[49]

Emergence Delirium. Most patients emerge from general anesthesia in a calm, tranquil manner. Some patients, however, emerge in a state of excitement, a condition characterized by restlessness, disorientation, crying, moaning, or irrational talking. In the extreme form of excitement, which is referred to as emergence delirium, the patient screams, shouts, and thrashes about wildly. It seems to be seen most frequently after tonsillectomy, thyroid surgery, circumcision, hysterectomy, and perineal and abdominal wall procedures.[51]

Hypoxia and resulting air hunger, as well as hypercarbia, may appear as restlessness, disorientation, slurred speech, and agitation. Hyponatremia, hypochloremia, and acid-base changes could all be seen during the immediate postoperative period and can be the cause of mental confusion. Pain is a common cause of restlessness and is commonly seen postoperatively. Urinary bladder and gastric distention, which may cause considerable discomfort, are easily overlooked.[51]

Drug reactions are commonly implicated as the cause of postoperative agitation. Such reactions are less common than they once were because the use of offending drugs is less prevalent. The most frequently implicated drugs are the anticholinergics, most notably scopolamine and atropine. They have been shown to have CNS-toxic effects that can include psychotic behavior, delirium, and motor disturbance. Ketamine is also associated with a high incidence of unpleasant agitation. Neuroleptic drugs such as droperidol, especially in high doses, may be associated with development of dyskinesia and involuntary muscle activity, as well as postoperative confusion.[49]

The patient's state of apprehension or anxiety can have a marked effect on emergence agitation; it is especially notable in apprehensive patients and, conversely, those seemingly unconcerned about forthcoming major surgery. Factors such as fear of disfigurement (e.g., caused by surgical procedure for removal of cancer) and feelings of suffocation also increase the likelihood of emergence excitement. Young patients tend to have an increased incidence of postoperative excitation, as do patients undergoing emergency procedures. Several psychiatric factors have been shown to increase the incidence of postoperative delirium, including a history of alcoholism, insomnia, depression, or debility.[51]

If emergence delirium occurs, the patient's status is thoroughly evaluated. Management includes determining an etiology, initiating specific therapy, and protecting patients from injuring themselves. When encountering a restless, confused postoperative patient, the first measure is to ensure that the agitation is not the result of hypoxia. Presuming pain to be the cause of agitation in a hypoxic patient and treating the excitement with opioids or sedatives may have disastrous consequences. Hypoxia must be quickly excluded from the differential diagnosis by pulse oximetry, arterial blood gas determination, or both.[2,3,50]

Hyponatremia may be suspected in the confused patient after prostate surgery, especially if the surgery was prolonged. A serum electrolyte determination can confirm the diagnosis. The treatment usually consists of fluid restriction and, rarely, hypertonic saline administration. Severe acid-base disturbances can be diagnosed and therapy directed by arterial blood gas determination. If pain appears to be the diagnosis after the exclusion of hypoxia, intravenous opioids may be administered in small increments. The CNS effects of the anticholinergics are usually dramatically reversed by the administration of physostigmine. The incidence of hallucinations with ketamine may be decreased by benzodiazepine or droperidol administration.[2] Gastric distention may be relieved by nasogastric aspiration, and urinary bladder distention is easily treated with catheterization.[2,4]

When dealing with perioperative anxiety, the best treatment is prevention. Some patients need reassurance that they will not experience intraoperative awareness and will receive pain medication, if needed, upon awakening.[52]

Occasionally one is faced with a restless postoperative patient who does not seem to be getting relief from opioid administration. Small intravenous doses of a short-acting benzodiazepine such as midazolam may be warranted. The anxiolytics are administered in reduced doses, because their respiratory depressant effects may be cumulative with existing opioids, sedatives, and residual general anesthetics. If overt psychotic behavior is apparent despite adequate treatment, psychiatric consultation should be obtained.[51]

The patient's respiratory function and airway patency are checked first, because restlessness is a well-known manifestation of hypoxia. Other causes of emergence delirium include a full bladder, cramped or sore muscles and joints from prolonged abnormal positioning on the operating table, pain, incomplete reversal of neuromuscular blocking agents, withdrawal from alcohol and other drugs, acid-base disturbances, and electrolyte abnormalities. The restless patient requires constant, careful observation. Gentle physical restraint may be required to prevent injury. Several nurses or other personnel may be needed. If hypoxia, pain, and a full bladder are ruled out, a change in positioning may have a quieting effect.[2]

Nausea and Vomiting. Nausea and vomiting, although usually not life-threatening, are probably the most unpleasant and lasting memories many patients have of their anesthesia. Although the incidence has decreased in recent years, nausea and vomiting still result in significant postoperative morbidity and patient discomfort. Nausea is described as a subjective, unpleasant mental experience, usually leading to vomiting. Retching is the rhythmic muscular activity that usually precedes vomiting. Vomiting is defined as the forceful expulsion of gastrointestinal contents through the mouth.[53]

Decidedly unpleasant, vomiting can also be dangerous. The physical exertion may increase postoperative bleeding and disrupt delicate suture lines. Tearing or rupture of the esophagus is probably rare but must be a concern in patients with a history of esophageal pathology. Aspiration of emesis is a life-threatening complication in a patient whose airway–protective reflexes are blunted by residual anesthetic or sedative drugs or damaged by surgical activity. If the vomiting is protracted, dangerous hypokalemia, hypochloremia, hyponatremia, and dehydration may develop. Nausea and vomiting are also the leading causes of unexpected hospitalization after surgery.[53,54]

The use of nitrous oxide is said to cause nausea and vomiting by gastric distention, sympathetic stimulation,

and changes in middle ear pressure. Adjunct drugs given preoperatively or in conjunction with the inhalation anesthetic may themselves be suspected of contributing to the high rate of emetic sequelae. The opioids, when given as premedications, may contribute to nausea and vomiting. Meperidine has also been known to cause nausea and vomiting. Some of the newer general anesthetics have resulted in less nausea and vomiting than their predecessors. Halothane, in subanesthetic doses, may even be antiemetic. When administered alone or in conjunction with the opioids, the anticholinergics can act as potent antiemetics.[55]

Muscle relaxants are thought not to influence postoperative vomiting. However, the reversal of muscle relaxants may contribute to postoperative vomiting. Neostigmine has potent muscarinic effects and may increase intestinal peristalsis and may even trigger spasm.[15,16]

Spinal anesthesia has long been known to trigger a substantial incidence of nausea and vomiting. During spinal anesthesia, a systolic blood pressure less than 80 mm Hg results in a significant incidence in emesis. The administration of 100% oxygen to these patients has substantially decreased the development of emesis.[56]

Gastric distention and irritation cause nausea and vomiting by direct stimulation of the vomiting center. The stomach may become distended during anesthesia by manual insufflation via mask induction. Swallowing air or blood may also result in significant stomach irritation. Acute appendicitis or bowel obstruction is notoriously associated with preoperative and postoperative emesis.

The site of the surgery may also influence the development of postoperative nausea and vomiting. Gastrointestinal procedures have a high frequency of postoperative emesis. Laparoscopic, ophthalmic, and otologic procedures have a high incidence. The duration of the procedure may affect the frequency. Finally, pain triggers nausea and vomiting in many patients.[55]

Patients with a history of motion sickness are most likely to experience postoperative emetic sequelae with each subsequent anesthetic. A certain number of patients experience nausea after fasting, even before the administration of any drugs. Many patients develop nausea upon their first movement and thus may have emesis during transport.[22,54] The female gender is also said to be associated with high incidence of postoperative emesis. The incidence of nausea and vomiting tends to decrease with advancing age.[55]

Other circumstances may act to increase the likelihood of postoperative emesis in any given patient. Patients with a full stomach from either a recent meal or swallowed blood are more likely to vomit on induction of or on emergence from anesthesia. Alcohol intoxication or illicit drug use may also increase the frequency of emesis. Vigorous nasopharyngeal or oropharyngeal suctioning can also elicit a strong gag reflex and trigger vomiting. In neurosurgical patients, especially those with closed head injury, increased intracranial pressure may trigger nausea and vomiting.[57]

The most effective treatment of postoperative nausea and vomiting is prevention. Several maneuvers merit mention as being fairly simple to perform and effective in their usefulness. Avoidance of gastric insufflation is paramount. In addition, prevent the swallowing of blood during oral, pharyngeal, or nasal surgery. If distention is suspected, it is decompressed intraoperatively.[2,4,46] A nasogastric tube is placed to empty fluid and gases from the stomach. Unfortunately, its presence may trigger gagging and subsequent vomiting. An oral airway may elicit the same response in a partially conscious patient and is removed at the first signs of gagging to prevent vomiting and subsequent aspiration.[57]

Many drugs have been shown to possess antiemetic qualities. Some are most effective when given prophylactically. However, many of the drugs are associated with negative or undesirable side effects, and as a result, prophylactic administration may be considered unjustified except under specific circumstances. Available antiemetics include anticholinergics, phenothiazines, antihistamines, butyrophenones, and antidopaminergics.[58]

It is important to remember the supportive care of the nauseated and vomiting patient. If vomiting is severe, electrolyte replacement must be considered. Prolonged vomiting may result in hypovolemia. Intravenous fluids may need to be increased to compensate for fluid losses. Opioids must never be withheld from the nauseated patient complaining of pain because pain itself may be the cause of the vomiting.[57,59]

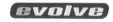 See the Clinical Applications for perianesthesia management and discussions on the Evolve website.

REFERENCES

1. Klein SM: Ambulatory anesthesia for the twenty-first century, *Surg Serv Manage* 6(9):45, 2000.
2. Drain CB: *Perianesthesia nursing: a critical care approach*, ed 4, Philadelphia, 2003, Saunders.
3. Barone CP, Pablo CS, Barone GW: Postanesthetic care in the critical care unit, *Crit Care Nurse* 24(1):38, 2004.
4. Fleisher LA: Risk of anesthesia. In Miller R, editor: *Anesthesia*, ed 6, Philadelphia, 2004, Churchill Livingstone.
5. Wilson M: Giving postanesthesia care in the critical care unit, *Dimen Crit Care Nurs* 19:38, 2000.
6. Arbour R: Sedation and pain management in critically ill adults, *Crit Care Nurse* 20(5):39, 2000.
7. Olson DM et al: Potential benefits of bispectral index monitoring in critical care. A case study, *Crit Care Nurse* 23(4):45, 2004.
8. Bhargava AK, Setlur R, Sreevastava D: Correlation of bispectral index and Guedel's stages of ether anesthesia, *Anesth Analg* 98:132, 2004.
9. Leslie K et al: Patients' knowledge of attitudes towards awareness and depth of anaesthesia monitoring, *Anaesth Intensive Care* 31:63, 2003.
10. Barash PG, Cullen BF, Stoelting RK: *Clinical anesthesia*, ed 4, Philadelphia, 2000, Lippincott.
11. Nissen D: *Mosby's Drug Consult 2005*, ed 9, St Louis, 2005, Elsevier.
12. Gahart BL, Nazareno AR: *2005 intravenous medications*, ed 21, St Louis, 2005, Elsevier.
13. Mokhlesi B, Corbridge T: Toxicology in the critically ill patient, *Clin Chest Med* 24:689, 2003.
14. Kirby RR et al: *Clinical anesthesia practice*, ed 2, Philadelphia, 2001, Saunders.
15. Katz RL: Muscle relaxants: clinical considerations, *Semin Anesth* 14:1, 1995.
16. Katz RL: Muscle relaxants: new drugs and special situations, *Semin Anesth* 14:245, 1995.
17. Sloan TB: Anesthetics and the brain, *Anesthesiol Clin North Am* 20:265, 2002.
18. ASPAN, Quinn DMD, Schick L: *Perianesthesia nursing core curriculum: preoperative, phase I and phase II PACU Nursing*, ed 1, Philadelphia, 2004, Saunders.
19. Stoelting RK, Miller RD: *Basics of anesthesia*, ed 5, New York, 2004, Churchill Livingstone.
20. Schutz, SL: Oxygen saturation monitoring by pulse oximetry. In McHale DJ, Carlson KK: *AACN procedure manual for critical care*, ed 4, Philadelphia, 2001, Saunders.
21. Watson C: Respiratory complications associated with anesthesia, *Anesthesiol Clin North Am* 20:275, 2002.
22. O'Brien D: Care of the perianesthesia patient. In Drain CB, editor: *Perianesthesia nursing: a critical care approach*, ed 4, Philadelphia, 2003, Saunders.
23. Faut-Callahan M, Slach JF: Pain management. In Waugaman WR, Foster SD, Rigor BM, editors: *Principles and practice of nurse anesthesia*, ed 3, Norwalk, 1999, Appleton & Lange.
24. Auburn D et al: Relationships between measurement of pain using visual analog score and morphine requirements during postoperative period, *Anesthesiology* 8:1415, 2003.
25. Golembiewski JA: Morphine and hydromorphone for postoperative analgesia: focus on safety, *J Perianesth Nurs* 18:120, 2003.
26. Reference deleted in proofs.
27. Blank T, Less DL: Cardiac physiology. In Miller R, editor: *Anesthesia*, ed 6, New York, 2004, Churchill Livingstone.
28. Burns SM: Delirium during emergence from anesthesia: a care study, *Crit Care Nurse* 23(1):66, 2003.
29. Sessler DI: Complications and treatment of mild hypothermia, *Anesthesiology* 95:531, 2001.
30. Tonnesen AS: Crystalloids and colloids. In Miller R, editor: *Anesthesia*, ed 6, New York, 2004, Churchill-Livingstone.
31. Cook KG: Assessment and management of anxiety in recovery room patients, *Curr Rev Recov Room Nurses* 7(5):51, 1993.
32. Soutar CR, McMahon K: A PACU patient classification system, *Surg Serv Manage* 6(9):39, 2000.
33. American Association of Critical-Care Nurses: Criteria for overflow patient care in PACUs, *AACN News* 17(8):16, 2000.
34. American Association of Critical-Care Nurses: *A joint position statement on ICU overflow patients*, 2000.
35. Litwack K: *Post anesthesia care nursing*, ed 2, St Louis, 1995, Mosby.
36. Grove TM: Management of problems in the post anesthesia care unit. II. Respiratory, cardiovascular and thermal regulation problems, *Curr Rev Post Anesth Care Nurs* 18:9, 1996.

37. Litwack K: *Post operative pulmonary complications,* Sacramento, 1995, CME Resource.

38. Hotchkiss MA, Drain CB: Assessment and management of the airway. In Drain CB, editor, *Perianesthesia nursing: a critical care approach,* ed 4, Philadelphia, 2003, Saunders.

39. Odom JL: Airway emergencies in the post anesthesia care unit, *Nurs Clin North Am* 28:483, 1993.

40. Ward D: Avoiding ventilatory emergencies, *Semin Anesth* 15(2):183, 1996.

41. Tarrac SE: Negative pressure pulmonary edema: a post-anesthesia emergency, *J Perianesth Nurs* 18:317, 2003.

42. Weitz HH: Perioperative cardiac complications, *Med Clin North Am* 85:1151, 2001.

43. Sloan SB, Weitz HH: Postoperative arrhythmias and conduction disorders, *Med Clin North Am* 85:1171, 2001.

44. Sessler DI: Perioperative heat balance, *Anesthesiology* 92:578, 2000.

45. De Witte J, Sessler DI: Perioperative shivering: physiology and pharmacology, *Anesthesiology* 96:467, 2002.

46. Hildebrand F et al: Pathophysiologic changes and effects of hypothermia on outcome in elective surgery and trauma patients, *Am J Surg* 187:363, 2004.

47. McHenry CR et al: Recognition, management, and prevention of specific operating room catastrophies, *J Am Coll Surg* 198:810, 2004.

48. Hall SC: General pediatric emergencies. Malignant hyperthermia syndrome, *Anesthesiol Clin North Am* 19:367, 2001.

49. Delinger K: Prolonged emergence and failure to regain consciousness. In Gravenstein N, Kirby R, editors: *Complications in anesthesiology,* ed 2, Philadelphia, 1996, Lippincott.

50. Benumof JL: *Airway management: principles and practice,* St Louis, 1996, Mosby.

51. O'Brien D: Acute postoperative delirium: definitions, incidence, recognition, and interventions, *J Perianesth Nurs* 17:384, 2002.

52. Klock A, Roxzen MF: Anesthesiolgist's role as perioperative physician, *Anesth Analg* 83(4):67, 1996.

53. Mazze R, Wharton RS: Fluid and electrolyte problems. In Gravenstein N, Kirby R, editors: *Complications in anesthesiology,* ed 2, Philadelphia, 1996, Lippincott.

54. Gan TJ et al: Consensus guidelines for managing postoperative nausea and vomiting, *Anesth Analg* 97:62, 2003.

55. Cameron D, Gan TJ: Management of postoperative nausea and vomiting in ambulatory surgery, *Anesthesiol Clin North Am* 21:347, 2003.

56. Borgeat A, Ekatodramis G, Schenker CA: Postoperative nausea and vomiting in regional anesthesia: a review, *Anesthesiology* 98:530, 2003.

57. Orkin FK: Postoperative nausea and vomiting. In Gravenstein N, Kirby R, editors: *Complication in anesthesiology,* ed 2, Philadelphia, 1996, Lippincott.

58. Feeley TW: The post anesthesia care unit. In Miller R: *Anesthesia,* ed 6, New York, 2004, Churchill-Livingstone.

59. Grove TM: Management of problems in the post anesthesia care unit. I. General considerations, pain, neurological problems, nausea, and vomiting, *Curr Rev Post Anesth Care Nurs* 18:1, 1996.

UNIT
III

CARDIOVASCULAR ALTERATIONS

CHAPTER 15

Cardiovascular Anatomy and Physiology

ANATOMY

Discussion of the anatomy of the heart and blood vessels in this text begins on a macroscopic level describing the major structures and then progresses to the cellular and molecular levels for each structure.

MACROSCOPIC STRUCTURE

Structures of the Heart. The heart is situated in the anterior thoracic cavity, just behind the sternum (Fig. 15-1). Several important structures are located behind the heart, including the esophagus, the aorta, the vena cava, and the vertebral column. The position of the heart in the chest is such that the chambers normally described as "right" and "left" are really anterior and posterior related to the position of the heart within the chest cavity.[1] The right ventricle constitutes the majority of the anterior surface (closest to the chest wall) and also the inferior surface (directly above the diaphragm). The left ventricle makes up the anterolateral (front and side) and posterior surfaces. The base of the heart is superior (atrial and great vessel level), and the tip (apex) is inferior (ventricular level) above the diaphragm. The base of the heart includes not only the superior portion of the heart itself but also the roots of the aorta, vena cava, and pulmonary vessels.

The increasing use of thoracic computed tomography (CT) in critical care has highlighted the anatomic inaccuracy of the terms right and left ventricle, because these terms do not relate to the position of the heart in the chest when described in standard anatomic position (i.e., upright and facing the observer).[1] However, at this time there is no move to change the traditional right/left nomenclature.

Size and Weight of the Heart. The average human heart is about the size of the clenched fist of that individual. In the adult, this averages 12 cm in length and 8 to 9 cm in breadth at the broadest part. In adult men, the weight of the normal heart averages 310 g, and that of women averages 255 g. There are no significant differences in ventricular wall thickness between men and women. Body weight is a better predictor of healthy heart weight than is body surface area or height. Pathologic conditions such as hypertension will increase the weight of the heart muscle secondary to ventricular hypertrophy.[2]

Layers of the Heart. There are four distinct layers of the heart, the pericardium, the epicardium, the myocardium, and the endocardium.

Pericardium. The heart and origin of the great vessels are surrounded by a double-layered sac called the *pericardium*. The pericardium is designed like a vacuum flask—two layers with a potential space between them. Ligaments anchor the outer pericardium to the diaphragm and great vessels so the heart is maintained in a fixed position within the thoracic cavity.[3] The pericardium also provides a physical barrier to infection. The outermost pericardium is a thick, fibrous envelope that is tough and inelastic.[3] Inside the fibrous layer is an inner serous sac that can be divided into two layers known as the parietal and visceral pericardium. The *parietal pericardium* forms an inner, serous lining to the tough, outer pericardium.[3] The *visceral pericardium* (also known as the *epicardium*) is flexible, attached directly to the heart, and folds with the surface contours of the heart.[3] The space between these two serous pericardial layers normally contains a very small amount of pericardial fluid (approximately 20 to 25 ml) that is secreted and reabsorbed and serves as a lubricant between the layers.[3] The fibrous, outer pericardial sac is noncompliant and unable to adapt to rapid increases in either cardiac size or the amount of fluid in the sac.[4] For example, blood can collect in this sac abnormally, as occurs in cardiac tamponade, or serum can collect in it, as in pericardial effusion. If the fluid collection in the sac impinges on ventricular filling, ventricular ejection, or coronary artery perfusion, a clinical emergency may exist that necessitates removal of the excess pericardial fluid to restore normal cardiac function.

Epicardial Fat. In adults a layer of adipose tissue is typically present beneath the visceral pericardium on top of the heart. This epicardial fat accumulates along the routes of the major coronary arteries and veins. The

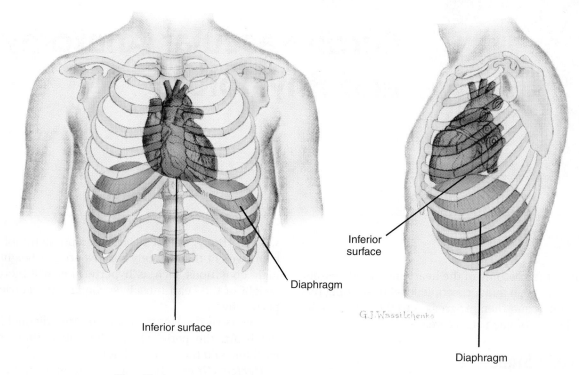

Fig. 15-1 Anatomic location of the heart within the thoracic cavity.

quantity of fat generally increases with age.[3] Women have a greater quantity of epicardial fat over the right ventricle compared with men.[3] If a person is overweight or obese with a large quantity of subcutaneous adipose tissue, there is usually more epicardial fat present. However, this is not always the case, and even slim patients can have large amounts of epicardial fat.[3] The fibrous, outer pericardium does not contain any fat deposits.[3]

Epicardium. The epicardium is tightly adhered to the heart and base of the great vessels and is identical to the visceral pericardium (see above). The coronary arteries lie on the top on the epicardium.[5]

Myocardium. The next layer of the heart—the myocardium, or mid-wall—is a thick, muscular layer. This layer includes all of the atrial and ventricular muscle fibers necessary for contraction. The fibers of the myocardium do not have the same thickness throughout the ventricular walls. The left ventricle is much thicker than the right ventricle or the atria. The fibers are organized so that the force of contraction is most efficient in ejecting blood toward the outflow tracts in a wringing motion from the apex towards the base (Fig. 15-2). The myocardium is the muscle that is damaged by a "heart attack" or transmural myocardial infarction.[6]

Endocardium. The innermost layer is the endocardium, which is a thin layer of endothelium and connective tissue lining the inside of the heart. Disruption in the endothelium as a result of surgery, trauma, or congenital abnormality can predispose the endocardium to infection. This infective endocarditis is a devastating dis-

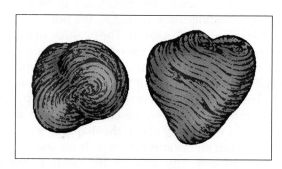

Fig. 15-2 Macroscopic structure of the spiral musculature of the ventricular walls.

ease that, if left untreated, can lead to massive valve damage or sepsis and death.[7]

Cardiac Chambers. The human heart has four chambers: the left and right atria and the left and right ventricles. The atria are thin-walled and normally low-pressure chambers. They function to receive blood from the vena cava and pulmonary arteries and to pump blood into their respective ventricles. Atrial contraction, also known as "atrial kick," contributes approximately 20% of blood flow to ventricular filling, whereas the other 80% occurs passively during diastole. The ventricles are the primary pumping forces of the heart. The healthy right ventricle is approximately 3 mm thick, whereas the normal left ventricle is 10 to 13 mm thick (Fig. 15-3). The right ventricle pumps blood into the low-pressured pulmonary circulation, which has a normal mean pressure

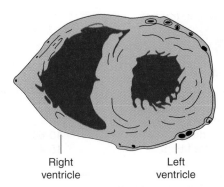

Fig. 15-3   A transverse section of the ventricles of the adult heart. The right ventricle forms the greater part of the anterior surface of the heart, and the wall of the left ventricle is three times as thick as the wall of the right ventricle. (From Quaal S: *Comprehensive intraaortic balloon pumping,* ed 2, St. Louis, 1993, Mosby.)

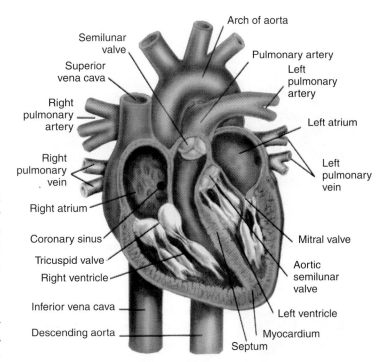

Fig. 15-4   Cross-sectional view of the heart. Note the position of the four cardiac valves. (From Thompson JM et al: *Mosby's clinical nursing,* ed 5, St Louis, 2002, Mosby.)

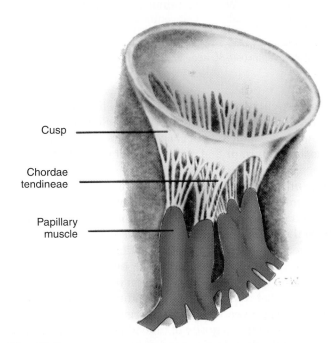

Fig. 15-5   The mitral valve and the relationship of the cusps, chordae tendineae, and the papillary muscles.

of approximately 15 mm Hg. The left ventricle must generate tremendous force to eject blood into the aorta (normal mean pressure of approximately 100 mm Hg). Because of left ventricular thickness and the great force it must generate, the left ventricle is considered the major pump of the heart. When the left ventricular muscle thins out as the result of dilation or disease, the effective pumping pressure is diminished, leading to increased left atrial pressure, pulmonary vasculature congestion, and, ultimately, systemic venous congestion.[8]

Cardiac Valves. Cardiac valves are composed of flexible, fibrous tissue. A normal valve has the translucent appearance of a rose petal. The valve structure allows blood to flow in only one direction. The opening and closing of the valves depends on the relative pressure gradients on either side of the valve. The four cardiac valves lie in an oblique plane of collagen described as the *fibrous skeleton.* Four adjacent rings of connective tissue contain and support the cardiac valves (Fig 15-4).

Atrioventricular Valves. The two atrioventricular (AV) valves are named for their location between the atria and the ventricles. These are the tricuspid (three cusps) valve on the right and the mitral (two cusps) valve on the left. The AV valves are open during ventricular diastole (filling) and prevent backflow of blood into the atria during ventricular systole (contraction). The *chordae tendineae* and *papillary muscles,* which attach to the tricuspid and mitral valves, give the valves stability and prevent valve leaflet eversion during systole (Fig. 15-5). Papillary muscles arise from the ventricular myocardium and derive their blood supply from the coronary arteries. Each papillary muscle gives rise to approximately 4 to 10 main chordae tendineae that divide into finer and finer cords as they approach and attach to the valve leaflets. The chordae tendineae are fibrous, avascular structures covered by a thin layer of endocardium. A dysfunction of the chordae tendineae or of a papillary muscle can cause incomplete closure of an AV valve, which results in backflow of blood into the atria and produces a murmur. For example, after an acute myocardial infarction (AMI), the papillary muscles may be at risk for rupture as a result of inadequate blood supply from the

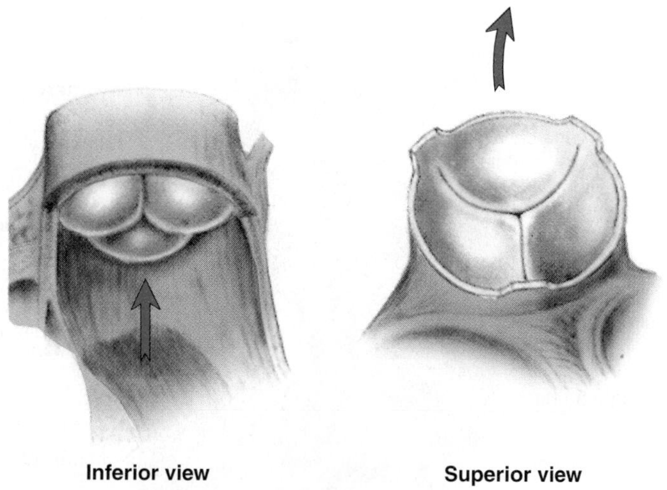

Inferior view   **Superior view**

Fig. 15-6 The aortic valve and the cuplike leaflets.

Table 15-1	Cardiac Valves and Their Locations	
Valve	**Type**	**Situated Between**
Tricuspid	AV	Right atrium, right ventricle
Pulmonic	SL	Right ventricle, pulmonary artery
Mitral	AV	Left atrium, left ventricle
Aortic	SL	Left ventricle, aorta

AV, Atrioventricular, *SL,* semilunar.

coronary circulation.[9] When a papillary muscle in the left ventricle ruptures, the mitral valve leaflets do not close completely. Clinically this causes acute mitral regurgitation and a murmur that can be auscultated with a stethoscope.

Semilunar Valves. The semilunar valves are the pulmonic and aortic valves. Each valve has three cuplike leaflets (Fig. 15-6). These valves separate the ventricles from their respective outflow arteries (Table 15-1). During ventricular systole (contraction), the semilunar valves open, allowing blood to flow out of the ventricles. As systole ends and the pressure in the outflow arteries exceeds that of the ventricles, the semilunar valves close, thus preventing blood regurgitation back into the ventricles. In the majority of individuals, the aortic valve has three leaflets. In about 1% of the population the aortic valve is bicuspid (two leaflet valve), which increases susceptibility to endocarditis and valve failure.[10,11] Aortic valve dysfunction—from any cause—not only affects the valve leaflets but also pathologically alters the shape of the left ventricle.

The Conduction System. To analyze electrical activity within the heart, it is helpful to understand the three main areas of impulse propogation and conduction: (1)

Table 15-2	Intrinsic Pacemaker Rates of Cardiac Conduction Tissue	
Location		**Rate (beats/min)**
SA node		60-100
AV node		40-60
Purkinje fibers		15-40

SA, Sinoatrial; *AV,* atrioventricular.

the sinoatrial (SA) node; the AV node; and (3) the conduction fibers within the ventricle, specifically the bundle of His, the bundle branches, and the Purkinje fibers.

The Sinoatrial Node. The SA node is considered the natural pacemaker of the heart because it has the highest degree of automaticity, producing the fastest intrinsic heart rate (Table 15-2). The node is a spindle-shaped structure located near the entrance of the superior vena cava, on the posterior aspect of the right atrium. Some normal variability in the position and shape of the node exists. The SA node is supplied from the right coronary system in 66% of people and from the left coronary system in 34%.[12] The SA node contains two types of cells—the specialized pacemaker cells found in the node center and the border zone cells. Both the pacemaker cells and the border zone cells have inherent depolarization capabilities (they automatically depolarize 60 to 100 times/min). The cells in the nodal center are responsible for the actual pace-making of the heart. The fibers in the border zone cells also contain intrinsic pacemaker properties, but depolarization is depressed by surrounding atrial tissue.

Once the center nodal cells depolarize, the impulse is conducted through the nodal border zone toward the atrium. Atrial depolarization occurs both cell to cell and through three specialized conduction pathways that exit the SA node (Fig. 15-7, *A*). These *internodal pathways* are directed to the AV node.[13,14] Also, a conduction pathway, known as *Bachmann's bundle,* travels from the right to the left atrium.

The Atrioventricular Node. The AV node is located posteriorly on the right side of the interatrial septum on the floor of the right atrium. Because the atria and ventricles are separated by nonconductive tissue, all electrical impulses initiated in the atria are conducted to the ventricles only via the AV node.[15,16] The AV node performs four essential functions to support cardiac conduction:

1. The AV node delays the conduction impulse from the atria (0.8 to 1.2 seconds) to provide time for the ventricles to fill during diastole.
2. The AV node controls the number of impulses that are transmitted from the atria to the ventricles.

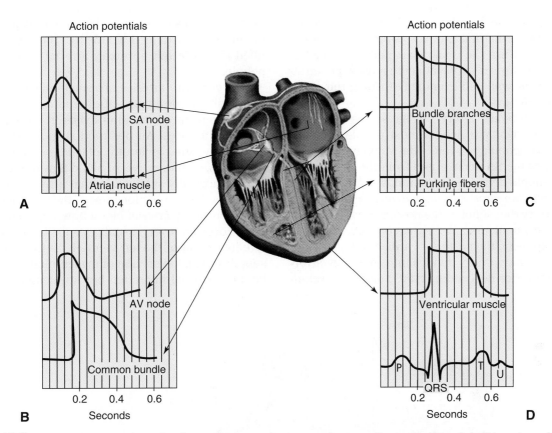

Action potentials

SA node

Atrial muscle

A   0.2   0.4   0.6

AV node

Common bundle

B   0.2   0.4   0.6   Seconds

Action potentials

Bundle branches

Purkinje fibers

0.2   0.4   0.6   **C**

Ventricular muscle

P   T   U

QRS

0.2   0.4   0.6   Seconds   **D**

Fig. 15-7   Heart with normal conduction pathways and transmembrane action potentials of **A,** SA node and atrial muscle; **B,** AV node and common bundle; **C,** bundle branches; and **D,** ventricular muscle. (From Thompson JM et al: *Mosby's clinical nursing,* ed 5, St Louis, 2002, Mosby.)

This prevents rapid irregular atrial heart rhythms from destabilizing the ventricles.

3. The AV node will act as a back-up pacemaker if the faster SA node fails. Normally, the intrinsic AV nodal rate is below the SA nodal rate (see Table 15-2). When an impulse from the SA node arrives at the AV node, the AV nodal tissue becomes depolarized and the AV pacemaker is reset (Fig. 15-7, *B*). This prevents the AV node from initiating its own pacemaker impulse that would compete with the SA node.

4. The AV node can conduct retrograde (backward) impulses through the node. If the SA and AV pacemaker cells fail to fire, an electrical impulse may be initiated in the ventricles and conducted backwards via the AV node. Retrograde conduction time is generally longer than that of antegrade (forward) conduction.

Bundle of His, Bundle Branches, and Purkinje Fibers. Electrical impulses are conducted in the ventricles through the bundle of His, the bundle branches, and the Purkinje fibers (Fig. 15-7, *C*). The bundle of His, bundle branches, and Purkinje fibers run through the subendocardium down the right side of the interventricular septum. About 12 mm from the AV node, the bundle of His divides into the right and left bundle branches.

The right bundle branch continues down the right side of the interventricular septum toward the right apex. The left bundle branch is thicker than the right and takes off from the bundle of His at almost a right angle. It then traverses the septum to the subendocardial surface of the left interventricular wall, where it divides into a thin, anterior branch and a thick, posterior branch. Functionally, when one of the left branches is blocked, it is referred to as a *hemiblock*. All of the bundle branches are subject to conduction defects (bundle branch blocks) that give rise to characteristic changes in the 12-lead ECG.

The right bundle branch and the two divisions of the left bundle branch eventually divide into the Purkinje fibers. These divide many times, terminating in the subendocardial surface of both ventricles. The Purkinje fibers have the fastest conduction velocity of all heart tissue. Ventricular muscle depolarization follows (Fig. 15-7, *D*).

Coronary Blood Supply. The coronary circulation consists of those vessels that supply the heart structures with oxygenated blood (coronary arteries) and then return the blood to the general circulation (coronary veins). The right and left coronary arteries arise at the base of the aorta immediately above the aortic valve (Fig. 15-8). After leaving the base of the aorta, the coronary arteries traverse the outside of the heart, above the epicardium, in the natural grooves (sulci) between the chambers. To perfuse the thick heart muscle, branches from these main arteries arise at acute angles, penetrating the muscular wall and eventually feeding the endocardium (Fig. 15-9).

The right coronary artery (RCA) serves the right atrium and the right ventricle in most people. In more than half of the population (66%) the sinus node artery, which supplies the SA node, arises from the RCA.[12] The AV node is supplied via the RCA in most of the population. The term *dominant coronary artery* is used to describe the artery that supplies the posterior part of heart. In 70% of the population, the right coronary artery is dominant, supplying the posterior cardiac wall.

The left coronary artery divides into two large arteries, the left anterior descending (LAD) and the circumflex (Cx). These vessels serve the left atrium and most of the left ventricle (Fig. 15-10). The SA node is supplied from the left coronary arterial system in 34% of people.[12]

The coronary arteries are small end-arteries and are susceptible to development of atherosclerotic plaque. A huge spectrum of variation exists in the disposition of coronary arteries. An obstruction in a coronary artery, caused by atherosclerotic plaque, plaque rupture, or thrombus, results in loss of blood flow to the myocardial muscle normally supplied by that artery. This can be fatal, depending on the location of the obstruction. Blockage of coronary arterial blood flow, especially in the left main coronary artery, usually results in death from massive infarction of the left ventricle. If the blocked artery supplies a smaller section of myocardium, the result may be a myocardial infarction but not death. Many clinical

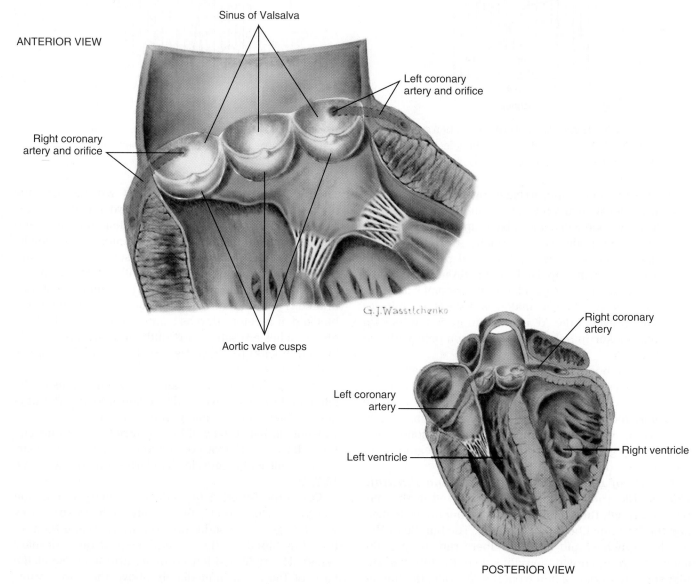

Fig. 15-8   Proximity of the right and left coronary arteries to the aortic valve and the sinus of Valsalva.

interventions are used to limit and prevent myocardial infarction and its sequelae.[6]

Several clinical situations merit a brief discussion here. During ventricular contraction, no blood flows to the cardiac tissues because of the contracted state of the cardiac muscle and resulting occlusion of arteries within the musculature. Coronary artery circulation is highest during early diastole, after the aortic valve has closed. During an episode of tachycardia, diastolic time is greatly diminished; hence coronary perfusion time is lessened. This offers an explanation for compromised coronary blood flow and fall in blood pressure during times of rapid heart rate.

Coronary Veins. The cardiac (coronary) veins follow the paths of the coronary arteries with one signifi-

cant difference. After blood passes through the coronary circulation, it is severely deoxygenated. The desaturated blood travels via the coronary veins that ultimately join together to become the *coronary sinus* (the largest cardiac vein) that empties into the back of the right atrium. The coronary venous blood then mixes with the systemic venous blood in the right atrium.

Physiologic Cardiac Shunts. A shunt occurs when there is mixing of deoxygenated blood (usually venous blood with reduced oxygen content) with arterial oxygenated blood. In the heart there is a specific situation where this is a normal physiologic process. The *thebesian veins* are small vessels that connect capillary beds directly with the cardiac chambers via irregular endothelium-lined sinuses within the myocardium. The thebesian veins add a small quantity of deoxygenated blood to the oxygenated blood in the left ventricle.

An example of an abnormal, or pathologic, intracardiac shunt is an opening in the ventricular septum, between the left and right sides of the heart. In the ventricle this septal opening, called a *ventricular septal defect* (VSD), allows mixing of blood from both ventricles. The clinical impact depends on the size of the intracardiac shunt. A VSD can be congenital, or ventricular septal rupture (VSR) can occur as a complication of a large anterior-wall myocardial infarction,[6] as described in Chapter 19.

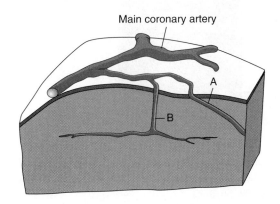

Fig. 15-9 Intramyocardial distribution of coronary arteries. *A,* Epicardial arteries rise at acute angles from main coronary vessels to supply epicardial surface of the heart. *B,* Smaller vessels branch at oblique angles from main coronary vessels that penetrate deeper into the myocardium and endocardium (intramural arteries). (Redrawn from Quaal S: *Comprehensive intraaortic balloon pumping,* ed 2, St Louis, 1993, Mosby.)

Major Cardiac Vessels

Aorta. The aorta is the largest artery in the body. It carries oxygenated blood from the left ventricle to the rest of the body. The aorta is separated from the left ventricle by the aortic valve. Just above the aortic valve there are two small openings that represent the origin of the right and left coronary arterial system (see Fig. 15-8).

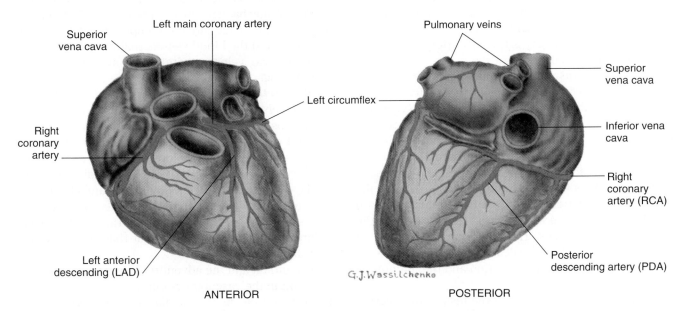

Fig. 15-10 Anterior and posterior views of the coronary artery circulation and major vessels.

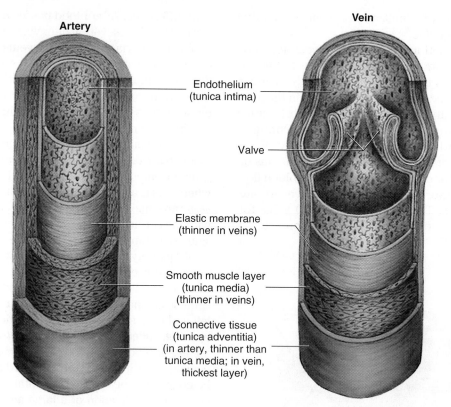

Artery

Vein

Endothelium
(tunica intima)

Valve

Elastic membrane
(thinner in veins)

Smooth muscle layer
(tunica media)
(thinner in veins)

Connective tissue
(tunica adventitia)
(in artery, thinner than
tunica media; in vein,
thickest layer)

Fig. 15-11   Cross section of an artery and vein showing the three layers: tunica intima, tunica media, and tunica adventitia. Note the difference in wall thickness between the artery and the vein and the lack of valves within the artery. (From Thompson JM et al: *Mosby's clinical nursing*, ed 5, St Louis, 2002, Mosby.)

These opening are known by several names, including the *coronary ostia* and the *sinus of Valsalva.*

Pulmonary Artery. The pulmonary artery carries deoxygenated blood from the right ventricle to the pulmonary arterioles. The pulmonary artery is separated from the right ventricle by the pulmonic valve. The main pulmonary artery divides into a right and a left branch that direct blood to the right and the left lung vasculature. The pulmonary artery is the only artery to carry deoxygenated blood in the body.

Pulmonary Veins. The four pulmonary veins return oxygenated blood from the lungs to the left atrium. These are the only veins in the body to carry oxygenated blood. The veins connect into the back wall of the left atrium (see Fig. 15-10). There are no valves that inhibit the flow of blood into the left atrium. Blood flow is accomplished by simple hydrostatic pressure gradients. The pressure must be lower in the left atrium than in the pulmonary circulation for flow to occur in a forward direction. Tissue from the left atria may grow into the pulmonary vein orifices. This opportunistic tissue is a frequent cause of atrial fibrillation. See Chapter 18 for more discussion on atrial fibrillation and the pulmonary veins.[17]

The Systemic Circulation. If the task of the heart is to generate enough pressure to pump the blood, it is the function of the vascular structures to act as conduits to carry vital oxygen and nutrients to each cell and also to carry away waste products. Also of primary importance is the ability to exchange those nutrients and waste products at the cellular level. The vascular system acts not only as a conducting system for the blood but also as a control mechanism for the pressure in the heart and vessels. So it is actually the complex interplay between the heart and the blood vessels that maintains adequate pressure and velocity within this system for optimal functioning.

The Arterial System. Arteries are constructed of three layers (Fig. 15-11). The innermost layer, or the intima, consists of a thin lining of endothelium and a small amount of elastic tissue. The smooth endothelial lining decreases resistance to blood flow and minimizes the chance for platelet aggregation. The media, or the middle layer, is made up of smooth muscle and elastic tissue. This muscular layer changes the lumen diameter when necessary. The adventitia, which is the outermost layer, is largely a connective tissue coat that helps strengthen and shape the vessels.

The intima and the adventitia layers remain relatively constant in the vascular system, whereas the elastin and smooth muscle in the media change proportions, depending on the size and type of the vessel. The aorta con-

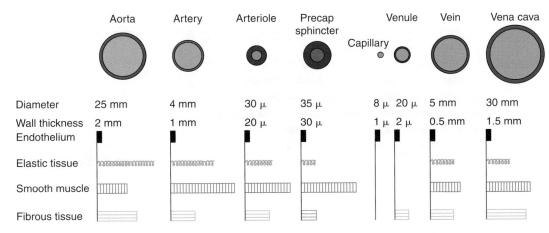

	Aorta	Artery	Arteriole	Precap sphincter	Capillary	Venule	Vein	Vena cava
Diameter	25 mm	4 mm	30 μ	35 μ	8 μ	20 μ	5 mm	30 mm
Wall thickness	2 mm	1 mm	20 μ	30 μ	1 μ	2 μ	0.5 mm	1.5 mm
Endothelium								
Elastic tissue								
Smooth muscle								
Fibrous tissue								

Fig. 15-12   Internal diameter, wall thickness, and relative amounts of the principal components of the vessel circulatory system. Cross sections of the vessels are not drawn to scale because of the huge range from aorta to vena cava to capillaries. (From Berne RM, Levy MN: *Cardiovascular physiology*, ed 8, St Louis, 2001, Mosby.)

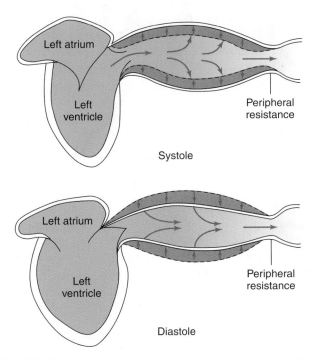

Fig. 15-13   Elastic and recoil properties of the aorta. (From Berne RM, Levy MN: *Cardiovascular physiology*, ed 8, St Louis, 2001, Mosby.)

tains the greatest amount of elastic tissue. This is necessary because of the sudden shifts in pressure created by the left ventricle. The arterioles, or smaller arteries, and precapillary sphincters have more smooth muscle than do the larger arteries and aorta because they function to change the luminal diameter when regulating blood pressure and blood flow to the tissues (Fig. 15-12).

Blood Flow and Blood Pressure. The pulsatile nature of arterial flow is caused by intermittent cardiac ejection and the stretch of the ascending aorta. The pressure wave initiated by left ventricular ejection (Fig. 15-13) travels considerably faster than does the blood itself. Thus when an examiner palpates a pulse, it is this propagation of the pressure wave that is perceived.

In the normal arterial system, the blood flow is described as laminar, or streamlined, because the fluid moves in one direction. However, there are small differences in the linear velocities within a blood vessel. The layer of blood immediately adjacent to the vessel wall moves relatively slowly because of the friction created as it comes in contact with the motionless vessel wall. In contrast, the more central blood in the lumen travels more rapidly (Fig. 15-14).

Clinical implications include conditions in which the vessel wall has an abnormality such as a small clot or plaque deposit. This disruption in the streamlined flow can set up eddy currents that may predispose the area to platelet aggregation and atherosclerosis.

Blood pressure (BP) measurement has several components. The systolic blood pressure (SBP) represents the ventricular volume ejection and the response of the arterial system to that ejection. The diastolic blood pressure (DBP) value indicates the ventricular resting state of the arterial system. The pulse pressure is the difference between the SBP and DBP. The mean arterial pressure (MAP) is the mean value of the area under the BP curve (Fig. 15-15). BP may be measured several ways. Direct measurement is accomplished by means of a catheter inserted into an artery. The BP is measured in mm Hg. The most common indirect method is by means of a stethoscope and sphygmomanometer (Fig. 15-16). Fig. 15-17 graphically summarizes blood pressures in various portions of the systemic circulatory system.

Vascular resistance is a reflection of arteriolar tone. The large amount of smooth muscle in the arterioles allows for relaxation or contraction of these vessels and causes changes in resistance and redistribution of blood flow. Resistance is the opposition to flow caused by the

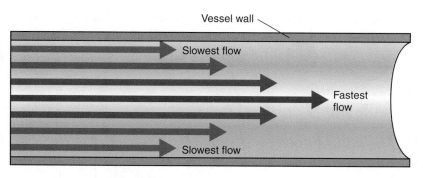

Fig. 15-14 Laminar flow in an artery.

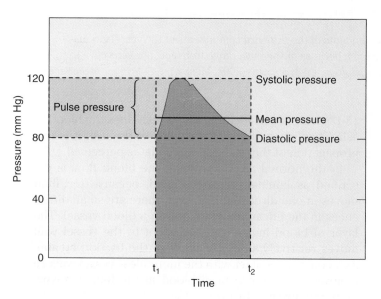

Fig. 15-15 Arterial systolic, diastolic, pulse, and mean pressures. (From Berne RM, Levy MN: *Cardiovascular physiology,* ed 8, St Louis, 2001, Mosby.)

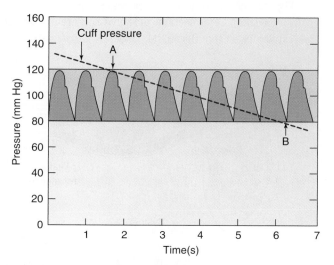

Fig. 15-16 Principles of blood pressure measurements with a sphygmomanometer. The oblique line represents pressure in the inflatable bag in the cuff. At cuff pressures greater than the systolic pressure (*to the left of* A), no blood progresses beyond the cuff and no sounds can be detected below the cuff with the stethoscope. At cuff pressures between the systolic and diastolic levels (*between* A *and* B), spurts of blood traverse the arteries under the cuff and produce Korotkoff sounds. At cuff pressures below the diastolic pressure (*to the right of* B), arterial flow past the region of the cuff is continuous and no sounds are audible. (From Berne RM, Levy MN: *Cardiovascular physiology,* ed 8, St Louis, 2001, Mosby.)

blood vessels. Most changes in resistance are caused by alterations in the tone of the arterial vessel walls, especially in the arterioles. The purpose of this mechanism is to maintain a constant blood pressure in the arterial system. The clinician can never assume that blood flow and blood pressure are identical. For example, poor blood flow to the tissues because of vasoconstricted peripheral arterioles causes the blood to back up and increases blood pressure. A higher blood pressure is a compensatory mechanism but does not necessarily mean there is adequate tissue perfusion.

It is also possible to calculate the resistance within the systemic vascular system, described by the phrase *systemic vascular resistance* (SVR). In the pulmonary circulation it is termed *pulmonary vascular resistance* (PVR). These derived values are based on calculations from other hemodynamic parameters as described in the section on hemodynamics in Chapter 17 and in the Appendix.

Precapillary Sphincters and the Microcirculation. Where present, the precapillary sphincters are small cuffs of smooth muscle that control blood flow at the junction of the arterioles and the capillaries. The precapillary sphincters allow selective blood flow into capillary beds, depending on their contractile state. The precapillary sphincters are not innervated by the autonomic nervous system as are the arterioles; rather, they respond to local or circulating vasoactive agents. This means that they do not have direct nervous connection to sympathetic input but respond to circulating epinephrine released by the adrenal glands.

As the blood reaches the capillary level, the pulsatile nature of arterial flow is dampened (see Fig. 15-17). Even

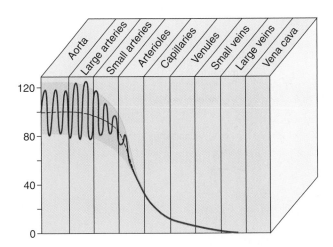

Fig. 15-17 Blood pressures in the different portions of the systemic circulatory system.

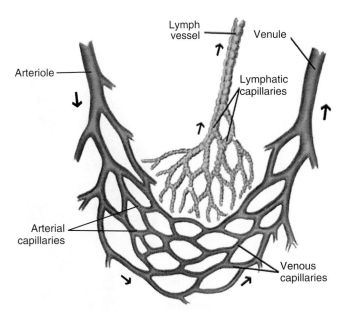

Fig. 15-18 Microcirculation. Note the branching nature and large cross-sectional area of the capillary bed. (From Thompson JM et al: *Mosby's clinical nursing*, ed 5, St Louis, 2002, Mosby.)

though the diameter of a capillary is less than that of the arteriole, the pressure and flow velocity in the capillary bed is low as a result of the large cross-sectional area of the branching capillary bed (Fig. 15-18). The capillary consists of a single cell layer of endothelium and is devoid of muscle or elastin (see Fig. 15-12). This allows solutes to diffuse in and out of the capillaries unimpeded by mechanical barriers. Capillaries normally retain large structures, such as red blood cells, but are highly permeable to smaller solutes, such as electrolytes.

The Venous System. As the blood leaves the capillary system, it passes through the venules and into the veins. Both venules and veins contain elastic tissue, smooth muscle, and fibrous tissue (see Fig. 15-12). The veins, however, contain a greater percentage of smooth muscle and fibrous tissue to accommodate the large venous volume and demand for reserve capacity. The majority of circulating blood is contained in the venous system. Veins are referred to as *capacitance vessels* (Fig. 15-19). Approximately 75% of the total blood volume is found in the veins.[18] This enables the body to tap into a huge reserve during times of need. For example, when a person changes from a supine to a sitting position, approximately 7 to 10 ml blood per kilogram of body weight will pool in the legs. Potentially, cardiac output could decrease by approximately 20% and stroke volume by 20% to 50%. However, normal arterial pressure and blood flow are maintained by a combination of reflex vasoconstriction and redistribution of blood from the venous capacitance vessels. In humans, these capacitance reservoirs are greatest in the spleen, the liver, and the intestines. Thus patients with decreased blood reserves, who are dehydrated or hypovolemic, require special caution during position changes, especially from supine to standing. Before helping such a patient to stand, one must allow him or her to "dangle" (sit on the side of the bed) to check for adequate venous reserves.

MICROSCOPIC STRUCTURE

To understand and appreciate the unique pumping ability of the heart, one must have knowledge of cardiac cell structure and function. This section reviews the anatomic mechanisms responsible for the contractile process in cardiac muscle cells.

Cardiac Fibers. Cardiac muscle fibers are typically found in a latticework arrangement. The fiber cells (myofibrils) divide, rejoin, and then separate again, but they retain distinct cellular walls and possess a single nucleus. This differs greatly from skeletal muscle, in which the cells have fused together to form a fiber and have many nuclei.

In general, cardiac myofibrils run on a longitudinal axis, and the fibers appear striped, or striated. When viewed under an electron microscope, these striations can actually be seen to be the contractile proteins (Fig. 15-20). The areas separating each myocardial cell from its neighbor are called *intercalated disks*, which are continuous with the sarcolemma, or cell membrane. The point where a longitudinal branch of the cell meets another cell branch is the tight junction (or gap junction), which offers much less of an impedance to electrical flow than does the sarcolemma. Because of this, depolarization occurs from one cell to another with relative ease. Also, the cardiac muscle is a functional syncytium, in which depolarization started in any cardiac cell quickly is spread to all of the heart.

Cardiac Cells. Each cardiac cell contains two types of intracellular contractile proteins, *actin* and *myosin*.

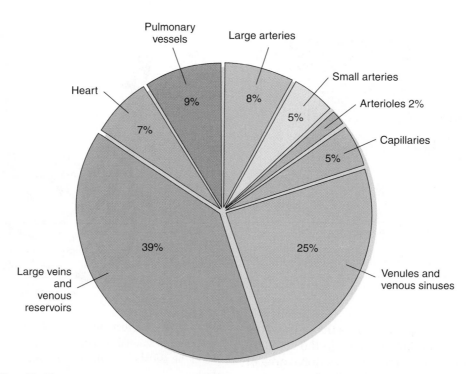

Fig. 15-19 Percentage of the total blood volume in each portion of the circulation system.

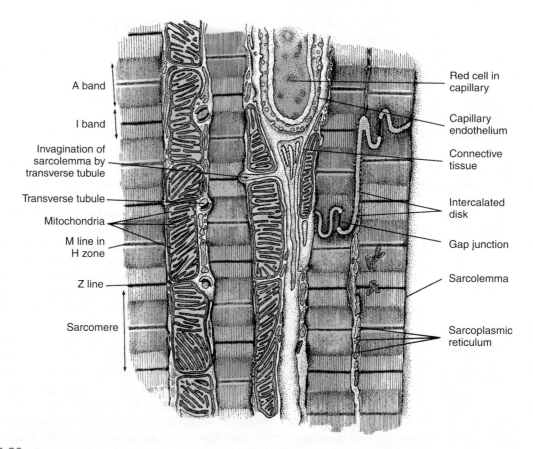

Fig. 15-20 Diagram of an electron micrograph of cardiac muscle showing the large numbers of mitochondria, the intercalated disks with tight junctions, the transverse tubules, and the longitudinal tubules (also known as the *sarcoplasmic reticulum*) (approximately ×30,000). (From Berne RM, Levy MN: *Cardiovascular physiology,* ed 8, St Louis, 2001, Mosby.)

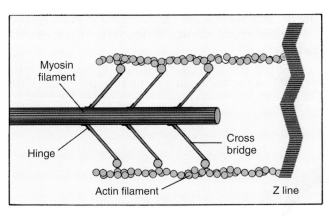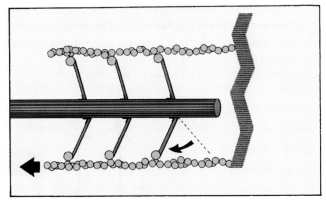

Fig. 15-21   Actin and myosin filaments and cross-bridges responsible for cell contraction.

Table 15-3	Definition of Terms Related to Cardiac Tissue Function
Term	**Definition**
Excitability	Ability of a cell or tissue to depolarize in response to a given stimulus
Conductivity	Ability of cardiac cells to transmit a stimulus from cell to cell
Automaticity	Ability of certain cells to spontaneously depolarize ("pacemaker potential")
Rhythmicity	Automaticity generated at a regular rate
Contractility	Ability of the cardiac myofibrils to shorten in length in response to an electrical stimulus (depolarization)
Refractoriness	State of a cell or tissue during repolarization when the cell or tissue either cannot depolarize regardless of the intensity of the stimulus or requires a much greater stimulus than is normally required

These proteins abound in the cell in organized longitudinal arrangements. When visualized by electron microscopy, the myosin filaments appear thick, whereas the almost double amounts of actin filaments appear thin. The actin filaments are connected to the Z bands (or discs) on one end, leaving the other end free to interact with the myosin cross-bridges.[19] In the resting muscle cell, the actin and myosin partially overlap. The ends of the myosin filament that overlap with the actin have tiny projections (Fig. 15-21). For contraction to occur, these projections interact with the actin to form cross-bridges (see Fig. 15-21). The portion of the muscle fiber between two Z bands is called a *sarcomere*. In a normal resting state, the sarcomere is about 2.0 to 2.2 mm.

Another extremely important intracellular structure necessary for successful contraction is the *sarcoplasmic reticulum* (SR). Calcium ions are stored in the SR and released for use after depolarization (Fig. 15-22). Deep invaginations into the sarcomere are called *transverse tubules*, or *T tubules*. The T tubules are essentially an extension of the cell membrane and thus function to conduct depolarization to structures deep within the cytoplasm, such as the SR. The cardiac cells abound with mitochondria, which contain respiratory enzymes necessary for oxidative phosphorylation. This enables the cell to keep up with the tremendous energy requirements of the repetitive contraction. When cardiac cells are damaged by trauma or ischemia, the myocardial cells release protein "biomarkers" that when measured by laboratory analysis can help determine the extent of injury. This is discussed in detail in Chapter 17.

PHYSIOLOGY

The study of the electrical and mechanical properties of cardiac tissue has fascinated scientists for more than 100 years. These properties include excitability, conductivity, automaticity, rhythmicity, contractility, and refractoriness. The following section relates these concepts specifically to cardiac cells (Table 15-3).

ELECTRICAL ACTIVITY

Transmembrane Potentials. Electrical potentials across cell membranes are present in essentially all cells of the body. Some cells, such as nerve and muscle cells, are specialized for conduction of electrical impulses along their membranes. This electrical potential, or transmembrane potential, refers to the relative electrical difference between the interior of a cell and that of the fluid surrounding the cell. *Ionic channels* are pores in cell membranes that allow for passage of specific ions at specific times or signals. Transmembrane potentials and ionic channels are extremely important in myocardial cells because they form the basis for electrical impulse conduction and muscular contraction. An understanding of the normal structure and function of cardiac ion channels is increasingly important as a basis for understand-ing the genesis of lethal cardiac dysrhythmias and devel-opment of cardiac drugs designed to treat these "chan-nelopathies."

Resting Membrane Potential. In a myocardial cell at rest, the normal resting membrane potential (RMP) is

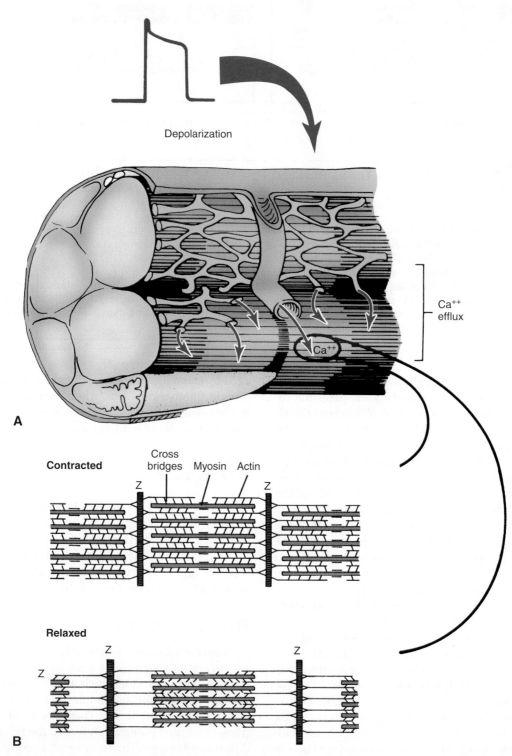

Fig. 15-22   A, Depolarization of a myocardial cell causes release of calcium from the sarcoplasmic reticulum and the transverse tubules. **B,** Calcium release allows for the cross-bridges on the myosin filaments to attach to the actin filaments to effect cell contraction. (From Quaal S: *Comprehensive intraaortic balloon pumping,* ed 2, St Louis, 1993, Mosby.)

approximately −80 to −90 millivolts (mV). This means that the interior of the cell is relatively negative compared with the exterior medium. The relative negativity of the cell interior is created by an uneven distribution of positively charged ions and negatively charged ions. When the cell is at rest, more positively charged ions are outside the cell than are inside the cell.

When the cell is at rest, the intracellular potassium (K^+) is very high, and intracellular sodium (Na^+) is low. Conversely, the extracellular K^+ is relatively low, compared with a high concentration of Na^+ (Table 15-4). Calcium (Ca^{++}) also has a much higher concentration outside the cell compared with inside when the cell is at rest.

Table 15-4	The Approximate Extracellular and Intracellular Concentrations of K^+, Na^+, and Ca^{++} in a Resting Myocardial Cell	
Ion	**Extracellular Concentration (mEq/L)**	**Intracellular Concentration (mEq/L)**
K+	4	135
Na^+	145	10
Ca^{++}	2	0.1

These large differences in individual ion concentrations create chemical gradients. A *chemical gradient* describes the tendency of an ion to move from an area of higher solute concentration to an area of lower concentration. However, an *electrical gradient* is also present, which causes the positively charged ions to move to an area of relative negativity. For example, the chemical gradient of K^+ forces it to move out of the cell because the intracellular concentration is so much higher than the outside medium. But, as a result of the relative negativity inside the cell (−80 to −90 mV), the electrical gradient works to retain the positively charged K^+ ion. An important factor influencing both gradients is membrane permeability, or the selectivity of the membrane to ionic movements. Even at rest, there is some slight movement of ions across the cell membrane. For example, the cell membrane is approximately 50 times more permeable to K^+ than it is to Na^+. Because K^+ movement out of the cell results in greater negativity inside the cell, K^+ is the principal ion responsible for maintaining the negative RMP.

Phases of the Action Potential. In a myocardial cell, when a sudden increase in the permeability of the membrane to Na^+ occurs, a rapid sequence of events follows that lasts a fraction of a second. This sequence of events is termed *depolarization*. The graphic representation of depolarization is the action potential (AP) (Fig. 15-23). The ionic currents cause changes in electrical potentials that are known as *AP phases 0, 1, 2, 3, and 4.* These phases give the AP a characteristic shape, as described below and shown in Fig. 15-7 and Table 15-5.

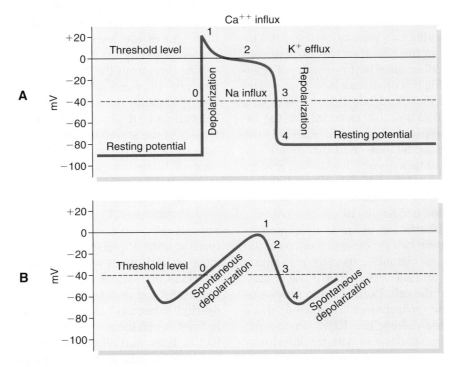

Fig. 15-23   Cardiac action potentials. **A,** Action potential phases 0 to 4 of a nonpacemaker cell. **B,** Action potential of a pacemaker cell. (From Thompson JM et al: *Mosby's clinical nursing,* ed 5, St Louis, 2002, Mosby.)

Table 15-5	Summary of Phases 0 through 4 of a Cardiac Cell Action Potential (AP)

Phase	Description	Ionic Movement	Mechanisms
0	Upstroke	Na^+ into cell	Fast Na^+ channels open
1	Overshoot		Fast Na^+ channels close
2	Plateau	Na^+, Ca^{++} into cell K^+ out	Multiple channels (Ca^{++}, Na^+, K^+) open to maintain membrane voltage
3	Repolarization	K^+ out of cell	Ca^{++} and Na^+ channels closed; K^+ channel remains open
4	RMP	Na^+ out, K^+ in	Na^+/K^+ pump

RMP, Resting membrane potential.

Phase 0. As the membrane is depolarized, Na^+ begins to enter the cell, thus causing the interior of the cell to become more positive. At approximately -65 mV, the membrane reaches threshold, the point at which the inward Na^+ current overcomes the efflux of K^+. This is accomplished by means of the fast Na^+ channels. With the fast Na^+ channels open, the inward rush of Na^+ is extremely rapid and briefly causes the inside of the cell to become slightly more positive than the outside of the cell. This series of events is graphically described as phase 0 of the AP and is reflected in the overshoot of the AP where the charge is 20 to 30 mV.

Phase 1 and Phase 2. When the rapid influx of Na^+ is terminated, a brief period of partial repolarization occurs as the AP slope returns toward the zero (phase 1 of the AP). The plateau that follows is described as phase 2. During this phase, another set of channels—the slow Na^+ and Ca^{++} channels—open and allow the influx of Ca^{++} and Na^+. Also during phase 2, K^+ tends to diffuse out of the cell, balancing the slow inward flux of Na^+ and Ca^{++}, thereby maintaining the plateau of the AP. The Ca^{++} entering the cell at this phase causes cardiac contraction, which is described later in this chapter. The inward flux of Ca^{++} during this phase can be influenced by many factors. For example, calcium channel–blocking drugs, such as verapamil and diltiazem, inhibit the inward Ca^{++} current into pacemaker tissue, especially the AV node. For this reason they are used therapeutically to slow the rate of atrial tachydysrhythmias and protect the ventricle from excessive atrial impulses. Calcium channel–blocking drugs are described in more detail in the cardiac drugs section of Chapter 19.

Phase 3. The repolarization phase is described as phase 3, and it depends on two processes. The first is the inactivation of the slow channels, thereby preventing further influx of Ca^{++} and Na^+. The other is the continued efflux of K^+ out of the cell. Both of these processes cause the intracellular environment to become more negative, thereby reestablishing the RMP. On the AP, phase 3 is seen as a gradual descent with the interior of the cell becoming more negative relative to the outside.

Phase 4. In phase 4, the AP returns to RMP of -80 to -90 mV. The excess Na^+ that entered the cell during depolarization is now removed from the cell in exchange for K^+ by means of the Na^+/K^+ pump. This mechanism returns the intracellular concentrations of Na^+ and K^+ to the levels before depolarization and is essential for normal ionic balance and preparation for the next depolarization (see Table 15-5).

Fiber Conduction and Excitability. Different parts of the conduction system require different electrical currents and create individual transmembrane action potentials, as shown in Fig. 15-7. In addition, ionic shifts within the endocardium, myocardium, and epicardium are not uniform, although the clinical significance of this finding is not clear at this time. Propagation of an AP along a cardiac fiber occurs as a result of ionic shifts discussed previously. As a local section of the cell becomes depolarized, reaches threshold, and completely depolarizes, it affects the adjacent area of the cell and begins depolarization in that area. Thus the AP propagates down the fiber in a wavelike fashion (Fig. 15-24). This is somewhat analogous to a trail of gunpowder. When the gunpowder is lit at one end, a small area ignites, burns, and then ignites the area of gunpowder immediately adjacent, and so on.

The time from the beginning of the AP until the time when the fiber can accept another AP is called the effective or *absolute refractory period*. During this period the cell cannot be depolarized regardless of the amount or intensity of the stimulus. This period lasts from the beginning of depolarization to approximately -50 mV during phase 3. Immediately after the absolute refractory period is the *relative refractory period*. At this time the cell is not fully repolarized but could depolarize with a strong enough stimulus (Fig. 15-25). This period lasts from approximately -50 mV during phase 3 to when the cell returns to RMP. At phase 4 the cell is fully repolarized and is again at RMP, ready to respond to the next stimulus. The concepts of relative versus absolute refractory periods are useful for understanding the genesis of ventricular dysrhythmias, as discussed in that section in Chapter 18. In brief, a cell cannot be stimulated to depolarize until it has at least partially recovered from the previous impulse. This means that an ectopic impulse cannot be propagated during the absolute refractory period.

Pacemaker Cell vs. Nonpacemaker Cell Action Potentials. The action potential, as just discussed, is

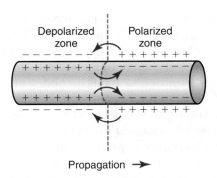

Fig. 15-24 Schematic representation of the propagation of an action potential along a cell membrane.

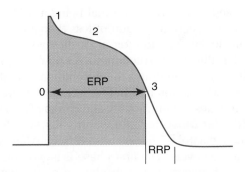

Fig. 15-25 The two parts of the refractory period. The effective (absolute) refractory period (ERP) extends from phase 0 to approximately 50 mV in phase 3. The remainder of the action potential is the relative refractory period (RRP). (From Conover MB: *Understanding electrocardiography,* ed 7, St Louis, 1996, Mosby.)

representative of the depolarization of nonpacemaker myocardial cells. The AP generated by a Purkinje fiber is similar to that of a ventricular myocardial cell except that phase 2 is usually more prolonged in the Purkinje fiber. Atrial myocardial cells exhibit a shortened plateau (phase 2) as compared with ventricular cells. The pacemaker cells of the SA node have an action potential that is very different from that of a myocardial or Purkinje cell. In the SA node the RMP is not as negative—approximately −65 mV. Also, rather than an RMP that remains constant, the cells slowly depolarize at a steady rate until threshold is reached (see Fig. 15-23, *B*). The lack of a steady-state RMP is largely the result of a steady Na^+ influx through the slow channels. This mechanism explains how the cells can spontaneously depolarize (automaticity). It also provides the basis for understanding alterations in the pacemaker cells. The frequency of the pacemaker cell discharge may be altered by changing the rate of depolarization or by raising or lowering the cellular RMP.

MECHANICAL ACTIVITY

Excitation-Contraction Coupling. The electrical activity discussed in the previous section is the stimulus for mechanical contraction. As the myocardial cell is depolarized, specifically during phase 2 of the AP, some Ca^{++} enters the cytoplasm through the cell membrane via special Ca^{++} channels. The majority of Ca^{++} enters the cytoplasm from stores in the SR. The cytoplasmic Ca^{++} then binds with troponin and tropomyosin, molecules that are present on the actin filaments, resulting in contraction. Occurring throughout the myocardium, the result is myocardial contraction. Once contraction has occurred, Ca^{++} is taken back up into the SR and the cytoplasmic concentration of Ca^{++} falls, leading to muscular relaxation. Both contraction and relaxation are active processes because they require energy from adenosine triphosphate (ATP) and because the Ca^{++} is removed from the cell by way of a Na^+/Ca^{++} pump. The role of this pump has not been fully established, but it clearly contributes to intracellular Ca^{++} regulation during diastole. The question of increased contractility also is not

completely elucidated. Variations in the strength of contraction may involve recruitment of more or fewer cross-bridges or a change in the calcium-binding properties of the contractile proteins. Ca^{++} sensitivity probably also increases as the muscle fiber is stretched. However, the role of Ca^{++} is much more complex than is presented here because it involves not only the mechanical events in the cell but also several metabolic and regulatory processes.

THE CARDIAC CYCLE

The cardiac cycle refers to one complete mechanical cycle of the heartbeat, beginning with ventricular contraction and ending with ventricular relaxation.

Ventricular Systole. Ventricular systole represents the ejection phase of the cardiac cycle. As the ventricles are electrically depolarized, the septum and papillary muscles tense first. This provides a stable outflow tract and competent AV valves. The ventricles begin to tense, beginning with the inner endocardium and continuing through the myocardium toward the outer epicardium. This increases the pressure within the ventricular chambers. This stage is known as *isovolumic contraction* because, even though the ventricular muscle is tensing, the ventricular volume does not change. When the intraventricular pressure exceeds that of the intraatrial pressure, the mitral and tricuspid valves close. As the ventricular tension increases, the intraventricular pressures exceed those of the aorta and pulmonary arteries, causing the aortic and pulmonic valves to open. The blood ejected from the ventricles each beat is called the *stroke volume.* In a healthy heart, more than half of the total ventricular blood volume is ejected; the blood that remains in the ventricles is the *residual* or *end-*systolic volume.

The ejection fraction (EF) is the ratio of the stroke volume ejected from the left ventricle per beat to the volume of blood remaining in the left ventricle at the end of diastole (left ventricular end-diastolic volume, or LVEDV). EF is expressed as a percent, normal being at least greater than 50%. An ejection fraction of less than 35% indicates poor ventricular function (as in cardiomyopathy), poor ventricular filling, obstruction to outflow (as in some valve stenosis conditions), or a combination of these. Both ejection fraction and LVEDV are widely used clinically as indexes of contractility and cardiac function.

Ventricular Diastole. After ventricular systole comes ventricular diastole. This is the ventricular filling phase of the cardiac cycle. The first phase is isovolumic relaxation, which occurs between closure of the semilunar (aortic and pulmonic) valves and the opening of the AV (mitral and tricuspid) valves. Immediately after is the rapid filling phase, in which the AV valves open and the majority of the ventricular filling occurs. The next phase is a reduced ventricular filling period. This is passive flow of blood from the periphery and pulmonary vasculature into the ventricles. The last part of ventricular diastolic filling occurs during atrial contraction, also described as *atrial kick*; it provides approximately 20% of total ventricular filling. With this, the cycle is complete and begins once again with systole (Fig. 15-26).

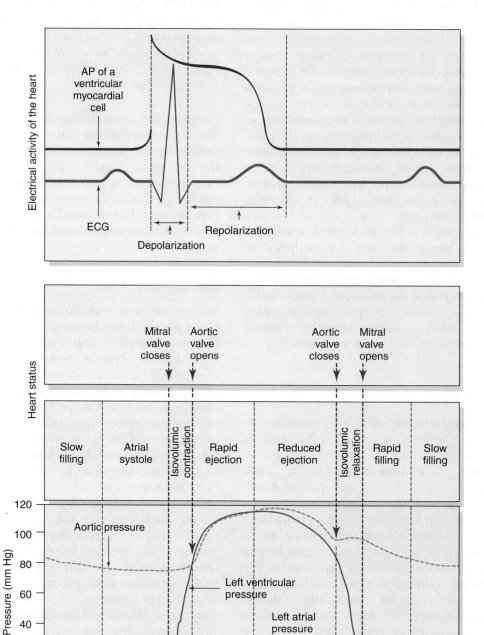

Fig. 15-26   The cardiac cycle.

INTERPLAY OF THE HEART AND VESSELS: CARDIAC OUTPUT

Cardiac output (CO) is defined as the volume of blood ejected from the heart over 1 minute. Therefore the determinants of CO are heart rate (HR) in beats/min and stroke volume (SV) in milliliters per beat. The equation is:

$$CO \times HR = SV$$

CO is normally expressed in liters per minute (L/min). The normal CO in the human adult is approximately 4 to 8 L/min. It is approximately 4 to 6 L/min at rest and increases with exercise. Cardiac output is a general term and can be made specific to body size by using the person's height and weight to determine the cardiac index (CI). CI is the CO divided by the individual's estimated body surface area, expressed in square meters (m^2). The normal range for CI is 2.5 to 4.5 L/min/m^2. Changes in either the SV or HR can change the CO. However, all three parameters must be individually assessed as described in the section on hemodynamics in Chapter 17.

An example of how this might be applied in a clinical situation for a person with an HR of 72 and an SV of 70 ml follows:

$$72 \text{ (beats/min)} \times 70 \text{ (ml/beat)} = 5.04 \text{ L/min}$$

If, however, the parameters change to an HR of 140 and an SV of 40 ml, the calculation would be as follows:

$$140 \text{ (beats/min)} \times 40 \text{ (ml/beat)} = 5.6 \text{ L/min}$$

Even though the CO is higher, clearly the faster heart rate is not an improvement in this situation. Because SV is so decreased in the second example, it indicates that cardiac decompensation is imminent. Stroke volume as a value is influenced by three primary factors: preload, afterload, and contractility (Fig. 15-27).

Preload. The concept of preload was introduced in the early 1900s when Ernest Starling described his findings in an isolated dog heart preparation. Starling found that as he increased the volume infused into a denervated heart, the cardiac output increased, until it reached a point at which further infusion actually caused the CO to decrease. This is now known as *Starling's law of the heart*, and it is graphically described as the *Starling curve* (Fig. 15-28). It can best be described on a molecular basis, using as a foundation the discussion of the actin and myosin cross-bridges in the myofibril. As the diastolic volume increases, it stretches the actin and myosin molecules in their resting state. As contraction occurs, contractility increases as a result of the increased stretch. However, if the stretch is excessive and causes the actin and myosin to be stretched beyond their cross-bridging limits (i.e., greater than 2.2 mm), contractility decreases. This is the basis for Starling's curve. With the advent of critical care units and sophisticated monitoring, this principle has acquired great significance in clinical practice. For example, after a myocardial infarction (MI), the ability of the left ventricle to pump may be impaired. It is desirable to optimize the contractility of the remaining viable heart muscle by "stretching"

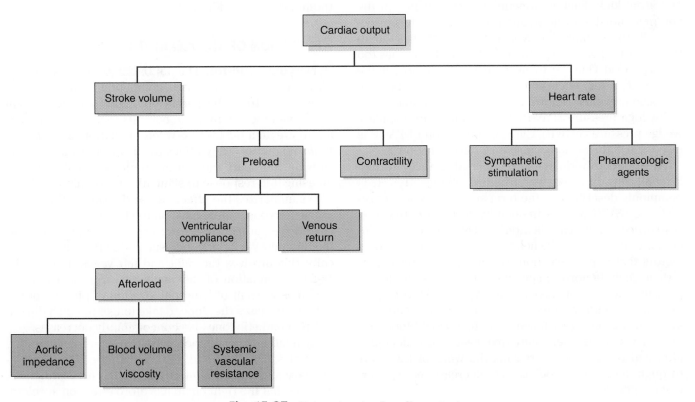

Fig. 15-27 Determinants of cardiac output.

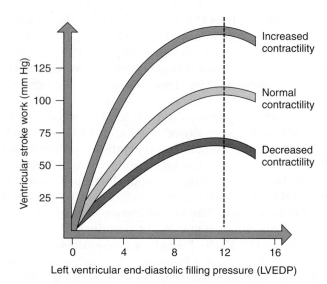

Fig. 15-28 Starling curve. As the left ventricular end-diastolic pressure (LVEDP) increases, so does ventricular stroke work or contractility. When left ventricular filling pressure exceeds a maximal point, contractility and cardiac output diminish.

Table 15-6	Summary of the Effects of the Parasympathetic and Sympathetic Nervous Systems on the Heart	
Function	**Parasympathetic**	**Sympathetic**
Automaticity	Decrease	Increase
Contractility	Decrease	Increase
Conduction velocity	Decrease	Increase
Chronotrophy (rate)	Decrease	Increase

it with added volume. But if the intravascular volume exceeds the stretch limit, CO diminishes.

Preload, then, is a function of the volume of blood presented to the left ventricle and also the compliance (the ability of the ventricle to stretch) of the ventricles at the end of diastole. It has been described as left ventricular end-diastolic pressure (LVEDP). Factors affecting the volume aspect include venous return, total blood volume, and atrial kick. Factors affecting the compliance of the ventricles are the stiffness and the thickness of the muscular wall. For example, the hypovolemic patient has too little preload, whereas the patient with heart failure has too much preload. One way to measure preload is through the pulmonary artery occlusion pressure (PAOP). This value was also previously known as either the pulmonary arterial wedge pressure (PAWP) or the pulmonary capillary wedge pressure (PCWP). Clinical application of PAOP is discussed in the hemodynamics section of Chapter 17.

Afterload. Afterload can be defined as the ventricular wall tension or stress during systolic ejection. It is commonly described by the term *systemic vascular resistance (SVR)* or, less frequently, *peripheral vascular resistance.* An increase in afterload usually means an increase in the work of the heart. Afterload is increased by factors that oppose ejection. Examples of increased afterload include aortic impedance (high diastolic aortic pressure, aortic stenosis), septal hypertrophy (obstruction in the outflow tract), vasoconstriction (increased systemic vascular resistance), and increased blood volume or viscosity. Therapeutic management to decrease afterload is aimed at decreasing the work of the heart through the use of vasodilators to decrease the myocardial oxygen demand.

An increase in afterload will evoke autoregulation where the ventricle adapts to changes in filling pressure without a continued increase in resting fiber length. For example, when systemic vascular resistance increases abruptly during vasoconstriction, ventricular diastolic pressure rises temporarily until the ventricle reaches a new equilibrium level of pressure.

Contractility. Contractility refers to the heart's contractile force. It is also referred to as *inotropy* (literally, *ino,* strength; *tropy,* enhancing), which can be positive (stronger contraction) or negative (weaker contraction). As discussed previously, contractility can be increased by Starling's mechanism. It also is altered by the sympathetic nervous system and by pharmacologic agents that mimic the sympathetic nervous system (i.e., sympathomimetics) (see Fig. 15-27).

REGULATION OF THE HEARTBEAT

Nervous Control. The autonomic nervous system (ANS) is composed of two competing neurologic systems of control. The parasympathetic nervous system (PNS) and the sympathetic nervous system (SNS) operate to create a balance between relaxation and *fight-or-flight* readiness. They affect cardiovascular function by slowing the heart rate during periods of calm and increasing it in response to sympathetic stimulation. Table 15-6 summarizes the effects these divisions of the autonomic nervous system have on the heart.

Parasympathetic fibers are concentrated mostly near the SA and AV conduction tissue and in the atria. Specifically, this involves the right and left vagus nerves (Fig. 15-29). Stimulation of the vagus nerve produces bradycardia as a result of hyperpolarization of phase 4 of the AP, which causes the slope to take longer to reach threshold. Sympathetic tone also concomitantly decreases.

Sympathetic nerve fibers have a greater impact on the ventricles. The right and left sympathetic chains probably have slightly different effects on the myocardium. It appears that the right chain has more effect on accelera-

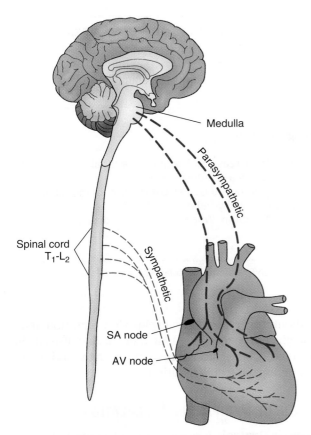

Fig. 15-29 Autonomic nervous system innervation of nodal tissue and myocardium by parasympathetic vagus nerve fibers and sympathetic chains. (Redrawn from Quaal S: *Comprehensive intraaortic balloon pumping*, ed 2, St Louis, 1993, Mosby.)

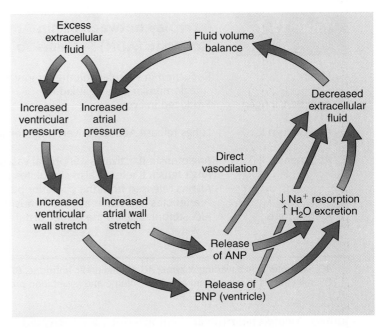

Fig. 15-30 The release of atrial peptide *(ANP)* from the atrium and brain natriuretic peptide *(BNP)* from the ventricle in response to volume overload.

tion properties, whereas the left chain has a greater influence on contractility.

Intrinsic Regulation. Supplementing the nervous control are several reflexes that serve as feedback mechanisms to the brain. These reflexes work to maintain even blood flow, oxygenation, and perfusion.

Baroreceptors. The *baroreceptors*, or pressure sensors, are located in the aortic arch and the carotid sinuses. They are more sensitive to wall changes (wall stretch) in these areas than to the absolute pressure. As the receptors sense a change in wall conformation, usually as a result of a decrease or increase in pressure, the autonomic nervous system is activated to either raise or lower the heart rate, respectively. For example, a drop in blood pressure alters the baroreceptor input to the vasomotor center in the medulla (brain stem), causing a reflex tachycardia. The baroreflex also initiates changes in venous tone to alter cardiac output according to need. Venoconstriction will increase blood return to the heart and augment stroke volume.

Chemoreceptors. The arterial *chemoreceptors*, or *carotid and aortic bodies*, are located in the carotid arteries and at the bifurcation of the aortic arch.[20] They possess a rich capillary blood supply and extensive in-

nervation of the peripheral nervous system. Their main function is to maintain homeostasis during hypoxemia.[20] The chemoreceptors signal changes in oxygen tension (Pao_2 less than 80 mm Hg), a drop in the pH level below 7.4, or a carbon dioxide tension ($Paco_2$) of greater than 40 mm Hg. Stimulation of the chemoreceptors normally also causes an increase in respiratory rate and depth.

Right Atrial Receptors. The *Bainbridge reflex* is attributed to receptors in the right atrium. When the pressure in the right atrium rises sufficiently to stimulate these stretch receptors, it causes a reflex tachycardia. The purpose of this reflex is possibly to protect the right side of the heart from an overload state and to quickly equalize filling pressures of the right and left sides of the heart.

Natriuretic Peptides. Another cardiac control mechanism involves the natriuretic peptide system (Fig. 15-30).[21] The heart secretes two major natriuretic peptides. The atrial myocardium secretes *atrial natriuretic peptide* (ANP), and the ventricular myocardium secretes *brain natriuretic peptide* (BNP). Both ANP and BNP are released in response to atrial and ventricular chamber stretch, respectively.[21] Both peptides cause vasodilatation, natriuresis (Na^+ and water loss via the kidneys) and inhibit the SNS and the renin-angiotensin-aldosterone system (RAAS).[21] Clinically, BNP levels are measured to confirm the diagnosis of acute heart failure.[22] A recombinant form of human BNP (Nesiritide [Natrecor]) is used therapeutically to mimic the clinical effects of BNP and treat symptoms of heart failure.[23]

Renin-Angiotensin-Aldosterone System. The RAAS system is activated by low blood pressure or intravascular volume depletion. The juxtaglomerular cells of the

Table 15-7	Interplay between Renin-Angiotensin-Aldosterone (RAAS) and Antidiuretic Hormone (ADH) Systems To Maintain Fluid Balance
Renin ↓	Reduction in vascular volume, or low arterial blood pressure will stimulate renin release from juxtaglomerular cells near kidney
Angiotensinogen ↓	Produced in liver
Angiotensin I ↓	Lungs release ACE to convert angiotensin I to angiotensin II
Angiotensin II ↓	Angiotensin II activates peripheral vascular receptors to increase SVR, and raise arterial BP
	Angiotensin II release also stimulates adrenal glands to release aldosterone
	ADH is released from the posterior pituitary when angiotensin II causes constriction of the renal arterioles and when hypothalamus detects intracellular dehydration.
Aldosterone	Aldosterone acts on the kidney distal tubules to retain sodium. When salt is retained, so is water.

ACE, Angiotensin-converting enzyme; *ADH,* antidiuretic hormone; *BP,* blood pressure; *SVR;* systemic vascular resistance.
Overall effect is to increase intravascular volume and raise blood pressure.

kidney, located near the afferent arteriole, are activated by low renal blood flow. As shown in Table 15-7, this stimulates release of the hormone renin. Renin converts the protein angiotensinogen to angiotensin I. When angiotensin I passes through the pulmonary vascular bed it is activated by an enzyme called ACE (angiotensin-converting enzyme) so it becomes Angiotensin II. Angiotensin II is a powerful agent with two principal actions. It activates peripheral vascular receptors to vasoconstrict the systemic arterial system and increase blood pressure, and it activates the release of aldosterone from the adrenal glands. Aldosterone works at the distal convoluted tubule in the kidney to retain sodium and thus water. Many drugs are used to manipulate the RAAS system to manage heart failure symptoms as described in Chapter 18 (see "Heart Failure") and Chapter 19 (see "Cardiac Drugs").

Respiratory Influences. Other influences involve the respiratory cycle and its effect on heart rate and stroke volume. Normally the heart rate varies slightly with the respiratory cycle. The heart usually accelerates on inspiration and decelerates with exhalation (see "Sinus Dysrhythmia" in Chapter 17). Also, left ventricular stroke volume decreases during normal inspiration. Possible reasons include normal fluctuations in sympathetic and vagal tone during respiration or any of the following alterations: decreased intrathoracic pressure contributing to increased venous return; the Bainbridge reflex; activation of stretch receptors in the lungs; interactions between the respiratory and cardiac centers in the medulla; increased capacity of the pulmonary vessels during lung inflation; decreased left ventricular compliance resulting from increased right ventricular return; increased impedance to left ventricular outflow related to the pleural pressure changes; or neural reflex mechanisms that are independent of mechanical influences. Thus many complex hemodynamic changes occur

throughout the respiratory cycle. Consideration must also be given to underlying lung and cardiac disease, intravascular volume status, respiratory rate, and added effects of mechanical ventilation.

CONTROL OF PERIPHERAL CIRCULATION

Intrinsic Control. Intrinsic, or local, control of the arterial peripheral circulation is most influential at the arteriolar level. The arterioles are the major resistance vessels because of the amount of smooth muscle in the vessel walls (see Fig. 15-12). The arteriole has the potential for either increasing or decreasing its lumen substantially. Several local factors influence this balance. One is pharmacologic stimuli, from locally released catecholamines, histamine, acetylcholine, serotonin, angiotensin, adenosine, and prostaglandins. These agents can be initiated by a variety of mechanisms, such as tissue injury, hypoxemia, or hormones. Other factors that influence circulation locally are temperature and carbon dioxide.

Extrinsic Control. Extrinsic control is mediated by two major mechanisms: the autonomic nervous system and peripheral vascular reflexes.

The ANS exerts dual antagonistic control over most organ systems via the sympathetic (constrict) and parasympathetic (dilate) fibers. Stimulation of the vasomotor center in the medulla causes increases in mean arterial pressure and heart rate by enhancing sympathetic outflow and possibly inhibiting parasympathetic outflow. The sympathetic outflow targets the resistance arterioles, causing vasoconstriction. Inhibition of these areas cause the opposite effect—vasodilation. Sympathetic fibers causing vasoconstriction supply the arteries, arterioles, and veins.

The capacitance vessels (veins) contain up to 75% of the blood volume.[18] Increasing venous tone (venoconstriction) will therefore increase the volume of blood re-

Table 15-8 **Regions in the Medulla Affecting Cardiovascular Activity**

Region	Activity
Dorsal lateral medulla (pressor region)	Vasoconstriction Cardiac acceleration Enhanced contractility
Ventromedial medulla (depressor region)	Direct spinal inhibition Inhibition of the pressor region

turning to the right side of the heart and augment stroke volume. The most richly innervated venous beds are those in the splanchnic and cutaneous (spleen and skin) circulations.[18] The venous and arterial vascular systems are interdependent. They both dilate and constrict in unison.[18] One does not act without the other. Table 15-8 summarizes the sympathetic receptors, including location and effects of stimulation.

Control of peripheral circulation is a combination of intrinsic and extrinsic mechanisms. Additional influences include emotions, temperature, and humoral substances.

A knowledge of normal cardiovascular anatomy and physiology is vital for a complete understanding of the changes that occur in cardiac disease states and provides an essential framework for understanding the principles of hemodynamic monitoring and current therapeutic interventions.

REFERENCES

1. Anderson RH, Razavi R, Taylor AM: Cardiac anatomy revisited, *J Anat* 205(3):159-177, 2004.
2. Frey N et al: Hypertrophy of the heart: a new therapeutic target? *Circulation* 109(13):1580-1589, 2004.
3. D'Avila A et al: Pericardial anatomy for the interventional electrophysiologist, *J Cardiovasc Electrophysiol* 14(4):422-430, 2003.
4. Goldstein JA: Cardiac tamponade, constrictive pericarditis, and restrictive cardiomyopathy, *Curr Probl Cardiol* 29(9):503-567, 2004.
5. Olivey HE, Compton LA, Barnett JV: Coronary vessel development the epicardium delivers, *Trends Cardiovasc Med* 14(6):247-251, 2004.
6. Antman EM et al: ACC/AHA guidelines for the management of patients with ST-elevation myocardial infarction—executive summary. A report of the American College of Cardiology/American Heart Association Task Force on Practice Guidelines (Writing Committee to revise the 1999 guidelines for the management of patients with acute myocardial infarction), *J Am Coll Cardiol* 44(3):671-719, 2004.
7. Horstkotte D et al: Guidelines on prevention, diagnosis and treatment of infective endocarditis—executive summary. The Task Force on Infective Endocarditis of the European Society of Cardiology, *Eur Heart J* 25(3):267-276, 2004.
8. Hunt SA et al: ACC/AHA guidelines for the evaluation and management of chronic heart failure in the adult—executive summary. A report of the American College of Cardiology/American Heart Association Task Force on Practice Guidelines (Committee to Revise the 1995 Guidelines for the Evaluation and Management of Heart Failure): Developed in collaboration with the International Society for Heart and Lung Transplantation; endorsed by the Heart Failure Society of America, *Circulation* 104(24):2996-3007, 2001.
9. Segal BL: Valvular heart disease, Part 2. Mitral valve disease in older adults, *Geriatrics* 58(10):26-31, 2003.
10. Robicsek F et al: The congenitally bicuspid aortic valve: how does it function? Why does it fail? *Ann Thorac Surg* 77(1):177-185, 2004.
11. Cripe L et al: Bicuspid aortic valve is heritable, *J Am Coll Cardiol* 44(1):138-143, 2004.
12. Berdajs D, Patonay L, Turina MI: The clinical anatomy of the sinus node artery, *Ann Thorac Surg* 76(3):732-735; discussion 735-736, 2003.
13. James TN: The internodal pathways of the human heart, *Prog Cardiovasc Dis* 43(6):495-535, 2001.
14. Bharati S: Anatomy of the atrioventricular conduction system, *Circulation* 103(12):E63-64, 2001.
15. James TN: Structure and function of the sinus node, AV node and His bundle of the human heart: part I—structure, *Prog Cardiovasc Dis* 45(3):235-267, 2002.
16. James TN: Structure and function of the sinus node, AV node and His bundle of the human heart: part II—function, *Prog Cardiovasc Dis* 45(4):327-360, 2003.
17. Perez-Lugones A et al: Evidence of specialized conduction cells in human pulmonary veins of patients with atrial fibrillation, *J Cardiovasc Electrophysiol* 14(8):803-809, 2003.
18. Peters J, Mack GW, Lister G: The importance of the peripheral circulation in critical illnesses, *Intensive Care Med* 27(9):1446-1458, 2001.
19. Pyle WG, Solaro RJ: At the crossroads of myocardial signaling: the role of Z-discs in intracellular signaling and cardiac function, *Circ Res* 94(3):296-305, 2004.
20. Prabhakar NR, Peng YJ: Peripheral chemoreceptors in health and disease, *J Appl Physiol* 96(1):359-366, 2004.
21. Suttner SW, Boldt J: Natriuretic peptide system: physiology and clinical utility, *Curr Opin Crit Care* 10(5):336-341, 2004.
22. Saul L, Shatzer M: B-type natriuretic peptide testing for detection of heart failure, *Crit Care Nurs Q* 26(1):35-39, 2003.
23. Colbert K, Greene MH: Nesiritide (Natrecor): a new treatment for acutely decompensated congestive heart failure, *Crit Care Nurs Q* 26(1):40-44, 2003.

CHAPTER 16

Cardiovascular Clinical Assessment

Physical assessment of the cardiovascular patient is a skill that must not be lost amidst the technology of the critical care setting. Data collected from a thorough, thoughtful history and examination contribute to both the nursing and the medical decisions for therapeutic interventions.

HISTORY

The patient history is important for providing data that contribute to the cardiovascular diagnosis and treatment plan. For a patient in acute distress, the history is curtailed to just a few questions about the patient's chief complaint, the precipitating events, and current medications (see the Data Collection feature on Cardiovascular History). For a patient without obvious distress, the history focuses on the following four areas:

1. Review of the patient's present illness.
2. Overview of the patient's general cardiovascular status, including previous cardiac diagnostic studies, interventional procedures, cardiac surgeries, and current medications (cardiac, noncardiac, and herbal).
3. Examination of the patient's general health status, including family history of coronary artery disease (CAD), hypertension, diabetes, peripheral arterial disease, or stroke.
4. Survey of the patient's lifestyle, including risk factors for CAD.

One of the unique challenges in cardiovascular assessment is identifying when "chest pain" is of cardiac origin and when it is not. The following safety information should always be considered:

- If there is any evidence of CAD or risk of heart disease, assume that the chest pain is caused by myocardial ischemia until proven otherwise.
- Questions to elicit the nature of the chest pain cover five basic areas: quality, location, duration of pain, factors that provoke the pain and factors that relieve the pain.[1] Questions that may help elicit this information are listed in Table 16-1.
- There may be little correlation between the severity of chest discomfort and the gravity of its cause. This is a result of the subjective nature of pain and the unique presentation of ischemic disease in women, elderly patients, and individuals with diabetes.
- Subjective descriptors vary greatly between individuals. Not all patients use the word pain; some may describe "pressure," "heaviness," "discomfort", or "indigestion."[1]
- There is not always a correlation between the location of chest discomfort and its source because of referred pain. For example, patients with gastroesophageal reflux disease (GERD) esophageal spasm can also present with visceral substernal chest pain that radiates to the left arm and jaw.[2,3]
- Other nonpainful symptoms that may signal cardiac dysfunction are dyspnea, palpitations, cough, fatigue, edema, ischemic leg pain, nocturia, syncope, and cyanosis.

In a recent metaanalysis of the evaluation of stable, intermittent chest pain, a patient's description of chest pain was found to be the most important predictor of underlying coronary disease.[4] In the evaluation of acute chest pain, the 12-lead electrocardiogram was the most useful bedside predictor for a diagnosis of ST-elevation myocardial infarction (STEMI).[4]

PHYSICAL EXAMINATION

A comprehensive physical assessment is fundamental to achievement of an accurate diagnosis. The nurse who has developed the skills of inspection, palpation, and auscultation will be confident when assessing patients with cardiovascular disease. Percussion is not employed when assessing the cardiovascular system.

DATA COLLECTION
Cardiovascular History

COMMON CARDIOVASCULAR SYMPTOMS
Chest pains
Palpitations
Dyspnea
Cough/hemoptysis
Nausea
Nocturia
Edema
Dizziness/syncope/visual changes
Claudication/extremity pain or paresthesias
Fatigue

PATIENT PROFILE
Baseline cognitive functioning
Health habits:
    Use of tea and coffee, over-the-counter drug use,
        smoking, exercise, sleep, and dietary habits
Use of illegal recreational drugs (e.g., cocaine)
Use of alcohol (occasional/daily)
Lifestyle pattern and responsibilities
Working, relaxing, coping, cultural habits
Social support systems
Recent life changes within the past 12 months
Emotional state
Evidence of psychologic stress, anger, anxiety, depression
Perception of illness and its meaning for the future

RISK FACTORS
Gender/age/cultural identity
Family history of premature CAD (age under 65 years)
Smoking history
Hypertension
Hyperlipidemia
Sedentary lifestyle
Diabetes mellitus
Obesity
Kidney failure

FAMILY HISTORY
CAD at age 65 years or younger
Myocardial infarction/early death of unknown etiology
Hypertension
Stroke
Diabetes mellitus
Lipid disorders
Collagen vascular disease

CARDIAC STUDIES OR INTERVENTIONS DONE IN THE PAST
Cardiac catheterization
Electrophysiology study
Cardiac ultrasound (echocardiogram)
12-Lead ECG

Exercise electrocardiography test (stress test)
Myocardial imaging with radiographic isotopes (thallium/
    dipyridamole) (Persantine/dobutamine)
Thrombolytic therapy
Percutaneous transluminal coronary angioplasty
Atherectomy
Stent placement
Valvuloplasty

MEDICAL HISTORY
Childhood
Murmurs, cyanosis, streptococcal infections, rheumatic
    fever

Adult
Diseases/abnormalities:
- Heart failure (right- or left-sided), CAD, heart valve disease, mitral valve prolapse, myocardial infarction, peripheral vascular disease, diabetes mellitus, hypertension, hyperlipidemia, dysrhythmias, murmurs, endocarditis, visual defects, recent weight changes, psychiatric illnesses, thrombophlebitis, deep vein thrombosis, systemic or pulmonary emboli

Surgical history
- Cardiovascular: Coronary artery bypass grafting, valvular placement, peripheral vascular bypasses or repairs, pacemaker, defibrillator implants (ICDs)
- Other body systems: Neurologic, gastrointestinal, musculoskeletal, pulmonary, renal, immunologic, hematologic

Allergies, especially to emergency medication (lidocaine, morphine), radiographic contrast agents, or iodine (shellfish)
Recent dental work or infection

CURRENT MEDICATION USAGE
ACE inhibitors
Anticoagulants
Antidysrhythmics
Antihypertensives
Antiplatelets
ARBs
β-blockers
Calcium channel blockers
Cholesterol-lowering agents
Digitalis
Diuretics
Nitrates
Hormone replacement therapy
Oral contraceptives
Potassium/calcium
Nonprescription medications/herbal remedies

CAD, Coronary artery disease; *ECG*, electrocardiogram; *ICDs*, implantable cardioverter defibrillators; *ACE*, angiotensin-converting enzyme; *ARB*, angiotensin receptor blocker.

INSPECTION

Face. The face is observed for the color of the skin (cyanotic, pale, or jaundiced) and for apprehensive or painful expressions. The skin, lips, tongue, and mucous membranes are inspected for pallor or cyanosis. *Central cyanosis* is a bluish discoloration of the tongue and sublingual area. Multiracial studies indicate that the tongue is the most sensitive site for observation of central cyanosis, which must be recognized and treated as a medical emergency. Pulse oximetry, arterial blood gas analysis, and treatment with 100% oxygen must be instituted immediately.

Thorax. Both the anterior and posterior thorax are inspected for skeletal deformities that may displace the heart and cause cardiac compromise. The skin on the chest wall and the abdomen is inspected for scars, bruises, wounds, and bulges associated with pacemaker or defibrillator implants. Respiratory rate, pattern, and effort are also observed and recorded.

Abdomen. The abdomen is assessed for signs of distention or ascites that may be associated with right-sided heart failure. Abdominal adiposity is a known risk factor for coronary artery disease.

Nail Beds and Cyanosis. The nail beds are inspected for signs of discoloration or cyanosis. *Clubbing* in the nail bed is a sign of longstanding central cyanotic heart disease or pulmonary disease with hypoxemia. Clubbing describes a nail that has lost the normal angle between the finger and the nail root; the nail becomes wide and convex. The terminal phalanx of the finger also becomes bulbous and swollen. Clubbing is rare and a sign of severe central cyanosis (Fig. 16-1).

Peripheral cyanosis, a bluish discoloration of the nail bed, is more commonly seen. Peripheral cyanosis occurs as a result of a reduction in the quantity of oxygen in the peripheral extremities secondary to arterial disease or decreased cardiac output. Clubbing never occurs as a result of peripheral cyanosis.

Lower Extremities. The legs are inspected for signs of peripheral arterial or venous vascular disease. The visible signs of arterial vascular disease include pale, shiny legs with sparse hair growth. Venous disease creates an edematous limb with deep red rubor, brown discoloration, and frequently leg ulceration. A comparison of arterial and venous disease is presented in Table 16-2.

Clubbing of Nail Beds

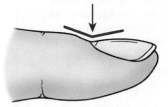

Normal nail shows a slight angle between root of nail bed and finger.

Normal Finger and Nail Bed

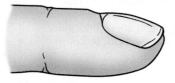

Early clubbing shows loss of angle at root of nail bed. Finger tip is of normal size.

Early Clubbing

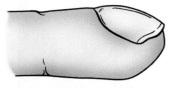

Moderate clubbing shows bulging of angle at root of nail bed. Distal finger/toe is enlarged.

Moderate Clubbing

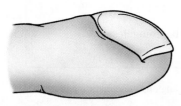

Advanced clubbing shows bulging and widening of nail bed. Distal finger/toe is bulbous.

Advanced Clubbing

Fig. 16-1 Clubbing of the nail beds.

Table 16-1	Clarifying Chest Pain Symptoms by Asking Specific Questions
Determine	**Typical Question**
Location, radiation	Where is it? Does it move or stay in one place?
Quality	What's it like?
Quantity	How severe is it? How frequent? How long does it last?
Chronology	When did it begin? How has it progressed? What are you doing when it occurs? What do you do to get rid of it?
Associated findings	Do you feel any other symptoms at the same time?
Treatment sought and effect	Have you seen a physician in the past for this same problem? What was the treatment?
Personal perception	What do you think this is from? Why do you think it happened now?

Posture. Body posture can indicate the amount of effort it takes to breathe. For example, sitting upright to breathe may be necessary for the patient with acute heart failure, and leaning forward may be the least painful position for the patient with pericarditis.

Weight. The weight in proportion to the height is assessed to determine whether the patient is obese or cachectic.

Mentation. The patient is observed for signs of confusion or lethargy that may indicate hypotension, low cardiac output (CO), or hypoxemia.

Jugular Veins. The jugular veins of the neck are inspected for a noninvasive estimate of intravascular volume and pressure. The external jugular veins are observed for jugular vein distention (JVD) (Fig. 16-2 and Box 16-1). *Jugular venous distention* occurs when central venous pressure is elevated, which occurs with fluid volume overload and right ventricular dysfunction. The right internal jugular vein can be used for measurement of central venous pressure (CVP) in centimeters of water (cm H_2O) (Fig. 16-3 and Box 16-2).[5-6]

Abdominojugular Reflux. The abdominojugular reflux sign can assist with the diagnosis of right ventricular failure. This noninvasive test is used in conjunction with measurement of jugular venous distention (see preceding paragraph). The procedure for assessing abdominojugular reflux is described in Box 16-3. A positive abdominojugular reflux sign is an increase in the jugular venous pressure (CVP equivalent) of greater than 3 cm sustained for at least 15 seconds.[7]

Thoracic Reference Points. The thoracic cage is divided with imaginary vertical lines (sternal, midclavicular, axillary, vertebral, and scapular), and the intercostal spaces (ICSs) are divided with horizontal lines to serve

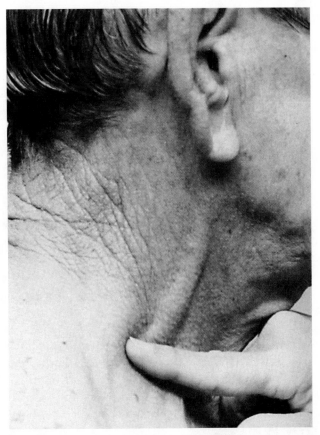

Fig. 16-2 Assessment of jugular vein distention (JVD). Applying light finger pressure over the sternocleidomastoid muscle, parallel to the clavicle, helps identify the external jugular vein by occluding flow and distending it. Release the finger pressure, and observe for true distention. If the patient's trunk is elevated to 30 degrees or more, JVD should not be present.

Table 16-2	Inspection and Palpation of Extremities: Comparison of Arterial and Venous Disease	
Characteristics	**Arterial Disease**	**Venous Disease**
Hair loss	Present	Absent
Skin texture	Thin, shiny, dry	Flaking, stasis, dermatitis, mottled
Ulceration	Located at pressure points, painful, pale, dry with little drainage; well-demarcated with eschar or dried; surrounded by fibrous tissue; granulation tissue scant and pale	Usually at the ankle; painless, pink, moist with large amount of drainage; irregular, dry, and scaly; surrounded by dermatitis; granulation tissue healthy
Skin color	Elevational pallor, dependent rubor	Brown patches, rubor, mottled cyanotic color when dependent
Nails	Thick, brittle	Normal
Varicose veins	Absent	Present
Temperature	Cool	Warm
Capillary refill	Greater than 3 seconds	Less than 3 seconds
Edema	None or mild, usually unilateral	Usually present foot to calf, unilateral or bilateral
Pulses	Weak or absent (0 to 1+)	Normal, strong, and symmetric

Modified from Krenzer ME: *AACN Clin Issues* 6(4):631, 1995.

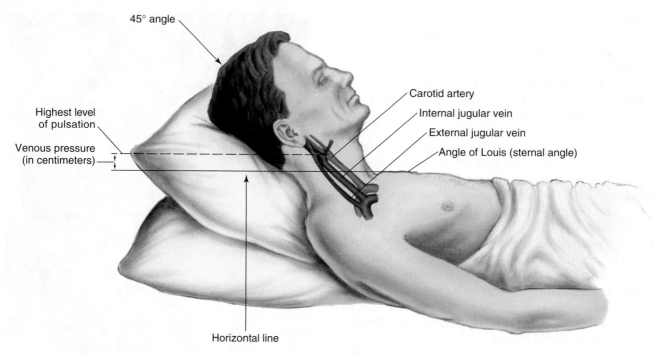

Fig. 16-3 Position of internal and external jugular veins. Pulsation in the internal jugular vein can be used to estimate central venous pressure. (Modified from Thompson JM et al: *Mosby's clinical nursing,* ed 5, St Louis, 2002, Mosby.)

Box 16-1

PROCEDURE FOR ASSESSING JUGULAR VEIN DISTENTION (JVD)

1. Patient reclines at a 30- to 45-degree angle.
2. Examiner stands on patient's right side and turns patient's head slightly toward the left.
3. If jugular vein is not visible, light finger pressure is applied across sternocleidomastoid muscle just above and parallel to clavicle. This pressure will fill external jugular vein by obstructing flow (see Fig. 16-2).
4. Once location of vein has been identified, pressure is released and presence of JVD assessed.
5. Because inhalation decreases venous pressure, JVD should be assessed at end-exhalation.
6. Any fullness in the vein extending more than 3 cm above sternal angle is evidence of increased venous pressure. Generally the higher the sitting angle of the patient when JVD is visualized, the higher the central venous pressure.
7. *Documentation:* JVD is reported by including angle of the head of the bed at the time JVD was evaluated (e.g., "presence of JVD with head of bed elevated to 45 degrees").

Box 16-2

PROCEDURE FOR ASSESSING CENTRAL VENOUS PRESSURE (CVP)

1. Patient reclines in bed. Highest point of pulsation in the internal jugular vein is observed during exhalation.
2. Vertical distance between this pulsation (at top of fluid level) and the sternal angle is estimated or measured in centimeters (cm).
3. This number is then added to 5 cm for an estimation of CVP. The 5 cm is the approximate distance of sternal angle above level of right atrium (see Fig. 16-3).
4. *Documentation:* Degree of elevation of patient is included in report (e.g., "CVP estimated at 13 cm, using internal jugular vein pulsation, with head of bed elevated 45 degrees").

as reference points in locating or describing cardiac findings (Fig. 16-4). The ribs are numbered from 1 (the first rib below the clavicle) to 12. The intercostal space between each rib is numbered the same as the rib that lies above it. The second rib is the easiest to locate, because

it is attached to the sternum at the angle of Louis. This angle (also called the sternal angle) is the bony ridge on the sternum that lies approximately 2 inches below the sternal notch (see Fig. 16-4, *A*). Once the second rib has been located, it can be used as a reference point to count off the other ribs and intercostal spaces.

Apical Impulse. The anterior thorax is inspected for the *apical impulse,* sometimes referred to as the *point of maximal impulse* (PMI). The apical impulse occurs as the left ventricle contracts during systole and rotates forward, causing the left ventricular apex of the heart to

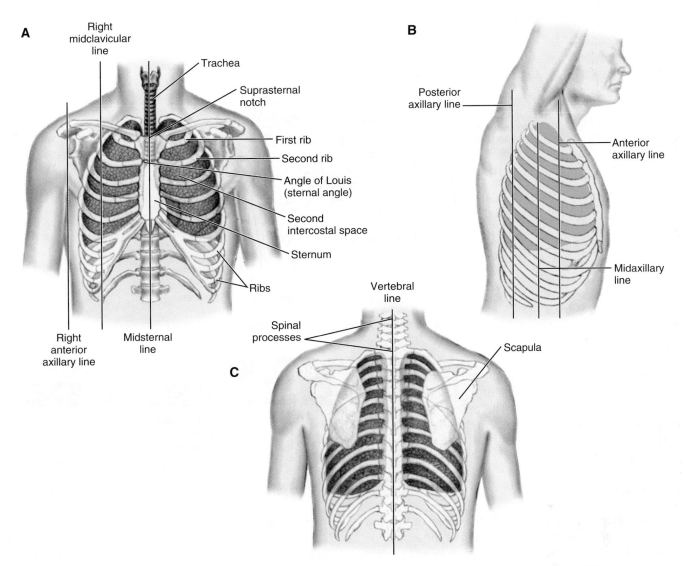

Fig. 16-4   Thoracic landmarks. **A,** Anterior thorax. **B,** Right lateral thorax. **C,** Posterior thorax.

Box 16-3

PROCEDURE FOR ASSESSING ABDOMINOJUGULAR REFLUX

1. Follow procedure for assessing JVD (see Box 16-1).
2. Observe the JVD in the right IJ vein before, during, and after midabdominal compression for 15 to 30 seconds.
3. The patient is asked to relax and breathe normally through an open mouth.
4. Firm pressure of approximately 20 to 35 mm Hg is applied to the midabdomen.
5. Ask the patient not to tense or hold his or her breath, (increases venous return to the heart and the test may be falsely positive).

RESULTS

6. A positive abdominojugular reflux is identified when abdominal compression causes a sustained JVD increase of 4 cm or more. This sign is indicative of right-sided heart failure.
7. A normal abdominojugular reflux includes no rise in JVD, a transient (less than 10 seconds) rise in JVD, or a rise in JVD less than or equal to 3 cm sustained throughout compression.

JVD, Jugular venous distention.

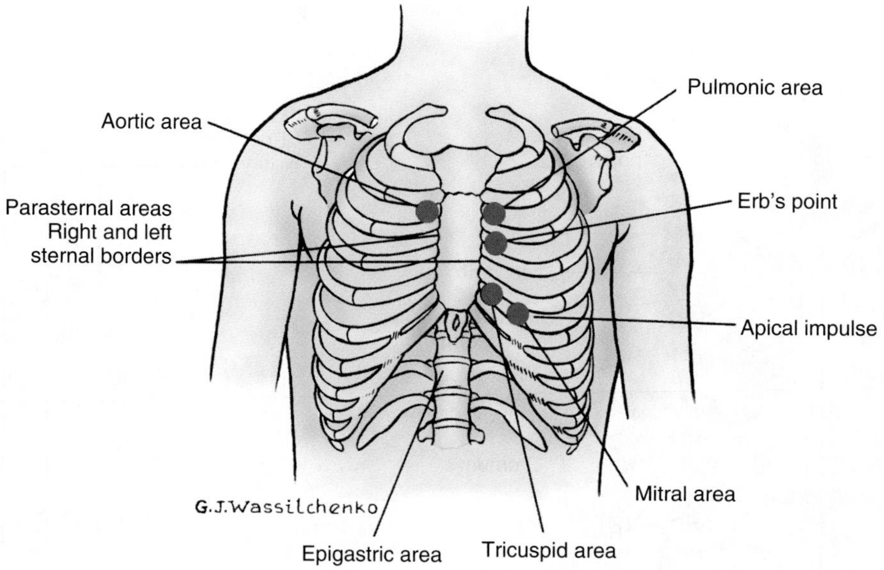

Fig. 16-5 Thoracic palpation and auscultation points.

hit the chest wall. The apical impulse is a quick, localized, outward movement normally located just lateral to the left midclavicular line at the fifth intercostal space in the adult patient (Fig. 16-5). The apical impulse is the only normal pulsation visualized on the chest wall. In the patient without cardiac disease, PMI may not be noticeable (Fig. 16-5).

PALPATION

Palpation is a technique that uses the sense of touch using the tips of the fingers and the palm of the hand.

Arterial Pulses. Seven pairs of bilateral arterial pulses are palpated. The examination incorporates bilateral assessment of the carotid, brachial, radial, ulnar, popliteal, dorsalis pedis, and posterior tibial arteries. The pulses are palpated separately and compared bilaterally to check for consistency. Pulse volume is graded on a scale of 0 to 3+ (Box 16-4). The abdominal aortic pulse can also be palpated.

Carotid Pulses. The carotid arteries are assessed at the medial mid-neck region. The touch is light because if blood flow through the carotid arteries is compromised by atherosclerotic plaque, firm palpation could cause total occlusion; thus only one carotid artery at a time is gently palpated.

Brachial, Ulnar, and Radial Pulses. The brachial pulse is assessed by gently palpating the inner aspect of the slightly bent elbow with the fingers. The radial pulse is palpated in the medial area of the wrist (thumb side). The ulnar artery is palpated at the opposite side of the wrist (little finger side). The radial and ulnar arterial pulses must be assessed before inserting an arterial line; this test, known as the *Allen Test*, is described in (Box 16-5).

Box 16-4

PULSE PALPATION SCALE

0	Not palpable
1+	Faintly palpable (weak and thready)
2+	Palpable (normal pulse)
3+	Bounding (hyperdynamic pulse)

Femoral Pulses. The femoral arteries are palpated by pressing deeply into the groin beneath the inguinal ligament, approximately midway between the anterior superior iliac spine and the symphysis pubis on both right and left sides.

Popliteal Pulses. The popliteal pulse is palpated behind the knee. The leg is very slightly bent, and the clinician's two hands gently cup the patient's knee with the thumbs on top of the knee cap. The pulse is palpated by the fingertips, behind the knee.

Dorsalis Pedis and Posterior Tibial Pulses. The pulses of the lower leg and foot are assessed both to determine flow to the limb but also to assess adequacy of CO to the extremities. The dorsalis pedis pulse is located on the upper aspect of the foot. The posterior tibial pulse is located behind the medial malleolus (inner ankle bone) of the lower leg.

Descending Aorta Pulse. When the patient is lying in a supine position, the abdominal aortic pulsation is located in the epigastric area and can be felt as a forward movement by using firm fingertip pressure above the umbilicus. If prominent or diffuse, the pulsation may indicate an abdominal aneurysm.

A diminished or absent pulse may indicate low CO or arterial stenosis or occlusion proximal to the site of the

Box 16-5

PROCEDURE FOR ASSESSMENT OF ARTERIAL BLOOD SUPPLY TO THE HAND—THE ALLEN TEST

Before a radial artery is punctured or cannulated, the Allen test is performed to assess blood flow to the hand and ensure that it is adequate.

If the patient is alert and cooperative, the procedure is as follows:

ALLEN TEST BY VISUAL INSPECTION

1. The patient is requested to repeatedly make a tight fist to squeeze the blood out of his or her hand.
2. The radial artery is compressed with firm thumb pressure by the examiner.
3. The patient is requested to open the hand, palm side up, while the radial artery is still occluded.
4. Pressure is released and the time it takes for the color to return to the hand is noted.

If the ulnar artery is patent, the color will return within 3 seconds. The patient may describe a tingling in the palm as blood flow returns. Delayed color return (a "failed" Allen test) implies that the ulnar artery is inadequate; therefore the radial artery is the only source of

blood flow to the hand and must not be punctured or cannulated.

ALLEN TEST WITH PULSE OXIMETRY

1. If the patient is unable to cooperate to make a fist, an alternative approach is to use a pulse oximeter that displays a pulse waveform.
2. Place the pulse oximeter on the middle finger and establish an adequate pulse amplitude display on the monitor.
3. Simultaneously compress the radial and ulnar arteries until the waveform clearly decreases or vanishes.
4. Release pressure off the ulnar artery only. If the ulnar artery is patent, the pulse amplitude recovers its normal appearance.
5. Repeat the procedure with the radial artery.
6. Only when there is adequate blood supply to the hand can arterial catheterization of the radial artery be accomplished safely.

Table 16-3   **Pitting Edema Scale**

| Scale | Edema | Indentation Depth | | Time to Baseline |
		Inches	Metric	
0	None present	0	0	
1+	Trace	0-1/4	<6.5 mm	Rapid
2+	Mild	1/4-1/2	6.5-12.5 mm	10-15 sec
3+	Moderate	1/2-1	12.5 mm-2.5 cm	1-2 min
4+	Severe	>1	>2.5 cm	2-5 min

>, Greater than; <, less than.

---

examination. An abnormally strong or bounding pulse suggests the presence of an aneurysm or an occlusion distal to the examination site. If a distal pulse cannot be palpated using light finger pressure, a Doppler ultrasound stethoscope is often helpful. It is important to mark the location of the audible signal with an indelible ink marker pen for future evaluation of pulse quality.

Capillary Refill. Capillary refill assessment is a maneuver that uses the patient's nail beds to evaluate both arterial circulation to the extremity and overall perfusion. The nail bed is compressed to produce blanching, and the release of the pressure should result in a return of blood flow and baseline nail color in less than 3 seconds. The severity of arterial insufficiency is directly proportional to the amount of time necessary to reestablish flow and color.

Edema. Edema is fluid accumulation in the extravascular spaces of the body. The dependent tissues within

the legs and sacrum are particularly susceptible. Note whether the edema is dependent, unilateral or bilateral, and pitting or nonpitting. The amount of edema is quantified by measuring the circumference of the limb or by pressing the skin of the feet, ankles, and shins against the underlying bone. Edema is a symptom associated with several diseases, and further diagnostic evaluation is required to determine the cause. Although no universal scale for pitting edema exists, typical scales use a 0 to 4+ system (Table 16-3).

AUSCULTATION

Blood Pressure Measurement. Blood pressure (BP) measurement is an essential component of every complete physical examination.[8] Hypertension is diagnosed as a systolic BP of 140 mm Hg or higher, or a diastolic BP of 90 mm Hg or above.[9] The incidence of hypertension in the United States has increased dramatically as a result of an aging population and obesity. In 1999 to 2000, 65 million adults in the United States were hypertensive, compared with 50 million in 1988 through 1994—an increase of 30%.[10]

In the critical care setting, systemic blood pressure can be measured directly or indirectly. Arterial monitoring devices (as discussed in Chapter 18) that directly measure arterial pressure by means of an invasive technique requiring placement of an arterial catheter are considered the gold standard.[8] Correct use of a stethoscope and sphygmomanometer and/or electronic measuring devices can produce indirect blood pressure values that closely reflect direct measurements (within 1 to 3 mm Hg). The following discussion reviews the essential elements of noninvasive BP monitoring.

Noninvasive Blood Pressure Monitoring. The most common peripheral locations for BP monitoring are the bilateral brachial arteries. BP is measured in both arms to rule out subclavian arterial stenosis. Normally the blood pressure between both arms varies only 5 to 10 mm Hg. A finding of more than 15 mm Hg difference between the bilateral arm pressures suggests arterial obstruction on the side with the lower pressure.[11] Asymmetry is documented so that all subsequent measurements are made on the arm with the higher pressure.

Correct position of the extremity being measured is essential. As long as the arm or leg is at the level of the heart, the blood pressure can be measured in any position. Falsely elevated readings are obtained if the arm is lower than the heart; falsely low pressures are measured if the arm is higher than the heart.[8]

Orthostatic Hypotension. Postural (orthostatic) hypotension occurs when the BP drops after upright posture is assumed. It is usually accompanied by complaints of dizziness, lightheadedness, or syncope. If a patient is seen with any of these symptoms, it is important to complete a full set of postural vital signs before increasing activity level (Box 16-6). The three most common causes of orthostatic vital sign changes (drop in BP and rise in heart rate) follow:

1. Intravascular volume depletion or fluid loss caused by bleeding, excessive diuresis, or fever.
2. Inadequate vascular vasoconstrictor mechanisms to constrict the arterial bed, which can occur in the elderly following prolonged immobility or as a result of spinal cord injury.
3. Autonomic insufficiency caused by administration of pharmacologic agents such as beta-blockers, ACE inhibitors, and calcium channel blockers.

Blood Pressure Cuff Size. Correct size and placement of the inflatable bladder (inside the nondistensible cuff) are crucial to obtaining an accurate blood pressure measurement.[8] Inflatable cuffs and bladders are available in many sizes; it is important to find the best fit to ensure accurate measurements. The bladder width should be 40% of the circumference of the limb (arm or leg) to be measured.[8] The length of the bladder should be long enough to encircle at least 80% of the width of the limb in adults.[8] Cuffs that are too small can give falsely high readings, and cuffs that are too large can give falsely low readings. It is also important that the meniscus of the mercury be at eye level when the BP is measured.[8] See Box 16-7 for key points to observe when obtaining standard BP readings.

Korotkoff Sounds. Obtaining systemic BP readings involves auscultation of *Korotkoff sounds,* the sounds created by turbulence of blood flow within a vessel

---

Box 16-6

MEASUREMENT OF POSTURAL (ORTHOSTATIC) VITAL SIGNS

GUIDELINES
1. Record blood pressure (BP) and heart rate (HR) in each position.
2. Do not remove cuff between measurements.
3. Record all associated signs and symptoms.
4. Clearly document patient position.

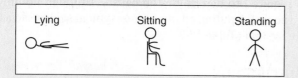

Lying   Sitting   Standing

TECHNIQUE
1. Keep patient as flat as possible for 10 minutes before initial assessment.
2. Obtain supine BP and HR measurements.

3. Patient sitting with legs hanging: measure immediately and after 2 minutes.
4. Patient standing: measure immediately and after 2 minutes. If BP and HR are stable but orthostasis is suspected, BP and HR can be repeated every 2 minutes. Note that this is rarely practical for the critically ill patient.

RESULTS
Normal Changes
HR increases by 5 to 20 beats/min (transiently).
Systolic BP drops 10 mm Hg.
Diastolic BP drops 5 mm Hg.

Positive Orthostasis
Drop in systolic BP by more than 20 mm Hg.
Drop in diastolic BP by more than 10 mm Hg within 3 minutes.

caused by constriction of the blood pressure cuff. The pressure in the cuff is inflated above the normal systolic pressure. As the pressure in the cuff is reduced, the Korotkoff sounds change in quality and intensity. These sounds are divided into five stages.[8] Systolic pressure is the highest point at which initial tapping occurs. Diastolic pressure is equated with the complete disappearance of Korotkoff sounds. There is often a muffling of diastolic sounds prior to complete disappearance of sounds. Because complete disappearance of the Korotkoff sounds corresponds more closely to intraarterial catheter measurement, this is the value that should be recorded.[8]

Auscultatory Gap. In elderly patients with systolic hypertension, the presence of an *auscultatory gap* is not uncommon. It is important to inflate the cuff above the patient's normal systolic pressure to avoid this gap and a subsequent underestimation of systolic blood pressure.[8] Using an initial palpation estimate of the systolic blood pressure prior to auscultation with a stethoscope is one recommended method to accurately determine the upper systolic blood pressure.[8]

Automated Blood Pressure Devices. Electronic automated devices are frequently used for measuring BP and have replaced the mercury sphygmomanometer in many places. The mercury used in the sphygmomanometer is nondegradable, and today it is considered an environmental pollutant that is difficult to dispose of safely. For this reason, mercury sphygmomanometers are being phased out of use in many hospitals. This is a controversial issue for many clinicians.[8]

In automated devices the systolic number is accurate, but the diastolic value is often calculated from the systolic pressure and the mean arterial pressure (MAP). Thus the diastolic value may not always be accurate.[8] Devices placed on the arm or leg are considered accurate (as long as the cuff size is correct) for systolic measurement and trending of blood pressure. There is considerable controversy about automated devices applied to the wrist or finger, and these should not be used to monitor blood pressure in any critically ill or cardiac patient.[8]

Automatic BP cuff placement should be rotated frequently to avoid excessive irritation to the extremity, especially when the automatic cuff is set to cycle more frequently than every 15 minutes.

Pulse Pressure. Pulse pressure describes the difference between the systolic and diastolic values. The normal pulse pressure is 40 mm Hg, or the difference between a systolic pressure of 120 and a diastolic pressure of 80 mm Hg. In the critically ill patient a low blood pressure is frequently associated with a narrow pulse pressure. For example, a patient with a BP of 90/72 mm Hg has a pulse pressure of 18 mm Hg. The narrowed pulse pressure is a temporary compensatory mechanism caused by arterial vasoconstriction secondary to volume depletion or heart failure. The narrow pulse pressure ensures that the mean arterial pressure (MAP)—78 in this example—remains in a therapeutic range to provide adequate organ perfusion.

In contrast, a hypotensive septic patient who exhibits vasodilation will have a wide pulse pressure and inadequate organ perfusion. If the BP is 90/36 mm Hg, the pulse pressure is 54 mm Hg, and the MAP calculates to an inadequate 54 mm Hg. In both these examples the systolic pressure is the same (90 mm Hg). The difference in pulse pressure is a function of intravascular volume and vascular tone.

Pulsus Paradoxus. In normal physiology the strength of the pulse fluctuates throughout the respira-

---

Box 16-8

PROCEDURE FOR MEASURING PULSUS PARADOXUS

MEASUREMENT WITH A SPHYGMOMANOMETER
1. The patient should be positioned supine in a comfortable position.
2. The breathing pattern should be of normal depth and rate to avoid excessive respiratory interference.
3. Blood pressure is measured following standard procedures (see Boxes 16-6 and 16-7). The sphygmomanometer cuff is inflated above systolic pressure, and Korotkoff sounds are auscultated over the brachial artery while the cuff is deflated at rate of approximately 2 to 3 mm Hg per heartbeat.
4. The peak systolic pressure during expiration should first be identified and reconfirmed (when Korotkoff sounds are heard only during expiration).
5. The cuff is then deflated slowly to establish the blood pressure at which Korotkoff sounds become audible during both inspiration and expiration (when the Korotkoff sounds are heard during both inspiration and expiration).
6. When the auscultated difference between these two levels exceeds 10 mm Hg during quiet respiration, a paradoxical pulse is present.

USING WAVEFORM ANALYSIS
7. A pulse oximetry sensor with a visible pulse waveform can be used as an additional measurement device.
8. In the critical care unit, an arterial waveform can be used to measure the systolic pressure difference between expiration and inspiration (if present).

Box 16-7

OBTAINING ACCURATE BLOOD PRESSURE READINGS

- Compare right and left measurement.
- Position extremity at the level of the heart.
- Document position of patient.
- Ensure proper cuff size.
- Measure readings at eye level at top of meniscus.

tory cycle. When the "pulse" is measured using the systolic blood pressure, the pressure decreases slightly during inspiration and rises slightly during respiratory exhalation. The normal difference is 2 to 4 mm Hg.8 In some clinical conditions such as cardiac tamponade, the BP decline is abnormally large during inspiration. Generally, an inspiratory decline of systolic BP of greater than 10 mm Hg is considered diagnostic of pulsus paradoxus.8,12-13 The traditional technique for measuring pulsus paradoxus using a sphygmomanometer and a blood pressure cuff is described in Box 16-8. If the patient is hypotensive, pulsus paradoxus will be more accurately assessed in the critical care unit by monitoring a pulse oximetry waveform, or by an indwelling arterial catheter waveform.

Pulsus Alternans. Pulsus alternans describes a regular pattern of pulse amplitude changes that alternate between stronger and weaker beats. This finding is suggestive of end-stage left ventricular heart failure.

Vascular Bruits. The carotid and femoral arteries are auscultated for bruits. A bruit, a high-pitched "sh-sh," is an extracardiac vascular sound that vacillates in volume with systole and diastole. An abnormal bruit is produced as blood flows through a partially occluded vessel. The auscultation of a bruit can expedite the diagnosis of suspected arterial obstruction.

Normal Heart Sounds. Auscultation of the heart is the most challenging part of the cardiac physical examination and, in an era of increasing technologic demands, is daunting to new clinicians. To summarize the advice given by most experts, the examiner must:

1. Auscultate systematically across the precordium.
2. Visualize the cardiac anatomy under each point of auscultation, expecting to hear the physiologically associated sounds.

3. Memorize the cardiac cycle to enhance the ability to hear abnormal sounds.
4. Practice, practice, practice.[14]

First and Second Heart Sounds. Normal heart sounds are referred to as the *first heart sound* (S_1) and the *second heart sound* (S_2). S_1 is the sound associated with mitral and tricuspid valve closure and is heard most clearly in the mitral and tricuspid areas. S_2 (aortic and pulmonic closure) can be heard best at the second intercostal space to the right and left of the sternum (see Fig. 16-5). Both sounds are high-pitched and heard best with the diaphragm of the stethoscope (Box 16-9). Each sound is loudest in an auscultation area located "down-

---

Box 16-9

CHARACTERISTICS OF HEART SOUNDS ONE (S_1) AND TWO (S_2)

S_1	S_2
High-pitched	High-pitched
Loudest in mitral area (apex)	Loudest in aortic area (base)
SPLIT S_1	**Split S_2**
Normal split less than 20 msec	Normal split less than 30 msec
Split heard best in tricuspid area	Split heard best in pulmonic area
Important to differentiate between split S_1 and S_4	↑Split with inhalation
Occurs immediately before carotid upstroke	↓Split with exhalation

↑, Increased; ↓, decreased.

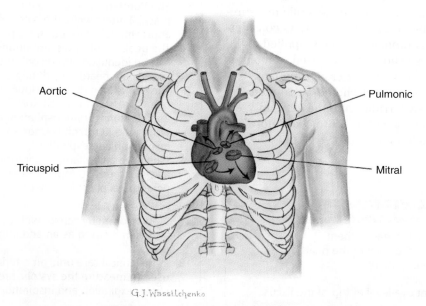

Fig. 16-6 Transmission of heart sounds to the thorax and their relationship to the anatomic position of the heart valves.

Aortic · Pulmonic · Tricuspid · Mitral

G.J.Wassilchenko

stream" from the actual valvular component of the sound, as shown in Fig. 16-6.

Physiologic Splitting of S₁ and S₂. Each normal heart sound has two components (right and left). Thus mitral valve closure and tricuspid valve closure are both responsible for S_1. Aortic valve and pulmonic valve closure are responsible for S_2. All the components of the split sounds are high-pitched and best heard with the diaphragm of the stethoscope (Fig. 16-7). Normally, sounds emitted from the left side are louder than the right because left ventricular contraction occurs milliseconds before right. *Physiologic splitting is accentuated by inspiration and usually disappears on expiration.* This splitting is most easily detected on inspiration because there is an increased blood return to the right side of the heart and a decreased amount of blood return to the left side of the heart. As a result, pulmonic valve closure is delayed because of the extra time needed for the increased blood volume to pass through the pulmonic valve, and aortic valve closure is early because of the relatively smaller amount of blood ejected from the left ventricle. The resulting heart sound is a split S_2 (you are able to hear the closure of each valve because there is more time between left and right contraction) (see Fig. 16-7).

Pathologic Splitting of S₁ and S₂. A variety of abnormalities can alter the intensity and timing of split heart sounds. For example, during auscultation in the pulmonic area, a pathological split is audible with a stethoscope if the pulmonic valve closure occurs after the aortic valve closes. Pathologic splitting of S_1 and S_2 is associated with specific cardiovascular conditions such as pulmonary hypertension, pulmonic stenosis, and right

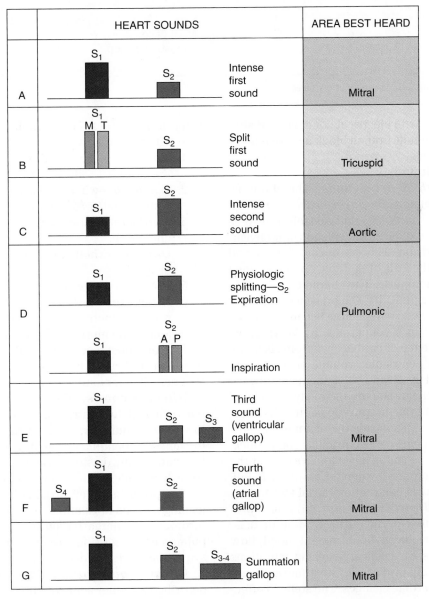

Fig. 16-7   Characteristics of normal and abnormal heart sounds and the auscultatory area where each is best heard.

Box 16-10

CHARACTERISTICS OF HEART SOUNDS THREE (S₃) AND FOUR (S₄)

S₃

Physiologic Causes

Related to diastolic motion and rapid filling of ventricles in early diastole

Can be normal in children and young adults (<40 yr)

Pathologic Causes

Ventricular dysfunction with an increase in end systolic volume (MI, heart failure, valvular disease, systemic or pulmonary hypertension)

Hyperdynamic states (anemia, thyrotoxicosis, mitral or tricuspid regurgitation)

Rhythmic Word Association

Kentucky

S_1 S_2 S_3

Synonyms

Ventricular gallop

Protodiastolic gallop

S₄

Related to diastolic motion and ventricular dilation with atrial contraction in late diastole

May occur with or without cardiac decompensation

Ventricular hypertrophy with a decrease in ventricular compliance (CAD, systemic hypertension, cardiomyopathy, aortic or pulmonary stenosis, increase in intensity with acute MI or angina)

Hyperkinetic states (anemia, thyrotoxicosis, arteriovenous fistula)

Acute valvular regurgitation

Tennessee

S_4 S_1 S_2

Atrial gallop

Presystolic gallop

MI, Myocardial infarction; *CAD,* coronary artery disease.

ventricular failure and with electrical conduction disturbances such as right bundle branch block and premature ventricular contractions.

Abnormal Heart Sounds

Third and Fourth Heart Sounds. The abnormal heart sounds are labeled as the *third heart sound* (S₃) and the *fourth heart sound* (S₄) and are referred to as *gallops* when auscultated during an episode of tachycardia. These low-pitched sounds occur during diastole and are best heard with the bell of stethoscope positioned lightly over the apical impulse. The characteristics of S₃ and S₄ are detailed in Box 16-10. The presence of S₃ may be normal in children and young adults because of rapid filling of the ventricle in a young, healthy heart. However, an S₃ in the presence of cardiac symptoms is an indication of increased ventricular volume suggestive of heart failure with fluid overload.[5,6] Not unexpectedly, the development of an S₃ heart sound is strongly associated with elevated levels of brain natriuretic peptide (BNP).

Auscultation of an S₄ also leads the examiner to suspect heart failure and decreased ventricular compliance. An S₄, also referred to as an "atrial gallop," occurs at the end of diastole (just before S₁) when the ventricle is full. It is associated with atrial contraction (atrial kick).

Heart Murmurs. *Heart valve murmurs* are prolonged extra sounds that occur during systole or diastole. Murmurs are produced by turbulent flood flow through the chambers of the heart causing vibrations that occur during systole or diastole. Most murmurs are caused by structural cardiac changes. The steps to effectively and accurately auscultate for cardiac murmurs are

listed in Box 16-11. Murmurs are characterized by specific criteria as follows:

1. ***Timing***—place in the cardiac cycle (systole/diastole).
2. ***Location***—where it is auscultated on the chest wall (mitral/aortic area).
3. ***Radiation***—how far the sound spreads across chest wall.
4. ***Quality***—whether the murmur is blowing, grating, or harsh.
5. ***Pitch***—whether the tone is high or low.
6. ***Intensity***—the loudness is graded on a scale using roman numerals I to VI; the higher the number, the louder the murmur, as shown in Box 16-12

The four most common valvular murmurs auscultated in adults are briefly discussed below. For more information on valvular anatomy refer to Chapter 15.

Mitral Stenosis. Mitral stenosis (MS) describes a narrowing of the mitral valve orifice. This produces a low-pitched murmur, which will vary in intensity and harshness depending on the degree of valvular stenosis. It occurs during diastole, is auscultated at the mitral area (fifth ICS, midclavicular line), and does not radiate. As the MS progresses, left atrial enlargement occurs, often leading to atrial fibrillation and development of left atrial thrombi. The increased left atrial pressure also creates pulmonary congestion, breathlessness, moist cough, and symptoms of right-sided heart failure.

Mitral Regurgitation. Mitral regurgitation (MR) is described as either acute or chronic. Causes of acute MR include rupture of a papillary muscle following an acute

Box 16-11

TECHNIQUE OF AUSCULTATION OF HEART SOUNDS AND MURMURS

1. Stethoscope
   a. *Diaphragm*
      Larger surface area
      Brings out higher frequency and filters out low frequency
      Use for listening to S_1/S_2 (split S_1/S_2), loud murmurs, pericardial friction rubs
   b. *Bell*
      Smaller surface area
      Filters out high-frequency sounds and accentuates low-frequency sounds
      Rest lightly on area (or else becomes a diaphragm)
2. Location: Heart sounds auscultated at A.P.T.M.
   A, *Aortic* area   (second right ICS along sternal border)
   P, *Pulmonic* area   (second left ICS along sternal border)
   T, *Tricuspid* area   (fourth left ICS along sternal border)
   M, *Mitral* area   (fifth ICS at MCL)
3. "Know your bases"
   • Base of the heart refers to the right and left second ICS beside the sternum S_2 where the aortic/pulmonic sounds are auscultated

• Apex/left ventricular area refers to the fifth ICS along the MCL
   —Most commonly referred to as the PMI
   —Also referred to as the mitral area
   —S_1 and mitral sounds are loudest here
• Erb's point: second aortic area (third left ICS along sternal border); pericardial friction rubs are heard best here
4. Palpation
   a. Location
   b. Palpate carotid pulse (or watch ECG to identify S_1/S_2)
5. Be "Quiet" and Patient!
   a. Listen for S_1/S_2 first, ignoring all other sounds
   b. "Inching technique"
   c. Once sure which is S_1/S_2, only then try to determine when the other sound comes in
   d. Is it systolic or diastolic?
   e. S_3 and S_4 are best heard with patient in left lateral decubitus position
      Note the location (suggests origin of sound)
      Note timing (S_4 comes just before S_1, and S_3 comes just after S_2)
6. Interpret the sounds based on clinical condition

ICS, Intercostal space; *MCL,* midclavicular line; *PMI,* point of maximal impulse.

Box 16-12

GRADING OF CARDIAC MURMURS

I/VI	Very faint; may be heard only in a quiet environment
II/VI	Quiet, but clearly audible
III/VI	Moderately loud
IV/VI	Loud; may be associated with a palpable thrill
V/VI	Very loud; thrill easily palpable
VI/VI	Very loud; may be heard with stethoscope off the chest
	Thrill palpable and visible

MI and rupture of one or more chordae tendinae. As a result, when the ventricle contracts during systole, a jet of blood is sent retrograde to the left atrium causing a sudden increase in left atrial pressure, acute pulmonary edema, and low cardiac output and leading to cardiogenic shock. Chronic mitral regurgitation is most often seen in the elderly as the valve structures sag and stretch over time. The murmur of MR is auscultated in the mitral area and occurs during systole. It is high-pitched and blowing, although the pitch and intensity will vary depending upon the degree of regurgitation. As MR progresses it radiates more widely, sometimes to under the left arm.

Aortic Stenosis. Aortic stenosis (AS) describes a narrowing of the aortic valve orifice. As a result the left ventricle (LV) faces increasing difficulty in ejecting blood to the aorta. The LV responds by increasing intraventricular pressure and adding muscle mass (LV hypertrophy) but over time, due to the pressure load and the stenotic aortic valve, the LV will fail and lose contractile force. The decreased blood volume entering the aorta during systole means that the coronary arteries do not fill efficiently, and chest pain is a common symptom of aortic stenosis. This chest pain can be difficult to differentiate from angina caused by coronary artery disease. Other symptoms include dizziness, syncope, and breathlessness caused by left-sided heart failure. Once symptoms occur, the clinical course is poor unless the aortic valve is replaced. Two years following onset of AS symptoms, survival can be less than 50% without aortic valve replacement. The murmur of aortic stenosis occurs during systole. It is auscultated at the aortic area (second intercostal space [ICS] [right sternal border—RSB]). AS produces a low-pitched murmur that does not radiate, although the tone of the murmur will vary depending on the degree of valvular obstruction. Since there is not a strong correlation between the loudness of the murmur, clinical symptoms, and the severity of the AS, it is advisable to perform an echocardiogram to visualize the valve, once an AS murmur is detected.

| Table 16-4 | Characteristics of Some Murmurs |

Defects	Timing in the Cardiac Cycle	Pitch, Intensity, Quality	Location, Radiation
SYSTOLIC MURMURS			
Mitral regurgitation	S_1 — S_2	High Harsh Blowing	Mitral area May radiate to axilla
Tricuspid regurgitation	S_1 — S_2	High Often faint, but varies Blowing	Tricuspid RLSB, apex, LLSB, epigastric areas Little radiation
Ventricular septal defect	S_1 — S_2	High Loud Blowing	Left sternal border
Aortic stenosis	S_1 ◇ S_2	Chhhh hh Medium Rough, harsh	Aortic area to suprasternal notch, right side of neck, apex
Pulmonary stenosis	S_1 ◇ S_2	Low to medium Loud Harsh, grinding	Pulmonic area No radiation
DIASTOLIC MURMURS			
Mitral stenosis	Atrial kick S_2 — S_1	Low Quiet to loud with thrill Rough rumble	Mitral area Usually no radiation
Tricuspid stenosis	Atrial kick S_2 — S_1	Medium Quiet; louder with inspiration Rumble	Tricuspid area or epigastrium Little radiation
Aortic regurgitation	S_2 — S_1	High Faint to medium Blowing	Aortic area to LLSB and aorta Erb's point
Pulmonic regurgitation	S_2 — S_1	Medium Faint Blowing	Pulmonic area No radiation

RLSB, Right lower sternal border; *LLSB,* left lower sternal border. Atrial kick is a synonym for atrial contraction.

Box 16-13

AUSCULTATION OF THE CARDIAC VALVES

AORTIC AREA
S_2 loud
Aortic systolic murmur

PULMONIC AREA
S_2 loud and split with inhalation
Pulmonic valve murmurs

ERB'S POINT
S_2 split with inhalation
Aortic diastolic murmur
Pericardial friction rub

TRICUSPID AREA
S_1 split
Right ventricular S_3 and S_4
Tricuspid valve murmurs
Murmur of ventricular septal defect

MITRAL AREA
S_1 loud
Left ventricular S_3 and S_4
Mitral valve murmurs

Box 16-14

DESCRIPTION OF INNOCENT MURMURS

- Always systolic
- Soft, short (grade I or grade II, low-pitched)
- Modified by change in position
- Normal S_2
- Most common at left sternal border

Aortic Insufficiency. Aortic regurgitation (AR), also commonly known as "aortic insufficiency" (AI) describes an incompetent aortic valve. It is often described in layperson's terms as a "leaking valve." Once the LV has ejected blood into the aorta the valve normally closes, maintains a tight seal, and prevents blood from moving back into the left ventricle. If the valve cusps do not maintain this seal, the sound of blood flowing back into the LV during diastole is heard as a high pitched, blowing murmur. This early diastolic murmur is not only initially audible at the aortic area (second ICS RSB), but as the aortic regurgitation progresses, it can be auscultated the length of the left sternal border. As with all valvular murmurs the pitch and intensity of the murmur will vary with the degree of regurgitation. For expected abnormal findings at each of the key auscultatory areas, see Box 16-13; and to see a comparison of the features of the most common valvular murmurs, see Table 16-4.

Innocent Murmurs. In children, adolescents, or healthy young adults, systolic "high flow" murmurs are common and are a result of vigorous ventricular contraction. These nonpathologic murmurs are termed *innocent murmurs.* They are always systolic, have a low to medium pitch (heard best with the bell of the stethoscope), and are grade I to II intensity with a blowing quality. They are often heard best in the tricuspid area and do not radiate (Box 16-14).

Murmurs Associated With Myocardial Infarction. At the bedside, the nurse is often the first person to aus-

cultate a new murmur. The holosystolic or pansystolic murmurs that can occur acutely as a complication of MI are good examples.

Papillary Muscle Rupture. The auscultation of a new, high-pitched, holosystolic, blowing murmur at the cardiac apex heralds mitral valve regurgitation secondary to papillary muscle dysfunction. This murmur may be soft (I/VI or II/VI) and occur only during ischemic episodes when the papillary muscle contractility is impaired, but its presence is associated with persistent pain, ventricular failure, and higher mortality. If the murmur is loud (V/VI or VI/VI), harsh, and radiating in all directions from the apex, the papillary muscle or chordae tendineae may have ruptured. The clinical auscultation of a new murmur should be confirmed by transthoracic or transesophageal echocardiography (TEE).[15] Papillary muscle rupture is an emergency situation necessitating immediate medical and surgical intervention.

Ventricular Septal Rupture. Ventricular septal rupture (VSR) is a rare emergency situation that can occur following an acute MI. VSR describes a new opening in the septum between the two ventricles. It creates a harsh, holosystolic murmur that is loudest (by auscultation) along the left sternal border. The clinical picture associated with acute ventricular septal rupture is that of acute ventricular failure and cardiogenic shock. Immediate diagnosis and treatment are necessary to prevent death.

Cardiac Rubs

Pericardial Friction Rub. A *pericardial friction rub* is a sound that can occur within 2 to 7 days of an MI. The friction rub results from pericardial inflammation *(pericarditis).* Classically a pericardia friction rub is a grating or scratching sound that is both systolic and diastolic, corresponding with cardiac motion within the pericardial sac. It is often associated with chest pain, which can be aggravated by deep inspiration, coughing, swallowing, and changing position. It is important to differentiate pericarditis from acute myocardial ischemia, and the detection of the pericardial friction rub through auscultation can assist in this differentiation, leading to effective diagnosis and treatment.

REFERENCES

1. Gibbons RJ et al: ACC/AHA 2002 Guideline update for the management of patients with chronic stable angina—summary article: a report of the American College of Cardiology/American Heart Association Task Force on Practice Guidelines (Committee on the Management of Patients with Chronic Stable Angina), *Circulation* 107(1): 149-158, 2003.

2. Wong WM, Fass R: Noncardiac chest pain, *Curr Treat Options Gastroenterol* 7(4):273-278, 2004.

3. Faybush EM, Fass R: Gastroesophageal reflux disease in noncardiac chest pain, *Gastroenterol Clin North Am* 33(1): 41-54, 2004.

4. Chun AA, McGee SR: Bedside diagnosis of coronary artery disease: a systematic review, *Am J Med* 117(5):334-343, 2004.

5. Drazner MH et al: Prognostic importance of elevated jugular venous pressure and a third heart sound in patients with heart failure, *N Engl J Med* 345(8):574-581, 2001.

6. Drazner MH, Rame JE, Dries DL: Third heart sound and elevated jugular venous pressure as markers of the subsequent development of heart failure in patients with asymptomatic left ventricular dysfunction, *Am J Med* 114(6):431-437, 2003.

7. Wiese J: The abdominojugular reflux sign, *Am J Med* 109(1):59-61, 2000.

8. Perloff D et al: Human blood pressure determination by sphygmomanometry, Dallas, 2001, American Heart Association.

9. Chobanian AV et al: Seventh report of the Joint National Committee on Prevention, Detection, Evaluation, and Treatment of High Blood Pressure, *Hypertension* 42(6):1206-1252, 2003.

10. Fields LE et al: The burden of adult hypertension in the United States 1999 to 2000: a rising tide, *Hypertension* 44(4):398-404, 2004.

11. Shadman R et al: Subclavian artery stenosis: prevalence, risk factors, and association with cardiovascular diseases, *J Am Coll Cardiol* 44(3):618-623, 2004.

12. Wu LA, Nishimura RA: Images in clinical medicine. Pulsus paradoxus, *N Engl J Med* 349(7):666, 2003.

13. Swami, A, Spodick DH: Pulsus paradoxus in cardiac tamponade: a pathophysiologic continuum, *Clin Cardiol* 26(5): 215-217, 2003.

14. Barrett MJ et al: Mastering cardiac murmurs: the power of repetition, *Chest* 126(2):470-475, 2004.

15. Antman EM et al: ACC/AHA guidelines for the management of patients with ST-elevation myocardial infarction—executive summary: a report of the American College of Cardiology/American Heart Association Task Force on Practice Guidelines (Writing Committee to Revise the 1999 Guidelines for the Management of Patients with Acute Myocardial Infarction), *Can J Cardiol* 20(10):977-1025, 2004.

CHAPTER 17

Cardiovascular Diagnostic Procedures

LABORATORY ASSESSMENT

Laboratory assessment of cardiovascular status is obtained through studies of blood serum. Accurate interpretation of these laboratory studies, along with the clinical picture, enables the critical care team to diagnose, treat, and assess the response to therapeutic interventions.

Laboratory studies of blood serum are performed to assess the following:

1. Electrolyte levels that can alter cardiac muscle contraction.
2. Cardiac biomarkers that reflect myocardial cellular integrity or infarction.
3. Hematologic status to evaluate risk of anemia and infection.
4. Coagulation times.
5. Serum lipid levels.
6. Status of other organ systems that can secondarily affect cardiac function.

ELECTROLYTES

Potassium. During depolarization and repolarization of nerve and muscle fiber, potassium and sodium exchange occurs intracellularly and extracellularly. The potassium gradient across the cell membrane determines conduction velocity and helps confine pacing activity to the sinus node. Thus either excess or deficiency of potassium can alter myocardial muscle function. Normal serum potassium levels are 3.5 to 4.5 mEq/L.

Hyperkalemia. Elevated serum potassium, termed *hyperkalemia*, can be caused by a variety of conditions that include excess potassium administration, extensive skeletal muscle destruction (rhabdomyolysis),[1-2] tumor lysis syndrome,[3] renal failure,[4] and some drugs.[5] Drugs that may induce hyperkalemia include potassium-sparing diuretics, angiotensin-converting enzyme (ACE) inhibitor drugs and angiotensin receptor–blocker (ARB) drugs.[5] Hyperkalemia elicits significant changes in the electrocardiogram (ECG) because it decreases the rate of ventricular depolarization, shortens repolarization, and also depresses atrioventricular (AV) conduction.[6] As

the serum levels of potassium rise above normal (greater than 4.5 mEq/L), evidence of these phenomena is clearly seen on the ECG (Fig. 17-1, *A*). Tall, peaked T waves are usually, although not uniquely, associated with early hyperkalemia and are followed by prolongation of the PR interval, loss of the P wave, widening of the QRS complex, and asystole. Severely elevated serum potassium (greater than 8 mEq/L) will cause a wide QRS tachycardia as shown in the 12-lead ECG in Fig. 17-1, *B*). If not corrected, severe hyperkalemia will lead to ventricular fibrillation or cardiac standstill.

This life-threatening condition can be acutely managed with an intravenous insulin/glucose infusion that drives the potassium inside the cell and temporarily out of the serum. Potassium is permanently removed from the serum by cation-exchange resin products, such as Kayexalate, placed into the gastrointestinal (GI) tract, or removed directly from the blood by hemodialysis. Coexisting low serum sodium, calcium, or pH levels potentiate the cardiac effects of hyperkalemia.

Hypokalemia. A low serum potassium level, called *hypokalemia* (less than 3.5 mEq/L), is commonly caused by GI losses, diuretic therapy with insufficient replacement, or chronic steroid therapy. Hypokalemia is also reflected by changes on the ECG (Fig. 17-2). The earliest ECG change is often premature ventricular contractions (PVCs), which can deteriorate into ventricular tachycardia or fibrillation (VT or VF) without appropriate potassium replacement.

Hypokalemia impairs myocardial conduction and prolongs ventricular repolarization. This can be seen by a prominent U wave (a positive deflection following the T wave on the ECG). The U wave is not totally unique to hypokalemia, but its presence is a signal for the clinician to check the serum potassium level. In the critical care unit, where patients are receiving diuretics and/or have nasogastric tubes to suction, the serum potassium is checked frequently by the critical care nurse and replaced intravenously to normal levels to prevent dysrhythmias. Great care must be taken when replacing potassium intravenously, to ensure it is diluted sufficiently and administered slowly to prevent accidental

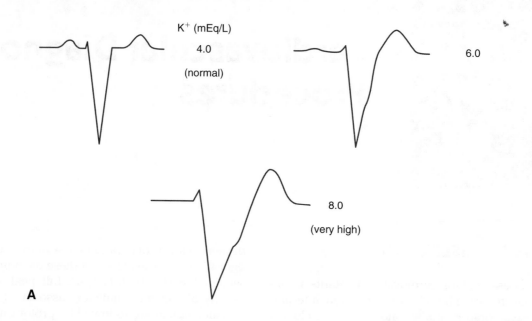

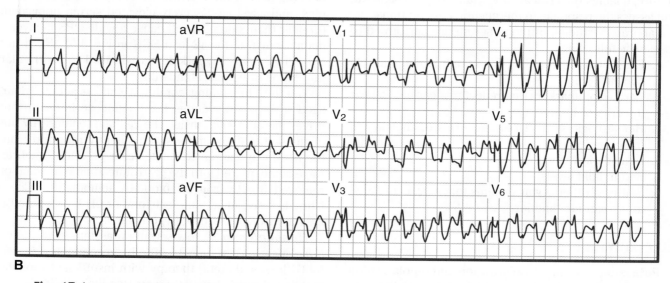

Fig. 17-1 Effects of hyperkalemia. **A,** Stages in hyperkalemia from normal potassium levels to plasma levels of 8 mEq/L. At approximately 6 mEq/L, the P wave flattens, the QRS broadens, and the ST segment disappears, with the S wave flowing into the tall, tented T wave. **B,** 12-Lead ECG of a patient with a serum potassium of 9.1 mEq/L.

overdose. Potassium is considered a "high-alert medication" and additional safety procedures are recommended for this drug (see the Patient Safety Alert feature on Medication Administration). If concomitant hypomagnesemia exists, successful replenishment of potassium deficit cannot be accomplished until the hypomagnesemia is reversed. See Box 17-1 for electrolyte values that affect cardiac contractility.

Calcium. Calcium (Ca^{++}) is an important cation in the body. Calcium metabolism is controlled by many factors including normal parathyroid hormone (PTH) function, calcitonin, and vitamin D acting on target or-

gans such as the kidney, bone, and the GI tract.[7] Calcium is an important mediator of many cardiovascular functions because of its effect on vascular tone, myocardial contractility, and cardiac excitability.[7]

Serum calcium values are recorded in three possible ways, depending on the hospital laboratory: milliequivalents per liter (mEq/L), milligrams per deciliter (mg/dl), or millimols per liter (mmol/L).

In the bloodstream, 55% of calcium is bound to protein (primarily albumin) and found in complexes with anions such as chloride and phosphate. As such it is not physiologically available to the body.[7] The remain-

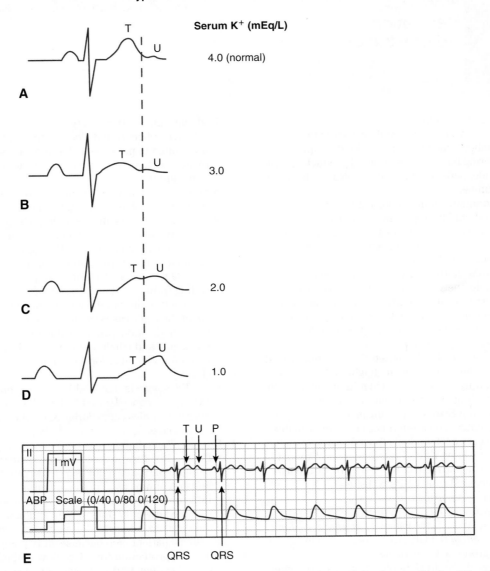

Fig. 17-2 Hypokalemia. **A,** At a normal serum concentration of 3.5 to 4.5 mEq/L, the amplitude of the T wave is appreciably greater than that of the U wave. **B,** By the time the serum potassium level has dropped to 3 mEq/L, the amplitudes of the T and U waves are approaching each other. **C** and **D,** With a further drop in the level of potassium, the U wave begins to tower over and fuse with the T wave. **E,** ECG tracing from a patient with a serum potassium of 2.6 mEq/L, with a prominent U wave.

ing 45% of calcium is biologically active and is called the *ionized calcium*.[7] The normal values for total and ionized serum calcium levels are listed in Box 17-1. The normal serum concentration of ionized calcium is maintained within very narrow limits; changes in ionized calcium level are responsible for the clinical effects of hypercalcemia and hypocalcemia. The only accurate way to determine the level of ionized calcium—described as physiologically active, "unbound" or "free"—is to measure the serum value with a laboratory assay. The mathematically calculated values that extrapolate from total calcium and serum albumin lev-

els are severely inaccurate and variable and should no longer be used.[7,8]

Hypercalcemia. Hypercalcemia is defined as increased amounts of ionized calcium (greater than 4.8 mg/dl or 1.30 mmol/L) or increased amounts of total serum calcium (greater than 10.5 mg/dl or 2.60 mmol/L). Serum calcium levels are increased by bone tumors; primary hyperparathyroidism caused by elevated PTH levels; excessive intake of supplemental calcium and vitamin D, usually in oral antacids; hypomagnesemia; and as a complication of kidney failure from decreased renal excretion of calcium.[7] Hypercalcemia affects

PATIENT SAFETY ALERT

Medication Administration

1. Accurate patient identification.
   - Use at least two patient identifiers (not patient's room number) whenever taking blood samples or administering medications or blood products. Examples include: patient name, date of birth, or hospital record number.
2. Effective communication among caregivers.
   - Hospitals should have (or implement) a process for taking verbal or telephone orders that requires a verification "read-back" of the complete order by the person receiving the order.
   - Because thousands of brand name and generic drugs are available, there is always potential for error. Similar drug names, either written or spoken, account for approximately 15% of all medication error reports to the *U.S. Pharmacopeia* (USP) Medication Errors Reporting program.
   - In March 2001 the USP released "Use Caution, Avoid Confusion," an updated list highlighting hundreds of confusing drug name sets and identifying more than 750 unique drug names that have been reported to the Medication Errors Reporting program. A poster and a laminated, quick-reference card are available for health care professionals free of charge from the USP by contacting USP's Practitioner and Product Experience department at 800-487-7776, or the list may be accessed from USP's website at www.usp.org/reporting/review/.
   - An organizational method to decrease the number of medication errors is the use of *computerized physician order entry* (CPOE), as advocated by the Leapfrog group: www.leapfroggroup.org.
   - Standardize the abbreviations, acronyms, and symbols used throughout the organization, including a list of abbreviations, acronyms, and symbols not to use.
   - Examples of problematic abbreviations include "U" for "units" and "μg" for "micrograms." When handwritten, "U" can be mistaken for a zero; in numerous case reports, an insulin dosage in "U" was interpreted as "0." Using the abbreviation "μg" instead of "mcg" for micrograms is also problematic; when handwritten, the symbol "μ" can look like an "m."
   - Use of "trailing zeros" (e.g., 2.0 vs. 2) and a "leading decimal point without a leading zero" (e.g., .2 instead of 0.2) are also dangerous prescription-writing practices. Misinterpretation of such abbreviations has caused and could lead to 10-fold dosing errors.
   - Information on similar medication issues is available on the web pages of the Joint Commission for the Accreditation of Healthcare Organizations (JCAHO): www.JCAHO.org.

3. High-alert medication safety.
   - Remove concentrated electrolytes (including but not limited to potassium chloride, potassium phosphate, and hypertonic sodium chloride) from patient care units.
   - Standardize and limit the number of drug concentrations available in the organization.
   - In the first 2 years after enacting a "sentinel event" reporting mechanism, the most common category was medication errors, and the most frequently implicated drug was potassium chloride (KCl). JCAHO reviewed 10 incidents of patient death resulting from misadministration of KCl. Eight were the result of direct infusion of concentrated KCl. In six of the eight cases the KCl was mistaken for another medication, primarily due to similarities in packaging and labeling. Most often, KCl was mistaken for sodium chloride, heparin, or furosemide (Lasix).
   - JCAHO suggests that health care organizations NOT make concentrated KCl available outside the pharmacy unless appropriate, specific safeguards are in place.
4. Infusion Pump Safety
   - Ensure free-flow protection on all general-use and patient-controlled analgesia (PCA) intravenous (IV) infusion pumps used in the organization.
   - Infusion pumps that do not provide protection from the free flow of IV fluid or medication into the patient are hazardous. USP reported six cases in which a patient died because an IV pump did not provide protection from free flow of the IV solution. (October 1991 to November 1999: four additional cases resulted in near-death.)
   - *Free flow* occurs when IV solution flows freely, under force of gravity, without being controlled by the infusion pump. Free flow typically occurs after the administration set is temporarily removed from the pump to transfer a patient to another area, change a patient's gown, or place a patient on a radiography table. Clinicians can greatly reduce this risk by using administration sets with set-based anti–free-flow mechanisms that prevent gravity free flow by closing off the IV tubing to prohibit flow when the administration set is removed from the pump.

The information in this feature can be accessed on the web pages of the following three safety organizations:
www.JCAHO.org
www.usp.org
www.leapfroggroup.org

Box 17-1

CHEMISTRY VALUES THAT AFFECT CARDIAC CONTRACTILITY AND CONDUCTION

NORMAL RANGES

	mEq/L	MG/DL	MMOL/L
Potassium (K^+)	3.5-4.5		
Ionized calcium (Ca) mmol/L		4.0-5.0	1.00-1.30
Total calcium (Ca^{++}) mmol/L		8.5-10.5	2.00-2.60
Magnesium (Mg^{++})	1.5-2.0	1.8-2.4	

NOTE: Laboratory values may be reported as either mEq/L, mg/dl, or mmol/L.

Each measurement parameter used will produce a different value. Some electrolytes are reported with more than one reference value.

Different clinical laboratories use different reference values.

Cited reference values may vary slightly from between hospital laboratories.

multiple organs, causes smooth muscle relaxation, and can lead to neurologic changes such as lethargy, confusion, and even coma.[7] Elevated serum calcium has the cardiovascular effect of strengthening contractility and shortening ventricular repolarization, demonstrated on the ECG by a shortened QTc interval.[7] Rhythm disturbances may include bradycardia; first-, second-, and third-degree heart block; and bundle branch block. Hypercalcemia can potentiate the effects of digitalis, precipitate digitalis toxicity, and cause hypertension.[7,9]

Management of hypercalcemia involves promotion of renal excretion of calcium by diuretics and high-volume intravenous (IV) normal saline at 200 to 300 ml/hour if tolerated by the cardiac, pulmonary, and renal systems. Patients who cannot tolerate this clinical regimen should be hemodialyzed using a low-calcium dialysate.[7]

Hypocalcemia. *Hypocalcemia* is defined as an *ionized calcium* level below normal (below 4 mg/dl or 1.05 mmol/L) or a low total serum calcium level. Hypocalcemia (measured by ionized calcium) is a common finding and is reported to occur in 26% to 88% of critically ill patients, depending on the admitting diagnosis.[10] The more severe the patient's illness, the greater the risk of developing hypocalcemia.[10] Transfusions of blood from the blood bank lower serum calcium levels because the citrate used as an anticoagulant in banked blood binds to the calcium. This is called *citrate chelation.* If citrate is used during hemodialysis or plasmapheresis, it will have the same calcium-binding (chelating) effect.[7] Phosphate also binds to calcium and will lower the serum calcium level.[7] Metabolic alkalosis often coexists with hypocalcemia.[7] The cardiovascular effects of hypocalcemia include decreased myocardial contractility, decreased car-

diac output, and hypotension. Rhythm disturbances with severe hypocalcemia are variable, ranging from bradycardia to ventricular tachycardia and asystole. When the ionized calcium is low, the ECG may show a prolonged QTc interval (Fig. 17-3). This predisposes a patient to the life-threatening ventricular dysrhythmia called *torsades de pointes.*

Management of hypocalcemia, especially when the ionized calcium is low, involves infusion of IV calcium chloride or IV calcium gluconate. Calcium chloride is generally used to raise calcium levels because it contains more calcium for the same volume.[7]

- Calcium chloride provides 27 mg elemental calcium per ml.
- Calcium gluconate provides 9 mg elemental calcium per ml.

Magnesium. Magnesium (Mg^{++}) is essential for many enzyme, protein, lipid, and carbohydrate functions in the body and is critical for the production and use of energy. The body stores most magnesium in bone (53%), muscle (27%), and soft tissues (19%); only a tiny proportion resides within the bloodstream—red blood cells contain 0.5% and serum contains 0.3%.[11] As with other electrolytes (see foregoing discussion of calcium), the ionized portion of the serum magnesium is the biologically active component that is available for biochemical processes. Serum magnesium is 67% ionized, 19% protein-bound and 14% complexed.[11] The serum magnesium is what is normally measured in a routine blood test. Serum magnesium can be reported either in mEq/L, mg/dl, or mmol/L, depending on the laboratory running the analysis. The normal serum range is from 1.5 to 2 mEq/L; 1.8 to 2.4 mg/dl; or 0.7 to 1.1 mmol/L. These represent the same serum level of magnesium despite different measurement guidelines used in the report. It is important to anticipate that normal reference values will vary between different hospital laboratories.

Hypermagnesemia. The incidence of hypermagnesemia is rare in comparison with hypomagnesemia, and it occurs secondary to kidney failure, tumor lysis syndrome, or iatrogenic overtreatment.

Hypomagnesemia. A total serum magnesium concentration below 1.5 mEq/L defines *hypomagnesemia.* It is commonly associated with other electrolyte imbalances, most notably alterations in potassium, calcium, and phosphorus. Low serum magnesium can stem from many causes. Hypomagnesemia is caused by insufficient intake in the diet or in total parental nutrition (TPN) and is associated with chronic alcohol abuse. In the critical care unit, aggressive diuresis with loop diuretics will lower both serum potassium and magnesium levels.[11] Diarrhea can be a significant cause of magnesium loss because lower GI fluids contain up to 15 mEq/L magnesium; vomiting or gastric suction causes less depletion because the upper GI fluids contain about 1 mEq/L.[11] Another cause of magnesium depletion is rapid administra-

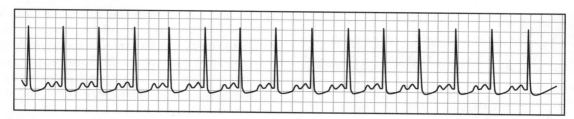

Fig. 17-3   Abnormal QT prolongation in a hypocalcemic patient. The patient is a 50-year-old woman admitted to the critical care unit with alcoholic liver disease and malnourishment. Total calcium is 5.1 mg/dl, and albumin is 1.3 mg/dl. The QT interval (0.55 second) is markedly prolonged for the heart rate (100/min). The QT interval varies with the heart rate and can be "corrected" using the formula $\sqrt{\dfrac{QT}{RR}} = QT_c$ (corrected QT). The corrected QT (QT_c) should be 0.44 second or less. The QT_c in the ECG tracing pictured is 0.55 second. Hypocalcemia lengthens ventricular repolarization. A quick method of assessing the QT interval is to remember that it is usually less than half of the RR interval. If it is more than half of the RR interval, it is prolonged. (From Yucha CB, Toto KH: *Crit Care Clin North Am* 6(4):747, 1994.)

tion of citrated blood products, which causes the citrate to bind to the magnesium, a condition known as *citrate chelation*. In chronic hypomagnesemia the serum levels will be replenished from the bone stores.[11]

Both hypokalemia and hypocalcemia are likely to be unresponsive to replacement therapy until the hypomagnesemia is corrected.[7,11] Expected cardiac-related changes with hypomagnesemia include hypertension and vasospasm, including coronary artery spasm. Some studies have linked magnesium depletion to sudden cardiac death, to an increased incidence of acute myocardial infarction (MI), and to the occurrence of ventricular dysrhythmias.[11]

In hypomagnesemia the ECG changes are similar to those seen with hypokalemia[11] (see Fig. 17-2) and hypocalcemia (see Fig. 17-3): prolonged PR and QTc intervals, presence of U waves, T-wave flattening, and a widened QRS complex. Cardiac dysrhythmias may be supraventricular or ventricular and include torsades de pointes. Dysrhythmias associated with hypomagnesemia may not respond to the usual antidysrhythmic drugs, but they often respond well to magnesium infusions. Magnesium sulfate (IV) is the treatment of choice for torsades de pointes. It is important to evaluate kidney function when administering magnesium to avoid precipitating hypermagnesium states.

CARDIAC BIOMARKER STUDIES

Cardiac Biomarkers. Cardiac biomarkers, previously described by the term *"cardiac enzymes,"* are proteins that are released from severely damaged myocardial tissue cells.[12,13] When myocardial cells are damaged, they release detectable proteins into the bloodstream so that a rise in biomarkers can be correlated with myocardial cellular damage. Biomarkers are divided into *cardiac-specific*—present only in cardiac muscle—and *nonspecific*—present in many muscles of the body. The biomarkers that are routinely measured include the cardiac-specific *troponin I (TnI)* and *CK-MB*, and the nonspecific muscle biomarkers *myoglobin, creatine ki-*

nase (CK), and *troponin T (TnT)*. See Table 17-1 for a summary of this information.[14] Unfortunately, in many hospitals the laboratory turnaround time for results of cardiac biomarkers is between 60 to 90 minutes, which limits the usefulness of the biomarkers in the emergency room when the patient is first admitted with symptoms of acute coronary syndrome.[14] If point-of-care testing at the bedside is used, the results are available more quickly and may be more helpful in the clinical decision-making process.[14]

CK and CK-MB. The traditional "gold standard" for diagnosing MI is the rise and fall of the serum MB fraction of the enzyme CK within 24 hours after the onset of symptoms. The CK-MB serum levels rise 4 to 8 hours after MI, peak at 15 to 24 hours, and remain elevated for 2 to 3 days (see Table 17-1). Serial samples are drawn routinely every at 6- or 8-hour intervals, and three samples are usually sufficient to support or rule out the diagnosis of MI. CK-MB is never an isolated test; it is always performed in conjunction with cardiac troponin levels.

Troponin T and Troponin I. The *troponins* are a structurally related group of proteins found in both cardiac and skeletal muscle. The three troponin proteins are: troponin C, cardiac troponin I (cTnI), cardiac troponin T (cTnT).

Troponin C is very similar in both cardiac and skeletal muscle, a fact that invalidates it as a marker of myocardial injury. Troponin I is found only in cardiac muscle, and troponin T displays significant amino acid differences between the cardiac and skeletal muscle complexes; both troponins are excellent markers of myocardial muscle damage. In cardiac muscle the troponin complexes (cTnI and cTnT) are mostly bound to the thin actin filament, which is disrupted when the muscle is deprived of oxygen (infarction). Small amounts of free cTnI and cTnT are also in the myocardial cell cytoplasm that produces the initial serum rise of troponin after cardiac cell wall disruption. cTnI is found only in cardiac muscle, and cardiac cTnT is structurally different from the general muscle (nonmyocardial); thus either or both

Table 17-1	Serum Biomarkers After Acute Myocardial Infarction (MI)		
Serum Biomarker	Time to Initial Elevation (Hours)*	Peak Elevation† (Hours)*	Return to Baseline (Hours/Days)*
Troponin I (TnI)	3-12	24	5-10 days
Troponin T (TnT)	3-12	12-48	5-14 days
CK-MB	3-12	24	2-3 days
Myoglobin	1-4	6-7	24 hours

CK, Creatine kinase.
*Time periods represent average reported values.
†Does not include patients who have had reperfusion therapy.

can be used as markers of acute MI, both in centralized laboratory tests and in bedside point-of-care testing.[14] Several different methods of laboratory assay are currently in use, which means that "normal" serum levels will vary between different clinical settings, although cardiac serum troponin levels (cTnI and cTnT) are low in the absence of myocardial muscle damage.

The initial elevation of troponin (cTnI and cTnT) and CK-MB occurs 3 to 6 hours after the acute myocardial damage has occurred. This means that if an individual comes to the emergency department as soon as chest pain is experienced, the enzymes will not have risen. For this reason, it is current clinical practice to diagnose an acute MI by 12-lead ECG and clinical symptoms, without the aid of checking for elevated cardiac biomarkers.[13]

Because cTnI is found only in cardiac muscle, it is a highly specific biomarker for myocardial damage, considerably more specific than CK-MB.[15] As a consequence, patients with a positive cTnI and a negative CK-MB usually "rule in" for an acute MI.[15] A negative cTnI result that remains negative many hours after an episode of chest pain is a strong indicator that the patient is not experiencing an acute MI.[16] Of course, even with a negative cTnI, symptoms of chest pain still indicate that the patient should have a comprehensive cardiac evaluation to determine if there is underlying coronary artery disease present that may later lead to complications.[12,13,16]

Lactate Dehydrogenase. Use of the troponins has replaced clinical measurement of *lactate dehydrogenase (LDH)* for identification of an MI that is several days old by the time a person first comes to the hospital. The cardiac-specific troponins remain elevated in the bloodstream for about a week following myocardial cell necrosis and thus can be used to diagnose a recent MI even though the acute manifestations of chest pain, ST-segment elevation, and CK-MB elevation are no longer present.

Myoglobin. Myoglobin is a nonspecific indicator of myocardial cell damage because it is identical in both cardiac and skeletal muscle. It is useful because it is the biomarker that rises earliest in the serum. Myoglobin begins to rise about 1 to 2 hours after myocardial injury. It is never used alone but can be used in conjunction with other more cardiac-specific biomarkers.

Cardiac Biomarkers and Reperfusion. Current management of ST-elevation myocardial infarction (STEMI) is to open the coronary artery obstructed by a thrombus and reperfuse the injured area as rapidly as possible.[13] Individuals who have recent onset of chest pain (within 12 hours) are candidates for reperfusion therapies, including fibrinolytic agents ("clot-busters"), cardiac catheterization with percutaneous coronary interventions (PCI) such as balloon angioplasty, atherectomy, or stent placement. If successful, these interventions may totally abort the MI or limit the amount of cardiac muscle damage, resulting in an early rise and fall of the cardiac biomarkers as illustrated in Fig. 18-12.[13] After reperfusion, the serum CK-MB level rises dramatically (generally doubles within 90 minutes) and peaks early (about 10 hours). Cardiac biomarker samples are drawn at admission, before administration of thrombolytic therapy or PCI, and then at 6- or 8-hour intervals for 18 to 24 hours to detect any biomarker rise and assess the return of effective myocardial reperfusion.

HEMATOLOGIC STUDIES

Hematologic laboratory studies that are routinely ordered for the management of patients with altered cardiovascular status are red blood cell (RBC or erythrocyte) level, hemoglobin (Hgb) level, hematocrit (Hct) level, and white blood cell (WBC or leukocyte) level.

Red Blood Cells. The normal amount of RBCs in a person varies with age, gender, environmental temperature, altitude, and exercise. Males produce 4.5 million to 6 million RBCs per cubic millimeter, whereas the normal level for females is 4 million to 5.5 million per cubic millimeter. *Anemia* is the clinical condition that occurs when not enough red blood cells are available to carry oxygen to the tissues. *Polycythemia* is the condition that occurs when excess RBCs are produced.

Hemoglobin. Hgb levels normally range from 14 to 18 g/dl in males and from 12 to 16 g/dl in females.

Hematocrit. Hct is the volume percentage of RBCs in whole blood—40% to 54% for males and 38% to 48% for females.

White Blood Cells. Most inflammatory processes that produce necrotic tissue within the heart muscle, such as rheumatic fever, endocarditis, and MI, increase the WBC level. White blood cells are also known as leukocytes, and a WBC test may be called a serum leukocyte count. The normal WBC level for both genders is 5,000 to 10,000 per cubic millimeter. The WBC level also increases in response to infection.

Platelets. The normal platelet count is 150,000 to 400,000 cells per cubic millimeter (cmm). Less commonly the normal platelet count range will be written as 150 to 400 × 10^9/L. Normally, the platelet count is the only laboratory value that is reported. Unfortunately, there is no routine test available for critical care patients that can evaluate platelet functionality. Platelets are important because they are the first cells to be activated when the coagulation system is stimulated. There are many drugs that inhibit platelet function and make the platelets "slippery" so that they do not clump together to activate the clotting process. Sometimes the antiplatelet action of a drug is its intended role, such as with aspirin used to prevent acute coronary syndrome, and sometimes it is an unintended side effect. If the platelet count is low this is termed *thrombocytopenia.*

Blood Coagulation Studies. Coagulation studies are ordered to determine blood-clotting effectiveness. Anticoagulants—most notably heparin, direct thrombin inhibitors, warfarin, and platelet inhibitory agents are administered daily in critical care units for a myriad of clinical reasons.[17-19] It is essential for the nurse to understand the laboratory tests that are used to monitor the effectiveness of therapeutic anticoagulation. In addition, many new anticoagulants are under development that will require close clinical surveillance of these specialized laboratory tests.[20]

Prothrombin Time. Most coagulation study results are reported as the length of time in seconds it takes for blood to form a clot in the laboratory test tube. The *prothrombin time (PT)* is no longer directly used to determine the therapeutic dosage of warfarin (Coumadin) necessary to achieve anticoagulation. The PT is not standardized between laboratories so the result of this test is always reported as a standardized *international normalized ratio (INR).*[21]

International Normalized Ratio. The INR was developed by the World Health Organization (WHO) in 1982 to standardize PT results among clinical laboratories worldwide.[21] Table 17-2 illustrates target INR ranges for different cardiovascular conditions that require anticoagulation.[21] It is recommended that the INR be used to guide anticoagulation therapy with warfarin rather than the PT, especially if the PT results are analyzed at more than one laboratory.[21]

When a patient is first started on warfarin, it is important to know that it can take 72 hours or more to achieve a therapeutic level of anticoagulation. This is because the half-life of prothrombin is between 60 and 72 hours.[21] This delay in anticoagulation effectiveness also occurs if a patient is being converted from heparin anticoagulation (monitored by *activated partial thromboplastin time* [aPTT] to warfarin anticoagulation (monitored by INR). To ensure a safe transition, a delay of 4 days or more must be anticipated and PT/INR values must be assessed before the heparin is discontinued.[21] For patients who are to undergo surgery and have a high risk of thromboembolism, and thus require anticoagulation, the steps are reversed. The warfarin is stopped 4 days before surgery and when the INR has returned to normal the patient is started on therapeutic unfractionated heparin (UFH) or low–molecular weight heparin (LMWH).[17]

If the patient becomes too anticoagulated with warfarin or like agents, the INR value will rise above normal therapeutic levels, increasing the risk of bleeding. If the INR is 3 to 5, the only treatment is to reduce the dosage of warfarin until the INR is within the desired range.[21] If the INR is 5 to 9, the suggested action is to temporarily stop the warfarin and to administer oral vitamin K (1 mg to 2.5 mg).[21] If the INR value is greater than 9, oral vita-

Table 17-2	Therapeutic Coagulation Values		
Test	**Clinical Condition**	**Normal Value**	**Therapeutic Anticoagulant Target Value**
INR	Normal coagulation	Less than 1.0	
INR	Chronic atrial fibrillation	2.0-3.0	
INR	Treatment of DVT/PE	2.0-3.0	
INR	Mechanical heart valve(s)	2.5-3.5	
aPTT	Normal coagulation	28-38 sec	1.5-2.5 times normal
PTT	Normal coagulation	60-90 sec	1.5-2.0 times normal
ACT*	Normal coagulation	0-120 sec	150-300 sec

INR, International normalized ratio; *aPPT,* activated partial thromboplastin time; *PTT,* partial thromboplastin time; *ACT,* activated coagulation time; *DVT,* deep vein thrombosis; *PE,* pulmonary embolism.
*ACT normal, therapeutic values may vary with type of activator used.

min K (3 to 5 mg) is recommended. If the INR is more than 20, the risk of a life-threatening hemorrhage is greatly increased and the patient should be given vitamin K 10 mg IV very slowly, following the individual hospital's procedure.[21] Fresh-frozen plasma (FFP) or prothrombin complex concentrate may also be given to lower the INR value and prevent bleeding.[21]

Activated Partial Thromboplastin Time. The *aPTT* is used to measure the effectiveness of IV or subcutaneous UFH administration. Coagulation monitoring is required with UFH, although not with subcutaneous LMWH, because of lower levels of plasma protein-binding.[20] In cases of over-anticoagulation with heparin the antidote is protamine sulfate.

Activated Coagulation Time. An additional test of heparin effect is the *activated coagulation time (ACT)*. The ACT can be performed outside of the laboratory setting in areas such as the cardiac catheterization laboratory, the operating room, or specialized critical care units. Normal and therapeutic values for all of these coagulation studies are shown in Table 17-2.

SERUM LIPID STUDIES

Four primary blood lipid levels are important in evaluating an individual's risk of developing and/or having progression of coronary artery disease: total cholesterol; low-density lipoprotein cholesterol (LDL-C); triglycerides; and high-density lipoprotein cholesterol (HDL-C). When levels of cholesterol low-density lipoproteins (LDLs) and triglycerides are elevated or the level of high-density lipoproteins (HDLs) is low, the patient is considered "at risk" for developing or having progression of coronary artery disease and is offered intensive interventions in diet therapy, exercise prescription, and/or drug therapy.[22,23]

Total Cholesterol. Cholesterol is a fatlike substance (lipid) that is present in cell membranes, produced by the liver, it is a precursor of bile acids and steroid hormones. The cholesterol level in the blood is determined partly by genetics and partly by acquired factors such as diet, calorie balance, and level of physical activity. Cholesterol in excess amounts (more than 200 mg/dl) in the serum forces the progression of atherosclerosis (atherogenesis). See Table 17-3 for desirable lipid levels to lower the risk of coronary artery disease (CAD) and to reduce morbidity and mortality in patients with established CAD.

Low-Density Lipoproteins. About 60% to 70% of the total serum cholesterol is carried in the bloodstream, complexed as *LDL-C*. Both the LDL-C and total serum cholesterol levels are directly correlated with risk for CAD, and high levels of each are significant predictors of future acute MI in persons with established coronary artery atherosclerosis. LDL-C is the major atherogenic lipoprotein and thus is the primary target for cholesterol-lowering efforts.[22-24] Current guidelines recommend maintaining an LDL-C level below 130 mg/dL for the patient with no history of atherosclerotic disease. A patient with known coronary artery disease but who is not high risk should aim for an LDL-C level below 100 mg/dL. The recommended target LDL-C level for high-risk patients with coronary artery disease (CAD) has recently been lowered to 70 mg/dL.[23]

Very–Low-Density Lipoproteins and Triglycerides. The *very–low-density lipoproteins (VLDLs)* contain 10% to 15% of the total serum cholesterol along with most of the triglycerides in fasting serum. Elevated triglyceride levels are often associated with reduced HDL-C levels.[22,23]

High-Density Lipoproteins. HDLs are particles that carry 20% to 30% of the total serum cholesterol. A low HDL-C level (less than 35 mg/dl) is another independent, significant risk factor for CAD. Several studies also support the finding that HDL-C helps protect against atherogenesis, and a level greater than 50 mg/dl may act as a "shield" against the risk of CAD.[22,23]

CHEMISTRY STUDIES THAT ASSESS OTHER ORGAN SYSTEMS

The chemistry studies that are the most useful in the diagnosis of cardiovascular abnormalities caused by other organs are those that provide information about glucose metabolism, thyroid function, kidney function, and liver metabolism.

Blood Glucose. The detection of increased blood glucose (more than 110 mg/dl) during a fasting state (serum drawn 12 hours after most recent ingestion of

Table 17-3	Desirable Lipid Levels
Lipid	**Desirable Level**
Total cholesterol	<200 mg/dl
LDL-C	<130 mg/dl without CAD
	<100 mg/dl with CAD but not considered "high-risk"
	<70 mg/dl with CAD and considered "high risk" for future coronary events
Triglycerides	<150 mg/dl
HDL-C	>40 mg/dl (male)
	>50 mg/dl (female)

Data from the Executive Summary of the Third Report of the National Cholesterol Education Program (NCEP) Expert Panel on Detection, Evaluation, and Treatment of High Blood Cholesterol in Adults (Adult Treatment Panel III), *JAMA* 285(19):2486-2497, 2001; and Grundy SM et al; Implications of recent clinical trials for the national Cholesterol Education Program (NCEP) Adult Treatment Panel III (ATP III) Guidelines, *Circulation* 110:227-239, 1993. *LDL-C,* Low-density lipoprotein-cholesterol; *HDL-C,* high-density lipoprotein-cholesterol; CAD, coronary artery disease; <less than; >more than.

food or drink) may indicate diabetes mellitus. Critically ill patients with elevated blood glucose are at increased risk for numerous complications unless the serum glucose is tightly controlled within the normal range.[25] Current guidelines from the American College of Endocrinology recommend maintaining the blood glucose in critically ill patients within the normal range below 110 mg/dL.[26] In many patients this will require administration of subcutaneous or IV insulin to lower blood sugar.[26] Additional information on cardiovascular risk in association with diabetes is presented in Chapter 19 and more extensive information about diabetes is discussed in Chapter 36.

Thyroid Hormone Levels. Thyroid hormone levels are not routinely ordered but can often be helpful diagnostically. Elevated levels of the thyroid hormones T_3 and T_4 may result in thyrotoxicosis and a hyperdynamic cardiovascular picture (palpitations, tachycardia, bounding pulses). Decreased levels of the thyroid hormones (hypothyroidism) may be an explanation for fatigue, dyspnea on exertion, decreased cardiac output (CO), and heart failure.

Blood Urea Nitrogen and Creatinine. Blood urea nitrogen (BUN) and creatinine are blood chemistries that reflect kidney function. With kidney dysfunction or failure, BUN and creatinine levels are increased. Kidney failure will also cause electrolyte imbalances of potassium, magnesium, and calcium, which alter cardiac conduction and contractility. Because elevated serum creatinine is often associated with diabetes, hypertension, and older age, it is a routine laboratory component of cardiovascular risk analysis. Kidney failure is also recognized as an independent risk factor for cardiovascular disease in hospitalized patients.[27,28]

Liver Enzymes. Liver function indexes seen on the chemistry report include alkaline phosphatase, bilirubin, aspartate aminotransferase (AST), and alanine aminotransferase (ALT). Abnormal liver function tests may alert the medical team to liver dysfunction caused by failure of the right side of the heart. "Normal" laboratory values vary from institution to institution, but elevation of values is always a cause for investigation.

DIAGNOSTIC PROCEDURES

CHEST RADIOGRAPHY

Basic Principles and Technique. Chest radiography is the oldest noninvasive method for visualizing images of the heart, and it remains a frequently used and valuable diagnostic tool. Information about cardiac anatomy and physiology can be obtained with ease and safety at a relatively low cost. In the critical care unit, the nurse may be the first person to view the chest radiograph of an acutely ill patient. Critical care nurses also have an important role in ensuring the quality of the film through

proper positioning and instruction of the patient. For these reasons the critical care nurse must have a basic understanding of chest x-ray techniques and interpretation as they apply to the cardiovascular system.

Tissue Densities. As x-rays travel through the chest from the emitting tube to the film plate, they are absorbed to a varying degree by the tissues through which they pass (Table 17-4). Very dense tissue, such as bone, absorbs almost all the x-rays, leaving the film unexposed, or white. The heart, the aorta, the pulmonary vessels, and the blood they contain are moderately dense structures, appearing as gray areas on the x-ray film. These vascular structures are surrounded by air-filled lung that allows the greatest penetration of x-rays, resulting in fully exposed (black) areas on the film. Thoracic structures can be studied best by examining their borders. Two structures with the same density, when located next to each other, have no visible border. If a structure is located next to a contrasting density (e.g., vascular structures next to an air-filled lung), even subtle changes in size and shape can be seen.

Standard Views. In most institutions a standard radiographic examination of the heart and lungs consists of posterior-anterior (PA) and left lateral films. The standard film is taken in the x-ray department with the patient in an upright position; the film exposed during a deep, sustained inhalation; and the x-ray tube aimed horizontally 6 feet from the film.[29] This is referred to as a *PA film* because the beam traverses the patient from posterior to anterior.

Portable Chest X-Ray. Because most patients in critical care units are too ill to go to the x-ray department, chest radiographs are routinely obtained by using portable x-ray machines, with the patient either sitting upright or lying supine, depending on the patient's clinical condition and the judgment of the nurse. The film plate is placed behind the patient's back and an anterior-posterior (AP) projection is used, in which the x-ray beam enters from the front of the chest.[30] In the supine film, with the patient lying flat on the bed, the x-ray tube can be only approximately 36 inches from the patient's chest because of ceiling height and x-ray equipment construction. This re-

Table 17-4	**Intrathoracic Structure X-Ray Densities**	
Metal or Bone (White)	**Fluid (Gray)**	**Air (Black)**
Ribs, clavicle, sternum, spine	Blood	Lung
Calcium deposits	Heart	
Surgical wires or clips	Veins	
Prosthetic valves	Arteries	
Pacemaker wires	Edema	

sults in a lower quality film from a diagnostic standpoint, because the images of the heart and great vessels are magnified and not as sharply defined. Whenever possible, the upright (AP) film is preferred to the supine (flat) one because it provides a more accurate image, it shows more of the lung since the diaphragm is lower, and the thoracic structures appear sharper and less magnified.

Nursing Interventions to Produce an Optimal Chest X-Ray.
The critical care nurse can have a big impact on the quality of the x-ray film. Key elements that the nurse can impact follow:

- The x-ray is taken when the patient has taken a deep breath (inspiration). During exhalation the lungs are less full of air, which can make the lung-tissue appear "cloudy" as if there is additional lung-water. The heart also appears larger during exhalation. This could lead to an erroneous diagnosis of heart failure. Alert patients are encouraged to take in a deep breath and hold it while the exposure is taken. For patients receiving mechanical ventilatory support, the exposure must be timed to coincide with maximal inhalation.[31]
- It is important to remove extrinsic tubing and other movable objects from the patient's thorax to permit optimal visualization of the chest. Hands or arms should not be across the chest during the x-ray.
- Have the patient sit upright in bed if the clinical condition allows for this position. Upright x-ray views have a sharper focus because the distance from the patient to the x-ray tube is closer to the standard 72 inches (6 feet).[31]
- Ensure the patient is "straight" in the bed rather than turned or twisted; this permits clearer visualization of the major thoracic structures.

Indications.
There is considerable debate over the optimal frequency of the "routine chest-x-ray" in the critical care unit.[30,32]

In some hospitals, to ensure that all portable x-rays have a clinical rationale, the physician requesting the film must complete a short form that states the reason for the chest x-ray (e.g., change in patient condition, new device implanted). In one hospital, when the above method was compared to the "routine daily chest-x-ray," it was found that this reduced the number of chest-x-rays by 22.5% over an 18-month period without any impact on patient clinical outcomes or mortality.[32] In contrast, other researchers have found that routine chest-x-rays generate clinically useful date up to 45% of the time.[30]

The American College of Radiology (ACR) expert panel made these recommendations on portable x-rays in the critical care unit[30]:

1. Daily chest-x-rays are recommended for patients with acute cardiopulmonary problems and those receiving mechanical ventilation.
2. Patients who require cardiac monitoring but are otherwise stable need only an admission film.

3. A chest x-ray is performed whenever a new thoracic device is placed or whenever there is a specific question about the patient's cardiopulmonary status that the chest x-ray could address.

Chest-X-Ray Analysis: Lines and Tubes.
Evaluation of a chest film is a systematic process. All thoracic invasive tubes and lines must be located and identified. Major thoracic structures, including the lungs, pleural space, mediastinum, diaphragm, and vascular structures, are assessed and compared with previous films, if available. Variations from previous films can alert the clinician to possible complications and provide information about the patient's hemodynamic status.

Central Venous Catheter.
Central venous catheters (CVC) are seen on the chest film as moderately radiopaque tubes extending centrally from a subclavian (SC), internal jugular (IJ), or femoral vein insertion site. The ideal location of the catheter tip is within the superior vena cava (SVC) so that it is close, but not inside, the right atrium. Central venous catheter misplacement during insertion ranges from 1% to 15% of cases.[30] The expertise of the clinician inserting the catheter and variations in patient anatomy are some of the reasons for the wide range of complications. The risk of pneumothorax is 5.6%.[30] In most hospitals a chest-x-ray is required following CVC insertion using the IJ or SC vein.

Pulmonary Artery Catheter.
A chest x-ray is required following insertion of a pulmonary artery catheter (PAC), also known as a Swan-Ganz catheter. The primary clinical reason for the chest-x-ray is to determine the position of the tip of the PAC. To wedge correctly, the noninflated catheter tip must lie within 2 centimeters (cm) of the hilar point of the lung and not extend beyond the proximal interlobar arteries.[30] The most serious potential complication is rupture of the pulmonary artery. This complication is rare but has a mortality of over 70% when it does occur.[30] For more information on pulmonary artery catheters, see that section later in this chapter.

Endotracheal Tube.
A chest x-ray is always requested following endotracheal intubation. This is because physical examination is not sufficiently sensitive to determine endotracheal tube (ETT) malposition. Although clinical physical assessment can recognize a misplaced ETT 2% to 5% of the time, suboptimal positioning is identified in 20% to 25% of cases by chest-x-ray.[30]

Enteric Tube.
Malposition of enteral feeding tubes occurs in 1% of cases and occurs more frequently with small-bore feeding tubes.[30] Because the consequences of delivering enteral nutrition into a nonenteric space are so severe for the patient, a chest x-ray is required following placement and before beginning tube feeds.

Chest Tube.
Chest tubes contain a radiopaque line that makes them clearly visible on the chest-x-ray. Chest tubes are located within either the pleural or mediastinal space. Pulmonary chest tubes are placed to treat pneu-

mothorax or hemothorax. Most pneumothoraces in the critical care unit are either iatrogenic (ventilator baro-trauma) or traumatic (complication of CVC placement), or occur following cardiothoracic surgery.[33] One or two mediastinal drainage tubes are commonly inserted during cardiac surgery. One may be positioned superiorly to drain the anterior mediastinum, and the other is directed inferiorly to drain the left posterolateral pericardial space.

Intraaortic Balloon Catheter. An intraaortic balloon pump (IABP) provides mechanical support for the failing heart. The catheter that is evaluated on the chest x-ray is a 26- to 28-mm inflatable balloon that surrounds a catheter inserted into the descending aorta, usually percutaneously via the femoral artery. A chest x-ray must be obtained immediately after insertion to evaluate the position of the IABP catheter.[33] The distal tip of the IABP catheter contains a small radiopaque marker that is helpful in determining its position on the chest film. The tip of the IABP catheter must lie below the origin of the left subclavian artery in the descending thoracic aorta (just below the aortic arch). Even when inserted properly, there is a risk of aortic dissection. Aortic dissection is a life threatening complication. It can be seen on the chest x-ray film as a loss of sharpness of the borders of the descending thoracic aorta.

Pacemaker or Implantable Defibrillator. A *pacemaker* and implantable cardioverter defibrillator (ICD) are cardiovascular devices that can be visualized on a chest film. There is considerable variety in the range of pacing electrodes that are encountered in critical care patients. If the pacemaker is permanently implanted, the entire system is seen on the chest film. If it is only a temporary pacemaker, the pulse generator is external to the body and is not seen on the chest-x-ray. The pacing electrodes are radiopaque and look like white wires extending transvenously into the right side of the heart. Pacing wires sutured on the epicardium during cardiac surgery are visible on the right atrium and/or right ventricle. Patients with a history of heart failure may have an additional pacing wire inserted into the coronary sinus (vein) to pace the left ventricle in addition to a right ventricular wire (i.e., biventricular pacing). Table 17-5 summarizes the most common cardiovascular devices and their correct position as seen on the chest x-ray.

Chest-X-Ray Analysis: Cardiac and Pulmonary. A wealth of physiologic data can be gleaned from a chest x-ray film. To be valid, this information must be interpreted in the context of a thorough physical examination and clinical knowledge of the patient's condition.

Cardiac Heart Size. Comparison of the cardiothoracic (CT) ratio (Fig. 17-4) can be used to assess heart size. The normal heart size is less than one third of the diameter of the chest viewed on the x-ray. Patients with chronic heart failure have cardiomegaly (enlarged heart).

Pulmonary Edema. Pulmonary edema is a common finding in the critically ill. The "wet lungs" appear on the chest x-ray as white, dense, cloudy areas. Pulmonary edema shows up very clearly on the chest x-ray, although in the absence of a clinical history the x-ray is not sufficient to determine if the pulmonary edema is from a cardiac or a pulmonary cause.[30] If the pulmonary edema is secondary to heart failure, sometimes described as "hydrostatic pulmonary edema," the distribution of fluid may be in a "bat-wing" distribution with the "white" areas concentrated in the hilar region (origin of the major pulmonary vessels). However, as the heart failure progresses the quantity of fluid in the alveolar spaces increases and the white, fluffy appearance is seen throughout the lung.

If the pulmonary edema is secondary to acute respiratory distress syndrome (ARDS), also known as *noncardiogenic pulmonary edema* or *permeability edema*, the distribution of fluid is randomly distributed. It may be described as diffuse bilateral infiltrates.[33]

Pneumonia. Hospital-acquired pneumonia (HAP) is a serious iatrogenic complication that may be detected on a chest x-ray. For the mechanically ventilated patient the risk is increased because the normal oropharyngeal defenses are bypassed by intubation. This leaves the patient vulnerable for development of ventilator-associated pneumonia (VAP), a complication with a reported incidence of between 12% to 29% of cases and a mortality of up to 50%.[30] On the chest x-ray, any appearance of a new or progressive opacity (dense, white area) is a cause for

Table 17-5	Cardiovascular Devices	
Device	**Function**	**Position**
Pulmonary artery catheter	Measures PAOP and right heart pressures	Tip in right or left pulmonary artery
CVC	CVP measurement, venous access	Superior vena cava
LA catheter	Left atrial pressure	Left atrium
Mediastinal chest tubes	Mediastinal fluid evacuation	Anterior mediastinum, posterior pericardium
Pacemaker leads	Cardiac pacing	Over right heart
IABP catheter	Assists LV function	Tip just below top of aortic arch

PAOP, Pulmonary artery occlusion pressure; *CVC,* central venous catheter; *CVP,* central venous pressure; *LA,* left atrium; *IAB,* intraaortic balloon; *LV,* left ventricle.

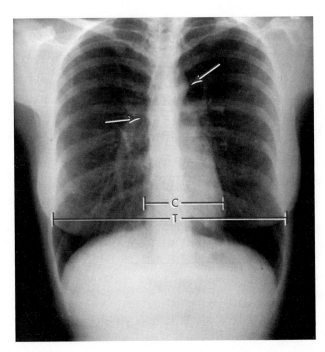

Fig. 17-4 Cardiothoracic (CT) ratio—a technique for estimating heart size on a PA (posterior-to-anterior) chest film. Normally the cardiac diameter is 50% or less of the thoracic diameter when measured during full inhalation. *C,* Maximal cardiac diameter; *T,* maximal thoracic diameter measured to the inside of the ribs. The width of the vascular pedicle *(arrows)* is a more accurate indicator of systemic blood volume.

concern and should be clinically investigated. More comprehensive information on pneumonia is provided in Chapter 23.

Pneumothorax. Pneumothorax, or air within the pleural cavity, is diagnosed by chest x-ray. Normally, the pleura are not visible because they are adjacent to the chest wall. As the pneumothorax increases in size, the nurse will be able to see the edge of the pleura as the trapped air separates it from the chest wall. The "pneumo" (air) appears black within the pleura. There are no lung markings in the pleural area, and the collapsed lung will appear increasingly dense (gray or white). The biggest risk is development of a *tension pneumothorax* that will shift the mediastinal structures. This is also visible on a chest x-ray. For more information on pneumothorax see Chapter 23.

DIGITAL RADIOGRAPHY

Digital radiography systems are being widely implemented in hospitals.[30] In a digital radiograph, the image is divided into discrete elements (pixels) that are assigned a specific value and stored for later display, either on a computer screen or by means of a laser printer. Pixel sizes vary; the smaller the pixel, the better the resolution. Digital systems have many advantages. No film

development is necessary, so the image can be displayed rapidly on a computer screen in the clinical area. The image can be expanded or compressed. This system also lends itself to computer-assisted diagnosis, which involves computer analysis of the image to detect and quantify pathologic findings. If a baseline film has been digitally recorded, the baseline film can be "subtracted" from the current film, highlighting any areas of change, such as increased heart size or new pulmonary infiltrates.

ELECTROCARDIOGRAPHY

Electrocardiography (ECG) is a complex subject about which much literature has been written and to which entire books have been devoted—and justifiably so. A detailed evaluation of an ECG can provide a wealth of cardiac diagnostic information and often provides the basis on which other, definitive diagnostic tests are selected. This section provides a comprehensive discussion of the many clinical factors that the critical care nurse considers when using ECG monitoring. Specific dysrhythmias commonly encountered in clinical practice are discussed in the section on dysrhythmia interpretation later in the chapter. The beginning section covers 12-lead ECG analysis and describes the skills needed to evaluate lead placement, left ventricular axis, and changes in the 12-lead ECG caused by ischemia or infarction. The intent is to provide a sound basis for understanding the value of the many clinical applications of electrocardiography.

ECG: Basic Principles. The ECG records electrical changes in heart muscle caused by an action potential. It does not record the mechanical contraction, which usually follows electrical depolarization immediately. A brief discussion of the cardiac action potential is included to reinforce the concept that it is the electrical changes that occur during electrical stimulation of the myocardial cell that produce the deflections seen on the ECG tracing (Fig. 17-5).

Phase 0. During phase 0 (depolarization), the electrical potential changes rapidly from a baseline of (minus) −90 mV to 20 mV and stabilizes at about 0 mV. Because this is a significant electrical change, it appears as a wave on the ECG as the QRS.

Phases 1 and 2. During phases 1 and 2, an electrical plateau is created, and it is during this plateau that mechanical contraction occurs. Because there is no significant electrical change, nothing shows on the ECG.

Phase 3. During phase 3 (repolarization), the electrical potential again changes, this time a little more slowly, from 0 mV back to (minus) −90 mV. This is another major electrical event, and it is reflected on the ECG as a T wave.

Phase 4. During phase 4 (resting period), the chemical balance is restored by the sodium pump, but since positively charged ions are exchanged on a one-for-one basis, no electrical activity is generated and no visible

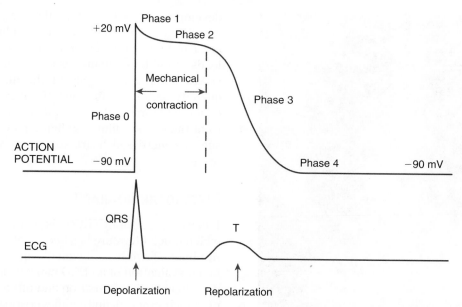

Fig. 17-5 Correlation of the action potential of a ventricular myocardial cell with the electrical events recorded on the surface ECG. Note that the ECG is "silent" during phase 2 of the action potential. Mechanical contraction is occurring, but no significant electrical activity is present.

change occurs on the ECG tracing. For more information on the cardiac action potential, see the section on the action potential in Chapter 15.

Electrocardiographic Leads. All electrocardiographs use a system of one or more leads. The basic 3-lead system consists of three bipolar electrodes that are applied to the chest wall and labeled right arm (RA), left arm (LA), and left leg (LL).[34] The term bipolar means that each created ECG lead has both a positive and a negative pole. One lead will also act as a ground. The function of the ground electrode is to prevent the display of background electrical interference on the ECG tracing. Leads do not transmit any electricity to the patient—they just sense and record it.

The positive electrode on the skin acts as a camera. If the wave of depolarization travels toward the positive electrode, an upward stroke, or *positive deflection*, is written on the ECG paper (Fig. 17-6, *A*). If the wave of depolarization travels away from the positive electrode, a downward line, or *negative deflection*, is recorded on the ECG (Fig. 17-6, *B*). When depolarization moves perpendicularly to the positive electrode, a biphasic complex occurs. Sometimes the complex may even appear almost flat, or isoelectric, if the electrical forces traveling in opposite directions are equal and have the effect of canceling out each other (Fig. 17-6, *C*). The size of the muscle mass being depolarized also has an effect, with the larger muscle mass (usually the left ventricle) having a greater influence on the tracing.

The wave of ventricular depolarization in the healthy heart travels from right to left and from head to toe. The appearance of the waveforms in different ECG leads will vary, depending on the location of the positive electrode.

12-Lead ECG Leads. The standard 12-lead ECG provides a picture of electrical activity in the heart using 10 different electrode positions to create 12 ECG images.[34] A standard 12-lead ECG contains six limb lead images and six chest (precordial) lead images. The limb lead tracings are obtained by placing electrodes on all four extremities. The exact location on the extremities does not matter as long as skin contact is good and bone is avoided. The machine interprets all extremity signals as coming from the connection of the extremity to the torso (i.e., from the shoulder or groin).

Leads I, II, and III are bipolar limb leads in that they consist of a positive and a negative electrode. The other three limb leads are labeled aV_R, aV_L, and aV_F, representing *augmented vector* right, left, and foot (Fig. 17-7, *A*). These unipolar leads consist of only a positive electrode, with the negative electrode calculated within the machine at roughly the center of the heart. Under these circumstances the ECG tracing would ordinarily be very small, so the machine enhances, or *augments*, it. The term *vector* refers to directional force.

The six standard precordial, or chest, leads are labeled "V" leads and are distributed in an arc around the left side of the chest. They are useful for viewing electrical forces traveling from right to left or front to back but are not helpful in evaluating vertical forces in the heart. For an accurate interpretation, all 12 leads must be considered (Fig. 17-7, *B*).

Right Ventricular Precordial Leads. At times, additional leads are helpful in evaluating the extent of myocardium involved in an acute MI. Both the right ventricle and the posterior wall of the heart are areas that are not clearly seen on a standard 12-lead ECG. The right ventri-

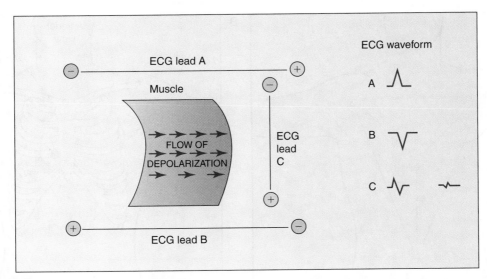

Fig. 17-6   Effect of lead position on the ECG tracing. *A,* Flow of depolarization toward the positive electrode results in a positive deflection on the ECG. *B,* Flow of depolarization away from the positive electrode results in a negative deflection on the ECG. *C,* Flow of depolarization perpendicular to the positive electrode results in a biphasic or nearly isoelectric deflection on the ECG. This basic principle applies to both the P wave and the QRS complex.

cle can be visualized more fully by adding right-sided chest leads (see Fig. 17-7, *B*). Labeled V_1R, V_2R, V_3R, V_4R, V_5R, and V_6R, they are added to the standard 12-lead ECG whenever right ventricular infarction is suspected. Right ventricular infarction is commonly accompanied by inferior and posterior wall infarction.[13] The use of the six right ventricular leads expands the diagnostic accuracy of the 12-lead ECG and is sometimes termed an *18-lead ECG.*[35]

Posterior Wall Leads. The posterior wall of the heart can be assessed using posterior chest leads (Fig. 17-7, *C*). These leads are labeled V_7, V_8, and V_9. Although posterior lead placement can be somewhat technically challenging, the information obtained is very useful clinically and may influence decisions regarding clinical management.[13] The use of the posterior leads expands the diagnostic accuracy of the 12-lead ECG and can be described as a 15-lead ECG.

Baseline Distortion. It is important that the tracing have a flat baseline, which is that portion of the tracing that is between the various waveforms. Two forms of artifact can distort the baseline: 60-cycle interference and muscular movement. Sixty-cycle interference (Fig. 17-8, *A*) results from leakage of electrical current somewhere within the system and appears as a generalized thickening of the baseline. It can usually be resolved by ensuring that all electrical equipment at the bedside is electrically grounded. Occasionally it may be necessary to unplug one piece of equipment at a time until the offending device is found. Muscular movement (Fig. 17-8, *B*) is displayed as a coarse, erratic disturbance of the baseline. In most cases, asking the patient to lie quietly while the ECG is being run is sufficient. If movement is caused by shiver-

ing or seizure activity, it is best to wait until the activity subsides before obtaining the 12-lead ECG. When baseline tremor is caused by Parkinson's disease or another neuromuscular disorder, a resolution may not be possible. It must be remembered that the artifact has an adverse effect on the accurate interpretation of the tracing and may at times mimic lethal ventricular dysrhythmias.

ECG Analysis

Specialized ECG Paper. ECG paper records the speed and magnitude of electrical impulses on a grid composed of small and large boxes (Fig. 17-9). Every large box has five small boxes in it. At a standard paper speed of 25 mm/second, on the horizontal axis, one small box (1 mm) is equivalent to 0.04 second, and one large box (5 mm) represents 0.20 second. Distances along the horizontal axis represent speed and are stated in seconds rather than in millimeters or number of boxes. The vertical axis represents the magnitude, or force, of the electrical signal. The vertical scale is standardized to a specific calibration as described below.

Calibration. At standard calibration, one small box equals 0.1 mm, and one large box equals 0.5 mm. It is important to look for the standardization mark, which is usually located at the beginning of the tracing (Fig. 17-10, *A*). The mark indicates that in response to a standard electrical signal of 1 mV, the calibration signal rises two large boxes to make a calibration mark. ECGs are sometimes run at different calibrations. If at standard calibration some complexes are so tall they run off the paper, the tracing is repeated at half standard (Fig. 17-10, *B*) and the calibration mark rises only one large box. If all of the complexes on a standard tracing are very small, it may be repeated at double standard, with the calibration

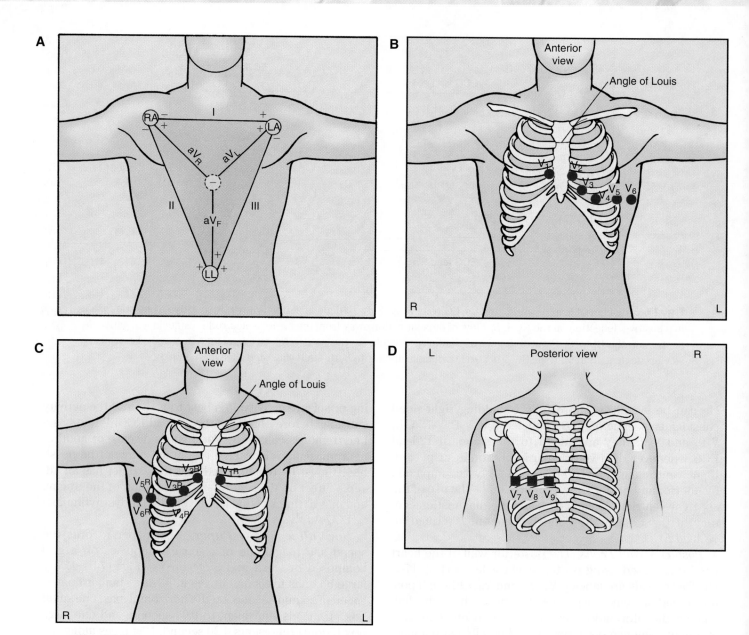

Fig. 17-7 **A,** Standard limb leads. Leads are actually located on the extremities: right arm *(RA),* left arm *(LA),* and left leg *(LL).* The right leg electrode serves as a ground. Leads I, II, and III are bipolar, using both a positive and a negative electrode. Leads aV_R, aV_L, and aV_F are augmented unipolar leads that use the calculated center of the heart as their negative electrode. **B,** Precordial leads. V_1 to V_6 are the six standard precordial leads and are placed as follows: V_1—fourth intercostal space, right sternal border; V_2—fourth intercostal space, left sternal border; V_3—equidistant between V_2 and V_4; V_4—fifth intercostal space, left midclavicular line; V_5—anterior axillary line, same horizontal level as V_4; V_6—midaxillary line, same horizontal level as V_4. **C,** The right precordial leads V_1R to V_6R are shown. They are not part of a standard 12-lead ECG but are used whenever a right ventricular infarction is suspected. Their placement is identical to V_3 to V_6, except on the right side of the chest rather than on the left. **D,** Posterior precordial leads V_7, V_8, and V_9. Placed on the patient's left posterior chest at the same horizontal level as V_4 (fifth intercostal space). V_7 is on the posterior axillary line, V_8 on the scapular line, and V_9 on the spinal border. These leads are added to the standard 12-lead ECG whenever a posterior wall infarction is suspected.

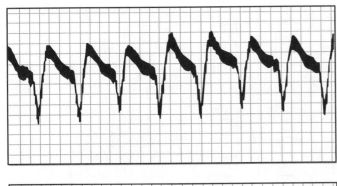

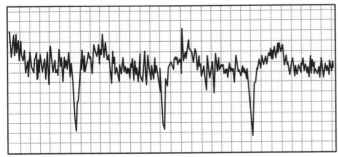

A

B

Fig. 17-8 **A,** Artifact—60 cycle interference. **B,** Artifact—muscular movement.

mark going up four large boxes (Fig. 17-10, *C*). In any case, the calibration must be clearly marked on the tracing, because some diagnostic conclusions are based on the magnitude of specific portions of the ECG complex.

Waveforms. The analysis of waveforms and intervals provide the basis for ECG interpretation (Fig. 17-11).

P Wave. The P wave represents atrial depolarization.

QRS Complex. The QRS complex represents ventricular depolarization, corresponding to phase 0 of the ventricular action potential. It is referred to as a *complex* because it actually consists of several different waves. Basically, the letter *Q* is used to describe an initial negative deflection; in other words, only if the first deflection from the baseline is negative will it be labeled a Q wave. The letter *R* applies to any positive deflection. If there are two positive deflections in one QRS complex, the second is labeled R′ (read "R prime") and is commonly seen in lead V$_1$ in right bundle branch block. The letter *S* refers to any subsequent negative deflections. Any combination of these deflections can occur and is collectively called the *QRS complex* (Fig. 17-12). The QRS duration is normally less than 0.10 second (2½ small boxes).

T Wave. The T wave represents ventricular repolarization, corresponding to phase 3 of the ventricular ac-

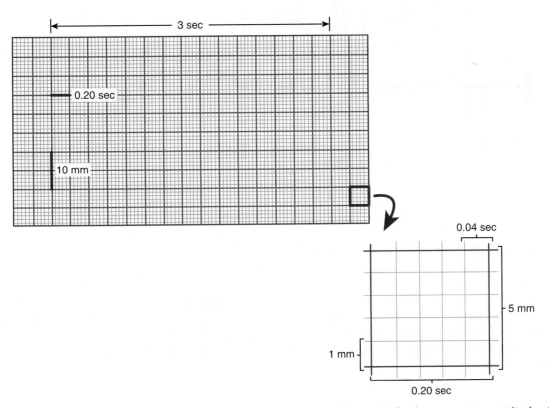

Fig. 17-9 ECG graph paper. The horizontal axis represents time, and the vertical axis represents magnitude of voltage. Horizontally, each small box is 0.04 second and each large box is 0.20 second. Vertically, each large box is 5 mm. Markings are present every 3 seconds at the top of the paper for ease in calculating heart rate.

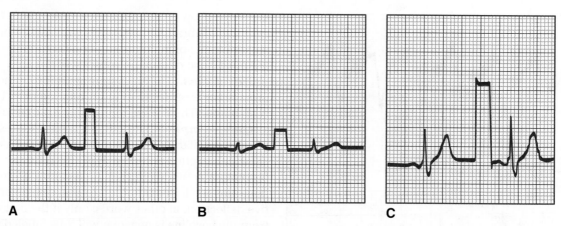

Fig. 17-10   A, Normal standardization mark, in which the machine is calibrated so that the standardization mark is 10 mm tall. **B,** Half standardization, used whenever QRS complexes are too tall to fit on the paper. **C,** Twice normal standardization, used whenever QRS complexes are too small to be adequately analyzed.

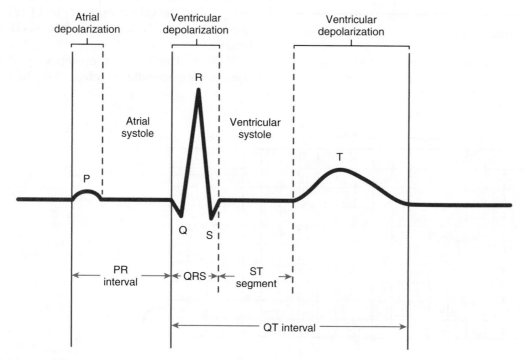

Fig. 17-11   Normal ECG waveforms, intervals, and correlation with events of the cardiac cycle. The *P wave* represents atrial depolarization, followed immediately by atrial systole. The *QRS* represents ventricular depolarization, followed immediately by ventricular systole. The *ST segment* corresponds to phase 2 of the action potential, during which time the heart muscle is completely depolarized and contraction normally occurs. The *T wave* represents ventricular repolarization. The *PR interval,* measured from the beginning of the P wave to the beginning of the QRS, corresponds to atrial depolarization and impulse delay in the AV node. The *QT interval,* measured from the beginning of the QRS complex to the end of the T wave, represents the time from initial depolarization of the ventricles to the end of ventricular repolarization.

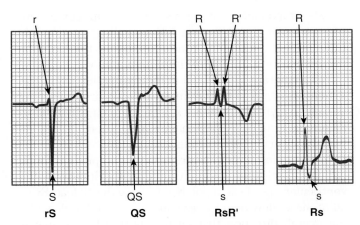

Fig. 17-12 Examples of QRS complexes. Small deflections are labeled with lowercase letters, whereas uppercase letters are used for larger deflections. A second upward deflection is labeled R′.

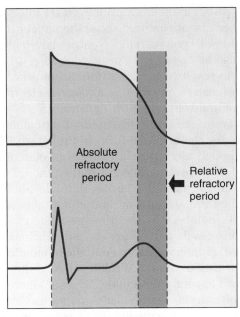

Fig. 17-13 Absolute and relative refractory periods correlated with the cardiac muscle's action potential and with an ECG tracing.

tion potential. The onset of the QRS to approximately the midpoint or peak of the T wave represents an absolute refractory period, during which the heart muscle cannot respond to another stimulus no matter how strong that stimulus might be (Fig. 17-13). From the midpoint to the end of the T wave, the heart muscle is in the relative refractory period. The heart muscle has not yet fully recovered, but it could be depolarized again if a strong enough stimulus were received. This can be a particularly dangerous time for ventricular ectopy to occur, especially if any portion of the myocardium is ischemic, because the ischemic muscle takes even longer to fully repolarize. This sets the stage for the disorganized, self-perpetuating depolarizations of various sections of the myocardium known as *ventricular fibrillation.*

Intervals Between Waveforms. Intervals between waveforms are also evaluated (see Fig. 17-11).

PR Interval. The PR interval is measured from the beginning of the P wave to the beginning of the QRS complex. Normally the PR interval is 0.12 to 0.20 seconds in length and represents the time between sinus node discharge and the beginning of ventricular depolarization. Because most of this time period results from delay of the impulse in the AV node, the PR interval is an indicator of AV nodal function.

In the electrophysiology laboratory and in some critical care units, these time values are described in milliseconds. There are 1000 milliseconds (msec) in one second. Thus the normal PR interval value can also be written as 120 to 200 msec.

ST Segment. The ST segment is the portion of the wave that extends from the end of the QRS to the beginning of the T wave. Its duration is not measured. Instead, its shape and location are evaluated.[34] The ST segment is normally flat and at the same level as the isoelectric

baseline. Any change from baseline is expressed in millimeters and may indicate myocardial ischemia (one small box equals 1 mm). ST-segment elevation (increase above baseline greater than 1 mm) is associated with acute myocardial injury, preinfarction, and pericarditis. ST-segment depression (decrease from baseline more than 1 mm) is associated with myocardial ischemia. The ST segment must be monitored carefully in high-risk patients such as described in the later section on continuous ST-segment monitoring.

QT Interval. The QT interval is measured from the beginning of the QRS complex to the end of the T wave and indicates the total time interval from the onset of depolarization to the completion of repolarization.[36] There is no established bedside monitoring lead recommended for measuring the QT interval.[34] On the 12-lead ECG, the QT interval is usually the longest in precordial leads V_3 and V_4.[34] The important point is that each clinician measures the QT interval using the same ECG lead.[34] At normal heart rates, the QT interval is less than half of the RR interval when measured from one QRS complex to the next. However, the length of a QT interval is a time interval that depends on heart rate and must be adjusted according to the heart rate to be evaluated in a clinically meaningful way.

Because the QT interval varies with the heart rate, it is often written as a "corrected" value. The corrected QT interval (QTc) is calculated by dividing the measured QT interval, in seconds, by the square root of the RR cycle length (see Fig. 17-3).[34,37] The normal QTc is less than 0.46 second (460 msec) in women and less than 0.45 second (450 msec) in men.[34] A prolonged QT interval is significant because it can predispose the patient to the development of polymorphic ventricular tachycardia, known also as *torsades de pointes*. A long QT interval can be the result of a *congenital* chromosomal abnormality, or it can be *acquired* as a result of electrolyte imbalance or antidysrhythmic drug therapy.[36]

Quinidine is an antidysrhythmic drug commonly responsible for the acquired form of prolonged QT interval,[36] although any class Ia drug (e.g., quinidine, procainamide, disopyramide) can lengthen the QT interval; Class III drugs (e.g., amiodarone, ibutilide, sotalol) also can prolong the QT interval and initiate an episode of torsades de pointes.[36] When drugs associated with a high risk of torsades de pointes are started, it is important to record the QT interval and to continue to monitor the QT interval during treatment. Prolongation of the absolute QT interval beyond 0.5 second (500 msec) increases the risk of polymorphic ventricular tachycardia.[36]

However, not all patients are at equal risk, and the reason some patients with a prolonged QT interval experience lethal ventricular dysrhythmias, whereas others do not, is not yet understood.[36] Researchers speculate that between 5% to 10% of patients with acquired long–QT syndrome (drug induced) also carry a genetic predisposition toward long–QT.[36]

The risk of torsades de pointes is intensified in both acquired and congenital long–QT syndrome in the presence of hypokalemia or hypomagnesemia. In addition, polymorphic ventricular tachycardia occurs most frequently in the presence of a slow ventricular rate whether due to heart block, a sinus pause, or sinus bradycardia.[36]

QT–interval monitoring is used as an indirect measure of ventricular repolarization.[34] One challenge is that it is often difficult on a bedside monitoring strip to determine precisely where the end of the QT interval occurs.[34]

Acute therapy is directed at increasing the heart rate, which will shorten the QT interval, and correcting drug and electrolyte abnormalities. It may also include placement of a temporary pacemaker and IV magnesium, especially if serum levels of magnesium are low.

Ventricular Axis. Electrical impulses spread through cardiac muscle tissue in many directions at once when the ventricular muscle is depolarized. Using the 12-lead ECG, all of these individual forces can be averaged to describe the overall direction that current is traveling, which is called the *mean vector*. The mean vector can be plotted on a circular graph known as the *hexaxial reference system* (Fig. 17-14), and a degree can be assigned to it. This degree represents the ventricular axis.

Parameters for ventricular axis are not always listed in the same way in every hospital.[38] Normal axis may be listed as 0 to 90 degrees for a "quick-look" or more accurately (minus) −30 to +110 degrees. Right-axis deviation (RAD) is present if the axis falls between +110 and +180 degrees. Left-axis deviation (LAD) is present if the axis falls between (minus) −30 and (minus) −90 degrees. See Fig. 17-14 to locate these points on the hexaxial reference wheel. If the axis plots in the upper left portion of the circle, also known as the *northwest quadrant*, it is called an *indeterminate axis*. This axis occurs rarely but can be seen when the wave of depolarization starts at the bottom of the ventricle—near the point of maximal impulse (PMI) or apex of the ventricle—and spreads upward toward the atria. Clinically this can be seen in beats of ventricular origin, such as premature ventricular contractions (PVCs) and some pacemaker-initiated beats.

Calculating Ventricular Axis. The ventricular axis is calculated using the six limb leads (leads I, II, III, and aV_R, aV_L, aV_F) in the three steps outlined below.

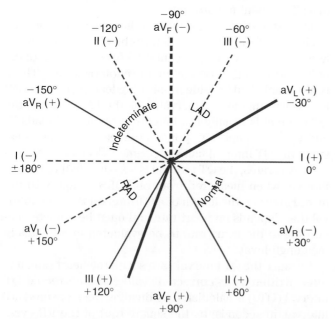

Fig. 17-14 Hexaxial reference system. *RAD,* Right axis deviation; *LAD,* left axis deviation.

Box 17-2

STEPS IN DETERMINING AXIS

1. Find the most isoelectric limb lead.
2. Using the hexaxial reference system, find the lead that is perpendicular to the one identified in step 1.
3. Determine whether the QRS is positive or negative in the perpendicular lead.
4. Look at the corresponding positive or negative pole of the perpendicular lead on the hexaxial reference system.
5. The degree listed on the hexaxial reference system is the axis.

STEP 1. Find the limb lead with the smallest QRS complex, or the one that is the most equiphasic (equal portions above and below the baseline). In Fig. 17-15, lead aV_F is the smallest.

STEP 2. Using the hexaxial reference system (see Fig. 17-14), locate the lead that is perpendicular to the one that had the smallest complex. For example, perpendicular to lead aV_F is lead I, so the mean vector lies parallel with lead I.

STEP 3. The third step is to determine whether the QRS complex is positive or negative in the lead parallel to the mean vector (in this case, lead I). If the QRS is positive, the mean vector is directed *toward* the positive electrode. If the QRS is negative, the mean vector is directed *away* from the positive electrode. In Fig. 17-15, the QRS deflection in lead I is upright, or positive. The positive pole of lead I is at the right midpoint of the hexaxial reference system and corresponds to a numeric degree of zero, which is within the normal range (Box 17-2).

Cardiac Monitor Lead Analysis. During continuous cardiac monitoring, adhesive, pregelled electrodes are used to obtain an ECG tracing that is similar to one lead of a 12-lead ECG. At a minimum, this requires three electrodes. One of the electrodes will act as a positive pole, one as a negative pole, and one as a ground. In most critical care units, five electrodes are used. Five leads allows the clinician to monitor two leads simultaneously or to allow selection of several different leads at any time through a lead selector switch on the monitor. Typical placement of the five electrodes in a multi-lead system is RA, LA, LL, and right leg (RL) with one chest lead that is generally placed in the V_1 position as illustrated in Fig. 17-16.

The selection of an ECG monitoring lead is not a decision to be made casually or according to habit. The chosen monitoring lead should be directly related to the patient's clinical condition and recent clinical history.[34] If the patient has experienced ST-segment elevation associated with acute coronary syndrome, percutaneous

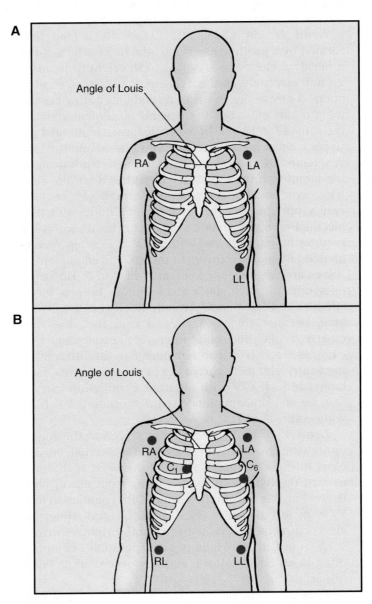

Fig. 17-16 **A,** Three electrodes and lead-wire cables allow monitoring of three of the limb leads (I, II, and III) and can also be rearranged to monitor MCL_1 and MCL_6 (see Fig. 15-18, *A*). **B,** Multilead monitoring system: five electrodes and lead-wire cables allow monitoring of any of the six standard limb leads (I, II, III, aV_R, aV_L, or aV_F) and any one precordial lead, either V_1 or V_6. C_1 indicates the proper position of the chest electrode for monitoring lead V_1, and C_6 indicates the proper position of the chest electrode for monitoring V_6. The cable attachments are color-coded for quick identification and placement. Accurate electrode placement is essential.

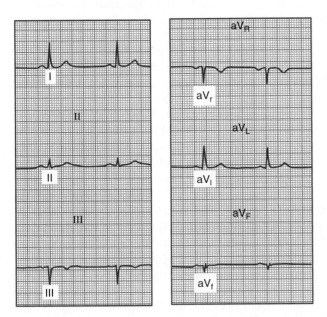

Fig. 17-15 Limb leads of normal ECG illustrating normal axis of 0 degrees.

catheter intervention (PCI), or recent cardiac surgery, the leads that exhibited ST-segment elevation should used to guide selection of the optimal ECG monitoring leads.[34]

Accurate lead placement is essential for accurate cardiac monitoring.[34] Lead placement must be verified at the beginning of each shift. Once a transient dysrhythmia has occurred, it is too late to change lead placement so that an accurate analysis can be performed.

Lead II. On a standard 12-lead ECG, lead II is formed by a positive electrode attached to the left leg, a negative electrode attached to the right arm, and a ground electrode on the right leg. It is not practical to connect electrodes to the arms and legs during continuous monitoring, but the general placement remains the same (Fig. 17-17). In the critical care unit, most patients have at least five electrodes placed and the lead is selected by choosing a lead via a selector button on the monitor. If the monitored heart has a normal electrical axis, lead II displays a waveform that is predominantly upright, has the greatest amplitude, and thus has the best signal-to-noise ratio. For this reason it is a popular monitoring lead and one that is often recommended by manufacturers of monitoring equipment. P waves are usually easy to identify in lead II. However, it is difficult to identify right bundle branch block (RBBB) and left bundle branch block (LBBB) in this lead, because this is a vertical lead that does not clearly display horizontal interventricular conduction changes. Lead II is also nondiagnostic in differentiating ventricular tachycardia (VT) from supraventricular tachycardia (SVT) with aberrant conduction. See p. 364 for key information on differentiating VT from wide-complex SVT.

Lead V₁. The V_1 electrode is placed at the fourth intercostal space to the right of the sternal border. Most of the electrical activity of the heart is directed toward the left ventricle, and away from the V_1 electrode. For this reason the normal QRS complex in lead V_1 is mostly negative (Fig. 17-18, *B*). Any abnormal electrical activity directed toward the right ventricle, such as in RBBB, results in an upright QRS complex, often in an RSR′ pattern, verbally described as "RSR prime."

V_1 is the optimum lead to select if the critical care nurse needs to analyze ventricular ectopy. V_1 provides information to facilitate differentiation between RBBB versus LBBB pattern, or distinguish between VT and SVT with aberrant conduction; determine whether PVCs originate in the right or left ventricle, and clarify when ST-segment changes are caused by the RBBB and when they are the result of ischemia. Lead V_1 is excellent for this purpose.

MCL₁. MCL₁ stands for "modified chest lead one." It is similar to a V_1 lead on a 5-lead or 12-lead ECG. The tracings are similar but not identical. In MCL₁ the negative electrode is placed on the right shoulder and the positive electrode is placed at the fourth intercostal space, just to the right of the sternum (Fig. 17-18, *A*). It is extremely important for this electrode to be placed accurately. MCL₁ is an uncommon lead choice today. It is only used if monitoring with a 3-lead system—where V_1 is not available—a rare situation within any critical care unit. The normal QRS complex in lead MCL₁ has a mostly negative deflection (see Fig. 17-18, *B*).

In contrast, the normal QRS complex in lead MCL₆ has a mostly positive deflection because of the position of the MCL₆ lead placement on the left lateral midaxillary chest wall (Fig. 17-18, *C*).

ECG Lead Selection for Optimal Bedside Monitoring. In the early years of critical care nursing, the primary goals of cardiac monitoring were heart rate surveillance, detection of "warning" ventricular dysrhythmias (mostly PVCs), and early detection of lethal dysrhythmias (ventricular fibrillation or asystole). Although these are still goals of ECG monitoring in the critical care unit, several more complex issues are now of concern. It is now known that not all wide QRS-complex tachycardias are ventricular in origin; sometimes they are supraventricular with aberrant ventricular conduction. Many patients are now undergoing reperfusion therapy involving balloon angioplasty, stent, or fibrinolysis, and these patients require continuous monitoring for ST-segment changes that may represent ischemia even in the absence of clinical symptoms. It is now important that the nurse admitting a patient to the critical care unit or telemetry unit make a well-planned choice of monitoring lead(s) tailored to the clinical needs of that particular patient. In addition, accuracy of lead placement is extremely important if these leads are to be used for specialized diagnostic purposes.[39] Limb electrodes need to be placed close to where the limb joins the torso. Diagnostic accuracy is diminished if limb electrodes are moved too close to the heart.

Continuous Dysrhythmia Monitoring. Patients with serious cardiac diseases such as acute MI, heart failure, and cardiomyopathy are at risk for the development of bundle branch blocks, complex ectopy, and wide-complex tachycardias. These patients need to be monitored with a precordial lead that documents interventricular conduction changes. This is lead V_1. Some 5-lead systems offer the clinician the choice of MCL₁ or V_1. The tracings in these two leads are not identical, and V_1 must be chosen over MCL₁ because it has a higher diagnostic accuracy. The six limb lead tracings also offer several monitoring choices that can be individualized to the clinical needs of the patient. Lead I and aV_F are selected to detect a sudden change in ventricular axis. If ST-segment monitoring is required, the lead is selected according to the area of ischemia. If the ischemic area is not known, leads V_3 and lead III are recommended to detect ST segment ischemia.[39] In inferior wall injury, leads II, III, and aV_F are chosen; if lateral ischemia is present, lead I or aV_L may be selected.

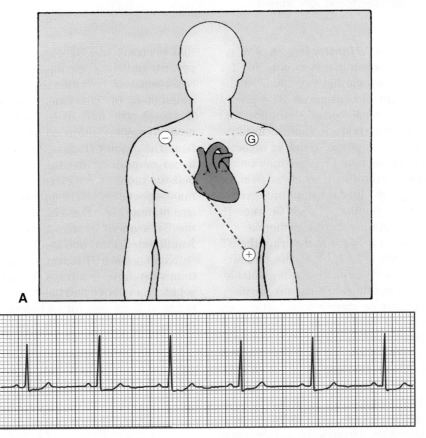

Fig. 17-17   Monitoring lead II. **A,** Electrode placement. The negative electrode is placed below the right shoulder; the positive electrode is placed on the lower left torso (preferably below the rib cage); the ground electrode is placed on the left shoulder. **B,** Typical ECG tracing in lead II.

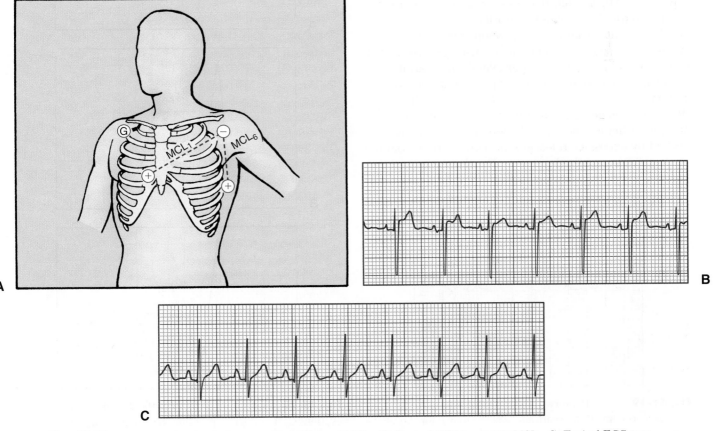

Fig. 17-18   **A,** Monitoring lead placement in MCL$_1$ and MCL$_6$. **B,** Typical ECG tracing in MCL$_1$. **C,** Typical ECG tracing in MCL$_6$.

Continuous ST-Segment Monitoring. A key responsibility of the critical care nurse is monitoring for ECG changes that signify myocardial ischemia. At the bedside this takes the form of continuous ST-segment monitoring using the traditional bedside monitor and ECG electrodes. Increasingly, bedside monitoring systems incorporate ST-segment analysis to detect myocardial ischemia or injury. ST-segment changes may be accompanied by classic symptoms such as chest pain, or may be "silent," without any clinical symptoms except ST depression on the ECG monitor.[40,41] See Chapter 18 for more information on silent myocardial ischemia.

The best way to choose a lead for monitoring the ST segment to detect ischemia is to look at the patient's 12-lead ECG during an episode of ischemia, if available. The standard 12-lead ECG obtained in an acute coronary syndrome before treatment or during a percutaneous coronary intervention (PCI) will reveal the leads that best demonstrate ischemia in that patient.[34] Under normal (nonischemic) conditions, the ST segment is at the same level as the TP segment, also known as the *isoelectric line* (Fig. 17-19).

Patients at risk of developing silent ischemia include anyone experiencing an acute coronary syndrome even if treated with thrombolytics, nitrates, or anticoagulation therapy. PCI patients are at risk for coronary artery reocclusion or spasm, reflected by ST-segment changes similar to those seen during PCI balloon inflation. Any patient admitted to the critical care unit with a history of a previous MI, angina, diabetes, or kidney failure is a candidate for ST-segment monitoring.

ST-segment deviation can develop secondary to nonischemic causes and can create a "false positive" alarm. Common culprits include hyperkalemia, pericarditis, hypokalemia, hypomagnesemia, hypothermia, ventricular aneurysm, hypothyroidism, pulmonary infarction, and drugs such as quinidine and digitalis. Patients with subarachnoid hemorrhage (SAH) demonstrate ST changes caused by excessive release of norepinephrine from the myocardial sympathetic nerves. The degree of myocardial necrosis and ST elevation is dependent upon the severity of neurologic injury.[42]

ST-segment deviation is measured as the number of millimeters of ST-segment vertical displacement from the isoelectric line, or from the patient's baseline. The measurement position is typically selected 60 to 80 msec from the J point (Fig. 17-20). This position is chosen to avoid monitoring the upstroke of the T wave. On the bedside monitor, ST elevation is displayed as a positive number, whereas ST depression is indicated by a negative number (see Fig. 17-20). To be clinically significant, the ST-segment change must be displaced by at least 1 millimeter (mm) and last for at least 60 seconds.

When setting ST alarm parameters, the individual patient's condition is always considered. The alarm may be set at 1 mm above and below the baseline ST level in patients at high risk for ischemia. In stable, low-risk patients, the suggested setting is 2 mm above or below the

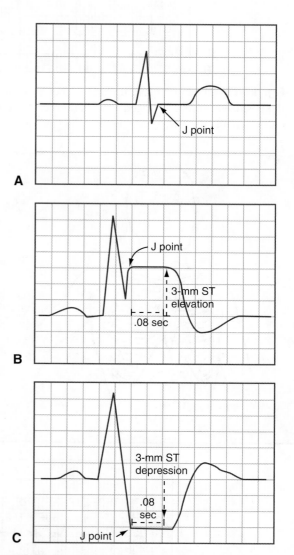

Fig. 17-20 **A,** Normal position of the J point. **B,** 3-mm ST elevation. **C,** 3-mm ST depression. ST changes are measured 60 to 80 msec (0.06-0.08 sec) after the J point.

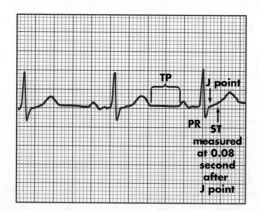

Fig. 17-19 The TP interval is used as the reference point for the isoelectric line if the heart rate is slow enough for the TP interval to be clearly seen. If not, the PR interval can be used.

isoelectric line.[34] The rationale for selection of wider ST alarm parameters in more stable patients is that this may reduce the number of false ST alarms.[34] This is important because stable patients tend to be more active, and when patients change position this can alter the isoelectric baseline. If there are too many false ST alarms, clinicians may be tempted to turn off or not pay attention to the ST alarm system. Poor electrode contact with the skin also is responsible for false ST-segment change alarms, emphasizing the need for adequate skin preparation before electrode placement.[34]

Some specific ECG patterns do not lend themselves to ST-segment monitoring; specifically, rhythms that are associated with a wide QRS and distortion of the ST segment. This includes left and right bundle branch block, paced rhythms, and idioventricular rhythms. Other rhythms that make ST-segment monitoring problematic include erratic atrial fibrillation or atrial flutter that obscures the isoelectric baseline.[34] Finally, agitated and restless patients make continuous ST-segment monitoring almost impossible.

Atrial Hypertrophy. Cardiac chamber enlargement can be suspected or diagnosed using the 12-lead ECG because muscle size influences the ECG tracing, although the echocardiogram is considered the gold standard for detecting cardiac chamber enlargement. Atrial hypertrophy on the 12-lead ECG is identified by the size and shape of the P waves and is usually seen best in lead II. Wide m-shaped P waves are seen in left atrial hypertrophy and are called *P mitrale*, because left atrial hypertrophy is often caused by mitral stenosis (Fig. 17-21, *A*). Tall, peaked P waves occur in right atrial hypertrophy and are referred to as *P pulmonale*, because this condition is often the result of chronic pulmonary disease (Fig. 17-21, *B*).

Ventricular Hypertrophy. Ventricular hypertrophy describes an increase in the size and muscle mass of one or both ventricles. Because a larger muscle is being depolarized, a greater amount of electrical activity is recorded on the ECG during depolarization. In ventricular hypertrophy, specific changes occur in the QRS complex. Upright QRS complexes become taller, and negative QRS complexes become even more negative. Often the QRS becomes slightly wider, because it takes longer to depolarize a larger muscle. The QRS axis often shifts toward the enlarged ventricle, because a greater portion of the total electrical activity of the heart occurs there. A diagnosis of LVH (left ventricular hypertrophy) and left bundle branch block (LBBB) on the 12-lead ECG is associated with increased cardiovascular mortality.[43,44] Although the 12-lead ECG can suggest hypertrophy, the echocardiogram is the most reliable diagnostic device, since it can visualize actual ventricular wall thickness and motion.[45]

Ischemia and Infarction. Ischemia occurs when the delivery of oxygen to the tissues is insufficient to meet metabolic demand. Cardiac ischemia in an unstable form occurs because of a sudden decrease in supply, such as when the artery is blocked by a thrombus or when coronary artery spasm occurs.[12,13] Stable angina can occur when a stenotic coronary artery is unable to adapt to sudden increase in demand created by exercise.[46] Ischemia is by nature a transient process. Either the balance of supply versus demand is restored and the muscle tissue recovers, or the imbalance becomes so great that the tissue can no longer survive and it infarcts and becomes necrotic. Many nursing and medical interventions are directed toward saving as much ischemic tissue as possible. Infarction refers to the actual death and disintegration of muscle cells and their eventual replacement by scar tissue. Once infarction has occurred, that process cannot be reversed.[13]

ECG Changes Indicating Ischemia and Infarction. Both ischemia and infarction cause changes in the way cardiac muscle cells respond to electrical stimuli, and these changes can usually be seen in a 12-lead ECG tracing.[47]

ST-segment elevation is seen when the positive electrode lies directly over an area of transmural (full-wall thickness) injury (Fig. 17-22, *A*). This represents a preinfarction state, and interventions to unblock the occluded coronary artery must be initiated to prevent death of myocardium.[13] ST elevation is a precursor to an *ST E*levation *M*yocardial *I*nfarction (STEMI).[13]

Not every myocardial infarction is heralded by ST elevation. When the patient has an MI without ST elevation, this is described as a *Non–ST E*levation *M*yocardial *I*nfarction (NSTEMI), but the diagnosis can be consider-

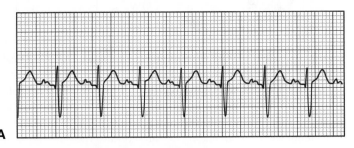

A

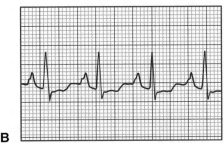

B

Fig. 17-21 Atrial hypertrophy. **A,** In left atrial hypertrophy, the P wave is broad and notched and is sometimes called *P mitrale*, because it is often associated with mitral valve disease. **B,** In right atrial hypertrophy, the P wave is tall and peaked and is sometimes called *P pulmonale*, because it is often associated with pulmonary disease.

Table 17-6	ECG Changes During Myocardial Infarction		
Location of Infarction	**Artery Involved**	**Leads Involved**	**ECG Changes**
Anterior wall	LAD	V_{3-4}	Q waves, ST ↑, T ↓
Inferior wall	RCA or LCx	II, III, aV_F	Q waves, ST ↑, T ↓
Ventricular septum	LAD	V_{1-2}	Q waves, ST ↑, T ↓
Lateral wall	LCx	V_{5-6}, I, aV_L	Q waves, ST ↑, T ↓
Posterior wall	RCA or LCx	V_{1-3} (ant); V_{7-9} (post)	Tall, upright R; ST ↓; Upright T with ST ↑ V_{7-9}
Right ventricle	Proximal RCA	V_4R (right)	ST ↑

LAD, Left anterior descending; ↑, elevated; ↓, depressed; *RCA,* right coronary artery; *LCx,* left circumflex; *ant,* anterior (see Fig. 17-7, *B,* for lead placement); *post,* posterior (see Fig. 17-7, *D,* for lead placement); *right,* right precordium (see Fig. 17-7, *C,* for lead placement).

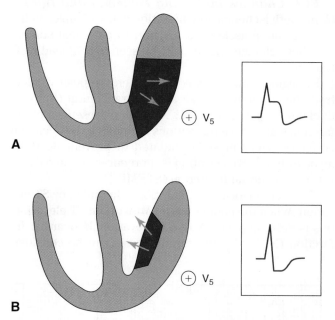

Fig. 17-22 **A,** Acute transmural ischemia. The electrical forces *(arrows)* responsible for the ST segment are directed outward through the entire thickness of the heart muscle wall, causing ST elevation in leads directly over the ischemic area. **B,** Acute subendocardial ischemia. The electrical forces responsible for the ST segment are deviated toward the inner layer of the heart, resulting in ST depression in leads directly over that area of the heart muscle wall.

ably more challenging without the signature ST changes seen on the ECG.[12]

ST-segment depression occurs when the reduction of blood flow is limited to the endocardium and some normal muscle tissue remains between the ischemic area and the positive electrode (Fig. 17-22, *B*). ST-segment depression is seen because the positive electrode is separated from the ischemic area by normal tissue. T waves most commonly flatten or become inverted.

Infarction involves actual necrosis (death) of muscle cells with eventual formation of scar tissue. These cells

can no longer be depolarized when an impulse reaches them. If the infarction involves the epicardial (outer) layer of the heart muscle or the entire thickness of the heart wall (transmural), the QRS complex changes. Abnormal Q waves typically develop in the leads overlying the affected area. Occasionally the entire QRS complex just becomes smaller, without actual development of Q waves.

Non–Q-wave Infarction. Not every acute MI results in a pathologic Q wave on the 12-lead ECG.[13] When the typical ECG changes are not present, the diagnosis depends on symptomatic clinical presentation, specific cardiac biomarkers (cTnI, cTnT, CK-MB), and non-ECG diagnostic tests such as cardiac catheterization.

Infarct Location by 12-Lead ECG. The location of the infarction can be roughly determined by noting the specific leads in which the ST-segment and T-wave changes are seen on the 12-lead ECG. See Table 17-6 for a summary of the anticipated 12-lead ECG changes.

Right ventricular infarction and posterior wall infarction are particularly difficult to identify on a standard 12-lead ECG, because none of the standard leads directly view these areas. A right ventricular infarction can be suspected and investigated in the setting of an acute inferior wall MI. To avoid missing this diagnosis, right-sided precordial leads (see Fig. 17-7, *B*) can be placed, and a 12-lead ECG obtained on any patient with a suspected inferior right ventricular wall MI.

A posterior wall MI may be suspected in a patient with an acute inferior wall MI when there is ST-segment depression in leads V_1, V_2, and V_3 on the standard 12-lead ECG. Tall upright R waves may also be present. Posterior wall involvement can be verified by adding posterior precordial leads V_7, V_8, and V_9 (see Fig. 17-7, *D*).[35]

Infarct ECG Progression. When blood flow in a coronary artery is suddenly occluded, the entire area of heart muscle normally perfused by that artery becomes ischemic. Collateral arterioles exist, which overlap and supply the perimeter of this area, and may prevent necrosis of some of the affected tissue. At the center of

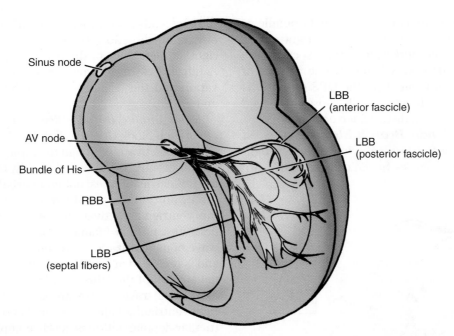

Fig. 17-23   Cardiac conduction system. *AV,* Atrioventricular; *RBB,* right bundle branch; *LBB,* left bundle branch. (Modified from Conover MB: *Understanding electrocardiography,* ed 7, St Louis, 1996, Mosby.)

the ischemic area, collateral blood flow is minimal or does not exist at all. Within a few hours, this tissue begins to necrose, or die. On the ECG tracing, this process is illustrated as follows. Within minutes of the onset of infarction, ST-segment elevation occurs in the leads directly overlying the affected heart wall. This ST-segment elevation persists for a period of hours to 1 day, gradually becoming less severe. Within the first few hours, T waves may become tall and symmetric. These are known as "hyperacute" T waves and indicate acute ischemia. Meanwhile, usually within 4 to 24 hours from the onset of the infarction, abnormal Q waves begin to develop in the affected leads and T waves begin to invert. Sometimes instead of actual Q waves developing, the R waves just become smaller. This still indicates necrosis of muscle tissue. The ST segments become isoelectric again in a few days, and the T wave becomes symmetric and deeply inverted in the affected leads. Occasionally these T-wave changes do not ever resolve. Usually, however, the T waves return to normal within several months. The Q waves may persist for the remainder of the patient's life, or they may get smaller over time and, in some individuals, disappear altogether. Table 17-7 summarizes the timing of these changes.

Intraventricular Ventricular Conduction Defects. Intraventricular conduction defects are the result of an abnormal pathway of conduction through the ventricles. Normally, conduction spreads from the AV node to the bundle of His and from there down the right and left bundle branches. The right bundle branch is long and thin and terminates in a mass of Purkinje fibers, which spread the wave of depolarization to the surrounding

Table 17-7	Timing of ECG Changes
Time Frame	**Change**
Immediate	ST-segment elevation in leads over the area of infarction
Within a few hours	Giant, upright T waves
Several hours	ST segment normalizes; T waves invert symmetrically
Several hours to days	Q waves or reduced R waves; voltage may remain low permanently

right ventricular muscle. After only a short distance, the left bundle branch divides into the left anterior fascicle, the left posterior fascicle, and the left septal fibers (Fig. 17-23). Each of these fascicles causes depolarization of separate areas of the left ventricle. If any part of the conduction system fails, the muscle cells in that area are still depolarized, but not as quickly. Depolarization must then spread from cell to cell, a slower process than activation through specialized conduction pathways.

On the ECG, intraventricular conduction defects cause a widening of the QRS because of the slower spread of depolarization. The affected muscle tissue begins the slower cell-to-cell depolarization just as the other areas in the ventricle are almost finished. This later depolarization is then tacked onto the end of the normal QRS, making it prolonged and altering its shape.

Any part of the conduction system can be affected. The term *bundle branch block* refers to complete interruption of conduction through either the right bundle or the entire left bundle branch. In complete right or left bundle branch block, the QRS is always 0.12 second (120 msec) or longer in duration. When only one fascicle of the left bundle branch is blocked, the QRS duration is within normal limits, although usually more prolonged than before the conduction disturbance occurred.

Right and Left Bundle Branch Blocks. The chest leads are the most useful in identifying complete right and left bundle branch blocks. Specifically, V_1 and V_6 are

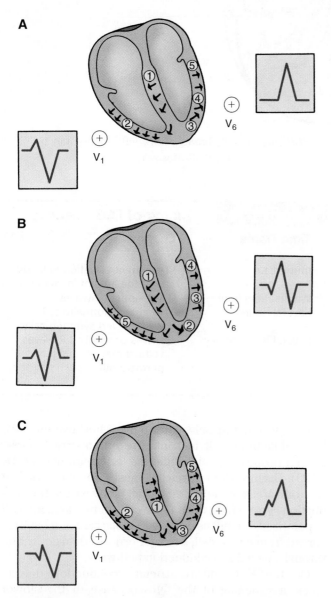

Fig. 17-24 **A,** Sequence of ventricular depolarization and resulting QRS complex, as seen in leads V_1 and V_6. **B,** Sequence of ventricular depolarization when right bundle branch block is present and resulting QRS complex, as seen in leads V_1 and V_6. **C,** Sequence of ventricular depolarization when left bundle branch block is present and resulting QRS complex, as seen in leads V_1 and V_6.

the best leads from which to identify forces traveling in a horizontal direction, because they are located on the right and left sides of the heart, respectively. Fig. 17-24, *A,* illustrates the normal sequence of ventricular activation and the usual shape of the QRS complex in V_1 and V_6.

Right Bundle Branch Block. In complete right bundle branch block (RBBB) (Fig. 17-24, *B*), the right ventricle is not activated through the rapid conduction system. Rather, it must be activated slowly, from one cell to the next. Electrical forces, not counterbalanced by opposing forces on the left, travel toward the right at the end of the ventricular activation. The septum is depolarized first, in a normal manner from left to right. Next, the wave of depolarization spreads through the left ventricle and is recorded in lead V_1 as a negative deflection. The final portion of the QRS complex is upright, indicating final forces traveling toward the right. This represents right ventricular depolarization that occurs after left ventricular depolarization is nearly complete. In lead V_6, the positive electrode is on the left side of the chest, so the waveforms are reversed. The final forces of the QRS are negative because they are traveling toward the right and away from the positive electrode of V_6. Note that the final negative deflection in V_6 is smaller than the final upright deflection in lead V_1, because the positive electrode in V_6 is at a greater distance from the right ventricle.

Left Bundle Branch Block. In complete left bundle branch block (LBBB) (Fig. 17-24, *C*), the conduction through the left ventricle must spread from cell to cell. Because a portion of the common left bundle normally initiates depolarization of the septum, the septum also is depolarized in an abnormal direction, from right to left. In lead V_1, this is recorded as an initial negative deflection. Next, the right ventricle is depolarized, seen as a small upright notch in the QRS as the forces travel briefly toward the positive electrode of V_1. Sometimes this notch is absent. The sequence of events has not changed, but the left ventricle is already beginning to be depolarized cell-to-cell and may offset the rightward forces of right ventricular depolarization. The final forces travel toward the left as the left ventricle is being depolarized. The left ventricle is a very large muscle mass, so these final forces are large and wide. In lead V_1, the final deflection is a deep, negative deflection (S wave), whereas in lead V_6, these final forces inscribe a tall, upright deflection (R wave).

Presence of an LBBB makes diagnosis of an acute anterior wall MI extremely difficult because the change in repolarization masks ST-segment elevation.[44] Perhaps related to this difficulty in interpreting injury, patients with acute coronary syndrome in the presence of LBBB and associated LV hypertrophy have a higher mortality than patients with acute coronary syndrome alone.[44]

Bundle branch blocks can easily be diagnosed at the bedside if the patient is being monitored with leads V_1

and V_6, respectively. A bundle branch block exists when the QRS complex is wider than 0.12 second, and when the complex did not originate from the ventricles, such as a PVC or paced beat. To determine which bundle branch is blocked, examine the last part of the QRS just before it returns to the baseline in leads V_1 and V_6. If upright in V_1 and negative in V_6, an RBBB exists. If negative in V_1 and upright in V_6, an LBBB is present.

Hemiblocks. Hemiblocks involve conduction failure of only part of the left bundle branch. In left anterior fascicular block (also called *left anterior hemiblock*), left ventricular depolarization begins in the left posterior fascicle and spreads anteriorly through Purkinje fibers distal to the block. The QRS is only slightly prolonged, up to 0.02 second longer than the patient's previous QRS. However, the axis changes dramatically and becomes more negative than minus 30 degrees (left-axis deviation). Other causes of left-axis deviation must be ruled out before a clinical diagnosis of left anterior hemiblock can be made (Boxes 17-3 and 17-4). In left posterior fascicular block (also called *left posterior hemiblock*), the anterior portion of the left ventricle is depolarized first. Conduction then spreads slowly to the right, inferiorly and posteriorly. Once again the QRS is slightly prolonged, although within normal limits. The axis then swings entirely the other direction and becomes greater than 110 degrees (right-axis deviation). Other causes of right-axis deviation must be ruled out before a definitive diagnosis of left posterior hemiblock can be made (see Box 17-4).

Box 17-3

CAUSES OF LEFT-AXIS DEVIATION

- Normal variation
- Mechanical shifts: exhalation; high diaphragm caused by pregnancy, ascites, or abdominal tumor
- Left anterior hemiblock
- Left ventricular hypertrophy
- Wolff-Parkinson-White syndrome
- Hyperkalemia
- Cardiomyopathy

Box 17-4

CAUSES OF RIGHT-AXIS DEVIATION

- Normal variation
- Mechanical shifts: inhalation, emphysema
- Left posterior hemiblock
- Right ventricular hypertrophy
- Lateral wall myocardial infarction
- Right bundle branch block
- Dextrocardia

Bifascicular Block. Blockage of either of the two branches of the left ventricular conduction system plus RBBB constitutes *bifascicular block*. Any combination of these conduction disturbances can occur and can evolve into complete heart block. Development of RBBB with left anterior fascicular block occurs in approximately 5% of patients with acute MI. The percentage for LBBB is similar. RBBB in combination with left posterior fascicular block is less common, probably because the left posterior fascicle is short and thick and has a dual blood supply from the left anterior descending and right posterior descending coronary arteries. Bifascicular block that develops during an acute MI warrants placement of a temporary pacemaker prophylactically in case conduction tissue ischemia progresses to complete heart block.

Dysrhythmia Interpretation. In clinical practice, the terms *dysrhythmia* and *arrhythmia* often are used interchangeably. The question of which word is the most accurate has been often discussed. Both terms are correct, and either may be used in practice. In this textbook, dysrhythmia is the more commonly used term. A dysrhythmia is any disturbance in the normal cardiac conduction pathway. Dysrhythmias can be detected on a 12-lead ECG, but very often they occur only sporadically. For this reason, patients in a critical care unit are monitored continuously, using a single- or dual-lead system, and rhythm strips are recorded routinely as well as any time the patient's rhythm changes. A systematic approach to evaluation of a rhythm strip is introduced first in this section, followed by specific criteria for common dysrhythmias encountered in clinical practice.

Heart Rate Determination. The first thing to assess when evaluating a rhythm strip is the ventricular rate. Regardless of the dysrhythmia involved, the ventricular rate holds the key to whether the patient can tolerate the dysrhythmia (i.e., maintain adequate blood pressure, cardiac output, and mentation). If the ventricular rate is consistently greater than 200 or less than 30, emergency measures must be started to correct the rate. A detailed analysis of the underlying rhythm disturbance can proceed later, when the immediate crisis is over. The three methods for calculating rate (Fig. 17-25, *A*) follow:

1. Number of RR intervals in 6 seconds times 10 (NOTE: ECG paper is usually marked at the top in 3-second increments, making a 6-second interval easy to identify.)
2. Number of large boxes between QRS complexes divided into 300
3. Number of small boxes between QRS complexes divided into 1500

In the healthy heart the atrial rate and the ventricular rate are the same. However, in many dysrhythmias, the atrial and ventricular rates are different; thus both must be calculated. To find the atrial rate, the PP interval, instead of the RR interval, is used in one of the three methods listed for determining rate.

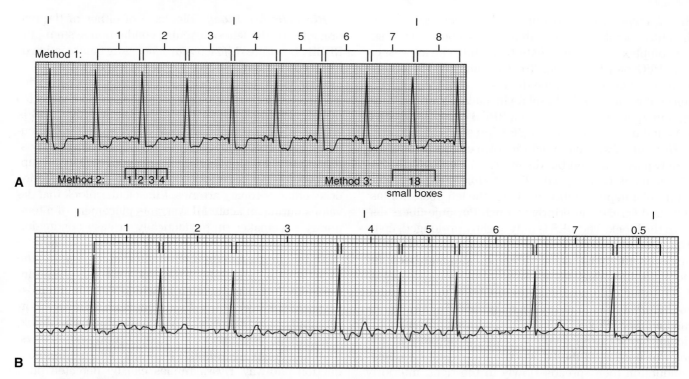

Fig. 17-25 **A,** Calculation of heart rate if the rhythm is regular. *Method 1:* number of RR intervals in 6 seconds multiplied by 10 (e.g., 8 × 10 = 80/min). *Method 2:* number of large boxes between QRS complexes divided into 300 (e.g., 300 ÷ 4 = 75/min). *Method 3:* number of small boxes between QRS complexes divided into 1500 (e.g., 1500 ÷ 18 = 84/min). **B,** Rate calculation if the rhythm is irregular. Only method 1 can be used (e.g., 7.5 intervals × 10 = 75/min).

The choice of method for calculating the heart rate depends on the regularity of the rhythm. If the rhythm is irregular, the first method (RRs in 6 seconds *multiplied by* 10) is the only method that can be used (Fig. 17-25, *B*). If the rhythm is regular, it is more accurate to use the second or third method. The second method can be easier to use when two consecutive R waves fall exactly on dark lines, and it provides a rapid estimate of rate. The third method is recommended when both R waves do not fall exactly on dark lines.

Rhythm Determination. The term *rhythm* refers to the regularity with which the P waves or R waves occur. Calipers assist in determining rhythm. One point of the calipers is placed on the beginning of one R wave while the other point is placed on the very next R wave. Leaving the calipers "set" at this interval, each succeeding RR interval is checked to be sure it is the same width as the first one measured.

In describing the rhythm, three terms are used. If the rhythm is *regular,* the RR intervals are the same, ±10%. For example, if there are 20 small boxes in an RR interval, an R wave could be off by two small boxes but the rhythm would still be considered regular. If the rhythm is *regularly irregular,* the RR intervals are not the same, but some sort of pattern is involved, which could be grouping, rhythmic speeding up and slowing down, or any other consistent pattern (Fig. 17-26, *A*). If the rhythm

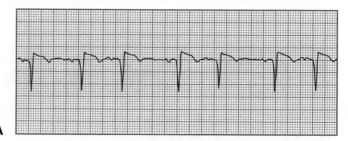

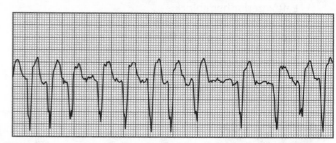

Fig. 17-26 **A,** Regularly irregular rhythm—irregular but with a consistent pattern, in that every other beat is premature. **B,** Irregularly irregular rhythm—irregular with no consistent pattern.

is *irregularly irregular,* the RR intervals are not the same and no pattern can be found (Fig. 17-26, *B*).

P-Wave Evaluation. The P wave is analyzed by answering the following questions. First, is the P wave present or absent? Second, is it related to the QRS? It is

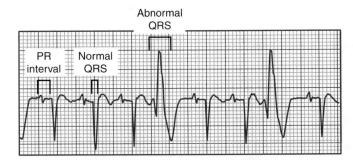

Fig. 17-27 PR interval measurement, from the beginning of the P wave to the beginning of the QRS complex. The PR interval on this tracing is 0.20 second; the QRS duration illustrates both normal and abnormal intervals. The narrow QRS complexes measure 0.08 second, which is normal. The wide QRS complexes measure 0.20 second and are caused by ventricular ectopy.

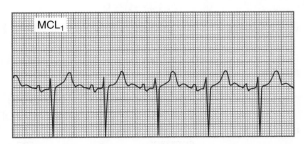

Fig. 17-28 Normal sinus rhythm. The rate is 70; the rhythm is regular. One P wave is present before each QRS complex. The PR interval is 0.18 second and does not vary throughout the strip. The QRS duration is 0.08 second. All evaluation criteria are within normal limits.

hoped that one P wave will be in front of every QRS. Sometimes two, three, or four P waves may be in front of every QRS. If this pattern is consistent, the P wave and QRS are still related, although not on a 1:1 basis.

PR-Interval Evaluation. The duration of the PR interval, which normally is 0.12 to 0.20 second (120 to 200 msec), is measured first. This is measured from the start of a visible P wave to the beginning of the following QRS (Fig. 17-27). Next, all PR intervals on the strip are verified to be sure they have the same duration as the original interval.

QRS Evaluation. The entire ECG strip must be evaluated to ascertain that the QRS complexes are consistently the same shape and width. The normal QRS duration is 0.06 to 0.10 second (60 to 100 msec). If more than one QRS shape is on the strip, each QRS must be measured. The QRS is measured from where it leaves the baseline to where it returns to the baseline (see Fig. 17-27).

QT Evaluation. The length of the QT varies with the heart rate. The QT interval is shorter when the heart rate is faster. A QT interval corrected for heart rate (QTc) that is longer than 0.50 second (500 msec) is of concern, as discussed in the earlier section on QT-interval monitoring.

Sinus Rhythms. The cardiac cycle begins when an impulse originates in the sinus node. As the wave of depolarization spreads through the atria, a P wave is inscribed on the ECG. The impulse is delayed briefly in the AV node, which corresponds to the PR interval on the ECG. After leaving the AV node, the wave of depolarization spreads rapidly through the bundle of His and the bundle branches and causes ventricular depolarization, which is recorded as a QRS complex by the ECG. Contraction immediately follows depolarization. Contraction is terminated by repolarization, which is demonstrated as a T wave on the ECG.

Normal Sinus Rhythm. If all of the events just discussed occur in their normal sequence with normal rates and intervals, the patient is in normal sinus rhythm. Specifically, the following are the criteria for normal sinus rhythm:

1. *Rate.* The intrinsic rate of the sinus node is 60 to 100 beats/min. *Intrinsic rate* is the normal rate at which a pacemaker site in the heart depolarizes automatically with no outside influences, such as drugs, fever, or exercise. In normal sinus rhythm, the rate must be whatever is "normal" for the sinus node, (i.e., 60 to 100 beats/min).
2. *Rhythm.* The rhythm must be regular, ±10%.
3. *P wave.* P waves must be present, and one and only one must precede every QRS complex.
4. *PR interval.* The PR interval represents delay in the AV node. In normal sinus rhythm, the PR interval is 0.12 to 0.20 second.
5. *QRS.* Size and shape do not matter in this complex, because it depends on lead placement and gain adjustments on the monitor. However, all QRS complexes must look alike. If conduction through the ventricles is normal, the QRS duration is 0.06 to 0.10 second. Fig. 17-28 is an example of normal sinus rhythm in V_1.

Sinus Bradycardia. Sinus bradycardia meets all of the criteria for normal sinus rhythm except that the rate is less than 60 (Table 17-8). It is normally seen in well-trained athletes at rest, or in many other individuals during sleep. Other conditions in which sinus bradycardia occurs include vagal stimulation, increased intracranial pressure, drug therapy with digoxin or beta-blockers, and ischemia of the sinus node caused by an acute MI. Sinus bradycardia is generally not treated unless the patient displays symptoms of hypoperfusion, such as hypotension, dizziness, chest pain, or changes in level of consciousness.

Sinus Tachycardia. Sinus tachycardia meets all the criteria for normal sinus rhythm except that the rate

Table 17-8	Sinus Rhythms			
Parameters	**Normal Sinus Rhythm**	**Sinus Bradycardia**	**Sinus Tachycardia**	**Sinus Dysrhythmia**
Rate	60-100/min	<60/min	>100/min	Variable
Rhythm	Regular	Regular	Regular	Irregular; respiratory variation
P wave	Present, with one per QRS	Present, with one per QRS	Present, with one per QRS	Present, with one per QRS
PR interval	0.12-0.20 sec and constant	0.12-0.20 sec and constant	0.12-0.20 sec and constant	0.12-0.20 sec and constant
QRS	0.06-0.10 sec	0.06-0.10 sec	0.06-0.10 sec	0.06-0.10 sec

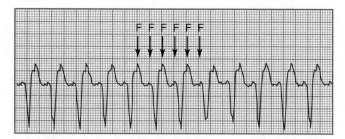

Fig. 17-29 Sinus tachycardia? In fact, this is atrial flutter with 2:1 conduction. Note how difficult it is to see the extra flutter waves *(F)* that are hidden in the QRS complexes.

is greater than 100 beats/min (see Table 17-8). Rates may be as high as 180 to 200 beats per minute in healthy, young adults during strenuous exercise. However, in the critical care setting, bed rest is prescribed for most patients. It is wise to be skeptical of any "sinus tachycardia" with a rate greater than 150 and to search for a triggering focus other than the sinus node. For example, atrial flutter waves might be difficult to see at first glance because of baseline distortion caused by the high ventricular rate (Fig. 17-29).

Sinus tachycardia can be caused by a wide variety of factors, such as exercise, emotion, pain, fever, hemorrhage, shock, heart failure, and thyrotoxicosis.[48] Illegal stimulant drugs such as cocaine, "ecstasy," and amphetamines can raise the resting heart rate significantly.[48] Many drugs used in critical care can also cause sinus tachycardia; common culprits are aminophylline, dopamine, hydralazine, atropine, and catecholamines such as epinephrine. Tachycardia is detrimental to anyone with ischemic heart disease because it decreases the time for ventricular filling, decreases stroke volume, and thus compromises cardiac output (CO). In addition, tachycardia increases heart work and myocardial oxygen demand, while decreasing oxygen supply by decreasing coronary artery filling time.

If the cause of the tachycardia can be determined (e.g., fever or pain), the cause is treated rather than trying to treat the heart rate directly.[48] Several drugs are available to decrease the heart rate if needed. Both cal-

cium channel blockers and beta-blockers are widely used for this purpose. However, a word of caution is warranted here. CO is determined by heart rate and stroke volume. If an injured heart can no longer maintain an adequate stroke volume, heart rate can be increased to maintain CO and supply an adequate blood flow to vital body tissues. If a drug is administered to force the sinus node to slow, severe and relatively immediate heart failure can result. The sinus node is controlled by many neural and humoral influences in the body, and the rate is set to try to meet the perceived demands; thus a close examination of the reason for the tachycardia is mandatory before treatment decisions are made.

Sinus Dysrhythmia. Sinus dysrhythmia, commonly called *sinus arrhythmia* in clinical practice, meets all of the criteria for normal sinus rhythm except that the rhythm is irregular (see Table 17-8). This irregularity coincides with the respiratory pattern; heart rate increases with inhalation and decreases with exhalation[49] (Fig. 17-30). Sinus dysrhythmia often occurs in children and young adults, and the incidence decreases with age. No treatment is required. To avoid being misled by other rhythm disturbances, one must examine all P waves closely to verify that they are all the same shape and that the PR intervals are all constant.

Atrial Dysrhythmias. Atrial dysrhythmias originate from an ectopic focus in the atria, somewhere other than the sinus node. The ectopic impulse occurs prematurely, before the normal sinus impulse is due to occur. The premature atrial depolarization may initiate a normal QRS complex, an abnormal or aberrant complex, or initiate a supraventricular tachycardia, clinically described as SVT. In recent years, huge advances have been made in the understanding of the pathogenesis and management of atrial dysrhythmias.

Premature Atrial Contractions. Premature atrial contractions (PACs) are isolated, early beats from an ectopic focus in the atria. The underlying rhythm is usually sinus. The regular sinus rhythm is interrupted by an early, abnormally-shaped atrial P wave. The early atrial wave usually looks different than the sinus P wave and may be inverted. The PR interval may be longer, shorter, or the

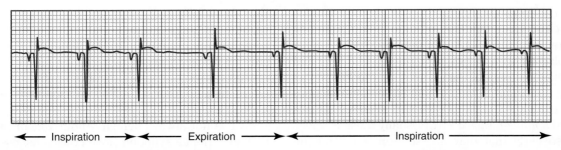

← Inspiration →← Expiration →← Inspiration →

Fig. 17-30 Sinus dysrhythmia. Note the increase in heart rate during inspiration and decrease in heart rate during expiration.

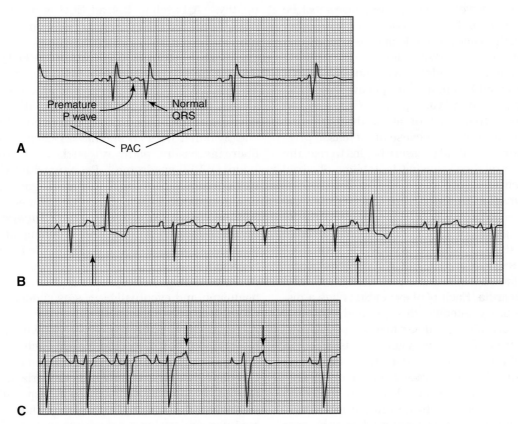

Fig. 17-31 Premature atrial contractions (PACs). **A,** Normally conducted PAC. The early P wave is indicated by the *arrow*, and the QRS that follows is of normal shape and duration. **B,** Nonconducted (blocked) PACs. The early P waves are indicated by *arrows*. Note how they distort the T waves, making them appear peaked, compared with the normal T waves seen after the third and fourth QRS complexes. **C,** Right bundle branch block aberration after a PAC.

same as the PR interval of a sinus impulse. The QRS that follows the ectopic atrial P wave can vary in shape depending on the degree of refractoriness of the AV node.

1. *Normal, narrow QRS:* If the atrial impulse arrives in the AV node after the AV node is fully repolarized, the impulse is conducted to the ventricles as a normal QRS. If the ventricles are also fully repolarized, conduction through the bundle branches is expected and a normal QRS is recorded on the ECG (Fig. 17-31, *A*).

2. *Wide QRS:* Occasionally, the early ectopic P wave can be conducted through the AV node, but part of

the conduction pathway through the ventricular bundle branches is blocked. Because the right bundle branch normally has the longest refractory period, it is usually the right bundle branch that is still blocked when the early impulse arrives. This produces a QRS that is wider than 0.12 second (120 msec) or wider than three small boxes on the ECG paper with a shape consistent with RBBB (Fig. 17-31, *B*). Conduction through the ventricles that is different from normal is referred to as *aberrant*. Consequently, these early, abnormally conducted PACs are described as *aberrantly conducted PACs*.

3. *Pause with no QRS:* Sometimes the ectopic P wave arrives so early that the AV node is still in its absolute refractory period. In this case, the wave of depolarization does not move past the AV node and no QRS follows. All that is seen on the ECG is an early, abnormal P wave followed by a pause until the next sinus P wave occurs (Fig. 17-31, *C*). This is called a *nonconducted PAC.* Usually these P waves are so early that they are superimposed on the T wave of the previous beat, making them difficult to find. The pause that follows is still clearly seen. Whenever an unexpected pause occurs in a rhythm, the T wave preceding the pause must be examined very carefully and compared with other T waves on the same strip to locate distortions that may reveal a hidden early P wave.

PACs can occur in individuals with normal hearts. PACs are accentuated by emotional upheaval, nicotine, caffeine, and digitalis. Mitral valve prolapse is associated with an increased frequency of atrial dysrhythmias. Heart failure can cause PACs because of increased pressure within the atria. As atrial pressure begins to rise, the atrial walls are stretched, causing irritability of atrial cells and the occurrence of PACs.

Supraventricular Tachycardia. The term supraventricular tachycardia (SVT) is clinically used to describe a varied group of dysrhythmias that originate above the AV node. SVT is not a very specific term. SVT includes sinus tachycardia, atrial tachycardia, multifocal atrial tachycardia, atrial flutter, atrial fibrillation, and junctional tachycardia. Each of these entities has a distinct pathophysiology, specific therapy, and expected outcome. SVT may also be described as a "narrow-complex tachycardia" defined as a QRS that is less than 0.12 second (120 milliseconds).[48] Once the specific dysrhythmia is identified, it is generally referred to by a specific name; for example, atrial fibrillation. In other words, the term SVT is used to describe a rapid, sustained atrial or junctional tachycardia when the exact mechanism is not yet known. Women are affected by episodic SVT at about twice the rate of men.[48]

In an acute situation a rapid dysrhythmia may be difficult to identify precisely. SVT can cause hemodynamic instability. It is important to differentiate ventricular tachycardia (VT) from SVT; then the focus can be directed toward rate control until the acute situation is resolved and hemodynamic stability is restored. At that point, a more careful analysis is needed to determine the specific dysrhythmia responsible for the SVT. The differentiation of SVT from VT requires specific knowledge of the relevant ECG criteria. This is discussed in detail later in this chapter.

SVT is not always benign. About 15% of people with SVT experience syncope (lose consciousness). Medications are used to limit the SVT rate, and prevent "blackouts" or syncope.[48] SVT that is persistent for weeks or months may lead to a tachycardia-mediated cardiomyopathy.[48] A baseline 12-lead ECG is helpful, and when possible a 12-lead ECG should be taken during the palpitations.[48]

SVT with Aberrant Conduction. If the QRS in SVT is wider than 0.12 second, it is important to differentiate between SVT with aberrant conduction and VT as described on p. 364 later in this chapter. SVT with aberrant conduction includes SVT with a bundle branch block and SVT that uses an anomalous congenital additional fiber (accessory pathway) such as Wolff-Parkinson-White (WPW) syndrome.[48] Patients with SVT with aberrant conduction are frequently misdiagnosed, and valuation by a specialist is highly recommended.[48]

Paroxysmal Supraventricular Tachycardia. *Paroxysmal* means starting and stopping abruptly. *Paroxysmal supraventricular tachycardia* (PSVT) refers to the sudden interruption of sinus rhythm by an atrial ectopic focus that fires repetitively at a rate of 150 to 250 beats/min and eventually stops as suddenly as it began (Fig. 17-32).

The rhythm of PSVT is perfectly regular, because the reentry loop has a specific length; each circuit through the loop requires exactly the same amount of time to complete. Reentry, either within the atria itself or involving the AV node, is the mechanism responsible for most supraventricular tachycardias, including PSVT. Other common underlying mechanisms include abnormal automaticity and triggered activity. P waves are present and abnormally shaped, although they may be difficult to identify because they often blend in with the previous T wave because of the rapid rate. It is most helpful if the beginning of the PSVT run is captured and recorded on ECG paper, because the early, abnormal P wave is often

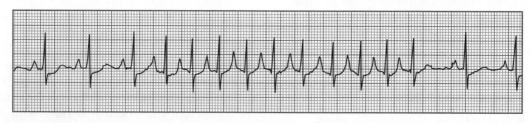

Fig. 17-32 Paroxysmal supraventricular tachycardia (PSVT). Note that the atrial rate during tachycardia is 158 beats/min. The run starts and stops abruptly.

easiest to identify in front of the first beat of the run. The PR interval should be the same for each cycle in the run, but it will probably be different from the PR interval of the patient's own normal sinus rhythm. Just as with PACs, the QRS complex is usually normal, because once the impulse passes through the AV node, conduction through the ventricles follows the usual pathway (Table 17-9). However, in PSVT, as discussed for SVT, aberrant conduction, often in the form of left or right bundle branch block, can occur with a wide QRS complex (greater than 0.12 second); this creates difficulty in differentiating relatively benign PSVT from its more serious counterpart, VT.

Sometimes, because of refractoriness in the AV node, not all of the ectopic P waves are conducted to the ventricles. Usually, at least every other P wave conducts a QRS, described as a 2:1 ratio, but occasionally the conduction relation may drop to three P waves for every QRS (3:1 ratio).

PSVT has essentially the same causal factors as PACs. PSVT has greater clinical significance, because it may be sustained for long periods and because it occurs at such a rapid rate. As stressed in the discussion of sinus tachycardia, rapid rates decrease ventricular filling time, increase myocardial oxygen consumption, and decrease oxygen supply. Heart failure, angina, or even myocardial infarction can result. PSVT usually responds rapidly to medical management, which initially includes the use of vagal maneuvers. Vagal maneuvers used in critical care include the following:[48]

1. Valsalva maneuver: asking the patient to "bear down" as if going to the bathroom.
2. Carotid sinus massage: performed on only one side of the neck over the carotid artery by a physician on a patient with a monitored ECG, and avoided on older patients who may have atherosclerotic disease of the carotid arteries.

If vagal maneuvers are unsuccessful at terminating the PSVT, the next step is generally the use of intravenous drugs, as long as the patient is hemodynamically stable.[48] The IV drug of choice to briefly block conduction through the AV node is adenosine (Adenocard). In PSVT, adenosine alone is often sufficient to restore normal sinus rhythm, but if not, it will unmask the ectopic P waves and confirm or provide strong clues to diagnose the SVT.[48] The usual dose is 6 mg given IV by rapid push followed by a normal saline bolus. If this does not create a temporary AV block or restore sinus rhythm, a 12 mg IV dose is administered. Potential dysrhythmic side effects of adenosine include a 1% to 15% chance of initiating atrial fibrillation.[48] Adenosine is contraindicated in patients with severe asthma.[48]

Other IV drugs that may be used to slow the rate in PSVT are amiodarone (Cordarone), a class III antidysrhythmic with a rapid onset and a short half-life.[48] Alternatively diltizam, a class IV calcium channel blocker in the nondihydropyridine group, can be used. The action of these drugs is to slow conduction through the AV node.[48] If IV drugs do not convert the PSVT or sustained SVT, or if the patient becomes hemodynamically unstable, the next step is electrical cardioversion.[48]

Multifocal Atrial Tachycardia. Multifocal atrial tachycardia (MAT) sometimes referred to as *chaotic atrial tachycardia*, occurs when there are numerous irritable atrial foci that intermittently fire and generate an impulse (Fig. 17-33). The atrial rate is greater than 100 beats per minute but generally does not exceed 160. The distinguishing feature on the ECG is that there are at least three different P-wave shapes, indicating at least three different irritable foci that can generate three different

Table 17-9	Atrial Dysrhythmias			
Parameter	Paroxysmal Supraventricular Tachycardia	Multifocal Atrial Tachycardia	Atrial Flutter	Atrial Fibrillation
Rate				
Atrial	150-250/min	100-160/min	250-350/min	>350/min (unable to count it)
Ventricular	Same or less	Same	250-350/min half or less	100-180/min (uncontrolled); <100/min (controlled)
Rhythm	Regular	Irregular	Atrial—regular; ventricular—may or may not be regular	Irregularly irregular
P wave	Present; abnormally shaped	Present; three or more different shapes	F waves	Fibrillatory baseline
PR interval	May be normal or prolonged	Variable	Conduction ratio: flutter waves per QRS	Absent
QRS	0.06-0.10 sec	0.06-0.10 sec	0.06-0.10 sec	0.06-0.10 sec

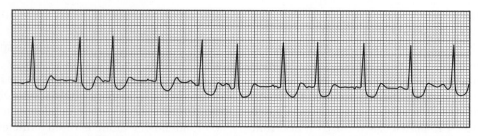

Fig. 17-33 Multifocal atrial tachycardia (MAT). Note that there are several differently shaped P waves and that the PR intervals vary.

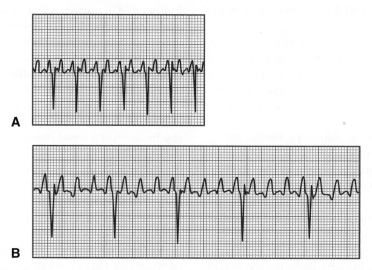

A

B

Fig. 17-34 **A,** Initial strip shows atrial flutter with 2 : 1 conduction through the AV node. **B,** During carotid sinus massage, the AV conduction rate is decreased, more clearly revealing the flutter waves.

atrial rates.[48] MAT is always irregular and is frequently misdiagnosed and confused with atrial fibrillation.[48] MAT is most commonly seen in elderly patients with chronic obstructive pulmonary disease (COPD). COPD causes chronic pulmonary hypertension, which in turn causes chronically elevated right atrial and right ventricular pressures. The abnormally high right atrial pressure causes stretching of the right atrial muscle cells and chronic irritability. Because the underlying cause cannot be resolved, this dysrhythmia is refractory to any treatment. There is no role for electrical cardioversion, antidysrhythmic drugs, or catheter ablation. Therapy is directed at limiting the effect of the COPD and correcting any electrolyte abnormalities.[48]

Atrial Flutter. Atrial flutter is recognized on the ECG by the *sawtooth* atrial pattern. These sawtooth-shaped atrial wavelets are not P waves; they are more appropriately called *F waves* (flutter waves), as shown in Fig. 17-34. Fortunately, the AV node does not allow conduction of all these impulses to the ventricles.

Pathogenesis of Atrial Flutter. Atrial flutter can be started by any isolated atrial impulse, but to be maintained, the atrial flutter requires a *reentry circular pathway* around macro structures in the atria. Typically these structures are in the right atrium and involve the

vena cava and the tricuspid valve in an area known as the *cavotricuspid isthmus.* The *reentry loop* typically circles counterclockwise around the tricuspid valve,[48] can run clockwise around the inferior vena cava (IVC), or can make a figure-eight loop around the IVC and the tricuspid valve.[50] To maintain a viable, self-perpetuating reentry pathway, the loop must avoid the SA node and be large enough to always meet tissue that is ready to be depolarized (accept a new electrical stimulus). The atrial reentry rate in atrial flutter is typically between 250 to 350 beats/min, producing the classic sawtooth or flutter wave pattern.[48] The atrial flutter wavelet always appears regular, because the circuit is always the same length and requires exactly the same amount of time to complete the reentry loop.

Atrial and Ventricular Rates in Atrial Flutter. When evaluating the rate of atrial flutter, it is important to calculate both atrial and ventricular rates. The ventricular rhythm is regular if the same number of flutter waves occurs between each QRS complex—in other words, if the degree of block at the AV node remains constant. Sometimes the refractoriness in the AV node changes from beat to beat, resulting in an irregular ventricular response. When describing atrial flutter, "PR interval" no longer applies; instead, it is a "conduction ratio," such as

3:1 or 4:1 (atrial waves-to-QRS complexes) that is used. In normal sinus rhythm, measuring the PR interval allows evaluation of the speed of conduction through the AV node; in atrial flutter, the number of flutter waves that bombard the AV node before one is allowed to pass through to the ventricles is a measure of AV nodal conduction. Once the impulse has passed the AV node, conduction through the ventricles is unaltered. The QRS duration remains normal or at least the same as it was in normal sinus rhythm (Table 17-9).

The major factor underlying atrial flutter symptoms is the ventricular response rate. If the atrial rate is 300 and the AV conduction ratio is 4:1, the ventricular response rate is 75 beats per minute and should be well tolerated. If, on the other hand, the atrial rate is 300 but the AV conduction ratio is 2:1, the corresponding ventricular rate of 150 may cause angina, acute heart failure, or other signs of cardiac decompensation. An atrial rate of 250 with a 1:1 AV conduction ratio yields a ventricular response rate of 250; the patient will be extremely symptomatic, and emergency measures are needed to decrease the ventricular rate.

Sometimes it is difficult to identify the flutter waves, especially if the conduction ratio is 2:1. Vagal maneuvers or adenosine can be useful diagnostic tools to allow better visualization of the flutter waves (see Fig. 17-34). Vagal maneuvers or IV adenosine (Adenocard) will not terminate atrial flutter but will create a temporary AV block to permit visualization of the atrial waveform and thereby facilitate accurate diagnosis.

Atrial Flutter Management. Pharmacologic cardioversion using ibutilide (Corvert) is effective at converting hemodynamically stable atrial flutter to sinus rhythm between 38% and 76% of the time.[48] The reasons for the variance in conversion in clinical studies is unknown, but it was not related to the length of time the patients had been in atrial flutter. For patients who responded to the ibutilide, the average conversion time after infusion was 30 minutes.[48] One of the complications of ibutilide is known to be polymorphic tachycardia—also known as *torsades de pointes*—but in studies with atrial flutter patients the rate of torsades de pointes was under 3%.[48]

Antidysrhythmic drugs are prescribed in two ways to treat atrial flutter: (1) to convert the rhythm to normal sinus rhythm (NSR); and (2) to slow conduction via the AV node. Of the specific drugs that may convert stable atrial flutter to sinus rhythm, the most effective is ibutilide (discussed in previous paragraphs); other, less effective agents include flecainide, propafenone, sotalol, procainamide, and amiodarone.[48] Other AV node–blocking medications are used to control the ventricular rate in atrial flutter but are ineffective at terminating the dysrhythmia. These include the calcium channel blockers, β-blockers and digoxin. Amiodarone shares both properties: it can slow conduction through the AV node and convert the atrial dysrhythmia. These drugs are effective

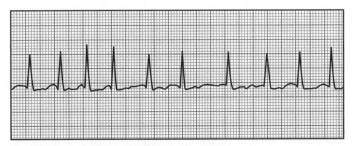

Fig. 17-35 Atrial fibrillation. Note the irregularly irregular ventricular rhythm.

as a mechanism to control the ventricular rate before electrical cardioversion.[48]

Nonpharmacologic interventions to convert atrial flutter to sinus rhythm are the most effective; these include electrical cardioversion and atrial overdrive pacing. The conversation rate with DC cardioversion is between 95% and 100%.[48] If atrial flutter has been present for more than 48 hours, up to one third of patients will have thrombi in the atria, and anticoagulation is mandated before either pharmacologic or electrical cardioversion. The risk of systemic emboli following cardioversion ranges from 2% to 7%.[48] Overdrive atrial pacing is often favored to convert atrial flutter following cardiac surgery. Epicardial wires that are placed at the time of surgery are connected to an external pacemaker. The overall success rate of atrial overdrive pacing is 83% (range 55% to 100%).[48]

For about 60% of patients, sudden onset of atrial flutter is associated with an acute disease process such as acute myocardial infarction or exacerbation of pulmonary disease, or follows cardiac or pulmonary surgery.[48] In this scenario, once the acute disease is managed the atrial flutter usually responds quickly to standard therapy and long-term drug management is not required. If at any time the patient with atrial flutter becomes hemodynamically unstable, electrical cardioversion is the recommended emergency intervention.[48]

For patients with atrial flutter unrelated to an acute disease process, permanent termination of the atrial flutter circuit can be achieved by *radiofrequency ablation* (RFA). RFA is a catheter procedure used to create a line of conduction block across one of more sections of the re-entry pathway. The most frequent location for RFA is a narrow band of tissue between the inferior vena cava and the tricuspid annulus known as the cavotricuspid isthmus).[48] Chapter 19 contains additional information on antidysrhythmic drugs on p. 553.

Atrial Fibrillation. Atrial fibrillation (AF) is the most frequently encountered dysrhythmia in the United States (Fig. 17-35). It affects an estimated 2.8 million individuals, with health care costs exceeding $1 billion.[51]

Atrial fibrillation is an SVT with non-sinus, uncoordinated atrial electrical activation that leads to a rapid deterioration in atrial mechanical function.[52] The ECG tracing in atrial fibrillation is notable for an uneven atrial baseline that lacks clearly defined P waves and instead shows rapid oscillations or fibrillatory wavelets that vary in size, shape, and frequency.[52] The atrial fibrillatory waves are particularly easy to identify in the inferior ECG leads II, III, AV_F.[52]

The ventricular response to atrial fibrillation is influenced by several factors: the efficiency of the AV node; autonomic nervous system activity—the level of sympathetic and parasympathetic (vagus nerve) tone; presence of medications that increase or slow conduction through the AV node-bundle branch conduction system; and various underlying heart conditions.[52] Atrial fibrillation displays irregular R-to-R intervals (different timing intervals between the QRS complexes) that do not show any logical pattern. The ability of the AV node and bundle branches to conduct or block the fibrillatory atrial impulses is key to the appearance of the QRS on the surface ECG. In AF, the QRS complex shape is usually narrow and normal in appearance, as long as the pathway through the ventricles is intact once the impulse leaves the AV node. The AV node acts as a filter to protect the ventricles from the hundreds of atrial impulses that occur each minute, although the AV node does not receive all of these atrial impulses. When the atrial muscle tissue immediately surrounding the AV node is in a refractory state, impulses generated in other areas of the atria cannot reach the AV node, which helps to explain the wide variation in RR intervals during atrial fibrillation (see Table 17-9).

Pathogenesis of Atrial Fibrillation. The pathogenesis of AF has traditionally been ascribed to random electrical foci firing in the atria. Recent research using high-density atrial mapping, high-speed video recordings, and ECG analysis has uncovered distinct spatial organization within the atria.[52,53] Atrial fibrillation is now known to involve several reentry circuits within the atria, and in some cases to originate at specific anatomical sites. The four pulmonary veins that drain into the left atrium are a trigger site for early atrial foci to both initiate and propagate reentry circuits to maintain atrial fibrillation.[53] The earliest atrial ectopic foci have been electrically mapped 2 to 4 cm within the pulmonary veins.[53] The affected pulmonary veins contain thin myocardial sleeves that project into the pulmonary veins from the left atrium. This ectopic tissue resembles discontinuous fingerlike projections about 5 millimeters (mm) thick that extend as far as 4.5 cm into one or more pulmonary veins. The tissue ultimately becomes part of the venous wall.[54] The spread of atrial fibrillation to the rest of the atria is thought to occur via multiple reentry *wavelets* that are maintained in perpetual motion by a "mother rotor," or dominant reentry circuit, that functions at a higher frequency, drives the atrial fibrillation, and originates from the ectopic pulmonary vein tissue.[53] When a single focus

can be identified, it is possible to encircle that area and isolate that site using RFA.[54] A catheter procedure to encircle and isolate the four pulmonary veins is being successfully used in many cardiac electrophysiology centers.

It is likely that there are several different types of atrial fibrillation, involving different mechanisms. As electrophysiologic mapping techniques become more advanced, the mystery surrounding the origin of AF will become less cloudy. What is now clear is that although atrial fibrillation may look disorganized on the ECG baseline, there is possibly an electrical pattern within the atria. Knowledge of this pattern will ultimately lead to new treatments that can help cure or control AF.

Types of Atrial Fibrillation. Atrial fibrillation is described by a number of additional labels that are associated with different clinical outcomes:

1. *Paroxysmal atrial fibrillation:* Atrial fibrillation that starts and stops abruptly is termed paroxysmal atrial fibrillation and is often described as "self-limiting."[52] Sometimes when the heart rate is really fast, it is not possible to identify the rhythm as AF and it may initially be labeled as an SVT. It is always helpful to catch the start or ending point of any SVT on an ECG rhythm strip so that the initial stimulus can be identified. A printed rhythm strip also permits a more precise analysis of the dysrhythmia once the patient's clinical condition has been stabilized. In the critical care unit it is important to document occurrence of paroxysmal atrial fibrillation by placing an ECG rhythm strip in the medical record and noting any associated clinical symptoms. The goal of treatment will be to convert the atrial fibrillation back to a sinus rhythm as soon as possible. Electrical or pharmacologic cardioversion is most effective when the AF has been present for less than 24 hours.[52]

2. *Recurrent atrial fibrillation:* When a patient has two or more episodes of paroxysmal AF, it is described as *recurrent*. There is often a period during which patients may go in and out of atrial fibrillation, before the electrical atrial remodeling is complete and AF becomes the dominant and persistent rhythm.

3. *Persistent atrial fibrillation:* When AF is sustained, or there are multiple bouts of paroxysmal AF, it is termed persistent or permanent. Research studies and clinical experience demonstrate that the longer a person remains in AF, the greater the degree of atrial electrical remodeling, and the more difficult it becomes to convert the atria back to sinus rhythm. Even after electrical cardioversion, when the ECG may show sinus rhythm, the mechanical function of the atria may take up to a week to return to normal.[53] It is estimated that 2.2 million Americans have persistent or paroxysmal AF.[52]

4. *Lone atrial fibrillation:* The expression *lone AF* is used to describe individuals under 60 years of age who have AF and according to clinical and diagnostic studies do not have structural heart disease.[52]

5. *Atrial fibrillation associated with underlying structural heart disease:* Some cardiac conditions are known to be associated with AF, particularly hypertension, especially with associated left ventricular hypertrophy, heart failure, valvular heart disease, acute MI, myocarditis, and pericarditis.[52,55] In developed countries, rheumatic heart disease—so prevalent at the beginning of the twentieth century—now plays a minor role.[55] When the atrial tissue of patients in persistent AF is examined histologically (tissue analysis), the atria show structural abnormalities beyond the changes known to be due to the underlying heart condition.[52] These changes are termed *electrical atrial remodeling.* The longer the person remains in AF, the less likely is a return to sinus rhythm.[52]

6. *Atrial fibrillation associated with other conditions:* Certain noncardiac conditions associated with an increased incidence of AF are diabetes, pulmonary embolism, pneumonia, and thyrotoxicosis. Generally, once the acute condition is treated the AF should resolve and not reoccur.[52] Hyperthyroidism is a correctable cause of atrial fibrillation that can be effectively reversed in most cases by correcting the thyrotoxic condition. If not recognized and treated, excess thyroid hormone makes rate control difficult, increases risk of a thromboembolic event, and causes higher morbidity and mortality.

7. *Neurogenic atrial fibrillation:* A condition where the autonomic nervous system triggers AF due to heightened vagal tone in susceptible individuals.[52]

8. *Silent atrial fibrillation:* In the critical care unit, all patients have ECG monitoring so detection of AF is not difficult. However, in recent clinical trial registries, between 10% and 50% of patients who were enrolled had clinically silent AF; this means that the AF was either asymptomatic or minimally symptomatic and the patient was unaware of the dysrhythmia.[55] The presence of silent AF is of concern because atrial fibrillation causes a deterioration in atrial mechanical function, formation of atrial emboli, increased risk of stroke, and is harder to convert to sinus rhythm the longer it is present.

9. *Cardiac surgery postoperative atrial fibrillation:* Atrial fibrillation occurs in approximately 30% of patients following coronary artery bypass surgery (CABG).[56] If the CABG surgery is combined with a mitral value replacement (MVR), the incidence of AF rises to 63.6%;[57] if the CABG is combined with aortic valve replacement (AVR), the incidence of AF is 48.8%.[57] Most AF develops on the second to third postoperative day, and affects both patients with and without prior history of atrial fibrillation.[56-57] Postoperative AF following cardiac surgery is associated with significant hemodynamic instability, increased length of hospital stay, decreased long-term survival, and increase in the risk of embolic stroke.[57] Patients who undergo minimally invasive cardiac surgery incur the same incidence of AF as patients who have traditional cardiac surgery procedures.[57]

Atrial Fibrillation Risk Factors. As more research has focused on the etiology of atrial fibrillation, a clearer picture of incidence and risk factors has emerged. AF is present in 0.4% of the population, although there is a huge variation based upon age. It occurs in less than 1% of persons less than 60 years, but the incidence rises to over 6% in those over 80 years of age.[52] Men have a higher risk of developing AF than women, and at an earlier age.[52] Average age of onset is 60.5 years for men and 65.5 years for women.[55] The incidence of reported "palpitations" or paroxysmal AF is higher in women.[55] Atrial fibrillation is the most common cardiac dysrhythmia in the United States and responsible for about one third of dysrhythmia—related hospital admissions.[55] According to epidemiologic data from the Framingham study, one in four men and women who are free of AF at 40 years of age will develop atrial fibrillation or flutter later in their life.[58] The risk is higher for people with a history of hypertension, heart failure, or myocardial infarction.[58]

Atrial Fibrillation Management. There is currently considerable debate about the most effective approach to treat atrial fibrillation. In the past the gold standard was to convert the patient out of the atrial fibrillation back to sinus rhythm. However, recent research has shown that for many patients staying out of atrial fibrillation is an unattainable goal. Furthermore, the long-term clinical outcome for the patient may be similar with either of the two following approaches:

1. Convert the atrial fibrillation back to sinus rhythm using pharmacologic or electrical cardioversion (rhythm control).
2. Allow the atrial fibrillation to persist and use pharmacologic measures to control the ventricular response rate (rate control).

RHYTHM CONTROL. For the hospitalized patient with *new-onset* atrial fibrillation with unstable hemodynamics, the focus is generally on rhythm control (conversion to sinus rhythm) using antidysrhythmic drugs or electrical cardioversion. Emergency drugs used to convert atrial fibrillation to sinus rhythm (also known as a chemical cardioversion) include amiodarone and ibutilide. Antidysrhythmic drugs used long-term to maintain the patient in sinus rhythm include amiodarone, disopyramide, flecainide, moricizine, procainamide, propafenone, quinidine, sotalol, and dofetilide or a combination of these medications as needed.[59] Even with drug therapy, recurrence of atrial fibrillation is likely.[59] Electrical cardioversion may be successful in converting the atria to sinus rhythm if attempted within a few days or weeks of the onset of atrial fibrillation. Its success is less likely if the AF has existed for a long time.[52] Without continued antidysrhythmic drug therapy, about 75% of cardioverted patients will be in atrial fibrillation at one year.60 This number changes to about 50% of patients (half in AF/half in sinus rhythm) with continued antidysrhythmic drug therapy.[60] One of the disadvantages to long-term antidysrhythmic drug treatment are drug side-effects and potential "prodysrhythmic" effect of certain medications.[59,61]

RATE CONTROL. The most frequently prescribed drugs used to control the ventricular rate in atrial fibrillation include calcium channel blockers, β-blockers, and digoxin. These drugs work to slow conduction through the AV node. They have no impact on the fibrillating atria. In the past it had always been assumed that "rate control" was an inferior strategy, because the patient stayed in atrial fibrillation, lost "atrial kick," and was presumed to have an increased risk of embolic stroke. Two multicenter trials have altered that perception: The *Atrial Fibrillation Follow-up: Investigation of Rhythm Management* (AFFIRM),[62] and the *RAte Control vs. Electrical Cardioversion for Persistent Atrial Fibrillation* (RACE).[63] These two trials found similar morbidity, mortality, and quality of life in patients treated long-term with either method: rhythm conversion or rate control.[59] For long-term management of atrial fibrillation, "rate control" is the recommended approach, and therapeutic anticoagulation to prevent embolic stroke is mandatory.[64] Antidysrhythmic medications used to manage atrial fibrillation are listed in the Pharmacologic Management table on Atrial Fibrillation in Chapter 19, p. 557.

Anticoagulation in Atrial Fibrillation. Both electrical and chemical (drug-induced) cardioversion entail the threat of precipitating emboli into the systemic circulation. During atrial fibrillation the atria do not contract; hence blood may pool and promote clots that attach to the atrial walls (mural thrombi). If cardioversion is successful and normal sinus rhythm is restored, the atria will again contract forcibly and, if thrombus formation has occurred, may send clots traveling through the pulmonary or systemic circulation.

To prevent embolic stroke it is important to pay attention to the "48-hour rule." Patients who have been in atrial fibrillation for 48 hours or longer (how long may not be known), must be adequately anticoagulated with an oral vitamin K antagonist (warfarin) to achieve a target INR of 2.5 (range between 2.0 and 3.0) for at least 3 weeks *before* elective cardioversion.[65] Following successful cardioversion patients should be anticoagulated for 4 weeks *after* cardioversion.[65]

Transesophageal echocardiography (TEE) is helpful in identifying the presence or absence of thrombi in the fibrillating atria and is recommended as a screening tool before elective cardioversion. It is especially helpful for patients in AF for less than 48 hours who, in the absence of atrial thrombi, may undergo cardioversion without anticoagulation.[65]

Patients who experience episodes of rapid atrial fibrillation for only a few hours or days at a time and then convert back to sinus rhythm spontaneously (paroxysmal atrial fibrillation) are at risk for embolic stroke and must be anticoagulated.[65] Especially vulnerable are those patients over 75 years of age with a history of transient ischemic attack (TIA) or stroke, a previous systolic embolism, moderately impaired left ventricular function, or symptoms of heart failure.[65]

Procedures to Treat Atrial Fibrillation. Several catheter and surgical interventions to treat atrial fibrillation are being explored. These include atrial pacing,[51,66] catheter isolation of the pulmonary veins, and Cox-Maze III surgery.[60,67]

The Cox-Maze III procedure (typically called the MAZE procedure) is an open-heart surgical operation designed to permanently cure atrial fibrillation.[52,60] It is suitable for only a tiny fraction of the individuals who have atrial fibrillation, generally those who have *lone atrial fibrillation* (see previous section on atrial fibrillation) without other structural heart disease. For carefully selected patients this surgery is successful over 90% of the time.[52,67] In general, these patients are younger. The cardiac surgeon makes a series of incisions that encircle the pulmonary veins to prevent initiation of atrial fibrillation by isolating the known foci near the pulmonary veins from the remainder of the atria; for some patients the mitral and tricuspid valve annuli may need to be isolated also.[52] Attempts to reproduce the success of the Maze procedure using specialized catheters in the cardiac catheterization laboratory are currently in development.[52] Other avenues include development of atrial pacemakers and defibrillators to convert atrial fibrillation.[52]

Junctional Dysrhythmias. Only certain areas of the AV node have the property of automaticity. The entire area around the AV node is collectively called the *junction;* hence impulses generated there are called *junctional.* After an ectopic impulse arises in the junction, it spreads in two directions at once. One wave of depolarization spreads upward into the atria and depolarizes them, causing the recording of a P wave on the ECG. This is called *retrograde (backward) conduction,* and the P wave is inverted when viewed in lead II. At the same time, another wave of depolarization spreads downward into the ventricles through the normal conduction pathway, producing a normal QRS complex. This is termed *antegrade (forward) conduction.*

Depending on timing, the P wave (1) may be seen in front of the QRS, with a short PR interval (less than 0.12 second), (2) may be obscured entirely by the QRS, or (3) may immediately follow the QRS.

Premature Junctional Contraction. If only a single ectopic impulse originates in the junction, it is simply called a *premature junctional contraction.* On the ECG the rhythm is regular from the sinus node, except for one early QRS complex of normal shape and duration. The P wave can be entirely absent. If a P wave can be found, it very closely precedes or follows the QRS. In lead II, the P wave appears inverted (having a negative deflection), because the atria are being depolarized from the AV node upward, which is the opposite direction from the wave of depolarization that occurs when triggered by the sinus node. If the P wave appears before the QRS, the PR interval is less than 0.12 second. Premature junctional contractions have virtually the same clinical significance as do PACs. However, if the patient is receiving digoxin, digitalis toxicity may be suspected. Although digoxin slows conduction through the AV node, it also increases automaticity in the junction.

Junctional Escape Rhythm. Sometimes the junction becomes the dominant pacemaker of the heart (Table 17-10). Normally the intrinsic rate of the junction is 40 to 60 beats/min. The intrinsic rate of the sinus node is 60 to 100 beats/min. Under normal conditions the junction never has a chance to "escape" and depolarize the heart because it is overridden by the sinus node. However, if the sinus node fails, the junctional impulses can depolarize completely and pace the heart. This is called a *junctional escape rhythm* and is a protective mechanism to prevent asystole in the event of sinus node failure. Generally, a junctional escape rhythm (Fig. 17-36) is well-tolerated hemodynamically, although efforts must be directed toward restoring sinus rhythm. Sometimes a pacemaker is inserted as a protective measure because of concern that the AV junction may also fail.

Junctional Tachycardia and Accelerated Junctional Rhythm. A junctional rhythm can also occur at a faster rate (see Table 17-10). As with sinus rhythm, the term *tachycardia* is reserved for rates greater than 100 per minute; thus junctional tachycardia is a junctional rhythm, usually regular, at a rate greater than 100. But what if the junctional rate is greater than 60 and less than 100 (faster than the intrinsic rate of the junction, yet not fast enough to be considered a tachycardia)? The phrase *accelerated junctional rhythm* applies to this situation. Accelerated junctional rhythm is usually well tolerated by the patient, mainly because the heart rate is within a reasonable range. Junctional tachycardia may not be tolerated as well, depending on the rate and the patient's underlying cardiac reserve. Once again, digitalis toxicity is strongly suspected, because digoxin enhances automaticity of the AV node. If digitalis toxicity is present, the optimal strategy is to measure the digoxin serum level and to withhold digoxin until the dysrhythmia resolves.

Ventricular Dysrhythmias. Ventricular dysrhythmias result from an ectopic focus in any portion of the ventricular myocardium. The usual conduction pathway through the ventricles is not used, and the wave of depolarization must spread from cell to cell. As a result, the QRS complex is prolonged and is always greater than

Table 17-10	Junctional Rhythms		
Parameter	Junctional Escape Rhythm	Accelerated Junctional Rhythm	Junctional Tachycardia
Rate	40-60/min	60-100/min	>100/min
Rhythm	Regular	Regular	Regular
P waves	May be present or absent; inverted in lead II	May be present or absent; inverted in lead II	May be present or absent; inverted in lead II
PR interval	<0.12 sec	<0.12 sec	<0.12 sec
QRS	0.06-0.10 sec	0.06-0.10 sec	0.06-0.10 sec

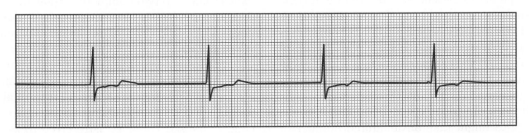

Fig. 17-36 Junctional escape rhythm. The ventricular rate is 38. P waves are absent, and the QRS is normal width.

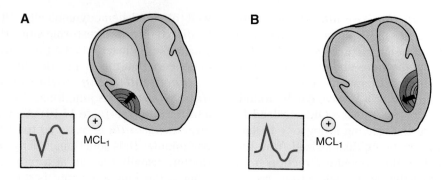

Fig. 17-37 **A,** Right ventricular premature ventricular contraction (PVC). The spread of depolarization is from right to left, away from the positive electrode in lead V_1 (MCL$_1$), resulting in a wide, negative QRS complex. **B,** Left ventricular PVC. The spread of depolarization is from left to right, toward the positive electrode in lead V_1 (MCL$_1$). The QRS complex is wide and upright.

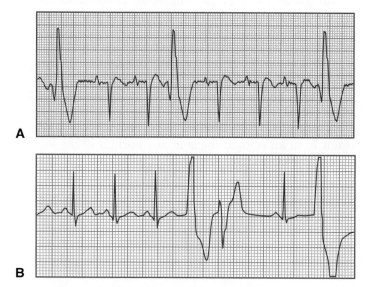

Fig. 17-38 **A,** Unifocal PVCs. **B,** Multifocal PVCs.

0.12 second. It is the width of the QRS, not the height, that is important in the diagnosis of ventricular ectopy.

Premature Ventricular Contractions. A single ectopic impulse originating in the ventricles is called a *premature ventricular contraction (PVC).* Some PVCs are very small in height but remain wider than 0.12 second. If in doubt, a different lead is evaluated. The shape of the QRS varies, depending on the location of the ectopic focus. If the ectopic focus is in the right ventricle, the impulse spreads from right to left, and the QRS resembles an LBBB pattern, because the left ventricle is the last to be depolarized. In V_1, this is a wide, negative QRS (Fig. 17-37, *A*). If the ectopic focus is in the left ventricular free wall, the wave of depolarization spreads from left to right (Fig. 17-37, *B*).

Because the ectopic focus could be any cell in the ventricle, the QRS might take an unlimited number of shapes or patterns. If all of the ventricular ectopic beats

look the same in a particular lead, they are called *unifocal*, which means that they probably all result from the same irritable focus (Fig. 17-38, *A*). Conversely, if the ventricular ectopics are of various shapes in the same lead, they are called *multifocal* (Fig. 17-38, *B*). Multifocal ventricular ectopics are more serious than unifocal ventricular ectopics, because they indicate a greater area of irritable myocardial tissue and are more likely to deteriorate into ventricular tachycardia or fibrillation. In general, ventricular dysrhythmias have more serious implications than do atrial or junctional dysrhythmias and occur only rarely in healthy individuals.

A PVC originates in a ventricular cell that has become abnormally permeable to sodium, usually as a result of damage of one kind or another. Because of this new permeability to sodium, the cell reaches depolarization threshold before an impulse is received from the sinus node. Once depolarization threshold is reached, the cell automatically depolarizes, thus beginning total ventricular depolarization. Ordinarily, the ventricular impulse does not conduct back through the AV node; hence the sinus node is not disturbed and continues to depolarize the atria, resulting in a normal P wave. Conduction from the sinus node will not proceed into the ventricles if they are in a refractory state. The next sinus beat, assuming there is no further ventricular ectopy, conducts normally through the AV node and into the ventricles.

Compensatory Pause. If the interval from the last normal QRS preceding the PVC to the one following it is exactly equal to two complete cardiac cycles (Fig. 17-39, *A*), a compensatory pause is present. It does not usually occur in PACs or premature junctional contractions, so when present, it is somewhat diagnostic of ventricular ectopy. If the normal sinus P wave that occurs immediately after the PVC finds the ventricles sufficiently recovered to accept another impulse, a normal QRS results and the PVC is sandwiched between two normal beats (Fig. 17-39, *B*). This PVC is referred to as *interpolated*, meaning *between*. Interpolated PVCs usually occur when

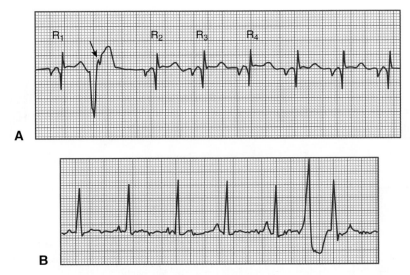

Fig. 17-39 A, PVC with a fully compensatory pause. The interval between the two sinus beats that surround the PVC (R_1 and R_2) is exactly two times the normal interval between sinus beats (R_3 and R_4). The fully compensatory pause occurs because the sinus node continues to pace despite the PVC. Note the sinus P wave *(arrow)* hidden in the ST segment of the PVC. This P wave did not conduct through to the ventricles because they had just been depolarized and were still in the absolute refractory period. **B,** Interpolated PVC. The PVC falls between two normal QRS complexes without disturbing the rhythm. Note that the RR interval between sinus beats remains the same.

either the PVC is very early or the normal sinus rate is relatively slow.

Occasionally the ventricular impulse spreads backwards across the AV node to depolarize the atria. When this occurs, the sinus node is reset and no full compensatory pause occurs.

Describing Ventricular Ectopy. PVCs can develop concurrently with any supraventricular dysrhythmia. Therefore it is not sufficient to describe a patient's rhythm as "frequent PVCs" or even "frequent unifocal PVCs." The underlying rhythm must always be described first (e.g., "sinus bradycardia with frequent unifocal PVCs" or "atrial fibrillation with occasional multifocal PVCs"). Timing of PVCs can also be described. When a PVC follows each normal beat, *ventricular bigeminy* is present (Fig. 17-40). If a PVC follows every two normal beats, it is called *ventricular trigeminy.*

In individuals with underlying heart disease, PVCs and/or episodes of self-terminating VT are potentially malignant. Nonsustained VT is defined as three or more consecutive premature ventricular beats at a rate faster than 110 per minute, lasting less than 30 seconds.

PVC Timing. The timing of PVCs can be important, especially if myocardial ischemia is present. The relative refractory period, represented on the ECG by the last half of the T wave, is a particularly vulnerable time for ectopy to occur because repolarization is not yet complete. Repolarization is even more delayed in ischemic tissue, so that various portions of the ventricular muscle are not repolarized simultaneously. If a PVC occurs at this critical point when only a part of the muscle is repolarized, individual segments of muscle can depolarize separately

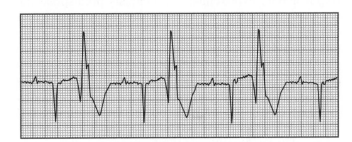

Fig. 17-40   Ventricular bigeminy.

from each other, resulting in ventricular fibrillation. This is called the *R-on-T phenomenon* (Fig. 17-41).

Two consecutive PVCs are described as a *couplet,* and three consecutive PVCs are called either a *triplet* or a *three-beat run of ventricular tachycardia.* More than three consecutive PVCs are considered ventricular tachycardia, but it is still useful to state how many beats of ventricular tachycardia occurred if the run was short (i.e., fewer than 20 beats).

Causes of PVCs. PVCs can result from many causes. They have been known to occur, although rarely, in healthy individuals with no evidence of heart disease. The critical care nurse has an important role in identifying factors that may be causing or at least contributing to PVCs. Acute ischemia is the most dangerous cause of ventricular ectopy. Ischemia causes cell membrane permeability to change, giving rise to early depolarization and the initiation of ectopic impulses. Ventricular ectopy that occurs during an acute ischemic event may require treatment with intravenous amiodarone or other antidysrhythmic drugs.

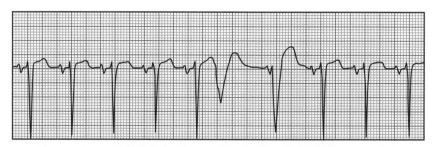

Fig. 17-41 R-on-T phenomenon.

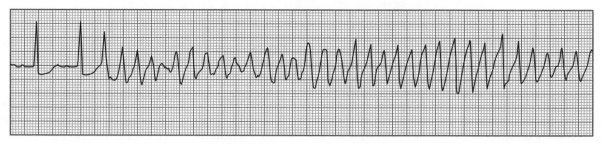

Fig. 17-42 Torsades de pointes.

Metabolic abnormalities are common causes of PVCs. Hypokalemia, hypoxemia, and acidosis predispose the cell membrane to instability and may cause ventricular ectopy. Treatment is directed toward identifying the metabolic disturbance and correcting it. Arterial blood gas values and serum potassium and magnesium levels are obtained if no recent results are available. The ability of oxygen and potassium values to change very rapidly in a critically ill patient must not be underestimated. If PVCs develop during suctioning of an intubated patient, a few additional breaths of 100% oxygen usually are sufficient to restore adequate oxygenation and to eliminate the ventricular ectopy.

Any form of heart disease can lead to ventricular ectopy. Patients with cardiomyopathy or ventricular aneurysms can have chronic, severe ventricular ectopy, which may prove to be refractory to any antidysrhythmic agent. Invasive procedures, such as insertion of a pulmonary artery catheter or cardiac catheterization, can cause PVCs by mechanically irritating the ventricular muscle. In these situations the ectopy usually resolves with removal or advancement of the catheter.

Certain drugs can cause ventricular ectopy. Digitalis toxicity is often accompanied by PVCs, which are somewhat resistant to conventional antidysrhythmic therapy. Some class I antidysrhythmic drugs can actually cause more serious dysrhythmias than those they were intended to treat. This is called a *prodysrhythmic effect* (also described as a *proarrhythmic effect*) and can sometimes be fatal. These drugs prolong the QT interval by lengthening the ventricular refractory period. This is a therapeutic effect, but when the QT prolongation becomes excessive, a characteristic form of polymorphic ventricular tachycardia called *torsades de pointes* devel-

ops (Fig. 17-42). In this dysrhythmia the ventricular tachycardia is very rapid and the QRS complexes appear to twist in a spiral pattern around the baseline. Clinically, torsades de pointes is poorly tolerated because of the extremely rapid rate. If not terminated, death will result. Sometimes torsades de pointes stops spontaneously, although the patient may experience a syncopal episode or seizure at the time of the dysrhythmia.

PVC Management. Not all ventricular ectopy requires treatment. In individuals without significant underlying heart disease, PVCs do not represent an increased risk for sudden death and are considered benign. If the patient complains of palpitations, therapy initially includes reassurance and elimination of such factors as caffeine or alcohol ingestion, emotional stress, and sympathomimetic drugs that increase ventricular irritability. If symptoms continue, mild tranquilizers can be administered or β-blockers can be given to reduce the response to sympathetic stimulation. Antidysrhythmic drugs such as Amiodarone or β-blockers are used during an acute MI when the damaged myocardium increases the risk of isolated PVCs becoming VT. In contrast, if the patient with PVCs has a healthy heart, antidysrhythmic drugs are used as a last resort because of the risk of prodysrhythmia (the drugs increase the incidence of VT). For further information on antidysrhythmic drugs, see p. 556.

Idioventricular Rhythm. At times, an ectopic focus in the ventricle can become the dominant pacemaker of the heart (Table 17-11). If both the sinus node and the AV junction fail, the ventricles depolarize at their own intrinsic rate of 20 to 40 times per minute. This is called an *idioventricular rhythm* and is protective in nature. Rather than trying to abolish the ventricular beats, the aim of treatment is to increase the effective heart rate

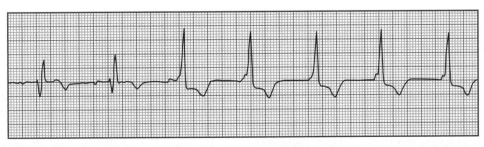

Fig. 17-43 Accelerated idioventricular rhythm (AIVR). The QRS duration is 0.14 second, and the ventricular rate is 65.

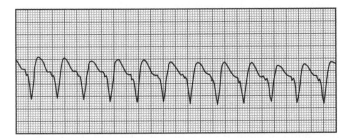

Fig. 17-44 Ventricular tachycardia.

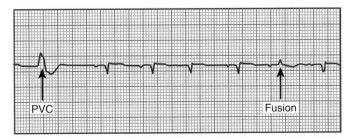

PVC

Fusion

Fig. 17-45 Ventricular fusion beat *(arrows)*. The QRS duration is only 0.08 second, and the shape represents both the normal QRS and the previous PVC.

Table 17-11	**Ventricular Rhythms**			
Parameter	**Idioventricular Rhythm**	**Accelerated Idioventricular Rhythm**	**Ventricular Tachycardia**	**Ventricular Fibrillation**
Rate	20-40/min	40-100/min	>100/min	None
Rhythm	Usually regular	Usually regular	Usually regular	Irregular
P waves	Absent or retrograde	Absent or retrograde	Absent or retrograde	None
PR interval	None	None	None	None
QRS	>0.12 sec	>0.12 sec	>0.12 sec	Fibrillatory waves

and reestablish a higher pacing site, such as the sinus node or the AV junction. Usually, a temporary pacemaker is used to increase heart rate until the underlying problems that caused failure of the other pacing sites can be resolved.

An accelerated idioventricular rhythm (AIVR) occurs when a ventricular focus assumes control of the heart at a rate greater than its intrinsic rate of 40 per minute but less than 100 per minute (Fig. 17-43). Although relatively benign in and of itself, this rhythm must be closely observed for any increase in rate, and the patient must be observed for hemodynamic deterioration. Usually it is not treated pharmacologically if well tolerated, although a transvenous temporary pacemaker should be inserted electively as a precaution against sudden hemodynamic deterioration. Intravenous lidocaine must never be administered to a patient with an idioventricular rhythm, because it suppresses the ventricular pacemaker and converts the rhythm to asystole.

Ventricular Tachycardia. Ventricular tachycardia (VT) is caused by a ventricular pacing site firing at a rate of 100 times or more per minute, usually maintained by a reentry mechanism within the ventricular tissue (Fig. 17-44). The complexes are wide, and the rhythm may be slightly irregular, often accelerating as the tachycardia continues (see Table 17-11). In most cases, the sinus node is not affected and it continues to depolarize the atria on schedule. P waves can sometimes be seen on the ECG tracing. They are not related to the QRS and may even appear to conduct a normal impulse to the ventricles if their timing is just right.

If the sinus impulse and the ventricular ectopic impulse meet in the middle of the ventricles, a fusion beat results. Fusion beats are narrower than ventricular beats and look like a cross between the patient's sinus QRS and the ventricular ectopic QRS (Fig. 17-45). When present, P waves and fusion beats are helpful in verifying the diagnosis of ventricular tachycardia as opposed to supraventricular tachycardia. A detailed discussion of the differentiation between VT and SVT is included in the section on differential diagnosis of a "wide QRS tachycardia" later in this chapter.

ETIOLOGY OF VENTRICULAR TACHYCARDIA. Over 90% of ventricular tachycardia occurs in the presence of structural cardiac disease, such as myocardial ischemia, congenital heart disease, valvular dysfunction, and cardiomyopathy. Other triggers include drug toxicity, electrolyte disturbances, and as an adverse reaction to certain antidysrhythmic drugs (prodysrhythmia). Only 10% of patients experience episodes of VT without known structural heart disease.[68]

Ventricular tachycardia is a serious dysrhythmia and must be treated quickly. The rapid ventricular rate makes this dysrhythmia poorly tolerated. In addition, the loss of the proper timing of atrial contraction, which would add volume to the ventricles just before contraction and enhance the force of contraction, is lost, thus greatly reducing cardiac output (CO). The fall in CO may cause the patient to lose consciousness. And finally, if not terminated quickly, VT is very likely to degenerate into ventricular fibrillation and death.

MANAGEMENT OF VENTRICULAR TACHYCARDIA. How ventricular tachycardia is clinically managed depends on whether the patient is stable or unstable, as well as whether a pulse and adequate blood pressure are present. Pulseless ventricular tachycardia is life-threatening. The patient will lose consciousness and will need immediate defibrillation as described in the American Heart Association (AHA) protocols for Advanced Cardiac Life Support (ACLS).[69]

Patients with stable VT who have a heart rate below 150 beats/min, palpable pulse, and stable blood pressure may be treated pharmacologically with amiodarone, β-blockers, lidocaine, procainamide, or overdrive pacing as described in the ACLS protocols.[69]

Once the acute episode is over, patients who have already experienced sustained ventricular tachycardia or cardiac arrest continue to be at risk for sudden cardiac death (SCD). An extensive clinical evaluation of these patients is warranted, including cardiac catheterization and electrophysiologic testing with programmed ventricular stimulation. Therapy is aimed at preventing a recurrence of sustained ventricular tachycardia/ventricular fibrillation (VT/VF). It may include treating the underlying cause, administering antidysrhythmic drugs, performing ablation of the reentrant pathway within the ventricle, or inserting an implantable cardioverter defibrillator (ICD).

ICDs can be programmed to deliver several bursts of overdrive pacing to terminate stable VT before cardioversion. This has the advantage of being more comfortable for the patient, since it prevents the discomfort of an internal shock if the overdrive pacing is successful. Most patients with an ICD are also managed with anti-dysrhythmic drugs. Antitachycardia (overdrive) pacing is an effective treatment if combined with defibrillation backup. It is risky without defibrillator support, since one of the complications of antitachycardiac pacing is acceleration of the ventricular tachycardia towards a faster, pulseless VT, polymorphic VT, or even ventricular fibrillation (VF). For more information on implantable cardioverter defibrillators, see Chapter 19, p. 515.

Ventricular Fibrillation. Ventricular fibrillation (VF) is the result of chaotic electrical activity in the ventricles from either repetitive, small areas of reentry or a series of rapid discharges from various foci within the ventricular myocardium. This causes the ventricles to be unable to contract completely and effectively. The ventricles merely quiver, and no forward flow of blood occurs. Without forward flow, no palpable pulse or audible apical heart tones are present. Clinically, VF is indistinguishable from asystole (absence of electrical activity). On the ECG, VF appears as a continuous, undulating pattern without clear P, QRS, or T waves (Fig. 17-46). When VF occurs in the setting of an acute ischemic event and is accompanied by a significant amount of myocardial damage, the survival rate is poor. Resuscitation is often unsuccessful; recurrence rates are high in those who are resuscitated. Ventricular fibrillation is seen on the ECG as either large, erratic undulations of the baseline (coarse VF) or as a mild tremor (fine VF). In VF the patient does not have a pulse, no blood is being pumped forward, and defibrillation is the only definitive therapy. Generally, coarse VF is more likely to be successfully defibrillated. Antidysrhythmic drugs such as intravenous amiodarone are administered if initial attempts at defibrillation fail. As with any cardiac arrest situation, supportive measures such as cardiopulmonary resuscitation (CPR), intubation, and correction of metabolic abnormalities are performed concurrently with definitive therapy.

Differential Diagnosis of a Wide QRS-Complex Tachycardia. Tachycardias that are triggered by an ectopic atrial or junctional focus are called *supraventricular*, meaning that they come from an irritable site above the ventricles.[48] Typical supraventricular tachycardia (SVT) has a narrow QRS complex (less than 0.12 second), because the electrical impulse enters the ventricle through the AV node and still follows the normal conduction pathway via the bundle branches through the

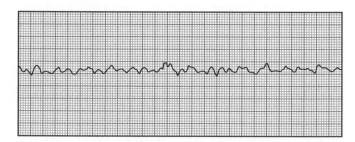

Fig. 17-46 Ventricular fibrillation.

ventricles. VT always has a wide QRS complex (greater than 0.12 second), because the impulse begins somewhere within the ventricles and must spread slowly—cell to cell—without the benefit of the usual conduction system. Therefore it is easy to distinguish between typical SVT and VT by QRS width alone. Unfortunately, not all SVTs result in a narrow QRS complex. The three situations in which an SVT presents with a wide QRS complex are as follows:

1. The patient may already have a right or left bundle branch block, resulting in a wide QRS even during sinus rhythm. Understandably, if that patient develops an atrial or junctional tachycardia, the bundle branch block remains unchanged and the QRS complex is still wide.

2. A supraventricular impulse may arrive in the ventricles so early that only part of the conduction system is repolarized. One of the bundle branches is still refractory, causing the wave of depolarization to spread abnormally (aberrantly) through the ventricles and resulting in a wide QRS complex.

3. Occasionally an anatomic variant occurs in which the patient has a small strip of muscle tissue connecting the atria with the ventricles and bypassing the AV node. This is called an *accessory pathway*, or *bypass tract*, the most common of which is *Wolff-Parkinson-White syndrome*, or WPW. This is not a problem in normal sinus rhythm, although it sometimes causes subtle ECG changes that allow it to be detected. However, when rapid atrial dysrhythmias occur, they can be conducted directly to a portion of the ventricular myocardium without normal AV delay. Depolarization through the ventricles then proceeds from cell to cell rather than through the normal pathway of the conduction system, resulting in a wide QRS-complex tachycardia that closely resembles VT.

Significance of VT versus SVT. Standard treatment for VT includes administration of intravenous amiodarone. In contrast, SVT is treated with a variety of drugs that work by blocking the AV node conduction pathway—diltiazem, verapamil, amiodarone, or digoxin. A problem occurs if the SVT has occurred as a result of the presence of an accessory pathway and the narrow complex tachycardia is treated with verapamil or other drugs that block the AV node but do not block the WPW accessory pathway. The consequences can be acute, severe hypotension or loss of consciousness requiring immediate cardioversion. For this reason, it is important in individuals who are relatively hemodynamically stable to be sure of the etiology of the tachycardia before treatment is initiated.

Regardless of the site of origin, a wide QRS-complex tachycardia may not be well tolerated, mainly because of the rapid heart rate that prevents adequate ventricular filling during diastole, as well as increasing myocardial oxygen demand while decreasing time available for coronary artery filling. Hemodynamic deterioration is evidenced by syncope, severe hypotension, or ischemic symptoms. In this case, emergency external cardioversion needs to be performed regardless of whether the tachycardia is of ventricular or supraventricular origin. Correct diagnosis of a wide QRS-complex tachycardia may have an impact on the long-term management of a patient as well. If atrial flutter or fibrillation is determined to be the underlying mechanism, long-term treatment probably includes amiodarone or a β-blocker to reduce the heart rate response when these dysrhythmias occur. If VT is determined to be the underlying mechanism in a patient without a history of ventricular dysrhythmias, a careful search for the cause (i.e., hypoxemia, electrolyte imbalance, excess sympathetic stimulation, or ischemia) is warranted. Depending on the clinical situation, the patient may require long-term antidysrhythmic therapy. If there is a history of VT or sudden cardiac death (SCD) and the patient is already on antidysrhythmic therapy, a recurrent episode of VT indicates that the current treatment regimen is not effective and the therapy needs to be changed. For more information on SCD, see Chapter 18, p. 455.

Clinical Differentiation of VT/SVT. Contrary to popular belief, hemodynamic stability or instability does not help to differentiate between VT and SVT with a wide QRS complex. In theory, an SVT is better tolerated, especially if atrial contraction is still occurring before each ventricular contraction (AV synchrony). However, clinically this is often variable. Ventricular tachycardia may be well tolerated, especially if the rate is less than 150 per minute. Some patients can be in sustained VT for hours without significant hemodynamic compromise. Conversely, because AV synchrony is lost in atrial fibrillation or atrial flutter, and the ventricular response rate may be very rapid, ventricular filling and, in turn, cardiac output can be severely compromised.

Careful physical examination can be of value in determining the source of the tachycardia. The jugular venous pulse can be assessed for the presence of cannon "*a* waves." When the atria contract at the same time as ventricular systole, the AV valves are closed and the blood in the atria is forced to regurgitate into the venous system. This is seen as a very large pulsation in the jugular vein. If it occurs sporadically (i.e., not with every beat), it is a sign of AV dissociation, or independent beating of the atria and ventricles. Heart sounds provide another diagnostic clue. Variation of the intensity of the first heart sound (S_1) from beat to beat favors VT, because this is also indicative of AV dissociation.

By far the most reliable means of diagnosing a wide QRS-complex tachycardia is through careful analysis of the ECG. Heart rate and rhythm are evaluated first, although they are not the only diagnostic indicators.

The QRS width is measured in more than one lead, because the lead with the widest QRS complex is the most reliable indicator of true QRS duration. (It is assumed that some portion of the QRS complex is isoelectric in leads where the QRS appears to be narrow.) QRS widths of less than 0.14 second favor SVT with aberrant conduction, whereas widths of greater than 0.14 second in an RBBB pattern or of greater than 0.16 second in an LBBB pattern favor VT.

The tracing is examined closely for the presence of P waves. If P waves can be identified and they do not correlate on a 1:1 basis with the QRS complexes, AV dissociation exists and strongly suggests VT.

Although P waves may be found in any lead, they are most likely to be visible in V_1 or lead II. When the sinus node remains in control of the atria and a ventricular ectopic focus is in control of the ventricles, it is likely that at some point the timing will be coordinated and, by chance, the sinus impulse will get to conduct through the AV node and begin to depolarize the ventricles just as the ventricular ectopic focus fires. The resulting QRS complex is a *fusion beat* (see Fig. 17-45), which looks like a blend of the patient's normal QRS and the wide QRS complex of the ventricular dysrhythmia. Fusion beats also strongly suggest VT.

Another helpful diagnostic criterion for VT is a QRS axis in the northwest quadrant of (minus) −90 degrees to −180 degrees (see Fig. 17-14). An axis in this quadrant means that the wave of depolarization is directed upward and to the right, exactly the opposite of normal ventricular depolarization. Even when ventricular conduction is abnormal, as in bundle branch blocks, ventricular depolarization begins at the level of the AV junction and spreads downward toward the apex, although conduction disturbances direct the current flow more to the

right or left than normal. Although not all VTs have an axis in the northwest quadrant, about one fourth of them do, and when present, an axis in the northwest quadrant confirms the diagnosis of VT. Fig. 17-47 illustrates how this abnormal axis can be rapidly identified from a five-lead ECG bedside monitor by noting the shape of the QRS in leads I and aV_F.

Finally, the shape of the QRS complex in the right precordial lead V_1 or MCL_1 and the left precordial lead V_6 or MCL_6 can be diagnostic of VT or of SVT with aberrant conduction. Fig. 17-48 summarizes these QRS patterns. In addition, if the QRS complex is either entirely positive from V_1 through V_6 or entirely negative, the diagnosis is VT. This phenomenon is known as *precordial concordance*.

Nursing Management. Proper electrode placement and appropriate lead selection have already been discussed but cannot be overemphasized. In addition to correct lead placement and selection, every effort must be made to record the wide QRS-complex tachycardia on a standard 12-lead ECG. Certainly, emergency treatment must not be delayed if the patient is hemodynamically unstable, but documenting the dysrhythmia by recording a "stat" 12-lead ECG must be given a high priority if time permits. VT and SVT are often nonsustained, and waiting for a physician's order or a technician to perform the test could result in failure to document the dysrhythmia at all, leaving the cause and subsequent therapy a mystery.

Atrioventricular Conduction Disturbance. Normally the sinoatrial (SA) node triggers electrical depolarization in the heart. From there, the impulse travels through three internodal tracts in the right atrium to the

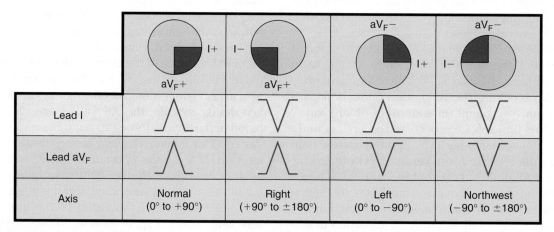

Fig. 17-47 Determination of QRS axis quadrant by noting predominant QRS polarity in leads I and aV_F. *Normal axis:* If QRS during tachycardia is primarily positive in both I and aV_F, the axis falls within the normal quadrant from 0 to 90 degrees. *Right axis deviation:* If the QRS complex is primarily negative in I and positive in aV_F, right axis deviation is present. *Left axis deviation:* If the QRS complex is predominantly positive in I and negative in aV_F, left axis deviation is present. *Indeterminate axis:* If QRS is primarily negative in both I and aV_F, a markedly abnormal "indeterminate," or "northwest," axis is present that is diagnostic of ventricular tachycardia. (From Drew B: *Heart Lung* 20[6]:615, 1991.)

atrioventricular (AV) node.[70] The left atrium is depolarized by a fiber known as Bachman's bundle.[70] The electrical impulse is briefly delayed in the AV node to allow the atria to contract and the mitral and tricuspid valves to close before the impulse is conducted to the bundle of His, the bundle branches, and the Purkinje fibers.[70]

On the ECG, the ability of the AV node to conduct is evaluated by measuring the PR interval and the relationship of P waves to QRS complexes (Table 17-12). The normal PR interval, measured from the beginning of the P wave to the beginning of the QRS complex, ranges from 0.12 to 0.20 second.

First-Degree AV Block. When all atrial impulses are conducted to the ventricles but the PR interval is greater than 0.20 second, a condition known as *first-degree AV block* exists (Fig. 17-49). First-degree AV block can be chronic or acute, and may be caused by a multitude of conditions. Long-standing first-degree block may occur related to fibrosis and sclerosis of the conduction system, lack of blood supply to the conduction system due to coronary artery disease, and also valvular heart disease, myocarditis, and various cardiomyopathies. First-degree heart block that develops acutely is of much greater concern. Causes include drug toxicity related to digoxin, beta-blockers or amiodarone administration, acute myocardial ischemia or infarction, hyperkalemia, edema following valvular heart surgery, and increased vagal tone.[70] First-degree AV block represents slowed

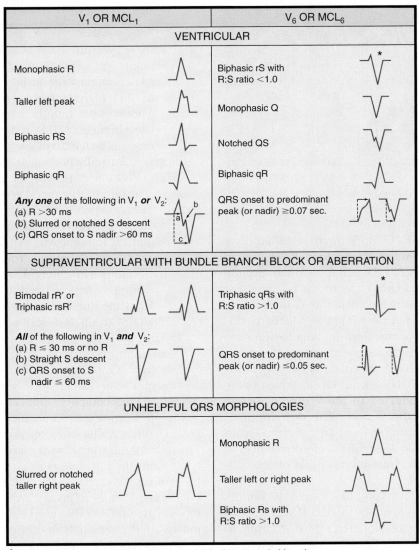

*Tachycardias with a right bundle branch block pattern in V_1 only

Fig. 17-48 Summary of morphologic clues in V_1 or MCL_1 *(left column)* and in V_6 or MCL_6 *(right column)* that are valuable in distinguishing supraventricular tachycardia with bundle branch block or aberration from ventricular tachycardia. If wide-complex tachycardia with taller right peak pattern (i.e., unhelpful morphology) develops in a patient monitored with a single MCL_1 lead, the nurse changes leads to determine whether the wide complex falls into one of the diagnostic patterns in V_6 (MCL_6). (From Drew B: *Heart Lung* 20[6]:614, 1991.)

Table 17-12		Atrioventricular (AV) Block		
Parameter	**First Degree**	**Second-Degree Mobitz I (Wenckebach)**	**Second-Degree Mobitz II**	**Third Degree (Complete)**
PR interval	>0.20 sec and constant	Increases with each consecutively conducted P wave	Constant	Varies randomly
P waves	1 P wave for each QRS	Intermittently not conducted, yielding more P waves than QRS complexes	Intermittently not conducted, yielding more P waves than QRS complexes	P waves independent and not related to QRS complexes
QRS	0.06-0.10 sec	0.06-0.10 sec	May be normal, but usually coexists with bundle branch block (>0.12)	0.06-0.10 sec if junctional escape pacemaker activates the ventricles >0.12 if ventricular escape pacemaker activates the ventricles

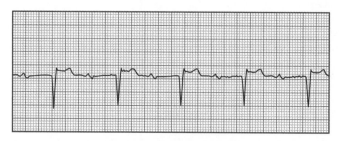

Fig. 17-49 First-degree AV block. The PR interval is prolonged to 0.44 second.

conduction through the AV node in over 90% of patients.[70] In a small percentage, the prolonged PR interval is caused by a delay within the atrial conduction pathways.[70] If the associated QRS is narrow it is likely that the only conduction abnormality is in the AV node. However, if the associated QRS complex is widened, it is likely that there is also damage to the bundle branches as a result of sclerosis, ischemia, or infarction.[70]

Second-Degree AV Block. Second-degree AV block can be broadly defined as a condition in which some atrial impulses are conducted to the ventricles, while others are "blocked" at the AV node. This description of intermittent AV conduction covers two patterns with markedly different clinical significance: second-degree AV block is divided into Mobitz type I (also known as *Wenckebach block*) and Mobitz type II.

MOBITZ TYPE I. In Mobitz type I block, the AV conduction times progressively lengthen until a P wave is not conducted. This typically occurs in a pattern of *"grouped beats"* and is observed on the ECG by a gradually lengthening PR interval, until ultimately the final P wave in the group fails to conduct. In Mobitz type I the QRS complex is generally of normal width and appearance.[70] Several factors must be present for Mobitz I (Wenckebach) to be diagnosed:

1. The sinus node is functional and generates impulses that conduct to the AV node at a constant rate. On the ECG the measured P-to-P interval is regular.
2. As each successive atrial impulse arrives earlier into the *relative refractory period* of the impaired AV node, more time is needed to conduct the impulse. On the ECG this is seen as an incremental increase in the length of each PR interval. The R-to-R interval usually becomes shorter with each beat.
3. The PR interval is shortest in the first beat.
   a. The initial PR interval is often, but not always, of normal length. If first-degree block coexists, the initial PR interval will be prolonged, but this initial PR interval will still have the shortest measured interval of the group.
   b. The initial PR interval is shorter because the AV node has experienced a "rest" or longer recovery time due to the final nonconducted P wave in the group as described below.
4. The final P wave of the group is not conducted. The atrial impulse arrives during the AV node's absolute refractory period and is not conducted. This is seen on the ECG by a P wave that is *not* followed by a QRS complex (Fig. 17-50).

Mobitz I block has a specific, repeating pattern that catches the eye. The expected groups are 3:2, 4:3 or 5:4. For example, if four P waves are conducted to the ventricles and the fifth one is not, a 5:4 conduction ratio is present (five P waves to four QRS complexes). The nonconducted P ends a "group." After the pause, the cycle repeats itself. The PR interval typically lengthens the most with the second beat of the cycle.[70]

Mobitz type I does not generally cause major hemodynamic compromise as long as the ventricular heart rate is maintained. However, in the presence of ischemia and infarction it can rapidly progress to a more severe level of block. If Mobitz type I occurs in the setting of an acute inferior wall infarction, close observation and, occasionally, placement of a temporary pacemaker as a precautionary measure is warranted.

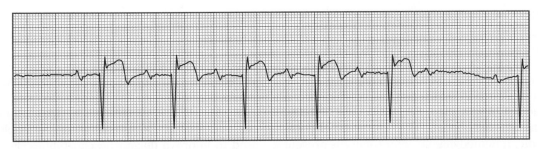

Fig. 17-50 Mobitz type I (Wenckebach) second-degree AV block. Note that the PR intervals gradually increase from 0.36 to 0.46 second until, finally, a P wave is not conducted to the ventricles.

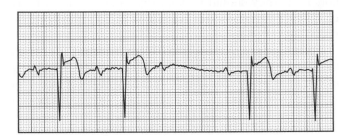

Fig. 17-51 Mobitz type II second-degree AV block. Note that the PR intervals remain constant.

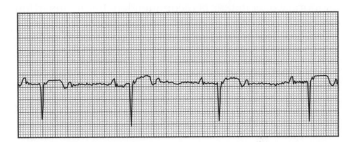

Fig. 17-52 2:1 AV block. Because no two consecutive P waves are conducted, it is not possible to determine with certainty whether this is Mobitz I or Mobitz II second-degree AV block.

MOBITZ TYPE II. Mobitz type II block is always anatomically located below the AV node in the bundle of His in the bundle branches or even in the Purkinje fibers.[70-71] This results in an *"all or nothing"* situation with respect to AV conduction. Sinus P waves either will or will not be conducted. When conduction does occur, all PR intervals are the same. Because of the anatomic location of the block, on the surface ECG the PR interval is constant and the QRS complexes are wide (Fig. 17-51).

Mobitz II block is more ominous clinically than Mobitz I and often progresses to complete AV block. In addition, if the block involves the Purkinje fibers an escape rhythm may not develop.[71] For this reason it is important to prepare for transcutaneous cardiac pacing (TCP) by bringing the TCP device (often combined with a defibrillator) to the bedside as a precaution. TCP refers to external pacing from outside the chest wall. When pacing is required, two large pacing electrodes are placed on the chest. There is always a diagram on the machine showing where to place the pads on the chest. Consider the possibility that the patient will need a temporary transvenous pacemaker inserted and possibly require a permanent pacemaker before hospital discharge.[72]

2:1 CONDUCTION. Occasionally, only every other P wave is conducted through the AV node (Fig. 17-52). This pattern could indicate either Mobitz type I or Mobitz type II, because consecutive conduction of P waves—which would reveal either a lengthening or constant PR—does not occur. In Mobitz I the conduction ratios may have decreased from 4:3 to 3:2 to 2:1, yet the site and type of block have not changed. The change in conduction ratio

may be caused by an increase in atrial rate, or it may change spontaneously.

In 2:1 conduction it is impossible to be certain whether the block is Mobitz type I or type II from the surface ECG. If it occurs along with other Mobitz I ratios, it is probably still Mobitz I. If it is an isolated occurrence with no other strips for comparison, the QRS width and the PR interval offer valuable clues to the site of the block. In Mobitz I the QRS is usually normal and the PR interval is usually prolonged. In Mobitz II the QRS is usually wide and the PR interval is usually normal.[70] Also, during an acute inferior MI, Mobitz type I AV block with 2:1 conduction is much more common than is type II.

Third-Degree AV Block. Third-degree, or complete, AV block is a condition in which no atrial impulses can conduct from the atria to the ventricles. The block can be located at the level of the AV node, or below the node within the bundle of His or the bundle branches. The opportunity for conduction is optimal, yet none occurs. It is hoped that a junctional or ventricular focus will depolarize spontaneously at its intrinsic rate of 20 to 40 beats/min and ventricular contraction will continue. If not, asystole occurs; there is no pulse, and death will result if intervention is not immediate.

On the ECG, P waves are present and usually occur at regular intervals. If a junctional focus is pacing the heart, normal QRSs are present but occur at a rate and timing interval totally independent of the P waves. The PR intervals vary widely, because the P wave and QRS are not related to each other. If a ventricular focus is pacing the heart, the QRS complex is wide and unrelated to the P waves (Fig. 17-53).

Management of AV Block. Clinically the consequences of AV block range from benign to life-threatening. First-degree AV block is seldom of immediate concern but bears close observation for progression of the conduction disturbance. Second-degree Mobitz I (Wenckebach) is usually benign, as long as the patient is not bradycardic. If hemodynamic compromise is present or deemed likely, a temporary pacemaker can be inserted prophylactically. Second-degree Mobitz II is more serious and often precedes complete AV block. Use of a temporary pacemaker is recommended, but its insertion can be elective if the patient remains hemodynamically stable. Complete heart block causes AV dissociation and is associated with a low cardiac output that requires use of a pacemaker. In complete heart block the patient may exhibit "cannon waves" as the dissociated atria contact against closed AV valves. An example of this phenomenon is shown on p. 401. If the patient is hemodynamically unstable, external transcutaneous cardiac pacing (TCP) can be used to maintain an adequate ventricular rate until a transvenous or permanent pacemaker can be inserted.[72,73]

Ambulatory ECG Tests. Before coming to the critical care unit a patient may have had other electrocardiographic (ECG) tests to determine the degree of cardiovascular disease. *Ambulatory electrocardiography* is a technique that records the ECG of patients while they perform their usual activities. It is designed to document abnormal cardiac rhythms that occur at random or that are induced by specific circumstances such as emotional stress or physical activity. Clinical indications include palpitations, dizziness, syncope, and pacemaker evaluation. Two types of recording systems are available: *continuous* and *intermittent.* Many intermittent systems have a short memory loop that permits capture of recent symptoms.

Continuous ECG Recording Systems. *Holter monitors* are the most widely used continuous recording systems. The patient wears skin electrodes and carries a small box that contains a digital or analog recorder. The monitor is carried by a shoulder strap or clipped to a belt or pocket for 24 hours and then is returned to the hospital or clinic for reading. This is a totally noninvasive procedure with no adverse effects. All Holter monitors record at least two leads to minimize inaccurate interpretation caused by artifact.

ECG Monitoring Leads. Usually five electrodes are placed. Two of them are positive electrodes, corresponding approximately to the V_1 and V_5 positions on a standard 12-lead ECG. Also placed are two negative electrodes and one ground. Occasionally, additional electrodes are used to improve diagnostic capabilities. For example, a separate lead can be used to detect pacemaker spikes if the patient is being monitored for pacemaker dysfunction. The skin electrodes are disposable, pregelled, and self-adhering. They should be kept dry—not because of any electrical danger but to prevent their falling off before the recording is completed.

Patient Education. If clear directions are provided to the patient, it will make a big difference to the quality of the final recording. The ambulatory monitor saves all of the ECG tracings for 24 hours. The final recording can display the time that an event occurred. Most also have an event marker, which the patient can press to indicate the onset of symptoms or another event that may be important. The patient is asked to keep a diary of activities, symptoms, and any medications that are taken.

Continuous recording systems are the most thorough form of ambulatory electrocardiography because they record every heartbeat for 24 hours. They do not require the active participation of the patient (although a detailed patient log is helpful) and therefore do not miss asymptomatic ECG changes or dysrhythmias that may be accompanied by a loss of consciousness. When dysrhythmias occur that correlate with symptoms, or symptoms occur in the absence of dysrhythmias, one of the primary goals of Holter monitoring has been achieved. Unfortunately, most patients do not have typical symptoms daily. If no significant dysrhythmias or symptoms occur during the 24-hour monitoring period, the test is unhelpful. The only activities that are restricted while wearing a Holter monitor are those that would get the chest electrodes or monitor wet, eliminating swimming and taking a shower or tub bath. Sponge baths are permitted as long as the chest electrodes are avoided.

Intermittent ECG Recording Systems. A portable monitor that does not record the ECG continuously

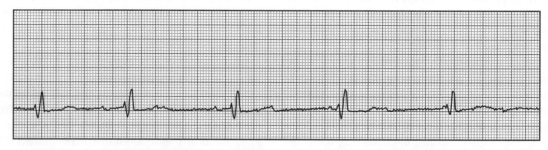

Fig. 17-53 Third-degree (complete) heart block.

can also be used to diagnose dysrhythmias. These may also be described as "event monitors." The patient wears electrodes, but the device is not constantly recording. The patient is instructed to press a button, when experiencing symptoms, to initiate the recording manually in real time. The big advantage of the intermittent recording system is the ability to leave the recorder in place up to 96 hours, as well as the ability to trigger recording when the symptoms occur.

External Loop Recorders. The external loop recorder records continuously but only keeps the most recent 4 minutes of ECG activity on the memory loop. The memory loop in the device means the patient can press a button and intermittently record a specific event such as heart palpitations during, or after, the event has occurred. At a later time the recorder is returned to the hospital or clinic for interpretation of the ECG. The recorder is small and can be clipped to a belt and worn for up to a month.

Patient Education. A well-informed patient can greatly enhance the quality of the recording. Many patients' symptoms do not occur every day and may be missed during a random 24-hour recording. Often symptoms tend to occur in association with specific activities. The patient is encouraged to be as active as possible. Keeping an accurate diary of activities is important, because it allows correlation of an identified dysrhythmia with a specific event.

Implantable ECG Recording Systems. For patients whose symptoms are not diagnosed with the traditional methods, or who require longer periods of follow-up to diagnose syncope or intermittent dysrhythmias, a small continuous *implantable loop recorder* may be inserted under the skin of the upper chest.[74] The recorder is about 2 inches by 1 inch by 1 inch. Insertion takes about 20 minutes under local anesthetic. It is especially useful if previous short-term ambulatory ECG recordings have failed to reveal an underlying problem. The inserted loop recorder continuously monitors the ECG rhythm for up to 14 months. Following a syncopal episode (loss of consciousness), the patient or a family member places a small, hand-held "activator" on the chest wall over the loop recorder to capture the most recent ECG data. The stored ECG is subsequently analyzed to determine if the syncopal episode was due to a dysrhythmia.[75,76] At this point, once a diagnosis is made, the implantable loop recorder can be safely removed.

Transtelephonic ECG Systems. Transtelephonic monitors are intermittent monitoring systems that are not attached to the patient all the time. These monitors consist of a small box, about 4 inches by 2 inches, with four metal electrodes on the bottom. The box is issued to the patient for a specific time, often 1 month, and the patient carries the box at all times. Whenever symptoms are experienced, the patient places the recording box in the center of the chest and places the four metal electrodes in firm contact with the skin.

An alternative method is to use two arm bracelets containing metal electrodes rather than direct chest placement. A button is depressed to activate the recording, which lasts 1 to 2 minutes. The recording is stored until it is convenient for the patient to make a telephone call to send in the recording to a central analysis facility. At that time, the patient's telephone is placed over a transmitter on the box and the recording is transmitted to the analysis facility, where it is printed out and analyzed as a readable ECG tracing.

Internet Remote Monitoring. The transtelephonic system (foregoing section) has been used for many years to remotely follow the function of implantable cardioverter defibrillators (ICDs) or pacemakers. New technology options mean that patients who have a recent model ICD or permanent pacemaker implanted may be able to have their device monitored via an internet-based, remote monitoring service. The patient dials a prearranged phone number to send the information to a protected site. This information is then downloaded by the dysrhythmia nurse or electrophysiologist to a secure Internet web page in the clinical setting. The clinician can view all the programmable details, plus any dysrhythmic events or malfunction of the ICD or the pacemaker. The quantity and quality of information transmitted is superior to that transmitted with older transtelephonic systems. The patient does not need to have a computer available because the information is transmitted using a small portable monitor and any standard telephone line.

Stress Tests: Exercise with ECG Monitoring. Exercise ECG, more commonly known as a "stress test" consists of the recording of an ECG tracing during a period of *physiologic stress* on the heart muscle and its blood supply to uncover and diagnose ischemia, which is not apparent at rest. Physiologic stress is created by asking the patient either to walk on a treadmill or to ride a stationary bicycle.

Physiology of Exercise on the Cardiovascular System. Exercise places unique demands on the cardiovascular system. Systemic oxygen consumption increases markedly, requiring the heart to increase CO to meet these demands. Myocardial contractility increases, resulting in greater stroke volume and systolic blood pressure. Heart rate is increased as a result of circulating catecholamines. Normally, as heart rate and stroke volume rise, cardiac output is increased dramatically and the tissue needs for oxygen are met. This enhanced myocardial performance is not without a penalty. Even at rest, the heart muscle extracts 70% of the oxygen available in the circulating blood. When the myocardial demand for oxygen increases during exercise, coronary blood flow must increase to maintain an adequate oxygen supply. In people with coronary artery disease, coronary blood flow cannot increase sufficiently to meet the high metabolic needs of the myocardium during exercise, and ischemia results.

Stress Test Protocols. The majority of exercise tests in the United States are performed using a treadmill on which both speed and slope can be varied, or using a stationary bicycle. A number of protocols have been developed using a treadmill. Two popular ones are the *Bruce protocol*, in which both grade and speed are varied every 3 minutes, and the *Balke protocol*, in which speed remains constant and grade is gradually increased every minute. Regardless of the protocol used, the ECG is monitored continuously. Blood pressure is also measured and recorded every minute.

Stress Test Heart Rate Criteria. The treadmill test is terminated when a desirable level, based on the patient's maximal stress test heart rate, is reached. The maximal predicted heart rate is estimated using the formula:

220 minus the patient's age

Increasing the heart rate to 85% to 90% of the predicted maximum is preferred, and in most patients this level of exercise is sufficient to unmask any significant coronary artery disease. The diagnostic value of the test is based on the maximal heart rate achieved, *not* on the length of time that the patient remains on the treadmill. A well-trained athlete might be able to stay on the treadmill for 15 minutes, whereas an elderly or sedentary person may tolerate it for only 3 to 5 minutes; yet if 85% of the predicted maximal heart rate is achieved, both tests are equally diagnostic. A person who is taking β-blockers may not be able to reach his or her target age-adjusted heart rate because of the bradycardiac effect of this class of drugs.

The test workload will also be described in METS (metabolic equivalents), of oxygen consumption.[77] The definition of 1 MET is 3.5 mls oxygen per kilogram (kg) per minute at rest for a 70 kg, 40-year-old male. The stress test result may be described as "poor exercise tolerance" (3 to 4 METS), or "good exercise tolerance" (10 to 11 METS).

Clinical Reasons to Stop the Treadmill Test. The test will also be aborted before maximal heart rate is reached if symptoms occur. Reasons to halt the test include the development of moderate to severe angina (chest pain), signs of pallor or poor perfusion, and also if the patient wishes to stop the test.[77] Other signs that would alert the nurse to stop the test include ST elevation equal to or greater than 1.0 mm (one small box); ST depression equal to or greater than 2.0 mm (2 small boxes); cardiac dysrhythmias or a marked shift in ventricular axis; increased symptoms such as breathlessness or fatigue and a fall in blood pressure of 10 mm Hg or more from baseline.[77] Blood pressure is expected to rise during exercise, but a systolic blood pressure greater than 250 mm Hg or a diastolic blood pressure greater than 115 mm Hg is considered high enough to stop the test.[77]

Predischarge Treadmill Tests. A low-level stress test is sometimes performed before discharge from the hospital on patients who have had an acute MI. In this case the heart rate is raised to only 120 or 130 beats per minute. ST-segment depression or elevation that occurs during the predischarge low-level stress test is a reliable indicator of additional myocardium at risk. However, exercise-induced angina or abnormal blood pressure responses to exercise often do not appear during a low-level stress test, so a "normal" predischarge stress test must be followed later by a test closer to maximal level.

Nursing Management. During the exercise test the patient is encouraged to continue as long as possible. However, the test is stopped if the patient requests because of symptoms such as fatigue, shortness of breath, leg cramps, significant ECG changes, blood pressure changes, or development of angina as described earlier. After the exercise test is completed, the patient is assisted into a supine position. The ECG, the pulse rate, and blood pressure are monitored for at least 10 more minutes to detect dysrhythmias or signs of ischemia. The patient is instructed to rest for the next 30 to 60 minutes after release from the exercise laboratory. Hot showers are to be avoided for 3 to 4 hours to prevent development of orthostatic hypotension. It is essential that nurses who monitor patients during this test are experienced and knowledgeable about all aspects of stress testing as well as emergency protocols. Emergency medications and a defibrillator must also be available in the test area.[78]

Patient Education. Many patients are anxious about undergoing exercise testing, and the anxiety is often multifactorial. Patients without known heart disease may be afraid that they will "fail" the test, find they have heart disease, and perhaps need open heart surgery. If the patient generally follows a sedentary lifestyle, anxiety may be caused by the fear of "collapsing" on the treadmill or spending several days recovering from exhaustion. Some are afraid that they will be forced to go beyond their endurance. Often, low-level exercise testing is performed before discharge on patients who have been hospitalized for an acute MI. These patients may be afraid that the strain on their heart is too great or that they will die during the test. Effective patient education can do much to allay these fears. In addition to describing the procedure itself, the nurse instructs the patient to fast for 3 hours before the test, refrain from smoking for at least 2 hours before the test, and wear comfortable shoes and loose-fitting clothes. Reassurance that the heart will be monitored closely during the test is also important.

ECHOCARDIOGRAPHY

Echocardiography uses *waves of ultrasound* to obtain and display images of cardiac structures. Normal human hearing occurs at a sound frequency of 20 to 20,000 cycles per second (hertz). Ultrasound uses sound frequencies greater than 20,000 hertz (Hz). When used to image cardiac structures, the best results are achieved using 1.5 megahertz to 10 megahertz (MHz). Usually 2.25 mHz is used with adults to allow optimal depth penetration, whereas 3 to 5 MHz is used in pediatric patients to provide a clearer image of the smaller structures.

Ultrasound is reflected best at interfaces between tissues that have different densities. In the heart these are the blood, cardiac valves, myocardium, and pericardium. Because all these structures differ in density, their borders can be seen on the echocardiogram.

Echocardiography is used to detect cardiac abnormalities such as mitral valve stenosis and regurgitation, prolapse of mitral valve leaflets, aortic stenosis and insufficiency, hypertrophic cardiomyopathy, atrial septal defect, thoracic aortic dissection, cardiac tamponade, and pericardial effusion.[79] The term echocardiogram describes a wide range of individual tests as described in the following sections.[79]

Transthoracic Echocardiography.
When a transthoracic echocardiogram (TTE) is performed, the patient is in either a supine, a left lateral, or a semirecumbent position. Which position is used depends on the patient's clinical condition and on which structures are to be examined. A transducer is placed on the skin, with lubricant between the transducer and the skin to improve contact and reduce artifact. The active element in the transducer is a piezoelectric crystal. *Piezoelectric* refers to the ability to transform electrical energy into mechanical (in this case, sound) energy. The transducer emits ultrasound waves and receives a signal from the reflected sound waves. Periods of sound transmission alternate with periods of sound reception.

Ultrasonic waves do not travel through air very well, and they cannot penetrate very dense structures, such as bone. In adults, the transducer is usually placed in the third or fourth intercostal space to the left of the sternum, because at that point the pericardium is in direct contact with the chest wall and the ultrasonic waves are not obstructed by either air or bone. Other positions are sometimes used if the standard location does not provide adequate visualization of the cardiac structures. In the critical care unit, the echocardiograph machine is usually brought to the bedside. The lighting in the room can be dimmed to improve the visual clarity of the images displayed on the screen. The nursing care consists of monitoring the patient during the procedure, which is usually performed by an echocardiography technician. TTE is completely noninvasive; the nurse explains this and the purpose of the test to the patient and family. The procedure is not uncomfortable, but it may be tiresome for certain patients because of the length of the procedure, which is usually 30 to 60 minutes.

Motion-Mode Echocardiography.
In Motion-mode (M-mode) TTE, a thin beam of ultrasound is directed through the heart (Fig. 17-54, *A*). Each interface is represented by a dot, and when recorded over time (like an ECG tracing), each dot becomes a line on an oscilloscope. A strip-chart recording can be made of this tracing as the heart beats. Because this is a recording of heart motion over time, this technique is called an *M-mode* (motion-mode) echocardiogram. A typical M-mode echo is shown in Fig. 17-54, *B*. M-mode echocardiograms are particularly useful in detecting small pericardial effusions and cardiac tamponade.

Two-Dimensional Echocardiogram.
The two-dimensional (2-D) echocardiogram uses crystals in the transducer to create a cross-sectional imaging plane. Sections of the heart are then viewed from a number of different angles (Fig. 17-55). The picture is displayed on an oscilloscope, and digital photographs are taken to serve as a permanent record. The 2-D echocardiogram images a whole "slice" of the heart at once and is used for direct measurement of LV volumes and wall mass.[79] The 2-D "slice" also permits visualization of the cardiac structures in relation to each other and readily identifies wall motion abnormalities.

Phonocardiogram.
Phonocardiography is combined with echocardiography to evaluate valvular dysfunction. *Phono* (sound), *cardio* (heart), *gram* (recording) together provide a graphic display of the sounds that occur in the heart and great vessels. The transducer is placed on the chest wall to record heart sounds that correspond to auscultation with a stethoscope. For more information on heart sounds, see Chapter 16, p. 310.

Color-Flow Doppler Echocardiography.
Doppler echocardiography provides a special kind of echocardiogram that assesses blood flow. It uses a pulsed or continuous wave of ultrasound that records frequency shifts of reflected sound waves, showing velocity and direction of blood flow relative to the transducer. Doppler signals are usually displayed in color. Known as *color-flow mapping* or *imaging*, this technique analyzes Doppler signals from multiple intracardiac sites simultaneously. The Doppler tracing for each site is displayed in a color-coded format superimposed on a real-time 2-D echocardiographic image. Flow toward the transducer is displayed in one color, whereas flow away from the transducer is displayed in a contrasting color. The brightness of the color is varied to signify varying flow velocities.

Doppler echocardiography is especially useful in individuals with valvular heart disease. The blood flow associated with regurgitation and stenosis can be detected, and estimates can be made of the severity of the disease. Doppler can accurately estimate RV systolic pressure.[79] When multiple valves are involved, the Doppler technique can clarify the extent of damage to the individual valves. Other uses for Doppler echocardiography include evaluation of congenital shunts, assessment of cardiac output, and measurement of volume flow. By

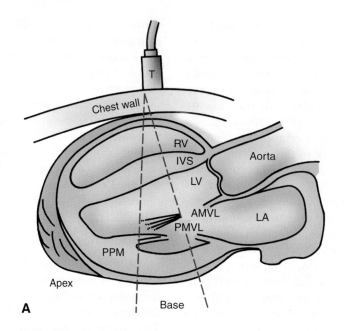

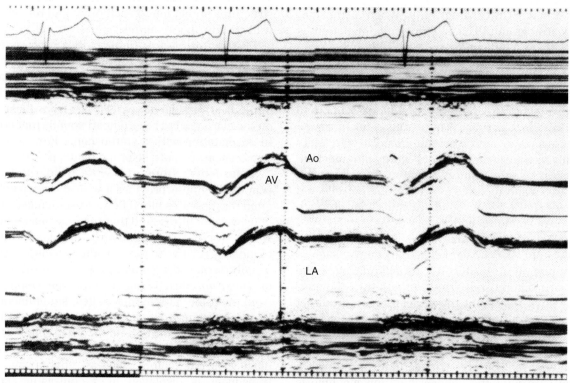

Fig. 17-54 **A,** Schematic presentation of cardiac structures traversed by two echobeams. **B,** Normal, M-mode echocardiogram at the level of the aorta, aortic valve leaflets, and left atrium. *T,* Transducer; *RV,* right ventricle; *IVS,* interventricular septum; *LV,* left ventricle; *AMVL,* anterior mitral valve leaflet; *LA,* left atrium; *PMVL,* posterior mitral valve leaflet; *PPM,* posterior papillary muscle; *Ao,* aorta; *AV,* aortic valve. (**B** from Kinney M et al: *Andreoli's comprehensive cardiac care,* ed 8, St Louis, 1995, Mosby.)

measuring flow velocity in the right ventricular outflow tract, mean pulmonary artery pressure can be estimated.

Transesophageal Echocardiography. Transesophageal echocardiography (TEE) is a technique in which the transducer (either single-plane, bi-plane, or multi-plane) is mounted on a flexible shaft similar to an endoscope and advanced into the esophagus, from where cardiac structures can be clearly visualized. The multi-plane transducer has a single array of crystals that can be rotated in a 180-degree arc, requiring less manipulation of the probe within the esophagus. Because of the close anatomic relationship between the heart and the esopha-

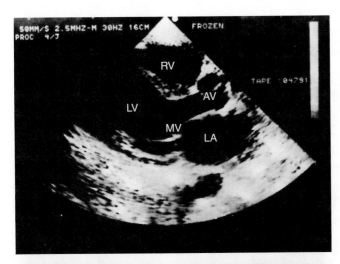

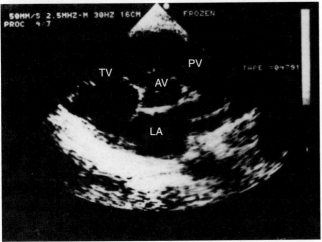

Fig. 17-55 Two-dimensional echocardiogram. Note that several sections of the heart can be viewed at one time, and it is easier to see the relationship of the chambers to one another. *RV,* Right ventricle; *LV,* left ventricle; *MV,* mitral valve; *LA,* left atrium; *TV,* tricuspid valve; *PV,* pulmonary vein. (From Kinney M et al: *Andreoli's comprehensive cardiac care,* ed 8, St Louis, 1995, Mosby.)

gus, TEE produces high-quality images of intracardiac structures and the thoracic aorta without the interference of the chest wall, bone, or air-filled lung.

The insertion procedure is similar to an upper GI endoscopy. The patient is asked to fast for a minimum of 6 hours before the TEE to prevent nausea and vomiting. For an elective TEE, medication is usually given to inhibit salivary secretions, reducing the risk of aspiration. Analgesic and sedative agents are administered to reduce fear and anxiety and to provide retrograde amnesia. Routine antibiotic prophylaxis against bacteremia and endocarditis is not necessary, although it is considered for high-risk patients such as those with prosthetic valves, previous endocarditis, or very poor dentition. The pharyngeal region is anesthetized with 2% viscous lidocaine (Xylocaine) and 10% lidocaine (Xylocaine)

spray to lessen the gag reflex and prevent retching and laryngospasm. The patient is usually placed in the left lateral decubitus position, although the supine position can be used in the critical care setting if necessary. A soft bite block is inserted between the teeth to prevent damage to the echoscope. As the echoscope is inserted, the patient is asked to swallow. The echoscope is advanced to 25 cm from the mouth, and imaging is begun (Fig. 17-56). TEE is also used intraoperatively during cardiac surgery for valve repair and replacement.[79] The images obtained by TEE are superior to TTE in a variety of ways. The entire thoracic aorta can be visualized clearly. Both atrial chambers are clearly seen with TEE, and the left atrial appendage is particularly well visualized, making TEE the procedure of choice for detection of left atrial thrombus. Diagnosis and quantification of atrial septal defects is possible with this method, and the addition of Doppler capabilities allows assessment of atrial shunting. TEE is useful in evaluating patients with valvular disorders including infective endocarditis to visualize vegetations on the valve leaflets.[79]

Manipulation of the TEE probe within the esophagus can cause a vasovagal response, producing bradycardia and hypotension. The most serious risk of the procedure is esophageal bleeding. Individuals with liver cirrhosis and/or esophageal varices, or patients on a heparin drip, are also at risk for esophageal bleeding. TEE must always be performed under ECG and BP monitoring, and if esophageal entry is difficult, it cannot be forced. In some hospitals TEE can represent 5% to 10% of all echocardiographic studies.[80] To remain competent at performing TEE safely, trained physicians must perform 10 to 25 TEE examinations per year to maintain the cognitive and technical skills necessary to maintain competence.[80] During TEE the patient's vital signs are closely monitored. Emergency resuscitation equipment must be present in case of a severe vasovagal episode (i.e., bradycardia, hypotension). Suction equipment must be at the bedside in the event that the patient vomits or has difficulty handling oral secretions.

Stress Echocardiography. Stress echocardiography is often used in the outpatient setting to identify stable angina. It provides a very accurate picture of the ischemic impact of coronary artery disease on the myocardium.[78,79] Stress echocardiography can diagnose both regional (ischemia) and global (cardiomyopathy) abnormalities.[79,80] It may also be used following myocardial infarction to evaluate the impact of necrosis on viable wall tissue.[79] Physiologic stress from increased exercise creates an imbalance between myocardial oxygen supply and demand. This causes ischemia and eventually results in wall-motion abnormalities, which are detectable with an echocardiogram. Stress can be applied to the heart by both physical and pharmacologic means.[79] One of two methods of physical exertion are generally employed; the patient can exercise on a treadmill or a stationary

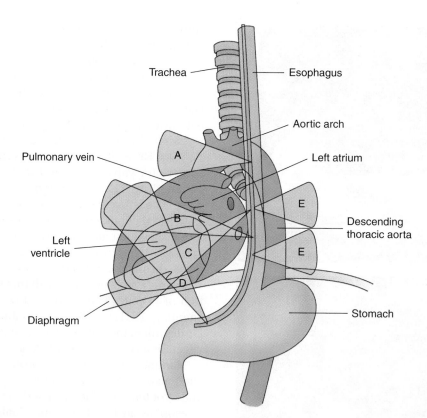

Fig. 17-56 Diagram of common scan planes during a transesophageal two-dimensional echocardiogram. *A,* Horizontal scan plane of aortic arch and distal portion of aorta. *B,* Basal short-axis (transverse), long-axis (sagittal) views, and short-axis views of both atria. *C,* Four-chamber and left atrioventricular long-axis views. Sagittal scan plane can image a cross section of the left ventricle. *D,* Transgastric short-axis view of left and right ventricles. *E,* Transverse and sagittal scan sections of descending aorta.

bicycle.[80] The protocols used for physical echocardiographic stress testing are very similar to those used in the ECG stress test setting (Table 17-13).

Dobutamine Stress Test. Pharmacologic stress is most frequently incited with a dobutamine infusion beginning at 5 mcg/kg/min and increasing as needed to 40 or 50 mcg/kg/min to achieve 85% of maximal heart rate.[80] Dobutamine causes myocardial ischemia through a dramatic increase in myocardial oxygen demand by an increase in heart rate, contractility, and systemic blood pressure. Potential side effects include hypotension, hypertension, dysrhythmias, nausea, headache, anxiety, and tremor.[80] Atropine is also administered if the dobutamine infusion alone does not cause an adequate increase in heart rate.[80] Because of the potential risks of dobutamine stress echocardiography, it is recommended that qualified physicians be engaged in at least 100 studies a year to maintain competence.[80] Vasodilating drugs that may sometimes be used are dipryidamole and adenosine.[79] For some centers, IV adenosine is the primary drug that is used, and dobutamine is the second choice.

Intravascular Ultrasound. Intravascular ultrasound (IVUS) is used as an adjunct diagnostic technique during coronary angiography or during a coronary percutaneous catheter procedure (PCI).[80,81] A miniature flexible ultrasound catheter that incorporates a high frequency transducer (20 to 40 MHz) provides high-resolution images of the coronary arterial wall. This technology is not an alternative to angiography but is used as a complementary diagnostic technique. IVUS permits an anatomic view of the interior of the coronary artery.[80,81] The cardiologist can visualize the exact location of atherosclerotic plaque, or see if a coronary stent has deployed (expanded) correctly against the vessel wall.[81]

Intracardiac Ultrasound. The use of intracardiac ultrasound is also increasing. Flexible ultrasound catheters can be directed into both the atria and ventricles. Diagnostic uses include direct visualization of intracardiac structures, replacement for TEE during interventional or selected surgical procedures, and views of the atrial or ventricular septum during a repair procedure.[80]

Hand-Carried Ultrasound Devices. Portable ultrasound, or handheld ultrasound is now used in many critical care units and emergency departments.[80] Portable ultrasound is designed to increase the accuracy of the bedside physical examination.

Table 17-13	Stress Testing Methods		
	Stress Electrocardiography (ECG)	**Stress Echocardiogram**	**Stress Radionuclide Imaging**
Exercise stress test	• 3-, 5-, or 12-lead ECG leads are attached to chest and limbs to monitor the ECG *during* the exercise protocol.	• The patient exercises according to protocol. • Echocardiogram is recorded immediately *after* exercise.	• The radiopharmaceutical (Thallium-201 or Tc-99m) is injected before exercise. • The patient exercises according to protocol. • Heart is scanned *after* exercise to view uptake of radiotracer.
Pharmacologic stress test	• Patient is at rest. • IV drugs stimulate heart rate and contractility: Starts with dopamine 5 mcg/kg/min and is increased as needed to increase heart rate. ECG is monitored *during* the drug infusions. • Other drugs include adenosine and dipryidamole.	• Patient is at rest. • IV drugs stimulate heart rate and contractility: Starts with dopamine 5 mcg/kg/min, and is increased as needed to increase heart rate. Echocardiogram is recorded *during* and *after* the drug infusions. • Other drugs include adenosine and dipryidamole.	• Patient is at rest. • IV drugs simulate exercise: Starts with dopamine 5 mcg/kg/min and is increased as needed to increase heart rate. • Radionuclide image is scanned both *during* and *after* pharmacologic stress. • Other drugs include: Adenosine and dipryidamole.
Clinical indications	• Used to rule out coronary artery disease (CAD). • Not as helpful if patient has a distorted ECG at baseline, due to LBBB, RBBB or internal ventricular pacemaker because ST-segment changes are obscured.	• Useful for patients with LBBB, RBBB, and implanted pacemaker, since the wall motion is visualized directly.	• Helpful for patients with LBBB, RBBB and implanted pacemaker. • Useful before CABG to determine if bypass graft will supply blood to an ischemic area. There is no benefit in grafting an artery to an infarcted area.
Clinical outcome of a "positive" test	• Chest pain develops. • ST-segment ECG changes.	• Chest pain develops. • Wall motion abnormalities are visualized.	• Areas of the heart that do not take up radiotracer are termed "cold spots." A "cold spot" is either *ischemic* or *infarcted*. • A follow-up scan later the same day (or the next day with some radiotracers) will show if the "cold spot" has "filled in"; if yes, this infers the area is ischemic; if it remains "cold," this means that the area is infarcted.

CAD, Coronary artery disease; *LBBB,* left bundle branch block; *RBBB,* right bundle branch block; *CABG,* coronary artery bypass graft.

MAGNETIC RESONANCE IMAGING

Magnetic resonance imaging (MRI) is a noninvasive imaging technique that can obtain specific biochemical information from body tissue without the use of ionizing radiation. The procedure does not present any known hazard to living cells. In many respects, the image created is superior to both x-ray film and ultrasonography, because bone does not interfere with magnetic resonance imaging.

Indications. Cardiac magnetic resonance imaging (CMRI) can provide information about tissue integrity, cardiac wall-motion abnormalities, aneurysms, ejection fraction, cardiac output, patency of proximal coronary arteries, and flow rates through coronary artery bypass grafts.[82,83] MRI is useful in diagnosing complications of myocardial infarction, such as pericarditis or pericardial effusion, valvular dysfunction, ventricular septal rupture, aneurysm, and intracardiac thrombus.

Blood that is actively flowing does not emit a magnetic resonance signal; thus it provides a natural dark contrast material in the lumen of proximal coronary arteries. As a result, abnormalities of lumen size such as narrowing—which may provide evidence of obstruction—can be visualized.

How Magnetic Resonance Imaging Works. The physics behind MRI scanning is quite complex, but the basic concept is fairly simple. Certain atoms within molecules act as tiny bar magnets with north and south poles. The nuclei spin around this axis like a spinning top. Under normal conditions these small atomic magnets are arranged at random. If a patient is placed within a strong magnetic field, many of the nuclei line up in the same direction as the magnetic force. When a radiofrequency wave is sent, some of the nuclei absorb this energy, causing them to fall out of alignment and wobble like a gyroscope that is winding down. This "wobbling" out of alignment is termed *resonance.* The process of returning to alignment with the magnetic field after the radiofrequency signal is turned off is called *relaxation.* These energy changes can be detected and recorded by the scanner.

Each type of atom has its own unique resonance and relaxation pattern. The easiest one to record at present is the hydrogen ion, although other atoms such as phosphorus, sodium, and carbon are also being studied. Because there are two hydrogen ions per molecule of water, magnetic resonance imaging is especially sensitive to changes in tissue water content. Myocardial ischemic injury results in predictable increases in regional myocardial water content, allowing differentiation between normal and ischemic tissue. Infarction leading to myocardial scarring results in tissue with a decreased water content, which can be identified on a magnetic resonance scan as an area of decreased signal intensity.

Magnetic resonance imaging works well for structures that have little or no motion, such as the brain. Cardiac applications have been limited because of the constant motion of the heart. In an attempt to overcome this limitation, various gating or slicing techniques have been used to time the images at exact phases of the cardiac cycle. The gating can be timed from the R wave of the ECG or from the arterial pulse tracing. Either method is satisfactory as long as the patient is in normal sinus rhythm. With any irregularity of the rhythm, the gating technique becomes much less helpful.

Metal Objects. Magnetic resonance imaging (MRI) is a very safe procedure. The main hazard of it is related to the presence of metal substances in the environment. Because the magnetism used is approximately 40,000 times stronger than the magnetic field of the earth, metal objects such as IV poles, infusion pumps, or oxygen tanks can become projectiles if they come close enough to the magnet's pull. No metal objects are permitted in the area of the MRI. The patient must be asked about the presence of any metallic implants (pacemaker), or other metal (residual bullet or shrapnel) that may be moved by the magnetic force during the scan. Aneurysm clips are composed of ferromagnetic materials and could experience significant torque when exposed to the magnetic field. Box 17-5 lists some guidelines about which implants are safe and which are not. Another consideration is that the magnetic field may cause a cardiac pacemaker or implantable cardioverter defibrillator (ICD) to turn off, or switch modes when exposed to the strong external magnetic field.

Challenges with Magnetic Resonance Imaging. MRI has significant limitations that affect patients in the critical care setting. One of the challenges is that patients must leave the unit and be transported to the nuclear medicine laboratory for MRI. Standard ventilators, monitoring equipment, and infusion pumps cannot be used because these machines contain metal parts. Special ventilators with nonmagnetic accessories are available, as well as nonmetal ECG, pulse oximetry sensors, and infusion pumps.

The narrow size of the magnet bore (tube or tunnel) requires that the patient be able to lie flat and motionless for up to 7 minutes at a time. The close quarters inside the magnet bore tend to provoke claustrophobia in anyone already predisposed to it, and sedation may be required. The patient who is claustrophobic needs considerable reassurance and education before lying supine and motionless inside the MRI tube.

Box 17-5

METALLIC IMPLANTS AND NUCLEAR MAGNETIC RESONANCE IMAGING

SAFE	**UNSAFE**
Nonferromagnetic aneurysm clips	Cardiac pacemaker
Hemostatic vascular slips	Implanted cardioverter defibrillator (ICD)
Staples	Pulmonary artery catheter
Carotid artery clamps*	Implanted drug infusion pump
Cochlear implants	Detectable metal in the eye
Wire sutures	Intracranial aneurysm clips
Vascular access ports	Bullets†
Plastic endotracheal tubes	
Chest tubes	
Catheters	
Orthopedic devices and prostheses	
Prosthetic heart valves‡	
Intravascular coils, stents, and filters§	

*Exceptions: Poppen-Blalock carotid artery clamp and clips made of 17-7PH stainless steel.

†Most are nonferromagnetic and therefore safe. However, steel shotgun pellets are replacing lead and are ferromagnetic, as are foreign-made ballistic material and shrapnel. Bullets are less likely to move if imbedded in scar tissue. The risk/benefit ratio must be considered.

‡Exception: Starr-Edwards Pre-6000 valve.

§Safe if they have been in place several weeks.

CARDIAC RADIONUCLIDE IMAGING STUDIES

There are several types of radionuclide imaging tests available. As with diagnostic ECG and echocardiography, many of the radionuclide tests can be performed both at rest and during exercise.[78]

Purpose of Radionuclide Scans. The purpose of a radionuclide scan is to determine whether there is a perfusion defect in cardiac muscle. A scan is indicated for the person with chest pain and known or suspected coronary artery disease. The radionuclide scan is especially helpful for the person who has a coexisting LBBB or a permanent pacemaker where the QRS shape is distorted. Both situations make interpretation of acute angina challenging to interpret on the 12-lead ECG accurately. This has opened a window of opportunity for radionuclide imaging, where the myocardial ability to receive blood flow is visualized directly.[84]

A radionuclide scan adds to the information that has been gained from both a cardiac catheterization study and a 12-lead ECG. Coronary artery anatomy and patency is important because regional myocardial blood supply is always from a specific coronary artery and any blockage of an artery can lead to a discrete myocardial perfusion defect, meaning that the blood supply to this area is either decreased (ischemic) or absent (infarcted). Although coronary arteriography defines the anatomy of the coronary arteries, it does not show whether the arteries actually perfuse the cardiac muscle.

Radionuclide Isotopes. The radioisotopes used in cardiac diagnostic imaging are very different from those used in oncology for tumor ablation. Diagnostic isotopes have a short half-life (minutes to hours) and are used in very small amounts to minimize radioactivity risk. Patients do not need to be isolated, and no specific precautions are required for blood, urine, stool, or other body fluids.

Thallium-201. Thallium-201 is a low-energy radioactive isotope. It is an analog of potassium and acts like potassium when injected into the bloodstream. Because thallium is similar to potassium, it is absorbed from the bloodstream by cardiac muscle cells as part of the sodium-potassium adenosine triphosphatase (ATPase) pump. Thallium uptake depends on two factors: (1) the patency of the coronary arteries; and (2) the amount of healthy myocardium with a functional sodium-potassium ATPase pump. If an area of myocardium is infarcted (dead tissue), it will not take up thallium. Once thallium has been injected, a specialized scintillation camera and associated computer system are used to scan the myocardium.

Technetium-99. Technetium-99 (Tc-99m) is also used frequently. It is often attached to other tracer substances for diagnostic imaging (Tc-99m-sestamibi or Tc-99m-tetrofosmin).[84] These substances are often described as *radiopharmaceuticals*.[84] Tc-99m tracers are highly suited to imaging myocardium during ACS because the tracers do not redistribute over time (they remain in myocardium), allowing a second scan to be performed many hours later if needed.[84] In clinical practice this is seldom practical, and use of radiopharmaceuticals in emergency situations is rare outside of research studies.[84] These tests are widely used when the patient's hemodynamic and cardiac condition is stable.

Exercise Radionuclide Scan Procedure. This test takes place in a specialized nuclear medicine department. The walls of the testing space are normally lined with lead to prevent any radioactivity dispersal to other areas. A patent IV is required. A radioisotope flow agent (Thallium 201 or Tc-99m) is injected into the bloodstream prior to exercise. Following the physical activity a specialized perfusion-scanning camera will scan the heart.

Before the *exercise radionuclide scan*, the procedure is fully explained to the patient, including a description of the equipment (ECG monitoring equipment, cardiovascular exercise treadmill or stationary bicycle, and an Anger gamma scintillation camera). The patient is usually fasting, because the scan involves vigorous exercise. Vasodilating medications that may alter the uptake of the radioisotope (nitrates, theophylline and related drugs) are held (not taken by the patient) before any baseline study. Other medications that will not affect the outcome of the study can be taken as usual. A patent IV line is inserted before the test. Once in the laboratory, the patient is asked to exercise vigorously for up to 1 minute or longer or until angina or fatigue develops. At this point the isotope is injected into the bloodstream. After the injection the patient is asked to exercise vigorously for another minute to stress the heart and circulate the radioisotope. As soon as possible after exercise (within 10 minutes), the patient is asked to lie on the examination table for the first perfusion scan by the scintillation camera. The camera examines the heart from three angles—anterior, left anterior oblique, and left lateral oblique—to increase accuracy. On the camera screen the heart image looks like a circle with a hole (doughnut shape). The myocardium appears, but the fluid-filled center does not.

Radionuclide Test Results. If no perfusion defect is seen, the test is complete for that patient. If a perfusion defect (dark area) is noted in the myocardium, the patient is asked to return for a repeat scan either 2 to 4 hours later, or the next day depending on the radioisotope tracer that was used. If a perfusion defect is present 4 hours later, this means the area is infarcted. This is sometimes described as a "cold spot," sometimes as a "fixed lesion." If the perfusion defect has taken up the radioisotope since the first test (redistribution), the area is ischemic. An ischemic defect is amenable to reperfusion therapy such as coronary artery bypass graft (CABG) surgery or a catheter based procedure to open a coronary artery.

Rest Radionuclide Scan Procedure. A patient who cannot tolerate a thallium/ECG stress test will have a pharmacologic radionuclide test. The test can be performed with Thallium-201 or Tc-99m. In the absence of physical exercise a dobutamine infusion is used to increase coronary artery and myocardial blood flow.[84] Other vasodilating medications that may be used include adenosine and dipryidamole.[84] The choice of agent is dependent on the preference of the physician conducting the study.

CARDIAC CATHETERIZATION AND CORONARY ARTERIOGRAPHY

Cardiac catheterization and coronary arteriography are routine diagnostic procedures for patients with known or suspected heart disease. Clinical indications for cardiac catheterization include myocardial ischemia, unstable angina, evolving myocardial infarction, heart failure with a history that suggests coronary artery disease or cardiac valvular disease, and congenital heart disease. Cardiac catheterization is used both to confirm physical findings and to provide a baseline for medical or surgical therapy.

Left-Heart Cardiac Catheterization. During catheterization of the left side of the heart, hemodynamic pressure measurements are taken in the aortic root, the left ventricle, and the left atrium. Radiopaque contrast (dye) is used to visualize the left ventricle (ventriculogram). This information is also used to calculated the LV ejection fraction. The coronary arteries are visualized and contrast dye is injected directly into each arterial system. The general term for vessel imaging is *angiogram* (veins and arteries), but the term generally used to describe the visualization of the coronary arteries is the more specific term *arteriogram*.

Right-Heart Cardiac Catheterization. Catheterization of the right side of the heart is performed using a thermodilution pulmonary artery catheter. Information obtained includes hemodynamic pressure measurements in the right atrium, the right ventricle, the pulmonary artery, and the pulmonary artery occlusion "wedge" position, as well as the measurement of cardiac output, calculated hemodynamic values, oxygen saturations, and an angiogram of the right-heart chambers using radiopaque contrast.

Procedure. Before the catheterization the patient meets with the cardiologist to discuss the purpose, benefit, and risks of the study. For many patients, cardiac catheterization is the first major invasive procedure after a diagnosis of possible cardiac disease. The patient is often very anxious and has many questions. It is important that both nursing and medical staff fully answer patients' questions about the catheterization experience.

The morning of the procedure the patient fasts except for ingesting prescribed cardiac medications. Light premedication is given before the patient goes to the catheterization laboratory. If there is a history of allergy, an antihistamine or corticosteroid may be administered to prevent an anaphylactic reaction to the radiopaque contrast. Throughout the cardiac catheterization the patient remains awake and alert. He or she is positioned on a hard table with a C-shaped or U-shaped camera arm overhead or to the side. This arm can be moved to view the heart from several different angles. Cardiac catheterization catheters, available in a variety of designs and sizes, are placed in the femoral vein and artery after the patient receives a local anesthetic. The choice of catheters is based on the cardiologist's experience and the diagnostic study required. The femoral artery is used to catheterize the left side of the heart, including the coronary arteries. The femoral vein is frequently used as the access vessel to pass catheters to the right side of the heart. During the study the patient receives heparin systemically to reduce the risk of emboli. Many patients also receive nitroglycerin to control chest pain, particularly when the coronary arteries are full of contrast material during the coronary arteriographic procedure. At this time the patient may also experience bradycardia or hypotension. To move the contrast dye more quickly and minimize the vagal effect on heart rate and blood pressure, the patient may be asked to cough. If the bradycardia persists, atropine or—occasionally—a transvenous pacemaker may be used. If hypotension continues, IV fluids are administered as a bolus. At the end of the study the femoral catheters are removed from the vessels. After the catheterization, once the patient is stable, the cardiologist meets with the patient and family to discuss the findings and plan of care.

Nursing Management

Femoral Artery Site Care. After the diagnostic catheters (and the sheaths through which they are inserted) are removed from the femoral artery and vein, pressure is applied to the femoral vessels until bleeding has stopped. After catheterization the patient remains flat for up to 6 hours (varies by institutional protocol and catheter size) to allow the femoral arterial puncture site to form a stable clot. Most bleeding occurs within the first 2 to 3 hours after the procedure. During this time the groin site is checked frequently for evidence of bleeding or hematoma. There are 3 methods that may be used to control bleeding at the femoral arterial puncture site following catheter/sheath removal. The most basic method is manual pressure, where a clinician holds pressure directly on the vein or artery until bleeding stops. The second method uses external mechanical compression over the site (C-Clamp or Femstop). The third method is to use an arteriotomy closure device. One closure device is designed to suture the artery closed as the sheath is removed; another option is placement of a collagen plug into the "track" of the sheath insertion site. The arteriotomy closure is performed by the cardiologist when the catheters/sheaths are removed. All of these methods are effective.[85] Following routine diagnostic cardiac catheterization procedures there is no difference in the rate of femoral arterial site complications between the different methods.[85] The patient is asked to lie still and not to bend at the hip. It usually takes about 40 minutes for a stable clot to form, but it can take longer in some patients, including those with a large body surface area.

Sometimes when the patient needs to void urine, this movement can dislodge the clot. If the patient cannot void in the supine position, a urinary catheter is usually inserted for women and a condom catheter is used for men.

Peripheral Pulses. The peripheral pulses located distal to the arterial access site are monitored closely by the critical care nurse. If the femoral artery has been used, pedal and posterior tibial pulses are assessed. If an alternative access site such as the radial artery is used, the radial pulse is assessed. Pulses are assessed every 15 minutes for the first hour after the catheterization and every 30 minutes to 1 hour thereafter. The affected limb is assessed for changes in color, temperature, pain, or paresthesia to detect early evidence of acute arterial occlusion.

Rehydration. The patient is encouraged to drink large amounts of clear liquids, and the IV fluid rate is increased to 100 ml/hour. Fluid is given for rehydration because the radiopaque contrast acts as an osmotic diuretic. This is also used to prevent *contrast-induced nephropathy* or damage to the kidney from the contrast dye used to visualize the heart structures. Patients who have elevated blood urea nitrogen (BUN) or creatinine levels before catheterization are at risk for acute renal failure from the dye. For these patients the quantity of contrast material is consciously limited and fluid boluses are given to preserve kidney function.

Angina. The patient is assessed for chest pain after the procedure. Usually, sublingual nitroglycerin is sufficient to relieve the pain, discomfort, or pressure. Not all patients describe their angina as "pain," and many other descriptors may be used. A 0-to-10 pain scale can be used to quantify the angina. A 12-lead ECG must be obtained immediately to identify the coronary arteries involved, and the cardiologist is notified. If the chest pain persists, this may indicate that a clot has formed in a coronary artery, and the patient may need to return to the cardiac catheterization laboratory for an interventional cardiology procedure. For more information, see percutaneous coronary interventions (PCI) in Chapter 19, p. 523.

Dysrhythmias. Dysrhythmias are always a concern after an invasive cardiovascular diagnostic procedure. They occur secondary to the underlying cardiac disease and the low potassium levels that can occur after excessive diuresis.

Patient Education. Because of the invasive nature of cardiac catheterization, many patients express considerable anxiety. Relevant information concerns the sensory details of the procedure, such as lying flat and motionless on a hard table for many hours and sometimes experiencing a feeling of warmth when the dye is injected. Pain is uncommon because opiate analgesics and sedative medications are always provided. Information about possible outcomes—both positive and negative—and possible complications must be provided to the patient. Also, postcatheterization requirements such as lying still and drinking large quantities of fluids are explained. The basic information can be provided using written material and videotapes, but it is vital to individualize the content and answer any specific concerns or questions. Patients are also asked to report any other unusual symptoms such as chest pain or nausea.

ELECTROPHYSIOLOGY STUDY

Indications. The electrophysiology study (EPS) is an invasive diagnostic tool used to record intracardiac electrical activity. A person may have an EPS performed because of a history of a syncopal episode (loss of consciousness), rapid, wide-complex tachycardia, or other cardiac electrical problems not diagnosed by the noninvasive diagnostic studies such as the 12-lead ECG, treadmill stress test, signal-averaged ECG, or Holter monitoring. The EPS is performed in a specially equipped cardiac catheterization laboratory.[86]

Before the electrophysiology study, written and verbal education is given to the patient and family to increase their sense of security and to decrease stress and anxiety. All antidysrhythmic medications are discontinued several days before the study so that any ventricular dysrhythmias may be readily induced during the EPS. Anticoagulants, especially warfarin, are also stopped before EPS. Premedication is administered before the study to induce a relaxed state, and during the procedure the patient is conscious but receives sedative agents (midazolam) at regular intervals. The patient fasts 6 hours before the EPS and during the procedure lies supine on a hard table with a C-shaped or U-shaped camera arm to the side or overhead to verify the position of the EPS catheters in the heart.

Electrophysiology equipment for stimulation of dysrhythmias and monitoring is usually nearby. A peripheral IV access and surface ECG leads are placed. Then electrophysiology catheters are inserted into the femoral vein and advanced to the right side of the heart under fluoroscopy. These catheters, similar to pacing catheters, are placed at specific anatomic sites within the heart to record the earliest electrical activity. The catheter placements are shown in Fig. 17-57, with catheter tip positioned at the following locations:

1. High right atrium (HRA) near to the SA node
2. AV node
3. Coronary sinus (CS) behind the left atrial/ventricular border

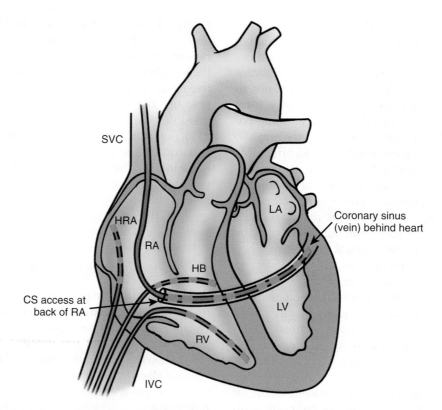

SVC

HRA

RA

HB

LA

Coronary sinus (vein) behind heart

CS access at back of RA

LV

RV

IVC

Placement of catheters in the heart in an electro-physiology study.

CS indicates coronary sinus: HB, His bundle; HRA, high right atrium; IVC, inferior vena cava; RV, right ventricle; SVC, superior vena cava.

Fig. 17-57 Catheter placement within the heart during electrophysiology study (EPS). *RA,* Right atrium; *LA,* left atrium.

4. His bundle (HB) near the tricuspid valve
5. Right ventricle (RV) near the apex

During EPS, *programmed electrical stimulation* is used to trigger the dysrhythmia. This technique delivers pulses of two to four early paced beats, via a specific catheter, to the selected area of myocardium. During the EPS, the electrophysiologist looks for a site of early electrical activation that stimulates the myocardium before the SA node. The goal of EPS is to discover the origin of dysrhythmias that cannot be evaluated from the surface ECG alone.

Atrial Measurements. Typical measurements during EPS include sinus node recovery time (SNRT) and sinoatrial conduction time (SACT), plus atrial pacing to measure both atrial and AV node refractory periods. Coronary sinus pacing is used to induce left atrial tachy-dysrhythmias.[86] Generally, atrial pacing is performed after the ventricular study to reduce the risk of putting the patient into atrial fibrillation/flutter secondary to retro-grade conduction up the His bundle-AV node.[86]

Ventricular Measurements. Programmed electrical stimulation is used to induce the ventricular dysrhythmia, especially in patients who have experienced sustained or nonsustained ventricular tachycardia, or survived a sudden cardiac death (SCD) episode. To measure the retrograde V-to-A interval and stimulate the myocardium, the RV catheter is selected to rapidly pace the right ventricle; then the catheter is moved to the right ventricular outflow tract (near the pulmonary valve) and the pacing stimulation is repeated. This protocol will produce VT in 92% of patients with a known history of VT or VF.[86]

Once the dysrhythmia is induced and diagnosed, it can be converted to normal sinus rhythm by 10 to 15 paced beats delivered at a rate faster than the VT, or by cardioversion/defibrillation, plus IV antidysrhythmic medications. At the end of the study, all of the electro-physiology catheters are removed before the patient returns to the nursing unit.[86]

Medical Management. After the EPS diagnosis, depending on the findings, the options for treatment are discussed with the patient and family. Many of the possible interventions may occur at the same time as the diagnosis.[86]

For example, if the diagnosis is WPW syndrome, the solution may be a radiofrequency catheter ablation of the accessory tract. If it is a bradydysrhythmia, a permanent pacemaker may be inserted. If the diagnosis is reentry ventricular tachycardia, the treatment may be insertion of an ICD. When an electrophysiology study is required for a patient with an ICD, the device can substitute for the EP catheters. In the latest generation of ICD generators, known as *tiered therapy devices* because of their three therapeutic components (pace termination, back-up bradycardia pacing, and cardioversion/defibrillation), it is not necessary for the patient to have EP catheters placed in the femoral vein. The EPS can be performed via the external ICD programmer in the EP laboratory. The ICD generator and leads perform programmed electrical stimulation in a manner similar to a full EPS. For more information on the therapeutic uses of the ICD, see Chapter 19, p. 515.

Nursing Management. The nursing care of the patient after removal of the EPS catheter is similar to the care provided for the cardiac catheterization patient. The nursing interventions focus on achieving hemostasis at the femoral puncture site, assessing pedal pulses and perfusion in the affected limb, monitoring for chest pain and dysrhythmias, and providing comprehensive patient education.[86]

In summary, the EPS can provide valuable information about intracardiac electrical abnormalities and reveal specialized diagnostic clues that can be used to guide medical and nursing management of the patient with life-threatening cardiac dysrhythmias.

SIGNAL-AVERAGED ECG

The signal-averaged ECG is used to identify individuals at risk for sudden cardiac death from ventricular dysrhythmias. This is a noninvasive test. The patient lies in a supine position and is asked to keep muscle movement to a minimum. Cardiac electrode leads are applied to the anterior and posterior chest walls, and the leads are connected to a signal-averaged ECG computer. This computer produces a high-resolution, high-magnification ECG signal. This "noise-free" ECG is then analyzed for both QRS duration and for the presence, duration, and measurement of late myopotentials. After computer analysis, the signal-averaged ECG is described as either negative (normal) or positive (abnormal). A positive signal-averaged ECG—in combination with other specific indicators—is a predictor of increased risk for sudden cardiac death.

Myocardium that is damaged, either by MI or by cardiomyopathy, produces late-activating myopotentials that may cause reentry ventricular dysrhythmias. The 12-lead ECG is not sufficiently sensitive to detect these low-amplitude, late potentials—hence the need for a high-resolution signal.

Many patients with a positive signal-averaged ECG (abnormal) display a normal signal-averaged ECG when placed on antidysrhythmic medications. The signal-averaged ECG is not analyzed in isolation. It is used in conjunction with other cardiac diagnostic tests, including the electrophysiology study. It is a helpful adjunct to the electrophysiology study but does not replace it.

HEAD UP–TILT TABLE TEST

A patient who is being evaluated for unexplained transient loss of consciousness (syncope) may undergo a head up–tilt table test (HUT). Etiology of syncope is divided into cardiac and noncardiac causes for the purposes of diagnosis. Diagnosis involves a comprehensive neurologic examination, evaluation of the carotid arteries, and if there is a history of dysrhythmias an EPS before the HUT. Cardiac causes of syncope (loss of consciousness) may include the following:

1. Postural orthostatic tachycardia syndrome (POTS) is described as a sinus tachycardia with a rate over 120 per minute, or a heart rate greater than 30 over baseline during the daytime and when standing. The heart rate falls dramatically when the person is lying down.[48] Blood pressure falls when the patient is standing (orthostatic hypotension) in many individuals. Patients are seen with palpitations, fatigue, exercise intolerance, symptoms of dizziness, lightheadedness, and presyncope or true syncopal episodes where they have lost consciousness.

2. *Vasodepressor syncope (VDS)*, or *neurocardiogenic syncope (NCS)*, also known as a vasovagal syndrome, describes a transient loss of consciousness caused by hypotension secondary to parasympathetic vasodilation, causing venous pooling which reduces cerebral perfusion and creates the syncopal episode.

The HUT is usually conducted in the radiology department. The patient lies supine on a table and is connected to an ECG monitor. A noninvasive blood pressure cuff is applied, and an IV line is established. The table head is elevated to between 40 and 80 degrees, as specified by a standard protocol. Blood pressure and heart rate measurements are determined every 3 minutes. A positive vasovagal response occurs if the patient loses consciousness as the head of the table is raised. However, not all susceptible individuals experience syncope under resting conditions. In this situation, low-dose isoproterenol (Isuprel) starting at 1 microgram per minute (mcg/min) to a maximum of 4 mcg/min may be infused to increase heart rate by 20% to 40%.[87] If the patient has a HUT-induced syncopal episode, secondary ventricular dysrhythmias may also occur. Therefore antidysrhythmic medications, a defibrillator, and ACLS trained clinicians must always be nearby.

Treatment of vasovagal syncope varies according to the cause. If increased circulating catecholamine levels are the problem, β-blockers are used to decrease catecholamine effect. If increased vagal tone is the cause, atropine-like drugs that block the parasympathetic nervous system may be prescribed. Tilt-training programs to train the patient's autonomic nervous system (ANS) to tolerate changes in posture are also available.[87] After treatment with appropriate medications, the HUT is repeated. For the patient who has experienced syncope of unknown cause, the HUT is a highly effective test if the EPS and neurologic examination are negative.

BEDSIDE HEMODYNAMIC MONITORING

Invasive hemodynamic monitoring is one of the major competencies required for the critical care nurse. Using invasive catheters and sophisticated monitors, the nurse evaluates a patient's cardiac function, circulating blood volume, and physiologic response to treatment. Knowledge of the theoretic base that underlies hemodynamic monitoring assists the clinician in developing decision-making skills to interpret and analyze trends and to formulate a nursing management plan appropriate for each individual patient. Research studies have shown that critical care nurses and physicians who frequently manage patients with invasive hemodynamic lines more accurately assess hemodynamic waveforms than clinicians who infrequently work in critical care.

Indications. The range of medical diagnoses for which hemodynamic monitoring can be used is enormous. Most of these medical diagnoses are linked by three nursing diagnoses:

1. Decreased Cardiac Output
2. Deficient Fluid Volume or Excess Fluid Volume
3. Ineffective Tissue Perfusion

These nursing diagnoses are based on pathophysiologic processes that alter one of the four hemodynamic mechanisms that support normal cardiovascular function: preload, afterload, heart rate, and contractility. Treatment of alterations in cardiac output, fluid volume, and tissue perfusion varies, based on the precipitating cause and medical diagnosis, as discussed later in this chapter in the section on pulmonary artery catheters. For information on pulmonary artery pressure monitoring, see pp. 401 to 412; for information on cardiac output, see p. 413.

There are different levels of hemodynamic monitoring intensity, depending on the clinical needs of the patient. The simplest level includes monitoring heart rhythm, central venous pressure (CVP), and arterial blood pressure—a combination that is commonly used after uncomplicated general surgery. If the patient has a low cardiac output (CO) after an acute MI, a more intense level of surveillance may be necessary. It might involve use of a thermodilution pulmonary artery catheter, which provides hemodynamic information that includes intracardiac pressures, direct measurement of CO, and—if necessary—continuous measurement of pulmonary arterial oxygen saturation (SvO_2).

Overview of Hemodynamic Monitoring
Equipment. A hemodynamic monitoring system has four component parts as shown in Fig. 17-58 and described in the following list:

1. An invasive catheter and high-pressure tubing connect the patient to the transducer.
2. The transducer receives the physiologic signal via the catheter and tubing and converts it into electrical energy.
3. The flush system maintains patency of the fluid-filled system and catheter.
4. The bedside monitor contains the amplifier/recorder, which increases the volume of the electrical signal and displays it on an oscilloscope and on a digital scale in millimeters of mercury (mm Hg).

Although many different types of invasive catheters can be inserted to monitor hemodynamic pressures, all such catheters are connected to similar equipment (see Fig. 17-58). Even so, there remains considerable variation in the way different hospitals configure their hemodynamic systems. The basic set-up consists of the following:

- A bag of 0.9% normal saline solution (some centers use D_5W) as a flush solution. In some hospitals the flush solution will contain 1 unit of heparin (range 0.25 to 2 units) per milliliter of solution; other hospitals do not use heparin in the flush solution because of concern over the development of heparin-induced thrombocytopenia (HIT).[88,89] A pressure infusion cuff covers the bag of flush solution and is inflated to 300 mm Hg.
- IV tubing; three-way stopcocks; and an in-line flow device attached for both continuous fluid infusion and manual flush. High-pressure tubing must be used to connect the invasive catheter to the transducer to prevent damping (flattening) of the waveform.
- A pressure transducer. Modern transducers are disposable, use a silicon chip, and are highly accurate.

Heparin. In some units the anticoagulant heparin is added to the infusion/flush setup to maintain catheter patency. Many critical care units empirically anticoagulate arterial and pulmonary artery (PA) catheters with flush solutions to decrease the risk of thrombus occluding the catheter lumen. Others do not use heparin because of concern over development of the autoimmune condition known as HIT or heparin-induced thrombocytopenia. This is sometimes described as a "heparin allergy" and is associated with a dramatic drop in platelet count and associated bleeding and thrombus.[88,89]

The flush solutions and tubing are usually changed every 96 hours. Again there is variety; some hospitals change flush solutions every 24 hours. For this reason it is essential to be familiar with the specific written procedures that concern hemodynamic monitoring equipment in each critical care unit.

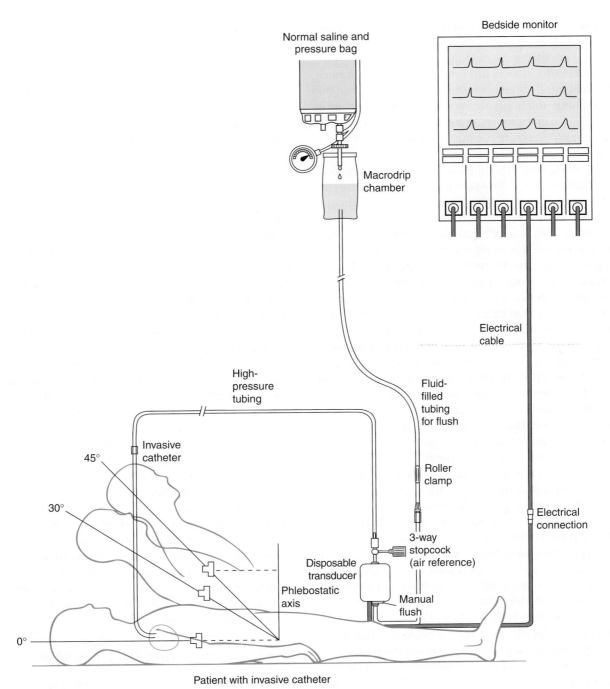

Fig. 17-58   The four parts of a hemodynamic monitoring include invasive catheter attached to high-pressure tubing to connect to the transducer; transducer; flush system, including a manual flush; and bedside monitor.

Calibration of Equipment.   To ensure accuracy of hemodynamic pressure readings, two baseline measurements are necessary:

1. Calibration of the system to atmospheric pressure, also known as "zeroing" the transducer.
2. Determination of the phlebostatic axis for transducer height placement; this is also termed "leveling" the transducer.[90]

Zeroing the Transducer.   To calibrate the equipment to atmospheric pressure, referred to as *zeroing the transducer,* the three-way stopcock nearest to the trans-

ducer is turned simultaneously to open the transducer to air (atmospheric pressure) and to close it to the patient and the flush system. The monitor is adjusted so that "0" is displayed, which equals atmospheric pressure. Atmospheric pressure is not actually "0"; it is 760 mm Hg at sea level. Using "0" to represent current atmospheric pressure provides a convenient baseline for hemodynamic measurement purposes.

Some monitors also require calibration of the upper scale limit while the system remains open to air. At the end of the calibration procedure, the stopcock is returned to the closed position and a closed cap is placed over the open port. At this point the patient's waveform and hemodynamic pressures are displayed.

Disposable transducers are now so accurate that once they are calibrated to atmospheric pressure, drift from the zero baseline is minimal. Although in theory this means that repeated calibration is unnecessary, clinical protocols in most units require the nurse to calibrate the transducer at the beginning of each shift for quality assurance.

Phlebostatic Axis. The phlebostatic axis is a physical reference point on the chest that is used as a baseline for consistent transducer height placement. To obtain the axis, a theoretic line is drawn from the fourth intercostal space (fourth ICP), where it joins the sternum, to a midaxillary line on the side of the chest. The midaxillary line is one half of the anterior-posterior depth of the lateral chest wall.[90] This point approximates the level of the atria, as shown in Fig. 17-58. It is used as the reference mark for both CVP and pulmonary artery catheter transducers. The level of the transducer "air reference stopcock" approximates the position of the tip of an invasive hemodynamic monitoring catheter within the chest.

Leveling the Transducer. Leveling the transducer is different from zeroing. This process aligns the transducer with the level of the left atrium. The purpose is to line up the *air-fluid interface* with the left atrium to correct for changes in *hydrostatic pressure* in blood vessels above and below the level of the heart.[90]

Some critical care units use a carpenter's level or laser-light-level to ensure that the transducer is parallel with the phlebostatic axis reference point. Whenever there is a change in patient position the transducer must be re-leveled to ensure accurate hemodynamic pressure measurements are obtained.[90] Errors in measurement can occur if the transducer is placed below the phlebostatic axis because the fluid in the system will weigh on the transducer, creating additional hydrostatic pressure, and produce a false high reading. For every inch the transducer is below the tip of the catheter, the fluid pressure in the system increases the measurement by 1.87 mm Hg. For example, if the transducer is positioned 6 inches below the tip of the catheter, this falsely elevates the displayed pressure by 11 mm Hg.

If the transducer is placed above this atrial level, gravity and lack of fluid pressure will give an erroneously low reading. Once again, for every inch the transducer is positioned above the catheter tip, the measurement is 1.87 mm Hg less than the true value. If several clinicians are taking measurements, the reference point can be marked on the side of the patient's chest to ensure accurate measurements.[90] See the Nursing Intervention Classification feature on Invasive Hemodynamic Monitoring for a summary of other nursing activities associated with hemodynamic monitoring.

Patient Position. Patient position in the hemodynamically monitored patient would not be an issue if critical care patients always lay flat in the bed. However, lying flat is not always a comfortable position, especially if the patient is alert or if the head of the bed needs to be elevated to decrease the work of breathing.

Head of Bed Position. Nurse researchers have determined that the CVP, pulmonary artery pressure (PAP), and pulmonary artery occlusion pressure (PAOP) (also called *pulmonary artery wedge pressure [PAWP]*) can be reliably measured at head-of-bed positions from 0 (flat) to 60 degrees if the patient is lying on his or her back (supine).[90] In general, if the patient is normovolemic and hemodynamically stable, raising the head of the bed does not affect hemodynamic pressure measurements. If the patient is so hemodynamically unstable or hypovolemic that raising the head of the bed negatively affects intravascular volume distribution, correcting the hemodynamic instability and leaving the patient in a supine position is always the first priority. In summary, the majority of patients do not need the head of the bed to be lowered to "0" to obtain accurate CVP, PAP, or PAOP readings.

Lateral Position. The landmarks for leveling the transducer are different if the patient is turned to the side. Researchers have evaluated hemodynamic pressure measurement readings with the patients in the 30- and 90-degree lateral positions with the head of the bed flat, and found the measurements to be reliable.[90] In the 30-degree angle position, the landmark to use for leveling the transducer is ½ the distance from the surface of the bed to the left sternal border.[90] In the 90-degree right-lateral position the transducer fluid-air interface was positioned at the fourth ICS mid-sternum. In the 90 degree left-lateral position the transducer was positioned at the left parasternal border (beside the sternum).[90] It is important to know that measurements can be recorded in nonsupine positions, because critically ill patients must be turned to prevent development of pressure ulcers and other complications of immobility.

INTRAARTERIAL BLOOD PRESSURE MONITORING

Indications. Intraarterial blood pressure monitoring is indicated for any major medical or surgical condition that compromises CO, tissue perfusion, or fluid volume status. The system is designed for continuous measurement of three blood pressure parameters—systole, diastole, and mean arterial blood pressure (MAP). In addition, the direct arterial access is helpful in the management of patients with acute respiratory failure who require frequent arterial blood gas (ABG) measurements.

Catheters. The size of the catheter used is proportionate to the diameter of the cannulated artery. In small arteries—such as the radial and dorsalis pedis—a 20-gauge, 3.8-cm to 5.1-cm, nontapered Teflon catheter is used most often. If the larger femoral or axillary arteries are used, a 19- or 20-gauge, 16-cm Teflon catheter is used.

NIC   Invasive Hemodynamic Monitoring

Definition: Measurement and interpretation of invasive hemodynamic parameters to determine cardiovascular function and regulate therapy as appropriate.

Activities

Assist with insertion and removal of invasive hemodynamic lines

Assist with Allen test for evaluation of collateral ulnar circulation before radial artery cannulation, if appropriate

Assist with chest x-ray examination after insertion of pulmonary artery catheter

Zero and calibrate equipment every 4 to 12 hours, as appropriate, with transducer at the level of the right atrium

Monitor blood pressure (systolic, diastolic, and mean), central venous/right atrial pressure, pulmonary artery pressure (systolic, diastolic, and mean), and pulmonary artery occlusion pressure

Monitor hemodynamic waveforms for changes in cardiovascular function

Compare hemodynamic parameters with other clinical signs and symptoms

Use closed-system cardiac output setup

Obtain cardiac output by administering cardiac output injectate within 4 seconds, and average three injections that are within less than 1 L of each other

Monitor pulmonary artery and systemic arterial waveforms; if damping occurs, check tubing for kinks or air bubbles, check connections, aspirate clot from tip of catheter, gently flush system, or assist with repositioning of catheter

Document pulmonary artery and systemic arterial waveforms

Monitor peripheral perfusion distal to catheter insertion site every 4 hours or as appropriate

Monitor for dyspnea, fatigue, tachypnea, and orthopnea

Monitor for forward progression of pulmonary catheter resulting in spontaneous wedge, and notify physician if it occurs

Refrain from inflating balloon more frequently than every 1 to 2 hours, or as appropriate

Monitor for balloon rupture (e.g., assess for resistance when inflating balloon and allow balloon to passively deflate after obtaining pulmonary artery occlusion pressure)

Prevent air emboli (e.g., remove air bubbles from tubing; if balloon rupture is suspected, refrain from attempts to reinflate balloon and clamp balloon port)

Maintain sterility of ports

Maintain closed-pressure system to ports, as appropriate

Perform sterile dressing changes and site care, as appropriate

Inspect insertion site for signs of bleeding or infection

Change IV solution and tubing every 24 to 72 hours, based on protocol

Monitor laboratory results to detect possible catheter-induced infection

Administer fluid and/or volume expanders to maintain hemodynamic parameters within specified range

Administer pharmacologic agents to maintain hemodynamic parameters within specified range

Instruct patient and family on therapeutic use of hemodynamic monitoring catheters

Instruct patient on activity restriction while catheters remain in place

From Dochterman JM, Bulecheck GM: *Nursing interventions classification (NIC),* ed 4, St Louis, 2004, Mosby.

Teflon catheters are preferred because of their lower risk of causing thrombosis.

The catheter insertion is usually percutaneous, although the technique varies with vessel size. Catheters are most often inserted in the smaller arteries, using a "catheter-over-needle" unit in which the needle is used as a temporary guide for catheter placement. With this method, once the unit has been inserted into the artery, the needle is withdrawn, leaving the supple plastic catheter in place. Insertion of a catheter into a larger artery usually necessitates use of the Seldinger technique. This procedure involves the following steps:

1. Entry into the artery using a needle
2. Passage of a supple guidewire through the needle into the artery
3. Removal of the needle
4. Passage of the catheter over the guidewire

5. Removal of the guidewire, leaving the catheter in the artery

If a catheter cannot be inserted into the artery using percutaneous methods, an arterial cutdown may be performed. This procedure is avoided, if possible, because it involves a skin incision to expose the artery directly and is associated with a higher risk of infection.

Insertion. Several major peripheral arteries are suitable for receiving a catheter and for long-term hemodynamic monitoring. The most frequently used site is the radial artery. If this artery is not available, the femoral, dorsalis-pedis, axillary, or brachial arteries may be used.

Allen Test. The major advantage of the radial artery is the supply of collateral circulation to the hand provided by the ulnar artery via the palmar arch in most of the population; thus other avenues of circulation are available if the radial artery becomes blocked after catheter placement. Before radial artery cannulation, collateral circulation must be assessed, either by using Doppler flow or by the Allen test. In the Allen test the radial and ulnar arteries are compressed simultaneously. The patient is asked to clench and unclench the hand until it blanches. One of the arteries is then released, and the hand should immediately flush from that side. The same procedure is repeated for the remaining artery.

Nursing Management. Intraarterial blood pressure monitoring is designed for continuous assessment of arterial perfusion to the major organ systems of the body. MAP is the clinical parameter most often used to assess perfusion, because MAP represents perfusion pressure throughout the cardiac cycle. Because one third of the cardiac cycle is spent in systole and two thirds in diastole, the MAP calculation must reflect the greater amount of time spent in diastole. The MAP formula when calculated by hand is:

$$\frac{(Diastole \times 2) + (Systole \times 1)}{3} = MAP$$

Thus a blood pressure of 120/60 mm Hg produces a MAP of 80 mm Hg. However, the bedside hemodynamic monitor may show a slightly different digital number because most computers calculate the area under the curve of the arterial line tracing (Table 17-14).

Perfusion Pressure. A MAP greater than 60 mm Hg is necessary to perfuse the coronary arteries A higher MAP may be required to perfuse the brain and the kidneys. A MAP between 70 and 90 mm Hg is ideal for the cardiac patient to decrease left ventricular (LV) workload. After a carotid endarterectomy or neurosurgery, a MAP of 90 to 110 mm Hg may be more appropriate to increase cerebral perfusion pressure. Systolic and diastolic pressures are monitored in conjunction with the MAP as a further guide to the accuracy of perfusion. Should cardiac output decrease, the body compensates by constricting peripheral vessels to maintain the blood pressure. In this situation the MAP may remain constant but the pulse pressure (difference between systolic and diastolic pressures) narrows. The following examples explain this point:

Mr. A: BP, 90/70 mm Hg; MAP, 76 mm Hg

Mr. B: BP, 150/40 mm Hg; MAP, 76 mm Hg

Both of these patients have a perfusion pressure of 76 mm Hg, but clinically they are very different. Mr. A is peripherally vasoconstricted, as is demonstrated by the narrow pulse pressure (90/70 mm Hg). His skin is cool to touch, and he has weak peripheral pulses. Mr. B has a wide pulse pressure (150/40 mm Hg), warm skin, and normally palpable peripheral pulses. Thus nursing assessment of the patient with an arterial line includes comparison of clinical findings with arterial line readings, including perfusion pressure and MAP.

Pulse Pressure. Another clinical example of hemodynamic nursing assessment is seen in patient JW 1 day after his CABG surgery. JW has recently been weaned from dopamine (Intropin) and sodium nitroprusside (Nipride) and has received a diuretic (20 mg of furosemide IV). He has voided 800 ml of urine via the Foley catheter during the last 2 hours. JW's MAP remains at 80 mm Hg, but his pulse pressure has narrowed by 30 mm Hg from 120/60 to 100/70 mm Hg. His heart rate has increased from 90 to 110 beats per minute. This clinical situation is not uncommon after furosemide (Lasix) administration, but the narrowed pulse pressure and increased heart rate may indicate hypovolemia. The nurse caring for JW will monitor the trend of the MAP. If the MAP begins to decrease and JW shows signs of a low CO, his physician will be notified. In most nonemergency situations, following the trend of the arterial pressure is more valuable than an isolated measurement.

Cuff Blood Pressure. If the arterial line becomes unreliable or dislodged, a cuff pressure can be used as a reserve system. In the normovolemic patient, little difference exists between the cuff blood pressure and arterial pressure. When the arterial catheter is functioning accurately, it is considered the gold standard.[91]

Slight pressure differences are to be expected between the cuff and the arterial catheter because the invasive catheter measures flow within the artery, whereas the arm cuff (mercury sphygmomanometer and stethoscope) measures pressure from the outside. In the normovolemic patient, differences of 5 to 10 mm Hg do not affect clinical management. If the patient has a low CO or is in shock, the cuff pressure is unreliable because of peripheral vasoconstriction, and an arterial line is inserted. If there is ever any doubt about the accuracy of the arterial waveform or pressure reading, a cuff blood pressure reading is always taken.

Arterial Pressure Waveform Interpretation. As the aortic valve opens, blood is ejected from the left ventricle and is recorded as an increase of pressure in the arterial system. The highest point recorded is called *systole.* After peak ejection (systole), force is decreased and pressure drops. A notch (the dicrotic notch) may be visible on the downstroke of this arterial waveform, representing closure of the aortic valve. The *dicrotic notch* signifies the beginning of diastole. The remainder of the downstroke represents diastolic runoff of blood flow into the arterial tree. The lowest point recorded is called *diastole.* A normal arterial pressure tracing is described in Fig. 17-59. Note that electrical stimulation (QRS) is always first and that the arterial pressure tracing follows the initiating QRS.

Decreased Arterial Perfusion. Specific problems with heart rhythm can translate into poor arterial perfusion if CO decreases. Poor perfusion may be seen as a single nonperfused beat after a premature ventricular

Table 17-14	Hemodynamic Pressures and Calculated Hemodynamic Values	
Hemodynamic Pressure	**Definition and Explanation**	**Normal Range**
Mean arterial pressure (MAP)	Average perfusion pressure created by arterial blood pressure during the cardiac cycle. The normal cardiac cycle is one third systole and two thirds diastole. These three components are divided by 3 to obtain the average perfusion pressure for the whole cardiac cycle.	70-100 mm Hg
Central venous pressure (CVP)	Pressure created by volume in the right side of the heart. When the tricuspid valve is open, the CVP reflects filling pressures in the right ventricle. Clinically, the CVP is often used as a guide to overall fluid balance.	2-5 mm Hg 3-8 cm water (H_2O)
Left atrial pressure (LAP)	Pressure created by volume in the left side of the heart. When the mitral valve is open, the LAP reflects filling pressures in the left ventricle. Clinically, the LAP is used after cardiac surgery to determine how well the left ventricle is ejecting its volume. In general, the higher the LAP, the lower the ejection fraction from the left ventricle.	5-12 mm Hg
Pulmonary artery pressure (PAP) (systolic, diastolic, mean) PA systolic (PAS) PA diastolic (PAD) PAP mean (PAP_M)	Pulsatile pressure in the pulmonary artery, measured by an indwelling catheter.	PAS 20-30 mm Hg PAD 5-10 mm Hg PAP_M 10-15 mm Hg
Pulmonary artery occlusion pressure (PAOP) (PCW, or PCWP, or PAWP)	Pressure created by volume in the left side of the heart. When the mitral valve is open, the PAOP reflects filling pressures in the pulmonary vasculature, and pressures in the left side of the heart are transmitted back to the catheter "wedged" into a small pulmonary arteriole.	5-12 mm Hg
Cardiac output (CO)	The amount of blood pumped out by a ventricle. Clinically, it can be measured using the thermodilution CO method, which calculates CO in liters per minute (L/min).	4-6 L/min (at rest)
Cardiac index (CI)	CO divided by body surface area (BSA), tailoring the CO to individual body size. A BSA conversion chart is necessary to calculate CI, which is considered more accurate than CO because it is individualized to height and weight. CI is measured in liters per minute per square meter BSA (L/min/m^2).	2.2-4.0 L/min/m^2
Stroke volume (SV)	Amount of blood ejected by the ventricle with each heartbeat. Hemodynamic monitoring systems calculate SV by dividing cardiac output (CO in L/min) by the heart rate (HR), then multiplying the answer by 1000 to change liters to milliliters (ml).	60-70 ml
Stroke volume index (SI)	SV indexed to BSA.	40-50 ml/m^2
Systemic vascular resistance (SVR)	Mean pressure difference across the systemic vascular bed, divided by blood flow. Clinically, SVR represents the resistance against which the left ventricle must pump to eject its volume. This resistance is created by the systemic arteries and arterioles. As SVR increases, CO falls. SVR is measured in either units or dynes/sec/cm^{-5}. If the number of units is multiplied by 80, the valve is converted to dynes/sec/cm^{-5}.	10-18 units or 800-1400 dynes/sec/cm^{-5}
Systemic vascular resistance index (SVRI)	SVR indexed to BSA.	2000-2400 dynes/sec/cm^{-5}
Pulmonary vascular resistance (PVR)	Mean pressure difference across pulmonary vascular bed, divided by blood flow. Clinically, PVR represents the resistance against which the right ventricle must pump to eject its volume. This resistance is created by the pulmonary arteries and arterioles. As PVR increases, the output from the right ventricle decreases. PVR is measured in either units or dynes/sec/cm^{-5}. PVR is normally one sixth of SVR.	1.2-3.0 units or 100-250 dynes/sec/cm^{-5}
Pulmonary vascular resistance index (PVRI)	PVR indexed to BSA.	225-315 dynes/sec/cm^{-5}/m^2

Continued

Table 17-14	Hemodynamic Pressures and Calculated Hemodynamic Values—cont'd	
Hemodynamic Pressure	**Definition and Explanation**	**Normal Range**
Left cardiac work index (LCWI)	Amount of work the left ventricle does *each minute* when ejecting blood. The hemodynamic formula represents pressure generated (MAP) multiplied by volume pumped (CO). A conversion factor is used to change mm Hg to kilogram-meter (kg-m). LCWI is always represented as an indexed volume (BSA chart). LCWI increases or decreases because of changes in either pressure (MAP) or volume pumped (CO).	3.4-4.2 kg-m/m²
Left ventricular stroke work index (LVSWI)	Amount of work the left ventricle performs with *each heartbeat.* The hemodynamic formula represents pressure generated (MAP) multiplied by volume pumped (SV). A conversion factor is used to change ml/mm Hg to gram-meter (g-m). LVSWI is always represented as an indexed volume. LVSWI increases or decreases because of changes in either pressure (MAP) or volume pumped (SV).	50-62 g-m/m²
Right cardiac work index (RCWI)	Amount of work the right ventricle performs *each minute* when ejecting blood. The hemodynamic formula represents pressure generated (PAP mean) multiplied by volume pumped (CO). A conversion factor is used to change mm Hg to kilogram-meter (kg-m). RCWI is always represented as an indexed value (BSA chart). Similar to LCWI, the RCWI increases or decreases because of changes in either pressure (PAP mean) or volume pumped (CO).	0.54-0.66 kg-m/m²
Right ventricular stroke work index (RVSWI)	Amount of work the right ventricle does *each heartbeat.* The hemodynamic formula represents pressure generated (PAP mean) multiplied by volume pumped (SV). A conversion factor is used to change mm Hg to gram-meter (g-m). RVSWI is always represented as an indexed value (BSA chart). Similar to LVSWI, the RVSWI increases or decreases because of changes in either pressure (PAP mean) or volume pumped (SV).	7.9-9.7 g-m/m²

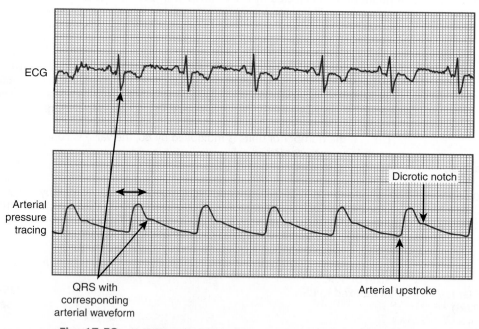

Fig. 17-59 Simultaneous ECG and normal arterial pressure tracing.

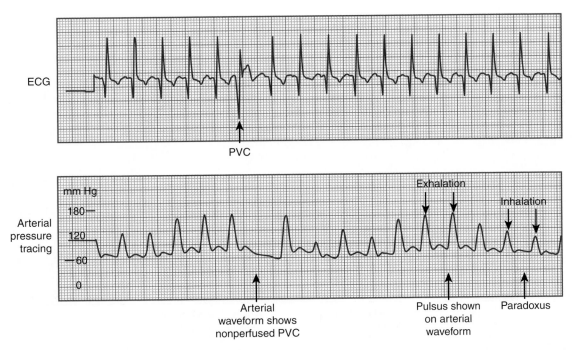

Fig. 17-60 Simultaneous ECG and arterial pressure tracings show normal arterial waveform with a nonperfused premature ventricular contraction (PVC). Arterial waveform also shows evidence of pulsus paradoxus in a patient who is mechanically ventilated.

contraction (PVC) (Fig. 17-60) or as multiple nonperfused beats (Fig. 17-61). In ventricular bigeminy, every second beat is poorly perfused (Fig. 17-62). A disorganized atrial baseline resulting from atrial fibrillation creates a variable arterial pulse because of the differences in stroke volume between each beat (Fig. 17-63). All of these examples illustrate that when two beats are close together, the left ventricle does not have time to fill adequately, and the second beat is poorly perfused or is not perfused at all.

Pulse Deficit. A pulse deficit occurs when the apical heart rate and the peripheral pulse are not equal. In the critical care unit this can be seen on the bedside monitor. Normally there is one arterial upstroke for each QRS, and if there are more QRS complexes than arterial upstrokes, a pulse deficit is present, as shown in Figs. 17-60 and 17-63. To identify a pulse deficit in an unmonitored patient, a stethoscope is placed over the apex of the heart. The heartbeat can be heard, but it cannot be felt as a radial pulse. To determine whether a pulse deficit is significant, it is necessary to evaluate the clinical impact on the patient and whether any change in MAP or pulse pressure has occurred. Generally, the more nonperfused beats, the more serious the problem.

Pulsus Paradoxus. Pulsus paradoxus is a decrease of more than 10 mm Hg in the arterial waveform that occurs during inhalation (inspiration). It is caused by a fall in CO as a result of increased negative intrathoracic pressure during inhalation. As pressure within the thorax falls, blood pools in the large veins of the lungs and

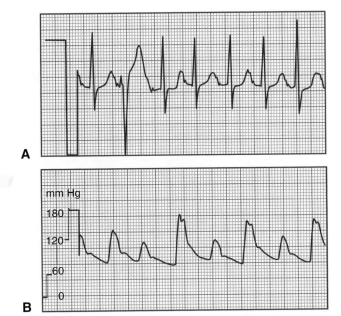

Fig. 17-61 Simultaneous **A,** ECG and **B,** arterial pressure tracings show pulsus alternans. A nonperfused premature ventricular contraction (PVC) is also present.

thorax, and stroke volume is decreased. The procedure for determining the presence of pulsus paradoxus is discussed in Box 16-8.

In certain clinical conditions the pulsus paradoxus is very obvious and can be clearly seen on an arterial waveform. It can be used as a clinical diagnostic test in a

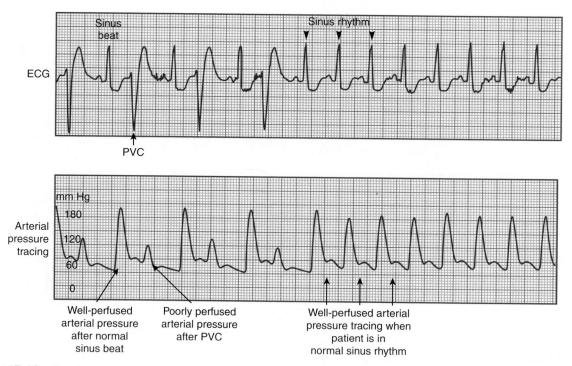

Fig. 17-62 Simultaneous ECG and arterial pressure tracings show ventricular bigeminy in which every other ventricular beat is poorly perfused on the arterial pressure waveform in the first part of the tracing. In the second half of the tracing, there is a well-perfused arterial pressure tracing as the patient converts to normal sinus rhythm.

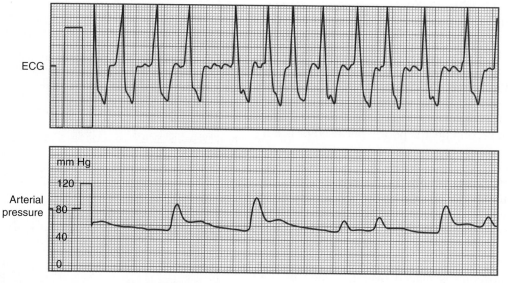

Fig. 17-63 Simultaneous ECG and arterial pressure tracings show atrial fibrillation, which results in irregular atrial pulsations. They create differences in beat-to-beat ventricular upstroke volume, resulting in diminished or absent ventricular output, as seen on the arterial waveform.

patient with cardiac tamponade, pericardial effusion, or constrictive pericarditis. Pulsus paradoxus commonly occurs in hypovolemic surgical patients who are mechanically ventilated with large tidal volumes (see Fig. 17-60).

Pulsus Alternans. In *pulsus alternans,* every other arterial pulsation is weak. This sometimes occurs in individuals with advanced left ventricular failure.

Damped Waveform. If the arterial monitor shows a low blood pressure, it is the responsibility of the nurse to determine whether it is truly a patient problem or a problem with the equipment, as described in Table 17-15. A low arterial blood pressure waveform is shown in Fig. 17-64. In this case the digital readout correlated well with the patient's own cuff pressure, confirming that the patient was hypotensive. This arterial waveform is more

Table 17-15	Nursing Measures to Ensure Patient Safety and to Troubleshoot Problems with Hemodynamic Monitoring Equipment		
Problem	**Prevention**	**Rationale**	**Troubleshooting**
Overdamping of waveform	Provide continuous infusion of solution containing heparin through an in-line flush device (1 unit of heparin for each milliliter of flush solution).	To ensure that recorded pressures and waveform are accurate because a damped waveform gives inaccurate readings.	Before insertion, completely flush the line and/or catheter. In a line attached to a patient, back flush through the system to clear bubbles from tubing or transducer.
Underdamping ("overshoot" or "fling")	Use short lengths of non-compliant tubing. Use "fast-flush square wave" test to demonstrate optimal system damping. Verify arterial waveform accuracy with the cuff blood pressure.	If the monitoring system is under-damped, both the systolic and diastolic values will be overestimated by both the waveform and the digital values. False high systolic values may lead to clinical decisions based on erroneous data.	Perform the "fast-flush square wave" test to verify optimal damping of the monitoring system.
Clot formation at end of catheter	Provide continuous infusion of solution containing heparin through an in-line flush device (1 unit of heparin for each milliliter of flush solution).	Any foreign object placed in the body can cause local activation of the patient's coagulation system as a normal defense mechanism. The clots that are formed may be dangerous if they break off and travel to other parts of the body.	If a clot in the catheter is suspected because of a damped waveform or resistance to forward flush of the system, gently aspirate the line using a small syringe inserted into the proximal stopcock. Then flush the line again once the clot is removed and inspect the waveform. It should return to a normal pattern.
Hemorrhage	Use Luer-Lok (screw) connections in line setup. Close and cap stopcocks when not in use. Ensure that the catheter is either sutured or securely taped in position.	A loose connection or open stop-cock creates a low-pressure sump effect, causing blood to back into the line and into the open air. If a catheter is accidentally removed, the vessel can bleed profusely, especially with an arterial line or if the patient has abnormal coagulation factors (resulting from heparin in the line) or has hypertension.	Once a blood leak is recognized, tighten all connections, flush the line, and estimate blood loss. If the catheter has been inadvertently removed, put pressure on the cannulation site. When bleeding has stopped, apply a sterile dressing, estimate blood loss, and inform the physician. If the patient is restless, an armboard may protect lines inserted in the arm.
Air emboli	Ensure that all air bubbles are purged from a new line setup before attachment to an indwelling catheter. Ensure that the drip chamber from the bag of flush solution is more than half full before using the in-line, fast-flush system. Some sources recommend removing all air from the bag of flush solution before assembling the system.	Air can be introduced at several times; including when central venous pressure (CVP) tubing comes apart, when a new line setup is attached, or when a new CVP or pulmonary artery (PA) line is inserted. During insertion of a CVP or PA line, the patient may be asked to hold his or her breath at specific times to prevent drawing air into the chest during inhalation. The in-line, fast-flush devices are designed to permit clearing of blood from the line after withdrawal of blood samples. If the chamber of the IV tubing is too low or empty, the rapid flow of fluid will create turbulence and cause flushing of air bubbles into the system and into the bloodstream.	Because it is impossible to get the air back once it has been introduced into the bloodstream, prevention is the best cure. If any air bubbles are noted, they must be vented through the in-line stopcocks and the drip chamber must be filled. The left atrial pressure (LAP) line setup is the only system that includes an air filter specifically to prevent air emboli.

Continued

Table 17-15		Nursing Measures to Ensure Patient Safety and to Troubleshoot Problems with Hemodynamic Monitoring Equipment—cont'd	
Problem	**Prevention**	**Rationale**	**Troubleshooting**
Normal waveform with *low* digital pressure	Ensure that the system is calibrated to atmospheric pressure. Ensure that the transducer is placed at the level of the phlebostatic axis.	To provide a 0 baseline relative to atmospheric pressure. If the transducer has been placed *higher* than the phlebostatic level, gravity and the lack of hydrostatic pressure will produce a false *low* reading.	Recalibrate the equipment if transducer drift has occurred. Reposition the transducer at the level of the phlebostatic axis. Misplacement can occur if the patient moves from the bed to the chair or if the bed is placed in a Trendelenburg position.
Normal wave form with *high* digital pressure	Ensure that the system is calibrated to atmospheric pressure. Ensure that the transducer is placed at the level of the phlebostatic axis.	To provide a 0 baseline relative to atmospheric pressure. If the transducer has been placed *lower* than the phlebostatic level, the weight of hydrostatic pressure on the transducer will produce a false *high* reading.	Recalibrate the equipment if transducer drift has occurred. Reposition the transducer at the level of the phlebostatic axis. This situation can occur if the head of the bed was raised and the transducer was not repositioned. Some centers require attachment of the transducer to the patient's chest to avoid this problem.
Loss of waveform	Always have the hemodynamic waveform monitored so that changes or loss can be quickly noted.	The catheter may be kinked, or a stopcock may be turned off.	Check the line setup to ensure that all stopcocks are turned in the correct position and that the tubing is not kinked. Sometimes the catheter migrates against a vessel wall, and having the patient change position restores the waveform.

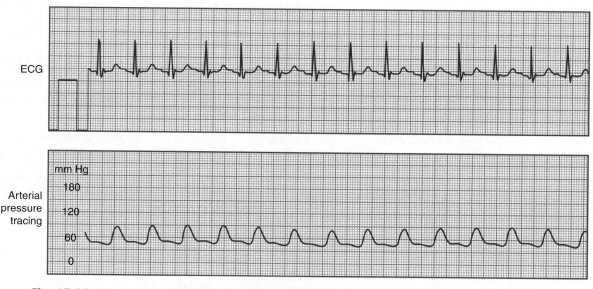

Fig. 17-64 Simultaneous ECG and arterial pressure tracings show a low arterial pressure waveform.

rounded, without a dicrotic notch, when compared with the normal waveform in Fig. 17-59. A damped (flattened) arterial waveform is shown in Fig. 17-65. In this case the patient's cuff pressure was significantly higher than the digital readout, thus representing a problem with equipment. A damped waveform occurs when communication from the artery to the transducer is interrupted and produces false values on the monitor and oscilloscope. Damping is caused by a fibrin "sleeve" that partially occludes the tip of the catheter, by kinks in the catheter or tubing, or by air bubbles in the system. Troubleshooting techniques (see Table 17-15) are used to find the origin of the problem and to remove the cause of damping.

Underdamped Waveform. Another cause of distortion of the arterial waveform is underdamping, often called *overshoot* or *fling.* This is recognized by a narrow upward systolic peak that produces a false high systolic reading when compared with the patient's cuff blood pressure as shown in Fig. 17-66. The overshoot is caused by an increase in dynamic response or increased oscillations within the system.

Fast-Flush Square Waveform Test. The monitoring system dynamic response can be verified for accuracy at the bedside by the *fast-flush square waveform,* or *dynamic frequency response,* test.[90] The nurse performs this test to ensure that the patient pressures and waveform shown on the bedside monitor are accurate.[90] The test makes use of the manual flush system on the transducer. Normally the flush device allows only 3 ml of fluid/hour. With the normal waveform displayed, the manual fast-flush is used to generate a rapid increase in pressure, which is displayed on the monitor oscilloscope. As shown in Fig. 17-67, the normal dynamic response waveform shows a square pattern with one or two oscillations before the return of the arterial wave-

form. If the system is overdamped, a sloped—rather than square—pattern is seen. If the system is underdamped, additional oscillations—or vibrations—are seen on the fast-flush square wave test. This test can be performed with any hemodynamic monitoring system. If air bubbles, clots, or kinks are in the system, the waveform becomes damped, or flattened, and this will be reflected in the square waveform result. This is an easy test to do, and it should be incorporated into nursing care procedures at the bedside when the hemodynamic system is first set up, at least once a shift, after opening the system for any reason, and whenever there is concern over the accuracy of the waveform.[90] If the pressure waveform is distorted or the digital display is inaccurate, the troubleshooting methods described in Table 17-15 can be implemented. The nurse caring for the patient with an arterial line must be able to assess whether a low MAP or narrowed perfusion pressure represents decreased arterial perfusion or equipment malfunction. Assessment of the arterial waveform on the oscilloscope, in combination with clinical assessment, and use of the square waveform test will yield the answer.

Alarms. All critically ill patients must have the hemodynamic monitoring alarms on and adjusted to sound an audible alarm if the patient should experience a change in blood pressure, heart rate, respiratory rate, or other significant monitored variable. The key issues con-

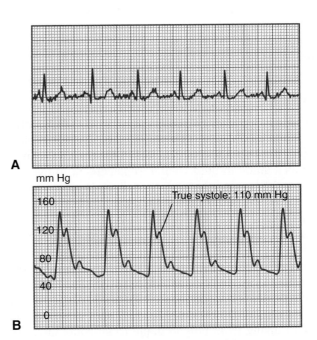

Fig. 17-66 Simultaneous **A,** ECG and **B,** arterial pressure tracings showing "overshoot," or "fling," caused by a heightened dynamic response in the monitoring system. The monitor recorded an arterial line blood pressure of 141/51 mm Hg. The patient's true blood pressure with cuff was 110/54 mm Hg. The 110 mm Hg cuff systolic is consistent with the arterial line tracing without "overshoot."

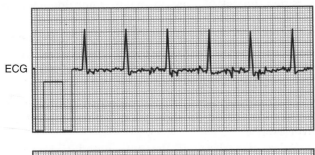

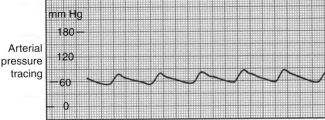

Fig. 17-65 Simultaneous ECG and arterial pressure tracings show a damped arterial pressure waveform.

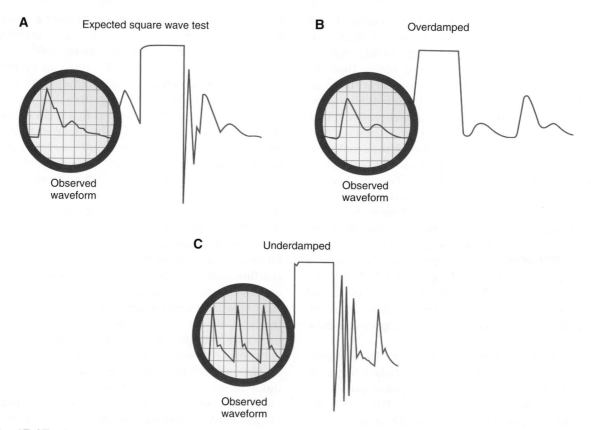

A Expected square wave test

Observed waveform

B Overdamped

Observed waveform

C Underdamped

Observed waveform

Fig. 17-67 Square Wave Test. **A,** Expected square wave test. **B,** Overdamped. **C,** Underdamped. (From Darovic GO: *Hemodynamic monitoring: invasive and noninvasive clinical application,* ed 3, Philadelphia, 2002, Saunders.)

cerning monitor alarms are presented in the Patient Safety Alert feature on Clinical Alarm Systems.

CENTRAL VENOUS PRESSURE MONITORING

Indications. Central venous pressure (CVP) monitoring is indicated whenever a patient has significant alteration in fluid volume (see Table 17-14). The CVP can be used as a guide in fluid volume replacement in hypovolemia and to assess the impact of diuresis after diuretic administration in the case of fluid overload. In addition, when a major IV line is required for volume replacement, a central venous catheter (CVC) is a good choice because large volumes of fluid can easily be delivered.

Central Venous Catheters. A range of CVC options are available as single-, double-, or triple-lumen infusion catheters, depending on the specific needs of the patient. Central venous catheters are made from a variety of materials ranging from polyurethane to silicone; most are soft and flexible.[92]

Insertion. The large veins of the upper thorax—subclavian (SC) and internal jugular (IJ)—are most commonly used for percutaneous CVC line insertion. The femoral vein in the groin is used when the thoracic veins are not accessible. All three major sites have advantages and disadvantages.

Internal Jugular Vein. The IJ is the most frequently used access site for CVC insertion. Compared to the other thoracic veins it is the easiest to canalize. If the IJ is not available the external jugular (EJ) may be accessed, although blood flow is significantly higher in the IJ, making it the preferred site. Another advantage of the IJ is that the risk of creating an iatrogenic pneumothorax is small. Disadvantages to the IJ are patient discomfort from the indwelling catheter when moving the head or neck and contamination of the IJ site from oral or tracheal secretions, especially if the patient is intubated or has a tracheostomy. This may be the reason why catheter-related infections are higher in the IJ compared to the SC position for indwelling catheters left in place over 4 days.[92]

Subclavian Vein. If the anticipated CVC dwelling time is prolonged over 5 days, the SC site is preferred. The SC position has the lowest infection rate and produces the least patient discomfort from the catheter. The disadvantages are that the SC vein is more difficult to access and carries a higher risk of iatrogenic pneumothorax or hemothorax, although the risk varies greatly, depending upon the experience and skill of the physician inserting the catheter.

Femoral Vein. The femoral vein is considered the easiest cannulation site because there are no curves in

PATIENT SAFETY ALERT

Clinical Alarm Systems

Clinical Alarm System Effectiveness

1. Implement regular preventive maintenance and testing of alarm systems.
2. Ensure that alarms are activated with appropriate settings and are sufficiently audible with respect to distances and competing noise within the unit.

Clinical Alarm Safety

Alarm Identification

1. Audible and visual indication should be present for any condition that poses a risk to the patient. Indicator should be visible from at least 10 feet (3 meters).
2. Cause of the alarm must be easily identifiable by health care practitioner.
3. Life-threatening conditions should be clearly differentiated from noncritical alarm situations.
4. High-priority alarms should override low-priority alarms.
5. Alarm must be sufficiently loud or distinctive to be heard over environmental noise of a busy critical care unit.
6. It should never be possible to turn the volume control to "off."

Disabling and Silencing Alarms

1. Alarm silence must have visual indicator to clearly show it is disabled.
2. Critical alarms should not be permanently overridden (turned "off").
3. New, life-threatening alarm conditions should override a silenced alarm.

Power

Battery units should initiate an alarm before a unit stops working effectively.

Alarm Limits

1. Alarm limits can be adjusted to meet clinical needs of patient. The system should default to standard settings between patients.
2. Alarm limits should preferably be displayed on the monitor.

Data from www.JCAHO.org and *Health Devices* 31:397-412, 2002.

the insertion route. The large diameter of the femoral vein carries a high blood flow that is advantageous for specialized procedures such as continuous renal replacement therapy (CRRT) or plasmapheresis. Disadvantages are that the patient cannot bend at the hip, because this interrupts blood flow through the catheter and may lead to thrombus formation; risk of retroperitoneal

bleed; and a higher rate of nosocomial infections, probably due to site location near the groin area.[92]

During insertion of the SC or IJ veins, the patient may be placed in a Trendelenburg position. Placing the head in a dependent position causes the IJ veins in the neck to become more prominent, facilitating line placement. To minimize the risk of air embolus during the procedure, the patient may be asked to "take a deep breath and hold it" any time the needle or catheter is open to air. The tip of the catheter is designed to remain in the vena cava and should not migrate into the right atrium. If the IJ or SC veins are not available, the femoral veins can be used for CVC access. The femoral veins are further away from the heart; thus, for accurate CVP measurements, the tip of the catheter must be advanced into the inferior vena cava near the right atrium. Because many patients are awake and alert when a CVC is inserted, a brief explanation about the procedure will minimize patient anxiety and result in cooperation during the insertion. This cooperation is important, because CVC insertion is a sterile procedure and because the supine or Trendelenburg position may not be comfortable for many patients. The ECG should be monitored during CVC insertion because of the associated risk of dysrhythmias.

All central catheters are designed for placement by percutaneous injection after skin preparation and administration of a local anesthetic. Usually a prepackaged CVC kit is used for the procedure. The standard CVC kit contains sterile towels, chorhexidine and alcohol skin prep, a needle introducer, a syringe, guidewire, and a catheter. The Seldinger technique, in which the vein is located by using a "seeking" needle and syringe, is the preferred method of placement. A guidewire is passed through the needle, the needle is removed, and the catheter is passed over the guidewire. Once the catheter is correctly placed in the vena cava, the guidewire is removed. Finally, an IV setup is attached and the catheter is sutured in place.

After thoracic CVC placement, a chest radiograph is obtained to verify placement and the absence of an iatrogenic hemothorax or pneumothorax, especially if the SC vein was accessed. The use of Doppler ultrasound guidance to find the vein and guide insertion may reduce the incidence of iatrogenic complications.[92] In the rare case that it is not possible to insert a CVC percutaneously, a surgical cutdown may be performed.

CVC Complications. The CVC is an essential tool in care of the critically ill patient, but it is associated with some risks, and for this reason it is the responsibility of all clinicians to be informed of these hazards and to follow hospital procedures to avoid iatrogenic complications. The most frequent CVC complications are air embolus, catheter associated thrombus formation, and infection.

Air Embolus. The risk of air embolus, although uncommon, is always present for the patient with a central venous line in place. Air can enter during insertion through a disconnected or broken catheter, or air can enter along the path of a removed CVC. This is more likely if the patient is in an upright position, because air can be pulled into the venous system with the increase in negative intrathoracic pressure during inhalation.[93] If a large volume of air (200 to 300 ml) is infused rapidly, it may become trapped in the right ventricular outflow tract, stopping blood flow from the right side of the heart to the lungs. If the air embolus is large, the patient will experience respiratory distress and cardiovascular collapse. Two clinical signs are specifically associated with a large venous air embolism "mill wheel murmur" and "gasp reflex."[93] A mill wheel murmur is a loud, churning sound heard over the middle chest, caused by the obstruction to right ventricular outflow. The gasp reflex is the automatic gasp for air that occurs during hypoxemia. Treatment involves administering 100% oxygen and placing the patient on the left side with the head downward (left lateral Trendelenburg position). This position displaces the air from the right ventricular outflow tract to the apex of the heart, where it can be either resorbed or aspirated. Precautions to prevent an air embolism in a CVP line include using only screw (Luer-Lock) connections, avoiding long loops of IV tubing, and using screw caps on the three-way stopcock.

Thrombus Formation. Clot formation (thrombus) at the CVC site is unfortunately not uncommon. Ultrasound studies have found asymptomatic thrombus formation to be in the range of 33% to 67% when the catheter is in place for over 7 days.[92] Symptomatic thrombi are reported in 0% to 5% of those cases.[92,94] Thrombus formation is not uniform; it may involve development of a *fibrin sleeve* around the catheter, or the thrombus may be attached directly to the vessel wall. Other factors that promote clot formation include rupture of vascular endothelium, interruption of laminar blood flow, and physical presence of the catheter, all of which activate the coagulation cascade. The risk of thrombus formation is higher if insertion was difficult or there were multiple needlesticks.[92] Gradual thrombus formation may lead to "sudden" CVC occlusion. Usually the CVC becomes more difficult to withdraw blood from, or the CVP waveform becomes intermittently damped over a period of hours or even 1 to 2 days and is reported as needing "frequent flushes" to remain patent. This situation is caused by the continued lengthening of a "fibrin sleeve" that extends along the catheter length from the insertion site past the catheter tip.[92,94] Some catheters are heparin-coated to reduce the risk of thrombus formation, although the risk of HIT, reported to be 0.4% with indwelling CVC, does not make this a benign option.[94] Sometimes CVC complications are additive; for example the risk of catheter-related infection is increased in the presence of thrombi. The thrombus likely serves as a culture medium for bacterial growth.[94]

Infection. Infection related to the use of central venous catheters is a major problem. Risk factors for catheter-related infections include extremes of age, impaired host defense mechanisms, severe illness, malnutrition, and presence of other invasive lines. It is estimated that more than 50,000 infections related to CVC use occur annually in the United States, with associated mortality between 10% and 20%.[94]

The incidence of infection is strongly correlated with the length of time the CVC has been left inserted. Catheters that are in place under 3 days almost never lead to infection, providing standard insertion and management procedures are followed. If the CVC remains between 3 and 7 days, the infection rate is 3% to 5%. Catheters remaining in one site over 7 days have an infection rate of 5% to 10%.[94]

CVC-related infection is noted either at the catheter insertion site or as a bloodstream infection (septicemia). Systemic manifestations of infection can be present without inflammation at the catheter site. To determine whether a suspect catheter is contaminated, after removal the tip is placed in a sterile container and cultured. No decrease in infections was found when catheters were routinely changed to prevent infectious, and this practice is no longer recommended.[95] A "suspect" CVC changed over guidewire risks a higher rate of infection.[95] Prevention is the best defense against complications resulting from infections. Most infections are transmitted via the skin. Therefore current insertion recommendations state that the physician should use good hand-washing procedures, clean the insertion site with 2% chlorhexidine, utilize sterile technique during catheter insertion, and maintain maximal sterile barrier precautions (see the Patient Safety Alert feature on Guidelines for Prevention and Management of Central Venous Catheter (CVC) Infections).[95-98]

All clinicians must use good hand-washing technique and follow aseptic procedures during site care and any time the CVC system is entered to withdraw blood, give medications, or change tubing.[95,98] The infusion of high-dextrose solutions such as total parental nutrition (TPN) may be associated with an increased risk of infection. Methods to lower TPN-related complications include use of a single-lumen CVC that is not accessed for other medications or laboratory samples.[99]

Incidence of infection is higher with use of occlusive dressings that do not allow removal of moisture. Therefore transparent, breathable dressings that allow removal of skin moisture are recommended. Site dressings that have antimicrobial properties are being used to try to lower infection rates. New developments in catheter design may also help to reduce central line infection. Catheters are available that are impregnated with an antimicrobial substance or have a silver-impregnated, tissue-barrier cuff attached to the catheter.[95] These catheters are designed to lower the rate of CVC infection.

Guidelines for Prevention and Management of Central Venous Catheter Infections

1. Use effective hand washing.
2. Educate and train health care providers who insert and maintain central venous catheters (CVCs).
3. Use maximal sterile barrier precautions during CVC insertion.
4. Use 2% chlorhexidine preparation for skin antisepsis.
5. Avoid routine replacement of CVCs as a strategy to prevent infection.
6. Insert antiseptic/antibiotic-impregnated short-term CVCs if rate of infection is high despite adherence to other strategies (education/training, maximal sterile barrier precautions, 2% chlorhexidine).
7. Confirm clinical suspicion of infection by taking cultures of blood and catheter samples.
8. Initially treat intravascular catheter infection with IV antimicrobial therapy, considering severity of patient's acute illness, underlying disease, and potential pathogens. Once the catheter-related pathogen is documented, narrow focus of antimicrobial therapy to treat specific organism(s).
9. Remove CVC if infected.

Data from O'Grady NP et al: *Am J Infect Control* 30:476-489, 2002; and Boyce JM, Pittet D: *Am J Infect Control* 30:1-46, 2002.

Nursing Management. In the critically ill patient the CVC is also used to monitor CVP and waveform. The CVP catheter is used to measure the filling pressures of the right side of the heart. During diastole, when the tricuspid valve is open and blood is flowing from the right atrium to the right ventricle, the CVP accurately reflects right ventricular end-diastolic pressure (RVEDP). The normal CVP is 2 to 5 mm Hg (3 to 8 cm H_2O).

Low CVP. A low CVP often occurs in the hypovolemic patient and suggests that insufficient blood volume is in the ventricle at end-diastole to produce an adequate stroke volume. Thus to maintain normal CO, the heart rate must increase. This increase produces the tachycardia often observed in hypovolemic states and increases myocardial oxygen demand.

The CVP is used in combination with the MAP and other clinical parameters to assess hemodynamic stability. In the hypovolemic patient, the CVP falls before a significant fall in MAP occurs, because peripheral vasoconstriction keeps the MAP normal. Thus the CVP is an excellent early-warning system for the patient who is bleeding, vasodilating, receiving diuretics, or being rewarmed after cardiac surgery.

High CVP. An elevated CVP occurs in cases of fluid overload. To circulate the excess blood volume, the heart must greatly increase its contractile force to move the large volume of blood. This increases the cardiac workload and increases myocardial oxygen consumption. The critical care nurse follows the trend of the CVP measurements to determine subsequent interventions for optimal fluid volume management.

CVP Limitations. The CVP is not a reliable indicator of left ventricular dysfunction. Left ventricular dysfunction, which can occur after an acute MI, increases filling pressures on the left side of the heart. The CVP, because it measures RVEDP, remains normal until the increase in pressure from the left side of the heart is reflected back through the pulmonary vasculature to the right ventricle. In this situation a pulmonary artery catheter that measures pressures on the left side of the heart is the monitoring method of choice. For more information on pulmonary artery pressure monitoring, see p. 401.

Water vs. Mercury CVP. CVP values are measured in millimeters of mercury (mm Hg), if bedside hardwire monitoring is used. If a patient is changed from hardwire monitoring using mm Hg to a water manometer and clinicians want to know the relationship between the two values, it involves a straightforward calculation based upon the following standard relationship: 1 mm Hg (mercury pressure) is equivalent to 1.36 cm H_2O (water pressure). It is important to recognize that although the numerical value in cm H_2O will be higher, the values are clinically equivalent for the specific patient. To convert water manometer pressure (cm H_2O) to mercury pressure: the water-pressure value is divided by 1.36 ($H_2O \div 1.36$). To convert mercury pressure (mm Hg) to water pressure: the mercury value is multiplied by 1.36 (mm Hg $\times$ 1.36).

Removal. Removal of the CVC is generally a nursing responsibility. Complications are infrequent, and the ones to anticipate are bleeding and air embolus. Recommended techniques to avoid air embolus during CVC removal include removing the catheter when the patient is supine in bed (not in a chair); and placing the patient flat or in reverse Trendelenburg position if the patient's clinical condition permits this maneuver.[93] Patients with heart failure, pulmonary disease, and neurologic conditions with raised intracranial pressure (ICP) should not be placed flat. If the patient is alert and able to cooperate, he or she is asked to take a deep breath to raise intrathoracic pressure during removal.[93] Following removal, to decrease the risk of air entering via a "track," an occlusive dressing is applied to the site.[93] If bleeding at the site occurs after removal, firm pressure is applied. If a patient has prolonged coagulation times, fresh-frozen plasma or platelets may be prescribed before CVC removal.

Patient Position. To achieve accurate CVP measurements, the phlebostatic axis is used as a reference point on the body, and the transducer or water manometer zero must be level with this point. If the phlebostatic axis is used and the transducer or water manometer is correctly aligned, any head-of-bed position of up to 60 degrees may be accurately used for CVP readings for most patients.[90] Elevating the head of the bed is especially helpful for the patient with respiratory or cardiac problems who will not tolerate a flat position.

CVP Waveform Interpretation. The normal right atrial (CVP) waveform has three positive deflections—called *a*, *c*, and *v waves*—that correspond to specific atrial events in the cardiac cycle (Fig. 17-68). The *a wave* reflects atrial contraction and follows the P wave seen on the ECG. The downslope of this wave is called the *x descent* and represents atrial relaxation. The *c wave* reflects the bulging of the closed tricuspid valve into the right atrium during ventricular contraction; this wave is small and not always visible, but corresponds to the QRS-T interval on the ECG. The *v wave* represents atrial filling and increased pressure against the closed tricuspid valve in early diastole. The downslope of the v wave is named the *y descent* and represents the fall in pressure as the tricuspid valve opens and blood flows from the right atrium to the right ventricle.

Cannon Waves. Dysrhythmias can change the pattern of the CVP waveform. In a junctional rhythm or after a PVC, the atria are depolarized after the ventricles if retrograde conduction to the atria occurs. This may be seen as a retrograde P wave on the ECG and as a large combined *ac wave* or *cannon wave* on the CVP waveform (Fig. 17-69). These cannon waves can be easily detected as large "pulses" in the jugular veins. Other pathologic conditions, such as advanced right ventricular failure or tricuspid valve insufficiency, allow regurgitant backflow of blood from the right ventricle to the right atrium during ventricular contraction, thus producing large v waves on the right atrial waveform. In atrial fibrillation, the CVP waveform has no recognizable pattern because of the disorganization of the atria.

Specialized Catheters. A CVC that incorporates a fiberoptic sensor to measure systemic venous oxygen saturation ($Scvo_2$) can be used as a traditional CVC and additionally used to follow the trend of venous oxygen saturation.[100] The physiology underlying use of this fiberoptic technology is discussed later in the chapter, in the section on Svo_2 monitoring.

LEFT ATRIAL PRESSURE MONITORING

Indications. Left atrial pressure (LAP) monitoring is used in rare cases after major cardiac surgery. Until the advent of the pulmonary artery catheter in the 1970s, LAP monitoring was used to assess hemodynamics on the left side of the heart. Today it is not used for routine monitoring but is a clinical choice on rare occasions in the postoperative management of the cardiac surgery

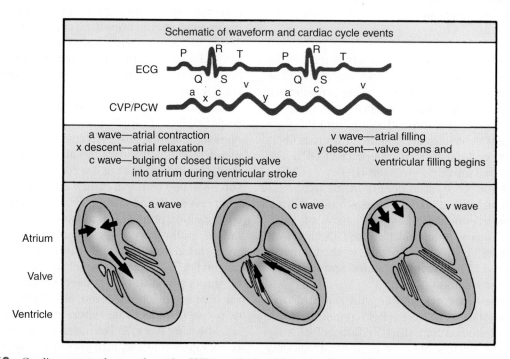

Fig. 17-68 Cardiac events that produce the CVP waveform with a, c, and v waves. The *a wave* represents atrial contraction. The *x descent* represents atrial relaxation. The *c wave* represents the bulging of the closed tricuspid valve into the right atrium during ventricular systole. The *v wave* represents atrial filling. The *y descent* represents opening of the tricuspid valve and filling of the ventricle.

patient who has significant pulmonary hypertension. In this situation, accurate left atrial pressures may be difficult to obtain with a pulmonary artery catheter.

Insertion. The LAP catheter is inserted into the left atrium during open heart surgery. The single-lumen catheter exits through the chest wall and is attached to a routine hemodynamic monitoring setup that contains an in-line air filter.

Nursing Management. The placement of the LAP catheter directly into the left atrium places the patient at particular risk for air or tissue emboli. Nursing care is planned to reduce these equipment-related risks. To reduce the risk of air emboli, an in-line air filter is added to the flush system that contains heparin. If the waveform becomes damped, noninvasive methods of troubleshooting—such as repositioning the patient—are performed. The catheter is not manually flushed, because to do so may increase the risk of emboli resulting from clot formation at the tip of the catheter. Pericardial tamponade is a potential complication of LAP catheter removal. Therefore mediastinal chest tubes are left in position until after the catheter is removed. Because of these risks, the LAP catheter is rarely left in place for more than 48 hours.

LAP Waveform Interpretation. The LAP waveform consists of two positive deflections, which are termed the *a* and *v waves*. The *a wave* represents atrial contraction, and the *v wave* represents filling of the left atrium against a closed mitral valve. Normal LAP pressure ranges from 5 to 12 mm Hg and is elevated with mitral valve disease or severe heart failure on the left side.

Pulmonary Artery Pressure Monitoring. The pulmonary artery (PA) catheter is the most invasive of the critical care monitoring catheters. It is also known as a *right heart catheter*, or a *Swan-Ganz catheter* (named after the catheter inventors). Recently the practice of routine use of PA catheters has been called into question and is considered controversial. Various reports describe a range of findings regarding clinical outcomes for patients with a PA catheter in place, including a reduction in new-onset organ failure,[101] an increase in morbidity,[102] no impact on morbidity,[103] an increase in cardiac events,[104] increase in complications,[105] and no benefit to the PA catheter as a guide for clinical interventions compared with less invasive methods.[106] The most important clinical advice is not to insert the PA catheter as a routine measure in every patient, but to determine whether the individual's clinical condition and management requires this level of intense monitoring.[107]

Approximately 1.5 million PA catheters are used in the United States annually[108]; 30% are used in cardiac surgery units, 30% in cardiac catheterization laboratories and coronary care units; 25% in high-risk surgery and trauma; and 15% in medical intensive care units.[108]

Indications. When specific hemodynamic and intracardiac data are required for diagnostic and treatment purposes, a thermodilution PA catheter may be inserted. This catheter is used for diagnosis and evaluation of heart disease, shock states, acute respiratory distress syndrome (ARDS), and medical conditions that compromise CO or fluid volume status. In addition, the PA catheter can be used to evaluate patient response to treatment, as described in Table 17-16. A significant

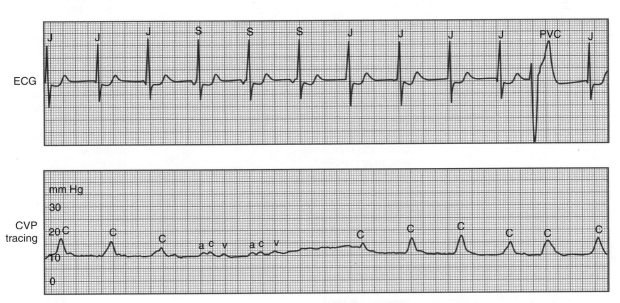

Fig. 17-69 Simultaneous ECG and CVP tracings. The CVP waveform shows large cannon waves (c waves) corresponding to the junctional beats or premature ventricular contractions *(lower strip).* As the patient converts to sinus rhythm, the CVP waveform has a normal configuration. *J,* Junctional rhythm followed by cannon waves on CVP waveform; *S,* sinus rhythm followed by normal CVP tracing with *a*, *c*, and *v* waves; *PVC,* premature ventricular contraction followed by cannon wave on CVP; *c,* cannon waves on CVP tracing; *ac,* normal right atrial pressure tracing.

Table 17-16   **Pulmonary Artery Catheters: Selected Indications for Use and Response to Treatment**

Diagnostic Indications*	Possible Cause	Associated Clinical Findings	Hemodynamic Profile†	Treatment and Expected Response

Hypovolemic shock	Trauma
	Surgery
	Bleeding
	Burns
	Excessive diuresis
		Cardiovascular (CV): sinus tachycardia, decreased blood pressure (BP) (systolic blood pressure [SBP] <90 mm Hg), weak peripheral pulses
		Pulmonary: lungs clear
		Renal: decreased urinary output
		Skin: normal skin temperature, no edema
		Neurologic: variable
			Low cardiac output (CO)
			Low cardiac index (CI) (2.2 L/min/m²)
			High systemic vascular resistance (SVR) (>1600 dynes/sec/cm⁻⁵)
			Low pulmonary artery pressure (PAP)
			Low pulmonary artery occlusion pressure (PAOP)
				Treatment: fluid challenge
				Expected hemodynamic response:
				  Decreased heart rate (HR)
				  Increased BP
				  Increased PAP
				  Increased PAOP
				  Increased central venous pressure (CVP)
				  Increased CO/CI
				  Decreased SVR

Septic shock	Sepsis	CV: sinus tachycardia, decreased BP (SBP <90 mm Hg), bounding peripheral pulses
		Pulmonary: lungs may be clear *or* congested, depending on the origin of the sepsis
		Renal: decreased urinary output
		Skin: warm and flushed
		Neurologic: variable
			High CO (>8 L/min)
			High CI
			Low SVR (<600 dynes/sec/cm⁻⁵)
			Low PAP
			Low PAOP
			Low CVP
				Treatment:
				  IV fluid to maintain hemodynamic function
				Fluid challenge
				Peripheral vasoconstricting agent (alpha) to increase SVR
				Antibiotics and laboratory cultures to find site of infection
				Consider rhAPC
				Expected hemodynamic response:
				  Decreased HR
				  Increased BP
				  Increased PAP
				  Increased PAOP
				  Increased CVP
				  Increased CO/CI
				  Increased SVR
				  $Svo_2 = 70\%$

Multisystem failure shock	Multiple organ dysfunction syndrome (MODS)	CV: normal sinus rhythm or sinus tachycardia, decreased BP, weak peripheral pulses
		Pulmonary: lungs may be clear *or* congested, depending on the site of sepsis; acidosis based on arterial blood gas (ABG) values, may require mechanical ventilation
		Renal: decreased urinary output, may have increased blood urea nitrogen (BUN) and increased creatinine levels
		Skin: cool and mottled
		Neurologic: variable, depending on fluid status and drugs used in treatment
			Low CO
			Low CI (<2.2 L/min/m²)
			High SVR (>1600 dynes/sec/cm⁻⁵)
			High or low PAP
			High or low PAOP
			High or low CVP
				Treatment:
				  Vasodilators to decrease SVR
				Antibiotics
				Support of body system as necessary (e.g., mechanical ventilation, hemodialysis)
				Expected hemodynamic response:
				  Decreased HR
				  Increased BP
				  Normalized PAP/PAOP/CVP
				  Decreased SVR, decreased pulmonary vascular resistance
				  Increased CO/CI

rhAPC, Recombinant human activated protein C.
*Patients undergoing major vascular or cardiac surgery may also have a PA catheter in situ to follow the trend of CO/CI, SVR/PVR, and fluid status during the first 24 hours after surgery.
†See Table 17-14 for definitions and the Appendix for normal values of hemodynamic parameters listed in this table.

Table 17-16		Pulmonary Artery Catheters: Selected Indications for Use and Response to Treatment—cont'd		
Diagnostic Indications	**Possible Cause**	**Associated Clinical Findings**	**Hemodynamic Profile**	**Treatment and Expected Response**
Cardiogenic shock	Left ventricular pump failure caused by acute myocardial infarction or severe mitral or aortic valve disease	CV: sinus tachycardia, possibly dysrhythmias, systolic BP <90 mm Hg, S_3 or S_4, weak peripheral pulses Pulmonary: lungs may have crackles or pulmonary edema Renal: decreased urinary output Skin: cool, pale, and moist Neurologic: may have decreased mentation caused by low BP and CO	Low CO Low CI (<2.2 L/min/m^2) High SVR (>1600 dynes/sec/cm^{-5}) High PAP High PAOP (>15 mm Hg) High CVP Low stroke volume index (SI) Low left cardiac work index (LCWI) Low left ventricular stroke work index (LVSWI)	Treatment: Intropic drugs to increase left ventricular contractility Vasodilators or intraaortic balloon pump (IABP) to decrease afterload Diuretics to decrease preload Optimization of heart rate and control of dysrhythmias Expected hemodynamic response: Decreased HR Increased BP Decreased PAP Decreased PAOP Decreased CVP Decreased SVR Increased CO/CI Increased SI Increased LCWI Increased LVSWI
Acute respiratory distress syndrome (ARDS) or noncardiogenic pulmonary edema	Trauma Sepsis Shock Inhaled toxins (smoke, chemicals, 100% oxygen) Aspiration of gastric contents Metabolic disorders	CV: sinus tachycardia, high or low BP, normal peripheral pulses Pulmonary: poor oxygenation and pulmonary edema, increased respiratory rate, or need for mechanical ventilation Renal: increased or decreased urinary output Skin: normal temperature Neurologic: anxiety or confusion associated with respiratory distress and poor oxygenation	Normal CO Normal CI Normal SVR Normal PAOP High PAP High PVR (>250 dynes/sec/cm^{-5}) Low right cardiac work index (RCWI) Low right ventricular stroke work index (RVSWI)	Treatment: Eliminate cause of ARDS Support pulmonary function as necessary Expected hemodynamic response: Decreased HR Normal BP Decreased PAP Decreased PVR Increased RCWI Increased RVSWI Normal CO/CI Normal SVR

advantage of the PA catheter over the previously described methods of monitoring is that it can simultaneously assess several hemodynamic parameters. These parameters include pulmonary artery systolic and diastolic pressures, pulmonary artery mean pressure, and pulmonary artery occlusion pressure (PAOP). Use of the PA catheter also makes it possible to measure CO and to calculate additional hemodynamic parameters.

Cardiac Output Determinants. CO is the product of heart rate (HR) multiplied by stroke volume (SV). Stroke volume is the volume of blood ejected by the heart each beat in milliliters.

$$\text{Heart Rate} \times \text{Stroke Volume} = \text{Cardiac Output}$$

The normal adult SV is 60 to 70 ml. The clinical factors that contribute to the heart's SV are preload, afterload, and contractility (Fig. 17-70). These three factors are monitored using the PA catheter. Another factor of CO is heart rate, which is recorded by the ECG leads or by clinical assessment.

Oxygen Supply and Demand. When the peripheral tissues need more oxygen (e.g., during exercise or fever), the normal, healthy heart can augment both HR and SV and greatly increase cardiac output. In the critically ill patient, when the tissues require more oxygen, these normal mechanisms are often nonfunctional, and it is the critical care nurse who assesses the need for and then optimizes hemodynamic function. The following discussion provides a basic understanding of the clinical factors that determine CO and the role of the critical care nurse in caring for the patient with an alteration in any of these factors.

Preload. Clinicians commonly describe the hemodynamic numbers related to preload as "filling pressures."

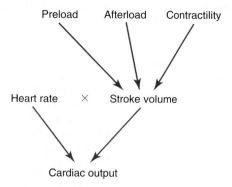

Fig. 17-70 Preload, afterload, and contractility all contribute to the heart's stroke volume. Stroke volume × Heart rate = Cardiac output.

These numbers include pulmonary artery diastolic pressure (PADP) and pulmonary artery occlusion pressure (PAOP) or "wedge" pressure, which measures preload in the left side of the heart, and CVP, which measures preload in the right side of the heart.

Preload is the *volume* in the ventricle at end-diastole. Because diastole is the filling stage of the cardiac cycle, the volume in the ventricle at end-diastole represents the presystolic volume available for ejection for that cardiac cycle. It is not possible to measure left ventricular volume directly in the critical care unit. However, the presence of blood within the ventricle creates pressures that can be measured by the PA catheter and transducer and can be displayed on the bedside monitor.

Measurement of Preload. When the PA catheter is correctly positioned, with the tip in one of the large branches of the pulmonary artery, the only valve between the PA catheter tip and the left ventricle is the mitral valve. During diastole, when the mitral valve is open, no obstruction exists between the tip of the PA catheter and the left ventricle (Fig. 17-71). The left ventricular preload volume creates left ventricular end-diastolic pressure (LVEDP). This is measured clinically by the PAOP. The PAOP and PADP are the values most often referred to in this chapter, because they are the values most often used in clinical practice. Normal LAP or PAOP is 5 to 12 mm Hg.

Frank-Starling Law of the Heart. Clinically the PAOP has significance because a change in left ventricular volume (preload) is reflected by a change in the

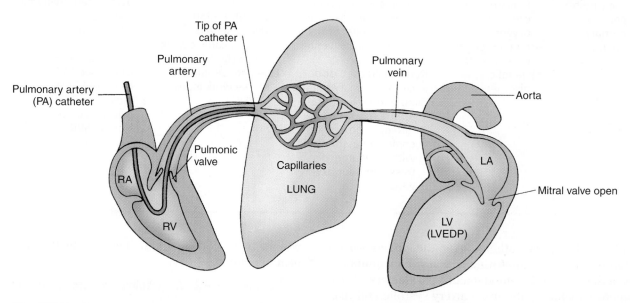

Fig. 17-71 Relationship of pulmonary artery occlusion pressure (PAOP) (wedge pressure) to left ventricular end-diastolic pressure (LVEDP)/preload. This diagram illustrates why, in the majority of clinical situations, the PAOP accurately reflects LVEDP, or preload. During diastole, when the mitral valve is open, there are no other valves or other obstructions between the tip of the catheter and the left ventricle (LV). Thus the pressure exerted by the volume in the LV is reflected back through the left atrium (LA), through the pulmonary veins, and to the pulmonary capillaries. *PA,* Pulmonary artery; *RA,* right atrium; *RV,* right ventricle.

measured PAOP (wedge pressure). Change in preload relies on a concept known as the *Frank-Starling law of the heart*. This concept states that the force of ventricular ejection is directly related to two elements:

1. Volume in the ventricle at end-diastole (preload)
2. Amount of myocardial stretch placed on the ventricle as a result

If the volume in the left ventricle is low, CO is also suboptimal. If intravenous fluids (volume) are infused, CO increases as LV volume and myocardial fiber stretch increase. This is true up to a point. Past this point, more fluid volume overdistends the ventricle and stretches the myocardial fibers so much that CO actually decreases. This scenario is seen clinically in the setting of acute heart failure with pulmonary edema. The impact of preload on CO is represented in Figs. 17-72 and 17-73, using the Frank-Starling Curve as a model.

Ejection Fraction. The relationship of preload to the CO is complex. This is because not all preload volume is ejected with every heartbeat. The percentage of preload volume ejected from the left ventricle per beat is measured during cardiac catheterization and is described as the ejection fraction (EF). A normal ejection fraction in a healthy heart is 70%. In clinical practice most cardiologists will accept an EF value of greater than 50% as normal. The volume ejected from the left ventricle with each beat is known as the stroke volume (SV) and can be calculated at the bedside by dividing the cardiac output by the heart rate per minute (CO ÷ HR).

Myocardial Dysfunction. A significant relationship exists between LVEDP and myocardial dysfunction. As a general rule, the higher the pressure inside the left ventricle, the greater the degree of myocardial dysfunction. The pressure rises at end-diastole (end of filling) because the compromised ventricle cannot eject all of the preload blood volume. In a patient with heart failure, the preload volume might be 100 ml. However, the stroke volume ejected may be only 30 ml. The ejection fraction in this patient is 30% (normal EF is greater than 50%). The remaining preload volume (70 ml in this example) will significantly elevate left ventricular pressures. When the mitral valve opens at the beginning of diastole, the pressure in the left atrium (LA) needs to be slightly higher than pressures in the LV to allow filling. The 70 ml remaining in the ventricle will produce high LV diastolic pressures. This will elevate the LA filling pressure and consequently elevate PAOP (wedge pressure). In this example, the LV is overstretched by excessive preload, and therefore CO will be below normal. A plan of care for this patient would include decreasing LV preload through (1) restriction of IV and oral fluids, (2) venodilation, and (3) diuresis. The myocardial dysfunction will lead to heart failure symptoms discussed in more detail in Chapter 18.

PADP/PAOP Relationship. LVEDP can be measured by two different methods using the PA catheter. The most accurate is the PAOP (wedge) method. The second method involves measuring PADP during diastole when the normal PADP is equal to or 1 to 3 mm Hg higher than the mean PAOP and LVEDP. It is physiologically impossible for the PAOP to ever be higher than the PADP. The clinician must recalibrate and troubleshoot the monitoring system if this appears to occur (see Table 17-15).

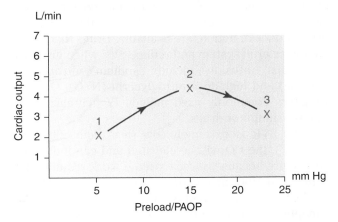

Fig. 17-72 Impact of preload on cardiac output. *1,* Poor cardiac output (CO) with low preload as a result of hypovolemia. *2,* Hypovolemia is corrected after the administration of 2 L of intravenous (IV) fluid. The preload volume in the ventricle is increased, and pulmonary artery occlusion pressure (PAOP) has risen. Because of the increased fiber stretch secondary to the increase in preload, CO has also risen. *3,* After the infusion of 2 more liters of IV solution, the myocardial fibers are overdistended, preload (PAOP) has increased, and CO has fallen as the volume in the left ventricle rises.

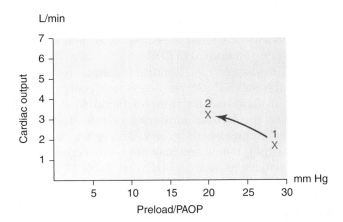

Fig. 17-73 Impact of preload and venodilation on cardiac output (CO). *1,* After an acute anterior wall myocardial infarction that has created significant left ventricular dysfunction, this patient has left ventricle (LV) pump failure with low CO and elevated filling pressures (pulmonary artery occlusion pressure [PAOP]). One of the clinical problems faced by this patient is too much preload. *2,* After administration of diuretics to remove volume and nitroglycerin to dilate the venous system, preload is reduced and CO rises.

Pulmonary Hypertension. It is important to be aware that specific clinical conditions can alter the normal PADP/PAOP relationship. If the patient has vascular lung disease that has elevated the PA pressures independently from the cardiac pressures, the PADP will not accurately reflect function of the left side of the heart. The clinical conditions that cause PA pressures to rise but PAOP to remain normal are primary pulmonary hypertension and ARDS. The numeric difference between the pulmonary artery diastolic pressure and the PAOP value is called a *gradient*. If a large gradient exists between the PAOP (wedge pressure) and pulmonary artery diastolic pressure when the PA catheter is inserted, the patient has pulmonary hypertension, as shown in Table 17-17, *illustration C*. Pulmonary hypertension is further discussed in Chapter 18, p. 471.

Heart Failure. In failure of the left side of the heart, both the PAOP and the PADP are elevated and approximately equal (see Table 17-17, *illustration B*). The heart failure may cause secondary pulmonary hypertension. In other words, over time the damage to the lung vasculature occurs because of exposure to high cardiac pressures.

Mitral Stenosis. Pathology of the mitral valve, either stenosis or regurgitation, alters the accuracy of PAOP (wedge) and PADP as parameters of left ventricular function. In mitral valve stenosis, left atrial pressure and PAOP are increased and cause pulmonary congestion; however, these elevated values are not reflective of LVEDP because a stenotic mitral valve decreases normal blood flow from the left atrium to the left ventricle, decreasing left ventricular preload and consequently lowering LVEDP. Therefore a nonstenotic mitral valve is essential for accurate readings because a narrowed mitral valve increases left atrial pressure, PAOP, and PADP in the presence of a normal LVEDP.

Mitral Regurgitation. If mitral regurgitation (MR) is present, the mean PAOP reading is artificially elevated because of abnormal backflow of blood from the left ventricle to the left atrium during systole. This PAOP reading is distinguished by very large v waves on the PAOP (wedge) tracing and may not be reflective of true left ventricular pressure (LVEDP) (see Table 17-17, *illustration F*).

The v waves can be dramatic in some patients. However, the size of the v wave is not related to the amount of MR, but to the compliance of the left atrium. If the MR is chronic and the left atrium is compliant, v waves may be small. By contrast, in the setting of acute MR after infarction of a papillary muscle, the noncompliant atrium contributes to the development of large v waves. Reading the PAOP tracing in the presence of MR is difficult. If there are large v waves (acute MR), v waves cannot be used to estimate LV preload. If the v wave is small (chronic MR), the mean PAOP or LAP can still estimate LV preload (LVEDP).

Afterload. *Afterload* is defined as the pressure the ventricle must generate to overcome the resistance to ejection created by the arteries and arterioles. It is a calculated measurement derived from information obtained from the PA catheter. As a response to increased afterload, ventricular wall tension rises. After a decrease in afterload, wall tension is lowered. The technical name for afterload is *systemic vascular resistance*.

Systemic Vascular Resistance. Resistance to ejection from the left side of the heart is estimated by calculating the systemic vascular resistance (SVR). The formula, normally calculated by the bedside computer, is as follows:

$$\frac{MAP - CVP}{CO} \times 80 = SVR$$

The normal value is 800 to 1200 dynes/sec/cm^{-5}. To index this value to the patient's body surface area, the cardiac index (CI) is placed in the formula in the same position as the CO. The critical care nurse frequently manipulates prescribed vasoactive drugs to therapeutically alter afterload. In general, the lower the SVR, the higher the CO.

Pulmonary Vascular Resistance. Resistance to ejection from the right side of the heart is estimated by calculating the pulmonary vascular resistance (PVR). The PVR value is normally one sixth of the SVR. Normal PVR is 100 to 250 dynes/sec/cm^{-5}. The formula for PVR is listed in the Appendix. In acute lung injury (ALI), the PVR increases above normal and the PA catheter is often used to monitor vasodilator therapy and fluid management.

Afterload Reduction. Pharmacologic manipulation of afterload to improve cardiac performance is commonly used with the critically ill patient. Many drugs, with different modes of action, are available. Drugs that vasodilate the arterial system and reduce SVR when given as a continuous infusion include sodium nitroprusside (Nipride) and high-dose nitroglycerin (NTG). Other vasodilators commonly used include IV hydralazine and oral ACE inhibitor drugs.

If the SVR is extremely low (less than 500 dynes/sec/cm^{-5}), the CO will be elevated and can induce cardiac failure because of the extreme work requirements. In this situation, medications may be used to "tighten up" the SVR. If the patient is refractory to dopamine, norepinephrine (Levophed) is used as a vasopressor to vasoconstrict the peripheral vasculature. The critical care nurse evaluates the effectiveness of the medication by increasing SVR into the therapeutic range. Frequent assessment of the peripheral circulation is required when drugs that increase SVR are used, since excessive vasoconstriction can negatively affect tissue perfusion.

Vasodilation of the pulmonary arterial vasculature is achieved by either a nitroglycerin drip (at doses that do not lower the systemic blood pressure) or prostaglandin infusions.

Table 17-17	Clinical Interpretation of Pulmonary Artery (PA) Waveforms		
PA Pressure	**Clinical Interpretation**	**mm Hg**	**Waveform Interpretation**
Pulmonary artery systolic (PAS) pressure	PAS pressure reflects the systolic pressure in the pulmonary vasculature. See waveform *A* for normal waveform. It is elevated in pulmonary hypertension because of idiopathic causes, in some congenital heart defects, and in lung disease.		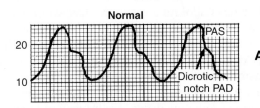
Pulmonary artery diastolic (PAD) pressure	In the patient with healthy lung vasculature, PAD pressure reflects left ventricular end-diastolic pressure (LVEDP), as shown in waveform *B*. Even if the patient experiences heart failure, the PAOP and PAD increase together.		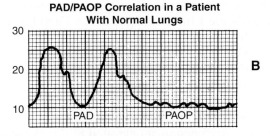
	In the presence of ARDS or pulmonary hypertension, PAD pressure is not an accurate reflection of pulmonary artery occlusion pressure (PAOP), as shown in waveform *C*.		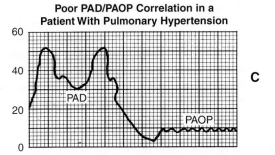
Mean pulmonary artery pressure (PAP mean or PAP_M)	PAP mean pressure is used in the calculation of pulmonary vascular resistance (PVR) and pulmonary vascular resist-ance index (PVRI), as described in Table 17-14. High mean pressures can be reflective of either cardiac or pulmonary disease. Low mean pressures are reflective of hypovolemia. See waveform *D* for PAP mean placement.		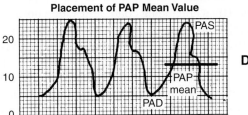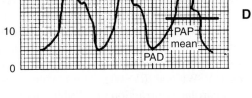
Pulmonary artery occlusion pressure (PAOP) or pulmonary artery wedge pressure (PAWP)	In the healthy patient, PAOP reflects blood in the left ventricle at end-diastole (LVEDP). The normal PAOP waveform is a left atrial waveform, as shown in waveform *E*. If a patient has mitral valve regurgitation, the v waves are larger than normal, increasing PAOP and possibly not reflecting true LVEDP, as shown in waveform *F*. PAOP is elevated in many cardiac disease states in which left ventricular function is compromised. PAOP is low in hypovolemic states.		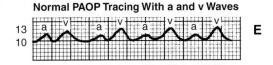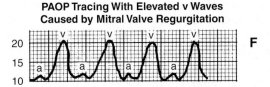

CASE STUDY

Mr. T had a large anterior wall myocardial infarction (MI) 2 days ago. As a result, he has symptoms of acute heart failure, an elevated SVR of 1840 dynes/sec/cm^{-5}, and a low cardiac output (CO) of 2.8 L/min. In a heart with decreased contractility after an MI, an afterload measurement above the normal range lowers CO. To optimize Mr. T's cardiac function, systemic vasodilators or "afterload-reducing drugs" are infused to lower SVR into the normal range. After the administration of sodium nitroprusside 1 to 4 mcg/kg/min, Mr. T's SVR decreased to 970 dynes/sec/cm^{-5} and his CO increased to 4.1 L/min. In this situation, decreasing the systemic vascular resistance to ejection greatly increased the amount of blood ejected from the left ventricle.

•••

In contrast, for the person with a normal heart without cardiac dysfunction, an elevated SVR may have minimal impact on CO. In summary, the importance of afterload on CO is related to the functional quality of the myocardium. Whether the heart muscle is globally damaged (cardiomyopathy) or regionally damaged (MI), small changes in SVR can produce significant changes in CO.

Contractility. Many factors have an impact on contractility, including preload volume as measured by PAOP, afterload (SVR), myocardial oxygenation, electrolyte balance, positive and negative inotropic drugs, and the amount of functional myocardium available to contribute to contraction. These factors can have a positive inotropic effect, thus enhancing contractility, or a negative inotropic effect, decreasing contractility. Significant factors related to contractility that can be measured by the PA catheter include preload filling pressures, afterload, and CO. Additional contractility numbers can be calculated and are displayed in the hemodynamic profile on the bedside monitor. These include left and right ventricular stroke work index values (LVSWI and RVSWI). These values estimate the force of cardiac contraction (see Table 17-14).

Preload has an impact on contractility by means of Starling's mechanism. As volume in the ventricle rises, contractility increases. If the ventricle is overdistended with volume, contractility falls (see Figs. 17-72 and 17-73). Afterload alters contractility by changes in resistance to ventricular ejection. If afterload is high, contractility is decreased. If afterload is low, contractility is augmented. Hypoxemia is known to act as a negative inotrope. The myocardium must have oxygen available to the cells to contract efficiently. Some cardiac drugs can also alter contractility. Calcium channel blocking agents may have a negative inotropic effect. In this case, if the cardiac depression is severe, calcium is the antidote because it is a positive inotrope.

Optimizing Contractility. Intravenous drugs such as dopamine and dobutamine are prescribed for their positive inotropic effect, whereas β-blockers such as propranolol (Inderal) have a negative inotropic effect and lower CO. The nurse considers the impact of these pharmacologic agents on contractility when following the trend of the patient's hemodynamic profile. No single hemodynamic number reflects contractility. However, if left ventricular contractility is increased in response to treatment, this is reflected by changes in PAOP (wedge) and by an increase in CO and LVSWI.

Pulmonary Artery Catheters. The traditional pulmonary artery (PA) catheter, invented by Swan and Ganz, has four lumens for measurement of right atrial pressure (RAP) or CVP, PA pressures, PAOP (wedge), and cardiac output (Fig. 17-74, *A*). Multifunction catheters may have additional lumens, which can be used for IV infusion (Fig. 17-74, *B*) and to measure continuous mixed venous oxygen saturation (Svo$_2$), right ventricular volume, and continuous cardiac output (Fig. 17-74, *C*). Other PA catheters include transvenous pacing electrodes to pace the heart if needed.

The PA catheter is 110 cm in length and is made of polyvinyl chloride. This supple material is ideal for flow-directional catheters. The most commonly used size is 7.5 or 8.0 Fr, although 5.0 and 7.0 Fr sizes are available. Each of the four lumens exits into the heart or pulmonary artery at a different point, graduated along the catheter length (see Fig. 17-74, *A*).

Right Atrial Lumen. The proximal lumen is situated in the right atrium and is used for IV infusion, CVP measurement, withdrawal of venous blood samples, and injection of fluid for CO determinations. This port is often described as the *right atrial port*, also called the *CVP port*.

Pulmonary Artery Lumen. The distal PA lumen is located at the tip of the PA catheter and is situated in the pulmonary artery. It is used to record PA pressures and can be used for withdrawal of blood samples to measure mixed venous blood gases (Svo$_2$).

Balloon Lumen. The third lumen opens into a balloon at the end of the catheter that can be inflated with 0.8 (7 Fr) to 1.5 (7.5 Fr) ml of air. The balloon is inflated during catheter insertion once the catheter reaches the right atrium to assist in forward flow of the catheter and to minimize right ventricular ectopy from the catheter tip. It is also inflated to obtain the PAOP, or "wedge," measurements when the PA catheter is correctly positioned in the pulmonary artery.

Thermistor Lumen. The fourth lumen is a thermistor (temperature sensor) used to measure changes in blood temperature. It is located 4 cm from the catheter tip and is used to measure thermodilution CO. The connector end of the lumen is attached directly to the CO computer.

Additional Features. If continuous Svo$_2$ is measured, the catheter has an additional fiberoptic lumen that exits at the tip of the catheter (see Fig. 17-74, *C*). If

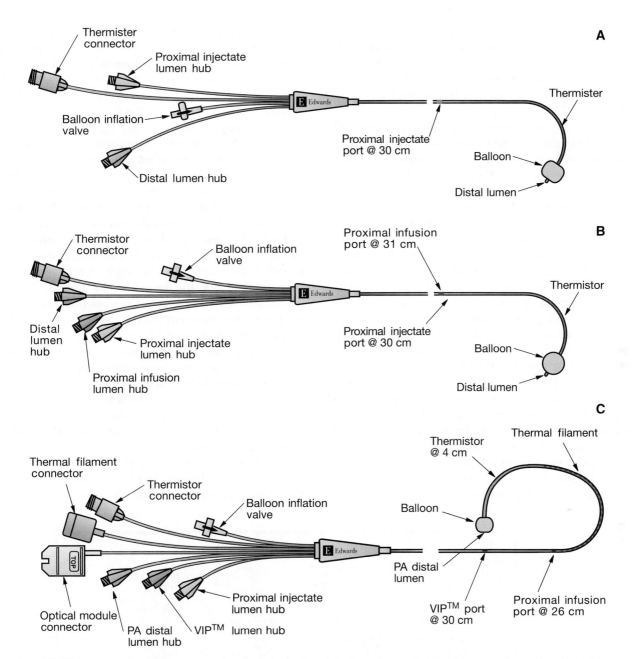

Fig. 17-74   Types of pulmonary artery catheters. **A,** Four-lumen catheter. **B,** Five-lumen catheter that includes an additional venous infusion port (VIP) into the right atrium. **C,** Seven-lumen catheter that includes a VIP port and two additional lumens for continuous cardiac output (CCO) and thermal filament, and continuous mixed venous oxygen saturation (SvO_2) monitoring (optical module connector). An additional option is to combine use of the CCO filament and the thermistor response time to calculate continuous end-diastolic volume (CEDV). (©2001 Edwards Lifesciences LLC. All rights reserved. Reprinted with permission ©Edwards Lifesciences, Swan-Ganz® is a trademark of Edwards Lifesciences Corporation, registered in the US Patent and Trademark Office.)

cardiac pacing is used, two PA catheter methods are available. One type of catheter has three atrial (A) and two ventricular (V) pacing electrodes attached to the catheter so that when it is properly positioned, the patient can be connected to a pacemaker and be AV-paced. The other catheter method uses a specific transvenous pacing wire that is passed through an additional catheter lumen and to exit into the right ventricle if ventricular

pacing is required. In addition, a right ventricular volumetric PA catheter is available that measures stroke volume in the RV.

Insertion. If a PA catheter is to be inserted into a patient who is awake, some brief explanations about the procedure are helpful to ensure that the patient understands what is going to happen. The initial insertion techniques used for placement of a PA catheter are similar to those described in the section on CVC insertion. In addition, because the PA catheter is positioned within the heart chambers and pulmonary artery on the right side of the heart, catheter passage is monitored using either fluoroscopy or waveform analysis on the bedside monitor (Fig. 17-75).

Before inserting the catheter into the vein, the physician—using sterile technique—tests the balloon for inflation and flushes the catheter with normal saline solution to remove any air. The PA catheter is then attached to the bedside hemodynamic line setup and monitor so that the waveforms can be visualized while the catheter is advanced through the right side of the heart (see Fig. 17-75). A larger introducer sheath (8.5 Fr)—which has the tip positioned in the vena cava and an additional IV side-port lumen—is often used to cannulate the vein first. This introducer sheath is known by several different names in clinical practice, including *sheath, cordis, introducer,* or *side-port.* This introducer sheath remains in place, and the supple PA catheter is threaded through it into the vena cava and into the right side of the heart.

Pulmonary Artery Waveform Interpretation. Each chamber of the heart has a distinctive waveform with recognizable characteristics. It is the responsibility of the critical care nurse to recognize each waveform displayed on the bedside monitor, both when the catheter enters the corresponding chamber during insertion and also during routine monitoring.[109]

Right Atrial Waveform. As the PA catheter is advanced into the right atrium during insertion, a right atrial waveform must be visible on the monitor, with recognizable a, c, and v waves (see Fig. 17-75). The normal mean pressure in the right atrium is 2 to 5 mm Hg. Before passage through the tricuspid valve, the balloon at the tip of the catheter is inflated for two reasons. First, it cushions the pointed tip of the PA catheter so that if the tip comes into contact with the right ventricular wall, it will cause less myocardial irritability and, consequently, fewer ventricular dysrhythmias. Second, inflation of the balloon assists the catheter to float with the flow of blood from the right ventricle into the pulmonary artery. It is because of these features and the balloon that PA catheters are described as *flow-directional catheters.*

Right Ventricular Waveform. The right ventricular waveform is distinctly pulsatile, with distinct systolic and diastolic pressures. Normal RV pressures are 20 to 30 mm Hg systolic and 0 to 5 mm Hg diastolic. Even with the balloon inflated, it is not uncommon for some ventricular ectopy to occur during passage through the RV. All patients who have a PA catheter inserted must have simultaneous ECG monitoring, with defibrillator and emergency resuscitation equipment nearby.

Pulmonary Artery Waveform. As the catheter enters the pulmonary artery, the waveform again changes. The diastolic pressure rises. Normal PA pressures range from 20 to 30 mm Hg systolic over 10 mm Hg diastolic. A dicrotic notch, visible on the downslope of the waveform, represents closure of the pulmonic valve.

Pulmonary Artery Occlusion Waveform. While the balloon remains inflated, the catheter is advanced

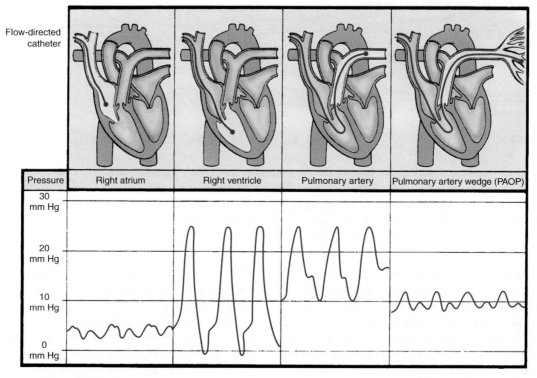

Fig. 17-75 Pulmonary artery (PA) catheter insertion with corresponding waveforms.

into the wedge position. This maneuver produces a pulmonary artery occlusion pressure (PAOP).[110] Here the waveform decreases in size and is nonpulsatile, reflective of a normal left atrial tracing with a and v wave deflections. This is known as a "wedge" tracing, because the balloon is "wedged" into a small pulmonary vessel. It is technically described as the *pulmonary artery occlusion pressure (PAOP)* (see Fig. 17-75). The balloon occludes the pulmonary vessel so that the PA lumen is exposed only to left atrial pressure and is protected from the pulsatile influence of the PA. When the balloon is deflated, the catheter should spontaneously float back into the PA. When the balloon is reinflated, the wedge tracing should be visible. The normal PAOP ranges from 5 to 12 mm Hg.

After insertion, the catheter is sutured to the skin and a chest radiograph is taken to verify placement. If the catheter is advanced too far into the pulmonary bed, the patient is at risk for pulmonary infarction. If the catheter is not sufficiently advanced into the PA, it will not be useful for PAOP (wedge) readings. However, in many critical care units, if the patient's PADP and PAOP (wedge) values approximate (within 0 to 3 mm Hg), the PADP is reliably used to follow the trend of LV filling pressure (preload). This prevents possible trauma from frequent balloon inflation; in such a situation the PA catheter would be consciously pulled back into a nonwedging position in the pulmonary artery.

After insertion of the catheter, the chest radiograph or fluoroscopy is used to verify PA catheter position to make sure that it is not looped or knotted in the RV and to rule out pneumothorax or hemorrhagic complications. A thin plastic cuff can be placed on the outside of the catheter when it is inserted to maintain sterility of that part of the PA catheter that exits from the patient. Then, if the catheter is not in the desired position or if it migrates out of position, the PA catheter can be repositioned. The plastic cuff is designed to keep the external catheter sterile for a short period after insertion.

Medical Management. Considerable controversy exists in the medical community over the routine use of PA catheters. Some physicians believe the complication rates associated with PA catheters are too high and discourage their use. Others firmly advocate their use and clinical benefit. Practice guidelines are available for physicians who routinely work with PA catheters.[111] Medical goals of hemodynamic monitoring include assessment of adequacy of perfusion in stable patients, early detection of decreased perfusion, titration of therapy to meet specific therapeutic outcomes, and differentiation of different organ system dysfunctions.

Nursing Management. The more knowledgeable the critical care nurse can become about use of the PA catheter, the more accurate and effective the nursing management interventions will be.[90,109] Factors that affect PA measurement are the head-of-bed position and lateral body position relative to transducer height placement, respiratory variation, and use of positive end-expiratory pressure (PEEP).

Patient Position. In the supine position, if the transducer is placed at the level of the phlebostatic axis, a head-of-bed position from flat up to 60 degrees is appropriate for most patients. PA and PAOP measurements in the lateral position may be significantly different from those taken when the patient is lying supine. At this point, if there is concern over the validity of pressure readings in a particular patient, it is more reliable to take measurements with the patient on his or her back, with the head of bed elevated from zero up to 60 degrees. A stabilization period of only 5 minutes is required before taking pressure readings after a patient changes position.[112]

Respiratory Variation. All PADP and PAOP (wedge) tracings are subject to respiratory interference, especially if the patient is on a positive-pressure, volume-cycled ventilator.[90] During inhalation the ventilator "pushes up" the PA tracing, which produces an artificially high reading (Fig. 17-76, *A*). During spontaneous respiration, negative intrathoracic pressure "pulls down" the waveform and can produce an erroneously low measurement (Fig. 17-76, *B*). To minimize the impact of respiratory variation, the PADP is read at end-expiration, which is the most stable point in the respiratory cycle. If the digital number fluctuates with respiration, a printed readout on paper can be obtained to verify true PADP. In some clinical settings, ECG or airway pressure and flow are recorded simultaneously with the PADP/PAOP tracing to identify end-expiration.[90]

PEEP. Some clinical diagnoses, such as ARDS, require the use of high levels of positive end-expiratory pressure (PEEP) set with the ventilator to treat refractory hypoxemia. If a PEEP of greater than 10 cm H_2O is used, PAOP (wedge) and PA pressures will be artificially elevated. Because of this impact of PEEP, in the past, patients in some critical care units were taken off the ventilator to record PA pressure measurements. It has since been shown that this practice closes alveoli, decreases the patient's oxygenation level, and may result in persistent hypoxemia. Because patients remain on PEEP for treatment, they remain on it during measurement of PA pressures. In this situation, the trend of PA readings is more important than one individual measurement.

Once again, the most important factor is not one individual measurement, or the absolute number obtained, but whether the trend of the measurements is being used as a basis for clinical interventions to support and improve cardiopulmonary function in the critically ill.

Avoiding Complications. Potential cardiac complications include ventricular dysrhythmias, endocarditis, valvular damage, cardiac rupture, and cardiac tamponade. Potential pulmonary complications include rupture of a pulmonary artery, pulmonary artery thrombosis,

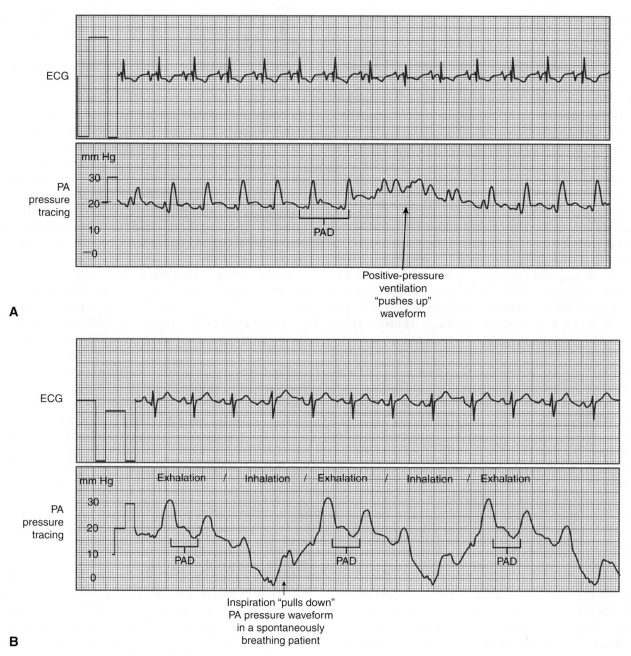

ECG

PA pressure tracing

mm Hg
30
20
10
—0

PAD

Positive-pressure ventilation "pushes up" waveform

A

ECG

PA pressure tracing

mm Hg
30
20
10
0

Exhalation / Inhalation / Exhalation / Inhalation / Exhalation

PAD   PAD   PAD

Inspiration "pulls down" PA pressure waveform in a spontaneously breathing patient

B

Fig. 17-76   Pulmonary artery (PA) waveforms that demonstrate the impact of ventilation of PA pressure readings. For accuracy, PA pressures are read at end-exhalation. **A,** Positive-pressure ventilation: the increase in intrathoracic pressure during inhalation "pushes up" the PA pressure waveform, creating a false high reading. **B,** Spontaneous breathing: the decrease in intrathoracic pressure during normal inhalation "pulls down" the PA waveform, creating a false low reading.

embolism or hemorrhage, and infarction of a segment of lung. The PA tracing is continuously monitored. This is to ensure that the catheter does not migrate forward into a spontaneous wedge or PAOP position. A segment of lung can suffer infarction if the wedged catheter occludes an arteriole for a prolonged period. If the catheter is spontaneously "wedged," the critical care nurse can gently pull the catheter back out of the wedge position if the institutional policy allows.[113]

Infection is always a risk with a PA catheter. The risks are similar to those discussed in the section on central venous catheters (Patient Safety Alert on CVC Infections).

PA Catheter Removal.   PA catheters can be safely removed from the patient by critical care nurses competent in this procedure.[90] Removal is not usually associated with major complications. The most common incidents are PVCs in about 2% of patients as the catheter is pulled through the RV.[90,114]

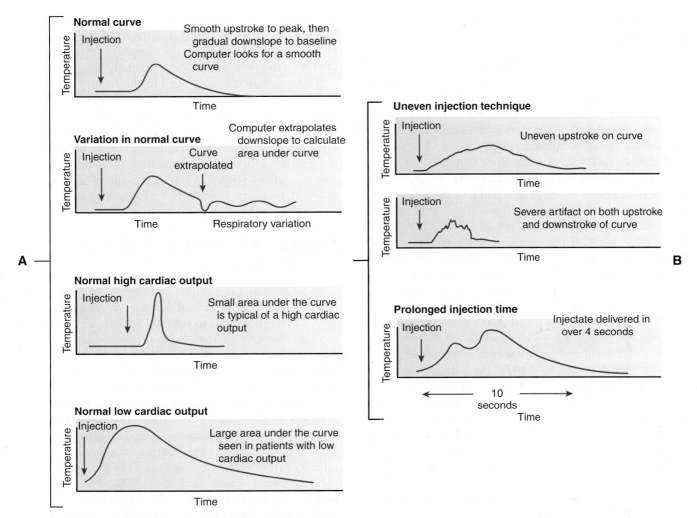

Fig. 17-77 **A,** Variations in the normal cardiac thermodilution bolus output curve. **B,** Abnormal cardiac output curves produce an erroneous cardiac output value.

Cardiac Output. The PA catheter measures cardiac output (CO) using either an intermittent (bolus) *or* a continuous CO method.

Thermodilution Cardiac Output Method. The bolus thermodilution method is performed at the bedside and results in CO calculated in liters per minute. Generally, three cardiac outputs that are within a 10% mean range are obtained at one time and then are averaged to calculate CO. A known amount (5-ml or 10-ml bolus) of iced or more typically room-temperature normal saline solution is injected into the proximal lumen of the catheter. The injectate exits into the right atrium (RA) and travels with the flow of blood past the thermistor (temperature sensor) located at the distal end of the catheter in the pulmonary artery. The injectate can be delivered by hand injection, using individual syringes of saline. Frequently a closed in-line system attached to a 500-ml bag of normal saline is used as a reservoir to deliver the individual injections.[115]

Sometimes the right atrial (proximal) port is clotted off and not usable. If another right atrial port is available,

this can be substituted. However, if a usable port is not available, to ensure accurate cardiac output data, a new pulmonary artery catheter is inserted.

Cardiac Output Curve. The thermodilution CO method uses the indicator-dilution principle, in which a known temperature is the indicator. It is based on the principle that the change in temperature over time is inversely proportional to blood flow. Blood flow can be diagrammatically represented as a cardiac output curve on which temperature is plotted against time (Fig. 17-77, *A*). Most hemodynamic monitors display this CO curve, which must then be interpreted to determine whether the CO injection is valid. The normal curve has a smooth upstroke, with a rounded peak and a gradually tapering downslope. If the curve has an uneven pattern, it may indicate faulty injection technique and the CO measurement must be repeated. Patient movement or coughing also alters the CO measurement (Fig. 17-77, *B*).

Injectate Temperature. If the CO is within the normal range, it is equally accurate whether iced or room temperature injectate is used. However, if the COs are extremely high or very low, iced injectate may be more accurate. To ensure accurate readings, the difference between injectate temperature and body temperature must be at least 10° C, and the injectate must be delivered within 4 seconds, with minimal handling of the syringe to prevent warming of the solution. This is particularly important if iced injectate is used. With all delivery systems, the injectate is delivered at the same point in the respiratory cycle, usually end-exhalation.

Patient Position and Cardiac Output. In the normovolemic, stable patient, reliable CO measurements can be obtained in a supine position (patient lying on his or her back) with the head of the bed elevated up to 45 degrees.[116] If the patient is hypovolemic or unstable, leaving the head of the bed in a flat position, or only slightly elevated, is the most clinically appropriate choice. CO measurements performed when the patient is turned to the side are not considered as accurate as those performed with the patient in the supine position.

Clinical Conditions That Alter Cardiac Output. Two clinical conditions produce errors in the thermodilution CO measurement: tricuspid valve regurgitation and ventricular septal rupture. If the patient has tricuspid valve regurgitation, the expected flow of blood from the right atrium to the pulmonary artery is disrupted by backflow from the right ventricle to the right atrium. This creates a lower CO measurement than the patient's actual output. If the person has an intracardiac left-to-right shunt, such as occurs following ventricular septal rupture, the thermodilution CO measures the large pulmonary volume and records a higher CO than the patient's true systemic output.

Continuous Invasive Cardiac Output Measurement. The bolus thermodilution method is reliable but performed intermittently. Continuous CO monitoring using a PA catheter is also used in clinical practice.[116] One method employs a thermal filament on the PA catheter to emit small energy signals (the indicator) into the bloodstream. These signals are then detected by the thermistor near the tip of the PA catheter, and the equivalent of an indicator curve is created and a CO value is calculated from this data.

Noninvasive Cardiac Output Measurement. One method of continuous CO measurement is impedance cardiography. Impedance cardiography works by emitting a low-voltage, high-frequency, alternating electrical current through the thorax via spot or band electrodes. The electrical impedance changes within the thorax are detected by the sensing electrodes. Because blood flow through the thoracic aorta causes shifts in impedance, this information can be used to calculate stroke volume and, from this, continuous CO can be measured.

Calculated Hemodynamic Profiles. For the patient with a thermodilution PA catheter in place, additional hemodynamic information can be calculated using routine vital signs, CO, and body surface area (BSA). These mea-

surements are calculated using specific formulas that are indexed to a patient's body size, using either the DuBois body area surface chart or the computer program associated with the new generation of hemodynamic monitors.

The calculated values used in the hemodynamic profiles are described in Table 17-14. Clinical use of these profiles is described in two case studies. In Hemodynamic Profile 1 (Box 17-6), the example is a step-by-step interpretation of the hemodynamic profile to familiarize the reader with use of calculated values. In Hemodynamic Profile 2 (Box 17-7), the example uses only values indexed to body weight and illustrates the impact of treatment on these values over time.

CONTINUOUS MONITORING OF VENOUS OXYGEN SATURATION

Indications. Continuous monitoring of venous oxygen saturation is indicated for the critically ill patient who has the potential to develop an imbalance between oxygen supply and metabolic tissue demand. This includes the patient in severe sepsis or shock, following high-risk cardiac surgery, and the patient with severe respiratory compromise, such as ARDS.

Continuous venous oxygen monitoring permits a calculation of the balance achieved between arterial oxygen supply (SaO_2) and oxygen demand at the tissue level by sampling desaturated venous blood from the pulmonary artery catheter distal tip. This sample is termed *mixed venous blood* saturation (SvO_2) because it is a mixture of all of the venous blood drained from many body tissues. Recently the same fiberoptic technology has been used in combination with a fiberoptic triple lumen CVC. In this situation the venous blood is sampled from the superior vena cava, just above the right atrium, and is abbreviated $ScvO_2$.

Under normal conditions the cardiopulmonary system achieves a balance between oxygen supply and demand. Four factors contribute to this balance:

1. Cardiac output (CO).
2. Hemoglobin (Hgb).
3. Arterial oxygen saturation (SaO_2).
4. Tissue metabolism (VO_2).

Three of these factors (CO, Hgb, and SaO_2) contribute to the supply of oxygen to the tissues. Tissue metabolism (VO_2) determines oxygen consumption or the quantity of oxygen extracted at tissue level that creates the demand for oxygen. The relationship of all these factors is illustrated in Fig. 17-78.

In addition to measurement of venous oxygen saturation, it is possible to calculate the actual quantity of oxygen (in mls /minute) that is provided to the tissues by the cardiopulmonary system, and also to assess the amount of oxygen consumed by the body tissues. These calculations rely on principles of oxygen transport physiology and are also the basis for calculation of SvO_2. These for-

Box 17-6

HEMODYNAMIC PROFILE 1

Mr. SR has a medical history of cardiomyopathy and chronic obstructive pulmonary disease (COPD). He is admitted to a coronary care unit because of an exacerbation of his biventricular heart failure. He has been complaining of anginal pain and shortness of breath. His nursing diagnoses are Decreased Cardiac Output and Impaired Gas Exchange.

Height	163 cm	PAD	27 mm Hg	PVR	322 dynes/sec/cm^{-5}
Weight	79 kg	PAP$_M$	36 mm Hg	PVRI	612 dynes/sec/cm^{-5}/m^2
Body surface area (BSA)	1.9 m^2	PAOP	26 mm Hg	LCW	2.1 kg-m
		CVP	24 mm Hg	LCWI	1.1 kg-m/m^2
HR	104 beats/min	CO	2.48 L/min	LVSW	2.4 g-m
ABP		CI	1.31 L/min/m^2	LVSWI	10.7 g-m/m^2
Systolic	88 mm Hg	SV	23.8 ml	RCW	1.21 kg-m
Diastolic	51 mm Hg	SI	12.5 ml/m^2	RCWI	0.64 kg-m/m^2
MAP	63 mm Hg	SVR	1257 dynes/sec/cm^{-5}	RVSW	11.7 g-m
PAS	55 mm Hg	SVRI	2388 dynes/sec/cm^{-5}/m^2	RVSWI	6.2 g-m/m^2

ANALYSIS OF HEMODYNAMIC PROFILE*

Profile	Analysis
HR (heart rate)	Heart rate of 104 beats/min is above normal limits (normal, 60-100 beats/min).
ABP (arterial blood pressure)	Narrow pulse pressure of 88/51 mm Hg with a low mean arterial pressure (MAP) of 63 mm Hg (normal MAP, 65-90 mm Hg).
Pulmonary artery pressure	Pulmonary artery pressures are elevated (55/27 mm Hg), consistent with diagnosis of cardiomyopathy, failure of left side of heart, and COPD (normal PAP, 25/10 mm Hg).
PAOP (pulmonary artery occlusion pressure)	Elevated PAOP (26 mm Hg), consistent with diagnosis of cardiomyopathy and failure of left side of heart (normal PAOP, 5-12 mm Hg).
CVP (central venous pressure)	Elevated CVP (24 mm Hg), consistent with diagnosis of cardiomyopathy, failure of right side of heart, and COPD (normal CVP, 4-6 mm Hg).
CO (cardiac output) and CI (cardiac index)	Poor CO and CI (CO, 2.48 L/min; CI, 1.31 L/min/m^2). Both values are below normal (normal CO, 4-6 L/min; normal CI, 2.2-4 L/min/m^2).
SV (stroke volume) and SI (stroke volume index)	SV and SI are low (SV, 23.8 ml/ SI, 12.5 ml/m^2). These results would be anticipated from the low cardiac output (normal SV, 60-70 ml; normal SI, 40-50 ml/min/m^2).
SVR (systemic vascular resistance) and SVRI (systemic vascular resistance index)	SVR and SVRI are at the upper normal range (SVR, 1257 dynes/sec/cm^{-5}, SVRI, 2388 dynes/sec/cm^{-5}/m^2). These values are not contributing to the low cardiac output at this time (normal SVR, 800-1400 dynes/sec/cm^{-5}; normal SVRI, 2000-2400 dynes/sec/cm^{-5}/m^2).
PVR (pulmonary vascular resistance) and PVRI (pulmonary vascular resistance index)	PVR and PVRI are elevated (PVR, 322 dynes/sec/cm^{-5}; PVRI 612 dynes/sec/cm^{-5}/m^2). High pulmonary vascular resistance may be contributing to the low cardiac output (normal PVR, 100-250 dynes/sec/cm^{-5}; normal PVRI, 225-315 dynes/sec/cm^{-5}/m^2).
LCWI (left cardiac work index) and LVSWI (left ventricular stroke work index)	Both LCWI and LVSWI are below normal (LCWI, 1.1 kg-m/m^2; LVSWI, 10.7 g-m/m^2), indicating that left ventricular myocardial damage may be present. This is consistent with Mr. SR's diagnosis of cardiomyopathy (normal LCWI, 3.4-4.2 kg-m/m^2; normal LVSWI, 50-62 g-m/m^2).
RCWI (right cardiac work index) and RVSWI (right ventricular stroke work index)	RCWI is normal, but RVSWI is below normal (RCWI, 0.64 kg-m/m^2; RVSWI, 6.2 g-m/m^2), indicating that right ventricular myocardial damage may be present. This is consistent with Mr. SR's diagnosis of cardiomyopathy and history of COPD (normal RCWI, 0.54-0.66 kg-m/m^2, normal RVSWI, 7.9-9.7, g-m/m^2).
Nursing impression	The hemodynamic data confirm the nursing clinical diagnosis of poor CO. The goal is to improve CO within the limits of Mr. SR's myocardial dysfunction and COPD. As CO improves and PA pressures decrease, the patient will have less pulmonary congestion, which will improve alveolar gas exchange.

*Formulas and normal values for the hemodynamics values are in Table 17-14 and the Appendix.

Box 17-7

HEMODYNAMIC PROFILE 2

1. ADMISSION

Mrs. JL has been admitted to the critical care unit with pulmonary edema. She has a history of anterior wall myocardial infarction and severe chronic obstructive pulmonary disease (COPD).

Height	159 cm	MAP	106 mm Hg	SI	9.9 ml/m²
Weight	45.8 kg	PAS	53 mm Hg	SVRI	5351 dynes/sec/cm⁻⁵/m²
Body surface area (BSA)	1.40 m²	PAD	27 mm Hg	PVRI	1046 dynes/sec/cm⁻⁵/m²
		PAPₘ	44 mm Hg	LCWI	1.9 kg-m/m²
HR	131 bpm	PAOP	27 mm Hg	LVSWI	14.3 g-m/m²
ABP		CVP	19 mm Hg	RCW	0.78 kg-m/m²
Systolic	160 mm Hg	CO	1.82 L/min	RCWI	5.9 g-m/m²
Diastolic	80 mm Hg	CI	1.3 L/min/m²		

Height	159 cm	MAP	106 mm Hg	SI	9.9 ml/m^2
Weight	45.8 kg	PAS	53 mm Hg	SVRI	5351 dynes/sec/cm^{-5}/m^2
Body surface area (BSA)	1.40 m^2	PAD	27 mm Hg	PVRI	1046 dynes/sec/cm^{-5}/m^2
		PAP$_M$	44 mm Hg	LCWI	1.9 kg-m/m^2
HR	131 bpm	PAOP	27 mm Hg	LVSWI	14.3 g-m/m^2
ABP		CVP	19 mm Hg	RCW	0.78 kg-m/m^2
Systolic	160 mm Hg	CO	1.82 L/min	RCWI	5.9 g-m/m^2
Diastolic	80 mm Hg	CI	1.3 L/min/m^2		

ANALYSIS OF HEMODYNAMIC PROFILE 1*

In the above hemodynamic profile, note the fast heart rate; high MAP; high PA and CVP filling pressures; low CI, SI, LVSWI, and RVSWI; and high SVRI and PVRI. These values are consistent with a diagnosis of failure of the left side of the heart, causing pulmonary edema, which may lead to cardiogenic shock. Treatment is focused on increasing the cardiac index by lowering SVRI and PVRI and using IV sodium nitroprusside and IV nitroglycerin in continuous infusion.

2. 3 HOURS LATER

Height	159 cm	MAP	83 mm Hg	SI	16.5 ml/m^2
Weight	45.8 kg	PAS	41 mm Hg	SVRI	3088 dynes/sec/cm^{-5}/m^2
Body surface area (BSA)	1.40 m^2	PAD	26 mm Hg	PVRI	300 dynes/sec/cm^{-5}/m^2
		PAP$_M$	33 mm Hg	LCWI	2.1 kg-m/m^2
HR	113 bpm	PAOP	26 mm Hg	LVSWI	18.6 g-m/m^2
ABP		CVP	11 mm Hg	RCWI	0.84 kg-m/m^2
Systolic	104 mm Hg	CO	2.61 L/min	RVSWI	7.4 g-m/m^2
Diastolic	69 mm Hg	CI	1.86 L/min/m^2		

ANALYSIS OF HEMODYNAMIC PROFILE 2

Results 3 hours later after sodium nitroprusside administration: note improving hemodynamics shown above as normal MAP and lower intracardiac filling pressures (PA and CVP). However, CI and SI remain low; and SVRI is above normal. Mrs. JL remains in severe left ventricular failure because of her low CI.

3. THE NEXT DAY

Height	159 cm	MAP	77 mm Hg	SI	22.5 ml/m^2
Weight	45.8 kg	PAS	31 mm Hg	SVRI	2423 dynes/sec/cm^{-5}/m^2
Body surface area (BSA)	1.40 m^2	PAD	15 mm Hg	PVRI	273 dynes/sec/cm^{-5}/m^2
		PAP$_M$	23 mm Hg	LCWI	2.4 kg-m/m^2
HR	104 beats/min	PAOP	15 mm Hg	LVSWI	22.9 g-m/m^2
ABP		CVP	4 mm Hg	RCWI	0.74 kg-m/m^2
Systolic	111 mm Hg	CO	3.28 L/min	RVSWI	7.1 g-m/m^2
Diastolic	60 mm Hg	CI	2.34 L/min/m^2		

ANALYSIS OF HEMODYNAMIC PROFILE 3

The following day Mrs. JL's hemodynamics have improved with continued use of sodium nitroprusside and nitroglycerin. CI is in the low-normal range, and SVRI and PVRI are in the high-normal range. LVSWI remains low, reflecting the patient's compromised left ventricle from the previous anterior wall myocardial infarction.

*See Box 17-6 for explanation of abbreviations and Table 17-14 and the Appendix for explanation of hemodynamic values.

mulas are explained in greater detail in Table 17-18 and are listed in the Appendix.

Catheters. There are two catheters, depending on where the fiberoptic tip is located, to measure venous oxygen saturation.

SvO₂ Catheter. The pulmonary arterial SvO₂ catheter contains the traditional four lumens plus a lumen containing two or three optical fibers. The fiberoptics are attached to an optical module that is connected to a small bedside computer. The optical module transmits a narrow band of light down one optical fiber. This light is reflected off the hemoglobin in the blood and returns to the optical module through the receiving fiberoptic. The SvO₂ signal is recorded on a continuous display.

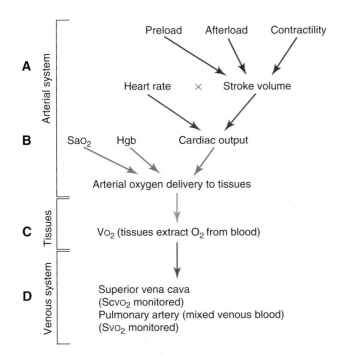

Fig. 17-78 The factors that contribute to the S_{VO_2} value. **A,** Cardiac output (CO) is determined by heart rate (S_{CVO_2} HR) × stroke volume (SV). **B,** The S_{aO_2}, Hgb, and CO all contribute to arterial oxygen delivery at the tissue level. **C,** Tissues extract and use the oxygen carried in the blood. This process of cellular oxygen consumption is termed V_{O_2}. **D,** Blood returns to the superior vena cava (recorded as S_{CVO_2}) and then to the pulmonary artery, where the mixed venous blood is recorded as S_{VO_2}.

S_{CVO_2} Catheter. The central venous S_{CVO_2} technology is incorporated into a multilumen central venous catheter (CVC). The fiberoptic catheter tip is positioned in a central vein such as the superior vena cava. The technology used to measure the venous saturation is identical in both catheters and the same continuous display module is used for both catheters.

The S_{CVO_2} catheter has been successfully used to guide hemodynamic fluid resuscitation in septic patients.[117] The relationship between the values obtained from the traditional pulmonary artery (S_{VO_2}) catheter and the central venous (S_{CVO_2}) catheter are very similar, although the S_{CVO_2} values are slightly higher. The trend of parallel measurements (up or down as patient condition changes) is in the same direction about 90% of the time.[100]

S_{VO_2}/S_{CVO_2} Calibration. The catheter is calibrated before insertion into the patient through a standardized color reference system, which is part of the catheter package. Insertion technique and sites are identical to those used for placement of conventional PA or CVC catheters. Waveform analysis and/or venous saturation measurement can be used for accurate placement. Once the catheter is inserted, recalibration is unnecessary un-less the catheter becomes disconnected from the optical module.

To recalibrate the fiberoptic module to verify accuracy when the catheter is already inserted in a patient, a mixed venous blood sample (S_{VO_2}) or central venous sample (S_{CVO_2}) must be withdrawn from the appropriate catheter tip and sent to the laboratory for oxygen saturation analysis. In many critical care units, this is a standard daily procedure to ensure that readings used to guide patient care remain accurate.[118]

Nursing Management. S_{VO_2} monitoring provides a continuous assessment of the balance of oxygen supply and demand for an individual patient. Nursing assessment includes evaluation of the S_{VO_2}/S_{CVO_2} value and evaluation of the four factors (S_{aO_2}, CO, Hgb, and V_{O_2}) that maintain the oxygen supply-demand balance.

Normal Values. Normal S_{VO_2} is approximately 75% in the healthy individual (range 60% to 80%). In critically ill patients, an S_{VO_2} value between 60% and 80% is evidence of adequate balance between oxygen supply and demand.

The normal values for the S_{CVO_2} catheter are slightly higher.[100] This is because the reading is taken before the blood enters the right heart chambers, where the *cardiac sinus* (vein) delivers venous blood drained from the myocardium into the right atrium. The heavily desaturated myocardial blood will decrease the oxygen saturation slightly. For this reason, S_{VO_2} values are always slightly lower than S_{CVO_2} readings in the same patient.

A clinical rule of thumb that is sometimes cited is to subtract 30 from the arterial oxygen saturation, and that should represent an acceptable venous oxygen saturation. For example:

$$S_{aO_2} \text{ is } 100\% - 30\% = 70\% \; S_{VO_2}/S_{CVO_2}$$
$$S_{aO_2} \text{ is } 95\% - 30\% = 65\% \; S_{VO_2}/S_{CVO_2}.$$

If the S_{VO_2}/S_{CVO_2} value changes by more than 10% and this change is maintained for more than 10 minutes, the clinician must determine which of the four factors is affecting S_{VO_2}.[118]

S_{VO_2}/S_{CVO_2} and Arterial Oxygen Saturation. A change in S_{VO_2}/S_{CVO_2} may be caused by a change in arterial oxygen saturation (S_{aO_2}). If the S_{aO_2} is increased because supplemental oxygen is being administered, the S_{VO_2} also will rise. If the oxygen supply is disrupted and S_{aO_2} is decreased, S_{VO_2} will fall. Decreased S_{VO_2} can be caused by any action or disease that reduces oxygen supply, including ARDS, endotracheal suctioning, removing a patient from the ventilator, or removing supplementary oxygen. Fig. 17-79 demonstrates a drop in S_{VO_2} during suctioning in a patient with ARDS. Transient decreases in S_{VO_2}/S_{CVO_2} related to a nursing action such as endotracheal suctioning are not usually a cause for concern. Some patients may be slow to resaturate up to the presuction level of S_{VO_2}/S_{CVO_2}. In this case, an

Table 17-18			Calculations of Oxygen Transport Physiology
Name	**Formula**	**Normal Value**	**Explanation**
Arterial oxygen saturation (Sao_2)	$\dfrac{HgbO_2}{(Hgb + HgbO_2)} \times 100$	>96%	Hgb, hemoglobin; $HgbO_2$ oxyhemoglobin. The arterial oxygen saturation represents the amount of oxyhemoglobin (oxygen bound to hemoglobin) divided by the total hemoglobin. Normally 96% of oxygen is bound to hemoglobin.
Blood oxygen content Cao_2 (arterial) Cvo_2 (venous)	(O_2 dissolved) + (O_2 saturation) ($Po_2 \times 0.003$) + ($1.34 \times Hgb \times So_2$)	19-20 ml/dl 12-15 ml/dl	Blood oxygen (O_2) content represents the amount of oxygen dissolved in 100 ml (1 dl) of blood. It can be calculated for both arterial blood (Cao_2) and for venous blood (Cvo_2). It is measured in ml/dl. It is the combination of both dissolved O_2 (Pao_2) and O_2 saturation (Sao_2).
Blood oxygen transport (also called "oxygen delivery")	$CO \times Cao_2 \times 10$ (arterial) $CO \times Cvo_2 \times 10$ (venous)	1000 ml/min 750 ml/min	Oxygen transport represents the amount of oxygen transported to or from the tissues each minute in milliliters (ml/min). Arterial O_2 transport is a measure of the O_2 delivered to the tissues. Venous O_2 transport reflects the venous return to the right side of the heart. Oxygen transport is calculated by multiplying the cardiac output (CO) by the oxygen content (Cao_2 or Cvo_2) and by the number 10. The difference between normal arterial and normal venous O_2 return represents oxygen consumption by the tissues.
Tissue oxygen consumption (Vo_2)	Arterial O_2 transport minus venous O_2 transport ($CO \times Cao_2 \times 10$) − ($CO \times Cvo_2 \times 10$)	250 ml/min	Oxygen consumption represents the amount of oxygen consumed by the tissues in 1 minute. To calculate Vo_2 it is necessary to know both arterial oxygen transport and venous oxygen transport values, which are calculated in ml/min. The difference represents oxygen consumption.
Arterial venous oxygen difference (A-Vo_2 difference)	Arterial O_2 content minus venous O_2 content $Cao_2 - Cvo_2$	3.0-5.5 ml/dl	The arterial venous oxygen difference represents the difference between the arterial oxygen content (Cao_2) and the venous oxygen content (Cvo_2). Because Cao_2 and Cvo_2 are measured in ml/dl, A-Vo_2 difference is also measured in ml/dl.
Mixed venous oxygen saturation (Svo_2)	Arterial O_2 transport minus tissue consumption equals venous return ($CO \times Cao_2 \times 10$) − Vo_2	60%-80%	Mixed venous oxygen saturation (Svo_2) represents the venous oxygen return that is bound (saturated) with hemoglobin. Saturation is measured in percent (%). The Svo_2 value is a function of the amount of oxygen delivered to the tissues minus the amount of oxygen consumed by the tissues (Vo_2) in milliliters per minute. The higher the amount (ml) of oxygen in the venous return, the greater the hemoglobin saturation will be.

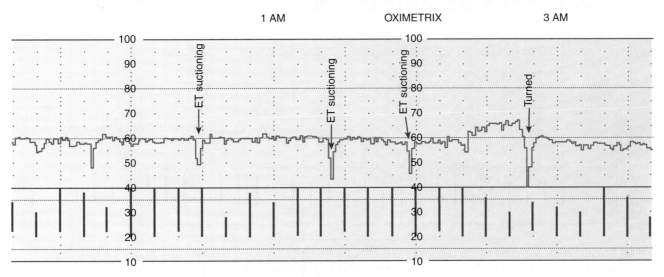

1 AM   OXIMETRIX   3 AM

Fig. 17-79   Fall in Svo_2 during endotracheal (ET) suctioning. The ET suction decreases Sao_2. The baseline Svo_2 is low (60%) because the patient has acute respiratory distress syndrome (ARDS) and is hypoxemic.

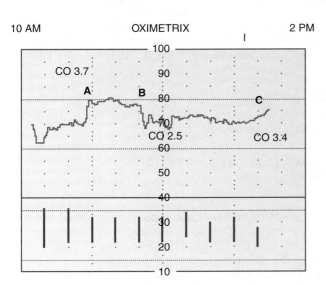

10 AM   OXIMETRIX   2 PM

Fig. 17-80   Impact of changes in cardiac output (CO) on Svo_2 values. *Point A:* Just before point A, Svo_2 readings are low because CO and pulmonary artery pressures were low as a result of excessive diuresis. Infusion of 500 ml of colloid solution and 1000 ml of lactated Ringer's solution crystalloid increased the Svo_2 and improved the CO, which rose to 3.7 L/min. *Point B:* A short run of ventricular tachycardia caused the CO to fall abruptly to 2.5 L/min and decreased the Svo_2 value. *Point C:* The beginning of an upward trend in Svo_2 is related to administration of fluids and to improvement in CO and in filling pressures. CO is now 3.4 L/min. The graph represents a 4-hour printout; the space between each dotted line represents 20 minutes.

appropriate nursing intervention is to wait until the venous oxygen saturation has again returned to baseline before initiating other nursing activities.

Svo₂/Scvo₂ and Cardiac Output. A change in $Svo_2/Scvo_2$ may also be caused by an alteration in CO. Four hemodynamic factors affect CO—preload, after-

load, contractility, and heart rate, as shown in Fig. 17-78. Changes in one or more of these individual factors affects CO. Fig. 17-80 shows an improvement in a patient's Svo_2 from 70% to 80% after volume administration that increased preload *(point A)*. Later this patient's CO fell abruptly during a short run of ventricular tachycardia *(point B)*. Any major loss of heart rate causes a decrease in CO. Alterations in contractility, preload, and afterload (SVR) also have the potential to alter CO. Because CO is an important component of the continuous Svo_2 value, several researchers have investigated whether Svo_2 could be substituted for thermodilution CO as a monitoring tool. Studies of adult patients after cardiac surgery and acute MI indicate that a sustained change in the Svo_2 value does not automatically mean there has been a change in CO. No consistent or reliable correlation was found between Svo_2 and CO in these clinical studies. Rather, a change in Svo_2 indicates a need to check a CO at the bedside to determine the cause of the change in venous oxygen saturation. The Svo_2 measurement is very sensitive and serves as an early warning for changes in patient condition, whether or not the change is the result of an alteration in CO. Therefore Svo_2 monitoring is an additional level of hemodynamic monitoring but does not replace thermodilution CO.

This principle is clearly illustrated in the Svo_2 Hemodynamic Profile 3 (Box 17-8), in which an increase in Svo_2 is not associated with a significant rise in CO. The rationale and explanation for this finding is also discussed in the section on assessment of oxygen consumption.

Svo₂/Scvo₂ and Hemoglobin. Hemoglobin (Hgb) is the transport mechanism for oxygen in the blood. If the Hgb level falls as a result of bleeding or red cell destruction, the body maintains oxygen transport by increasing CO and using oxygen reserves in the venous blood return. Therefore the body can compensate effi-

Box 17-8

Hemodynamic Profile 3

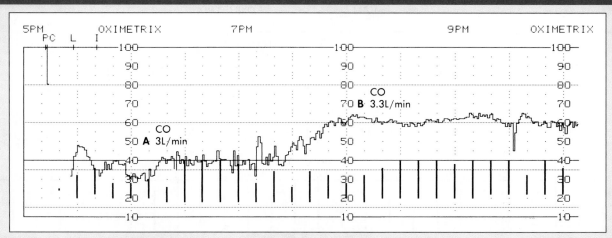

Mr. EH has just been admitted to the cardiovascular critical care unit after open heart surgery. At *point A* (see figure above) he has an extremely low mixed venous oxygen saturation (Svo_2) of 40%. An Svo_2 below 40% indicates that the oxygen supply is not adequate to meet the demands of the body tissues, resulting in metabolic acidosis. To determine the reason for the low Svo_2 one must know the hemoglobin (Hgb), the arterial oxygen saturation (Sao_2), the cardiac output (CO), and the tissue oxygen consumption (Vo_2). EH'S Hgb value is 11.6 g/dL (normal male Hgb, 13.5-18.0 g/dL), which is acceptable after major surgery; the Sao_2 is 99.6% (normal, 97%), which is high because this patient is receiving mechanical ventilation with 70% oxygen immediately after surgery; and the CO is low at 3.15 L/min (normal, 4-6 L/min). EH is receiving dopamine 5 mcg/kg/min for his low CO. He is shivering and cold because his body temperature is only 35.2° C after the surgery. Using the values described above—Hgb 11.6 g/dL; Sao_2, 99.6%; and CO 3.15 L/min—it is possible to calculate the tissue oxygen consumption (Vo_2) for EH.

ARTERIAL SUPPLY	VENOUS RETURN
CO (Pao_2 × 0.003) + (1.34 × Hgb × Sao_2) 10—CO (Pvo_2 × 0.0031) + (1.34 × Hgb × Svo_2) 10 = Vo_2	

(To calculate arterial oxygen supply, the oxygen in the venous return, Vo_2 and the difference between the arterial and venous oxygen content [A-Vo_2 difference], insert EH's values **[in bold]** into the above formula.)

ARTERIAL SUPPLY	VENOUS RETURN	Vo_2	A-Vo_2 DIFFERENCE
3.15 (354 × 0.003) + (1.34 × **11.6** × **0.99**) 10—**3.15 (20** × 0.003) + (1.34 × **11.6** × **0.38**) 10			
3.15 (1.0) + 15.3) 10	**3.15** (0.06 + 5.90) 10		
3.15 (16.3) 10	**3.15** (5.90) 10		
505 ml/min (see illustration above)	183 ml/min	= 322 ml/min	10.4 ml/dl

At *point A* (see illustration) the arterial oxygen supply to the tissues is 505 ml/min (normal, 1000 ml/min), whereas the oxygen returned in the venous blood is only 183 ml/min (normal, 750 ml/min). EH's Vo_2 is elevated at 322 ml/min (normal, 250 ml/min). The clinical goals for this patient would be to (1) increase the CO and (2) use sedation or muscle relaxants to decrease oxygen consumption by controlling the shivering. The difference between the oxygen content in the arterial and the venous blood (A-Vo_2 difference) is very large at 10.4 ml/dl (normal, 3.5-5.0 ml/dl). These calculated values confirm the nursing diagnosis of Ineffective Tissue Perfusion with a decreased cardiac output.

Two hours later, at *point B* (see illustration), EH's Svo_2 has improved to a low-normal value of 60%. Additional inotropic drugs have been administered. At this time the Hgb is 10.8 g/dl, Sao_2 is 99.6%, and CO remains low at 3.3 L/min. Thus the improvement in Svo_2 has not been caused by a dramatic increase in CO. When EH's oxygen consumption is calculated at *point B,* it becomes evident that the decrease in physical activity after sedation with morphine to reduce shivering has improved the Svo_2. EH's values are emphasized in bold.

ARTERIAL SUPPLY	VENOUS RETURN
CO (Pao_2 × 0.003) + (1.34 × Hgb × Sao_2) 10—CO (Pvo_2 × 0.003) + (1.34 × Hgb × Svo_2) 10 = Vo_2	

ARTERIAL SUPPLY	VENOUS RETURN	Vo_2	A-Vo_2 DIFFERENCE
3.3 (266 × 0.003) + (1.34 × **10.8** × **0.99**) 10—**3.3 (28** × 0.003) + (1.34 × **10.8** × **0.60**) 10			
3.3 (0.82 + 14.32) 10	**3.3** (0.86 + 8.6) 10		
3.3 (15.1) 1	**3.3** (9.4) 10		
498 ml/min	300 ml/min	= 198 ml/min	5.7 ml/dl

At *point B* (see illustration), EH's arterial oxygen supply is still low at 498 ml/min, and the oxygen in his mixed venous blood return remains low at 300 ml/min. Vo_2 is now lower than normal (typical after sedation)—198 ml/min. At this time the A-Vo_2 difference is almost within the normal limits at 5.7 ml/dl. These findings are confirmed by the low-normal Svo_2 value of 60% at *point B.* This case study illustrates the point that tissue oxygen consumption (O_2 demand) can be as important as cardiac output (CO) and oxygenation (O_2 supply) in determining mixed venous oxygen saturation (Svo_2) in the patient with a compromised cardiovascular system.

See Table 17-18 for explanation of abbreviations and Box 17-7 and the Appendix for explanation of hemodynamic values.

Table 17-19	Alterations in Oxygen Consumption (Vo_2)	
Condition or Activity	**% Increase Over Resting Vo_2**	**% Decrease Under Resting Vo_2**
CLINICAL CONDITIONS THAT INCREASE Vo_2		
Fever	10% (for each 1° C over normal)	
Skeletal injuries	10%-30%	
Work of breathing	40%	
Severe infection	60%	
Shivering	50%-100%	
Burns	100%	
Routine postoperative procedures	7%	
Nasal intubation	25%-40%	
Endotracheal tube suctioning	27%	
Chest trauma	60%	
Multiple organ dysfunction syndrome	20%-80%	
Sepsis	50%-100%	
Head injury, with patient sedated	89%	
Head injury, with patient not sedated	138%	
Critical illness in emergency department	60%	
NURSING ACTIVITIES THAT INCREASE Vo_2		
Dressing change	10%	
Electrocardiogram	16%	
Agitation	18%	
Physical examination	20%	
Visitor	22%	
Bath	23%	
Chest x-ray examination	25%	
Position change	31%	
Chest physiotherapy	35%	
Weighing on sling scale	36%	
CONDITIONS THAT DECREASE Vo_2		
Anesthesia		25%
Anesthesia in burned patients		50%

From White KM et al: *Heart Lung* 19(5):550, 1990.

ciently for anemia. In the healthy person, Hgb must be extremely low before Svo_2 falls. However, in an anemic patient with a compromised cardiovascular system who cannot adequately increase CO, Svo_2/$Scvo_2$ declines as venous oxygen reserves are depleted by the body.

Svo_2/$Scvo_2$ and Oxygen Consumption. Oxygen consumption (Vo_2) describes the amount of oxygen the body tissues consume for normal function in 1 minute. If the body's metabolic demands increase because of exercise or increased metabolic rate, the body increases CO to augment oxygen supply and also uses reserve oxygen in the venous system. Normal oxygen delivery to the tissues is 1000 ml (1 L) of oxygen per minute. At rest a person might consume one quarter of available oxygen, or 250 ml of oxygen per minute. This leaves a venous oxygen reserve of 750 ml of oxygen per minute (see Table 17-18). Thus for the normal individual, the combination of increased CO and use of considerable venous oxygen reserve provides adequate compensation for increased

metabolic needs. However, for the critically ill patient with either cardiac or respiratory dysfunction, an increase in activity leading to increased oxygen consumption may overwhelm the cardiopulmonary system and oxygen reserves.

In the critically ill patient, routine nursing procedures can increase Vo_2 by 10% to 36% (Table 17-19). The critical care nurse can observe the effect of increased Vo_2 during routine nursing care and under conditions that increase metabolic rate. Activities such as turning, giving a backrub, or getting a patient out of bed are often accompanied by a sudden, temporary decrease in the patient's continuous Svo_2/$Scvo_2$ reading. Once the movement is finished, most patients resaturate up to their preactivity venous saturation level within a few minutes. In critically ill patients, it may take up to 5 minutes for resaturation (rise in Svo_2/$Scvo_2$) to occur. In this situation, the appropriate nursing action is to observe the patient clinically, in conjunction with monitoring Svo_2/$Scvo_2$, and to

Table 17-20	Svo_2 Measurements	
Svo_2 Measurement	**Physiologic Basic for Change in Svo_2/$Scvo_2$**	**Clinical Diagnosis and Rationale**
High Svo_2 (80%-95%)	Increased oxygen supply Decreased oxygen demand	Patient receiving more oxygen than required by clinical condition Anesthesia, which causes sedation and decreased muscle movement Hypothermia, which lowers metabolic demand (e.g., with cardiopulmonary bypass) Sepsis caused by decreased ability of tissues to use oxygen at a cellular level False high positive because PA catheter is wedged in a pulmonary arteriole (Svo_2 only)
Normal Svo_2/$Scvo_2$ (60% to 80%)	Normal oxygen supply and metabolic demand	Balanced oxygen supply and demand Anemia or bleeding with compromised cardiopulmonary system
Low Svo_2/$Scvo_2$ (less than 60%)	Decreased oxygen supply caused by: Low hemoglobin (Hgb) Low arterial saturation (Sao_2) Low cardiac output (CO) Increased oxygen consumption (Vo_2)	Hypoxemia resulting from decreased oxygen supply or lung disease Cardiogenic shock caused by left ventricular pump failure Metabolic demand exceeds oxygen supply in conditions that increase muscle movement and increase metabolic rate, including physiologic states such as shivering, seizures, and hyperthermia and nursing interventions such as being weighed on a bedscale and turning

postpone additional maneuvers until the venous saturation has returned to baseline.

Many clinical conditions that dramatically increase Vo_2 are often seen in critical care units. Conditions such as sepsis, multiple organ dysfunction syndrome (MODS), burns, head injury, and shivering can more than double the normal oxygen tissue requirements (see Table 17-19). Such dramatic increases in Vo_2 translate into a low Svo_2/$Scvo_2$ value, even if the CO is normal, as discussed in the following case study.

CASE STUDY

An example of the impact of increased oxygen consumption and low CO on Svo_2 is shown in the case study in Box 17-8. Patient EH has just been admitted to the critical care unit and is cold and shivering after cardiopulmonary bypass and cardiac surgery. At *point A* (see illustration in Box 17-8), Svo_2 is low at 40%. The low Svo_2 is caused by postoperative shivering, which has greatly increased EH's oxygen consumption. The oxygen consumption (Vo_2) is high at 322 ml/min (normal 250 ml/min). An additional factor is that EH has a low CO (normal 4 to 6 L/min). EH's CO is 3 L/min, which provides below-normal flow and oxygen delivery to the tissues. The oxygen delivery is low at only 505 ml/min (normal is 1000 ml/min). The increased Vo_2 and the low CO both contribute to the low Svo_2.

At *point B* (see illustration in Box 17-8), the shivering has stopped after analgesia and sedation; consequently, the tissue oxygen consumption (Vo_2) has decreased to

198 ml/min, which is within normal range. As a result, the Svo_2 has risen to 60%. However, EH's CO remains low. Thus the very low Svo_2 at *point A* was caused by increased oxygen consumption resulting from shivering and was not related to the low CO. However, because an Svo_2 of 60% is considered a "low-normal value," nursing interventions would now focus on improving the CO to increase the Svo_2 value.

•••

Normal Svo_2/$Scvo_2$. If Svo_2/$Scvo_2$ is within the normal range of 60% to 80% and the patient is not clinically compromised, one can assume that oxygen supply and demand are balanced for that individual. The situation becomes out of balance when either a decrease in oxygen delivery (Sao_2) occurs because of changes in CO or Hgb or an increase in oxygen demand (increased Vo_2) occurs.

Low Svo_2/$Scvo_2$. If Svo_2/$Scvo_2$ falls below 60% and is sustained, the clinician must assume that oxygen supply is not equal to demand (Table 17-20). It is helpful to assess the cause of decreased Svo_2/$Scvo_2$ in a logical sequence that reflects knowledge of the meaning of the venous saturation value. The following is one such assessment sequence:

1. Clinically assess the patient.
2. Assess whether the decreased Svo_2/$Scvo_2$ is caused by low oxygen supply. Verify the effectiveness of the ventilator or oxygen mask, or check arterial oxygen saturation (Sao_2) from arterial blood gas values.
3. Assess cardiac function by performing a CO measurement.

4. Assess Hgb value by checking recent laboratory results or by withdrawing a blood sample for laboratory analysis.
5. Assess whether the decreased $Svo_2/Scvo_2$ is the result of a recent patient movement or nursing action that may have temporarily increased Vo_2.

If $Svo_2/Scvo_2$ falls below 40%, the balance of oxygen supply and demand may not be adequate to meet tissue needs at the cellular level. At some point the cells change from an aerobic to anaerobic mode of metabolism, which results in the production of lactic acid and is representative of a shock state in which cellular injury or cell death may result. At this point every attempt must be made to determine the cause of the low $Svo_2/Scvo_2$ and to correct the oxygen supply-demand imbalance. To avoid the risk of lactic acidosis it is helpful to watch the trend of the $Svo_2/Scvo_2$ and to intervene early with a goal of maintaining the venous oxygen saturation above 70%.[117]

High Svo₂. In certain clinical conditions, $Svo_2/Scvo_2$ may increase to an above-normal level (greater than 80%). This occurs during times of low oxygen demand (decreased Vo_2) such as during anesthesia or hypothermia. In certain cases of septic shock, the tissue cells cannot use the oxygen supplied to them, and as a consequence, the oxygen is not extracted from the blood at the tissue level. In this situation the venous oxygen reserve remains elevated and $Svo_2/Scvo_2$ is higher than normal (see Table 17-20). Finally, if the pulmonary artery Svo_2 catheter drifts into a wedged position, the Svo_2 increases because the fiberoptic tip of the catheter comes into contact with newly oxygenated blood.

SUMMARY

The range of diagnostic tools available to the bedside critical care nurse will continue to expand. As critical care patient needs become more complex and nursing responsibilities augment, incorporation of appropriate diagnostic information into the nursing management plan will only increase in importance.

REFERENCES

1. Criddle LM: Rhabdomyolysis. Pathophysiology, recognition, and management, *Crit Care Nurse* 23(6):14-28, 2003.
2. Malinoski DJ, Slater MS, Mullins RJ: Crush injury and rhabdomyolysis, *Crit Care Clin* 20(1):171-192, 2004.
3. Davidson MB et al: Pathophysiology, clinical consequences, and treatment of tumor lysis syndrome, *Am J Med* 116(8):546-554, 2004.
4. Gennari FJ, Segal AS: Hyperkalemia: an adaptive response in chronic renal insufficiency, *Kidney Int* 62(1):1-9, 2002.
5. Palmer BF: Managing hyperkalemia caused by inhibitors of the renin-angiotensin-aldosterone system, *N Engl J Med* 351(6):585-592, 2004.
6. Diercks DB et al: Electrocardiographic manifestations: electrolyte abnormalities, *J Emerg Med* 27(2):153-160, 2004.
7. Ariyan CE, Sosa JA: Assessment and management of patients with abnormal calcium, *Crit Care Med* 32(4 Suppl):S146-154, 2004.
8. Dickerson RN et al: Accuracy of methods to estimate ionized and "corrected" serum calcium concentrations in critically ill multiple trauma patients receiving specialized nutrition support, *JPEN J Parenter Enteral Nutr* 28(3):133-141, 2004.
9. Ma G et al: Electrocardiographic manifestations: digitalis toxicity, *J Emerg Med* 20(2):145-152, 2001.
10. Zivin JR et al: Hypocalcemia: a pervasive metabolic abnormality in the critically ill, *Am J Kidney Dis* 37(4):689-698, 2001.
11. Noronha JL, Matuschak GM: Magnesium in critical illness: metabolism, assessment, and treatment, *Intensive Care Med* 28(6):667-679, 2002.
12. Braunwald E et al: ACC/AHA guideline update for the management of patients with unstable angina and non-ST-segment elevation myocardial infarction—2002: summary article: a report of the American College of Cardiology/American Heart Association Task Force on Practice Guidelines (Committee on the Management of Patients with Unstable Angina), *Circulation* 106(14):1893-1900, 2002. Full text available online at www.ahajournals.org.
13. Antman EM et al: ACC/AHA guidelines for the management of patients with ST-elevation myocardial infarction—executive summary: a report of the American College of Cardiology/American Heart Association Task Force on Practice Guidelines (Writing Committee to Revise the 1999 Guidelines for the Management of Patients with Acute Myocardial Infarction), *Circulation* 110:588-636, 2004. Full text available online at www.ahajournals.org.
14. Novis DA et al: Biochemical markers of myocardial injury test turnaround time: a College of American Pathologists Q-Probes study of 7020 troponin and 4368 creatine kinase-MB determinations in 159 institutions, *Arch Pathol Lab Med* 128(2):158-164, 2004.
15. Lin JC et al: Rates of positive cardiac troponin I and creatine kinase MB mass among patients hospitalized for suspected acute coronary syndromes, *Clin Chem* 50(2):333-338, 2004.
16. Smith SW et al: Outcome of low-risk patients discharged home after a normal cardiac troponin I, *J Emerg Med* 26(4):401-406, 2004.
17. Hirsh J, Raschke R: Heparin and low-molecular-weight heparin: the Seventh ACCP Conference on Antithrombotic and Thrombolytic Therapy, *Chest* 126(3 Suppl):188S-203S, 2004.
18. Ansell J et al: The pharmacology and management of the vitamin K antagonists: the Seventh ACCP Conference on Antithrombotic and Thrombolytic Therapy, *Chest* 126(3 Suppl):204S-233S, 2004.
19. Patrono C et al: Platelet-active drugs: the relationships among dose, effectiveness, and side effects: the Seventh ACCP Conference on Antithrombotic and Thrombolytic Therapy, *Chest* 126(3 Suppl):234S-264S, 2004.
20. Hirsh J, Heddle N, Kelton JG: Treatment of heparin-induced thrombocytopenia: a critical review, *Arch Intern Med* 164(4):361-369, 2004.
21. Hirsh J et al: American Heart Association/American College of Cardiology Foundation guide to warfarin therapy, *Circulation* 107(12):1692-1711, 2003.
22. Executive Summary of the Third Report of The National Cholesterol Education Program (NCEP) Expert Panel on Detection, Evaluation, and Treatment of High Blood Cho-

lesterol in Adults (Adult Treatment Panel III), *JAMA* 285(19):2486-2497, 2001. Full text available online at www.ahajournals.org.

23. Grundy SM et al: Implications of recent clinical trials for the National Cholesterol Education Program Adult Treatment Panel III guidelines, *Circulation* 110(2):227-239, 2004.

24. Grundy SM et al: Clinical management of metabolic syndrome: report of the American Heart Association/National Heart Lung, and Blood Institute/American Diabetes Association Conference on Scientific Issues Related to Management, *Circulation* 10(4):551-556, 2004. Full text available online at www.ahajournals.org.

25. van den Berghe G et al: Intensive insulin therapy in the critically ill patients, *N Engl J Med* 345(19):1359-1367, 2001.

26. Garber AJ et al: American College of Endocrinology position statement on inpatient diabetes and metabolic control, *Endocr Pract* 10(1):77-82, 2004.

27. Anavekar NS et al: Relation between renal dysfunction and cardiovascular outcomes after myocardial infarction, *N Engl J Med* 351(13):1285-1295, 2004.

28. Go AS et al: Chronic kidney disease and the risks of death, cardiovascular events, and hospitalization, *N Engl J Med* 351(13):1296-1305, 2004.

29. ACR practice guideline for the performance of pediatric and adult chest radiography, 2002, American College of Radiology; available online at www.acr.org.

30. Trotman-Dickenson B: Radiology in the intensive care unit (Part I), *J Intensive Care Med* 18(4):198-210, 2003.

31. ACR practice guideline for the performance of pediatric and adult bedside radiography (Portable chest radiography), 2002, American College of Radiology; Available online at www.acr.org.

32. Krinsley JS: Test-ordering strategy in the intensive care unit, *J Intensive Care Med* 18(6):330-339, 2003.

33. Trotman-Dickenson B: Radiology in the intensive care unit (part 2), *J Intensive Care Med* 18(5):239-252, 2003.

34. Drew BJ et al: Practice standards for electrocardiographic monitoring in hospital settings, *Circulation* 110(17):2721-2746, 2004. Full text available online at www.ahajournals.org.

35. Hinkle C, Stegall G: The possibility of obtaining 15- and 18-lead ECGs on all patients with myocardial infarction, *Crit Care Nurse* 20(2):125-126, 2000.

36. Roden DM: Drug-induced prolongation of the QT interval, *N Engl J Med* 350(10):1013-1022, 2004.

37. Dekker JM et al: Heart rate-corrected QT interval prolongation predicts risk of coronary heart disease in black and white middle-aged men and women: the ARIC study, *J Am Coll Cardiol* 43(4):565-571, 2004.

38. Tilley P, Petersen D: Pulling axis together, *Dimens Crit Care Nurs* 22(5):210-215, 2003.

39. AACN: *ST segment monitoring: AACN Practice Alert,* 2004, American Association of Critical Care Nurses; available online at www.aacn.org.

40. Pelter MM, Adams MG, Drew BJ: Transient myocardial ischemia is an independent predictor of adverse in-hospital outcomes in patients with acute coronary syndromes treated in the telemetry unit, *Heart Lung* 32(2):71-78, 2003.

41. Booker KJ et al: Frequency and outcomes of transient myocardial ischemia in critically ill adults admitted for noncardiac conditions, *Am J Crit Care* 12(6):508-516, 2003.

42. Tung P et al: Predictors of neurocardiogenic injury after subarachnoid hemorrhage, *Stroke* 35(2):548-551, 2004.

43. Zimetbaum PJ et al: Electrocardiographic predictors of arrhythmic death and total mortality in the multicenter unsustained tachycardia trial, *Circulation* 110(7):766-769, 2004.

44. Pope JH et al: The impact of electrocardiographic left ventricular hypertrophy and bundle branch block on the triage and outcome of ED patients with a suspected acute coronary syndrome: a multicenter study, *Am J Emerg Med* 22(3):156-163, 2004.

45. Cheitlin MD et al: ACC/AHA/ASE 2003 guideline update for the clinical application of echocardiography—summary article: a report of the American College of Cardiology/American Heart Association Task Force on Practice Guidelines (ACC/AHA/ASE Committee to Update the 1997 Guidelines for the Clinical Application of Echocardiography), *J Am Soc Echocardiogr* 16(10):1091-1110, 2003. Full text available online at www.ahajournals.org.

46. Gibbons RJ et al: ACC/AHA 2002 guideline update for the management of patients with chronic stable angina—summary article: a report of the American College of Cardiology/American Heart Association Task Force on Practice Guidelines (Committee on the Management of Patients with Chronic Stable Angina), *Circulation* 107(1):149-158, 2003. Full text available online at www.ahajournals.org.

47. Birnbaum Y, Drew BJ: The electrocardiogram in ST elevation acute myocardial infarction: correlation with coronary anatomy and prognosis, *Postgrad Med J* 79(935):490-504, 2003.

48. Blomstrom-Lundqvist C et al: ACC/AHA/ESC guidelines for the management of patients with supraventricular arrhythmias—executive summary: a report of the American College of Cardiology/American Heart Association Task Force on Practice Guidelines and the European Society of Cardiology Committee for Practice Guidelines (Writing Committee to Develop Guidelines for the Management of Patients with Supraventricular Arrhythmias) developed in collaboration with NASPE-Heart Rhythm Society, *J Am Coll Cardiol* 42(8):1493-1531, 2003. Full text available online at www.jacc.org.

49. Yasuma F, Hayano J: Respiratory sinus arrhythmia: why does the heartbeat synchronize with respiratory rhythm? *Chest* 125(2):683-690, 2004.

50. Zhang S et al: Lower loop reentry as a mechanism of clockwise right atrial flutter, *Circulation* 109(13):1630-1635, 2004.

51. Irwin ME: Cardiac pacing device therapy for atrial dysrhythmias, *AACN Clin Issues* 15(3):377-390, 2004.

52. Fuster V et al: ACC/AHA/ESC guidelines for the management of patients with atrial fibrillation. A report of the American College of Cardiology/American Heart Association Task Force on Practice Guidelines and the European Society of Cardiology Committee for Practice Guidelines and Policy Conferences (Committee to Develop Guidelines for the Management of Patients with Atrial Fibrillation) developed in collaboration with the North American Society of Pacing and Electrophysiology, *Circulation* 104(17):2118-2150, 2001. Full text available online at www.ahajournals.org

53. Everett TH, Olgin JE: Basic mechanisms of atrial fibrillation, *Cardiol Clin* 22(1):9-20, 2004.

54. Finta B, Haines DE: Catheter ablation therapy for atrial fibrillation, *Cardiol Clin* 22(1):127-145, 2004.

55. Crystal E, Connolly SJ: Atrial fibrillation: guiding lessons from epidemiology, *Cardiol Clin* 22(1):1-8, 2004.

56. Eagle KA et al: American College of Cardiology; American Heart Association., ACC/AHA 2004 guideline update for coronary artery bypass graft surgery—summary article: a Report of the American College of Cardiology/American Heart Association Task Force on Practice Guidelines (Committee to Update the 1999 Guidelines

for Coronary Artery Bypass Graft Surgery), *Circulation* 110(14):1168-1176, 2004. Full text available online at www.ahajournals.org.

57. Kern LS: Postoperative atrial fibrillation: new directions in prevention and treatment, *J Cardiovasc Nurs* 19(2):103-115, 2004.

58. Lloyd-Jones DM et al: Lifetime risk for development of atrial fibrillation: the Framingham Heart Study, *Circulation* 110(9):1042-1046, 2004.

59. Kellen JC: Implications for nursing care of patients with atrial fibrillation: lessons learned from the AFFIRM and RACE studies, *J Cardiovasc Nurs* 19(2):128-137, 2004.

60. Weiss EM, Buescher T: Atrial fibrillation: treatment options and caveats, *AACN Clin Issues* 15(3):362-376, 2004.

61. Corley SD et al: Relationships between sinus rhythm, treatment, and survival in the Atrial Fibrillation Follow-Up Investigation of Rhythm Management (AFFIRM) Study, *Circulation* 109(12):1509-1513, 2004.

62. Wyse DG et al: A comparison of rate control and rhythm control in patients with atrial fibrillation, *N Engl J Med* 347(23):1825-1833, 2002.

63. Van Gelder IC et al: A comparison of rate control and rhythm control in patients with recurrent persistent atrial fibrillation, *N Engl J Med* 347(23):1834-1840, 2002.

64. Snow V et al: Management of newly detected atrial fibrillation: a clinical practice guideline from the American Academy of Family Physicians and the American College of Physicians, *Ann Intern Med* 139(12):1009-1017, 2003.

65. Singer DE et al: Antithrombotic therapy in atrial fibrillation: the Seventh ACCP Conference on Antithrombotic and Thrombolytic Therapy, *Chest* 126(3 Suppl):429S-456S, 2004.

66. Daoud EG et al: Temporary atrial epicardial pacing as prophylaxis against atrial fibrillation after heart surgery: a meta-analysis, *J Cardiovasc Electrophysiol* 14(2):127-132, 2003.

67. Gillinov AM et al: Contemporary surgical treatment for atrial fibrillation, *Pacing Clin Electrophysiol* 26(7 Pt 2): 1641-1644, 2003.

68. Chiu C, Sequeira IB: Diagnosis and treatment of idiopathic ventricular tachycardia, *AACN Clin Issues* 15(3):449-461, 2004.

69. Hazinski MF, Cummins RO, Field JM: *Handbook of emergency cardiovascular care for healthcare providers,* Dallas, Tex, 2000, American Heart Association.

70. Paul S: Understanding advanced concepts in atrioventricular block, *Crit Care Nurse* 21(1):56-66, 2001.

71. Adams-Hamoda MG, Pelter MM: Heart blocks, *Am J Crit Care* 12(1):77-78, 2003.

72. Gregoratos G et al: ACC/AHA/NASPE 2002 guideline update for implantation of cardiac pacemakers and antiarrhythmia devices—summary article: a Report of the American College of Cardiology/American Heart Association Task Force on Practice Guidelines (ACC/AHA/NASPE Committee to Update the 1998 Pacemaker Guidelines), *Circulation* 106:2145-2161, 2002. Full text available online at www.ahajournals.org.

73. Timothy PR, Rodeman BJ: Temporary pacemakers in critically ill patients: assessment and management strategies, *AACN Clin Issues* 15(3):305-325, 2004.

74. Sivakumaran S et al: A prospective randomized comparison of loop recorders versus Holter monitors in patients with syncope or presyncope, *Am J Med* 115(1):1-5, 2003.

75. Krahn AD et al: Use of the implantable loop recorder in evaluation of patients with unexplained syncope, *J Cardiovasc Electrophysiol* 14(9 Suppl):S70-S73, 2003.

76. Krahn AD et al: Insertable loop recorder use for detection of intermittent arrhythmias, *Pacing Clin Electrophysiol* 27(5):657-664, 2004.

77. Gibbons RJ et al: ACC/AHA 2002 guideline update for exercise testing—summary article: a report of the American College of Cardiology/American Heart Association Task Force on Practice Guidelines (Committee to Update the 1997 Exercise Testing Guidelines), *Circulation* 106(14): 1883-1892, 2002. Full text available online at www. ahajournals.org.

78. Rodgers GP et al: American College of Cardiology/American Heart Association Clinical Competence Statement on Stress Testing: a Report of the American College of Cardiology/American Heart Association/American College of Physicians-American Society of Internal Medicine Task Force on Clinical Competence, *Circulation* 102(14): 1726-1738, 2000. Full text available online at www. ahajournals.org.

79. Cheitlin MD et al: ACC/AHA/ASE 2003 guideline update for the clinical application of echocardiography—summary article: a report of the American College of Cardiology/American Heart Association Task Force on Practice Guidelines (ACC/AHA/ASE Committee to Update the 1997 Guidelines for the Clinical Application of Echocardiography), *Circulation* 108(9):1146-1162, 2003. Full text available online at www.ahajournals.org.

80. Fearon WF, Yeung AC: Evaluating intermediate coronary lesions in the cardiac catheterization laboratory, *Rev Cardiovasc Med* 4(1):1-7, 2003.

81. Quinones MA et al: ACC/AHA clinical competence statement on echocardiography: a report of the American College of Cardiology/American Heart Association/American College of Physicians-American Society of Internal Medicine Task Force on clinical competence, *J Am Soc Echocardiogr* 16(4):379-402, 2003. Full text available online at www.ahajournals.org.

82. Constantine G et al: Role of MRI in clinical cardiology, *Lancet* 363(9427):2162-2171, 2004.

83. Shan K et al: Role of cardiac magnetic resonance imaging in the assessment of myocardial viability, *Circulation* 109(11):1328-1334, 2004.

84. Klocke FJ et al: ACC/AHA/ASNC guidelines for the clinical use of cardiac radionuclide imaging—executive summary: a report of the American College of Cardiology/American Heart Association Task Force on Practice Guidelines (ACC/AHA/ASNC Committee to Revise the 1995 Guidelines for the Clinical Use of Cardiac Radionuclide Imaging), *J Am Coll Cardiol* 42(7): 1318-1333, 2003. Full text available online at www.jacc. org.

85. Nikolsky E et al: Vascular complications associated with arteriotomy closure devices in patients undergoing percutaneous coronary procedures: a meta-analysis, *J Am Coll Cardiol* 44(6):1200-1209, 2004.

86. Attin M: Electrophysiology study: a comprehensive review, *Am J Crit Care* 10(4):260-273, 2001.

87. Sealey B, Lui K: Diagnosis and management of vasovagal syncope and dysautonomia, *AACN Clin Issues* 15(3): 449-461, 2004.

88. Warkentin TE, Greinacher A: Heparin-induced thrombocytopenia: recognition, treatment, and prevention: the Seventh ACCP Conference on Antithrombotic and Thrombolytic Therapy, *Chest* 126(3 Suppl):311S-337S. Available online at www.accp.org.

89. Warkentin TE: An overview of the heparin-induced thrombocytopenia syndrome, *Semin Thromb Hemost* 30(3): 273-283, 2004.

90. AACN: *Pulmonary artery pressure monitoring: AACN Practice Alert,* 2004, American Association of Critical Care Nurses; available online at www.aacn.org.

91. Perloff D et al: *Human blood pressure determination by sphygmomanometry,* ed 6, Dallas, Tex, 2001, American Heart Association.

92. Polderman KH, Girbes AR: Central venous catheter use. Part 1: mechanical complications, *Intensive Care Med* 28(1):1-17, 2002.

93. Dumont CP: Procedures nurses use to remove central venous catheters and complications they observe: a pilot study, *Am J Crit Care* 10(3):151-155, 2001.

94. Polderman KH, Girbes AR: Central venous catheter use. Part 2: infectious complications, *Intensive Care Med* 28(1):18-28, 2002.

95. O'Grady NP et al: Guidelines for the prevention of intravascular catheter-related infections, *Infect Control Hosp Epidemiol* 23(12):759-769, 2002.

96. Chaiyakunapruk N et al: Chlorhexidine compared with povidone-iodine solution for vascular catheter-site care: a meta-analysis, *Ann Intern Med* 136(11):792-801, 2002.

97. Hu KK et al: Using maximal sterile barriers to prevent central venous catheter-related infection: a systematic evidence-based review, *Am J Infect Control* 32(3): 142-146, 2004.

98. Boyce JM, Pittet D: Guideline for hand hygiene in healthcare settings. Recommendations of the Healthcare Infection Control Practices Advisory Committee and the HIPAC/SHEA/APIC/IDSA Hand Hygiene Task Force, *Am J Infect Control* 30(8):S1-46, 2002.

99. Dimick JB et al: Risk of colonization of central venous catheters: catheters for total parenteral nutrition vs. other catheters, *Am J Crit Care* 12(4):328-335, 2003.

100. Reinhart K et al: Continuous central venous and pulmonary artery oxygen saturation monitoring in the critically ill, *Intensive Care Med* 30(8):1572-1578, 2004.

101. Ivanov R, Allen J, Calvin JE: The incidence of major morbidity in critically ill patients managed with pulmonary artery catheters: a meta-analysis, *Crit Care Med* 28(3): 615-619, 2000.

102. Connors AF Jr et al: Outcomes following acute exacerbation of severe chronic obstructive lung disease. The SUPPORT investigators (Study to Understand Prognoses and Preferences for Outcomes and Risks of Treatments), *Am J Respir Crit Care Med* 154(4 Pt 1):959-967, 1996.

103. Richard C et al: Early use of the pulmonary artery catheter and outcomes in patients with shock and acute respiratory distress syndrome: a randomized controlled trial, *JAMA* 290(20):2713-2720, 2003.

104. Polanczyk CA et al: Right heart catheterization and cardiac complications in patients undergoing noncardiac surgery: an observational study, *JAMA* 286(3):309-314, 2001.

105. Rhodes A et al: A randomised, controlled trial of the pulmonary artery catheter in critically ill patients, *Intensive Care Med* 28(3):256-264, 2002.

106. Sandham JD et al: A randomized, controlled trial of the use of pulmonary-artery catheters in high-risk surgical patients, *N Engl J Med* 348(1):5-14, 2003.

107. Jacka MJ et al: The appropriateness of the pulmonary artery catheter in cardiovascular surgery, *Can J Anaesth* 49(3):276-282, 2002.

108. Bernard GR et al: Pulmonary artery catheterization and clinical outcomes: National Heart, Lung, and Blood Institute and Food and Drug Administration Workshop Report. Consensus Statement, *JAMA* 283(19):2568-2572, 2000.

109. Aitken LM: Expert critical care nurses' use of pulmonary artery pressure monitoring, *Intensive Crit Care Nurs* 16(4):209-220, 2000.

110. Pinsky MR: Hemodynamic monitoring in the intensive care unit, *Clin Chest Med* 24(4):549-560, 2003.

111. Practice guidelines for pulmonary artery catheterization: an updated report by the American Society of Anesthesiologists Task Force on Pulmonary Artery Catheterization, *Anesthesiology* 99(4):988-1014, 2003.

112. Bridges EJ: Monitoring pulmonary artery pressures: just the facts, *Crit Care Nurse* 20(6):59-78, 2000.

113. Antle DE: Ensuring competency in nurse repositioning of the pulmonary artery catheter, *Dimens Crit Care Nurs* 19(2):44-51, 2000.

114. Baldwin IC, Heland M: Incidence of cardiac dysrhythmias in patients during pulmonary artery catheter removal after cardiac surgery, *Heart Lung* 29(3):155-160, 2000.

115. Gawlinski A: Measuring cardiac output: intermittent bolus thermodilution method, *Crit Care Nurse* 20(2):118-120, 122-124, 2000.

116. Giuliano KK et al: Backrest angle and cardiac output measurement in critically ill patients, *Nurs Res* 52(4):242-248, 2003.

117. Rivers E et al: Early goal-directed therapy in the treatment of severe sepsis and septic shock, *N Engl J Med* 345(19):1368-1377, 2001.

118. Jesurum J: Protocols for Practice—Svo$_2$ Monitoring, *Crit Care Nurse* 24(4):73-76, 2004.

CHAPTER 18

Cardiovascular Disorders

Cardiovascular disease remains the leading cause of mortality in the United States. There are 2,400,000 deaths from cardiovascular causes in the United States each year or 60% of "total mortality."[1] The estimated direct and indirect national cost is $133.2 billion.[1] Cardiovascular diseases are the leading cause of death for both women and men.[1] An understanding of the pathology of cardiovascular disease processes and current clinical management allows the critical care nurse to accurately anticipate and plan interventions. This chapter focuses on cardiac disorders commonly seen in the critical care environment.

CORONARY ARTERY DISEASE

DESCRIPTION AND ETIOLOGY

Atherosclerosis is a progressive disease that affects arteries throughout the body. In the heart, atherosclerotic changes are clinically known as *coronary artery disease* (CAD). This disease process is also known by the term *coronary heart disease* (CHD) because ultimately other heart structures will become involved in the disease process. The atherosclerotic vascular changes that lead to CAD may have begun in childhood.[2] Research and epidemiologic data collected during the past 50 years have demonstrated a strong association between specific risk factors and the development of CAD.[1] These risk factors are further delineated into nonmodifiable and modifiable coronary risk factors (Box 18-1).

RISK FACTORS FOR CORONARY ARTERY DISEASE

Age, Gender, and Race. The severe effects of CAD occur as a person ages. In general, CAD symptoms are seen in middle and old age.[1] Traditionally CAD has been regarded as a male disease, but it is increasingly obvious that in modern society it affects both genders.[1] The average age for a person having a first heart attack is 68.8 years for men and 70.4 years for women.[1] Starting at age 75 the prevalence of cardiovascular disease is higher in

women than in men.[3] In fact, CAD rates in postmenopausal women are two to three times higher than those of women the same age before menopause.[1] Nonwhite populations of both genders have higher CAD mortality rates than do white populations of similar socioeconomic status.[1]

Family History. A positive family history is one in which a close blood relative has had a myocardial infarction or stroke before the age of 60. This family history suggests a genetic or lifestyle predisposition to the development of coronary artery disease.

Hyperlipidemia. Hyperlipidemia is a leading factor responsible for severe atherosclerosis and the development of CAD. Determining total serum cholesterol and triglyceride levels represents a helpful start in the evaluation process.[3,4] A lipid panel blood test will measure the following values:

- High-density lipoprotein (HDL) cholesterol
- Low-density lipoprotein (LDL) cholesterol
- Very–low-density lipoprotein (VLDL) cholesterol
- Triglycerides

Treatment of hyperlipidemia has advanced beyond the concept of lowering total cholesterol to treatment of specific lipoprotein abnormalities.[3-6] The current target levels for specific serum lipids are listed in Table 18-1.

Total Cholesterol. The total cholesterol is the sum of the HDL, LDL, and VLDL cholesterol in the bloodstream. It is used as a starting point for lipid testing. If the total cholesterol is over 200 mg/dl, that is an indication to investigate the lipid profile and other risk factors for development of CAD.

HDL Cholesterol. HDL cholesterol is frequently described as the "good" cholesterol because higher serum levels exert a protective effect against acute atherosclerotic events. All the reasons are not completely understood, but one recognized physiologic effect is the ability of HDL to promote the efflux of cholesterol from cells. This process may minimize the accumulation of foam cells in the artery wall and thus decrease the risk of developing atherosclerosis.[7] High HDL levels confer both antiinflammatory and antioxidant benefits on the arterial wall.[7] In contrast, a low HDL level is an independent risk

Box 18-1

CORONARY ARTERY DISEASE RISK FACTORS

NONMODIFIABLE
Age
Gender
Family history
Race

MODIFIABLE
Elevated serum lipids
Hypertension
Cigarette smoking
Prediabetes or diabetes mellitus
Diet high in saturated fat, cholesterol, and calories
Elevated homocysteine level
Metabolic syndrome
Obesity
Physical inactivity
Postmenopause *(modification is controversial)*

Table 18-1 — Lipid Guidelines and CAD Risk

Lipid	Target Value*
Total cholesterol	Below 200 mg/dl
HDL cholesterol	Above 40 mg/dl for men
	Above 50 mg/dl for women
LDL cholesterol	Below 70 mg/dl if very high risk
	Below 100 mg/dl if high risk
	Below 130 mg/dl if low risk
VLDL cholesterol	Below 30 mg/dl
Triglycerides	Below 150 mg/dl

*Values outside the target range increase CAD risk
HDL, High-density lipoprotein; *LDL,* low-density lipoprotein; *VLDL,* very–low-density lipoprotein.

factor for the development of CAD and other atherosclerotic conditions. HDL cholesterol is generally higher in women and is raised by physical exercise and by stopping smoking. In patients with low HDL cholesterol, when lifestyle changes are ineffective the HDL level can be raised by drugs such as extended release nicotinic acid (niacin), and fibrates.

LDL Cholesterol. LDL cholesterol is usually described as the "bad" cholesterol because high levels are associated with an increased risk of acute coronary syndrome, stroke, and peripheral arterial disease. High LDL levels initiate the atherosclerotic process by infiltrating the vessel wall and binding to the matrix of cells beneath the endothelium.[7] LDL cholesterol also exerts an inflammatory effect on the arterial vessel wall.[7] A high LDL cholesterol level is initially managed by nonpharmacologic lifestyle changes such as weight loss, smoking cessation, low fat diet, physical exercise, and attainment of a normal body size as measured by the body mass index (BMI). If lifestyle changes are insufficient to reduce the LDL cholesterol level in the bloodstream, the drug category of choice is a "*statin.*" There are numerous research studies that have conclusively demonstrated that lowering the LDL cholesterol with statins for either primary or secondary prevention is highly effective in lowering mortality due to CAD.[1,3] The goal of therapy is that it be tailored to treat the individual cardiovascular risk profile. The target LDL cholesterol is determined according to the individual's risk profile as described in Table 18-1. Patients with highest risk are advised to maintain LDL cholesterol below 70 mg/dl; those at high risk, a level below 100 mg/dl; and those at low risk, LDL below 130 mg/dl. Controversy exists as to whether the tiered LDL goals in the current guidelines are sufficiently low to prevent coronary atherosclerosis developing in per-

sons without CAD. Some cardiologists advocate a reduction of the LDL goal to 50 to 70 mg/dl range for everyone, not only those with a known cardiovascular disease.[8]

VLDL Cholesterol. VLDL cholesterol is not usually measured, although a normal value is about 30 mg/dl.[4] The value can be estimated by subtracting the sum of the HDL and LDL from the total cholesterol. When triglycerides are elevated the VLDL cholesterol will also be high.

Triglycerides. Triglycerides are serum lipids that constitute an additional and separate atherogenic risk factor. Triglycerides are carried by VLDL cholesterol in the bloodstream.[5] An optimal triglyceride level is below 150 mg/dl, and the more elevated the triglyceride serum level the higher the risk of developing coronary artery disease. A value from 150 to 199 mg/dl is borderline high; from 200 to 500 mg/dl is high; and a value above 500 mg/dl signals a high risk of atherogenic complications and a strong risk for the presence or development of type 2 diabetes.

Lipoprotein(a). LDL cholesterol can be further analyzed by the category of lipid particles that make up the total LDL value. Researchers have investigated the function of several lipid particles to determine their role in the development of premature atherosclerotic CAD. One particle that has been extensively studied is *lipoprotein(a)* abbreviated Lp(a), and described verbally as "LP little a." Lp(a) is manufactured in the liver and circulates in the bloodstream bound to a large glycoprotein named *apolipopotein(a),* abbreviated as apo(a).[9] The Lp(a)-apo(a) lipid particle is elevated in the presence of inflammation and will stimulate both atheroma and clot formation in inflamed arteries.[9] This is thought to be because the apo(a) is structurally similar to plasminogen, a protein essential for clot formation.

Lp(a) levels are 90% genetically determined. Elevated Lp(a) plasma levels constitute the most frequently encountered genetic lipid disorder in families with premature CAD.[9] Testing for Lp(a) is reserved for high-risk patient populations such as those with a strong family history of premature atherosclerotic disease, and for patients with premature CAD who do not exhibit the expected cardiac risk factors. Reduction of Lp(a) levels to below 30 mg/dl is the therapeutic goal. This is generally achieved by ingesting high doses (3 to 4 g/day) of extended-release nicotinic acid (niacin). Unfortunately, the Lp(a) level is not reduced by statins, drugs that traditionally lower LDL levels. Nor is Lp(a) reduced by physical exercise, a low fat diet, weight loss, or tight blood-glucose control.[9] At the present time, lifestyle changes are recommended; research is ongoing, but a cure is not yet discernable.

High-Fat Diet. A diet rich in saturated fats will lead to elevated cholesterol levels in the blood. The first line of treatment to lower elevated serum cholesterol is a low-fat, high-fiber diet and increased physical exercise.[5,6] If these measures are not effective, lipid-lowering drugs are indicated.[1] This sounds simple in theory, but less than half of the people who qualify for lipid reduction therapy are actually taking their medications; only a third of treated patients reach their LDL target; and half of patients prescribed a lipid-lowering drug have stopped taking it six months later.[1] Although the drugs are very helpful for some, they are clearly not a panacea for everyone.

Obesity. Obesity is a disease of modern times. It is often associated with a sedentary life style. It also increases susceptibility to the development of other risk factors, such as hypertension, decreased insulin sensitivity, and hyperlipidemia, with increased LDL and low HDL cholesterol.[10] In the United States, 122 million adults are overweight or obese.[11] Body weight is defined using the body mass index.

Body Mass Index (BMI) is a mathematic formula used to assess body weight relative to height. BMI is used to evaluate the threat of excess pounds as a risk factor for coronary artery disease and permits comparisons of people of different gender, age, height, and body type.[1] BMI is calculated as the weight in kilograms divided by the square of the height in meters (kg/m^2). The BMI calculation in both metric and pounds/inches is shown in Box 18-2. A normal BMI is between 18.5 and 25 kg/m^2. A BMI between 25 and 30 kg/m^2 indicates the person is overweight. A BMI greater than 30 kg/m^2 is the definition of obesity.[4]

The distribution pattern of fat on the body is a CAD risk factor. The more weight carried in the abdominal area, producing a large waist, the greater the risk of coronary artery disease. Excess abdominal adiposity (apple body shape) indicates additional fat around the abdominal organs as compared with individuals who have a smaller waist and larger hips (pear body shape). A waist size greater than 40 inches in men and 35 inches in women increases CAD risk. Physical exercise has been

shown to assist with weight reduction, lower risk from CAD, and decrease the risk of developing type 2 diabetes.

Physical Inactivity. Regular vigorous physical activity using large muscle groups promotes physiologic adaptation to aerobic exercise that can prevent the development of coronary artery disease and reduce symptoms in patients with established cardiovascular disease.[12] Exercise will also reduce the incidence of many other diseases including type 2 diabetes, osteoporosis, obesity, depression, and cancers of the colon and breast.[12] Multiple research trials have demonstrated the positive effects of physical activity on the other major cardiac risk factors.[12] Exercise alters the lipid profile by decreasing LDL cholesterol and triglycerides and increasing HDL cholesterol.[12] Exercise reduces insulin resistance at the cellular level, thus lowering the risk of developing type 2 diabetes, especially if combined with a weight-loss program.[12] Epidemiologic studies indicate that physical athletics as a young person do not confer protection in later years. Lifelong physical activity is

---

Box 18-2

HOW TO CALCULATE AND INTERPRET BODY MASS INDEX (BMI)

USE A CALCULATOR
Metric: Divide body weight in kg by height in meters; divide the result again by height in meters.
Formula:

$$BMI = \frac{Weight\ in\ kilograms}{(Height\ in\ meters) \times (Height\ in\ meters)}$$

Example: A person weighs 100 kg and is 1.91 meters tall

$$BMI = \frac{100\ Kilograms}{(1.91\ Meters) \times (1.91\ Meters)} = 27.7$$

Pounds/Inches Multiply weight in pounds by 703; divide the result by height in inches, then divide again by height in inches.
Formula:

$$BMI = \frac{Weight\ in\ pounds}{(Height\ in\ inches) \times (Height\ in\ inches)} \times 703$$

Example: A person weighs 222 pounds and is 6 feet 3 inches (75 inches) tall

$$BMI = \frac{222\ pounds}{(75\ inches) \times (75\ inches)} \times 703 = 27.7$$

HOW TO INTERPRET THE BODY MASS INDEX (BMI) RESULT

BMI (KG/M^2)	WEIGHT STATUS
Under 18.5	Underweight
18.5 to 24.9	Normal weight
25 to 29.5	Overweight
Over 30	Obese

necessary to prevent atherosclerotic coronary artery disease and stroke.[12]

Hypertension. Normal blood pressure is described as a systolic blood pressure (SBP) below 120 mm Hg and a diastolic blood pressure (DBP) below 80 mm Hg. *Hypertension* is defined as the elevation of either SBP greater than 140 mm Hg or DBP higher than 90 mm Hg. *Controlled hypertension* describes a situation in which administration of antihypertensive medications maintains the patient's blood pressure (BP) within the normal range.

Hypertension is a cardiac risk factor because the high systolic pressure damages the arterial endothelium, leading to vascular inflammation that encourages formation of plaque. Hypertension is divided into stages for the purposes of treatment as shown in Table 18-2.

Prehypertension reflects a systolic pressure of 120 to 139 mm Hg, or a diastolic pressure above 85 mm Hg.[1,11] In the United States this affects a huge number of people: one in five adults is prehypertensive.

Hypertension is diagnosed when the BP is above 140/90 mm Hg. Hypertension affects another one in four adults in the United States. Once the BP is above 140/80, hypertension is described as either stage 1 or stage 2 (see Table 18-2).

Hypertension is often described as the "silent killer," because 30% of those affected are unaware they have seriously elevated BP.[1] In the United States, 65 million people are hypertensive (35 million women and 30 million men). Of those who know that they are hypertensive, 34% are on medication and have their BP controlled; 25% are on medication but do not have their BP under control; and 11% are hypertensive but are not taking any medication.[1] It is essential that patients understand that sustained elevation of BP leads inexorably towards atherosclerosis, heart failure, kidney failure, stroke, and heart attack.[11] So widespread is hypertension in industrialized societies that even a normotensive person at age 55 has a 90% lifetime risk of developing hypertension. This implies that even normotensive persons should adopt interventions to maintain a normal BP.[11]

Table 18-2	Blood Pressure Guidelines and CAD Risk	
	Systolic BP*	**Diastolic BP***
Normal (optimal)	Less than 120	Less than 80
Prehypertension	120-139	80-89
Stage 1 hypertension	140-159	90-99
Stage 2 hypertension	160 or higher	100 or higher

*Values above normal increase risk of CAD and heart failure.
CAD, Coronary artery disease; *BP,* blood pressure.

According to recent guidelines, the goal of treatment for the hypertensive person without other risk factors is to achieve a BP below 140/80 mm Hg. For the hypertensive person who already has diabetes or kidney disease the target BP is lower, below 130/80 mm Hg. A normal BP is below 120/80 mm Hg.[11]

Lifestyle interventions that can normalize BP include physical exercise, low salt diet, limiting alcohol intake, and achievement of normal body weight. Most patients are started on a diuretic, and if this is insufficient may be placed on angiotensin converter enzyme inhibitor (ACEI) drugs, angiotensin receptor blocker (ARB) drugs, beta-blockers, or calcium channel blockers. Most patients will require at least two medications each from different drug classifications to normalize their BP.[11] A discussion of hypertensive emergencies with acute organ damage is included as the last section of this chapter.

Cigarette Smoking. The greater the number of cigarettes smoked per day, the greater the risk of developing CAD, acute MI, and stroke.[1,13,14] Cigarette smoking unfavorably alters serum lipid levels, decreases HDL cholesterol level, and increases LDL cholesterol and triglyceride levels. In the United States, smoking remains commonplace; 25.2% of men and 20.2% of women over 18 years of age smoke cigarettes. Passive, secondhand smoke exposure also increases cardiovascular risk, and 34.7% of nonsmoking adults are exposed to environmental tobacco smoke at home or at work.[1,13-15] Within 1 year of giving up cigarettes, an ex-smoker's risk of developing CAD decreases by 50%. With 15 smoke-free years the person's risk falls to almost that of a lifetime non-smoker.[1] Nicotine is addictive, and giving up smoking is difficult. People need tremendous help and support to be able to "kick the habit." The good news is that many do quit, and since 1965 smoking in the United States has declined by over 40% among adults.[1] See Chapter 24 for patient education guidelines on how to stop smoking.

Diabetes Mellitus. Individuals with diabetes mellitus (types 1 and 2) have a higher incidence of coronary heart disease than the general population. Elevated blood glucose is a known risk factor for development of vascular inflammation associated with atherosclerosis. The target range for normoglycemia is 70 to 110 mg/dl. It is recommended that patients in the intensive care unit (ICU) have blood glucose maintained within the normal range to decrease complications.[16]

A fasting blood glucose between 110 and 125 mg/dl represents a prediabetic state and is a risk factor for the development of diabetes and CAD as listed in Table 18-3. The upper limit for normal fasting plasma glucose is 126 mg/dl. Patients with diabetes have an increased risk of developing coronary artery disease and have worse clinical outcomes following acute coronary syndrome events.[17] In a recent multinational study of patients who were seen at hospitals with symptoms of acute coronary syndrome, almost one in four had a known history of diabetes.[18] More detailed information on type 2 diabetes and the use of insulin and oral medications to control blood glucose and combat insulin resistance is included in Chapters 35 and 36.

Chronic Kidney Disease. Chronic kidney disease is considered a "risk equivalent" for coronary artery disease.[3,19] This means patients with chronic kidney disease have as much risk of experiencing a coronary event as if they already had CAD.[3,20] The risk of death for the patient with acute myocardial infarction rises as the serum creatinine rises.[20] In one study the in-hospital mortality rates for patients with an acute MI was 2% for patients with normal kidney function, 6% for those with mild kidney failure, 14% for those with moderate kidney failure, 21% for those with severe kidney failure, and 30% for patients with end-stage kidney disease.[20]

Metabolic Syndrome. The metabolic syndrome is a combination of several key risk factors that unite to greatly increase the risk of developing CAD and type 2 diabetes. An estimated 47 million adults in the United States (23.7%) manifest measurable signs of metabolic syndrome.[1,5] The following are risk factors:

1. Waist circumference greater than 40 inches (102 cm) in men and greater than 35 inches (88 cm) in women[21]
2. Serum triglyceride level greater than 150 mg/dl ($\geq$1.7 mmol/L)[21]
3. High-density lipoprotein (HDL) cholesterol level less than 40 mg/dl ($\leq$1.04 mmol/L) in men; less than 50 mg/dl ($\leq$1.29 mmol/L) in women[21]
4. Blood pressure 130/85 mm Hg or higher, which is diagnostic for prehypertension or hypertension[21]
5. Fasting glucose level of 100 to 110 mg/dl, which is diagnostic of prediabetes. A fasting blood glucose level greater than 126 mg/dl is diagnostic of diabetes.[21]

It is perhaps obvious that individuals with the signs of metabolic syndrome are at increased risk of developing coronary artery disease; even so, it is surprising to what degree this holds true. In the Framingham epidemiologic study, presence of the factors associated with metabolic syndrome predicted 25% of all new-onset CAD and almost 50% of new-onset diabetes.[21]

Table 18-3	Fasting Blood Glucose and CAD Risk
	Fasting Plasma Glucose*
Normal blood glucose	70 mg/dl to 110 mg/dl
Prediabetic	110 mg/dl to 125 mg/dl
Diabetic	126 mg/dl or higher

*Values above normal increase risk of CAD and kidney failure.
CAD, Coronary artery disease.

Women and Heart Disease—Premenopause and Postmenopause. Serious CAD symptoms occur approximately 5 years later in women than in men.[22] The average age for the first acute myocardial infarction (MI) in men is 65.8 years and in women 70.4 years.[1] Incidence of coronary artery disease in women is two to three times higher in postmenopausal women compared with women who are premenopausal.[1] Thus in the past it had seemed logical to prescribe hormone replacement therapy (HRT) to treat the symptoms of menopause. However, well-designed research trials discovered an increase in cardiovascular events in the first year of HRT (estrogen plus progestin) replacement therapy, although cardiac events declined after the first year.[22,23] Subsequent studies have confirmed this result.[22] In 2004 the estrogen-only HRT trial was stopped by the National Institutes of Health (NIH) because of an increased risk of stroke in the women taking estrogen. For these reasons, HRT is no longer recommended for prevention of atherosclerotic cardiovascular disease.[24]

Cardiovascular disease kills more than half a million women annually in the United States. To emphasize the magnitude of the problem, this represents more deaths than the next seven fatal diseases for women combined and also exceeds the number of cardiovascular-related deaths in men each year.[25] Mortality rates for women after an acute MI are also higher than for men: 38% to 25%, respectively. Some of the reasons for the higher mortality are that women wait longer before seeking medical help, have smaller coronary arteries, are older when symptoms occur, and experience very different symptoms than men of the same age.[26]

Hyperhomocysteinemia. Homocysteine plays an essential part in protein metabolism. It is a derivative of methionine, an amino acid found in dietary protein. Homocysteine is metabolized in the body by two metabolic pathways; one pathway requires folate and vitamin B_6, and the other is dependent upon vitamin B_{12}.[27] A person missing these vitamins will not be able to metabolize homocysteine. *Hyperhomocysteinemia*, or elevated levels of homocysteine in the bloodstream, is either acquired or occurs as a genetic error of metabolism.[27] High levels are of concern because of the association with atherosclerotic coronary artery disease, stroke, and peripheral arterial disease. An optimal level of plasma homocysteine is believed to be between 5 and 15 micromoles per liter (mmol/L).[27,28] Between 5% and 7% of the population may have mild homocysteinemia. Plasma levels associated with hyperhomocysteinemia are shown in Table 18-4.[27] Atherosclerotic cardiovascular risks from elevated homocysteine levels are reduced by consumption of a varied diet. Typical sources of vitamin B_6, B_{12}, and folic acid, which provide folate, are shown in Table 18-5. Individuals at high risk may need to take daily multiple vitamin supplements containing vitamins B_6, B_{12}, and folic acid.[28]

Table 18-4	Blood Homocysteine Guidelines and CAD Risk
	Homocysteine Plasma Level*
Normal homocysteine	5 to 15 mmol/L
Moderate risk	16 to 30 mmol/L
Intermediate risk	30 to 100 mmol/L
High risk	Over 100 mmol/L

From Reeder SJ et al: Homocysteine: the latest risk factor for heart disease, *Dimens Crit Care Nurs* 19(1):22-28, 2000.
*Values above normal level increase CAD risk.
CAD, Coronary artery disease.

Table 18-5	Vitamin B₆, B₁₂, and Folic Acid Food Sources

Vitamin	Recommended Dietary Allowance	Sources
B_6	2 mg	Chicken, fish, liver, pork, kidney, eggs, unmilled rice, soybeans, and whole-wheat foods
B_{12}	6 mcg	Peanuts, walnuts, and animal products
Folic acid	400 mcg	Citrus fruits, tomatoes, vegetables, and grain products

From Reeder SJ et al: Homocysteine: the latest risk factor for heart disease, *Dimens Crit Care Nurs* 19(1):22-28, 2000.

Vascular Inflammation. The link between vascular inflammation and atherosclerotic disease is now well established.[29] However, measurement of this link has been more controversial.[29] Many researchers believe the development of atherosclerotic plaque occurs in response to inflammation. Noxious inflammatory agents circulate in the bloodstream and stimulate chemical mediators that directly modify the arterial wall (see following section on pathophysiology). The initial inflammatory stimuli include increased blood sugar, elevated blood lipids, nicotine, and hypertension. However, other clinical conditions such as connective tissue disorders and systemic infection will also produce an inflammatory state, and it is not clear what the impact of inflammation produced by these stimuli is, if any, on the vessels.[29] It is hoped that measurement of inflammatory chemical markers will some day allow prediction of acute coronary events.

Table 18-6	C-Reactive Protein and CAD Risk
	hs-CRP Level*
Low risk	Below 1 mg/L
Moderate risk	1-3 mg/L
High risk	Above 3 mg/L

Data from Pearson TA et al: Markers of inflammation and cardiovascular disease, application to clinical and public health practice: a statement for HealthCare Professionals from the Centers for Disease Control and Prevention and the American Heart Association, *Circulation* 107(3):499-511, 2003.
*Values above normal level increase CAD risk, but test results are not valid in presence of infection or other inflammatory condition. A test result greater than 10 mg/L suggests a noncoronary source of inflammation or infection.
CAD, Coronary artery disease.

C-Reactive Protein. The inflammatory marker most frequently cited is *C-reactive protein* (CRP). It is measured as *high-sensitivity C-reactive protein* (hs-CRP).[29] The higher the hs-CRP value, the greater the risk of a coronary event, especially if all other potential causes of systemic inflammation such as infection can be ruled out. Value ranges for hs-CRP are shown in Table 18-6. If other systemic inflammatory conditions such as bronchitis or a urinary tract infection are present, the hs-CRP test loses all predictive value.[29] C-Reactive protein and other inflammatory markers are used to estimate the probability of future acute coronary events.[29,30] During acute coronary syndrome events, there is widespread activation of neutrophils in the cardiac circulation (measured from the coronary sinus), which suggests that inflammation is not limited to one unstable plaque.[31] Debate continues as to whether CRP is simply a marker of vascular inflammation or whether it also contributes to the proinflammatory state.[7]

Multifactorial Risk. The major risk factors for developing CAD have been extensively documented in large epidemiologic studies: smoking, family history, adverse lipid profile, and elevated blood pressure.[3] Certain medical conditions are considered "risk equivalents" of CAD. A *risk equivalent* means the person has the same risk of having an acute MI as if they actually had coronary heart disease already.[3] Two noncardiac medical conditions are considered risk equivalents for CAD: diabetes mellitus and chronic kidney disease. Peripheral arterial disease (PAD) and cerebral vascular disease are atherosclerotic conditions that are also considered CAD risk equivalents.

Coronary artery disease has multifactorial causation; the greater the number of risk factors, the greater the risk of developing CAD.[1,3,21,32] The best time for an individual to make lifestyle changes is before symptoms of coronary artery disease occur. Patients with two or more risk factors, or one or more of the "CAD risk equivalent diseases" have the greatest potential to benefit from risk factor reduction and lifestyle change.[3]

Primary vs. Secondary Prevention of CAD. If a person has symptoms of CAD or has previously had an acute coronary syndrome event, the goal of any lifestyle change or medication is termed *secondary prevention*, or preventing another heart attack. If an individual matches the risk profile described in the previous pages, but does *not* have symptoms of CAD or has *not* had an acute MI, the treatment plan is described as *primary prevention*. The constellation of cardiac risk factors is now well established and is predictive for development of CAD for most populations in the developed industrial world.

PATHOPHYSIOLOGY OF CAD

Coronary heart disease is a progressive atherosclerotic disorder of the coronary arteries that results in narrowing or complete occlusion. *Atherosclerosis* affects the medium-size arteries that perfuse the heart and other major organs. Normal arterial walls are composed of three layers: the *intima* (inner lining), the *media* (middle muscular layer), and the *adventitia* (outer coat).

Development of Atherosclerosis. It is now well understood that atherosclerosis is a chronic inflammatory disorder that is characterized by an accumulation of macrophages and T lymphocytes in the arterial intimal wall. High LDL is one of the triggers of vascular inflammation. The inflammation injures the wall, allowing the LDL cholesterol to move into the vessel wall below the endothelial surface.[7] In addition, blood monocytes adhere to endothelial cells and migrate into the vessel wall. Within the artery wall, some monocytes differentiate into macrophages that unite with, and then internalize, LDL cholesterol. The *foam cells* that result are the marker cells of atherosclerosis.[7]

Elevated LDL cholesterol levels promote low-level endothelial inflammation that allows lipoproteins to infiltrate the intimal vessel wall. Once infiltrated under the endothelium, the LDL tends to stay within the vessel wall rather than return to the circulation.[7] This is in contrast to the actions of HDL cholesterol. HDL enters the vessel wall, helps efflux cholesterol from cells, and then returns to the circulation.[7] The actions of HDL may help minimize the number of foam cells in the artery wall.[7]

Atherosclerotic Plaque Rupture. When "mature" atherosclerotic plaque develops, it is not uniform in composition. It has a lipid liquid center filled with procoagulant factors. A connective tissue *fibrous cap* covers the top of the fluid lipid center.[3,29-31] The abrupt rupture of this cap allows procoagulant lipids to flood into the vessel lumen and rapidly form a coronary thrombosis as shown in Table 18-7. As the enlarging clot blocks blood flow through the coronary artery a "heart attack" will oc-

cur unless there is adequate collateral circulation from other coronary vessels. Symptoms and suggested cardiac interventions at appropriate stages in development of CAD are listed in Table 18-7.

Plaques that are likely to rupture are saturated with macrophages and other inflammatory cells. These *vulnerable plaques* are usually nonobstructive and are situated at bends or branch-points in the arterial tree.[3] It is not yet known what factors cause the fibrous cap to rupture or erode. As deep fissures in the cap expose the procoagulant factors to the blood plasma, an unstoppable cycle is put into motion. When platelets in the bloodstream are exposed to collagen, necrotic debris, von Willebrand factor, and thromboxane, a clot is formed that can occlude the coronary artery. Highly fibrotic plaques do not rupture. The type of atherosclerotic plaque that is prone to rupture has a weak fibrous cap and a large amount of liquid cholesterol within the core (see Table 18-7).[31]

Plaque Regression. A reduction in blood cholesterol decreases atherosclerotic plaque size by decreasing the amount of liquid cholesterol within the plaque core.[5] Lowering cholesterol levels will not change the dimensions of the fibrous or calcified portions of the plaque. However, lower cholesterol levels reduce vascular inflammation and make vulnerable plaque less likely to rupture.

If diet is not effective in lowering blood cholesterol, lipid-lowering drugs are prescribed to lower the LDL cholesterol level below 100 mg/dl for patients at risk of coronary artery disease and to aim for an LDL level below 70 mg/dl for individuals with the highest risk profile.[5] Drugs, diet, and exercise are used to lower the triglyceride level to less than 150 mg/dl, and to raise HDL-cholesterol above 40 mg/dl for men and above 50 mg/dl for women.[3,5,6,32]

ACUTE CORONARY SYNDROMES

The term *acute coronary syndrome* (ACS) is used to describe the array of clinical presentations of coronary artery disease that range from unstable angina to acute MI, as shown in Table 18-7.[1,3,33] It is important to recognize that the general public and media describe an acute myocardial infarction as a "heart attack." The following section will initially discuss stable manifestations of CAD (stable angina) followed by a description of the acute manifestations (unstable angina and acute MI).

Angina. Angina pectoris, or chest pain, caused by myocardial ischemia is not a separate disease, but rather a symptom of CAD. It is caused by a blockage or spasm of a coronary artery, leading to diminished myocardial blood supply. The lack of oxygen causes myocardial ischemia, which is felt as chest pain. Angina may occur anywhere in the chest, neck, arms, or back, but the most commonly described location is pain or pressure behind

Table 18-7	Timeline of Atherogenesis from a Normal Artery through Acute Myocardial Infarction Depicted by Longitudinal Section of an Artery, Plus Associated Symptoms and Interventions

Atherogenesis-Thrombogenesis	Associated Symptoms	Cardiac Intervention
A. Normal artery, normal vessel wall	A. No symptoms	A-C. Primary prevention of CAD recommended: low-fat diet, take regular physical exercise, avoid smoking, and achieve normal BMI
B. Lipids in bloodstream	B. No symptoms	
C. Extracellular lipid accumulates in the intima of the artery (atheroma).	C. No symptoms	
D. Evolves to become a fatty-fibrous (atherosclerotic) lesion. Some lesions will contain a lipid interior covered by a fibrous cap.	D. May experience chest pain symptoms with exercise that are relieved by rest or NTG (stable angina). May have no symptoms at all until the lesion fills over 75% of the vessel lumen.	D. PCI if stable angina present and CAD diagnosed by cardiac catheterization
E. Rupture of the cap allows the lipid in the center to be released into the bloodstream, stimulating clot formation (thrombogenesis).	E. Chest pain not relieved by rest, or NTG (ACS—unstable angina)	E. Call 911--immediate transport to a hospital, preferably one with experience treating ACS
F. Fresh clot blocks the vessel. Spasm of the artery may also occur near the thrombus.	F. Chest pain unrelieved by rest or NTG—severity, location of angina and associated symptoms vary greatly between individuals (ACS—acute MI)	F. Emergency intervention to open the artery: fibrinolytic or catheter-based procedure (PCI)
G. Vessel is open, but the atherosclerotic lesion remains.	G. No symptoms	G. Secondary prevention of CAD to prevent repeat MI; beta-blockers to prevent arrhythmias; ACE-1 drugs to prevent ventricular remodeling and heart failure; elective PCI

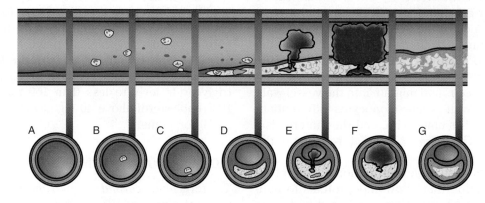

ACE-1, Angiotensin-converting enzyme 1; ACS, acute coronary syndrome; BMI, body mass index; CAD, coronary artery disease; MI, myocardial infarction; NTG, nitroglycerin; PCI, percutaneous coronary intervention. Unnumbered figure modified from Antman EM et al.: Circulation 110:588-636, 2004.

the sternum. The pain often radiates to the left arm but can also radiate down both arms and to the back, the shoulder, the jaw, and/or the neck (Fig. 18-1). Angina symptoms are not the same for all individuals. The presenting characteristics can be highly individualized, as described in Box 18-3. It is essential that patients and families are taught that angina does not always present in the dramatic "Hollywood Heart Attack" scenario seen on television and in movies, where the person clutches the throat or chest and exhibits extreme distress.[3]

Women and Angina. Many women experience a variety of different symptoms both prior to an acute MI and during the acute event as shown in Box 18-4.[34] The recognition and publicity about the fact that many women do not experience "crushing chest pain" is important if women's symptoms are not to be trivialized by clinicians.[35] Ultimately, it is important that all patients are made aware of *angina symptom equivalents* such as unexpected shortness of breath, breaking out in a cold sweat, or sudden fatigue, nausea, or lightheadedness.[3]

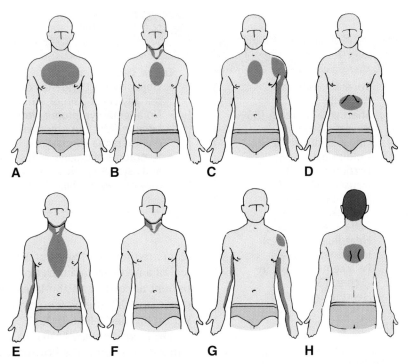

Fig. 18-1 Common sites for anginal pain. **A,** Upper part of chest. **B,** Beneath sternum, radiating to neck and jaw. **C,** Beneath sternum, radiating down left arm. **D,** Epigastric. **E,** Epigastric, radiating to neck, jaw, and arms. **F,** Neck and jaw. **G,** Left shoulder. **H,** Intrascapular.

Box 18-3

CHARACTERISTICS OF ANGINA PECTORIS

LOCATION
Beneath sternum, radiating to neck and jaw
Upper chest
Beneath sternum, radiating down left arm
Epigastric
Epigastric, radiating to neck, jaw, and arms
Neck and jaw
Left shoulder, inner aspect of both arms
Intrascapular

DURATION
Less than 5 minutes
Less than 5 minutes (stable)
Longer than 5 minutes or worsening symptoms without relief from rest of medication indicates unstable or pre-infarction symptoms (unstable)

QUALITY
Sensation of pressure or heavy weight on the chest
Feeling of tightness, like a vise
Visceral quality (deep, heavy, squeezing, aching)

Burning sensation
Shortness of breath, with feeling of suffocation
Most severe pain ever experienced

RADIATION
Medial aspect of left arm
Jaw
Left shoulder
Right arm

PRECIPITATING FACTORS
Exertion/exercise
Cold weather
Exercising after a large, heavy meal
Walking against the wind
Emotional upset
Fright, anger
Coitus

MEDICATION RELIEF
Usually within 45 seconds to 5 minutes of sublingual nitroglycerin administration

---

Stable Angina. *Stable angina* is predictable and caused by similar precipitating factors each time; typically it is exercise-induced. Patients become used to the pattern of this type of angina and may describe it as "my usual chest pain." Pain control is achieved by rest and by sublingual nitroglycerin within 5 minutes. Stable angina is the result of fixed lesions (blockages) of more than 75% of the coronary artery lumen. Ischemia and chest pain occur when myocardial demand from exertion exceeds the fixed blood oxygen supply.[4]

Box 18-4

CARDIOVASCULAR SYMPTOMS EXPERIENCED BY WOMEN BEFORE ACUTE MYOCARDIAL INFARCTION

SYMPTOMS 1 MONTH BEFORE ACUTE MI	SYMPTOMS DURING ACUTE MI
Unusual fatigue (71%)	Shortness of breath (58%)
Sleep disturbance (48%)	Weakness (55%)
Shortness of breath (42%)	Unusual fatigue (43%)
Indigestion (39%)	Cold sweat (39%)
Anxiety (36%)	Dizziness (39%)
Heart racing (27%)	Nausea (36%)
Arms weak/heavy (25%)	Arm heaviness or weakness (35%)
Changes in thinking or memory (24%)	Ache in arms (32%)
Vision change (23%)	Heat/flushing (32%)
Loss of appetite (22%)	Indigestion (31%)
Hands/arms tingling (22%)	Pain centered high in chest (31%)
Difficulty breathing at night (19%)	Heart racing (23%)

From McSweeney JC et al: Women's early warning symptoms of acute myocardial infarction, *Circulation* 108(21):2619-2623, 2003.

MI, Myocardial infarction.

Box 18-5

SILENT ISCHEMIA

CLINICAL CHARACTERISTICS
- Objective ECG evidence of myocardial ischemia without any chest pain or symptoms
- No anginal symptoms after a previous myocardial infarction (MI), but objective ECG evidence of myocardial ischemia continues
- Symptoms of angina with some episodes of ischemia, and asymptomatic with other ischemic events; patient may or may not have had a previous MI

Unstable Angina. *Unstable angina* is defined as a change in a previously established stable pattern of angina. It is part of the continuum of ACS. Unstable angina usually is more intense than stable angina, may awaken the person from sleep, or may necessitate more than nitrates for pain relief. A change in the level or frequency of symptoms requires immediate medical evaluation. Severe angina that persists for more than 5 minutes, is worsening in intensity, and is not relieved by one nitroglycerin tablet is a medical emergency and the patient or a family member must call 911 immediately.[3] The 911 (Emergency Medical Services) system is available to 90% of the population of the United States.[3] In a recent study, patients with an acute MI who used 911 and were transported to the hospital by ambulance had significantly faster receipt of initial reperfusion therapies.[36] Family and friends are discouraged from driving a person experiencing unstable angina to the hospital and instead are encouraged to call 911. Patients should be instructed never to drive themselves but to call the Emergency Medical Services (EMS) via 911.

Unstable angina is an indication of atheroslcerotic plaque instability. It can signal atherosclerotic plaque rupture and thrombus formation that can lead to myocardial infarction. The patient who comes to the emergency department with recent onset of unstable angina but who has nonspecific or nonelevated ST-segment changes on the 12-lead ECG may be admitted to the critical care unit as a "rule-out MI." If the symptoms are typical of a myocardial infarction, it is important to treat the patient according to the latest published guidelines, because not all patients who experience an MI have ST elevation on the 12-lead ECG.[33]

Variant Angina. Variant, or Prinzmetal's, angina is caused by spasm of a coronary artery.[37] Spasm can occur with or without atherosclerotic lesions. Variant angina commonly occurs when the individual is at rest and is often cyclic, occurring at the same time every day. It usually is associated with ST-segment elevation. Smoking, alcohol, and illegal stimulant drug use (cocaine) may precipitate spasm. The diagnosis is made during a cardiac catheterization study. To force the artery to spasm, 50 mcg of ergonovine intravenously (IV) is administered every 5 minutes, until a maximum dose of 400 mcg has been administered or the signs and symptoms of coronary artery spasm appear. Signs of spasm include ST-segment elevation and chest pain. Nitroglycerin will rapidly reverse the effects of ergonovine.[37] Coronary artery spasm can occur both with and without CAD. The prognosis is excellent when there is no significant coronary artery stenosis. Coronary artery spasm is treated with nitroglycerin or calcium channel blockers to vasodilate the coronary arteries.

Silent Ischemia. Silent ischemia describes a situation where objective evidence of ischemia is observed on an ECG monitor but the person does not complain of anginal symptoms. Silent ischemia can occur in many clinical situations, as described in Box 18-5. One third of patients who are having a heart attack do not report chest pain as a symptom.[3] Diabetic patients are at particular risk from silent ischemia. Many patients who have had type 2 diabetes for over 10 years have developed *autonomic neuropathy,* which decreases their ability to experience chest pain. In addition, diabetic patients may misinterpret angina equivalent symptoms such as nausea, vomiting, and diaphoresis as signaling a disruption in glucose control rather than a sign of myocardial ischemia.[3]

Box 18-6

FACTORS TO CONSIDER WHEN ASSESSING CHEST PAIN

- Onset (Was it sudden or gradual?)
- Duration (Did pain last seconds or minutes? How soon after onset did the patient call for help?)
- Precipitating factors (Was the patient up and moving around?)
- Location (Was pain substernal? Was it located in same area as previous pain?)
- Radiation (Did pain radiate to the jaw, neck, arm, or shoulder?)
- Quality (Was pain similar to previous anginal pain? Less painful or more painful?)
- Intensity (On a scale of 1 to 10, where would the patient rate the pain?)
- Relieving factors (What made the pain better: changing position, nitroglycerin, oxygen, the presence of the nurse?)
- Aggravating factors (Did things such as the environment, telephone calls, or waiting for help worsen the pain?)
- Associated symptoms (Was the pain accompanied by nausea, vomiting, diaphoresis, or dyspnea?)
- Emotional response (Was there an emotional response that intensified the pain: anxiety, fear, anger?)

NURSING DIAGNOSES — Coronary Artery Disease and Angina

- Acute Pain related to transmission and perception of cutaneous, visceral, muscular, or ischemic impulses
- Ineffective Cardiopulmonary Tissue Perfusion related to decreased myocardial oxygen supply and/or increased myocardial oxygen demand
- Activity Intolerance related to cardiopulmonary dysfunction
- Powerlessness related to lack of control over current situation
- Anxiety related to threat to biologic, psychologic, and/or social integrity
- Deficient Knowledge: Discharge Regimen related to lack of previous exposure to information (See Patient Education feature on Coronary Artery Disease and Angina)

MEDICAL MANAGEMENT

Accurate assessment of chest pain symptoms is essential if unstable angina is to be recognized and treated effectively. Factors to consider when assessing chest pain are listed in Box 18-6. An important reason to ask questions about the chest pain is to differentiate between stable and unstable angina. The change from stable to unstable angina is potentially life-threatening for the patient. If the ST segments are elevated or there is a newly documented left bundle branch block on the 12-lead ECG, the patient will be treated for acute MI.[3] However, if these classic ECG signs are missing and the chest pain continues, the current pharmacologic treatments of choice are aspirin, vasodilation by nitroglycerin, intravenous antiplatelet agents such as the glycoprotein (GP) IIb/IIIa-inhibitors and IV infractionated heparin.[33] Low–molecular weight heparin (LMWH) combined with fibrinolysis is an alternative to heparin–fibrinolysis for patients under 75 years of age with a serum creatinine below 2.5 mg/dl for men and below 2 mg/dl for women.[3]

Another option is to take the patient directly to the cardiac catheterization laboratory for direct visualization of the coronary arteries by the cardiologist. Recanalization of the coronary arteries is recommended, provided the institution performs more than 200 procedures annually or the individual physician performs more than 75 interventional procedures annually.[3,33]

NURSING MANAGEMENT

Nursing management of the patient with coronary artery disease and angina incorporates a variety of nursing diagnoses (see the Nursing Diagnosis feature on Coronary Artery Disease and Angina). Nursing interventions focus on early identification of myocardial ischemia, control of chest pain, recognition of complications, maintenance of a calm environment, and patient and family education.

Recognize Myocardial Ischemia. Complaints of chest discomfort (angina) must be evaluated quickly, since angina is an indicator of myocardial ischemia (see Box 18-6). The patient is asked to rate the intensity of the chest discomfort on a scale of 1 to 10. The words "chest pain" are not to be used exclusively, since some patients describe their angina as "pressure" or "heaviness." It is important to document the characteristics of the pain and the patient's heart rate and rhythm, blood pressure, respirations, temperature, skin color, peripheral pulses, urine output, mentation, and overall tissue perfusion. A 12-lead ECG is used to identify the area of ischemic myocardium. The major concern is that the chest pain may represent preinfarction angina, and early identification is essential so that the patient can be immediately treated. This may include transfer to the cardiac catheterization laboratory for a coronary arteriogram and opening of a blocked artery. Or, if the hospital does not have a cardiac catheterization laboratory, GP IIb/IIIa receptor–blockers may be infused to prevent the evolution of the acute MI before transfer.[3,33]

Relieve Chest Pain. In the critical care unit, control of angina is achieved by a combination of supplemental oxygen, nitrates, analgesia, and surveillance of the angina and of the effects of pharmacologic therapy.

1. *Oxygen:* all patients with acute ischemic pain are administered supplemental oxygen to increase myocardial oxygenation. Use of pulse oximetry is recommended to guide therapy and maintain oxygen saturation above 90%.[3] Those patients who develop symptoms of acute heart failure may require emergency intubation and mechanical ventilation to correct significant hypoxemia.[3,33]

2. *Nitrates:* a combination of intravenous and sublingual nitroglycerin is used to vasodilate the coronary arteries and decrease pain. After nitrate administration, the critical care nurse closely observes the patient for relief of chest pain, for return of the ST segment to baseline, and for the potential development of unwanted side effects such as hypotension and headache. Avoid administration of a nitrate if the SBP is below 90 mm Hg or if a male patient has recently taken a phosphodiesterase inhibitor drug (e.g., Viagra).[3,33]

3. *Analgesia:* Morphine 2 to 4 mg IV is the analgesic opiate of choice for preinfarction angina. It both relieves pain and decreases fear and anxiety. After administration, the critical care nurse assesses the patient for pain relief and the development of unwanted side effects such as hypotension and respiratory depression.[3,33]

4. *Aspirin:* Chewing an oral nonenteric-coated aspirin (162 to 325 mg) at the beginning of chest pain has been shown to reduce mortality. The nonenteric formulation is preferred because it increases absorption in the mouth when chewed, not swallowed.[3,33]

Maintain a Calm Environment. Patients admitted to a critical care unit with unstable angina experience extreme anxiety and fear of death. The critical care nurse is faced with the challenge of ensuring that the elements of a calm environment that will alleviate the patient's fear and anxiety are maintained, while being ready at all times to respond to an acute emergency, such as a cardiac arrest, or to assist with emergency intubation or insertion of hemodynamic monitoring catheters. Additional aspects of acute cardiac care are listed in the Nursing Interventions Classification feature on Cardiac Care: Acute.

NIC Cardiac Care: Acute

Definition: Limitation of complications for a patient recently experiencing an episode of an imbalance between myocardial oxygen supply and demand resulting in impaired cardiac function

Activities

Evaluate chest pain (e.g., intensity, location, radiation, duration, and precipitating and alleviating factors)

Provide immediate and continuous means to summon nurse, and let the patient and family know calls will be answered immediately

Monitor cardiac rhythm and rate

Auscultate heart sounds

Recognize the frustration and fright caused by inability to communicate and exposure to strange machinery and environment

Auscultate lungs for crackles or other adventitious sounds

Monitor neurologic status

Monitor intake/output, urine output, and daily weight

Select best ECG lead for continuous monitoring

Obtain 12-lead ECG

Determine cardiac serum biomarkers, CK-MB, or troponins T or I

Monitor kidney function (e.g., blood urea nitrogen and serum creatinine levels)

Monitor liver function (ALT/AST/LDH)

Monitor lab values for electrolytes, which may increase the risk of dysrhythmias (e.g., serum potassium and magnesium)

Obtain chest x-ray

Monitor trends in blood pressure and hemodynamic parameters, if available (e.g., central venous pressure and pulmonary artery occlusion ["wedge"] pressure)

Provide small, frequent meals

Limit intake of caffeine, sodium, cholesterol, food high in fat

Monitor the effectiveness of oxygen therapy

Monitor determinants of oxygen delivery (e.g., PaO_2 and hemoglobin levels and cardiac output)

Maintain an environment conducive to rest and healing

Instruct the patient to avoid activities that result in the Valsalva maneuver (e.g., straining during bowel movement)

Administer medications that will prevent episodes of the Valsalva maneuver (e.g., stool softeners, antiemetics)

Refrain from taking rectal temperatures

Prevent peripheral thrombus formation (e.g., if patient is immobile, turn every 2 hours and administer low-dose anticoagulants)

Administer medications to relieve/prevent pain and ischemia, as needed

Monitor effectiveness of medication

Adapted from Dochterman JM, Bulechek GM: Nursing interventions classification (NIC), ed 4, St Louis, 2004, Mosby.

Patient Education. In the critical care unit, the patient's ability to retain educational information is severely affected by stress and pain. Patient education topics that should be discussed when the clinical condition has stabilized are listed in the Patient Education feature on Coronary Artery Disease and Angina. It is essential to teach avoidance of the *Valsalva maneuver*, which is defined as forced expiration against a closed glottis. This can be explained to the patient as "bearing down" when going to the bathroom or breath-holding when repositioning in bed. The Valsalva maneuver causes an increase in intrathoracic pressure that decreases venous return to the right side of the heart and is associated with low blood pressure and symptomatic bradycardia.

Once the anginal pain is controlled, longer-term patient and family education can begin. Points to cover include risk factor modification, signs and symptoms of angina, when to call the physician, medications, and dealing with emotions and stress. However, because the acute hospital length of stay for uncomplicated angina is usually less than 3 days, referral to a cardiac rehabilitation program for a controlled exercise program and risk factor modification after discharge is perhaps the most helpful teaching intervention a critical care nurse can provide. Clinical practice guidelines for the management of coronary artery disease and stable angina are listed in the Evidence-Based Collaborative Practice feature.

MYOCARDIAL INFARCTION

DESCRIPTION AND ETIOLOGY

Myocardial infarction (MI) is the term used to describe irreversible myocardial necrosis (cell death) that results from an abrupt decrease or total cessation of coronary blood flow to a specific area of the myocardium.[1] In the hospital this is often referred to as an "acute MI," indicating both the sudden onset and the life-threatening nature of the event. Increasingly, an acute MI is described in relation to whether there was ST elevation on the diagnostic 12-lead ECG. Thus it may be labeled a *non–ST elevation acute MI* (NSTEMI),[33] or an a *ST elevation acute MI* (STEMI).[3]

The three mechanisms that block the coronary artery and are responsible for the acute reduction in oxygen delivery to the myocardium are the following:

1. Plaque rupture
2. New coronary artery thrombosis
3. Coronary artery spasm close to the ruptured plaque

Myocardial tissue can best be salvaged within the first 2 hours (120 minutes) after the onset of anginal symptoms as illustrated in Fig. 18-2.[3] The earlier the myocardium is revascularized, the better the survival.[33] Unfortunately, many persons do not seek treatment until the acute phase has passed.[3]

PATHOPHYSIOLOGY

Ischemia. The outer region of the infracted myocardial area is the *zone of ischemia*, as illustrated in Fig. 18-3. It is composed of viable cells. Priority interventions are targeted to save this viable muscle. Repolarization in this zone is temporarily impaired but eventually will be restored to normal. Repolarization of the cells in this area manifests as T-wave inversion (Fig. 18-4, *B*).

Injury. The infarcted zone is surrounded by injured but still potentially viable tissue in an area known as the *zone of injury* (see Fig. 18-3). Cells in this area do not fully repolarize because of the deficient blood supply. This is recorded on the ECG as elevation of the ST segment (Fig. 18-4, *C*).

PATIENT EDUCATION

Coronary Artery Disease and Angina

- Angina: describe signs and symptoms such as pain, pressure, and heaviness in chest, arms, or jaw
- Preinfarction or unstable angina: any chest pain that is not relieved within 5 min by a sublingual nitroglycerin (NTG) tablet provides reason to call 911 (emergency services)
- Use of the pain scale from 1 to 10: notify critical care nurse or emergency personnel of any changes in pain intensity
- Use of sublingual NTG for angina: pain intensity should decrease on the pain scale after NTG administration. At home, NTG must be kept in a dark, air-tight container, or it loses its potency. To ensure potency, the NTG supply must be replaced about every 6 months. Active NTG has a slight burning sensation when placed under the tongue.
- Avoidance of the Valsalva maneuver
- Risk factor modification tailored to the patient's individual risk factor profile:
  —Decrease fat intake to 30% of total calories a day
  —Stop smoking
  —Reduce salt intake
  —Control hypertension
  —Treat diabetes and control blood glucose levels, if patient is diabetic
  —Increase physical activity; achieve ideal body weight
- Refer to cardiac rehabilitation program
- Medication teaching: indications, side effects
- Follow-up care after discharge
- Symptoms to report to a health care professional
- Discuss how to handle emotional stress and anger

EVIDENCE-BASED COLLABORATIVE MANAGEMENT
Coronary Artery Disease and Stable Angina

Summary of Evidence-Based Recommendations for Management of Coronary Artery Disease and Stable Angina

Strong Evidence the Following Lifestyle Interventions Are Helpful To Prevent CAD
- Diet
  —Low-salt, high-fiber, fruit, vegetables, grains
  —All dietary fat less than 30% of total calories
  —Multivitamin if homocysteine level elevated
  —Limit sugary foods
  —Limit calories if overweight
  —Omega-3 fatty acids included in diet
- Exercise
  —Start by walking, more and increase physical exercise from there
  —Refer to cardiac rehabilitation program
- Obesity
  —Achieve healthy body weight
- Addiction
  —Stop cigarette smoking
  —Limit alcohol intake

Strong Evidence the Following Diagnostic Procedures Are Helpful for the Patient With Angina:
- When a patient is first seen with chest pain, quickly obtaining a detailed history of symptoms, focused physical examination, and risk factor assessment can help determine whether the probability of coronary artery disease (CAD) is low, intermediate, or high.
- Initial laboratory tests include hemoglobin, fasting blood glucose, lipid panel.
- Baseline 12-lead ECG at rest, even if chest pain not present.
- Obtain 12-lead ECG during any episode of chest pain.
- Chest x-ray if symptoms of heart failure are present.
- Exercise 12-lead ECG if condition stable and symptoms suggestive of CAD; or if condition stable with complete right bundle branch block or complete left bundle branch block that makes the ECG difficult to interpret for ischemia.
- Cardiac echocardiography for patients with a systolic murmur suggestive of aortic stenosis
- Cardiac echocardiography to determine extent of left ventricular (LV) hypertrophy or dysfunction
- Stress cardiac echocardiography recommended for patient with greater than 1 mm ST-segment depression at rest (stress may be by physical exercise or by pharmacologic stimulation)

- Coronary angiography (typically as part of a cardiac catheterization procedure) is recommended for patients at high risk of adverse coronary events

Initial Pharmacologic and Lifestyle Treatment Recommendations
- The goal of treatment is to eliminate chest pain.
- The ten most important elements of CAD and stable angina management can be remembered using the A-to-E mnemonic:
  A   Aspirin and anti-anginals
  B   Beta-blocker and blood pressure
  C   Cholesterol and cigarettes
  D   Diet and diabetes
  E   Education and exercise

The above translates to the following: daily (low-dose) 75-325 mg aspirin; oral nitrates, sublingual nitroglycerin for episodes of angina; beta-blockers to decrease LV workload and decrease blood pressure to less than 130/80 mm Hg; and diet or lipid reduction drug therapy (statin) to lower low-density lipoprotein cholesterol (LDL-C) to below 100 mg/dl (LDL-C to below 70 mg/dl if patient at very high risk), increase HDL-C above 40 mg/dl for men, and above 50 mg/dl for women, and reduce triglycerides below 150 mg/dl. Always ask about tobacco use, recommend strongly stopping smoking, encourage nicotine replacement therapy (nicotine patches or gum) as needed; low fat, calorie appropriate diet, nutritional consult as needed; fasting blood glucose 70-100 mg/dl; hemoglobin $A1_C$ below 7%; education about risk factor modification and the CAD disease process; recommend daily exercise for 30-60 minutes (ideal) or at least 3-4 times a week; achieve a BMI between 18.5-24.9 kg/m^2, waist less than 40 inches for men and 35 inches for women. Treat depression if present, hormone replacement therapy is not recommended as a treatment for symptoms of coronary heart disease.

Interventional vs. Surgical Recommendations for Stable High-Risk Patients
Patients are "risk stratified" according to their symptoms and the results of cardiac diagnostic tests.
- Percutaneous catheter interventions (PCI)
  —Angioplasty, atherectomy, stent
  —PCI is more frequently performed than open heart surgery for relief of anginal symptoms
- Coronary artery bypass surgery
  —For patients with left main occlusion or multivessel disease
  —For patients with two-vessel disease with significant proximal LAD stenosis and LV ejection fraction below 50%.

From Gibbons RJ et al: ACC/AHA 2002 guideline update for the management of patients with chronic stable angina-summary article, *Circulation* 107(1):149-158, 2003; and Mosca L et al: Evidence-based guidelines for cardiovascular disease prevention in women, *Circulation* 109(5):672-693, 2004.

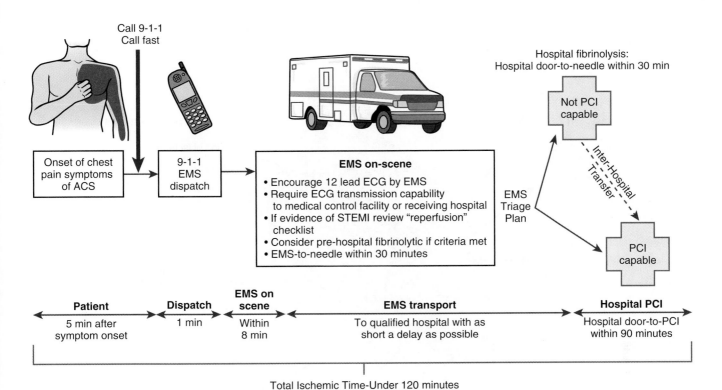

Fig. 18-2   Prehospital Chest Pain/ACS Evaluation and Treatment Options. (Adapted from Antman EM et al: ACC/AHA guidelines for the management of patients with ST-elevation myocardial infarction—executive summary: a report of the American College of Cardiology/American Heart Association Task Force on Practice Guidelines (Writing Committee to Revise the 1999 Guidelines for the Management of Patients with Acute Myocardial Infarction), *Circulation* 110(5):588-636, 2004.)

Infarction. The area of dead muscle (necrosis) in the myocardium is known as the *zone of infarction* (Fig. 18-3). On the ECG, evidence of this zone is seen by new pathologic Q waves, which reflect a lack of depolarization from the cardiac surface involved in the MI (Fig. 18-4, *D*). As healing takes place, the cells in this area are replaced by scar tissue.

Transmural MI or Q-Wave MI. Myocardial infarctions are classified according to their location on the myocardial surface and the muscle layers affected. Not all infarctions cause necrosis in all layers, as shown in Fig. 18-5. A transmural MI involves all three cardiac layers—the *endocardium*, the *myocardium*, and the *epicardium*. A transmural (full thickness) MI usually provokes significant ECG changes, as shown in Fig. 18-4. This is also described as a *Q-wave MI.* It is important to be aware that not every acute MI produces a recognizable series of Q waves on the 12-lead ECG. In addition, some patients who had a demonstrated Q wave on a 12-lead ECG as a result of an acute MI lose the Q wave months or years later. The reasons for this are not yet known, but it may represent the development of collateral circulation.

12-Lead ECG Changes. The ECG changes produced by a transmural infarction demonstrate alteration in both myocardial depolarization (QRS complex) and repolarization (ST segment). The changes in repolarization are seen by the presence of new Q waves. These new, pathologic Q waves are deeper and wider than tiny q waves found on the normal 12-lead ECG.[3]

MI Location. The location of infarction is determined by correlating the ECG leads with Q waves and the ST-segment T-wave abnormalities (Table 18-8). Infarction most commonly affects the left ventricle and the interventricular septum; however, the right ventricle can also be infracted and many patients who sustain an inferior MI have some right ventricular damage. The ECG manifestations that are used to diagnose an MI and pinpoint the area of damaged ventricle include inverted T waves, ST-segment elevation, and pathologic Q waves in specific lead groupings as described below.

Anterior Wall Infarction. Anterior wall infarction results from occlusion of the proximal left anterior descending (LAD) artery (see Table 18-8). ST-segment elevation is expected in leads V_1 through V_4 on the 12-lead ECG as shown in Fig. 18-6. If the left main coronary ar-

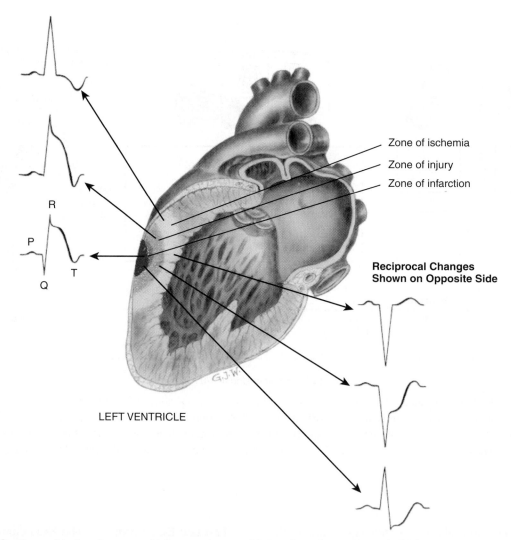

P R Q T

LEFT VENTRICLE

Zone of ischemia
Zone of injury
Zone of infarction

Reciprocal Changes
Shown on Opposite Side

Fig. 18-3   Zone of ischemia, zone of injury, and zone of infarction, shown through ECG waveforms and reciprocal waveforms corresponding to each zone.

Table 18-8	Correlations Among Ventricular Surfaces, Electrocardiographic Leads, and Coronary Arteries	
Surface of Left Ventricle	**ECG Leads**	**Coronary Artery Usually Involved**
Inferior	II, III, aV$_F$	Right coronary artery
Lateral	V$_5$-V$_6$, I, aV$_L$	Left circumflex
Anterior	V$_2$-V$_4$	Left anterior descending
Anterior lateral	V$_1$-V$_6$, I, aV$_L$	Left main coronary artery
Septal	V$_1$-V$_2$	Left anterior descending
Posterior	V$_1$-V$_2$ V$_7$-V$_9$ (direct)	Left circumflex or right coronary artery (reciprocal changes)

I lateral	aVR	V$_1$ septal	V$_4$ anterior
II inferior	aVL lateral	V$_2$ septal	V$_5$ lateral
III inferior	aVF inferior	V$_3$ anterior	V$_6$ lateral

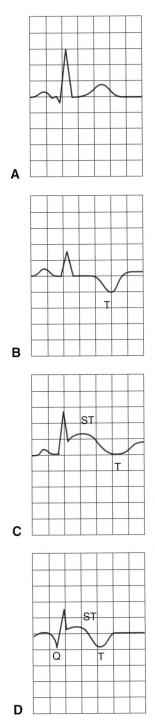

A

B

C

D

Fig. 18-4 ECG changes indicative of ischemia, injury, and infarction (necrosis) of the myocardium. **A,** Normal ECG. **B,** Ischemia indicated by inversion of the T wave. **C,** Ischemia and current of injury indicated by T-wave inversion and ST-segment elevation. The ST segment may be elevated above or depressed below the baseline, depending on whether the tracing is from a lead facing toward or away from the infarcted area and depending on whether epicardial or endocardial injury occurs. Epicardial injury causes ST elevation in leads facing the epicardium. **D,** Ischemia, injury, and myocardial necrosis. The Q wave indicates necrosis of the myocardium.

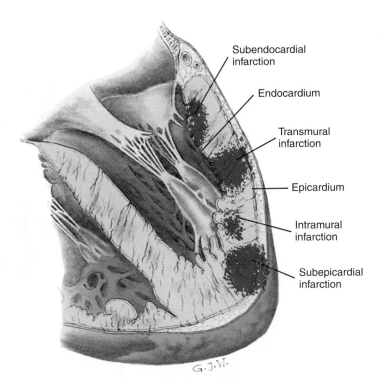

Fig. 18-5 Location of infarctions in myocardium.

tery is occluded, the ECG manifestations will involve almost all of the precordial leads V_1-V_6 and leads I and aV_L (see Table 18-8). These specific groups of ECG changes that help to locate the part of the heart that is infarcting are termed *indicative changes.* A large anterior wall MI may be associated with left ventricular (LV) pump failure, cardiogenic shock, or death.[3]

Left Lateral Wall Infarction. Left lateral wall infarction occurs as a result of occlusion of the circumflex coronary artery. On a 12-lead ECG, new Q waves and ST-segment T-wave changes are seen in leads I, aV_L, V_5, and V_6 as shown in Fig. 18-7. In reality, few patients present with only lateral wall ECG changes, and some anterior wall leads (V_3 and V_4) may also show evidence of injury or infarction.

Inferior Wall Infarction. Inferior wall infarction occurs with occlusion of the right coronary artery (RCA). This infarction is manifested by ECG changes in leads II, III, and aV_F as shown in Fig 18-8. Conduction disturbances are expected with an inferior wall MI and are related to the anatomy of the coronary arterial supply. Because the RCA perfuses the sinoatrial (SA) node in just over half of the population and also supplies the proximal bundle of His and atrioventricular (AV) node in over 90% of individuals, heart block and other conduction disturbances should be anticipated. Inferior wall MI carries a mortality of about 6%. If the right ventricle is involved, mortality rises to 25% to 30%.[3]

Right Ventricular Infarction. Infarction of the right ventricle (RV) occurs when there is a blockage in a

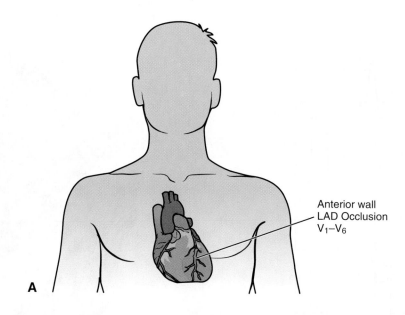

Anterior wall
LAD Occlusion
V_1–V_6

A

LIMB LEADS   PRECORDIAL LEADS

Lead I	AV_R	V_1	V_4
Lead II	AV_L	V_2	V_5
Lead III	AV_F	V_3	V_6

B

Example of an Acute Anterior Wall MI

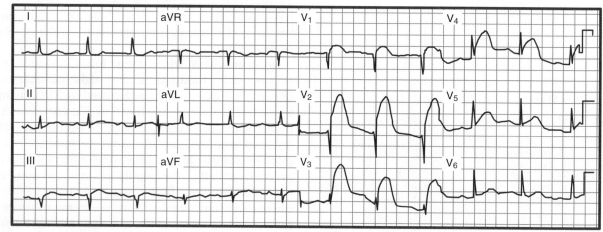

C

Fig. 18-6   12-lead ECG—Changes with anterior wall STEMI. **A,** MI location on cardiac wall. **B,** ECG leads with expected ST-segment elevation. **C,** 12-lead ECG from patient experiencing left anterior wall STEMI.

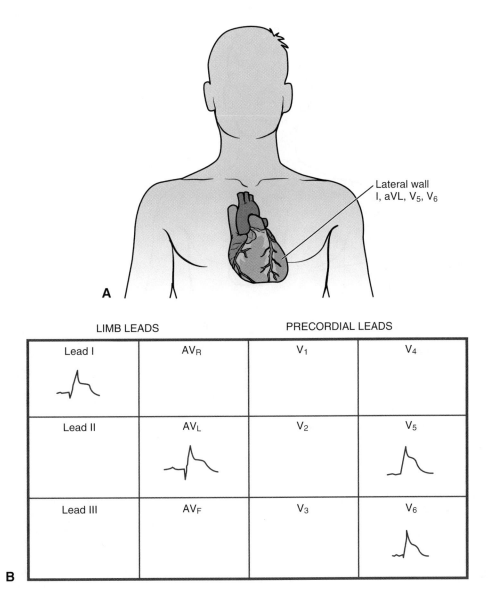

Lateral wall
I, aVL, V$_5$, V$_6$

A

LIMB LEADS		PRECORDIAL LEADS	
Lead I	AV$_R$	V$_1$	V$_4$
Lead II	AV$_L$	V$_2$	V$_5$
Lead III	AV$_F$	V$_3$	V$_6$

B

Fig. 18-7 12-lead ECG—Changes with lateral wall STEMI. **A,** MI location on cardiac wall. **B,** ECG leads with expected ST-segment elevation.

proximal section of the right coronary artery. This places all of the right ventricle and the inferior wall at risk. RV ischemia can be demonstrated in up to half of inferior wall STEMIs, although only 10% to 15% show the hemodynamic abnormalities associated with classic RV infarction.[3] If massive RV infarction occurs the patient can suffer cardiogenic shock, which carries over 50% mortality in this population.[38]

To detect a RV infarct, specific ECG lead placement is used. Electrodes are placed over the right precordium (chest) in a mirror image of the conventional left-sided leads. It is important to write R on the 12-lead ECG (for example: V$_1$R = V$_6$R) in front of all of the recorded RV chest leads to ensure that the lead location is clear. The

limb leads are not affected. See Fig. 17-7, *C,* for the correct position of the right-sided precordial leads to diagnose an acute RV MI.[39] The ECG voltage is much lower in the V$_1$R = V$_6$R leads, and ST elevation when it is detected is usually seen in V$_4$R as shown in Fig. 18-9. The RV has a very thin wall, which means that ST elevation is only detected in the RV leads during the acute phase of the infarction.[3]

Posterior Wall Infarction. Infarction in the posterior wall can occur because of a blockage either in the right coronary artery or in the circumflex artery. This is because both arteries supply this section of the heart, although the RCA is generally the dominant vessel. A posterior wall MI is difficult to detect but may be identified by

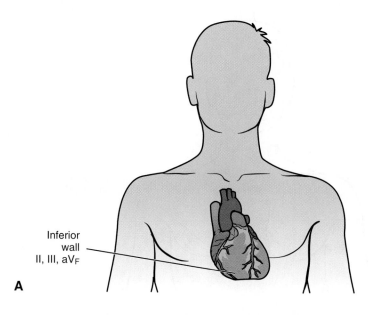

A

LIMB LEADS   PRECORDIAL LEADS

Lead I	aV$_R$	V$_1$	V$_4$
Lead II	aV$_L$	V$_2$	V$_5$
Lead III	aV$_F$	V$_3$	V$_6$

B

Example of an Acute Inferior Wall MI

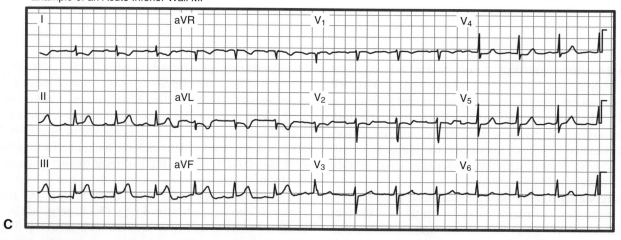

C

Fig. 18-8 12-lead ECG—Changes with inferior wall STEMI. **A,** MI location on cardiac wall. **B,** ECG leads with expected ST-segment elevation. **C,** 12-lead ECG from patient experiencing inferior wall STEMI.

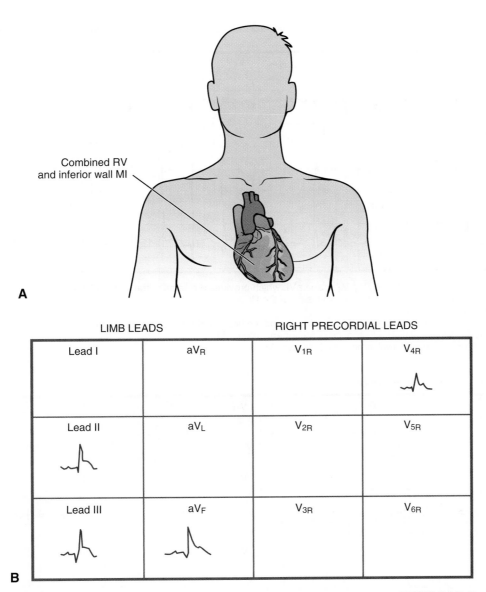

Fig. 18-9 12-lead ECG—Changes with inferior-right ventricular STEMI. **A,** Picture of RV Wall MI. **B,** Acute inferior wall MI (RCA occluded).

Continued

either specific leads placed in the left scapular area or by very tall R waves in leads V_1 and V_2, as shown in Fig. 18-10. See Fig. 17-7, *D*, for the correct placement of the left posterior leads used to diagnose an acute posterior MI.

Non–ST Segment Elevation MI. The 12-lead ECG is a highly useful diagnostic tool. For many years it was considered the "gold standard" when diagnosing an acute MI. Now it is known that the *ST segment* is not elevated in every acute MI. One reason for the lack of ST-segment elevation may be that the infarction and subsequent necrosis are not full-thickness. Because some of the muscle in the area can still be depolarized, ST elevation may not occur. This type of MI is also less likely to develop Q waves on a subsequent 12-lead ECG once the acute phase has passed. This situation is diagnostically

known as a *Non–ST Segment Elevation MI* (NSTEMI).[33] This condition has previously been described by several names including *nontransmural MI; non–Q-wave MI* or *subendocardial MI.* Because patients who sustain a NSTEMI do have CAD it is important that they be treated aggressively to minimize the size of the infarcted area. Without the visual clue of the ST-segment elevation on the 12-lead ECG, the patients cannot receive immediate IV fibrinolytic agents, but they can be appropriately managed in an interventional catheterization laboratory and receive GPIIb/IIIa-inhibitor therapy as illustrated in the timeline in Fig. 18-2. The 12-lead ECG plays a vital role in identifying the treatment plan for an acute coronary syndrome. ST elevation is helpful when present, but it would be a mistake to believe that if the ST is not elevated the

Example of an Acute Inferior Wall and RV Wall MI, Shows ST elevation in leads II, III, AVF and reciprocal changes (ST depression) in anterior and lateral leads.

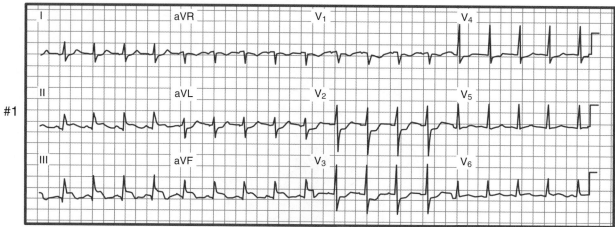

Reciprocal changes seen in V$_1$, V$_2$, V$_3$, V$_4$, I, and aVL which provides a clue as to the extent of the MI.
Angiographic changes associated with an occlusion of the RCA.
These findings can range from:
- Proximal occlusion (near origin of RCA) which will produce both inferior MI, posterior MI and RV MI
- Middle RCA occlusion which will produce posterior and inferior MI
- Distal RCA occlusion which will produce inferior wall MI

C

Example of an Acute RV MI in right precordial leads.

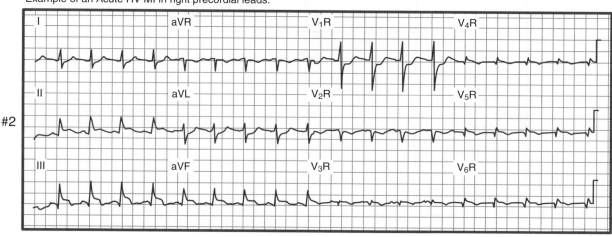

ECG shows ST elevation in right precordial leads (V$_3$R to V$_6$R) indicating RV wall injury/infarct.
Note limb leads are identical in both ECGs.

D   **These two 12-lead ECGs are from the same patient with RV MI**

Fig. 18-9, cont'd   C, Example of an acute inferior RV wall MI with conventional 12 lead. **D,** Example of an acute RV wall MI with right-sided 12-lead ECG. Both 12-lead ECGs are taken from the same patient.

patient is not in danger of myocardial infarction, as shown in Fig. 18-11. In this case the definitive diagnosis may be made either in the cardiac catheterization laboratory or by elevation of specific cardiac biomarkers.

Cardiac Biomarkers during MI. In the presence of damaged or necrosed myocardial muscle cells, cardiac biomarkers are released. These biomarkers are also called "cardiac enzymes." To confirm the diagnosis of acute MI, the serum biomarkers CK-MB and either tro-

ponin I or troponin T are measured. If the coronary artery is opened by fibrinolytic therapy or a percutaneous catheter intervention (PCI) the biomarkers exhibit a more rapid rise and dramatic fall as shown in Fig. 18-12. Information on biomarkers is also shown in Table 17-1.

Complications with Acute MI. Many patients experience complications occurring either early or late in the postinfarction course. These complications may result from electrical dysfunction or from a pump problem.

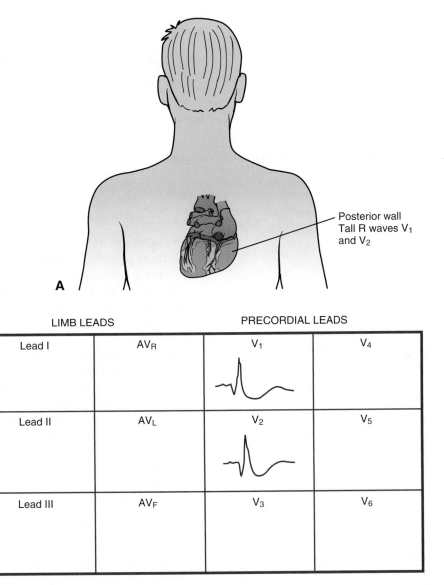

Fig. 18-10   12-lead ECG—Changes with STEMI. **A,** MI location on cardiac wall. **B,** ECG leads with expected ST-segment elevation in posterior wall STEMI.

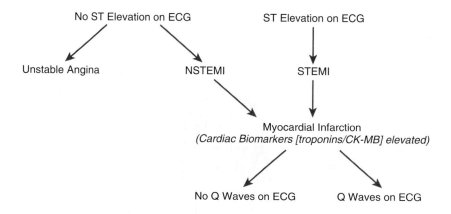

Fig. 18-11 Acute coronary syndrome. Adapted from Braunwald E et al.: *Circulation* 106(14):1893-1900, 2002. Full text available online at http://www.ahajournals.org.

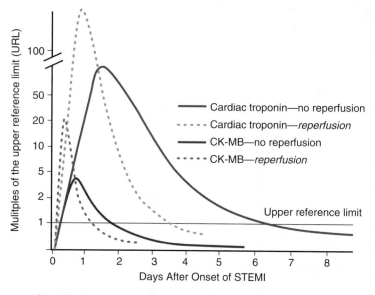

Fig. 18-12 Cardiac biomarkers during MI. (From ACC/AHA guidelines for the management of patients with ST-elevation myocardial infarction—executive summary: a report of the American College of Cardiology/American Heart Association Task Force on Practice Guidelines [Writing Committee to Revise the 1999 Guidelines for the Management of Patients with Acute Myocardial Infarction], *Circulation* 110[9]:e82-292, 2004).

Electrical dysfunctions include bradycardia, bundle branch blocks, and varying degrees of heart block. Pumping complications cause heart failure, pulmonary edema, and cardiogenic shock.[3]

Sinus Bradycardia and Sinus Tachycardia. Sinus bradycardia (heart rate less than 60 beats/min) oc-

curs in 30% to 40% of patients who sustain an acute MI.[3] It is more prevalent with an inferior wall infarction in the first hour following STEMI.[3] Symptomatic bradycardia with hypotension and low cardiac output is treated with atropine 0.6 to 1.0 mg IV push, repeated every 5 minutes to a maximum dose of 0.04 mg/kg (e.g., 2 mg for a person who weighs 50 kg).[3]

Sinus Tachycardia. Sinus tachycardia (heart rate more than 100 beats/min) most often occurs with an anterior wall MI. Anterior infarctions impair left ventricular pumping ability, thereby reducing the ejection fraction and the stroke volume. In an attempt to maintain cardiac output, the heart rate increases. Sinus tachycardia must be corrected, because it greatly increases myocardial oxygen consumption leading to further ischemia.

Atrial Dysrhythmias. Premature atrial contractions (PACs) occur frequently in patients who sustain an acute myocardial infarction. Atrial fibrillation is also common and may occur spontaneously or be preceded by PACs. With onset of atrial fibrillation the loss of organized atrial contraction decreases cardiac output by up to 20%. A global registry of patients with acute coronary syndrome (ACS) found that almost 8% of ACS patients have preexisting atrial fibrillation, while just over 6% develop new-onset atrial fibrillation during their hospitalization for ACS.[40] Patients with atrial fibrillation—both new-onset and preexisting—have higher morbidity than patients without atrial fibrillation during an acute coronary syndrome. Specifically, ACS patients with new-onset atrial fibrillation experience a greater number of in-hospital adverse events such as reinfarction, shock, pulmonary edema, bleeding, and stroke.[40] Atrial

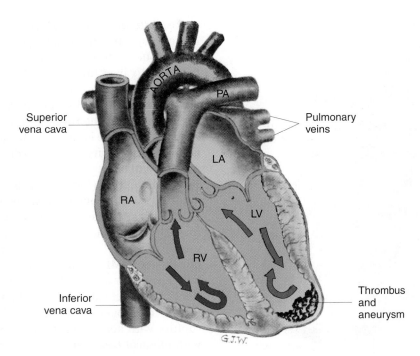

Fig. 18-13 Ventricular aneurysm after acute myocardial infarction (MI). *PA,* Pulmonary artery; *LA,* left atrium; *RA,* right atrium; *LV,* left ventricle; *RV,* right ventricle.

fibrillation during the hospitalization significantly affects risk of death in the setting of an acute MI; it increases in-hospital mortality by 20% and long-term mortality by 34%.[3]

Ventricular Dysrhythmias. Premature ventricular contractions (PVCs) are seen in almost all patients within the first few hours after a myocardial infarction. They are initially controlled by administering oxygen to reduce myocardial hypoxia and by correcting acid-base or electrolyte imbalances. In the setting of an acute MI, PVCs are pharmacologically treated if they have the following characteristics: frequent (more than 6 per minute), closely coupled (R-on-T phenomenon), multiform in shape, and occur in bursts of three or more, increasing the risk of sustained ventricular tachycardia. Ventricular fibrillation (VF) is a life-threatening dysrhythmia associated with high mortality in acute MI. Increasingly, β-blockers are prescribed after an acute MI to decrease mortality from ventricular dysrhythmias.[3]

AV Heart Block During MI. Heart block occurs in 6% to 14% of patients with STEMI, and those patients have increased mortality.[3] In STEMI, AV block most often occurs after an inferior wall infarction. Because the right coronary artery supplies the AV node in 90% of the population, RCA occlusion leads to ischemia and infarction of the AV node cells. The development of sudden heart block is much less common now that most patients receive fibrinolysis or PCI to open the occluded vessel. In the majority of cases, transcutaneous pacing is the primary intervention; transvenous pacemakers are used less frequently.[3]

Ventricular Aneurysm After MI. A ventricular aneurysm (Fig. 18-13) is a noncontractile, thinned left ventricular wall, which results from an acute transmural infarction. It most often occurs in the setting of an acute left anterior descending (LAD) artery occlusion with a wide area of infarcted myocardium.[3] The most effective prevention is early reperfusion of the myocardium, accomplished by opening the thrombosed coronary artery. In one study the rate of ventricular aneurysm was reduced from 18% in untreated patients to 7% when the coronary artery was opened by fibrinolysis.[3] The most common complications of a ventricular aneurysm are acute heart failure, systemic emboli, angina, and ventricular tachycardia (VT). Treatment is directed toward management of these complications and surgical repair by left ventricular aneurysmectomy. The affected area may be described as hypokinetic (contracts poorly), *akinetic* (noncontractile scar tissue), or *dyskinetic* (scar tissue that moves in the opposite direction to the normal contractile myocardium). The prognosis depends on the size of the aneurysm, the level of overall left ventricular dysfunction, and the severity of coexisting CAD.

Ventricular Septal Rupture After MI. Postinfarction rupture of the ventricular septal wall is a rare but potentially lethal complication of an acute anterior wall MI. (Fig. 18-14). *Ventricular septal rupture,* also known as *acquired ventricular septal defect* (VSD) is an abnormal communication between the right and left ventricle. This complication occurs in less than 1% of all myocardial infarctions, and the incidence has declined, since most STEMI patients have the blocked coronary artery

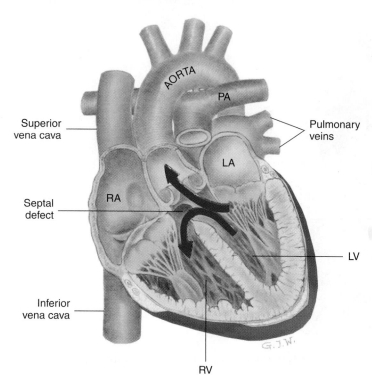

Fig. 18-14 Ventricular septal rupture after acute myocardial infarction (MI). See Fig. 18-13 for explanation of abbreviations.

opened.[3] Nevertheless, rupture of the ventricular septum carries an extremely high mortality.[41] Reports of 35% to 73% mortality are typical.[42,43] Most patients with septal rupture also have signs and symptoms of cardiogenic shock. Ventricular septal rupture manifests as severe chest pain, syncope, hypotension, and sudden hemodynamic deterioration caused by shunting of blood from the high-pressure left ventricle into the low-pressure right ventricle through the new septal opening. A holosystolic murmur (often accompanied by a thrill) can be auscultated and is best heard along the left sternal border. A diagnosis of postinfarction ventricular septal rupture can be made at the bedside with use of oxygen saturation assessment via a pulmonary artery catheter or by transesophageal echocardiography (TEE). Rupture of the septum is a medical and surgical emergency. The patient's condition is stabilized with vasodilators and an intraaortic balloon pump (IABP) to decrease afterload.[43] The goal of afterload reduction in this patient population is to decrease the amount of blood being shunted to the right side of the heart and consequently to increase the flow of blood to the systemic circulation. If the septal rupture is very small, and the patient's condition is sufficiently stable to wait for scar tissue to form before surgical repair, survival improves. Unfortunately, when the septal opening is large, the massive left to right shunt across the septum makes the chances of survival dismal with or without surgery.[42,43]

Papillary Muscle Rupture After MI. Papillary muscle rupture can occur when the infarct involves the area around one of the papillary muscles that support the mitral valve. Infarction of the papillary muscles results in ineffective mitral valve closure, and blood is forced back into the low-pressure left atrium during ventricular systole. The rupture may be partial or complete. Complete rupture is catastrophic and precipitates severe acute mitral regurgitation, cardiogenic shock, and high risk of death.

Partial rupture (Fig. 18-15) also results in mitral regurgitation, but the condition can be stabilized with aggressive medical management using the IABP and vasodilators. Urgent surgical intervention is required to replace the mitral valve.[44] As with other structural complications during acute MI, the incidence is decreased in patients who have their myocardium reperfused early.[3] Of the patients with acute MI who are admitted to the critical care unit in cardiogenic shock, 10% have papillary muscle rupture with acute mitral regurgitation. Mortality is 71% with medical treatment, and 40% with surgical intervention to replace or repair the mitral valve.[3]

Cardiac Wall Rupture After MI. Of the deaths that occur after myocardial infarction, 1% to 6% can be attributed to cardiac rupture.[3] Cardiac wall rupture has two peak times of incidence. The first occurs within the first 24 hours and the second between the third and fifth postinfarction day when leukocyte scavenger cells are removing necrotic debris, thus thinning the myocardial wall.[3] The onset is sudden and usually catastrophic. Bleeding into the pericardial sac results in cardiac tamponade, cardiogenic shock, pulseless electrical activity (PEA), and death. Survival is rare. If rupture occurs in the hospital, emergency pericardiocentesis is required to relieve the tamponade until a surgical repair can be attempted. The best prevention is early reperfusion of the myocardium.[3]

Pericarditis After MI. Pericarditis is inflammation of the pericardial sac. It can occur during a transmural MI or after an acute MI. Pericarditis may occur in 5% to 20% of transmural infarctions, but is only treated if it is clinically significant.[45] The damaged epicardium becomes rough and inflamed and irritates the pericardium lying adjacent to it, precipitating pericarditis. Pain is the most common symptom of pericarditis, and a pericardial friction rub is the most common initial sign. The friction rub is best auscultated with a stethoscope at the sternal border and is described as a grating, scraping, or leathery scratching. Pericarditis frequently produces a pericardial effusion.[45] Once the effusion (fluid) occurs, the friction rub may disappear. On the 12-lead ECG, pericarditis may manifest as elevation of the ST segment in all of the typically upright leads.[46] Pericarditis is treated with nonsteroidal antiinflammatory drugs. Pericarditis that occurs as a late complication of acute MI is known as *Dressler's syndrome.*[45,47]

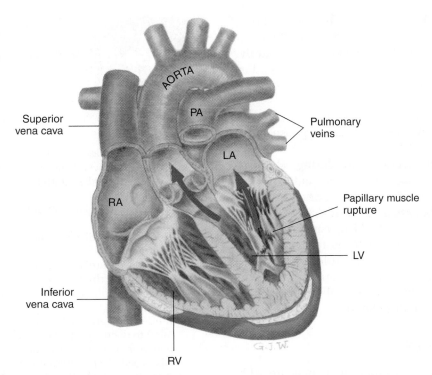

Fig. 18-15 Papillary muscle rupture after acute myocardial infarction (MI). See Fig. 18-13 for explanation of abbreviations.

Heart Failure and Acute MI. Almost 20% of patients with acute STEMI also have acute heart failure on admission to the hospital. These patients have often waited longer to come to the hospital and are older and more likely to be female. Compared with acute MI patients without heart failure, these patients have a higher risk of adverse in-hospital events and have longer lengths of stay and higher in-hospital mortality.[48] More detailed information about heart failure is presented later in this chapter on p. 459.

MEDICAL MANAGEMENT

Quality outcomes research shows that compliance with the recent research guidelines developed by the American College of Cardiology and the American Heart Association (ACC/AHA) decreases in-hospital mortality following acute MI.[49,50] Patients admitted to hospitals that adhere to the AHA/ACC guidelines for treatment of either STEMI or NSTEMI have 8.3% in-hospital mortality compared with 15.3% mortality for patients managed at hospitals where the most recent guidelines are not fully used.[49,50] The guidelines are research-based and are designed to improve the outcome of patients admitted to the hospital with an acute MI. Clinical guidelines address the issues of interventions to open the coronary artery, anticoagulation, prevention of dysrhythmias, tight glucose control, and prevention of ventricular remodeling following STEMI.[3]

Recanalization of the Coronary Artery. The essential immediate interventions are either fibrinolytic therapy or percutaneous coronary intervention (PCI) to open the occluded artery for the patient with an acute STEMI.[3] All clinical guidelines emphasize the need for patients with symptoms of acute coronary syndrome to be rapidly triaged and treated.[3]

Anticoagulation. In the acute phase following an STEMI, if the patient has not received fibrinolytic therapy or PCI to recanalize (open) the coronary artery, anticoagulation with heparin is required.[3] It is also prudent to administer IV unfractionated heparin (UFH), or subcutaneous (SQ) low–molecular weight heparin (LMWH) if the person is at risk for thrombus development.[3] Patients at risk for thrombotic emboli include those with an anterior wall infarction, atrial fibrillation, previous embolus, cardiomyopathy, or cardiogenic shock. An initial heparin bolus of 60 units/kilogram IV followed by a continuous heparin drip at 12 units/kg/hour to maintain an activated partial thromboplastin time (aPTT) between 50 and 70 seconds (1.5 to 2.0 times control) is recommended. Alternatively LMWH may be used at doses that will provide full anticoagulation.[3] When the risk of systemic embolic complications remains high, especially in atrial fibrillation, the patient should be anticoagulated with warfarin (Coumadin).[3]

Dysrhythmia Prevention. The antidysrhythmic with the best safety record following STEMI is amiodarone. The reduction in death related to decreased dysrhythmias after MI is 13%.[3] Beta-blockers are another class of antidysrhythmics that are recommended for all patients following STEMI. Beta-blockers prevent ventricular dysrhythmias, lower blood pressure, and prevent reinfarction, especially in patients with left ventricular dysfunction.[3]

Tight Glucose Control. Achievement of normal serum blood glucose both during the acute phase and after MI improves survival.[3]

Prevention of Ventricular Remodeling. Many patients are at risk for development of heart failure following STEMI. The category of vasodilating drugs known as *angiotensin-converting enzyme inhibitors* (ACEIs) or angiotensin receptor–blockers (ARB) can stop or limit the ventricular remodeling that leads to heart failure. Either an ACEI drug or, if this not tolerated, an ARB medication is indicated for all patients following STEMI.[3] Information about the clinical effects of heart failure is covered later in this chapter.

NURSING MANAGEMENT

Nursing management of the patient with an acute MI incorporates a variety of nursing diagnoses (see the Nursing Diagnoses feature on Myocardial Infarction). Nursing interventions focus on achieving a balance among myocardial oxygen supply and demand, preventing complications, and providing patient and family education.

Balance of Myocardial Oxygen Supply and Demand. In the acute period, if severe heart muscle damage has occurred, myocardial oxygen supply is increased by the administration of supplemental oxygen to prevent tissue hypoxia. Many clinical signs manifest this imbalance (Box 18-7). Drugs play an increasingly important role in balancing supply and demand, and it is the critical care nurse who both administers and monitors the effectiveness of these agents. For the patient with a low cardiac output, positive inotropic drugs such as dobutamine, dopamine, and milrinone are prescribed. These inotropic agents are used to increase cardiac contractility in the healthy areas of the heart (thus increasing oxygen supply), while avoiding damage to the recently infarcted areas. Myocardial oxygen supply can be further enhanced by the use of coronary artery vasodilators. Nitroglycerin is recommended for the first 48 hours to increase vasodilation and prevent myocardial ischemia.[3] Research evidence supports the administration of early β-blockade therapy to decrease myocardial workload and to prevent dysrhythmias. Administration of β-blockade reduces mortality by 14% in the first 7 days after an MI, and by 23% long-term.[3] However, if the patient is in cardiogenic shock, β-blockers are held until the cardiac output has improved.[3] Other interventions to decrease cardiac work and myocardial oxygen consumption include bed rest with bedside commode privileges when the patient is clinically stable.

NURSING DIAGNOSES **Myocardial Infarction**

- Acute Pain related to transmission and perception of cutaneous, visceral, muscular, or ischemic impulses
- Decreased Cardiac Output related to alterations in preload
- Decreased Cardiac Output related to alterations in afterload
- Decreased Cardiac Output related to alterations in contractility
- Decreased Cardiac Output related to alterations in heart rate or rhythm
- Activity Intolerance related to cardiopulmonary dysfunction
- Ineffective Cardiopulmonary Tissue Perfusion related to decreased myocardial oxygen supply and/or increased myocardial oxygen demand
- Disturbed Sleep Pattern related to fragmented sleep
- Anxiety related to threat to biologic, psychologic, and/or social integrity
- Ineffective Coping related to situational crisis and personal vulnerability
- Powerlessness related to lack of control over current situation or disease progression
- Deficient Knowledge: Discharge Regimen related to lack of previous exposure to information (See Patient Education feature on Myocardial Infarction)

Prevention of Complications. A thorough grasp of the range of potential complications that can occur following STEMI is essential. Cardiac monitoring for early detection of ventricular dysrhythmias is ongoing. Assessment for signs of continued ischemic pain is important, because angina is a warning sign of myocardium at risk. In response to angina, a 12-lead ECG is taken to determine if there is an extension of the infarct, nitroglycerin is administered, and the physician is notified immediately so that interventions may be initiated to limit the size of the MI. Heart failure is a serious complication following STEMI. Therefore whenever the patient's blood pressure is stable, treatment with ACEI is initiated. These vasodilators are used to prevent the left ventricular remodeling and dilation that occur in many patients after an acute MI. Hypotension is a potential complication of ACEI, especially with the first dose. It is an important nursing responsibility to monitor blood pressure and patient symptoms after taking this medication. Surveillance to detect both obvious and subtle signs of bleeding is also a priority because so many acute MI pa-

Box 18-7

CLINICAL MANIFESTATIONS OF ACUTE MYOCARDIAL INFARCTION

- Tachycardia with or without ectopy
- Bradycardia
- Normotension or hypotension
- Tachypnea
- Diminished heart sounds, especially S_1
- If left ventricular dysfunction present, may have S_3 and/or S_4
- Systolic murmur
- Pulmonary crackles
- Pulmonary edema
- Air hunger
- Orthopnea
- Frothy sputum
- Decreased cardiac output
- Decreased urine output
- Decreased peripheral pulses
- Slow capillary refill
- Restlessness
- Confusion
- Anxiety
- Agitation
- Denial
- Anger

PATIENT EDUCATION — Myocardial Infarction

- Pathophysiology of coronary artery disease, angina, and acute myocardial infarction
- Angina: describe signs and symptoms, such as pain, pressure, or heaviness in chest, arms, or jaw
- Use of the pain scale from 1 to 10: notify critical care nurse or emergency personnel of any changes in chest pain intensity
- Avoid the Valsalva maneuver
- Risk factor modification tailored to the patient's individual risk factor profile:
  —Decrease fat intake <30% of total calorie a day
  —Reduce total serum cholesterol to <200 mg/dl
  —Reduce LDL cholesterol to below 70 mg/dl
  —Stop smoking
  —Reduce salt intake
  —Control hypertension
  —Control diabetes if patient is diabetic
  —Increase physical activity
  —Achieve ideal body weight if patient is overweight
- Refer to cardiac rehabilitation program
- Medication teaching: indications, side effects
- Follow-up care after discharge
- Symptoms to report to a health care professional
- Discuss how to handle emotional stress and anger

tients receive antiplatelet, anticoagulant, and fibrinolytic medications.[3]

In the first 24 hours, the stable patient with acute MI may be given only a light diet, because appetite is often poor in such patients. It is no longer considered necessary to restrict iced fluids or caffeine. While the patient is in bed, an upright position is preferred to foster better lung expansion. Deep breathing decreases the risk of atelectasis. An upright position also decreases venous return, lowers preload, and decreases cardiac work. The patient is taught to avoid increasing intraabdominal pressure (Valsalva maneuver). Stool softeners are given to the patient to lessen the risk of constipation from analgesics and bed rest and also to decrease the risk of straining. The nurse controls the critical care unit environment by decreasing noise, diminishing sensory overload, and allowing adequate rest periods.

PATIENT EDUCATION

Once the acute phase has passed, education for the patient and family is focused on risk factor reduction, manifestations of angina, when to call a physician or emergency services, medications, and resumption of physical and sexual activity (see the Patient Education feature on Myocardial Infarction). If possible, a referral is made to a cardiac rehabilitation program so that this education can be reinforced outside the acute care hospital environ-

ment.[51] Clinical practice guidelines for multidisciplinary care of the patient with an acute myocardial infarction are listed in the Evidence-Based Collaborative Practice feature on Acute Coronary Syndrome and Acute Myocardial Infarction.

SUDDEN CARDIAC DEATH

DESCRIPTION

Between 400,000 to 460,000 people die suddenly from a cardiac cause each year.[1] This number represents 60% of all cardiac deaths.[1] These statistics represent deaths that occur outside the hospital with symptoms that last less than 1 hour, or occur in a hospital emergency room.[1,52] Sudden cardiac death represents just over 5% of total annual mortality from all causes.[53]

When the onset of symptoms is rapid, the most likely mechanism of death is ventricular tachycardia (VT), which degenerates into ventricular fibrillation (VF). This syndrome is called *sudden cardiac death (SCD)*. In spite of aggressive cardiopulmonary resuscitation (CPR)

EVIDENCE-BASED COLLABORATIVE PRACTICE

Acute Coronary Syndrome and Acute Myocardial Infarction (Non-STEMI and STEMI)

Prevention of Acute Coronary Syndrome

The term ACS is used to define the life-threatening consequences of CAD, notably unstable angina, non-STEMI and STEMI:

- Unstable angina is a term that denotes chest pain that is not relieved by SL nitroglycerin or rest within 5 minutes.
- Non-STEMI is an acute MI *without* ST elevation on the 12-lead ECG.
- STEMI is an acute MI *with* ST elevation on the 12-lead ECG.

All of the recommendations are "class I," meaning there is strong research evidence to support these recommendations.

Recommendations That Decrease the Risk of Developing Non-STEMI and STEMI

- Primary care providers should evaluate CAD risk factors for all patients every 3 to 5 years.
- The 10-year risk of ACS and acute MI should be assessed for all patients who have more than two major risk factors.
- An intensive risk factor modification program is recommended for patients with established CAD, or high-risk equivalents such as diabetes or chronic kidney disease.

Recommendations That Patients Be Educated about Emergency ACS Symptoms

- Patients who have previously diagnosed CAD should take one SL nitroglycerin, and patient (if alone) or friends or relatives should call 911 if chest pain/discomfort is unrelieved or worsening in 5 minutes.
- The same recommendation applies to patients without known CAD. If pain is unrelieved with rest or worsening at 5 minutes, patient (if alone) or friends or relatives should call 911.
- Patients with chest discomfort should be transported to the hospital via ambulance rather than be driven by friends or relatives.
- Family members should be advised to take a CPR course before an ACS emergency. This will teach CPR skills, demonstrate use of an AED, and educate participants about the "chain of survival" concept.

Recommendations for Prehospital EMS-Paramedic First Responders

- First responders such as EMS-paramedics can provide early defibrillation and ACLS for patients in cardiac arrest.
- EMS personnel should administer 162 to 325 mg nonenteric aspirin (chewed, not swallowed) to patients with chest pain suspected of having a STEMI.
- A prehospital fibrinolysis protocol is reasonable for patients with STEMI when there are physicians in the ambulance, or when there is a well-organized EMS service with full-time paramedics plus 12-lead ECG transmission capability and online medical direction.
- Patients over 75 years of age or those with cardiogenic shock should be transported to a hospital with the ability to provide fibrinolytics, emergency PCI, or emergency CABG. PCI or CABG, when needed, should be provided within 18 hours of the onset of cardiogenic shock.
- Patients with STEMI who have a contraindication to fibrinolytic therapy should be brought to a hospital capable of emergency PCI or CABG. At the scene the **door-to-departure time should be less than 30 minutes.** PCI should be initiated **within 90 minutes** from initial medical contact.

Recommendations for Initial Emergency Clinical Management

- Hospitals should establish multidisciplinary teams to facilitate rapid triage of patients who present to the ED with chest pain.
- Use of written protocols is recommended to standardize care. An immediate cardiology consult is advised if the patient symptoms fall outside the written protocol.

STEMI

- Fibrinolytics for STEMI: Time from coming into contact with the health care system (paramedics or ED) and receiving fibrinolytics should be **less than 30 minutes.** A brief, focused neurologic examination to determine prior stroke or presence of cognitive defects is necessary prior to administration of fibrinolytics.
- PCI for STEMI: Time from coming into contact with the health care system (paramedics or ED) to balloon inflation PCI should be **less than 90 minutes.**

From Braunwald E et al: ACC/AHA 2002 guideline update for the management of patients with unstable angina and non–ST-segment elevation myocardial infarction—summary article: a report of the American College of Cardiology/American Heart Association Task Force on Practice Guidelines (Committee on the Management of Patients with Unstable Angina), *J Am Coll Cardiol* 40(7):1366-1374, 2002; Antman EM et al: ACC/AHA guidelines for the management of patients with ST-elevation myocardial infarction—executive summary: a report of the American College of Cardiology/American Heart Association Task Force on Practice Guidelines (Writing Committee to Revise the 1999 Guidelines for the Management of Patients with Acute Myocardial Infarction), *Circulation* 110:588-636, 2004. Full text available online at www.ahajournals.org.

ACS, Acute coronary syndrome; *AED,* automated external defibrillator; *ACLS,* advanced cardiac life support; *CABG,* coronary artery bypass graft surgery; *CAD,* coronary artery disease; *CPR,* cardiopulmonary resuscitation; *ECG,* electrocardiogram; *ED,* emergency department; *EMS,* emergency medical services; *MI,* myocardial infarction; *non-STEMI,* non–ST elevation myocardial infarction; *PCI,* percutaneous coronary intervention; *SL,* sublingual; *STEMI,* ST elevation myocardial infarction.

Non-STEMI

- If the level of risk for the patient with Non-STEMI is not immediately apparent, a "chest pain unit" within the ED permits close surveillance by competent clinicians without immediate hospital admission.
- Glycoprotein IIb/IIIa inhibitors for Non-STEMI, in addition to aspirin and heparin, are indicated when cardiac catheterization or PCI are planned.
- PCI may be indicated for Non-STEMI.

Recommendations for Initial Emergency Physical Assessment

Vital Signs

- HR, BP, RR, temperature SpO2, ECG monitor to detect presence of dysrhythmias

Physical Assessment

- Assess for warm or cool skin, color, capillary refill, peripheral pulses
- Auscultate heart for cardiac murmur or new S_3 or S_4
- Auscultate lungs for air entry plus crackles, wheezes
- Observe for breathlessness, frothy pink sputum (pulmonary edema)
- Ask patient, family, significant others for relevant history

Recommendations for Emergency Diagnostics

12-Lead ECG

- The 12-lead ECG should be shown to the ED physician within 10 minutes of the patient's arrival in the ED for all patients with chest discomfort or angina equivalent symptoms.
- If the first ECG is normal but the patient continues to have symptoms of chest pain/discomfort, the 12-lead ECG should be repeated at 5- to 10-minute intervals, **or** continuous 12-lead ECG monitoring can be used.
- In patients with inferior wall infarction, RV infarction must be suspected and right-sided ECG leads then recorded. V_4R is diagnostic lead of choice to diagnose ST elevation in the RV.

Laboratory Studies

- Laboratory tests should be drawn as part of the general management of STEMI but should not delay the administration of reperfusion therapy.

Cardiac Biomarkers

- Cardiac-specific troponins are recommended for patients with coexistent skeletal muscle injury. Clinicians are advised not wait for results of the biomarker assay before initiating reperfusion therapy. Point-of-care (handheld) biomarker assay results are permissible, but subsequent biomarker assays should be via quantitative laboratory analysis.

Imaging Studies

- Portable chest x-ray: obtaining the chest x-ray must not delay reperfusion therapy unless a major complication such as aortic dissection is suspected.
- Portable echocardiography (TTE or TEE) or MRI scan to distinguish aortic dissection from STEMI, for patients in whom the symptoms are not clear

Recommendations for Routine Care

Prevent Hypoxia

- Supplemental oxygen administered to maintain SaO2 above 90%

Coronary Vasodilation

- Nitroglycerin 0.04 mg SL every 5 minutes for three doses. If chest pain/discomfort is ongoing, start peripheral IV. Administer IV nitroglycerin for relief of chest pain, control of hypertension, or relief of pulmonary congestion.

Pain Control

- Morphine sulphate 2-4 mg IV in 2-mg increments at 5- to 15-minute intervals for STEMI pain control

Aspirin

- Aspirin 162 mg to be chewed for rapid buccal absorption

Beta-Blockers

- Oral beta-blocker therapy administered to STEMI patients without contraindications to beta-blockade, irrespective of fibrinolytic or primary PCI reperfusion

Recommendations for Emergency Interventions for STEMI

Fibrinolytic Drugs

- Fibrinolytic drugs administered to STEMI patients with ST elevation greater than 0.1 mV (1 mm or one small box) in two contiguous precordial (chest) leads **or** two adjacent limb leads, new LBBB or presumed new LBBB, and onset of symptoms less than 12 hours ago
- Before administration of fibrinolytic therapy, rule out neurologic contraindications.
- Rule out facial trauma, uncontrolled hypertension, or ischemic stroke within the last 3 months
- If contraindications to fibrinolysis are present, PCI is the preferred method of reperfusion.

PCI

- Emergency diagnostic coronary angiography to identify blocked coronary artery before PCI
- Emergency PCI is recommended over fibrinolytic therapy if symptom onset was longer ago than 3 hours
- Emergency PCI can be performed within 12 hours of symptom onset for patients with new LBBB, or presumed new LBBB.

BP, Blood pressure, *HR*, heart rate; *IV*, intravenous; *LBBB*, left bundle branch block; *MRI*, magnetic resonance imaging; *SaO2*, arterial oxygen saturation; *SpO2*, oxygen saturation from external pulse-oximeter; *TEE*, transesophageal echocardiogram; *TTE*, transthoracic echocardiogram; *RR*, respiratory rate; *RV*, right ventricle.

Continued

EVIDENCE-BASED COLLABORATIVE PRACTICE

Acute Coronary Syndrome and Acute Myocardial Infarction—cont'd

PCI—cont'd
- Emergency PCI balloon inflation within 90 minutes of arrival at the hospital
- If cardiogenic shock develops less than 36 hours after MI, in patients younger than 75 years with ST elevation, or patients with new LBBB, "rescue PCI" is recommended within 18 hours of shock onset.

Cardiac Surgery
- Emergency CABG surgery is undertaken for specific indications in STEMI:
  - Failed PCI with persistent pain or hemodynamic instability
  - Recurrent ischemia refractory to medical therapy in patients with suitable anatomy who are not candidates for PCI
  - Post-MI ventricular septal rupture (VSR) or papillary muscle rupture, both of which frequently lead to cardiogenic shock
  - Cardiogenic shock less than 36 hours after MI, in patients younger than 75 years with ST elevation, or patients with new LBBB who have multivessel or left main disease
  - Recurrent ventricular dysrhythmias with 50% or greater left main coronary artery lesion and/or triple vessel disease

Recommendations for Secondary Prevention of Complications

Medications
- ACE Inhibitors—prevent ventricular remodeling
- Beta-blockers—prevent ventricular dysrhythmias
- Diuretics—if heart failure has developed
- Antihyperlipidemics—if total cholesterol, LDL, or triglycerides elevated

Recommendations for Management of Complications Following STEMI

Cardiogenic Shock
- IABP for patients with hypotension (BP 90 mm Hg or SBP 30 mm Hg below baseline)

Ventricular Arrhythmias
- VF or pulseless VT is managed by standard ACLS criteria (unsynchronized monophasic shock of 200 joules; if unsuccessful a second shock of 200-300 joules, if unsuccessful a third shock of 360 joules).
- Patients with hemodynamically significant VT more than 2 days post-STEMI who have ongoing ventricular dysrhythmias are considered for implantation of an ICD.
- Patients with an EF between 30%-40% at 1 month after STEMI should undergo an electrophysiology study (EPS), and if they are inducible to VT/VF, an ICD is recommended to reduce risk of SCD.
- Patients with an EF below 30% at one month after STEMI are at high risk of SCD.

AV block
- Transvenous pacemaker inserted (emergency) or permanent pacemaker (later elective) for symptomatic second- or third-degree AV block
- All patients after STEMI who require permanent pacing should also be evaluated for ICD indications.

Provide Relevant Education

Medications
- Written and verbal instructions about medication dosages, administration, and side effects

Emergency Information
- Give patient and family information about calling 911 if pain/angina equivalent symptoms persist or are worse after 5 minutes.
- Family members of high-risk patients are advised to take a CPR class and learn about AED.

Risk Factors
- Smoking cessation, hypertension control, weight control, normal blood glucose; low-fat diet; normal lipid panel
- Increase physical activity, no new HRT for women

Cardiac Rehabilitation
- Participation in a cardiac rehabilitation program will help the patient continue the process of risk factor and lifestyle modification.

ACE, Angiotensin-converting enzyme; *EF*, ejection fraction; *HRT*, hormone replacement therapy; *IABP*, intraaortic balloon pump; *ICD*, implantable cardioverter defibrillator; *LDL*, low-density lipoprotein cholesterol; *SCD*, sudden cardiac death; *VF*, ventricular fibrillation; *VSR*, *v*entricular septal rupture; *VT*, ventricular tachycardia.

---

initiated outside the hospital, few who sustain an out-of-the-hospital cardiac arrest survive to hospital discharge. Strategies that have been shown to improve resuscitation survival involve huge community-wide programs to teach laypersons CPR plus how to use an automated external defibrillator (AED). With such a program in place, plus accessible AED units and rapid emergency medical services (EMS) support, survival to hospital discharge has been shown to improve.[54]

ETIOLOGY

Most SCD incidents occur in patients with preexisting ventricular dysfunction secondary to cardiac disease.

Box 18-8

CAUSES OF SUDDEN CARDIAC DEATH

ACQUIRED SCD RISK
The vast majority of SCD patients are older adults and have a history of coronary artery disease, MI, and subsequent heart failure.

Heart Failure
Ejection fraction less than 30%
Heart structure is abnormal (systolic or diastolic ventricular dysfunction)
Coronary artery disease and a history of MI that has produced scar tissue is the most common cause of VT/VF leading to SCD
Cardiomyopathy (dilated or ischemic)
Patients who are inducible for VT/VF in EPS are at highest risk
Risk decreased by implantation of ICD and antidysrhythmic drug therapy

GENETIC SCD RISK
Genetic cardiovascular disease accounts for 40% of SCD in young adults.

Brugada Syndrome
ECG signs: Coved ST elevation (greater than 2 mm) in right precordial leads, although ECG variations also occur
Heart structure appears normal
High risk of VT or VF in otherwise young healthy adults
VT/VF often occurs at night, at rest
Represents 4% of all SCD; average age 41 years
Represents up to 20% of genetic SCD patients
Hereditary: autosomal-dominant genetic transmission

Five times more common in males
Patients who are inducible in EPS are at increased risk
Risk reduced by implantation of an ICD

Wolff-Parkinson-White Syndrome
Congenital accessory conduction pathway connects the atria and ventricles
Accessory pathway is *in addition* to the normal conduction system
Accessory pathway allows very rapid transmission of impulses allowing "preexcitation" of the ventricle that can degenerate into VT/VF, especially if atrial dysrhythmias are present
WPW usually identified when patient is a teenager or young adult
WPW often recognized during exercise by palpitations or breathlessness
Can be cured in many cases by radiofrequency ablation of the accessory pathway

Hypertrophic Cardiomyopathy
Risk of VT/VF with exercise
If a patient has the hypertrophic subaortic obstructive cardiomyopathy (HOCM) form, this can be cured in many cases by alcohol ablation of the enlarged ventricular septum
For other HCM patients, risk is reduced by implantation of an ICD

Long QT Syndrome
Risk of VT/VF with exercise
Risk reduced by implantation of an ICD

CV, Cardiovascular; *EPS,* electrophysiology study; *HCM,* hypertrophic cardiomyopathy; *ICD,* implantable cardioverter defibrillator; *MI,* myocardial infarction; *SCD,* sudden cardiac death; *VF,* ventricular fibrillation; *VT,* ventricular tachycardia; *WPW,* Wolff-Parkinson-White.

Specific SCD risk factors include extensive coronary atherosclerosis with or without a history of an acute MI, dilated or hypertrophic cardiomyopathy, valvular heart disease, autonomic nervous system abnormalities; electrical system abnormalities such as AV block, Wolff-Parkinson-White (WPW) syndrome, prolonged QT syndrome, Brugada syndrome, and patients taking medications that prolong the QT interval.[55-57] An ejection fraction less than 30% and a history of ventricular dysrhythmias are powerful predictors of SCD. Other risk factors as listed in Box 18-8. Unfortunately, many individuals are unaware of their risk, or there are other risk factors that have not yet been considered. In one longitudinal analysis, 48% of the sudden cardiac death victims had not been previously diagnosed with cardiac disease.[52]

MEDICAL MANAGEMENT

Depending on the length of time the patient was unconscious as a result of the cardiac arrest, cognitive defects may be present because of the lack of cerebral blood flow. The cardiac arrest may also have damaged the myocardium and other tissues. Therapy is tailored to the needs of the patient. Survivors receive antidysrhythmic agents and have an internal cardioverter defibrillator (ICD) unit implanted.[58-60] Prevention focuses on identification and treatment of high-risk cardiac patients (see "Implantable Cardioverter Defibrillator" and "Antidysrhythmic Drugs" in Chapter 19).

HEART FAILURE

DESCRIPTION AND ETIOLOGY

The number of patients with heart failure is increasing in the United States. Currently over 2 million Americans have a diagnosis of heart failure (HF), and about 500,000 new cases are diagnosed each year.[61] Each year, 300,00 patients die of HF and patients spend over 6.5 million days in the hospital.[61] Heart failure is primarily a disease of the elderly. Approximately 6% to 10% of people over 65 years of age have a diagnosis of HF; for patients who are hospitalized with this diagnosis, 80% of them are over 80 years old. The number of patients diagnosed with HF is increasing. The total inpatient and outpatient costs for HF exceed $38 billion each year, a sum that represents over 5% of the total United States health care budget.[61]

PATHOPHYSIOLOGY

Heart failure is a response to cardiac dysfunction, a condition in which the heart cannot pump blood at a volume required to meet the body's needs. Any condition that impairs the ability of the ventricles to fill or eject blood can cause HF. Coronary artery disease with resultant necrotic damage to the left ventricle is the underlying cause of HF in most patients. Other major conditions that lead to HF include valvular dysfunction, infection (myocarditis or endocarditis), cardiomyopathy, and uncontrolled hypertension.[61]

ASSESSMENT AND DIAGNOSIS

Heart failure is typically classified using the New York Heart Association (NYHA) criteria. Patients are assigned into four groups, I through IV, depending on their degree of symptoms and the amount of patient effort required to elicit symptoms (Table 18-9). Research-based clinical guidelines suggest adding a second level of classification that emphasizes the progressive nature of HF through various stages, with increasing symptom distress and intensified clinical interventions (Table 18-10).[61] Heart failure can manifest itself in many different ways depending on how far the ventricular remodeling and dysfunction has advanced. Heart failure may be discovered secondary to a known clinical syndrome such as acute MI, or because of decreased exercise tolerance, fluid retention, or admission to the critical care unit for an unrelated condition.[61] For patients with fluid retention, the most reliable clinical sign of fluid volume overload is jugular venous distention (JVD).[61] The procedure used to estimate JVD is described in Chapter 16 (see Fig. 16-2 and Box 16-1).

The first step in diagnosis is to determine the underlying structural abnormality creating the ventricular dysfunction and symptoms. Various imaging tests are available to visualize cardiac anatomy and laboratory tests are used to evaluate the impact of hormonal or electrolyte imbalance. The results of these tests permit the cardiology team to design a treatment plan to control symptoms and possibly correct the underlying cause. All patients do not have the same type of heart failure, as described below.

Left Ventricular Failure. Failure of the left ventricle is defined as a disturbance of the contractile function of the left ventricle, resulting in a low cardiac output state.

Table 18-9	New York Heart Association Functional Classification of Heart Failure

Class	Definition
I	Normal daily activity does not initiate symptoms.
II	Normal daily activities initiate onset of symptoms, but symptoms subside with rest.
III	Minimal activity initiates symptoms; patients are usually symptom-free at rest.
IV	Any type of activity initiates symptoms, and symptoms are present at rest.

This leads to vasoconstriction of the arterial bed that raises systemic vascular resistance (SVR), a condition also described as "high afterload," and creates congestion and edema in the pulmonary circulation and alveoli. Clinical manifestations include decreased peripheral perfusion with weak or diminished pulses; cool, pale extremities; and in later stages, peripheral cyanosis (Table 18-11). Over time, with progression of the disease state the fluid accumulation behind the dysfunctional left ventricle elevates pulmonary pressures, contributes to pulmonary congestion and edema, and produces dysfunction of the right ventricle, resulting in failure of the right side of the heart.

Right Ventricular Failure. Failure of the right side of the heart is defined as ineffective right ventricular contractile function. Pure failure of the right ventricle may result from an acute condition such as a pulmonary embolus or a right ventricular infarction, but it is most commonly caused by failure of the left side of the heart (see above). The common manifestations of right ventricular failure are the following: jugular venous distention, elevated central venous pressure (CVP), weakness, peripheral or sacral edema, hepatomegaly (enlarged liver), jaundice, and liver tenderness. Gastrointestinal (GI) symptoms include poor appetite, anorexia, nausea, and an uncomfortable feeling of fullness (see Table 18-11).

Systolic Heart Failure. Systolic dysfunction describes an abnormality of the heart muscle that markedly decreases contractility during systole (ejection) and thus lessens the quantity of blood that can be pumped out of the heart. Patients with a diagnosis of systolic heart failure have signs and symptoms of HF combined with a below-normal ejection fraction (EF). Left ventricular systolic dysfunction is the classic picture that most clinicians picture when thinking about heart failure. In addition to the signs and symptoms of left heart failure (see above) the patient will have a low EF.

Table 18-10	Progression of Heart Failure			
Stage	**Structural Heart Disorder**	**Symptoms**	**Management**	**NYHA Class**
A	No, but at risk because of: Hypertension CAD Diabetes mellitus	None	Preventive treatment of known risk factors: Hypertension Lipid disorders Cigarette smoking Diabetes mellitus Discourage alcohol and illicit drug use	I
B	Yes, but without symptoms: Previous MI Family history of CM Asymptomatic valvular disease/CM	None	Treat all risk factors. When indicated, use the following: ACE inhibitors Beta-blockers	II
C	Yes, with prior or current symptoms	Shortness of breath Fatigue Reduced exercise tolerance	Treat all risk factors, plus HF symptoms: Diuretics ACE inhibitors Beta-blockers Digitalis Dietary salt restriction	III
D	Yes, with refractory HF symptoms despite maximal specialized interventions (pharmacologic, medical, nursing) Recurrently hospitalized for HF symptoms	Marked symptoms at rest despite maximal medical therapy	Refractory HF requires interventions from previous stages (A-C), plus the following: Continuous intravenous inotropic support Mechanical assist devices Heart transplantation Hospice care	IV

Adapted from Hunt SA et al: *Circulation* 104:2996-3007, 2001. Full text available online at http://www.ahajournals.org.
HF, Heart failure; *CAD*, coronary artery disease; *MI*, myocardial infarctions, *CM*, cardiomyopathy; *ACE*, angiotensin-converting enzyme.

Table 18-11	Clinical Manifestations of Failure of Right and Left Sides of Heart			
Left Ventricular Failure		**Right Ventricular Failure**		
Signs	**Symptoms**	**Signs**	**Symptoms**
Tachypnea Tachycardia Cough Bibasilar crackles Gallop rhythms (S_3 and S_4) Increased pulmonary artery pressures Hemoptysis Cyanosis Pulmonary edema	Fatigue Dyspnea Orthopnea Paroxysmal nocturnal dyspnea Nocturia	Peripheral edema Hepatomegaly Splenomegaly Hepatojugular reflux Ascites Jugular venous distention Increased central venous pressure Pulmonary hypertension	Weakness Anorexia Indigestion Weight gain Mental changes

There is some debate as to how low the EF has to be to qualify as systolic heart failure but the range is generally below 50%;[62] some clinicians cite numbers below 45% or even below 40%.[63,64] Symptoms of systolic heart failure include dyspnea, exercise intolerance, and fluid volume overload.

Coronary artery disease (CAD) and its sequelae represent the underlying cause in two thirds of patients with systolic heart failure.[61] The remaining patients with systolic dysfunction have nonischemic cardiomyopathy, (interchangeably described as *dilated cardiomyopathy*)[65] which results from an identifiable cause such as hypertension, thyroid disease, cardiac valvular disease, alcohol use, or myocarditis.[61] If the cause is unknown, systolic dysfunction is described as *idiopathic dilated cardiomyopathy*.[61] The incidence of systolic heart failure in the general population is 3%; it increases with age and is more common in men.[64] Clinical findings that are required to make a diagnosis of systolic heart failure include the following[61]:

- Signs and symptoms of heart failure.
- Left ventricular systolic dysfunction with an ejection fraction below normal.

In systolic heart failure the ventricular chambers change their shape, a detrimental development known as *ventricular remodeling*. The negative impact on the cardiac cells is different from the dysfunction and loss of myocytes from myocardial ischemia and infarction. Ventricular remodeling is modulated by catecholamines and activation of neuro-hormonal compensatory mechanisms (described in the following paragraphs). The heart chamber walls ultimately become dilated, thinned, and poorly contractile.

There are significant hemodynamic changes that occur as systolic dysfunction progresses. In systolic heart failure, the left ventricular end-diastolic volume is high, which in turn raises the left ventricular end-diastolic pressure when compared to a normal heart. This increase in intracardiac volume and pressure causes a rise in left atrial and pulmonary venous pressures. This means that all blood flowing into the heart via the pulmonary vascular bed is exposed to increased hydrostatic pressure, necessary just to fill the congested heart. The increase in pulmonary vascular pressure causes transudation of fluid from the pulmonary capillaries into the alveolar interstitium, and this fluid is ultimately forced through the walls of the alveoli, causing pulmonary edema. The pulmonary complications of HF are described in greater detail below. The elevated left heart pressures eventually raise pressures in the right side of the heart and lead to secondary right heart failure. Right heart pressures are elevated in nearly 80% of patients with chronically elevated left heart pressures.[61]

Diastolic Heart Failure. Diastolic dysfunction describes an abnormality of the heart muscle that makes it unable to relax, stretch, or fill during diastole. The ejection fraction can be normal or abnormal (low), and the patient may be symptomatic or symptom-free.[62,66] Between 20% and 40% of patients with HF are believed to have diastolic muscle dysfunction.[61] The principal causes are similar to systolic heart failure (see above): coronary artery disease, myocardial ischemia, atrial fibrillation, uncontrolled hypertension in 75% of cases, and left ventricular hypertrophy (LVH) in about 40%.[66] Some conditions that are known to markedly alter diastolic function include hypertrophic cardiomyopathy (HCM), restrictive cardiomyopathy, and infiltrative diseases such as amyloidosis and neoplastic infiltrate.[61,65] The incidence of diastolic heart failure is highest in patients

older than 75 years and disproportionately affects elderly women.[61] It is postulated that the process of ageing negatively impacts diastolic function, imposing stiffness and fibrosis on both the cardiac muscle and cardiovascular vessels.[61]

Clinical findings that are required to make a diagnosis of diastolic heart failure include the following[61-63]:

- Signs and symptoms of heart failure.
- Normal or only mildly abnormal left ventricular systolic dysfunction.
- Abnormal left ventricular relaxation, filling, diastolic distensibility or diastolic stiffness.

Diastolic heart failure is caused by dysfunction during the diastolic phase of the cardiac cycle. In affected patients, the heart muscle takes longer to relax compared with a normal heart, the ventricular chamber does not distend to accept the fill-volume, and the myocardium remains stiff throughout diastole.[66,67] Normally, diastole is the filling stage of the cardiac cycle when the ventricle relaxes completely. The abnormal hemodynamics of diastolic heart failure can be elicited by diagnostic tests such as cardiac catheterization and a stress-echocardiogram (see chapter 17).[66] An ejection fraction above the range of 40%-50% is considered normal for this population.

In diastolic heart failure, the left ventricular end-diastolic pressure (LVEDP) is high, whereas the left ventricular end-diastolic volume (LVEDV) is paradoxically low, when compared to normal hearts.[62] Another diagnostic clue is that many patients with diastolic heart failure have normal intracardiac pressures at rest, but during exercise the LVEDP and pulmonary vascular pressures rise rapidly.[62] This is because the noncompliant, stiff ventricle cannot increase stroke volume during exercise; thus cardiac output remains low even though physical demand is high. Not unexpectedly, patients with diastolic heart failure often experience a sudden rise in blood pressure and sinus tachycardia during exercise; they are exercise-intolerant and experience fatigue, dyspnea, pulmonary venous congestion, and even pulmonary edema.[62,63,66]

Systolic vs. Diastolic Heart Failure. It turns out to be impossible to accurately determine whether a patient has systolic or diastolic heart failure from clinical assessment alone.[62] This is because both types of HF produce similar signs and symptoms. The level of symptoms and quality of life are variable between individuals, and between men and women, even when the EF and presumed cardiac dysfunction is the same.[68] This may be because the majority of symptoms come from the neuro-hormonal compensatory mechanisms (see below) rather than the cardiac output. An elevated B-natriuretic peptide (BNP) level (greater than 100 picograms/ml) is very useful to diagnose heart failure in patients with fluid overload and shortness of breath.[69] The BNP value tends to be higher in patients with a diagnosis of systolic heart failure compared with diastolic heart failure, although this differentiation is not reliable enough to be used to differentiate the two types of heart failure in clinical practice.[69] The more severe the heart failure, the higher the BNP level. The primary use of the BNP test is to diagnose if heart failure is present.

The definitive diagnosis of the type of HF is often made using Doppler echocardiography. An echocardiogram performed at rest and during exercise (stress echo) permits visualization of heart wall movement during both systole and diastole. Calculation of the EF can be determined using Doppler echocardiography or during a cardiac catheterization. These diagnostic tests also show that there are patients who exhibit combined systolic and diastolic heart failure.[62]

The annual mortality rate in diastolic heart failure is 5% to 8%, markedly less than the 10% to 15% annual mortality for patients with systolic heart failure. To put this in perspective, age-matched controls without any heart failure experience an annual mortality rate of just 1%.[62,66]

It is not possible to distinguish whether a patient has systolic or diastolic heart failure simply by looking at the medications they are prescribed. The same drugs are used to treat the two types of HF although the underlying rationales may be different.[63] For example, β-blockers are used in diastolic heart failure to slow the heart rate, to prolong diastole to give more time for ventricular filling, and to modify the ventricular response to exercise, especially for patients who have a preserved ejection fraction.[63] When β-blockers are prescribed for treatment of systolic heart failure the intent is to preserve long-term inotropic (contractile) function and prevent ventricular remodeling.[63] Diuretics are used to treat both types of HF, although a smaller dosage is generally needed in diastolic heart failure.[63] Angiotensin-converting enzyme (ACE) inhibitors and angiotensin receptor–blockers (ARB) are also used to treat both types of HF. The medications used to treat heart failure are further discussed in Chapter 19 (see the Pharmacologic Management Table on Heart Failure, p. 561).

Acute vs. Chronic Heart Failure. Acute versus chronic heart failure refers to the rapidity with which the syndrome develops, the presence and activation of compensatory mechanisms, and the presence or absence of fluid accumulation in the interstitial space (see Table 18-10). In clinical practice guidelines, the terms *acute* and *chronic* have replaced the older name, "congestive heart failure" (CHF), because not all heart failure involves pulmonary congestion.[61] However, the description of a patient with CHF remains commonly employed in clinical practice.

Acute heart failure has a sudden onset, with no compensatory mechanisms. The patient may experience acute pulmonary edema, low cardiac output, or even cardiogenic shock. Patients with chronic heart failure are hypervolemic, have sodium and water retention, and have structural heart chamber changes such as dilation or hypertrophy.[61]

Chronic heart failure is ongoing, with symptoms that may be made tolerable by medication, diet, and a reduced activity level. The deterioration into acute heart failure can be precipitated by the onset of dysrhythmias, acute ischemia, sudden illness, or cessation of medications. This may necessitate admission to a critical care unit.

NEURO-HORMONAL COMPENSATORY MECHANISMS IN HEART FAILURE

When the heart begins to fail and the cardiac output is no longer sufficient to meet the metabolic needs of the tissues, the body activates several major compensatory mechanisms: the sympathetic nervous system, the renin-angiotensin-aldosterone system (RAAS), and, if hypertension is present, the development of ventricular hypertrophy (see Table 18-10). This process ultimately reshapes the ventricle in a process described as *ventricular remodeling*. These pathophysiologic processes, and the pharmacologic measures taken to limit ventricular remodeling, are described in the following paragraphs.

1. *Sympathetic nervous system:* The sympathetic nervous system compensates for low cardiac output by increasing heart rate (HR) and blood pressure (BP). As a result, levels of circulating catecholamines are increased, resulting in peripheral vasoconstriction. In addition to raising BP and HR, catecholamines cause shunting of blood from nonvital organs, such as the skin, to vital organs, such as the heart and brain. This mechanism, although initially helpful, may become a negative factor if elevation of HR increases myocardial oxygen demand while shortening the amount of time for diastolic filling and coronary artery perfusion.

2. *Renin-angiotensin-aldosterone system:* Activation of RAAS in heart failure promotes fluid retention.[61,70] The RAAS is activated by low cardiac output that causes the hormone *renin* to be secreted by the kidneys. A physiologic chain of events is then set in motion that leads to volume overload. The renin acts on *angiotensinogen* in the bloodstream and converts it to *angiotensin I;* when angiotensin passes through the lung tissues it is activated by an enzyme named *ACE* that converts the angiotensin I to *angiotensin II,* a powerful vasoconstrictor that increases SVR, raises BP and increases the workload of the left ventricle; the increased SVR further lowers cardiac output. The mineralocorticoid hormone *aldosterone* is released from the adrenal glands and stimulates sodium retention via the distal tubules of the kidney. In addition, in response to the low cardiac output the renal arterioles constrict, decrease glomerular filtration, and increase reabsorption of sodium from the proximal and distal tubules. To break the RAAS cycle of fluid retention in heart failure, two types of drugs are prescribed to interrupt the steps. To inhibit the conversion of angiotensin I to angiotensin II, a drug in the ACE-inhibitor (ACEI) category is prescribed (see the

Pharmacologic Management Tables on Characteristics of Selected Vasodilators and Heart Failure in Chapter 19). These agents prevent arterial vasoconstriction, decrease blood pressure and SVR, and decrease the amount of ventricular remodeling that often occurs with HF. Or, a drug that inhibits angiotensin II directly may be prescribed instead. The drugs in this category are termed *angiotensin receptor–blockers* (ARB).[71] Aldactone (Spirolactone)

is a drug from a different category that is also prescribed to break the RAAS cycle. Aldactone is a *mineralocorticoid receptor antagonist* that will inhibit (block) the retention of sodium from the distal tubules of the kidney.[70,72] Fig. 18-16 shows the mechanism of action by which these drugs act on the RAAS.

3. *Ventricular hypertrophy:* Ventricular hypertrophy is the final compensatory mechanism. It is also

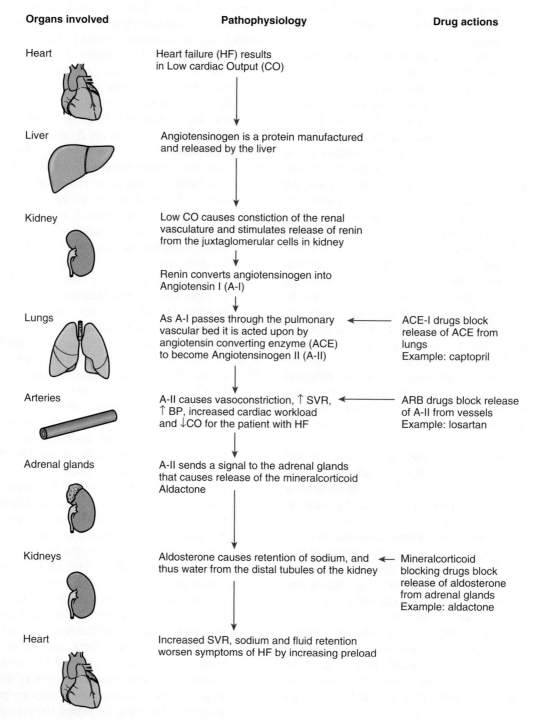

Organs involved	Pathophysiology	Drug actions
Heart	Heart failure (HF) results in Low cardiac Output (CO)	
Liver	Angiotensinogen is a protein manufactured and released by the liver	
Kidney	Low CO causes constiction of the renal vasculature and stimulates release of renin from the juxtaglomerular cells in kidney	
	Renin converts angiotensinogen into Angiotensin I (A-I)	
Lungs	As A-I passes through the pulmonary vascular bed it is acted upon by angiotensin converting enzyme (ACE) to become Angiotensinogen II (A-II)	ACE-I drugs block release of ACE from lungs Example: captopril
Arteries	A-II causes vasoconstriction, ↑ SVR, ↑ BP, increased cardiac workload and ↓CO for the patient with HF	ARB drugs block release of A-II from vessels Example: losartan
Adrenal glands	A-II sends a signal to the adrenal glands that causes release of the mineralcorticoid Aldactone	
Kidneys	Aldosterone causes retention of sodium, and thus water from the distal tubules of the kidney	Mineralcorticoid blocking drugs block release of aldosterone from adrenal glands Example: aldactone
Heart	Increased SVR, sodium and fluid retention worsen symptoms of HF by increasing preload	

Fig. 18-16 Renin-angiotensin-aldosterone system (RAAS), role in heart failure, and interaction of specific drugs.

strongly associated with preexisting hypertension. Because myocardial hypertrophy increases the force of contraction, hypertrophy helps the ventricle overcome an increase in afterload. When this mechanism is no longer efficient for the ventricle, it will remodel by dilation.

4. *Ventricular remodeling:* As a result of the above mechanisms, the shape of the ventricle changes, or is "remodeled," to resemble a round bowl. A dilated ventricle has poor contractility and is enlarged without hypertrophy. Research trial evidence indicates that synergistic use of drugs from different categories—ACEI or ARB, Aldactone, plus β-blockade—can halt or reduce the progression of heart failure remodeling.[71,73,74]

Pulmonary Complications of Heart Failure. The clinical manifestations of acute heart failure result from tissue hypoperfusion and organ congestion and are progressive, as described above. The severity of clinical manifestations also progresses as heart failure worsens. Initially manifestations appear only with exertion but eventually occur at rest as well.[61]

Shortness of Breath in Heart Failure. The patient experiences the feeling of shortness of breath first with exertion, but as heart failure worsens, symptoms are also present at rest. Recently a diagnostic blood test has become available to assist clinicians in differentiating whether a patient's shortness of breath is caused by cardiac failure or by pulmonary complications. B-type natriuretic peptide (BNP) is released from the cardiac ventricles in response to increased wall tension. Heart failure increases LV wall tension because of the excess preload in the ventricles. When the BNP blood level is greater than 100 picograms per milliliter (pg/ml), the dyspnea is probably related to cardiac rather than pulmonary failure.[75,76] The more severe the heart failure, the higher the BNP test result.[77] If the patient has concomitant kidney disease, the BNP clinical diagnostic point to diagnose heart failure rises to greater than 200 pg/ml.[78] Breathlessness in HF is described by the following terms:

1. *Dyspnea:* the patient's sensation of shortness of breath; it results from pulmonary vascular congestion and decreased lung compliance.
2. *Orthopnea:* describes difficulty in breathing when lying flat because of an increase in venous return that occurs in the supine position.
3. *Paroxysmal nocturnal dyspnea:* a severe form of orthopnea in which the patient awakens from sleep gasping for air.
4. *Cardiac asthma:* dyspnea with wheezing, a nonproductive cough, and pulmonary crackles that progress to the gurgling sounds of pulmonary edema.

Pulmonary Edema in Heart Failure. Pulmonary edema, or protein-laden fluid in the alveoli, inhibits gas exchange by impairing the diffusion pathway between the alveolus and the capillary. It is caused by increased left atrial and ventricular pressures and results in an excessive accumulation of serous or serosanguineous fluid in the interstitial spaces and alveoli of the lungs. The formation of pulmonary edema has two stages. The first stage is not as severe and is characterized by interstitial edema, engorgement of the perivascular and peribronchial spaces, and increased lymphatic flow as illustrated in Fig. 18-17, *B.* The later stage is characterized by alveolar edema resulting from fluid moving into the alveoli from the interstitium (Fig. 18-17, *C*). Eventually, blood plasma moves into the alveoli faster than the lymphatic system can clear it, thereby interfering with diffusion of oxygen, depressing the arterial partial pressure of oxygen (Pao_2), and leading to tissue hypoxia (Fig. 18-17, *D*).

Heart failure patients in pulmonary edema are extremely breathless and anxious and have a sensation of suffocation. They expectorate pink, frothy liquid and feel as if they are drowning. They may sit bolt upright, gasp for breath, or thrash about. The respiratory rate is elevated, and accessory muscles of ventilation are used, with nasal flaring and bulging neck muscles. Respirations are characterized by loud inspiratory and expiratory gurgling sounds. Diaphoresis is profuse, and the skin is cold, ashen, and sometimes cyanotic, reflecting low cardiac output, increased sympathetic stimulation, peripheral vasoconstriction, and desaturation of arterial blood.

Arterial Blood Gases in Pulmonary Edema. Arterial blood gas (ABG) values are variable. In the early stage of pulmonary edema, respiratory alkalosis may be present because of hyperventilation, which eliminates CO_2. As the pulmonary edema progresses and gas exchange becomes impaired, acidosis (pH <7.35) and hypoxemia ensue. A chest x-ray usually confirms an enlarged cardiac silhouette, pulmonary venous congestion, and interstitial edema.

Cardiogenic vs. Noncardiogenic Pulmonary Edema. In the critical care unit, when a patient develops pulmonary edema it is often a challenge to determine whether the cause is cardiac, known as *cardiogenic pulmonary edema,* or whether the origin is pulmonary or systemic in origin. The latter is referred to as *noncardiogenic pulmonary edema* or, more commonly, *acute respiratory distress syndrome* (ARDS). Options to determine the cause of the pulmonary edema include use of the serum BNP level[78] or insertion of a pulmonary artery catheter. The PA catheter is used to determine the patients "wedge" pressure. It is essential to understand the different etiologies because the treatment of each form of pulmonary edema is very specific. For more information on management of ARDS, see Chapter 23.

Dysrhythmias and Heart Failure. A ventricular EF below 30% and the presence of NYHA class III or IV heart failure are strongly associated with ventricular dysrhythmias and an increased risk of death.[79,80] Because sustained ventricular tachycardia or fibrillation (VT/VF) initiate sudden cardiac death, high-risk patients with severe heart failure are prescribed both antidysrhythmic drugs and have an implantable cardioverter defibrillator (ICD) inserted.[80-82]

Many patients with heart failure also have atrial fibrillation. Digoxin is frequently prescribed in atrial fibrillation to control ventricular heart rate. Digoxin does not prolong life but makes patients feel less symptomatic. Digoxin may also work synergistically with specific β-blockers (carvedilol) and make the symptoms more tolerable for patients with severe heart failure.[80,83]

MEDICAL MANAGEMENT

The goals of the medical management of heart failure are to relieve heart failure symptoms, enhance cardiac performance, and correct known precipitating causes of acute heart failure.

Relief of Symptoms and Enhancement of Cardiac Performance. In the acute phase of advanced heart failure the patient may have a pulmonary artery catheter in place so that LV function can be followed closely. Control of symptoms involves management of fluid overload and improvement of cardiac output by decreasing systemic vascular resistance and increasing contractility. Diuretics are administered to decrease preload and to eliminate excess fluid from the body.[72] If pulmonary edema develops, additional diuretics are used. Morphine is given to facilitate peripheral dilation and decrease anxiety. Afterload is decreased by vasodilators, such as sodium nitroprusside (SNP or Nipride) and nitroglycerin. Nitrates are used to decrease preload and vasodi-

late the coronary arteries if CAD is an underlying cause of the acute heart failure. For some patients an IABP is also required.[84] Contractility is initially increased by continuous infusion of positive inotropic drugs (dopamine), or by combination inodilators such as dobutamine or milrinone. Nesiritide (Natrecor) or BNP IV is indicated for the relief of patients with acutely decompensated heart failure who have dyspnea at rest. Nesiritide lowers pulmonary artery pressures and "wedge" pressure, which decreases symptoms of dyspnea.[85,86]

Once the acute heart failure is controlled, the patient is weaned off IV medications, which are gradually replaced by oral agents. Before the transition out of the critical care unit, the heart failure patient will receive ACE inhibitors to inhibit LV chamber remodeling and slow LV dilation.[61,70,73] If the patient does not tolerate ACE inhibitors, the ARB category of drugs may be substituted.[71] Low dosage β-blockers such as carvedilol may also be prescribed, although strict surveillance is required to anticipate and avoid untoward negative inotropic effects.[80,87] Digoxin may be added to the regimen, especially if the person has concomitant atrial fibrillation.[83] Nonpharmacologic interventions that are increasingly used include cardiac resynchronization therapy (CRT).[88] CRT is biventricular pacing where the right and left ventricles each have a pacing lead in contact with the myocardium. The RV lead is inside the right ventricle, while the LV lead is positioned into a left wall tributary of the coronary sinus vein.[88-90] In newer permanent pacemaker models, both RV and LV leads are paced to synchronize the ventricles and improve heart failure symptoms.

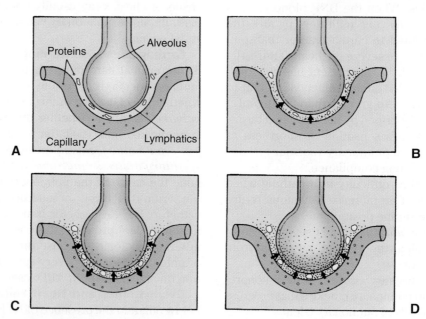

Fig. 18-17   As pulmonary edema progresses, it inhibits oxygen and carbon dioxide exchange at the alveolar capillary interface. **A,** Normal relationship. **B,** Increased pulmonary capillary hydrostatic pressure causes fluid to move from the vascular space into the pulmonary interstitial space. **C,** Lymphatic flow increases in an attempt to pull fluid back into the vascular or lymphatic space. **D,** Failure of lymphatic flow and worsening of left-sided heart failure results in further movement of fluid into the interstitial space and the alveoli.

Correct Precipitating Causes. Once symptoms of HF are controlled, diagnostic studies such as cardiac catheterization, echocardiogram, and thallium scan are undertaken to uncover the cause of the heart failure and tailor long-term management to treat the cause. Some structural problems such as valvular disease may be amenable to surgical correction.

Palliative Care for End-Stage Heart Failure. Because heart failure is a progressive disease, some patients will not recover.[61] At some point, many NYHA Class IV heart failure patients will become candidates for palliative care.[91]

NURSING MANAGEMENT

Nursing management of the patient with heart failure incorporates a variety of nursing diagnoses (see the Nursing Diagnoses feature on Acute Heart Failure). Nursing management interventions are designed to achieve optimum cardiopulmonary function, promote comfort and emotional support, monitor the effectiveness of pharmacologic therapy, ensure nutritional intake is sufficient, and provide patient and family education.

Optimize Cardiopulmonary Function. The patient's ECG is evaluated for any dysrhythmias that may be present or may develop as a result of drug toxicity or electrolyte imbalance. Patients with heart failure are prone to digoxin toxicity secondary to decreased renal perfusion, as well as to electrolyte imbalances. Breath sounds are

NURSING DIAGNOSES	Acute Heart Failure

- Impaired Gas Exchange related to ventilation/perfusion mismatching or intrapulmonary shunting
- Decreased Cardiac Output related to alterations in preload
- Decreased Cardiac Output related to alterations in contractility
- Decreased Cardiac Output related to alterations in heart rate or rhythm
- Activity Intolerance related to cardiopulmonary dysfunction
- Anxiety related to threat to biologic, psychologic, and/or social integrity
- Ineffective Coping related to situational crisis and personal vulnerability
- Disturbed Sleep Pattern related to circadian desynchronization
- Deficient Knowledge: Discharge Regimen related to lack of previous exposure to information (See Patient Education feature on Acute Heart Failure)

auscultated frequently to determine adequacy of respiratory effort and to assess for onset or worsening of pulmonary congestion. Oxygen through a nasal cannula is administered to relieve dyspnea. Diuretics or vasodilators are used to decrease excessive preload and afterload.[72,85] If the patient is not hypotensive, morphine may be administered to decrease hyperventilation and anxiety. If the patient's ventilatory status worsens, the nurse must be prepared for endotracheal intubation and mechanical ventilation. Obtaining daily weights is important until the weight stabilizes at a "dry" weight. Generally, the daily weight is used in fluid management and a weekly weight is optimally used for tracking body weight (muscle, fat).

Promote Comfort and Emotional Support. During periods of breathlessness, activity must be restricted; bed rest usually is prescribed for the patient, who is positioned with the head of the bed elevated to allow for maximal lung expansion. The arms can be supported on pillows so that no undue stress is placed on the shoulder muscles. The legs may be placed in a dependent position to encourage venous pooling, thereby decreasing venous return. Rest periods must be carefully planned and adhered to, while independence within the patient's activity prescription is fostered. Vital signs are recorded before an activity is begun and after it is completed. Signs of activity intolerance, such as dyspnea, fatigue, sustained increase in pulse, and onset of dysrhythmias, are documented and reported to the physician. Activity is gradually increased according to patient tolerance. Skin breakdown is a risk because of the combination of bed rest, inadequate nutrition, peripheral edema, and decreased perfusion to the skin and subcutaneous tissue. Frequent position changes and mobilization are helpful to provide comfort and prevent this complication.

Monitor the Effects of Pharmacologic Therapy. Patients experiencing acute heart failure require aggressive pharmacologic therapy.[80,86,92,93] The nurse must know the action, side effects, therapeutic levels, and toxic effects of the diuretics and venodilators used to decrease preload, the positive inotropic agents used to increase ventricular contractility, the vasodilators used to decrease afterload, and any antidysrhythmics used to control heart rate and prevent dysrhythmias. The patient's hemodynamic response to these agents is closely monitored. Fluid intake and output balances are tabulated daily, or even hourly, in the critical care unit.

Nutritional Intake. Patients experiencing heart failure often experience decreased appetite and nausea; therefore small, frequent meals may be more appropriate than the standard three large meals. Food must be as tasty as possible; favorite foods as well as food from home may be incorporated into the diet as long as the foods are compatible with nutritional restrictions such as low sodium to decrease the risk of fluid retention. Each patient must be assessed for nutritional imbalance individually. Some people with heart failure are well nourished, some are obese, and some are malnourished before they enter the hospital.

PATIENT EDUCATION

Acute Heart Failure

- Heart failure: pathophysiology of heart failure
- Fluid balance: low-salt diet to reduce fluid retention; intake and output measurement; signs of fluid overload, such as peripheral edema
- Daily weight: increase or loss of 1 to 2 pounds in a few days is a sign of fluid gain or loss, not true weight gain or loss
- Breathlessness: increasing shortness of breath, wheezing, and sleeping upright on pillows are symptoms that must be monitored and reported to a health care professional
- Activity: activity conservation with rest periods as heart failure progresses
- Medications: medications are complex, and information must be in writing, as well as oral
  - Preload: purpose of diuretics, increased urine output, and control of fluid volume
  - Afterload: purpose of vasodilators or ACE inhibitors in decreasing the workload of the heart
  - Heart rate: purpose of digoxin to control atrial fibrillation—a frequent dysrhythmia in heart failure
  - Contractility: with the exception of digoxin, no oral contractility drugs are approved by the Food and Drug Administration
  - Anticoagulation: patients with distended atria and enlarged ventricles or with atrial fibrillation may be prescribed anticoagulants (warfarin [Coumadin]); risks of bleeding, importance of correct dosages, prothrombin times, international normalized ratio, and nutritional-pharmacologic interactions are emphasized
- Follow-up care
- Symptoms to report to a health care professional

Box 18-9

COLLABORATIVE MANAGEMENT

HEART FAILURE

A collaborative heart failure management team provides an integrated approach to care to achieve clinical stability for the patient.

1. **Ensure systematic assessment and management**
   - To achieve an absence of "congestion" and to stabilize patient's condition at the best "stage" possible when in hospital (see Tables 18-10 and 18-11).
   - To maintain same stability once discharged home and to avoid hospital readmission.

2. **Counsel and educate patient/family after discharge from hospital. Patients and families should understand the following:**
   - Heart failure disease process.
   - Heart failure medications, dosages, medication schedule, drug side effects.
   - Fluid balance related to salt restriction (2-g sodium diet), daily weight, diuretic regimen.
   - When to call health care provider.
   - Risk of additional complications: sudden cardiac death, progressive heart failure, need for other cardiac procedures (pacemaker; ICD, PCI) or cardiac surgery (bypass graft, valve replacement). Some patients may require a mechanical assist device or heart transplantation.
   - Purpose of "advance directive" for health care decisions.

3. **Promote patient compliance with treatment regimen.**
   - Patients need support from concerned companions and health care professionals.
   - Patient should remain physically active and involved with life.

4. **Facilitate hospital discharge; implement outpatient models of health care delivery.**
   - Close communication between inpatient and outpatient health care providers is essential.

Data from Grady KL et al: *Circulation* 102:2443-2456, 2000; and Hunt S et al: *Circulation* 104(24):2996-3007, 2001.
ICD, Implantable cardioverter-defibrillator; *PCI,* percutaneous coronary intervention.

PATIENT EDUCATION

The nurse assesses both the patient's and families' understanding of the pathophysiology and individual risk factor profile for heart failure.[94] Primary topics of education include the importance of a low-salt diet, daily weight, fluid restrictions, and written information about the multiple medications used to control the symptoms of heart failure (see the Patient Education feature on Acute Heart Failure).[61,95] Many patients with a diagnosis of heart failure also require education about lifestyle changes such as smoking cessation, weight loss, energy conservation, and how to incorporate exercise and sodium restriction into their daily life.[73,96,97] Achieving the optimal outcomes for the patient with heart failure requires contributions from a team of educated health care clinicians.[61,73,95,97] Collaborative multidisciplinary

goals, developed from clinical practice guidelines for management of the patient with symptoms of acute heart failure, are listed in Box 18-9.

CARDIOMYOPATHY

DESCRIPTION AND ETIOLOGY

Cardiomyopathy is a disease of the heart muscle: *cardio* (heart), *myo* (muscle), and *pathy* (pathology). Cardiomyopathies are classified on the basis of structural abnormalities and, if known, genotype. The cardiomyo-

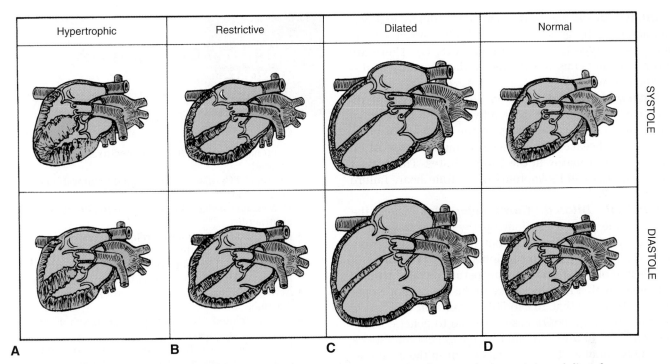

Hypertrophic	Restrictive	Dilated	Normal	
				SYSTOLE
				DIASTOLE
A	**B**	**C**	**D**	

Fig. 18-18 Types of cardiomyopathies and the differences in ventricular diameter during systole and diastole, compared with a normal heart. **A,** Hypertrophic. **B,** Restrictive. **C,** Dilated. **D,** Normal.

pathic categories are hypertrophic, restrictive, and dilated as illustrated in Fig. 18-18.

Hypertrophic Obstructive Cardiomyopathy. Hypertrophic cardiomyopathy (HCM) is a genetically inherited disease that affects the myocardial sarcomere.[98,99] As HCM progresses the left ventricle becomes stiff, noncompliant, and hypertrophied, sometimes in an asymmetrical fashion.[98] Today it is apparent that HCM occurs in two forms. The most well known, but less frequent, manifestation is a stiff, noncompliant myocardial muscle with LV hypertrophy and bizarre cellular hypertrophy of the upper ventricular septum. This LV septal hypertrophy obstructs outflow through the aortic valve, especially during exercise (see Fig. 18-18, *A*). It also pulls the papillary muscle out of alignment, causing mitral regurgitation. This form of HCM used to be known as *idiopathic hypertrophic subaortic stenosis (IHSS)*; however, because IHSS does not describe all patients with hypertrophied hearts, the more general term *HCM* is now used.[98] Other patients with HCM have generalized LV hypertrophy, but the septum is not more enlarged than the rest of the myocardium.[98] HCM causes significant diastolic dysfunction because the muscle-bound, stiff, noncompliant heart muscle cannot fill adequately during diastole.

Two advances in diagnostic medicine have propelled understanding of the differences between these two forms of HCM. The two-dimensional transthoracic echocardiogram (TTE) is often useful as the first diagnostic test to identify HCM.[98] The TTE enables visualization of the septal anatomy, septal movement, plus ventricular wall thickness and motion. The second advance is due to the advent of diagnostic genetics. Genetic test-

ing for HCM is generally performed at a center with expertise in this area.[98] HCM is inherited as an autosomal dominant trait, and the clinical expression is caused by mutations in any of one of 10 genes. Each different gene encodes different protein components of the myocardial sarcomere.[98] Genetic analysis is an area of ongoing research that will undoubtedly help clarify other aspects of this cardiomyopathy within the next decade.

Symptoms are similar to those seen with heart failure plus the symptoms of myocardial ischemia, supraventricular tachycardia (SVT), VT syncope, and stroke.[100] Symptoms are generally more intense with physical exercise, especially in the obstructive form of HCM where the aortic outflow tract is obstructed by the enlarged LV septum. There is also a known association between HCM and sudden cardiac death (SCD). For this reason, limitation of physical activity may be recommended. Causes of SCD are thought to stem from ventricular dysrhythmias and also atrial fibrillation.[98] Episodes of paroyxsmal atrial fibrillation occur in 20% to 25% of HCM patients.[98] The atrial dysrhythmias are related to increased age and atrial enlargement.[98] Pharmacologic management includes beta-blockers to decrease LV workload, medications to control and prevent atrial and ventricular dysrhythmias, anticoagulation if atrial fibrillation or left ventricular thrombi are present, and finally drugs to manage heart failure. Interventional procedures include insertion of an ICD to decrease the risk of SCD, and percutaneous alcohol ablation of the intraventricular septum to decrease the size of the septal wall.[98,99] Surgical procedures such as septal myectomy and mitral valve replacement are options now used less frequently.[98]

Dilated Cardiomyopathy. Dilated cardiomyopathy is characterized by gross dilation of both ventricles without muscle hypertrophy (see Fig. 18-18, *C*). There are several distinct causes of dilated cardiomyopathy, as discussed below.

Ischemic Dilated Cardiomyopathy. Ischemic dilated cardiomyopathy is caused by repeated myocardial injury or infarction secondary to the sequelae of coronary artery disease. It is the most common cause of dilated cardiomyopathy in the United States. The patient will have signs and symptoms of systolic heart failure and a low EF.[64]

Familial Dilated Cardiomyopathy. When the cause of the dilated cardiomyopathy is unknown, it is termed *idiopathic*. In some, but not all cases, the occurrence is linked to genetic inheritance. Scientific advances in molecular genetics now permit detailed studies of families with a high incidence of dilated cardiomyopathy. It is believed that 10% to 50% of *familial idiopathic dilated cardiomyopathy* cases are due to genetic transmission.[101-103] In affected families, the genetic mutations are highly variable. The variations occur in the gene that codes for the sarcomere contractile protein in the heart. The heritable trait can be expressed as either autosomal-dominant or recessive gene inheritance.[101-103] Preliminary research studies indicate that the genetic picture is highly individual between different family groups, even if the clinical picture appears similar.[101-103]

Other Causes of Dilated Cardiomyopathy. There are many other nonischemic, nongenetic known causes of dilated cardiomyopathy. Injury can be caused by valvular heart dysfunction that has placed extreme pressure or volume on the chambers; also, viral or bacterial infections such as myocarditis can lead to inflammatory changes that permanently remodel the heart.[104] Other noncardiac causes include infiltration by systemic collagens as in amyloidosis or sarcoidosis.[105]

In dilated cardiomyopathy the myocardial muscle fibers contract poorly, resulting in global left ventricular dysfunction, low cardiac output, atrial and ventricular dysrhythmias, blood pooling that leads to ventricular thrombi and embolic episodes, and finally, refractory heart failure and premature death. The goals of the medical management of dilated cardiomyopathy are similar to those for systolic heart failure: improvement of pump function, removal of excess fluid, control of heart failure symptoms, anticipation and management of complications, and prevention of sudden cardiac death (SCD).

Restrictive Cardiomyopathy. Restrictive cardiomyopathy (RCM) is the least commonly encountered cardiomyopathy in industrialized societies (see Fig. 18-18, *B*). As with the other cardiomyopathies, this form can be idiopathic or can occur secondary to a known cause.[106,107] RCM results in ventricular wall rigidity as a consequence of myocardial fibrosis. The overall effect is the diastolic inhibition of ventricular filling. Diastolic

---

NURSING DIAGNOSES | **Cardiomyopathy**

- Decreased Cardiac Output related to alterations in preload
- Decreased Cardiac Output related to alterations in afterload
- Decreased Cardiac Output related to alterations in contractility
- Decreased Cardiac Output related to alterations in heart rate or rhythm
- Impaired Gas Exchange related to ventilation/perfusion mismatching or intrapulmonary shunting
- Activity Intolerance related to cardiopulmonary dysfunction
- Anxiety related to threat to biologic, psychologic, and/or social integrity
- Powerlessness related to lack of control over current situation and/or disease progression
- Deficient Knowledge: Discharge Regimen related to lack of previous exposure to information (see Patient Education feature on Cardiomyopathy)

---

heart failure, low cardiac output, dyspnea, orthopnea, and liver engorgement are the most common clinical manifestations of restrictive cardiomyopathy. Medical management includes beta-blockers to slow the heart rate and allow more time for ventricular filling, diuretics to remove excess fluid, and a low-sodium diet.

NURSING MANAGEMENT

Nursing management of the patient with cardiomyopathy incorporates a variety of nursing diagnoses related to the symptoms of heart failure. These nursing diagnoses are reviewed in the Nursing Diagnoses feature on Cardiomyopathy. Nursing interventions are individualized according to the type of cardiomyopathy and are focused on achievement of a stable fluid balance, monitoring the effects of pharmacologic therapy, safely increasing mobility, and providing patient and family education. As with heart failure, a collaborative team of compassionate, knowledgeable professionals is required to provide effective care and education for these challenging patients.[95]

PATIENT EDUCATION

Education is tailored to the type of cardiomyopathy and to any associated conditions (see the Patient Education feature on Cardiomyopathy).

Cardiomyopathy

Cardiomyopathy produces symptoms of heart failure; patient education covers many of the same issues discussed for heart failure:

- Cardiomyopathy: explain pathophysiology of cardiomyopathy and heart failure
- Fluid balance: low-salt to reduce fluid retention; intake and output measurement; signs of fluid overload, such as peripheral edema
- Daily weight: increase or loss of 1 to 2 pounds in a few days is a sign of fluid gain or loss, not true weight gain or loss
- Breathlessness: increasing shortness of breath, wheezing, and sleeping upright on pillows are symptoms that must be monitored and reported to a health care professional.
- Activity: activity conservation with rest periods as heart failure progresses
- Medications: medications are complex, and information must be in writing, as well as oral
  - —Preload: purpose of diuretics, increased urine output, and control of fluid volume
  - —Afterload: purpose of vasodilators or ACE inhibitors in decreasing the workload of the heart
  - —Heart rate: purpose of digoxin to control atrial fibrillation, a frequent dysrhythmia in heart failure; purpose of amiodarone to control ventricular and atrial dysrhythmia common in heart failure
  - —Contractility: with the exception of digoxin, no oral contractility drugs are approved by the Food and Drug Administration
  - —Decrease sympathetic response: purpose of carvedilol (beta-blocker) to lower cardiac response to adrenergic stimulation
  - —Anticoagulation: patients with distended atria, enlarged ventricles, or atrial fibrillation may be prescribed anticoagulants (Coumadin) and/or aspirin; risk of bleeding, importance of correct dosages, prothrombin times, international normalized ratio, and nutritional-pharmacologic interactions are emphasized
- Follow-up care
- Symptoms to report to a health care professional

PULMONARY HYPERTENSION

DESCRIPTION AND ETIOLOGY

Pulmonary arterial hypertension (PAH) is a progressive, ultimately fatal disease of the pulmonary vasculature. Because it affects arterial vessels it is discussed with the cardiovascular diseases that affect the arteries. PAH may arise as an isolated condition or be associated with other diseases. The World Health Organization (WHO) classifies pulmonary hypertension into groups based on mechanism of illness and morphologic changes in the vessels rather than the traditional grouping of primary and secondary causes.[108] Some of the causes of PAH likely to be seen in a critical care unit are discussed below. Whatever the etiology, the presence of pulmonary arterial hypertension significantly increases morbidity and mortality of any underlying cardiac or pulmonary disease.

Idiopathic or Primary Pulmonary Hypertension. If the cause of the pulmonary arterial hypertension is unknown or genetic it is termed *idiopathic pulmonary hypertension* or *primary pulmonary hypertension* (PPH).[109] The incidence of PPH is very low, estimated at 1 to 2 cases per million.[109] PPH has an insidious onset and diagnosis is difficult due to the nonspecific nature of the symptoms. Frequently, by the time a firm diagnosis is made, the patient is highly symptomatic. Without treatment, according to the U.S. National Institutes of Health (NIH) the median survival after diagnosis is 68% at one year, falls to 48% after 3 years, and is reduced to 34% at 5 years.[109,110]

Pulmonary Arterial Hypertension and Respiratory Hypoxemic Disorders. Pulmonary arterial hypertension can occur as a result of chronic respiratory diseases that cause hypoxemia. All patients with PAH feel short of breath with exercise, but this group of patients is dyspneic even at rest. Chronic obstructive pulmonary disease (COPD), interstitial lung disease, and sleep-disordered breathing are chronic respiratory diseases that can lead to PAH.[111] Pulmonary function tests and sleep apnea studies are performed as part of the diagnosis for this group of patients.[109,112]

Pulmonary Arterial Hypertension and Thromboembolic Disorders. Pulmonary arterial hypertension can happen acutely in response to a large pulmonary embolus that blocks flow to the pulmonary vascular bed. PAH can also occur following multiple microembolic thrombi that obstruct the smaller pulmonary arteries. If the risk of pulmonary emboli is recognized in the hypercoagulable patient, this condition is potentially preventable.[113] Current guidelines recommend that when PAH is diagnosed, a ventilation-perfusion scan (VQ scan) be performed to determine the presence or absence of pulmonary emboli.[114]

Pulmonary Venous Hypertension. Pulmonary venous hypertension causes PAH by a very different mechanism than other forms of pulmonary hypertension. It occurs as a result of elevated pressures in the left side of the heart that subsequently raise the pulmonary venous pressure. Patients with pulmonary venous hypertension have a history of coronary artery disease (CAD), acute MI, valvular disease, heart failure, or dilated cardiomyopathy. PAH develops as the high pressures in left heart failure are communicated across the pulmonary vascular bed to the right ventricle. This is a common etiology of PAH, since 80% of patients with chronically high left heart pressures also have elevated right heart pressures.[61]

Other, less frequent causes of pulmonary arterial hypertension that may be seen in critical care units include systemic vascular collagen diseases, congenital heart disease, human immunodeficiency virus (HIV) infection, drugs such as the fenfluramines used in weight loss and liver failure with portal hypertension.

PATHOPHYSIOLOGY

The pulmonary vascular bed is normally a high-flow, low-pressure, low-resistance system that easily adjusts to changes in cardiac output, oxygen demand, and exercise. In the presence of pulmonary arterial hypertension these characteristics are lost. Progressive and sustained elevation of pulmonary pressures with increased pulmonary vascular resistance (PVR) leads to increased pressure on the right ventricle, increased RV workload, RV hypertrophy, and ultimately to RV heart failure and death. Although the etiology of PPH is unknown, it is thought to be a disorder of the pulmonary vascular endothelium. That it is an imbalance between several metabolically active prostaglandins secreted by the endothelium is one theory.[109] Overproduction of substances that cause vasoconstriction such as *thromboxane* and *endothelin;* or a decrease in endothelial factors that cause vasodilation, specifically endothelial *prostacyclin* and *nitric oxide* (NO); or a combination of these factors may be the catalyst.

ASSESSMENT AND DIAGNOSIS

The diagnosis of PAH is difficult and of PPH even more so. Pulmonary hypertension is often a diagnosis of exclusion when all other diagnostic theories are exhausted. The clinical symptoms of PAH are nonspecific in the early stages of the disease and reflect the inability of the pulmonary vascular bed to accommodate increased cardiac output with exercise. Initial signs and symptoms include pallor, dyspnea with exertion, and fatigue. As the disease progresses the severity of symptoms increases to include chest pain and syncope with exertion.

The most helpful noninvasive test is the echocardiogram. Diagnostic findings in PAH include right atrial and right ventricular enlargement, reduced right ventricular function, displacement of the intraventricular septum, and tricuspid regurgitation (TR).[110] Presence of a pericardial effusion is a negative prognostic finding associated with earlier mortality.[110]

The most helpful invasive diagnostic test is a right-sided cardiac catheterization, because this will provide verifiable numbers. To diagnose PAH, the pulmonary artery mean pressure must be greater than 25 mm Hg at rest and above 30 mm Hg with exercise. An elevated right atrial pressure (RAP) is a poor long-term prognostic

sign.[110] An important component of the cardiac catheterization study used to diagnose PAH is an evaluation of the ability of the pulmonary vessels to vasodilate in response to administration of a pulmonary arterial vasodilator such as inhaled nitrous oxide (NO), IV adenosine, or IV epoprostenol (prostacyclin).[109,110] The response of the pulmonary vasculature to this vasoreactivity test will determine how helpful pulmonary arterial vasodilating medications will be.

If PAH is diagnosed when the condition is advanced, the pulmonary pressures may almost equal the systemic aortic pressure and the pulmonary arterioles may not vasodilate in response to drugs. In this scenario the enlarged right ventricle will put pressure on the intraventricular septum and compress the left ventricle. The smaller, compressed LV means that cardiac output is greatly reduced.[115] Interpretation of PA pressures, cardiac catheterization, and echocardiogram are discussed in detail in Chapter 17.

MEDICAL MANAGEMENT

Medical management is focused on early diagnosis, use of appropriate pharmacologic therapies, and prevention of complications.

Medications. The medication regimen options include calcium channel blockers, prostacyclin, anticoagulants, diuretics, and oxygen.

Calcium-channel blockers may lengthen survival in a few patients with PAH who demonstrate a significant vasodilator response, but the majority of PAH patients are nonresponders and are more effectively managed with one of the newer drugs developed specifically to treat PAH.[110,116]

Prostacyclin acts directly on the pulmonary vasculature to vasodilate the arteries. Epoprostenol (Flolan) was the first prostacyclin available. It is administered IV and has a half-life of only 2 to 3 minutes, and interruptions in therapy must be avoided. In research studies, PPH patients treated with epoprostenol had improved survival rates at 1 year (87%), 2 years (72%), 3 years (63%), and 5 years (54%) compared with nontreated historical controls.[110] Patients who are critically ill and have functional class IV symptoms, should be started on epoprostenol, because it is the most rapidly effective therapy.[116] Treprostinil sodium (Remodulin) is a more recently approved prostacyclin analogue. It is administered via a subcutaneous (SC) infusion catheter and pump and has a half life of 3 hours.[109] One oral medication is available: bosentan (Tracleer) blocks the endothelial vasoconstrictor *endothelin* to promote pulmonary vasodilation. These drugs do not cure the PAH but all vasodilate the pulmonary vascular bed, control symptoms, and prolong life in responsive patients. Research to develop other therapies such as phosphodiesterase inhibitors, selective endothelin A receptor antagonists, and prostacyclin analogs with alternative delivery routes (inhaled, oral), to treat pulmonary hypertension are ongoing.[116,117]

Anticoagulation is an essential component of the pharmacologic management. The 1-year, 3-year, and 5-year survival rates in PAH patients who are anticoagulated with warfarin (Coumadin) are 91%, 62%, and 47%, respectively, compared to 52%, 31%, and 31% in nonanticoagulated PAH patients.[110]

For patients who are refractory to pharmacologic management a heart-lung transplant may be an option.[118] Detailed information on heart-lung transplant is provided in Chapter 41.

NURSING MANAGEMENT

Nursing management of the patient with pulmonary arterial hypertension incorporates a variety of nursing diagnoses related to the symptoms of breathlessness and right-sided heart failure. These nursing diagnoses are reviewed in the Nursing Diagnoses feature on Pulmonary Arterial Hypertension. Nursing interventions are individualized according to how advanced the symptoms of PAH are. Interventions are focused on lowering PA pressures, administration of pharmacologic therapy, monitoring of the effects and safety of all medications, treating pain that can occur at the site of injection, and providing patient and family education.[109]

PATIENT EDUCATION

Before discharge from the hospital the person with PAH needs to know the underlying reason for their disease process (if known). All patients must be provided with a written medication list with the name and purpose of all their drugs. Specific education may be directed to management of a tunneled IV catheter or SC pump for administration of a prostacyclin analog drug. The name of the health care professional to contact for questions related to the PAH is also important (see the Patient Education feature Pulmonary Arterial Hypertension). A collaborative team of empathetic, educated professionals is essential to provide effective care for these challenging patients (see the Evidence-Based Collaborative Practice feature on Pulmonary Arterial Hypertension).

ENDOCARDITIS

DESCRIPTION AND ETIOLOGY

Infective endocarditis (IE) is an infection on the endothelial surface of the heart, specifically thrombotic-

EVIDENCE-BASED COLLABORATIVE MANAGEMENT

Pulmonary Arterial Hypertension

Recommendations for Early Detection and Screening for Pulmonary Arterial Hypertension

- Relatives of patients with familial pulmonary arterial hypertension (PAH) are recommended to undergo prenatal genetic testing before any pregnancy.
- Pregnancy is not recommended for female patients with PAH.
- If PAH is suspected, a 12-lead ECG is required as an early screening test to rule out other possible cardiac anomalies. The ECG is not diagnostic for PAH.
- If PAH is suspected, a chest x-ray can reveal features supportive of a PAH diagnosis.
- If PAH is suspected, Doppler echocardiography is recommended to noninvasively evaluate RV systolic pressures and to assess for anatomic abnormalities such as RA or RV enlargement, LV involvement, and intracardiac shunting.

Recommendations for Diagnostic Tests to Further Evaluate PAH

- In patients with unexplained PAH, testing for connective tissue disease and HIV is recommended.
- In patients with probable connective tissue PAH, a V/Q scan is recommended.
- Pulmonary function tests are recommended to rule out other causes of lung disease.
- Lung biopsy is not recommended. It carries a high risk and low diagnostic yield.
- Right-sided heart catheterization is recommended.
- Serial assessments of functional class and endurance on a 6-minute walk are recommended.

Recommendations for Management of PAH

- Patients with PAH should undergo acute vasoreactivity testing using a short-acting agent such as IV epoprostenol or adenosine, or inhaled NO.

- Patients with PAH, in the absence of right-sided heart failure, demonstrating a favorable acute response to a vasodilator (defined as a fall in mPAP of at least 10 mm Hg to 40 mm Hg, with an increased or unchanged CO), should be considered candidates for a trial of therapy with an oral calcium channel blocker.
- Calcium channel blockers should not be used empirically to treat PAH in the absence of demonstrated acute vasoreactivity.
- Patients with idiopathic PAH should receive anticoagulation with warfarin (Coumadin).
- In patients with PAH occurring in association with other underlying processes, such as scleroderma or congenital heart disease, anticoagulation should be considered.
- In patients with PAH, supplemental oxygen should be used as necessary to maintain oxygen saturations >90% at all times.

Recommendations for Medications to Treat PAH

- Patients with PAH in functional class II who have failed calcium channel blocker therapy may benefit from treatment. However, limited data are available, and no specific drug is recommended.
- Patients with PAH in functional class III who have failed calcium channel blocker drugs are candidates for long-term therapy with one of the following drugs:
- Endothelin-receptor antagonists
  —Bosentan (oral)
  —Sitaxsentan (oral)
- Prostanoids
  —Epoprostenol (IV)
  —Treprostinil (SC)
  —Iloprost (inhaled)
- Patients with PAH in functional class IV who have failed calcium channel blocker therapy are candidates for long-term therapy with IV epoprosternol (treatment of choice).

From McGoon M et al: Screening, early detection, and diagnosis of pulmonary arterial hypertension: ACCP evidence-based clinical practice guidelines, *Chest* 126(suppl 1):14S-34S, 2004; Badesch DB et al: Medical therapy for pulmonary arterial hypertension: ACCP evidence-based clinical practice guidelines, *Chest* 126(suppl 1):35S-62S, 2004.

CO, Cardiac output; *ECG*, electrocardiogram; *IV*, intravenous; *LV*, left ventricle; *mPAP*, mean pulmonary artery pressure; *NO*, nitrous oxide; *PAH*, pulmonary arterial hypertension; *RA*, right atrium; *RV*, right ventricle; *SC*, subcutaneous; *V/Q*, ventilation-perfusion.

---

fibrin vegetations on the cardiac valves. The older term of bacterial endocarditis is no longer employed because nonbacterial organisms can also be the infective source. The incidence of IE is rising, with 5,000 to 20,00 new cases diagnosed per year. IE is the fourth most common cause of life-threatening infectious syndromes (after urosepsis, pneumonia, and intraabdominal sepsis). The risk of acquiring IE is higher among patients with congenital heart disease, valvular heart disease, and pros-

thetic heart valves. In patients with intravenous drug abuse (IVDA), the incidence of IE is 60 times that of age-matched controls.[119] Development of IE depends on two factors:

1. Susceptible lesion in the vascular endothelium.
2. An organism to establish the infection.

The source of the organism may be unknown, or it may be traced to an invasive procedure, such as a biopsy, urogenital procedure, or dental work, or a preexisting condition such as valvular heart disease (Box 18-10).

PATHOPHYSIOLOGY

Infective endocarditis is consequent to a bacterial or fungal organism in the bloodstream that successfully colonizes the cardiac endothelium. It is fatal if not treated. Bacterial infections are the most common, with almost a third of all IE originating from *Staphylococcus aureus*.[119] The thrombotic vegetations are colonized by bacteria and encased in a fibrin shell, which protects them from destruction by phagocytic neutrophils. It is because of this extensive protective mechanism that antibiotic therapy must be so intensive and prolonged.[120]

ASSESSMENT AND DIAGNOSIS

Initial symptoms include fever, sometimes accompanied by rigor (shivering). Blood cultures are drawn during periods of elevated temperature to detect the infective organism. At least 10 milliliters (mls) of venous blood should be placed in each of the blood culture containers to ensure that the organism will be detected.[119] Culture-negative endocarditis occurs in about 5% of patients, usually related to recent or current antibiotic treatment.[119] White blood cell (WBC) counts are typically elevated in response to the infection.

Cough and pleuritic chest pain are present in 40% to 60% of cases. Thus the first noninvasive test is often a chest x-ray to detect nodular infiltrates, identified in over 70% of symptomatic patients.[119] The other essential noninvasive test is an echocardiogram of the heart valves to visualize vegetations. A transthoracic echocardiogram (TTE) may be initially performed, but a transesophageal echo (TEE) is even more valuable because of the clarity of the heart valve images. Color-flow mapping is especially useful to visualize the severity of valvular regurgitation if present.[119] Stroke is a major complication of endocarditis, involving vegetations dislodged from the mitral and aortic valves: 10% of patients with aortic valve IE and 18% of patients with mitral valve IE will suffer a stroke, based on a case series of 700 patients.[121] In over half of these cases, stroke was the presenting symptom.[121] Septic emboli may be visible on the fingers and toes. The risk of death increases with the development of emboli and decreased arterial perfusion to vital organs. Other patients may be seen with symptoms of acute heart failure. It is important to be aware that acute HF is the most frequent cause of death in patients with infective endocarditis.[119,121] Clinical manifestations of endocarditis that may be discovered on physical examination are listed in Box 18-11.

MEDICAL MANAGEMENT

Treatment requires prolonged IV therapy with adequate doses of antimicrobial agents tailored to the specific IE microbe and patient circumstances. The antibiotic management of native valve endocarditis (NVE) is frequently different from treatment of prosthetic valve endocarditis (PVE) or IVDA endocarditis. Best outcomes are achieved if therapy is initiated before hemodynamic compromise.[119] In many cases, antimicrobial drugs are not sufficient to cure the IE. Cardiac surgery to excise the damaged native or prosthetic valve is necessary in 30% to 40% of symptomatic patients. Usually valve surgery is delayed until the patient is stable.[119] An increasing number of patients with uncomplicated IE are being discharged to home earlier than in the past and are continuing the IV antimicrobial therapy via a surgically or peripherally implanted long-term central venous catheter at home.[120]

NURSING DIAGNOSES   Endocarditis

- Decreased Cardiac Output related to alterations in preload
- Decreased Cardiac Output related to alterations in afterload
- Decreased Cardiac Output related to alterations in contractility
- Decreased Cardiac Output related to alterations in heart rate or rhythm
- Activity Intolerance related to cardiopulmonary dysfunction
- Acute Pain related to transmission and perception of cutaneous, visceral, muscular, or ischemic impulses
- Risk for Infection risk factor: invasive procedures
- Anxiety related to threat to biologic, psychologic, and/or social integrity
- Deficient Knowledge: Discharge Regimen related to lack of previous exposure to information (see Patient Education feature on Endocarditis)

PATIENT EDUCATION   Endocarditis

- Pathophysiology of endocarditis
- Medications: importance of long-term intravenous antibiotics
- Temperature: daily temperature
- Infection control: prophylactic antibiotics related to dental work or other invasive procedures, when current medical crisis controlled
- Activity tolerance: increase activity as tolerated; rest periods as needed
- Heart failure: if symptoms of heart failure are present, education is given on fluid and sodium restriction, fluid balance, diuretic management, daily weight, and controlling breathlessness
- Follow-up care after discharge
- Symptoms to report to a health care professional

NURSING MANAGEMENT

Nursing management of the patient with infective endocarditis incorporates a variety of nursing diagnoses (see the Nursing Diagnoses feature on Endocarditis). Nursing interventions focus on timely antimicrobial administration to resolve the infection, prevent complications, provide pain medication, and individualize patient education.

Resolve the Infection. Infective endocarditis requires a long course of intravenous antibiotics, usually 6 weeks. This is begun in the hospital and continued at home with an indwelling central catheter once the patient is in stable condition.[120] Nursing assessment includes monitoring for signs of worsening infection, such as persistent temperature elevation, malaise, weakness, easy fatigability, and night sweats, or new emboli on hands or feet (see the Patient Education feature on Endocarditis).

Prevent Complications. Between 20% and 50% of patients with IE experience embolic events, affecting the brain, lungs, or major abdominal organs.[119,122] The nursing assessment is attuned to the early detection of new neurologic complications such as changes in level of consciousness, visual changes, or complaints of headache. Shortness of breath or chest pain with hemoptysis is always reported. Evaluation of liver and kidney function is essential to monitor the health of those organs. As valvular dysfunction accelerates, acute heart failure develops. Cardiac assessment includes auscultation of heart sounds to detect the presence of, or change in, a cardiac murmur. This could be caused either by worsening HF or by pulmonary emboli.

PATIENT EDUCATION

The person with infective endocarditis needs to know the manifestations of infection, how to take an oral temperature, and what medical procedures increase risk of a recurrence of IE. A written list of all medications must be supplied (see the Patient Education feature on Endocarditis). It is essential to reinforce the necessity of the patient providing other health care professionals such as the dentist or podiatrist with a comprehensive endocarditis history.[119] The patient with known IVDA has a unique set of challenges to overcome.[123] Multidisciplinary support for the patient to meet the challenge of opiate withdrawal and psychologic dependence is essential to prevent a relapse.[123] Many clinicians participate in the care of a patient with infective endocarditis.

VALVULAR HEART DISEASE

DESCRIPTION AND ETIOLOGY

Valvular heart disease describes structural and/or functional abnormalities of single or multiple cardiac valves. The result is an alteration in blood flow across the valve.

The two types of valvular lesions are stenotic and regurgitant. These are described here with reference to the specific cardiac valves involved.

Usually, if a person is admitted to the critical care unit with valve disease, he or she either is experiencing acute heart failure or is being admitted for cardiac surgical valvular replacement. In the past in the United States, most valvular lesions were rheumatic in origin; that is, damage was a direct result of group A beta-hemolytic streptococcal pharyngitis. Today, as a result of aggressive treatment of "strep throat," this is rarely a problem. Now the elderly are more likely to be seen with symptoms of heart failure and "*degenerative*" valve changes. These may be described as *myxomatous* leaflet degeneration or annular calcification.[124,125]

PATHOPHYSIOLOGY

Mitral Valve Stenosis. Mitral stenosis (MS) describes a progressive narrowing of the mitral valve orifice. Symptoms occur when the normal valve size is reduced to 2 cm^2 or less.[2,125] Symptoms occur at rest when the valve area is reduced below 1 cm^2.[125] Narrowing is caused by aging valve tissue or by acute rheumatic valvulitis (Table 18-12, *A*). The diffuse valve leaflets fibrose and fuse, reducing mobility and thickening the chordae tendineae. As a result, the mitral valve can no longer open or close passively in response to left atrial and ventricular pressure changes. Thus, blood flow across the valve is impeded. Mitral stenosis increases the risk of developing atrial fibrillation because of the high pressures in the left atrium that will stimulate left atrial remodeling and enlargement. Development of atrial fibrillation will significantly increase symptoms and may increase the need for surgical replacement of the valve.

Mitral Valve Regurgitation. Mitral regurgitation may occur secondary to rheumatic disease, aging of the valve, or it can be caused by endocarditis, or papillary muscle dysfunction (Table 18-12, *B*). In mitral valve regurgitation (MR) the valve annulus, leaflets, chordae tendineae, and papillary muscles may all be dysfunctional, or the dysfunction may be isolated to just one component of the valve. Mitral valve regurgitation results in retrograde flow of blood into the left atrium with each ventricular contraction. MR is always described as either chronic or acute because of the very different impact upon the left-sided chambers.

With *chronic MR*, the left atrium will have dilated to accommodate the additional regurgitant volume, whereas the left ventricle will have hypertrophied (increased muscle) to maintain an adequate stroke volume and cardiac output. By contrast, *acute MR* is precipitated by papillary muscle rupture secondary to an acute MI.[125] This is a medical emergency. This left atrium cannot accommodate the sudden increase in volume and pressure, and use of an IABP and inotropic drug support are often required. Once the patient's condition has stabilized, surgical replacement or repair of the incompetent valve is performed.[126]

Aortic Valve Stenosis. Aortic stenosis (AS) describes a narrowing of the aortic valve area. AS can result from aging, rheumatic valvulitis, or deterioration of a congenital bicuspid valve.[127] (Table 18-12, *C*). When the aortic valvular opening is reduced to less than 1.5 cm^2 this is classified as mild AS, and on cardiac catheterization or Doppler echocardiography there will be a "*gradient*" of about 25 mm Hg across the valve.[124] The gradient represents the difference in systolic pressure between the LV and the aorta. A significant pressure difference is a diagnostic hallmark of valvular stenosis.[124] If the valve orifice has narrowed to 1 cm^2 or less, the gradient will be greater than 50 mm Hg and the diagnosis will be upgraded to severe AS.[124] The impedance of LV ejection into the aorta results in increased left ventricular systolic pressure, left ventricular hypertrophy, and eventually left ventricular dilation. When symptoms such as angina, dyspnea, syncope, and other indicators of heart failure develop, it is critical to intervene to prevent further damage to the left ventricle. Aortic valve replacement is usually indicated.

Aortic Valve Regurgitation. Aortic regurgitation (AR), also know as aortic insufficiency (AI) can occur as a result of rheumatic fever, systemic hypertension, Marfan syndrome, syphilis, rheumatoid arthritis, aging valve tissue, or discrete subaortic stenosis (Table 18-12, *D*). Aortic valve incompetence results in a reflux of blood back into the left ventricle during ventricular diastole. To accommodate this extra volume, the left ventricle initially dilates and then hypertrophies in an attempt to empty more completely and to meet the needs of the peripheral circulation. Aortic valve replacement is recommended for symptomatic patients with well-preserved or moderate LV dysfunction.[128]

Tricuspid Valve Stenosis. Tricuspid stenosis (TS) is rarely an isolated lesion (Table 18-12, *E*). TS often occurs in conjunction with mitral or aortic disease. Its origin most often is rheumatic fever or a complication of IVDA and resultant endocarditis.[129] Tricuspid stenosis increases the pressure work of the usually low-pressure right atrium, resulting in right atrial hypertrophy. In addition, the right atrium dilates in an attempt to accommodate the residual right atrial volume and the incoming venous return. As a result, systemic venous congestion occurs—the consequences of which include jugular venous congestion, liver failure, hepatomegaly, ascites, and peripheral edema.

Tricuspid Valve Regurgitation. Tricuspid regurgitation usually results from advanced failure of the left side of the heart that eventually affects the right side of the

Table 18-12	Valvular Dysfunction		
	Pathophysiology	**Clinical Manifestations**	**Physical Signs**

MITRAL VALVE STENOSIS

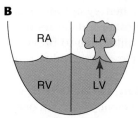

Mitral valve stenosis

 indicates stenosis

	Pathophysiology	Clinical Manifestations	Physical Signs
	Left atrium must generate more pressure to propel blood beyond the lesion Rise in left atrial pressure and volume reflected retrograde into pulmonary vessels Right ventricular hypertrophy Right ventricular failure	Dyspnea on exertion Fatigue and weakness Pronounced respiratory symptoms—orthopnea, paroxysmal nocturnal dyspnea Mild hemoptysis with bronchial capillary rupture Susceptibility to pulmonary infections	Chest radiograph—pulmonary congestion, redistribution of blood flow to upper lobes ECG—atrial fibrillation and other atrial dysrhythmias Auscultation—diastolic murmur, accentuated S_1, opening snap Catheterization—elevated pressure gradient across valve; increased left atrial pressure, pulmonary artery wedge pressure, and pulmonary artery pressure; low cardiac output

MITRAL VALVE REGURGITATION

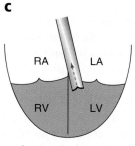

Mitral valve regurgitation

indicates backward flow from a valve that is leaking or regurgitant

	Pathophysiology	Clinical Manifestations	Physical Signs
	Left ventricular dilation and hypertrophy Left atrial dilation and hypertrophy	Weakness and fatigue Exertional dyspnea Palpitations Severe symptoms precipitated by left ventricular failure, with consequent low output and pulmonary congestion	Chest radiograph—left atrial and left ventricular enlargement, variable pulmonary congestion ECG—P mitrale, left ventricular hypertrophy, atrial fibrillation Auscultation—murmur throughout systole Catheterization—opacification of left atrium during left ventricular injection, v waves, increased left atrial and left ventricular pressures Variable elevations of pulmonary pressures

AORTIC VALVE STENOSIS

Aortic valve stenosis

indicates stenosis

	Pathophysiology	Clinical Manifestations	Physical Signs
	Left ventricular hypertrophy Progressive failure of ventricular emptying Pulmonary congestion Failure of right side of heart, with systemic venous congestion Sudden cardiac death	Exertional dyspnea Exercise intolerance Syncope Angina Heart failure (left ventricular failure)	Chest radiograph—poststenotic aortic dilation, calcification ECG—left ventricular hypertrophy Auscultation—systolic ejection murmur Catheterization—significant pressure gradient, increased left ventricular end-diastolic pressure

Table 18-12	Valvular Dysfunction—cont'd		
	Pathophysiology	**Clinical Manifestations**	**Physical Signs**

AORTIC VALVE REGURGITATION

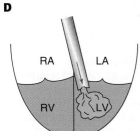

RA   LA
RV   LV

Aortic valve regurgitation

 indicates backward flow from a valve that is leaking or regurgitant

	Pathophysiology	Clinical Manifestations	Physical Signs
	Increased volume load imposed on left ventricle Left ventricular dilation and hypertrophy	Fatigue Dyspnea and exertion Palpitations	Chest radiograph—boot-shaped elongation of cardiac apex ECG—left ventricular hypertrophy Auscultation—diastolic murmur Catheterization—opacification of left ventricle during aortic injection Peripheral signs—hyperdynamic myocardial action and low peripheral resistance

TRICUSPID VALVE STENOSIS

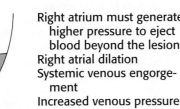

RA   LA
RV   LV

Tricuspid valve stenosis

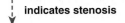 **indicates stenosis**

	Pathophysiology	Clinical Manifestations	Physical Signs
	Right atrium must generate higher pressure to eject blood beyond the lesion Right atrial dilation Systemic venous engorgement Increased venous pressure	Venous distention Peripheral edema Ascites Hepatic engorgement Anorexia	Chest radiograph—right atrial enlargement ECG—right atrial enlargement (P pulmonale) Auscultation—diastolic murmur Catheterization—elevated right atrial pressure with large a waves; pressure gradient across the tricuspid valve

TRICUSPID VALVE REGURGITATION

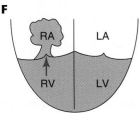

RA   LA
RV   LV

Tricuspid valve regurgitation

indicates backward flow from a valve that is leaking or regurgitant

	Pathophysiology	Clinical Manifestations	Physical Signs
	Right ventricular hypertrophy and dilation	Decreased cardiac output Neck vein distention Hepatic engorgement Ascites Edema Pleural effusions	Chest radiograph—right atrial and ventricular enlargement ECG—right ventricular hypertrophy and right atrial enlargement, atrial fibrillation Auscultation—murmur throughout systole Catheterization—elevated right atrial pressure and v waves

ECG, Electrocardiogram.

heart, severe pulmonary hypertension, or as a complication of infective endocarditis[110,129] (Table 18-12, *F*).

Pulmonic Valve Disease. Pulmonary valve disease is not a common disorder in adults. It is most often related to congenital anomalies and produces failure of the right side of the heart.

Mixed Valvular Lesions. Many persons have mixed lesions (i.e., an element of both stenosis and regurgitation). Mixed lesions can accentuate the severity of a condition. For example, when combined, aortic stenosis and aortic regurgitation increase left ventricular volume and pressure and thereby multiply the degree of left ventricular work.

MEDICAL MANAGEMENT

Management of valvular disorders includes pharmacologic therapy to control symptoms of heart failure and then cardiac surgical repair or replacement of the affected valve.[124,125] When surgery is not feasible, balloon dilation is a rare option selected for individuals too ill to undergo a major cardiac surgical procedure.

NURSING MANAGEMENT

Nursing management of the patient with valvular disease incorporates a variety of nursing diagnoses (see the Nursing Diagnoses feature on Valvular Heart Disease). Nursing management interventions focus upon achievement of adequate cardiac output, maintenance of fluid balance, and patient and family education.

Cardiac Output. Low cardiac output is a common finding in patients with valvular heart disease. It can occur because of decreased forward flow through a stenotic valve, because of bidirectional flow across an incompetent valve, or because of associated heart failure. Vital signs and the effect of positive inotropic and afterload-reducing agents are assessed and documented. If the patient has hemodynamic catheters inserted, cardiac output and hemodynamic parameters are measured and evaluated. Patient care activities are carefully planned to provide adequate rest periods to prevent fatigue.

Fluid Balance. Fluid status is evaluated by auscultation of breath sounds for crackles, heart sounds for presence of an S_3, daily weight to trend a "sudden weight gain," and presence of peripheral edema. The appearance of pulmonary crackles or an S_3 heart sound confirms volume overload. The jugular vein is assessed for signs of increased distention. Diuretics and vasodilators

Box 18-12

COLLABORATIVE MANAGEMENT

VALVULAR HEART DISEASE
1. **Assess valvular dysfunction**
   - Clinical assessment
     Auscultation for heart murmurs
     Signs/symptoms of heart failure; dyspnea is usually the earliest symptoms (see Table 18-7)
     - *Echocardiogram:* valve motion, ventricular wall motion
     - *Cardiac catheterization:* valve/ventricular wall motion, ejection fraction
2. **Consider valve surgery**
   - If heart failure symptoms appear, surgery is indicated
   - Valve replacement
3. **Provide patient/family education**
   - Anticoagulation (if mechanical valve or atrial fibrillation present)
   - Heart failure medications (if heart failure is present)
   - *Infection prevention:* endocarditis prophylaxis
   - *Postoperative:* specialized education related to sternal incision

Data from Bonow RO et al: *J Heart Valve Dis* 7:672-707, 1998.

are administered to counteract excess fluid retention. The patient is weighed daily, and fluid intake and output are monitored and recorded.

PATIENT EDUCATION

Patient education for the patient with acute or chronic heart failure secondary to valvular dysfunction includes (1) information related to diet, (2) fluid restrictions, (3) the actions and side effects of heart failure medications, (4) the need for prophylactic antibiotics before undergoing any invasive procedures such as dental work, and (5) when to call the health care provider to report a negative change in cardiac symptoms (see the Patient Education feature on Valvular Heart Disease). Many patients will also require information about valvular heart surgery. Achieving the optimal outcomes for the patient with valve disease requires contributions from a team of educated health care clinicians. Collaborative multidisciplinary priorities are listed in Box 18-12. See the section on heart valve replacement in Chapter 19 for more information on surgical management.

ATHEROSCLEROTIC DISEASES OF THE AORTA

DESCRIPTION

Two aortic conditions are described—aortic aneurysm and aortic dissection. Both disease states are the result

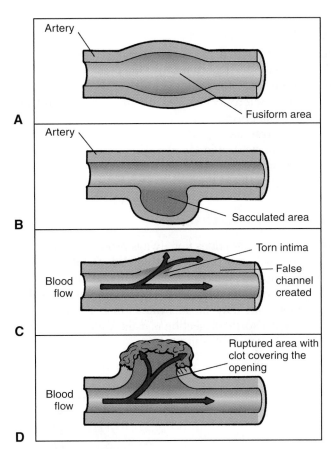

Fig. 18-19 Four types of vascular injury. **A,** Fusiform aneurysm, in which an entire segment of an artery is dilated, thus taking on a spindle or bulbous shape. Fusiform aneurysms occur most often in the abdominal aorta secondary to atherosclerosis. **B,** Sacculated aneurysm, which involves only one side of an artery and usually is located in the ascending aorta. **C,** Dissection, which occurs because of a tear in the intima, resulting in the shunting of blood between the intima and media of a vessel. **D,** Pseudoaneurysm, which can result from arterial trauma, such as that caused by an arterial introducer sheath or intraaortic balloon catheter (IABC), where the arterial opening does not heal normally and is covered by a clot that may rupture at any time.

of progressive atherosclerotic disease and systemic arterial hypertension.

Aortic Aneurysm. An aortic aneurysm (AA) is a localized dilation of the arterial wall that results in an alteration in vessel shape and blood flow. Fig. 18-19, *A* and *B*, displays the two types of vascular aneurysms. Aortic aneurysm is diagnosed most commonly in older adults. Abdominal aortic aneurysm is four times more common than is thoracic aneurysm.

Aortic Dissection. An aortic dissection occurs when a column of blood separates the vascular layers. This creates a *false lumen*, which communicates with the true lumen through a tear in the intima as illustrated in Fig. 18-19, *C*.

ETIOLOGY

Most patients with an aortic aneurysm (90%) have a history of systemic hypertension. Other causes of aortic aneurysm include the following:

1. Atherosclerotic changes in the thoracic and abdominal aorta
2. Blunt trauma
3. Marfan syndrome
4. Pregnancy
5. Injury or dissection

ASSESSMENT AND DIAGNOSIS

An aortic aneurysm does not always produce symptoms. It may be detected during routine abdominal examination as a palpable, pulsatile mass located in the umbilical region of the abdomen to the left of the midline. A thoracic aneurysm may be identified on a routine chest x-ray film. An aortic dissection is usually identified emergently by the onset of acute pain.

Aortic Aneurysm. An aneurysm less than 4 cm in diameter can be managed on an outpatient basis with frequent blood pressure monitoring and ultrasound testing to document any changes in the size of the aneurysm. The patient is encouraged to lose weight if obesity is a factor, and hypertension is treated to decrease hemodynamic stress on the site. An aortic aneurysm greater than 5 cm requires surgical repair, or placement of an aortic stent to eliminate the risk of rupture (Box 18-13).

Aortic Dissection. Aortic dissections are classified according to the site of the tear. Two classification systems are used in clinical practice. These use either the letters *A* and *B* or numerals *I*, *II*, or *III*, as shown in Fig. 18-20. The classic clinical manifestation is the sudden onset of intense, severe, tearing pain, which may be localized initially in the chest, abdomen, or back. As the aortic tear (dissection) extends, pain radiates to the back or distally toward the lower extremities. Many patients have hypertension upon initial presentation and the focus is upon control of blood pressure and early

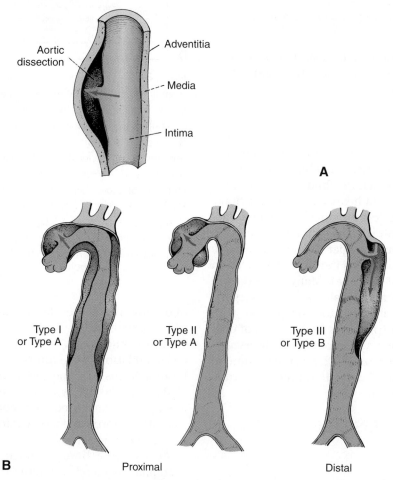

Fig. 18-20   Aortic dissection. **A,** Separation of vascular layers. **B,** Classification of aortic dissection. (Modified from Price SA, Wilson LM: *Pathophysiology: clinical concepts of disease processes,* ed 5, St Louis, 1997, Mosby.)

operation. Patients who present with hypotension, poor organ perfusion, and shock do not experience higher in-hospital mortality provided immediate and successful surgical repair can be achieved.[130] The International Registry of Aortic Dissection (IRAD) records indicate that acute aortic dissection is more common in men (72%), than women (32%), but because women present at an older age and with greater delay, they experience a higher in-hospital mortality.[131] Morbidity and mortality associated with aortic dissection increase with advanced age.[132] Cardiovascular warning signs may include severe hypertension, fleeting peripheral pulses, limb ischemia, or a new murmur indicative of aortic regurgitation; the most frequent acute neurologic changes include altered mental status and coma.[130-132] An ascending aortic dissection produces pain in the central chest or midscapular region of the back. A descending aortic dissection usually manifests by pain that radiates down the back, abdomen, or legs. The location of the dissection may be estimated according to the site of pain, although this does not eliminate the need for diagnostic procedures. The two most helpful initial diagnostic tests are the transthoracic echocardiogram (TTE) and computed tomography (CT) because both permit rapid visualization of the thoracic structures. The chest x-ray is only helpful if the mediastinum is already widened. Diagnostic findings that identify high-risk patients include a widened mediastinum or an excessively dilated aorta. The definitive invasive diagnostic procedure is an aortogram (aortic angiogram with radiopaque contrast).

MEDICAL MANAGEMENT

Medical management of an aortic aneurysm depends upon what symptoms are seen and hemodynamics. If the patient is stable, management is focused upon controlling hypertension and educating the patient about the need for corrective surgery before the aneurysm is more than 5 cm wide. If the patient is seen with an acute aortic dissection, management involves immediate control of hypertension with intravenous drugs and control of pain with opiates. Progression of the dissection is evaluated by the patient's report of worsening or new pain. If the patient presents with hypotension or in cardiogenic shock, blood pressure support measures to maintain tissue perfusion are initiated. In such cases emergency surgery may be performed. Surgery is usually required for dissections that involve the ascending aorta to prevent death from cardiac tamponade. This includes type A, or type I and type II dissections. The surgical procedure includes resection of the affected area, followed by graft placement and restoration of blood flow to major branches of the aorta. Replacement of the aortic valve is performed if the dissection involves the valve. Dissections that involve the descending aorta (type B, or type III) do not always require surgery.

NURSING MANAGEMENT

Nursing management of the patient with aortic aneurysm or aortic dissection incorporates a variety of nursing diagnoses (see the Nursing Diagnoses feature on Aortic Aneurysm and Aortic Dissection). Nursing inter-

---

Box 18-13

INDICATIONS FOR AORTIC ANEURYSM REPAIR

Aneurysm greater than 5 cm
Aneurysm progressively increasing in size
Impending rupture
Symptoms resulting from cerebral or coronary ischemia or peripheral (limb) ischemia
Pericardial tamponade
Uncontrollable pain
Aortic insufficiency

NURSING DIAGNOSES Aortic Aneurysm and Aortic Dissection

- Decreased Cardiac Output related to alterations in preload
- Acute Pain related to transmission and perception of cutaneous, visceral, muscular, or ischemic impulses
- Ineffective Peripheral Tissue Perfusion related to decreased peripheral blood flow
- Activity Intolerance related to cardiopulmonary dysfunction
- Ineffective Cardiopulmonary Tissue Perfusion related to decreased myocardial oxygen supply and/or increased myocardial oxygen demand
- Risk for Infection: invasive procedures
- Anxiety related to threat to biologic, psychologic, and/or social integrity
- Ineffective Renal Tissue Perfusion related to decreased renal blood flow
- Activity Intolerance related to cardiopulmonary dysfunction
- Deficient Knowledge: Discharge Regimen related to lack of previous exposure to information (see Patient Education feature on Aortic Aneurysm and Aortic Dissection)

EVIDENCE-BASED COLLABORATIVE PRACTICE

Aortic Aneurysm and Aortic Dissection

Recommendations for Prevention of Atherosclerotic Aortic Aneurysm and Dissection

- Hypertension is a major risk factor. There are no specific recommendations related to BP control and aortic disease. Reduction of BP to below 130/80 mm Hg is consistent with recommendations for other atherosclerotic diseases (coronary and cerebrovascular).
- Cigarette smoking is a major risk factor for aortic disease. Stopping smoking is essential.
- Aortic dissection also occurs as a complication of blunt chest trauma from high-speed motor vehicular trauma.

Recommendations for Treatment of Aortic Dissection

- Admission to the critical care unit for monitoring of heart rate and BP.
- Reduction of systolic BP using IV beta-blockers (Esmolol) or beta-blocker alpha-blocker combination (Labetalol). Beta-blockers are recommended because they reduce the force of blood ejected from the ventricle against the weakened aortic wall.
- When further systolic BP reduction is necessary, IV vasodilators (sodium nitroprusside) are added in addition to beta-blockers.
- Intubation and mechanical ventilation are recommended when there is profound hemodynamic instability.
- Pain relief (morphine sulphate) and sedation are recommended.
- Diagnosis of aortic dissection is made by clinical signs and location of the site of the tear and false lumen. CT is the most common diagnostic test in an emergency. MRI is often used for chronic stable dissections. TTE followed by TEE may also be used.
- Treatment recommendations depend upon classification of the dissection:
  —Type A (type I, type II) dissections that involve the aortic arch are repaired surgically to prevent aortic rupture or cardiac tamponade.
  —Type B (type III) dissections are recommended for medical treatment. Surgery or endovascular repair are recommended only in cases of persistent chest pain, aortic expansion, periaortic hematoma, or mediastinal hematoma.
- Type A aortic dissection is a high-risk diagnosis with overall hospital mortality of 25%. Patients with type A dissections who are admitted to the hospital with hypotension have a higher risk of adverse events.

Recommendations For Treatment of Elective Abdominal Aortic Aneurysm

- Formation of AAA or dissection before the sixth decade of life is uncommon.
- Based upon current evidence, 5.5 cm aneurysm size is the best threshold for repair in the "average" patient. Individual anatomy, patient age, and physical size must also be considered.
- Until the results of long-term randomized trials are available, the choice between endoluminal repair (stent) versus open abdominal surgery will depend upon patient and physician preferences.

From Erbel R et al: Diagnosis and management of aortic dissection, *Eur Heart J* 22(18):1642-1681, 2001; Brewster DC et al: Guidelines for the treatment of abdominal aortic aneurysms. Report of a subcommittee of the Joint Council of the American Association for Vascular Surgery and Society for Vascular Surgery, *J Vasc Surg* 37(5):1106-1117, 2003; Trimarchi S et al: Contemporary results of surgery in acute type A aortic dissection: the International Registry of Acute Aortic Dissection experience, *J Thorac Cardiovasc Surg* 129(1):112-122, 2005.

AAA, Abdominal aortic aneurysm; *BP,* blood pressure; *IV,* intravenous; *CT,* computed tomography; *MRI,* magnetic resonance imaging; *TTE,* transthoracic echocardiography; *TEE,* transesophageal echocardiography.

ventions are directed toward control of hypertension, pain control, and education of the patient and family.

Hypertension Management. The cardiovascular status is assessed hourly, including monitoring blood pressure in both arms, checking peripheral pulses bilaterally, auscultating for an aortic murmur, and monitoring the ECG for ischemic changes or dysrhythmias. Patients usually require an arterial line and receive potent antihypertensive drugs such as labetalol, which combines (1) beta-blocking activity to reduce cardiac output and lower blood pressure and (2) peripheral alpha-blocking activity to vasodilate the arteries and decrease blood pressure.

Pain Control. Acute pain is a classic sign of aortic dissection. Opiates and sedatives are administered to control pain, decrease anxiety, and increase comfort. Because these drugs can mask the pain of further dissection, they are administered judiciously. The patient's neurovascular status is assessed hourly. Documentation includes the presence and distribution of pain, pallor, paresthesia, paralysis, and pulselessness.

PATIENT EDUCATION

In the acute period, education is limited to an explanation of the critical care environment and the importance

PATIENT EDUCATION

Aortic Aneurysm and Aortic Dissection

- Pathophysiology of atherosclerotic aortic disease: aortic aneurysm or aortic dissection
- Hypertension control: hypertension increases risk of aneurysm rupture or increasing the aortic dissection
- Pain control: use of 1 to 10 pain scale; provide information about availability of pain medications for acute pain
- Preprocedure teaching for aortic angiogram, CT scan, or transesophageal echocardiogram
- Preoperative teaching for aortic surgical repair
- Risk factor modification: after the acute episode, if the cause of the aortic aneurysm or aortic dissection is atherosclerosis, an individual risk factor profile is developed for each patient. Strategies to discuss include the following: decrease fat intake to less than 30% of total calories a day, achieve total blood cholesterol of less than 200 mg/dl, stop smoking, reduce salt intake, control hypertension, treat diabetes if patient is diabetic, increase physical activity, achieve ideal body weight
- Symptoms to report to a health care professional: pain, signs and symptoms of infection
- Follow-up care after discharge

of blood pressure control. If additional procedures such as an aortogram, CT scan, or surgery are to be performed, the critical care nurse assists with these explanations (see the Patient Education feature on Aortic Aneurysm and Aortic Dissection). Recommendations for prevention and treatment of atherosclerotic aortic aneurysm and dissection are listed in the Evidence-Based Collaborative Practice feature on Aortic Aneurysm and Aortic Dissection.

PERIPHERAL ARTERIAL DISEASE

DESCRIPTION

Peripheral vascular disease (PVD) is divided into arterial and venous diseases of the peripheral vessels. Venous disease is a chronic condition that is managed on an outpatient basis and does not require admission to a critical care unit. By contrast, peripheral arterial disease (PAD) may require critical care admission for either an acute thrombotic occlusion or following a vascular surgical procedure. PAD can occur in any peripheral artery. It is especially painful in the arteries that supply the lower

extremities. The following descriptions relate to arterial peripheral vascular disease.

ETIOLOGY

Atherosclerosis is a common cause of chronic arterial occlusion in older adults. Peripheral arterial disease affects just over 4% of people under 40 years of age but has an impact on almost 15% of those over 70 years.[133] Risk factors are the same for both PAD and coronary artery disease (CAD). Most patients diagnosed with PAD have at least one risk factor that predisposes them to development of CAD.[133] Diabetes, smoking, hypertension, hyperlipidemia, and male gender all increase the risk of peripheral arterial occlusion.[133] As with CAD, the presence of kidney disease also increases the incidence of concomitant PAD.[134]

PATHOPHYSIOLOGY

The most commonly affected vessels in the lower extremities are the superficial femoral artery and the popliteal artery in the legs, followed by the distal aorta and iliac arteries.

ASSESSMENT AND DIAGNOSIS

Ankle Brachial Index. The "ankle-brachial index" (ABI) is a noninvasive test used to estimate the severity of arterial disease in the leg by comparing it to the measured arterial pressure in the arm. The systolic BP is measured on the arm and on the leg (just above the ankle). A BP cuff is used to occlude the pressure and the SBP is measured at both the posterior tibial pulse and the dorsalis pedis pulse location.[135] The SBP can be palpated with the fingers, or auscultated using a handheld 5- to 7-megahertz (MHz) Doppler. To calculate the ABI, the arm SBP is divided into the ankle SBP number.[135] A normal ABI value is between 0.9 and 1.0 and signifies that the peripheral arteries are normal. Patients with an ABI value between 0.71 and 0.9 have mild PAD; those with an ABI between 0.41 to 0.7 have moderate PAD; an ABI less than 0.4 indicates severe PAD.[135] Generally as the ABI value decreases, symptoms of peripheral ischemia increase.[135]

As with other atherosclerotic conditions, PAD is typically asymptomatic until the disease process is well advanced. Clinicians who rely on history of leg pain alone will miss 85% to 90% of PAD in the early stages.[135] The ABI can be used as a screening tool to detect the presence of PAD before symptoms occur.[135] Prevention measures can then be discussed with the patient.

Intermittent Claudication. Arterial occlusion obstructs blood flow to the distal extremity. The lack of blood flow produces ischemic muscle pain known as *in-*

termittent claudication. This cramping, aching pain while walking is often the first symptom of peripheral occlusive disease. The pain is relieved by rest and may remain stable in occurrence and intensity for many years. Symptoms do not occur until more than 75% of the vessel lumen is occluded. Arterial pulses are diminished, transiently present (vessel spasm), or absent distal to the site of occlusion. Diabetic patients have a much higher incidence of peripheral vascular disease than do the general population.

Rest Pain. As peripheral arterial disease progresses, many patients develop pain at rest. Pain at rest threatens the viability of the limb and requires immediate catheter or surgical intervention to relieve the blockage and restore circulation to the extremity.

Acute Occlusion. The symptoms of acute occlusion from thrombosis are sudden onset of severe pain, loss of pulses, collapse of superficial veins, coldness, pallor, and impaired motor and sensory function. As with rest pain, acute occlusion requires immediate intervention to open the artery.

Atrophic Tissue Changes. Skin changes associated with peripheral arterial disease include thickening of the nails and drying of the skin. Hair loss is common on the lower leg, feet, and toes. A temperature gradient may be present as a line of demarcation between areas that have adequate arterial perfusion and areas that are poorly perfused. Wasting of muscle or soft tissue may also be seen. As the atherosclerotic arterial disease progresses, skin ulcerations and gangrene can occur.

MEDICAL MANAGEMENT

Medical therapy is geared toward controlling or eliminating risk factors, providing good foot care, and suggesting alterations in lifestyle to promote rest and pain relief. Pharmacologic management may include the use of anticoagulants, vasodilators, or antiplatelet agents. If these therapies do not produce positive results, the patient may be a candidate for percutaneous transluminal angioplasty (PTA), stent placement, or vascular bypass surgery. PTA or stent placement is effective if the lesion (blockage) is discrete and localized. However, if the arterial disease is diffuse, bypass surgery is usually performed. If gangrene (cell death) is present, limb or partial limb amputation is required.

EVIDENCE-BASED COLLABORATIVE PRACTICE
Peripheral Arterial Disease

Peripheral arterial disease (PAD) affects about 27 million people in Europe and the USA (16% of the population ages 55 years and older). An international multidisciplinary group of clinicians has summarized evidence from clinical trials to begin the process of developing clinical guidelines.

Recommendations To Increase Awareness of PAD and Its Consequences

- Patients who are at highest risk of developing PAD are those who smoke cigarettes, have diabetes, and are elderly. In screening asymptomatic patients in high-risk groups, 30% to 50% of patients have PAD and do not know it.
- Other PAD risk factors include hypertension, hyperlipidemia, male sex, elevated homocysteine levels, elevated plasma fibrinogen levels, elevated blood glucose, prior MI, heart failure, and history of TIA or stroke.
- Patients with symptomatic PAD are at increased risk of stroke and are six times more likely to die within 10 years than those without PAD.
- Many patients are not aware of the link between PAD and cardiac and cerebrovascular atherosclerotic disease.

Recommendations To Improve the Identification of Patients With Symptomatic PAD

- Because PAD is asymptomatic in the early stages of the disease the ankle-brachial index (ABI) is recommended as a screening tool in high-risk patients. See text for information on how to measure the ABI.
- If the diagnosis is not made until the patient complains of intermittent claudication (pain with walking), the disease is already at an advanced stage.

Recommendations To Treat Risk Factors Associated With PAD

- Stop smoking (if patient smokes). This is not easy to do. A report from the American Lung Association reveals that although 70% of smokers surveyed would like to quit smoking, only 34% attempt to quit per year, and an average of only 2.5% succeed.
- If hyperlipidemic achieve a normal lipid panel: reduce total serum cholesterol to below 200 mg/dl and LDL-C to less than 100 mg/dl.
- Studies have not specifically examined the effect of controlling hypertension and diabetes on rates of PAD. However, extrapolating from the cardiac literature, researchers recommend reducing BP to below 130/80 mg Hg and maintaining blood glucose within the normal range (70-110 mg/dl; hemoglobin A1$_C$ at or below 7%).
- Low-dose aspirin or another platelet-inhibitor drug is recommended.
- Exercise rehabilitation is recommended. The goal is to increase the ability of the patient to walk longer distances without leg pain.

From Belch JJ et al: Critical issues in peripheral arterial disease detection and management: a call to action, *Arch Intern Med* 163(8):884-892, 2003.

PAD, Peripheral arterial disease; *TIA*, transient ischemic attack; *MI*, myocardial infarction; *BP*, blood pressure; *ABI*, ankle brachial index; *LDL-C*, low-density lipoprotein cholesterol.

NURSING MANAGEMENT

Nursing management of the patient with peripheral arterial insufficiency incorporates a variety of nursing diagnoses (see the Nursing Diagnoses feature on Peripheral Arterial Disease). Nurses assess the quality of the peripheral arterial pulses, intervene to maintain skin integrity and control pain, and educate the patient and family about peripheral vascular disease.

Arterial Pulses. Assessments of peripheral pulses, limb color, and temperature are all critical in the evaluation of an ischemic limb. Many hospitals use a standard scale to improve documentation of pulses. If the pulse cannot be palpated, a Doppler may be used to assess blood flow.

Skin Integrity. Care is taken to protect the limb from injury and development of pressure ulcers. Healing is often impaired because of poor arterial blood flow or diabetes. Feet may be protected from injury by cotton or lamb's wool placed between the toes or by a bed cradle. However, for an acute ischemic limb, removal of the thrombus is the only treatment that will salvage ischemic tissue.

Pain Control. The term for pain during exercise in the presence of peripheral arterial disease is *intermittent claudication*. Leg pain that occurs following exercise, caused by increased muscle oxygen demand, can be effectively managed by stopping the exertion. However, pain at rest (without exercise) is a warning sign of an anoxic limb. The pain of an acute ischemic limb is extreme, and morphine is used for pain control. Ultimately, removal of the arterial obstruction is the only method to eliminate the pain.

PATIENT EDUCATION

Education topics include risk factor modification that emphasizes similar lifestyle changes to those recommended for patients with coronary artery disease, including smoking cessation, promoting exercise, maintenance of ideal body weight, inspection of the feet and legs, foot care, avoidance of foot trauma, and medications (see the Patient Education feature on Peripheral Arterial Disease). Many patients with PAD underestimate their risk of stroke or acute MI and do not understand that the risk factors for PAD are the same for all of the cardiovascular atherosclerotic diseases.[136] Walking is good exercise for increasing blood flow to the lower extremities and is highly recommended for the person with peripheral arterial disease.[137]

If a surgically implanted prosthetic bypass graft is in place, teaching must include information about infective endocarditis precautions. If the patient is diabetic, education about diabetes management is also included in the teaching plan. The Patient Education feature lists the salient points to include when teaching patients and families about peripheral arterial disease. Symptoms of peripheral arterial disease are listed in the Evidence-Based Collaborative Practice feature on Peripheral Arterial Disease.

CAROTID ARTERY DISEASE

DESCRIPTION

The bifurcation of the carotid arteries is a common site of atherosclerotic plaque development (Fig. 18-21). Because these arterioles carry the blood supply to the brain, when they are obstructed, the presenting symptoms are neurologic. Carotid artery disease is a readily treatable obstruction to prevent a "stroke." Blood supply to the brain is provided by two separate arterial systems: the vertebral arteries, and the internal carotid arteries, branches of which anastomose to form the *circle of Willis*. Any abrupt interruption in circulation for 4 to 6 minutes can produce permanent brain damage. When circulation to an area is impaired gradually, collateral circulation is often able to develop and maintain an adequate supply of blood to that area of the brain. With an abrupt interruption in blood supply, an area of brain tissue will become ischemic and often become permanently damaged.

ETIOLOGY

The most common cause of carotid artery disease in the United States is atherosclerosis.[138] Other rare causes include fibromuscular dysplasia, irradiation, and arteritis. The risk factors for development of atherosclerotic carotid artery disease and stroke are similar to those for

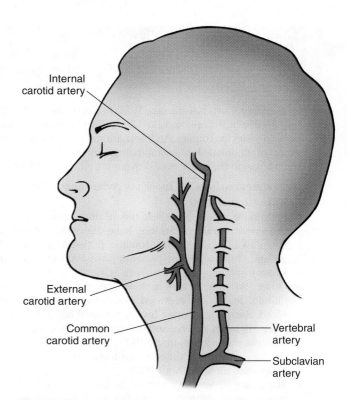

Fig. 18-21 Carotid arteries (common, internal, and external). Atherosclerotic plaque develops in the common carotid artery at the bifurcation into the internal and external carotid arteries. Plaque also develops in the common, internal, and external carotid arteries.

CAD and PAD. Thus patients with any of these conditions must be educated about the other disease processes. The modifiable risk factors include uncontrolled hypertension (SBP over 160 mm Hg), atrial fibrillation, current smoker, diabetes with uncontrolled blood glucose, and hyperlipidemia.[139] Women taking hormone replacement therapy after menopause also experience an increased risk of stroke.[139] The incidence of carotid stenosis increases with age. Asymptomatic carotid artery stenosis with greater than 50% occlusion is present is 10% of men and 7% of women over 50 years of age, and the risk of stroke doubles with each successive decade after age 55.[139] The presence of coexisting CAD also increases incidence of stroke; 8% of men and 11% of women will have a stroke within 6 years of succumbing to an acute MI.[139]

The major mechanisms by which atherosclerosis in the carotid arteries creates ischemic symptoms are embolization and thrombosis. Ulcerated carotid lesions with accumulated platelet and fibrin thrombi travel, along with cholesterol deposits, to become emboli to the brain. Stenotic areas in the carotid arteries are prone to thrombosis because of sluggish flow across the lesions. Doppler studies can examine the carotid arteries noninvasively. If a stroke is suspected an emergency CT scan is the appropriate diagnostic test.[138]

Carotid artery disease can remain asymptomatic for many years. Once emboli are dislodged, the manifestations of carotid artery disease are neurologic, and include hemiparesis, dysphasia, dysarthria, global aphasia, diplopia, vertigo, syncope, confusion, and monocular blindness. Neurologic symptoms that resolve completely within a short time are classified as *transient ischemic attacks (TIA)*. Symptoms that do not resolve are described as *completed strokes*.[138,139] If a patient has recently experienced a TIA, the risk of stroke is increased.[138,139] Additional information on the management of the patient experiencing a stroke is discussed in Chapter 27.

MEDICAL MANAGEMENT

Medical management is focused on lowering the atherosclerotic risk factors over which the patient has control. This includes regulation of hypertension, smoking cessation, seeking medical attention for treatable cardiac abnormalities such as atrial fibrillation, reducing weight, and reducing the cholesterol level to less than 200 mg/dl. Antithrombotic therapy (warfarin, aspirin, or other antiplatelet therapy) must be prescribed for patients with atrial fibrillation with a comprehensive individualized assessment of the relative risk of embolism versus the risk of bleeding complications.[139]

Asymptomatic patients who have carotid stenosis pose a quandary. In these patients the risk of stroke needs to be weighed against the risks of surgery—specifically, the increased risk of stroke during surgery. Current clinical guidelines suggest that patients with carotid stenosis greater than 60% will benefit from carotid surgi-

cal endarterectomy when performed by a surgeon with a history of less than 3% operative morbidity and mortality.[139] The role of stent placement in the carotid artery is also under investigation.[139] The goal of these therapies is to prevent a stroke. Asymptomatic patients with carotid artery stenosis need to be informed of both the risks involved with any procedure and their risk for future cerebrovascular events such as stroke.

NURSING MANAGEMENT

Nursing management is focused on assessment of adequate cerebral perfusion represented by vital signs, respiratory pattern, level of consciousness, pupil reaction, pupil size, and possible cranial nerve deficits manifested by difficulty in swallowing, loss of gag reflex, changes in speech, and loss of facial symmetry. The National Institutes of Health (NIH) stroke scale is used to predict patient outcome on both initial and ongoing assessment of TIA and stroke-related symptoms.[140] The nurse educates the patient and family about the causes of the current event and provides information on preventing further cerebrovascular events. Several nursing diagnoses are associated with management of the patient with carotid artery disease (see the Nursing Diagnoses feature on Carotid Artery Disease).

Neurologic Assessment. Neurologic assessment of the patient with carotid artery disease is divided into two

EVIDENCE-BASED COLLABORATIVE PRACTICE

Carotid Arterial Disease

Recommendations for Prevention of Carotid Artery Disease

1. Stop smoking (if patient smokes), and avoid exposure to environmental tobacco smoke (also called second-hand tobacco smoke). Risk of stroke increases 1.5 to 2.2 times as a result of cigarette smoking.
2. Achieve a normal BP. Target BP is below 140/90 mm Hg. However, if patient has coexisting diabetes, kidney disease, or heart failure the target is 130/80 mm Hg or lower. Oral antihypertensive drugs are prescribed if the target BP is not met with diet and exercise alone. Reduction in blood pressure greatly reduces stroke incidence.
3. Achieve and maintain normal weight. The target weight-to-height ratio is a BMI between 18.5 and 24.9 kg/m². A BMI above 25 kg/m² defines obesity. Obese patients are also identified as having a large waist circumference: greater than 40 inches (men) and greater than 35 inches (women).
4. Have serum lipids checked, and attain a normal lipid profile. Many patients are prescribed lipid-lowering drugs to achieve the goals listed below:
   —Total cholesterol below 200 mg/dl
   —LDL-C below 100 mg/dl if has CV disease or diabetes (all patients with carotid arterial disease will fall into this category)
   —LDL-C below 130 mg/dl if no evidence of CV disease or diabetes
   —Triglycerides below 150 mg/dl
5. Normal fasting blood glucose between 70-110 mg/dl. If diabetic, the hemoglobin A1$_C$ should be close to normal, or below 7%.
6. Eat a healthy diet. Reduce saturated fat and add fruits and vegetables. Add omega-3 fatty acids as part of the treatment regimen to lower elevated triglycerides.
7. Take regular exercise. Optimal goal is 30-60 minutes daily or at least 3 times weekly.
8. Aspirin 75-325 orally, or other platelet-inhibitor medications are frequently prescribed as part of a prevention regimen.
9. The "statin" class of drugs has been shown to reduce the risk of stroke in patients with coronary artery disease and also in patients with elevated serum cholesterol.

Recommendations When There Are Signs and Symptoms of Carotid Artery Disease

10. There is no recommendation on the treatment of asymptomatic narrowing of the carotid artery. A stenotic carotid artery may be detected by the presence of a bruit on a clinical exam. Results of noninvasive diagnostic tests help the clinician and patient determine if surgical carotid endarterectomy is warranted.
11. Data from the Framingham study has shown a higher risk of acute MI and vascular death in patients with carotid bruit compared to those without a carotid bruit. However, routine testing for presence of asymptomatic coronary arterial disease or other vascular disease before carotid endarterectomy has not been recommended.
12. If the patient has had a previous stroke, a TIA, or if there are signs and symptoms of cardiac disease, a thorough cardiovascular work-up is warranted.
13. A symptomatic patient with a carotid artery stenosis between 70% and 99% is a typically a candidate for carotid endarterectomy surgery.
14. All patients who have carotid endarterectomy should also follow all of the prevention recommendations.

From Biller J et al: Guidelines for carotid endarterectomy, *Stroke* 29(2):554-562, 1998; Adams RJ et al: Coronary risk evaluation in patients with transient ischemic attack and ischemic stroke, *Stroke* 34(9):2310-2322, 2003; Pearson TA et al: AHA Guidelines for primary prevention of cardiovascular disease and stroke: 2002 update, *Circulation* 106(3):388-391, 2002; Goldstein LB et al: Primary prevention of ischemic stroke, *Stroke* 32(1):280-299, 2001; Statins after ischemic stroke and transient ischemic attack, *Stroke* 35(4):1023, 2004.

BP, Blood pressure; *BMI*, body mass index; *CV*, cardiovascular; *LDL-C*, low-density lipoprotein cholesterol; *mg/dl*, milligrams per deciliter; *MI*, myocardial infarction, *TIA*, transient ischemic attack.

---

parts: (1) level of consciousness, mental alertness, and cerebral perfusion; and (2) cranial nerve function.

A neurologic assessment is performed to make sure that the patient has not suffered a TIA or stroke. Thus questions to ascertain level of consciousness relate to time and place and reason for hospital admission. Mental alertness is assessed by the ability with which the patient responds to these and other questions. In addition, the person is asked to move all four limbs on command. To assess specific cranial nerves, the patient is asked to make a grimace, which should demonstrate bilateral facial symmetry; to stick out the tongue to ensure it is midline; and to swallow and speak, which should be done without difficulty. (See "Cranial Nerves" in Chapter 25 and "Rapid Neurologic Examination" in Chapter 26.)

PATIENT EDUCATION

If a patient is admitted to a critical care unit who has known carotid artery disease and has not had a cerebrovascular event, preventive education is essential. It is important to discuss the mechanism of stroke in carotid artery disease. A stroke is most often caused by an embolic thrombus that has traveled in the bloodstream to a specific area of the brain. The thrombus may have originated in the atria during an episode of atrial fibrillation, or in the carotid arteries. In the carotid arteries a thrombus can develop across the narrowed carotid artery lumen, reducing flow and causing widespread cerebral hypoperfusion. Many patients who have atherosclerotic carotid artery disease also have CAD or PAD and are diabetic or hypertensive.[139] The major areas of patient education are listed in the Patient Education feature on Carotid Artery Disease. Recommendations for prevention of carotid artery disease are listed in the Evidence-Based Collaborative Practice feature on Carotid Artery Disease.

VENOUS THROMBOEMBOLISM

DESCRIPTION

Venous thromboembolism (VTE) comprises two directly related conditions: deep vein thrombosis (DVT) and pulmonary embolism (PE). *Deep vein thrombosis (DVT)* describes a clot (thrombus) that forms in a large vein in the leg, pelvis, and less commonly, the arm. It is often (but not always) accompanied by inflammation, pain, tenderness, and redness at the site of the thrombus. The concern is that the thrombus may migrate as a VTE via the venous circulation to the pulmonary vascular bed, causing a pulmonary embolism, the development of pulmonary hypertension, or possibly death.[141-144]

ETIOLOGY

At least 250,000 episodes of *VTE* leading to hospitalization or death occur in the United States annually.[145] Patients in the critical care unit face additional risks secondary to invasive procedures, immobility, and vascular inflammation.[146,147] Other risk factors for *VTE* include age older than 40, obesity, immobility, trauma, spinal cord injury, certain cancers, major surgery, and sepsis.[148-150] The VTE incidence is similar for both men and women, unless a woman is taking hormone replacement therapy (HRT) or a contraceptive pill, which increases her risk.[145] Inherited coagulation disorders and hypercoagulability, also described as *genetic thrombophilia,* confer a propensity for clotting and increase the DVT risk profile in patients with this genetic inheritance.[151]

Three major predisposing factors are traditionally described as *Virchow's triad:* these are stasis of blood, endothelial injury, and hypercoagulability. Usually two of these three conditions must be present for thrombosis to occur. Patients in critical care units generally have one or more risk factors that predispose them to the devel-

opment of a venous thrombus.[152] The risk of developing a DVT ranges from 13% to 31% when critically ill patients do not receive appropriate prophylaxis.[152] The incidence of DVT increases with age and markedly increases the patient's risk of fatal pulmonary embolism (see "Pulmonary Embolism" in Chapter 23).

ASSESSMENT AND DIAGNOSIS

Development of DVT may be insidious. Many patients with DVT are asymptomatic. Pain, if present, is described as an aching or throbbing sensation, which worsens with ambulation. A positive *Homans' sign*, which is pain in the calf on dorsiflexion of the foot, heightens the suspicion of a DVT but is not considered a reliable marker. If DVT is present in the upper extremity, the entire arm swells. Other clinical manifestations include redness with swelling, increased skin temperature, dilation of superficial veins, and mottling and cyanosis caused by stagnant blood flow.

When DVT is suspected, a noninvasive venous ultrasound test is usually used to evaluate vein patency.[153] If the thrombus is large and the vein is easy to visualize, the presence of a DVT can be confirmed by this method alone. However, when the results of the ultrasound are inconclusive, the addition of the D-dimer blood test increases diagnostic accuracy.[153-158] The D-dimer test measures the presence of cross-linked fibrin derivatives in the serum. It is a sensitive marker of thrombosis but it lacks specificity. This means if the normal D-dimer serum value is elevated, it signifies the presence of clots, but the thrombi could be anywhere in the body. The ultrasound can help to localize the location of the DVT. Together, these two tests represent a useful and powerful diagnostic strategy.[153] Another helpful consideration is when the D-dimer value is normal (not elevated); in this case a DVT (or other thrombosis) can safely be ruled out.[153-158]

If pulmonary embolism is suspected, physicians either use CT of the thorax or, less frequently, a ventilation-perfusion (VQ) lung scan (36% to 32% respectively) as the initial method of evaluation.[159] Pulmonary angiography is uncommon as a first-line diagnostic study.[159]

Current guidelines recommend evaluating the risk factors for each patient on an individual basis; maintaining a high index of suspicion and using thromboprophylaxis for at-risk patients; and, if VTE is suspected, using clinical assessment, venous ultrasound and the D-dimer assay to confirm or negate the presence of venous thromboembolism.[143]

MEDICAL MANAGEMENT

Prevention of VTE. Major therapeutic emphasis is placed on prophylaxis for critically ill patients at high risk of VTE.[144,148] Preventive measures include prophylactic anticoagulation with either subcutaneous low–molecular weight heparin (LMWH) or unfractionated heparin, increasing mobility, or use of sequential compression devices (SCD) placed on the lower extremities.

Management of Diagnosed VTE. The patient is confined to bed rest with elevation of the limb, and anticoagulation therapy is initiated. Analgesics are prescribed to reduce discomfort.

Anticoagulation. Anticoagulants are prescribed to reduce further clotting. The risks and benefits of therapeutic anticoagulation are discussed with the patient and family before therapy begins. In the acute phase the VTE can be treated with either intravenous heparin or subcutaneous LMWH. Subsequently, oral warfarin (Coumadin) may be used. Antiplatelet therapy with aspirin or other drugs is added to prevent VTE reoccurrence. Antiplatelet therapy alone does not provide protection against development of VTE.[143] None of the aforementioned antithrombotics dissolve the existing clot, but they will prevent new thrombi from forming. Lytic therapy is generally reserved for massive pulmonary embolism. Patients receiving anticoagulation therapy require careful assessment for bleeding tendencies, including obtaining frequent bleeding studies— activated partial thromboplastin time (aPTT), international normalized ratio (INR), or prothrombin time (PT). Stool and urine are tested for presence of occult blood; gums are inspected for bleeding; when endotracheal suctioning is required, it is important to be gentle and to assess for presence of blood in the aspirate. Once the patient begins to ambulate, full-length, custom-fitted elastic stockings are ordered. Complaints or observation of dyspnea or chest pain must be quickly evaluated to assess the risk of pulmonary embolism. Medical management with anticoagulants is adequate for most patients; however, those at risk for pulmonary embolism (i.e., patients with cancer, bleeding disorders, or spinal cord injury) may require surgical intervention for protection. Possible procedures include venous embolectomy and insertion of an inferior vena cava filter.[160]

NURSING MANAGEMENT

The focus of nursing management is always to prevent the development of DVT; for the patient with DVT the interventions are to rest the affected extremity, prevent complications that may result from VTE, and monitor anticoagulant therapy. Several nursing diagnoses are used in the management of the patient with VTE (see the Nursing Diagnoses feature on Venous Thromboembolism).

Prevention of Thromboembolism. Normally the simple action of walking helps return blood to the right side of the heart and prevents venous stasis that may lead to development of venous thrombi. For critically ill patients, immobility is often imposed because of the severity of the illness. Once stable, most patients are assisted out of bed and helped to walk to restore the circulatory pump.

Activity With DVT. For the patient who has developed a DVT, physical activity is limited to prevent dislodgement of emboli. During the acute phase, self-care activities are limited and bed rest is maintained. Range-of-motion exercises can be performed with any unaffected limb. The patient is instructed to avoid bending at the knees or hips because this impedes venous return. Antiembolism stockings that have been custom-fitted can also be used. It is not clear when it is "safe" to resume normal activity, such as walking, after DVT. Usually it is resumed after a Doppler study shows no evidence of DVT in the extremity and after symptoms have abated. Prevention strategies again become important, since the patient remains at risk for a recurrence. In general, early ambulation after surgery or other procedures and avoidance of bed rest are the most effective prevention strategies.

Risk of Pulmonary Embolism. The patient with a VTE is closely monitored for signs of pulmonary embolism and instructed to report immediately any chest pain, dyspnea, hemoptysis, or tachypnea. Risk factors for VTE are nearly identical to those for pulmonary embolism. For patients who must remain immobile because of their clinical condition, external pneumatic compression devices, antiembolism stockings, and low-dose heparin are commonly used.[145,152]

Anticoagulation. Anticoagulant therapy is monitored by obtaining daily coagulation values—aPTT if the patient is receiving IV heparin,[161] and daily INR if the patient is receiving warfarin (Coumadin).[162] There is not a

---

NURSING DIAGNOSES Venous Thromboembolism

- Activity Intolerance related to prolonged immobility or deconditioning
- Acute Pain related to transmission and perception of cutaneous, visceral, muscular, or ischemic impulses
- Powerlessness related to lack of control over current situation and/or disease progression
- Anxiety related to threat to biologic, psychologic, and/or social integrity
- Deficient Knowledge: Discharge Regimen related to lack of previous exposure to information (see Patient Education feature on Venous Thromboembolism)

test in clinical use to evaluate LMWH effectiveness.[161] Signs of bleeding are monitored and any symptoms are treated promptly. For the critically ill patient, hemoglobin levels and hematocrit are monitored daily, and stools are assessed for occult blood. Avoidable mechanical trauma is minimized. The alert patient should be instructed to use a soft toothbrush and, if needed, an electric razor.

PATIENT EDUCATION

Patient education emphasizes VTE prevention for all patients who are immobile in the critical care unit for any length of time. This includes explanations about activity prophylaxis such as early ambulation after major surgery, external pneumatic compression boots, and low-dose heparin.

For patients who have a diagnosed DVT, education is focused on immobilization of the limb, avoidance of trauma to the limb, and elevation of the limb to decrease venous pooling and increase blood flow. If the patient is anticoagulated, the risks and benefits of this therapy are discussed, as well as the risk of VTE and pulmonary embolus. The patient is instructed to report any chest pain, shortness of breath, or respiratory distress (see the Pa-

tient Education feature on Venous Thromboembolism). A collaborative team of clinicians, aware of current clinical recommendations, is essential to provide effective care for all critical care patients at risk for VTE (see the Evidence-Based Collaborative Practice feature on Venous Thromboembolism).

PATIENT EDUCATION

Venous Thromboembolism

- Pathophysiology of deep vein thrombosis
- Discuss risk of pulmonary embolus, need for antiembolism stockings or pneumatic compression devices on legs; avoid trauma to legs and report any chest pain, breathlessness, or increased respiratory rate
- Medications: anticoagulants (heparin or Coumadin) to prevent formation of new thrombus at the site; aspirin to decrease platelet aggregation

---

EVIDENCE-BASED COLLABORATIVE PRACTICE
Venous Thromboembolism

Summary of Evidence-Based Recommendations for Venous Thromboembolism Prevention

Strong Evidence of the Following:

- Aspirin **alone** should not be used for VTE prophylaxis for any patient group.
- For moderate-risk general surgery patients, prophylaxis with low-dose unfractionated heparin 5000 units every 12 hours (IV or SQ) **or** low–molecular weight heparin (LMWH) less than 3400 units once daily SQ.
- For moderate-risk general surgery patients, prophylaxis with low-dose unfractionated heparin 5000 units every 8 hours (IV or SQ) **or** low-molecular weight heparin (LMWH) greater than 3400 units once daily SQ.
- For highest-risk general surgery patients with multiple risk factors, the recommendation is to combine pharmacologic and mechanical prevention methods.
  —Pharmacologic prophylaxis: low-dose unfractionated heparin 5000 units every 8 hours **or** low–molecular weight heparin (LMWH) greater than 3400 units once daily.

  —Mechanical prophylaxis: graduated-compression stockings **or** intermittent pneumatic compression devices.
- Oral vitamin K agonists (warfarin) are used to achieve a target INR of 2.5 (INR range 2-3).
- All patients admitted to the critical care unit must be assessed for their risk of VTE.
- Most critically ill patients will require thromboprophylaxis against VTE.
- Some of the patients at highest risk for VTE include those undergoing open urologic surgery, gynecologic surgery, or total hip or knee procedures; all trauma patients with at least one risk factor; and medical patients with acute heart failure or acute respiratory failure. Others included in this group are immobile patients confined to bed who have at least one risk factor such as age over 40 years or history of prior VTE.
- Rates of DVT in critical care patients not receiving prophylaxis range from 10% to 80%.

From Greets WH et al: Prevention of venous thromboembolism; the seventh AACP conference on antithrombotic and thrombolytic therapy, *Chest* 126(3 Suppl): 338S-400S, 2004.

DVT, Deep vein thrombosis; *INR*, international normalized ratio; *IV*, intravenous; *SQ*, subcutaneous; *VTE*, venous thromboembolism.

HYPERTENSIVE EMERGENCY

DESCRIPTION

Hypertensive emergency is relatively uncommon. It is seen in less than 1% of patients who are hypertensive but when present, it is life-threatening and demands early recognition and management to minimize morbidity and mortality. Formerly known by the names *hypertensive crisis* or *malignant hypertension*, with the advent of so many categories of antihypertensive medications this condition can be effectively managed in the critical care setting. Two forms of acute hypertension are recognized:

1. *Hypertensive emergencies* pose a risk of end-organ damage and are life-threatening. The target organ can be the heart (acute MI), the brain (stroke), or the kidney (renal failure).
2. *Hypertensive urgencies* are characterized by a serious elevation in blood pressure but do not put the patient at risk for end-organ damage.

ETIOLOGY

Hypertensive emergency may occur in patients with no history of the condition or can be precipitated by noncompliance with or inadequate drug therapy. In patients with no known history of hypertension, causes of hypertensive emergency include the following:

1. Acute renal failure
2. Acute central nervous system (CNS) events: hypertension frequently accompanies subarachnoid hemorrhage (SAH), intracerebral hemorrhage, or a stroke
3. Acute aortic dissection: hypertension frequently precedes dissection
4. Pregnancy-induced eclampsia: intense arterial vascular constriction, which raises blood pressure and also decreases blood supply to the placenta
5. Pheochromocytoma: an adrenal tumor that produces epinephrine and norepinephrine and raises blood pressure as a result of the circulating catecholamines
6. Drug-induced hypertension: illegal drugs, particularly cocaine or amphetamines
7. Drug-food interactions: hypertensive response to tyramine-containing foods or beverages (beer or aged cheese) during treatment with a monoamine oxidase inhibitor (MAOI). This is rare today because most patients are prescribed other antidepressant medications.

PATHOPHYSIOLOGY

The exact trigger of a hypertensive crisis is often not known. However, the majority of patients suffer from known hypertension before the event, and the sudden rise in blood pressure is often related to the underlying disease process. Clinical manifestations of hypertensive emergency are listed in Table 18-13.

ASSESSMENT AND DIAGNOSIS

Hypertensive emergency can be manifested by any of the following symptoms, depending on the target organ involved:

Table 18-13	Hypertensive Emergencies
Emergency	**Examples of Causes**
CARDIOVASCULAR COMPROMISE	
Chest pain	Unstable angina, myocardial infarction, aortic dissection
Acute heart failure	Myocardial infarction, severe hypertension
Hypertension after vascular surgery	Aortic aneurysmectomy, carotid endarterectomy, coronary artery bypass grafting
CENTRAL NERVOUS SYSTEM (CNS) COMPROMISE	
Papilledema	Increased intracranial pressure—mass lesion Malignant hypertension—any cause
Headache, agitation, lethargy, confusion	Hypertensive encephalopathy—any cause, subarachnoid hemorrhage, stroke
Coma	Stroke, advanced hypertensive encephalopathy, trauma, tumor
Seizures	Advanced hypertensive encephalopathy, CNS tumor, eclampsia, stroke (less common)
Focal neurologic deficit	Stroke, CNS tumor, hypertensive encephalopathy
Acute renal failure	Malignant hypertension, vasculitis, scleroderma, glomerulonephritis
Catecholamine excess	Pheochromocytomas, monoamine oxidase inhibitor (MAOI) in combination with certain drugs and foods; abrupt withdrawal of antihypertensive medications such as clonidine, guanabenz, or beta-blockers

CNS, Central nervous system.

1. CNS compromise, identified by headache, blurred vision, change in level of consciousness, or coma
2. Cardiovascular compromise, identified by the chest pain of an acute coronary syndrome or aortic dissection
3. Acute renal failure, identified by a sudden absence of urine output
4. Catecholamine excess

Worsening of symptoms may indicate hypertensive encephalopathy. Diagnostic studies include blood pressure measurement in both arms and placement of an intraarterial line for close monitoring of blood pressure. A 12-lead ECG is taken to evaluate for evidence of acute MI or left ventricular hypertrophy.

MEDICAL MANAGEMENT

Hypertensive Emergencies. Hypertensive emergencies are defined as an acute BP elevation greater than 180/120 mm Hg complicated by impending or progressive target organ dysfunction.[11] Hypertensive emergencies with the risk of end organ damage necessitate admission of the patient to the critical care unit, where IV antihypertensive therapy can be administered and blood pressure can be monitored continuously by means of an arterial line. Several IV medications, in many different drug classes, are available for acute reduction of blood pressure. Ideally the drug should be targeted to the specific condition. *Sodium nitroprusside* (SNP or Nipride) is frequently the first drug used to lower BP in hypertensive emergency. SNP is useful because of its half-life of seconds. It is not suitable for long-tem use because of development of a toxic metabolite that causes cyanide-like toxicity.[163]

Short-acting beta-blockers that are effective are *labetalol* and *esmolol*. Beta-blockers are especially effective if aortic dissection is present. For patients with heart failure, the intravenous ACE inhibitor *enalaprilat* lowers BP. For hypertensive patients with chest pain, the vasodilator nitroglycerin (NTG) is used. For patients with renal compromise, the dopamine receptor antagonist (DA-1) *fenoldopam* will lower BP and increase blood flow to the kidneys.[163] *Hydralazine* is the IV agent of choice in eclampsia because it does not cross the placental barrier. The calcium channel blocker *nicardipine* has been used for patients with CNS compromise, although SNP, *labetalol*, and *enalaprilat* are also employed.[164] The alpha-blocker *phentolamine* is used for patients in pheochromocytoma crisis.[165] Sometimes, combinations of the aforementioned agents are used to more effectively bring the hypertension under control. The intravenous diuretic *furosemide* (Lasix) is used if fluid retention is present.

PATIENT EDUCATION — **Hypertensive Emergency**

- Pathophysiology of hypertensive crisis
- Normal and abnormal blood pressure values
- Self-monitoring of blood pressure at home
- Connection between hypertension and other atherosclerotic diseases such as coronary artery disease, peripheral arterial disease (PAD), and cerebrovascular disease
- Warning signs of a "heart attack," or myocardial infarction
- Warning signs of a "brain attack," or stroke
- Warning signs of intermittent claudication or PAD
- Risk factors modification: after the acute episode, if the cause of the carotid artery disease is atherosclerosis, an individual risk factor profile is developed for each patient. Strategies to discuss include the following: decrease fat intake to less than 30% of total calories a day, achieve total blood cholesterol of less than 200 mg/dl, stop smoking, reduce salt intake, control hypertension, control diabetes if patient is diabetic, increase physical activity, achieve and maintain ideal body weight
- Medications: antihypertensive medications, rationale, and side effects
- Signs and symptoms to report to a health care professional
- Follow-up care after discharge

NURSING DIAGNOSES — **Hypertensive Emergency**

- Ineffective Cerebral Tissue Perfusion related to vasospasm or hemorrhage
- Ineffective Cardiopulmonary Tissue Perfusion related to acute myocardial ischemia
- Anxiety related to threat to biologic, psychologic, and/or social integrity
- Deficient Knowledge: Discharge Regimen related to lack of previous exposure to information (see Patient Education feature on Hypertensive Emergency)

EVIDENCE-BASED COLLABORATIVE PRACTICE

Hypertensive Emergencies

Definition

Hypertensive emergency is defined as an acute BP elevation greater than 180/120 mm Hg complicated by impending or progressive target organ dysfunction.

Recommendations

1. Early identification of hypertensive emergency in the emergency department and admission to an intensive care unit is recommended.
2. Patients with hypertensive emergency should have continuous BP monitoring.
3. IV drugs are used to reduce BP (not necessarily to normal) to prevent or limit target organ damage.
4. Initial goal is to reduce BP by no more than 25%. For example, reduce systolic pressure to 160 and diastolic pressure to 100-110 mm Hg in the 2 to 6 hours following admission.
5. Decreasing the BP gradually is recommended to avoid cerebral, coronary, and renal ischemia.
6. Drugs that cause rapid falls in blood pressure are not recommended in the management of acute hypertensive emergency. For this reason, short-acting nifedipine is not endorsed (sublingual or IV).
7. Further gradual reductions in BP can be achieved in the following 24-48 hours.

Special Situations: Hypertension and Acute Ischemic Stroke

8. For patients admitted with an ischemic stroke, there is no clinical evidence to support rapid reduction in BP. For patients with a SBP greater than 220 mm Hg or

a DBP between120 to 140 mm Hg, BP should be lowered cautiously by 10% to 15% only.

9. If the DBP is above 140 mm Hg, sodium nitroprusside (SNP) is recommended to cautiously lower the SDP by about 10%.
10. SBP greater than 185 mm Hg and/or DBP greater than 110 mm Hg contraindicates the use of thrombolytic therapy (t-PA) within the first three hours of an acute ischemic stroke. The BP must be lowered prior to the administration of t-PA.
11. Careful monitoring of the patient for signs of neurologic deterioration related to the lower pressure is mandated in all situations.

Special Situation: Hypertension and Aortic Dissection

12. Patients with aortic dissection should have their systolic BP lowered to below 100 mm Hg if tolerated.

Ultimate BP Target Goal

13. Goal of therapy for all patients is a target BP of 140/90 mm Hg or lower before discharge from the hospital. Some patients will require oral medications to achieve this target.
14. Target BP is 130/80 mm Hg or lower for patients with known hypertension, kidney failure, diabetes, or cardiovascular disease. Almost all patients with these conditions will require oral medications to achieve their target BP. Many patients will require two or more oral drugs.

From Chobanian AV et al: Seventh report of the Joint National Committee on Prevention, Detection, Evaluation, and Treatment of High Blood Pressure, *Hypertension* 42(6):1206-1252, 2003.

BP, Blood pressure; *DBP*, diastolic blood pressure; *IV*, intravenous; *SBP*, systolic blood pressure; *t-PA*, tissue plasminogen activator.

There is no published guideline that addresses how quickly the BP should be reduced during hypertensive emergency. There is also variability depending on the target organ that is affected. When the brain is the target organ, it is important to be aware that cerebral hypoperfusion can occur if BP is lowered too rapidly. Current guidelines for treating stroke do not recommend a rapid reduction of blood pressure.[138] This is because the BP will spontaneously decrease during the first 3 days after a stroke.[166] For the patient with coronary artery disease experiencing hypertensive emergency, the need to maintain adequate diastolic blood pressure to allow for coronary artery filling is paramount.[167] If vasodilator therapy drops the diastolic pressure too far—when coronary artery filling occurs—myocardial ischemia may result.[167] Thus the question of how much to decrease the blood

pressure in hypertensive emergency is not simply a matter of reading the number on the monitor from the patient's arterial line, but involves an assessment of the underlying pathology and an appreciation of the physiologic requirements of the target organ that has been affected. For more information on specific agents see "Vasodilator Drugs" in Chapter 19.

Hypertensive Urgencies. Hypertensive urgencies may not necessitate admission to a critical care unit, because organ damage is not evident and the patient may be treated with rapid-acting oral antihypertensive agents. As above, there are many drug categories available including ACEI, ARBs, calcium channel blockers, and beta-blockers. Other oral drugs that are available, but less often prescribed in the critical care phase of management, include clonidine, guanabenz, prazosin, and minoxidil. A loop diuretic (furosemide) is generally prescribed in addition to the antihypertensive agents.

NURSING MANAGEMENT

The focus of nursing management for the patient with hypertensive crisis is to return the blood pressure to the desired range without introducing other complications as a result of the therapy. Then, once the hypertension is controlled, identify the factors that resulted in this life-threatening condition. Several nursing diagnoses are associated with hypertensive crisis (see the Nursing Diagnoses feature on Hypertensive Emergency).

During the acute phase the patient is observed closely for clinical manifestations in other organ systems, including the neurologic, cardiac, and renal systems.[167] Neurologic compromise may be manifested by mental confusion, stupor, seizures, coma, or stroke. Cardiac compromise may be exhibited by aortic dissection, myocardial ischemia, or dysrhythmias. Acute renal failure may not be evident immediately, but urine output, BUN, and serum creatinine values are evaluated over several days to determine whether the kidneys were affected by the hypertensive episode. When short-acting intravenous antihypertensive agents are administered, the blood pressure is closely monitored. If potent antihypertensive drugs such as sodium nitroprusside or labetalol are being used, an arterial line must be inserted and the drugs must be infused through an infusion pump.

PATIENT EDUCATION

Patient education during the acute phase of a hypertensive emergency is limited to an explanation of the need to control blood pressure and the purpose of the equipment used in the critical care unit. Once the hypertensive crisis is resolved, the focus of education is on lifestyle changes related to risk factor modification. Hypertension is emphasized as a risk factor for atherosclerotic arterial disease of the heart, brain and peripheral arterial system. For a more complete discussion of hypertension as a cardiovascular risk factor see p. 430 at the beginning of this chapter. The major points to discuss with the patient are listed in the Patient Education feature on Hypertensive Emergency. Management of hypertensive emergencies/urgencies are listed in the Evidence-Based Collaborative Practice feature.

SUMMARY

The number of patients with cardiovascular disease continues to grow.[1] Fortunately, considerable research and clinical progress has occurred that has clarified the diagnosis management of many cardiac conditions. To be able to participate fully in the collaborative management of patients with CV disorders, it is essential that the critical care nurse understand the spectrum of interventions from basic nursing care procedures to the most recent advances in therapy.

REFERENCES

1. American Heart Association: *Heart disease and stroke statistics—2004 Update.* Dallas, Texas, 2004, American Heart Association.
2. Kavey RE et al: American Heart Association guidelines for primary prevention of atherosclerotic cardiovascular disease beginning in childhood, *Circulation* 107(11):1562-1566, 2003.
3. Antman EM et al: ACC/AHA guidelines for the management of patients with ST-elevation myocardial infarction—executive summary: a report of the American College of Cardiology/American Heart Association Task Force on Practice Guidelines (Writing Committee to Revise the 1999 Guidelines for the Management of Patients with Acute Myocardial Infarction), *Circulation* 110:588-636, 2004. Full text available online at www.ahajournals.org.
4. Gibbons RJ et al: ACC/AHA 2002 guideline update for the management of patients with chronic stable angina—summary article: a report of the American College of Cardiology/American Heart Association Task Force on Practice Guidelines (Committee on the Management of Patients with Chronic Stable Angina), *Circulation* 107(1):149-158, 2003.
5. Executive summary of the third report of the National Cholesterol Education Program (NCEP) Expert Panel on Detection, Evaluation, and Treatment of High Blood Cholesterol in Adults (Adult Treatment Panel III), *JAMA* 285(19):2486-2497, 2001. Full text available online at www.ahajournals.org.
6. Grundy SM et al: Implications of recent clinical trials for the National Cholesterol Education Program Adult Treatment Panel III guidelines, *Circulation* 110(2):227-239, 2004.
7. Barter PJ et al: Antiinflammatory properties of HDL, *Circ Res* 95(8):764-772, 2004.
8. O'Keefe JH Jr et al: Optimal low-density lipoprotein is 50 to 70 mg/dl: lower is better and physiologically normal, *J Am Coll Cardiol* 43(11):2142-2146, 2004.
9. Futterman LG, Lemberg L: Lp(a) lipoprotein—an independent risk factor for coronary heart disease after menopause, *Am J Crit Care* 10(1):63-67, 2001.
10. Mokdad AH et al: The continuing epidemics of obesity and diabetes in the United States, *JAMA* 286(10):1195-1200, 2001.
11. Chobanian AV et al: Seventh report of the Joint National Committee on Prevention, Detection, Evaluation, and Treatment of High Blood Pressure, *Hypertension* 42(6):1206-1252, 2003.
12. Thompson PD et al: Exercise and physical activity in the prevention and treatment of atherosclerotic cardiovascular disease: a statement from the Council on Clinical Cardiology (Subcommittee on Exercise, Rehabilitation, and Prevention) and the Council on Nutrition, Physical Activity, and Metabolism (Subcommittee on Physical Activity), *Circulation* 107(24):3109-3116, 2003. Full text available online at www.ahajournals.org.

13. Brook RD et al: Air pollution and cardiovascular disease: a statement for healthcare professionals from the Expert Panel on Population and Prevention Science of the American Heart Association, *Circulation* 109(21):2655-2671, 2004. Full text available online at www.ahajournals.org.

14. Sargent RP, Shepard RM, Glantz SA: Reduced incidence of admissions for myocardial infarction associated with public smoking ban: before and after study, *BMJ* 328(7446): 977-980, 2004.

15. Houterman S, Verschuren WM, Kromhout D: Smoking, blood pressure and serum cholesterol-effects on 20-year mortality, *Epidemiology* 14(1):24-29, 2003.

16. Garber AJ et al: American College of Endocrinology position statement on inpatient diabetes and metabolic control, *Endocr Pract* 10(1):77-82, 2004.

17. McGuire DK et al: Association of diabetes mellitus and glycemic control strategies with clinical outcomes after acute coronary syndromes, *Am Heart J* 147(2):246-252, 2004.

18. Franklin K et al: Implications of diabetes in patients with acute coronary syndromes: the Global Registry of Acute Coronary Events, *Arch Intern Med* 164(13):1457-1463, 2004.

19. Sarnak MJ et al: Kidney disease as a risk factor for development of cardiovascular disease: a statement from the American Heart Association Councils on Kidney in Cardiovascular Disease, High Blood Pressure Research, Clinical Cardiology, and Epidemiology and Prevention, *Hypertension* 42(5):1050-1065, 2003.

20. Wright RS et al: Acute myocardial infarction and renal dysfunction: a high-risk combination, *Ann Intern Med* 137(7):563-570, 2002.

21. Grundy SM et al: Clinical management of metabolic syndrome: report of the American Heart Association/National Heart, Lung, and Blood Institute/American Diabetes Association conference on scientific issues related to management, *Circulation* 109(4):551-556, 2004. Full text available online at www.ahajournals.org.

22. Grady D et al: Cardiovascular disease outcomes during 6.8 years of hormone therapy: Heart and Estrogen/progestin Replacement Study follow-up (HERS II), *JAMA* 288(1): 49-57, 2002.

23. Hulley S et al: Randomized trial of estrogen plus progestin for secondary prevention of coronary heart disease in postmenopausal women. Heart and Estrogen/progestin Replacement Study (HERS) Research Group, *JAMA* 280(7):605-613, 1998.

24. Anderson GL et al: Effects of conjugated equine estrogen in postmenopausal women with hysterectomy: the Women's Health Initiative randomized controlled trial, *JAMA* 291(14): 1701-1712, 2004.

25. Mosca L et al: Evidence-based guidelines for cardiovascular disease prevention in women, *Circulation* 109(5):672-693, 2004.

26. Lefler LL, Bondy KN: Women's delay in seeking treatment with myocardial infarction: A meta synthesis, *J Cardiovasc Nurs* 19(4):251-268, 2004.

27. Reeder SJ et al: Homocysteine: the latest risk factor for heart disease, *Dimens Crit Care Nurs* 19(1):22-28, 2000.

28. Aronow WS: Homocysteine. The association with atherosclerotic vascular disease in older persons, *Geriatrics* 58(9):22-24, 27-28, 2003.

29. Pearson TA et al: Markers of inflammation and cardiovascular disease: application to clinical and public health practice: a statement for healthcare professionals from the Centers for Disease Control and Prevention and the American Heart Association, *Circulation* 107(3):499-511, 2003.

30. Speidl WS et al: High-sensitivity C-reactive protein in the prediction of coronary events in patients with premature coronary artery disease, *Am Heart J* 144(3):449-455, 2002.

31. Buffon A et al: Widespread coronary inflammation in unstable angina, *N Engl J Med* 347(1):5-12, 2002.

32. Smith SC Jr et al: ACC/AHA guidelines for percutaneous coronary intervention (revision of the 1993 PTCA guidelines)—executive summary: a report of the American College of Cardiology/American Heart Association task force on practice guidelines (Committee to revise the 1993 Guidelines For Percutaneous Transluminal Coronary Angioplasty) endorsed by the Society for Cardiac Angiography and Interventions, *Circulation* 103(24): 3019-3041, 2001. Full text available online at www. ahajournals.org.

33. Braunwald E et al: ACC/AHA guideline update for the management of patients with unstable angina and non–ST-segment elevation myocardial infarction—summary article: a report of the American College of Cardiology/American Heart Association Task Force on Practice Guidelines (Committee on the Management of Patients with Unstable Angina), *Circulation* 106(14):1893-1900, 2002. Full text available online at www.ahajournals.org.

34. McSweeney JC et al: Women's early warning symptoms of acute myocardial infarction, *Circulation* 108(21):2619-2623, 2003.

35. Bairey Merz N et al: Women's ischemic syndrome evaluation: current status and future research directions: report of the National Heart, Lung and Blood Institute workshop: October 2-4, 2002—executive summary, *Circulation* 109(6):805-807, 2004. Full text available online at www.ahajournals.org.

36. Canto JG et al: Use of emergency medical services in acute myocardial infarction and subsequent quality of care: observations from the National Registry of Myocardial Infarction 2, *Circulation* 106(24):3018-3023, 2002.

37. Keller KB, Lemberg L: Prinzmetal's angina, *Am J Crit Care* 13(4):350-354, 2004.

38. Jacobs AK et al: Cardiogenic shock caused by right ventricular infarction: a report from the SHOCK registry, *J Am Coll Cardiol* 41(8):1273-1279, 2003.

39. Lanza M: Right ventricular myocardial infarction: when the power fails, *Dimens Crit Care Nurs* 21(4):122-126, 2002.

40. Mehta RH et al: Comparison of outcomes of patients with acute coronary syndromes with and without atrial fibrillation, *Am J Cardiol* 92(9):1031-1036, 2003.

41. Birnbaum Y et al: Ventricular septal rupture after acute myocardial infarction, *N Engl J Med* 347(18):1426-1432, 2002.

42. Crenshaw BS et al: Risk factors, angiographic patterns, and outcomes in patients with ventricular septal defect complicating acute myocardial infarction. GUSTO-I (Global Utilization of Streptokinase and TPA for Occluded Coronary Arteries) Trial Investigators, *Circulation* 101(1):27-32, 2000.

43. Deja MA et al: Post infarction ventricular septal defect—can we do better? *Eur J Cardiothorac Surg* 18(2):194-201, 2000.

44. Birnbaum Y et al: Mitral regurgitation following acute myocardial infarction, *Coron Artery Dis* 13(6):337-344, 2002.

45. Maisch B et al: Guidelines on the diagnosis and management of pericardial diseases executive summary; the Task

Force on the Diagnosis and Management of Pericardial Diseases of the European Society of Cardiology, *Eur Heart J* 25(7):587-610, 2004.

46. Wang K, Asinger RW, Marriott HJ: ST-segment elevation in conditions other than acute myocardial infarction, *N Engl J Med* 349(22):2128-2135, 2003.

47. Paelinck B, Dendale PA: Images in clinical medicine. Cardiac tamponade in Dressler's syndrome, *N Engl J Med* 348(23):e8, 2003.

48. Wu AH et al: Hospital outcomes in patients presenting with congestive heart failure complicating acute myocardial infarction: a report from the Second National Registry of Myocardial Infarction (NRMI-2), *J Am Coll Cardiol* 40(8):1389-1394, 2002.

49. Szekendi MK: Compliance with acute MI guidelines lowers inpatient mortality, *J Cardiovasc Nurs* 18(5):356-359, 2003.

50. Eagle KA et al: Adherence to evidence-based therapies after discharge for acute coronary syndromes: an ongoing prospective, observational study, *Am J Med* 117(2):73-81, 2004.

51. Balady GJ et al: Core components of cardiac rehabilitation/secondary prevention programs: a statement for healthcare professionals from the American Heart Association and the American Association of Cardiovascular and Pulmonary Rehabilitation Writing Group, *Circulation* 102(9):1069-1073, 2000. Full text available online at www.ahajournals.org.

52. Fox CS et al: Temporal trends in coronary heart disease mortality and sudden cardiac death from 1950 to 1999: the Framingham Heart Study, *Circulation* 110(5):522-527, 2004.

53. Chugh SS et al: Current burden of sudden cardiac death: multiple source surveillance versus retrospective death-certificate based review in a large U.S. community, *J Am Coll Cardiol* 44(6):1268-1275, 2004.

54. Hallstrom AP et al: Public-access defibrillation and survival after out-of-hospital cardiac arrest, *N Engl J Med* 351(7):637-646, 2004.

55. Priori SG et al: Task Force on Sudden Cardiac Death of the European Society of Cardiology, *Eur Heart J* 22(16):1374-1450, 2001.

56. Antzelevitch C et al: Brugada Syndrome. Report of the Second Consensus Conference. Endorsed by the Heart Rhythm Society and the European Heart Rhythm Association, *Circulation* 111(5):659-670, 2005.

57. Antezano ES, Hong M: Sudden cardiac death, *J Intensive Care Med* 18(6):313-329, 2003.

58. Gregoratos G et al: ACC/AHA/NASPE 2002 guideline update for implantation of cardiac pacemakers and antiarrhythmia devices—summary article: a report of the American College of Cardiology/American Heart Association Task Force on Practice Guidelines (ACC/AHA/NASPE Committee to Update the 1998 Pacemaker Guidelines), *Circulation* 106(16):2145-2161, 2002. Full text available online at www.ahajournals.org.

59. Steinbeck G: Evolution of implantable cardioverter defibrillator indications: comparison of guidelines in the United States and Europe, *J Cardiovasc Electrophysiol* 13(suppl 1):S96-99, 2002.

60. Epstein AE: An update on implantable cardioverter-defibrillator guidelines, *Curr Opin Cardiol* 19(1):23-25, 2004.

61. Hunt SA et al: ACC/AHA Guidelines for the evaluation and management of chronic heart failure in the adult—executive summary: a report of the American College of Cardiol-ogy/American Heart Association Task Force on Practice Guidelines (Committee to Revise the 1995 Guidelines for the Evaluation and Management of Heart Failure): Developed in collaboration with the International Society for Heart and Lung Transplantation; Endorsed by the Heart Failure Society of America, *Circulation* 104(24):2996-3007, 2001. Full text available online at www.ahajournals.org.

62. Zile MR, Brutsaert DL: New concepts in diastolic dysfunction and diastolic heart failure: Part I: diagnosis, prognosis, and measurements of diastolic function, *Circulation* 105(11):1387-1393, 2002.

63. Zile MR, Brutsaert DL: New concepts in diastolic dysfunction and diastolic heart failure: Part II: causal mechanisms and treatment, *Circulation* 105(12):1503-1508, 2002.

64. Henry LB: Left ventricular systolic dysfunction and ischemic cardiomyopathy, *Crit Care Nurs Q* 26(1):16-21, 2003.

65. Bolliger K, Sadar AM: Care and management of the patient with right heart failure secondary to diastolic dysfunction: an advanced practice perspective and case review, *Crit Care Nurs Q* 26(1):22-27, 2003.

66. Aurigemma GP, Gaasch WH: Clinical practice. Diastolic heart failure, *N Engl J Med* 351(11):1097-1105, 2004.

67. Zile MR, Baicu CF, Gaasch WH: Diastolic heart failure—abnormalities in active relaxation and passive stiffness of the left ventricle, *N Engl J Med* 350(19):1953-1959, 2004.

68. Riedinger MS et al: Quality of life in patients with heart failure: do gender differences exist? *Heart Lung* 30(2):105-116, 2001.

69. Maisel AS et al: Bedside B-type natriuretic peptide in the emergency diagnosis of heart failure with reduced or preserved ejection fraction. Results from the Breathing Not Properly (BNP) multinational study, *J Am Coll Cardiol* 41(11):2010-2017, 2003.

70. Thohan V, Torre-Amione G, Koerner MM: Aldosterone antagonism and congestive heart failure: a new look at an old therapy, *Curr Opin Cardiol* 19(4):301-308, 2004.

71. Patten RD, Soman P: Prevention and Reversal of LV Remodeling with Neurohormonal Inhibitors, *Curr Treat Options Cardiovasc Med* 6(4):313-325, 2004.

72. Paul S: Balancing diuretic therapy in heart failure: loop diuretics, thiazides, and aldosterone antagonists, *Congest Heart Fail* 8(6):307-312, 2002.

73. Paul S: Ventricular remodeling, *Crit Care Nurs Clin North Am* 15(4):407-411, 2003.

74. Dimopoulos K et al: Meta-analyses of mortality and morbidity effects of an angiotensin receptor blocker in patients with chronic heart failure already receiving an ACE inhibitor (alone or with a beta-blocker), *Int J Cardiol* 93(2-3):105-111, 2004.

75. McCullough PA, Sandberg KR: B-type natriuretic peptide and renal disease, *Heart Fail Rev* 8(4):355-358, 2003.

76. Maisel AS et al: Impact of age, race, and sex on the ability of B-type natriuretic peptide to aid in the emergency diagnosis of heart failure: results from the Breathing Not Properly (BNP) multinational study, *Am Heart J* 147(6):1078-1084, 2004.

77. Maisel AS et al: Rapid measurement of B-type natriuretic peptide in the emergency diagnosis of heart failure, *N Engl J Med* 347(3):161-167, 2002.

78. McCullough PA et al: Uncovering heart failure in patients with a history of pulmonary disease: rationale for the early use of B-type natriuretic peptide in the emergency department, *Acad Emerg Med* 10(3):198-204, 2003.

79. Buxton AE et al: Relation of ejection fraction and inducible ventricular tachycardia to mode of death in patients with coronary artery disease: an analysis of patients enrolled in the multicenter unsustained tachycardia trial, *Circulation* 106(19):2466-2472, 2002.

80. Stroe AF, Gheorghiade M: Carvedilol: beta-blockade and beyond, *Rev Cardiovasc Med* 5(suppl 1):S18-27, 2004.

81. Zhang J: Sudden cardiac death: implantable cardioverter defibrillators and pharmacological treatments, *Crit Care Nurs Q* 26(1):45-49, 2003.

82. Whang W et al: Heart failure and the risk of shocks in patients with implantable cardioverter defibrillators: results from the Triggers of Ventricular Arrhythmias (TOVA) study, *Circulation* 109(11):1386-1391, 2004.

83. Khand AU et al: Carvedilol alone or in combination with digoxin for the management of atrial fibrillation in patients with heart failure? *J Am Coll Cardiol* 42(11):1944-1951, 2003.

84. Chen EW et al: Relation between hospital intra-aortic balloon counterpulsation volume and mortality in acute myocardial infarction complicated by cardiogenic shock, *Circulation* 108(8):951-957, 2003.

85. Burger AJ et al: Effect of nesiritide (B-type natriuretic peptide) and dobutamine on ventricular arrhythmias in the treatment of patients with acutely decompensated congestive heart failure: the PRECEDENT study, *Am Heart J* 144(6):1102-1108, 2002.

86. Colbert K, Greene MH: Nesiritide (Natrecor): a new treatment for acutely decompensated congestive heart failure, *Crit Care Nurs Q* 26(1):40-44, 2003.

87. Abraham WT, Iyengar S: Practical considerations for switching beta-blockers in heart failure patients, *Rev Cardiovasc Med* 5(suppl 1):S36-S44, 2004.

88. Albert NM: Cardiac resynchronization therapy through biventricular pacing in patients with heart failure and ventricular dyssynchrony, *Crit Care Nurse* 23(suppl 3):2-13, 2003.

89. Abraham WT, Hayes DL: Cardiac resynchronization therapy for heart failure, *Circulation* 108(21):2596-2603, 2003.

90. Young JB et al: Combined cardiac resynchronization and implantable cardioversion defibrillation in advanced chronic heart failure: the MIRACLE ICD Trial, *JAMA* 289(20):2685-2694, 2003.

91. Goodlin SJ et al: Consensus statement: Palliative and supportive care in advanced heart failure, *J Card Fail* 10(3):200-209, 2004.

92. Rudisill PT, Kennedy C, Paul S: The use of beta-blockers in the treatment of chronic heart failure, *Crit Care Nurs Clin North Am* 15(4):439-446, 2003.

93. Fonarow GC et al: Organized Program to Initiate Lifesaving Treatment in Hospitalized Patients with Heart Failure (OPTIMIZE-HF): rationale and design, *Am Heart J* 148(1):43-51, 2004.

94. Callahan HE: Families dealing with advanced heart failure: a challenge and an opportunity, *Crit Care Nurs Q* 26(3):230-243, 2003.

95. Grady KL et al: Team management of patients with heart failure: a statement for healthcare professionals from the Cardiovascular Nursing Council of the American Heart Association, *Circulation* 102(19):2443-2456, 2000.

96. Coviello JS, Nystrom KV: Obesity and heart failure, *J Cardiovasc Nurs* 18(5):360-366, 2003.

97. Sneed NV, Paul SC: Readiness for behavioral changes in patients with heart failure, *Am J Crit Care* 12(5):444-453, 2003.

98. Maron BJ et al: American College of Cardiology/European Society of Cardiology clinical expert consensus document on hypertrophic cardiomyopathy: a report of the American College of Cardiology Foundation Task Force on Clinical Expert Consensus Documents and the European Society of Cardiology Committee for Practice Guidelines, *J Am Coll Cardiol* 42(9):1687-1713, 2003.

99. Nishimura RA, Holmes DR Jr: Clinical practice. Hypertrophic obstructive cardiomyopathy, *N Engl J Med* 350(13):1320-1327, 2004.

100. Elliott P, McKenna WJ: Hypertrophic cardiomyopathy, *Lancet* 363(9424):1881-1891, 2004.

101. Kamisago M et al: Mutations in sarcomere protein genes as a cause of dilated cardiomyopathy, *N Engl J Med* 343(23):1688-1696, 2000.

102. Li D et al: Novel cardiac troponin T mutation as a cause of familial dilated cardiomyopathy, *Circulation* 104(18):2188-2193, 2001.

103. Murphy RT et al: Novel mutation in cardiac troponin I in recessive idiopathic dilated cardiomyopathy, *Lancet* 363(9406):371-372, 2004.

104. Noutsias M et al: Current insights into the pathogenesis, diagnosis and therapy of inflammatory cardiomyopathy, *Heart Fail Monit* 3(4):127-135, 2003.

105. Syed J, Myers R: Sarcoid heart disease, *Can J Cardiol* 20(1):89-93, 2004.

106. Ammash NM et al: Clinical profile and outcome of idiopathic restrictive cardiomyopathy, *Circulation* 101(21):2490-2496, 2000.

107. Felker GM et al: Underlying causes and long-term survival in patients with initially unexplained cardiomyopathy, *N Engl J Med* 342(15):1077-1084, 2000.

108. Farber HW, Loscalzo J: Pulmonary arterial hypertension, *N Engl J Med* 351(16):1655-1665, 2004.

109. Eells PL: Advances in prostacyclin therapy for pulmonary arterial hypertension, *Crit Care Nurse* 24(2):42-54, 2004.

110. McLaughlin VV et al: Prognosis of pulmonary arterial hypertension: ACCP evidence-based clinical practice guidelines, *Chest* 126(suppl 1):78S-92S, 2004.

111. Presberg KW, Dincer HE: Pathophysiology of pulmonary hypertension due to lung disease, *Curr Opin Pulm Med* 9(2):131-138, 2003.

112. Atwood CW Jr et al: Pulmonary artery hypertension and sleep-disordered breathing: ACCP evidence-based clinical practice guidelines, *Chest* 126(suppl 1):72S-77S, 2004.

113. Fedullo PF et al: Chronic thromboembolic pulmonary hypertension, *Clin Chest Med* 22(3):561-581, 2001.

114. Rubin LJ: Diagnosis and management of pulmonary arterial hypertension: ACCP evidence-based clinical practice guidelines—executive summary, *Chest* 126(suppl 1):4S-6S, 2004.

115. Runo JR, Loyd JE: Primary pulmonary hypertension, *Lancet* 361(9368):1533-1544, 2003.

116. Huffman MD, McLaughlin VV: Pulmonary arterial hypertension: new management options, *Curr Treat Options Cardiovasc Med* 6(6):451-458, 2004.

117. Galie N, Manes A, Branzi A: Prostanoids for pulmonary arterial hypertension, *Am J Respir Med* 2(2):123-137, 2003.

118. Doyle RL et al: Surgical treatments/interventions for pulmonary arterial hypertension: ACCP evidence-based clinical practice guidelines, *Chest* 126(suppl 1):63S-71S, 2004.

119. Horstkotte D et al: Guidelines on prevention, diagnosis and treatment of infective endocarditis—executive summary; the Task Force on Infective Endocarditis of the European Society of Cardiology, *Eur Heart J* 25(3):267-276, 2004.

120. Andrews MM, von Reyn CF: Patient selection criteria and management guidelines for outpatient parenteral antibiotic therapy for native valve infective endocarditis, *Clin Infect Dis* 33(2):203-209, 2001.

121. Sexton DJ, Spelman D: Current best practices and guidelines. Assessment and management of complications in infective endocarditis, *Cardiol Clin* 21(2):273-282, vii-viii, 2003.

122. Anderson DJ et al: Stroke location, characterization, severity, and outcome in mitral vs aortic valve endocarditis, *Neurology* 61(10):1341-1346, 2003.

123. Broyles LM, Korniewicz DM: The opiate-dependent patient with endocarditis: addressing pain and substance abuse withdrawal, *AACN Clin Issues* 13(3):431-451, 2002.

124. Segal BL: Valvular heart disease, Part 1. Diagnosis and surgical management of aortic valve disease in older adults, *Geriatrics* 58(9):31-35, 2003.

125. Segal BL: Valvular heart disease, Part 2. Mitral valve disease in older adults, *Geriatrics* 58(10):26-31, 2003.

126. Wiegand DL: Advances in cardiac surgery: valve repair, *Crit Care Nurse* 23(2):72-91, 2003.

127. Robicsek F et al: The congenitally bicuspid aortic valve: how does it function? Why does it fail? *Ann Thorac Surg* 77(1):177-185, 2004.

128. Hicks GL Jr, Massey HT: Update on indications for surgery in aortic insufficiency, *Curr Opin Cardiol* 17(2):172-178, 2002.

129. Bonow RO et al: ACC/AHA Guidelines for the Management of Patients with Valvular Heart Disease—executive summary: a report of the American College of Cardiology/American Heart Association Task Force on Practice Guidelines (Committee on Management of Patients with Valvular Heart Disease), *J Heart Valve Dis* 7(6):672-707, 1998. Full text available online at www.ahajournals.org.

130. Girardi LN et al: Management strategies for type A dissection complicated by peripheral vascular malperfusion, *Ann Thorac Surg* 77(4):1309-1314, 2004.

131. Nienaber CA et al: Gender-related differences in acute aortic dissection, *Circulation* 109(24):3014-3021, 2004.

132. Mehta RH et al: Acute type B aortic dissection in elderly patients: clinical features, outcomes, and simple risk stratification rule, *Ann Thorac Surg* 77(5):1622-1628, 2004.

133. Selvin E, Erlinger TP: Prevalence of and risk factors for peripheral arterial disease in the United States: results from the National Health and Nutrition Examination Survey 1999-2000, *Circulation* 110(6):738-743, 2004.

134. O'Hare AM et al: High prevalence of peripheral arterial disease in persons with renal insufficiency: results from the National Health and Nutrition Examination Survey 1999-2000, *Circulation* 109(3):320-323, 2004.

135. Belch JJ, Topol EJ, Agnelli G et al: Critical issues in peripheral arterial disease detection and management: a call to action, *Arch Intern Med* 163(8):884-892, 2003.

136. McDermott MM et al: Knowledge and attitudes regarding cardiovascular disease risk and prevention in patients with coronary or peripheral arterial disease, *Arch Intern Med* 163(18):2157-2162, 2003.

137. Gardner AW et al: Response to exercise rehabilitation in smoking and nonsmoking patients with intermittent claudication, *J Vasc Surg* 39(3):531-538, 2004.

138. Adams HP Jr et al: Guidelines for the early management of patients with ischemic stroke: a scientific statement from the Stroke Council of the American Stroke Association, *Stroke* 34(4):1056-1083, 2003.

139. Goldstein LB et al: Primary prevention of ischemic stroke: a statement for healthcare professionals from the Stroke Council of the American Heart Association, *Stroke* 32(1):280-299, 2001.

140. Schlegel D et al: Utility of the NIH Stroke Scale as a predictor of hospital disposition, *Stroke* 34(1):134-137, 2003.

141. Fedullo PF, Tapson VF: Clinical practice. The evaluation of suspected pulmonary embolism, *N Engl J Med* 349(13):1247-1256, 2003.

142. Horlander KT, Mannino DM, Leeper KV: Pulmonary embolism mortality in the United States, 1979-1998: an analysis using multiple-cause mortality data, *Arch Intern Med* 163(14):1711-1717, 2003.

143. British Thoracic Society: Guidelines for the management of suspected acute pulmonary embolism, *Thorax* 58(6):470-483, 2003.

144. Greets WH et al: Prevention of venous thromboembolism; the seventh AACP conference on antithrombotic and thrombolytic therapy, *Chest* 126(suppl 3):338S-400S, 2004.

145. Moores L, Bilello KL, Murin S: Sex and gender issues and venous thromboembolism, *Clin Chest Med* 25(2):281-297, 2003.

146. Cook D et al: Prevention and diagnosis of venous thromboembolism in critically ill patients: a Canadian survey, *Crit Care* 5(6):336-342, 2001.

147. Cook D et al: Clinically important deep vein thrombosis in the intensive care unit: a survey of intensivists, *Crit Care* 8(3):R145-R152, 2004.

148. Rogers FB et al: Practice management guidelines for the prevention of venous thromboembolism in trauma patients: the EAST practice management guidelines work group, *J Trauma* 53(1):142-164, 2002.

149. Green D: Diagnosis, prevalence, and management of thromboembolism in patients with spinal cord injury, *J Spinal Cord Med* 26(4):329-334, 2003.

150. Dellinger RP et al: Surviving Sepsis Campaign guidelines for management of severe sepsis and septic shock, *Crit Care Med* 32(3):858-873, 2004.

151. Caprini JA et al: Laboratory markers in the diagnosis of venous thromboembolism, *Circulation* 109(12 Suppl 1):I4-I8, 2004.

152. Geerts W et al: Venous thromboembolism and its prevention in critical care, *J Crit Care* 17(2):95-104, 2002.

153. Zierler BK: Ultrasonography and diagnosis of venous thromboembolism, *Circulation* 109(12 Suppl 1):I9-14, 2004.

154. Kelly J et al: Plasma D-dimers in the diagnosis of venous thromboembolism, *Arch Intern Med* 162(7):747-756, 2002.

155. Frost SD, Brotman DJ, Michota FA: Rational use of D-dimer measurement to exclude acute venous thromboembolic disease, *Mayo Clin Proc* 78(11):1385-1391, 2003.

156. Eichinger S et al: D-dimer levels and risk of recurrent venous thromboembolism, *JAMA* 290(8):1071-1074, 2003.

157. Wells PS et al: Evaluation of D-dimer in the diagnosis of suspected deep-vein thrombosis, *N Engl J Med* 349(13):1227-1235, 2003.

158. Stein PD et al: D-dimer for the exclusion of acute venous thrombosis and pulmonary embolism: a systematic review, *Ann Intern Med* 140(8):589-602, 2004.

159. Stein PD, Kayali F, Olson RE: Trends in the use of diagnostic imaging in patients hospitalized with acute pulmonary embolism, *Am J Cardiol* 93(10):1316-1317, 2004.

160. Streiff MB: Vena caval filters: a review for intensive care specialists, *J Intensive Care Med* 18(2):59-79, 2003.

161. Hirsh J, Raschke R: Heparin and low-molecular-weight heparin: the Seventh ACCP Conference on Antithrombotic

and Thrombolytic Therapy, *Chest* 126(suppl 3):188S-203S, 2004.

162. Ansell J et al: The pharmacology and management of the vitamin K antagonists: the Seventh ACCP Conference on Antithrombotic and Thrombolytic Therapy, *Chest* 126(suppl 3):204S-233S, 2004.

163. Devlin JW et al: Fenoldopam versus nitroprusside for the treatment of hypertensive emergency, *Ann Pharmacother* 38(5):755-759, 2004.

164. Mayer S: Management of hypertension in neurologic emergencies. In *SCCM 33rd Critical Care Congress,* Orlando, Florida, 2004, Society of Critical Care Medicine.

165. Tuncel M, Ram VC: Hypertensive emergencies: etiology and management, *Am J Cardiovasc Drugs* 3(1):21-31, 2003.

166. Hickey JV, Salmeron ET, Lai JM: Twenty-four-hour blood pressure variability after acute ischemic stroke, *Crit Care Nurs Q* 25(2):1-12, 2002.

167. Sladen R: Therapeutic options for the treatment of acute hypertension. In *SCCM 33rd Critical Care Congress,* Orlando, Florida, 2004, Society of Critical Care Medicine.

CHAPTER 19

Cardiovascular Therapeutic Management

TEMPORARY PACEMAKERS

Pacemakers are electronic devices that can be used to initiate the heartbeat when the heart's intrinsic electrical system cannot effectively generate a rate adequate to support cardiac output. Pacemakers can be used temporarily, either supportively or prophylactically, until the condition responsible for the rate or conduction disturbance resolves. Pacemakers also can be used on a permanent basis if the patient's condition persists despite adequate therapy. The use of permanent pacemakers as a form of device-based therapy is gaining popularity.[1]

This section emphasizes temporary pacemakers, because the critical care nurse is responsible for preventing, assessing, and managing pacemaker malfunctions when these devices are used in the clinical setting. A brief discussion of permanent pacemakers is provided, and similarities between implanted and temporary pacemakers are presented where appropriate.

INDICATIONS

The clinical indications for instituting temporary pacemaker therapy are similar regardless of the cause of the rhythm disturbance that necessitates the placement of a pacemaker (Box 19-1). Such causes range from drug toxicities and electrolyte imbalances to sequelae related to acute myocardial infarction or cardiac surgery.

Therapeutic Indications. Dysrhythmias that are unresponsive to drug therapy and result in compromised hemodynamic status are a definite indication for pacemaker therapy. The goal of therapy in the case of bradydysrhythmia is to increase the ventricular rate and thus enhance cardiac output. Alternately, "overdrive" pacing can be used to decrease the rate of a rapid supraventricular or ventricular rhythm. This rapid pacing of the heart, or overdrive pacing, functions either to prevent the "breakthrough" ectopy that can result from a slow rate or to interrupt an ectopic focus and allow the natural pacemaker to regain control. Temporary pacing may be used in the treatment of symptomatic bradycardia or progressive heart block that occurs secondary to myocardial ischemia or drug toxicity. After cardiac surgery, temporary pacing can be used to improve a transiently depressed, rate-dependent cardiac output. In addition, conduction disturbances that can occur after valvular surgery can be managed effectively with temporary pacing.

Diagnostic Indications. Several diagnostic uses for temporary pacing have evolved during the past several years. Electrophysiology studies (EPS) are now performed in cardiac catheterization laboratories equipped with specialized pacing equipment. During an electrophysiology study, special pacing electrodes are used to diagnose the patient's potential for dysrhythmias.[2] These electrodes are used to induce dysrhythmias in patients with recurrent symptomatic tachydysrhythmias. This allows the physician to closely evaluate the particular dysrhythmia and to determine appropriate therapy. For those patients whose tachydysrhythmia is found to be refractory to conventional antidysrhythmic therapy, radiofrequency (RF) current catheter ablation of the responsible tissue can be done safely and effectively in the electrophysiology laboratory. After a mapping procedure localizes the site of dysrhythmia formation, short bursts of radiofrequency current are delivered through the catheter, destroying the offending tissue with heat. Radiofrequency ablation is more effective than its predecessor, direct current (DC) ablation, because it delivers a more precise, localized ablation current that lowers the incidence of complications and does not require general anesthesia.[3] Ablation has been shown to be an effective treatment for patients with symptomatic supraventricular tachycardias that result from atrioventricular (AV) node reentry or accessory pathways, such as Wolff-Parkinson-White syndrome.[4]

The atrial electrogram (AEG) is simply an amplified recording of atrial activity that can be obtained through the use of an atrial pacing electrode or an esophageal "pill" electrode and a standard electrocardiogram (ECG) machine. It often is used after cardiac surgery to facilitate the diagnosis of supraventricular dysrhythmias in patients with temporary atrial epicardial wires already in place.[5]

THE PACEMAKER SYSTEM

A pacemaker system is a simple electrical circuit consisting of a pulse generator and a pacing lead (an insulated electrical wire) with one, two, or three electrodes.

Pacing Pulse Generator. The pulse generator is designed to generate an electrical current that travels through the pacing lead and exits through an electrode (exposed portion of the wire) that is in direct contact with the heart. This electrical current initiates a myocardial depolarization. The current then seeks to return by one of several ways to the pulse generator to complete the circuit.

The power source for a temporary external pulse generator is the standard 9-volt alkaline battery inserted into the generator. Implanted permanent pacemaker batteries are generally long-lived lithium cells.

Pacing Lead Systems. The pacing lead used for temporary pacing may be bipolar or unipolar. In a bipolar system, two electrodes (positive and negative) are located within the heart, whereas in a unipolar system, only one electrode (negative) is in direct contact with the myocardium. In both unipolar and bipolar systems, the current flows from the negative terminal of the pulse generator, down the pacing lead to the negative electrode, and into the heart. The current is then picked up by the positive electrode (ground) and flows back up the lead to the positive terminal of the pulse generator.

The bipolar lead used in transvenous pacing has two electrodes on one catheter (see Fig. 19-1, *D*). The distal, or negative, electrode is at the tip of the pacing lead and is in direct contact with the heart, usually inside the right atrium or ventricle. Approximately 1 cm from the negative electrode is a positive electrode. The negative electrode is attached to the negative terminal, and the positive electrode is attached to the positive terminal of the pulse generator, either directly or via a bridging cable (see Fig. 19-1).

An epicardial lead system is often used for temporary pacing after cardiac surgery. The bipolar epicardial lead system has two separate insulated wires (one negative and one positive electrode) that are loosely secured with sutures to the cardiac chamber to be paced. Both leads are in contact with the myocardial tissue, so either wire may be used as the negative, or pacing, electrode. The remaining wire is then used as the positive, or ground, electrode.

A unipolar pacing system (epicardial or transvenous) has only one electrode (the negative electrode) making contact with the heart. In the case of a permanent pacemaker, the positive electrode can be created by the metallic casing of the subcutaneously implanted pulse generator (Fig. 19-2). Or, as is the case with a unipolar epicardial lead system, the positive electrode can be formed by a piece of surgical steel wire sewn into the subcutaneous tissue of the chest or the metal portion of a surface ECG electrode.

Both systems have advantages and disadvantages. Because the unipolar pacing system has a wide sensing area as a result of the relatively long distance between the negative and positive electrodes, it has better sensing capabilities than does a bipolar system. However, this feature makes the unipolar system more susceptible to sensing extraneous signals, such as the electrical artifact created by normal muscle movements (myopotentials) or external electromagnetic interference (EMI), which may result in inappropriate inhibition of the pacing stimulus. This problem is generally of more concern in permanent pacing systems, in which the "can" of the pacemaker generator may be used as a part of the pacing circuit. Because the can is located near a large muscle mass, upper body movement can result in the inappropriate sensing of myopotentials.[6]

PACING ROUTES

Several routes are available for temporary cardiac pacing (Box 19-2). Permanent pacing usually is accomplished transvenously, although in situations in which a thoracotomy is otherwise indicated, such as in cardiac surgery, the physician may elect to insert permanent epicardial pacing wires.

Transcutaneous cardiac pacing involves the use of two large skin electrodes, one placed anteriorly and the other posteriorly on the chest, connected to an external pulse generator. It is a rapid, noninvasive procedure that nurses can perform in the emergency setting and is recommended as a primary intervention in the Advanced Cardiac Life Support (ACLS) algorithm for the treatment of symptomatic bradycardia.[7] Improved technology related to stimulus delivery and the development of large electrode pads that help disperse the energy have helped reduce the pain associated with cutaneous nerve and muscle stimulation. Discomfort may still be an issue in

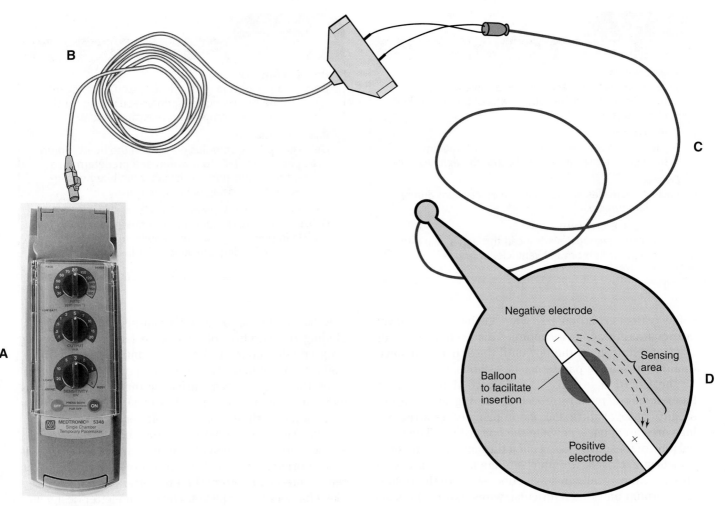

Fig. 19-1   The components of a temporary bipolar transvenous catheter. **A,** Single-chamber temporary (external) pulse generator. **B,** Bridging cable. **C,** Pacing lead. **D,** Enlarged view of the pacing lead tip. (**A** Courtesy Medtronic Inc., Minneapolis, Minn.)

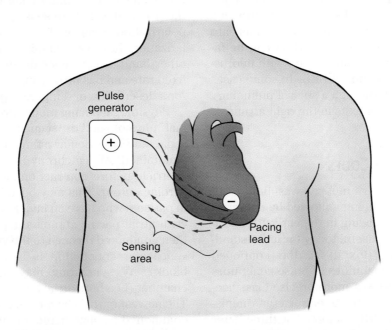

Fig. 19-2   The components of a permanent unipolar transvenous pacing system.

Box 19-2

ROUTES FOR TEMPORARY PACING

TRANSCUTANEOUS
Emergency pacing is achieved by depolarizing the heart through the chest by means of two large skin electrodes.

TRANSTHORACIC
A pacing wire is inserted emergently by threading it through a transthoracic needle into the right ventricle.

EPICARDIAL
Pacing electrodes are sewn to the epicardium during cardiac surgery.

TRANSVENOUS (ENDOCARDIAL)
The pacing electrode is advanced through a vein into the right atrium or right ventricle, or both.

Box 19-3

PACEMAKER TERMINOLOGY

FIXED-RATE (ASYNCHRONOUS)
Delivers a pacing stimulus at a set (fixed) rate regardless of the occurrence of spontaneous myocardial depolarization; occurs in non-sensing modes

DEMAND (SYNCHRONOUS)
Delivers a pacing stimulus only when the heart's intrinsic pacemaker fails to function at a predetermined rate; the pacing stimulus is either inhibited or triggered by the sensing of intrinsic activity

ATRIOVENTRICULAR (AV) SEQUENTIAL (DUAL-CHAMBER)
Delivers a pacing stimulus to both the atrium and ventricle in physiologic sequence with sufficient AV delay to permit adequate ventricular filling

some patients, particularly when higher energy levels are required to achieve capture. This route is generally used as a short-term therapy until the situation resolves or another route of pacing can be established.

The insertion of temporary epicardial pacing wires has become a routine procedure during most cardiac surgical cases. Ventricular and in many cases atrial pacing wires are loosely sewn to the epicardium. The terminal pins of these wires are pulled through the skin before the chest is closed. If both chambers have pacing wires attached, the atrial wires exit subcostally to the right of the sternum and the ventricular wires exit in the same region but to the left of the sternum. These wires can be removed several days after surgery by gentle traction at the skin surface with minimal risk of bleeding.[6]

Temporary transvenous endocardial pacing is accomplished by advancing a pacing electrode wire through a vein, often the subclavian or internal jugular, and into the right atrium or right ventricle. Insertion can be facilitated either through direct visualization with fluoroscopy or by the use of the standard ECG. In some cases the pacing wire is inserted through a special pulmonary artery catheter via a port that exits in the right atrium or ventricle.

FIVE-LETTER PACEMAKER CODES

In the 1960s, pacemaker terminology was limited to "fixed-rate" and "demand" pacing, followed by the introduction of "AV sequential" pacing in the early 1970s. Although these terms are still useful today for understanding pacemaker function (Box 19-3), the continued expansion of functional capabilities of pulse generators made it necessary to develop a more precise classification system. Therefore in 1974 the Inter-Society Commission for Heart Disease (ICHD) adopted a three-letter code for describing the various pacing modalities available. The code has since undergone several revisions, including the addition of two more letters representing programming characteristics and antitachycardia functions, to accommodate the development of newer devices that are rate-responsive or that combine pacing and cardioversion/defibrillation capabilities (see Table 19-1 for a description of the five-letter code).[8] The original three-letter code, however, remains adequate to describe temporary pacemaker function.

The original code is based on three categories, each represented by a letter. The first letter refers to the cardiac chamber that is paced. The second letter designates which chamber is sensed, and the third letter indicates the pacemaker's response to the sensed event. These three letters are used to describe the mode of pacing. For example, a VVI pacemaker paces the ventricle when the pacemaker fails to sense an intrinsic ventricular depolarization. Sensing of a spontaneous ventricular depolarization, however, inhibits ventricular pacing. On the other hand, a VOO pacemaker paces the ventricle at a fixed rate and has no sensing capabilities (see Table 19-2 for a description of temporary pacing modes).

Physiologic pacing modes are those in which the normal physiologic, or sequential, relationship between atrial and ventricular stimulation and contraction is maintained. AV synchrony increases the volume in the ventricle before contraction and thus helps to improve cardiac output. This may be achieved with atrial pacing in patients who have an intact conduction system, where each atrial pacing stimulus depolarizes the atria and is then conducted through to the ventricles. When atrial-to-ventricular conduction is impaired (i.e., during heart block), AV synchrony may be maintained via dual-chamber (i.e., both atrial and ventricular) pacing modes. The newest of these is the DDD mode, which is the most common dual-chambered mode used today.[6] In DDD pacing, atrial and ventricular leads are used for both pac-

Table 19-1		NASPE/BPEG Generic (NPG) Code			
Position	**I**	**II**	**III**	**IV**	**V**
	Chamber(s) Paced	**Chamber(s) Sensed**	**Response to Sensing**	**Programmability**	**Antitachydysrhythmia Function(s)**
	0 = None	0 = None	0 = None	0 = None	0 = None
	A = Atrium	A = Atrium	T = Triggered	P = Simple programmability (rate, output, sensitivity)	P = Pacing (antitachydysrhythmia)
	V = Ventricle	V = Ventricle	I = Inhibited	M = Multiprogrammability	S = Shock
	D = Dual (A + V)	D = Dual (A + V)	D = Dual (T + I)	C = Communicating	D = Dual (P + S)
	S* = Single (A or V)	S = Single (A or V)			

Modified from Bernstein AD et al: The NASPE/BPEG generic pacemaker code for antibradycardia and adaptive rate pacing and antitachyarrhythmia devices, *PACE* 10:794, 1987.
*Used by manufacturer only.
NOTE: Positions I through III are used exclusively for antibradysrhythmia function.
NASPE, North American Society of Pacing and Electrophysiology; *BPEG,* British Pacing and Electrophysiology Group.

Table 19-2	Examples of Temporary Pacing Modes
Pacing Mode	**Description**
ASYNCHRONOUS	
AOO	Atrial pacing, no sensing
VOO	Ventricular pacing, no sensing
DOO	Atrial and ventricular pacing, no sensing
SYNCHRONOUS	
AAI	Atrial pacing, atrial sensing, inhibited response to sensed P waves
VVI	Ventricular pacing, ventricular sensing, inhibited response to sensed QRS complexes
DVI	Atrial and ventricular pacing, ventricular sensing; both atrial and ventricular pacing are inhibited if a spontaneous ventricular depolarization is sensed
UNIVERSAL	
DDD	Both chambers are paced and sensed; inhibited response of the pacing stimuli to sensed events in their respective chamber; triggered response to sensed atrial activity to allow for rate-responsive ventricular pacing

ing and sensing. In response to sensed activity, the pacemaker inhibits the pacing stimulus so that a sensed P wave in the atrium will inhibit the atrial spike and a sensed R wave in the ventricle will inhibit the ventricular pacing spike. In addition, a sensed P wave may also be used to "trigger" a ventricular pacing stimulus when normal conduction through the AV node is impaired. Although the DDD mode is more complicated to program and interpret than earlier modes, it offers the most options for maintaining physiologic pacing.

PACEMAKER SETTINGS

The controls on all external temporary pulse generators are similar, and their function must be thoroughly understood so that pacing can be initiated quickly in an emergency situation and troubleshooting facilitated should problems with the pacemaker arise.

The *rate control* (Fig. 19-3) regulates the number of impulses that can be delivered to the heart per minute. The rate setting depends on the physiologic needs of the

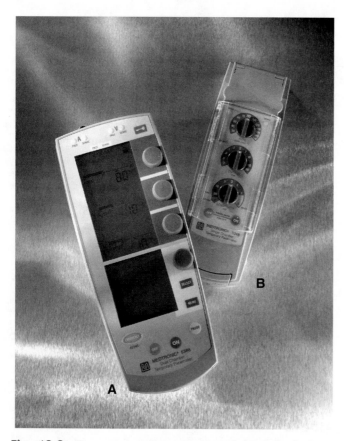

Fig. 19-3 Temporary pulse generators (external). **A,** Dual-chamber pulse generator. **B,** Single-chamber pulse generator. (Courtesy Medtronic Inc, Minneapolis, Minn.)

Box 19-4

TEMPORARY PACEMAKER TESTING FOR PACING THRESHOLDS

1. Adjust pacemaker rate setting so that patient is 100% paced. It may be necessary to increase the pacing rate to achieve this setting.
2. Gradually decrease output (milliampere, mA) setting until 1:1 capture is lost. Pacing threshold is located where capture is lost.
3. Slowly increase output setting until 1:1 capture is reestablished. With a properly positioned pacing electrode, the pacing threshold should be less than 1.0 mA.
4. Set output (mA) setting two to three times higher than measured threshold because thresholds tend to fluctuate over time.
5. Evaluate pacing thresholds for both atrial and ventricular leads separately if patient is connected to a dual-chamber pulse generator.

Box 19-5

TEMPORARY PACEMAKER SENSITIVITY THRESHOLDS

- Set the sensitivity control to its most sensitive setting.
- Adjust the pulse generator rate to 10 beats/min less than the patient's intrinsic rate (the flash indicator should flash regularly).
- Reduce the generator output to the minimal value to prevent the risk of competing with the intrinsic rhythm.
- Gradually increase the sensitivity value until the sense indicator stops flashing and the pace indicator starts flashing.
- Decrease sensitivity until the sense indicator begins to flash again; this is the sensitivity threshold.
- Adjust the sensitivity setting on the generator to half the threshold value; restore generator output and rate to their original values.

---

patient, but in general it is maintained between 60 and 80 beats/min. Pacing rates for overdrive suppression of tachydysrhythmias may greatly exceed these values. Some generators have special controls for overdrive pacing that allow for rates of up to 800 stimuli per minute. If the pacemaker is operating in a dual-chamber mode, the ventricular rate control also regulates the atrial rate.

The *output dial* regulates the amount of electrical current (measured in milliamperes [mA]) that is delivered to the heart to initiate depolarization. The point at which depolarization occurs is termed *threshold* and is indicated by a myocardial response to the pacing stimulus (capture). Threshold can be determined by gradually decreasing the output setting until 1:1 capture is lost. The output setting is then slowly increased until 1:1 capture is reestablished; this threshold to pace is less than 1 mA with a properly positioned pacing electrode. The output, however, is set two to three times higher than threshold because thresholds tend to fluctuate over time (see Box 19-4 for the procedure for measuring pacing thresholds). Separate output controls for both the atrium and the ventricle are used with a dual-chamber pulse generator.

The *sensitivity control* regulates the ability of the pacemaker to detect the heart's intrinsic electrical activ-

ity. Sensitivity is measured in millivolts (mV) and determines the size of the intracardiac signal that the generator will recognize. If the sensitivity is adjusted to its most sensitive setting—a setting of 0.5 to 1.0 mV—the pacemaker can respond even to low-amplitude electrical signals coming from the heart. On the other hand, turning the sensitivity to its least sensitive setting (adjusting the dial to a setting of 20 mV or to the area labeled *async*) will result in the inability of the pacemaker to sense any intrinsic electrical activity and cause the pacemaker to function at a fixed rate. A sense indicator (often a light) on the pulse generator signals each time intrinsic cardiac electrical activity is sensed. A pulse generator may be designed to sense atrial or ventricular activity, or both (see Box 19-5 for the procedure for measuring sensitivity). The sensitivity is set at half the value of the sensitivity threshold to ensure that all appropriate intrinsic cardiac signals are sensed. For example, if the measured sensitivity threshold is 3 mV, the generator is set at 1.5 mV. The pacemaker's sensing ability can be quickly evaluated by observing for a change in pacing rhythm in response to spontaneous depolarizations.

The *AV interval control* (available only on dual-chamber generators) regulates the time interval between the atrial and ventricular pacing stimuli. This interval is analogous to the PR interval that occurs in the intrinsic ECG. Proper adjustment of this interval to between 150 and 250 milliseconds (msec) preserves AV synchrony and permits maximal ventricular stroke volume and enhanced cardiac output.

Temporary DDD pacemakers have several other digital controls that are unique to this newer type of temporary pulse generator (see Fig. 19-3, *B*). The *lower rate*, or *base rate*, determines the rate at which the generator will pace when intrinsic activity falls below the set rate of the pacemaker. The *upper rate* determines the fastest ventricular rate the pacemaker will deliver in response to sensed atrial activity. This setting is needed to protect the patient's heart from being paced in response to rapid atrial dysrhythmias. The *pulse width*, which can be adjusted from 0.05 to 2 msec, controls the length of time that the pacing stimulus is delivered to the heart. There also is an *atrial refractory period*, programmable from 150 to 500 msec, which regulates the length of time after either a sensed or paced ventricular event, during which the pacemaker cannot respond to another atrial stimulus. An emergency button is also available on some models to allow for rapid initiation of asynchronous (DOO) pacing during an emergency.

Finally, on all temporary pacemakers, an on/off switch is provided with a safety feature that prevents the accidental termination of pacing. On new generators there is also a locking feature to prevent unintended changes to the prescribed settings.

PACING ARTIFACTS

All patients with temporary pacemakers require continuous ECG monitoring. The pacing artifact is the spike that is seen on the ECG tracing as the pacing stimulus is delivered to the heart. A *P wave* is visible after the pacing artifact if the atrium is being paced (Fig. 19-4, *A*). Similarly, a *QRS complex* follows a ventricular pacing artifact (Fig. 19-4, *B*). With dual-chamber pacing, a pacing artifact precedes both the P wave and the QRS complex (Fig. 19-4, *C*).

Not all paced beats look alike. For example, the artifact (spike) produced by a unipolar pacing electrode is larger than that produced by a bipolar lead (Fig. 19-5). Furthermore, the QRS complex of paced beats appears different, depending on the location of the pacing elec-

trode. If the pacing electrode is positioned in the right ventricle, a left bundle branch block (LBBB) pattern is displayed on the ECG. On the other hand, a right bundle branch block (RBBB) pattern is visible if the pacing stimulus originates from the left ventricle.

PACEMAKER MALFUNCTIONS

Most pacemaker malfunctions can be categorized as abnormalities of either pacing or sensing.

Problems with pacing can involve the failure of the pacemaker to deliver the pacing stimulus, a pacing stimulus that fails to depolarize the heart, or the incorrect number of pacing stimuli per minute.

Pacing Abnormalities. Failure of the pacemaker to deliver the pacing stimulus results in the disappearance of the pacing artifact, even though the patient's intrinsic rate is less than the set rate on the pacer (Fig. 19-6). This can occur either intermittently or continuously and can be attributed to failure of the pulse generator or its battery, a loose connection between the various components of the pacemaker system, broken lead wires, or stimulus inhibition as a result of EMI. Tightening connections, replacing the batteries or the pulse generator itself, or removing the source of EMI may restore pacemaker function.

If the pacing stimulus fires but fails to initiate a myocardial depolarization, a pacing artifact will be present but will not be followed by the expected P wave or QRS complex, depending on the chamber being paced (Fig. 19-7). This "loss of capture" most often can be attributed either to displacement of the pacing electrode or to an increase in threshold (electrical stimulus necessary to elicit a myocardial depolarization) as a result of drugs, metabolic disorders, electrolyte imbalances, or fibrosis or myocardial ischemia at the site of electrode placement. In many cases, increasing the output (mA) may elicit capture. For transvenous leads, repositioning the patient to the left side may improve lead contact and restore capture.

Pacing also can occur at inappropriate rates. For example, impending battery failure in a permanent pacemaker can result in a gradual decrease in the paced rate, or "rate drift." Inappropriate stimuli from a pacemaker also may result in a pacemaker-mediated tachycardia. This usually occurs as a result of sensing inappropriate signals in a dual chamber pacemaker that is in a trigger mode, such as DDD. The tachycardia can be terminated by placing a magnet over the generator to transiently suspend sensing.[9]

Sensing Abnormalities. Sensing abnormalities include both undersensing and oversensing. *Undersensing* is the inability of the pacemaker to sense spontaneous myocardial depolarizations. This results in competition between paced complexes and the heart's intrinsic rhythm. This malfunction can be demonstrated on the

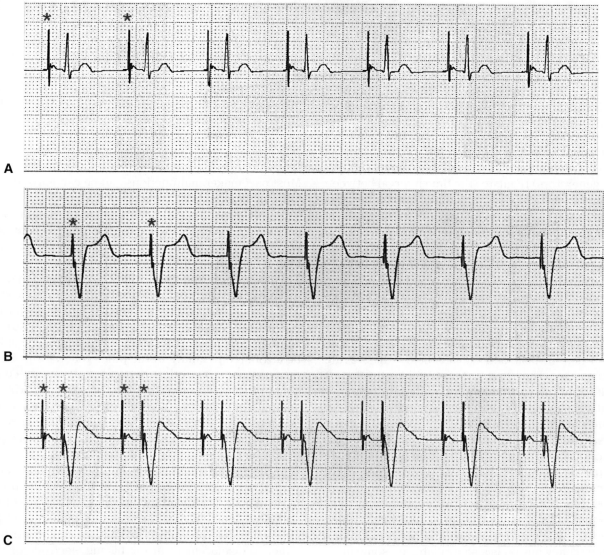

Fig. 19-4 Pacing examples. **A,** Atrial pacing. **B,** Ventricular pacing. **C,** Dual-chamber pacing. The * represents a pacemaker impulse.

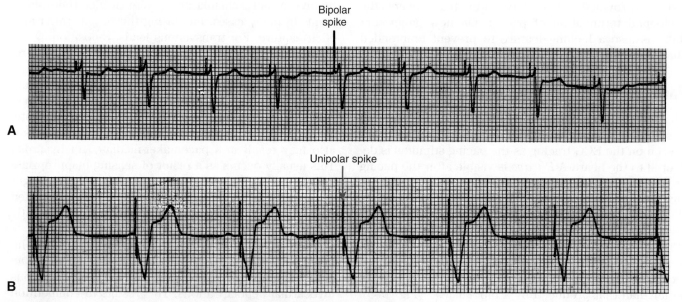

Fig. 19-5 Bipolar and unipolar pacing. **A,** Bipolar pacing artifact. **B,** Unipolar pacing artifact. (Modified from Conover MB: *Understanding electrocardiography* ed 8, St Louis, 2003, Mosby.)

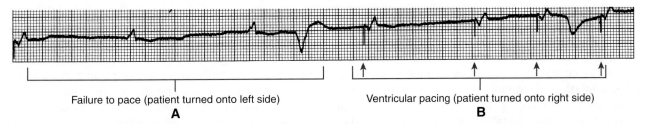

Failure to pace (patient turned onto left side)
A

Ventricular pacing (patient turned onto right side)
B

Fig. 19-6 Pacemaker malfunction: failure to pace. **A,** Patient with a transvenous pacemaker is turned onto the left side. Immediately, there is a failure to pace (loss of pacer artifacts on ECG). The patient's heart rate is extremely low without pacemaker support. **B,** The nurse turns the patient onto the right side, the transvenous electrode floats into contact with the right ventricular wall, and pacing is resumed. (From Kesten KS, Norton CK: *Pacemakers: patient care, troubleshooting, rhythm analysis,* Baltimore, 1985, Resource Applications.)

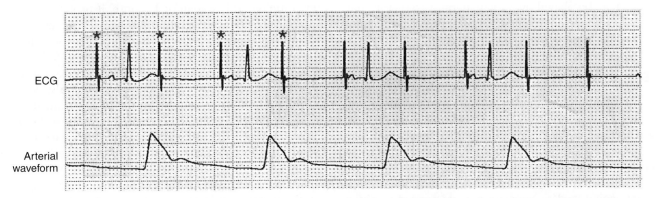

ECG

Arterial
waveform

Fig. 19-7 Pacemaker malfunction: failure to capture. Atrial pacing and capture occur after pacer spike(s) 1, 3, 5, and 7. The remaining pacer spikes fail to capture the tissue, resulting in loss of the P wave, no conduction to the ventricles, and no arterial waveform. The * represents a pacemaker impulse.

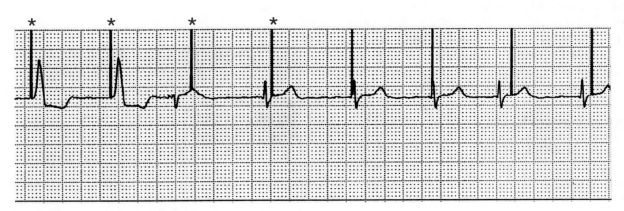

Fig. 19-8 Pacemaker malfunction: undersensing. Notice that after the first two paced beats, a series of intrinsic beats occur; the pacemaker unit fails to sense these intrinsic QRS complexes. These spikes do not capture the ventricle because they occur during the refractory period of the cardiac cycle. The * represents a pacemaker impulse.

ECG by pacing artifacts that occur *after* or are unrelated to spontaneous complexes (Fig. 19-8). Undersensing can result in the delivery of pacing stimuli into a relative refractory period of the cardiac depolarization cycle. A ventricular pacing stimulus delivered into the downslope of the T wave (R-on-T phenomenon) is a real danger with this type of pacer aberration, since it may precipitate a lethal dysrhythmia. The nurse must act quickly to determine the cause and initiate appropriate interventions. Often the cause can be attributed to inadequate wave amplitude (or height of the P or R wave). If this is the case, the situation can be promptly remedied by increasing the sensitivity (moving the sensitivity dial toward its lowest setting). Other possible causes include inappropriate (i.e., asynchronous) mode selection, lead displacement or fracture, loose cable connections, and pulse generator failure.

Oversensing results from the inappropriate sensing of extraneous electrical signals, leading to unnecessary triggering or inhibiting of stimulus output, depending on the pacer mode. The source of these electrical signals can range from the presence of tall, peaked T waves to EMI in the critical care environment. Because most temporary pulse generators are programmed in demand modes, oversensing results in unexplained pauses in the ECG tracing as the extraneous signals are sensed and inhibit pacing. Often, simply moving the sensitivity dial toward 20 mV stops the pauses. With permanent pacemakers, a magnet may be placed over the generator to restore pacing in an asynchronous mode until appropriate changes in the generator settings can be programmed.

MEDICAL MANAGEMENT

The physician determines the pacing route based on the patient's clinical situation. Generally transcutaneous pacing is used in emergent situations until a transvenous lead can be secured. If the patient is undergoing heart surgery, epicardial leads may be electively placed at the end of the operation. The physician places the transvenous or epicardial pacing lead(s), repositioning as needed to obtain adequate pacing and sensing thresholds. Decisions regarding lead placement may later limit the pacing modes available to the clinician. For example, to perform dual-chamber pacing, both atrial and ventricular leads must be placed. In emergent situations, however, interventions are focused on establishing ventricular pacing, and atrial lead placement may not be feasible. After lead placement, the initial settings for output and sensitivity are determined, the pacing rate and mode are selected, and the patient's response to pacing is evaluated.

NURSING MANAGEMENT

Nursing responsibilities associated with the care of a patient with a temporary pacemaker are associated with several nursing diagnoses (see the Nursing Diagnoses feature on Temporary Pacemaker) and can be combined into four primary areas: assessment and prevention of pacemaker malfunction, protection against microshock, surveillance for complications such as infection, and patient education.

Prevention of Pacemaker Malfunction. Continuous ECG monitoring is essential to facilitate prompt recognition of and appropriate intervention for pacemaker malfunction. In addition, proper care of the pacing system can do a great deal to prevent pacing abnormalities.

The temporary pacing lead and bridging cable must be properly secured to the body with tape to prevent the accidental displacement of the electrode, which can re-

sult in failure to pace or sense. The external pulse generator can be secured to the patient's waist with a strap or placed in a telemetry bag for the mobile patient. For the patient on a regimen of bed rest, the pulse generator can be suspended with twill tape from an intravenous (IV) pole mounted overhead on the ceiling. This not only will prevent tension on the lead while the patient is moved (given adequate length of bridging cable) but also will alleviate the possibility of accidental dropping of the pulse generator.

The nurse inspects for loose connections between the lead(s) and pulse generator on a regular basis. In addition, replacement batteries and pulse generators must always be available on the unit. Although the battery has an anticipated life span of 1 month, it probably is sound practice to change the battery if the pacemaker has been operating continually for several days. Newer generators provide a low-battery signal 24 hours before complete loss of battery function to prevent inadvertent interruptions in pacing. The pulse generator must always be labeled with the date that the battery was replaced.

Microshock Protection. It is important to be aware of all sources of EMI within the critical care environment that could interfere with the pacemaker's function. Sources of EMI in the clinical area include electrocautery, defibrillation current, radiation therapy, magnetic resonance imaging devices, and transcutaneous electrical nerve stimulation (TENS) units. In most cases, if EMI is suspected of precipitating pacemaker malfunction, converting to the asynchronous mode (fixed rate) will maintain pacing until the cause of the EMI is removed.

NURSING DIAGNOSES | Temporary Pacemaker

- Decreased Cardiac Output related to alterations in heart rate
- Ineffective Cardiopulmonary Tissue Perfusion related to acute myocardial ischemia
- Risk for Infection risk factor: invasive monitoring devices
- Anxiety related to threat to biologic, psychologic, and/or social integrity
- Disturbed Body Image related to functional dependence on life-sustaining technology
- Deficient Knowledge: Discharge Regimen related to lack of previous exposure to information (see Patient Education feature on Temporary Pacemaker)

Because the pacing electrode provides a direct, low-resistance path to the heart, the nurse takes special care while handling the external components of the pacing system to avoid conducting stray electrical current from other equipment. Even a small amount of stray current transmitted via the pacing lead could precipitate a lethal dysrhythmia. The possibility of "microshock" can be minimized by the wearing of rubber gloves when handling the pacing wires and by proper insulation of terminal pins of pacing wires when they are not in use. The latter can be accomplished either by using caps provided by the manufacturer or by improvising with a plastic syringe or section of disposable rubber glove. The wires are to be taped securely to the patient's chest to prevent accidental electrode displacement. Additional safety measures include using a nonelectric or a properly grounded electric bed, keeping all electrical equipment away from the bed, and permitting the use of only rechargeable electric razors.

Infection Risk. Infection at the lead insertion site is a rare but serious complication associated with temporary pacemakers. The site(s) is carefully inspected for purulent drainage, erythema, and edema, and the patient is observed for signs of systemic infection. Site care is performed according to the institution's policy and procedure. Although most infections remain localized, endocarditis can occur in patients with endocardial pacing leads. A less common complication associated with transvenous pacing is myocardial perforation, which can result in rhythmic hiccoughs or cardiac tamponade.

PATIENT EDUCATION

Patient teaching for the person with a temporary pacemaker emphasizes prevention of complications (see the Patient Education feature on Temporary Pacemaker). The patient is instructed not to handle any exposed portion of the lead wire and to notify the nurse if the dressing over the insertion site becomes soiled, wet, or dislodged. The patient also is advised not to use any electrical devices brought in from home that could interfere with pacemaker functioning. Furthermore, patients with temporary transvenous pacemakers need to be taught to restrict movement of the affected extremity to prevent lead displacement.

PERMANENT PACEMAKERS

Over 200,000 permanent pacemakers are implanted annually in the United States, and critical care nurses are likely to encounter these devices in their clinical practice.[6] Originally designed to provide an adequate ventricular rate in patients with symptomatic bradycardia, the goal of pacemaker therapy today is to simulate, as much as possible, normal physiologic cardiac depolarization and conduction. Sophisticated generators now permit rate-responsive pacing, either in response to sensed atrial activity (DDD) or in response to a variety of physiologic sensors (body motion, QT interval, and minute ventilation). In patients who do not have a functional sinus node that can increase their heart rate, rate-responsive pacemakers have been shown to improve exercise capacity and quality of life.[10] Table 19-3 describes the types of rate-responsive pacing generators currently in clinical use.

The patient who has a permanent pacemaker implanted has an anticipated length of hospital stay of 1 to 5 days. The longer length of stay is for patients with seri-

---

PATIENT EDUCATION — Temporary Pacemaker

- Description of pacemaker therapy
- Care of the pacemaker system:
  Minimize handling of leads or cables
  Notify nurse if dressing becomes wet or loose
- Activity restrictions (minimize upper extremity movement with transvenous leads)
- Electrical safety precautions (no electric razors)
- Symptoms to report (dizziness)

Table 19-3	Permanent Pacemaker Rate Response Pacing Modes
Pulse Generator	**Description**
AAIR	AAI features, plus rate-responsive pacing; used for patients with a symptomatic bradycardia with a paceable atrium and intact atrioventricular (AV) conduction
VVIR	VVI features, plus rate-responsive pacing; used for patients with an atrium that is unpaceable as a result of chronic atrial fibrillation or other atrial dysrhythmia
DDDR	DDD features, plus rate-responsive pacing; used for patients with a symptomatic bradycardia in which the atrium is paceable but AV conduction is, or may become, unreliable

ous complications such as myocardial infarction or shock.

Recent technologic advances in the computer industry have had a major impact on today's permanent pacemakers. Microprocessors have allowed for the development of increasingly smaller generators despite the incorporation of more complex features. Today's generators are not only smaller but also more energy-efficient and more reliable than previous models. An example of a modern pacemaker is shown in Fig. 19-9. A new trend in permanent pacemakers has been the use of these devices as a type of nonpharmacologic therapy for treatment of conditions such as heart failure and atrial fibrillation.

Cardiac Resynchronization Therapy. About one third of patients with severe heart failure have ventricular conduction delays (prolonged QRS duration or bundle branch block). Such conduction delays have been shown to create a lack of synchrony between the contraction of the left and right ventricles. The hemodynamic consequences of this dyssynchrony include impaired ventricular filling and decreased ejection fraction, cardiac output, and mean arterial pressure.[11] Cardiac resynchronization therapy (CRT) uses atrial pacing plus stimulates both the left and right ventricles (biventricular pacing), in an attempt to optimize atrial and ventricular mechanical activity. The CRT device uses three pacing leads, one each in the right atrium and the right ventricle, and a specially designed transvenous lead that is inserted via the coronary sinus to pace the left ventricle.[12] Because many heart failure patients are also at risk for sudden cardiac death (SCD), biventricular pacing is now available on some implantable cardioverter-defibrillators. A number of clinical trials have shown symptom and structural cardiac improvement with this new therapy.[13,14]

Atrial Arrhythmia Suppression. There is a growing incidence of atrial fibrillation, and atrial pacing has been proposed as a possible preventative therapy for this dysrhythmia in selected patients.[6] Atrial pacing in patients with bradycardias has been shown to lower the recurrence of atrial fibrillation, especially when compared with ventricular pacing.[10] For patients with paroxysmal atrial fibrillation, investigational strategies include pacing both atriums (bi-atrial pacing) and chronically pacing the atrium at a rate higher than the patient's basal sinus rate.[15] In addition, most pacemakers can now be programmed to "mode switch" to a non-P wave tracking mode when rapid atrial rates are sensed.[6]

MEDICAL MANAGEMENT

Permanent pacemakers may be implanted with the patient under local anesthesia in either the operating room or the cardiac catheterization laboratory. Generally, transvenous leads are inserted via the cephalic or subclavian vein and positioned in the right atrium and/or the right ventricle, under fluoroscopy. Satisfactory lead placement is determined by testing stimulation and sensitivity thresholds with a pacing system analyzer. The lead(s) is then attached to the generator, which is inserted into a surgically created "pocket" in the subcutaneous tissue below the clavicle.

NURSING MANAGEMENT

Nursing management for patients after permanent pacemaker implant includes monitoring for complications related to insertion, as well as for pacemaker malfunction. Postoperative complications are rare but include cardiac perforation and tamponade, pneumothorax, hematoma, lead displacement, and infection.[6]

Identification of permanent pacemaker malfunction is the same as that described previously for temporary pacemakers. To evaluate pacemaker function, the nurse must know at least the pacemaker's programmed mode of pacing and the lower rate setting. With permanent pacemakers, settings are adjusted noninvasively through a specialized programmer that uses pulsed magnetic fields or a radiofrequency signal. If a pacemaker problem is suspected, ECG strips are obtained and the physician notified so that the pacemaker settings can be reprogrammed as needed. If the patient experiences symptoms of decreased cardiac output, he or she may require support with temporary transcutaneous pacing until the problem is corrected.

Critical care nurses also may be involved in monitoring patients with permanent pacemakers after discharge.

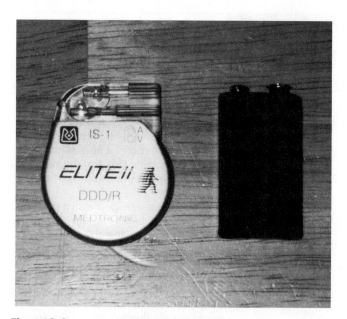

Fig. 19-9 A permanent pacemaker (Medtronic Elite II) placed next to a 9-volt battery for comparison of size. This dual-chamber generator is 7.5 mm thick and weighs only 26 g.

Some units are equipped with transtelephonic monitoring equipment that allows patients to transmit information via the telephone using a monitoring device in their home. Transmission of the patient's ECG can provide information to confirm proper pacemaker function (capture and sensing), as well as determination of battery status (rate).

The foregoing discussion provides an introduction to the basic concepts of pacemaker therapy. It is essential, however, that the nurse who cares for patients with either permanent or temporary pacemakers be familiar with even the most sophisticated modes of pacemaker function. Only by keeping "pace" with current technology can the nurse accurately interpret pacer function and thereby safely and effectively care for patients with pacemakers.

IMPLANTABLE CARDIOVERTER DEFIBRILLATOR

An implantable cardioverter defibrillator (ICD) is an electronic device that is used in the treatment of tachydysrhythmias. The ICD is capable of identifying and terminating life-threatening ventricular dysrhythmias. Initially an ICD was only recommended for patients who had survived an episode of cardiac arrest caused by ventricular fibrillation (VF) or ventricular tachycardia (VT).[10] A number of clinical trials that compared ICD therapy for such secondary prevention of SCD with antidysrhythmic drug therapy found improved survival with the ICD.[16] As a result, ICD use was expanded to include primary prevention of SCD in patients with coronary artery disease (CAD), previous myocardial infarction, or left ventricular dysfunction when VT or VF was inducible during EPS. Recent trials have shown improved survival with ICD implantation in high risk patients (i.e., those with previous myocardial infarction and an ejection fraction <30%) even without evidence of VT/VF on an EPS.[17] These results are likely to further increase the number of patients who receive an ICD (see "Sudden Cardiac Death" in Chapter 18).

ICD SYSTEM

The ICD system contains (1) sensing electrodes to recognize the dysrhythmia and (2) defibrillation electrodes or patches that are in contact with the heart and can deliver a "shock." These electrodes are connected to a generator that is surgically placed in the subcutaneous tissue either in the upper left abdominal quadrant or in the pectoral region (Fig. 19-10). The early model generators could defibrillate or cardiovert only lethal dysrhythmias. Current generation devices deliver a "tiered" therapy with programmable antitachycardia pacing, bradycardia back-up pacing, low-energy cardioversion, and high-energy defibrillation options. With tiered therapy, antitachycardia pacing is used as the first line of treatment in some cases of VT. If the VT can be pace-terminated successfully, the patient will not receive a "shock" from the generator and may not even realize that the ICD terminated the dysrhythmia. If programmed bursts of pacing do not terminate the VT, the ICD will "cardiovert" the rhythm. If the dysrhythmia deteriorates into VF, the ICD is programmed to defibrillate at a higher energy. If the dysrhythmia terminates spontaneously, the device will not discharge (Fig. 19-10). Occasionally, the electrical rhythm may deteriorate to asystole or a slow idioventricular rhythm. In such cases the bradycardia back-up pacing function is activated.

New product development for ICDs has resulted in dual-chamber devices with leads in both the atria and the ventricles. The introduction of atrial leads allows for dual chamber pacing to optimize hemodynamic performance, as well as atrial sensing to more accurately discriminate between atrial and ventricular tachycardias and decrease the incidence of inappropriate shocks. Implantable defibrillators with atrial capabilities may also be used to deliver therapies such as cardioversion or antitachycardia pacing to patients with atrial tachydysrhythmias, but research is needed to evaluate the exact role of this therapy.[10] Other developments in ICD technology include improved diagnostic and telemetry functions, such as the ability to provide real-time electrograms obtained from the ICD electrodes.

ICD INSERTION

The ICD has progressed not only in the area of programmable functions but also in the insertion design. Initially, all ICDs were implanted surgically either (1) during open heart surgery, with electrode patches sewn directly onto the epicardium, or (2) by means of a thoracotomy incision, with the electrode patches attached to the outside of the pericardium. Today's smaller generators, combined with the use of transvenous leads, obviate the need for major surgery. Transvenous electrode leads are inserted into the subclavian vein and advanced into the right side of the heart, where contact with the endocardium is achieved. To improve defibrillation efficacy, an additional subcutaneous patch may be placed with some models. The endocardial leads are used for sensing, pacing, and cardioversion/defibrillation. They are connected to the generator by tunneling through the subcutaneous tissue; thus thoracotomy is avoided. The endocardial lead system offers several advantages: it is less invasive, requires shorter hospitalization, and is associated with significantly lower implantation mortality.[10] Technical advances and the development of smaller ICDs have made it feasible to implant these devices in the pectoral position, similar to that used for permanent pacemakers.

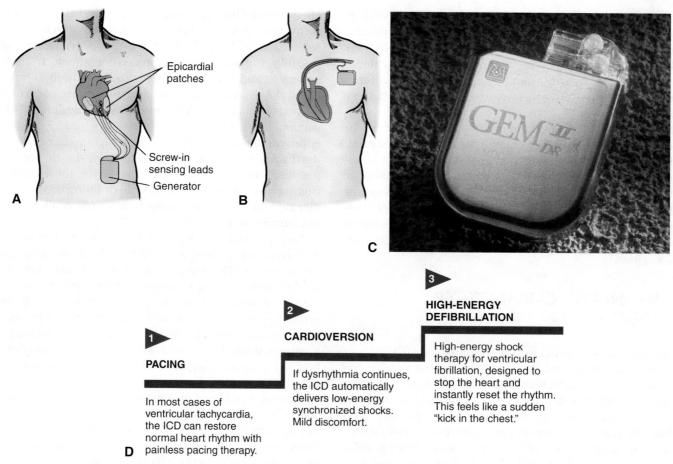

Fig. 19-10   **A,** Placement of an implantable cardioverter defibrillator (ICD) and epicardial lead system. The generator is placed in a subcutaneous "pocket" in the left upper abdominal quadrant. The epicardial screw-in sensing leads monitor the heart rhythm and connect to the generator. If a life-threatening dysrhythmia is sensed, the generator can pace-terminate the dysrhythmia or deliver electrical cardioversion or defibrillation through the epicardial patches. With this system, the leads/patches must be placed during open-chest (sternal or thoracotomy) surgery. **B,** In the transvenous lead system, open-chest surgery is not required. The pacing/cardioversion/defibrillation functions are all contained in a lead (or leads) inserted into the right atrium and ventricle. New generators are small enough to place in the pectoral region. **C,** An example of a dual-chamber ICD (Medtronic Gem II DR) with tiered therapy and pacing capabilities. **D,** Tiered therapy is designed to use increasing levels of intensity to terminate ventricular dysrhythmias. (Courtesy Medtronic Inc, Minneapolis, Minn.)

MEDICAL MANAGEMENT

Medical management of the ICD patient begins before implantation, with a thorough evaluation of the patient's dysrhythmia and underlying cardiac function. A number of noninvasive studies are available to help identify patients at risk for SCD. These include signal-averaged electrocardiography, echocardiography, baroreceptor sensitivity testing, and heart rate variability studies. Generally, patients identified at risk for SCD undergo an electrophysiology study to identify the origin of the dysrhythmia and to determine the effect of antidysrhythmic agents in suppressing or altering the rate of the dysrhythmia. Further assessment of cardiac status is made to determine whether additional interventions (cardiac

surgery, angioplasty) are indicated to improve cardiac function. This part of the work-up may include cardiac catheterization, stress testing, and echocardiography. Based on the aforementioned evaluation, decisions are made regarding the implantation approach (i.e., thoracotomy at the time of surgery or nonthoracotomy) and the type of therapy required (antitachypacing, cardioversion, defibrillation).

ICD Programming. An electrophysiologist generally performs initial programming of the device at the time of implantation. During implantation, defibrillation threshold measurements are obtained. This involves inducing the dysrhythmia and then evaluating the device's ability to terminate the dysrhythmia. Once it is determined that the ICD functions adequately, further follow-up is conducted on an outpatient basis to monitor the number of discharges and the battery life of the device.

NURSING MANAGEMENT

If the ICD system was implanted during open heart surgery, the postoperative nursing management is similar to that for any patient undergoing cardiac surgery. If an endocardial lead system is implanted, the nursing management is less intense and the hospital stay is shorter. The nursing diagnoses and management of the patient with an ICD are listed in the Nursing Diagnoses feature on Implantable Cardioverter Defibrillator. In the case of a ventricular dysrhythmia, it is important to know the type of ICD implanted, how the device functions, and whether it is activated (i.e., on). If the patient experiences a shockable rhythm, the nurse should be prepared to defibrillate in event that the device fails. When performing external defibrillation, the paddles/patches should not be placed directly over the ICD generator. In addition, standard paddle placement may need to be altered in patients with ICDs to achieve successful defibrillation.[7] Most patients will continue to take some antidysrhythmic medications to decrease the number of "shocks" required and to slow the rate of the tachycardia. Complications associated with the ICD include infection from the implanted system, broken leads, and the sensing of supraventricular tachydysrhythmias resulting in unneeded discharges.

PATIENT EDUCATION

To facilitate a positive psychologic adjustment to the ICD, education of the patient and family about the device is vital (see the Patient Education feature on Implantable Cardioverter Defibrillator). Preoperative teaching for the ICD patient includes information about how the device works and what to expect during the implantation procedure. After implantation, education is focused on aspects of living with an ICD. Patients need information pertaining to scheduled device follow-up and instructions about what to do if they experience a "shock." Many institutions also have successfully used family support groups for this patient population.

FIBRINOLYTIC THERAPY

Fibrinolytic therapy is an important clinical intervention for the patient experiencing acute ST elevation myocardial infarction (STEMI). Before the introduction of fibrinolytic agents, the medical management of acute myocardial infarction (MI) was focused on decreasing myocardial oxygen demands to minimize myocardial necrosis and thus preserve ventricular function. Today, efforts to limit the size of infarction are directed toward the timely reperfusion of the jeopardized myocardium by restoring blood flow in the culprit vessel (the open artery theory). The use of fibrinolytic therapy to accomplish this objective is predicated on the theory that the significant event in acute coronary syndromes (unstable angina, acute MI) is the rupture of an atherosclerotic plaque with thrombus formation (Fig. 19-11). The thrombus, which is composed of aggregated platelets bound together with fibrin strands, occludes the coronary artery, depriving the myocardium of oxygen previously supplied by that artery. The administration of a fibrinolytic agent results in the lysis of the acute thrombus, thus recanalizing, or opening, the obstructed coronary artery and restoring blood flow to the affected tissue. Once perfusion is restored, adjunctive measures are taken to prevent further clot formation and reocclusion.

ELIGIBILITY CRITERIA

Certain criteria have been developed, based on research findings, to determine the patient population that would most likely benefit from the administration of fibrinolytic therapy. In general, patients with recent onset of chest pain (less than 12 hours' duration) and persistent ST elevation (greater than 0.1 mV in two or more contiguous leads) are considered candidates for fibrinolytic therapy.[18] Patients who present with bundle branch blocks that may obscure ST-segment analysis and a history suggestive of an acute MI are also considered candidates for therapy (see"Myocardial Infarction," p. 439).

Exclusion criteria are usually based on the increased risk of bleeding incurred by the use of fibrinolytics. Patients who have stable clots that might be disrupted by fibrinolytic therapy (those secondary to recent surgery, trauma, or a cerebrovascular accident) are generally not considered candidates for fibrinolytic therapy. Other common criteria for the use of fibrinolytic therapy are included in Box 19-6.

Currently fibrinolytic therapy is not indicated for patients with unstable angina or non-ST elevation myocardial infarction (NSTEMIs). It is believed that these conditions

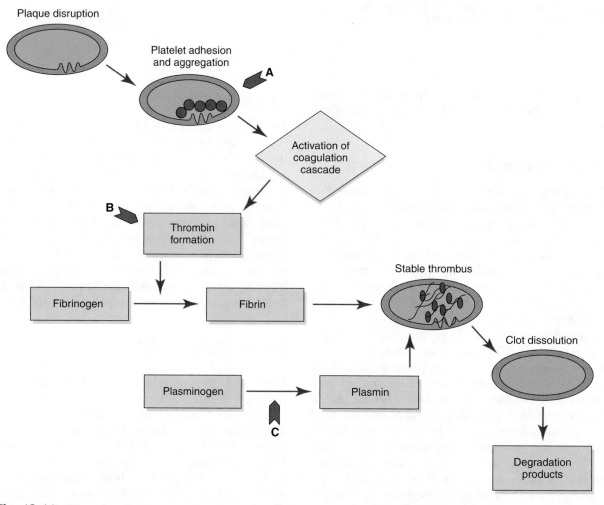

Fig. 19-11 Thrombus formation and site of action of medications used in the treatment of acute myocardial infarction. *A,* Site of action of antiplatelet agents such as aspirin and glycoprotein IIb/IIIa inhibitors. *B,* Heparin bonds with antithrombin III and thrombin to create an inactive complex. *C,* Fibrinolytic agents convert plasminogen to plasmin, an enzyme responsible for degradation of fibrin clots.

result from plaque rupture with the formation of an only partially occlusive thrombus. Since fibrinolysis breaks up the clot and releases thrombin, this could paradoxically increase the material necessary for further thrombosis.[7] Instead, these patients are treated with antiplatelet agents (aspirin) and antithrombin drugs (heparin).

Box 19-6

FIBRINOLYTIC THERAPY SELECTION CRITERIA

- No more than 12 hours from onset of chest pain; less if possible
- ST-segment elevation on ECG or new-onset left bundle branch block
- Ischemic chest pain of 30 minutes' duration
- Chest pain unresponsive to sublingual nitroglycerin
- No conditions that might cause a predisposition to hemorrhage

---

FIBRINOLYTIC AGENTS

Five fibrinolytic agents are currently available for intravenous treatment of acute STEMI. All of these agents stimulate lysis of the clot by converting inactive plasminogen to plasmin, an enzyme responsible for degradation of fibrin (see Fig. 19-11). Streptokinase and urokinase were the first generation of fibrinolytic agents and had their primary effect on circulating plasminogen. Urokinase is no longer available because of manufacturing problems.[19] Newer fibrinolytic agents (alteplase, reteplase, tenecteplase) have more effect on clot plasminogen than circulating plasminogen and are therefore considered "clot-selective." A comparison of currently approved fibrinolytic agents is provided in the Pharmacologic Management table on Fibrinolytic Agents for Use in Acute Myocardial Infarction. Because patients with an area of plaque disruption are still at risk for clot formation and reocclusion, fibrinolytic therapy is used in conjunction with anticoagulants (heparin) and antiplatelet

---

Pharmacologic Management: Fibrinolytic Agents for Use in Acute Myocardial Infarction

DRUG	DOSAGE	ACTIONS	SPECIAL CONSIDERATIONS
Clot-Specific t-PA (alteplase)	IV: 100 mg over 90 min with the first 15 mg given as a bolus	Binds to fibrin at the clot and promotes activation of plasminogen to plasmin	Short half-life, so heparin is usually given with the drug as a bolus and then followed with an infusion Aspirin is begun with administration of the drug and continued daily
r-PA (reteplase)	IV: 10 units given as a bolus, repeated in 30 min	Binds to fibrin at the clot and promotes activation of plasminogen to plasmin	Heparin is started with administration of the drug and continued for 24 hours Aspirin is begun with administration of the drug and continued daily
TNKase (tenecteplase)	IV: 30-50 mg based on body weight, given as a single bolus	Binds to fibrin at the clot and promotes activation of plasminogen to plasmin	Heparin is started with administration of the drug Aspirin is begun with administration of the drug and continued daily
Non–Clot-Specific SK (streptokinase)	IV: 1.5 million units given over 60 min	Catalyzes the conversion of plasminogen to plasmin, which causes lysis of fibrin Has systemic lytic effects	May cause allergic reactions and hypotension Heparin may be administered IV or SQ Aspirin is begun with administration of the drug and continued daily
APSAC (anistreplase)	IV: 30 units via slow bolus over 2-5 min	A molecular combination of streptokinase and plasminogen with actions similar to streptokinase Has systemic lytic effects	May cause allergic reactions and hypotension Long half-life, so heparin is usually started 4-6 hr after APSAC Aspirin is begun with administration of the drug and continued daily

IV, Intravenous; *APSAC*, anisoylated plasminogen-streptokinase activator complex; *r-PA*, recombinant plasminogen activator; *t-PA*, tissue plasminogen activator; *SQ*, subcutaneous.

agents (aspirin). Intravenous heparin and oral aspirin are prescribed either during or immediately after fibrinolytic therapy. The timing of these interventions may vary, based on the specific fibrinolytic agent used and institutional protocols. With clot-specific agents such as alteplase and reteplase, immediate administration of heparin is recommended to prevent reocclusion. The nonspecific plasminogen activators *streptokinase* and *APSAC* (anisoylated plasminogen-streptokinase activator complex) produce a prolonged lytic state, so heparin is not of clear benefit. If administered, heparin therapy is usually continued for 24 to 72 hours, whereas daily aspirin is continued indefinitely.[18]

Streptokinase. *Streptokinase* (SK) is a fibrinolytic agent derived from beta-hemolytic streptococci, which when combined with plasminogen, catalyzes the conversion of plasminogen to plasmin—the enzyme responsible for clot dissolution in the body. SK can be administered either intravenously or by an intracoronary approach, which necessitates cardiac catheterization. The efficacy of both routes has been established, although use of the intracoronary route is not considered practical for treatment of acute MI.[18]

Side Effects. The three major problems associated with the use of SK are its systemic lytic effects coupled with a long half-life, potential antigenic effects if readministered, and hypotension. Because the anticoagulant action of SK is systemic (non–clot specific) and prolonged (half-life 20 to 25 minutes), bleeding is the most common complication; thus the patient requires careful observation during the 12 hours immediately after administration (Box 19-7). In addition, because SK is a bacterial protein, it can produce a variety of allergic reactions, including anaphylaxis, especially when administered to a patient who either has received SK therapy previously or has had a recent streptococcal infection. It is necessary to be familiar with the possible allergic manifestations (Box 19-8), as well as cognizant of the fact that as a result of delayed antibody formation, symptoms may develop

several days after infusion. Diphenhydramine (Benadryl) or steroids are often prescribed before SK administration to blunt this unwanted effect. Hypotension is sometimes associated with the rapid administration of SK. This fall in blood pressure usually responds to volume replacement but occasionally requires vasopressor support.

Tissue Plasminogen Activator. Marketed under the name *Activase*, tissue plasminogen activator (t-PA) or alteplase is a naturally occurring enzyme (thus nonantigenic) that is clot-specific and has a very short half-life (3 to 4 minutes). It converts plasminogen to plasmin after binding to the fibrin-containing clot. This clot-specificity results in an increased concentration and activity of plasmin at the site of the clot where it is needed. It was hoped that this characteristic of t-PA would prevent the induction of a systemic lytic state that occurs with SK therapy. The results of studies comparing the adverse effects of SK and t-PA, however, show similar incidences of bleeding after administration.[20] Tissue plasminogen activator was approved specifically for intravenous administration. Several different dosing regimens have been proposed and tested in the clinical setting, but accelerated-dose t-PA is now considered the most effective in establishing early patency of the occluded vessel.[21]

Anistreplase. Anistreplase, also known as anisoylated plasminogen-streptokinase activator complex (APSAC; Eminase), was approved by the FDA in 1990 for use in the treatment of acute MI. Often referred to as a second-generation streptokinase, it has certain advantages over SK that are related specifically to duration of action and ease of administration. Because it is inactive on administration, APSAC can be given rapidly as a bolus injection. The half-life of APSAC is markedly increased (90 minutes), so concomitant heparin therapy, if used, should begin at least 6 hours after administration to decrease the risk of bleeding associated with the prolonged fibrinolytic activity (see the Pharmacologic Management Table on Thrombolytic Agents for Use in Acute Myocardial Infarction). Disadvantages, which are similar to those of SK, include the potential for allergic reactions and hypotension. APSAC has efficacy similar to streptokinase in terms of clot lysis but is much more expensive.

Box 19-7

SIGNS OF INADEQUATE HEMOSTASIS RELATED TO FIBRINOLYTIC THERAPY

- Bleeding or hematoma at puncture sites
- Hematuria, hematemesis, hemoptysis, melena, epistaxis
- Bruising or petechiae (pinpoint hemorrhages)
- Flank ecchymoses with complaints of low back pain (suggestive of retroperitoneal bleeding)
- Gingival bleeding
- Change in neurologic status (intracranial bleeding)
- Deterioration in vital signs, decreased hematocrit values (internal bleeding)

Box 19-8

POSSIBLE ALLERGIC MANIFESTATIONS RELATED TO STREPTOKINASE THERAPY

- Anaphylaxis
- Urticaria
- Itching
- Nausea
- Flushing
- Fever
- Chills

Recombinant Plasminogen Activator. Recombinant plasminogen activator (r-PA), or reteplase, is a variant of the natural human enzyme t-PA. Reteplase is less fibrin-selective and has a longer half-life than t-PA, making it suitable for bolus administration rather than as a continuous infusion. This new-generation plasminogen activator is given as a double bolus and then followed with a heparin infusion. Unlike t-PA, reteplase does not require weight-based dosing. Studies have shown that reteplase is as effective as t-PA in the treatment of acute MI and is easier to administer.[22]

Tenecteplase. Tenecteplase (TNKase) is the newest of the fibrinolytic agents. It is a genetically engineered variant of alteplase with slower plasma clearance and better fibrin-specificity. A recent study found that TNKase was as effective as alteplase, with similar rates of bleeding complications between the two agents.[23] TNKase requires only a single bolus injection, which may help facilitate more rapid treatment both in and out of the hospital.

The benefit of fibrinolytic therapy correlates with the degree of restoration of normal blood flow in the infarct-related artery. Coronary artery patency is defined by angiographic perfusion grades developed by the Thrombolysis in Myocardial Infarction (TIMI) study group in 1985 (Box 19-9).[24] Achievement of TIMI grade 3 flow is associated with the best long-term survival. Studies also indicate that rapid restoration of normal blood flow within 90 minutes of treatment results in improved left ventricular function and reduced mortality.[20] All of the currently available fibrinolytics have been shown to achieve TIMI 3 flow in 55% to 60% of patients at 90 minutes.[21]

The area of fibrinolytic therapy is rapidly evolving, and drug dose ranges and regimens are subject to change when research findings are updated. Several new fibrinolytic agents currently under investigation include lanoteplase (n-PA) and staphylokinase.[21] Whereas current fibrinolytic agents target the fibrin portion of the clot, future treatment strategies are focusing on the platelet portion of the clot (see Fig. 19-11). Recent clinical trials evaluating the combination of antiplatelet IIb/IIIa–receptor antagonists with fibrinolytic agents (at half-dose) found equivalent outcomes to fibrinolytics alone.[25-26] There is speculation that such combination therapy could be administered to patients who must be transported to another facility for percutaneous intervention. This "facilitated" approach to revascularization could combine the benefits of rapid administration of drug therapy with the proven efficiency of catheter-based intervention.[27]

EVIDENCE OF REPERFUSION

Several phenomena may be observed after the reperfusion of an artery that has been completely occluded by a thrombus (Box 19-10). Recognition of these noninvasive markers of recanalization is essential for documenting the patient's response to fibrinolytic therapy.

Pain and Reperfusion Dysrhythmias. Initially, when there is reperfusion, ischemic chest pain ceases abruptly as blood flow is restored. Another reliable indicator of reperfusion is the appearance of various "reperfusion" dysrhythmias. Premature ventricular contractions, bradycardias, heart block, ventricular tachycardia, and, rarely, ventricular fibrillation may occur. The reason for the occurrence of these dysrhythmias remains unclear but is thought to be the result of restored flow to ischemic tissue. Generally reperfusion dysrhythmias are self-limiting or nonsustained, and aggressive antidysrhythmic therapy is not required. However, vigilant monitoring of the patient's ECG is essential because a stable condition may deteriorate rapidly and the dysrhythmias may require emergency treatment.

ST Segment. Another noninvasive marker of recanalization is the rapid resolution of the previously elevated ST segments, which indicates restoration of blood flow to previously ischemic myocardial tissue. For this reason a monitoring lead should be chosen that clearly demonstrates ST elevation before initiation of therapy[28] (see "Continuous ST-Segment Monitoring" on p. 342).

Creatine Kinase. The serum concentration of creatine kinase (formerly known as *creatine phosphokinase*) rises rapidly and markedly after reperfusion of the ischemic myocardium. This phenomenon is termed *washout*, because it is thought to result from the rapid readmission of creatine kinase—an enzyme released by damaged myocardial cells—into the circulation after restoration of blood flow to previously unperfused areas of the heart (see "Cardiac Biomarkers" on p. 324).

Box 19-9

FLOW IN THE INFARCT-RELATED ARTERY AS DESCRIBED IN THE THROMBOLYSIS IN MYOCARDIAL INFARCTION (TIMI) TRIAL[24]

TIMI 3	Normal or brisk flow through the coronary artery
TIMI 2	Partial flow, slower than in normal vessels
TIMI 1	Sluggish flow with incomplete distal filling
TIMI 0	No flow beyond the point of occlusion

Box 19-10

NONINVASIVE EVIDENCE OF REPERFUSION

- Cessation of chest pain
- Reperfusion dysrhythmias, primarily ventricular
- Return of elevated ST segments to baseline
- Early and marked peaking of creatine kinase (CK) and troponins

Residual Coronary Stenosis. Fibrinolytic therapy has been determined to be a successful strategy for re-opening occluded coronary arteries in the setting of acute MI. This results in the salvage of myocardium by limiting infarct size, significantly reducing morbidity and mortality associated with cardiogenic shock and ventricular fibrillation. However, residual coronary stenosis resulting from the atherosclerotic process remains, even after successful fibrinolysis. Subsequent prevention of reocclusion is critical to preserving myocardial function and preventing the risk of late complications. Therefore fibrinolytic therapy is recognized as an emergency procedure to restore patency until more definitive therapy can be initiated to effectively reduce the degree of stenosis (an interventional catheter procedure) or to bypass the offending occlusion (coronary artery bypass surgery).

NURSING MANAGEMENT

Nursing management of the patient undergoing fibrinolytic therapy begins with identifying potential candidates. In many institutions, checklists are used to facilitate rapid identification of patients who are candidates for fibrinolytics. The nurse prepares the patient for fibrinolytic therapy by starting intravenous lines and obtaining baseline laboratory values and vital signs. Assessment of the patient continues throughout administration of the fibrinolytic agent for clinical indicators of reperfusion and complications related to therapy. Several nursing diagnoses are linked to the management of the patient receiving fibrinolytic therapy (see the Nursing Diagnoses feature on Postfibrinolytic Therapy).

The most common complication related to thrombolysis is bleeding, not only as a result of the fibrinolytic therapy itself but also because the patients routinely receive anticoagulation therapy for several days to minimize the possibility of rethrombosis. Therefore the nurse must continually monitor for clinical manifestations of bleeding (see Box 19-7). Mild gingival bleeding and oozing around venipuncture sites is common and not a cause of concern. Should serious bleeding occur, such as intracranial or internal bleeding, all fibrinolytic and heparin therapies are discontinued and volume expanders or coagulation factors, or both, are administered.

In addition to accurate assessment of the patient for evidence of bleeding, nursing management includes preventive measures to minimize the potential for bleeding. For example, patient handling is limited, injections are avoided if at all possible, and additional pressure is provided to ensure hemostasis at venipuncture and arterial puncture sites. Intravenous lines are placed before administering lytic therapy, and a heparin lock may be used for obtaining laboratory specimens during treatment.

PATIENT EDUCATION

Education for the patient receiving fibrinolytic therapy includes information regarding the actions of fibrinolytic agents, with emphasis on precautions to minimize bleeding (see the Patient Education feature on Postfibrinolytic Therapy). For example, the patient is cautioned against vigorous tooth brushing and told to refrain from using straight-edge razors. In addition, information is provided regarding ongoing risk factor management in the prevention of atherosclerotic CAD.

NURSING DIAGNOSES   Postfibrinolytic Therapy

- Ineffective Cardiopulmonary Tissue Perfusion related to acute myocardial ischemia
- Acute Pain related to transmission and perception of cutaneous, visceral, muscular, or ischemic impulses
- Anxiety related to threat of biologic, psychologic, and/or social integrity
- Deficient Fluid Volume related to absolute loss
- Deficient Knowledge: Discharge Regimen related to lack of previous exposure to information (see Patient Education feature on Postfibrinolytic Therapy)

PATIENT EDUCATION   Postfibrinolytic Therapy

- Pathophysiology of atherosclerosis
- Risk factor management
- Description of fibrinolytic agent and how it works
- Measures to minimize bleeding and bruising associated with fibrinolytic therapy
- Recognition and actions to take for recurrent ischemic symptoms
- Information regarding prescribed medications (antiplatelet agents, anticoagulants)

CATHETER INTERVENTIONS FOR CORONARY ARTERY DISEASE

During the past three decades, there has been a growing trend toward percutaneous catheter-based interventions for the treatment of coronary artery disease (CAD). Percutaneous transluminal coronary angioplasty (PTCA) was first introduced in 1977 as an alternative to coronary artery bypass surgery. The advantages of PTCA included avoiding the risks involved with cardiac surgery (general anesthesia, thoracotomy, extracorporeal circulation, and mechanical ventilation) and significantly decreasing convalescence time. Disadvantages included acute complications related to the procedure itself, restenosis or renarrowing of the vessel after the procedure, and difficulty in accessing certain lesions.[29] Research in this area has continued, and a growing number of interventional devices have been developed to address the limitations of conventional angioplasty. Today options for percutaneous coronary intervention (PCI) include not only PTCA but also atherectomy, laser angioplasty, and stent placement, used either alone or in conjunction with angioplasty. Patients undergoing percutaneous catheter-based interventions have an anticipated length of hospital stay of 1 to 3 days.

INDICATIONS FOR CATHETER-BASED INTERVENTIONS

Indications for catheter-based interventions have been considerably broadened since the initial application of balloon angioplasty. Whereas once only patients with single-vessel CAD were considered for PTCA, now patients with multivessel disease, even those who have previously undergone saphenous vein graft (SVG) and internal mammary artery (IMA) graft or fibrinolytic therapy for acute MI, may be candidates for catheter intervention. Trials comparing fibrinolytics to catheter-based reperfusion in the setting of acute MI have shown an advantage for percutaneous catheter interventions over drug therapy in preventing death, reinfarction, or stroke, even though there may be delays related to transporting patients to facilities with interventional capabilities.[27]

Earlier restrictions regarding the characteristics and location of the atherosclerotic lesion have also changed with operator experience and improved technology. Left main coronary lesions have been successfully dilated under certain conditions. Also, no longer is the presence of an eccentric (uneven distribution of plaque), moderately calcified, or nonproximal lesion an absolute contraindication. Furthermore, it is now sometimes possible to traverse and dilate a totally occluded vessel. Lesion morphology related to shape, size, location, and amount of calcification has been more clearly defined through clinical experience and is now used to guide the selection of specific catheter-based interventions[30] (see "Coronary Artery Disease," p. 427).

Surgical Backup. Initially most institutions required that patients preparing to undergo PTCA be candidates for coronary artery bypass surgery. Complications such as dissection, where plaque within the vessel cracks during balloon inflation and results in abrupt closure of the vessel, could arise during the procedure, requiring the patient to undergo emergency coronary artery bypass surgery. Today the majority of dissections are effectively treated with stent placement, with less than 2% of patients requiring emergency bypass surgery. As a result, most institutions have evolved to an informal surgical back-up plan, such as the first available operating room. Nevertheless, the availability of cardiac surgical services on site is still recommended.[30]

PERCUTANEOUS TRANSLUMINAL CORONARY ANGIOPLASTY

Percutaneous transluminal coronary angioplasty (PTCA) involves the use of a balloon-tipped catheter that, when advanced through an atherosclerotic lesion (atheroma), can be inflated intermittently for the purpose of dilating the stenotic area and improving blood flow through it (Fig. 19-12). The high balloon-inflation pressure stretches the vessel wall, fractures the plaque, and enlarges the vessel lumen. A successful angioplasty procedure is one in which the stenosis is reduced to less than 50% of the vessel lumen diameter, although most clinicians aim for less than 20% final diameter stenosis.[30] Procedural success is influenced by patient variables such as age, cardiac function, and comorbidities such as diabetes, as well

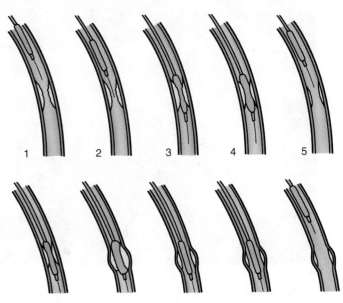

Fig. 19-12 Percutaneous transluminal coronary angioplasty (PTCA) used to open a stenotic vessel occluded by atherosclerosis.

as by characteristics of the lesion itself. Lesions that are discrete (less than 1 cm in length), concentric, easily accessible, and have little or no calcification are most likely to be treated successfully with PTCA. Once seen as a "rescue" procedure to reduce a severe stenosis that persisted following fibrinolytic therapy, PTCA is now preferred as the initial method of treatment for acute MI (primary angioplasty).[27]

Procedure. PTCA is performed in the cardiac catheterization laboratory under fluoroscopy. Introducer catheters, or "sheaths," are inserted percutaneously into the femoral artery and vein. The venous sheath can be used to perform a right heart catheterization with a pulmonary artery (PA) catheter or to insert a pacing catheter, or both. A catheter with pacing capabilities may be indicated if dilation of the right coronary artery or circumflex artery is anticipated because the blood supply to the conduction system of the heart may be interrupted, requiring emergency pacing. The pacing catheter also serves as an anatomic landmark for locating the lesions to be dilated. The patient is systemically heparinized to prevent clots from forming on or in any of the catheters, with dosing adjusted to achieve a target activated clotting time. A special guiding catheter designed to engage the coronary ostia is inserted through the arterial sheath and advanced in a retrograde manner through the aorta. Nitroglycerin or calcium channel blockers may be given at this time to prevent coronary artery spasm and to maximize coronary vasodilation during the procedure. A guidewire is then advanced down the coronary artery and negotiated across the oc-

cluding atheroma. The balloon catheter is advanced over this guidewire and positioned across the lesion. The balloon is inflated and deflated repetitively (each inflation not to exceed 90 seconds) until evidence of dilation is demonstrated on an angiogram (Fig. 19-13). In cases that require prolonged balloon inflations, an autoperfusion angioplasty catheter is available with side holes that allow passive blood flow through the central lumen to the distal coronary artery if adequate systemic blood pressure is present.

The patient is transferred to the coronary care or angioplasty unit after the procedure for care and observation. The arterial sheath is attached to a continuous heparinized saline flush, and intravenous fluids must be infused through the venous sheath to maintain luminal patency. Heparin is usually discontinued immediately to facilitate early sheath removal. If the patient's postangioplasty course is uneventful, the sheaths are removed within 2 to 4 hours of the procedure. After sheath removal, the patient may be discharged home 6 to 12 hours later.

Complications. As stated earlier, serious complications can result from angioplasty that necessitate emergency intervention. These complications include persistent coronary artery spasm, coronary artery dissection, and acute coronary thrombosis. Stents have proven efficacious in the repair of coronary dissections, decreasing the need for emergency bypass surgery. Prevention of acute closure related to coronary thrombosis was historically treated with short-term anticoagulation with intravenous heparin plus aspirin to inhibit platelet aggrega-

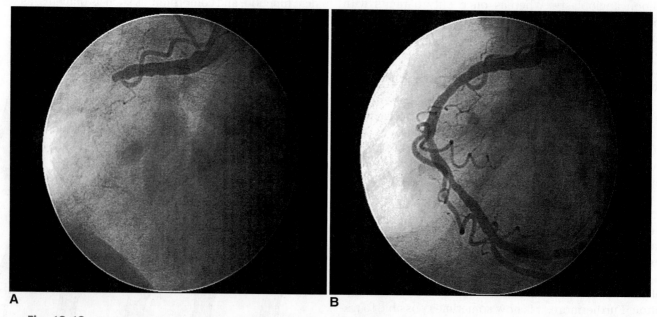

A   **B**

Fig. 19-13   **A,** Coronary arteriogram of an acute proximal total occlusion of the right coronary artery (RCA). Patient had sudden onset of chest pain at home and was emergently admitted to the cardiac catheterization laboratory. **B,** The same vessel (RCA) shown in **A** after successful coronary atherectomy and intracoronary thrombolytic therapy to open the occluded artery. Symptoms of chest pain resolved after the procedure.

tion. Recently, more potent antiplatelet agents (glycoprotein IIb/IIIa inhibitors) have become available to reduce the formation of intracoronary thrombosis after percutaneous intervention. Initially used only in patients with high risk for abrupt closure after percutaneous interventions, these agents now have been found to have benefit across the spectrum of interventional procedures, from PTCA to atherectomy to stenting.[30]

Abciximab (ReoPro) was the first of the glycoprotein IIb/IIIa inhibitors approved by the Food and Drug Administration (FDA) as an adjunct to PTCA for the prevention of abrupt closure of arteries in high-risk patients. Following that two additional agents, *eptifibatide* (Integrilin) and *tirofiban* (Aggrastat), were also approved. These drugs block the enzyme *glycoprotein IIb/IIIa*, which is essential for platelet aggregation. Indications and dosing of these agents is provided in the Pharmacologic Management table on Glycoprotein IIB/IIIA Inhibitors. The major complication of glycoprotein IIb/IIIa inhibitors is bleeding, and nursing management requires careful assessment of all potential bleeding sites, especially at the femoral sheath site. Extra precautions are used to immobilize the sheath insertion site, either with a sheet tuck to the affected leg or a leg restraint.[31]

Other complications that can occur in the period immediately after angioplasty include bleeding and hematoma formation at the site of vascular cannulation; compromised blood flow to the involved extremity; contrast-induced renal failure; dysrhythmias; and vasovagal response (hypotension, bradycardia, and diaphoresis) during manipulation or removal of introducer sheaths.

Restenosis. Although PTCA has relatively high success rates in initially opening occluded vessels, this technique by itself has major limitations, including a high frequency of restenosis. Restenosis within the first year after intervention occurs in over one third of patients who undergo PTCA and is diagnosed when patients experience a recurrence of anginal symptoms.[32] Restenosis is influenced by the final lumen diameter achieved by the procedure, the severity of elastic recoil of the vessel walls in response to the balloon inflation, and the amount of intimal hyperplasia that occurs as the vessel heals over the treated area. Patient characteristics may also increase the risk of restenosis, such as a history of diabetes mellitus or unstable angina.[33] Once the phenomenon of restenosis was recognized, devices were sought to more completely remove plaque and open the vessel at the time of the intervention. Coronary atherectomy, laser angioplasty, and placement of endovascular prostheses (stents) are interventional technologies developed to address the problems of acute closure and restenosis associated with PTCA.[29]

ATHERECTOMY

Atherectomy is the excision and removal of the atherosclerotic plaque by cutting, shaving, or grinding, using specialized coronary catheters. Initially atherectomy devices were used alone in an attempt to avoid the trauma to the vessel that was known to occur with balloon angioplasty and more efficiently remove the atherosclerotic plaque, thereby decreasing the rate of restenosis. Later, as restenosis was also found to occur with these devices, balloon angioplasty was added as an adjunctive

Pharmacologic Management: Glycoprotein IIB/IIIA Inhibitors

DRUG	INDICATIONS/DOSE	COMMENTS
Abciximab (ReoPro)	**ACS:** 0.25 mg/kg IVP, then 10 mcg/min until PCI **PCI:** 0.25 mg/kg IVP, then 0.125 mcg/kg/min × 12 hr	Used concomitantly with heparin and aspirin May affect platelet function for up to 48 hr post infusion
Eptifibatide (Integrilin)	**ACS:** IV bolus or 180 mcg/kg followed with an infusion of 2 mcg/kg/min for up to 72 hrs; if the patient undergoes PCI, the dose is decreased to 0.5 mcg/kg/min and continued for 24 hr postprocedure, for a total of 96 hr **PCI:** 135 mcg/kg IVP, followed by an infusion of 0.5 mcg/kg/min × 24 hr	Concomitant heparin and aspirin may be administered Platelet function returns to baseline within 6-8 hr Contraindicated in patients with significant renal dysfunction
Tirofiban (Aggrastat)	**ACS (with or without PCI):** 0.4 mcg/kg/min for 30 min, then continued at 0.1 mcg/kg/min for 48-108 hr post ACS or for patients undergoing PCI	Administered in combination with heparin for patients undergoing PCI Platelet function returns to baseline within 4-8 hr Dosage should be reduced in patients with severe renal dysfunction

ACS, Acute coronary syndrome; *IVP,* intravenous push; *PCI,* percutaneous coronary intervention; *IV,* intravenous.

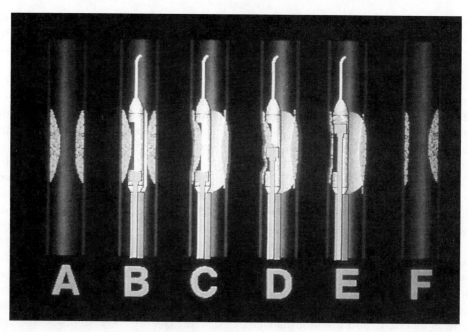

Fig. 19-14 Directional coronary atherectomy (DCA) device. **A,** Atheroma (plaque) in vessel lumen. **B,** DCA device in position. **C,** Inflation of low-pressure support balloon that pushes the plaque into the "window" of the device (the ability to turn the atherocath in different directions within the artery explains the name of the DCA device). **D,** The cutter begins to shear away plaque. **E,** The plaque is pushed into the nose cone (collection chamber) of the atherocath. **F,** Vessel lumen shows decreased plaque after removal of catheter.

Table 19-4	Atherectomy Devices	
Device	**Design**	**Uses**
Directional coronary atherectomy	Rotating, cup-shaped cutter within a windowed cylindric housing; plaque that protrudes into window is shaved off and collected within nose cone of cutter housing (see Fig. 19-14)	Ostial lesions Eccentric lesions in large vessels Proximal, discrete lesions In-stent restenosis
Rotational ablation catheter (Rotablator)	A high-speed, rotating, diamond-studded burr; "sanding effect"; generates microparticles that pass distally into microcirculation	In-stent restenosis Calcified lesions
Transluminal extraction catheter	Motorized cutting head with triangular blades; excised plaque removed by suction	Long, diffuse lesions Occluded saphenous vein graft

therapy to optimize the diameter of the vessel lumen and offset the intimal hyperplasia that would occur secondary to the procedure.[34]

Three atherectomy devices are described in Table 19-4: directional coronary atherectomy (DCA), rotational ablation (Rotablator), and transluminal extraction catheter. All three devices are FDA-approved for use in coronary as well as peripheral arteries. Because these devices use different mechanisms, they may offer special advantages for different types of lesions. The current trend is to use a "lesion-specific" approach in the selection of a device for catheter intervention.

Directional Coronary Atherectomy. The mechanism of action of the DCA catheter is shown in Fig.

19-14. Because DCA extracts pieces of atheroma that can be studied microscopically (rather like a biopsy specimen), it has provided significant research toward the understanding of both the pathogenesis of CAD and the restenosis process caused by intimal hyperplasia after catheter interventions. Because of this device's ability to direct the cutting mechanism toward the plaque, it is well suited for lesions that involve a bifurcation or major side branch, as well as eccentric lesions. DCA may also be used to remove plaque (debulk) lesions before stenting.[29]

Rotablator. The Rotablator device has a diamond-coated burr that drills through the plaque, creating tiny particles. This particulate matter is carried through the blood stream and disposed of by the reticuloendothelial system. This device is the preferred treatment for heavily calcified lesions, since the burr drill preferentially ablates calcified plaque and is deflected by the elastic elements of the vessel wall.[35] Improved lumen diameter may be achieved when angioplasty is used after the Rotablator procedure (adjunctive angioplasty).[34] Rotational atherectomy may be used to debulk severely calcified lesions before stent placement and to remove in-stent restenosis.[29]

Transluminal Extraction Catheter. The transluminal extraction catheter (TEC) consists of a motorized cutting head with triangular blades that rotate at 700 revolutions/min to shave atherosclerotic lesions. As the plaque is excised, a suction device incorporated into the catheter is used to remove the plaque from the vessel. This device has been successful in the treatment of long, diffuse lesions and of stenosis that occurs in bypass grafts. Unlike PTCA and DCA, the TEC may also be used to establish reperfusion through total occlusions.[34] TEC atherectomy may be performed first to debulk the lesion and then is followed by angioplasty and/or stenting to further decrease the amount of residual stenosis.

Procedure. The procedure for atherectomy is similar to that described for PTCA. The sheaths required are larger to facilitate passage of the larger atherectomy catheters. As a result, postprocedure complications related to the sheaths may be increased. Patients undergoing Rotablator procedures may also have an increased need for continued nitroglycerin to treat vasospasm in the postprocedure period.[35]

LASER ANGIOPLASTY

Laser is an acronym for *l*ight *a*mplification by *s*timulated *e*mission of *r*adiation. Laser plaque ablation in coronary arteries, using the excimer laser, has been studied in a number of clinical trials. The excimer laser is a contact cutter, meaning that it ablates only tissue that it touches. The catheter is advanced by a guidewire system similar to that used in angioplasty. The excimer laser, which uses high-energy pulsed ultraviolet light—so-called *cold laser*—to vaporize plaque, is particularly suited for complex lesions, including chronic total occlusions and lengthy or calcified lesions.[33] The excimer laser is also used to treat in-stent restenosis, in conjunction with angioplasty.[29]

CORONARY STENTS

A significant development in interventional cardiology has been the coronary stent prosthesis. This is a self-expanding or balloon-expandable stent that is introduced into the coronary artery over a guidewire in a region that has been previously dilated with PTCA to prevent acute closure and restenosis, as well as to obtain a larger vascular lumen diameter. Stent implantation was

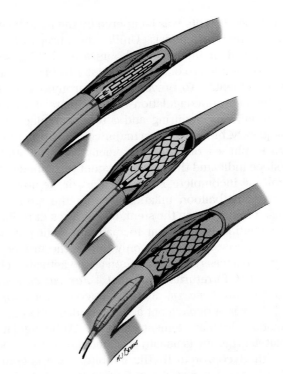

Fig. 19-15 Intracoronary stent (balloon expandable stent). (From Bevans M, McLimore E: *J Cardiovasc Nurs* 7(1):34, 1992.)

initially limited to large vessels (greater than 3 mm) with proximal, discrete lesions. Improvements in stent design and operator technique now allow for their deployment in smaller vessels with diffuse disease, vessels with lesions at bifurcations, and vessels with thrombus. Stents are now used in as many as 80% to 90% of all interventional procedures.[29] Indications for stenting have been expanded to include not only treatment of acute closure but also primary stenting to optimize the results of other treatments (PTCA, atherectomy, fibrinolytics) and prevent restenosis.

Procedure. The procedure for stent placement is similar to that used in other catheter interventions. Access to the coronary arteries is obtained via a femoral sheath, which allows for placement of a catheter over a guidewire. A stent is positioned at the target side and is expanded, and the catheter is removed, leaving the stent in place. Intravascular ultrasound is being used by some clinicians to evaluate the vessel lumen diameter after stent deployment.[30] Information obtained from ultrasound has provided a better estimate of residual plaque than that provided by angiography, since contrast material may surround the lattice-work of the stent, giving the appearance of a large lumen even when the stent is not fully open. Multiple stents may be implanted sequentially within a vessel to fully cover the area of the lesion.

Numerous stents are now available. Over 65 stents are now approved for routine use, with numerous others in various stages of development.[36] Most stents are balloon-expandable Fig. 19-15.

Early use of stents was hampered by the incidence of subacute stent thrombosis. Unlike the abrupt closure that occurred in the first 24 hours after PTCA, stent thrombosis tended to occur in the first 2 to 14 days after stent placement.[36] To prevent acute thrombosis of the stent, intense anticoagulation and antiplatelet therapy were initially used during and after stent placement. Consequently, bleeding was a major complication during the early phases of stent placement. Clinical studies have since indicated that subacute stent thrombosis was a result of incomplete stent opening or deployment. High-pressure balloon inflations within the stents are now used to fully open the stent, and as a result reduced anticoagulation is sufficient to maintain stent patency. Physicians now use heparin only during the procedure and remove access sheaths as soon as the activated clotting time (ACT) returns to normal.[37] *For patients who cannot tolerate heparin*, another anticoagulant *may be used*.[38] Newer anticoagulant agents are described in the Pharmacologic Management table on Anticoagulants. Antiplatelet therapy is usually initiated during the procedure with glycoprotein IIb/IIIa inhibitors and is continued for 12 to 24 hours, depending on the agent used.[37] Oral antiplatelet therapy is routinely prescribed at discharge and includes agents such as ticlopidine or clopi-dogrel for 2 to 4 weeks and aspirin indefinitely. Ticlopidine, although proven to be effective, has serious and sometimes fatal side effects including neutropenia. Clopidogrel, which is similar to ticlopidine but does not cause as much bone marrow suppression, is now used more often.[30] Conventional medications for treatment of CAD, such as IV nitroglycerin and calcium channel blockers, may also be prescribed.

In-Stent Restenosis. Stents have been shown to decrease the incidence of restenosis when compared with balloon angioplasty, most likely as a result of achieving the largest possible lumen diameter at the time of the intervention.[33] Stents did not, however, prove to be a "cure" for restenosis as was once hoped. Restenosis within the stent is caused by intimal hyperplasia and can occur in a diffuse pattern throughout the stent or as discrete lesions within the body of the stent or at the stent margins.[37] In-stent restenosis may be treated effectively with repeat balloon angioplasty, laser angioplasty, or rotoablation.[39]

Much research has been focused on ways to prevent in-stent restenosis and includes both pharmacologic and nonpharmacologic approaches. Two recent advances in the treatment of restenosis include the use of radiation applied to the inside of the coronary vessel

Pharmacologic Management: Anticoagulants

CLASSIFICATION/DRUG	MECHANISM OF ACTION	INDICATIONS	SPECIAL CONSIDERATIONS
Heparin Heparin sodium	Enhances activity of antithrombin III, a natural anticoagulant	Prevention of clotting in patients with MI and those undergoing PCI or cardiac surgery	Effectiveness of treatment may be monitored by aPTT or ACT Response is variable due to binding with plasma proteins Effects may be reversed with protamine sulfate Risk of developing HIT
Low–Molecular Weight Heparin Dalteparin (Fragmin) Enoxaparin (Lovenox)	Enhances activity of anti-thrombin III	Prophylaxis and treatment of thromboembolic complications following surgery Prevention of clots in patients with unstable angina and MI	More predictable response than heparin, since drug is not largely bound to protein aPTT not particularly useful in monitoring treatment
Direct Thrombin Inhibitor Lepirudin (Refludan) Bivalirudin (Angiomax)	Directly inhibits thrombin	Prophylaxis and treatment of thrombosis in patients with HIT Prevention of clots in patients with unstable angina or PCI	aPTT may be monitored daily Dose should be adjusted for patients with renal insufficiency No reversal agent available

aPTT, Activated partial thromboplastin time; *ACT*, activated clotting time; *MI*, myocardial infarction; *PCI* percutaneous coronary intervention; *HIT*, heparin-induced thrombocytopenia.

(brachytherapy) and stents that have the ability to deliver drugs locally at the site of the intervention (drug-eluting stents).[33]

Brachytherapy. The delivery of intracoronary radiation has been studied using beta and gamma radiation, and both have been shown to be effective at reducing restenosis rates when compared to placebo.[40-41] However, this type of therapy has several limitations, including the added procedural time and the need for specialized equipment and personnel. As a result, this therapy is not available at all centers that perform PCI.[33]

Drug-Eluting Stents. Stents coated with drugs that inhibit cell growth have also been shown to effectively lower restenosis rates. A drug coated with sirolimus (an immunosuppressive drug used to prevent organ transplant rejection) was recently approved by the FDA. In clinical trials this stent was shown to significantly decrease restenosis when compared with bare metal stents[42-43] Another stent coated with paxlitaxel (an anticancer agent) has also shown promising results.[44]

NURSING MANAGEMENT

Nursing management and diagnoses after angioplasty, atherectomy, or stent insertion focuses on accurate assessment of the patient's condition and prompt intervention (see the Nursing Diagnoses feature on Post PTCA, Coronary Atherectomy, and Stent). The nurse at the bedside is in the unique position to continuously monitor for clinical manifestations of potential problems and take quick and appropriate action to minimize the deleterious effects of complications related to the interventional catheter procedure.

Angina. It is essential that the nurse observe the patient for recurrent angina, a clinical indication of myocardial ischemia. Angina may be accompanied by elevated ST segments on the bedside monitor or the 12-lead ECG. Angina during interventional cardiology procedures is an expected occurrence at the time of balloon inflation or manipulation within the coronary artery. Intraprocedure angina is caused by the temporary interruption of blood flow through the involved artery, which should subside with deflation or removal of the balloon or nitroglycerin administration, or both. Angina after a coronary interventional procedure may be a result of transient coronary vasospasm, or it may signal a more serious complication. In any case, the nurse must act quickly to assess for manifestations of myocardial ischemia and initiate clinical interventions as indicated. The physician usually orders intravenous nitroglycerin to be titrated to alleviate chest pain. Continued angina despite maximal vasodilator therapy generally rules out transient coronary vasospasm as the source of ischemic pain, and redilation or emergency coronary artery bypass surgery must be considered. The risk is that a clot in the coronary artery, usually occurring at a site where the intimal wall has been dissected, will cause an acute occlusion.

Femoral Site Care. While the sheath is in place or after its removal, bleeding or hematoma at the sheath insertion site may occur as a result of the effects of heparin. The nurse observes the patient for bleeding or swelling at the puncture site and frequently assesses adequacy of circulation to the involved extremity. The nurse also assesses the patient for back pain, which can indicate retroperitoneal bleeding from the internal arterial puncture site. The patient is instructed to keep the involved leg straight and not to elevate the head of the bed any more than 30 degrees while the sheath is in place (to prevent dislodgment) and for several hours after its removal (to prevent bleeding). After sheath removal, direct pressure is applied to the puncture site for 15 to 30 minutes; a sandbag may be ordered if direct pressure is inadequate for hemostasis. For stents or atherectomy, which require a larger sheath size, a C-clamp or femoral compression device may be used to apply continued pressure for 1 to 2 hours to ensure adequate hemostasis.

Patients usually are allowed to resume ambulation 6 to 8 hours later, depending on institution protocol. Excessive bleeding or hematoma formation can become a serious problem because it may result in hypotension or compromised blood flow to the involved extremity. For this reason, pulses are usually monitored every 15 minutes for the first 2 hours immediately after the procedure, and then every 1 to 2 hours until the sheaths are removed.

NURSING DIAGNOSES

Post-PTCA, Coronary Atherectomy, and Stent

- Ineffective Cardiopulmonary Tissue Perfusion related to acute myocardial ischemia
- Ineffective Altered Peripheral Tissue Perfusion related to decreased peripheral blood flow
- Activity Intolerance related to prolonged immobility or deconditioning
- Acute Pain related to transmission and perception of cutaneous, visceral, muscular, or ischemic impulses
- Anxiety related to threat to biologic, psychologic, and/or social integrity
- Deficient Knowledge: Discharge Regimen related to lack of previous exposure to information (see Patient Education feature on Post-PTCA Coronary Atherectomy, and Stent)

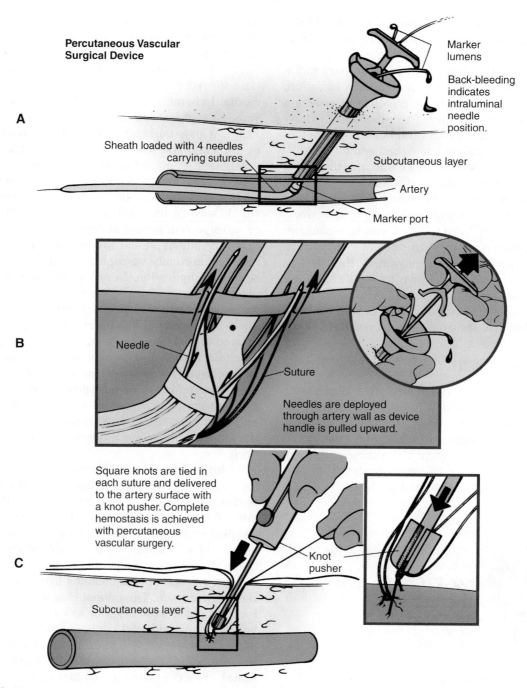

Percutaneous Vascular Surgical Device

Marker lumens

Back-bleeding indicates intraluminal needle position.

A

Sheath loaded with 4 needles carrying sutures

Subcutaneous layer

Artery

Marker port

B

Needle

Suture

Needles are deployed through artery wall as device handle is pulled upward.

Square knots are tied in each suture and delivered to the artery surface with a knot pusher. Complete hemostasis is achieved with percutaneous vascular surgery.

C

Knot pusher

Subcutaneous layer

Fig. 19-16 Example of a percutaneous vascular surgical device used to close the femoral artery after catheter interventions for coronary artery disease. **A,** Insertion of device into femoral artery. **B,** After the interventional procedure, the device is removed by pulling upward to allow needles—in the device—to close the artery. **C,** The sutured artery is secured with a knot pusher. (Courtesy Perclose, Inc, Redwood City, Calif.)

After sheath removal, pulses are again monitored at 15-minute intervals for a brief period.

Recently, new vascular hemostatic devices have been developed to address the problem of achieving hemostasis at the femoral access site after sheath removal. Perclose has marketed a percutaneous vascular surgical device that is inserted into the femoral artery in the same position as a conventional introducer sheath (Fig. 19-16, A). The device contains needles and sutures that are used to suture the artery closed after the interventional procedure (Fig. 19-16, B). At the end of the procedure, when the artery is sealed, the needles are removed by the cardiologist and the sutures are knotted firmly (Fig. 19-16, C). VasoSeal and Angioseal are vascular hemostatic devices that use a collagen plug, injected through a preloaded syringe system into the supraarterial space,

Post-PTCA, Coronary Atherectomy, and Stent

- Pathophysiology of atherosclerosis
- Risk factor modification (diet, exercise, smoking cessation, weight loss)
- Information about prescribed medications (e.g., antiplatelet agents, nitrates, calcium channel blockers)
- Symptoms to report to the health care professional (chest pain, shortness of breath, bleeding)
- Follow-up appointments

PTCA, Percutaneous transluminal coronary angioplasty.

Box 19-11

INDICATIONS FOR BALLOON VALVULOPLASTY

AORTIC
Nonsurgical candidates with incapacitating symptoms
Patients with aortic stenosis who require urgent non-cardiac surgery
Patients with severe heart failure or cardiogenic shock because of aortic stenosis whose conditions need to be stabilized until valve replacement is deemed safer
Patients with poor left ventricular function, low cardiac output, and small gradient across a stenotic aortic valve whose need for aortic valve replacement requires assessment

MITRAL
As an alternative to open mitral commissurotomy

to promote hemostasis at the arterial puncture site.[45,46] Gentle pressure is maintained over the puncture site for approximately 5 minutes, until hemostasis is achieved. When devices such as these are used, time to ambulation and discharge can be significantly shortened. The collagen plug is completely absorbed after 90 days, but until that time the site cannot be used for another procedure.

PATIENT EDUCATION

Typically patients undergoing elective angioplasty, atherectomy, or laser procedures are hospitalized for approximately 24 hours. Stent procedures may require a slightly longer hospital stay. All patients require education about their medication regimen and about risk-factor modification (see the Patient Education feature on Post PTCA, Coronary, Atherectomy, and Stent). Because of the abbreviated hospital stay, the nurse often has time to do little more than identify the offending risk factors and initiate basic instruction. Patients are referred to local cardiac rehabilitation centers for more extensive teaching and follow-up to facilitate understanding and compliance with risk factor modification.

Another point of instruction that must be addressed is the patient's knowledge deficit related to discharge medications. Patients often are sent home on a regimen of antiplatelet drugs, as well as a nitrate such as isosorbide to promote vasodilation. In addition, if the patient has demonstrated evidence of a vasospastic component to the disease, calcium channel blockers are prescribed. It is essential that the patient clearly understand the rationale for therapy, as well as potential side effects of each drug. It is important that patients be provided with written information and a number to call if problems occur.

BALLOON VALVOTOMY

After the development of percutaneous balloon angioplasty for CAD, it became reasonable to consider adaptation of this technique as a nonsurgical intervention for stenotic cardiac valves. Percutaneous balloon valvotomy has become an accepted alternative to surgical approaches in selected patients with mitral valve stenosis. Aortic valvotomy has a limited role in adults, since restenosis and clinical deterioration occur within 6 to 12 months in most patients and it is associated with significant morbidity and mortality (Box 19-11).[47]

Balloon valvotomy is performed in the cardiac catheterization laboratory. The procedure is similar to a routine cardiac catheterization, including cannulation of the femoral artery and vein with percutaneous introducer sheaths. The balloon dilation catheter is then threaded over a guidewire across the stenotic valvular orifice. The valves may be approached either retrograde via the aorta or antegrade across the interatrial septum. In the antegrade transseptal approach, the balloon catheter is passed across the interatrial septum, which results in the creation of a small atrial septal defect.[48] Subsequent inflations of the balloon increase the valve opening by separating fused commissures, cracking calcified leaflets, and stretching valve structures. Inflations are continued until the balloon "waist" disappears, which indicates full inflation. Regurgitant flow can result, particularly after mitral valvotomy, and may result in the need for emergency valve replacement if severe. The risks of balloon valvotomy are similar to those inherent in most catheterization procedures and include cardiac perforation, thromboembolic events, dysrhythmias, and vascular complications caused by the sheath.[49] The postprocedure nursing management is similar to that for other percutaneous cardiac catheter procedures.

CLINICAL APPLICATION

Cardiovascular Concepts

Mrs. C is a 68-year-old white woman with a history of coronary artery disease (CAD) and hypertension. She has an 8-year history of exertional angina, which became unstable 3 weeks ago. A myocardial infarction was ruled out, and a cardiac catheterization procedure was performed, revealing significant obstruction in the left anterior descending (LAD) artery and in the right coronary artery (RCA) with an ejection fraction of 35%. She underwent coronary artery bypass grafting (CABG) to the LAD using the internal mammary artery and to the RCA using a saphenous vein graft.

She returned to the critical care unit on a nitroglycerin drip at 66 mcg/min. Her vital signs on admission are blood pressure (BP) 98/52 mm Hg (mean of 65 mm Hg); heart rate (HR) 100 (sinus tachycardia with frequent premature ventricular contractions); respiratory rate (RR) 12 breaths/min via the ventilator; temperature 36.2° C; central venous pressure (CVP) 6 mm Hg; pulmonary artery pressure (PAP) 24/10 mm Hg; pulmonary artery occlusion pressure (PAOP) 9 mm Hg. A thermodilution cardiac output (CO) of 4.5 L/min is obtained, and calculated values indicated a cardiac index (CI) of 2 L/min/m^2 and a systemic vascular resistance (SVR) of 1048 dynes/sec/cm^{-5}. Urine output is 700 ml/hr and chest tube output is minimal. Laboratory values on arrival are potassium 3.4 mEq/L, magnesium 1.8 mg/L, hematocrit 30.0%.

1. What are possible causes for Mrs. C's low cardiac index?
2. What are potential causes for the ventricular ectopy?

Mrs. C is given 2 L of crystalloid and 500 ml of hetastarch (Hespan). Her potassium and magnesium are replaced. A dopamine drip is initiated at 6 mcg/kg/min. A warming blanket is applied. Repeat vital signs show BP 96/48 mm Hg; HR 120 (sinus tachycardia); RR 14; temperature 36.9° C; CVP 12 mm Hg; PAP 30/15 mm Hg; PAOP 13 mm Hg; CO 4.2 L/min; CI 1.9 L/min/m^2; SVR 990 dynes/sec/cm^{-5}. Urine output has decreased to 30 ml/hr. Chest tube output is less than 40 ml/hr. Recent laboratory values show hematocrit 29.0%, potassium 4.6 mEq/L, magnesium 2.5 mEq/L, pH 7.29, Pao$_2$ 100, Paco$_2$ 35, HCO$_3$ 18, O$_2$ sat 98%. The cardiac surgeon requests that an intraaortic balloon pump be brought to the bedside.

3. What effects would the dopamine drip have in this dosage range?
4. What is the most likely reason for Mrs. C's acidosis?
5. What are the primary physiologic effects of the intraaortic balloon?
6. What potential complications should the nurse monitor for while the patient is on the intraaortic balloon pump (IABP)?

The intraaortic balloon is inserted and Mrs. C's vital signs improve: BP 110/43 mm Hg; HR 96 (sinus rhythm); CVP 10 mm Hg; PAP 28/14 mm Hg; PAOP 12 mm Hg; CO 5.8 L/min; CI 2.9 L/min/m^2; SVR 827 dynes/sec/cm^{-5}. She is extubated the following morning, and the IABP is weaned and removed on postoperative day 3.

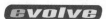 See the Evolve website for the discussion of this Clinical Application.

CARDIAC SURGERY

The nursing management of the patient undergoing cardiac surgery is demanding yet exciting work that requires the talents of an experienced team of critical care nurses. The following discussion introduces basic cardiac surgical techniques and principles of cardiopulmonary bypass and highlights the key points about postoperative care of the adult patient who requires either valve replacement or coronary artery revascularization.

CORONARY ARTERY BYPASS SURGERY

Since its introduction more than two decades ago, coronary artery bypass surgery has been proven both safe and effective in relieving medically uncontrolled angina pectoris in most patients. With improved medical management of CAD, including improvements in percutaneous revascularization techniques, much debate has been generated regarding the efficacy of medical vs. surgical therapy for CAD (see "Medical Management" for coronary artery disease, p. 523; "Catheter Interventions for Coronary Artery Disease" earlier in this chapter).

The combined results of three major randomized trials support the view that coronary artery bypass grafting (CABG) affords dramatic improvement of symptoms and quality of life. CABG is more effective than medical therapy for improving survival in patients with left main–vessel or triple-vessel disease or with double-vessel disease involving the left anterior descending artery (LAD), as well as more effective for relieving exercise-induced ischemia or chronic ischemia leading to left ventricular (LV) dysfunction. Medical therapy is recommended when ischemia is prevented by antianginal drugs that are well tolerated by the patient.[50] Surgical revascularization has been shown to be more efficacious than angioplasty in patients with diabetes mellitus.[51] CABG also offers advantages over percutaneous revascularization in patients with multivessel disease. When arterial grafts are used, CABG has superior long-term patency rates, surpassing those of angioplasty or stents.[52] In addition, bypass surgery may allow for more complete revascularization since it can be used on vessels that are not amenable to treatment with a percutaneous approach, such as those with total occlusions or excessive tortuosity. (For more information, see the Clinical Application feature on Cardiovascular Concepts.)

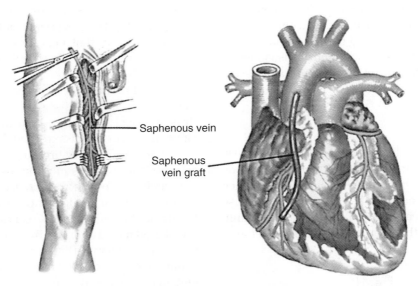

Fig. 19-17 Saphenous vein graft.

The anticipated length of stay for coronary artery bypass surgery ranges from 5 to 9 days. The longer length of stay is for patients who undergo cardiac catheterization and CABG surgery.

Myocardial revascularization involves the use of a conduit, or channel, designed to bypass an occluded coronary artery. Currently, the two most common conduits are the saphenous vein graft (SVG) and the internal mammary artery (IMA). SVG involves the anastomosis of an excised portion of the saphenous vein proximal to the aorta and distal to the coronary artery below the obstruction (Fig. 19-17). Traditionally the SVG was obtained through an open incision, but recent technology has allowed for the endoscopic harvesting of this vessel. This minimally invasive technique of graft procurement decreases postoperative pain and reduces scarring.[53]

The IMA, which usually remains attached to its origin at the subclavian artery, is swung down and anastomosed distal to the coronary artery (Fig. 19-18). Both the right IMA (RIMA) and the left IMA (LIMA) may be used as conduits. Of note, emergency coronary artery bypass surgery may preclude the use of the IMA because of the extra time required to mobilize the artery, as well as the inability to effect cardioplegia through this conduit. However, the current trend is to use arterial conduits such as the IMA when possible, because their long-term patency rates are superior to those of the SVG.[54]

The right gastroepiploic artery (GEA) has also been introduced as an alternate conduit for CABG. The GEA, which is a branch of the gastroduodenal artery, is pulled up to the pericardial cavity and anastomosed to a distal portion of the coronary artery (Fig. 19-19). Although it is a little smaller in diameter than the IMA, studies indicate that patency rates are excellent.[55] Because of its size and anatomic location, the GEA is well suited for bypassing the right coronary artery, the circumflex artery, or the pos-

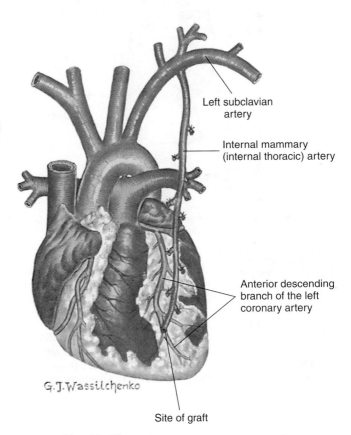

Fig. 19-18 Internal mammary artery graft.

terior descending artery. The technical aspects of obtaining this conduit, however, may limit its widespread use.

The potential benefit of long-term patency associated with arterial conduits has revived interest in the use of radial artery (RA) grafts. First introduced as a potential conduit for myocardial revascularization in the 1970s, RA grafts were abandoned because of a high incidence of early graft occlusion and vasospasm. Current early patency rates of 90% or better have been attributed to improved harvesting techniques and the use of postoperative calcium channel blockers to minimize vasospasm.[56] A comparison of conduits used for myocardial revascularization is provided in Table 19-5.

VALVULAR SURGERY

Valvular disease results in various hemodynamic dysfunctions that usually can be managed medically as long as the patient remains symptom-free. There is reluctance to intervene surgically early in the course of this disease because of the surgical risks and long-term complications associated with prosthetic valve replacement.

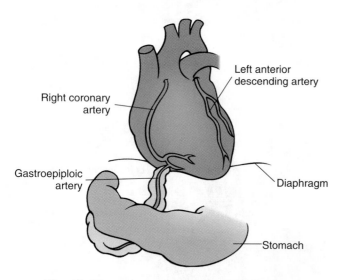

Fig. 19-19 Gastroepiploic artery graft.

These consequences, however, must be weighed against the possibility of irreversible deterioration in left ventricular function that may develop during the compensated asymptomatic phase. (See "Valvular Heart Disease," p. 476.)

Surgical therapy for aortic valve disease is limited at this time to aortic valve replacement (AVR). However, three surgical procedures are available to treat mitral valve disease: commissurotomy, valve repair, and valve replacement. Commissurotomy is performed for mitral stenosis and involves incising fused leaflets and debriding calcium deposits to increase valve mobility. In the setting of mitral regurgitation, valve repair may be attempted, often with the use of a ring to reduce the size of the dilated mitral annulus, thus enhancing leaflet coaptation (annuloplasty). Both forms of valve reconstruction avoid the complications inherent with a prosthetic valve and may obviate the need for long-term anticoagulation.[57] If reconstruction of the mitral valve is not possible, it is replaced (mitral valve replacement [MVR]).

Valvular surgery has an anticipated length of hospital stay from 5 to 9 days. The longer length of stay is for patients who undergo cardiac catheterization in addition to valvular surgery. Prosthetic valves are designed with an orifice, through which blood flows, and an occluding structure that opens and closes. The two categories of prosthetic valves are mechanical valves and biologic valves, or tissue valves. *Mechanical valves* are made from combinations of metal alloys, pyrolite carbon, Dacron, and Teflon and have rigid occluding devices (Fig. 19-20). Their construction renders them highly durable, but all patients with mechanical valves require anticoagulation to reduce the incidence of thromboembolism. *Biologic valves* are constructed from animal or

Table 19-5	Conduits Used for Coronary Artery Bypass Grafts	
Type of Graft	**Advantages**	**Disadvantages**
Saphenous vein	Easily harvested Length allows for multiple grafts No anatomic limitations to graft sites	Long-term patency is not as good as that of arterial grafts Requires at least two anastomosis sites Associated with leg edema postoperatively
Internal mammary artery	Improved patency over venous grafts Only requires one anastomosis	Requires extensive dissection Not accessible for emergency bypass Associated with increased chest-wall discomfort postoperatively Anatomic limitations to bypassing some areas of the heart
Gastroepiploic artery	Improved patency over venous grafts Only requires one anastomosis Associated with increased gastrointestinal complications postoperatively	Technically difficult to harvest Not accessible for emergency bypass Anatomic limitations to bypassing some areas of the heart
Radial artery	Improved patency over venous grafts Easily harvested	Requires adequate collateral flow to hand via ulnar artery May be associated with higher rates of vasospasm Requires two anastomosis sites

human cardiac tissue and have flexible occluding mechanisms. Because of their low thrombogenicity, tissue valves offer the patient freedom from therapeutic anticoagulation. Their durability, however, is limited by their tendency toward early calcification (see Box 19-12 for a description of various valvular prostheses).

The first mechanical valve had a ball-in-cage design. The Starr-Edwards is the only type of this valve still seen today. Later valves used a tilting disk mechanism to occlude blood flow. The Björk-Shiley tilting disk valve was discontinued in the United States because of mechanical failure, but patients with this valve are still alive today. The majority of valves used today have a bi-leaflet design, the first of which was introduced by St. Jude Medical in 1977. One of the primary goals in mechanical valve research is to design a valve that would alleviate the causes of thrombosis—surface roughness, turbulent flow and stagnation in valve pivots. Two of the newest valves on the market, the ATS and On-X valves, offer several new improvements in this area.[58]

The choice of a valvular prosthesis depends on many factors. Because mechanical valves are more durable, for example, they may be chosen over a tissue valve for a young person who is anticipated to have a relatively long life span ahead. Similarly, a bioprosthesis (tissue valve) may be chosen for an elderly patient; the valve has a reduced longevity, but this disadvantage is offset by the older patient's decreased life expectancy.[47] For patients with medical contraindications to anticoagulation or for patients whose past compliance with drug therapy has been questionable, a tissue valve is generally selected. Technical considerations, such as the size of the annulus (or the anatomic ring in which the valve sits), also can influence the choice of valve (a bioprosthesis may be too big for a small aortic root).

CARDIOPULMONARY BYPASS

Cardiopulmonary bypass (CPB) is a mechanical means of circulating and oxygenating a patient's blood while di-

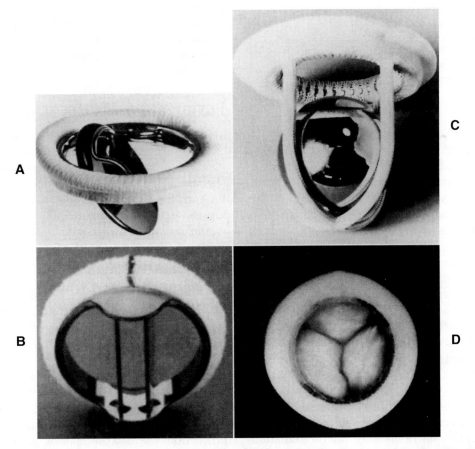

Fig. 19-20 Prosthetic valves. **A,** The Björk-Shiley tilting-disk valve with pyrolytic-carbon disk, Stellite cage, and Teflon cloth sewing ring. The valve opens to 60 degrees. **B,** The Starr-Edwards caged-ball valve model 6320 with completely cloth-covered Stellite cage and hollow Stellite ball, with specific gravity close to that of blood. **C,** The St. Jude Medical mechanical heart valve, a mechanical-central flow disk. **D,** The Hancock II porcine aortic valve. The flexible Derlin stent and sewing ring are covered in Dacron cloth. (**A, B,** and **D** from Eagle K et al: *The practice of cardiology,* ed 2, Boston, 1989, Little, Brown; **C,** courtesy St Jude Medical, Inc., Copyright 1993, St Paul, Minn.)

CLASSIFICATION OF PROSTHETIC CARDIAC VALVES

MECHANICAL VALVES
Caged-ball: a ball moves freely within a three- or four-sided metallic cage mounted on a circular sewing ring
  • Starr-Edwards
Tilting-disk: a free-floating, lens-shaped disk mounted on a circular sewing ring
  • Björk-Shiley (discontinued)
  • Medtronic Hall
  • Omniscience
  • Monostrut
Bi-leaflet: two semicircular leaflets, mounted on a circular sewing ring that opens centrally
  • St. Jude Medical
  • Duromedics
  • CarboMedics
  • On-X ATS

BIOLOGIC (TISSUE) VALVES (BIOPROSTHESES)
Porcine heterograft: a porcine aortic valve mounted on a semiflexible stent and preserved in glutaraldehyde
  • Hancock
  • Carpentier-Edwards
  • Toronto Stentless (St. Jude)
  • Free Style Stentless (Medtronic)
Homograft: a human heart valve (aortic or pulmonic) harvested from a donated heart and cryopreserved; may or may not be mounted on a support ring

verting most of the circulation from the heart and lungs during cardiac surgical procedures. The extracorporeal circuit consists of cannulas that drain off venous blood, an oxygenator that oxygenates the blood by one of several methods, and a pump head that pumps the arterialized blood back to the aorta through a single cannula. The patient is systemically heparinized before initiation of bypass to prevent clotting within the bypass circuit.

Systemic hypothermia during bypass can reduce tissue oxygen requirements to 50% of normal, which affords the major organs additional protection from ischemic injury. Lowering the body temperature to about 28° C (82.4° F) is accomplished through a heat exchanger incorporated into the pump. The blood is warmed back up to normal body temperature before bypass is discontinued.

The technique of hemodilution also is used to enhance tissue oxygenation by improving blood flow through the systemic and pulmonary microcirculation during bypass. *Hemodilution* refers to the dilution of autologous (patient's own) blood with the isotonic crystalloid solution used to prime the pump. Capillary perfusion is enhanced by hemodilution, because the reduced viscosity (stickiness) of the blood decreases both resistance to flow through the capillaries and the possibility

of microthrombi formation. At the completion of CPB, the large quantities of "pump blood" that remain in the bypass circuit can be collected and used for initial postoperative volume replacement.

In response to findings that the low cardiac output syndrome often seen postoperatively might be a result of intraoperative myocardial ischemia or necrosis, efforts have been directed toward providing additional protection to the myocardium during bypass. Rapidly stopping the heart in diastole by perfusing the coronary arteries with a cold potassium cardioplegic ("heart-paralyzing") agent has been the method of choice for intraoperative myocardial protection. Continued research in this area has resulted in the emergence of blood as a vehicle for the cardioplegic components to enhance the supply of oxygen and nutrients to the arrested myocardial cells.[59] Warm (normothermic) cardioplegia is also being investigated and is believed by some to result in less ventricular dysfunction postoperatively.[60] Regardless of the type of cardioplegic solution used, it must be reinfused at regular intervals during bypass to keep the heart in an arrested state and to minimize myocardial oxygen requirements.

Numerous clinical sequelae can result from CPB (Table 19-6). Knowledge of these physiologic effects allows the nurse to anticipate problems and intervene effectively.

POSTOPERATIVE MANAGEMENT

Medical and nursing management of the postoperative cardiac surgery patient are often overlapping. The physician prescribes therapeutic interventions and identifies specific hemodynamic endpoints that are individualized for each patient. The nurse is then responsible for applying these therapies to maintain the patient's hemodynamic parameters within the desired range. For example, orders may be written to maintain the patient's blood pressure, filling pressures, cardiac output, and systemic vascular resistance within a desired range, using a combination of volume, vasodilator, and inotropic infusions. In most institutions, standard protocols are used to facilitate the postoperative nursing diagnoses and management of cardiac surgical patients (see the Nursing Diagnoses feature on Status Post Open Heart Surgery).

Cardiovascular Support. Postoperative cardiovascular support often is indicated because of a low output state resulting from preexisting heart disease, a prolonged CPB pump run, and/or inadequate myocardial protection. Cardiac output can be maximized by adjustments in heart rate, preload, afterload, and contractility.

Heart Rate. In the presence of low cardiac output, the heart rate can be appropriately regulated by means of temporary pacing or drug therapy. Temporary epicardial pacing usually is instituted when the heart rate of the adult patient who has had cardiac surgery drops to

Table 19-6	Physiologic Effects of Cardiopulmonary Bypass (CPB)
Effects	**Causes**
Intravascular fluid deficit (hypotension)	Third spacing Postoperative diuresis Sudden vasodilation (drugs, rewarming)
Third spacing (weight gain, edema)	Decreased plasma protein concentration Increased capillary permeability
Myocardial depression (decreased cardiac output)	Hypothermia Increased systemic vascular resistance Prolonged CPB pump run Preexisting heart disease Inadequate myocardial protection
Coagulopathy (bleeding)	Systemic heparinization Mechanical trauma to platelets Depressed release of clotting factors from liver as a result of hypothermia
Pulmonary dysfunction (decreased lung mechanics and impaired gas exchange)	Decreased surfactant production Pulmonary microemboli Interstitial fluid accumulation in lungs
Hemolysis (hemoglobinuria)	Red blood cells damaged in pump circuit
Hyperglycemia (rise in serum glucose)	Decreased insulin release Stimulation of glycogenolysis
Hypokalemia (low serum potassium)	Intracellular shifts during bypass and postoperative diuresis
Hypomagnesemia (low serum magnesium)	Postoperative diuresis secondary to hemodilution
Neurologic dysfunction (decreased level of consciousness, motor/sensory deficits)	Inadequate cerebral perfusion Microemboli to brain (air, plaque fragments, fat globules)
Hypertension (transient rise in blood pressure)	Catecholamine release and systemic hypothermia causing vasoconstriction

less than 80 beats/min. In the case of tachycardia, intravenous beta-blockers (esmolol) or calcium channel blockers (diltiazem) may be used in the acute postoperative period to slow supraventricular rhythms with a ventricular response that exceeds 110 beats/min. Because ventricular ectopy can result from hypokalemia, serum potassium levels are maintained in the high-normal range (4.5 to 5 mEq/L) to provide some margin for error. Maintaining serum magnesium in a therapeutic range (2 mEq/L) has also been shown to reduce the incidence of dysrhythmias in the postoperative period.[61]

Atrial fibrillation occurs in a third of patients after cardiac surgery, with a peak occurrence in the first 2 to 3 days after surgery. This rhythm may induce hemodynamic compromise, prolong hospitalization, and increase the patient's risk of stroke. Prophylactic administration of antidysrhythmic agents such as beta-blockers has been shown to decrease the incidence of atrial fibrillation and its clinical sequelae.[61]

Preload. In most patients, reduced preload is the cause of low postoperative cardiac output. If a pulmonary artery catheter has been inserted during surgery, monitoring pulmonary artery occlusion pressure (PAOP), also known as the "wedge pressure," can provide a more convenient and accurate guide to left ventricular preload than can monitoring central venous pressure (CVP) alone. To enhance preload, volume may be administered in the form of crystalloid, colloid, or packed red cells. It is not uncommon to achieve the greatest hemodynamic stability in cardiac surgery patients when filling pressures (pulmonary artery diastolic pressure [PADP] or PAOP) are in the range of 18 to 20 mm Hg (normally 5 to 12 mm Hg).

Afterload. Partly as a result of the peripheral vasoconstrictive effects of hypothermia, many patients who have had cardiac surgery demonstrate postoperative hypertension. Although transient, postoperative hypertension can precipitate or exacerbate bleeding from the mediastinal chest tubes. In addition, the high systemic vascular resistance (SVR, or afterload) resulting from the intense vasoconstriction can increase left ventricular workload. Therefore vasodilator therapy with intravenous sodium nitroprusside or nitroglycerin often is used to reduce afterload and thus control hypertension and improve cardiac output.

A small percentage of patients may experience hypotension after cardiopulmonary bypass, associated with peripheral vasodilation and a low SVR. This is believed to be in part because of the systemic inflammatory response that occurs in response to CPB. Therapy for these patients usually includes volume loading and vasopressors such as phenylephrine or vasopressin to tighten the peripheral vasculature and maintain an adequate mean arterial pressure.[62]

NURSING DIAGNOSES **Status Post Open Heart Surgery**

- Decreased Cardiac Output related to alterations in preload
- Decreased Cardiac Output related to alterations in afterload
- Decreased Cardiac Output related to alterations in contractility
- Decreased Cardiac Output related to alterations in heart rate or rhythm
- Impaired Gas Exchange related to ventilation/perfusion mismatching or intrapulmonary shunting
- Ineffective Airway Clearance related to excessive secretions of abnormal viscosity of mucus
- Activity Intolerance related to cardiopulmonary dysfunction
- Deficient Fluid Volume related to absolute loss
- Risk for Infection: invasive procedures
- Acute Pain related to transmission and perception of cutaneous, visceral, muscular, or ischemic impulses
- Anxiety related to threat to biologic, psychologic, and/or social integrity
- Disturbed Sleep Pattern related to fragmented sleep
- Deficient Knowledge: Discharge Regimen related to lack of previous exposure to information (see Patient Education feature on Status After Open Heart Surgery)

Contractility. If these adjustments in heart rate, preload, and afterload fail to produce significant improvement in cardiac output, contractility can be enhanced with positive inotropic support or intraaortic balloon pumping (IABP), thus augmenting circulation (see "Intraaortic Balloon Pump" and "Inotropic Drugs" later in this chapter).

Temperature Regulation. Hypothermia can contribute to depressed myocardial contractility in the patient who has had cardiac surgery. In addition, hypothermia may contribute to postoperative bleeding, because functioning of clotting factors is depressed during hypothermia. After surgery, patients may be rewarmed using warmed air or water blankets. To prevent subsequent excessive temperature elevations, care must be taken to remove the blankets promptly when the body temperature reaches 98.6° F (37° C).

Control of Bleeding. Postoperative bleeding from the mediastinal chest tubes can be caused by inadequate hemostasis, disruption of suture lines, or coagulopathy associated with CPB or hypothermia. Bleeding is more likely to occur with IMA grafts as a result of the extensive chest-wall dissection required to free the IMA. If bleeding in excess of 150 ml/hour occurs early in the postoperative period, clotting factors (fresh-frozen plasma, fibrinogen, and platelets) and additional protamine (used to reverse the effects of heparin) may be administered, along with prompt blood replacement. Other medications used in the treatment of postoperative bleeding are described in the Pharmacologic Management table on Postoperative Bleeding.

In some institutions, autotransfusion devices, which facilitate the collection and reinfusion of shed mediastinal blood, may be used to replace red blood cell loss.[63] A number of chest drainage systems are configured for ei-

Pharmacologic Management: Postoperative Bleeding

DRUG	DOSE	ACTION/SIDE EFFECTS
Amicaproic acid (Amicar)	Loading dose: 5 g over 1 hr, followed by a continuous infusion of 1 g/hr for 8 hr or until bleeding is controlled	Inhibits conversion of plasminogen to plasminogen to plasmin to prevent fibrinolysis, helping to stabilize clots
Desmopressin acetate (DDAVP)	0.3 mg/kg IV over 20-30 min	Improves platelet function by increasing levels of factor VIII Side effects include facial flushing, tachycardia, headache, and hypotension
Protamine sulfate	25-50 mg IV slowly over 10 min	Neutralizes the anticoagulant effect of heparin Can cause hypotension, bradycardia, and allergic reactions

IV, Intravenous.

ther intermittent or continuous autotransfusion. These systems contain a special reservoir section where blood is collected directly from the chest tubes (Fig. 19-21). The accumulated blood is then passed through a microaggregate filter before reinfusion into the patient. Once bleeding slows and autotransfusion is no longer required, the chest tubes are connected directly to the chest tube drainage system (see the Nursing Interventions Classification [NIC] feature on Autotransfusion).

The use of prophylactic positive end-expiratory pressure (PEEP) in conjunction with mechanical ventilation may be helpful in controlling bleeding in some cases by increasing intrathoracic pressure enough to effect tamponade of oozing mediastinal blood vessels. Rewarming the patient reverses the depressed manufacture and release of clotting factors that result from hypothermia. However, persistent mediastinal bleeding—usually in excess of 500 ml in 1 hour or 300 ml/hour for 2 consecutive hours despite normalization of clotting studies—is an indication for reexploration of the surgical site.

Chest Tube Patency. Chest tube stripping to maintain patency of the tubes is controversial because of the

NIC   Autotransfusion

Definition: Collecting and reinfusing blood that has been lost intraoperatively or postoperatively from clean wounds

Activities

Screen for appropriateness of salvage (contraindications include sepsis or infection or tumor at the site, blood containing an irrigant that is not injectable, hemostatic agents, or microcrystalline collagen)
Determine the risk/benefit ratio
Obtain patient's informed consent
Instruct patient regarding procedure
Use appropriate blood retrieval system
Label collection device with the patient's name, hospital number, date, and time that collection was begun
Monitor patient and system frequently during retrieval

Maintain integrity of the system before, during, and after blood retrieval
Screen blood for appropriateness of reinfusion
Maintain integrity of blood between salvage and reinfusion
Prepare blood for reinfusion
Document time of initiation of collecting, condition of blood, type and amount of anticoagulants, and retrieval volume
Reinfuse transfusion within 6 hr of retrieval
Maintain Universal Precautions

From Dochterman TM: *Nursing interventions classification (NIC),* ed 4, St Louis, 2004, Mosby.

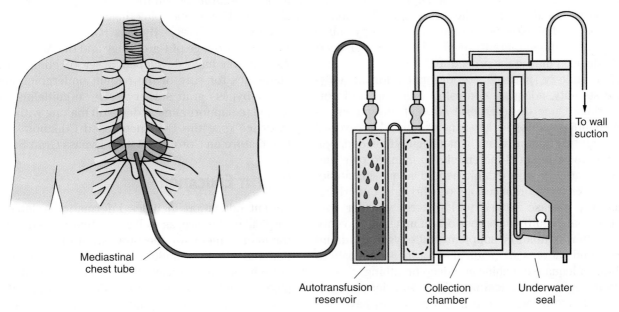

Fig. 19-21   Components of an autotransfusion system.

high negative pressure generated by routine methods of stripping. It is believed to result in tissue damage that can actually contribute to bleeding. This risk, however, must be carefully weighed against the very real danger of cardiac tamponade if blood is not effectively drained from around the heart. Therefore chest tube stripping often is advocated in instances of excessive postoperative bleeding. However, the technique of "milking" the chest tubes is advisable for routine postoperative care, because this technique generates less negative pressure and decreases the risk of bleeding.

Cardiac Tamponade. Cardiac tamponade may occur after surgery if blood accumulates in the mediastinal space, impairing the heart's ability to pump. Signs of tamponade include elevated and equalized filling pressures (CVP, PADP, PAOP), decreased cardiac output, decreased blood pressure, jugular venous distention, pulsus paradoxus, muffled heart sounds, sudden cessation of chest tube drainage, and a widened cardiac silhouette on chest x-ray film. Interventions for tamponade may include emergency sternotomy in the intensive care unit or a return to the operating room for surgical evacuation of the clot.

Pulmonary Care. Until recently, overnight intubation to facilitate lung expansion and optimize gas exchange was common in patients who had cardiac surgery. Newer protocols that facilitate early extubation (within the first 4 to 8 hours) have now been implemented in most institutions.[64,65] Early extubation requires a multidisciplinary approach that incorporates anesthesiologists, surgeons, nurses, and respiratory therapists. Potential candidates must be identified before surgery so that the anesthetic regimen can be modified to support early extubation. One approach is to use short-acting anesthetic agents such as propofol (Diprivan) at the end of the surgery and minimize the use of opioids. Another option is to administer neostigmine and glycopyrrolate at the end of the surgery to reverse the neuromuscular blockade used during the procedure.

After surgery, patients are evaluated for hemodynamic stability, adequate control of bleeding, and normothermia. Once these criteria are met, the patient is weaned off propofol or given neuromuscular reversal agents, and ventilator weaning can begin. If needed, opioids are given in small increments to manage pain and anxiety. Patients who exhibit hemodynamic instability or intraoperative complications or who have underlying pulmonary disease related to long-term valvular dysfunction may require longer periods of mechanical ventilation. After extubation, supplemental oxygen is administered, and patients are medicated for incisional pain to facilitate adequate coughing and deep breathing.

Neurologic Complications. The transient neurologic dysfunction often seen in patients who have had cardiac surgery probably can be attributed to decreased cerebral perfusion and to cerebral microemboli, both related to the CPB pump run. Compounding these are environmental factors, such as sensory deprivation and sensory overload associated with being in a critical care unit. The term *postcardiotomy delirium* has been used to describe this postoperative syndrome that initially may be seen as only a mild impairment of orientation but that may progress to agitation, hallucinations, and paranoid delusions.[66]

Treatment of delirium may require the use of medications such as benzodiazepines or haloperidol (Haldol). In addition, environmental modifications such as noise reduction, restoring normal day/night lighting patterns, and placing familiar objects at the bedside may help to calm and reorient the patient. Liberalizing visitation policies to allow family members a prolonged presence at the bedside is also highly desirable. Nursing management is organized to maximize optimal sleep patterns whenever possible.

Infection. Postoperative fever is fairly common after CPB. However, persistent temperature elevation to more than 101° F (38.3° C) must be investigated. Sternal wound infections and infective endocarditis are the most devastating infectious complications, but leg wound infection, pneumonia, and urinary tract infection also can occur. Infection rates are greater in diabetic patients. Recent studies have shown that maintaining blood glucose between 80 and 110 mg/dl in the perioperative period through a continuous insulin infusion may decrease the risk of infection in this population.[67]

Kidney Involvement. Hemolysis caused by trauma to the red blood cells in the extracorporeal circuit results in hemoglobinuria, which can damage kidney tubules. Therefore small amounts of furosemide (Lasix) usually are given to promote urine flow if the urine output is low (less than 25 to 30 ml/hour) and "pink-tinged."

Coronary Artery Bypass Graft Guidelines. The American College of Cardiology and the American Heart Association have developed a set of clinical practice guidelines for care of the patient undergoing coronary artery bypass graft surgery.[50] These guidelines are designed to support clinical decision making with research evidence (see the Evidence-Based Collaborative Practice feature on Coronary Artery Bypass Graft Surgery).

PATIENT EDUCATION

Patient education includes information related to the surgical procedure, as well as content related to risk factor management for the prevention of atherosclerosis. Patients who have undergone valve surgery may also require information regarding the need for antibiotic prophylaxis before invasive procedures and specifics pertaining to their anticoagulation regimen (see the Patient Education feature on Status Post Open Heart Surgery).

EVIDENCE-BASED COLLABORATIVE PRACTICE

Coronary Artery Bypass Graft Surgery

Summary of Evidence and Evidence-Based Review Recommendations for Management of the CABG Surgery Patient

Strong Evidence To Support the Following:

CABG criteria for stable and unstable angina

- CABG should be performed in patients who have significant left main coronary artery stenosis.
- CABG should be performed in patients who have left main equivalent: significant (greater than or equal to 70%) stenosis of the proximal left anterior descending (LAD) artery and proximal left circumflex artery.
- CABG is useful in patients who have three-vessel disease. Survival benefit is greater in patients with abnormal left ventricular (LV) function; such as when LV ejection fraction (LVEF) is less than 0.50 (50%) and/or there are large areas of demonstrable myocardial ischemia.
- CABG is beneficial for patients with 1- or 2-vessel disease plus extensive ischemia and LVEF less than 0.50 (50%).
- CABG is beneficial for patients with disabling or unstable angina despite maximal noninvasive therapy, when surgery can be performed with acceptable risk. If the angina is not typical, objective evidence of ischemia should be obtained.
- CABG is recommended for unstable angina/non–ST elevation myocardial infarction (NSTEMI) in patients in whom emergency percutaneous coronary intervention (PCI) revascularization is not optimal or possible and who have ongoing ischemia not responsive to maximal nonsurgical therapy.

CABG criteria during ST elevation myocardial infarction

- Emergency or urgent CABG in patients with ST elevation myocardial infarction (STEMI) should be undertaken in the following circumstances:
  1. Failed angioplasty with persistent pain or hemodynamic instability in patients with coronary anatomy suitable for surgery
  2. Persistent or recurrent ischemia refractory to medical therapy in patients who have coronary anatomy suitable for surgery, who have a significant area of myocardium at risk, and who are not candidates for PCI
  3. At the time of surgical repair of postinfarction ventricular septal rupture or mitral valve insufficiency
  4. Cardiogenic shock in patients less than 75 years old with ST-segment elevation or left bundle-branch block or posterior MI who develop shock within 36 hours of MI and are suitable for revascularization that can be performed within 18 hours of shock, unless further support is futile because of the patient's wishes or contraindications/unsuitability for further invasive care

CABG criteria with life-threatening ventricular dysrhythmias

- Life-threatening ventricular dysrhythmias in the presence of greater than or equal to 50% left main stenosis and/or 3-vessel coronary disease.

CABG plus valve surgery criteria

- Patients undergoing CABG who also have severe aortic stenosis (AS) should undergo aortic valve replacement (AVR). Severe AS is measured by a mean gradient greater than or equal to 50 mm Hg or Doppler velocity greater than or equal to 4 meters per second.

Reduction in intraoperative complications

- Significant atherosclerosis of the ascending aorta mandates a surgical approach that will minimize the possibility of arteriosclerotic emboli and stroke.
- Blood cardioplegia should be considered in patients undergoing cardiopulmonary bypass (CPB) accompanying coronary artery bypass graft (CABG) surgery for acute myocardial infarction (MI) or unstable angina.
- In every patient undergoing CABG, the left internal mammary artery (IMA) should be given primary consideration for revascularization of the left anterior descending (LAD) artery.

Transmyocardial revascularization

- Transmyocardial surgical laser revascularization, either alone or in combination with CABG surgery, is reasonable in patients with angina refractory to medical therapy who are not candidates for PCI or surgical revascularization.

Reduction in risk of infection

- Preoperative antibiotic administration should be used in all patients to reduce the risk of postoperative infection.
- A deep sternal wound infection should be treated with aggressive surgical debridement and early revascularized muscle flap coverage, unless there are complicating circumstances.

Prevention of postoperative dysrhythmias

- Preoperative or early postoperative administration of beta-blockers in patients without contraindications should be used as the standard therapy to reduce the incidence and/or clinical sequelae of atrial fibrillation after CABG surgery.

Antiplatelet therapy

- Aspirin is the drug of choice for prophylaxis against early saphenous vein graft (SVG) closure.
- If clinical circumstances permit, clopidogrel should be withheld for 5 days before the performance of CABG surgery.

Pharmacologic management of hyperlipidemia

- All CABG surgery patients should receive statin therapy unless otherwise contraindicated.

---

1. Eagle A et al; ACC/AHA 2004 guideline update for coronary artery bypass graft surgery: a report of the American College of Cardiology/American Heart Association Task Force on Practice Guidelines (Committee to Update the 1999 Guidelines for Coronary Artery Bypass Graft Surgery), *Circulation* 110(14:):e340-437, 2004.

Continued

Smoking cessation is important

- All smokers should receive educational counseling and be offered smoking cessation therapy after CABG surgery.
- Pharmacologic therapy including nicotine replacement and bupropion (in select patients) should be offered to patients indicating a willingness to quit.

Cardiac rehabilitation is beneficial

- Cardiac rehabilitation should be offered to all eligible patients after CABG.

Moderate Evidence to Support the Following:

Assessment of preoperative risk

- Preoperative statistical risk models may be used to obtain objective estimates of cardiac surgical operative mortality.
- After myocardial infarction that leads to clinically significant right ventricular dysfunction, it is reasonable to delay surgery for 4 weeks to allow recovery.

CABG risk-benefit analysis for stable and unstable angina

- CABG can be beneficial for patients who have proximal or nonproximal LAD stenosis with 1- or 2-vessel disease. Decision depends on extent of ischemia and LVEF (see section on *strong evidence* above).

CABG during ST elevation myocardial infarction

- CABG may be performed as primary reperfusion in patients who have suitable anatomy, who are not candidates for or who have had failed fibrinolysis or PCI, and who are not in the early hours (6 to 12 hours) of evolving STEMI. In patients who have had a STEMI or an NSTEMI, CABG mortality is elevated for the first 3 to 7 days after infarction, and the benefit of revascularization must be balanced against this increased risk. Beyond 7 days after infarction, the revascularization criteria described in *strong evidence* section is applicable.

CABG Plus Valve Surgery Criteria

- For patients with a preoperative diagnosis of clinically significant mitral regurgitation (MR), concomitant mitral valve repair or replacement at the time of CABG is probably indicated.
- For patients undergoing CABG who have moderate aortic stenosis (AS), concomitant aortic valve replacement (AVR) is probably indicated. Moderate AS is measured by a mean transvalve gradient of 30 to 50 mm Hg or Doppler velocity 3 to 4 meters per second.
- Patients undergoing CABG who have mild AS may be considered candidates for AVR if the risk of the combined procedure is acceptable. Mild AS is measured by mean gradient less than 30 mm Hg or Doppler velocity less than 3 meters per second.

Reduction in risk of thrombus formation

- Following cardiac surgery, patients with atrial fibrillation that is recurrent or that persists more than 24 hours should receive warfarin anticoagulation for 4 weeks.
- Long-term (3 to 6 months) anticoagulation is indicated for the patient with recent anteroapical infarct and persistent wall-motion abnormality after CABG surgery.
- Preoperative screening with echocardiography is considered for patients who have had a recent anterior MI to detect left ventricular thrombus; if present, the timing or surgical approach may be altered.

Reduction in Risk of Carotid Disease and Stroke

- Carotid endarterectomy is probably indicated before CABG surgery or concomitant to CABG, in patients with a symptomatic carotid stenosis or in asymptomatic patients with a unilateral or bilateral internal carotid stenosis of 80% or more.
- Carotid screening is probably indicated in the following subsets: age greater than 65 years, left main coronary stenosis, peripheral arterial disease, history of smoking, history of transient ischemic attack or stroke, or carotid bruit on examination.

Cardiac Biomarker Elevation and Outcome

- Assessment of cardiac biomarkers in the first 24 hours after CABG may be considered. Patients with the highest elevations of creatine kinase-MB (greater than 5 times upper limits of normal) are at increased risk of subsequent events.

Adjuncts to Myocardial Protection

- Use of prophylactic intraaortic balloon pump (IABP) support as an adjunct to myocardial protection is probably indicated in patients with evidence of ongoing myocardial ischemia and/or patients with a subnormal cardiac index.

Reduction in risk of infection

- Risk for deep sternal wound infection is reduced by aggressive control of perioperative hyperglycemia with a continuous, intravenous insulin infusion.

Prevention of postoperative dysrhythmias

- Preoperative administration of amiodarone reduces the incidence of postcardiotomy atrial fibrillation and is an appropriate prophylactic therapy for patients at high risk for postoperative atrial fibrillation who have contraindications to therapy with beta-blockers (refer to *strong evidence* section above).
- Digoxin and nondihydropyridine calcium channel blockers are useful for control of ventricular rate but at present have no indication for prophylactic use.
- Low-dose sotalol can be considered to reduce the incidence of atrial fibrillation after CABG in patients who are not candidates for traditional beta-blockers.

Very Little or no Evidence To Support the Following:

Hormonal replacement therapy

- Initiation of hormone replacement therapy (HRT) is not recommended for women undergoing CABG surgery.

CABG not recommended for stable angina without significant coronary arterial disease

- CABG is not recommended for patients with stable angina who have borderline 1- or 2-vessel disease (50%-60% occlusion), not involving left main, or proximal LAD; patients who have mild symptoms that are unlikely due to myocardial ischemia; patients who have not received an adequate trial of medical therapy; patients who have only a small area of viable myocardium; or patients who have no demonstrable ischemia on noninvasive testing.

Coronary Artery Bypass Graft Surgery—cont'd

CABG during ST elevation myocardial infarction
- Emergency CABG should not be performed in patients with persistent angina and a small area of myocardium at risk who are hemodynamically stable or when successful epicardial reperfusion but unsuccessful microvascular reperfusion would result.

CABG and poor LV function risk-benefit analysis
- CABG should not be performed in patients with poor LV function without evidence of intermittent ischemia and without evidence of significant revascularizable viable myocardium.

CABG and life-threatening ventricular dysrhythmias
- CABG is not recommended in ventricular tachycardia with myocardial scarring and no evidence of ischemia.

PATIENT EDUCATION

Status Post Open Heart Surgery

- Pathophysiology of disease (either coronary artery or valvular disease)
- Risk factor modification to prevent CAD (smoking cessation, regular exercise, weight loss)
- Postoperative incisional care
- Activity limitations (no lifting, pushing, or pulling of anything >10 lb for 6-8 weeks; no driving for 6-8 weeks)
- Recommended exercise progression after surgery
- Recommended diet after surgery
- Information regarding prescribed medications (including prescribed pain medication)
- Anticipated mood changes after surgery
- Follow-up appointment for clinic or primary physician
- Additional information for valve patients:
  Symptoms of endocarditis
  Antibiotic prophylaxis before invasive procedures
  Information regarding anticoagulant therapy and follow-up

RECENT ADVANCES

Surgical Treatment of Cardiac Dysrhythmias. The increasing success of radiofrequency ablation has limited the use of surgery for intractable supraventricular and ventricular tachydysrhythmias. If catheter ablation of the dysrhythmia is not feasible or has proved ineffective, the patient may be evaluated for surgical treatment. During surgery the origin of the dysrhythmia first is localized with specialized pacing electrodes (referred to as *intraoperative mapping*). The offending area of myocardium is then either excised or eliminated by cryosurgery (freezing) or laser. This procedure is most successful in patients who have an organized type of tachydysrhythmia originating from a defined area, such as a scar or aneurysm.[68]

The *maze procedure* is a surgical intervention for patients with atrial fibrillation or atrial flutter that has not responded to medical therapy. A series of cuts is made in the atrial tissue to create an electrical maze that disrupts the re-entrant pathways and directs the sinus impulse through the AV node.[69] The goal of treatment is not only to prevent the recurrence of atrial tachydysrhythmias but also to restore sinus rhythm and AV synchrony, if possible. If the sinus node is no longer functioning, a pacemaker may be implanted to restore an AV sequential rhythm. Initial success rates for the maze procedure have been promising, and research is now focused on the development of specialized ablation catheters to facilitate a less invasive approach to this procedure.[70,71]

Minimally Invasive Cardiac Surgery. Over the past decade, new techniques have been developed to address some of the problems associated with traditional cardiac surgery procedures. Most of these procedures are accomplished without a median sternotomy, using a series of holes or "ports" in the chest and/or small thoracotomy incisions. CABG or valve surgery can then be performed using a thoracoscope for visualization and specially designed instruments.[57] These procedures may be performed without cardiopulmonary bypass ("off-pump" or "beating heart") or with a less invasive, catheter-based system of cardiopulmonary bypass with access via the femoral artery and vein.[72]

A variety of incisional approaches can be used for "beating heart" surgery. In minimally invasive direct coronary artery bypass graft (MIDCABG) surgery, a small left anterior thoracotomy incision is used to directly harvest the left internal mammary artery (LIMA), which is then anastomosed to the left anterior descending artery. Alternative approaches may use a segment of saphenous vein or radial artery, one end of which is attached to the LIMA and the other to accessible coronary arteries.[72] Some surgeons may opt for a standard median sternotomy approach to allow for bypassing distal vessels.

Several techniques are used to stabilize the operative area during a beating heart procedure. A number of immobilization devices have been developed to stabilize cardiac wall motion at the site of the anastomosis. In addition, drugs that temporarily decrease the heart rate (such as esmolol or diltiazem) or cause transient cardiac asystole (such as adenosine) may also be used to further limit cardiac motion.[72]

These minimally invasive techniques have been applied to two different groups of patients: low-risk patients with single anterior lesions or uncomplicated valve repair; and high-risk patients who are not candidates for conventional bypass. Results from minimally invasive surgery have been encouraging, with advantages including decreased neurologic, renal, and pulmonary complications, shorter length of critical care unit and hospital stays, and decreased cost.[73] Studies comparing off-pump surgery with conventional surgery have shown comparable graft patency and similar or less surgical morbidity with off-pump procedures.[74,75] Minimally invasive procedures will continue to be refined with the advent of robotic equipment for use in cardiac surgery, currently under clinical investigation at a small number of centers. Robotic-assisted surgery allows for viewing of a computer-enhanced image while manipulating instruments via small portholes, using robotic arms that are controlled by the surgeon.[76]

Transmyocardial revascularization (TMR) is an investigational procedure for patients with severe CAD that is not amenable to traditional revascularization procedures.[77] In this procedure a laser is used to create full-thickness channels in the ventricular wall to increase blood flow to ischemic areas. This allows the myocardium to be perfused with oxygenated blood directly from the ventricular cavity. TMR is performed in an effort to improve myocardial oxygenation, thus reducing angina and improving the patient's functional status.

The surgical version of this procedure involves an anterolateral thoracotomy for exposure of the left ventricle. The procedure is performed on a beating heart without the use of cardiopulmonary bypass. Approximately 20 to 40 channels are created in the myocardial wall, with laser bursts timed to occur when the ventricle is full of blood. Bleeding is controlled with manual pressure at the laser site. The procedure is performed under general anesthesia. After surgery, patients are monitored in the critical care unit to allow for detection and treatment of dysrhythmias, myocardial ischemia, and bleeding.[77]

In clinical trials, TMR has been strongly correlated with improvement in anginal symptoms and improved activity tolerance when compared with maximal medical therapy, although there was no change in mortality.[78] TMR has also been shown to be a useful adjunct to cardiac surgery for patients in whom complete surgical revascularization is not feasible.[79]

Although future trends in the surgical management of cardiac disease are difficult to predict, the critical care nurse must continue to be prepared to meet the challenge of providing a high level of nursing management at the bedside. A solid knowledge base and keen assessment skills are prerequisites for the accurate anticipation of problems and prompt intervention necessary to stabilize the patient and prevent the occurrence of life-threatening complications.

MECHANICAL CIRCULATORY ASSIST DEVICES

Mechanical circulatory assist devices are used in the treatment of heart failure when conventional pharmacologic therapy has proved ineffective. The primary goals of mechanical assist devices are to decrease myocardial workload and maintain adequate perfusion to vital organs. If the cardiac failure is reversible, a short duration of ventricular assistance is used to allow the myocardium time to recover. If the condition is irreversible, a mechanical assist device may be used as a bridge to transplant for qualified candidates or as a destination therapy in those who have no other surgical options. (See "Heart Transplantation," p. 1098.)

INTRAAORTIC BALLOON PUMP

The intraaortic balloon pump (IABP) currently is the most widely used temporary mechanical circulatory assist device for supporting failing circulation (Box 19-13). Its therapeutic effects are based on the hemodynamic principles of diastolic augmentation and afterload reduction.

The most commonly used intraaortic balloon (IAB) catheter consists of a single, sausage-shaped polyurethane balloon that is wrapped around the distal end of a vascular catheter and positioned in the descending thoracic aorta just distal to the takeoff of the left subclavian artery. The second generation of IAB catheters are more

---

Box 19-13

INDICATIONS FOR THE USE OF INTRAAORTIC BALLOON PUMP

- Left ventricular failure after cardiac surgery
- Unstable angina refractory to medications
- Recurrent angina after acute MI
- Complications of acute MI
  Cardiogenic shock
  Papillary muscle dysfunction/rupture with mitral regurgitation
  Ventricular septal rupture
  Refractory ventricular dysrhythmias

MI, Myocardial infarction.

flexible and can be wrapped to a smaller diameter than its predecessors and therefore can be inserted into the femoral artery percutaneously rather than surgically. When attached to a bedside pumping console and properly synchronized to the patient's cardiac cycle, the intraaortic balloon inflates during diastole and deflates just before systole.

Initially, as the balloon is inflated in diastole concurrent with aortic valve closure, the blood in the aortic arch above the level of the balloon is displaced retrograde (backward) toward the aortic root, augmenting diastolic coronary arterial blood flow and increasing myocardial oxygen supply (Fig. 19-22, *A*). The blood volume in the aorta below the level of the balloon is propelled forward toward the peripheral vascular system, which may enhance renal perfusion. Subsequently, the deflation of the balloon just before the opening of the aortic valve creates a potential space or vacuum in the aorta, toward which blood flows unimpeded during ventricular ejection (Fig. 19-22, *B*). This decreased resistance to left ventricular ejection, or decreased afterload, facilitates ventricular emptying and reduces myocardial oxygen demands. The overall physiologic effect of IABP therapy is an improvement in the balance between myocardial oxygen supply and demand.[80] Contraindications to balloon pumping include aortic aneurysm, aortic valve insufficiency, and severe peripheral vascular disease.

Medical Management. The intraaortic balloon may be inserted in the operating room, the cardiac catheterization laboratory, or the critical care unit. The IAB catheter is usually inserted percutaneously through the femoral artery and advanced to the correct position in the descending thoracic aorta. The physician may insert the balloon through an introducer sheath or perform a sheathless insertion to minimize the degree of vessel occlusion created by the catheter. If percutaneous catheter placement is not feasible, the catheter may be placed via surgical cutdown or a direct thoracic approach. After insertion, the balloon is attached to the console and filled with the prescribed volume of helium, and pumping is initiated. If the balloon fails to unwrap completely during filling, the physician may rapidly inflate and deflate the balloon manually, using a syringe.

Nursing Management. The management of the pumping console and its timing functions may be performed by the nurse caring for the patient or delegated to specially trained personnel on the unit. In either situation, several important nursing diagnoses and management responsibilities relate to the management of the patient receiving IABP therapy (see the Nursing Diagnoses feature on Intraaortic Balloon Pump [IABP]).

Dysrhythmias. The ECG and arterial pressure tracing are constantly monitored to verify the timing and effect of balloon counterpulsations (Fig. 19-23). For coun-

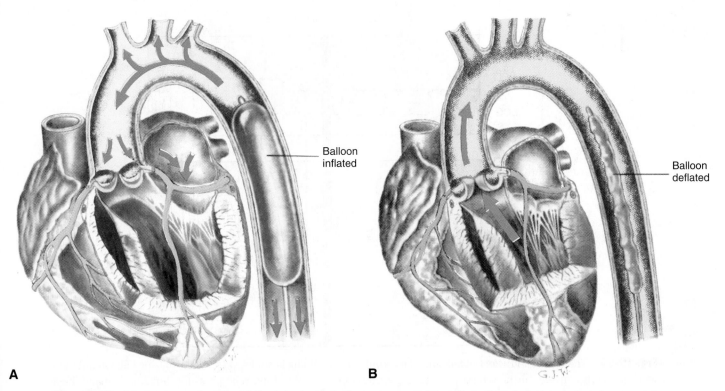

Fig. 19-22 Mechanisms of action of the intraaortic balloon pump. **A,** Diastolic balloon inflation augments coronary blood flow. **B,** Systolic balloon deflation decreases afterload.

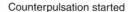

NURSING DIAGNOSES

Intraaortic Balloon Pump

- Decreased Cardiac Output related to alterations in preload
- Decreased Cardiac Output related to alterations in afterload
- Decreased Cardiac Output related to alterations in contractility
- Decreased Cardiac Output related to alterations in heart rate or rhythm
- Activity Intolerance related to cardiopulmonary dysfunction
- Ineffective Cardiopulmonary Tissue Perfusion related to acute myocardial ischemia
- Ineffective Peripheral Tissue Perfusion related to decreased peripheral blood flow
- Risk for Infection risk factor: invasive procedures
- Disturbed Sleep Pattern related to circadian desynchronization
- Disturbed Body Image related to functional dependence on life-sustaining technology
- Deficient Knowledge: Discharge Regimen related to lack of previous exposure to information (see Patient Education feature on Intraaortic Balloon Pump)

terpulsation to occur, the pump must receive a trigger signal to identify the beginning of a new cardiac cycle. The trigger can be the R wave of the ECG, the upstroke of the arterial pressure waveform, or a pacemaker spike.[80] Dysrhythmias can adversely affect the timing of balloon inflation and deflation; thus rhythm disturbances must be detected and treated promptly. Current balloon pumps have automatic timing features that use internal algorithms to adjust inflation and deflation in response to changes in the patient's heart rate or rhythm. Mean arterial pressure is ideally maintained at about 80 mm Hg with adequate pumping.

Peripheral Ischemia. The most common complication of IABP support is lower extremity ischemia secondary to occlusion of the femoral artery, either by the catheter itself or by emboli from thrombus formation on the balloon.[81] While ischemic complications have decreased with sheathless insertion techniques and the introduction of smaller balloon catheters (8.0 Fr vs. 9.5 Fr.), evaluation of peripheral circulation remains an important nursing assessment.[82] Consequently, the presence and quality of peripheral pulses distal to the catheter insertion site are assessed frequently, along with color, temperature, and capillary refill of the involved extremity. Doppler localization of peripheral pulses may be required if pulses are difficult to palpate on the cannulated extremity. Signs of diminished perfusion must be reported immediately. Anticoagulation such as a heparin infusion may be prescribed to de-

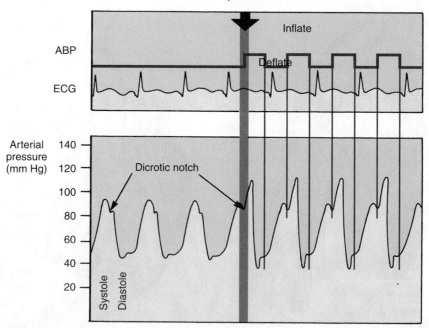

Fig. 19-23 The timing and effect of balloon counterpulsations. Timing is adjusted by synchronizing balloon inflation with the dicrotic notch on the arterial waveform, resulting in an elevated diastolic pressure. Inflation is maintained throughout diastole to augment coronary perfusion. Deflation occurs just before the next systole, resulting in a reduced systolic pressure and decreased afterload. (From Guzzetta CE, Dossey BM: *Cardiovascular nursing: holistic practice*, St Louis, 1992, Mosby.)

crease the incidence of thrombosis. Other vascular complications associated with IABP include acute aortic dissection and the development of pseudoaneurysms at the catheter insertion site.

Balloon Perforation. Another potential complication of IAB therapy is balloon perforation. Perforation occurs secondary to repeated contact of the balloon membrane with calcified plaque in the aorta as the balloon inflates and deflates. The patient is monitored for evidence of a balloon leak, such as a gas leak alarm from the pump console and the presence of blood in the IAB tubing. If a balloon leak is detected, pumping is stopped and the physician immediately notified so that the balloon can be removed. If the balloon is not promptly removed or pumping is attempted after the perforation, the IAB may become entrapped as the blood hardens within the catheter, creating a mass. If this occurs, the balloon must be surgically removed.

Balloon Catheter Position. The balloon catheter must be maintained in proper position to optimize its effectiveness and minimize complications. The balloon may migrate proximally and occlude the left subclavian artery, or it may move distally, compromising renal circulation. Therefore careful assessment of the left radial pulse and urinary output is essential. Measures to prevent accidental displacement of the balloon catheter include ensuring that the patient observes complete bed rest, with the head of the bed elevated no more than 30 degrees, and avoids any flexion of the involved hip.

Preventing Complications. Log rolling, in which the patient is moved from side to side every 2 hours, is used to maintain skin integrity and to prevent pulmonary atelectasis. Some institutional protocols call for implementation of continuous lateral rotation therapy to help facilitate pulmonary toilet in the patient with an IAB. Because thrombocytopenia may occur as a result of mechanical destruction of the platelets by the pumping action of the balloon, platelet counts are closely monitored and the patient is observed for evidence of bleeding. Because infection of the insertion site is a potential complication, the IAB dressing is changed in accordance with the hospital policy for other invasive lines.

Psychologic Needs. Finally, the psychologic needs of the patient must not be overlooked. Sleep deprivation is not at all uncommon, partly caused by the continuous nursing management requirements for the patient but also related to the noise level in the unit, including the sounds made by the balloon pumping device. In addition, anxiety related to fear of not recovering and loss of control because of forced immobility are common occurrences. Pharmacologic agents such as midazolam (Versed) may be used to decrease patient anxiety and promote rest.

IABP Weaning. Weaning from the balloon pump is considered when hemodynamic stability has been achieved with no, or only minimal, pharmacologic support. One weaning procedure consists of slowly decreasing the pumping frequency from every beat to every eighth beat, as tolerated.[80] To prevent thrombus formation on the balloon surface, the IABP must remain at a minimal pumping ratio (or volume) until its removal.

Patient Education. Patient education for the patient with an IAB is presented in the Patient Education feature on Intraaortic Balloon Pump (IABP). Many of the IABP manufacturers provide helpful educational booklets designed for patients and families.

VENTRICULAR ASSIST DEVICES

The ventricular assist device (VAD) is designed to support a failing natural heart with flow assistance. Diversion of varying amounts of systemic blood flow around a failing ventricle by means of a pump reduces cardiac workload while maintaining adequate perfusion to sustain end-organ function. VADs can be used to support a failing right ventricle, left ventricle, or both.[83]

Ventricular assist devices are currently indicated for three types of clinical applications. The first category of patients includes those who, despite aggressive medical therapy, continue to demonstrate persistent cardiac failure but who have the potential for regaining normal heart function if the heart is given time to rest. This category, termed *bridge to recovery*, consists of patients who have acute postsurgical myocardial dysfunction, are in refractory cardiogenic shock after acute MI, or have acute viral myocarditis. The second category, termed *bridge to transplant*, includes those patients with decompensated chronic heart failure who need circulatory support until heart transplantation can be performed. The third category, termed *destination therapy*, was only recently approved by the FDA. These are severe heart failure patients who are not transplant candidates, for whom the VAD may provide improved survival and quality of life.[84]

There are currently five FDA-approved ventricular assist devices.[85] All consist of a pumping chamber, cannula, and some type of power source.[86] Device selection is based on individual VAD capabilities and institutional preference (Table 19-7). External VADs are used primar-

---

PATIENT EDUCATION   **Intraaortic Balloon Pump**

- Description of the IABP and how it works
- Activity restrictions (minimize leg movement)
- Symptoms to report to the health care professional (pain in the back, leg, chest)

Table 19-7	Ventricular Assist Devices	
Type	**Indications**	**Description**
EXTERNAL		
Abiomed BVS 5000	Short-term univentricular or biventricular support	A two-chamber pump connected to the patient via tubing The pumps contain bladders that fill by gravity and trigger ejection when they are full. They are mounted on an IV pole and positioned at a level relative to the patient. Systemic anticoagulation is required.
Thoratec	Short-term univentricular or bi-ventricular support	A pneumatically driven pump that contains a plastic blood sac and two mechanical valves The device senses when the sac is full and triggers the ejection of blood. The pump is located on the patient's abdomen and connected to a large console, which limits mobility. Systemic anticoagulation is required.
IMPLANTABLE		
Heartmate IP	Long-term left-ventricular support as bridge to transplant	A pneumatically driven pump that is implanted in the abdomen and contains two porcine valves Textured surfaces in the blood chamber promote an endothelial lining, so patients may be maintained on aspirin. The pump is attached to an external console that rests on a wheeled cart and has limited battery capabilities.
Heartmate VE	Long-term left-ventricular support as bridge to transplant or destination therapy	An electrically driven pump that is implanted in the abdomen and contains two porcine valves Textured surfaces (as above) allow patients to be maintained on aspirin. The pump is connected to a direct power source via a cable and may be operated by battery for 6-8 hours.
Novacor LVAS	Long-term left-ventricular support as bridge to transplant. Under investigation for destination therapy	An electrically driven pulsatile pump implanted in the upper abdomen A percutaneous driveline connects to an external controller and can operate on battery for short periods of time (4 hours). Systemic anticoagulation is required.

ily for short-term support, while smaller implantable VADS are used for long-term therapy. The left ventricular assist device (LVAD) is used most commonly because left ventricular (LV) failure occurs more often than does right ventricular (RV) failure. Use of biventricular support (bi-VAD) may be needed in the acute phase, because RV failure often follows LV failure. Outflow cannulas that divert blood from the heart to the LVAD for LV support are surgically placed in either the left atrium or the LV apex, depending on the indication for the device. For example, if the patient is "pending recovery" of the natural heart, preservation of LV function mandates left atrial cannulation. The right atrium is cannulated for outflow for RV support. Inflow back to the heart from the pump is accomplished by cannulation of the aorta or femoral artery for the LVAD and pulmonary artery for the right ventricular assist device (RVAD) (see Fig. 19-24 for cannula placement in bi-VAD configuration of the Abiomed pump). Flow rates between 1 and 6 L/min are used to maintain adequate cardiac output while decreasing ventricular workload.

Nursing Management. Nursing diagnosis and management for a patient with a VAD include monitoring for hemodynamic changes as well as for complications related to the device (see the Nursing Diagnoses feature on Ventricular Assist Device [VAD]). The same interventions to optimize cardiac output by manipulation of heart rate, preload, afterload, and contractility that are used with cardiac surgery patients apply to patients with a VAD. Adequate filling volumes are required to maintain pump flow. Afterload reduction may be needed to improve output from the unassisted ventricle when univentricular support is used. Complications common to all types of VADs include bleeding, infection, thromboembolism, and device failure, although rates of complications vary among the different models.[85]

Device Failure. Because of the life-saving nature of this therapy, device failure is a life-threatening event. Because VAD designs vary considerably, troubleshooting methods for device failure are unique to each device. The nurse must be aware of signs of device malfunction

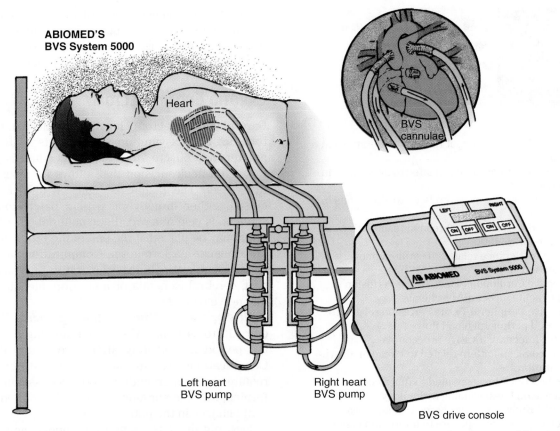

ABIOMED'S
BVS System 5000

Heart

BVS
cannulae

LEFT   RIGHT
ON OFF   ON OFF

AB ABIOMED   BVS System 5000

Left heart
BVS pump

Right heart
BVS pump

BVS drive console

Fig. 19-24   Diagram of a bi-ventricular support (BVS) system. (Courtesy Abiomed, Inc, Danvers, Mass.)

as well patient factors (volume status, dysrhythmias, RV failure) that may affect VAD function.

Anticoagulation. The requirement for anticoagulation varies with the type of VAD, the flow rate, and institutional protocol. If patients are anticoagulated with heparin, nurses are responsible for maintaining the activated clotting time (ACT) within a therapeutic range and monitoring for complications of bleeding. If bleeding occurs, additional coagulation studies such as activated partial thromboplastin time (aPTT), prothrombin time (PT), International Normalized Ratio (INR), and fibrinogen and platelet counts may be performed. Continued bleeding may necessitate holding the heparin infusion and administering fresh-frozen plasma and platelets. If patients are not anticoagulated, the risk of thrombi obstructing a VAD cannula increases, as does the risk of an embolic event.

Infection. Patients with a VAD are at considerable risk for infection. The most common infection is pneumonia secondary to immobility and the need for ventilatory support. Other infectious risks are posed by the presence of invasive catheters and the surgically implanted VAD. Infection is prevented by using strict aseptic technique with all invasive tubing and dressing changes. Site care varies, depending on institutional protocols and the type of VAD that is used. Nurses monitor patients for infection by obtaining temperatures, in-

specting insertion sites and incisions, and following daily leukocyte counts. If an infection is suspected, pancultures (blood, urine, and sputum) are taken to guide appropriate antibiotic therapy.

Weaning. Weaning is accomplished by gradually decreasing flow rates to allow the patient's ventricle to contribute more to total blood flow. Controversy exists with regard to anticoagulation; however, during weaning of VAD flow rates to less than 2 L/min, ACTs are maintained between 160 and 480 seconds with heparin, depending on institutional protocols. This minimizes the potential for thrombus formation in the extracorporeal circuit during weaning but also increases the risk of bleeding and therefore necessitates close monitoring.

Patient Education. The rapid and acute nature of cardiogenic shock limits the nurse's ability to prepare patients and families for VAD insertion. Despite the critical nature of the illness, nurses explain the reason for the use of the VAD and provide information about the critical care environment and equipment (see the Patient Education feature on Ventricular Assist Device). Technologic advances and approval of devices for destination therapy will likely increase the number of VAD patients discharged to home. These patients and their families will require education related to care of the device, as well as reinforcement on components of heart failure management.

VASCULAR SURGERY

Vascular surgery may be used as a treatment for arterial occlusive disease or to correct structural abnormalities such as aneurysms. Because atherosclerosis is a diffuse disease that affects not only the peripheral vessels but also the coronary arteries, patients undergoing arterial vascular surgery are at high risk for perioperative cardiac events. The nursing care of patients after vascular surgery focuses not only on observations for surgical complications such as hematoma or reocclusion, but also on prompt recognition and appropriate treatment of complications that may arise from the impact of the procedure on preexisting cardiac, pulmonary, or kidney disease.

CAROTID ENDARTERECTOMY

Carotid endarterectomy may be beneficial in both symptomatic and asymptomatic patients with stenoses greater than 60% to 70%.[87] The procedure is performed through a neck incision that allows for visualization of the vessel. The plaque is removed and the vessel is closed, either directly or with a patch composed of saphenous vein or a prosthetic material. A Jackson-Pratt drain may be placed at the end of the procedure to minimize hematoma formation. Complications after carotid endarterectomy include perioperative myocardial infarction, cerebral ischemia or infarction, bleeding, and cranial nerve damage.

Postoperative Nursing Management. Patients require 12 to 24 hours of intensive nursing assessment in the period immediately after carotid endarterectomy. Complications are rare but may be life-threatening and require rapid intervention. Serial assessments are performed, and the surgeon is promptly notified of significant changes in the patient's status.

Neurologic Assessment. Frequent neurologic assessments are performed as the patient awakens from anesthesia and then hourly for the first 12 hours. This assessment should include level of consciousness, orientation, pupil response, motor function, and evaluation of cranial nerve function (swallowing/gag reflexes, hoarseness, tongue movement, and facial drooping).[88] Compression, traction, or inadvertent severing can damage nerves that lie in or near the surgical field. The most common injuries are damage to the laryngeal and hypoglossal nerves. Most cranial nerve dysfunction resolves within a short time.

Bleeding. Bleeding is assessed by observation of the dressing for drainage or swelling and measurement of output from the neck drain if present. If hematoma formation occurs internally, it may impinge on the trachea, so the patient is also monitored for signs of a compromised airway. In addition to monitoring respiratory rate and oxygen saturation, the patient is assessed for tracheal deviation and for symptoms of upper airway obstruction such as stridor or wheezing. A small venous hematoma may respond to manual pressure, but larger arterial hematomas that expand rapidly require emergent return to the operating room for reexploration and evacuation.[87]

Cardiovascular Monitoring. Continuous ECG monitoring is generally used after carotid endarterectomy, using ST-segment monitoring to detect myocardial ischemia. Bradycardia is common secondary to baroreceptor stimulation during the operative procedure but is usually hemodynamically tolerated as long as the patient's blood pressure is adequate. Manipulation of the carotid bulb during the surgery often results in hemodynamic instability in the immediate postoperative period. An arterial line is generally placed to allow for prompt detection and treatment of either hypotension or hypertension. Adequate blood pressure control in the postoperative period is of paramount importance. Hypertension will increase the risk of bleeding at the suture line and is generally treated with short-acting vasodilators such as sodium nitroprusside. A relative hypotension compared with the patient's baseline will result in inadequate cerebral perfusion and potential neurologic deficits, so vasopressors such as phenylephrine may be used to maintain an adequate blood pressure.

ABDOMINAL AORTIC ANEURYSM REPAIR

An abdominal aortic aneurysm is generally repaired when the aneurysm is 5 cm or greater in size. The procedure is performed under general anesthesia and involves surgical access either through a midline abdominal incision or via a flank incision (retroperitoneal approach). Clamping the aorta proximal and distal to the dilated area isolates the aneurysm. The aneurysmal portion of the aorta is replaced with a prosthetic graft, which is then enclosed within the aneurysmal sac.[89]

Postoperative complications include myocardial ischemia or infarction, bleeding, acute renal failure, and distal embolization. Rarely, colon or spinal cord ischemia may occur secondary to interruption of blood flow during aortic cross-clamping or embolization. After the procedure, patients are generally monitored in the critical care unit for 24 to 48 hours, with a total length of hospital stay of 5 to 9 days.

Postoperative Management. Nursing assessment of vital signs along with assessment of peripheral perfusion is performed frequently in the early postoperative period. Continuous ECG monitoring with ST-segment analysis is used to detect myocardial ischemia. An arterial line is placed to allow for prompt detection and treatment of hypotension or hypertension. Hypertension increases the risk of bleeding at the suture lines and is often treated with short-acting vasodilators such as sodium nitroprusside. Hypotension may result in compromised perfusion to organs or the extremities and is treated with volume replacement and vasopressors as needed. Hourly assessment of urine output is performed to evaluate kidney function. If urine output is less than 30 ml/hour, diuretics or low-dose dopamine may be used after correction of hypovolemia. The dressing is assessed for bleeding, and potential signs of internal hemorrhage from the graft site (hypotension, complaints of back pain) are further evaluated with serial hematocrits. Patients without preoperative pulmonary conditions are generally rapidly weaned from ventilatory support, with supplemental oxygen given as needed to maintain an acceptable oxygen saturation.

Endovascular Stent Grafts. The endoluminal placement of stent grafts is a newer, less invasive approach for repair of an aortic aneurysm. In this procedure a sutureless vascular graft is implanted into the abdominal aorta through a femoral arteriotomy (Fig. 19-25). The stent isolates the aneurysmal wall from intraluminal blood pressure to prevent further expansion or rupture of the aneurysm.[89] It is hoped that this approach will reduce morbidity associated with more invasive surgery and decrease costs by shortening length of stay.

PERIPHERAL VASCULAR PROCEDURES

Progression of peripheral arterial disease can lead to critical limb ischemia. This may initially manifest itself as intermittent claudication but, if left untreated, can progress to rest pain, ulceration, or even gangrene. Initial treatment focuses on lifestyle modification, such as smoking cessation, adequate diabetic control, effective treatment of hypertension, and dyslipidemia management. Pharmacologic interventions such as antiplatelet agents may be used. If these nonoperative strategies fail, patients may be considered for surgical or interventional revascularization via surgical bypass, percutaneous transluminal angioplasty (PTA), or stent placement.[90]

Surgical Revascularization. *Arteriosclerosis obliterans* is a condition in which atherosclerosis produces progressive obstruction of medium-to-larger arteries. These lesions commonly occur at bifurcations of the abdominal aorta and the iliac, femoral, popliteal or tibial, and peroneal arteries. The surgical procedure performed is based on the site of the vascular lesion(s) and the patient's operative risk. For example, aortofemoral bypass grafting is the preferred operation for treatment of aortoiliac occlusive disease in low-risk patients because it results in the highest patency rates. But axillobifemoral bypass or unilateral femorofemoral bypass may be selected in higher-risk patients, since both of these procedures can be performed under regional anesthesia.[90] Types of peripheral vascular procedures are shown in Fig. 19-26.

Choice of Conduit. Conduits available for peripheral vascular bypass include vein grafts (reversed saphenous vein, arm vein, or human umbilical vein) and synthetic grafts made of polytetrafluoroethylene. As in coronary artery bypass grafting, the type of conduit used has an impact on the patency rate of the graft. In general, veins are the preferred conduit because of better patency rates (60% to 80% at 5 years) and lower potential for infection.[90]

Nursing Management. The primary focus of nursing care in the immediate postoperative period is assessment of the adequacy of perfusion to the limb supplied by the graft and identification of surgical complications. Pulse checks are performed frequently, and the surgeons

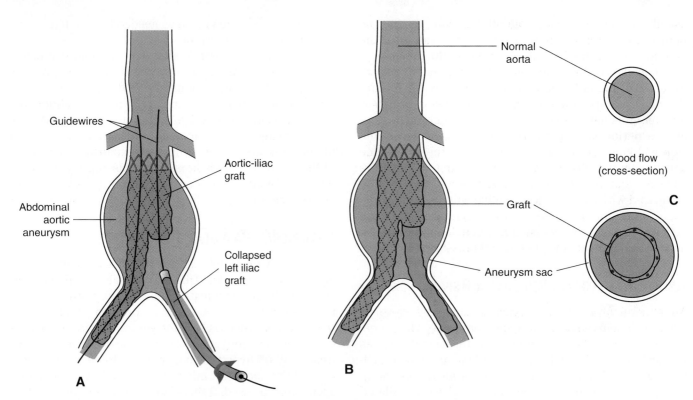

Fig. 19-25 Placement of an endovascular aortic stent. **A,** With fluoroscopic guidance the collapsed stent is inserted through an incision in the femoral or iliac artery over a guidewire. **B,** The positioned stent is opened with a balloon and anchored to the vessel by several small hooks. **C,** The stent isolates the aneurysmal wall from intraluminal blood pressure.

are notified of any decrease in the strength of the Doppler signal. Because distal perfusion is compromised in this patient population, nursing measures to prevent skin breakdown (sheepskin, frequent repositioning, foot cradles) are implemented. If the graft was placed above the renal arteries, kidney function may be impaired as a result of interruption of renal blood flow during graft placement. Urine output is therefore assessed hourly and supported with fluids, diuretics, and low-dose dopamine as needed. ST-segment monitoring is performed to detect episodes of myocardial ischemia throughout the perioperative period.

Percutaneous Interventions. Percutaneous transluminal angioplasty (PTA) can be performed to treat occlusions or narrowing in the peripheral vasculature via catheters similar to those used in PTCA. As with coronary angioplasty, advances in catheter design and the development of intravascular stents have resulted in a dramatic increase in the number of percutaneous procedures performed. PTA was traditionally limited to the treatment of short, focal stenoses or occlusions but is now routinely used to treat more extensively diseased segments, as an emergency treatment to attempt limb salvage before surgical bypass or as an alternative for patients who are poor surgical candidates. Intravascular stents may be used in combination with PTA, depending on the lesion morphology and location. Complications of interventional vascular procedures include hematoma formation at the site of the arteriotomy, formation of a pseudoaneurysm, distal embolization, and thrombotic occlusion.

EFFECTS OF CARDIOVASCULAR DRUGS

Multiple medications are used in the treatment of critically ill cardiovascular patients. The critical care nurse is responsible for preparation and administration of these drugs and often is required to titrate the dose on the basis of the patient's hemodynamic response. The medications used to treat cardiovascular disease are rapidly changing and expanding as more is learned about the pathophysiology of cardiac disease and as improved formulas are developed by pharmaceutical companies. The critical care nurse who has a general understanding of the mechanisms of action of the various drug classifications can readily apply this knowledge to new drugs within the same classification. The following discussion provides a concise review of drugs commonly administered to support cardiovascular function in the critical care setting. The emphasis is on intravenously administered medications that are used for the acute rather than the chronic management of cardiovascular conditions.

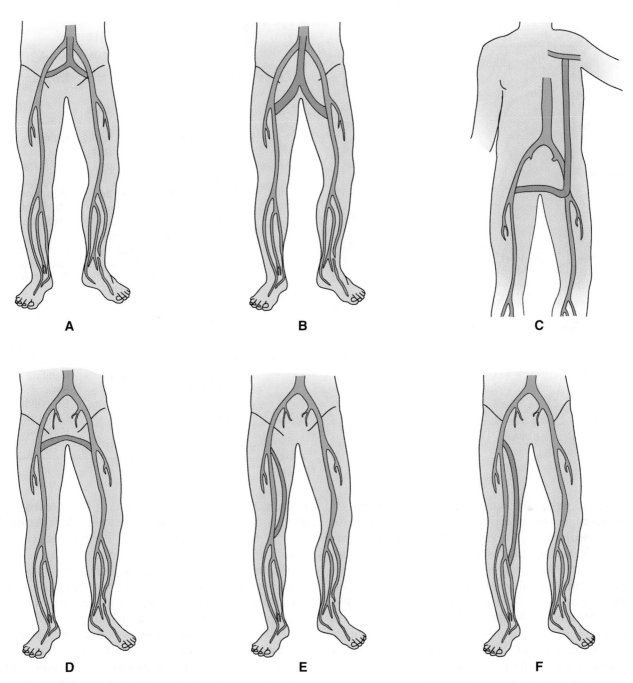

Fig. 19-26   Peripheral arterial bypass procedures. **A,** Aortoiliac bypass. **B,** Aortobifemoral bypass. **C,** Axillobifemoral bypass. **D,** Femorofemoral bypass. **E,** Femoropopliteal bypass. **F,** Femorotibial bypass.

ANTIDYSRHYTHMIC DRUGS

Antidysrhythmic drugs comprise a diverse category of pharmacologic agents used to terminate or prevent an array of abnormal cardiac rhythms. These drugs commonly are classified according to their primary effect on the action potential of cardiac cells (Fig. 19-27). The classification scheme shown in Table 19-8 is the most commonly used system. Classification of newer agents is more difficult, because some of these agents have characteristics of more than one class and others have no characteristics of the current system.

Class I Drugs.   Class I agents are sodium channel blockers that decrease the influx of sodium ions through "fast" channels during phase 0 depolarization. This prolongs the absolute (effective) refractory period, thus decreasing the risk of premature impulses from ectopic foci. In addition, these drugs depress automaticity by slowing the rate of spontaneous depolarizations of pacemaker cells during the resting phase (phase 4).

Class I drugs can be further subdivided into three

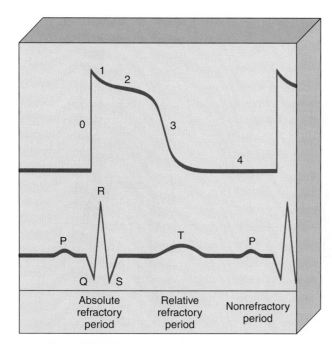

Fig. 19-27 The phases of the cardiac action potential and their relationship to the heart's refractory periods. *Phase 0,* Depolarization—rapid influx of sodium. *Phase 1,* Rapid repolarization—rapid efflux of potassium ions and decreased sodium conductance. *Phase 2,* Plateau—slow influx of sodium and calcium ions. *Phase 3,* Repolarization—continued efflux of potassium ions. *Phase 4,* Resting phase—restoration of ionic balance by sodium and potassium pumps.

Table 19-8	Classification of Antidysrhythmic Agents	
Class	**Action**	**Drugs**
I	Blocks sodium channels ("stabilizes" cell membrane)	
IA	Blocks sodium channels and delays repolarization, thus lengthening the duration of the action potential	Quinidine Procainamide Disopyramide
IB	Blocks sodium channels and accelerates repolarization, thus shortening the duration of the action potential	Lidocaine Mexiletine Tocainide
IC	Blocks sodium channels and slows conduction through the His-Purkinje system, thus prolonging the QRS duration	Flecainide Encainide Propafenone
II	Blocks β-receptors	Esmolol Metoprolol Propranolol
III	Slows repolarization and prolongs the duration of the action potential	Amiodarone Ibutilide Sotalol Dofetilide
IV	Blocks calcium channels	Diltiazem Verapamil

groups according to their potency as sodium channel inhibitors and their effect on phase 3 repolarization. Class IA agents—*quinidine, procainamide,* and *disopyramide*—block not only the fast sodium channels but also phase 3 repolarization and thereby prolong the action potential duration. Clinically this may result in measurable increases in the QRS duration and lengthening of the QT interval. All class IA agents may depress myocardial contractility, with disopyramide having the most potent negative inotropic effect.[91] Drugs in class IB have only a moderate effect on sodium channels and actually accelerate phase 3 repolarization to shorten the action potential duration; *lidocaine, mexiletine,* and *tocainide* belong in this group. Class IC agents are the most potent sodium channel blockers, with little effect on repolarization. Class IC drugs increase both the PR and the QRS intervals. Included in this group are *encainide, flecainide,* and *propafenone.* The results of the Cardiac Arrhythmia Suppression Trial (CAST) indicated that treatment with encainide and flecainide may be associated with increased mortality, and thus the use of these agents in clinical practice has been decreased.[92]

Class II Drugs. Class II drugs are beta-adrenergic blockers (beta-blockers). These agents inhibit dysrhythmias mediated by the sympathetic nervous system by competing with endogenous catecholamines for available receptor sites. As a result, spontaneous depolariza-

tion during the resting phase (phase 4) is depressed and atrioventricular conduction is slowed. Drugs in this class can be further subdivided into cardioselective (those that block only β₁-receptors) and noncardioselective (those that block both β₁- and β₂-receptors). Knowledge of the effects of adrenergic-receptor stimulation allows for anticipation of not only the therapeutic responses brought about by beta-blockade but also the potential adverse effects of these agents (Table 19-9). For example, bronchospasm can be precipitated by noncardioselective beta-blockers in a patient with chronic obstructive pulmonary disease (COPD) secondary to blocking the effects of β₂-receptors in the lungs. Beta-blockers also are negative inotropes and must be used cautiously in patients with left ventricular dysfunction. Although numerous beta-blockers are available, only *esmolol, metoprolol,* and *propranolol* are available as intravenous agents for the treatment of acute dysrhythmias. Of these, esmolol (Brevibloc) offers significant advantages for the critically ill patient because of its short half-life (approximately 9 minutes). It is used in the treatment of supraventricular tachycardias, such as atrial fibrillation and atrial flutter.

Class III Drugs. Class III agents include *amiodarone, dofetilide, ibutilide,* and *sotalol.* These agents markedly slow the rate of phase 3 repolarization, increasing the effective refractory period and the action potential dura-

Table 19-9	Effects of Adrenergic Receptors	
Receptor	Location	Response to Stimulation
Alpha (α)	Vessels of skin, muscles, kidneys, and intestines	Vasoconstriction of peripheral arterioles
Beta$_1$ (β_1)	Cardiac tissue	Increased heart rate Increased conduction Increased contractility
Beta$_2$ (β_2)	Vascular and bronchial smooth muscle	Vasodilation of peripheral arterioles Bronchodilation

tion. Although their effect on the action potential is similar, these drugs differ greatly in their mechanism of action and their side effects. At this time, sotalol is approved only for oral use. Intravenous amiodarone was originally approved for treatment of serious ventricular dysrhythmias that were refractory to other medications. Because of its effectiveness, it is now used for both atrial and ventricular dysrhythmias.[7] Dofetilide (Tikosyn) is a new class III antidysrhythmic agent used for the conversion to and maintenance of normal sinus rhythm in patients with highly symptomatic atrial fibrillation/flutter. Because dofetilide prolongs the refractoriness of both atrial and ventricular tissue, prolongation of the QT interval can occur, which is associated with an increased risk of torsades de pointes.[93] Therapy with dofetilide is initiated in a hospital setting under close monitoring. Ibutilide (Covert) is a short-term antidysrhythmic agent used for the rapid conversion of acute atrial fibrillation or atrial flutter to sinus rhythm. The drug is administered as a 10-minute infusion in a carefully monitored clinical setting. The most serious side effect of ibutilide is its potential for inducing life-threatening dysrhythmias, especially torsades de pointes.[92]

Class IV Drugs. Class IV agents are calcium channel blockers that inhibit the influx of calcium through slow calcium channels during the plateau phase (phase 2). This effect occurs primarily in tissue in which slow calcium channels predominate, primarily in the sinus and AV nodes and the atrial tissue. *Verapamil* was the first drug in this category available as an intravenous antidysrhythmic. It depresses sinus and AV node conduction and is effective in terminating supraventricular tachycardias caused by AV nodal reentry. Recently *diltiazem* (Cardizem) has become available in IV form and is thought to be as effective as verapamil in treating supraventricular dysrhythmias, with fewer hypotensive side effects. Because accessory pathways are not affected by calcium channel blockade, both of these

agents must be avoided in the treatment of atrial fibrillation for patients with Wolff-Parkinson-White syndrome.[7]

Unclassified Antidysrhythmics. *Adenosine* (Adenocard) is an antidysrhythmic agent that remains unclassified under the current system. Adenosine occurs endogenously in the body as a building block of adenosine triphosphate (ATP). Given in intravenous boluses, adenosine slows conduction through the AV node, causing transient AV block. It is used clinically to convert supraventricular tachycardias and to facilitate differential diagnosis of rapid dysrhythmias. Because of its short half-life, the drug is administered intravenously as a rapid bolus, followed by a saline flush. The bolus is delivered as centrally as possible so that the drug reaches the heart before it is metabolized.[7] Side effects are transient because the drug is rapidly taken up by the cells and is cleared from the body within 10 seconds.

Magnesium is also unclassified under the present system. Although its action as an antidysrhythmic agent is not entirely understood, clinical studies suggest that it may reduce the incidence of both ventricular and supraventricular dysrhythmias in selected patient populations. It is considered the treatment of choice in patients with torsades de pointes. For acute treatment, 1 to 2 g of magnesium is administered over 1 to 2 minutes. In patients with confirmed hypomagnesemia, this bolus may be followed with a 24-hour infusion.[7]

Side Effects. Antidysrhythmic drugs carry the risk of serious side effects, some of which may be life-threatening. The major side effects of the intravenous antidysrhythmic agents are listed in the Pharmacologic Management table on Selected Antidysrhythmic Agents. The most severe complication is the potential for a "prodysrhythmic" effect. This may result in a worsening of the underlying dysrhythmia, the occurrence of a new dysrhythmia, or the development of a bradydysrhythmia. For example, torsades de pointes is a prodysrhythmia caused by a number of drugs. The development of a prodysrhythmia is unpredictable; thus the nurse plays an important role in evaluating ECG changes, monitoring drug levels, and assessing patient symptoms. Antidysrhythmic agents may also alter the amount of energy required for defibrillation and pacing. For example, increases in an antidysrhythmic drug dose may increase the amount of output (mA) required to depolarize the myocardium.

Treatment of Atrial Fibrillation. Over 2 million people in the United States have atrial fibrillation, and extensive research has been done on the treatment of this disorder. The goals of pharmacologic therapy for atrial fibrillation include reestablishing and maintaining sinus rhythm, decreasing the rapid ventricular response during episodes of atrial fibrillation, and preventing the risk of thromboembolism. The Pharmacologic Management table on Atrial Fibrillation reviews current drugs used in the treatment of atrial fibrillation. Recent clinical trials suggest that rate control is equivalent to restoration of sinus rhythm in terms of mortality.[94]

Pharmacologic Management: Selected Antidysrhythmic Agents

DRUG/SITE OF ACTION	INDICATIONS	DOSAGE	MAJOR SIDE EFFECTS
Sinus Node, Atria, or AV Node			
Adenosine	SVT, PSVT	6 mg IV rapid push; if unsuccessful, repeat with 12 mg over 1-2 sec; follow with IV fluid 10 ml flush (NS or D5W)	Transient; flushing, dyspnea, hypotension
Digoxin	AFib, AF, PSVT	0.5-1 mg loading dose in divided doses; maintenance dose of 0.125-0.375 mg daily	Bradycardia, heart block Toxicity: CNS and GI symptoms
Diltiazem	SVT, AFib, AF	Bolus dose of 0.25 mg/kg IV over 2 min, followed by an infusion of 5-15 mg/hr	Bradycardia, hypotension, AV block
Esmolol	ST, SVT	Loading dose of 500 mcg/kg/min over 1 min, followed by an infusion of 50 mcg/kg/min for 4 min; repeat procedure every 5 min, increasing infusion by 25-50 mcg/kg/min to maximum of 200 mcg/kg/min	Hypotension, bradycardia, heart failure
Ibutilide	AFib, AF	0.010-0.025 mg/kg infused over 10 min (may repeat once) or 1 mg diluted in 50 ml infused over 10 min (may repeat once)	Minimal side effects except for rare polymorphic VT (torsades de pointes)
Propranolol	SVT	1-3 mg IV every 5 min not to exceed 0.1 mg/kg	Bradycardia, heart block, heart failure
Verapamil	AF, PSVT	5-10 mg IV, may repeat in 15-30 min	Hypotension, bradycardia, heart failure
Ventricle			
Lidocaine	PVCs, VT, VF	1-1.5 mg/kg bolus, followed by continuous infusion of 1-4 mg/min	CNS toxicity, nausea, vomiting with repeated doses
Atria and Ventricle			
Amiodarone	VT/VT arrest	300 mg IV push; may repeat with 150 mg in 3-5 min (maximum dose of 2.2 g/24 hr)	Hypotension, abnormal liver function tests
	Stable, VT, AFib, AF	150 mg IV over 10 min, followed by 360 mg over 6 hr (1 mg/min); maintenance infusion of 0.5 mg/min	
Procainamide	AF, SVT, PVCs, VT	Loading dose of 12-17 mg/kg at a rate of 20 mg/min, followed by infusion of 1-4 mg/min	Hypotension, GI effects Widening of QRS and QT lengthening

SVT, Supraventricular tachycardia; *PSVT*, paroxysmal supraventricular tachycardia; *IV*, intravenous; *NS*, normal saline; *AFib*, atrial fibrillation; *CNS*, central nervous system; *GI*, gastrointestinal; *AF*, atrial flutter; *AV*, atrioventricular; *ST*, sinus tachycardia; *PVCs*, premature ventricular contractions; *VT*, ventricular tachycardia; *VF*, ventricular fibrillation.

INOTROPIC DRUGS

Critically ill patients with compromised cardiac function often require the use of medications to enhance myocardial contractility (positive inotropes). Clinically available inotropes include cardiac glycosides, sympathomimetics, and phosphodiesterase inhibitors. These agents increase myocardial contractility, resulting in improved cardiac output, more complete emptying of the ventricles, and decreased filling pressures.

Cardiac glycosides include digitalis and its derivatives. Although these drugs have been used for centuries, their slow onset of action and risk of toxicity make them more appropriate for the management of chronic heart failure. Because digoxin also causes slowing of the sinus rate and a decrease in AV conduction, it may be administered intravenously in the acute care setting to control supraventricular dysrhythmias.

Sympathomimetic agents stimulate adrenergic receptors, thereby simulating the effects of sympathetic nerve stimulation. Included in this category are naturally occurring catecholamines (epinephrine, dopamine, and norepinephrine), as well as synthetic catecholamines (dobutamine and isoproterenol). The cardiovascular effects of these drugs, which vary according to their selectivity for specific receptor sites, are often dose-dependent as well. Table 19-10 describes the cardiovascular effects of sympathomimetic drugs at various dosages.

Dopamine (Intropin) is one of the most widely used drugs in the critical care setting. It is a chemical precursor of norepinephrine, which, in addition to both α- and β-receptor stimulation, can activate dopaminergic recep-

Pharmacologic Management: Atrial Fibrillation

TREATMENT GOAL	CLASSIFICATION/DRUG	SPECIAL CONSIDERATIONS
Conversion/maintenance of sinus rhythm	**Class IA** Quinidine Procainamide (Pronestyl) Disopyramide (Norpace)	Class IA drugs prolong QT intervals and may cause torsades de pointes. Rate control should be achieved before initiation of therapy.
	Class IC Flecainide (Tambocor) Propafenone (Rhythmol)	Class IC drugs are prodysrhythmic in patients with CAD or previous MI and should be avoided in these patients.
	Class III Amiodarone (Cordarone) Dofetilide (Tikosyn) Ibutilide (Corvert) Sotalol (Betapace)	Amiodarone and sotalol also have beta-blocking properties and may help with rate control. Treatment with dofetilide requires careful monitoring for prodysrhythmic effects. Ibutilide is an intravenous agent and is used for conversion only.
Control of ventricular rate	**Beta-Blockers** Esmolol (Brevibloc) Metoprolol (Lopressor) Propranolol (Inderal)	Intravenous esmolol or may be used in acute settings to control ventricular rate. Oral agents are used for maintenance therapy. Beta-blockers provide good rate control during exercise.
	Calcium Channel Blockers Diltiazem (Cardizem) Verapamil (Isoptin)	Intravenous calcium channel blockers may be used in emergency situations, followed by oral agents for maintenance therapy.
	Digitalis Compounds Digoxin (Lanoxin)	Digoxin does not effectively control rate with exercise, so it may be used in combination with other drugs.
Prevention of thromboembolism	**Anticoagulants** Heparin Warfarin (Coumadin)	Heparin may be used in emergency situations, prior to cardioversion. Warfarin is used long-term, with monitoring to achieve an INR of 2.0-3.0.
	Antiplatelet Agents Aspirin	May be used in patients with contraindications to warfarin or low-risk patients under age 65.

CAD, Coronary artery disease; *MI*, myocardial infarction; *INR*, international normalized ratio.

Table 19-10   Physiologic Effects of Sympathomimetic Agents

Drug	Dosage	Receptor Activated*				Cardiovascular Effects		
		Alpha	Beta₁	Beta₂	Dopa	CO	HR	SVR
Dobutamine	<5 mcg/kg/min	0	↑↑↑	↑	0	↑↑	↑	0/↓
	5-20 mcg/kg/min	0	↑↑↑	↑↑	0	↑↑↑	↑↑	↓
	>20 mcg/kg/min	0	↑↑↑	↑↑	0	↑↑↑	↑↑↑	↓↓
Dopamine	<3 mcg/kg/min	0	↑	↑	↑↑↑	0/↑	0/↑	0
	3-10 mcg/kg/min	↑	↑↑↑	↑	↑↑↑	↑↑↑	↑	↑
	11-20 mcg/kg/min	↑↑↑	↑↑↑	↑	↑↑	↑↑	↑↑	↑↑↑
	>20 mcg/kg/min	↑↑↑↑	↑↑	0	0	↑	↑	↑↑↑
Epinephrine	<2 mcg/min	0	↑	↑↑	0	0/↑	0/↑	↓
	2-8 mcg/min	↑↑	↑↑↑	↑↑	0	↑↑↑	↑	↑
	9-20 mcg/min	↑↑↑	↑↑	↑↑	0	↑↑	↑↑	↑↑
Isoproterenol	1-7 mcg/min	0	↑↑↑	↑↑↑	0	↑↑↑	↑↑↑	↓↓↓
Norepinephrine	<2 mcg/min	↑↑↑	↑↑	0	0	↑	0/↑	↑↑↑
	2-16 mcg/min	↑↑↑↑	↑↑	0	0	↓	↑	↑↑↑↑
Phenylephrine	10-100 mcg/min	↑↑↑↑	0	0	0	0	↓	↑↑↑

*Refer to Table 19-9 for actions of receptors.
CO, Cardiac output; *HR*, heart rate; *SVR*, systemic vascular resistance; 0, no effect; ↑, increased; ↓, decreased (the number of arrows indicates the degree of effect [e.g., ↑, mild and ↑↑↑, strong effect]).

tors in the renal and mesenteric blood vessels. The actions of this drug are entirely dose-related.[95] At low dosages of 1 to 2 mcg/kg/min, dopamine stimulates dopaminergic receptors, causing renal and mesenteric vasodilation. However, it is now clear that this increase in urine output does not confer protection against development of acute renal failure. The resultant increase in renal perfusion increases urinary output. Moderate dosages result in stimulation of β_1-receptors to increase myocardial contractility and improve cardiac output. At dosages greater than 10 mg/kg/min, dopamine predominantly stimulates α-receptors, resulting in vasoconstriction that often negates both the β-adrenergic and dopaminergic effects.

Dobutamine (Dobutrex) is a synthetic catecholamine with predominantly β_1 effects. It also produces some β_2 stimulation, resulting in a mild vasodilation. Dobutamine is as effective as dopamine in increasing myocardial contractility and is useful in the treatment of heart failure, especially in hypotensive patients who cannot tolerate vasodilator therapy. The usual dosage range is 2.5 to 20 mg/kg/min, titrated on the basis of hemodynamic parameters.

Epinephrine (Adrenalin) is produced by the adrenal gland as part of the body's response to stress. This agent has the ability to stimulate both α- and β-receptors, depending on the dose administered (see Table 19-10). At doses of 1 to 2 mg/min, epinephrine binds with β-receptors to increase heart rate, cardiac conduction, contractility, and vasodilation, thereby increasing cardiac output. As the dosage is increased, α-receptors are stimulated, resulting in increased vascular resistance and blood pressure. At these doses, epinephrine's impact on cardiac output depends on the heart's ability to pump against the increased afterload. Epinephrine accelerates the sinus rate and may precipitate ventricular dysrhythmias in the ischemic heart. Other side effects include restlessness, angina, and headache.

Norepinephrine (Levophed) is similar to epinephrine in its ability to stimulate β- and α-receptors, but it lacks the β_2 effects. At low infusion rates, β_1-receptors are activated to produce increased contractility and thus augment cardiac output. At higher doses the inotropic effects are limited by marked vasoconstriction mediated by α-receptors. Clinically norepinephrine is used most often as a vasopressor to elevate blood pressure in shock states.

Isoproterenol (Isuprel) is a pure β-receptor stimulant with no α effects. It produces dramatic increases in heart rate, conduction, and contractility via beta$_1$ stimulation and vasodilation via β_2 stimulation. Isoproterenol also produces vasodilation of the pulmonary arteries and bronchodilation. It greatly increases the automaticity of cardiac cells and frequently precipitates dysrhythmias, such as premature ventricular contractions and even ventricular tachycardia. These effects limit its usefulness in most patients.

Phosphodiesterase Inhibitors. Phosphodiesterase inhibitors are inotropic agents that also are potent vasodilators (inodilators). Drugs in this classification inhibit the enzyme *phosphodiesterase*, resulting in increased levels of cyclic adenosine monophosphate (AMP) and intracellular calcium. Amrinone (Inocor) and milrinone (Primacor) were the first of these agents approved for use in the United States. Increases in cardiac output occur as a result of increased contractility (inotropic effects) and decreased afterload (vasodilative effects). Filling pressures tend to decrease, whereas the heart rate and blood pressure remain fairly constant. Amrinone may cause thrombocytopenia, so platelet counts are monitored and patients observed for hemorrhagic complications. Milrinone is associated with a lower rate of thrombocytopenia but can induce ventricular dysrhythmias (premature ventricular complexes, ventricular tachycardia) in a significant number of patients.[96]

VASODILATOR DRUGS

Vasodilators are pharmacologic agents that improve cardiac performance by various degrees of arterial or venous dilation, or both. The goal of vasodilator therapy may be a reduction of preload or afterload, or both. Afterload reduction is accomplished by vasodilation of arterial vessels. This results in decreased resistance to left ventricular ejection and may improve cardiac output without increasing myocardial oxygen demands. Reduction of preload is accomplished by dilating venous vessels to increase capacitance. This results in decreased filling pressures for a failing heart. These drugs may be classified into four groups on the basis of mechanism of action (see the Pharmacologic Management table on Characteristics of Selected Vasodilators).

Direct Smooth Muscle Relaxants. Direct-acting vasodilators include *sodium nitroprusside* (Nipride), *nitroglycerin* (Tridil), and *hydralazine* (Apresoline). These drugs produce relaxation of vascular smooth muscle via the activation of nitric oxide, resulting in decreased peripheral vascular resistance. Hypotension may occur as a result of peripheral vasodilation, and headaches may be caused by cerebral vasodilation. Compensatory mechanisms can occur in response to the drop in blood pressure. These include baroreceptor activation that causes reflex tachycardia and activation of the renin-angiotensin-aldosterone system (RAAS) (see Fig. 18-16), with resultant sodium and water retention.

Sodium nitroprusside (Nipride) is a potent, rapidly acting venous and arterial vasodilator, particularly suitable for rapid reduction of blood pressure in hypertensive emergencies and perioperatively. It also is effective for afterload reduction in the setting of severe heart failure. The drug is administered by continuous intravenous infusion, with the dosage titrated to maintain the desired blood pressure and systemic vascular resistance (SVR). Prolonged administration can result in thiocyanate toxicity, manifested by nausea, confusion, and tinnitus.[97]

Intravenous nitroglycerin (Tridil) causes both arterial and venous vasodilation, but its venous effect is

Pharmacologic Management: Characteristics of Selected Vasodilators

DRUG CLASSIFICATION	DOSAGE	PRELOAD	AFTERLOAD	SIDE EFFECTS
Direct Smooth Muscle Relaxants				
Sodium nitroprusside (Nipride)	0.25-6 mcg/kg/min IV infusion	Moderate	Strong	Hypotension, thiocyanate toxicity, reflex tachycardia
Nitroglycerin (Tridil)	5-300 mcg/min IV infusion	Strong	Mild	Headache, reflex tachycardia, hypotension
Calcium Channel Blockers				
Nicardipine (Cardene)	5 mg/hr IV, titrated to 15 mg/hr	None	Strong	Hypotension, headache, reflex tachycardia
Nifedipine (Procardia)	10-30 mg PO	None	Strong	Hypotension, headache, reflex tachycardia
ACE Inhibitors				
Captopril (Capoten)	6.25-100 mg PO every 8-12 hr	Moderate	Moderate	Hypotension, chronic cough, neutropenia
Enalapril (Vasotec)	0.625 mg IV over 5 min, then every 6h	Moderate	Moderate	Hypotension, elevation of liver enzymes
Alpha-Adrenergic Blockers				
Labetalol (Normodyne)	20-80 mg IV bolus every 10 min, then 1-2 mg/min infusion	Moderate	Moderate	Orthostatic hypotension, bronchospasm, AV block
Phentolamine (Regitine)	1-2 mg/min infusion	Moderate	Moderate	Hypotension, tachycardia

IV, Intravenous; *PO*, by mouth; *ACE*, angiotensin-converting enzyme; *AV*, atrioventricular.

more pronounced. It is used in the critical care setting for the treatment of acute heart failure (HF) because it reduces cardiac filling pressures, relieves pulmonary congestion, and decreases cardiac workload and oxygen consumption. In addition, nitroglycerin dilates the coronary arteries and is a useful adjunct in the treatment of unstable angina and acute MI. The initial dosage is 10 mcg/min, and the infusion is titrated upward to achieve the desired clinical effect: a reduction or elimination of chest pain, decreased PAOP (wedge pressure), or a decrease in blood pressure. Nitroglycerin also is administered prophylactically to prevent coronary vasospasm after coronary angioplasty, atherectomy, stent insertion, or fibrinolytic therapy. The most common side effects of this drug include hypotension, flushing, and headache.[98]

Hydralazine (Apresoline) is a potent arterial vasodilator. It seldom is given as a continuous infusion, but rather in intravenously administered dosages of 5 to 10 mg every 4 to 8 hours. Occasionally, hydralazine is given as an intermediate drug in the transition between the weaning of a continuous infusion and the initiation of oral antihypertensive medications. The major side effect is reflex tachycardia mediated by the sympathetic nervous system. This may be diminished by the concomitant administration of beta-blockers.

Calcium Channel Blockers. Calcium channel blockers are a chemically diverse group of drugs with differing pharmacologic effects (see the Pharmacologic Management table on Calcium Channel Blockers).

Nifedipine (Procardia) and nicardipine (Cardene) are *dihydropyridines*. Drugs in this group of calcium channel blockers (with the suffix "pine") are used primarily as arterial vasodilators. These drugs reduce the influx of calcium in the arterial resistance vessels. Both coronary and peripheral arteries are affected. They are used in the critical care setting to treat hypertension. Nifedipine is available in an oral form only but in the past was prescribed sublingually during hypertensive emergencies. Reports of adverse events associated with sublingual nifedipine have prompted the FDA to discourage its use.[99] Nicardipine recently became available as an intravenous calcium channel blocker, and as such it offers more accurate titration for effective control of hypertension. Side effects of nifedipine and nicardipine are related to vasodilation and include hypotension, reflex tachycardia, flushing, headache, and ankle edema.

Diltiazem (Cardizem) is from the *benzothiazine* group of calcium channel blockers. Verapamil (Calan, Isoptin) is part of the *phenylalkylamine* group. The different classifications account for the variety of action between these calcium channel blockers. These drugs dilate coronary arteries but have little effect on the peripheral vasculature. They are used in the treatment of angina, especially that which has a vasospastic component, and as antidysrhythmics in the treatment of supraventricular tachycardias.

ACE Inhibitors. Angiotensin-converting enzyme (ACE) inhibitors produce vasodilation by blocking the

Pharmacologic Management: Characteristics of Calcium Channel Blockers

DRUG	ACTIONS	DOSAGE	SPECIAL CONSIDERATIONS
Dihydropyridines			
Nicardipine (Cardene)	Short-term control of hypertension	5 mg/hr IV, titrated to 15 mg/hr	Hypotension, headache, nausea
Nifedipine (Procardia)	Hypertension	10-30 mg PO	Hypotension, headache, reflex tachycardia
Benzothiazepines			
Diltiazem (Cardizem)	SVT, AFib, AF, angina	Bolus dose of 0.25 mg/kg IV over 2 min, followed by an infusion of 5-15 mg/hr	Bradycardia, hypotension, AV block
Phenylalkylamines			
Verapamil (Calan, Isoptin)	AF, PSVT	5-10 mg IV, may repeat in 15-30 min	Hypotension, bradycardia, heart failure

IV, Intravenous; *PO,* by mouth; *SVT,* supraventricular tachycardia, *AFib,* atrial fibrillation; *AF,* atrial flutter; *AV,* atrioventricular; *PSVT,* paroxysmal supraventricular tachycardia.

conversion of angiotensin I to angiotensin II. Because angiotensin is a potent vasoconstrictor, limiting its production decreases peripheral vascular resistance. In contrast to the direct vasodilators and nifedipine, ACE inhibitors do not cause reflex tachycardia or induce sodium and water retention. However, these drugs may cause a profound fall in blood pressure, especially in patients who are volume-depleted. Blood pressure must be monitored carefully, especially during initiation of therapy.

Captopril (Capoten) and enalapril (Vasotec) are used in patients with heart failure to decrease SVR (afterload) and PAOP (preload). Captopril is available in an oral form only but has a relatively rapid onset of action (approximately 1 hour). Enalapril is available in an intravenous form and may be used to decrease afterload in more emergent situations.

B-Type Natriuretic Peptide. *Nesiritide* (Natrecor) is a new vasodilator used in the treatment of acute heart failure. This agent is a recombinant form of human brain natriuretic peptide (BNP), the hormone released by cardiac cells in response to ventricular distention. The primary effects of nesiritide include decreasing filling pressures (PAOP, CVP), reducing vascular resistance (SVR, PVR), and increasing urine output. Compared with traditional vasodilator therapy for acute heart failure, nesiritide reportedly is as effective with fewer side effects (e.g., headache).[100] The recommended dose is an IV bolus of 2 mcg/kg, followed by a continuous infusion of 0.01 mcg/kg/min. The primary side effect is hypotension. If this occurs, nesiritide may need to be discontinued for a time and then restarted at a lower dose after the patient has stabilized.[101]

Alpha-Adrenergic Blockers. Peripheral adrenergic blockers block α-receptors in arteries and veins, resulting in vasodilation. Orthostatic hypotension is a common side effect and may result in syncope. Long-term therapy also may be complicated by fluid and water retention.

Labetalol (Normodyne), a combined peripheral alpha-blocker and cardioselective beta-blocker, is used in the treatment of acute stroke and hypertensive emergencies. Because the blockade of β_1-receptors permits the decrease of blood pressure without the risk of reflexive tachycardia and increased cardiac output, this drug also is useful in the treatment of acute aortic dissection.[102]

Phentolamine (Regitine) is a peripheral alpha-blocker that causes decreased afterload via arterial vasodilation. It is given as a continuous infusion at a rate of 1 to 2 mg/min and is titrated to achieve the required reduction in blood pressure and SVR. Phentolamine is the drug of choice in the treatment of pheochromocytoma.[97] This drug also is used to treat the extravasation of dopamine. If this occurs, 5 to 10 mg is diluted in 10 ml normal saline and administered intradermally into the infiltrated area.

DA-1-Receptor Agonists. Fenoldopam (Corlopam) is the first of a new class of vasodilators called *selective, specific dopamine DA-1-receptor agonists.*[98] The drug is a potent vasodilator that affects both peripheral, renal and mesenteric arteries. It is administered via continuous IV infusion beginning at 0.1 mcg/kg/min and titrated up to the desired blood pressure effect with a maximum recommended dose of 0.5 mcg/kg/min. It can be administered as an alternative to sodium nitroprusside or other antihypertensives in the treatment of hypertensive emergencies. Fenoldopam can be used safely for patients with renal dysfunction or for those at high risk for renal insufficiency after cardiac catheterization, cardiac surgery, or PCI.[103]

Vasopressors. Vasopressors are sympathomimetic agents that mediate peripheral vasoconstriction through stimulation of α-receptors (see Table 19-10). This results in increased systemic vascular resistance and thus elevates blood pressure. Some of these drugs (epinephrine and norepinephrine) also have the ability to stimulate β-receptors. Vasopressors are not widely used in the treatment of critically ill cardiac patients, because the dramatic increase in afterload is taxing to a damaged heart. Occasionally, vasopressors may be used to maintain organ perfusion in shock states. For example, phenylephrine (Neo-Synephrine) or norepinephrine (Levophed) may be administered as a continuous intravenous infusion to maintain organ perfusion by increasing systemic vascular resistance in severe sepsis or septic shock.

Vasopressin, also known as antidiuretic hormone (ADH) has recently become popular in the critical care setting for its vasoconstrictive effects. At higher doses, vasopressin directly stimulates contraction of vascular smooth muscle, resulting in vasoconstriction of capillaries and small arterioles. A one-time dose of 40 units intravenously is recommended in the ACLS guidelines a first-line drug therapy for VF or pulseless VT that is refractory to initial defibrillation.[7] A recent study suggests that vasopressin may also be effective in the treatment of asystole as well.[104] Continuous infusions of 0.02 units/min up to 0.1 units/min have been used in the treatment of vasodilatory shock in patients with refractory hypotension following CPB.[62] Patients must be monitored for side effects such as heart failure (due to the antidiuretic effects) and myocardial ischemia. Vasopressin should be infused through a central line to avoid the risk of peripheral extravasation and resultant tissue necrosis.[62]

DRUG TREATMENT OF HEART FAILURE

Nearly 5 million Americans have heart failure, making it a major chronic health issue.[84] The goals of treatment in heart failure include alleviating symptoms, slowing the progression of the disease, and improving survival.[105] Results from a number of randomly controlled clinical trials have resulted in guidelines for the pharmacologic treatment of heart failure.[106] More information about heart failure is available on p. 459. The Pharmacologic Manage-

Pharmacologic Management: Heart Failure

CLASSIFICATION/ DRUG	MECHANISM OF ACTION	EFFECTS	SPECIAL CONSIDERATIONS
ACE Inhibitors Captopril (Capoten) Enalapril (Vasotec) Lisinopril (Prinivil)	Interferes with the renin-angiotensin-aldosterone system by preventing conversion of angiotensin I to angiotensin II.	Decreases afterload Decreases preload Reverses ventricular remodeling	Agents appear equivalent in treatment of heart failure Monitor closely for hypotension when initiating therapy May be contraindicated in patients with renal insufficiency
Angiotensin Receptor Blockers Losartan (Cozaar) Valsartan (Diovan)	Interferes with the renin-angiotensin-aldosterone system by blocking the effect of angiotensin II at the angiotensin II receptor site	Decreases afterload Decreases preload Reverses ventricular remodeling	Reserved for patients who cannot tolerate ACE inhibitors due to side effects such as severe cough or angioedema
Beta-Blocker Metoprolol (Lopressor) Carvedilol (Coreg)	Counteracts the SNS response activated in heart failure by blocking receptor sites. Metoprolol is a cardioselective beta-blocker, while carvedilol blocks both α- and β-receptor sites.	Slows heart rate Prevents dysrhythmias Decreases blood pressure Reverses ventricular remodeling	Not initiated during decompensated stage of heart failure Use cautiously in patients with reactive airway disease, poorly controlled diabetes, bradydysrhythmias or heart block Carvedilol dose is increased slowly, while monitoring for symptoms secondary to vasodilation, such as dizziness or hypotension
Aldosterone Antagonist Spironolactone (Aldactone)	Counteracts the effects of aldosterone, which include sodium and water retention	Decreases preload Decreases myocardial hypertrophy	May increase serum potassium.
Inotropes Digoxin (Lanoxin)	Affects the Na^+/K^+-ATPase pump in myocardial cells to increase the strength of contraction	Increases contractility Increases cardiac output Prevents atrial dysrhythmias	Risk of toxicity is increased with hypokalemia.

ACE, Angiotensin-converting enzyme; *SNS*, sympathetic nervous system; *Na⁺/K⁺-ATPase*, sodium, potassium, adenosine triphosphatase.

ment table on Heart Failure reviews the drugs currently recommended for the treatment of heart failure.

REFERENCES

1. Schron EB, Domanski MJ: Implantable devices benefit patients with cardiovascular disease, *J Cardiovasc Nurs* 18(5):337, 2003.
2. Attin M: Electrophysiology study: A comprehensive review, *Am J Crit Care* 10(4):260, 2001.
3. Tracy CM et al: ACC/AHA clinical competence statement on invasive electrophysiology studies, catheter ablation, and cardioversion, *J Am Coll Cardiol* 36(5): 1725, 2000.
4. Gilbert CJ: Common supraventricular tachycardias: mechanisms and management, *AACN Clin Issues* 12(1):100, 2001.
5. Hutchinson ML: Ask the experts: correct procedures for performing atrial electrograms, *Crit Care Nurse* 21(5):69, 2001.
6. Boyle J, Rost MK: Present status of cardiac pacing: a nursing perspective, *Crit Care Nurs Q* 23(1):1, 2000.
7. American Heart Association: ECC Guidelines. Part 6. Advanced cardiovascular life support, *Circulation* 102(8): I-136, 2000.
8. Bernstein AD et al: The NASPE/BPEG generic pacemaker code for antibradycardia and adaptive rate pacing and antitachyarrhythmia devices, *Pacing Clin Electrophysiol* 10:794, 1987.
9. Reynolds J, Apple S: A systematic approach to pacemaker assessment, *AACN Clin Issues* 12(1):114, 2001.
10. Gregoratos G et al: ACC/AHA/NASPE 2002 guideline update for implantation of cardiac pacemakers and antiarrhythmia devices: summary article, *Circulation* 106:2145, 2002.
11. Albert NM: Cardiac resynchronization therapy through biventricular pacing in patients with heart failure and ventricular dyssynchrony, *Crit Care Nurse Suppl* 23(3):2, 2003.
12. Flanagan J et al: Heart failure patients with ventricular dyssynchrony: management with a cardiac resynchronization therapy device, *Prog Cardiovasc Nurs* 18:184, 2003.
13. Abraham WT et al: Cardiac resynchronization in chronic heart failure, *N Engl J Med* 344:1845, 2002.
14. Bradley DJ et al: Cardiac resynchronization and death from progressive heart failure: a meta-analysis of randomized controlled trials, *JAMA* 289:730, 2003.
15. Obias-Manno D: Unconventional applications of pacemaker therapy, *AACN Clin Issues* 12(1):127, 2001.
16. Connolly SJ et al: Meta-analysis of the implantable cardioverter defibrillator secondary prevention trials: AVID, CASH and CIDS studies: Antiarrhythmic vs Implantable Defibrillator study, Cardiac Arrest Study Hamburg, Canadian Implantable Defibrillator Study, *Eur Heart J* 21:2071, 2000.
17. Moss AJ et al for the MADIT II Investigators: Prophylactic implantation of a defibrillator in patients with myocardial infarction and reduced ejection fraction, *N Engl J Med* 346:877, 2002.
18. Antman EM et al: ACC/AHA guidelines for the management of patients with ST-elevation myocardial infarction, *J Am Coll Cardiol* 44:671, 2004.
19. Bussard ME: Reteplase: nursing implications for catheter-directed thrombolytic therapy for peripheral vascular occlusion, *Crit Care Nurse* 22(3):57, 2002.
20. Gylys K, Gold M: Acute coronary syndromes: new developments in pharmacological treatment strategies, *Crit Care Nurse Suppl* 20(2):3, 2000.
21. Kline-Rogers E, Martin JS, Smith DD: New era of reperfusion in acute myocardial infarction, *Crit Care Nurse* 19(1):21, 1999.
22. GUSTO III Investigators: A comparison of reteplase with alteplase for acute myocardial infarction, *N Engl J Med* 337(16):1118, 1997.
23. Assent-2 Investigators: Single bolus tenecteplase compared with front-loaded alteplase in acute myocardial infarction: the ASSENT-2 double-blind randomized trial, *Lancet* 354(9180):716, 1999.
24. The TIMI Study Group: The thrombolysis in myocardial infarction (TIMI) trial: phase I findings, *N Engl J Med* 312:932, 1985.
25. The GUSTO V Investigators: Reperfusion therapy for acute myocardial infarction with fibrinolytic therapy or combination low dose fibrinolytic therapy and platelet glycoprotein IIb/IIIa inhibition: the GUSTO V trial, *Lancet* 357:1905, 2001.
26. Lincoff AM et al: Mortality at 1 year with combination platelet glycoprotein IIb/IIIa inhibition and reduced dose fibrinolytic therapy versus conventional fibrinolytic therapy for acute myocardial infarction: the GUSTO V randomized trial, *JAMA* 288:2130, 2002.
27. Topol EJ: Current status and future prospects for acute myocardial infarction therapy, *Circulation* 108(suppl III):III-6, 2003.
28. Leeper B: Continuous ST segment monitoring, *AACN Clin Issues* 14(2):145, 2003.
29. Arjomand H et al: Percutaneous coronary intervention; historical perspectives, current status and future directions, *Am Heart J* 146(5):787, 2003.
30. Smith SC et al: ACC/AHA guidelines for percutaneous coronary intervention (revision of the 1993 PTCA guidelines)-executive summary: a report of the ACC/AHA task force on practice guidelines, *Circulation* 103(24):3019, 2001.
31. Juran NB et al: Nursing interventions to decrease bleeding at the femoral access site after percutaneous coronary intervention, *Am J Crit Care* 8(5):303, 1999.
32. Kuntz RE, Baim DS: Prevention of coronary restenosis: the evolving evidence base for radiation therapy, *Circulation* 101(18):2130, 2000.
33. Rajagopal V, Rockson SG: Coronary restenosis: a review of mechanisms and management, *Am J Med* 115:547, 2003.
34. Senerchia CC: Highlights from the past decade of interventional device research, *Crit Care Nurs Clin North Am* 11(3):311, 1999.
35. Thorbs N et al: Coronary rotational atherectomy: a nursing perspective, *Crit Care Nurse* 20(2):77, 2000.
36. Futterman LG, Lembeur L: Update on the management of acute myocardial infarction: facilitated percutaneous coronary intervention, *Am J Crit Care* 9(1):70, 2000.
37. Mixon TA, Dehmer GJ: Patient care before and after percutaneous coronary interventions, *Am J Med* 115:642, 2003.
38. Hilt T, Bayat M: Drugs used to limit blood surface interactions, *Crit Care Nurs Clin North Am* 14(1):7, 2002.
39. Mehran R et al: Treatment of in-stent restenosis with excimer laser coronary angioplasty versus rotational atherectomy: comparative mechanisms and results, *Circulation* 101:2484, 2000.
40. Leon MB et al: Localized intracoronary gamma-radiation therapy to inhibit the recurrence of stenosis after stenting, *N Engl J Med* 344:250, 2001.

41. Popma JJ et al: Randomized trial of 90Sr/90Y beta-radiation versus placebo control for treatment of in-stent restenosis, *Circulation* 106:1090, 2002.

42. Morice MC et al: A randomized comparison of a sirolimus-eluting stent with a standard stent for coronary revascularization, *N Engl J Med* 347:561, 2003.

43. Sousa JE et al: New frontiers in cardiology: drug-eluting stents: Part I, *Circulation* 107:2274, 2003.

44. Park SJ et al: Apaclitaxel-eluting stent for the prevention of coronary restenosis, *N Engl J Med* 348:1537, 2003.

45. Schickel SI et al: Achieving femoral artery hemostasis after cardiac catheterization: a comparison of methods, *Am J Crit Care* 8(6):406, 1999.

46. Hamel WJ: Suppose a Perclose, *Prog Cardiovasc Nurs* 14(4):136-142, 1999.

47. Bonow RO et al: ACC/AHA guidelines for the management of patients with valvular heart disease, *Circulation* 98(18):1949, 1998.

48. Holloway S, Feldman T: An alternative to valvular surgery in the treatment of mitral stenosis: balloon mitral valvotomy, *Crit Care Nurse* 17(3):27, 1997.

49. Hung JS et al: Complications of Inoue balloon mitral commissurotomy: impact of operator experience and evolving technique, *Am Heart J* 138(1):114, 1999.

50. Eagle KA et al: ACC/AHA 2004 guideline update for coronary artery bypass graft surgery, *Circulation* 110(14): e340, 2004.

51. Grundy SM et al: Diabetes and cardiovascular disease, *Circulation* 100(10):1134, 1999.

52. Stables R: Coronary artery bypass surgery versus percutaneous coronary intervention with stent implantation in patients with multivessel coronary artery disease (the stent or surgery trial): a randomized controlled trial, *Lancet* 360(9338):965, 2002.

53. O'Hanlon JV: Minimally invasive saphenous vein harvesting, *Crit Care Nurs Q* 23(1):42, 2000.

54. Mack MJ: Advances in the treatment of coronary artery disease, *Ann Thorac Surg* 76:S2240, 2003.

55. Tavilla G et al: Long-term follow-up of coronary artery bypass grafting in three-vessel disease using exclusively pedicled bilateral internal thoracic and right gastroepiploic arteries, *Ann Thorac Surg* 77(3):794, 2004.

56. Schouchoff B: Radial artery: an alternative revascularization conduit, *Crit Care Nurs Q* 23(1):28, 2000.

57. Wegund DL: Advances in cardiac surgery: valve repair, *Crit Care Nurs* 23(2):72, 2003.

58. Gott VL et al: Mechanical heart valves: 50 years of evolution, *Ann Thorac Surg* 76:S2230, 2003.

59. Louagie YA et al: Continuous cold blood cardioplegia improves myocardial protection: a prospective randomized study, *Ann Thorac Surg* 77(2):664, 2004.

60. Ferreira R et al: Comparison between warm blood and crystalloid cardioplegia during open heart surgery, *Int J Card* 90(2):253, 2003.

61. Kern LS: Postoperative atrial fibrillation: new directions in prevention and treatment, *J Cardiovasc Nurs* 19(2):103, 2004.

62. Albright TN et al: Vasopressin in the cardiac surgery intensive care unit, *Am J Crit Care* 11(4):326, 2002.

63. Reger TB, Roditski D: Bloodless medicine and surgery for patients having cardiac surgery, *Crit Care Nurs* 21(4):35, 2001.

64. Nicholson DJ et al: Postoperative pulmonary function in coronary artery bypass graft surgery patients undergoing early tracheal extubation: a comparison between short-term mechanical ventilation and early extubation, *J Cardiothorac and Vasc Anesth* 16(1):27, 2002.

65. Sakallaris BR et al: Same day transfer of patients to the cardiac telemetry unit after surgery: the Rapid After Bypass Back Into Telemetry (RABBIT) program, *Crit Care Nurse* 20(2):50, 2000.

66. Segatore M, Dutkiewicz M, Adams D: The delirious cardiac surgical patient: theoretical aspects and principles of management, *J Cardiovasc Nurs* 12(4):32, 1998.

67. Van den Berghe G et al: Outcome benefit of intensive insulin therapy in the critically ill: Insulin dose versus glycemic control, *Crit Care Med* 31(2):359, 2003.

68. Bourke JP et al: Surgery for postinfarction ventricular tachycardia in the pre-implantable cardioverter defibrillator era: early and long-term outcomes in 100 consecutive patients, *Heart* 82:156, 1999.

69. Bubien R, Sanchez JE: Atrial fibrillation: treatment rational and clinical utility of nonpharmacologic therapies, *AACN Clin Issues* 12(1):140, 2001.

70. Damiano RJ et al: The long-term outcome of patients with coronary artery disease and atrial fibrillation undergoing the Cox maze procedure, *J Thorac and Cardiovasc Surg* 126(6):2016, 2003.

71. Raman J et al: Surgical radiofrequency ablation of both atria for atrial fibrillation: results of a multicenter trial, *J Thorac and Cardiovasc Surg* 126(5):1357, 2003.

72. Chen-Scarabelli C: Beating heart coronary artery bypass surgery, *Crit Care Nurse* 22(5):44, 2002.

73. Munro N: Cardiac bypass without the pump, *RN* 66(10): 28, 2003.

74. Puskas JD et al: Off-pump vs conventional coronary artery bypass grafting: early and 1-year graft patency, cost, and quality of life outcomes: a randomized trial, *JAMA* 291(15):1841, 2004.

75. Mack MJ et al: Comparison of coronary bypass surgery with and without cardiopulmonary bypass in patients with multivessel disease, *J Thorac Cardiovasc Surg* 127(1): 167, 2004.

76. Pike NA, Gundry SR: Robotically assisted cardiac surgery: minimally invasive techniques to totally endoscopic heart surgery, *J Cardiovasc Nurs* 18(5):382, 2003.

77. Lindsay MR: Transmyocardial laser revascularization revisited, *Crit Care Nurs Q* 26(1):69, 2003.

78. Kleiman NS et al: Evolving revascularization approaches for myocardial ischemia, *Am J Cardiol* 92(suppl):9N, 2003.

79. Wehberg KE et al: Improved patient outcomes when transmyocardial revascularization is used as adjunctive revascularization, *Heart Surg Forum* 6(5):328, 2003.

80. Metules T: IABP therapy: getting patients treatment fast, *RN* 66(5):56, 2003.

81. Meco M et al: Mortality and morbidity from intra-aortic balloon pumps: risk analysis, *J Cardiovasc Surg* 43(1):12, 2002.

82. Cohen M et al: Comparison of outcomes after 8 vs 9.5 French size intra-aortic balloon counterpulsation catheters based on 9,332 patients in the Prospective Benchmark Registry, *Catheter Cardiovasc Interv* 56(2):163, 2002.

83. Stahl MA, Richards NM: Ventricular assist devices: Developing and maintaining a training and competency program, *J Cardiovasc Nurs* 16(3):34, 2003.

84. Stevenson LW: Left ventricular assist devices: bridges to transplantation, recovery, and destination for whom? *Circulation* 108:309, 2003.

85. Delgado DH et al: Mechanical circulatory assistance: state of the art, *Circulation* 106:2046, 2002.

86. Cianci P et al: Current and potential applications of left ventricular assist devices, *J Cardiovasc Nurs* 18(1):17, 2003.

87. Biller J et al: Guidelines for carotid endarterectomy: a statement for health professionals from a special writing group of the stroke council American Heart Association, *Circulation* 97(5):501, 1998.

88. Kallenbach AM, Rosenblum J: Carotid endarterectomy: creating the pathway to 1-day stay, *Crit Care Nurse* 20(4):23, 2000.

89. Jones MA, Hoffman LA, Makaroun MS: Endovascular grafting for repair of abdominal aortic aneurysm, *Crit Care Nurse* 20(4):38, 2000.

90. DeSanctis JT: Percutaneous interventions for lower extremity peripheral vascular disease, *Am Fam Physician* 64(12):1965, 2001.

91. Wooten JM, Earnest J, Reyes J: Review of common adverse effects of selected antiarrhythmic drugs, *Crit Care Nurs Q* 22(4):23, 2000.

92. Haugh KH: Antidysrhythmic agents at the turn of the 21st century, *Crit Care Nurs Clin North Am* 14(1):53, 2002.

93. Diaz AL, Clifton GD: Dofetilide: a new class III antiarrhythmic for the management of atrial fibrillation, *Prog Cardiovasc Nurs* 16:126, 2001.

94. Prasun MA, Kocheril AG: Treating atrial fibrillation: rhythm control or rate control, *J Cardiovasc Nurs* 18(5): 369, 2003.

95. Kee VR: Hemodynamic pharmacology of intravenous vasopressors, *Crit Care Nurse* 23(4):79, 2003.

96. Branum K: Decompensated heart failure, *AACN Clin Issues* 14(4):498, 2003.

97. Bisognano JD, Weder AB: Effective treatment of severe hypertension, *Prog Cardiovasc Nurs* 14(4):150, 1999.

98. Chase SL: The newest critical care drugs: part one, *RN* 62(5):34, 1999.

99. Grossman E et al: Should a moratorium be placed on sublingual nifedipine capsules given for hypertensive emergencies and pseudoemergencies? *JAMA* 276(16):1328, 1996.

100. Publication committee for the VMAC Investigators: Intravenous nesiritide vs nitroglycerin for treatment of decompensated congestive heart failure: a randomized controlled trial. VMAC study, *JAMA* 287:1531, 2002.

101. Prahash A, Lynch T: B-type natriuretic peptide: a diagnostic, prognostic, and therapeutic tool in heart failure, *Am J Crit Care* 13(1):46, 2004.

102. Harrington C: Managing hypertension in patients with stroke: are you prepared for labetalol infusion? *Crit Care Nurse* 23(3):30, 2003.

103. Thompson EJ, King SL: Acetylcysteine and Fenoldopam: promising new approaches for preventing effects of contrast nephrotoxicity, *Crit Care Nurse* 23(3):39, 2003.

104. Wenzel B et al: A comparison of vasopressin and epinephrine for out-of-hospital cardiopulmonary resuscitation, *N Eng J Med* 113(2):105, 2004.

105. Jessup M, Brozena S: Medical progress: heart failure, *N Engl J Med* 348(20):2007, 2003.

106. Hunt SH et al: ACC/AHA guidelines for the evaluation and management of chronic heart failure in the adult—executive summary (A report of the ACC/AHA task force on practice guidelines), *J Am Coll Cardiol* 38:2101, 2001.

PULMONARY ALTERATIONS

CHAPTER 20

Pulmonary Anatomy and Physiology

The pulmonary system consists of the thorax, conducting airways, respiratory airways, and pulmonary blood and lymph supply. The primary functions of the pulmonary system are ventilation and respiration. *Ventilation* is the movement of air in and out of the lungs. *Respiration* is the process of gas exchange, that is, the movement of oxygen from the atmosphere into the blood stream and the movement of carbon dioxide from the blood stream into the atmosphere. The anatomic structures that constitute the pulmonary system are intimately related to function, and structural abnormalities can readily translate into pulmonary disorders; thus an applicable knowledge of anatomy and physiology is imperative in caring for the patient with pulmonary dysfunction.

THORAX

The thorax contains the major organs of respiration. It consists of the thoracic cage, lungs, pleura, and muscles of ventilation. Together these structures form the ventilatory pump, which performs the work of breathing.

THORACIC CAGE

The thoracic cage is a cone-shaped structure that is rigid but flexible. It must be somewhat rigid to protect the underlying structures, yet it also must be flexible to accommodate inhalation and exhalation. The cage consists of 12 thoracic vertebrae, each with a pair of ribs. Posteriorly, each rib is attached to its own vertebra, but anteriorly, attachment varies (Fig. 20-1). The first seven pairs of ribs are attached directly to the sternum. The eighth, ninth, and tenth pairs are attached by cartilage to the ribs above. The eleventh and twelfth ribs have no anterior attachment, and for this reason, they sometimes are referred to as *floating ribs*. The second rib is attached to the sternum at the angle of Louis, which is the raised ridge that can be felt just below the suprasternal notch.[1]

LUNGS

The lungs are cone-shaped organs that have a total volume of approximately 3.5 to 8.5 liters. The superior portion is known as the *apex*, and the inferior portion is known as the *base*. The apical portion of each lung rises a few centimeters above the clavicle (see Fig. 20-1). Each lung is firmly attached to the thoracic cavity at the hilum and at the pulmonary ligament.[2]

Lobes and Segments. The lungs are divided into lobes and segments (Fig. 20-2), with the lobes being separated by pleural membrane–covered fissures. The right lung, which is larger and heavier than the left, is divided into upper, middle, and lower lobes. The left lung is divided into only an upper and a lower lobe.[2] A portion of the left lung, the lingula, corresponds anatomically with the right middle lobe. The horizontal fissure divides the right upper lobe from the right middle lobe. The oblique fissure divides the right upper and middle lobes from the lower lobe and the left upper lobe from the lower lobe. The lobes are divided into 18 segments, each of which has its own bronchus branching immediately off a lobar bronchus. Ten segments are located in the right lung and eight in the left lung.[1]

Mediastinum. The area between the two lungs, the mediastinum, contains the heart, great vessels, lymphatics, and the esophagus. A portion of the mediastinal area contains the root of the lungs, also known as the hilum, in which the visceral and parietal pleura form a sheath around the mainstem bronchi, the major blood vessels, and the nerves that enter and exit the lungs.[2]

PLEURA

The pleura is a thin membrane that lines the outside of the lungs and the inside of the chest wall. The visceral pleura adheres to the lungs, extending onto the hilar bronchi and into the major fissures. The parietal pleura lines the inner surface of the chest wall and mediastinum.[2] The two pleural surfaces are separated by an airtight space, which contains a thin layer of lubricating fluid. Pleural fluid allows the visceral and parietal pleural

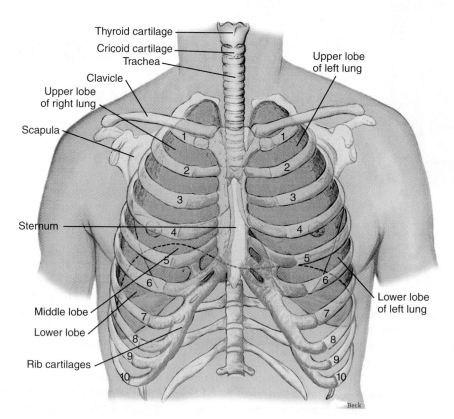

Thyroid cartilage
Cricoid cartilage
Trachea
Clavicle
Upper lobe
of right lung
Scapula
Sternum
Middle lobe
Lower lobe
Rib cartilages

Upper lobe
of left lung

Lower lobe
of left lung

Beck

Fig. 20-1 Ventilatory structures of the chest wall and lungs, showing ribs *(numbered)* and lobes of the lungs. Each intercostal space takes the number of the rib above it. The *dotted line* indicates the location of the diaphragm at inhalation and exhalation. Note the apex of each lung rising above the clavicle. (From Thibodeau GA: *Anthony's textbook of anatomy and physiology,* ed 13, St Louis, 1990, Mosby.)

membranes to glide against each other during inhalation and exhalation.[1,3] The pleural space has the capacity to hold much more fluid than its normal volume of a few milliliters.[1]

Intrapleural Pressure. The pleural space has a pressure within it termed the *intrapleural pressure,* which differs from the intrapulmonary (pressure within the lungs) and atmospheric pressures.[4] Under normal conditions intrapleural pressure is less than intrapulmonary pressure and less than atmospheric pressure, with a normal range of −4 to −10 cm H_2O during exhalation and inhalation, respectively.[3] A deep inhalation can generate intrapleural pressures of −12 to −18 cm H_2O. This negative intrapleural pressure results from forces within the chest wall that exert pressure to pull the parietal pleura outward and away from the visceral pleura while the elastic fibers within the lungs exert pressure to pull the visceral pleura inward away from the parietal pleura. The constant "pull" of the two pleural membranes in opposite directions from each other causes the pressure within the space to be subatmospheric.[4] It is the negative pressure in the pleural space that keeps the lungs inflated (Box 20-1). If atmospheric pressure enters the

pleural space, all or part of a lung will collapse, producing a pneumothorax.[1]

MUSCLES OF VENTILATION

The muscles of ventilation (Fig. 20-3) are governed by the regulatory activity of the central nervous system, which sends messages to the muscles to stimulate contraction and relaxation. This muscular activity controls inhalation and exhalation. Muscles that increase the size of the chest are termed *muscles of inhalation;* those that decrease the size of the chest are termed *muscles of exhalation.*[5]

Inhalation. The main muscle of inhalation is the diaphragm. The diaphragm is a dome-shaped fibromuscular septum that separates the thoracic and abdominal cavities. It is connected to the sternum, ribs, and vertebrae. During normal, quiet breathing the diaphragm does approximately 80% of the work of breathing. On inhalation the diaphragm contracts and flattens, pushes down on the viscera, and displaces the abdomen outward. Diaphragmatic contraction also lifts and expands the rib cage to some extent.[1,5,6]

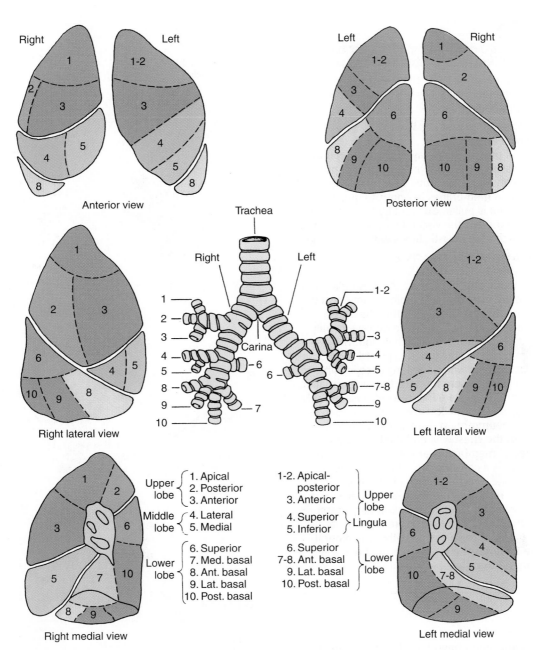

Fig. 20-2 Lungs divided into lobes and segments. Note the differences between the right and left lungs. (From Wilkens RL, Stoller JK, Scanlon CL: *Egan's fundamentals of respiratory care*, ed 8, St Louis, 2003, Mosby.)

The action of the diaphragm is governed by the medulla, which sends its impulses through the phrenic nerve. The phrenic nerve arises from the cervical plexus through the fourth cervical nerve, with secondary contributions by the third and fifth cervical nerves. For this reason and because the diaphragm does most of the work of inhalation, trauma involving levels C3 to C5 causes ventilatory dysfunction.[5]

Other muscles of inhalation include those that lift the rib cage. The most important of these are the external intercostal muscles, which elevate the ribs and expand the chest cage outward. In addition, the scalene, anterior serratus, and sternocleidomastoid muscles also participate to elevate the first two ribs and sternum.[1,5,6]

Exhalation. Exhalation in the healthy lung is a passive event requiring very little energy. Exhalation occurs when the diaphragm relaxes and moves back up toward the lungs. The intrinsic elastic recoil of the lungs assists with exhalation. Because exhalation is a passive act, there are no true muscles of exhalation other than the internal intercostal muscles, which assist the inward movement of the ribs. During exercise, however, exhalation becomes a more active event, requiring some participation of the accessory muscles of ventilation. Several

Box 20-1

WHY THE LUNGS STAY INFLATED

The lungs stay inflated because the pressure surrounding them (intrapleural) is always less than the pressure within them (intrapulmonary).

WHY IS THE INTRAPLEURAL PRESSURE LESS THAN THE INTRAPULMONARY PRESSURE?

The intrapleural pressure is always (1) less then intrapulmonary pressure, (2) less than atmospheric pressure, and (3) considered negative because of the "pull" of the two pleural membranes in opposite directions. The parietal pleura is pulled outward by forces within the chest wall, whereas the visceral pleural is pulled inward by the force of the elastic fibers within the lungs.

WHY DO THE TWO PLEURAL MEMBRANES "PULL" IN OPPOSITE DIRECTIONS?

The parietal pleura, attached to the chest, is pulled outward because the elastic fibers within the intercostal muscles exert outward pressure on the ribs. These fibers are in a relaxed state when the rib cage is fully expanded, such as during a deep inhalation. The visceral pleura, attached to the lungs, is pulled inward because the elastic fibers within the lungs, responsible for elastic recoil, exert pressure to make the lungs smaller. Elastic fibers in the lungs are in a relaxed position only when the lung is at its smallest configuration, such as occurs with a pneumothorax. Hence, because of the opposite pull of the chest wall and the lung and because the pleural membranes are attached to these structures, there is a constant pull of the two membranes in opposite directions. The subatmospheric pressure, which results within the pleural space, plus the greater-than-atmospheric intrapulmonary pressure within the lungs allows the lungs to remain inflated. Anything that causes the pressure within the pleural space to rise to atmospheric pressure or above will cause the lung(s) to collapse—a pneumothorax.

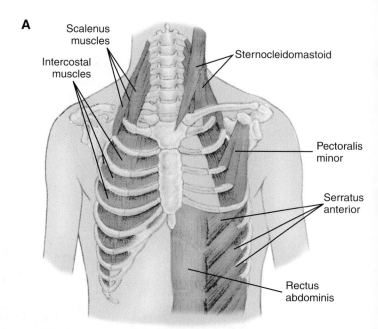

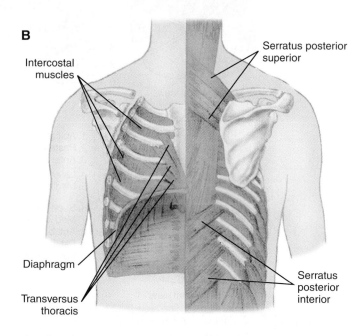

Fig. 20-3 Muscles of ventilation. **A,** Anterior view. **B,** Posterior view.

muscles of the abdomen have long been thought to contribute to active exhalation.[4,5]

Accessory Muscles. The accessory muscles of ventilation usually are considered to be those muscles that enhance chest expansion during exercise but that are not active during normal, quiet breathing. These muscles include the scalene, sternocleidomastoid, and other chest and back muscles, such as the trapezius and the pectoralis major.[1,5,6]

CONDUCTING AIRWAYS

The conducting airways consist of the upper airways, the trachea, and the bronchial tree (Fig. 20-4). The purpose of the conducting airways is threefold. The first is to warm and humidify the inhaled air. The second is to

act as a protective mechanism that prevents the entrance of foreign matter into the gas exchange areas. The third is to serve as a passageway for air entering and leaving the gas exchange regions of the lungs.[1-3]

UPPER AIRWAYS

The upper airways consist of the nasal and oral cavities, the pharynx, and the larynx (see Fig. 20-4). Their main contribution to ventilation is the conditioning of inspired air. *Conditioned air* is air that has been warmed, humid-

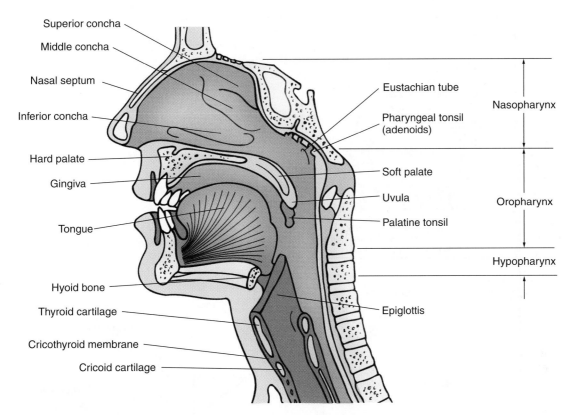

Fig. 20-4   Structures of the upper airways. Note the placement of the epiglottis. (From Ellis PD, Billings DM: *Cardiopulmonary resuscitation: procedures for basic and advanced life support*, St Louis, 1980, Mosby.)

ified, and cleansed of some irritants. Warming and humidifying, which are essential to achieving a nonirritant effect on the lower airways, occur mainly within the nose through a dense vascular network that lines the nasal passages. The air is cleansed by the coarse hairs that line the nasal passages by filtering large inhaled particles.[1,3]

Epiglottis. Also located in the upper airways is the epiglottis. It protects the lower airways by closing the opening to the trachea during swallowing so that food passes into the esophagus and not the trachea. The epiglottis is a thin, leaf-shaped, elastic cartilage, located directly posterior to the root of the tongue, that is, attached to the thyroid cartilage (see Fig. 20-4). It opens widely during inhalation, permitting air to pass through the trachea into the lower airways.[1]

TRACHEA

The trachea is a hollow tube approximately 11 cm (4.5 inches) in length and 2.5 cm (1 inch) in diameter (Fig. 20-5). It begins at the cricoid cartilage and ends at the bifurcation (the major carina) from which the two mainstem bronchi arise. The carina is approximately at the level of the aortic arch, the fifth thoracic vertebra,[7] or just below the level of the angle of Louis.[1] The trachea consists of smooth muscle supported anteriorly by 16 to

20 C-shaped, cartilaginous rings. These prevent tracheal collapse during bronchoconstriction and strong coughing. The posterior wall of the trachea lies contiguous with the anterior wall of the esophagus. Having no cartilaginous support, this wall is composed only of muscle tissue, which is separated from the anterior esophageal wall by loose connective tissue (see Fig. 20-5, *insert*).[1]

BRONCHIAL TREE

The two mainstem bronchi are structurally different (see Fig. 20-5). The left bronchus is slightly narrower than the right, and because of its position above the heart, the left bronchus angles directly toward the left lung at approximately 45 to 55 degrees from the midline. The right bronchus is wider and angles at 20 to 30 degrees from the midline. Because of this angulation and the forces of gravity, the most common site of aspiration of foreign objects is through the right mainstem bronchus into the lower lobe of the right lung.[2,3]

Bronchi. Each branching of the tracheobronchial tree produces a new generation of tubes (Fig. 20-6). The main-stem bronchi are the first generation; the next branch, the five lobar bronchi, is the second generation. The third generation includes the 18 segmental bronchi. The fourth through approximately the ninth generations are referred to as the small bronchi, beginning with the

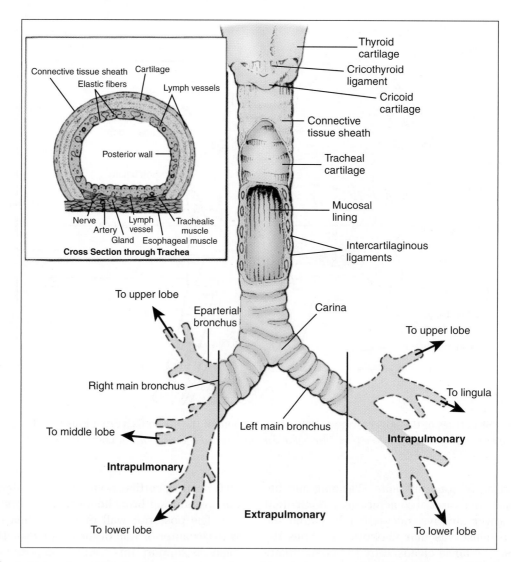

Fig. 20-5 Anterior view of the trachea and primary bronchi and a cross section through a part of the trachea, including a C-shaped cartilaginous element. (From Martin DE: *Respiratory anatomy and physiology,* St Louis, 1988, Mosby.)

subsegmental bronchi. In these bronchi, diameters decrease; however, because the number of bronchi increases with each generation, the total cross-sectional area increases with each generation. This great increase in the cross-sectional area of the lung is extremely significant in that it allows easy ventilation in spite of the decreasing airway lumens.[1]

Bronchioles. The final subdivision of the conducting airways is the bronchioles. These are tubes with a diameter less than 1 mm and without connective tissue and cartilage within their walls. Their walls do, however, contain smooth muscle.[2] When smooth-muscle constriction occurs, these airways may close completely from lack of structural support. The terminal bronchioles form the last branch of the conducting airways, after which the gas exchange areas of the lungs begin. There are more than 32,000 terminal bronchioles.[1]

Defense System. The main defense system within the airways is the mucociliary escalator, or mucous blanket, a combination of mucus and cilia. The mucus, which floats atop the cilia (Fig. 20-7), traps foreign particles. Ciliary movement then propels the entire mucous blanket and any trapped particles upward toward the pharynx at an average speed of 1 mm/min in the smaller bronchioles and 12 mm/min in the larger airways and trachea.[8] Once the pharynx is reached, the mucus is either swallowed or cleared. The submucous glands of the airways produce approximately 100 ml of mucus per day, with all but about 10 ml resorbed through the bronchial lining.[7] The mucociliary escalator is so efficient that almost no particles larger than 3 μm reach the alveoli. The cough reflex is another protective mechanism in the lungs. Excessive amounts of foreign particles in the trachea and bronchi can initiate the cough reflex. Once ini-

Conducting Airways				Respiratory Unit
Trachea	Segmental bronchi	Subsegmental bronchi (bronchioles)		Alveolar ducts
		Nonrespiratory	Respiratory	
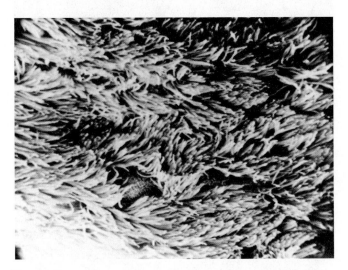				
Generations	8	16	24	26

Fig. 20-6   Conducting and respiratory airways. Note the branching with increasing generations. (From Thompson JM et al: *Mosby's clinical nursing*, ed 5, St Louis, 2002, Mosby.)

Fig. 20-7   Scanning electron micrograph of the luminal surface and cilia of a bronchiole from a normal adult male (×2000). (From Ebert RV, Terracio MJ: *Am Rev Respir Dis* 112:491, 1975.)

tiated, the rapid expulsion of air carries away any foreign particles with it.[9]

RESPIRATORY AIRWAYS

The respiratory airways consist of the respiratory bronchioles and the alveoli. The respiratory airways also are known as the *terminal respiratory units*, or the *acini*. It is in these areas of the lungs that gas exchange takes place.

RESPIRATORY BRONCHIOLES

Each terminal bronchiole gives rise to two respiratory bronchioles, each branching two to four more times.[2] The respiratory bronchioles form the transition zone of the lungs, acting as both conducting airways and gas exchange units. While air is moving through them, alveolar outpouchings on their surfaces allow gas exchange to take place (see Fig. 20-6).[1]

ALVEOLI

Each respiratory bronchiole gives rise to several alveolar ducts, which terminate in clusters of 10 to 16 alveoli (see Fig. 20-6). Thus each terminal respiratory unit contains approximately 100 alveolar ducts and 2000 alveoli.[10] The alveolus is the primary site of gas exchange and the end point in the respiratory tract. Approximately 300 million alveoli are in the two lungs. The alveoli are composed of several types of cells, including types I and II alveolar epithelial cells and alveolar macrophages.[1,3]

Type I Alveolar Epithelial Cells. Type I alveolar epithelial cells comprise approximately 90% of the total alveolar surface within the lungs (Fig. 20-8). They are the chief structural cells of the alveolar wall and play a major role in the maintenance of the gas-blood barrier and gas exchange. Type I cells are extremely susceptible to injury and become inflamed when exposed to inhaled toxins.[1,8]

Collateral Air Passages. A variety of collateral air passages are located within the lower regions of the

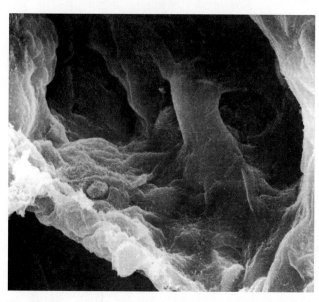

Fig. 20-8 Detail of an alveolar surface composed chiefly of type I alveolar epithelial cells (picture width—1 cm equals 3.46 µm). (From Martin DE: *Respiratory anatomy and physiology*, St Louis, 1988, Mosby.)

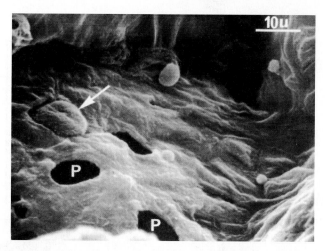

Fig. 20-9 Scanning electron micrograph of the surface of a human alveolus, showing pores of Kohn *(P)* and a macrophage *(arrow)* (×1500). (Courtesy Dr. MS Wang.)

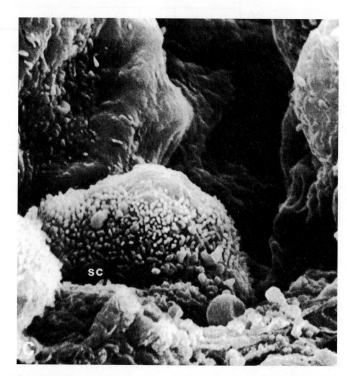

Fig. 20-10 Type II alveolar epithelial cell. Note the presence of brush microvilli on all except the bald top of the round luminal surface. Type II cells produce surfactant. (Picture width: 1 cm equals 0.85 µm.) (From Martin DE: *Respiratory anatomy and physiology*, St Louis, 1988, Mosby.)

lungs. Within the walls of the type I cells are the pores of Kohn (Fig. 20-9), which allow collateral movement of air between alveoli. The canals of Lambert are collateral air pathways that exist between the alveoli and the respiratory and terminal bronchioles.[8] They are of particular benefit when a respiratory bronchiole is blocked or collapsed, since they allow gas to pass into alveoli distal to the blockage. Thus collateral air passages are of significant benefit in any pathologic condition of the lung that results in obstruction of airflow into a portion of the lungs. In contrast, however, these pores and canals also allow the movement of microorganisms through lung tissue.[1,2]

Type II Alveolar Epithelial Cells. Type II alveolar epithelial cells occur in much greater numbers than type I cells, but because of their minute size, they comprise a smaller portion of the total alveolar wall. After injury to the alveolar wall, type II cells rapidly divide to line the surface; later they transform into type I cells. The most important function of the type II cells is their ability to produce, store, and secrete pulmonary surfactant (Fig. 20-10).[1,3,8]

Surfactant. Surfactant is a phospholipid composed of fatty acids bound to lecithin. Like other surfactants, such as detergents and soaps, pulmonary surfactant functions to lower surface tension of the alveoli. Whereas with detergents and soaps this decrease in surface tension cleans clothes, within the lungs it stabilizes the alveoli, increases lung compliance, and eases the work of breathing. When pulmonary disease disrupts the normal synthesis and storage of surfactant, the lungs become less compliant and the work of breathing increases. Severe loss of surfactant results in alveolar instability and collapse and impairment of gas exchange.[11]

Defense System. Alveolar macrophages are monocytes that originate in the bone marrow and are released into the blood stream (Fig. 20-11).[1-3] On entering the pulmonary capillary circulation, they move through the capillary membrane wall into the interstitial space and through

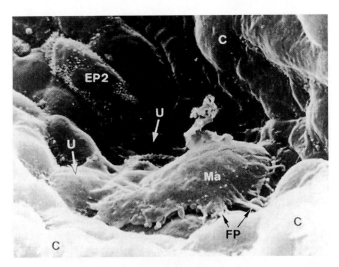

Fig. 20-11 Scanning electron micrograph of a healthy human lung, showing an alveolar macrophage *(Ma)* attached to the epithelium partly by filopodia *(FP)* and forming an undulating membrane *(U)* in the direction of forward movement to the left. Several capillaries *(C)* are evident, and a type II alveolar epithelial cell *(EP2)* can be seen in the background. (Original magnification ×3700.) (From Gehr P, Bachofen M, Weibel ER: *Respir Physiol* 32[2]:121, 1978.)

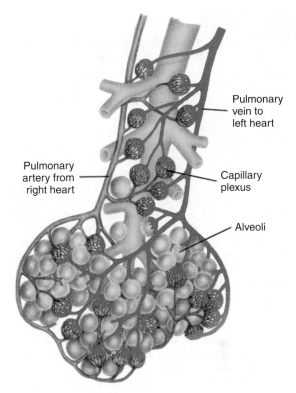

Fig. 20-12 Terminal ventilation and perfusion units of the lung. Pulmonary arterial blood is venous *(dark gray)*, and pulmonary venous blood is oxygenated *(blue)*. (From Thompson JM et al: *Mosby's clinical nursing*, ed 5, St Louis, 2002, Mosby.)

to the alveoli. Once in the alveoli, the monocytes transform into macrophages and assume a phagocytic role. They move from alveolus to alveolus through the pores of Kohn, keeping the alveoli clean and sterile through phagocytosis and microbial killing activity, which includes the secretion of hydrogen peroxide, lysozyme, and other substances that kill microorganisms.[2,3]

PULMONARY BLOOD AND LYMPH SUPPLY

Two vascular systems and one lymphatic system make up the pulmonary blood and lymph supply. The pulmonary circulation is the vascular system that forms the gas exchange network surrounding the alveoli. The bronchial circulation is the vascular system that perfuses the tracheobronchial tree.[1]

PULMONARY CIRCULATION

The pulmonary circulatory system begins at the pulmonary artery, which receives venous blood from the right side of the heart. The pulmonary artery then divides into left and right branches and continues to branch until it forms the capillaries that surround the alveoli (Fig. 20-12). After gas exchange takes place, the blood is returned to the left side of the heart through the pulmonary veins.[1,2]

Pulmonary Artery Pressures. The pulmonary circulation is, by far, the largest vascular bed within the body

and is the only one that receives the entire cardiac output. Just as the systemic circulation has a systolic and a diastolic blood pressure, so does the pulmonary circulation. However, because of the relative lack of smooth muscle within the vessels of the pulmonary circulation, the pressures are vastly lower than within the systemic circulation.[1,3] Pulmonary artery systolic (PAS) pressure averages 25 mm Hg, pulmonary artery diastolic (PAD) pressure averages 10 mm Hg, and pulmonary artery mean (PAM) pressure is 15 mm Hg.[12] Because of the low pulmonary artery pressures, right ventricular wall thickness needs to be only approximately one third of left ventricular wall thickness. However, just as hypertension can occur within the systemic circulation, it also can occur within the pulmonary circulation (Box 20-2).[13]

ALVEOLAR-CAPILLARY MEMBRANE

The vessels of the alveolar-capillary membrane form a network around each alveolus that is so dense it forms an almost continuous sheet of blood covering the alveoli.[2] The interior diameter of each capillary segment is just large enough to allow red blood cells to squeeze by in single file so that their cell membranes touch the capillary walls (Fig. 20-13).[4] In this way, oxygen and carbon

Box 20-2

PULMONARY HYPERTENSION

Pulmonary hypertension is defined as increased pressure (PAS greater than 30 mm Hg and PAM greater than 18 mm Hg) within the pulmonary arterial system. It occurs when the cross-sectional area of the pulmonary bed decreases as a result of vasoconstriction and/or structural changes in the vascular bed. These changes may be a result of a variety of pathophysiologic conditions, including impedance to pulmonary venous drainage (e.g., mitral stenosis); increased pulmonary blood flow (e.g., septal defect); impedance to flow through large pulmonary arteries (e.g., pulmonary embolus) or small pulmonary blood vessels (e.g., collagen vascular diseases); and impedance to flow from hypoxic vasoconstriction.

The pulmonary hypertension resulting from hypoxic vasoconstriction, although caused in part by vasospasm, is largely a result of alterations in the structure of the blood vessels of the pulmonary circulation, which results in an increase in the medial thickness and a reduction in the size of the vascular lumen. Pulmonary hypertension increases the afterload of the right ventricle and, when chronic, can result in right ventricular hypertrophy (cor pulmonale) and failure.

PAS, Pulmonary artery systolic; *PAM,* pulmonary artery mean.

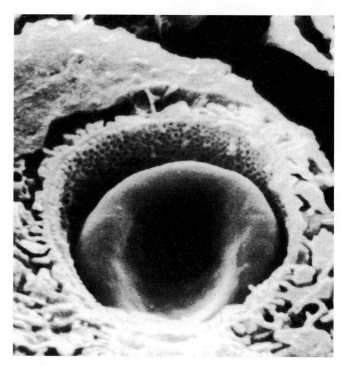

Fig. 20-13 Scanning electron micrograph of a red blood cell in a capillary. Note that the diameters of both are similar. In many instances the red blood cells course through even smaller capillaries, often through capillaries that are one-half the diameter of the red blood cell. This is possible because the cells are pliable, mainly as a result of their biconcave disk shape. (From Martin DE: *Respiratory anatomy and physiology,* St Louis, 1988, Mosby.)

dioxide need not pass through significant amounts of plasma when diffusing into and out of the alveoli, making a highly efficient vehicle for gas exchange. Each red blood cell spends approximately three fourths of a second in the alveolar-capillary network and is exposed to the alveolar gas of two or three alveoli.[1] In that short time, hemoglobin is brought from its normal venous blood saturation level of 75% to its arterial saturation of more than 96%.[4] Actually, hemoglobin levels have been shown to reach normal within only a 0.25-second exposure to alveolar gas; thus under conditions such as in tachycardia, in which the red blood cells spend less time within the pulmonary capillary network, normal oxygenation can still occur.[3]

Membrane Layers. The alveolar-capillary membrane is less than 0.5 μm thick[14] and is composed of several layers of cells: the alveolar epithelium, the alveolar basement membrane, the interstitial space, the capillary basement membrane, and the capillary endothelium (Fig. 20-14). Oxygen and carbon dioxide traverse easily across these layers, which present no barrier to diffusion because the membrane is very thin.[3]

BRONCHIAL CIRCULATION

The bronchial circulation, also known as the *systemic blood supply to the lungs,* is the system that perfuses the tracheobronchial tree, the visceral pleura, interstitial

and connective tissue, some arteries and veins, lymph nodes, and the nerves within the thoracic cavity. The bronchial arteries that perfuse structures in the left side of the thorax branch off the aorta, and those that perfuse the right-sided structures branch from the intercostal, subclavian, or internal mammary artery. After perfusing the specific lung structures, most of the venous blood returns to the right side of the heart; however, some venous blood from the bronchial circulation returns directly into the pulmonary veins and the left atrium.[1]

Physiologic Shunting. The left atrium normally contains pure oxygenated blood, with a hemoglobin saturation at 100%. The mixing of venous blood from the bronchial circulation with the oxygenated blood in the left atrium decreases the saturation of left atrial blood to a range between 96% and 99%. For this reason, while a person is breathing room air, the oxygen saturation of arterial blood is less than 100%. The dumping of venous blood into the left atrium is known as an *anatomic shunt.* The thebesian veins, which drain the right coronary circulation, are also responsible for the addition of venous blood to the left atrium. These two systems constitute the normal anatomic shunt, which comprises approximately 3% to 5% of the total cardiac output.[15]

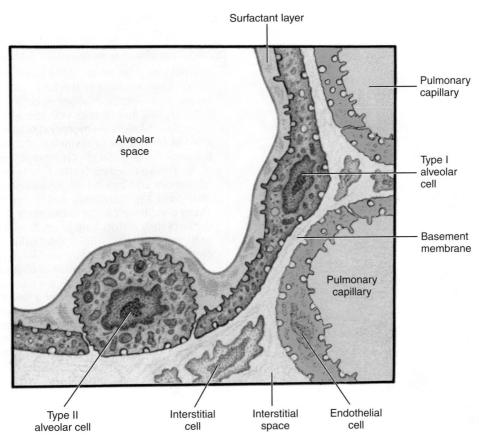

Surfactant layer

Pulmonary capillary

Alveolar space

Type I alveolar cell

Basement membrane

Pulmonary capillary

Type II alveolar cell

Interstitial cell

Interstitial space

Endothelial cell

Fig. 20-14   Layers of the alveolar-capillary membrane. (From Thompson JM et al: *Mosby's clinical nursing,* ed 5, St Louis, 2002, Mosby.)

LYMPHATIC CIRCULATION

The lungs are more richly supplied with lymphatic tissue than any other organ, perhaps because of their constant exposure to the external environment. The lymphatic vessels parallel much of the pulmonary vasculature and the tracheobronchial tree to the level of the terminal and respiratory bronchioles. Lymphatic vessels also are located within the connective tissue of lung parenchyma and within the pleural membranes. These vessels eventually drain into the primary lymph nodes located at the hila of the lungs. The lymphatic system in the lungs serves two purposes. As part of the immune system, it is responsible for removing foreign particles and cell debris from the lungs and for producing both antibody and cell-mediated immune responses. It also is responsible for removing fluid from the lungs and for keeping the alveoli clear.[1-3]

VENTILATION

Air moves into and out of the lungs because of the difference between intrapulmonary pressure (pressure inside the lungs) and atmospheric pressure (Fig. 20-15). The movement of air into the lungs is known as *inhalation,* whereas the movement of air out of the lungs is known as *exhalation.* At the command of the central nervous system, the muscles of ventilation contract, the thorax and lungs expand, and intrapulmonary pressure falls. When the pressure falls below atmospheric pressure, air enters the lungs and inhalation occurs. At the end of inhalation, the muscles of ventilation relax, the thorax contracts and the lungs are compressed, and intrapulmonary pressure rises. When the pressure rises above atmospheric pressure, air exits the lungs and exhalation occurs.[4,16]

WORK OF BREATHING

The work of breathing is the amount of work that must be performed to overcome the elastic and resistive properties of the lungs. The elastic properties are determined by lung recoil, chest wall recoil, and the surface tension of the alveoli. The resistive properties are determined by airway resistance.[1,16,17] Normally the work of breathing occurs during inhalation. Even exhalation, however, can be a strain when lung recoil, chest wall recoil, and/or airway resistance is abnormal.[4,16]

During normal, quiet ventilation only 1% to 2% of basal oxygen consumption is required by the pulmonary sys-

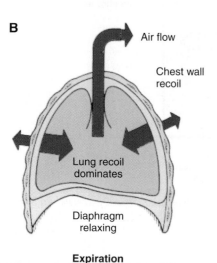

A

Air flow

Chest wall recoil

Muscular contraction dominates

Lung recoil

Diaphragm contracting

Inspiration

B

Air flow

Chest wall recoil

Lung recoil dominates

Diaphragm relaxing

Expiration

Fig. 20-15 The process of inhalation and exhalation. **A,** During inhalation the muscles of ventilation contract, the thorax and lungs expand, and air enters the lungs. **B,** During exhalation the muscles of ventilation relax, the thorax and lungs are compressed, and air exits the lungs. (Modified from McCance KL, Huether SE, editors: *Pathophysiology: the biologic basis for disease in adults and children*, ed 5, St Louis, 2002, Mosby.)

tem.[17] During heavy exercise the amount of energy required by the pulmonary system can become progressively greater. Thus the work of breathing can be a factor that limits exercise in the patient with pulmonary disease. Pathologic conditions of the pulmonary system can drastically change the energy requirement for ventilation. Pulmonary diseases that decrease lung compliance (e.g., atelectasis, pulmonary edema), decrease chest wall compliance (e.g., kyphoscoliosis), increase airway resistance (e.g., bronchitis and asthma), or decrease lung recoil (e.g., emphysema) can increase the work of breathing so much that one third or more of the total body energy is used for ventilation (Box 20-3).[4,16]

BOX 20-3

HOW LUNG DISEASE CAN ALTER VENTILATION

Normal muscular action of the diaphragm, flexibility of the rib cage, elasticity of the lungs, and airway diameter are instrumental in allowing easy inhalation and exhalation. Any interference with these actions impairs normal ventilation. Pulmonary diseases can be categorized as obstructive or restrictive, depending on how the underlying cause affects normal ventilation.

Restrictive diseases "restrict" lung or chest wall movement and include diffuse interstitial lung fibrosis, atelectasis, kyphoscoliosis, and severe chest wall pain. These conditions can be either acute or chronic, and because they restrict lung or chest wall expansion, or both, patients have smaller tidal volumes but an increased ventilatory rate to maintain minute ventilation.

Obstructive diseases result in obstruction to normal airflow. The classic examples are emphysema, in which airflow is decreased because of a decrease in lung recoil, and asthma, in which airflow is decreased because of diffuse airway narrowing. Emphysema results in lungs that inflate easily but, lacking the normal elastic recoil, do not compress to assist with exhalation. Patients with emphysema may have little difficulty inhaling but struggle to exhale.

PULMONARY VOLUMES AND CAPACITIES

Pulmonary ventilation can be described in terms of volumes and capacities (Fig. 20-16). Tidal volume (V_T) is the amount of air inhaled and exhaled with each breath. Inspiratory reserve volume (IRV) is the maximum amount of air that can be inhaled over and above the normal tidal volume. Expiratory reserve volume (ERV) is the maximum amount of air that can be exhaled beyond the normal tidal volume. The residual volume (RV) is the amount of air left in the lungs after a complete exhalation. Inspiratory capacity (IC) is the sum of the tidal volume and the inspiratory reserve. Functional residual capacity (FRC) is the sum of the expiratory reserve volume and the residual volume. Vital capacity (VC) is the sum of the inspiratory reserve volume, the tidal volume, and the expiratory reserve volume. Total lung capacity (TLC) is the sum of all four volumes and represents the maximal amount of air that can be inhaled.[3,16]

Physiologic Dead Space. The portion of total ventilation that participates in gas exchange is known as *alveolar ventilation.* The portion of ventilation that does not is known as *wasted ventilation.* The areas in the lungs that are ventilated but in which no gas exchange occurs are known as *dead space regions.* The conducting airways are referred to as *anatomic dead space* because they are ventilated but not perfused; thus they are not able to participate in gas exchange. In addition, some ventilation goes to unperfused alveoli. Without perfu-

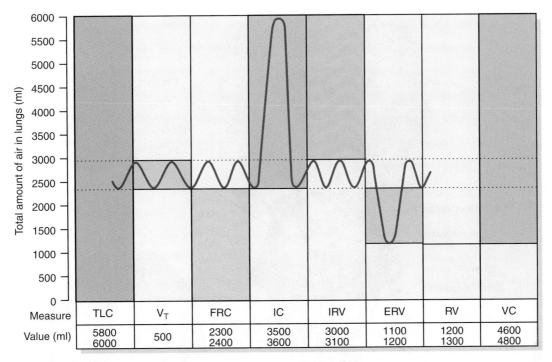

Fig. 20-16 Lung volume measurements. All values are approximately 25% less in women. *TLC*, Total lung capacity; *V*$_T$, tidal volume; *FRC*, functional residual capacity; *IC*, inspiratory capacity; *IRV*, inspiratory reserve volume; *ERV*, expiratory reserve volume; *RV*, residual volume; *VC*, vital capacity.

Measure	TLC	V$_T$	FRC	IC	IRV	ERV	RV	VC
Value (ml)	5800 6000	500	2300 2400	3500 3600	3000 3100	1100 1200	1200 1300	4600 4800

sion, gas exchange cannot take place and thus the ventilation is wasted. These unperfused alveoli are known as *alveolar dead space.* Anatomic dead space plus alveolar dead space is termed *physiologic dead space.*[3,15,16]

REGULATION OF VENTILATION

Regulation of ventilation by the brain is complex and not completely understood. Ventilation is regulated by a triad comprising a controller (located within the central nervous system), a group of effectors (muscles of ventilation), and a variety of sensors that include chemoreceptors (central and peripheral) and mechanoreceptors (located in chest wall and lungs). Efferent nerve fibers convey impulses from the controller to the effectors, whereas afferent nerve fibers carry impulses from some of the sensors to the controller (Fig. 20-17).[18]

Controller. The central nervous system houses what is known as the *controller of ventilation.* Actually, the controller is not located in one specific area; rather, it is in several areas that work together to provide coordinated ventilation. The brainstem regulates automatic ventilation, the cerebral cortex allows voluntary ventilation, and neurons housed in the spinal cord process information from the brain and from the peripheral receptors, allowing them to send final information to the muscles of ventilation.[18]

Brainstem. In the brainstem, both the medulla oblongata and the pons are involved in ventilation. Four different groups of neurons are thought to participate in the regulation of inhalation and exhalation. The dorsal respiratory group, located in the medulla, is responsible for the basic rhythm of ventilation. Cells in this area are believed to automatically fire and trigger inhalation. The pneumotaxic center in the pons is responsible for limiting inhalation and thus triggering exhalation. This response also facilitates control of the rate and pattern of respiration. The ventral respiratory group, located in the medulla, is responsible for both inspiration and expiration during periods of increased ventilation. The apneustic center in the lower pons is thought to work with the pneumotaxic center to regulate the depth of inspiration.[18]

Cerebral Cortex. The cerebral cortex functions by allowing voluntary ventilation to override the automatic controls of the medulla and pons. Voluntary ventilatory control is most important during such behavioral states as crying, laughing, singing, and talking. During these states, voluntary control may override the automatic control, which responds chiefly to chemical stimuli and to changes in lung inflation.[3,18]

Effectors. The effectors of ventilation are the muscles of ventilation (see Fig. 20-3). In considering their function in the control of ventilation, however, the most important issue is that they function in a coordinated fashion. The central nervous system regulates this function.[18]

Sensors. The main sensors for the regulation of ventilation are the central and peripheral chemoreceptors (see Fig. 20-17). These chemoreceptors respond to

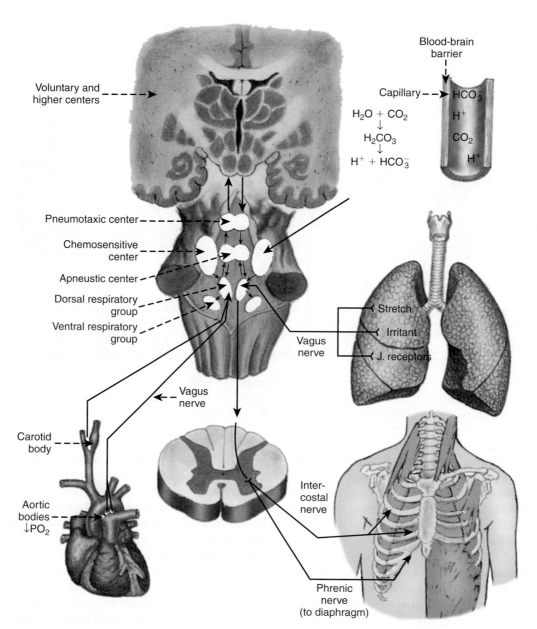

Voluntary and higher centers

Blood-brain barrier

Capillary

$$H_2O + CO_2$$
$$\downarrow$$
$$H_2CO_3$$
$$\downarrow$$
$$H^+ + HCO_3^-$$

HCO_3^-

H^+

CO_2

H^+

Pneumotaxic center

Chemosensitive center

Apneustic center

Dorsal respiratory group

Ventral respiratory group

Vagus nerve

Stretch

Irritant

J. receptors

Vagus nerve

Carotid body

Aortic bodies
↓PO₂

Inter-costal nerve

Phrenic nerve (to diaphragm)

Fig. 20-17 Respiratory control system. (From McCance KL, Huether SE, editors: *Pathophysiology: the biologic basis for disease in adults and children,* ed 4, St Louis, 2002, Mosby.)

changes in the chemical composition of the blood or other fluid around them. Other sensors that are found in the lung include the irritant receptors, stretch receptors, and the juxtacapillary (J) receptors.[3,18]

Central Chemoreceptors. The central chemoreceptors are located near the ventral surface of the medulla in the chemosensitive area (see Fig. 20-17). These chemoreceptors are surrounded by cerebral extracellular fluid and respond primarily to changes in the hydrogen ion concentration of that fluid. Ventilation increases when the hydrogen ion concentration rises and decreases when the hydrogen ion concentration falls. A rise in the partial pressure of carbon dioxide ($Paco_2$) causes the movement of carbon dioxide across the blood-brain barrier into the cerebrospinal fluid, stimulating the move-

ment of hydrogen ions into the brain's extracellular fluid. These hydrogen ions then stimulate the chemoreceptors, and ventilation is increased. Consequently, the increase in ventilation causes exhalation of excess carbon dioxide, the $Paco_2$ falls, and ventilation returns to normal. Central chemoreceptors are not affected by changes in the partial pressure of oxygen (Pao_2).[18]

Peripheral Chemoreceptors. The peripheral chemoreceptors are located above and below the aortic arch and at the bifurcation of the common carotid arteries (see Fig. 20-17). The most important action of the peripheral chemoreceptors is their response to changes in the Pao_2, because they are the primary receptors that increase ventilation in response to arterial hypoxemia. Thus immediate hyperventilation, one of the principal

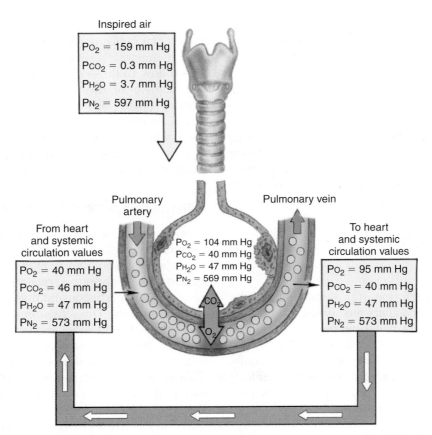

Fig. 20-18   Process of respiration. (From Thompson JM et al: *Mosby's clinical nursing,* ed 5, St Louis, 2002, Mosby.)

compensatory mechanisms in response to hypoxemia, is governed by these chemoreceptors. The peripheral chemoreceptors also respond to changes in Pa_{CO_2} and hydrogen ion concentration. An increase in either results in an increase in ventilation. Studies indicate that the peripheral chemoreceptors probably are more involved with short-term response to carbon dioxide, whereas the central chemoreceptors are responsible for the long-term response to carbon dioxide.[18]

Other Receptors. Irritant receptors lie between airway epithelial cells and function to stimulate bronchoconstriction and hyperpnea in response to inhaled irritants. Stretch receptors, which are located in the airways, are stimulated by changes in lung volume. They inhibit inhalation and are thought to protect the lung from overinflation (Hering-Breuer reflex). J receptors lie in the alveolar walls close to the capillaries. They are stimulated by engorgement of the pulmonary capillaries and an increase in the interstitial fluid volume. Stimulation of the J receptors is thought to cause rapid, shallow breathing.[1]

RESPIRATION

Respiration refers to the movement of oxygen and carbon dioxide. Gas exchange that takes place at the lung level through the alveolar-capillary membrane is referred to as *external respiration.* The diffusion of gases

in and out of the cells at the tissue level is referred to as *internal respiration.*[3]

DIFFUSION

Oxygen and carbon dioxide move throughout the body by diffusion. Diffusion moves molecules from an area of high concentration to an area of low concentration. The difference in the concentrations of the gases is referred to as the *driving pressure.* The greater the driving pressure of the gas through the membrane, the greater the diffusion.[3] Within the lungs, diffusion occurs because of the difference in the driving pressure between the pulmonary capillaries and the alveoli. Oxygen is in high concentration within the alveoli and thus exerts a higher driving pressure as compared with the pulmonary capillaries; therefore oxygen moves by diffusion from the alveoli into the pulmonary capillaries. On the other hand, carbon dioxide is in higher concentration and thus has a higher driving pressure within the pulmonary capillaries as compared with the alveoli; therefore carbon dioxide diffuses out of the capillaries into the alveoli, where it is exhaled (Fig. 20-18).[4] The driving pressure of oxygen is lower at higher altitudes because the effects of gravity on the gases are lessened[19] and is higher when supplemental oxygen is administered.[20]

In addition to the driving pressure of the gases, several other factors affect the rate of diffusion. These include the thickness of the alveolar-capillary membrane,[3] the surface area of the membrane,[21] and the diffusion coefficient of the gas.[20] An increase in the thickness of the alveolar-capillary membrane (e.g., pulmonary edema, fibrosis)[3] or a decrease in the surface area of the membrane (e.g., pneumonectomy, lobectomy, pulmonary embolus, emphysema)[21] will decrease the rate of diffusion. The diffusion coefficient of each gas is determined by its solubility. The higher the diffusion coefficient, the faster the gas diffuses. Carbon dioxide has a much higher diffusion coefficient than oxygen, thus carbon dioxide diffuses 20 times more rapidly than does oxygen.[20]

VENTILATION/PERFUSION RELATIONSHIPS

Ventilation (V) and perfusion (Q) should be equally matched at the alveolar capillary membrane level for optimal gas exchange to take place, but because of normal regional variations in the distribution of ventilation and perfusion, this is not the case. Normally alveolar ventilation is approximately 4 L/min, and pulmonary capillary perfusion is approximately 5 L/min. Thus the normal ventilation to perfusion (V/Q) ratio is 4:5, or 0.8.[15,20]

DISTRIBUTION OF VENTILATION

The distribution of ventilation throughout the lungs is not even. This is the result of a variety of factors, including the configuration of the thorax and the effects of gravity on intrapleural pressure. The thorax allows more lung expansion at the base than at the apex, which permits more ventilation to the base and limits ventilation to the apex. Gravity also produces regional variations in intrapleural pressure. At rest the negative intrapleural pressure at the apex is greater than at the base, and thus alveoli in the apexes are larger and have more air left in them at the end of expiration. Because the alveoli are larger, they are less compliant and more difficult to inflate. On inhalation the alveoli at the base expand more because they have less pressure to overcome.[3,15,16] In the upright person, the base of the lung receives about four times more ventilation than does the apex.[16] In the supine person, gravity produces the same effects in the dependent zones of the lungs (posterior regions).[3,15,16]

DISTRIBUTION OF PERFUSION

The distribution of perfusion through the lungs is related to gravity and intraalveolar pressures. Because of the effects of gravity, the pressure in the capillaries in the lungs is higher in the bases than in the apexes. This promotes preferential blood flow to the gravity-dependent areas of the lungs. Intraalveolar pressures also vary throughout the different regions of the lungs, with the highest pressure in the apexes and the lowest pressure

in the bases. Thus in some areas of the lungs, the intraalveolar pressure has the potential of exceeding capillary hydrostatic pressure, resulting in an absence of blood flow to these areas. On the basis of this concept the lung can be divided into three zones. Zone 1 is the nondependent portion of the lung, which has the potential of no perfusion. Zone 2 is the middle portion of the lung, which receives varying blood flow. Zone 3 is the gravity-dependent area of the lung, which receives a constant blood flow (Fig. 20-19).[3,15]

VENTILATION/PERFUSION MISMATCHING

A variety of factors can affect the matching of ventilation to perfusion in the lungs, and their relationship can be considered as a continuum (Fig. 20-20). At one end of the continuum the alveolus is receiving ventilation but is not receiving any perfusion and thus is unable to participate in gas exchange. This situation is referred to as *alveolar dead space*. On the other end of the continuum, the alveolus is receiving perfusion but is not receiving any ventilation and thus is unable to participate in gas exchange. This situation is referred to as *intrapulmonary shunting*. In this case the blood is returned to the left side of the heart unoxygenated.[21] Between these two extremes exist an infinite number of ventilation/perfusion mismatches. Situations in which ventilation exceeds perfusion (V/Q >0.8) are considered to be *dead space–producing*, whereas situations in which perfusion exceeds ventilation (V/Q <0.8) are considered to be *shunt-producing*. Although minor mismatching of ventilation may not significantly affect gas exchange, significant alterations in the relationship result in hypoxemia.[15,21]

Hypoxic Vasoconstriction. The distribution of perfusion is also affected by the amount of oxygen in the alveoli. Although most blood vessels in the body dilate in response to hypoxia, the pulmonary vessels constrict when the Pa_{O_2} is less than 60 mm Hg. This event is known as *hypoxic vasoconstriction*, and it generally occurs when a portion of the pulmonary capillaries perfuses unventilated or underventilated alveoli. It is thought to be a compensatory response used to limit the returning of unoxygenated blood to the left side of the heart. If the response is prolonged and generalized throughout the lungs, pulmonary hypertension will result.[3]

GAS TRANSPORT

Gas transport refers to the movement of oxygen and carbon dioxide to and from the tissue cells. The transportation vehicle is the blood stream, which is moved by the pumping action of the heart (cardiac output). At the tissue level, both oxygen and carbon dioxide move into and out of the cell by diffusion. Oxygen diffuses into the cell because of the pressure gradient that exists between oxygen

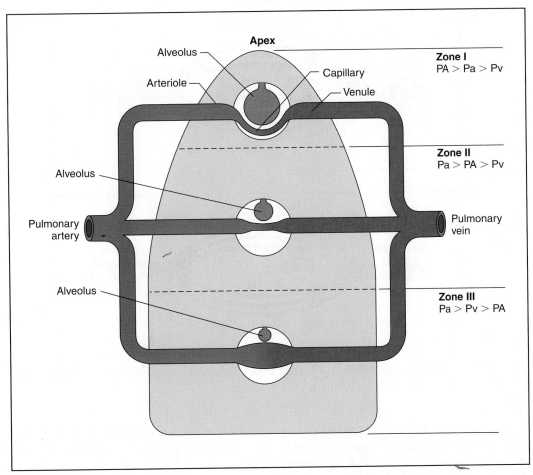

Fig. 20-19   The effects of gravity and alveolar pressure on pulmonary blood flow. Note the three different lung zones. (From McCance KL, Huether SE, editors: *Pathophysiology: the biologic basis for disease in adults and children,* ed 4, St Louis, 2002, Mosby.)

in the capillary and oxygen in the cell (Fig. 20-21, *A*). Carbon dioxide diffuses into the capillary because of the pressure gradient that exists between carbon dioxide in the cell and carbon dioxide in the capillary (Fig. 20-21, *B*).[3]

OXYGEN CONTENT

Oxygen is transported to the tissues by the blood in two ways. It is either dissolved in plasma (PaO_2) or bound to hemoglobin molecules (oxygen saturation [SaO_2]). Most of the oxygen is transported by hemoglobin, with the portion of oxygen dissolved in plasma equal to approximately 3% of the total oxygen within the blood.[22] The pressure exerted by the oxygen dissolved in plasma is important because this oxygen diffuses across the capillary membrane into the cells first and serves as the vehicle for the unloading of the oxygen from the hemoglobin molecule. As molecules of dissolved oxygen leave the plasma and diffuse into the cells, the molecules of oxygen move off the hemoglobin, dissolve into the plasma, and, in turn, diffuse into the cells.[19] For this process to begin, a pressure gradient must exist between the oxygen level in the capillary and the oxygen level in the cell.

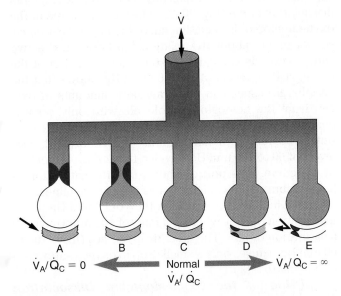

Fig. 20-20   Continuum of ventilation/perfusion relationships. *A,* Intrapulmonary shunting. *B,* V/Q mismatching—shunt-producing situation. *C,* Normal V/Q ratio. *D,* V/Q mismatching—dead space–producing situation. *E,* Alveolar dead space. (From Misasi RS, Keyes JL: *Crit Care Nurse* 16[3]:23, 1996.)

A

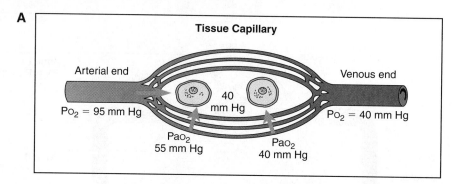

Tissue Capillary

Arterial end

$Po_2 = 95$ mm Hg

40 mm Hg

Pao_2 55 mm Hg

Pao_2 40 mm Hg

Venous end

$Po_2 = 40$ mm Hg

B

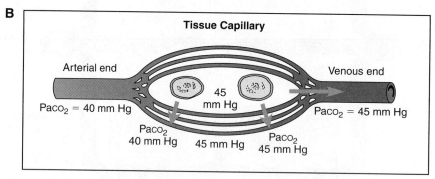

Tissue Capillary

Arterial end

$Paco_2 = 40$ mm Hg

45 mm Hg

$Paco_2$ 40 mm Hg

45 mm Hg

$Paco_2$ 45 mm Hg

Venous end

$Paco_2 = 45$ mm Hg

Fig. 20-21 Internal respiration. **A,** Diffusion of oxygen from a tissue capillary into a tissue cell. **B,** Diffusion of carbon dioxide from a tissue cell into a tissue capillary.

Oxygen Content Formula. The amount of oxygen in the arterial blood can be calculated using the arterial oxygen content (Cao_2) formula. The amount of oxygen in the venous blood can be calculated using the venous oxygen content (Cvo_2) formula (see Appendix).[22]

Oxyhemoglobin Dissociation Curve. The relationship between dissolved oxygen and hemoglobin-bound oxygen is illustrated graphically as the oxyhemoglobin dissociation curve (Fig. 20-22). The sigmoid shape of the oxyhemoglobin dissociation curve illustrates several essential points about the relationship between the two ways oxygen is carried. The steep lower portion of the curve, at Pao_2 levels of 10 to 60 mm Hg, shows that the peripheral tissues can withdraw large amounts of oxygen from the hemoglobin molecule with only a small change in Pao_2, thus preserving the gradient for the continued unloading of hemoglobin.[19,22] The area at Pao_2 levels of 60 to 100 mm Hg is called the *flat upper portion* of the curve. This portion shows that the saturation of hemoglobin remains high even as the Pao_2 declines. For example, in a healthy person, a Pao_2 of 60 mm Hg yields a saturation of 89%, whereas a Pao_2 of 100 mm Hg yields a saturation of 98%. The great drop in Pao_2 (from 100 to 60 mm Hg) causes only a small drop in oxygen saturation (from 98% to 89%).[20,22]

Shifting of the Oxyhemoglobin Dissociation Curve. Under normal circumstances, hemoglobin has a steady and predictable affinity for oxygen. The combination of oxygen and hemoglobin based on this affinity is responsible for the position of the oxyhemoglobin dissociation curve wherein a given Pao_2 yields a predictable oxygen saturation.[19,22] Occasionally events occur that alter the affinity hemoglobin has for oxygen. These events include changes in pH, $Paco_2$, temperature, and 2,3-diphosphoglycerate (2,3-DPG) (Box 20-4). Any time this affinity is altered, the position of the oxyhemoglobin dissociation curve shifts (see Fig. 20-22). Shifts in the position of the curve mean there is a change in the way oxygen is taken up by the hemoglobin molecule at the alveolar level, as well as a change in the way oxygen is delivered at the tissue level.[20,22]

Shift to the Right. When the curve is shifted to the right (see Fig. 20-22, *curve C*), there is a lower oxygen saturation for any given Pao_2; in other words, hemoglobin has less affinity for oxygen. Although the saturation is lower than expected, a right shift enhances oxygen delivery at the tissue level because hemoglobin unloads more readily. Factors that cause this change in oxygen-hemoglobin affinity and shift the curve to the right include fever, increased $Paco_2$, acidosis, and an increase in 2,3-DPG.[20,22]

Shift to the Left. When the curve is shifted to the left (see Fig. 20-22, *curve A*), quite the reverse occurs: there is a higher arterial saturation for any given Pao_2 because hemoglobin has an increased affinity for oxygen. Although the saturation is higher, oxygen delivery to the tissues is impaired because hemoglobin does not unload as easily. Factors that contribute to the effect include hypothermia, alkalemia, decreased $Paco_2$, and decreased 2,3-DPG.[20,22]

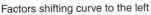

Factors shifting curve to the left
1. ↑ pH
2. ↓ P_{CO_2}
3. ↓ Temperature
4. ↓ 2, 3-DPG:
   a. Hexokinase deficiency
   b. Hypothyroidism
   c. Bank blood
5. Some congenital hemoglobinopathies:
   a. Hemoglobin Ranier
   b. Hemoglobin Hiroshima
   c. Hemoglobin San Francisco
6. Carboxyhemoglobin

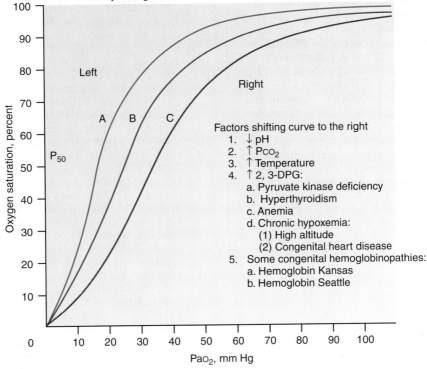

Factors shifting curve to the right
1. ↓ pH
2. ↑ P_{CO_2}
3. ↑ Temperature
4. ↑ 2, 3-DPG:
   a. Pyruvate kinase deficiency
   b. Hyperthyroidism
   c. Anemia
   d. Chronic hypoxemia:
     (1) High altitude
     (2) Congenital heart disease
5. Some congenital hemoglobinopathies:
   a. Hemoglobin Kansas
   b. Hemoglobin Seattle

Fig. 20-22   Oxyhemoglobin dissociation curve. *A,* The curve is shifted to the left because of hemoglobin's increased affinity for oxygen. *B,* The standard oxyhemoglobin dissociation curve. *C,* The curve is shifted to the right because of hemoglobin's decreased affinity for oxygen. (Modified from Kinney MR et al, editors: *AACN's clinical reference for critical care nursing,* ed 4, St Louis, 1998, Mosby).

Abnormalities of Hemoglobin. Hemoglobin carries approximately 97% of the total amount of oxygen held within the bloodstream. This great carrying capacity depends on hemoglobin that is normal in amount and molecular structure. Most hemoglobin abnormalities affect the oxygen-carrying capability of this molecule. The most common abnormality involving hemoglobin is a decrease in amount. This can be an acute or a chronic situation (anemia). Abnormal hemoglobin structure also can pose problems, such as hemoglobin S, which is responsible for sickle cell anemia. Hemoglobin S has less affinity for oxygen than does normal hemoglobin. Normal hemoglobin can become abnormal hemoglobin under certain conditions. Methemoglobin and carboxyhemoglobin are two such examples. Methemoglobin occurs when the iron atoms within the hemoglobin molecule are oxidized from the ferrous state to the ferric state. Methemoglobin does not carry oxygen. Carboxyhemoglobin occurs when carbon monoxide combines with hemoglobin. Carbon monoxide uses the same binding site as does oxygen and has a much greater affinity for hemoglobin.[19]

CARBON DIOXIDE CONTENT

Carbon dioxide, one of the end products of aerobic cellular metabolism, is produced continuously within the cells. On its way from the cells to the lungs, carbon dioxide is transported within the plasma and the erythrocytes. Carbon dioxide is transported, physically dissolved as the Pa_{CO_2} (5%), bound to blood proteins (including hemoglobin) in the form of carbaminohemoglobin compounds (5% to 10%), and combined with water to form carbonic acid (80% to 90%), some of which dissociates into hydrogen ions and bicarbonate.[4] In the

Box 20-4

What Is 2,3–DPG?

2,3-Diphosphoglycerate (2,3-DPG), an organic phosphate found primarily in red blood cells, has the ability to alter the affinity of hemoglobin for oxygen. When the level of 2,3-DPG increases within the red blood cells, hemoglobin's affinity for oxygen is decreased (a shift in the oxyhemoglobin curve to the right), thus making more oxygen available to the tissues. Increased synthesis of 2,3,-DPG apparently is an important component of the adaptive responses in healthy persons to an acute need for more tissue oxygen. Tissue hypoxia acts as the stimulus for production of 2,3-DPG, and increased amounts have been found in patients with anemia, right-to-left shunts, and congestive heart failure and in persons residing at high altitudes.

A decrease in the amount of 2,3-DPG is detrimental to tissue oxygenation because this decrease causes hemoglobin's affinity for oxygen to increase (a shift in the oxyhemoglobin curve to the left). Situations resulting in decreased 2,3-DPG levels include hypophosphatemia, septic shock, and the use of banked blood. Blood preserved with acid citrate dextrose loses most of its red cell 2,3-DPG within several days. Blood preserved with citrate phosphate dextrose maintains its 2,3-DPG levels for several weeks. Transfusion of blood with low 2,3-DPG will not be beneficial for tissue oxygenation until the 2,3-DPG level is restored, which may take 18 to 24 hours.

lungs these methods of carbon dioxide carriage are reversed as the carbon dioxide leaves the plasma and erythrocytes for exhalation.[20]

REFERENCES

1. Ruppel GL, White D: The respiratory system. In Wilkins RL, Stoller JK, Scanlan CL, editors: *Egan's fundamentals of respiratory care,* ed 8, St Louis, 2003, Mosby.
2. Sobonya RE: Normal anatomy and development of the lung. In Baum GL, Wolinsky E, editors: *Textbook of pulmonary diseases,* ed 5, Philadelphia, 1994, Little Brown.
3. Brashers VL: Structure and function of the pulmonary system. In McCance KL, Huether SE, editors: *Pathophysiology: the biologic basis for disease in adults and children,* ed 4, St Louis, 2002, Mosby.
4. Guyton AC, Hall JE: *Textbook of medical physiology,* ed 10, Philadelphia, 2000, Saunders.
5. Flaminiano LE, Celli BD: Respiratory muscle testing, *Clin Chest Med* 22:661, 2001.
6. Anderson WM, Zavecz JH: The chest wall, diaphragm, and mediastinum. In Bone RC, editor: *Pulmonary and critical care medicine,* ed 6, St Louis, 1998, Mosby.
7. Cosenza JL, Norton LC: Secretion clearance: state of the art from a nursing perspective, *Crit Care Nurse* 6(4):23, 1986.
8. Welsh DA, Mason CM: Host defense in respiratory infections, *Med Clin North Am* 85:1329, 2001.
9. Irwin RS: Managing cough as a defense mechanism and as a symptom. A consensus panel report of the American College of Chest Physicians, *Chest* 114(suppl 2):133S, 1998.
10. Albertine KH, Williams MC, Hyde DM: Anatomy of the lungs. In Murray JF, Nadel JA, editors: *Textbook of respiratory medicine,* ed 3, Philadelphia, 2000, Saunders.
11. Anzueto A: Surfactant supplementation in the lung, *Respir Care Clin North Am* 8:211, 2002.
12. Hughes WW: The cardiovascular system. In Wilkins RL, Stoller JK, Scanlan CL, editors: *Egan's fundamentals of respiratory care,* ed 8, St Louis, 2003, Mosby.
13. Arroliga AC: Pulmonary vascular disease. In Wilkins RL, Stoller JK, Scanlan CL, editors: *Egan's fundamentals of respiratory care,* ed 8, St Louis, 2003, Mosby.
14. West JB, Wagner PD: Ventilation, blood flow, and gas exchange. In Murray JF, Nadel JA, editors: *Textbook of respiratory medicine,* ed 3, Philadelphia, 2000, Saunders.
15. Misasi RS, Keyes JL: Matching and mismatching ventilation and perfusion in the lung, *Crit Care Nurse* 16(3):23, 1996.
16. Ruppel GL: Ventilation. In Wilkins RL, Stoller JK, Scanlan CL, editors: *Egan's fundamentals of respiratory care,* ed 8, St Louis, 2003, Mosby.
17. Rodarte JR, Shardonofsky FR: Respiratory system mechanics. In Murray JF, Nadel JA, editors: *Textbook of respiratory medicine,* ed 3, Philadelphia, 2000, Saunders.
18. Caruana-Montaldo B, Gleeson K, Zwillich CW: The control of breathing in clinical practice, *Chest* 117:205, 2000.
19. Wilson WC, Shapiro B: Perioperative hypoxia. The clinical spectrum and current oxygen monitoring methodology, *Anesthesiol Clin North Am* 19:769, 2001.
20. Scanlan CL, Wilkins: Gas exchange and transport. In Wilkins RL, Stoller JK, Scanlan CL, editors: *Egan's fundamentals of respiratory care,* ed 8, St Louis, 2003, Mosby.
21. Henig NR, Pierson DJ: Mechanisms of hypoxemia, *Respir Care Clin North Am* 6:501, 2000.
22. Berry BE, Pinard AE: Assessing tissue oxygenation, *Crit Care Nurse* 22(3):22, 2002.

CHAPTER 21

Pulmonary Clinical Assessment

A ssessment of the patient with pulmonary dysfunction is a systematic process that incorporates both an inquiry into the chronology of the present illness, better known as a *history*, and an investigation of the current physical manifestations, better known as a *physical examination*. The purpose of the assessment is twofold: first, to recognize changes in the patient's pulmonary status that would necessitate nursing or medical intervention; and second, to determine the ways in which the patient's pulmonary dysfunction is interfering with his or her self-care activities. Once completed, the assessment serves as the foundation for developing the management plan for the patient. The assessment process can be brief or can involve a detailed history and examination, depending on the nature and immediacy of the patient's situation. Whatever the setting, the nurse should develop and practice a sequential pattern of assessment to avoid omitting portions of the examination.

HISTORY

Taking a thorough and accurate history is extremely important to the assessment process. The patient's history provides the foundation and direction for the rest of the assessment. The overall goal of the patient interview is to expose key clinical manifestations that will facilitate the identification of the underlying cause of the illness. This information will then assist in the development of an appropriate management plan.[1]

The initial presentation of the patient determines the rapidity and direction of the interview. For a patient in acute distress (Box 21-1), the history should be curtailed to just a few questions about the patient's chief complaint and precipitating events. For a patient in no obvious distress, the history should focus on five different areas: (1) review of the patient's present illness, (2) overview of the patient's general respiratory status, (3) examination of the patient's general health status, (4) survey of the patient's family and social background, and (5) description of the patient's current symptoms.[1] Specific items regard-

ing each of these areas are outlined in the Data Collection feature on Pulmonary History.

Symptoms that are common in the pulmonary patient include dyspnea, cough, wheezing, edema, palpitations, fatigue, chest pain, hemoptysis, and sputum abnormalities. Information should be elicited regarding the location, onset and duration, characteristics, setting, aggravating and alleviating factors, associated symptoms, and efforts to treat the symptoms. If the cough is productive, the patient should be asked questions about the color, amount, odor, and consistency of the sputum.[2-5]

PHYSICAL EXAMINATION

Four techniques are used in physical assessment: inspection, palpation, percussion, and auscultation. *Inspection* is the process of looking intently at the patient. *Palpation* is the process of touching the patient to judge the size, shape, texture, and temperature of the body surface or underlying structures. *Percussion* is the process of creating sound waves on the surface of the body to determine abnormal density of any underlying areas. *Auscultation* is the process of concentrated listening with a stethoscope to determine characteristics of body functions.[6,7]

INSPECTION

Inspection of the patient should focus on three different areas: (1) observation of the tongue and sublingual area, (2) assessment of chest wall configuration, and (3) evaluation of respiratory effort. If possible, patients should be positioned upright, with their arms resting at their sides.[3] Inspection generally begins during the interview process.[2]

Tongue and Sublingual Area. The tongue and sublingual area should be observed for a blue, gray, or dark purple tint or discoloration indicating the presence of central cyanosis. *Central cyanosis* is a sign of hypoxemia, or inadequate oxygenation of the blood, and is considered to be life-threatening. It occurs when the

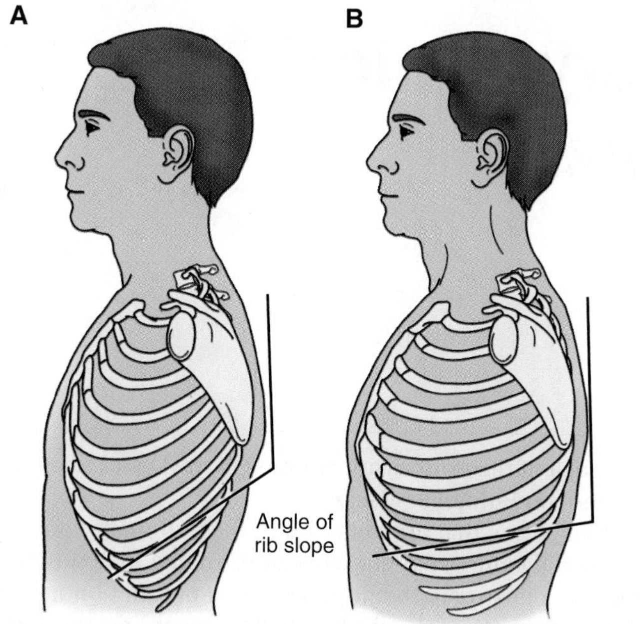

A

B

Angle of
rib slope

Fig. 21-1 Chest wall configuration. **A,** Normal configuration. **B,** Increased anteroposterior diameter. Note contrast in the angle of the slope of the ribs. (From Barkauskas V et al: *Health and physical assessment,* ed 3, St Louis, 2002, Mosby.)

> **Box 21-1**
>
> **MANIFESTATIONS OF RESPIRATORY DECOMPENSATION**
>
> **INADEQUATE AIRWAY**
> Stridor
> Noisy respirations
> Supraclavicular and intercostal retractions
> Flaring of nares
> Labored breathing with use of accessory muscles
>
> **INADEQUATE VENTILATION**
> Absence of air exchange at nose and mouth (breathlessness)
> Minimal/absent chest wall motion
> Manifestations of obstructed airway
> Central cyanosis
> Decreased or absent breath sounds (bilateral, unilateral)
> Restlessness, anxiety, confusion
> Paradoxical motion involving significant portion of chest wall
> Decreased Pao_2, increased $Paco_2$, decreased pH
>
> **INADEQUATE GAS EXCHANGE**
> Tachypnea
> Decreased Pao_2
> Increased dead space
> Central cyanosis
> Chest infiltrates on x-ray evaluation

amount of reduced hemoglobin (unsaturated hemoglobin) exceeds 5 g/dL. The fingers and toes may also appear discolored, an indication of the presence of peripheral cyanosis.[8]

Chest Wall Configuration. Assessment of chest wall configuration incorporates observations about the size and shape of the patient's chest. Normally, the ratio of anteroposterior (AP) diameter to lateral diameter ranges from 1:2 to 5:7 (Fig. 21-1, *A*).[2,4,5] An increase in the AP diameter is suggestive of chronic obstructive pulmonary disease (COPD).[2,4,5] The shape of the chest should be inspected for any structural deviations. Some of the more frequently seen abnormalities are pectus excavatum, pectus carinatum, barrel chest, and spinal deformities. In *pectus excavatum* (funnel chest), the sternum and lower ribs are displaced posteriorly, creating a funnel or pit-shaped depression in the chest. This causes a decrease in the AP diameter of the chest and may interfere with respiratory function. In *pectus carinatum* (pigeon breast), the sternum projects forward, causing an increase in the AP diameter of the chest. The *barrel chest* also results in an increase in AP diameter of the chest and is characterized by displacement of the sternum forward and the ribs outward (Fig. 21-1, *B*). Spinal deformities such as *kyphosis, lordosis,* and *scoliosis* also may be present and can interfere with respiratory function.[9]

Respiratory Effort. Evaluation of respiratory effort incorporates observations on the rate, rhythm, symmetry, and quality of ventilatory movements.[2] Normal breathing at rest is effortless and regular and occurs at a

rate of 12 to 20 breaths per minute.[3] There are a number of abnormal respiratory patterns (Fig. 21-2). Some of the more commonly seen patterns in patients with pulmonary dysfunction are tachypnea, hyperventilation, and air trapping. *Tachypnea* is manifested by an increase in the rate and decrease in the depth of ventilation. *Hyperventilation* is manifested by an increase in both the rate and depth of ventilation. Patients with COPD often experience obstructive breathing, or *air trapping.* As the patient breathes, air becomes trapped in the lungs and ventilations become progressively more shallow until the patient actively and forcefully exhales.[10]

Additional Assessment Areas. Other focuses for the careful assessment are patient position, active effort to breathe, use of accessory muscles, presence of intercostal retractions, unequal movement of the chest wall, flaring of nares, and pausing midsentence to take a breath.[2,4,5] The presence of other iatrogenic features, such as chest tubes, central venous lines, artificial airways, and nasogastric tubes should be noted because they may affect assessment findings.

PALPATION

Palpation of the patient should focus on three different aspects: (1) confirmation of the position of the trachea, (2) assessment of thoracic expansion, and (3) evaluation

DATA COLLECTION

Pulmonary History

CHIEF COMPLAINT

Cough
- Onset and duration
  Sudden or gradual
  Episodic or continuous
- Characteristics
  Dry or wet
  Hacking, hoarse, barking, or congested
  Productive or nonproductive
- Sputum
  Present or absent
  Frequency of production
  Appearance—color (clear, mucoid, purulent, blood-tinged, mostly bloody), foul odor, frothy
  Amount
- Pattern
  Paroxysmal
  Related to time of day, weather, activities, talking, or deep breathing
  Change over time
- Severity
  Causes fatigue
  Disrupts sleep or conversation
  Produces chest pain
- Associated symptoms
  Shortness of breath
  Chest pain or tightness with breathing
  Fever
  Upper respiratory tract signs (sore throat, congestion, increased mucus production)
  Noisy respirations or hoarseness
  Gagging or choking
  Anxiety, stress, or panic reactions
- Efforts made to treat
  Prescription or nonprescription drugs
  Vaporizers
  Effective or ineffective

Shortness of Breath (SOB) or Dyspnea on Exertion (DOE)
- Onset and duration
  Sudden or gradual
  Gagging or choking episode a few days before onset
- Pattern
  Related to position—improves when sitting up or with head elevated; number of pillows used to alleviate problems
  Related to activity—exercise or eating; extent of activity that produces dyspnea
  Related to other factors—time of day, season, or exposure to something in the environment
  Harder to inhale or harder to exhale
- Severity
  Extent activity is limited
  Breathing itself causes fatigue
  Anxiety about getting enough air

- Associated symptoms
  Pain or discomfort—exact location in respiratory tree
  Cough, diaphoresis, swelling of ankles, or cyanosis
- Efforts made to treat
  Prescription or nonprescription drugs
  Oxygen
  Effective or ineffective

Chest Pain
- Onset and duration
  Gradual or sudden
  Associated with trauma, coughing, or lower respiratory tract infection
- Associated symptoms
  Shallow breathing
  Uneven chest expansion
  Fever
  Cough
  Radiation of pain to neck or arms
  Anxiety about getting enough air
- Efforts made to treat
  Heat, splinting, or pain medication
  Effective or ineffective

PATIENT'S PERCEPTION OF THE PROBLEM
- Degree of concern about the symptoms
- Opinion of its cause

PATIENT HISTORY: FACTORS RELATING TO RESPIRATORY DISORDERS (CAUSES OR AGGRAVATING FACTORS)
- Tobacco use—both present and past
  Type of tobacco—cigarettes, cigars, pipes, or smokeless
  Duration and amount—age started, inhale when smoking, amount used in the past and present
  Pack years—number of packs per day multiplied by number of years patient has smoked
  Efforts to quit—previous attempts and current interest
- Work environment
  Nature of work
  Environmental hazards: chemicals, vapors, dust, pulmonary irritants, or allergens
  Use of protective devices
- Home environment
  Location
  Possible allergens: pets, house plants, plants and trees outside the home, or other environmental hazards
  Type of heating
  Use of air conditioning or humidifier
  Ventilation
  Stairs to climb

MEDICAL HISTORY
- Infectious respiratory diseases
  Strep throat
  Mumps
  Tonsillitis

Continued

DATA COLLECTION

Pulmonary History—cont'd

MEDICAL HISTORY—CONT'D

- Thoracic trauma or surgery
- Previous diagnosis of pulmonary disorders—dates of hospitalization
- Chronic pulmonary disease—date, treatment, and compliance with therapy
    Tuberculosis
    Bronchitis
    Emphysema
    Bronchiectasis
    Asthma
    Cystic fibrosis
    Sinus infection
- Other chronic disorders—cardiovascular, cancer, musculoskeletal, neurologic
    Nasal surgery or injury
    Obstruction of one or both nares
    Mouth breathing often necessary (especially at night)
    History of nasal discharge

- Nosebleeds
    Affects one or both nostrils
    Aggravated by crusting
- Previous tests
    Allergy testing
    Pulmonary function tests
    Tuberculin and fungal skin tests
    Chest x-rays

FAMILY HISTORY

- Tuberculosis
- Cystic fibrosis
- Emphysema
- Allergies
- Asthma
- Atopic dermatitis
- Smoking by household members
- Malignancy

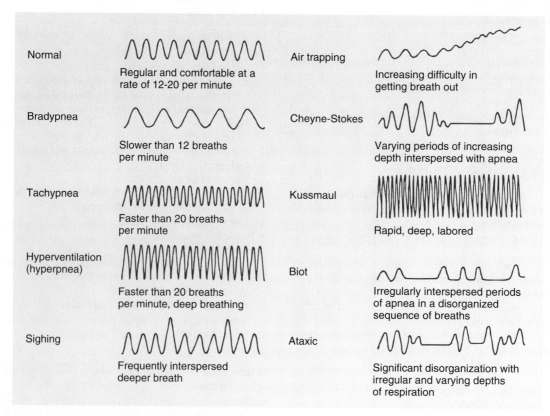

Fig. 21-2   Patterns of respiration. (From Seidel HM et al: *Mosby's guide to physical examination,* ed 5, St Louis, 2003, Mosby.)

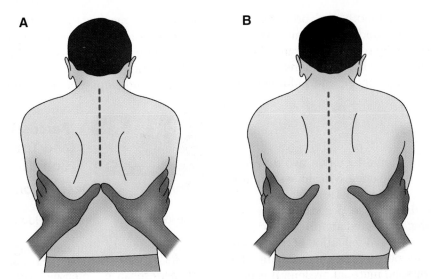

Fig. 21-3   Assessment of thoracic expansion. **A,** Exhalation. **B,** Inhalation. (From Wilkins RL, Stoller JK, Scanlon CL, editors: *Egan's fundamentals of respiratory care,* ed 8, St Louis, 2003, Mosby.)

of fremitus. In addition, the thorax should be assessed for any areas of tenderness, lumps, or bony deformities. The anterior, posterior, and lateral areas of the chest should be evaluated in a systematic fashion.[2]

Position of Trachea. Confirmation of the position of the trachea is performed to verify that the trachea is midline. It is assessed by placing the fingers in the suprasternal notch and moving upward.[10] Deviation of the trachea to either side can indicate a pneumothorax, unilateral pneumonia, diffuse pulmonary fibrosis, a large pleural effusion, or severe atelectasis. With atelectasis the trachea shifts to the same side as the problem, and with pneumothorax the trachea shifts to the opposite side of the problem.[9]

Thoracic Expansion. Assessment of thoracic expansion involves measuring the degree and symmetry of respiratory movement. It is assessed by placing the hands on the anterolateral chest with the thumbs extended along the costal margin, pointing to the xiphoid process, or on the posterolateral chest with the thumbs on either side of the spine at the level of the tenth rib (Fig. 21-3). The patient is instructed to take a few normal breaths and then a few deep breaths. Chest movement is assessed for equality, which signifies symmetry of thoracic expansion.[3,9,10] Asymmetry is an abnormal finding that can occur with pneumothorax, pneumonia, or other disorders that interfere with lung inflation. The degree of chest movement is felt to ascertain the extent of lung expansion. The thumbs should separate 3 to 5 cm during deep inspiration.[5,10] Lung expansion of a hyperinflated chest is less than that of a normal one.[5,10]

Tactile Fremitus. Assessment of tactile fremitus is performed to identify, describe, and localize any areas of increased or decreased fremitus. Fremitus refers to the palpable vibrations felt through the chest wall when the

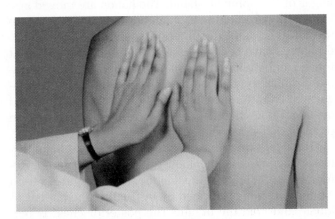

Fig. 21-4   Assessment of tactile fremitus, showing simultaneous application of the fingertips of both hands to compare sides. (From Barkauskas V et al: *Health and physical assessment,* ed 3, St Louis, 2002, Mosby.)

patient speaks. It is assessed by placing the palmar surface of the hands against opposite sides of the chest wall and having the patient repeat the word "ninety-nine" (Fig. 21-4). The hands are moved systematically around the thorax until the anterior, posterior, and both lateral areas have been assessed.[9,10] If only one hand is used, it is moved from one side of the chest to the corresponding area on the other side of the chest until all areas have been assessed.[10]

Fremitus varies from patient to patient and depends on the pitch and intensity of the voice. Fremitus is described as normal, decreased, or increased. With normal fremitus, vibrations can be felt over the trachea but are barely palpable over the periphery.[2] With decreased fremitus, there is interference with the transmission of vibrations. Examples of disorders that decrease fremitus include pleural effusion, pneumothorax, bronchial obstruction, pleural thickening, and emphysema. With increased fremitus, there is an increase in the transmission of vibrations. Examples of disorders that increase fremitus include pneumonia, lung cancer, and pulmonary fibrosis.[5]

PERCUSSION

Percussion of the patient should focus on two different concerns: (1) evaluation of the underlying lung structure and (2) assessment of diaphragmatic excursion. Although not an often-used technique, percussion is a useful method for confirming suspected abnormalities.

Underlying Lung Structure. Evaluation of the underlying lung structure is performed to estimate the amounts of air, liquid, or solid material present. It is performed by placing the middle finger of the nondominant hand on the chest wall. The distal portion, between the last joint and the nail bed, is then struck with the middle finger of the dominant hand. The hands are moved systematically around the thorax, side-to-side, to compare similar areas until the anterior, posterior, and both lateral areas have been assessed (Fig. 21-5). Five different tones can be elicited: resonance, hyperresonance, tympany, dullness, and flatness. These tones are distinguished by differences in intensity, pitch, duration, and quality. Table 21-1 describes the different percussion tones and their associated conditions.[3,9]

Diaphragmatic Excursion. Assessment of diaphragmatic excursion is accomplished by measuring the difference in the level of the diaphragm on inspiration and expiration. It is performed by instructing the patient to inhale and hold the breath. The posterior chest is percussed downward, over the intercostal spaces, until the dull sound produced by the diaphragm is heard. The spot is marked. The patient is then instructed to take a few breaths in and out, exhale completely, and then hold his or her breath. The posterior chest is percussed again, and the new area of dullness over the diaphragm is then

located and marked. The difference between the two spots is noted and measured (Fig. 21-6). Normal diaphragmatic excursion is 3 to 5 cm.[10] It is decreased in such disorders or conditions as ascites, pregnancy, hepatomegaly, and emphysema. It is increased in pleural effu-

Table 21-1	Percussion Tones and Their Associated Conditions	
Tone	**Description**	**Condition**
Resonance	Intensity—loud Pitch—low Duration—long Quality—hollow	Normal lung Bronchitis
Hyperresonance	Intensity—very loud Pitch—very low Duration—long Quality—booming	Asthma Emphysema Pneumothorax
Tympany	Intensity—loud Pitch—musical Duration—medium Quality—drumlike	Large pneumothorax Emphysematous blebs
Dullness	Intensity—medium Pitch—medium-high Duration—medium Quality—thudlike	Atelectasis Pleural effusion Pulmonary edema Pneumonia Lung mass
Flatness	Intensity—soft Pitch—high Duration—short Quality—extremely dull	Massive atelectasis Pneumonectomy

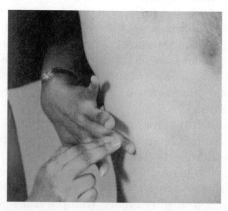

Fig. 21-5 Percussion of the thorax. (From Barkauskas V et al: *Health and physical assessment,* ed 3, St Louis, 2002, Mosby.)

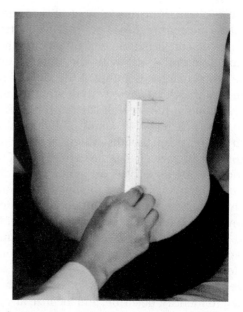

Fig. 21-6 Assessment of diaphragmatic excursion. (From Barkauskas V et al: *Health and physical assessment,* ed 3, St Louis, 2002, Mosby.)

sion or disorders that elevate the diaphragm, such as atelectasis or paralysis.[9]

AUSCULTATION

Auscultation of the patient should focus on three different areas: (1) evaluation of normal breath sounds, (2) identification of abnormal breath sounds, and (3) assessment of voice sounds. Auscultation requires a quiet environment, proper positioning of the patient, and a bare chest.[11] Breath sounds are best heard with the patient in the upright position.[5]

Normal Breath Sounds. Evaluation of normal breath sounds is performed to assess air movement through the pulmonary system and to identify the presence of abnormal sounds. It is performed by placing the diaphragm of the stethoscope against the chest wall and instructing the patient to breathe in and out slowly with his or her mouth open.[2] Both the inspiratory and expiratory phases should be assessed. Auscultation should be done in a systematic sequence, side-to-side, top-to-bottom, posteriorly, laterally, and anteriorly (Fig. 21-7).[5]

Normal breath sounds are different, depending on their location. They are classified into three categories: vesicular, bronchovesicular, and bronchial. Table 21-2 describes the characteristics of normal breath sounds and their associated conditions.[2,5,11]

Table 21-2	Characteristics of Normal Breath Sounds
Sound	**Characteristics**
Vesicular	Heard over most of lung field; low pitch; soft and short exhalation and long inhalation
Bronchovesicular	Heard over main bronchus area and over upper right posterior lung field; medium pitch; exhalation equals inhalation
Bronchial	Heard only over trachea; high pitch; loud and long exhalation

Modified from Thompson JM et al: *Mosby's clinical nursing,* ed 5, St. Louis, 2002, Mosby

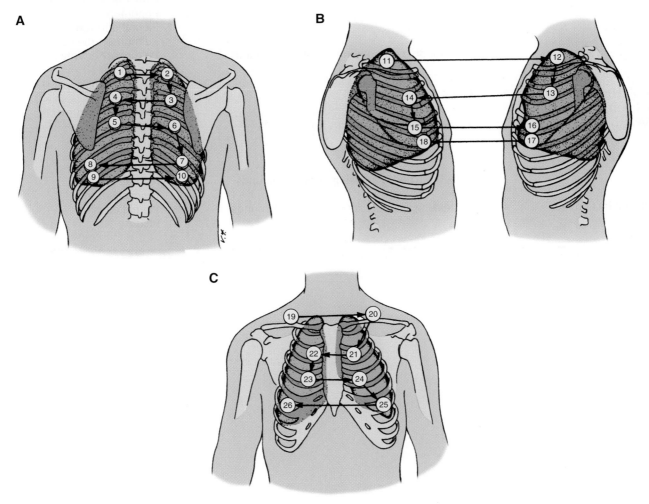

Fig. 21-7 Auscultation sequence. **A,** Posterior. **B,** Lateral. **C,** Anterior. (From Perry AG, Potter PA: *Clinical nursing skills and techniques,* ed 5, St Louis, 2003, Mosby.)

Abnormal Breath Sounds. Identification of abnormal breath sounds occurs once the normal breath sounds have been clearly delineated. There are three categories of abnormal breath sounds: absent or diminished breath sounds; displaced bronchial breath sounds; and adventitious breath sounds. Table 21-3 describes the various abnormal breath sounds and their associated conditions.[2,5,11]

An *absent* or *diminished breath sound* indicates that there is little or no airflow to a particular portion of the lung (either a small segment or an entire lung).[11] *Displaced bronchial breath sounds* are normal bronchial

Table 21-3	Abnormal Breath Sounds and Their Associated Conditions	
Abnormal Sound	**Description**	**Condition**
Absent breath sounds	No airflow to particular portion of lung	Pneumothorax Pneumonectomy Emphysematous blebs Pleural effusion Lung mass Massive atelectasis Complete airway obstruction
Diminished breath sounds	Little airflow to particular portion of lung	Emphysema Pleural effusion Pleurisy Atelectasis Pulmonary fibrosis
Displaced bronchial sounds	Bronchial sounds heard in peripheral lung fields	Atelectasis with secretions Lung mass with exudates Pneumonia Pleural effusion Pulmonary edema
Crackles (rales)	Short, discrete popping or crackling sounds	Pulmonary edema Pneumonia Pulmonary fibrosis Atelectasis Bronchiectasis
Rhonchi	Coarse, rumbling, low-pitched sounds	Pneumonia Asthma Bronchitis Bronchospasm
Wheezes	High-pitched, squeaking, whistling sounds	Asthma Bronchospasm
Pleural friction rub	Creaking, leathery, loud, dry, coarse sounds	Pleural effusion Pleurisy

sounds heard in the peripheral lung fields instead of over the trachea. This condition is usually indicative of fluid or exudate present in the alveoli.[11] *Adventitious breath sounds* are extra or added sounds heard in addition to the other sounds already discussed. They are classified as crackles, rhonchi, wheezes, and friction rubs. *Crackles* (also called *rales*) are short, discrete popping or crackling sounds produced by fluid in the small airways or alveoli or by the snapping open of collapsed airways during inspiration. They can be heard on inspiration and expiration and may clear with coughing.[2,5,11] Crackles can be further classified as fine, medium, or coarse, depending on pitch.[3,5] *Rhonchi* are coarse, rumbling, low-pitched sounds produced by airflow over secretions in the larger airways or narrowing of the large airways. They are heard mainly on expiration and sometimes can be cleared with coughing. Rhonchi can be further classified as bubbling, gurgling, or sonorous, depending on the characteristics of the sound.[11] *Wheezes* are high-pitched, squeaking, whistling sounds produced by airflow through narrowed small airways. They are heard mainly on expiration but may be heard throughout the ventilatory cycle. Depending on their severity, wheezes can be further classified as mild, moderate, or severe.[11] A *pleural friction rub* is a creaking, leathery, loud, dry, coarse sound produced by irritated pleural surfaces rubbing together. It is usually heard best in the lower anterolateral chest area during both inspiration and expiration. Pleural friction rubs are caused by inflammation of the pleura.[2,5]

Voice Sounds. Assessment of voice sounds is particularly useful in detecting lung consolidation or lung compression. Three abnormal types of voice sounds are bronchophony, whispering pectoriloquy, and egophony. *Bronchophony* describes a condition in which the spoken voice is heard on auscultation with higher intensity and clarity than usual. Normally the spoken word is muffled when heard through the stethoscope. It is assessed by placing the diaphragm of the stethoscope against the posterior side of the patient's chest and instructing the patient to say "ninety-nine." Bronchophony is present when the sound heard is clear, distinct, and loud. *Whispering pectoriloquy* describes a condition of unusually clear transmission of the whispered voice on auscultation. Normally the whispered word is unintelligible when heard through the stethoscope. It is assessed by placing the stethoscope against the posterior side of the patient's chest and instructing the patient to whisper "one, two, three." Whispering pectoriloquy is present when the sound heard is clear and distinct. *Egophony* describes a condition in which the voice sounds increase in intensity and develop a nasal bleating quality on auscultation. It is assessed by placing the stethoscope against the posterior side of the patient's chest and instructing the patient to say "e-e-e." Egophony is present when the "e" sound changes to an "a" sound.[2,4,11]

ASSESSMENT FINDINGS OF COMMON DISORDERS

Table 21-4 presents a variety of common pulmonary disorders and their associated assessment findings.

Table 21-4	Assessment Findings Frequently Associated With Common Lung Conditions	
Condition	**Breath Sounds**	**Description**
NORMAL LUNG 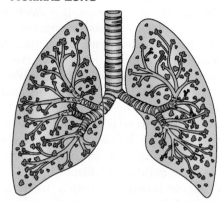	Inspiration > expiration Pitch—low Intensity—soft Adventitious sounds—none	Tracheobronchial tree and alveoli are clear; pleurae are thin and close together; chest wall is mobile
ASTHMA 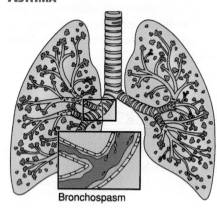 Bronchospasm	Inspiration = expiration Pitch—moderate Intensity—soft Adventitious sounds—expiratory sibilant wheezes	Asthma is characterized by intermittent episodes of airway obstruction caused by bronchospasm, excessive bronchial secretion, or edema of bronchial mucosa; resultant airway resistance, especially during expiration, produces symptoms of wheezing, dyspnea, and chest tightness
ATELECTASIS 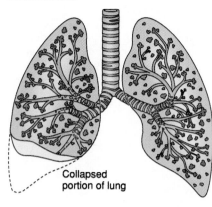 Collapsed portion of lung	*Over empty area* Inspiration > expiration Pitch—low or absent Intensity—soft or absent Adventitious sounds—fine, high-pitched crackles over terminal portion of inspiration if bronchus patent NOTE: Over consolidated lung—bronchial breath sounds, crackles, and wheezes	Atelectasis is collapse of alveolar lung tissue, and findings reflect presence of a small, airless lung; this condition is caused by complete obstruction of a draining bronchus by a tumor, thick secretions, or an aspirated foreign body, or by compression of lung

From Barkauskas V et al: *Health and physical assessment,* ed 3, St. Louis, 2002, Mosby.
NOTE: Although some disease conditions are bilateral, one diseased lung and one normal lung are illustrated for each condition to provide contrast. When an abnormality is illustrated, the pathologic condition is illustrated on the left side and the normal lung is on the right side of the illustration.

Inspection	Palpation	Percussion	Auscultation
Good, symmetric rib and diaphragmatic movement Anteroposterior diameter < transverse diameter Respirations 12-20/min and regular	Trachea—midline Expansion—adequate, symmetric Tactile fremitus—moderate and symmetric No lesions or tenderness	Resonant Diaphragmatic excursion—3-5 cm	Breath sounds—vesicular Vocal resonance—muffled Adventitious sounds—none, except for a few transient crackles at bases
Cyanosis Air trapping with audible wheezing Use of accessory muscles of respiration Increased respiratory rate	Tactile fremitus—decreased	Hyperresonant	Breath sounds—distant Vocal resonance—decreased Adventitious sounds—wheezes
Less chest motion on affected side Affected side retracted, with ribs appearing close together Cough Rapid, shallow breathing	Trachea—shifted to affected side Expansion—decreased on affected side Tactile fremitus—decreased or absent	Dull to flat over collapsed lung Hyperresonant over remainder of affected hemithorax	Breath sounds—decreased or absent Vocal resonance—varies in intensity, usually reduced or absent in affected area Adventitious sounds—fine, high-pitched crackles may be heard over terminal portion of inspiration

Continued

Table 21-4	Assessment Findings Frequently Associated with Common Lung Conditions—cont'd	
Condition	**Breath Sounds**	**Description**
BRONCHIECTASIS 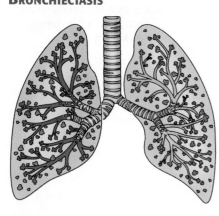	Inspiration > expiration Pitch—low Intensity—soft Adventitious sounds—crackles (sometimes disappear after coughing) 	Bronchiectasis is abnormal dilation of bronchi or bronchioles or both
BRONCHITIS—ACUTE 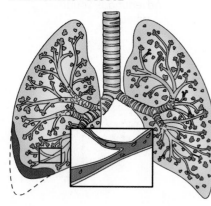	Inspiration > or = expiration Pitch—low Intensity—soft Adventitious sounds—localized crackles, expiratory sibilant wheezes 	Acute bronchitis is inflammation of bronchial tree characterized by partial bronchial obstruction and secretions or constrictions; it results in abnormally deflated portions of lung
EMPHYSEMA 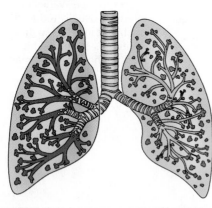	Inspiration = expiration Pitch—low to very low Intensity—soft to very soft Adventitious sounds—occasional rhonchi and/or sibilant wheezes; fine inspiratory crackles 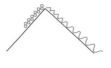	Emphysema is a permanent hyperinflation of lung beyond terminal bronchioles, with destruction of alveolar walls; airway resistance is increased, especially on expiration

Inspection	Palpation	Percussion	Auscultation
If mild, respirations are normal If severe, tachypnea Less expansion of affected side Cough with purulent sputum	Trachea—midline or deviated toward affected side Expansion—decreased on affected side Tactile fremitus—increased	Resonant or dull	Breath sounds—usually vesicular Vocal resonance—usually muffled Adventitious sounds—crackles
If severe, tachypnea and cyanosis Rasping cough with mucoid sputum	Tactile fremitus—normal to increased	Resonant	Breath sounds—vesicular Vocal resonance—moderate Adventitious sounds—localized crackles, sibilant wheezes
Dyspnea with exertion Barrel chest Tachypnea Use of accessory muscles of respiration	Expansion—limited Tactile fremitus—decreased	Resonant to hyperresonant Diaphragmatic excursion—decreased	Breath sounds—decreased intensity; often prolonged expiration Vocal resonance—muffled or decreased Adventitious sounds—occasional wheezes; often fine crackles in late inspiration

Continued

Table 21-4	Assessment Findings Frequently Associated with Common Lung Conditions—con'td	
Condition	**Breath Sounds**	**Description**
PLEURAL EFFUSION AND THICKENING 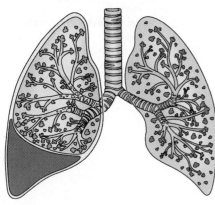	Inspiration > expiration Pitch—low to absent Intensity—soft to absent Adventitious sounds—occasional pleural friction rub 	Pleural effusion is a collection of fluid in pleural space; if pleural effusion is prolonged, fibrous tissue may also accumulate in pleural space; clinical picture depends on amount of fluid or fibrosis present and rapidity of development; fluid tends to gravitate to most dependent areas of thorax, and adjacent lung is compressed
PNEUMONIA WITH CONSOLIDATION 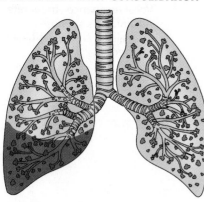	Inspiration = expiration Pitch—high Intensity—loud Adventitious sounds—inspiratory crackles in terminal third of inspiration 	Pneumonia with consolidation occurs when alveolar air is replaced by fluid or tissue; physical findings depend on amount of parenchymal tissue involved
PNEUMOTHORAX 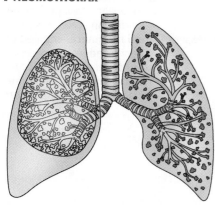	Inspiration > expiration Pitch—low to absent Intensity—soft to absent Adventitious sounds—none 	Pneumothorax implies air in pleural space The three types of pneumothorax are (1) closed—air in pleural space does not communicate with air in lung; (2) open—air in pleural space freely communicates with air in lung; air in pleural space is atmospheric; and (3) tension—air in pleural space communicates with air in lungs only on inspiration; air pressure in pleural space is greater than atmospheric pressure Physical signs depend on degree of lung collapse and presence or absence of pleural effusion

Inspection	Palpation	Percussion	Auscultation
Tachypnea Decreased in definition of intercostals spaces on affected side Dyspnea	Trachea—deviation toward normal side Expansion—decreased on affected side Tactile fremitus—decreased or absent	Dull to flat No diaphragmatic excursion on affected side	Breath sounds—decreased or absent Vocal resonance—muffled or absent; if fluid compresses lung, sounds may be bronchial over compression, and bronchophony, egophony, and whisper pectoriloquy may be present Adventitious sounds—pleural friction rub sometimes present
Tachypnea Guarding and less motion on affected side	Expansion—limited on affected side Tactile fremitus—usually increased, but may be weak if a bronchus leading to affected area is plugged	Dull to flat	Breath sounds—increased in intensity; bronchovesicular or bronchial breath sounds over affected area Vocal resonance—increased bronchophony, egophony, whisper pectoriloquy present Adventitious sounds—inspiratory crackles terminal third of inspiration
Restricted lung expansion on affected side If large, tachypnea Bulging in intercostal spaces on affected side Cyanosis	Trachea—deviated toward normal side Expansion—decreased on affected side Tactile fremitus—absent	Hyperresonant Decreased diaphragmatic excursion	Breath sounds—usually decreased or absent; if open pneumothorax, have an amorphous quality Vocal resonance—decreased or absent Adventitious sounds—none

Continued

Table 21-4	Assessment Findings Frequently Associated with Common Lung Conditions—cont'd	
Condition	**Breath Sounds**	**Description**
PULMONARY FIBROSIS—DIFFUSE 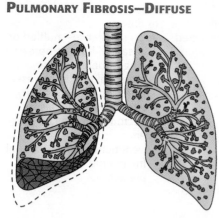	Inspiration = expiration Pitch—low to absent Intensity—soft to absent Adventitious sounds—crackles 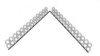	Pulmonary fibrosis is presence of excessive amount of connective tissue in lungs; consequently, lungs are smaller than normal and less compliant, lower lobes are usually affected most

Inspection	Palpation	Percussion	Auscultation
Dyspnea on exertion Tachypnea Thoracic expansion diminished Cyanosis	Trachea—deviated to most affected side	Resonant to dull	Breath sounds—reduced or absent, bronchovesicular or bronchial Vocal resonance—increased, whisper pectoriloquy may be present Adventitious sounds—crackles on inspiration

REFERENCES

1. Gehring PE: Physical assessment begins with a history, *RN* 54(11):26, 1991.
2. O'Hanlon-Nichols T: Basic assessment series: the adult pulmonary system, *Am J Nurs* 98(2):39, 1998.
3. Brenner M, Welliver J: Pulmonary and acid-base assessment, *Nurs Clin North Am* 25:761, 1990.
4. Finesilver C: Pulmonary assessment: what you need to know, *Prog Cardiovasc Nurs* 18:83, 2003.
5. Wilkins RL: Bedside assessment of the patient. In Wilkins RL, Stoller JK, Scanlan CL, editors: *Egan's fundamentals of respiratory care,* ed 8, St Louis, 2003, Mosby.
6. Stiesmeyer JK: A four-step approach to pulmonary assessment, *Am J Nurs* 93(8):22, 1993.
7. Fitzgerald MA: The physical exam, *RN* 54(11):34, 1991.
8. Carpenter KD: A comprehensive review of cyanosis, *Crit Care Nurse* 13(4):66, 1993.
9. Barkauskas V et al: *Health and physical assessment,* ed 3, St Louis, 2002, Mosby.
10. Seidel HM et al: *Mosby's guide to physical examination,* ed 5, St Louis, 2003, Mosby.
11. Boyda EK et al: *Pulmonary auscultation,* St Paul, 1987, 3M Health Care Group.

CHAPTER 22

Pulmonary Diagnostic Procedures

*T*o complete the assessment of the critically ill pulmonary patient, a review of the patient's laboratory studies and diagnostic tests is performed. Although many procedures exist for diagnosing pulmonary disease, their application in the critically ill patient is limited. Only those studies and tests that are currently used in the critical care setting are presented here. Bedside monitoring devices are also discussed.

LABORATORY STUDIES

ARTERIAL BLOOD GASES

Interpretation of arterial blood gas (ABG) levels can be difficult, especially if one is under pressure to do it quickly and accurately. One method that can help ensure accuracy when analyzing arterial blood gas levels is to follow the same steps of interpretation each time. A specific method to be used each time that blood gas values must be interpreted is presented here (Box 22-1).

Step 1. Look at the Pao_2 level and answer the question, "Does the Pao_2 show hypoxemia?" The Pao_2 is a measure of the partial pressure of oxygen dissolved in arterial blood plasma, with "P" standing for "partial pressure" and "a" standing for "arterial." Sometimes Pao_2 is shortened to Po_2. It is reported in millimeters of mercury (mm Hg). Pao_2 reflects 3% of total oxygen in the blood.[1]

The normal range in Pao_2 for persons breathing room air at sea level is 80 to 100 mm Hg. However, the normal range is age-dependent in two groups: infants and persons aged 60 years and older. The normal level for infants breathing room air is 40 to 70 mm Hg.[2] The normal level for persons 60 years and older decreases with age as changes occur in the ventilation/perfusion (V/Q) matching in the aging lung.[3] The correct Pao_2 for older persons can be ascertained as follows: 80 mm Hg (the lowest normal value) minus 1 mm Hg for every year that a person is over the age of 60. Using this formula, a 65-year-old individual can have a Pao_2 as low as 75 mm Hg and still be within the normal range (formula for 5 years over 60 years of age: 80 mm Hg − 5 mm Hg = 75

mm Hg). An acceptable range for an 80-year-old person is 60 mm Hg (formula for 20 years over the age of 60: 80 mm Hg − 20 mm Hg = 60 mm Hg). At any age, a Pao_2 lower than 40 mm Hg represents a life-threatening situation that necessitates immediate action.[1,4] In addition, a Pao_2 less than the predicted lowest value indicates hypoxemia, which means that a lower-than-normal amount of oxygen is dissolved in plasma.

There are several reasons to analyze the Pao_2 level before those of other blood gas components. First, a Pao_2 of less than 40 mm Hg severely compromises tissue oxygenation and calls for the immediate administration of supplemental oxygen and/or mechanical ventilation. Second, the test results for the Pao_2 level can be quickly analyzed. If the Pao_2 level is more than the lowest value for the patient's age, it is normal.

Step 2. Look at the pH level and answer the question, "Is the pH on the acid or alkaline side of 7.40?" The pH is the hydrogen ion (H^+) concentration of plasma. Calculation of pH is accomplished by using the partial pressure of carbon dioxide ($Paco_2$) and the plasma bicarbonate level (HCO_3^-). The formula used is the Henderson-Hasselbalch equation (Box 22-2).[4]

The normal pH of arterial blood is 7.35 to 7.45, with the mean being 7.40. If the pH level is less than 7.40, it is on the acid side of the mean. A pH level less than 7.35 is known as *acidemia*, and the overall condition is called *acidosis*. If the pH level is greater than 7.40, it is on the alkaline side of the mean. A pH level greater than 7.45 is known as *alkalemia*, and the overall condition is called *alkalosis*.[1,4]

Step 3. Look at the $Paco_2$ level and answer the question, "Does the $Paco_2$ show respiratory acidosis, alkalosis, or normalcy?" The $Paco_2$ is a measure of the partial pressure of carbon dioxide dissolved in arterial blood plasma, and it is reported in mm Hg. It is the acid-base component that reflects the effectiveness of ventilation in relation to the metabolic rate.[1,4] In other words, the $Paco_2$ value indicates whether the patient can ventilate well enough to rid the body of the carbon dioxide produced as a consequence of metabolism.

The normal range for $Paco_2$ is 35 to 45 mm Hg. This range does not change as a person ages. A $Paco_2$ value of

Box 22-1

STEPS FOR INTERPRETATION OF BLOOD GAS LEVELS

STEP 1
Look at the Pa_{O_2} level and answer the question, *"Does the Pa_{O_2} level show hypoxemia?"*

STEP 2
Look at the pH level and answer the question, *"Is the pH level on the acid or alkaline side of 7.40?"*

STEP 3
Look at the Pa_{O_2} level and answer the question, *"Does the Pa_{CO_2} level show respiratory acidosis, alkalosis, or normalcy?"*

STEP 4
Look at the HCO_3^- level and answer the question, *"Does the HCO_3^- level show metabolic acidosis, alkalosis, or normalcy?"*

STEP 5
Look back at the pH level, and answer the question, *"Does the pH show a compensated or an uncompensated condition?"*

Box 22-2

THE HENDERSON-HASSELBALCH EQUATION FOR BLOOD pH

The blood pH depends on the ratio of bicarbonate to dissolved carbon dioxide. As long as the ratio is 20:1, the pH will be 7.4.

$$pH = pK* + \log \frac{base}{acid}$$

$$pH = pK + \log \frac{HCO_3^-}{CO_2}$$

$$pH = 6.1 + \log \frac{24 \text{ mEqL}}{40 \times 0.03 \text{ mEq/L}}$$

$$pH = 6.1 + \log 20$$

$$pH = 6.1 + 1.3$$

$$pH = 7.4$$

*pK is the pH at which the substance is half dissociated and half undissociated—value here is 6.1; HCO_3^- normal 24 mEq/L; CO_2 normal for arterial blood is 40 mm Hg and must be converted to mEq/L to be used in this equation. Therefore the 40 mm Hg is multiplied by .03 to convert to mEq/L.

Box 22-3

UNCOMPENSATED ABGs

EXAMPLE 1
Pa_{O_2}:   90 mm Hg
pH: 7.25
Pa_{CO_2}:   50 mm Hg
HCO_3^-:   22 mEq/L
Interpretation: Uncompensated respiratory acidosis

EXAMPLE 2
Pa_{O_2}:   90 mm Hg
pH: 7.25
Pa_{CO_2}:   40 mm Hg
HCO_3^-:   17 mEq/L
Interpretation: Uncompensated metabolic acidosis

greater than 45 mm Hg defines *respiratory acidosis*, which is caused by alveolar hypoventilation. Hypoventilation can result from chronic obstructive pulmonary disease (COPD), oversedation, head trauma, anesthesia, drug overdose, neuromuscular disease, or hypoventilation with mechanical ventilation.[1]

Ventilatory failure results whenever the Pa_{CO_2} level exceeds 50 mm Hg. Acute ventilatory failure occurs when the Pa_{CO_2} level is greater than 50 mm Hg and the pH level is less than 7.30. It is referred to as *acute* because the pH is abnormal, thereby not allowing enough time for the body to compensate by returning the pH to the normal range. Chronic ventilatory failure is defined as a Pa_{CO_2} value of greater than 50 mm Hg, with a pH level of greater than 7.30.[1]

A Pa_{CO_2} value that is less than 35 mm Hg defines *respiratory alkalosis*, which is caused by alveolar hyperventilation. Hyperventilation can result from hypoxia, anxiety, pulmonary embolism, pregnancy, and hyperventilation with mechanical ventilation or as a compensatory mechanism to metabolic acidosis.[2,4]

Step 4. Look at the HCO_3^- level and answer the question, "Does the HCO_3^- show metabolic acidosis, alkalosis, or normalcy?" The bicarbonate (HCO_3^-) is the acid-base component that reflects kidney function. The bicarbonate is reduced or increased in the plasma by renal mechanisms. The normal range is 22 to 26 mEq/L.[2,4]

A bicarbonate level of less than 22 mEq/L defines *metabolic acidosis*, which can result from ketoacidosis, lactic acidosis, renal failure, or diarrhea. The cumulative effect is a gain of acids or a loss of base. A bicarbonate level that is greater than 26 mEq/L defines *metabolic al-*

kalosis, which can result from fluid loss from the upper gastrointestinal tract (vomiting or nasogastric suction), diuretic therapy, severe hypokalemia, alkali administration, or steroid therapy.[2,4]

Step 5. Look back at the pH level and answer the question, "Does the pH show a compensated or an uncompensated condition?" If the pH level is abnormal (less than 7.35 or greater than 7.45), the Pa_{CO_2} value or the HCO_3^- level, or both, will also be abnormal. This is an uncompensated condition because the body has not had enough time to return the pH to its normal range.[1,4] See Box 22-3 for two examples of uncompensated ABGs. If the pH level is within normal limits and both the Pa_{CO_2} value and the HCO_3^- level are abnormal, the condition is compensated because the body has had enough time to restore the pH to within its normal range.[1,4] Differentiating the primary disorder from the compensatory response can be difficult. The primary disorder is the abnormality that caused the pH level to shift initially. It is determined according to the pH level; thus, the primary disorder is considered to be the one on whichever side of 7.40 the pH level occurs.[1,4] See Box 22-4 for two examples of compensated ABGs. Partial compensation may also be present and is evidenced by abnormal pH, $Paco_2$, and HCO_3^- levels, indications that the body is attempting to return the pH to its normal range.[1,4]

Table 22-1 summarizes the changes in the acid-base components that accompany various acid-base disorders.[1,2] In addition to the parameters previously discussed, other factors must be considered when reviewing a patient's ABGs, including oxygen saturation, oxygen content, expected Pao_2, base excess and deficit, and anion gap analysis. Table 22-2 summarizes conditions that may potentiate acid-base abnormalities.[1,4]

Oxygen Saturation. Oxygen saturation is a measure of the amount of oxygen bound to hemoglobin, compared with hemoglobin's maximal capability for binding oxygen. It can be assessed as a component of the ABG (Sao_2) or can be measured noninvasively using a pulse oximeter (Spo_2).[1,5] Oxygen saturation is reported as a percentage or as a decimal, with normal being greater than 95% when the patient is on room air. Normally, the saturation level cannot reach 100% (on room air) because of the physiologic shunting.[1,2] However, when supplemental oxygen is administered, oxygen saturation may approach 100% so closely that it is reported as 100%.

Proper evaluation of the oxygen saturation level is vital. For example, an Sao_2 of 97% means that 97% of the

---

Box 22-4

COMPENSATED ABGS

EXAMPLE 1

Pao_2:	90 mm Hg
pH:	7.37
$Paco_2$:	60 mm Hg
HCO_3^-:	38 mEq/L

Interpretation: Compensated respiratory acidosis with metabolic alkalosis. (The acidosis is considered the main disorder and the alkalosis the compensatory response, because the pH is on the acid side of 7.40)

EXAMPLE 2

Pao_2:	90 mm Hg
pH:	7.42
$Paco_2$:	48 mm Hg
HCO_3^-:	35 mEq/L

Interpretation: Compensated metabolic alkalosis with respiratory acidosis. (The alkalosis is considered the main disorder and the acidosis the compensatory response, because the pH is on the alkaline side of 7.40.)

Table 22-1 — Arterial Blood Gas Assessment

Disorder	pH	$Paco_2$	HCO_3^-
RESPIRATORY ACIDOSIS			
Uncompensated	<7.35	>45 mm Hg	22-26 mEq/L
Partially compensated	<7.35	>45 mm Hg	>26 mEq/L
Compensated	7.35-7.39	>45 mm Hg	>26 mEq/L
RESPIRATORY ALKALOSIS			
Uncompensated	>7.45	<35 mm Hg	22-26 mEq/L
Partially compensated	>7.45	<35 mm Hg	<22 mEq/L
Compensated	7.41-7.45	<35 mm Hg	<22 mEq/L
METABOLIC ACIDOSIS			
Uncompensated	<7.35	35-45 mm Hg	<22 mEq/L
Partially compensated	<7.35	<35 mm Hg	<22 mEq/L
Compensated	7.35-7.39	<35 mm Hg	<22 mEq/L
METABOLIC ALKALOSIS			
Uncompensated	>7.45	35-45 mm Hg	>26 mEq/L
Partially compensated	>7.45	>45 mm Hg	>26 mEq/L
Compensated	7.41-7.45	>45 mm Hg	>26 mEq/L
COMBINED RESPIRATORY AND METABOLIC ACIDOSIS	<7.35	>45 mm Hg	<22 mEq/L
COMBINED RESPIRATORY AND METABOLIC ALKALOSIS	>7.45	<35 mm Hg	>26 mEq/L

available hemoglobin is bound with oxygen. The word "available" is essential to evaluating the SaO_2 level, because the hemoglobin level is not always within normal limits and oxygen can bind only with what is available. A 97% saturation level associated with 10 g of hemoglobin does not deliver as much oxygen to the tissues as does a 97% saturation associated with 15 g of hemoglobin. Thus assessing only the SaO_2 level and finding it within normal limits must not lead one to believe that the patient's oxygenation status is normal. The hemoglobin level must also be evaluated before a decision on oxygenation status can be made.[1,6]

Oxygen Content. Oxygen content (CaO_2) is a measure of the total amount of oxygen carried in the blood, including the amount dissolved in plasma (measured by the PaO_2) and the amount bound to the hemoglobin molecule (measured by the SaO_2). CaO_2 is reported in milliliters of oxygen carried per 100 ml of blood. The normal value is 20 ml of oxygen per 100 ml of blood. To calculate the oxygen content, the PaO_2, the SaO_2, and the hemoglobin level are used (see Appendix). A change in any one of these parameters will affect the CaO_2.[1]

The value of assessing the CaO_2 is best illustrated by the examples in Table 22-3. Here, the ABG parameters that are used most commonly to evaluate oxygenation

status (PaO_2 and SaO_2) are both normal. Assessing only the PaO_2 and the SaO_2 would lead to the invalid conclusion that Patient B's oxygenation status is normal. However, consideration of the hemoglobin and the CaO_2 reveals that the oxygenation of Patient B's blood is significantly abnormal.

Expected PaO_2. When a patient receives supplemental oxygen, the PaO_2 level is expected to rise. There is value in knowing the level to which the PaO_2 should rise in normal subjects on a given FiO_2 and comparing that with the level to which the PaO_2 actually does rise in patients with pulmonary disease, because this illustrates how well the lung is functioning. Calculating the expected PaO_2 is accomplished by multiplying the FiO_2 value by 5.[7] Thus the expected PaO_2 on an FiO_2 of 30% is at least 150 mm Hg (30×5), whereas the expected PaO_2 on an FiO_2 of 50% is 250 mm Hg (50×5). These expected PaO_2 values represent the oxygen level achievable with healthy lungs. Pulmonary disease can radically decrease the expected PaO_2 level. It is impossible to apply the "FiO_2 value $\times$ 5" rule to achieve the expected PaO_2 value when the patient is on a system that delivers oxygen by liters per minute. For these situations, Table 22-4 shows the FiO_2 levels that correspond to various oxygen delivery systems.[8]

Table 22-5 illustrates three examples of what can occur when the expected PaO_2 level does not reach normal. Patient A shows a normal expected PaO_2; thus it is assumed that his or her lungs are performing normally. The fact that the expected PaO_2 has been reached means that he or she may not require supplemental oxygen. Patient B has not reached the expected PaO_2, but at least he or she is not hypoxemic. The administration of supplemental oxygen should bring the PaO_2 level above 80 mm Hg. However, because the expected PaO_2 level has not been achieved, it must be assumed that removal of oxygen will result in hypoxemia.[1] Patient C has not reached the expected PaO_2 and is therefore having trouble with oxygenation.

Base Excess and Base Deficit. Base excess and base deficit reflect the nonrespiratory contribution to acid-base balance and are reported in milliequivalents per liter above or below the normal range of -2 mEq/L to $+2$ mEq/L. A negative base level is reported as a *base*

Table 22-2	Causes of Acid-Base Disorders
Disorders	**Potential Cause**
Respiratory acidosis	Hypoventilation resulting from COPD
	Oversedation
	Head trauma
	Anesthesia
	Drug overdose
	Neuromuscular disease
	Hypoventilation with mechanical ventilation
Respiratory alkalosis	Hypoxia
	Anxiety
	Pulmonary embolism
	Hyperventilation with mechanical ventilation
Metabolic acidosis	*High anion gap:* Diabetic or alcoholic ketoacidosis, renal failure (uremia), rhabdomyolysis, toxin ingestion, methanol or salicylates
	Nonanion gap: Diarrhea, renal tubular acidosis, ureterosigmoidoscopy, ileostomy
Metabolic alkalosis	Steroid therapy
	Vomiting, gastrointestinal suction
	Diuretic therapy
	Potassium deficit
	Sodium bicarbonate intake

COPD, Chronic obstructive pulmonary disease.

Table 22-3	Assessing Oxygenation Status			
Patient	**PaO_2 Level (mm Hg)**	**SaO_2 Level (%)**	**Hgb Level (g%)**	**CaO_2 Level (vol%)**
A	100	97	15	19.8
B	100	97	10	13.3

Table 22-4	Guidelines for Estimating Fio_2 with Low-Flow Oxygen Devices	
100% O_2 Flow Rate (L)		**Fio_2 (%)**
NASAL CANNULA OR CATHETER		
1		24
2		28
3		32
4		36
5		40
6		44
OXYGEN MASK		
5-6		40
6-7		50
7-8		60
MASK WITH RESERVOIR BAG		
6		60
7		70
8		80
9		90
10		99+

From Scanlon CL, Wilkins RL, Stoller JK, editors: *Eagan's fundamentals of respiratory care,* ed 8, St Louis, 2003, Mosby.
NOTE: Normal ventilatory pattern assumed.

Table 22-5	The Expected Pao_2 Compared with the Actual Pao_2		
Patient*	**Fio_2 Level (%)**	**Expected Pao_2 Level (mm Hg)**	**Actual Pao_2 Level (mm Hg)**
A	30	150	160
B	50	250	85
C	50	250	60

*Patients are all younger than 60 years.

deficit, which correlates with *metabolic acidosis*, whereas a positive base level is reported as a *base excess*, which correlates with *metabolic alkalosis*.[4]

Anion Gap. Calculation of the anion gap can give a more complete analysis of metabolic disturbances that occur in the critically ill patient. The anion gap is computed by subtracting the major plasma anions—chloride and bicarbonate—from the major plasma cation—sodium (Box 22-5).[4,9] The remainder is made up of minor plasma anions such as organic ions, phosphates, and negatively charged proteins. The normal anion gap is 8

Box 22-5
ANION GAP

Formula: Extracellular fluid cations minus extracellular fluid anions plus measured bicarbonate level

OR

Sodium (Na^+) − (chloride [Cl^-] + Bicarbonate [HCO_3^-]) = 8-16 mEq/L

EXAMPLE

Na^+, 145; Cl^-, 105; HCO_3^-, 15

$145 - 105 + 15 = 145 - 120 = 25$

Interpretation: High anion-gap metabolic acidosis

to 16 mEq/L.[4] Any process that significantly increases the minor plasma anions creates a high–anion-gap metabolic acidosis. Elevation of the anion gap is seen with processes such as diabetic or alcoholic ketoacidosis, lactic acidosis, renal failure, and uremia , and toxins such as salicylates and methanol.[4,9] A non–anion-gap metabolic acidosis can occur through the loss of bicarbonate and the retention of the chloride ion (hyperchloremic metabolic acidosis).[4,9] Clinically a non–anion-gap acidosis is associated with diarrhea, renal failure, hyperalimentation, and ureterosigmoidoscopy.[1,4] Therefore anion-gap calculation helps to simplify and determine the cause of metabolic acidosis.

CLASSIC SHUNT EQUATION AND OXYGEN TENSION INDICES

The efficiency of oxygenation can be assessed by measuring the degree of intrapulmonary shunting that occurs in a patient at any one time, using the classic shunt equation and oxygen tension indices. *Intrapulmonary shunting* (QS/QT [the portion of cardiac output not exchanging with alveolar blood divided by the total cardiac output]) refers to venous blood that flows to the lungs without being oxygenated because of nonfunctioning alveoli.[1] Other names for this condition include shunt effect, low V/Q, wasted blood flow, and venous admixture.[2] Direct determination of intrapulmonary shunting requires the use of the classic shunt equation (see Appendix), which is both invasive and cumbersome. A shunt greater than 10% is considered abnormal and indicative of a shunt-producing disorder. A shunt greater than 30% is a serious and potentially life-threatening condition, which requires pulmonary intervention.[1]

Often times, intrapulmonary shunting is estimated by using the oxygen tension indices. One advantage to these methods is the ease of performance, though they have been found to be unreliable in critically ill patients.[1,2] An estimate of intrapulmonary shunting can be

Table 22-6		Calculation of Intrapulmonary Shunting			
FiO$_2$	Pao$_2$ Level (mm Hg)	PAo$_2$ Level (mm Hg)	Pao$_2$/Fio$_2$	a/A Ratio (%)	A-a Gradient (mm Hg)
0.21	40	97	190	0.41	57
0.50	80	300	160	0.27	220
1.0	150	610	60	0.25	460

Data from Murray JF, Nadel JA: *Textbook of respiratory medicine,* Philadelphia, 1988, Saunders.

determined by computing the difference between the alveolar and arterial oxygen concentrations. Normally, alveolar and arterial Po$_2$ values are approximately equal. When they are not, it indicates that venous blood is passing malfunctioning alveoli and returning unoxygenated to the left side of the heart.[1] The most common oxygen tension indices used to estimate intrapulmonary shunting are the Pao$_2$/Fio$_2$ ratio, the Pao$_2$/PAo$_2$ ratio, and the A-a gradient (P[A-a]o$_2$).

Pao$_2$/Fio$_2$ Ratio. The Pao$_2$/Fio$_2$ ratio is clinically the easiest formula to calculate because it does not call for the computation of the alveolar PO$_2$. Normally the Pao$_2$/Fio$_2$ ratio is greater than 286, with the lower the value the worse the lung function.[1,2]

Pao$_2$/PAo$_2$ Ratio. The Pao$_2$/PAo$_2$ ratio (arterial/alveolar O$_2$ ratio) is normally greater than 60%. The disadvantage to using this formula is that it calls for the computation of the alveolar PO$_2$ (see Appendix), but the advantage is that it is unaffected by changes in the Fio$_2$, as long as the underlying lung condition is stable.[1,2]

Alveolar-Arterial Gradient. The A-a gradient (P[A-a]o$_2$) is normally less than 20 mm Hg on room air for patients younger than 61 years. This estimate of intrapulmonary shunting is the least reliable clinically but is used often in clinical decision making. One of the major disadvantages to using this formula is that it is greatly influenced by the amount of oxygen the patient is receiving.[1,2]

Serial determinations of the estimates of intrapulmonary shunting provide the practitioner with objective data on which to base clinical decisions.[1] Table 22-6 illustrates the change in intrapulmonary shunting in the hypoxemic patient using the previously described oxygen tension indices to estimate severity of shunting.

DEAD SPACE EQUATION

The efficiency of ventilation can be measured using the clinical dead space (V$_D$/V$_T$) equation (see Appendix). The formula measures the fraction of tidal volume not participating in gas exchange. Dead space greater than 0.6 indicates a dead space–producing disorder and is considered abnormal. The major limitations to using this formula are that it requires the measurement of exhaled carbon dioxide to complete and that the work of breathing by patients must remain stable during the collection.[1]

SPUTUM STUDIES

Careful analysis of sputum specimens is crucial for the rapid identification and treatment of pulmonary infections. The most difficult aspect of sputum examination is proper collection of the specimen. In general, collection of a good sputum sample requires a conscious, cooperative, and sufficiently hydrated patient.[2] When the patient has difficulty producing sputum, heated, nebulized saline may help to loosen secretions for expectoration.[2] Chest physiotherapy combined with nebulization improves the success rate. Collection of a sputum specimen is best done in the morning, because a greater volume of secretions is present as a result of nighttime pooling. Brushing the teeth and rinsing the oropharyngeal airway is recommended to reduce contamination before collecting a sample.[1]

Many critically ill patients cannot cough effectively, and thus sputum collection by other means is required. These methods include tracheobronchial aspiration, transtracheal aspiration, and the use of a fiberoptic bronchoscopy with a protected brush catheter. Because each method has its own benefits and risks, the patient's clinical condition determines the appropriate technique.[1,10]

Many critically ill patients have endotracheal or tracheostomy tubes already in place. Collecting sputum specimens from these patients requires special attention to technique (Box 22-6). Deep specimens are obtained to avoid collecting specimens that contain resident upper airway flora that may have migrated down the tube. Colonization of the lower airways with upper airway flora can occur within 48 hours of intubation.[11]

Once a sputum specimen is obtained, it is examined for volume, physical properties, mucopurulence, and color. Next, a microscopic examination is done to identify the source of the specimen. If a bacterial infection is suspected, a Gram's stain followed by a culture and sensitivity (C&S) is performed.

Box 22-6

PROCEDURE FOR COLLECTION OF TRACHEAL OR ENDOTRACHEAL SPUTUM SPECIMEN

1. Clear the endotracheal or tracheostomy tube of all local secretions, avoiding deep airway penetration.
2. Attach a sputum trap to a sterile suction catheter, and advance the catheter into the trachea while trying to avoid contact with the endotracheal tube or tracheostomy tube.
3. After the catheter is fully advanced, apply suction until secretions return to the sputum trap. When enough secretions are collected, discontinue suctioning and remove the catheter.
4. Do not apply suction while the catheter is being withdrawn, because this can contaminate the sample with sputum from the upper airway. Do not flush the catheter with sterile water, because this dilutes the sample.
5. If the catheter becomes plugged with secretions, place it in a sterile container and send it to the laboratory. The specimen must be transported immediately or refrigerated if a delay is necessary.

DIAGNOSTIC PROCEDURES

BRONCHOSCOPY

Fiberoptic bronchoscopy is a relatively safe procedure done at the bedside, and is most often used as both a diagnostic and therapeutic tool. Diagnostic indications include hemoptysis, infectious pneumonia, difficult intubation, pulmonary injury after chest trauma, acute burn inhalation injury, aspiration lung injuries, and acute upper airway obstruction. Therapeutic indications include the aspiration of foreign bodies; removal of obstructing secretions; atelectasis; difficult intubation; and resection of small, benign growths from the airway.[1,2]

Before the bronchoscopy, a complete patient history and examination, including a chest x-ray examination, are performed.[2] Preprocedure evaluation of the patient also includes clotting studies (prothrombin time [PT], partial thromboplastin time [PTT], and platelet count) and evaluation of the arterial blood gas levels.[2] Hypoxemic patients need supplemental oxygen during the procedure. The patient must have nothing by mouth for 6 to 8 hours before the bronchoscopy to reduce the risk of aspiration.[2]

Although a topical anesthetic can be used alone, it is generally supplemented by an intravenous sedative and/or analgesic. A benzodiazepine for sedative effects and/or a narcotic analgesic are administered intravenously during the procedure.[1] Preprocedure medications for a diagnostic bronchoscopy may include atropine and intramuscular codeine. Atropine lessens the vasovagal response and reduces the secretions, whereas codeine decreases the cough reflex. When a bronchoscopy is performed therapeutically to remove secretions, decreased cough and gag reflexes are present, which may impair secretion clearance.[1,2] Maintenance of the airway is essential to prevent complications.

Complications of the procedure may be related to the procedure itself, the anesthetic, or an ancillary procedure. Minor complications include laryngospasm, bronchospasm, epistaxis, fever, vomiting, altered pulmonary mechanics, and hemodynamic instability. Major complications include anaphylaxis, infection, hypotension, cardiac dysrhythmias, pneumothorax, hemorrhage, respiratory failure, hypoxemia, and cardiopulmonary arrest.[1,2]

THORACENTESIS

Thoracentesis is a simple, usually uncomplicated procedure done at the bedside for the removal of fluid or air from the pleural space. It is used most often as a diagnostic measure; it may also be performed therapeutically for the drainage of a pleural effusion or empyema.[1] No absolute contraindications to thoracentesis exist, although there are some risks that generally contraindicate the procedure in all but emergency situations. These risk factors include unstable hemodynamics, coagulation defects, mechanical ventilation, the presence of an intraaortic balloon pump, or patients who are uncooperative. In most clinical situations, diagnostic thoracentesis can be delayed until these risk factors are eliminated.[2]

The patient is placed in a sitting position with legs over the side of the bed and hands and arms supported on a padded overbed table. If the patient's condition precludes sitting, the side-lying position with the back flush with the edge of the bed and the affected side down can be used.[1] The patient is cautioned not to move or cough during the procedure.[2] During the thoracentesis, the site of the needle insertion is usually determined by previous chest x-ray examination, computed tomography (CT) scan, or chest percussion. A local anesthetic is used to minimize patient discomfort during insertion of the thoracentesis needle.[2]

Complications associated with thoracentesis include pain, pneumothorax, and reexpansion pulmonary edema. Pneumothorax can occur as a result of introduction of air into the pleural space, puncture of the lung, or rupture of the visceral pleura.[12] Reexpansion pulmonary edema can occur when a large amount of effusion fluid (approximately 1000 to 1500 ml) is removed from the pleural space. Removal of the fluid increases the negative intrapleural pressure, which can lead to edema when the lung does not reexpand to fill the space. The patient experiences severe coughing and shortness of breath. The onset of these symptoms is an indication to discontinue the thoracentesis.[13]

BEDSIDE PULMONARY FUNCTION TESTS

Pulmonary function tests (PFTs) are designed to quantify respiratory function and are an essential component of a thorough pulmonary evaluation. PFTs are used for a variety of purposes, including preoperative assessment, evaluating lung mechanics, diagnosing and tracking pulmonary diseases, and monitoring therapy. Results are individualized according to age, gender, and body size.[14]

A complete pulmonary function test consists of four components: lung volumes, mechanics of breathing, diffusion, and arterial blood gases. PFTs may take as long as 2 hours to complete. Because of the severity of illness encountered in the critical care area, all four components are rarely completed. Most often, measurements of pulmonary function in the critically ill are limited to those areas that give the practitioner information about the patient's need for or ability to wean from mechanical ventilation. This section covers the areas tested most often at the bedside of critically ill individuals.

Measurement of lung volumes and capacities (Box 22-7) provides valuable information about the origin of a disease process. Four lung volumes and four lung capacities can be measured. Measurement of volumes at the bedside is limited to tidal volume and vital capacity. Generally, a vital capacity of 10 to 15 ml/kg is a minimally accepted value for weaning, with a respiratory rate of less than 24 breaths per minute.[15]

The assessment of the mechanics of breathing includes measurement of the flow of gas, lung and chest compliance, respiratory muscle strength, and tissue resistance. In the critical care area, dynamic and static compliance are measured at the bedside. *Compliance* is a measure of the distensibility of the lungs (how easily they are inflated). Dynamic compliance is measured during the breathing cycle. A value of 46 to 66 ml/cm H_2O is normal (see Appendix). It should be noted that measurement of dynamic compliance does not distinguish among resistance forces. Therefore conditions that increase resistance alter the dynamic compliance value. Dynamic compliance decreases with any decrease in lung compliance or increase in airway resistance, such as occurs with bronchospasm and retained secretions. Static compliance is measured under no-flow conditions so that resistance forces are removed. Static compliance decreases with any decrease in lung compliance, such as occurs with pneumothorax, atelectasis, pneumonia, pulmonary edema, and chest wall restrictions. A normal value is 57 to 85 ml/cm of H_2O (see Appendix).[16]

Assessment of inspiratory muscle strength can be evaluated through the measurement of maximal inspiratory pressure (MIP) and negative inspiratory pressure (NIP). Both should be more negative than -20 to -25 cm H_2O. Other names for these same tests are negative inspiratory effort (NIE), peak inspiratory pressure

---

Box 22-7

LUNG VOLUMES AND CAPACITIES

Tidal volume (V_T): The volume of air exhaled after a normal resting inhalation: $V_T \times$ respiratory rate = minute ventilation. Normal is 500 ml.

Inspiratory reserve volume (IRV): The amount of additional air that can be taken in after a normal inhalation. Normal is 3000-3100 ml.

Inspiratory capacity (IC): The maximal amount of air that can be inhaled after a normal exhalation. Normal is 3500-3600 ml.

Expiratory reserve volume (ERV): The additional amount of air that can be exhaled after a normal resting exhalation. Normal is 1100-1200 ml.

Vital capacity (VC): The maximal amount of air that can be exhaled after a maximal inhalation. Normal is 4600-4800 ml.

Residual volume (RV): The amount of air left in the lung after maximal exhalation. Normal is 1200-1300 ml.

Functional residual capacity (FRC): The amount of air left in the lung after a normal exhalation. The total of the ERV and RV. Normal is 2300-2400 ml.

Total lung capacity (TLC): The maximal volume of air in the lung after a maximal inspiration. The total of all lung volumes. Normal is 5800-6000 ml.

(PIP), and peak inspiratory force (PIF). Both the MIP and NIP require a cooperative patient and can provide useful information about spontaneous breathing ability. Maximal expiratory pressure (MEP) can be measured to test the ability to cough in patients with neuromuscular dysfunction. Other common methods used to assess respiratory muscle strength are maximum voluntary ventilation (MVV), minute ventilation (V_E), and breathing pattern.[15,17]

Dynamic pulmonary function tests are designed to evaluate the function of the respiratory muscles, thorax, and lungs. These tests are timed breathing studies that evaluate the degree of respiratory impairment and include forced vital capacity (FVC), peak expiratory flow rate (PEFR), forced expiratory volume in 1 second (FEV_1), and forced expiratory volume divided by the forced vital capacity (FEV_1/FVC). Forced expiratory flow ($FEF_{25\%-75\%}$) is the mean rate of air flow over the middle half of the FVC and is a good index of airway resistance. When these studies are performed at the bedside, they require the use of spirometry for volume measurement. The tests can be performed with intubated or nonintubated patients. In the intubated patient, the spirometer is attached to the end of the endotracheal tube. In the nonintubated patient, a nose clip is placed on the patient and the patient is instructed to breathe through a spirometer tube. The patient is seated on the side of the bed if possible.[16] Table 22-7 provides a description of each of these parameters.

Table 22-7	Bedside Pulmonary Function Tests
Test	**Description**
Respiratory rate (f)	Number of breaths per minute
Tidal volume (V_T)	Volume of air exhaled after a normal resting inhalation
Minute ventilation (V_E)	Volume of air expired per minute (tidal volume $\times$ respiratory rate = minute ventilation)
Maximal voluntary ventilation (MVV)	Maximal amount of air that can be moved into and out of the lungs in 1 minute
Forced vital capacity (FVC)	Maximal amount of air that can be forcefully exhaled from the lungs after maximal inhalation
Maximal inspiratory pressure (MIP)	Maximal negative pressure generated on inhalation
Maximal expiratory pressure (MEP)	Maximal positive pressure generated on exhalation
Peak expiratory flow rate (PEFR)	Maximal flow rate achieved during forced exhalation
Forced expiratory flow at midpoint of vital capacity ($FEF_{25\%-75\%}$)	Measure of the average flow rate during the middle 50% of exhalation
Forced expiratory flow at 1 second (FEV_1)	Volume of air exhaled in first second of forced exhalation

Box 22-8

STEPS FOR INTERPRETATION OF A CHEST X-RAY FILM

STEP 1
Look at the different densities (black, gray, and white), and answer the question, *"What is air, fluid, tissue, and bone?"*

STEP 2
Look at the shape or form of each density, and answer the question, *"What normal anatomic structure is this?"*

STEP 3
Look at both right and left sides, and answer the question, *"Are the findings the same on both sides, or are there differences (both physiologic and pathophysiologic)?"*

STEP 4
Look at all the structures (bones, mediastinum, diaphragm, pleural space, and lung tissue), and answer the question, *"Are there any abnormalities present?"*

STEP 5
Look for all tubes, wires, and lines, and answer the question, *"Are the tubes, wires, and lines in the proper place?"*

VENTILATION/PERFUSION SCANNING

Ventilation/perfusion scanning is indicated when a serious alteration of the normal ventilation/perfusion (V/Q) relationship is suspected. V/Q studies are ordered most often to diagnose and follow a suspected pulmonary embolus. V/Q scanning is approximately 90% accurate in determining this diagnosis. Comparing the perfusion scan with the results of a clinical examination may improve this percentage somewhat.

The V/Q scan consists of both a ventilation scan and a perfusion scan. The ventilation scan is performed by having the patient inhale a radiolabeled gas and air mixture through a mask. The perfusion scan is performed by intravenously injecting the patient with a radioisotope. Scintillation cameras record the gamma radiation images produced by the isotope as it is breathed or perfused into the lung. When an obstruction of the isotope's flow into an area of the lung occurs, the diminished radioactivity is reflected in the camera image of that zone.[1,2]

Because the results are less than 100% accurate in predicting pulmonary emboli, most V/Q scans are interpreted in one of four ways. The scan is interpreted as normal when the perfusion scan is normal, and the prob-

ability of pulmonary embolism approaches zero. A low probability interpretation is given when there are small V/Q mismatches, focal V/Q matches with no corresponding radiographic abnormalities, or when the perfusion defects are considerably smaller than the radiographic abnormalities. This finding is associated with a 12% chance of pulmonary embolus.[17] An intermediate or indeterminate probability reading is used when there are severe diffuse airflow obstructions; perfusion defects corresponding in size and position to radiographic abnormalities; and a single, moderate V/Q mismatch without a corresponding radiographic abnormality. There is a 30% probability of pulmonary embolus with this finding.[18] A high probability interpretation is used when the perfusion defects are substantially larger than the radiographic abnormalities or when there is one or more large or two or more moderate V/Q mismatches with no corresponding radiographic abnormalities. This finding is seen infrequently but has a predictive value of 85%.[14]

CHEST RADIOGRAPHY

Chest radiography is an important diagnostic procedure for any critically ill patient. Chest x-ray examinations aid in the diagnosis of various disorders and complications and assist in the evaluation of treatment.[1]

When interpreting a chest x-ray film, a systematic method is used for viewing it (Box 22-8). Areas of the film that are assessed include bones, mediastinum, di-

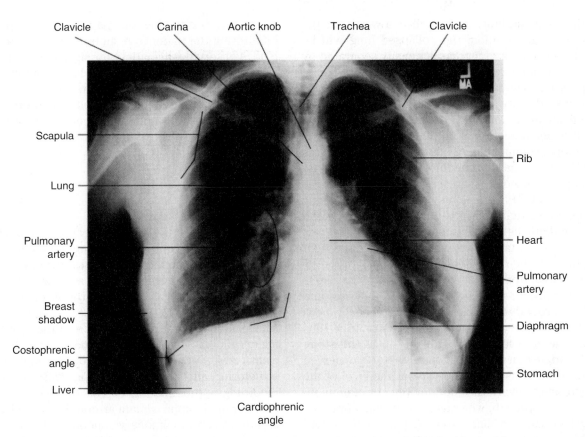

Clavicle   Carina   Aortic knob   Trachea   Clavicle

Scapula

Lung

Pulmonary artery

Breast shadow

Costophrenic angle

Liver

Rib

Heart

Pulmonary artery

Diaphragm

Stomach

Cardiophrenic angle

Fig. 22-1   Location of structures on a normal chest x-ray film. (From Dettenmeir PA: *Radiographic assessment for nurses,* St Louis, 1995, Mosby.)

aphragm, pleural space, and lung tissue. See Fig. 22-1 for an example of a normal chest x-ray film.

Bones. The clavicles, ribs, thoracic and cervical spine, and scapulae are assessed. The clavicles should be symmetric, and the ribs should be an equal distance apart. Intervertebral disk spaces should be evident, indicating an adequately exposed inspiratory film.[18] The thoracic and cervical spine should be straight without signs of curvature. The scapulae usually appear as areas of added density in the upper lung fields. There should be no evidence of fractures, calcification and lesions (increased density), or demineralization (decreased density).[18]

Mediastinum. The structures assessed in the mediastinal area are the aortic knob and the trachea. The trachea should be midline with a slight deviation to the right as it approaches the carina.[1] Shifting of the mediastinal structures can occur with atelectasis and removal of all or a portion of a lung (toward the area of involvement), pneumothorax (away from the area of involvement), pleural effusion, and tumors.[1,18,19]

Diaphragm. The diaphragm should be clearly visible with sharp costophrenic angles (where the chest wall and the tapered edges of the diaphragm meet).[1] The level of the diaphragm (on deep inspiration) should appear at the tenth or eleventh rib,[1] with the right side 1 to 2 cm higher than the left side.[18] A gastric air bubble may be found under the left side of the diaphragm.[1] An elevated diaphragm may be seen in pregnancy, obesity, conditions that cause air or fluid to accumulate in the peritoneal space, and intestinal obstruction.[1] An elevated hemidiaphragm is associated with a number of conditions, including phrenic nerve injury, previous chest surgery, subphrenic abscess, trauma, stroke, tumor, pneumonia, and radiation therapy.[1] Flattening of the diaphragm can be a sign of increased air in the lungs, such as occurs with chronic obstructive pulmonary disease (COPD) or a pleural effusion.[18] Obliteration or "blunting" of the costophrenic angle can occur with pleural effusion, atelectasis, or pneumothorax.[18,19]

Pleural Space. Identification of the pleural space on a chest x-ray film is an abnormal finding. The pleural space is not visible unless air (pneumothorax) or fluid (pleural effusion) enters it. As fluid accumulates in the pleural space, it surrounds the lung and eventually compresses it. With a pleural effusion, blunting of the costophrenic angle may be evident first, with flattening of the diaphragm and obscuring of the heart borders occurring as the effusion grows.[19] With a pneumothorax, the pleural edges become evident as one looks through and between the images of the ribs on the film. A thin line appears just parallel to the chest wall, indicating where the lung markings have pulled away from the chest wall.[18,19] In addition, the collapsed lung will be manifested as an area of increased density separated by an area of radiolucency (blackness).

Lung Tissue. The lung tissue is viewed for any areas of increased density or increased radiolucency that could indicate an abnormality. Increased density can be the result of accumulation of fluid in the lungs (e.g., water, pus, blood, edema fluid) or collapse of lung tissue (as occurs with atelectasis or pneumothorax). Increased radiolucency is caused by increased air in the lungs, as may occur with COPD.[19] In some patients a fine line may be present on the right side at about the level of the sixth rib in the midlung field. This is a normal finding and represents the horizontal fissure, which separates the right upper lobe from the right middle lobe.[19]

Tubes, Wires, and Lines. The chest x-ray film also is assessed for proper placement of all tubes, wires, and lines. When properly positioned, an endotracheal tube is 2 to 3 cm above the carina, and a nasogastric tube runs the length of the esophagus, with the tip in the stomach.[18] The origin of a central venous catheter is observed as a thin, continuous radiopaque line at the level of the jaw, progressing toward the superior vena cava in an internal jugular approach, whereas a subclavian approach originates in the clavicular area. A pulmonary artery catheter is viewed running through the right atrium and right ventricle into the pulmonary artery.[18] Additional items that may be present include temporary or permanent pacing wires, a permanent pacing generator, an implantable cardioverter defibrillator (ICD), a peripherally inserted central catheter (PICC), chest tubes (pleural or mediastinal), electrocardiography (ECG) electrodes, and surgical markers and clips.[18-19]

NURSING MANAGEMENT

Nursing management of a patient undergoing a diagnostic procedure involves a variety of interventions, which include preparing the patient psychologically and physically for the procedure, monitoring the patient's responses to the procedure, and assessing the patient after the procedure. Preparing the patient includes teaching the patient about the procedure, answering any ques-

tions, and positioning the patient for the procedure. Monitoring the patient's responses to the procedure includes observing the patient for signs of pain, anxiety, or respiratory distress (see Box 22-1) and monitoring vital signs, breath sounds, and oxygen saturation. Assessing the patient after the procedure includes observing for complications of the procedure and medicating the patient for any postprocedural discomfort.

BEDSIDE MONITORING

CAPNOGRAPHY

Capnography is the measurement of exhaled carbon dioxide gas and can be used to monitor a patient's ventilatory status. A capnograph is also known as an *end-tidal* CO_2 monitor, because the CO_2 is measured near the end of the exhalation.[20] Most often, the gas sample is analyzed through infrared gas analysis.[20] Frequently the CO_2 is measured via the exhalation port of the ventilator tubing; as the gas passes through the sensor, the data are transferred to the display unit. A display unit produces a waveform, called a *capnogram* (Fig. 22-2), and a numeric recording approximating the $Paco_2$. The ability of the capnograph to approximate arterial $Paco_2$ is altered with abnormal cardiopulmonary function.[21] Clinical application of capnography can provide information in a number of areas, including estimation of $Paco_2$ levels, assessment of dead space (increased V/Q), assessment of pulmonary blood flow, and endotracheal tube placement.[21]

Normally alveolar and arterial CO_2 concentrations are equal in the presence of normal ventilation/perfusion relationships. In a patient who is hemodynamically stable, the end-tidal CO_2 ($Petco_2$) can be used to estimate the $Paco_2$, with the $Petco_2$ levels 1 to 5 mm Hg less than $Paco_2$ levels.[22] The practitioner must determine first that a normal V/Q relationship exists before correlation of the $Petco_2$ and the $Paco_2$ can be assumed.[21-23]

Assessment of changes in physiologic dead space can be carried out with end-tidal CO_2 monitoring, based on the degree of difference between the $Paco_2$ and the $Petco_2$. As the severity of pulmonary impairment increases, so does the disparity between the $Paco_2$ and the $Petco_2$, as indicated by an increased gradient. A gradient

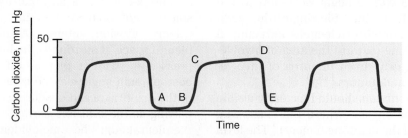

Fig. 22-2 Normal findings on a capnogram. *A→B* indicates the baseline; *B→C,* expiratory upstroke; *C→D,* alveolar plateau; *D,* partial pressure of end-tidal carbon dioxide; *D→E,* inspiratory downstroke. (From Frakes M: Measuring end-tidal carbon dioxide: clinical applications and usefulness, *Crit Care Nurse* 21[5]:23, 2001.)

of greater than 5 mm Hg can be seen with underperfused alveolar-capillary units (dead space–producing situations) and nonperfused alveolar-capillary units (alveolar dead space). Increased dead space ventilation is a result of decreased pulmonary blood flow or cardiac output and lung disease. This leads to an abnormality in the transfer of CO_2 from the blood to the lung. The result is a $PetCO_2$ level that is lower than the $PaCO_2$ because of the mixing of carbon dioxide between perfused and nonperfused units. The end result is an increased or widened $PaCO_2$-to-$PetCO_2$ gradient.[21,22]

The noninvasive measurement of $PetCO_2$ allows for the assessment of adequacy of cardiopulmonary resuscitation and endotracheal tube placement. Decreased pulmonary blood flow is associated with lower $PetCO_2$ values, reflected clinically by decreased cardiac output, as in the case of cardiopulmonary resuscitation.[20,22] During endotracheal intubation, a low $PetCO_2$ reading would indicate that the tube is positioned in the stomach, because the amount of carbon dioxide in the esophagus is expected to be low.[20,22]

Capnography and $PetCO_2$ analysis have many diverse applications in the critical care area; however, the practitioner must never assume the $PetCO_2$ values reflect $PaCO_2$ values without waveform analysis.[20,21,23]

SUBLINGUAL CAPNOMETRY

Sublingual carbon dioxide ($P_{SL}CO_2$) measurement is a new noninvasive technology available for monitoring patients at risk for hypoperfusion. Unrelieved hypoperfusion has been closely linked with development of multisystem organ dysfunction syndrome (MODS).[24,25] Traditionally, clinicians have relied on changes in vital signs or invasive therapies to indicate changes in perfusion status. Implementation of sublingual capnometry monitoring may assist in the identification of patients at risk for hypoperfusion.

Sublingual capnometry employs the gastrointestinal circulation as a means of indicating oxygen debt and cellular acidosis. The gastrointestinal circulation is sensitive to changes in blood flow and retention of carbon dioxide potentially leading to lactic acidosis because of anaerobic metabolism.[24,25] Traditionally serum lactate levels and changes in vital signs lag behind the development of oxygen debt and lactic acidosis. Oxygen debt and the sequalae are key in development of MODS.[24] Mixed venous blood has been shown to be sensitive to change in oxygen level however measurement requires insertion of an invasive catheter.

Sublingual capnometry has demonstrated a 90% confidence level in reflecting carbon dioxide level.[25] In addition, in animal models as a rise in $P_{SL}CO_2$ corrrelates with a decrease in arterial blood pressure and cardiac index. $P_{SL}CO_2$ is noninvasive, portable, and technically similar to taking an oral temperature for a patient. The system has three primary components: a disposable PCO_2 sensor, a fiberoptic cable that connects a disposable PCO_2 sensor, a fiberoptic cable that connects the disposable sensor to a blood gas analyzer, and a blood gas–monitoring instrument (Fig. 22-3). The optical fiber is coated with a silicone membrane that consists of a CO_2-sensitive fluorescent dye and is permeable to CO_2. The mucosal CO_2 passes through the silicone membrane and comes in contact with the dye. The dye is permeated by light and comes in contact with the blood gas instrument, which emits light in correlation with the amount of CO_2 detected.[24,25] The sensor is placed under the tongue with the sensor facing the mucosal membrane, and within five minutes the numeric $P_{SL}CO_2$ is displayed. Oral intubation has not been shown to affect the validity of the readings.

An absolute normal has not been established although an elevated level of $P_{SL}CO_2$ has been reported in nonsurvivors, as have elevated serum lactate levels.[24] $P_{SL}CO_2$ has also been shown to detect hypoperfusion before changes in vital signs or other laboratory values, in part because of the sensitivity of the gut circulation. Reports have demonstrated readings within two standard deviations of the mean.[24] Protocols addressing the frequency of monitoring and interpretation of the data are currently in development. Monitoring changes in this parameter should alert clinicians to more closely monitor the perfusion status of the patient. Implementation and ongoing monitoring may alert the patient care team to new threats of hypoperfusion and potentially avoid the development of MODS. The study of $P_{SL}CO_2$ use in prehospital care has been reported.[24] Research studies related to patient outcome utilizing this technology must be developed.

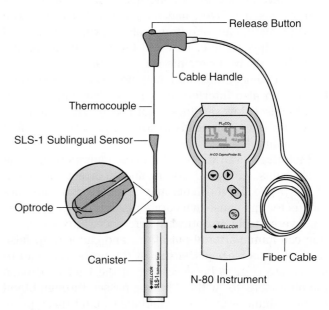

Fig. 22-3 The *CapnoProbe* SL System, highlighting the location of the CO_2-sensing optrode. (Reprinted by permission of Nellcor Puritan Bennett, Inc, Pleasanton, CA.)

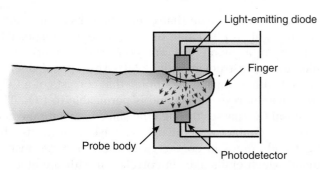

Fig. 22-4 Pulse oximeter finger probe. (From Wilkins RL, Stoller JK, Scanlon CL, editors: *Egan's fundamentals of respiratory care*, ed 8, St Louis, 2003, Mosby.)

PULSE OXIMETRY

Pulse oximetry is a noninvasive method for monitoring oxygen saturation (SpO_2). It is indicated in any situation in which the patient's oxygenation status requires continuous observation. It consists of a microprocessor and a probe that attaches to the patient (finger, ear, toe, or nose). The probe consists of two light-emitting diodes and a photodetector (Fig. 22-4). The diodes transmit red and infrared light wavelengths through the pulsating vascular bed to the photodetector on the other side. The photodetector converts the light signals into an electric signal, which is then sent to the microprocessor, which converts it to a digital reading. The pulse oximeter is considered very accurate, readings vary less than 4% to 5% at a saturation greater than 70%. However, several physiologic and technical factors limit the monitoring system.[1]

Physiologic Limitations. Physiologic limitations include elevated levels of abnormal hemoglobins, presence of vascular dyes, and poor tissue perfusion. The pulse oximeter cannot differentiate between normal and abnormal hemoglobin. Elevated levels of abnormal hemoglobin falsely elevate the SpO_2. Vascular dyes such as methylene blue, indigo carmine, indocyanine green, and fluorescein also interfere with pulse oximetry and can lead to falsely low readings. Poor tissue perfusion to the area with the probe leads to loss of pulsatile flow and signal failure.[1,2,5]

Technical Limitations. Technical limitations include bright lights, excessive motion, and incorrect placement of the probe. Bright lights may interfere with the photodetector and cause inaccurate results. The probe must be covered to limit optical interference. Excessive motion can mimic arterial pulsations and can lead to false readings. Incorrect placement of the probe can lead to inaccurate results, because part of the light can reach the photodetector without having passed through blood (optical shunting).[1,2,5] Interventions to limit these problems include using the proper probe in the appropriate spot (e.g., not using a finger probe on the ear), applying the probe according to the directions, and ensuring that the area being monitored has adequate perfusion.[1,2,5]

REFERENCES

1. Des Jardin T, Burton G: *Clinical manifestations and assessment of respiratory disease,* ed 4, St Louis, 2002, Mosby.
2. Michota FA: *Diagnostic procedures handbook,* ed 2, Hudson, 2001, Lexi-comp.
3. Hardie JA et al: Reference values for arterial blood gases in the elderly, *Chest* 125:2053, 2004.
4. Whittier WL, Rutecki GW: Primer on clinical acid-base problem solving, *Dis Mon* 50:122, 2004.
5. Attin M et al: An educational project to improve knowledge related to pulse oximetry, *Am J Crit Care* 11:529, 2002.
6. Berry B, Pinard A: Assessing tissue oxygenation, *Crit Care Nurse* 22(3):22, 2002.
7. Schallom L, Ahrens T: Clinical application: using oxygenation profiles to manage patients, *Crit Care Nurs Clin North Am* 11:437, 1999.
8. Moses S: *Family practice notebook,* Retrieved from the Internet at http://www.fpnotebook.com/REN53.htm, 2004.
9. Wilson WC: Clinical approach to acid-base analysis. importance of the anion gap, *Anesthesiol Clin North Am* 19:907, 2001.
10. Janson S: Biologic markers of airway inflammation in asthma, *AACN Clin Issues* 11:232, 2000.
11. Kollef MH: Prevention of hospital-associated pneumonia and ventilator-associated pneumonia, *Crit Care Med* 6:1396, 2004.
12. Nakamoto DA, Haaga JR: Emergent ultrasound interventions, *Radiol Clin North Am* 42:457, 2004.
13. Jones PW: Ultrasound-guided thoracentesis: is it a safer method? *Chest* 123:418, 2003.
14. Douce FH: Pulmonary function testing. In Scanlan CL, Wilkins RL, Stoller JK, editors: *Egan's fundamentals of respiratory care,* ed 8, St Louis, 2003, Mosby.
15. Hanneman S: Weaning from short-term mechanical ventilation, *Crit Care Nurse* 24(1):70, 2004.
16. Kallet RH, Katz JA: Respiratory system mechanics in acute respiratory distress syndrome, *Respir Care Clin North Am* 9:297, 2003.
17. Epstein SK: Weaning parameters, *Respir Care Clin North Am* 6:253, 2000.
18. Siela D: Using chest radiography in the intensive care unit, *Crit Care Nurse* 22(4):18, 2002.
19. Reed J: *Chest radiology: plain film patterns and differential diagnosis,* ed 5, St Louis, 2003, Mosby.
20. Frakes M: Measuring end-tidal carbon dioxide: clinical applications and usefulness, *Crit Care Nurse* 21(5):23, 2001.
21. Ahrens T et al: End-tidal carbon dioxide measurements as a prognostic indicator of outcome in cardiac arrest, *Am J Crit Care* 10:391, 2001.
22. Ahrens T, Sona C: Capnography application in acute and critical care, *AACN Clin Issues* 14:123, 2003.
23. St. John R: End-tidal carbon dioxide monitoring, *Crit Care Nurse* 23(4):83, 2003.
24. Boswell S, Scalea T: Sublingual capnometry an alternative to gastric tonometry for the management of shock resuscitation. *AACN Clin Issues* 14:176, 2003.
25. Reilly P, Howell D: What's the $P_{SL}CO_2$? – The role of sublingual carbon dioxide measurement in patient care. *NTI News-AACN* 20(8):1, 2003.

CHAPTER 23

Pulmonary Disorders

*U*nderstanding the pathology of the disease, the areas of assessment on which to focus, and the usual medical management allows the critical care nurse to more accurately anticipate and plan nursing interventions. This chapter focuses on pulmonary disorders commonly seen in the critical care environment.

ACUTE RESPIRATORY FAILURE

DESCRIPTION

Acute respiratory failure (ARF) is a clinical condition in which the pulmonary system fails to maintain adequate gas exchange.[1] It is the most common organ failure seen in the intensive care unit today,[2,3] with a mortality rate of 22% to 75%.[2] Mortality varies directly with the number of additional organ failures.[2] Additional risk factors for mortality included history of liver, renal, or hematologic dysfunction, presence of shock, and age greater than 55 years.[3]

ARF results from a deficiency in the performance of the pulmonary system.[1,4] It usually occurs secondary to another disorder that has altered the normal function of the pulmonary system in such a way as to decrease the ventilatory drive, decrease muscle strength, decrease chest wall elasticity, decrease the lung's capacity for gas exchange, increase airway resistance, or increase metabolic oxygen requirements.[5]

ARF can be classified as hypoxemic normocapnic respiratory failure (type I) or hypoxemic hypercapnic respiratory failure (type II), depending on analysis of the patient's arterial blood gases (ABGs). In type I respiratory failure, the patient presents with a low PaO_2 and a normal $PaCO_2$, whereas in type II respiratory failure, PaO_2 is low and $PaCO_2$ is high.[4]

ETIOLOGY

The etiologies of ARF may be classified as *extrapulmonary* or *intrapulmonary*, depending on the component of the respiratory system that is affected. Extrapulmonary causes include disorders that affect the brain, the spinal cord, the neuromuscular system, the thorax, the pleura, and the upper airways. Intrapulmonary causes include disorders that affect the lower airways and alveoli, the pulmonary circulation, and the alveolar-capillary membrane.[6] Table 23-1 lists the different etiologies of ARF and their associated disorders.

PATHOPHYSIOLOGY

Hypoxemia is the result of impaired gas exchange and is the hallmark of acute respiratory failure. Hypercapnia may be present, depending on the underlying cause of the problem. The main causes of hypoxemia are alveolar hypoventilation, ventilation/perfusion (V/Q) mismatching, and intrapulmonary shunting.[7] Type I respiratory failure usually results from V/Q mismatching and intrapulmonary shunting, whereas type II respiratory failure usually results from alveolar hypoventilation, which may or may not be accompanied by V/Q mismatching and intrapulmonary shunting.[1]

Alveolar Hypoventilation. Alveolar hypoventilation occurs when the amount of oxygen being brought into the alveoli is insufficient to meet the metabolic needs of the body.[6] This can be the result of increasing metabolic oxygen needs or decreasing ventilation.[5] Hypoxemia caused by alveolar hypoventilation is associated with hypercapnia and commonly results from extrapulmonary disorders.[1,7]

Ventilation/Perfusion (V/Q) Mismatching. V/Q mismatching occurs when ventilation and blood flow are mismatched in various regions of the lung in excess of what is normal. Blood passes through alveoli that are underventilated for the given amount of perfusion, leaving these areas with a lower-than-normal amount of oxygen. V/Q mismatching is the most common cause of hypoxemia and is usually the result of alveoli that are partially collapsed or partially filled with fluid.[6-8]

Intrapulmonary Shunting. The extreme form of V/Q mismatching, intrapulmonary shunting, occurs when blood reaches the arterial system without participating in gas exchange. The mixing of unoxygenated (shunted)

Table 23-1	Etiologies of Acute Respiratory Failure
Affected Area	**Disorders***

EXTRAPULMONARY

Brain	Drug overdose
	Central alveolar hypoventilation syndrome
	Brain trauma or lesion
	Postoperative anesthesia depression
Spinal cord	Guillain-Barré syndrome
	Poliomyelitis
	Amyotrophic lateral sclerosis
	Spinal cord trauma or lesion
Neuromuscular system	Myasthenia gravis
	Multiple sclerosis
	Neuromuscular-blocking antibiotics
	Organophosphate poisoning
	Muscular dystrophy
Thorax	Massive obesity
	Chest trauma
Pleura	Pleural effusion
	Pneumothorax
Upper airways	Sleep apnea
	Tracheal obstruction
	Epiglottitis

INTRAPULMONARY

Lower airways and alveoli	Chronic obstructive pulmonary disease (COPD)
	Asthma
	Bronchiolitis
	Cystic fibrosis
	Pneumonia
Pulmonary circulation	Pulmonary emboli
Alveolar-capillary membrane	Acute lung injury (ALI)
	Inhalation of toxic gases
	Near-drowning

*Not an inclusive list.

blood and oxygenated blood lowers the average level of oxygen present in the blood. Intrapulmonary shunting occurs when blood passes through a portion of a lung that is not ventilated. This may be the result of (1) alveolar collapse secondary to atelectasis or (2) alveolar flooding with pus, blood, or fluid.[6,7]

If allowed to progress, hypoxemia can result in a deficit of oxygen at the cellular level. As the tissue demands for oxygen continue and the supply diminishes, an oxygen supply/demand imbalance occurs and tissue hypoxia develops. Decreased oxygen to the cells contributes to impaired tissue perfusion and the development of lactic acidosis and multiple organ dysfunction syndrome.[8]

ASSESSMENT AND DIAGNOSIS

The patient with ARF may experience a variety of clinical manifestations, depending on the underlying cause and the extent of tissue hypoxia. The clinical manifestations commonly seen in the patient with ARF are usually related to the development of hypoxemia, hypercapnia, and acidosis (Table 23-2).[9] Because the clinical symptoms are so varied, they are not considered reliable in predicting the degree of hypoxemia or hypercapnia[8] or the severity of ARF.[3]

Diagnosing and following the course of respiratory failure is best accomplished by ABG analysis. ABG analysis confirms the level of $Paco_2$, Pao_2, and blood pH. ARF is generally accepted as being present when the Pao_2 is less than 60 mm Hg and/or the $Paco_2$ is greater than 45 mm Hg. In patients with chronically elevated $Paco_2$ levels, these criteria must be broadened to include a pH less than 7.35.[9]

A variety of additional tests are performed depending on the patient's underlying condition. These include bronchoscopy for airway surveillance or specimen retrieval, chest radiography, thoracic ultrasound, thoracic computed tomography, and selected lung function studies.[10]

MEDICAL MANAGEMENT

Medical management of the patient with ARF is aimed at treating the underlying cause, promoting adequate gas exchange, correcting acidosis, initiating nutrition support, and preventing complications. Medical interventions to promote gas exchange are aimed at improving oxygenation and ventilation.

Oxygenation. Actions to improve oxygenation include supplemental oxygen administration and the use of positive airway pressure. The purpose of oxygen therapy is to correct hypoxemia, and although the absolute level of hypoxemia varies in each patient, most treatment approaches aim to keep the arterial hemoglobin oxygen saturation greater than 90%.[9] The goal is to keep the tissues' needs satisfied but not produce hypercapnia or oxygen toxicity.[9] Supplemental oxygen administration is effective in treating hypoxemia related to alveolar hypoventilation and V/Q mismatching. When intrapulmonary shunting exists, supplemental oxygen alone is ineffective.[11] In this situation, positive pressure is necessary to open collapsed alveoli and facilitate their participation in gas exchange. To avoid intubation, positive pressure can be delivered noninvasively via a nasal or oronasal mask.[12] One recent study found that a full-face oronasal mask is better tolerated than a nasal mask.[13] For further information on noninvasive ventilation, see Chapter 24.

Ventilation. Interventions to improve ventilation include the use of noninvasive and invasive mechanical

Table 23-2	Clinical Manifestations of Acute Respiratory Failure

	Signs and Symptoms		
Organ System	**Hypoxemia**	**Hypercapnia**	**Acidosis**
Central nervous	Restlessness Agitation Irritability Confusion Personality changes Impaired judgment Memory loss Sleep disturbance Bizarre behavior Decreased level of consciousness	Headache Drowsiness Decreased level of consciousness Papilledema Blurred vision Confusion Seizures Sleep disturbances	Drowsiness Confusion Decreased level of consciousness
Cardiovascular	Tachycardia Bounding pulse Hypertension (systolic) Wide pulse pressure Dysrhythmias Palpitations Chest pain	Same as hypoxemia Flushing of the skin	Weak pulse Hypotension Dysrhythmias (bradycardia)
Pulmonary	Tachypnea Hyperventilation Dyspnea Shortness of breath Active accessory muscles (neck and shoulders) Active abdominal movement during respiration Ascites, edema, neck vein distention Intercostals' retractions, tracheal tugging, flaring nares	Same as hypoxemia	Same as hypoxemia
Renal	Decreased urinary output Polycythemia Hypertension Edema	Decreased urinary output Hypochloremia Edema Hypertension	Hypochloremic metabolic alkalosis
Gastrointestinal	Decreased bowel sounds Abdominal distention Anorexia Nausea Vomiting Constipation Gastrointestinal bleeding	Same as hypoxemia	Same as hypoxemia
Skin	Pallor Cyanosis Clammy Cool Plethora	Flushed Clammy	Sympathetic nervous system responses (cool, clammy, pale)

Modified from Vaughan P: *Crit Care Nurs* 1(6):46, 1981.

ventilation. Depending on the underlying cause and the severity of the ARF, the patient may be initially treated with noninvasive ventilation.[12] However, one study found that those patients with a pH of less than 7.25 at initial presentation had an increased likelihood of the need for invasive mechanical ventilation.[14] The selection of ventilatory mode and settings depends on the patient's underlying condition, severity of respiratory failure, and body size. Initially the patient is started on volume ventilation in the assist/control mode. In the patient with chronic hypercapnia, the settings should be adjusted to keep the arterial blood gas values within the parameters expected to be maintained by the patient after extubation.[15] For further information on mechanical ventilation see Chapter 24.

Pharmacology. Medications to facilitate dilation of the airways may also be of benefit in the treatment of the patient with ARF. Bronchodilators, such as beta$_2$- agonists and anticholinergic agents, aid in smooth muscle relaxation and are of particular benefit to patients with airflow limitations. Methylxanthines, such as aminophylline, are no longer recommended because of their negative side effects. Steroids also are often administered to decrease airway inflammation and enhance the effects of the beta$_2$-agonists. Mucolytics and expectorates are also no longer used since they have been found to be of no benefit in this patient population.[16]

Sedation is necessary in many patients to assist with maintaining adequate ventilation. It can be used to comfort the patient and decrease the work of breathing, particularly if the patient is fighting the ventilator. Analgesics should be administered for pain control.[17] In some patients, sedation does not decrease spontaneous respiratory efforts enough to allow adequate ventilation. Neuromuscular paralysis may be necessary to facilitate optimal ventilation. Paralysis also may be necessary to decrease oxygen consumption in the severely compromised patient.[18]

Acidosis. Acidosis may occur in the patient for a number of reasons. Hypoxemia causes impaired tissue perfusion, which leads to the production of lactic acid and the development of metabolic acidosis. Impaired ventilation leads to the accumulation of carbon dioxide and the development of respiratory acidosis. Once the patient is adequately oxygenated and ventilated, the acidosis should correct itself. The use of sodium bicarbonate to correct the acidosis has been shown to be of minimal benefit to the patient and thus is no longer recommended even in the presence of severe acidosis (pH<7.2).[19]

Nutrition Support. The initiation of nutrition support is of utmost importance in the management of the patient with ARF. The goals of nutrition support are to meet the overall nutritional needs of the patient while avoiding overfeeding, to prevent nutrition delivery–related complications, and to improve patient outcomes.[20] Failure to provide the patient with adequate nutrition support results in the development of malnutrition. Both malnutrition and overfeeding can interfere with the performance of the pulmonary system, further perpetuating ARF. Malnutrition decreases the patient's ventilatory drive and muscle strength, whereas overfeeding increases carbon dioxide production, which then increases the patient's ventilatory demand, resulting in respiratory muscle fatigue.[21]

The enteral route is the preferred method of nutrition administration. If the patient cannot tolerate enteral feedings or cannot receive enough nutrients enterally, he or she will be started on parenteral nutrition. Because the parenteral route is associated with a higher rate of complications, the goal is to switch to enteral feedings as soon as the patient can tolerate them.[20,21] Nutrition support should be initiated before the third day of mechanical ventilation for the well-nourished patient and within 24 hours for the malnourished patient.[20,21]

Complications. The patient with acute respiratory failure may experience a number of complications including ischemic-anoxic encephalophathy,[22] cardiac dysrhythmias,[23] venous thromboembolism,[24] and gastrointestinal bleeding.[25] Ischemic-anoxic encephalopathy results from hypoxemia, hypercapnia, and acidosis.[22] Dysrhythmias are precipitated by hypoxemia, acidosis, electrolyte imbalances, and the administration of β$_2$-agonists.[23] Maintaining oxygenation, normalizing electrolytes, and monitoring drug levels will facilitate the prevention and treatment of encephalopathy and dysrhythmias.[22,23] Venous thromboembolism is precipitated by venous stasis resulting from immobility and can be prevented through the use of graduated compression stockings and low-dose unfractionated heparin or low–molecular-weight heparin.[24] Gastrointestinal bleeding can be prevented through the use of histamine$_2$-antagonists, cytoprotective agents, or proton pump inhibitors.[25] In addition, the patient is at risk for the complications associated with an artificial airway, mechanical ventilation, enteral and parenteral nutrition, and peripheral arterial cannulation.

NURSING MANAGEMENT

Nursing management of the patient with acute respiratory failure incorporates a variety of nursing diagnoses (see the Nursing Diagnoses feature on Acute Respiratory Failure). Nursing care is directed by the specific etiology of the respiratory failure, although some common interventions are used. The nurse has a significant role in optimizing oxygenation and ventilation, providing comfort and emotional support, and maintaining surveillance for complications. Nursing interventions to optimize oxygenation and ventilation include positioning, preventing desaturation, and promoting secretion clearance.

Positioning. Positioning of the patient with ARF depends on the type of lung injury and the underlying cause of hypoxemia. For those patients with V/Q mismatching, positioning is used to facilitate better matching of ventilation with perfusion to optimize gas exchange.[26] Because gravity normally facilitates preferential ventilation and perfusion to the dependent areas of the lungs, the best gas exchange would take place in the dependent areas of the lungs.[11] Thus the goal of positioning is to place the least affected area of the patient's lung in the most dependent position. Patients with unilateral lung disease should be positioned with the healthy lung in a dependent position.[26,27] Patients with diffuse lung disease may benefit from being positioned with the right lung down,

---

NURSING DIAGNOSES — Acute Respiratory Failure

- Impaired Gas Exchange related to alveolar hypoventilation
- Impaired Gas Exchange related to ventilation/perfusion mismatching or intrapulmonary shunting
- Ineffective Breathing Pattern related to musculoskeletal fatigue or neuromuscular impairment
- Risk for Aspiration
- Imbalanced Nutrition: Less Than Body Requirements related to lack of exogenous nutrients or increased metabolic demand
- Risk for Infection
- Impaired Spontaneous Ventilation related to respiratory muscle fatigue or metabolic factors
- Acute Confusion related to sensory overload, sensory deprivation, and sleep pattern disturbance
- Anxiety related to threat to biologic, psychologic, and/or social integrity
- Disturbed Body Image related to functional dependence on life-sustaining technology
- Compromised Family Coping related to critically ill family member
- Deficient Knowledge: Discharge Regimen related to lack of previous exposure to information (see Patient Education special feature on Acute Respiratory Failure)

PATIENT EDUCATION — Acute Respiratory Failure

- Pathophysiology of disease
- Specific etiology
- Precipitating factor modification
- Importance of taking medications
- Breathing techniques (e.g., pursed-lip breathing, diaphragmatic breathing)
- Energy conservation techniques
- Measure to prevent pulmonary infections (e.g., proper nutrition, hand washing, immunization against *Streptococcus pneumoniae* and influenza viruses)
- Signs and symptoms of pulmonary infections (e.g., sputum color change, shortness of breath, fever)
- Cough enhancement techniques (e.g., cascade cough, huff cough, end-expiratory cough, augmented cough)

---

because it is larger and more vascular than the left lung.[27,28] For those patients with alveolar hypoventilation, the goal of positioning is to facilitate ventilation. These patients benefit from nonrecumbent positions such as sitting or a semierect position.[29] In addition, semirecumbency has been shown to decrease the risk of aspiration and inhibit the development of nosocomial pneumonia.[30] Frequent repositioning (at least every 2 hours) is beneficial in optimizing the patient's ventilatory pattern and V/Q matching.[31]

Preventing Desaturation. A number of activities can prevent desaturation from occurring. These include performing procedures only as needed, hyperoxygenating the patient before suctioning, providing adequate rest and recovery time between various procedures, and minimizing oxygen consumption. Interventions to minimize oxygen consumption include limiting the patient's physical activity, administering sedation to control anxiety, and providing measures to control fever.[29] The patient should be continuously monitored with a pulse oximeter to warn of signs of desaturation.

Promoting Secretion Clearance. Interventions to promote secretion clearance include providing adequate

systemic hydration, humidifying supplemental oxygen, coughing, and suctioning. Postural drainage and chest percussion and vibration have been found to be of little benefit in the critically ill patient[32,33] and thus are not discussed here.

To facilitate deep breathing, the patient's thorax should be maintained in alignment and the head of the bed elevated 30 to 45 degrees. This position best accommodates diaphragmatic descent and intercostal muscle action.

Once the patient is extubated, deep breathing and incentive spirometry should be started as soon as possible. Deep breathing involves having the patient take a deep breath and hold it for approximately 3 seconds or longer. Incentive spirometry involves having the patient take at least 10 deep, effective breaths per hour using an incentive spirometer. These actions help prevent atelectasis and reexpand any collapsed lung tissue. The chest should be auscultated during inflation to ensure that all dependent parts of the lung are well ventilated and to help the patient understand the depth of breath necessary for optimal effect. Coughing should be avoided unless secretions are present because it promotes collapse of the smaller airways.

Patient Education. Early in the patient's hospital stay, the patient and family should be taught about acute respiratory failure, its etiologies, and its treatment. As the patient moves toward discharge, teaching should focus on the interventions necessary for preventing the reoccurrence of the precipitating disorder (see the Patient Education feature on Acute Respiratory Failure). If the

EVIDENCE-BASED COLLABORATIVE PRACTICE

Smoking Cessation Guidelines

The following are the key recommendations of the updated guideline, *Treating Tobacco Use and Dependence*, based on the literature review and expert panel opinion:

1. Tobacco dependence is a chronic condition that often requires repeated intervention. However, effective treatments exist that can produce long-term or even permanent abstinence.
2. Because effective tobacco dependence treatments are available, every patient who uses tobacco should be offered at least one of these treatments:
   - Patients *willing* to try to quit tobacco use should be provided treatments identified as effective in this guideline.
   - Patients *unwilling* to try to quit tobacco use should be provided a brief intervention designed to increase their motivation to quit.
3. It is essential that clinicians and health care delivery systems (including administrators, insurers, and purchasers) institutionalize the consistent identification, documentation, and treatment of every tobacco user seen in a health care setting.
4. Brief tobacco dependence treatment is effective, and every patient who uses tobacco should be offered at least brief treatment.
5. There is a strong dose-response relation between the intensity of tobacco dependence counseling and its effectiveness. Treatments involving person-to-person contact (via individual, group, or proactive telephone counseling) are consistently effective, and their effectiveness increases with treatment intensity (e.g., minutes of contact).
6. Three types of counseling and behavioral therapies were found to be especially effective and should be used with all patients attempting tobacco cessation:
   - Provision of practical counseling (problem solving/ skills training)

   - Provision of social support as part of treatment (intratreatment social support)
   - Help in securing social support outside of treatment (extratreatment social support)
7. Numerous effective pharmacotherapies for smoking cessation now exist. Except in the presence of contraindications, these should be used with all patients attempting to quit smoking.
   - Five *first-line* pharmacotherapies were identified that reliably increase long-term smoking abstinence rates:
     - Bupropion SR
     - Nicotine gum
     - Nicotine inhaler
     - Nicotine nasal spray
     - Nicotine patch
   - Two *second-line* pharmacotherapies were identified as efficacious and may be considered by clinicians if first-line pharmacotherapies are not effective:
     - Clonidine
     - Nortriptyline
   - Over-the-counter nicotine patches are effective relative to placebo, and their use should be encouraged.
8. Tobacco dependence treatments are both clinically effective and cost-effective relative to other medical and disease prevention interventions. As such, insurers and purchasers should ensure that the following occurs:
   - All insurance plans include as a reimbursed benefit the counseling and pharmacotherapeutic treatments identified as effective in this guideline
   - Clinicians are reimbursed for providing tobacco dependence treatment just as they are reimbursed for treating other chronic conditions

From Fiore MC, Bailey WC, Cohen SJ, et al: *Treating Tobacco Use and Dependence* (Clinical Practice Guideline), Rockville, MD, June 2000, U.S. Department of Health and Human Services, Public Health Service.

---

patient smokes, he or she should be encouraged to stop smoking and be referred to a smoking cessation program (see the Evidence-Based Collaborative Practice feature on Smoking Cessation Guidelines). In addition, the importance of participating in a pulmonary rehabilitation program should be stressed. Additional information for the patient can be found at the American Lung Association website (www.lungusa.org).

Collaborative management of the patient with acute respiratory failure is outlined in Box 23-1.

ACUTE LUNG INJURY

DESCRIPTION

Acute lung injury (ALI) is a systemic process that is considered to be the pulmonary manifestation of multiple organ dysfunction syndrome.[34] It is characterized by noncardiac pulmonary edema and disruption of the alveolar-capillary membrane as a result of injury to either the pulmonary vasculature or the airways.[35]

Box 23-1

COLLABORATIVE MANAGEMENT

ACUTE RESPIRATORY FAILURE
- Identify and treat underlying cause
- Administer oxygen therapy
- Intubate patient
- Initiate mechanical ventilation
- Administer medications
  - Bronchodilators
  - Steroids
  - Sedatives
  - Analgesics
- Position patient to optimize ventilation/perfusion matching
- Suction as needed
- Provide adequate rest and recovery time between various procedures
- Correct acidosis
- Initiate nutritional support
- Maintain surveillance for complications
  - Encephalopathy
  - Cardiac dysrhythmias
  - Venous thromboembolism
  - Gastrointestinal bleeding
- Provide comfort and emotional support

Box 23-2

RISK FACTORS FOR ALI

DIRECT INJURY
Aspiration
Near-drowning
Toxic inhalation
Pulmonary contusion
Pneumonia
Oxygen toxicity
Transthoracic radiation

INDIRECT INJURY
Sepsis
Nonthoracic trauma
Hypertransfusion
Cardiopulmonary bypass
Severe pancreatitis
Embolism—air, fat, amniotic fluid
Disseminated intravascular coagulation (DIC)
Shock states

ARDS, Acute respiratory distress syndrome.

Many different diagnostic criteria have been used to identify ALI, which has led to confusion, particularly among researchers. In an attempt to standardize the identification of this disorder, the American-European Consensus Committee on ARDS recommended the following criteria be used to diagnose ALI:
- Acute in onset
- Ratio of partial pressure of oxygen (PaO_2) to fraction of inspired oxygen (FiO_2) less than or equal to 300 mm Hg (regardless of positive end-expiratory pressure [PEEP] level)
- Bilateral infiltrates on chest radiography
- Pulmonary artery occlusion pressure (PAOP) less than or equal to 18 mm Hg or no clinical evidence of left atrial hypertension[36,37]

The severest form of ALI is called acute (formerly called "adult") respiratory distress syndrome (ARDS).[36] ARDS is identified by the same diagnostic criteria as ALI except that the ratio of PaO_2 to FiO_2 is less than or equal to 200 mm Hg. As the etiology, pathophysiology, and treatment of ALI is the same as for ARDS, the discussion will use the broader term of ALI.[37]

ETIOLOGY

A wide variety of clinical conditions is associated with the development of ALI. These are categorized as *direct* or *indirect*, depending on the primary site of injury (Box 23-2).[35,38] Direct injuries are those in which the lung epithelium sustains a direct insult. Indirect injuries are those in which the insult occurs elsewhere in the body and mediators are transmitted via the blood stream to the lungs. Sepsis, aspiration of gastric contents, diffuse pneumonia, and trauma were found to be major risk factors for the development of ALI.[37]

The mortality rate for ALI is estimated to be 30% to 40%.[37]

PATHOPHYSIOLOGY

The progression of ALI can be described in three phases: exudative, fibroproliferative, and resolution. ALI is initiated with stimulation of the inflammatory-immune system as a result of a direct or indirect injury (Fig. 23-1). Inflammatory mediators are released from the site of injury, resulting in the activation and accumulation of the neutrophils, macrophages, and platelets in the pulmonary capillaries. These cellular mediators initiate the release of humoral mediators that cause damage to the alveolar-capillary membrane.[38]

Exudative Phase. Within the first 72 hours after the initial insult, the exudative phase or acute phase ensues. Once released, the mediators cause injury to the pulmonary capillaries, resulting in increased capillary membrane permeability leading to the leakage of fluid filled with protein, blood cells, fibrin, and activated cellular and humoral mediators into the pulmonary interstitium. Damage to the pulmonary capillaries also causes the development of microthrombi and elevation of pulmonary

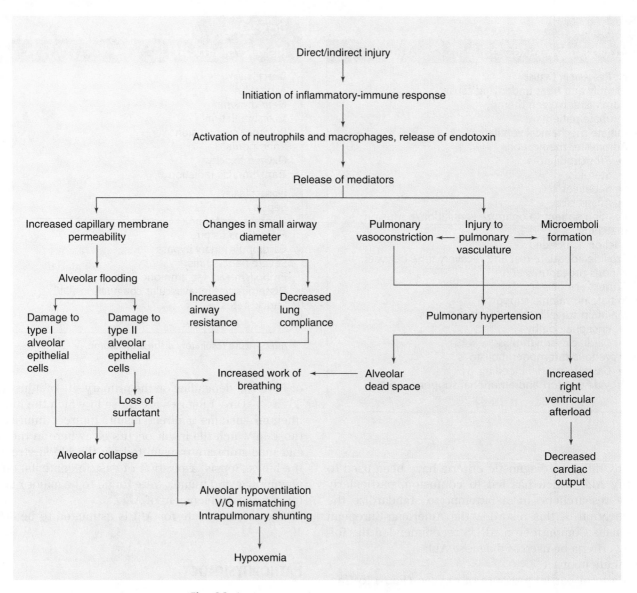

Fig. 23-1 Pathophysiology of acute lung injury.

artery pressures. As fluid enters the pulmonary interstitium, the lymphatics are overwhelmed and unable to drain all the accumulating fluid, resulting in the development of interstitial edema. Fluid is then forced from the interstitial space into the alveoli, resulting in alveolar edema. Pulmonary interstitial edema also causes compression of the alveoli and small airways. Alveolar edema causes swelling of the type I alveolar epithelial cells and flooding of the alveoli. Protein and fibrin in the edema fluid precipitate the formation of hyaline membranes over the alveoli. Eventually, the type II alveolar epithelial cells are also damaged, leading to impaired surfactant production. Injury to the alveolar epithelial cells and the loss of surfactant lead to further alveolar collapse.[38,39]

Hypoxemia occurs as a result of intrapulmonary shunting and V/Q mismatching secondary to compression, col-

lapse, and flooding of the alveoli and small airways. Increased work of breathing occurs as a result of increased airway resistance, decreased functional residual capacity (FRC), and decreased lung compliance secondary to atelectasis and compression of the small airways. Hypoxemia and the increased work of breathing lead to patient fatigue and the development of alveolar hypoventilation. Pulmonary hypertension occurs as a result of damage to the pulmonary capillaries, microthrombi, and hypoxic vasoconstriction leading to the development of increased alveolar dead space and right ventricular afterload. Hypoxemia worsens as a result of alveolar hypoventilation and increased alveolar dead space. Right ventricular afterload increases and leads to right ventricular dysfunction and a decrease in cardiac output.[38]

Fibroproliferative Phase. This phase begins as disordered healing starts in the lungs. Cellular granulation

Table 23-3	Physiology and Associated Physical Examination of Patient With ALI	
Phase	**Physiology**	**Physical Examination**
Exudative phase	Parenchymal surface hemorrhage Interstitial or alveolar edema Compression of terminal bronchioles Destruction of type 1 alveolar cells	Restless, apprehensive, tachypneic Respiratory alkalosis Pao_2 normal CXR: normal Chest examination: moderate use of accessory muscles, lungs clear Pulmonary artery pressures: elevated Pulmonary artery occlusion pressure: normal or low
Fibroproliferative phase	Destruction of type 2 alveolar cells Gas exchange compromised Increased peak inspiratory pressure Decreased compliance (static and dynamic) Refractory hypoxemia: • Intraalveolar atelectasis • Increased shunt fraction • Decreased diffusion Decreased functional residual capacity Interstitial fibrosis Increased dead space ventilation	Pulmonary artery pressures: elevated Increased workload on right ventricle Increase use of accessory muscles Fine crackles or rales Increasing agitation related to hypoxia CXR: interstitial or alveolar infiltrates; elevated diaphragm Hyperventilation; hypercarbia Decreased Svo_2 Widening alveolar-arterial gradient Increased work of breathing Worsening hypercarbia and hypoxemia Lactic acidosis (related to aerobic metabolism) Alteration in perfusion: • Increased heart rate • Decreased blood pressure • Change in skin temperature and color • Decreased capillary filling End-organ dysfunction: • Brain: change in mentation, agitation, hallucinations • Heart: decreased cardiac output→ angina, CHF, papillary muscle dysfunction, dysrhythmias, MI • Renal: decreased urinary or GFR • Skin: mottled, ischemic • Liver: elevated SGOT, bilirubin, alkaline phosphatase, PT/PTT; decreased albumin

Modified from Phillips JK: *Crit Care Clin North Am* 11:233, 1999.
ALI, Acute lung injury; *Pao₂,* arterial oxygen pressure; *CXR,* chest radiograph; *Svo₂,* venous oxygen saturation; *HF,* heart failure; *MI,* myocardial infarction; *GFR,* glomerular filtration rate; *SGOT,* serum glutamate oxaloacetate transaminase; *PT,* prothrombin time; *PTT,* partial thromboplastin time.

and collagen deposition occur within the alveolar-capillary membrane. The alveoli become enlarged and irregularly shaped (fibrotic) and the pulmonary capillaries become scarred and obliterated. This leads to further stiffening of the lungs, increasing pulmonary hypertension, and continued hypoxemia.[38,39]

Resolution Phase. Recovery occurs over several weeks as structural and vascular remodeling take place to reestablish the alveolar-capillary membrane. The hyaline membranes are cleared and intraalveolar fluid is transported out of the alveolus into the interstitium. The type II alveolar epithelial cells multiply, some of which differentiate to type I alveolar epithelial cells, facilitating the restoration of the alveolus. Alveolar macrophages remove cellular debris.[38,39]

ASSESSMENT AND DIAGNOSIS

Initially the patient with ALI may be seen with a variety of clinical manifestations, depending on the precipitating event. As the disorder progresses, the patient's signs and symptoms can be associated with the phase of ALI that he or she is experiencing (Table 23-3). During the exudative phase, the patient presents with tachypnea, restlessness, apprehension, and moderate increase in accessory muscle use. During the fibroproliferative phase, the patient's signs and symptoms progress to agitation, dyspnea, fatigue, excessive accessory muscle use, and fine crackles as respiratory failure develops.[40,41]

Arterial blood gas analysis reveals a low Pao_2, despite increases in supplemental oxygen administration (refractory hypoxemia).[40] Initially the $Paco_2$ is low as a result of hyperventilation, but eventually the $Paco_2$ increases as the patient fatigues. The pH is high initially but decreases as respiratory acidosis develops.[40,41]

Initially the chest x-ray film may be normal, because changes in the lungs do not become evident for up to 24 hours. As the pulmonary edema becomes apparent, diffuse, patchy interstitial and alveolar infiltrates appear. This progresses to multifocal consolidation of the lungs, which appears as a "whiteout" on the chest x-ray film.[40]

MEDICAL MANAGEMENT

Medical management of the patient with ALI involves a multifaceted approach. This strategy includes treating the underlying cause, promoting gas exchange, supporting tissue oxygenation, and preventing complications. Given the severity of hypoxemia, the patient is intubated and mechanically ventilated to facilitate adequate gas exchange.[42]

Ventilation. Traditionally the patient with ALI was ventilated with a mode of volume ventilation, such as assist/control ventilation (A/CV) or synchronized intermittent mandatory ventilation (SIMV), with tidal volumes adjusted to deliver 10 to 15 ml/kg. Current research now indicates that this approach may have actually led to further lung injury. It is now known that repeated opening and closing of the alveoli cause injury to the lung units (atelectrauma), resulting in inhibited surfactant production, and increased inflammation (biotrauma), resulting in the release of mediators and an increase in pulmonary capillary membrane permeability. In addition, excessive pressure in the alveoli (barotrauma) or excessive volume in the alveoli (volutrauma) leads to excessive alveolar wall stress and damage to the alveolar-capillary membrane, resulting in air escaping into the surrounding spaces.[42] Thus several different approaches have been developed to facilitate the mechanical ventilation of the patient with ALI.

Low Tidal Volume. Low tidal volume ventilation uses smaller tidal volumes (6 to 10 ml/kg) to ventilate the patient, in an attempt to limit the effects of barotrauma and volutrauma. The goal is to provide the maximum tidal volume possible while maintaining an airway pressure less than 30 cm H_2O. To allow for adequate carbon dioxide elimination, the respiratory rate is increased to 20 to 30 breaths/min.[42,43]

Permissive Hypercapnia. Permissive hypercapnia uses low tidal volume ventilation in conjunction with normal respiratory rates, in an attempt to limit the effects of atelectrauma and biotrauma. Normally, to maintain normocapnia the patient's respiratory rate would have to be increased to compensate for the small tidal volume. In ALI though, increasing the respiratory rate can lead to worsening alveolar damage. Thus the patient's carbon dioxide level is allowed to rise, and the patient becomes hypercapnic. As a general rule, the patient's $Paco_2$ should not rise faster than 10 mm Hg per hour and overall should not exceed 80 to 100 mg Hg. Because of the negative cardiopulmonary effects of severe acidosis, the arterial pH is generally maintained at 7.20 or greater. To maintain the pH, the patient is given intravenous sodium bicarbonate or the respiratory rate and/or tidal volume are increased. Permissive hypercapnia is contraindicated in patients with increased intracranial pressure, pulmonary hypertension, seizures, and cardiac failure.[44]

Pressure Control Ventilation. In pressure control ventilation (PCV) mode, each breath is delivered or augmented with a preset amount of inspiratory pressure as opposed to tidal volume, which is used in volume ventilation. Thus the actual tidal volume the patient receives varies from breath to breath. PCV is used to limit and control the amount of pressure in the lungs and decrease the incidence of volutrauma. The goal is to keep the patient's plateau pressure (end-inspiratory static pressure) lower than 30 cm H_2O. A known problem with this mode of ventilation is that as the patient's lungs get stiffer, it becomes harder and harder to maintain an adequate tidal volume and severe hypercapnia can occur.[42,43]

Inverse Ratio Ventilation. Another alternative ventilatory mode that is used in managing the patient with ALI is inverse ratio ventilation (IRV), either pressure-controlled or volume-controlled. IRV prolongs the inspiratory (I) time and shortens the expiratory (E) time, thus reversing the normal I:E ratio. The goal of IRV is to maintain a more constant mean airway pressure throughout the ventilatory cycle, which helps keep alveoli open and participating in gas exchange. It also increases FRC and decreases the work of breathing. In addition, as the breath is delivered over a longer period of time, the peak inspiratory pressure in the lungs is decreased. A major disadvantage to IRV is the development of auto-positive end-expiratory pressure (PEEP). As the expiratory phase of ventilation is shortened, air can become trapped in the lower airways, creating unintentional PEEP (also known as auto-PEEP), which can cause hemodynamic compromise and worsening gas exchange. Patients on IRV usually require heavy sedation with neuromuscular blockade to prevent them from fighting the ventilator.[42,43]

Oxygen Therapy. Oxygen is administered at the lowest level possible to support tissue oxygenation. Continued exposure to high levels of oxygen can lead to oxygen toxicity, which perpetuates the entire process. The goal of oxygen therapy is to maintain an arterial hemoglobin oxygen saturation of 90% or greater using the lowest level of oxygen—preferably less than 0.50.[35]

Positive End-Expiratory Pressure (PEEP). Because the hypoxemia that develops with ALI is often refractory or unresponsive to oxygen therapy, it is necessary to facilitate oxygenation with PEEP. The purpose of using PEEP in the patient with ALI is to improve oxygenation while reducing FiO_2 to less toxic levels. PEEP has several positive effects on the lungs including opening collapsed alveoli, stabilizing flooded alveoli, and increasing FRC. Thus PEEP decreases intrapulmonary shunting and increases compliance. PEEP also has several negative effects including (1) decreasing cardiac output (CO) as a result of decreasing venous return secondary to increased intrathoracic pressure and (2) barotrauma, as a result of gas escaping into the surrounding spaces secondary to alveolar rupture. The amount of PEEP a patient requires is determined by evaluating both arterial hemoglobin oxygen saturation and cardiac output. In most cases a PEEP of 10 to 15 cm H_2O is adequate. If PEEP is too high, it can result in overdistention of the alveoli, which can impede pulmonary capillary blood flow, decrease surfactant production, and worsen intrapulmonary shunting. If PEEP is too low, it allows the alveoli to collapse during expiration, which can result in more damage to alveoli.[42]

Tissue Perfusion. Adequate tissue perfusion depends on an adequate supply of oxygen being transported to the tissues. An adequate CO and hemoglobin level is critical to oxygen transport. CO depends on heart rate, preload, afterload, and contractility. A variety of fluids and medications are used to manipulate this parameter. Newer approaches to fluid management include maintaining a very low intravascular volume (pulmonary artery occlusion pressure of 5 to 8 mm Hg) with fluid restriction and diuretics, while supporting the CO with vasoactive and inotropic medications. The goal is to decrease the amount of fluid leakage into the lungs.[45]

Investigational Therapies. A number of investigational studies of other therapies for the treatment of ALI are underway. These therapies include drugs to block or neutralize the various mediators released as part of the inflammatory-immune response and methods to limit the damage to the lungs. A number of different kinds of drugs are being tested including activated protein C, antiadhesion molecules, atrial natriuretic peptide (ANP), corticosteroids, cytokine antagonists, ketoconazole, lisofylline, N-acetylcysteine, and prostaglandin E_1.[46] Methods to limit damage to the lungs include extracorporeal/intracorporeal gas exchange, surfactant therapy, partial liquid ventilation, and extracorporeal carbon dioxide removal. The use of inhaled nitric oxide is also being investigated to help reverse pulmonary vasoconstriction and improve perfusion of ventilated regions of the lungs.

Surfactant Therapy. One of the newer drugs currently being tested in adults with severe ALI is exogenous surfactant. The two main types of exogenous surfactant available are natural, which includes bovine, porcine, or human amniotic fluid preparations, and synthetic. The advantage of natural surfactant is that it has surfactant-associated proteins and thus may have better spreading and lung defense properties. The disadvantage is that the foreign proteins in natural surfactants can be antigenic. Currently, dosage recommendations are 3 to 15 mg/kg, although dosages up to 300 mg/kg are often needed to overcome the various surfactant inhibitors present in ALI. Three routes of administration have been tried: direct tracheal instillation through an endotracheal tube, bronchial instillation via a bronchoscope, and aerosolized delivery. Direct instillation through an endotracheal tube ensures delivery of the entire dose to the trachea but requires large volumes to be effective. In addition, it is difficult to achieve reasonable alveolar deposition and spreading from tracheal instillation. Bronchial instillation through a bronchoscope delivers large doses to distal regions of the lung but requires a complex procedure and long treatment time and thus may not be well tolerated by the patient. Aerosolized delivery of surfactant has the advantage of being administered continuously and directly into the alveoli, but the slower delivery of a loading dose may delay effectiveness. In addition, aerosols delivered through a ventilator circuit can be inefficient, with as little as 5% of the dose making its way through the endotracheal tube to the lung parenchyma. Though proven to be extremely beneficial in neonates, exogenous surfactant has not yet been proven to be of any benefit to adult patients.[47]

Inhaled Nitric Oxide. Nitric oxide is a potent bronchodilator and selective pulmonary vasodilator that has been used in the treatment of ALI and other disorders resulting in pulmonary hypertension. When inhaled, nitric oxide is distributed to the well-ventilated regions of the lungs, resulting in vasodilation and increased blood flow to these areas. This leads to improved matching of ventilation to perfusion and enhanced oxygenation. Though optimal dosing guidelines for nitric oxide have not yet been established, dosage ranges of 2 to 20 parts per million (ppm) have been reported to be effective. Several different types of delivery systems have been developed to facilitate the precise delivery of the drug via the ventilator. Toxic effects include the production of nitric dioxide, which can cause pulmonary parenchymal damage, and methemoglobinemia, which can interfere with the delivery of oxygen to the cells. Adverse effects include platelet inhibition, increased left ventricular filling pressure caused by increased right ventricular stroke volume, and rebound hypoxemia and pulmonary hypertension upon discontinuing administration of the gas.[48]

Partial Liquid Ventilation. Partial liquid ventilation involves the instillation of perfluorocarbon into the lungs via an endotracheal tube. Perfluorocarbon is a liquid that has a low surface tension and a high solubility for oxygen and carbon dioxide. Once instilled, the liquid flows down into the dependent regions of the lungs, where it facilitates the patency of functioning alveoli and helps open collapsed alveoli. The low surface tension of perfluorocarbon decreases alveolar surface tension, which increases alveolar compliance and, in turn, decreases airway pressures. The high solubility of the liquid enhances gas exchange through the liquid. Partial liquid ventilation is accomplished by instilling a volume of perfluorocarbon equal to the patient's functional residual capacity (approximately 30 ml/kg) into the patient's lungs and then instituting conventional gas ventilation.[49]

Extracorporeal/Intracorporeal Gas Exchange. Extracorporeal and intracorporeal gas exchanges are last-resort techniques currently being used in the treatment of severe ALI when conventional therapy has failed. These methods allow the lungs to rest by facilitating the removal of carbon dioxide and providing oxygen external to the lungs via an "artificial lung," or membrane/fiber oxygenator. Extracorporeal membrane oxygenation (ECMO), extracorporeal carbon dioxide removal (ECCO$_2$R), and intravascular oxygenation (IVOX) are three different techniques that currently employ this type of technology. ECMO is similar to cardiopulmonary bypass in that blood is removed from the body and pumped through a membrane oxygenator, where CO$_2$ is removed and O$_2$ is added, and then returned to the body. ECCO$_2$R is a variation of ECMO with the primary focus of removal of CO$_2$. IVOX facilitates oxygenation and ventilation using a fiber oxygenator that is implanted in the inferior vena cava. All of these techniques pose serious bleeding problems to the patient, and none of them has been shown to improve patient outcome.[50]

NURSING MANAGEMENT

Nursing management of the patient with ALI incorporates a variety of nursing diagnoses (see the Nursing Diagnoses feature on Acute Lung Injury). Nursing interventions include optimizing oxygenation and ventilation, providing comfort and emotional support, and maintaining surveillance for complications.

Optimizing Oxygenation and Ventilation. Nursing interventions to optimize oxygenation and ventilation include positioning, preventing desaturation, and promoting secretion clearance. For further discussion on these interventions see "Nursing Management" of acute respiratory failure earlier in this chapter. One additional nursing intervention that can be used to improve the oxygenation and ventilation of the patient with ALI is prone positioning.

Prone Positioning. A number of studies have shown that prone positioning the patient with ALI results in an improvement in oxygenation. Although a number of theories propose how prone positioning improves oxygenation, the discovery that with ALI there is greater damage to the dependent areas of the lungs probably provides the best explanation. It was originally thought that ALI was a diffuse homogenous disease that affected all areas of the lungs equally. It is now known that the dependent lung areas are more heavily damaged than the nondependent lung areas. Turning the patient prone improves perfusion to less damaged parts of lungs and im-

proves V/Q matching and decreases intrapulmonary shunting. Prone positioning appears to be more effective when initiated during the early phases of ALI.[51] For more information on prone positioning see Chapter 24.

Collaborative management of the patient with ALI is outlined in Box 23-3.

PNEUMONIA

DESCRIPTION

Pneumonia is an acute inflammation of the lung parenchyma that is caused by an infectious agent that can lead to alveolar consolidation. Pneumonia can be classified as community-acquired (CAP) or hospital-acquired (HAP). Community-acquired pneumonia is acquired outside of the hospital.[52] Severe CAP requires admission to the intensive care unit and accounts for about 10% of all patients with pneumonia. The mortality for this patient group is in excess of 50%.[53] Hospital-acquired pneumonia is acquired while in the hospital for at least 48 hours.[54] Ventilator-associated pneumonia (VAP) is a subgrouping of HAP that refers to development of pneumonia after the insertion of an artificial airway. VAP represents 80% of all HAP cases.[54]

ETIOLOGY

The spectra of etiologic pathogens of pneumonia vary with the type of pneumonia as do the risk factors for the disease.

NURSING DIAGNOSES | Acute Lung Injury

- Impaired Gas Exchange related to ventilation/perfusion mismatching or intrapulmonary shunting
- Decreased Cardiac Output related to alterations in preload
- Imbalanced Nutrition: Less Than Body Requirements related to lack of exogenous nutrients or increased metabolic demand
- Risk for Aspiration
- Risk for Infection
- Anxiety related to threat to biologic, psychologic, and/or social integrity
- Disturbed Body Image related to functional dependence on life-sustaining technology
- Compromised Family Coping related to critically ill family member

---

Box 23-3

COLLABORATIVE MANAGEMENT

ACUTE LUNG INJURY
- Administer oxygen therapy
- Intubate patient
- Initiate mechanical ventilation
  - Permissive hypercapnia
  - Pressure control ventilation
  - Inverse ratio ventilation
- Use PEEP
- Administer medications
  - Bronchodilators
  - Sedatives
  - Analgesics
  - Neuromuscular blocking agents
- Maximize cardiac output
  - Preload
  - Afterload
  - Contractility
- Prone patient
- Suction as needed
- Provide adequate rest and recovery time between various procedures
- Initiate nutritional support
- Maintain surveillance for complications
  - Encephalopathy
  - Cardiac dysrhythmias
  - Venous thromboembolism
  - Gastrointestinal bleeding
  - Atelectrauma
  - Biotrauma
  - Volutrauma
  - Barotrauma
  - Oxygen toxicity
- Provide comfort and emotional support

Box 23-4

SEVERE ACUTE RESPIRATORY SYNDROME

Severe acute respiratory syndrome (SARS) is a form of serious community-acquired pneumonia caused by the SARS-associated coronavirus (SARS-CoV). It was first reported in February 2003, and over the following months spread to more than two dozen countries before it was contained.

The virus is transmitted by respiratory droplets.

The onset of symptoms usually occurs within 10 days of either (1) travel to an area with documented or suspected community transmission of SARS; or (2) close contact with either a person with a respiratory illness who traveled to a SARS area or a known suspect SARS case.

The incubation period for SARS is typically 2 to 7 days, although in some cases it may be as long as 14 days. The patient may first be seen with a wide spectrum of respiratory symptoms, anywhere from mild to severe. The illness usually begins with a high fever (temperature greater than 100.4° F [>38.0° C]) which may be accompanied with chills, headache, a general feeling of discomfort, and body aches. Respiratory symptoms may include a dry, nonproductive cough, shortness of breath, difficulty breathing, and hypoxemia.

Evidence of pneumonia (focal, unilateral area of consolidation) on chest x-ray film may also be present. Laboratory findings include low white blood cell and platelet counts, raised lactate dehydrogenase, and slightly raised creatinine kinase and C-reactive protein levels.

Patients suspected to be infected with the SARS virus should be placed immediately in negative pressure isolation. All health care personnel should wear an N-95 respirator mask and implement full barrier precautions when entering the patient's room. Antibiotics have not proven to be effective. Treatment of SARS is largely supportive with antipyretics, supplemental oxygen, and ventilatory support as needed.

Data from Manocha S, Walley KR, Russell JA: Severe acute respiratory syndrome (SARS): a critical care perspective, *Crit Care Med* 31:2684, 2003; and Peiris JS et al: The severe acute respiratory syndrome, *N Engl J Med* 349:2431, 2003.

Severe CAP. Pathogens that can cause severe CAP include *Streptococcus pneumoniae*, *Legionella* species, *Haemophilus influenzae*, *Staphylococcus aureus*, *Mycoplasma pneumoniae*, respiratory viruses, *Chlamydia pneumoniae*, and *Pseudomonas aeruginosa*.[55] A number of factors increase the risk for developing CAP including alcoholism, chronic obstructive pulmonary disease (COPD), and comorbid conditions such as diabetes, malignancy, and coronary artery disease.[52] Impaired swallowing and altered mental status also contribute to the development of CAP, because they result in an increased exposure to the various pathogens due to chronic aspiration of oropharyngeal secretions.[52] Severe acute respiratory syndrome is discussed in Box 23-4.

HAP. Pathogens that can cause HAP include *S. aureus*, *S. pneumoniae*, *P. aeruginosa*, *Acinetobacter baumannii*, *Klebsiella spp.*, *Proteus spp.*, *Serratia spp.*, fungi, and respiratory viruses.[54] Two of the pathogens most frequently associated with VAP are *S. aureus* and *P. aeruginosa*.[56] Risk factors for HAP can be categorized as host-related, treatment-related, and infection control–related (Box 23-5).[57]

PATHOPHYSIOLOGY

Development of acute pneumonia implies a defect in host defenses, a particularly virulent organism, or an overwhelming inoculation event. Bacterial invasion of the lower respiratory tract can occur by inhalation of aerosolized infectious particles, aspiration of organisms colonizing the oropharynx, migration of organisms from adjacent sites of colonization, direct inoculation of organisms into the lower airway, spread of infection to the lungs from adjacent structures, spread of infection to the lung through the blood, and reactivation of latent infection (usually in the setting of immunosuppression). The most common mechanism appears to be aspiration of oropharyngeal organisms.[58] Table 23-4 lists the precipitating conditions that can facilitate the development of pneumonia.

Fig. 23-2 depicts the pathophysiology of HAP. Colonization of the patient's oropharynx with infectious organisms is a major contributor to the development of HAP. Normally the oropharynx has a stable population of resident flora that may be anaerobic or aerobic. When stress occurs, such as with illness, surgery, or infection, pathogenic organisms replace normal resident flora. Previous antibiotic therapy also affects the resident flora population, making replacement by pathologic organisms more likely. The pathogens are then able to invade the sterile lower respiratory tract.[56]

Disruption of the gag and cough reflexes, altered consciousness, abnormal swallowing, and artificial airways all predispose the patient to aspiration and colonization of the lungs and subsequent infection. Histamine$_2$ agonists, antacids, and enteral feedings also contribute to this problem because they raise the pH of the stomach and promote bacterial overgrowth. The nasogastric tube then acts as a wick, facilitating the movement of bacteria from the stomach to the pharynx, where the bacteria can be aspirated.[52]

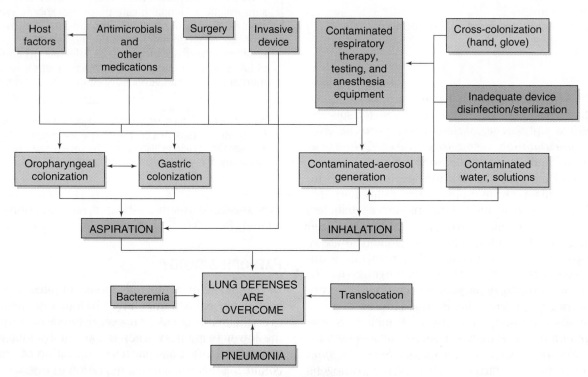

Fig. 23-2 Pathophysiology of pneumonia. (From Tablan OC et al: *Am J Infect Control* 22:247, 1994.)

Table 23-4	Precipitating Conditions of Pneumonia
Condition	**Etiologies**
Depressed epiglottal and cough reflexes	Unconsciousness, neurologic disease, endotracheal or tracheal tubes, anesthesia, aging
Decreased cilia activity	Smoke inhalation, smoking history, oxygen toxicity, hypoventilation, intubation, viral infections, aging, COPD
Increased secretion	COPD, viral infections, bronchiectasis, general anesthesia, endotracheal intubation, smoking
Atelectasis	Trauma, foreign body obstruction, tumor, splinting, shallow ventilations, general anesthesia
Decreased lymphatic flow	Heart failure, tumor
Fluid in alveoli	Heart failure, aspiration, trauma
Abnormal phagocytosis and humoral activity	Neutropenia, immunocompetent disorders, patients receiving chemotherapy
Impaired alveolar macrophages	Hypoxemia, metabolic acidosis, cigarette smoking history, hypoxia, alcohol use, viral infections, aging

COPD, Chronic obstructive pulmonary disease.

Infection results in pulmonary inflammation with or without significant exudates. Increased capillary permeability occurs, leading to increased interstitial and alveolar fluid. V/Q mismatching and intrapulmonary shunting occurs, resulting in hypoxemia as lung consolidation progresses. Untreated pneumonia can result in ARF and initiation of the inflammatory-immune response. In addition, the patient may develop a pleural effusion. This is the result of the vascular response to inflammation, whereby capillary permeability is increased and fluid from the pulmonary capillaries diffuses into the pleural space.[52,58]

Prevention of VAP is discussed under the mechanical ventilation section of Chapter 24.

ASSESSMENT AND DIAGNOSIS

The clinical manifestations of pneumonia will vary with the offending pathogen. The patient may first be seen with a variety of signs and symptoms including dyspnea, fever, and cough (productive or nonproductive).[59] Coarse crackles on auscultation and dullness to percussion may also be present.[59]

Chest radiography is used to evaluate the patient with suspected pneumonia. The diagnosis is established by the presence of a new pulmonary infiltrate. The radiographic pattern of the infiltrates will vary with the organism.[59] A sputum Gram's stain and culture are done to facilitate the identification of the infectious pathogen. In 50% of cases, though, a causative agent is not identified.[52] A diagnostic bronchoscopy may be needed, particularly if the diagnosis is unclear or current therapy is not working.[53] In addition, a complete blood count with differential, chemistry panel, blood cultures, and arterial blood gases are obtained.[55]

MEDICAL MANAGEMENT

Medical management of the patient with pneumonia should include antibiotic therapy, oxygen therapy for hypoxemia, mechanical ventilation if acute respiratory failure develops, fluid management for hydration, nutritional support, and treatment of associated medical problems and complications. For patients having difficulty mobilizing secretions, a therapeutic bronchoscopy may be necessary.[53,54]

Antibiotic Therapy. Although bacteria-specific antibiotic therapy is the goal, this may not always be possible because of difficulties in identifying the organism and the seriousness of the patient's condition. The time involved obtaining cultures should be balanced against the need to begin some treatment based on patient condition. Empiric therapy has become a generally acceptable approach. In this approach, choice of antibiotic treatment is based on the most likely etiologic organism while avoiding toxicity, superinfection, and unnecessary cost. If available, Gram's stain results should be used to guide choices of antibiotics. Antibiotics should be chosen that offer broad coverage of the usual pathogens in the hospital or community. Failure to respond to such therapy may indicate that the chosen antibiotic regimen does not appropriately cover all of the etiologic pathogens or that a new source of infection has developed.[54,55]

Independent Lung Ventilation. In patients with unilateral pneumonia or severely asymmetric pneumonia, this alternative mode of mechanical ventilation may be necessary to facilitate oxygenation. As the alveoli in the affected lung become flooded with pus, the lung becomes less compliant and difficult to ventilate. This results in a shifting of ventilation to the good lung without

NURSING DIAGNOSES Pneumonia

- Ineffective Airway Clearance related to excessive secretions or abnormal viscosity of mucus
- Impaired Gas Exchange related to ventilation/perfusion mismatching or intrapulmonary shunting
- Imbalanced Nutrition: Less Than Body Requirements related to lack of exogenous nutrients or increased metabolic demand
- Risk for Aspiration
- Risk for Infection
- Anxiety related to threat to biologic, psychologic, and/or social integrity
- Powerlessness related to lack of control over current situation or disease progression
- Compromised Family Coping related to critically ill family member

Box 23-6

COLLABORATIVE MANAGEMENT

PNEUMONIA
- Administer oxygen therapy
- Initiate mechanical ventilation as required
- Administer medications
  - Antibiotics
  - Bronchodilators
- Position patient to optimize ventilation/perfusion matching
- Suction as needed
- Provide adequate rest and recovery time between various procedures
- Maintain surveillance for complications
  - Acute respiratory failure
- Provide comfort and emotional support

a concomitant shift in perfusion and thus an increase in V/Q mismatching. Independent lung ventilation (ILV) allows each lung to be ventilated separately, thus controlling the amount of flow, volume, and pressure each lung receives. A double-lumen endotracheal tube is inserted, and each lumen is usually attached to a separate mechanical ventilator. The ventilator settings are then customized to the needs of each lung to facilitate optimal oxygenation and ventilation.[60]

NURSING MANAGEMENT

Nursing management of the patient with pneumonia incorporates a variety of nursing diagnoses (see the Nursing Diagnoses feature on Pneumonia). Nursing interventions include optimizing oxygenation and ventilation, preventing the spread of infection, providing comfort and emotional support, and maintaining surveillance for complications. In addition, the patient's response to the antibiotic therapy should be monitored for adverse effects.

Optimizing Oxygenation and Ventilation. Nursing interventions to optimize oxygenation and ventilation include positioning, preventing desaturation, and promoting secretion clearance. For further discussion on these interventions see "Nursing Management" of acute respiratory failure earlier in this chapter.

Preventing the Spread of Infection. Prevention should be directed at eradicating pathogens from the environment and interrupting the spread of organisms

from person to person. Significant progress has been made in removing contaminants from the patient environment through proper disinfection of respiratory equipment and increased use of disposable supplies. Other possible environmental sources of pathogens include suctioning equipment and indwelling lines. These invasive tools must be given proper aseptic care.[56]

Proper hand hygiene is the single most important measure available to prevent the spread of bacteria from person to person (see the Evidence-Based Collaborative Practice feature on Hand Hygiene Guidelines). In addition, meticulous oral care, including suctioning of the secretions pooling above the cuff of the artificial airway, is critical to decreasing the bacterial colonization of the oropharynx.[30]

Collaborative management of the patient with pneumonia is outlined in Box 23-6.

ASPIRATION PNEUMONITIS

DESCRIPTION

The presence of abnormal substances in the airways and alveoli as a result of aspiration is misleadingly called *aspiration pneumonia*. This term is misleading because the aspiration of toxic substances into the lung may or may not involve an infection. *Aspiration pneumonitis* is a more accurate title, because injury to the lung can result from the chemical, mechanical, and/or bacterial characteristics of the aspirate.

ETIOLOGY

A number of factors have been identified that place the patient at risk for aspiration (Box 23-7). Gastric contents and oropharyngeal bacteria (see "Pneumonia" earlier in

EVIDENCE-BASED COLLABORATIVE PRACTICE
Hand Hygiene Guidelines

- Wash hands with soap and water when visibly dirty or contaminated with blood and other body fluids.
  - When washing hands with soap and water, wet hands first with water, apply an amount of product recommended by the manufacturer to hands, and rub hands together vigorously for at least 15 seconds, covering all surfaces of the hands and fingers. Rinse hands with water and dry thoroughly with a disposable towel. Use towel to turn off the faucet. Avoid using hot water, because repeated exposure to hot water may increase the risk of dermatitis.
- If hands are not visibly soiled, use an alcohol-based hand rub for routinely decontaminating hands.
  - When decontaminating hands with an alcohol-based hand rub, apply product to palm of one hand and rub hands together, covering all surfaces of hands and fingers, until hands are dry (follow the manufacturer's recommendations regarding the volume of product to use).

- Decontaminate hands before and after having direct contact with patients.
- Decontaminate hands before and after donning gloves.
  - Wear gloves when contact with blood or other potentially infectious materials, mucous membranes, or nonintact skin could occur.
  - Change gloves during patient care if moving from a contaminated body site to a clean body site.
  - Remove gloves after caring for a patient. Do not wear the same pair of gloves for the care of more than one patient, and do not wash gloves between uses with different patients.
- Decontaminate hands after contact with inanimate objects (including medical equipment).
- Do not wear artificial fingernails or extenders when having direct contact with patients at high risk (e.g., those in critical care units or operating rooms).
- Keep natural nails tips less than ¼-inch long.

From Advisory Committee and the HICPAC/SHEA/APIC/IDSA Hand Hygiene Task Force: Recommendations of the Healthcare Infection Control Practices, *MMWR* 51(RR16):1, 2002.

Box 23-7
RISK FACTORS FOR ASPIRATION

- Altered level of consciousness
- Depressed gag, cough, or swallowing reflexes
- Presence of feeding tubes (all types)
- Presence of artificial airways
- Ileus or gastric distention
- History of gastrointestinal disorders:
  - Dysphagia
  - Achalasia
  - Gastroesophageal reflux disease
  - Esophageal strictures

this chapter) are the most common things aspirated by the critically ill patient.[61,62] The effects of gastric contents on the lungs will vary based on the pH of the liquid. If the pH is less than 2.5, the patient will develop a severe chemical pneumonitis resulting in hypoxemia. If the pH is greater than 2.5, the immediate damage to the lungs will be lessened but the elevated pH may have promoted bacterial overgrowth of the stomach.[61,62] Once the bacteria-laden gastric contents are aspirated into the lungs, overwhelming bacterial pneumonia can develop.[62]

PATHOPHYSIOLOGY

The type of lung injury that develops after aspiration is determined by a number of factors including the quality of the aspirate and the status of the patient's respiratory defense mechanisms.

Acid Liquid. The aspiration of acid (pH <2.5) liquid gastric contents results in the development of bronchospasm and atelectasis almost immediately. Over the next 4 hours, tracheal damage, bronchitis, bronchiolitis, alveolar-capillary breakdown, interstitial edema, and alveolar congestion and hemorrhage occur.[63] Severe hypoxemia develops as a result of intrapulmonary shunting and V/Q mismatching. As the disorder progresses, necrotic debris and fibrin fill the alveoli, hyaline membranes form, and hypoxic vasoconstriction occurs, resulting in elevated pulmonary artery pressures.[62,63] The clinical course will follow one of three patterns: (1) rapid improvement in 1 week; (2) initial improvement followed by deterioration and development of ARDS or pneumonia; or (3) rapid death from progressive ARF.[63]

Acid Food Particles. The aspiration of acid (pH <2.5) nonobstructing food particles can produce the most severe pulmonary reaction because of extensive pulmonary damage.[63] Severe hypoxemia, hypercapnia, and acidosis occur.[62,63]

Nonacid Liquid. The aspiration of nonacid (pH >2.5) liquid gastric contents is similar to acid liquid aspiration initially, but minimal structural damage occurs.[63] Intrapulmonary shunting and V/Q mismatching usually start to reverse within 4 hours, and hypoxemia clears within 24 hours.[62,63]

Nonacid Food Particles. The aspiration of nonacid (pH >2.5) nonobstructing food particles is similar to acid aspiration initially, with significant edema and hemorrhage occurring within 6 hours. After the initial reaction, the response changes to a foreign body–type reaction with granuloma formation occurring around the food particles within 1 to 5 days.[63] In addition to hypoxemia, hypercapnia and acidosis occur as a result of hypoventilation.[62,63]

ASSESSMENT AND DIAGNOSIS

Clinically, the patient presents with signs of acute respiratory distress, and gastric contents may be present in the oropharynx. The patient will have shortness of breath, coughing, wheezing, cyanosis, and signs of hypoxemia. Tachypnea, tachycardia, hypotension, fever, and crackles also are present. Copious amounts of sputum are produced as alveolar edema develops.[61,62]

ABGs reflect severe hypoxemia. Chest x-ray film changes appear 12 to 24 hours after the initial aspiration, with no one pattern being diagnostic of the event. Infiltrates will appear in a variety of distribution patterns depending on the position of the patient during aspiration and the volume of the aspirate. If bacterial infection becomes established, leukocytosis and positive sputum cultures occur.[62]

MEDICAL MANAGEMENT

Management of the patient with aspiration lung disorder includes both emergency and follow-up treatment. When aspiration is witnessed, emergency treatment should be instituted to secure the airway and minimize pulmonary damage. The upper airway should be immediately suctioned to remove the gastric contents.[61,62] Direct visualization by bronchoscopy is indicated to remove large particulate aspirate[61] or to confirm an unwitnessed aspiration event.[63] Bronchoalveolar lavage is not recommended because this practice disseminates the aspirate in lungs and increases damage. Prophylactic antibiotics are not recommended either.[63]

After airway clearance, attention should be given to supporting oxygenation and hemodynamics. Hypoxemia should be corrected with supplemental oxygen or mechanical ventilation with PEEP, if necessary.[61-63] Hemodynamic changes result from fluid shifts into the lungs that can occur after massive aspirations. Monitoring intravascular volume is essential, and judicious amounts of replacement fluids should be instituted to maintain adequate urinary output and vital signs.[63]

Initially antibiotic therapy is not indicated. If symptoms fail to resolve within 48 hours, empiric antibiotic therapy should be initiated. Corticosteroids have not demonstrated to be of any benefit in the treatment of aspiration pneumonitis and thus are not recommended either.[62]

NURSING MANAGEMENT

Nursing management of the patient with aspiration lung disorder incorporates a variety of nursing diagnoses (see the Nursing Diagnoses feature on Aspiration). Nursing interventions include optimizing oxygenation and ventilation, preventing further aspiration events, providing comfort and emotional support, and maintaining surveillance for complications.

Optimizing Oxygenation and Ventilation. Nursing interventions to optimize oxygenation and ventilation include positioning, preventing desaturation, and promoting secretion clearance. For further discussion on these interventions see "Nursing Management" of acute respiratory failure earlier in this chapter.

Preventing Aspiration. One of the most important interventions for preventing aspiration is identifying the patient at risk for aspiration. Actions to prevent aspiration include confirming feeding tube placement, checking for signs and symptoms of feeding intolerance, elevating the head of the bed at least 30 degrees or turning the patient on his or her right side if remaining flat is essential, ensuring proper inflation of artificial airway cuffs, and frequent suctioning of the oropharynx of an intubated patient to prevent secretions from pooling above the cuff of the tube.[64]

Collaborative management of the patient with aspiration pneumonitis is outlined in Box 23-8.

Box 23-8

COLLABORATIVE MANAGEMENT

ASPIRATION PNEUMONITIS
- Administer oxygen therapy
- Secure the patient's airway
- Place patient in slight Trendelenburg position
- Turn patient to right lateral decubitus position
- Suction patient's oropharyngeal area
- Initiate mechanical ventilation as required
- Maintain surveillance for complications
  - Pneumonia
  - Acute respiratory failure
  - Acute lung injury
- Provide comfort and emotional support

Box 23-9

RISK FACTORS FOR PULMONARY THROMBOEMBOLISM

PREDISPOSING FACTORS
Venous stasis
    Atrial fibrillation
    Decreased cardiac output (CO)
    Immobility
Injury to vascular endothelium
    Local vessel injury
    Infection
    Incision
    Atherosclerosis
Hypercoagulability
    Polycythemia

PRECIPITATING CONDITIONS
Previous pulmonary embolus
Cardiovascular disease
    Heart failure
    Right ventricular infarction
    Cardiomyopathy
    Cor pulmonale
Surgery
    Orthopedic
    Vascular
    Abdominal
Cancer
    Ovarian
    Pancreatic
    Stomach
    Extrahepatic bile duct system
Trauma (injury or burns)
    Lower extremities
    Pelvis
    Hips
Gynecologic status
    Pregnancy
    Postpartum
    Birth control pills
    Estrogen replacement therapy

PULMONARY EMBOLISM

DESCRIPTION

A pulmonary embolism (PE) occurs when a clot (thrombotic embolus) or other matter (nonthrombotic embolus) lodges in the pulmonary arterial system, disrupting the blood flow to a region of the lungs. The majority of thrombotic emboli arise from the deep leg veins, particularly the iliac, femoral, and popliteal veins.[65] Other sources include the right ventricle, the upper extremities, and the pelvic veins. Nonthrombotic emboli arise from fat, tumors, amniotic fluid, air, and foreign bodies. This section of the chapter focuses on thrombotic emboli.

ETIOLOGY

A number of predisposing factors and precipitating conditions put a patient at risk for developing a PE (Box 23-9). Of the three predisposing factors (i.e., hypercoagulability, injury to vascular endothelium, and venous stasis [Virchow's triad]), endothelial injury appears to be the most significant.[65]

PATHOPHYSIOLOGY

A massive PE occurs with the blockage of a lobar or larger artery, resulting in occlusion of more than 40% of the pulmonary vascular bed. Blockage of the pulmonary arterial system has both pulmonary and hemodynamic consequences. The effects on the pulmonary system are increased alveolar dead space, bronchoconstriction, and compensatory shunting. The hemodynamic effects include an increase in pulmonary vascular resistance and right ventricular workload.[66]

Increased Dead Space. An increase in alveolar dead space occurs because an area of the lung is receiving ventilation without being perfused. The ventilation to this area is known as *wasted ventilation*, because it does not participate in gas exchange. This effect leads to alveolar dead space ventilation and an increase in the work of breathing. To limit the amount of dead space ventilation, localized bronchoconstriction occurs.[66]

Bronchoconstriction. Bronchoconstriction develops as a result of alveolar hypocarbia, hypoxia, and the release of mediators. Alveolar hypocarbia occurs as a consequence of decreased carbon dioxide in the affected area and leads to constriction of the local airways, increased airway resistance, and redistribution of ventilation to perfused areas of the lungs. A variety of mediators are released from the site of the injury, either from the clot or the surrounding lung tissue, which further causes constriction of the airways. Bronchoconstriction promotes the development of atelectasis.[66]

Compensatory Shunting. Compensatory shunting occurs as a result of the unaffected areas of the lungs having to accommodate the entire cardiac output. This creates a situation in which perfusion exceeds ventilation and blood is returned to the left side of the heart without participating in gas exchange. This leads to the development of hypoxemia.[66]

Hemodynamic Consequences. The major hemodynamic consequence of a PE is the development of pulmonary hypertension, which is part of the effect of a mechanical obstruction when more than 50% of the vascular bed is occluded. In addition, the mediators released at the injury site and the development of hypoxia cause pulmonary vasoconstriction, which further exacerbates pulmonary hypertension. As the pulmonary vascular resistance increases, so does the workload of the right ventricle as reflected by a rise in PA pressures. Consequently, right ventricular failure occurs, which can lead to decreases in left ventricular preload, CO, and blood pressure, and shock.[66]

ASSESSMENT AND DIAGNOSIS

The patient with a pulmonary embolism may have any number of presenting signs and symptoms, with the most common being tachycardia and tachycapnia. Additional signs and symptoms that may be present include dyspnea, apprehension, increased pulmonic component of the second heart sound (P_1), fever, rales, pleuritic chest pain, cough, evidence of a deep vein thrombosis, and hemoptysis.[66] Syncope and hemodynamic instability can occur as a result of right ventricular failure.[65]

Initial laboratory studies and diagnostic procedures that may be done are ABG analysis, D-dimer, electrocardiogram (ECG), chest radiography and echocardiography (ECHO). ABGs may show a low PaO_2, indicating hypoxemia; a low $PaCO_2$, indicating hypocarbia; and a high pH, indicating a respiratory alkalosis. The hypocarbia with resulting respiratory alkalosis is caused by tachypnea.[65] An elevated D-dimer will occur with a PE and a number of other disorders. A normal D-dimer will not occur with a PE and thus can be used to rule a PE out as the diagnosis.[67] The most frequent ECG finding seen in the patient with a PE is sinus tachycardia.[65] The classic ECG pattern associated with a PE—S wave in lead I, and Q wave with inverted T wave in lead III—is seen in fewer than 20% of patients.[65] Other ECG findings associated with a PE include right bundle branch block, new onset atrial fibrillation, T-wave inversion in the anterior or inferior leads[65] and ST-segment changes.[66] Chest x-ray findings vary from normal to abnormal and are of little value in confirming the presence of a PE. Abnormal findings include cardiomegaly, pleural effusion, elevated hemidiaphragm, enlargement of the right descending pulmonary artery (Palla's sign), a wedge-shaped density above the diaphragm (Hampton's hump), and the presence of atelectasis.[65] An ECHO, either transthoracic or transesophageal, is also useful in the identification of a PE, because it can provide visualization of any emboli in the central pulmonary arteries. In addition, it can be used for assessing the hemodynamic consequences of the PE on the right side of the heart.[67]

Differentiating a PE from other illnesses can be difficult because many of its clinical manifestations are found in a variety of other disorders.[65] Thus a variety of other tests may be necessary, including a V/Q scintigraphy, pulmonary angiogram, and deep vein thrombosis (DVT) studies.[65-67] Given the advent of more sophisticated computed tomography (CT) scanners, the spiral CT is also being used to diagnose a PE.[67,68] A definitive diagnosis of a PE requires confirmation by a high-probability V/Q scan, an abnormal pulmonary angiogram or CT, or strong clinical suspicion coupled with abnormal findings on lower extremity DVT studies.[67]

MEDICAL MANAGEMENT

Medical management of the patient with a pulmonary embolism involves both prevention and treatment strategies. Prevention strategies include the use of prophylactic anticoagulation with low-dose or adjusted-dose heparin, low–molecular-weight heparin, or oral anticoagulants. The use of graduated compression stockings and intermittent pneumatic leg compression have also been demonstrated as effective methods of prophylaxis in low-risk patients.[69]

Treatment strategies include preventing the recurrence of a PE, facilitating clot dissolution, reversing the effects of pulmonary hypertension, promoting gas exchange, and preventing complications. Medical interventions to promote gas exchange include supplemental oxygen administration, intubation, and mechanical ventilation.[66]

Prevention of Recurrence. Interventions to prevent the recurrence of a PE include the administration of unfractionated or low–molecular-weight heparin and warfarin (Coumadin).[69] Heparin is administered to prevent further clots from forming and has no effect on the existing clot. The heparin should be adjusted to maintain the activated partial thromboplastin time (aPTT) in the range of 1.5 to 2.3 times control.[69] Warfarin should be started at the same time, and when the international normalized ratio (INR) reaches 3.0, the heparin should be discontinued. The INR should be maintained between 2.0 and 3.0. The patient should remain on warfarin for 3 to 12 months depending on his or her risk for thromboembolic disease.[69]

Interruption of the inferior vena cava is reserved for patients in whom anticoagulation is contraindicated. The procedure involves placement of a percutaneous venous filter (e.g., Greenfield filter) into the vena cava, usually below the renal arteries. The filter prevents further thrombotic emboli from migrating into the lungs.[69]

Clot Dissolution. The administration of thrombolytic agents in the treatment of PE has had limited success. Currently, thrombolytic therapy is reserved for the patient with a massive PE and concomitant hemodynamic instability. Either recombinant tissue-type plasminogen activator (rt-PA) or streptokinase may be used. The therapeutic window for using thrombolytic therapy is 14 days.[70]

Although often considered as a last resort, a pulmonary embolectomy may be performed to surgically remove the clot. Generally it is performed as an open procedure while the patient is on cardiopulmonary bypass.[71]

Reversal of Pulmonary Hypertension. To reverse the hemodynamic effects of pulmonary hypertension, additional measures may be taken. These include the administration of inotropic agents and fluid. Fluids should be administered to increase right ventricular preload, which would stretch the right ventricle and increase contractility, thus overcoming the elevated pulmonary arterial pressures. Inotropic agents also can be used to increase contractility to facilitate an increase in CO.[66]

NURSING MANAGEMENT

Prevention of pulmonary embolism should be a major nursing focus, because the majority of critically ill patients are at risk for this disorder. Nursing actions are aimed at preventing the development of DVT, which is a major complication of immobility and a leading cause of PE. These measures include the use of antiembolic stockings and/or pneumatic compression stockings, elevation of the legs, active/passive range of motion exercises, adequate hydration, and progressive ambulation. For more discussion on DVT see "Deep Vein Thrombosis" in Chapter 18 ("Cardiovascular Disorders").

Nursing management of the patient with a PE incorporates a variety of nursing diagnoses (see the Nursing Diagnoses feature on Pulmonary Embolus). Nursing interventions include optimizing oxygenation and ventilation, monitoring for bleeding, providing comfort and emotional support, and maintaining surveillance for complications.

Optimizing Oxygenation and Ventilation. Nursing interventions to optimize oxygenation and ventilation include positioning, preventing desaturation, and promoting secretion clearance. For further discussion on these interventions see "Nursing Management" of acute respiratory failure earlier in this chapter.

Monitoring for Bleeding. The patient receiving anticoagulant or thrombolytic therapy should be observed for signs of bleeding. The patient's gums, skin, urine, stool, and emesis should be screened for signs of overt or covert bleeding. In addition, monitoring the patient's INR or aPTT is critical to managing the anticoagulation therapy.

Patient Education. Early in the patient's hospital stay, the patient and family should be taught about pulmonary embolus, its etiologies, and its treatment (see the Patient Education feature on Pulmonary Embolus). As the patient moves toward discharge, teaching should focus on the interventions necessary for preventing the reoccurrence of deep vein thrombosis and subsequent

NURSING DIAGNOSES — **Pulmonary Embolus**

- Impaired Gas Exchange related to ventilation/perfusion mismatching or intrapulmonary shunting
- Acute Pain related to transmission and perception of cutaneous, visceral, muscular, or ischemic impulses
- Risk for Aspiration
- Anxiety related to threat to biologic, psychologic, and/or social integrity
- Powerlessness related to lack of control over current situation or disease progression
- Compromised Family Coping related to critically ill family member
- Deficient Knowledge: Discharge Regimen related to lack of previous exposure to information (see Patient Education special feature on Pulmonary Embolus)

PATIENT EDUCATION — **Pulmonary Embolus**

- Pathophysiology of disease
- Specific etiology
- Precipitating factor modification
- Measure to prevent deep vein thrombosis (e.g., avoid tight-fitting clothes, crossing legs, and prolonged sitting or standing; elevate legs when sitting; exercise)
- Signs and symptoms of deep vein thrombosis (e.g., redness, swelling, sharp or deep leg pain)
- Importance of taking medications
- Signs and symptoms of anticoagulant complications (e.g., excessive bruising, discoloration of the skin, changes in color of urine or stools)
- Measures to prevent bleeding (e.g., use soft-bristle toothbrush, caution when shaving)

emboli, signs and symptoms of deep vein thrombosis and anticoagulant complications, and measures to prevent bleeding. If the patient smokes, he or she should be encouraged to stop smoking and be referred to a smoking cessation program.

Collaborative management of the patient with a pulmonary embolus is outlined in Box 23-10.

STATUS ASTHMATICUS

DESCRIPTION

Asthma is a chronic obstructive pulmonary disease that is characterized by partially reversible airflow obstruction, airway inflammation, and hyperresponsiveness to a variety of stimuli.[72] Status asthmaticus is a severe asthma attack that fails to respond to conventional therapy with bronchodilators, which may result in acute respiratory failure.[73]

ETIOLOGY

The precipitating cause of the attack is usually an upper respiratory infection, allergen exposure, or a decrease in antiinflammatory medications. Other factors that have been implicated include overreliance on bronchodilators, environmental pollutants, lack of access to health care, failure to identify worsening airflow obstruction, and noncompliance with the health care regimen.[72]

PATHOPHYSIOLOGY

An asthma attack is initiated when exposure to an irritant or trigger occurs, resulting in the initiation of the inflammatory-immune response in the airways. Bronchospasm occurs along with increased vascular permeability and increased mucus production. Mucosal edema and thick, tenacious mucus further increase airway responsiveness. The combination of bronchospasm, airway inflammation, and hyperresponsiveness results in narrowing of the airways and airflow obstruction. These changes have significant effects on the pulmonary and cardiovascular systems.[72]

Pulmonary Effects. As the diameter of the airways decreases, airway resistance increases, resulting in increased residual volume, hyperinflation of the lungs, increased work of breathing, and abnormal distribution of ventilation. V/Q mismatching occurs, which results in hypoxemia. Alveolar dead space also increases as hypoxic vasoconstriction occurs, resulting in hypercapnia.[72]

Cardiovascular Effects. Inspiratory muscle force also increases in an attempt to ventilate the hyperinflated lungs. This results in a significant increase in negative intrapleural pressure, leading to an increase in venous return and pooling of blood in the right ventricle. The stretched right ventricle causes the intraventricular septum to shift, thereby impinging on the left ventricle. In addition, the left ventricle has to work harder to pump blood from the markedly negative pressure in the thorax to elevated pressure in systemic circulation. This leads to a decrease in cardiac output and a fall in systolic blood pressure on inspiration (pulsus paradoxus).[72]

ASSESSMENT AND DIAGNOSIS

Initially the patient may present with a cough, wheezing, and dyspnea. As the attack continues, the patient develops tachypnea, tachycardia, diaphoresis, increased accessory muscle use, and pulsus paradoxus greater than 25 mm Hg. Decreased level of consciousness, inability to speak, significantly diminished or absent breath sounds, and inability to lie supine herald the onset of acute respiratory failure.[73-75]

Initial ABGs indicate hypocapnia and respiratory alkalosis caused by hyperventilation. As the attack continues and the patient starts to fatigue, hypoxemia and hypercapnia develop.[73] Lactic acidosis also may occur as a result of lactate overproduction by the respiratory muscles. The end result is the development of respiratory and metabolic acidosis.[74]

Deterioration of pulmonary function tests despite aggressive bronchodilator therapy is diagnostic of status asthmaticus and indicates the potential need for intubation. A peak expiratory flow rate (PEFR) less than 40% of predicted or an FEV_1 (maximum volume of gas that the patient can exhale in 1 second [forced expiratory volume in 1 second]) less than 20% of predicted indicates severe airflow obstruction, and the need for intubation with mechanical ventilation may be imminent.[75]

MEDICAL MANAGEMENT

Medical management of the patient with status asthmaticus is directed toward supporting oxygenation and ventilation. Bronchodilators, corticosteroids, oxygen therapy, and intubation and mechanical ventilation are the mainstays of therapy.[73]

Bronchodilators. Inhaled beta$_2$-agonists and anticholinergics are the bronchodilators of choice for status asthmaticus. Beta$_2$-agonists promote bronchodilation and can be administered by nebulizer or metered-dose inhaler (MDI). Usually larger and more frequent doses are given, and the drug is titrated to the patient's response. Anticholinergics that inhibit bronchoconstriction are not very effective by themselves, but in conjunction with beta$_2$-agonists, they have a synergistic effect and produce a greater improvement in airflow. The routine use of xanthines is not recommended in the treatment of status asthmaticus because they have been shown to have no therapeutic benefit.[72-75]

A number of studies have focused on the bronchodilator abilities of magnesium. Although it has been demonstrated that magnesium is inferior to beta$_2$-agonists as a bronchodilator, in patients who are refractory to conventional treatment, magnesium may be beneficial. A bolus of 1 to 4 g of intravenous magnesium given over 10 to 40 minutes has been reported to produce desirable effects.[72,73,75]

A number of studies of other studies are evaluating the effects of leukotriene inhibitors such as zafirlukast, montelukast, and zilueton in the treatment of status asthmaticus. Leukotrienes are inflammatory mediators known to cause bronchoconstriction and airway inflammation. Research suggests that these agents may beneficial as bronchodilators in those patients who are refractory to beta$_2$-agonists.[75]

Systemic Corticosteroids. Intravenous or oral corticosteroids also are used in the treatment of status asthmaticus. Their antiinflammatory effects limit mucosal edema, decrease mucus production, and potentiate beta$_2$-agonists. It usually takes 6 to 8 hours for the effects of the corticosteroids to become evident.[73] The use of inhaled corticosteroids for the treatment of status asthmaticus remains undecided at this time.[72,75] Initial studies indicate they may be beneficial in certain patient populations.[75]

Oxygen Therapy. Initial treatment of hypoxemia is with supplemental oxygen. High-flow oxygen therapy is administered to keep the patient's SaO$_2$ greater than 92%.[72]

Another therapy currently under investigation is the use of heliox. A mixture of helium and oxygen, heliox has a lower density and higher viscosity than an oxygen and air mixture. Heliox is believed to reduce the work of breathing and improve gas exchange because it flows more easily through constricted areas. Studies have shown that it reduces air trapping and carbon dioxide and helps relieve respiratory acidosis.[72]

Intubation and Mechanical Ventilation. Indications for mechanical ventilation include cardiac or respiratory arrest, disorientation, failure to respond to bronchodilator therapy, and exhaustion.[72,74,75] A large endotracheal tube (8 mm) should be used to decrease airway resistance and to facilitate suctioning of secretions. Ventilating the patient with status asthmaticus can be very difficult. High inflation pressures should be avoided because they can result in barotrauma. The use of PEEP should be monitored closely because the patient is prone to developing air trapping. Patient-ventilator asynchrony also can be a major problem. Sedation and neuromuscular paralysis may be necessary to allow for adequate ventilation of the patient.[72,74]

NURSING MANAGEMENT

Nursing management of the patient with status asthmaticus incorporates a variety of nursing diagnoses (see the Nursing Diagnoses feature on Status Asthmaticus). Nursing interventions include optimizing oxygenation and ventilation, providing comfort and emotional support, and maintaining surveillance for complications.

Optimizing Oxygenation and Ventilation. Nursing interventions to optimize oxygenation and ventilation include positioning, preventing desaturation, and promoting secretion clearance. For further discussion on these interventions see "Nursing Management" of acute respiratory failure earlier in this chapter.

Patient Education. Early in the patient's hospital stay, the patient and family should be taught about asthma, its triggers, and its treatment (see the Patient Education feature on Status Asthmaticus). As the patient moves toward discharge, teaching should focus on the interventions necessary for preventing the recurrence of status asthmaticus, early warning signs of worsening airflow obstruction, correct use of an inhaler

NURSING DIAGNOSES Status Asthmaticus

- Impaired Gas Exchange related to alveolar hypoventilation
- Impaired Gas Exchange related to ventilation/perfusion mismatching or intrapulmonary shunting
- Ineffective Breathing Pattern related to musculoskeletal fatigue or neuromuscular impairment
- Ineffective Airway Clearance related to excessive secretions or abnormal viscosity of mucus
- Risk for Infection
- Anxiety related to threat to biologic, psychologic, and/or social integrity
- Disturbed Body Image related to actual change in body structures, function, or appearance
- Compromised Family Coping related to critically ill family member
- Deficient Knowledge: Discharge Regimen related to lack of previous exposure to information (see Patient Education special feature on Status Asthmaticus)

PATIENT EDUCATION

Status Asthmaticus

- Pathophysiology of disease
- Specific etiology
- Early warning signs of worsening airflow obstruction (20% drop in peak expiratory flow rate [PEFR] below predicted or personal best, increase in cough, shortness of breath, chest tightness, wheezing)
- Treatment of attacks
- Importance of taking prescribed medications and avoidance of over-the-counter asthma medications
- Correct use of an inhaler (with and without spacer device)
- Correct use of a peak flow meter
- Removal or avoidance of environmental triggers (e.g., pollen; dust; mold spores; cat and dog dander; cold, dry air; strong odors; household aerosols; tobacco smoke; air pollution)
- Measures to prevent pulmonary infections (e.g., proper nutrition and hand washing, immunization against *Streptococcus pneumoniae* and influenza viruses)
- Signs and symptoms of pulmonary infection (e.g., sputum color change, shortness of breath, fever)
- Importance of participating in pulmonary rehabilitation program

Box 23-11

COLLABORATIVE MANAGEMENT

STATUS ASTHMATICUS
- Administer oxygen therapy
- Intubate patient
- Initiate mechanical ventilation
- Administer medications
  - Bronchodilators
  - Corticosteroids
  - Sedatives
- Maintain surveillance for complications
  - Acute respiratory failure
- Provide comfort and emotional support

and a peak flowmeter, measures to prevent pulmonary infections, and signs and symptoms of a pulmonary infection. If the patient smokes, he or she should be encouraged to stop smoking and be referred to a smoking cessation program. In addition, the importance of participating in a pulmonary rehabilitation program should be stressed.

Collaborative management of the patient with status asthmaticus is outlined in Box 23-11.

AIR LEAK DISORDERS

DESCRIPTION

Air leak disorders consist of those conditions that result in extraalveolar air accumulation. These disorders are commonly classified into two categories: pneumothorax[76] and barotrauma/volutrauma.[77] A pneumothorax occurs as the result of the accumulation of air or other gas in the pleural space,[6] whereas barotrauma and volutrauma occur as the result of the accumulation of air in the interstitial space.[77] Either excessive pressure in the alveoli (barotrauma) or excessive volume in the alveoli (volutrauma) can lead to excessive alveolar wall stress and damage to the alveolar-capillary membrane, resulting in air escaping into the surrounding spaces.[42] The individual disorders comprising these two categories are described in Table 23-5.

ETIOLOGY

The two main causes of air leak disorders are (1) disruption of the parietal or visceral pleura, which allows air to enter the pleural space,[76] and (2) rupture of alveoli, which allows air to enter the interstitial space.[77] Disruption of the parietal pleura occurs as the result of penetrating trauma to the chest wall, which allows atmospheric air to enter the pleural space (traumatic open pneumothorax).[76] Disruption of the visceral pleura occurs as the result of air entering the pleural space from the lung. This may be caused by blunt chest wall trauma (traumatic closed pneumothorax), diagnostic or therapeutic procedures (traumatic iatrogenic pneumothorax), diseases of the pulmonary system (secondary spontaneous pneumothorax), or ruptured subpleural blebs (primary spontaneous pneumothorax).[76] Alveolar rupture occurs as the result of a change in the pressure gradient between the alveoli and the surrounding interstitial space. An increase in alveolar pressure or a decrease in interstitial pressure can lead to overdistention of the alveoli, rupture, and air leakage into the interstitial space. One of the most common causes of barotrauma and volutrauma is mechanical ventilation.[77]

PATHOPHYSIOLOGY

The pathologic consequences of pneumothorax and barotrauma/volutrauma are different.

Pneumothorax. Regardless of the etiology, once air enters the pleural space, the affected lung becomes compressed. As the lung collapses, the alveoli become underventilated, causing V/Q mismatching and intrapulmonary shunting. If the pneumothorax is large, hypoxemia en-

Table 23-5	Air Leak Disorders
Type	**Description**

PNEUMOTHORAX

SPONTANEOUS

Primary	Disruption of the visceral pleura that allows air from the lung to enter the pleural space; occurs spontaneously in patients *without* underlying lung disease
Secondary	Disruption of the visceral pleura that allows air from the lung to enter the pleural space; occurs spontaneously in patients *with* underlying lung disease

TRAUMATIC

Open	Laceration in the parietal pleura that allows atmospheric air to enter the pleural space; occurs as a result of penetrating chest trauma
Closed	Laceration in the visceral pleura that allows air from the lung to enter the pleural space; occurs as a result of blunt chest trauma
Iatrogenic	Laceration in the visceral pleura that allows air from the lung to enter the pleural space; occurs as a result of therapeutic or diagnostic procedures, such as central line insertion, thoracentesis, and needle aspirations
Tension	Occurs when air is allowed to enter the pleural space but not exit it; as pressure increases inside the pleural space, the lung collapses and the mediastinum shifts to the unaffected side; may be a result of a spontaneous or traumatic pneumothorax

VOLUTRAUMA

Pulmonary interstitial emphysema	Air in the pulmonary interstitial space
Subcutaneous emphysema	Air in the subcutaneous tissues
Pneumomediastinum	Air in the mediastinal space
Pneumopericardium	Air in the pericardial space
Pneumoperitoneum	Air in the peritoneal space
Pneumoretroperitoneum	Air in the retroperitoneal space

sues and acute respiratory failure quickly develops. In addition, increased pressure within the chest can lead to shifting of the mediastinum, compression of the great vessels, and decreased cardiac output.[76]

Barotrauma/Volutrauma. Once air enters the interstitial space, it travels though the pulmonary interstitium (pulmonary interstitial emphysema), out through the hilum, and into the mediastinum (pneumomediastinum), pleural space (pneumothorax),[78] subcutaneous tissues (subcutaneous emphysema),[77] pericardium (pneumopericardium),[42] peritoneum (pneumoperitoneum),[80] and retroperitoneum (pneumoretroperitoneum).[78] Except for pneumothorax, the resultant disorders are usually fairly benign. Pneumomediastinum has been associated with decreased venous return and upper airway obstruction, and pneumopericardium has been associated with cardiac tamponade.[42]

ASSESSMENT AND DIAGNOSIS

The clinical manifestations of a pneumothorax depend on the degree of lung collapse. When a pneumothorax is large, decreased respiratory excursion on the affected side may be noticed, along with bulging intercostal muscles. The trachea may deviate away from the affected side. Percussion reveals hyperresonance with decreased or absent breath sounds over the affected area. ABGs will demonstrate hypoxemia and hypercapnia.[76] A chest x-ray film will confirm the pneumothorax with increased translucency evident on the affected side (Fig. 23-3).[78]

The clinical manifestations of barotrauma and volutrauma are much more subtle. Subcutaneous emphysema is manifested by crepitus, usually around the face, neck, and upper chest.[77] Stabbing substernal pain with position changes and increased ventilation is the most commonly reported symptom of a pneumomediastinum.[81] In addition, a clicking or crunching sound synchronous with the heart sounds may be heard over the apex of the heart (Hamman's sign).[82] A friction rub may be heard with a pneumopericardium.[82] Barotrauma is also confirmed with an x-ray film. Extraalveolar air as evidenced by increased translucency will be present in the affected area (e.g., chest, abdomen).[78]

MEDICAL MANAGEMENT

Medical management of the patient with air leak disorders will vary depending on the severity of the specific disorder. Usually only a pneumothorax would require treatment, and that would depend on the size. A pneumothorax of less than 15% usually requires no treatment other than supplemental oxygen administration, unless

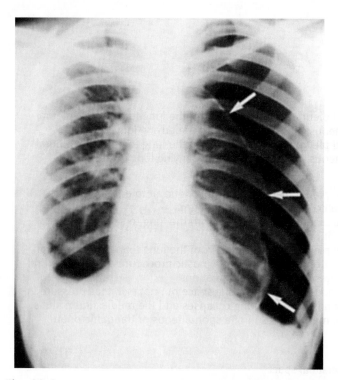

Fig. 23-3 Left-sided tension pneumothorax. Note the shift of the heart and mediastinum to the right. (From Des Jardin T, Burton GC: *Clinical management and assessment of respiratory disease,* ed 3, St. Louis, 1995, Mosby.)

complications occur or underlying lung disease or injury is present.[76]

A pneumothorax greater than 15% requires intervention to evacuate the air from the pleural space and facilitate reexpansion of the collapsed lung. Interventions include aspiration of the air with a needle, placement of a percutaneous catheter attached to a Heimlich valve, insertion of a thoracic vent, and insertion of a chest tube with underwater-seal suction drainage. A small one-way valve device that is easily secured to a catheter placed in the chest, the Heimlich valve allows air to exit from the pleural space but not enter it. A thoracic vent is similar to a Heimlich valve in that it is a one-way valve, but it comes attached to the catheter. Chest tubes are usually inserted in the fourth or fifth intercostal space on the midaxillary line. Once the tubes are inserted and connected to an underwater chest drainage system with at least 20 cm of suction, a chest x-ray examination should be performed to confirm reexpansion of the lung.[76]

Two conditions that require emergency intervention for immediate relief are a tension pneumothorax and a tension pneumopericardium.

Tension Pneumothorax. A tension pneumothorax develops when air enters the pleural space on inhalation and cannot exit on exhalation. As pressure inside the pleural space increases, it results in collapse of the lung and shifting of the mediastinum and trachea to the unaffected side (see Fig. 23-3). The resultant effect is decreased venous

return and compression of the unaffected lung. Clinical signs include diminished breath sound, hyperresonance to percussion, tachycardia, and hypotension. Treatment comprises administering supplemental oxygen and inserting a large-bore needle or catheter into the second intercostal space at the midclavicular line of the affected side. This action relieves the pressure within the chest. The needle should remain in place until the patient is stabilized and a chest tube is inserted.[76]

Tension Pneumopericardium. A tension pneumopericardium develops when air enters the pericardial space and has no outlet for exiting. As pressure inside the pericardium increases, it results in compression of the heart and the development of cardiac tamponade. A pericardiocentesis should be performed immediately to relieve the pressure within the pericardial sac.[42,82]

NURSING MANAGEMENT

Nursing management of the patient with air leak disorders incorporates a variety of nursing diagnoses (see the Nursing Diagnoses feature on Air Leak Disorders). Nursing interventions should focus on optimizing oxygenation and ventilation, maintaining the chest tube system, providing comfort and emotional support, and maintaining surveillance for complications.

Optimizing Oxygenation and Ventilation. Nursing interventions to optimize oxygenation and ventilation include positioning, preventing desaturation, and promoting secretion clearance. For further discussion on these interventions see "Nursing Management" of acute respiratory failure earlier in this chapter.

Maintaining the Chest Tube System. Maintaining the chest tube system (Box 23-12) involves careful atten-

Box 23-12

CHEST TUBE REVIEW

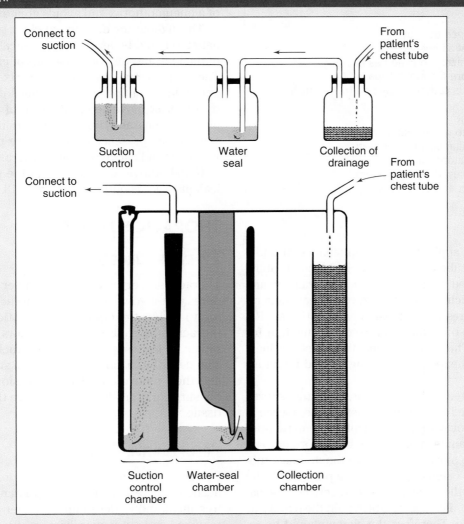

Three-bottle chest drainage system and corresponding chambers of Pleur-Evac chest drainage system. (From Daitch JS: Postanesthesia care after thoracic surgery. In Frost EAM, editor: *Post anesthesia care unit: current practices,* ed 2, St Louis, 1990, Mosby.)

Chest tubes are inserted into the pleural space to remove fluid or air and thus reinstate the negative intrapleural pressure and reexpand a collapsed lung. Once a chest tube is inserted, it is connected to a water-seal drainage system. Water-seal drainage systems have evolved from separate glass bottles of one, two, or three containers into a self-contained disposable plastic unit. The drainage system is aseptically prepared for use, with sterile water placed in the water seal and suction control chambers. Usually the water-seal chamber is filled to the 2-cm level and the suction-control chamber is filled to the desired level of suction. The water-seal chamber acts as a one-way valve, allowing air to escape from the chest but not enter it. Once the chest tubes are placed, the suction control chambers is attached to an external suction regulator, which is adjusted until gentle bubbling occurs in the chamber. Any fluid draining from the chest will be evident in the collection chamber. Connection points of the drainage tubing are sealed with tape, and an occlusive dressing is applied over the chest tube insertion site. Nursing measures are aimed at maintaining the patency and sterility of the system.

tion to the suction applied and to maintenance of unobstructed drainage tubes. Kinks and large loops of tubing should be prevented because they impede drainage and air evacuation, which in turn may prevent timely lung reexpansion or may result in a tension pneumothorax. Retained drainage also becomes an excellent medium for bacterial growth. The water-seal chamber must routinely be observed for unexpected bubbling caused by an air leak in the system.

When unexpected bubbling is present, the source must be identified. To determine whether the source is within the system or within the patient, systematic brief clamping of the drainage tube should be performed. The nurse should place a padded clamp on the drainage tubing as close to the occlusive dressing as possible. If the air bubbling stops, the air leak is located between the patient and the clamp. The leak can be within the patient or at the insertion site. Therefore the clamp should be removed and the chest tube site exposed. The tube should be inspected at the site where it enters the chest to ensure that all the eyelets are within the patient. If an eyelet port is outside the chest, it can be a source of an air leak and must be occluded, which may require the attention of the physician. When the insertion site has been eliminated as a leakage source, the chest dressing should be reapplied, completely and securely covering the site. If the air bubbling does not stop when a clamp is placed on the chest tube, the leak is located between the clamp and the drainage collector. By releasing the clamp and moving it down the tubing a few inches to a point where the bubbling stops, the leak will be located. Once located, the area of the leak can be taped to reestablish a seal, or the system can be replaced.

Sterile petroleum gauze and a bottle of sterile water should be available at all times. If the chest tube system is inadvertently interrupted, the tube should be placed a few centimeters into the bottle of water while the drainage system is reestablished. Sterile petroleum gauze is applied to the chest wall if the chest tube is accidentally removed. Implementing both of these techniques immediately minimizes or prevents the formation of a pneumothorax and avoids greater complications.

Throughout the duration of chest tube placement, the patient should be assessed periodically for reexpansion of the lung and for complications of chest tube drainage. The nurse should assess the thorax and lungs, paying particular attention to any tracheal deviation, asymmetry of chest movement, presence of subcutaneous emphysema, characteristics of breathing, quality of lung sounds, and presence of tympany or percussion sounds, which are indicative of pneumothorax.

Collaborative management of the patient with an air leak disorder is outlined in Box 23-13.

THORACIC SURGERY

TYPES OF SURGERY

Thoracic surgery refers to a number of surgical procedures that involve opening the thoracic cavity (thoracotomy) and/or the organs of respiration. Indications for thoracic surgery range from tumors and abscesses to repair of the esophagus and thoracic vessels.[83] Table 23-6 describes a variety of thoracic surgical procedures and their indications. This discussion focuses only on the surgical procedures that involve the removal of lung tissue.

PREOPERATIVE CARE

Before surgery, a complete evaluation of the patient is needed to determine the appropriateness of surgery as a treatment and to determine whether lung tissue can be removed without jeopardizing respiratory function. This is especially important when a lobectomy or pneumonectomy is being considered. When resection is being undertaken for tumor treatment, preoperative care includes evaluation of the type and extent of the tumor and the physical condition of the patient.[83]

The evaluation of the patient's physical status should focus on the adequacy of cardiopulmonary function. The preoperative evaluation should include pulmonary function tests to determine the patient's ability to manage with less lung tissue. Cardiac function also should be evaluated. Uncontrolled dysrhythmias, acute myocardial infarction, severe chronic heart failure, and unstable angina are all contraindications to surgery.[84]

SURGICAL CONSIDERATIONS

The type and location of surgery will dictate the type of surgical approach that is used. The most common approach is the posterolateral thoracotomy, which allows for exposure of both the lung and mediastinum. Other

Table 23-6   Thoracic Surgeries

Procedure	Definition	Indications
Pneumonectomy 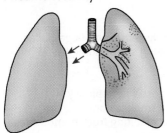	Removal of entire lung with or without resection of the mediastinal lymph nodes	Malignant lesions Unilateral tuberculosis Extensive unilateral bronchiectasis Multiple lung abscesses Massive hemoptysis Bronchopleural fistula
Lobectomy 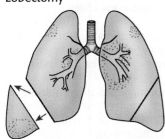	Resection of one or more lobes of lung	Lesions confined to a single lobe Pulmonary tuberculosis Bronchiectasis Lung abscesses or cysts Trauma
Segmental resection 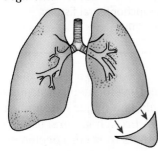	Resection of bronchovascular segment of lung lobe	Small peripheral lesions Bronchiectasis Congenital cysts or blebs
Wedge resection 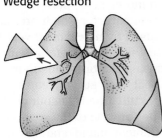	Removal of small wedge-shaped section of lung tissue	Small peripheral lesions (without lymph node involvement) Peripheral granulomas Pulmonary blebs
Bronchoplastic reconstruction (also called sleeve resection) 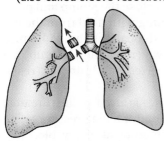	Resection of lung tissue and bronchus with end-to-end reanastomosis of bronchus	Small lesions involving the carina or major bronchus without evidence of metastasis May be combined with lobectomy

Continued

Table 23-6	Thoracic Surgeries—cont'd	
Procedure	**Definition**	**Indications**
Lung volume reduction surgery	Resection of the most damaged portions of lung tissue, allowing more normal chest wall configuration	Severe emphysema
Bullectomy	Resection of a large bulla (an airspace that is greater than one centimeter in diameter that formed as a result of pulmonary tissue destruction)	Severe emphysema with large bullae compressing surrounding tissue
Open lung biopsy	Resection of a small portion of the lung for biopsy	Failure of closed lung biopsy Removal of small lesions
Decortication	Removal of fibrous membrane from pleural surface of lung	Fibrothorax resulting from hemothorax or empyema
Drainage of empyema	Drainage of pus in the pleural space	Acute and chronic infections
Partial rib resection	Removal of one or more ribs to allow healing of underlying lung tissue	Chronic empyemic infections
Video-assisted thoracoscopy (VATS)	Endoscopic procedure performed through small incisions in the chest	Evaluation of pulmonary, pleural, mediastinal, or pericardial conditions Biopsy of lung, pleural, or mediastinal lesions Recurrent spontaneous pneumothorax Evacuation of emphysema, hemothorax, pleural effusion, or pericardial effusion Blebectomy/bullectomy Pleurodesis Sympathectomy Closure of bronchopleural fistula Lysis of adhesions

approaches that are used include anterolateral thoracotomy, and median sternotomy.[83]

Special care is taken to avoid drainage of blood or secretions into the unaffected lung during surgery, because such an occurrence could cause hypoxemia and cardiac dysfunction. A double-lumen endotracheal tube is used during the surgery to protect the unaffected lung from secretions and necrotic tumor fragments. To decrease the incidence of hypoxemia during the procedure, 5 to 10 cm H_2O of PEEP is maintained to the deflated lung. In addition, the deflated lung is intermittently ventilated during the procedure.[85]

COMPLICATIONS AND MEDICAL MANAGEMENT

A number of complications are associated with a lung resection. These include acute respiratory failure, bronchopleural fistula, hemorrhage, cardiovascular disturbances, and mediastinal shift.

Acute Respiratory Failure. In the postoperative period, acute respiratory failure may result from atelectasis or pneumonia. Atelectasis can occur as a result of anesthesia, the surgical procedure, immobilization, and pain. Treatment should be aimed at correcting the underlying problems and supporting gas exchange. Supplemental oxygen and mechanical ventilation with PEEP may be necessary.[85]

Bronchopleural Fistula. Development of a postoperative bronchopleural fistula is a major cause of mortality after a lung resection. A bronchopleural fistula develops when the suture line fails to secure occlusion of the bronchial stump and an opening develops. This can result from an imperfect stump closure, perforation of the stump (e.g., with a suction catheter), high pressure within the airways (e.g., caused by mechanical ventilation),[86] or infection.[87] During surgery, careful attention is given to isolating and closing the bronchus in an attempt to secure a lasting seal with subsequent stump healing.[83] In addition, early extubation is encouraged to eliminate the possibility of perforation of the stump and high airway pressures.[86] Clinical manifestations of a bronchopleural fistula include shortness of breath and coughing up serosanguineous sputum. Immediate surgery is usually necessary to close the stump and prevent flooding of the remaining lung with fluid from the residual space.[87] If this occurs, the patient should be placed with the operative side down (remaining lung up) and a chest tube should be inserted to drain the residual space.[83]

Hemorrhage. Hemorrhage is an early, life-threatening complication that can occur after a lung resection. It can result from bronchial or intercostal artery bleeding or disruption of a suture or clip around a pulmonary vessel.[86] Excessive chest tube drainage can signal excessive bleeding. During the immediate postoperative period, chest tube drainage should be measured every 15 minutes; this frequency should be decreased as the patient stabilizes. If chest tube loss is greater than 100 ml/hour, fresh blood is noted, or a sudden increase in drainage occurs, hemorrhage should be suspected.

Cardiovascular Disturbances. Cardiovascular complications after thoracic surgery include dysrhythmias and pulmonary edema. Resections of a large lung area or a pneumonectomy may be followed by a rise in central venous pressure. With the loss of one lung, the right ventricle must empty its stroke volume into a vascular bed that has been reduced by 50%. This means a higher pressure system is created, which increases right ventricular workload and precipitates right ventricular failure. Depending on previous heart function, acute decompensation of both ventricles can result. Measures are aimed at supporting cardiac function and avoiding intravascular volume excess. These measures include optimizing preload, afterload, and contractility with vasoactive agents.[86]

POSTOPERATIVE NURSING MANAGEMENT

Nursing care of the patient who has had thoracic surgery incorporates a number of nursing diagnoses (see the Nursing Diagnoses feature on Thoracic Surgery). Nursing interventions include optimizing oxygenation and ventilation, preventing atelectasis, monitoring chest tubes, assisting the patient to return to an adequate activity level, providing comfort and emotional support, and maintaining surveillance for complications (also see p. 620).

Optimizing Oxygenation and Ventilation. Nursing interventions to optimize oxygenation and ventilation include positioning, preventing desaturation during procedures, and promoting secretion clearance.

Preventing Atelectasis. Nursing interventions to prevent atelectasis include proper patient positioning and early ambulation, deep-breathing exercises, incentive spirometry (IS), and pain management. The goal is to promote maximal lung ventilation and prevent hypoventilation.

Patient Positioning and Early Ambulation. The nurse should consider the surgical incision site and the type of surgery when positioning the patient. After a lobectomy, the patient should be turned onto the nonoperative side to promote V/Q matching. When the good lung is dependent and blood flow is greater to the area with better ventilation, V/Q matching is better. V/Q mismatching results when the affected lung is positioned down because of the increase in blood flow to an area with less ventilation. The patient should be turned frequently to promote secretion removal but should have the affected lung dependent as little as possible. The patient who has had a pneumonectomy should be positioned supine or on the operative side during the initial period. Turning onto the operative side promotes splint-

NURSING DIAGNOSES **Thoracic Surgery**

- Ineffective Breathing Pattern related to decreased lung expansion
- Impaired Gas Exchange related to ventilation/perfusion mismatching or intrapulmonary shunting
- Impaired Gas Exchange related to alveolar hypoventilation
- Acute Pain related to transmission and perception of cutaneous, visceral, muscular, or ischemic impulses
- Anxiety related to threat to biologic, psychologic, and/or social integrity
- Disturbed Body Image related to actual change in body structures, function, or appearance
- Compromised Family Coping related to critically ill family member

ing of the incision and facilitates deep-breathing exercises. Tilting the patient slightly toward the unaffected side is possible, but the surgeon should indicate when free side-to-side positioning is safe.[87]

When sitting at the bedside or ambulating, patients must be encouraged to keep the thorax in straight alignment while they breathe deeply. This position best accommodates diaphragmatic descent and intercostal muscle action. The sitting or standing position provides enhanced ventilation to areas of the lung that are dependent in the supine position, thus accommodating maximal inflation and promoting gas exchange. Ambulation is essential in restoring lung function and should be initiated as soon as possible.[88]

Deep Breathing and Incentive Spirometry. Deep breathing and incentive spirometry should be performed regularly by patients who have undergone a thoracotomy. Deep breathing involves having the patient take a deep breath and holding it for approximately 3 seconds or longer. Incentive spirometry involves having the patient take at least 10 deep, effective breaths per hour using an incentive spirometer. These activities help reexpand collapsed lung tissue, thus promoting early resolution of the pneumothorax in patients with partial lung resections. The chest should be auscultated during inflation to ensure that all dependent parts of the lung are well ventilated and to help the patient understand the depth of breath necessary for optimal effect. Coughing, which should be encouraged only when secretions are present, assists in mobilizing secretions for removal.[88]

Pain Management. Pain can be a major problem after thoracic surgery. Pain can increase the workload of the heart, precipitate hypoventilation, and inhibit mobilization of secretions. Clinical manifestations of pain include tachypnea, tachycardia, elevated blood pressure, facial grimacing, splinting of the incision, hypoventilation, moaning, and restlessness. Several alternatives for pain management after thoracic surgery can be used. The two most common methods are systemic narcotic administration and epidural narcotic administration. Systemic narcotics can be administered intravenously or via patient-controlled analgesia (PCA) method. In addition, the patient should be assisted with splinting the incision with a pillow or blanket when deep breathing and coughing. Splinting stabilizes the area and reduces pain when moving, deep breathing, or coughing.[89]

Maintaining the Chest Tube System. Chest tubes are placed after most thoracic surgery procedures to remove air and fluid. The drainage will initially appear bloody, becoming serosanguineous and then serous over the first 2 to 3 days postoperatively. Approximately 100 to 300 ml of drainage will occur during the first 2 hours postoperatively, which will decrease to less than 50 ml/hour over the next several hours. Routine stripping of chest tubes is not recommended because excessive negative pressure can be generated in the chest. If blood clots are present in the drainage tubing or an obstruction is present, the chest tubes may be carefully milked. The chest tube may be placed to suction or water seal.[90]

During auscultation of the lungs, air leaks should be evaluated. In the early phase, an air leak is commonly heard over the affected area, because the pleura have not yet tightly sealed. As healing occurs, this leak should disappear. An increase in an air leak or the appearance of a new air leak should prompt investigation of the chest drainage system to discover whether air is leaking into the system from outside or whether the leak is originating from the incision. Increased air leaks not related to the thoracic drainage system may indicate disruption of sutures.[86]

Assisting Patient to Return to Adequate Activity Level. Within a few days after surgery, range of motion exercises for the shoulder on the operative side should be performed. The patient frequently splints the operative side and avoids shoulder movement because of pain. If immobility is allowed, stiffening of the shoulder joint can result. This is referred to as *frozen shoulder* and may require physical therapy and rehabilitation to regain satisfactory range of motion of the shoulder joint.[87]

Usually on the day after surgery, the patient is able to sit in a chair. Activity should be systematically increased, with attention to the patient's activity tolerance. With adequate pulmonary function before surgery and a surgical approach designed to preserve respiratory function, full return to previous activity levels is possible. This may take as long as 6 months to 1 year, depending on the tissue resected and the patient's general condition.[83]

LONG-TERM MECHANICAL VENTILATOR DEPENDENCE

DESCRIPTION

Long-term mechanical ventilator dependence (LTMVD) is a secondary disorder that occurs when a patient requires assisted ventilation longer than expected given the patient's underlying condition;[91] usually the patient will have also failed at least one weaning attempt.[92] It is the result of complex medical problems that do not allow the weaning process to take place in a normal and timely manner.

ETIOLOGY AND PATHOPHYSIOLOGY

A wide variety of physiologic and psychologic factors contribute to the development of LTMVD. Physiologic factors include those conditions that result in decreased gas exchange, increased ventilatory workload, increased ventilatory demand, decreased ventilatory drive, and increased respiratory muscle fatigue (Box 23-14).[93] Psychologic factors include those conditions that result in loss of breathing pattern control, lack of motivation and confidence, and delirium (Box 23-15). The development of LTMVD also is affected by the severity and duration of the patient's current illness and any underlying chronic health problems.[94]

MEDICAL AND NURSING MANAGEMENT

The goal of medical and nursing management of the patient with LTMVD is successful weaning. The Third National Study Group on Weaning from Mechanical Ventilation, sponsored by the American Association of Critical-Care Nurses, proposed the Weaning Continuum Model that divides weaning into three stages: preweaning, weaning process, and weaning outcome.[95] It is within this framework that the management of the long-term ventilator-dependent patient is described. In addition, the common nursing diagnoses for this patient population are listed in the Nursing Diagnoses feature on Long-Term Mechanical Ventilation.

Preweaning Stage. For the long-term ventilator-dependent patient, the preweaning phase consists of resolving the precipitating event that necessitated ventilatory assistance and preventing the physiologic and psychologic factors that can interfere with weaning. Before any attempts at weaning, the patient should be assessed for weaning readiness, an approach should be determined, and a method should be selected.[96]

Weaning Preparedness. The patient should be physiologically and psychologically prepared to initiate the weaning process by addressing those factors that can interfere with weaning. Aggressive medical management to prevent and treat ventilation/perfusion mis-

Box 23-14

PHYSIOLOGIC FACTORS CONTRIBUTING TO LTMVD

Decreased gas exchange
- Ventilation/perfusion mismatching
- Intrapulmonary shunting
- Alveolar hypoventilation
- Anemia
- Acute heart failure

Increased ventilatory workload
- Decreased lung compliance
- Increased airway resistance
- Small endotracheal tube
- Decreased ventilatory sensitivity
- Improper positioning
- Abdominal distention
- Dyspnea

Increased ventilatory demand
- Increased pulmonary dead space
- Increased metabolic demands
- Improper ventilator mode/settings
- Metabolic acidosis
- Overfeeding

Decreased ventilatory drive
- Respiratory alkalosis
- Metabolic alkalosis
- Hypothyroidism
- Sedatives
- Malnutrition

Increased respiratory muscle fatigue
- Increased ventilatory workload
- Increased ventilatory demand
- Malnutrition
- Hypokalemia
- Hypomagnesemia
- Hypophosphatemia
- Hypothyroidism
- Critical illness polyneuropathy
- Inadequate muscle rest

LTMVD, Long-term mechanical ventilation dependence.

Box 23-15

PSYCHOLOGIC FACTORS CONTRIBUTING TO LTMVD

Loss of breathing pattern control
- Anxiety
- Fear
- Dyspnea
- Pain
- Ventilator asynchrony
- Lack of confidence in ability to breathe

Lack of motivation and confidence
- Inadequate trust in staff
- Depersonalization
- Hopelessness
- Powerlessness
- Depression
- Inadequate communication

Delirium
- Sensory overload
- Sensory deprivation
- Sleep deprivation
- Pain
- Medications

LTMVD, Long-term mechanical ventilation dependence.

NURSING DIAGNOSES   Long-Term Mechanical Ventilation Dependence

- Impaired Spontaneous Ventilation related to respiratory muscle fatigue or neuromuscular impairment
- Dysfunctional Ventilatory Weaning Response related to physical, psychosocial, or situational factors
- Risk for Aspiration
- Imbalanced Nutrition: Less Than Body Requirements related to lack of exogenous nutrients or increased metabolic demand
- Risk for Infection
- Acute Confusion related to sensory overload, sensory deprivation, and sleep pattern disturbance
- Disturbed Body Image related to functional dependence on life-sustaining technology
- Anxiety related to threat to biologic, psychologic, and/or social integrity
- Powerlessness related to lack of control over current situation or disease progression
- Compromised Family Coping related to critically ill family member

matching, intrapulmonary shunting, anemia, cardiac failure, decreased lung compliance, increased airway resistance, acid-base disturbances, hypothyroidism, abdominal distention, and electrolyte imbalances should be initiated. In addition, interventions to decrease the work of breathing should be implemented, such as replacing a small endotracheal tube with a larger tube or a tracheostomy, suctioning airway secretions, administering bronchodilators, optimizing the ventilator settings and trigger sensitivity, and positioning the patient in straight alignment with the head of the bed elevated at least 30 degrees. Enteral or parenteral nutrition should be started and the patient's nutritional state optimized. Physical therapy should be initiated for the patient with critical illness polyneuropathy because increased mobility facilitates weaning. A means of communication should be established with the patient. Sedatives can be administered to provide anxiety control, but the avoidance of respiratory depression is critical.[97]

Weaning Readiness. Although a variety of different methods for assessing weaning readiness have been developed, none has proven to be very accurate in predicting weaning success in the patient with LTMVD. One study did indicate that the presence of left ventricular dysfunction, fluid imbalance, and nutritional deficiency increased the duration of mechanical ventilation. Another study suggested that the upward trending of the albumin level may be predictive of weaning success. Because so many variables can affect the patient's ability to wean, any assessment of weaning readiness should incorporate these variables. Cardiac function, gas exchange, pulmonary mechanics, nutritional status, electrolyte and fluid balance, and motivation should all be considered when making the decision to wean. This assessment should be ongoing to reflect the dynamic nature of the process.[98]

Weaning Approach. Although weaning the patient requiring short-term mechanical ventilation is a relatively simple process that can usually be accomplished with a nurse and respiratory therapist, weaning the patient with LTMVD is a much more complex process that usually requires a multidisciplinary team approach. Multidisciplinary weaning teams that use a coordinated and collaborative approach to weaning have demonstrated improved patient outcomes and decreased weaning times. The team should consist of a physician, a nurse, a respiratory therapist, a dietitian, a physical therapist, and a case manager, a clinical outcomes manager, or a clinical nurse specialist. Additional members, if possible, should include an occupational therapist, a speech therapist, a discharge planner, and a social worker. Working together, the team members should develop a comprehensive plan of care for the patient that is efficient, consistent, progressive, and cost-effective.[99] Several studies have demonstrated successful weaning through the use of nurse and respiratory therapist managed protocols.[100]

Collaborative management of the patient requiring long-term mechanical ventilation is outlined in Fig. 23-4.

Weaning Method. A variety of weaning methods are available, but no one method has consistently proven to be superior to the others. These methods include T-tube (T-piece), constant positive airway pressure (CPAP), pressure support ventilation (PSV), and synchronized intermittent mandatory ventilation (SIMV). One recent multicenter study lends evidence to support the use of PSV for weaning over T-tube or SIMV weaning. Often these weaning methods are used in combination with each other, such as SIMV with PSV, CPAP with PSV, or SIMV with CPAP.[92]

Weaning Process Stage. For the long-term ventilator patient, the weaning process phase consists of initiating the weaning method selected and minimizing the physiologic and psychologic factors that can interfere with weaning.[95] It is imperative that the patient not become exhausted during this phase, because this can result in a setback in the weaning process.[97] During this phase the patient is assessed for weaning progress and signs of weaning intolerance.[92]

Weaning Initiation. Weaning should be initiated in the morning while the patient is rested. Before starting the weaning process, the patient is provided with an explanation of how the process works, a description of the sensations to expect, and reassurances that he or she will be closely monitored and returned to the original ventilator mode and settings if any difficulty occurs.[92] This information should be reinforced with each weaning attempt.

T-tube and CPAP weaning are accomplished by removing the patient from the ventilator and then placing the patient on a T-tube or by placing the patient on CPAP mode for a specified duration of time, known as a weaning trial, for a specified number of times per day. When the weaning trial is over, the patient is placed on the assist-control mode (continuous mandatory ventilation mode on the Puritan-Bennett 7200 ventilator) of the ventilator and allowed to rest to prevent respiratory muscle fatigue. Gradually the duration of time spent weaning is increased, as is the frequency, until the patient is able to breathe spontaneously for 24 hours. If PSV is used in conjunction with CPAP, the PSV is initially set to provide the patient with an assisted tidal volume of 10 to 12 ml/kg, and this is gradually weaned until a level of 6 to 8 cm H_2O of pressure support is achieved. SIMV and PSV weaning are accomplished by gradually decreasing the number of breaths or the amount of pressure support the patient receives by a specified amount until the patient is able to breathe spontaneously for 24 hours.[92]

Weaning Progress. Weaning progress can be evaluated using various methods. Evaluation of weaning progress when using a weaning method that gradually withdraws ventilatory support, such as SIMV or PSV, can be accomplished by measuring the percentage of the minute ventilation requirement that is provided by the ventilator. If the percentage steadily decreases, weaning is progressing. Evaluation of weaning progress when using a weaning method that removes ventilatory support, such as T-tube or CPAP, can be accomplished by measuring the amount of time the patient remains free from support. If the time steadily increases, weaning is progressing.[92]

Weaning Intolerance. Once the weaning process has begun, the patient should be continuously assessed for signs of intolerance. When present, these signs indicate when to place the patient back on the ventilator or to return the patient to the previous ventilator settings. Commonly used indicators include dyspnea, accessory muscle use, restlessness, anxiety, change in facial expression, changes in heart rate and blood pressure, rapid, shallow breathing, and discomfort.[98] Table 23-7

LONG TERM DEPENDENCE ON MECHANICAL VENTILATION*

	WEANING PHASE	EXTENDING WEANING PHASE	POST WEANING PHASE — EXTUBATION/ DECANNULATION	POST WEANING PHASE — VENTILATOR FACILITY PLACEMENT	POST WEANING PHASE — TERMINAL WEANING
DATE Criteria: —Vent >3 days —Medically stable —Unsuccessful initial weaning attempt					
CONSULTS	Pulmonary Physician/Intensivist Wean Team assessment	Consider Psychiatric evaluation Wean Team rounds qweek	SNF Pulmonary Coordinator	Placement Coordinator	Chaplain
DIAGNOSTICS/ MONITORING	As ordered ECG monitoring Continuous SpO₂ monitoring VS with weaning and q2-4h	As ordered ↑↑ VS with weaning and q8-12h	As ordered D/C ECG monitoring Spot check SpO₂ qam VS q8-12h	As ordered D/C ECG monitoring Continuous SpO₂ monitoring VS q8-12h	D/C diagnostics ECG monitoring D/C SpO₂ monitoring D/C routine VS
TREATMENTS	Pressure reduction therapy or lateral rotation therapy	↑		↑	↑
MEDICATIONS	Anxiety management Dyspnea management Pain management Sleep management Stress ulcer prophylaxis DVT prophylaxis Additional medications as ordered Bronchodilators as ordered	↑↑↑↑↑↑↑ Antidepressant therapy	↑↑↑↑↑↑↑↑	↑↑↑↑↑↑↑↑	Pain control Dyspnea control D/C all other medications
RESPIRATORY	Continue mechanical ventilation Maintain endotracheal tube Initiate/progress weaning trials to extubation or tracheostomy inserted Monitor for weaning intolerance Monitor for airway/cuff problems Monitor secretions/suction prn	↑ Place tracheostomy Progress weaning trials to T-piece ↑↑↑	D/C mechanical ventilation Extubate or button trach/decannulate IS q1-2h WA; advancing to q4h WA Monitor for respiratory distress ↑↑	Place on home ventilator Tracheostomy Continue/progress weaning trials till transfer Monitor for weaning intolerance ↑↑	D/C mechanical ventilation Tracheostomy D/C weaning trials
ACTIVITY	Maintain HOB 30°-45° Provide regular sleep periods Initiate PROM q4h WA Dangle/OOB in chair qd	Sleep 6-8 hours/night ↑ OOB in chair 2-3x/d Ambulate with PT/RT assist Bath patient prior to 2200	↑↑ D/C PROM Progressive ambulation ↑	↑↑ Continue PROM q4h WA ↑↑↑	↑ Complete bed rest D/C all activity
PHYSICAL THERAPY	PT evaluation Initiate/progress therapy to qd Strengthening/balance	PT reevaluation Progress therapy to 2x/d (if needed) Transfer/pre-gait training	Progress to 3h/d if going to Rehab ↑↑	Continue PT plan ↑	D/C therapy
				Addressograph	

*This clinical pathway is a tool to assist health care providers in achieving quality patient outcomes by providing appropriate and timely patient care. It is not intended to establish a community standard of care, replace a clinician's medical judgment, establish a protocol for all patients, or exclude alternative therapies.

SNF, Skilled nursing facility; *ECG,* electrocardiogram; *D/C,* discontinue; *VS,* vital signs; *DVT,* deep vein thrombosis; *WA,* when awake; *HOB,* head of bed; *PROM,* passive range of motion; *OOB,* out of bed; *PT,* physical therapy; *RT,* respiratory therapy; *ST,* speech therapy; *OT,* occupational therapy; *P-M,* Passy-Muir; *M-F,* Monday through Friday; *UE,* upper extremity; *ADLs,* activities of daily living; *RD,* registered dietitian; *I&O,* intake and output; *IV,* intravenous; *PEG,* percutaneous endoscopic gastrostomy; *PICC,* peripherally inserted central catheter; *LCSW,* licensed clinical social worker; *SO,* significant other; *CM,* case manager; *WT,* weight.

Continued

Fig. 23-4 Interdisciplinary plan of care: long-term mechanical ventilation dependence.

LONG TERM DEPENDENCE ON MECHANICAL VENTILATION*

DATE	WEANING PHASE	EXTENDING WEANING PHASE	EXTUBATION/ DECANNULATION	POST WEANING PHASE	
				VENTILATOR FACILITY PLACEMENT	TERMINAL WEANING
SPEECH THERAPY		ST evaluation for P-M valve and swallowing; Initiate/progress P-M valve to at least 60 min	ST reevaluation for swallowing; Initiate swallowing therapy if positive for aspiration	ST reevaluation; Continue ST plan	D/C therapy
OCCUPATIONAL THERAPY	OT evaluation; Initiate/progress therapy to 3x/wk; Initiate self-hygiene/grooming	OT reevaluation; Progress therapy to qd (M-F); Hygiene, grooming, and sitting; Graded UE strengthening	↑↑; Dress and bathing training; Stand for ADLs	↑ Continue OT plan	D/C therapy
NUTRITION	RD evaluation; Initiate/progress nutritional support to enteral feedings; Monitor I&O qd; Weigh patient qwk; Insert small-bore feeding tube; Maintain IV access	RD reevaluation; Continue enteral feedings/start oral feedings if negative for aspiration; ↑↑; Place PEG; Insert PICC	Progress to total oral feedings if negative for aspiration; D/C feeding tube and IV access when no longer needed	↑ Continue RD plan; Maintain PEG; Maintain PICC	D/C nutritional support; D/C I&O; D/C weights
SOCIAL SERVICES	LCSW evaluation; Identify sources of support and prior level of functioning; Support for SO; Conduct initial SO conferences	LCSW reevaluation; Maintain communication with SO; ↑; Conduct follow-up SO conference	↑↑; ↑; Conduct SO conferences as needed	↑; Continue LCSW plan; ↑; Conduct transfer SO conference	↑↑; ↑↑
TEACHING	Orient patient/SO to environment/procedures/equipment; Explain weaning plan to patient/SO		Initiate/complete disease management education; Explain discharge plan to patient/SO	Orient patient/SO to environment/procedures/equipment; Explain transfer plan to patient/SO	Explain terminal weaning to patient (as appropriate)/SO
DISCHARGE PLANNING	CM evaluation; Clarify payor issues; Transfer to long-term ventilator unit	CM reevaluation; Initiate referral process (as indicated); Initiate transfer summary form; Transfer to acute care no earlier than 72h after D/C ventilator	↑; Complete referral process; Complete transfer summary form; Discharge to SNF/rehab/home (with home care) no earlier than 72h after D/C tracheostomy	↑; Arrange transportation; Transfer/discharge to ventilator facility	
EXPECTED OUTCOMES — To be reviewed qwk at WT rounds	• LTMV-WT evaluation completed • Skin remains intact • Anxiety controlled • Rests at regular periods • OOB in chair qd • Participates in PT qd • Participates in OT 3x/wk • Meets needs on enteral nutrition • Initial SO conference done • Transferred to 2 West • Weaned to T-piece/tracheostomy completed <21 days after intubation • Absence of complications	• Skin remains intact • Anxiety controlled • Rest 6 hours at night • OOB in chair 2x/d • Participates in PT 2x/d • Participates in OT qd (M-F) • Uses P-M valve for 60 min • Swallowing evaluated before oral feeding initiated • Meets needs on enteral nutrition • Follow-up SO conference done • Transferred to 4T • Weaned to T-piece • Absence of complications	• Extubated/decannulated without difficulty • Trach buttoned prior to decannulation • Discharged no earlier than 72h after decannulation • Patient education completed • Discharged without delay • Absence of complications	• Transferred/discharged without delay • Absence of complications	• SO conference done • Dyspnea controlled • Life support withdrawn without problems

Fig. 23-4, cont'd

Table 23-7	Weaning Intolerance Indications and Interventions	
Indicator	**Etiology**	**Intervention**

PULMONARY SIGNS (EMOTIONAL)

Altered breathing pattern	Inadequate understanding of	Build trust in staff; consistent care providers
Dyspnea intensity	weaning process	Encouragement; concrete goals for extubation
Change in facial expression	Inability to control breathing	Involve patient in process and planning daily activities
	pattern	Efficient communication established
	Environmental factors	Organize care; avoid interruptions during weaning
		Adequate sleep
		Calm, caring presence of nurse; nonsedating anxiolytics
		Measure dyspnea
		Fan; music
		Biofeedback; relaxation; breathing control
		Family involvement; normalizing daily activities

PULMONARY SIGNS (PHYSIOLOGIC)

Accessory muscle use	Airway obstruction	Suction/air-mask bag unit ventilation; manually ventilate patient
Prolonged expiration	Secretions/atelectasis	
Asynchronous movements of chest and abdomen	Bronchospasm	Bronchodilators
	Patient position/kinked	Sitting upright in bed or chair or per patient preference
Retractions	ET tube	
Facial expression changes	Increased workload or muscle	
Dyspnea	fatigue	
Shortened inspiratory time	Caloric intake	Dietary assessment
Increased breathing frequency, decreased V_T	Electrolyte imbalances	Assess electrolytes; give replacements as necessary
	Inadequate rest	Rest between weaning trials (i.e., SIMV frequency rate >5)
	Patient/ventilator interactions	Assess ventilator settings (i.e., flow rate, trigger sensitivity)
	Increased V_E requirement	Muscle training if appropriate
	Infection	Check for infection (treat if indicated)
	Overfeeding	Appropriate caloric intake
	Respiratory alkalosis	Baseline ABGs achieved (ventilate according to pH)
	Anxiety	Coaching to regularize breathing pattern; give nonsedating anxiolytics
	Pain	Judicious use of analgesics

CNS CHANGES

Restless/irritable	Hypoxemia/hypercarbia	Increase Fio_2
Decreased responsiveness		Return to mechanical ventilation
		Discern etiology and treat

CV DETERIORATION

Excessive change in BP or HR	Heart failure	Diuretics as ordered
	Increase venous return	Beta-blockers
Dysrhythmias	Ischemia	Increase Fio_2
Angina		Return to mechanical ventilation
Dyspnea		Discern etiology and treat

Modified from Knebel AR: *Am J Crit Care* 1(3):19, 1992.
ET, Endotracheal; *SIMV,* synchronized intermittent mandatory ventilation; V_E, respiratory minute volume; V_T, tidal volume; *ABGs,* arterial blood gases; *Fio_2,* fraction of inspired oxygen; *CNS,* central nervous system; *CV,* cardiovascular; *BP,* blood pressure; *HR,* heart rate.

list the different weaning intolerance indicators and actions that can be taken to control or prevent them.

Facilitative Therapies. Additional therapies may be needed to facilitate weaning in the patient who is having difficulty making weaning progress. These therapies include ventilatory muscle training and biofeedback. Inspiratory muscle training is used to enhance the strength and endurance of the respiratory muscles. Biofeedback can be used to promote relaxation and assist in the management of dyspnea and anxiety.[92]

Weaning Outcome Stage. Two outcomes are possible for a patient with LTMVD: weaning completed and incomplete weaning.[91]

Weaning Completed. Weaning is deemed successful when a patient is able to breathe spontaneously for 24 hours without ventilatory support. Once this occurs, the patient may be extubated or decannulated at any time, though this is not necessary for weaning to be considered successful.[91]

Incomplete Weaning. Weaning is deemed incomplete when a patient has reached a plateau (5 days at the same ventilatory support level without any changes) in the weaning process despite managing the physiologic and psychologic factors that impede weaning. Thus the patient is unable to breathe spontaneously for 24 hours without full or partial ventilatory support. Once this occurs, the patient should be placed in a subacute ventilator facility or discharged home on a ventilator with home care nursing follow-up.[91]

REFERENCES

1. Christie HA, Goldstein LS: Respiratory failure and the need for ventilatory support. In Wilkins RL, Stoller JK, Scanlan CL, editors: *Egan's fundamentals of respiratory care*, ed 8, St Louis, 2003, Mosby.
2. Flaatten H et al: Outcome after acute respiratory failure is more dependent on dysfunction in other vital organs than on severity of the respiratory failure, *Crit Care* 7:R72, 2003.
3. Vincent JL et al: The epidemiology of acute respiratory failure in critically ill patient, *Chest* 121:1602, 2002.
4. Balk R, Bone RC: Classification of acute respiratory failure, *Med Clin North Am* 67:551, 1983.
5. Curtis JR, Hudson LD: Emergent assessment and management of acute respiratory failure in COPD, *Clin Chest Med* 15:481, 1994.
6. Raju P, Manthous CA: The pathogenesis of respiratory failure, *Respir Care Clin North Am* 6:195, 2000.
7. West JD, Wagner PD: Ventilation, blood flow and gas exchange. In Murray JF, Nadel JA, editors: *Textbook of respiratory medicine*, ed 3, Philadelphia, 2000, Saunders.
8. Misasi RS, Keyes JL: The pathophysiology of hypoxia, *Crit Care Nurse* 14(4):55, 1994.
9. Sigillito RJ, DeBlieux: Evaluation and initial management of the patient in respiratory distress, *Emerg Med Clin North Am* 21:239, 2003.
10. Dakin J, Griffiths M: The pulmonary physician in critical care 1: pulmonary investigations for acute respiratory failure, *Thorax* 57:79, 2002.
11. Misasi RS, Keyes JL: Matching and mismatching ventilation and perfusion in the lung, *Crit Care Nurse* 16(3):23, 1996.
12. Peter JV et al: Noninvasive ventilation in acute respiratory failure—a meta-analysis update, *Crit Care Med* 30:555, 2002.
13. Kwok H et al: Controlled trial of oronasal versus nasal mask ventilation in the treatment of acute respiratory failure, *Crit Care Med* 31:468, 2003.
14. Soo Hoo GW, Hakimian N, Santiago SM: Hypercapnic respiratory failure in COPD patients: response to therapy, *Chest* 117:169, 2000.
15. Gali B, Goyal DG: Positive pressure mechanical ventilation, *Emerg Med Clin North Am* 21:453, 2003.
16. Palm KM, Decker WW: Acute exacerbation of chronic obstructive pulmonary disease, *Emerg Med Clin North Am* 21:331, 2003.
17. Jacobi J et al: Clinical practice guidelines for the sustained use of sedatives and analgesics in the critically ill adult, *Crit Care Med* 30:119, 2002.
18. Murray MJ et al: Clinical practice guidelines for sustained neuromuscular blockade in the adult critically ill patient, *Crit Care Med* 30:142, 2002.
19. Holmes CL: The evaluation and management of shock, *Clin Chest Med* 24:775, 2003.
20. Parrish CR, McCray S: Nutrition support for the mechanically ventilated patient, *Crit Care Nurse* 23(1):79, 2003.
21. Sloan DS: Nutritional support of the critically ill and injured patient, *Crit Care Clin* 20:135, 2004.
22. Misra S, Ganzini L: Delirium, depression, and anxiety, *Crit Care Clin* 19:771, 2003.
23. Seidlitz M: Cardiac problems in the post acute ventilated patient, *Clin Chest Med* 22:175, 2001.
24. Williams MT et al: Venous thromboembolism in the intensive care unit, *Crit Care Clin* 19:185, 2003.
25. Cash BD: Evidence-based medicine as it applies to acid suppression in the hospitalized patient, *Crit Care Med* 30:S373, 2002.
26. Wong WP: Use of body positioning in the mechanically ventilated patient with acute respiratory failure: application of Sackett's rules of evidence, *Physiother Theory Pract* 15(1):25, 1999.
27. Force TR et al: Patient position and motion strategies, *Respir Care Clin North Am* 4:665, 1998.
28. Lasater-Erhand M: The effect of patient position on arterial saturation, *Crit Care Nurse* 15(5):31, 1995.
29. Cosenza JJ, Norton LC: Secretion clearance: state-of-the-art from a nursing perspective, *Crit Care Nurse* 6(4):23, 1986.
30. Collar HR et al: Prevention of ventilator-associated pneumonia: an evidence-based systematic review, *Ann Intern Med* 138:494, 2003.
31. Krishnagopalan S et al: Body positioning of intensive care patients: clinical practice versus standards, *Crit Care Med* 30:2588, 2002.
32. Stiller K: Physiotherapy in intensive care: towards an evidence-based practice, *Chest* 118:1801, 2000.
33. Jones A, Rowe BH: Bronchopulmonary hygiene physical therapy in bronchietasis and chronic obstructive pulmonary disease: a systematic review, *Heart Lung* 29:125, 2000.
34. Khadaroo RG, Marshall JC: ARDS and the multiple organ dysfunction syndrome. Common mechanisms of a common systemic process, *Crit Care Clin* 18:127, 2002.
35. Michaels AJ: Management of posttraumatic respiratory failure, *Crit Care Clin* 20:83, 2004.
36. Bernard GR et al: The American-European consensus conference on ARDS: definitions, mechanisms, relevant outcomes, and clinical trial coordination, *Am J Respir Crit Care Med* 149:818, 1994.
37. Neff MJ: The epidemiology and definition of the acute respiratory distress syndrome, *Respir Care Clin North Am* 9:273, 2003.
38. Dechert RE: The pathophysiology of acute respiratory distress syndrome, *Respir Care Clin North Am* 9:283, 2003.
39. Cheng IW, Matthay MA: Acute lung injury and the acute respiratory distress syndrome, *Crit Care Clin* 19:693, 2003.
40. Udobi KF: Acute respiratory distress syndrome, *Am Fam Physician* 67:315, 2003.
41. Perina DG: Noncardiogenic pulmonary edema, *Emerg Med Clin North Am* 21:385, 2003.
42. Hass CF: Lung protective mechanical ventilation in acute respiratory distress syndrome, *Respir Care Clin North Am* 9:363, 2003.

43. Rouby, JJ et al: Mechanical ventilation in patients with acute respiratory distress syndrome, *Anesthesiology* 101: 228, 2004.

44. Hickling KG: Permissive hypercapnia, *Respir Care Clin North Am* 8: 155, 2002.

45. Roseberg AL: Fluid management in patients with acute respiratory distress syndrome, *Respir Care Clin North Am* 9:481, 2003.

46. Widemann HP et al: Emerging system pharmacologic approaches in acute respiratory distress syndrome, *Respir Care Clin North Am* 9:495, 2003.

47. Anzueto A: Surfactant supplementation in the lung, *Respir Care Clin North Am* 8:211, 2002.

48. Hurford WE: Inhaled nitric oxide, *Respir Care Clin North Am* 8:261, 2002.

49. Kacmarek RM: Liquid ventilation, *Respir Care Clin North Am* 8:187, 2002.

50. Alpard SK, Zwischenberger JB: Extracorporeal gas exchange, *Respir Care Clin N Am* 4:711, 1998.

51. Piedalue F, Albert RK: Prone positioning in acute respiratory distress syndrome, *Respir Care Clin N Am* 9:495, 2003.

52. Pimentel L, McPherson SJ: Community-acquired pneumonia in the emergency department: a practical approach to diagnosis and management, *Emerg Med Clin North Am* 21:395, 2003.

53. Baudouin SV: The pulmonary physician in critical care. 3: critical care management of community acquired pneumonia, *Thorax* 57:267, 2002.

54. Rello J, Diaz E: Pneumonia in the intensive care unit, *Crit Care Med* 31:2544, 2003.

55. Niederman MS et al: Guidelines for the management of adults with community-acquired pneumonia, *Am J Respir Crit Care Med* 163:1730, 2001.

56. Alcon A, Fabregas N, Torres A: Hospital-acquired pneumonia: etiologic considerations, *Infect Dis Clin North Am,* 17:679, 2003.

57. Harris JR, Miller TH: Preventing nosocomial pneumonia: evidence-based practice, *Crit Care Nurse* 20(1):51, 2000.

58. Longworth DL, Schmitt SK: Pulmonary infections. In Wilkins RL, Stoller JK, Scanlan CL, editors: *Egan's fundamentals of respiratory care,* ed 8, St Louis, 2003, Mosby.

59. Mabie M, Wunderink RG: Use and limitation of clinical and radiologic diagnosis of pneumonia, *Semin Respir Infect* 18:72, 2003.

60. Thomas AR, Bryce TL: Ventilation in the patient with unilateral lung disease, *Crit Care Clin* 14:743, 1998.

61. Johnson JL, Hirsch CS: Aspiration pneumonia, *Postgrad Med* 113(3):99, 2003.

62. Marik PE: Aspiration pneumonitis and aspiration pneumonia, *N Engl J Med* 344:665, 2001.

63. Tietjen PA, Kaner RJ, Quinn CE: Aspiration emergencies, *Clin Chest Med* 15:117, 1994.

64. Goodwin RS: Prevention of aspiration pneumonia: a research-based protocol, *Dimen Crit Care Nurs* 15(2): 58, 1996.

65. Sadosty AT, Boie ET, Stead LG: Pulmonary embolism, *Emerg Med Clin North Am* 21:363, 2003.

66. Wood KE: Major pulmonary embolism: review of a pathophysiologic approach to the golden hour of hemodynamically significant pulmonary embolism, *Chest* 121:877, 2002.

67. Kearon C: Diagnosis of pulmonary embolism, *CMAJ* 168: 183, 2003.

68. Trowbridge RL et al: The effects of helical computed tomography on diagnostic and treatment strategies in patients with suspected pulmonary complications, *Am J Med* 116:84, 2004.

69. Ramzi DW, Leeper KV: DVT and pulmonary embolism: part II. Treatment and prevention, *Am Fam Physician* 69:2841, 2004.

70. Agnelli G, Becattini C, Kirschstein T: Thrombolysis vs heparin in the treatment of pulmonary embolism: a clinical outcome–based meta-analysis, *Arch Intern Med* 162: 2537, 2002.

71. Yalamanchili K et al: Open pulmonary embolectomy for treatment of major pulmonary embolism, *Ann Thorac Surg* 77:819, 2004.

72. Rodrigo GJ, Rodrigo C, Hall JB: Acute asthma in adults: a review, *Chest* 125:1081, 2004.

73. Higgins JC: The "crashing asthmatic," *Am Fam Physician* 67:997, 2003.

74. Phipps P, Garrard CS: The pulmonary physician in critical care. 12: acute severe asthma in the intensive care unit, *Thorax* 58:81, 2003.

75. Siwik JP, Nowak RM, Zoratti EM: The evaluation and management of acute, severe asthma, *Med Clin North Am* 5:1049, 2002.

76. Strange C: Pleural diseases. In Scanlan CL, Wilkins RL, Stoller JK, editors: *Egan's fundamentals of respiratory care,* ed 8, St Louis, 2003, Mosby.

77. Adams AB, Simonson DA, Dries DJ: Ventilator-induced lung injury, *Respir Care Clin North Am* 9:343, 2003.

78. O'Donovan PB, Stoller JK: A synopsis of thoracic imaging. In Wilkins RL, Stoller JK, Scanlan CL, editors: *Egan's fundamentals of respiratory care,* ed 8, St Louis, 2003, Mosby.

79. Reference deleted in proofs.

80. Mularski RA, Sippel JM, Osborne, ML: Pneumoperitoneum: a review of nonsurgical causes, *Crit Care Med* 28:2638, 2000.

81. Miura H et al: Clinical features of medical pneumomediastinum, *Ann Thorac Cardiovasc Surg* 9:188, 2003.

82. Brander L et al: Continuous left hemidiaphragm sign revisited: a case of spontaneous pneumopericardium and literature review, *Heart* 88:e5, 2002.

83. Dawes BSG: Thoracic surgery. In Rothrock JC, Smith DA, McEwen DR, editors: *Alexander's care of the patient in surgery,* ed 12, St Louis, 2003, Mosby.

84. Tamul PC, Peruzzi WT: Assessment and management of patients with pulmonary disease, *Crit Care Med* 32:S137, 2004.

85. Cohen E: Management of one-lung ventilation, *Anesthesiol Clin North Am* 19:475, 2001.

86. Kopec SE: The postpneumonectomy state, *Chest* 114: 1158, 1998.

87. Brenner Z, Addona C: Caring for the pneumonectomy patient: challenges and changes, *Crit Care Nurse* 15(5):65, 1995.

88. Brooks, JA: Postoperative nosocomial pneumonia: nurse-sensitive interventions, *AACN Clin Issues* 12:305, 2001.

89. Hazelrigg SR, Cetindag IB, Fullerton J: Acute and chronic pain syndromes after thoracic surgery, *Surg Clin North Am* 82:849, 2002.

90. Cerfolio RJ: Advances in thoracostomy tube management, *Surg Clin North Am* 82:833, 2002.

91. Knebel AR et al: Weaning from mechanical ventilation: concept development, *Am J Crit Care Nurs* 3:416, 1994.

92. Burns SM: *Weaning from long-term mechanical ventilation,* Aliso Viejo, Calif, 1998, American Association of Critical-Care Nurses.

93. Rossi A, Poggi R, Roca J: Physiologic factors predisposing to chronic respiratory failure, *Respir Care Clin North Am* 8:379, 2002.

94. MacIntyre NR: Psychological factors in weaning from mechanical ventilatory support, *Respir Care* 40:277, 1995.
95. Knebel AR et al: Weaning from mechanical ventilatory support: refinement of a model, *Am J Crit Care Nurs* 7:149, 1998.
96. Chatila WM, Criner GJ: Complications of long-term mechanical ventilation, *Respir Care Clin North Am* 8:419, 2002.
97. Goldstone J: The pulmonary physician in critical care. 10: difficult weaning, *Thorax* 57:986, 2002.
98. Scheinhorn DJ, Chao DC, Stearn-Hassenpflug M: Liberation from prolonged mechanical ventilation, *Crit Care Clin* 18:569, 2002.
99. Grap MJ et al: Collaborative practice: development, implementation, and evaluation of a weaning protocol for patients receiving mechanical ventilation, *Am J Crit Care* 12:454, 2003.
100. Tietsort J, McPeck M, Rinaldo-Gallo S: Respiratory care protocol development and impact, *Respir Care Clin North Am* 10:223, 2004.

CHAPTER 24

Pulmonary Therapeutic Management

OXYGEN THERAPY

Normal cellular function depends on an adequate supply of oxygen being delivered to the cells to meet their metabolic needs. The goal of oxygen therapy is to provide a sufficient concentration of inspired oxygen to permit full use of the oxygen-carrying capacity of the arterial blood, thus ensuring adequate cellular oxygenation given an adequate cardiac output (CO) and hemoglobin (Hgb) concentration.[1,2]

PRINCIPLES OF THERAPY

Oxygen is an atmospheric gas that must also be considered a drug, because—like most other drugs—oxygen has both detrimental and beneficial effects. Oxygen is one of the most commonly used and misused drugs. As a drug, it must be administered for good reason and in a proper, safe manner. Oxygen is generally ordered in liters per minute (L/min); as a concentration of oxygen expressed as a percent, such as 40%; or as a fraction of inspired oxygen (FiO_2), such as 0.4.

The primary indication for oxygen therapy is hypoxemia.[3] The amount of oxygen administered depends on the pathophysiologic mechanisms affecting the patient's oxygenation status. In most cases the amount required should provide an arterial partial pressure of oxygen (PaO_2) of greater than 60 mm Hg or an arterial hemoglobin saturation (SaO_2) of greater than 90% during both rest and exercise.[2] The concentration of oxygen given to an individual patient is a clinical judgment based on the many factors that influence oxygen transport, such as Hgb concentration, CO, and the arterial oxygen tension.[1,2]

Once oxygen therapy has begun, the patient is continuously assessed for level of oxygenation and the factors affecting it. The patient's oxygenation status is evaluated several times daily until the desired oxygen level is reached and has stabilized. If the desired response to the amount of oxygen delivered is not achieved, the oxygen supplementation is adjusted and the patient's condition reevaluated. It is important to use this dose-response method so that the lowest possible level of oxygen is administered that will still achieve a satisfactory PaO_2 or SaO_2.[2,3]

METHODS OF DELIVERY

Oxygen therapy can be delivered by many different devices (Table 24-1). Common problems with these devices include system leaks and obstructions, device displacement, and skin irritation. These devices are classified as low-flow, reservoir, or high-flow systems.[3]

Low-flow Systems. A low-flow oxygen delivery system provides supplemental oxygen directly into the patient's airway at flows of less than or equal to 8 L/min. Because this flow is insufficient to meet the patient's inspiratory volume requirements, it results in a variable FiO_2 as the inspired oxygen is mixed with room air. The patient's ventilatory pattern will also affect the FiO_2 of a low-flow system. As the patient's ventilatory pattern changes, the inspired oxygen concentration varies because of differing amounts of room air gas mixing with the constant flow of oxygen. A nasal cannula is an example of a low-flow device.[3]

Reservoir Systems. A reservoir system incorporates some type of device to collect and store oxygen between breaths. When the patient's inspiratory flow exceeds the oxygen flow of the oxygen delivery system, the patient is able to draw from the reservoir of oxygen to meet his or her inspiratory volume needs. Thus there is less mixing of the inspired oxygen with room air. A reservoir oxygen delivery system can deliver a higher FiO_2 than a low-flow system. Examples of reservoir systems are simple face masks, partial rebreathing masks, and nonrebreathing masks.[3]

High-flow Systems. With a high-flow system, the oxygen flows out of the device into the patient's airways in amounts sufficient to meet all inspiratory volume requirements. This type of system is not affected by the patient's ventilatory pattern. An air-entrainment mask is an example of a high-flow system.[1,3]

Complications of Oxygen Therapy. Oxygen, like most drugs, has adverse effects and complications re-

Table 24-1		Oxygen Therapy Systems			
Category	**Device**	**Flow**		**Fio₂ Range (%)**	**Fio₂ Stability**
Low-flow	Nasal cannula	¹/₄-8 L/min (adults) ≤2 L/min (infants)		22-45	Variable
	Nasal catheter	¹/₄-8 L/min		22-45	Variable
	Transtracheal catheter	¹/₄-4 L/min		22-35	Variable
Reservoir	Reservoir cannula	¹/₄-4 L/min		22-35	Variable
	Simple mask	5-12 L/min		35-50	Variable
	Partial rebreathing mask	6-10 L/min (prevent bag collapse on inspiration)		35-60	Variable
	Nonrebreathing mask	6-10 L/min (prevent bag collapse on inspiration)		55-70	Variable
	Nonrebreathing circuit (closed)	3 × V_E (prevent bag collapse on inspiration)		21-100	Fixed
High-flow	Air-entrainment mask (AEM)	Varies, should provide output flow >60 L/min		24-50	Fixed
	Air-entrainment nebulizer	10-15 L/min input; should provide output flow of at least 60 L/min		28-100	Fixed

Modified from Wilkins RL, Stoller JK, Scanlan CL, editors: *Egan's fundamentals of respiratory care,* ed 8, St Louis, 2003, Mosby.
V_E, Minute volume.

sulting from its use. The old adage "if a little is good, a lot is better" does not apply to oxygen. The lung is designed to handle a concentration of 21% oxygen, with some adaptability to higher concentrations, but adverse effects and oxygen toxicity can result if a high concentration is administered for too long.[4]

Oxygen Toxicity. The most detrimental effect of breathing a high concentration of oxygen is the development of oxygen toxicity. It can occur in any patient breathing oxygen concentrations of greater than 50% for more than 24 hours. Patients most likely to develop oxygen toxicity are those who require intubation, mechanical ventilation, and high oxygen concentrations for extended periods.[1,3]

Hyperoxia, or the administration of higher-than-normal oxygen concentrations, produces an overabundance of oxygen free radicals. These radicals are responsible for the initial damage to the alveolar-capillary membrane. Oxygen free radicals are toxic metabolites of oxygen metabolism. Normally, enzymes neutralize the radicals, which prevent any damage from occurring. During the administration of high levels of oxygen, the large number of oxygen free radicals produced exhausts the supply of neutralizing enzymes. Thus damage to the lung parenchyma and vasculature occurs, resulting in the initiation of acute lung injury (ALI).[1,4]

A number of clinical manifestations are associated with oxygen toxicity. The first symptom is substernal chest pain that is exacerbated by deep breathing. A dry cough and tracheal irritation follow. Eventually, definite pleuritic pain occurs on inhalation, followed by dyspnea. Upper airway changes may include a sensation of nasal stuffiness, sore throat, and eye and ear discomforts. Chest radiographs and pulmonary function tests show

Advantages	Disadvantages	Best Use
Use on adults, children, infants; easy to apply; disposable, low cost; well tolerated	Unstable, easily dislodged; high flows uncomfortable; can cause dryness/ bleeding; polyps, deviated septum may block flow	Stable patient needing low Fio_2; home care patient requiring long-term therapy
Use on adults, children, infants; good stability; disposable, low cost	Difficult to insert; high flows increase back pressure; needs regular changing; polyps, deviated septum may block insertion; may provoke gagging, air swallowing, aspiration	Procedures where cannula difficult to use (bronchoscopy); long-term care for infants
Lower O_2 usage/cost; eliminates nasal/ skin irritation; improved compliance; increased exercise tolerance; increased mobility; enhanced image	High cost; surgical complications; in- fection; mucus plugging; lost tract	Home care or ambulatory patients who need increased mobility or who do not accept nasal oxygen
Lower O_2 usage/cost; increased mobility; less discomfort because of lower flows	Unattractive, cumbersome; poor compliance; must be regularly re- placed; breathing pattern affects performance	Home care or ambulatory patients who need increased mobility
Use on adults, children, infants; quick, easy to apply; disposable, inexpensive	Uncomfortable; must be removed for eating; prevents radiant heat loss; blocks vomitus in unconscious patients	Emergencies, short-term therapy requiring moderate Fio_2
Same as simple mask; moderate to high Fio_2	Same as simple mask; potential suf- focation hazard	Emergencies, short-term therapy re- quiring moderate to high Fio_2
Same as simple mask; high Fio_2	Same as simple mask; potential suf- focation hazard	Emergencies, short-term therapy re- quiring high Fio_2
Full range of Fio_2	Potential suffocation hazard; requires 50 psi air/O_2; blender failure common	Patients requiring precise Fio_2 at any level (21%-100%)
Easy to apply; disposable, inexpensive; stable, precise Fio_2	Limited to adult use; uncomfortable, noisy; must be removed for eating; Fio_2 >0.40 not ensured; Fio_2 varies with back pressure	Unstable patients requiring precise low Fio_2
Provides temperature control and extra humidification	Fio_2 <28% or >0.40 not ensured; Fio_2 varies with back pressure; high infection risk	Patients with artificial airways re- quiring low to moderate Fio_2

no abnormalities until symptoms are severe. Complete, rapid reversal of these symptoms occurs as soon as normal oxygen concentrations return.[4]

Carbon Dioxide Retention. In patients with severe chronic obstructive pulmonary disease (COPD), carbon dioxide (CO_2) retention may occur as a result of administering oxygen in higher concentrations. A number of possible theories have been proposed for this phenomenon. One theory states that in patients with COPD the normal stimulus to breathe (increasing CO_2 levels) is muted and decreasing oxygen levels become the stimulus to breathe. When oxygen is administered and hypoxemia corrected, the stimulus to breathe is abolished and hypoventilation develops, resulting in a further increase in the arterial partial pressure of carbon dioxide ($Paco_2$).[3] Another theory is that the administration of oxygen abolishes the compensatory response of hypoxic pulmonary vasoconstriction. This results in an increase in perfusion of underventilated alveoli and the development of dead space, producing ventilation/perfusion mismatching. As alveolar dead space increases, so does the retention of CO_2.[3,5] One further theory states that the rise in CO_2 is related to the proportion of deoxygenated hemoglobin to oxygenated hemoglobin (Haldane effect). Because deoxygenated hemoglobin carries more CO_2 than oxygenated hemoglobin, when oxygen is administered it increases the amount of oxygenated hemoglobin, which results in an increase in the release of CO_2 at the lung level.[5] Because of the risk of CO_2 accumulation, all chronically hypercapnic patients require careful low-flow oxygen administration.[3] (see the Clinical Application feature on Pulmonary Concepts.)

Absorption Atelectasis. Another adverse effect of high concentrations of oxygen is absorption atelectasis.

CLINICAL APPLICATION

Pulmonary Concepts

Mr. B is a 63-year-old obese man. He has a long history of chronic obstructive pulmonary disease (COPD) associated with smoking two packs of cigarettes a day for 40 years. Over the past week Mr. B has experienced a "flu-like" illness with fever, chills, malaise, anorexia, diarrhea, nausea, vomiting, and a productive cough with thick, brown, purulent sputum. His admission chest x-ray film reveals infiltrates in the right upper lobe, right middle lobe, right lower lobe, and left lower lobe. Gram stain of Mr. B's sputum contains numerous gram-positive diplococci. His baseline vital signs are BP 110/60; HR 114 (sinus tachycardia); RR 30; T 101.3° F. His baseline arterial blood gas (ABG) values on a 50% nonrebreather mask are PaO_2 50; $PaCO_2$ 33; pH 7.52; HCO_3^- 28; O_2 saturation (sat) 88%. Mr. B is diagnosed with community-acquired pneumonia.

1. Which of Mr. B's symptoms support the diagnosis of pneumonia?
2. Why is Mr. B's pneumonia referred to as "community-acquired" pneumonia?
3. Interpret Mr. B's current acid-base status.
4. Why does Mr. B's $PaCO_2$ measure 33?
5. What is the most probable cause of Mr. B's hypoxemia?

Mr. B is started on the antibiotic therapy and systemic and nebulized bronchodilators, his oxygen concentration is increased to 100%, and he is systemically hydrated with intravenous fluids. Six hours after admission, Mr. B's condition continues to deteriorate. Crackles and rhonchi are now heard throughout both lung fields, respirations are shallow, and he is no longer able to produce an effective cough. Mr. B is extremely agitated, is diaphoretic, and has marked cyanosis around his lips. His vital signs are BP 90/60; HR 130 (sinus tachycardia with occasional premature ventricular contractions); RR 30; T 103.1° F. His ABG values on a 100% nonrebreather mask are PaO_2 40; $PaCO_2$ 70; pH 7.22; HCO_3^- 28; O_2 sat 78%.

6. Given Mr. B's medical diagnosis, what is the most probable cause of his acute respiratory failure?
7. What is the most likely cause of Mr. B's agitation?
8. Interpret Mr. B's current acid-base status.
9. Outline the medical treatments you would anticipate for Mr. B.
10. What effect would turning Mr. B to his right side have on his oxygenation status?
11. List three priority nursing diagnoses for Mr. B.

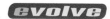 For the discussion and continuation of this Clinical Application, see the Evolve website.

Breathing high concentrations of oxygen washes out the nitrogen that normally fills the alveoli and helps hold them open (residual volume). As oxygen replaces the nitrogen in the alveoli, the alveoli start to shrink and collapse because oxygen is absorbed into the blood stream faster than it can be replaced in the alveoli, particularly in areas of the lungs that are minimally ventilated.[1,3]

NURSING MANAGEMENT

Nursing interventions for the management of the patient receiving oxygen therapy are outlined in the Nursing Interventions Classification feature on Oxygen Therapy.

ARTIFICIAL AIRWAYS

PHARYNGEAL AIRWAYS

Pharyngeal airways are used to maintain airway patency by keeping the tongue from obstructing the upper airway. The two types of pharyngeal airways are *oropharyngeal* and *nasopharyngeal*. Complications of these airways include trauma to the oral or nasal cavity, obstruction of the airway, laryngospasm, gagging, and vomiting.[6,7]

Oropharyngeal Airway. An oropharyngeal airway is made of plastic and is available in a variety of sizes. The proper size is selected by holding the airway against the side of the patient's face and ensuring that it extends from the corner of the mouth to the angle of the jaw. If the airway is improperly sized, it will occlude the airway.[6,7] An oral airway is placed by inserting a tongue depressor into the patient's mouth to displace the tongue downward and then passing the airway into the patient's mouth, slipping it over the patient's tongue (Fig. 24-1).[7] When properly placed, the tip of the airway lies above the epiglottis at the base of the tongue. It should be used only in an unconscious patient who has an absent or diminished gag reflex.[6,7]

Nasopharyngeal Airway. A nasopharyngeal airway is usually made of plastic or rubber and is available in a variety of sizes. The proper size is selected by holding the airway against the side of the patient's face and ensuring that it extends from the tip of the nose to the earlobe.[6,7] A nasal airway is placed by lubricating the tube and inserting it midline along the floor of the naris into the posterior pharynx.[7] When properly placed, the tip of the airway lies above the epiglottis at the base of the tongue.[6,7]

ENDOTRACHEAL TUBES

An endotracheal tube (ETT) is the most commonly used artificial airway for providing short-term airway manage-

NIC   Oxygen Therapy

Definition: Administration of oxygen and monitoring of its effectiveness

Activities

Clear oral, nasal, and tracheal secretions, as appropriate

Restrict smoking

Maintain airway patency

Set up oxygen equipment and administer through a heated, humidified system

Administer supplemental oxygen, as ordered

Monitor the oxygen liter flow

Monitor position of oxygen delivery device

Instruct patient about importance of leaving oxygen delivery device on

Periodically check oxygen delivery device to ensure that the prescribed concentration is being delivered

Ensure replacement of oxygen mask/cannula whenever the device is removed

Monitor patient's ability to tolerate removal of oxygen while eating

Change oxygen delivery device from mask to nasal prongs during meals, as tolerated

Observe for signs of oxygen-induced hypoventilation

Monitor for signs of oxygen toxicity and absorption atelectasis

Monitor oxygen equipment to ensure that it is not interfering with the patient's attempts to breathe

Monitor patient's anxiety related to need for oxygen therapy

Monitor for skin breakdown from friction of oxygen device

Provide for oxygen when patient is transported

Instruct patient to obtain a supplementary oxygen prescription before air travel or trips to high altitude, as appropriate

Consult with other health care personnel about use of supplemental oxygen during activity and/or sleep

Instruct patient and family about use of oxygen at home

Arrange for use of oxygen devices that facilitate mobility and teach patient accordingly

Convert to alternate oxygen delivery device to promote comfort, as appropriate

From Dochterman JM, Bulechek GM: *Nursing interventions classification (NIC),* ed 4, St Louis, 2004, Mosby.

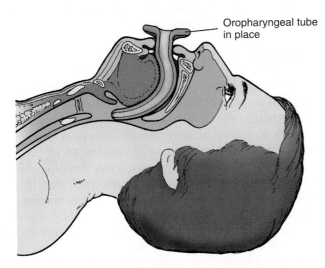

Oropharyngeal tube in place

Fig. 24-1 Oropharyngeal airway placement. (From Marshak AB: Emergency life support. In Wilkins RL, Stoller JK, Scanlan CL editors: *Egan's fundamentals of respiratory care,* ed 8, St Louis, 2003, Mosby.)

ment. Indications for endotracheal intubation include maintenance of airway patency, protection of the airway from aspiration, application of positive-pressure ventilation, facilitation of pulmonary toilet, and use of high oxygen concentrations.[8] An ETT may be placed through the orotracheal or nasotracheal route.[9,10] In most situations involving emergency placement, the orotracheal route is used because the approach is simpler and affords use of a larger diameter endotracheal tube.[10,11] Nasotracheal intubation provides greater patient comfort over time and is preferred in situations in which the patient has a jaw fracture.[9,11,12] The advantages of orotracheal intubation and nasotracheal intubation are presented in Table 24-2.

ETTs are available in a variety of sizes, sized according to the inner diameter of the tube, and have a radiopaque marker that runs the length of the tube. On one end of the tube is a cuff that is inflated using the pilot balloon. Because of the high incidence of cuff-related problems, low-pressure, high-volume cuffs are preferred. On the other end of the tube is a 15-mm adaptor that facilitates the connection of the tube to a manual resuscitation bag (MRB), T-tube, or ventilator (Fig. 24-2).[13]

Intubation. Before intubation, the necessary equipment is gathered and organized to facilitate the procedure. Readily available equipment should include a suction system with catheters and tonsil suction, an MRB with a mask connected to 100% oxygen, a laryngoscope handle with assorted blades, a variety of sizes of ETTs, and a stylet. Before the procedure is initiated, all equipment is inspected to ensure it is in working order. The patient should be prepared for the procedure, if possible, with an intravenous catheter in place, and should be monitored with a pulse oximeter. The patient is sedated before the procedure (as clinical condition allows), and a topical anesthetic is applied to facilitate placement of

Table 24-2	Advantages of Orotracheal, Nasotracheal, and Tracheostomy Tubes		
Orotracheal Tubes	**Nasotracheal Tubes**	**Tracheostomy Tubes**
Easier access Avoid nasal and sinus complications Allow for larger diameter tube, which facilitates: • Work of breathing • Suctioning • Fiberoptic bronchoscopy	Easily secured and stabilized Reduced risk of unintentional extubation Well tolerated by patient Enable swallowing and oral hygiene Facilitate communication Avoid need for bite block	Easily secured and stabilized Reduced risk of unintentional decannulation Well tolerated by patient Enable swallowing, speech, and oral hygiene Avoid upper airway complications Allow for larger diameter tube, which facilitates: • Work of breathing • Suctioning • Fiberoptic bronchoscopy

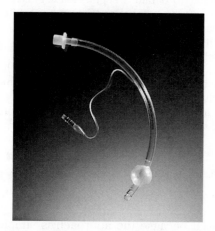

Fig. 24-2   Endotracheal tube. (Courtesy Nellcor Puritan Bennett, Pleasanton, California.)

the tube. In some cases a paralytic agent may be necessary if the patient is extremely agitated.[8,11]

The procedure is initiated by positioning the patient with the neck flexed and head slightly extended in the "sniff" position. The oral cavity and pharynx are suctioned, and any dental devices are removed. The patient is preoxygenated and ventilated using the MRB and mask with 100% oxygen. Each intubation attempt is limited to 30 seconds. Once the ETT is inserted, the patient is assessed for bilateral breath sounds and chest movement. Absence of breath sounds is indicative of an esophageal intubation, whereas breath sounds heard over only one side is indicative of a mainstem intubation. A disposable end-tidal CO_2 detector is used to initially verify correct airway placement, after which the cuff of the tube is inflated and the tube is secured. Finally, a chest radiograph is obtained to confirm placement.[8,10,11] The tip of the endotracheal tube should be approximately 3 to 4 cm above the carina when the patient's head is in the neutral position (Fig. 24-3).[10] Once final adjustment of the position is complete, the level of insertion (marked in centimeters on the side of the tube) at the teeth is noted.[8,10] A number of complications can occur during the intubation procedure, including nasal and

oral trauma, pharyngeal and hypopharyngeal trauma, vomiting with aspiration, and cardiac arrest.[14,15] Hypoxemia and hypercapnia can also occur, resulting in bradycardia, tachycardia, dysrhythmias, hypertension, and hypotension.[8,12]

Complications. A number of complications can occur while the ETT is in place, including nasal and oral inflammation and ulceration, sinusitis and otitis, laryngeal and tracheal injuries, and tube obstruction and displacement. A number of complications can occur days to weeks after the ETT is removed, including laryngeal and tracheal stenosis and a cricoid abscess (Table 24-3). Delayed complications usually require some form of surgical intervention to correct.[14,15]

TRACHEOSTOMY TUBES

A tracheostomy tube is the preferred method of airway maintenance in the patient requiring long-term intubation. Although no ideal time to perform the procedure has been identified, it is commonly accepted that if the patient has been intubated or is anticipated to be intubated for more than 2 to 3 weeks, a tracheotomy should be performed.[16] A tracheotomy is also indicated in several other situations, including upper airway obstruction or trauma and in patients with neuromuscular diseases.[16]

A tracheostomy tube provides the best route for long-term airway maintenance because it avoids the oral, nasal, pharyngeal, and laryngeal complications associated with an ETT. The tube is shorter, of wider diameter, and less curved than an ETT; thus the resistance to air flow is less, and breathing is easier. Additional advantages of a tracheostomy tube include easier secretion removal, increased patient acceptance and comfort, the possibility of the patient being able to eat and talk, and the facilitation of ventilator weaning.[11,16] Table 24-2 presents a list of the advantages of a tracheostomy tube.

Tracheostomy tubes are made of plastic or metal and may be single-lumen or double-lumen. Single-lumen tubes consist of the tube and a built-in cuff, which is connected to a pilot balloon for inflation purposes, and an obturator, which is used during tube insertion. The double-

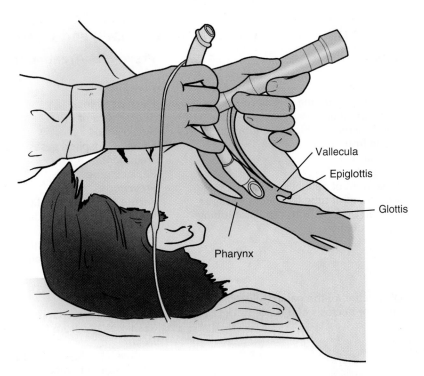

Fig. 24-3   Endotracheal tube placement. (Modified from Ellis PD, Billings DM: *Cardiopulmonary resuscitation: procedures for basic and advanced life support*, St Louis, 1980, Mosby.)

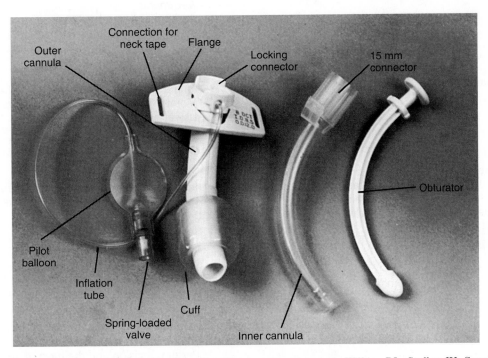

Fig. 24-4   Tracheostomy tube. (From Scanlan CL: Airway management. In Wilkins RL, Stoller JK, Scanlan CL, editors: *Egan's fundamentals of respiratory care*, ed 8, St Louis, 2003, Mosby.)

lumen tubes consist of the tube with the attached cuff, the obturator, and an inner cannula that can be removed for cleaning and then reinserted or, if disposable, replaced by a new sterile inner cannula. The inner cannula can quickly be removed if it becomes obstructed, making the system safer for patients with significant secre-tion problems. Single-lumen tubes provide a larger internal diameter for airflow than do double-lumen tubes, thus reducing airflow resistance and allowing the patient to ventilate through the tube with greater ease. Plastic tracheostomy tubes also have a 15-mm adaptor on the end (Fig. 24-4).[17]

Table 24-3	Endotracheal Tubes: Complications, Causes, and Treatment	
Complications	**Causes**	**Prevention/Treatment**
Tube obstruction	Patient biting tube Tube kinking during repositioning Cuff herniation Dried secretions, blood, or lubricant Tissue from tumor Trauma Foreign body	*Prevention:* Place bite block Sedate patient PRN Suction PRN Humidify inspired gases *Treatment:* Replace tube
Tube displacement	Movement of patient's head Movement of tube by patient's tongue Traction on tube from ventilator tubing Self-extubation	*Prevention:* Secure tube to upper lip Restrain patient's hands as needed Sedate patient PRN Ensure that only 2 inches of tube extend beyond lip Support ventilatory tubing *Treatment:* Replace tube
Sinusitis and nasal injury	Obstruction of the paranasal sinus drainage Pressure necrosis of nares	*Prevention:* Avoid nasal intubations Cushion nares from tube and tape/ties *Treatment:* Remove all tubes from nasal passages Administer antibiotics
Tracheoesophageal fistula	Pressure necrosis of posterior tracheal wall, resulting from overinflated cuff and rigid nasogastric tube	*Prevention:* Inflate cuff with minimal amount of air necessary Monitor cuff pressures every 8 hours *Treatment:* Position cuff of tube distal to fistula Place gastrostomy tube for enteral feedings Place esophageal tube for secretion clearance proximal to fistula
Mucosal lesions	Pressure at tube and mucosal interface	*Prevention:* Inflate cuff with minimal amount of air necessary Monitor cuff pressures every 8 hours Use appropriate size tube *Treatment:* May resolve spontaneously Perform surgical intervention
Laryngeal or tracheal stenosis	Injury to area from end of tube or cuff, resulting in scar tissue formation and narrowing of airway	*Prevention:* Inflate cuff with minimal amount of air necessary Monitor cuff pressures every 8 hours Suction area above cuff frequently *Treatment:* Perform tracheostomy Place laryngeal stent Perform surgical repair
Cricoid abscess	Mucosal injury with bacterial invasion	*Prevention:* Inflate cuff with minimal amount of air necessary Monitor cuff pressures every 8 hours Suction area above cuff frequently *Treatment:* Perform incision and drainage of area Administer antibiotics

PRN, As needed.

Tracheotomy. A tracheostomy tube is inserted via either an open procedure or a percutaneous procedure. An open procedure is usually performed in the operating room, whereas a percutaneous procedure can be done at the patient's bedside.[18] A number of complications can occur during the tracheotomy procedure, including misplacement of the tracheal tube, hemorrhage, laryngeal nerve injury, pneumothorax, pneumomediastinum, and cardiac arrest.[15]

Complications. A number of complications can occur while the tracheostomy tube is in place, including stomal infection, hemorrhage, tracheomalacia, tracheoesophageal fistula, tracheoinnominate artery fistula, and tube obstruction and displacement. A number of complications can occur days to weeks after the tracheostomy tube is removed; these include tracheal stenosis and a tracheocutaneous fistula (Table 24-4). Delayed complications usually require some form of surgical intervention to correct.[19]

NURSING MANAGEMENT

The patient with an endotracheal or tracheostomy tube requires some additional measures to address the effects associated with tube placement on the respiratory and other body systems (see the Nursing Interventions Classification feature on Artificial Airway Management). Nursing interventions in the management of the patient with an artificial airway include humidification, cuff management, suctioning, and communication. Because the tube bypasses the upper airway system, warming and humidifying of air must be performed by external

---

NIC   Artificial Airway Management

Definition: Maintenance of endotracheal and tracheostomy tubes and preventing complications associated with their use

Activities

Provide an oropharyngeal airway or bite block to prevent biting on the endotracheal tube, as appropriate

Provide 100% humidification of inspired gas/air

Provide adequate systemic hydration via oral or intravenous fluid administration

Inflate endotracheal/tracheostoma cuff using minimal occlusive volume technique or minimal leak technique

Maintain inflation of the endotracheal/tracheostoma cuff at 15 to 20 mm Hg during mechanical ventilation and during and after feeding

Suction the oropharynx and secretions from the top of the tube cuff before deflating cuff

Monitor cuff pressures every 4 to 8 hr during expiration using a three-way stopcock, calibrated syringe, and mercury manometer

Check cuff pressure immediately after delivery of any general anesthesia

Change endotracheal tapes/ties every 24 hr, inspect the skin and oral mucosa, and move ET tube to the other side of the mouth

Loosen commercial endotracheal tube holders at least once a day, and provide skin care

Auscultate for presence of lung sounds bilaterally after insertion and after changing endotracheal/tracheostomy ties

Note the centimeter reference marking on endotracheal tube to monitor for possible displacement

Assist with chest x-ray examination, as needed, to monitor position of tube

Minimize leverage and traction on the artificial airway by suspending ventilator tubing from overhead support, using flexible catheter mounts and swivels, and supporting tubes during turning, suctioning, and ventilator disconnection and reconnection

Monitor for presence of crackles and rhonchi over large airways

Monitor for decrease in exhale volume and increase in inspiratory pressure in patients receiving mechanical ventilation

Institute endotracheal suctioning, as appropriate

Institute measures to prevent spontaneous decannulation: secure artificial airway with tape/ties; administer sedation and muscle paralyzing agent as appropriate; and use arm restraints, as appropriate

Provide additional intubation equipment and ambu bag in a readily available location

Provide trachea care every 4 to 8 hr as appropriate: clean the inner cannula, clean and dry the area around the stoma, and change tracheostomy ties

Inspect skin around tracheal stoma for drainage, redness, and irritation

Maintain sterile technique when suctioning and providing tracheostomy care

Shield the tracheostomy from water

Provide mouth care and suction oropharynx, as appropriate

Tape the tracheostomy obturator to head of bed

Tape a second tracheostomy (same type and size) and forceps to head of bed

Institute chest physiotherapy, as appropriate

Ensure that endotracheal/tracheostomy cuff is inflated during feedings, as appropriate

Elevate head of the bed or assist patient to a sitting position in a chair during feedings, as appropriate

From Dochterman JM, Bulechek GM: *Nursing interventions classification (NIC),* ed 4, St Louis, 2004, Mosby

Table 24-4	Tracheostomy Tubes: Complications, Causes, and Treatment	
Complications	**Causes**	**Prevention/Treatment**
Hemorrhage	Vessel opening after surgery Vessel erosion caused by tube	*Prevention:* Use appropriate size tube Treat local infection Suction gently Humidify inspired gases Position tracheal window not lower than third tracheal ring *Treatment:* Pack lightly Perform surgical intervention
Wound infection	Colonization of stoma with hospital flora	*Prevention:* Perform routine stoma care *Treatment:* Remove tube, if necessary Perform aggressive wound care and debridement Administer antibiotics
Subcutaneous emphysema	Positive-pressure ventilation Coughing against a tight, occlusive dressing or sutured or packed wound	*Prevention:* Avoid suturing or packing wound closed around tube *Treatment:* Remove any sutures or packing if present
Tube obstruction	Dried blood or secretions False passage into soft tissues Opening of cannula positioned against tracheal wall Foreign body Tissue from tumor	*Prevention:* Suction PRN Humidify inspired gases Use double-lumen tube Position tube so that opening does not press against tracheal wall *Treatment:* Remove/replace inner cannula Replace tube
Tube displacement	Patient movement Coughing Traction on ventilatory tubing	*Prevention:* Use commercial tube holder Suture tube in place Use tubes with adjustable neck plates for patients with short necks Support ventilatory tubing Sedate patient PRN Restrain patient as needed *Treatment:* Cover stoma and manually ventilate patient via mouth Replace tube
Tracheal stenosis	Injury to area from end of tube or cuff, resulting in scar tissue formation and narrowing of airway	*Prevention:* Inflate cuff with minimal amount of air necessary Monitor cuff pressures every 8 hours *Treatment:* Perform surgical repair
Tracheoesophageal fistula	Pressure necrosis of posterior tracheal wall, resulting from overinflated cuff and rigid nasogastric tube	*Prevention:* Inflate cuff with minimal amount of air necessary Monitor cuff pressures every 8 hours *Treatment:* Perform surgical repair
Tracheoinnominate artery fistula	Direct pressure from the elbow of the cannula against the innominate artery Placement of tracheal stoma below fourth tracheal ring Downward migration of the tracheal stoma, resulting from traction on tube High-lying innominate artery	*Prevention:* Position tracheal window not lower than third tracheal ring *Treatment:* Hyperinflate cuff to control bleeding Remove tube and replace with endotracheal tube and apply digital pressure through stoma against the sternum Perform surgical repair
Tracheocutaneous fistula	Failure of stoma to close after removal of tube	*Treatment:* Perform surgical repair

PRN, As needed.

means. Because the cuff of the tube can cause damage to the walls of the trachea, proper cuff inflation and management is imperative. In addition, the normal defense mechanisms are impaired and secretions may accumulate; thus suctioning may be needed to promote secretion clearance. Because the tube does not allow air flow over the vocal cords, developing a method of communication is also very important. Last, observing the patient to ensure proper placement of the tube and patency of the airway is essential. Patient safety issues are addressed in the Patient Safety Alert feature on Artificial Airways.

Humidification. Humidification of air normally is performed by the mucosal layer of the upper respiratory tract. When this area is bypassed, such as occurs with both endotracheal and tracheostomy tubes, or when supplemental oxygen is used, humidification by external means is necessary. Various humidification devices add water to inhaled gas to prevent drying and irritation of the respiratory tract, to prevent undue loss of body water, and to facilitate secretion removal.[20,21] The humidification device should provide inspired gas conditioned (heated) to body temperature and saturated with water vapor.[22]

Cuff Management. Because the cuff of the endotracheal or tracheostomy tube is a major source of the complications associated with artificial airways, proper cuff management is essential. To prevent the complications associated with cuff design, only low-pressure, high-volume cuffed tubes are used in clinical practice.[13,23] Even with these tubes, cuff pressures can be generated that are high enough to lead to tracheal ischemia and injury. Both cuff inflation techniques and cuff pressure monitoring are critical components of the care of the patient with an artificial airway.[10,23]

Cuff Inflation Techniques. Two different cuff inflation techniques currently are being used: the minimal leak (ML) technique and the minimal occlusion volume (MOV) technique. The ML technique consists of injecting air into the cuff until no leak is heard and then withdrawing the air until a small leak is heard on inspiration. Problems with this technique include difficulty maintaining positive end-expiratory pressure (PEEP) and aspiration around the cuff. The MOV technique consists of injecting air into the cuff until no leak is heard at peak inspiration. The problem with this technique is that it generates higher cuff pressures than does the ML technique. The selection of one technique over the other is determined by individual patient needs. If the patient needs a seal to provide adequate ventilation and/or is at high risk for aspiration, the MOV technique is used. If these are not concerns, usually the ML technique is used.[10-11,22,23]

Cuff Pressure Monitoring. Cuff pressures are monitored at least every shift with a cuff pressure manometer. Cuff pressures should be maintained at 20 to 25 mm Hg (24 to 30 cm H_2O), because greater pressures decrease blood flow to the capillaries in the tracheal wall and lesser pressures increase the risk of aspiration. Pressures in excess of 22 mm Hg (30 cm H_2O) should be reported to the physician. In addition, cuffs are not routinely deflated, because this increases the risk of aspiration.[10,22,23]

Foam Cuff Tracheostomy Tubes. One tracheostomy tube on the market has a cuff made of foam that is self-inflating (Fig. 24-5). It is deflated during insertion; afterwards the pilot port is opened to atmospheric pressure (room air), and the cuff self-inflates. Once inflated, the foam cuff conforms to the size and shape of the patient's trachea, thereby reducing the pressure against the tracheal wall. The pilot port is either left open to atmospheric pressure or attached to the mechanical ventilator tubing, thus allowing the cuff to inflate and deflate with

PATIENT SAFETY ALERT | **Artificial Airways**

In the event of unintentional extubation or decannulation, the patient's airway should be opened with the head tilt–chin lift maneuver and maintained with an oropharyngeal or nasopharyngeal airway. If the patient is not breathing, he or she should be manually ventilated with a manual resuscitation bag and face mask with 100% oxygen. In the case of a tracheostomy, the stoma should be covered to prevent air from escaping through it.

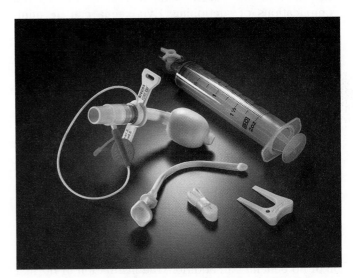

Fig. 24-5 Foam cuff tracheostomy tube. (Courtesy Smiths Medical, Inc., London, UK.)

the cycling of the ventilator. Routine maintenance of a foam cuff tracheostomy tube includes aspirating the pilot port every 8 hours to measure cuff volume, to remove any condensation from the cuff area, and to assess the integrity of the cuff. Removal is accomplished by deflating the cuff; this can be complicated if the plastic sheath covering the foam is perforated. When perforation occurs, the foam may not be deflatable because the air cannot be totally aspirated.[24]

Suctioning. Suctioning is often required to maintain a patent airway in the patient with an endotracheal or tracheostomy tube. Suctioning is a sterile procedure that is performed only when the patient needs it and not on a routine schedule.[10,22] Indications for suctioning include coughing, secretions in the airway, respiratory distress, presence of rhonchi on auscultation, increased peak airway pressures on the ventilator, and decreasing SaO_2 or PaO_2.[11] A number of complications are associated with suctioning, including hypoxemia, atelectasis, bronchospasms, dysrhythmias, increased intracranial pressure, and airway trauma.[11]

Complications. Hypoxemia can result from disconnecting the oxygen source from the patient and/or removing the oxygen from the patient's airways when the suction is applied. Atelectasis is thought to occur when the suction catheter is larger than one half of the diameter of the ETT. Excessive negative pressure occurs when suction is applied, promoting collapse of the distal airways. Bronchospasms are the result of the stimulation of the airways with the suction catheter. Cardiac dysrhythmias, particularly bradycardias, are attributed to vagal stimulation. Airway trauma occurs with impaction of the catheter in the airways and excessive negative pressure applied to the catheter.[10,11]

Suctioning Protocol. A number of protocols regarding suctioning have been developed. Several different practices have been found helpful in limiting the complications of suctioning. Hypoxemia can be minimized by giving the patient three hyperoxygenation breaths (breaths at 100% FiO_2) with the ventilator, before the procedure and again after each pass of the suction catheter.[10,25] If the patient exhibits signs of desaturation, hyperinflation (breaths at 150% tidal volume) should be added to the procedure.[10] Atelectasis can be avoided by using a suction catheter with an external diameter less than one half of the internal diameter of the ETT. Using no greater than 120 mm Hg of suction will decrease the chances of hypoxemia, atelectasis, and airway trauma.[10] Limiting the duration of each suction pass to 10 to 15 seconds[10] and the number of passes to three or less also will help minimize hypoxemia, airway trauma, and cardiac dysrhythmias.[26] The process of applying intermittent (instead of continuous) suction has been shown to be of no benefit.[27] In addition, the instillation of normal saline to help remove secretions has not proven to be of any benefit[28] and may actually contribute to the development of hypoxemia[10,29] and lower airway colonization, resulting in hospital-acquired pneumonia.[10,30]

Closed Tracheal Suction System. One device to facilitate suctioning a patient on the ventilator is the closed tracheal suction system (CTSS) (Fig. 24-6). This device consists of a suction catheter in a plastic sleeve that attaches directly to the ventilator tubing. It allows the patient to be suctioned while remaining on the ventilator. Advantages of the CTSS include the maintenance of oxygenation and PEEP during suctioning, the reduction of hypoxemia-related complications, and the protection of staff members from the patient's secretions. The CTSS is convenient to use, requiring only one person to perform the procedure.

Concerns related to the CTSS include autocontamination, inadequate removal of secretions, and increased risk of unintentional extubation resulting from the extra weight of the system on the ventilator tubing. Autocontamination has been shown not to be an issue if the catheter is cleaned properly after every use. Inadequate removal of secretions may or may not be a problem, and further investigation is required to settle this issue.[11] Though recommendations for changing the catheter vary, one study indicated that the catheter could be changed on an as-needed basis without increasing the incidence of hospital-acquired pneumonia.[31]

Communication. One of the major stressors for the patient with an artificial airway is impaired communication. This is related to the inability to speak, insufficient explanations from staff members, inadequate understanding, fear of being unable to communicate, and difficulty with communication methods.[32] A number of interventions can facilitate communication in the patient with an endotracheal or tracheostomy tube. These include performing a complete assessment of the patient's ability to communicate, teaching the patient how to communicate, using a variety of methods to communicate, and facilitating the patient's ability to communicate by providing the patient with his or her eyeglasses or hearing aid.[33]

A number of methods are available to facilitate communication in this patient population. These include the use of verbal and nonverbal language and a variety of devices to assist the short-term and long-term ventilator-assisted patient. Nonverbal communication may include the use of sign language, gestures, lip-reading, pointing, facial expressions, or eye blinking. Simple devices available include pencil and paper; Magic Slates; magnetic boards with plastic letters; picture, alphabet, or symbol boards; and flash cards. More sophisticated devices include typewriters, computers, talking tracheostomy and endotracheal tubes, and external handheld vibrators. Regardless of the method selected, the patient must be taught how to use the device.[10,33]

Passy-Muir Valve. One of the newer devices used to assist the mechanically ventilated patient with a tra-

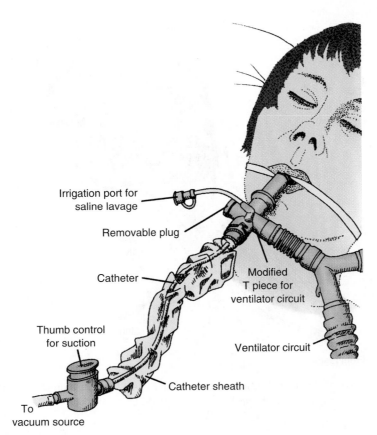

Irrigation port for
saline lavage

Removable plug

Catheter

Thumb control
for suction

To
vacuum source

Catheter sheath

Modified
T piece for
ventilator circuit

Ventilator circuit

Fig. 24-6   Closed tracheal suction system. (From Sills JR: *Entry-level respiratory therapist exam guide,* St Louis, 2000, Mosby.)

cheostomy to speak is the Passy-Muir valve. This one-way valve opens on inhalation, allowing air to enter the lungs through the tracheostomy tube, and closes on exhalation, forcing air over the vocal cords and out the mouth, thus permitting the patient to speak (Fig. 24-7). Before placing the valve on a tracheostomy tube, the cuff must be deflated to allow air to pass around the tube, and the tidal volume of the ventilator has to be increased to compensate for the air leak. In addition to assisting the patient to communicate, the Passy-Muir valve can assist the ventilator-dependent patient with relearning normal breathing patterns. The valve is contraindicated in patients with laryngeal and pharyngeal dysfunction, excessive secretions, and poor lung compliance.[34]

Oral Hygiene. Patients with artificial airways are extremely susceptible to developing hospital-acquired pneumonia due to microaspiration of subglottic secretions. Subglottic secretions are fluids from the oropharyngeal area that pool above the inflated cuff of the endotracheal tube or tracheostomy tube. These secretions are full of microorganisms from the patient's mouth. As the cuff of the artificial airway does not create a tight seal in the patient's airway, these secretions seep around the cuff and into the patient's lungs, thus promoting the development of hospital-acquired pneumonia.[35] Though bacteria are normally present in a patient's mouth, in the

critically ill patient there are increased amounts of bacteria and more resistant bacteria. Decreased salivary flow, poor mucosal status,[36] and dental plaque all contribute to this problem.[37]

Proper oral hygiene has the potential to decrease the incidence of hospital acquired pneumonia.[38,39] However, recent studies have shown that routine oral care is not a priority intervention for many nurses.[38,39] Currently there is no evidence-based protocol for oral care. Research studies are lacking, particularly with regard to frequency and effectiveness of different procedures.[40] Most experts agree, though, that oral care should consist of brushing the patient's teeth with a soft toothbrush to reduce plaque, brushing the patient's tongue and gums with a foam swab to stimulate the tissue, and performing deep oropharyngeal suction to remove any secretions that have pooled above the patient's cuff.[38,39]

Extubation/Decannulation. Once the airway is no longer needed, it is removed. Extubation is the process of removing an ETT. It is a simple procedure that can be accomplished at the bedside (see the Nursing Intervention Classification feature on Endotracheal Extubation).[10,11] Before deflating the cuff of an endotracheal or tracheostomy tube in preparation for removal, it is very important to ensure that secretions are cleared from above the tube cuff. Complications of extubation include

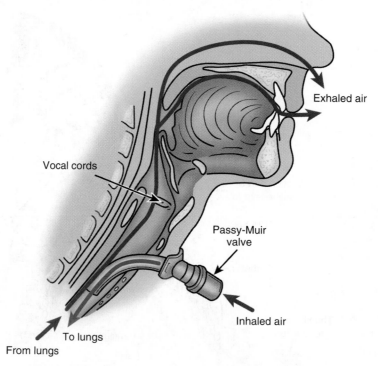

Exhaled air

Vocal cords

Passy-Muir
valve

Inhaled air

To lungs

From lungs

Fig. 24-7 Passy-Muir valve mechanism of action. (From Hodder RV: A 55-year-old patient with advanced COPD, tracheostomy tube, and sudden respiratory distress, *Chest* 121:279, 2002.)

NIC	Endotracheal Extubation

Definition: Purposeful removal of the endotracheal tube from the nasopharyngeal or oropharyngeal airway

Activities

Position the patient for best use of ventilatory muscles, usually with the head of the bed elevated 75 degrees
Instruct patient about the procedure
Hyperoxygenate the patient and suction the endotracheal airway
Suction the oral airway
Deflate the endotracheal cuff and remove the endotracheal tube
Encourage the patient to cough and expectorate sputum

Administer oxygen as ordered
Encourage coughing and deep breathing
Suction the airway, as needed
Monitor for respiratory distress
Observe for signs of airway occlusion
Monitor vital signs
Encourage voice rest for 4 to 8 hr as appropriate
Monitor ability to swallow and talk

From Dochterman JM, Bulechek GM: *Nursing interventions classification (NIC)*, ed 4, St Louis, 2004, Mosby.

---

sore throat, stridor, hoarseness, odynophagia, vocal cord immobility, pulmonary aspiration, and cough.[15] Decannulation is the process of removing a tracheostomy tube. It is also a simple process that can be performed at the bedside. After the removal of the tracheostomy tube, the stoma is usually covered with a dry dressing, with the expectation that the stoma will close within several days.[10,11] Difficulty removing the tracheostomy tube as a result of a tight stoma is usually the only complication associated with decannulation.[15]

INVASIVE MECHANICAL VENTILATION

INDICATIONS

Mechanical ventilation is indicated for a variety of physiologic and clinical reasons. Physiologic objectives include supporting cardiopulmonary gas exchange (alveolar ventilation and arterial oxygenation), increasing lung volume (end-expiratory lung inflation and functional residual capacity), and reducing the work of breathing.

Clinical objectives include reversing hypoxemia and acute respiratory acidosis, relieving respiratory distress, preventing or reversing atelectasis and respiratory muscle fatigue, permitting sedation and/or neuromuscular blockade, decreasing oxygen consumption, reducing intracranial pressure, and stabilizing the chest wall.[41]

TYPES OF VENTILATORS

The two main types of ventilators currently available are positive-pressure ventilators and negative-pressure ventilators. Negative-pressure ventilators are applied externally to the patient and decrease the atmospheric pressure surrounding the thorax to initiate inspiration. They generally are not used in the critical care environment. Positive-pressure ventilators use a mechanical drive mechanism to force air into the patient's lungs through an endotracheal or tracheostomy tube.[42]

Ventilator Mechanics. The ventilator must complete four phases of ventilation to properly ventilate the patient: (1) change from exhalation to inspiration; (2) inspiration; (3) change from inspiration to exhalation; and (4) exhalation. The ventilator uses four different variables to begin, sustain, and terminate each of these phases. These variables are described in terms of *volume, pressure, flow,* and *time.*[43]

Trigger. The phase variable that initiates the change from exhalation to inspiration is called the *trigger.* Breaths may be pressure-triggered or flow-triggered, based on the sensitivity setting of the ventilator and the patient's inspiratory effort; or time-triggered, based on the rate setting of the ventilator. A breath that is initiated by the patient is known as a *patient-triggered* or *patient-assisted* breath, whereas a breath that is initiated by the ventilator is known as a *machine-triggered* or *machine-controlled* breath. A *time-triggered breath* is a machine-controlled breath in which the ventilator initiates a breath after a preset amount of time has elapsed. It is controlled by the rate setting on the ventilator (thus a rate of 10 breaths/min yields one breath every 6 seconds). *Flow-triggered* and *pressure-triggered* breaths are patient-assisted breaths in which the patient initiates the breath by decreasing the flow or pressure (respectively) within the breathing circuit. Flow-triggering (also known as *flow-by*) is controlled by adjusting the flow-sensitivity setting of the ventilator, whereas pressure-triggering is controlled by adjusting the pressure-sensitivity setting. Many ventilators offer the different types of triggers in combination with each other. Thus a breath may be both time-triggered and flow-triggered, depending on the patient's ability to interact with the ventilator and initiate a breath.[42,43]

Limit. The variable that maintains inspiration is called the *limit* or *target.* Inspiration can be pressure-limited, flow-limited, or volume-limited. A pressure-limited breath is one in which a preset pressure is attained and maintained during inspiration. A flow-limited breath is one in which a preset flow is reached before the end of inspiration. A volume-limited breath is one in which a preset volume is delivered during the inspiration. However, the limit variable does not end inspiration; it only sustains it.[42,43]

Cycle. The variable that ends inspiration is called the *cycle.* The four classifications of positive-pressure ventilators are based on the cycle variable: volume-cycled, pressure-cycled, flow-cycled, and time-cycled. *Volume-cycled ventilators* are designed to deliver a breath until a preset volume is delivered. *Pressure-cycled ventilators* deliver a breath until a preset pressure is reached within the patient's airways. *Flow-cycled ventilators* deliver a breath until a preset inspiratory flow rate is achieved. *Time-cycled ventilators* deliver a breath over a preset time interval.[42,43]

Baseline. The variable that is controlled during exhalation is called the *baseline.* Pressure is almost always used to adjust this variable. The patient exhales to a certain baseline pressure that is set on the ventilator. It may be set at zero, which is atmospheric pressure, or above atmospheric pressure, which is known as *positive end-expiratory pressure (PEEP).*[42,43]

MODES OF VENTILATION

The term *ventilator mode* refers to how the machine will ventilate the patient. In other words, selection of a particular mode of ventilation determines how much the patient will participate in his or her own ventilatory pattern. The choice depends on the patient's situation and the goals of treatment. The mode is determined by the combination of phase variables selected. A large variety of modes are available (Table 24-5).[42-44] Many of these modes may be used in conjunction with each other. Because brands of ventilators vary in their ability to perform certain functions, not all modes are available on all ventilators.[43]

VENTILATOR SETTINGS

A variety of settings on the ventilator allow the ventilator parameters to be individualized to the patient and also allow selection of the desired ventilation mode (Table 24-6). In addition, each ventilator has a patient-monitoring system that allows all aspects of the patient's ventilatory pattern to be assessed, monitored, and displayed.[41,42,45]

COMPLICATIONS

Mechanical ventilation is often lifesaving, but similar to other interventions, it is not without complications. Some complications are preventable, whereas others can be minimized but not eradicated. Physiologic complications

Table 24-5	Modes of Mechanical Ventilation	
Mode of Ventilation	**Clinical Application**	**Nursing Implications**
Continuous mandatory (volume or pressure) ventilation (CMV) also known as assist-control (A/C) ventilation: delivers gas at preset tidal volume or pressure (depending on selected cycling variable) in response to patient's inspiratory efforts and will initiate breath if patient fails to do so within preset time	Volume controlled– (VC-) CMV is used as the primary mode of ventilation in spontaneously breathing patients with weak respiratory muscles Pressure controlled– (PC-) CMV is used in patients with decreased lung compliance or increased airway resistance particularly when the patient is at risk for volutrauma	Hyperventilation can occur in patients with increased respiratory rates Sedation may be necessary to limit the number of spontaneous breaths Patient on VC-CMV should be monitored for volutrauma Patient on PC-CMV should be monitored for hypercapnia
Pressure-regulated volume control ventilation (PRVCV): a variation of CMV that combines both volume and pressure features; delivers a preset tidal volume using the lowest possible airway pressure; airway pressure will not exceed preset maximum pressure limit	PRVCV is used in patients with rapidly changing pulmonary mechanics (airway resistance and lung compliance), thus limiting potential complications	
Pressure-controlled inverse ratio ventilation (PC-IRV): PC-CMV mode in which the inspiratory-to-expiratory (I:E) time ratio is greater than 1:1	PC-IRV is used in patients with hypoxemia refractory to PEEP; the longer inspiratory time increases functional residual capacity and improves oxygenation by opening collapsed alveoli, and the shorter expiratory time induces auto-PEEP that prevents alveoli from recollapsing	Requires sedation and/or pharmacologic paralysis because of discomfort Increased intrathoracic pressure can result in excessive air trapping and decreased cardiac output
Intermittent mandatory (volume or pressure) ventilation (IMV) also known as synchronous intermittent mandatory ventilation (SIMV): delivers gas at preset tidal volume or pressure (depending on selected cycling variable) and rate while allowing patient to breathe spontaneously; ventilator breaths are synchronized to patient's respiratory effort	Volume controlled– (VC-) IMV is used both as a primary mode of ventilation in a wide variety of clinical situations and as a weaning mode Pressure controlled– (PC-) IMV is used in patients with decreased lung compliance or increased airway resistance when the need to preserve the patient's spontaneous effects is important	May increase the work of breathing and promote respiratory muscle fatigue Patient should be monitored for hypercapnia, particularly with PC-IMV
Adaptive support ventilation (ASV): ventilator automatically adjusts settings to maintain 100 ml/min/kg of minute ventilation; pressure support	ASV is a computerized mode of ventilation that increases or decreases ventilatory support based on patient needs; can be used with any patient requiring volume controlled ventilation	Not intended as a weaning mode Adapts to changes in patient position
Constant positive airway pressure (CPAP): positive pressure applied during spontaneous breaths; patient controls rate, inspiratory flow, and tidal volume	CPAP is a spontaneous breathing mode used in patients to increase functional residual capacity and improve oxygenation by opening collapsed alveoli at end expiration; it is also used for weaning	Side effects include decreased cardiac output, volutrauma, and increased intracranial pressure No ventilator breaths are delivered in PEEP and CPAP mode unless used with CMV or IMV Patient needs to be monitored for hypercapnia
Airway pressure release ventilation (APRV): two different levels of CPAP (inspiratory and expiratory) are applied for set periods of time, allowing spontaneous breathing to occur at both levels	APRV is a spontaneous breathing mode used in patients to maintain alveolar recruitment without imposing additional peak inspiratory pressures that could lead to barotraumas	

PEEP, Positive end-expiratory pressure.

Table 24-5	Modes of Mechanical Ventilation—cont'd	
Mode of Ventilation	**Clinical Application**	**Nursing Implications**
Pressure support ventilation (PSV): preset positive pressure used to augment patient's inspiratory efforts; patient controls rate, inspiratory flow, and tidal volume	PSV is a spontaneous breathing mode used as the primary mode of ventilation in patients with stable respiratory drive to overcome any imposed mechanical resistance (e.g., artificial airway) PSV can also be used with IMV to support spontaneous breaths	Patient should be monitored for hypercapnia Advantages include reduced patient work of breathing and improved patient-ventilator synchrony
Volume-assured pressure support ventilation (VAPSV) also known as pressure augmentation (PA): a variation of PSV with a set tidal volume to ensure that patient receives minimum tidal volume with each pressure support breath	VAPSV is a spontaneous breathing mode used to treat acute respiratory illness and to facilitate weaning	Advantages include increased patient comfort, decreased work of breathing and decreased respiratory muscle fatigue, and promotion of respiratory muscle conditioning
Independent lung ventilation (ILV): each lung is ventilated separately	ILV is used in patients with unilateral lung disease, bronchopleural fistulas, and bilateral asymmetric lung disease	Requires a double-lumen endotracheal tube, two ventilators, sedation, and/or pharmacologic paralysis
High-frequency ventilation (HFV): delivers a small volume of gas at a rapid rate High-frequency positive-pressure ventilation (HFPPV): delivers 60-100 breaths/min High-frequency jet ventilation (HFJV): delivers 100-600 cycles/min High-frequency oscillation (HFO): delivers 900-3000 cycles/min	HFV is used in situations in which conventional mechanical ventilation compromises hemodynamic stability, with bronchopleural fistulas, during short-term procedures, and with diseases that create a risk of volutrauma	Patients require sedation and/or pharmacologic paralysis Inadequate humidification can compromise airway patency Assessment of breath sounds is difficult

associated with mechanical ventilation include ventilator-induced lung injury, cardiovascular compromise, gastrointestinal disturbances, patient-ventilator dyssynchrony, and hospital-acquired pneumonia.

Ventilator-Induced Lung Injury. Mechanical ventilation can cause two different types of injury to the lungs; air leaks and biotrauma.[46] Air leaks related to mechanical ventilation are the result of excessive pressure in the alveoli (barotrauma), excessive volume in the alveoli (volutrauma), or shearing due to repeated opening and closing of the alveoli (atelectrauma).[47] Barotrauma, volutrauma, and atelectrauma can lead to excessive alveolar wall stress and damage to the alveolar-capillary membrane, resulting in air leaking into the surrounding spaces. Once in the space, the air travels out through the hilum and into the mediastinum (pneumomediastinum), pleural space (pneumothorax), subcutaneous tissues (subcutaneous emphysema), pericardium (pneumopericardium), peritoneum (pneumoperitoneum), and retroperitoneum (pneumoretroperitoneum). The resultant disorders vary from the fairly benign to the potentially lethal—the most lethal of which include a pneumothorax or a pneumopericardium resulting in cardiac tamponade.[48] Barotruma, volutrauma, and atelectrauma can also cause the release of cellular mediators and the initiation of the inflammatory-immune response. This type of ventilator-induced injury is known as biotrauma.[49] Biotrauma can result in the development of acute lung injury.[50] To limit ventilator-induced lung injury, the plateau pressure (pressure needed to inflate the alveoli) should be kept less than 32 cm H_2O, PEEP should be used to avoid end-expiratory collapse and reopening, and the tidal volume should be set at 6 to 10 ml/kg.[46,49]

Cardiovascular Compromise. Positive-pressure ventilation increases intrathoracic pressure, which decreases venous return to the right side of the heart. Impaired venous return decreases preload, which results in a decrease in CO.[48,51] As a secondary consequence, hepatic and renal dysfunction may occur. In addition, positive-pressure ventilation impairs cerebral venous return. In patients with impaired autoregulation, positive-pressure ventilation can result in increased intracranial pressure.[51]

Gastrointestinal Disturbances. A number of gastrointestinal disturbances also can occur as a result of

Table 24-6	Ventilator Settings	
Parameter	**Description**	**Typical Settings**
Respiratory rate (f)	Number of breaths the ventilator delivers per minute	6-20 breaths/min
Tidal volume (V$_T$)	Volume of gas delivered to patient during each ventilator breath	10-12 ml/kg 6-8 ml/kg in acute lung injury (ALI)
Oxygen concentration (Fio$_2$)	Fraction of inspired oxygen delivered to patient	May be set between 21% and 100%; adjusted to maintain Pao$_2$ level greater than 60 mm Hg or Spo$_2$ level greater than 90%
Positive end expiratory pressure (PEEP)	Positive pressure applied at the end of expiration of ventilator breaths	3-5 cm H$_2$O
Pressure support (PS)	Positive pressure used to augment patient's inspiratory efforts	5-10 cm H$_2$O
Inspiratory flow rate and time	Speed with which the tidal volume is delivered	40-80 L/min Time: 0.8-1.2 second
I:E ratio	Duration of inspiration to duration of expiration	Rate: 1:2 to 1:1.5 unless inverse ratio ventilation is desired
Sensitivity	Determines the amount of effort the patient must generate to initiate a ventilator breath; it may be set for pressure-triggering or flow-triggering	Pressure trigger: 0.5-1.5 cm H$_2$O below baseline pressure Flow trigger: 1-3 L/min below baseline flow
High pressure limit	Regulates the maximal pressure the ventilator can generate to deliver the tidal volume; when the pressure limit is reached, the ventilator terminates the breath and spills the undelivered volume into the atmosphere	10-20 cm H$_2$O above peak inspiratory pressure

positive-pressure ventilation. Gastric distention occurs when air leaks around the endotracheal or tracheostomy tube cuff and overcomes the resistance of the lower esophageal sphincter.[43,48] Vomiting can occur as a result of pharyngeal stimulation from the artificial airway.[15] These problems can be prevented by inserting a nasogastric tube and ensuring appropriate cuff inflation.[43,48] In addition, hypomotility and constipation may occur as a result of immobility and the administration of paralytic agents, analgesics, and sedatives.[48]

Patient-Ventilator Dyssynchrony. Because the normal ventilatory pattern is usually initiated by the establishment of negative pressure within the chest, the application of positive pressure can lead to patient difficulties in breathing on the ventilator. To achieve optimal ventilatory assistance, the patient should breathe in synchrony with the machine. The selected mode of ventilation, the settings, and the type of ventilatory circuitry used can also increase the work of breathing and lead to the patient breathing out of synchrony with the ventilator. Patient-ventilatory dyssynchrony can result in a decrease in effectiveness of mechanical ventilation, the development of auto-PEEP, and psychologic distress in the patient. Patients who are not breathing in synchrony with the ventilator appear to be fighting or "bucking" the ventilator. To minimize this problem, the ventilator is adjusted to accommodate the patient's spontaneous breathing pattern and to work with the patient. If this is not possible, the patient may need to be sedated and/or pharmacologically paralyzed.[43,52]

Ventilator-Associated Pneumonia. Ventilator-associated pneumonia (VAP) is a subgroup of hospital-acquired pneumonia that refers to development of pneumonia while undergoing mechanical ventilation (see the Evidence-Based Collaborative Practice feature on Ventilator-Associated Pneumonia). There is great potential for the development of pneumonia after the placement of an artificial airway, because the tube bypasses or impairs many of the lung's normal defense mechanisms. Once an artificial airway is placed, contamination of the lower airways follows within 24 hours. This results from a number of factors that directly and indirectly promote airway colonization. The use of respiratory therapy devices (e.g., ventilators, nebulizers, and intermittent positive-pressure breathing machines) also can increase the risk of pneumonia. The severity of the patient's illness, presence of acute lung injury, or malnutrition significantly increases the likelihood that an infection will ensue. In addition, such therapeutic measures as nasogastric tubes, antacids, and histamine$_2$-antagonists facilitate the development of pneumonia. Nasogastric tubes promote aspiration by acting as a wick for stomach contents, whereas antacids and histamine inhibitors increase the pH level

EVIDENCE-BASED COLLABORATIVE PRACTICE

American Association of Critical Care Nurses Practice Alert: Ventilator-Associated Pneumonia

Expected Practice

☑ All patients receiving mechanical ventilation, as well as those at high risk for aspiration (e.g., decreased level of consciousness; with enteral tube in place), should have the head of the bed (HOB) elevated at an angle of 30 to 45 degrees unless medically contraindicated.

☑ Use an endotracheal tube (ET) with a dorsal lumen above the endotracheal cuff to allow drainage by continuous suctioning of tracheal secretions that accumulate in the subglottic area.

☑ Do not routinely change, on the basis of duration of use, the patient's ventilator circuit.

Supporting Evidence

■ Critically ill patients who are intubated for >24 hours are at 6 to 21 times the risk of developing ventilator-associated pneumonia (VAP),[1-3] and those intubated for <24 hours are at 3 times the risk of VAP.[4] Other risk factors for VAP include decreased level of consciousness, gastric distention, presence of gastric or small intestine tubes, and a trauma or COPD diagnosis. VAP is reported to occur at rates of 10 to 35 cases/1000 ventilator days, depending on the clinical situation.[3]

■ Aspiration of oral and/or gastric fluids is presumed to be an essential step in the development of VAP. Pulmonary aspiration is increased by supine positioning and pooling of secretions above the ET tube cuff.[1,5,6]

■ Morbidity and mortality associated with the development of VAP is high, with mortality rates ranging from 20% to 41%.[4,7,8] Development of VAP increases ventilator days, critical care lengths of stay (LOS), and hospital LOS by 4, 4, and 9 days, respectively,[2-7] and results in >$40,000 additional costs/VAP case.[2,6]

■ Compared to supine positioning, studies have shown that simple positioning of the HOB to 30 degrees or higher significantly reduces gastric reflux and VAP (8% versus 34%, respectively),[4,9-12] yet national surveys and reports in the literature describe poor compliance rates with HOB elevation in critical care units.[4,13-15]

■ Studies show that the use of special ET tubes which remove secretions pooled above the cuff with continuous suction decrease VAP by 45% to 50%.[16-19]

■ Studies on the frequency of ventilator circuit changes have found no increase in VAP with prolonged use.[20-22]

■ National regulatory and expert consensus groups include these interventions as critical to decrease VAP.[1,23-25]

What You Should Do

■ Always keep mechanically ventilated patients' HOB elevated to 30 degrees or higher, unless medically contraindicated; use an ET tube with continuous suction above the cuff, do not routinely change ventilator circuits.

■ Ensure that your critical care unit has written practice documents such as a policy, procedure, or standard of care that includes these practice alerts.

■ Determine your unit's rate of compliance with the HOB elevation directive, and use an ET tube with continuous suction above the cuff.

■ If compliance is <90%, develop a plan to improve compliance[13]:

→ Consider forming a multidisciplinary task force (nurses, physicians, respiratory therapist, clinical pharmacist) or a unit core group of staff to address VAP practice changes.

→ Educate staff about the significance of nosocomial pneumonias in critically ill patients and how these interventions can reduce VAP.

→ Incorporate content into orientation programs and initial and annual competency verifications.

→ Develop a variety of communication strategies to alert and remind staff of the importance of these VAP interventions.

→ Develop documentation standards for HOB elevation that include rationale for when the HOB is not elevated.

→ Incorporate HOB elevation to at least 30 degrees in any unit standing orders (include those for monitoring into your critical care scorecard), quality improvement plan, and/or process improvement activities to ensure that practice changes continue.

References

1. Weinstein R et al: Guidelines for prevention of healthcare-associated pneumonia, *MMWR Morb Mortal Wkly Rep*, in press.

2. Rello J et al: Epidemiology and outcomes of ventilator-associated pneumonia in a large US database, *Chest* 122:2115-2121, 2002.

3. Craven D: Epidemiology of ventilator-associated pneumonia, *Chest* 117:186S-187S, 2000.

4. Kollef M: Ventilator-associated pneumonia: a multivariate analysis, *JAMA* 270:1965-1970, 1993.

5. Torres A et al: Pulmonary aspiration of gastric contents in patients receiving mechanical ventilation: The effect of body position, *Ann Intern Med* 116:540-542, 1992.

6. Craven D et al: Nosocomial pneumonia: emerging concepts in diagnosis, management and prophylaxis, *Curr Opin Crit Care* 8:421-429, 2002.

7. Bercault N, Boulain T: Mortality rate attributable to ventilator-associated nosocomial pneumonia in an adult intensive care unit: a prospective case-control study, *Crit Care Med* 29:2303-2309, 2001.

8. Heyland D et al: The attributable morbidity and mortality of ventilator-associated pneumonia in the critically ill patient, *Am J Resp Crit Care Med* 159:1249-1256, 1999.

9. Ibanez J et al: Gastroesophageal reflux in intubated patients receiving enteral nutrition: effect of supine and semi recumbent positions, *JPEN J Parenter Enteral Nutr* 16:419-422, 1992.

Continued

EVIDENCE-BASED COLLABORATIVE PRACTICE

American Association of Critical Care Nurses
Practice Alert: Ventilator-Associated Pneumonia—cont'd

10. Orozco-Levi M et al: Semi-recumbent position protects from pulmonary aspiration but not completely from gastroesophageal reflux in mechanically ventilated patients. *Am J Respir Crit Care Med* 152:1387-1390, 1995.

11. Drakulovic M et al: Supine body position as a risk factor for nosocomial pneumonia in mechanically ventilated patients: a randomized trial, *Lancet* 354:1851-1854, 1999.

12. Dotson R, Robinson R, Pingleton S: Gastroesophageal reflux with nasogastric tubes: effect of nasogastric tube size, *Am J Respir Crit Care Med* 149:1659-1662, 1994.

13. Zack J et al: Effect of an educational program aimed at reducing the occurrence of ventilator-associated pneumonia, *Crit Care Med* 30:2407-2412, 2002.

14. Berenholtz S, Pronovost P: Barriers to translating evidence into practice, *Curr Opin Crit Care* 9:321-325, 2003.

15. Grap M et al: Use of backrest elevation in critical care: pilot study, *Am J Crit Care* 8:475-480, 1999.

16. Valles J et al: Continuous aspiration of subglottic secretions in preventing ventilator-associated pneumonia, *Int Care Med* 122:179-186, 1995.

17. Mahul P et al: Prevention of nosocomial pneumonia in intubated patients: respective role of mechanical subglottic secretion drainage and stress ulcer prophylaxis, *Int Care Med* 18:20-25, 1992.

18. Kollef M, Skubas N, Sundt T: A randomized clinical trial of continuous aspiration of subglottic secretions in cardiac surgery patients, *Chest* 116:1339-1346, 1999.

19. Cook D et al: Influence of airway management on ventilator-associated pneumonia: evidence from randomized trials, *JAMA* 279:761-787, 1998.

20. Dreyfuss D et al: Prospective study of nosocomial pneumonia and of patient circuit colonization during mechanical ventilation with circuit changes every 48 hours versus no change, *Am Rev Respir Dis* 143:738-743, 1991.

21. Kotilainen H, Keroack M: Cost analysis and clinical impact of weekly ventilator circuit changes in patients in intensive care unit, *Am J Infect Control* 25:117-120, 1997.

22. Kollef M et al: Mechanical ventilation with or without 7-day circuit changes: a randomized controlled trial, *Ann Intern Med* 123:168-174, 1995.

23. Joint Commission on Accreditation of Healthcare Organizations. ICU Core Measures—draft statement, www.jcaho,org/pms/core+measures/candidate+core+measure+set.htm, accessed September 26, 2003.

24. Parrish C, Krenitsky J, McCray C: Nutritional support for the mechanically ventilated patient. In AACN's *Protocols for Practice, Care of the Mechanically Ventilated Patient* series, Aliso Viejo, Calif, 1998, AACN.

25. Collard H, Saint S: Prevention of ventilator-associated pneumonia, Agency for Health Care Policy and Research (AHCPR) website: www.ahcpr.gov/clinic/ptsafety/chap17a.htm.

Other VAP Articles of Interest

Hixon S, Sole M, King T: Nursing strategies to prevent ventilator-associated pneumonia, *AACN Clin Issues* 9:76-90, 1998.

Pfeifer L et al: Preventing ventilator-associated pneumonia, *Am J Nurs* 101:24AA-24GG, 2001.

of the stomach, thus promoting the growth of bacteria that can then be aspirated.[53] Managing the patient with pneumonia is discussed in Chapter 23.

WEANING

Weaning is the gradual withdrawal of the mechanical ventilator and the reestablishment of spontaneous breathing. Weaning should begin only after the original process requiring ventilator support for the patient has been corrected and patient stability has been achieved. Other factors to consider when weaning are length of time on ventilator, sleep deprivation, and nutritional status. Major factors that affect the patient's ability to wean include the ability of the lungs to participate in ventilation and respiration, cardiovascular performance, and psychologic readiness.[54] This discussion focuses on weaning the patient from short-term (3 days or less) mechanical ventilation. Managing the patient requiring long-term mechanical ventilation is discussed in Chapter 23.

Readiness To Wean. Once the decision is made to wean the patient, the patient is assessed for readiness to wean. Evaluation of the patient includes the patient's level of consciousness, physiologic and hemodynamic stability, adequacy of oxygenation and ventilation, spontaneous breathing capability, and respiratory rate and pattern. In addition, pulmonary mechanics may be measured. Two strong predictors for weaning readiness are vital capacity (VC)/kg greater than 15 ml and negative inspiratory pressure (NIP) of -30 cm H_2O or less.[55]

Once readiness to wean has been established, the patient is prepared for the weaning trial. The patient is positioned upright to facilitate breathing and suctioned to ensure airway patency. In addition, the process is ex-

NIC | Mechanical Ventilatory Weaning

Definition: Assisting the patient to breathe without the aid of a mechanical ventilator

Activities

Monitor degree of shunt, vital capacity, V_d/V_T, mandatory minute ventilation, inspiratory force, and FEV_1 for readiness to wean from mechanical ventilation based on agency protocol

Monitor to ensure that patient is free of significant infection before weaning

Monitor for optimal fluid and electrolyte status

Collaborate with other health team members to optimize patient's nutritional status, ensuring that 50% of the diet's nonprotein caloric source is fat rather than carbohydrate

Position patient for best use of ventilatory muscles and to optimize diaphragmatic descent

Suction the airway, as needed

Administer chest physiotherapy, as appropriate

Consult with other health care personnel in selecting a method for weaning

Alternate periods of weaning trials with sufficient periods of rest and sleep

Avoid delaying return of patient with fatigued respiratory muscles to mechanical ventilation

Set a schedule to coordinate other patient care activities with weaning trials

Promote the best use of the patient's energy by initiating weaning trials after the patient is well rested

Monitor for signs of respiratory muscle fatigue (e.g., abrupt rise in $Paco_2$, rapid, shallow ventilation, paradoxic abdominal wall motion), hypoxemia, and tissue hypoxia while weaning is in process

Administer medications that promote airway patency and gas exchange

Set discrete, attainable goals with the patient for weaning

Use relaxation techniques, as appropriate

Coach the patient during difficult weaning trials

Assist the patient to distinguish spontaneous breaths from mechanically delivered breaths

Minimize excessive work of breathing that is nontherapeutic by eliminating extra dead space, adding pressure support, administering bronchodilators, and maintaining airway patency, as appropriate

Avoid pharmacologic sedation during weaning trials, as appropriate

Provide some means of patient control during weaning

Stay with the patient and provide support during initial weaning attempt

Tell patient about ventilator setting changes that increase the work of breathing, as appropriate

Provide the patient with positive reinforcement and frequent progress reports

Consider using alternative methods of weaning as determined by patient's response to the current method

Instruct the patient and family about what to expect during various stages of weaning

Prepare discharge arrangements through multidisciplinary involvement with patient and family

From Dochterman JM, Bulechek GM: *Nursing interventions classification (NIC)*, ed 4, St Louis, 2004, Mosby.

plained to the patient, and the patient is offered reassurance and diversional activities. Nursing activities to facilitate weaning are listed in the Nursing Intervention Classification feature on Mechanical Ventilatory Weaning. The patient is assessed immediately before the start of the trial and frequently during the weaning period for signs of weaning intolerance (Box 24-1).[54-56]

Weaning Methods. A number of methods can be used to wean a patient from the ventilator. The method selected depends on the patient, his or her pulmonary status, and the length of time on the ventilator. The three main methods for weaning are (1) T-tube (T-piece) trials, (2) synchronized intermittent mandatory ventilation (SIMV), and (3) pressure support ventilation (PSV).[54-56]

T-*Piece.* T-piece weaning trials consist of alternating periods of ventilatory support (usually on assist/control [A/C] or continuous mandatory ventilation [CMV]) with periods of spontaneous breathing. The trial is initiated by removing the patient from the ventilator and having the patient breathe spontaneously on a T-piece oxygen delivery system. After a set amount of time, the patient is placed back on the ventilator. The goal is to progressively increase the duration of time spent off the ventilator. During the weaning process, the patient is observed closely for respiratory muscle fatigue.[49-51] Constant positive airway pressure (CPAP) may be added to prevent atelectasis and improve oxygenation.[56]

SIMV. The goal of SIMV weaning is the gradual transition from ventilatory support to spontaneous breathing. It is initiated by placing the ventilator in the SIMV mode and slowly decreasing the rate until zero (or close to zero) is reached. The rate is usually decreased one to three breaths at a time, and an arterial blood gas (ABG) sample is usually obtained 30 minutes afterward. This method of weaning can increase the work of breathing, and thus the patient must be closely monitored for signs of respiratory muscle fatigue.[54-56]

PSV. PSV weaning consists of placing the patient on the pressure support mode and setting the pressure support at a level that facilitates the patient's achieving a spontaneous tidal volume of 10 to 12 ml/kg. PSV augments the patient's spontaneous breaths with a positive-pressure "boost" during inspiration. During the weaning process, the level of pressure support is gradually de-

Box 24-1

WEANING INTOLERANCE INDICATORS

- Decrease in level of consciousness
- Systolic blood pressure increased or decreased by 20 mm Hg
- Diastolic blood pressure greater than 100 mm Hg
- Heart rate increased by 20 beats/min
- Premature ventricular contractions greater than 6/min, couplets, or runs of ventricular tachycardia
- Changes in ST segment (usually elevation)
- Respiratory rate greater than 30 breaths/min or less than 10 breaths/min
- Respiratory rate increased by 10 breaths/min
- Spontaneous tidal volume less than 250 ml
- $Paco_2$ increased by 5 to 8 mm Hg and/or pH less than 7.30
- Spo_2 less than 90%
- Use of accessory muscles of ventilation
- Complaints of dyspnea, fatigue, or pain
- Paradoxic chest wall motion
- Diaphoresis

creased in increments of 3 to 6 cm H_2O, while maintaining a tidal volume of 10 to 15 ml/kg, until a level of 5 cm H_2O is achieved. If the patient is able to maintain adequate spontaneous respirations at this level, extubation is considered. PSV also can be used with SIMV weaning to help overcome the resistance in the ventilator system.[54-56]

NURSING MANAGEMENT

Nursing management of the patient on a ventilator is outlined in the Nursing Intervention Classification feature on Mechanical Ventilation. Routine assessment of a patient on a ventilator includes monitoring the patient for both patient-related and ventilator-related complications. It includes a total patient assessment, with particular emphasis on the pulmonary system, placement of the ETT, and observation for subcutaneous emphysema and synchrony with the ventilator. Assessment of the ventilator includes a review of all the ventilator settings and alarms. A clear understanding of the alarms and their related problems is important (Table 24-7). In addition, the peak inspiratory pressure, exhaled tidal vol-

---

NIC   Mechanical Ventilation

Definition: Use of an artificial device to assist a patient to breathe

Activities

Monitor for respiratory muscle fatigue

Monitor for impending respiratory failure

Consult with other health care personnel in selection of a ventilator mode

Initiate setup and application of the ventilator

Instruct the patient and family about the rationale and expected sensations associated with use of mechanical ventilators

Routinely monitor ventilator settings

Monitor for decrease in exhale volume and increase in inspiratory pressure

Ensure that ventilator alarms are on

Administer muscle-paralyzing agents, sedatives, and narcotic analgesics, as appropriate

Monitor the effectiveness of mechanical ventilation on patient's physiologic and psychologic status

Initiate calming techniques, as appropriate

Provide patient with a means for communication (e.g., paper and pencil or alphabet board)

Check all ventilator connections regularly

Empty condensed water from traps, as appropriate

Use aseptic technique, as appropriate

Monitor ventilator pressure reading and breath sounds

Stop NG feedings during suctioning and 30 to 60 min before chest physiotherapy

Silence ventilator alarms during suctioning to decrease frequency of false alarms

Monitor patient's progress on current ventilator settings and make appropriate changes as ordered

Monitor for adverse effects of mechanical ventilation: infection, barotraumas, and reduced cardiac output

Position to facilitate ventilation/perfusion matching ("good lung down"), as appropriate

Collaborate with physician to use CPAP or PEEP to minimize alveolar hypoventilation, as appropriate

Perform chest physical therapy, as appropriate

Perform suctioning, based on presence of adventitious sounds and/or increased ventilatory pressures

Promote adequate fluid and nutritional intake

Provide routine oral care

Monitor effects of ventilator changes on oxygenation: ABG, Sao_2, Svo_2, end-tidal CO_2, Q_S/Q_T, and $A-aDO_2$ levels and patient's subjective response

Monitor degree of shunt, vital capacity, V_t/V_d, mandatory minute ventilation (MMV) inspiratory force, and FEV_1 for readiness to wean from mechanical ventilation based on agency protocol

From Dochterman JM, Bulechek GM: *Nursing interventions classification (NIC)*, ed 4, St Louis, 2004, Mosby.

Table 24-7	Troubleshooting Ventilator Alarms	
Problem	**Causes**	**Interventions**
Low exhaled V_T	Altered settings; any condition that triggers high or low pressure alarm; patient stops spontaneous respirations; leak in system preventing V_T from being delivered; cuff insufficiently inflated; leak through chest tube; airway secretions; decreased lung compliance; spirometer disconnected or malfunctioning	Check settings; evaluate patient, check respiratory rate; check all connections for leaks; suction patient's airway; check cuff pressure; calibrate spirometer
Low inspiratory pressure	Altered settings; unattached tubing or leak around ET tube; ET tube displaced into pharynx or esophagus; poor cuff inflation or leak; tracheal-esophageal fistula; peak flows that are too low; low V_T's; decreased airway resistance resulting from decreased secretions or relief of bronchospasm; increased lung compliance resulting from decreased atelectasis; reduction in pulmonary edema; resolution of ALI; change in position	Reset alarm; reconnect tubing; modify cuff pressures; tighten humidifier; check chest tube; adjust peak flow to meet or exceed patient demand and correct for the patient's V_T; reposition or change ET tube
Low exhaled minute volume	Altered settings; leak in system; airway secretions; decreased lung compliance; malfunctioning spirometer; decreased patient-triggered respiratory rate resulting from drugs; sleep; hypocapnia; alkalosis; fatigue; change in neurologic status	Check settings; assess patient's respiratory rate, mental status, and work of breathing; evaluate system for leaks; suction airway; assess patient for changes in disease state; calibrate spirometer
Low PEEP/CPAP pressure	Altered settings; increased patient inspiratory flows; leak; decreased expiratory flows from ventilator	Check settings and correct; observe for leaks in system; if unable to correct problem, increase PEEP settings
High respiratory rate	Increased metabolic demand; drug administration; hypoxia; hypercapnia; acidosis; shock; pain; fear; anxiety	Evaluate ABGs; assess patient; calm and reassure patient
High pressure limit	Improper alarm setting; airway obstruction resulting from patient fighting ventilator (holding breath as ventilator delivers V_T); patient circuit collapse; tubing kinked; ET tube in right mainstem bronchus or against carina; cuff herniation; increased airway resistance resulting from bronchospasm, airway secretions, plugs, and coughing; water from humidifier in ventilator tubing; decreased lung compliance resulting from tension pneumothorax; change in patient position; ALI; pulmonary edema; atelectasis; pneumonia; or abdominal distention	Reset alarms; clear obstruction from tubing; unkink and reposition patient off of tubing; empty water from tubing; check breath sounds; reassure patient and sedate if necessary; check ABGs for hypoxemia; observe for abdominal distention that would put pressure on the diaphragm; check cuff pressures; obtain chest x-ray and evaluate for ET tube position, pneumothorax, and pneumonia; reposition ET tube; give bronchodilator therapy
Low-pressure oxygen inlet	Improper oxygen alarm setting; oxygen not connected to ventilator; dirty oxygen intake filter	Correct alarm setting; reconnect or connect oxygen line to a 50-psi source; clean or replace oxygen filter
I : E ratio	Inspiratory time longer than expiratory time; use of an inspiratory phase that is too long with a fast rate; peak flow setting too low while rate too high; machine too sensitive	Change inspiratory time or adjust peak flow; check inspiratory phase, or hold; check machine sensitivity
Temperature	Sensor malfunction; overheating resulting from too low or no gas flow; sensor picking up outside airflow (from heaters, open doors or windows, air conditioners); improper water levels	Test or replace sensor; check gas flow; protect sensor from outside source that would interfere with readings; check water levels

Modified from Flynn JBM, Bruce NP: *Introduction to critical care nursing skills,* St. Louis, 1993, Mosby.
V_T, Tidal volume; *ET,* endotracheal; *ALI,* acute lung injury; *PEEP,* positive end-expiratory pressure; *CPAP,* constant positive airway pressure.

Invasive Mechanical Ventilation

A number of measures are required to maintain a trouble-free ventilator system. These include maintaining a functional manual resuscitation bag connected to oxygen at the bedside, ensuring that the ventilator tubing is free of water, positioning the ventilator tubing to avoid kinking, maintaining the patency of ventilator tubing and connections, changing ventilator tubing per hospital policy, and monitoring the temperature of the inspired air. In the event that the ventilator malfunctions, the patient is removed from the ventilator and ventilated manually with an MRB. In addition, alarms should be sufficiently audible with respect to distances and competing noise within the unit.

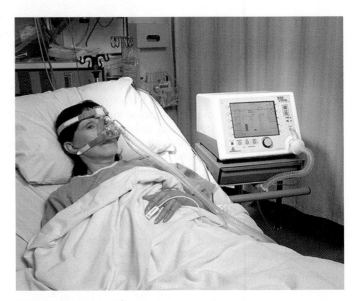

Fig. 24-8 BiPAP® Vision Face Mask in use. (Courtesy Respironics Inc, Murrysville, Pa.).

ume, and arterial blood gases are also monitored. Patient safety issues are addressed in the Patient Safety Alert feature on Invasive Mechanical Ventilation.

Bedside evaluation of VC, minute ventilation, ABG values, and other pulmonary function tests may be warranted, according to the patient's condition. The use of pulse oximetry can facilitate continuous, noninvasive assessment of oxygenation. Static and dynamic compliance should also be monitored to assess for changes in lung compliance (see Appendix).

Semirecumbency. Positioning of the patient requiring mechanical ventilation is also important. Semirecumbent positioning (elevation of the head of the bed to 45 degrees) may help reduce the incidence of gastroesophogeal reflux and lead to a decreased incidence of VAP. Thus the head of the patient's bed should be elevated to 45 degrees at all times unless contraindicated (e.g., hemodynamic instability).[53,57] However, this intervention does increase the risk of skin sheer on the coccyx, and extra surveillance is mandatory for prevention of pressure ulcers.[57]

NONINVASIVE MECHANICAL VENTILATION

Noninvasive mechanical ventilation is a relatively new method of ventilation that uses a mask instead of an ETT to administer positive-pressure ventilation. Advantages of this type of ventilation include decreased frequency of hospital-acquired pneumonia, increased comfort, and the noninvasive nature of the procedure, which allows easy application and removal. It is indicated in both type I and type II acute respiratory failure and when intubation is not an option. Contraindications to noninvasive mechanical ventilation include hemodynamic instability, dysrhythmias, apnea, uncooperativeness, intolerance of the mask, and the inability to maintain a patent airway, clear secretions, and properly fit the mask.[58] One recent study found that a full-face mask is better tolerated than a nasal mask.[59]

Noninvasive mechanical ventilation can be applied using a nasal or facial mask and ventilator or a BiPAP (trademark of Respironics) machine (Fig. 24-8). This mode of therapy uses a combination of PSV (ventilator) or inspiratory positive airway pressure (IPAP) (BiPAP machine) and PEEP (ventilator) or expiratory positive airway pressure (EPAP) (BiPAP machine) to assist the spontaneously breathing patient with ventilation. On inspiration, the patient receives PSV or IPAP to increase tidal volume and minute ventilation, which results in increased alveolar ventilation, a decreased $PaCO_2$ level, relief of dyspnea, and reduced accessory muscle use. On expiration, the patient receives PEEP or EPAP to increase functional residual capacity, which results in an increased PaO_2 level. Humidified supplemental oxygen is administered to maintain a clinically acceptable PaO_2 level, and timed breaths may be added if necessary.[60]

NURSING MANAGEMENT

Routine assessment of patient on a ventilator includes monitoring the patient for both patient-related and ventilator-related complications. As with invasive mechanical ventilation, the patient must be closely monitored while receiving noninvasive mechanical ventilation. Respiratory rate, accessory muscle use, and oxygenation status are continually assessed to ensure that the patient

NIC   Respiratory Monitoring

Definition: Collection and analysis of patient data to ensure airway patency and adequate gas exchange

Activities

Monitor rate, rhythm, depth, and effort of respirations

Note chest movement, watching for symmetry, use of accessory muscles, and supraclavicular and intercostal muscle retractions

Monitor for noisy respirations, such as crowing or snoring

Monitor breathing patterns: bradypnea, tachypnea, hyperventilation, Kussmaul respirations, Cheyne-Stokes respirations, apneustic breathing, Biot respirations, and ataxic patterns

Palpate for equal lung expansion

Percuss anterior and posterior thorax from apices to bases bilaterally

Note location of trachea

Monitor for diaphragmatic muscle fatigue (paradoxic motion)

Auscultate breath sounds, noting areas of decreased/absent ventilation and presence of adventitious sounds

Determine the need for suctioning by auscultating for crackles and rhonchi over major airways

Auscultate lung sounds after treatments to note results

Monitor pulmonary function test values, particularly vital capacity, maximal inspiratory force, forced expiratory volume in 1 second (FEV_1) and FEV_1/forced vital capacity, as available

Monitor mechanical ventilator readings, noting increases in inspiratory pressures and decreases in tidal volume, as appropriate

Monitor for increased restlessness, anxiety, and air hunger

Note changes in SaO_2, SvO_2, end-tidal CO_2, and changes in arterial blood gas values, as appropriate

Monitor patient's ability to cough effectively

Note onset, characteristics, and duration of cough

Monitor patient's respiratory secretions

Monitor for dyspnea and events that improve and worsen it

Monitor for hoarseness and voice changes every hour in patients with facial burns

Monitor for crepitus, as appropriate

Monitor chest x-ray reports

Open the airway, using the chin-lift or jaw-thrust technique, as appropriate

Place the patient on side, as indicated, to prevent aspiration; log roll if cervical aspiration suspected

Institute resuscitation efforts, as needed

Institute respiratory therapy treatments (e.g., nebulizer), as needed

From Dochterman JM, Bulechek GM: *Nursing interventions classification (NIC)*, ed 4, St Louis, 2004, Mosby.

---

is tolerating this method of ventilation. Continued pulse oximetry with a set alarm parameter is initiated (see the Nursing Intervention Classification feature on Respiratory Monitoring).[60]

The key to ensuring adequate ventilatory support is a properly fitted mask. Either a nasal mask or a full-face mask may be used, depending on the patient. A properly fitted mask minimizes air leakage and discomfort for the patient. Transparent dressings placed over the pressure points of the face help minimize air leakage and prevent facial skin necrosis from the mask. The BiPAP machine is able to compensate for air leaks.[61]

The patient is positioned with the head of the bed elevated at 45 degrees to minimize the risk of aspiration and facilitate breathing. Insufflation of the stomach is a complication of this mode of therapy and places the patient at risk for aspiration. Thus the patient is closely monitored for gastric distention, and a nasogastric tube is placed for decompression as necessary. Often patients are very anxious and have high levels of dyspnea before the initiation of noninvasive mechanical ventilation. Once adequate ventilation has been established, anxiety and dyspnea are usually sufficiently relieved. Heavy sedation should be avoided, but if needed, it would consti-

PATIENT SAFETY ALERT   Noninvasive Mechanical Ventilation

The patient requiring noninvasive mechanical ventilation with a full-face mask should never be restrained. The patient has to be able to remove the mask in the event that the mask becomes displaced or the patient vomits. A displaced mask can force the patient's bottom jaw inward and occlude the patient's airway.

tute the need for intubation and invasive mechanical ventilation. Spending 30 minutes with the patient after the initiation of noninvasive ventilation is important because the patient needs reassurance and must learn how to breathe on the machine.[59,61] Patient safety issues are addressed in the Patient Safety Alert, Noninvasive Mechanical Ventilation.

POSITION THERAPY

Position therapy can help match ventilation and perfusion through the redistribution of oxygen and blood flow in the lungs, which improves gas exchange. Using the concept that there is preferential blood flow to the gravity-dependent areas of the lungs, position therapy is used to place the least damaged portion of the lungs into a dependent position. Thus the least damaged portions of the lungs receive preferential blood flow, resulting in less ventilation/perfusion mismatching.[62] Currently there are two different approaches to position therapy; prone positioning and rotation therapy. Which position works best with each specific pulmonary disorder is still under investigation.

PRONE POSITIONING

Prone positioning is a relatively new therapeutic modality used to improve oxygenation in ALI. It involves turning the patient completely over onto his or her stomach into the facedown position. Although a number of theories have been proposed to explain how prone positioning improves oxygenation, the discovery that ALI causes greater damage to the dependent areas of the lungs probably provides the best explanation. It was originally thought that ALI was a diffuse homogenous disease that affected all areas of the lungs equally. It is now known that the dependent lung areas are more heavily damaged than the nondependent lung areas. Turning the patient prone improves perfusion to less damaged areas of the lungs and improves ventilation/perfusion matching and

decreases intrapulmonary shunting.[63] In addition, prone positioning can be used to facilitate the mobilization of secretions and provide pressure relief.[64] Prone positioning is contraindicated in patients with increased intracranial pressure, hemodynamic instability, spinal cord injuries, and abdominal surgery. Patients who are unable to tolerate a facedown position are also not appropriate candidates for this type of therapy.[63]

Currently no standard for the length of time a patient should remain in the prone position has been established. A review of the research on this subject revealed a wide variation, anywhere from 30 minutes to 40 hours.[64] The therapy is considered successful if the patient has an improvement in PaO_2 of greater than 10 mm Hg within 30 minutes of being placed in the prone position.[63,64] Thus the positioning schedule (length of time in prone position and frequency of turning) is usually based on the patient's tolerance of the procedure, the success of the procedure in improving the patient's PaO_2, and whether the patient is able to sustain improvements in PaO_2 when turned back to the supine position.[64] Prone positioning is discontinued when the patient no longer demonstrates a response to the position change.[63]

The biggest limitation to prone positioning is the actual mechanics of turning the patient. A number of procedures have been discussed in the literature that advise using either pillows to support the patient or the Vollman Prone Positioner (Hill-Rom, Inc.).[64] The latter is a steel frame with four cushions to support the patient's forehead, chin, chest, and pelvic area (Fig. 24-9). The device is applied to the patient in the supine position and then used to turn the patient to the prone position (Fig. 24-10).[64] Regardless of the method used, the abdomen must be allowed to hang free to facilitate diaphragmatic descent.[63,64]

Before turning the patient to the prone position, the patient's eyes are lubricated and taped closed, the pa-

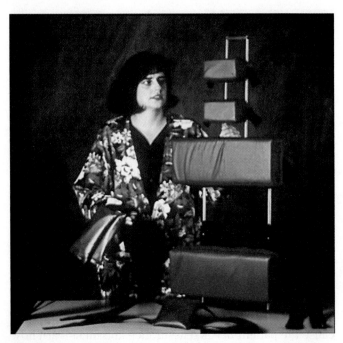

Fig. 24-9 Vollman prone positioner. (Courtesy Kathleen Vollman and Hill-Rom Services, Inc., Batesville, Ind.)

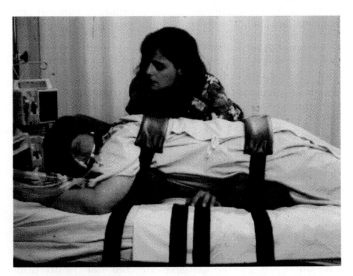

Fig. 24-10 Patient in prone position. (Courtesy Kathleen Vollman and Hill-Rom Services, Inc., Batesville, Ind.)

tient's tubes and drains are secured, and the procedure is explained to the patient and family. A team is organized to implement the turning procedure, and one member is positioned at the head of the bed to maintain the patient's airway. Complications of the procedure include dislodgment or obstruction of tubes and drains, hemodynamic instability, massive facial edema, pressure ulcers, aspiration, and corneal ulcerations.[63]

ROTATION THERAPY

The use of automated turning beds to provide rotation therapy is often found in the critical care setting. Kinetic therapy (KT) and continuous lateral rotation therapy (CLRT) are two forms of rotation therapy. KT is defined as the continuous turning of a patient from side to side with a 40-degree or greater rotation. CLRT is defined as the continuous turning of a patient from side to side with a less-than-40-degree rotation.[65] There are two different types of beds that can perform this type of therapy; an oscillation bed and a kinetic bed. An oscillation bed is one in which the mattress inflates and deflates to provide rotation and a kinetic bed is one which the entire platform of the bed rotates.[66]

Rotation therapy is thought to improve oxygenation through better matching of ventilation to perfusion[67] and to prevent pulmonary complications associated with bed rest and mechanical ventilation.[68] Studies have found, however, that to achieve such benefits, rotation must be aggressive and the patient must be at least 40 degrees per side, with a total arc of at least 80 degrees,[69] for at least 18 hours a day.[68] Thus continuous lateral rotation therapy has been shown to be of minimal pulmonary benefit to the critically ill patient. However, kinetic therapy has been shown to decrease the incidence of VAP particularly in neurologic and postoperative patients.[69] One recent study demonstrated that kinetic therapy decreased the incidence of both VAP and lobar atelectasis in a variety of medical, surgical, and trauma patients[68] (see the Evidence-Based Collaborative Practice feature on Recommendations for Physiotherapy in the ICU).

EVIDENCE-BASED COLLABORATIVE PRACTICE

Summary of Evidence and Evidence-Based Recommendations for Physiotherapy in the ICU

Strong evidence of the following:
- Physiotherapy is the treatment of choice for patients with acute lobar atelectasis.
- Prone positioning improves oxygenation for some patients with severe acute respiratory failure or ALI.
- Positioning in side-lying position (affected lung uppermost) improves oxygenation for some patients with unilateral lung disease.
- Hemodynamic status should be monitored during physiotherapy to detect any deleterious side effects of treatment.
- Sedation before physiotherapy will decrease or prevent adverse hemodynamic or metabolic responses.
- Preoxygenation, sedation, and reassurance are necessary before suction to avoid suction-induced hypoxemia.
- Rotation therapy (kinetic therapy) decreases the incidence of pulmonary complications.

Moderate evidence of the following:
- Multimodality physiotherapy has a short-lived beneficial effect on respiratory function.
- MH may have a short-lived beneficial effect on respiratory function, but hemodynamic status, airway pressure, or V_T should be monitored to detect any deleterious side effects of treatment.
- ICP and CPP should be monitored on appropriate patients during physiotherapy to detect any deleterious side effects of treatment.

Very limited or no evidence of the following:
- Routine physiotherapy in addition to nursing care prevents pulmonary complications commonly found in ICU patients.
- Physiotherapy is effective in the treatment of pulmonary conditions commonly found in ICU patients (with the exception of acute lobar atelectasis).
- Physiotherapy facilitates weaning, decreases length of stay in the ICU or hospital, and reduces mortality or morbidity.
- Positioning (with the exception of examples cited above), percussion, vibrations, suction, or mobilization are effective components of physiotherapy for ICU patients.
- Limb exercises prevent loss of joint range or soft-tissue length, or improve muscle strength and function, for ICU patients.

From Stiller K: Physiotherapy in intensive care: towards an evidence-based practice, *Chest* 118:1801, 2000.
ALI, Acute lung injury; *MH,* manual hyperinflation; V_T, tidal volume; *ICP,* intracranial pressure; *CPP,* cerebral perfusion pressure; *ICU,* intensive care unit.

Complications of the procedure include dislodgment or obstruction of tubes, drains, and lines; hemodynamic instability; and pressure ulcers. Lateral rotation does not replace manual repositioning to prevent pressure ulcers.[70] Repositioning changes the relationship of the patient's posterior surface to the mattress. This gives the skin a chance to reperfuse and to ventilate. In addition, repositioning shifts weight-bearing points. To prevent pressure ulcers the patient should be positioned 30 degrees from the surface of the mattress regardless of the degree of rotational turn. One study found that patients receiving rotational therapy actually developed pressure ulcers of the sacrum, occiput, and heels.[71]

PHARMACOLOGY

A number of pharmacologic agents are used in the care of the critically ill patient with pulmonary dysfunction. The Pharmacologic Management table on Pulmonary Disorders reviews the various agents and any special considerations necessary for administering them.[72]

BRONCHODILATORS AND ADJUNCTS

Medications to facilitate removal of secretions and dilate airways are of major benefit in the treatment of various pulmonary disorders. Mucolytics are administered to help liquefy secretions, which facilitates their removal.[73,74] Bronchodilators, such as beta₂-agonists[75] and anticholinergic agents,[76] aid in smooth muscle relaxation and are of particular benefit to patients with airflow limitations.[74] Steroids also are often used in conjunction with beta₂-agonists to decrease airway inflammation and enhance their effects.[74,77]

NEUROMUSCULAR BLOCKING AGENT

Sedation is necessary in many patients to assist with maintaining adequate ventilation. It can be used to comfort the patient and decrease the work of breathing, particularly if the patient is fighting the ventilator. For further discussion on sedation see Chapter 9. In some patients, sedation does not decrease spontaneous respiratory efforts enough to allow adequate ventilation, and patient-ventilator dyssynchrony may develop. Neuromuscular paralysis may be necessary to facilitate optimal ventilation. Paralysis also may be necessary to decrease oxygen consumption in the severely compromised patient.[78,79]

Nursing management of the patient receiving a neuromuscular blocking agent should incorporate a number of additional interventions. Because paralytic agents only halt skeletal muscle movement and do not inhibit pain or awareness, they must be administered with a sedative or anxiolytic agent. Pain medication is administered if the patient has a pain-producing illness or surgery. Providing reorientation and explanations for all procedures is crit-

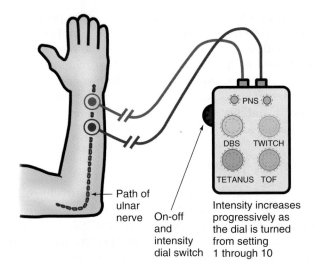

Fig. 24-11 Peripheral nerve stimulator (PNS). Note placement of electrodes along ulnar nerve. *TOF,* Train-of-four.

ical because the patient can still hear but not move or see. The patient is also at high risk for developing the complications of immobility. Interventions related to the prevention of skin breakdown, atelectasis, and deep vein thrombosis are also implemented. Patient safety is another concern, because the patient cannot react to the environment. Special precautions are taken to protect the patient at all times.[80]

Peripheral Nerve Stimulator. Long-term use of neuromuscular blocking agents can result in prolonged neuromuscular blockade and skeletal muscle weakness. To avoid this complication, the patient's level of paralysis is carefully monitored using a peripheral nerve stimulator (PNS). The PNS delivers an electrical stimulus (single twitch, post-tetanic count, double-burst stimulation, or train-of-four) to a preselected nerve (ulnar, facial, posterior tibial, or peroneal) via electrodes (needle, ball, or pregelled), and the response is monitored to gauge the level of paralysis.[80]

Usually the ulnar nerve is used, with pregelled electrodes being placed 2 to 3 inches proximal to the crease of the wrist (Fig. 24-11). The train-of-four (TOF) stimulation test, which delivers four electrical stimuli in a row at a time, is the most common test used. When the ulnar nerve is stimulated with TOF, the expected response is four twitches (adduction) of the thumb medially across the palm of the hand. The number of twitches correlates to the level of paralysis; four twitches indicates less than 75% blockade; three twitches is approximately 75% blockade; two twitches is approximately 80% blockade; one twitch is approximately 90% blockade; and zero twitches indicates 100% blockade. Usually the neuromuscular blocking agent is titrated to maintain an 80% blockade, or two out of four twitches. The goal is to administer the smallest dose possible of the paralytic agent to avoid prolonged weakness after the therapy is discontinued.[80]

Pharmacologic Management: Pulmonary Disorders

DRUG	DOSAGE	ACTIONS	SPECIAL CONSIDERATIONS
Neuromuscular Blocking Agents (NMBAs)			
Vecuronium (Norcuron)	Loading dose: 0.08-0.1 mg/kg IV IV infusion: 0.8-1.2 mcg/kg/min	Used to paralyze patient to decrease oxygen demand and avoid ventilator dyssynchrony	Administer sedative and analgesic agents concurrently, because NMBAs have no sedative or analgesic properties
Pancuronium (Pavulon)	Loading dose: 0.06-0.1 mg/kg IV IV infusion: 0.02-0.04 mg/kg/h		
Pipecuronium (Arduan)	Loading dose: 0.8-0.1 mg/kg IV IV infusion: not recommended		Evaluate the level of paralysis q4h using a peripheral nerve stimulator
Rocuronium (Zemuron)	Loading dose: 0.6-1 mg/kg IV IV infusion: 9-12 mcg/kg/min		Monitor patients for immobility complications
Atracurium (Tracrium)	Loading dose: 0.3-0.4 mg/kg IV IV infusion: 4-12 mcg/kg/min		Protect patients from the environment because they are unable to respond
Cisatracurium (Nimbex)	Loading dose: 0.1-0.2 mg/kg IV IV infusion: 2-8 mcg/kg/min		Prolonged muscle paralysis may occur after discontinuation of the paralytic agent
Doxacurium (Nuromax)	Loading dose: 0.05-0.1 mg/kg IV IV infusion: 0.3-0.5 mcg/kg/min		
Mivacurium (Mivacron)	Loading dose: 0.15-0.25 mg/kg IV IV infusion: 3-15 mcg/kg/min		
Mucolytics			
Acetylcysteine (Mucomyst)	Nebulizer: 20% solution, 3-5 ml tid-qid; or 10% solution, 6-10 ml tid-qid	Used to decrease the viscosity and elasticity of mucus by breaking down disulfide bonds within the mucus	May be administered with a bronchodilator, because drug can cause bronchospasms and inhibit ciliary function
			Treatment is considered effective when bronchorrhea develops and coughing occurs
			Antidote for acetaminophen overdose
Beta₂-Agonists			
Epinephrine (Adrenalin)	Nebulizer: 1% solution, 2.5-5 mg (0.25-0.5 ml) qid	Used to relax bronchial smooth muscle and dilate airways and prevent bronchospasms	May cause skeletal muscle tremors
Racemic epinephrine	Nebulizer: 2.25% solution, 5.625-11.25 mg (0.25-0.5 ml) qid		Higher doses may cause tachycardia, palpitations, increased blood pressure, dysrhythmias, and angina
Isoetharine 1% (Bronkosol)	Nebulizer: 1% solution, 2.5-5 mg (0.25-0.5 ml) qid MDI: 1-2 puffs (340 mcg/puff) qid		May increase serum glucose and decrease serum potassium levels
Terbutaline (Brethaise, Brethine)	MDI: 2 puffs (200 mcg/puff) q4-6h		Treatment is considered effective when breath sounds improve and dyspnea is lessened
Metaproterenol (Alupent, Metaprel)	Nebulizer: 5% solution, 15 mg (0.3 ml) tid-qid MDI: 2-3 puffs (650 mcg/puff) tid-qid		Only approximately 10% of the administered dose reaches the site of action within the lungs
Albuterol (Proventil, Ventolin)	Nebulizer: 5% solution, 2.5 mg (0.5 ml) tid-qid MDI: 2 puffs (90 mcg/puff) tid-qid		
Bitolterol (Tomalate, Produral)	Nebulizer: 0.2% solution, 2.5 mg (1.25 ml) bid-qid MDI: 2 puffs (370 mcg/puff) q8h		
Levalbuterol (Xopenex)	Nebulizer: 0.625 mg q6-8h		

MDI, Metered-dose inhaler.

Pharmacologic Management: Pulmonary Disorders—cont'd

DRUG	DOSAGE	ACTIONS	SPECIAL CONSIDERATIONS
Anticholinergic Agents			
Ipratropium (Atrovent)	Nebulizer: 0.02% solution, 0.5 mg (2.5 ml) q6-8h	Used to block the constriction of bronchial smooth muscle and reduce mucus production	Relatively few adverse effects because systemic absorption is poor
Xanthines			
Theophylline	Loading dose: 5 mg/kg IV IV infusion: 0.5-0.7 mg/kg/hr	Used to dilate bronchial smooth muscle and reverse diaphragmatic muscle fatigue	Administer loading dose over 30 min
Aminophylline	Loading dose: 6 mg/kg IV IV infusion: 0.5-0.7 mg/kg/hr		Monitor serum blood levels; therapeutic level is 10-20 mg/dl
			Administer with caution in patients with cardiac, renal, or hepatic disease
			Signs of toxicity include central nervous system excitation, seizures, confusion, irritability, hyperglycemia, headache, nausea, hypotension, and dysrhythmias
Inhaled Corticosteroids			
Beclomethasone (Vanceril, Beclovent)	MDI: 2 puffs (42 mcg/puff) tid-qid	Used to decrease airway inflammation and enhance effectiveness of beta-agonists	Suppresses inflammatory response and interferes with ability to fight infection
Flunisolide (Aero Bid)	MDI: 2 puffs (250 mcg/puff) bid		Oral candidiasis is a side effect that can be minimized by having patients rinse their mouths after treatment
Triamcinolone (Azmacort)	MDI: 2 puffs (100 mcg/puff) tid-qid		

Use of the PNS for estimating the degree of paralysis is not without its problems. Poor skin contact, improper electrode placement, edema in the extremity being monitored, and malfunction of the device can lead to overestimation of the degree of blockade. The patient appears to have a zero-out-of-four twitch response, but evidence of muscle movement is present. More problematic is underestimation of the degree of blockade. Direct stimulation of the muscle or mistaking finger responses (instead of the thumb) can result in a false-positive twitch response. This can lead to the unnecessary administration of additional doses of the paralytic agent. It is imperative that the patient's twitch response be correlated with clinical observations of patient movement.[80]

REFERENCES

1. O'Connor BS, Vender JS: Oxygen therapy, *Crit Care Clin* 11:67, 1995.
2. Kruse JA: Oxygen therapy. In Kruse JA, Fink MP, Carlson RW: *Saunders manual of critical care*, Philadelphia, 2003, Saunders.
3. Heuer AJ, Scanlan CL: Medical gas therapy. In Wilkins RL, Stoller JK, Scanlan CL, editors: *Egan's fundamentals of respiratory care*, ed 8, St Louis, 2003, Mosby.
4. White AC: The evaluation and management of hypoxemia in the chronic critically ill patient, *Clin Chest Med* 22:123, 2001.
5. Rossi A, Poggi R, Roca J: Physiologic factors predisposing to chronic respiratory failure, *Respir Care Clin North Am* 8:379, 2002.
6. Marshak AB: Emergency life support. In Wilkins RL, Stoller JK, Scanlan CL, editors: *Egan's fundamentals of respiratory care*, ed 8, St Louis, 2003, Mosby.
7. Greenberg RS: Facemask, nasal, and oral airway devices, *Anesthesiol Clin North Am* 20:833, 2002.
8. Shuster M, Nolan J, Barnes TA: Airway and ventilation management, *Cardiol Clin* 20:23, 2002.
9. Rodricks MB, Deutschman CS: Emergent airway management: indications and methods in the face of confounding conditions, *Crit Care Clin* 16:389, 2000.
10. Henneman E, Ellstrom K, St. John RE: *Airway management*, Aliso Viejo, Calif, 1999, American Association of Critical-Care Nurses.
11. Simmons KF, Scanlan CL: Airway management. In Wilkins RL, Stoller JK, Scanlan CL, editors: *Egan's fundamentals of respiratory care*, ed 8, St Louis, 2003, Mosby.
12. Blanda M, Gallo UE: Emergency airway management, *Emerg Med Clin North Am* 21:1, 2003.

13. Colice GL: Technical standards for tracheal tubes, *Clin Chest Med* 12:433, 1991.

14. Loh KS, Irish JC: Traumatic complications of intubation and other airway management procedures, *Anesthesiol Clin North Am* 20:953, 2002.

15. Feller-Kopman D: Acute complications of artificial airways, *Clin Chest Med* 24:445, 2003.

16. Heffner JE: Tracheotomy application and timing, *Clin Chest Med* 24:389, 2003.

17. Walts PA, Murthy SC, DeCamp MM: Techniques of surgical tracheostomy, *Clin Chest Med* 24:413, 2003.

18. Weilitz PB, Dettenmeier PA: Back to basics: test your knowledge of tracheostomy tubes, *Am J Nurs* 94(2):46, 1994.

19. Sue RD, Susanto I: Long-term complications of artificial airways, *Clin Chest Med* 24:457, 2003.

20. Branson RD: Humidification for patients with artificial airways, *Respir Care* 44:630, 1999.

21. Fink J: Humidity and bland aerosol therapy. In Wilkins RL, Stoller JK, Scanlan CL, editors: *Egan's fundamentals of respiratory care*, ed 8, St Louis, 2003, Mosby.

22. Heffner JE, Hess D: Tracheostomy management in the chronically ventilated patient, *Clin Chest Med* 22:55, 2001.

23. Wright SE, VanDahm K: Long-term care of the tracheostomy patient, *Clin Chest Med* 24:473, 2003.

24. Bivona: *Fome-Cuf users manual*, Gary, Ind, 1991, Bivona.

25. Grap MJ et al: Endotracheal suctioning: ventilator vs. manual delivery of hyperoxygenation breaths, *Am J Crit Care* 5:192, 1996.

26. Stone KS: Ventilator versus manual resuscitation bag as the method of delivering hyperoxygenation before endotracheal suctioning, *AACN Clin Issues Crit Care Nurs* 1:289, 1990.

27. Czarnik RE et al: Differential effects of continuous versus intermittent suction on tracheal tissue, *Heart Lung* 20:144, 1991.

28. Raymond SJ: Normal saline instillation before suctioning: helpful or harmful? A review of the literature, *Am J Crit Care* 4:267, 1995.

29. Kinloch D: Instillation of normal saline during endotracheal suctioning: effects on mixed venous oxygen saturation, *Am J Crit Care* 8:231, 1999.

30. Hagler DA, Traver GA: Endotracheal saline and suction catheters: sources of lower airway contamination, *Am J Crit Care* 3:444, 1994.

31. Kollef MH et al: Mechanical ventilation with or without daily changes of in-line suction catheters, *Am J Respir Crit Care Med* 156:466, 1997.

32. Jablonski RS: The experience of being mechanically ventilated, *Qual Health Res* 4:186, 1994.

33. Williams ML: An algorithm for selecting a communication technique with intubated patients, *Dimens Crit Care Nurs* 11:222, 1992.

34. Hodder RV: A 55-year-old patient with advanced COPD, tracheostomy tube, and sudden respiratory distress, *Chest* 120:279, 2002.

35. Napolitano LM: Hospital-acquired and ventilator-associated pneumonia: what's new in diagnosis and treatment? *Am J Surg* 186:4S, 2003.

36. Dennesen P et al: Inadequate salivary flow and poor oral mucosal status in intubated intensive care patients, *Crit Care Med* 31:781, 2003.

37. Fourrier F et al: Colonization of dental plaque: a source of nosocomial infections in intensive care unit patients, *Crit Care Med* 26:301, 1998.

38. Binkley et al: Survey of oral care practices in U.S. intensive care units, *Am J Infect Control* 32:161, 2004.

39. Munro CL, Grap MJ: Oral health and care in the intensive care unit: state of the science, *Am J Crit Care* 13:25, 2004.

40. Grap MF et al: Oral care interventions in critical care: frequency and documentation, *Am J Crit Care* 12:113, 2003.

41. Gali B, Goyal DG: Positive-pressure mechanical ventilation, *Emerg Med Clin North Am* 21:453, 2003.

42. Chatburn RL, Volsko TA: Mechanical ventilators. In Wilkins RL, Stoller JK, Scanlan CL, editors: *Egan's fundamentals of respiratory care*, ed 8, St Louis, 2003, Mosby.

43. Pilbeam SP: *Mechanical ventilation: physiological and clinical applications*, ed 3, St Louis, 1998, Mosby.

44. Pierce LNB: *Traditional and nontraditional modes of mechanical ventilation*, Aliso Viejo, Calif, 1998, American Association of Critical-Care Nurses.

45. Shelledy DC, Peters JI: Initiating and adjusting ventilatory support. In Wilkins RL, Stoller JK, Scanlan CL, editors: *Egan's fundamentals of respiratory care*, ed 8, St Louis, 2003, Mosby.

46. Adams AB, Simonson DA, Dries DJ: Ventilator-induced lung injury, *Respir Care Clin North Am* 9:343, 2003.

47. Whitehead T, Slutsky AS: The pulmonary physician in critical care. 7: Ventilator-induced lung injury, *Thorax* 57:635, 2002.

48. Chatila WM, Criner GJ: Complications of long-term mechanical ventilation, *Respir Care Clin N Am* 8:631, 2002.

49. Marini JJ, Gattinoni L: Ventilatory management of acute respiratory distress syndrome: a consensus of two, *Crit Care Med* 32:250, 2004.

50. Gajic O et al: Ventilator-associated lung injury in patients without acute lung injury at the onset of mechanical ventilation, *Crit Care Med* 32:1817, 2004.

51. Pannu N, Mehta RL: Mechanical ventilation and renal function: an area for concern? *Am J Kidney Dis* 39:616, 2002.

52. Sassoon CS, Foster GT: Patient-ventilator asynchrony, *Curr Opin Crit Care* 7:28, 2001.

53. Kollef MH: Prevention of hospital-associated pneumonia and ventilator-associated pneumonia, *Crit Care Med* 32:1396, 2004.

54. Shelledy DC: Discontinuing ventilatory support. In Wilkins RL, Stoller JK, Scanlan CL, editors: *Egan's fundamentals of respiratory care*, ed 8, St Louis, 2003, Mosby.

55. Hannemann SK: *Weaning from short-term mechanical ventilation*, Aliso Viejo, Calif, 1998. American Association of Critical-Care Nurses.

56. Hess D: Ventilator modes used in weaning, *Chest* 120(6 Suppl):474S, 2001.

57. Cook DJ: Toward understanding evidence uptake: semirecumbency for pneumonia prevention, *Crit Care Med* 30:1472, 2002.

58. Liesching T, Kwok H, Hill NS: Acute applications of noninvasive positive-pressure ventilation, *Chest* 124:699, 2003.

59. Kwok H et al: Controlled trial of oronasal versus nasal mask ventilation in the treatment of acute respiratory failure, *Crit Care Med* 31:468, 2003.

60. Peter JV: Noninvasive ventilation in acute respiratory failure—a meta-analysis update, *Crit Care Med* 30:555, 2002.

61. Vines DL: Noninvasive positive-pressure ventilation. In Wilkins RL, Stoller JK, Scanlan CL, editors: *Egan's fundamentals of respiratory care,* ed 8, St Louis, 2003, Mosby.

62. Misasi RS, Keyes JL: Matching and mismatching ventilation and perfusion in the lung, *Crit Care Nurse* 16(3):23, 1996.

63. Piedalue F, Albert RK: Prone positioning in acute respiratory distress syndrome, *Respir Care Clin North Am* 9:495, 2003.

64. Klein DG: Prone positioning in patients with acute respiratory distress syndrome: the Vollman Prone Positioner, *Crit Care Nurse* 19(4):66, 1999.

65. Marik PE, Fink MP: One good turn deserves another! *Crit Care Med* 30:2146, 2002.
66. Stiller K: Physiotherapy in intensive care: towards an evidence-based practice, *Chest* 118:1801, 2000.
67. McLean B: Rotational kinetic therapy for ventilation/perfusion mismatch, *Crit Care Nurs Eur* 1:113, 2001.
68. Ahrens T et al: Effect of kinetic therapy on pulmonary complications, *Am J Crit Care Nurs* 13:376, 2004.
69. Collard HR: Prevention of ventilator-associated pneumonia: an evidenced-based systematic review, *Ann Intern Med* 138:494, 2003.
70. Powers J, Daniels D: Turning points: implementing kinetic therapy in the ICU, *Nurs Manage* 35(5):1, 2004.
71. Russell T, Logsdon A: Pressure ulcers and lateral rotation beds: a case study, *J Wound Ostomy Continence Nurs* 30:143, 2003.
72. *2004 Mosby's drug consult*, ed 14, St Louis, 2004, Mosby.
73. Duarte AG, Fink JB, Dhand R: Inhalation therapy during mechanical ventilation, *Respir Care Clin North Am* 7:233, 2001.
74. Rau JL: Airway pharmacology. In Wilkins RL, Stoller JK, Scanlan CL, editors: *Egan's fundamentals of respiratory care*, ed 8, St Louis, 2003, Mosby.
75. Dutta EJ, Li JT: Beta-agonists, *Med Clin North Am* 86:991, 2002.
76. Rodrigo GJ, Rodrigo C: The role of anticholinergics in acute asthma treatment: an evidence-based evaluation, *Chest* 121:1977, 2002.
77. Sutherland ER et al: Inhaled corticosteroids reduce the progression of airflow limitation in chronic obstructive pulmonary disease: a meta-analysis, *Thorax* 58:937, 2003.
78. Jacobi J et al: Clinical practice guidelines for the sustained use of sedatives and analgesics in the critically ill adult, *Crit Care Med* 30:119, 2002.
79. Murray MJ: Clinical practice guidelines for sustained neuromuscular blockade in the adult critically ill patient, *Crit Care Med* 30:142, 2002.
80. Loyola R, Dreher HM: Management of pharmacologically induced neuromuscular blockade using peripheral nerve stimulation, *Dimens Crit Care Nurs* 22:157, 2003.

NEUROLOGIC
ALTERATIONS

Neurologic Anatomy and Physiology

*T*he nervous system is mankind's "executive suite," charged with direction of all human body systems as well as providing the unique ability for thought, emotion, understanding of complex information, and integration of numerous stimuli. As the recipient of all sensory information for analysis, the nervous system generates intellectual and motor responses aimed at maintaining integrity of life structures. Critical care nurses must attain a basic understanding of the anatomy and physiology of this complex system, because it serves as the basis for innervation and proper functioning of all other systems. This chapter reviews the anatomic divisions and functions of the central nervous system, including the cellular microstructure, protective encasement, an overview of networked functions, and mechanisms aimed at maintenance of structural and physiologic integrity. The cranial nerves, a component of the peripheral nervous system, are presented in table format at the end of the chapter.

DIVISIONS OF THE NERVOUS SYSTEM

The nervous system is the most highly organized system of the body, with all of its parts functioning as an inseparable unit. For review, this system may be classified by anatomic location or according to function.

ANATOMIC DIVISIONS

The central nervous system (CNS) is made up of the brain and spinal cord. The peripheral nervous system (PNS) comprises the 12 pairs of cranial nerves, the 32 pairs of spinal nerves, and all other nerves serving a variety of functions throughout the body.

PHYSIOLOGIC DIVISIONS

The somatic, or voluntary, nervous system is composed of fibers that connect the CNS with structures of the skeletal muscles and the skin. The autonomic, or involuntary, nervous system is composed of fibers that connect the CNS with smooth muscle, cardiac muscle, internal organs, and glands. It includes both sympathetic and parasympathetic branches.

Most activities of the nervous system originate from sensory receptors, such as visual, auditory, or tactile receptors. This sensory information is transmitted to the CNS by afferent fibers (sensory fibers). Efferent fibers (motor fibers) transmit the CNS response to the periphery to produce a motor response, such as contraction of skeletal muscles, contraction of the smooth muscles of organs, or secretion by endocrine glands. To better understand the macrostructure and functions of the nervous system, it is essential to look first at the microstructure, or cellular level.

MICROSTRUCTURE OF THE NERVOUS SYSTEM

Two types of cells make up the nervous system: neurons and the neuroglia. Neurons are the cells primarily charged with the functional work of the nervous system, including receipt of information, integration, and networked shuttling of data, and transmission or conduction of nerve impulses to recipient cells. Neuroglial cells serve as the support infrastructure of the nervous system, providing both protection and a structural foundation for neurons, as well as participating in neuronal repair.

NEUROGLIA

Neuroglial cells consist of four types: *astroglia (astrocytes)*, *oligodendroglia*, *ependyma*, and *microglia* (Fig. 25-1). These cells provide the neuron with structural support, nourishment, and protection (Table 25-1).[1] In the nervous system there are six to ten times more neuroglial cells than neurons. Neuroglia retain their mitotic abilities and are the primary source of CNS neoplasms.[1-3]

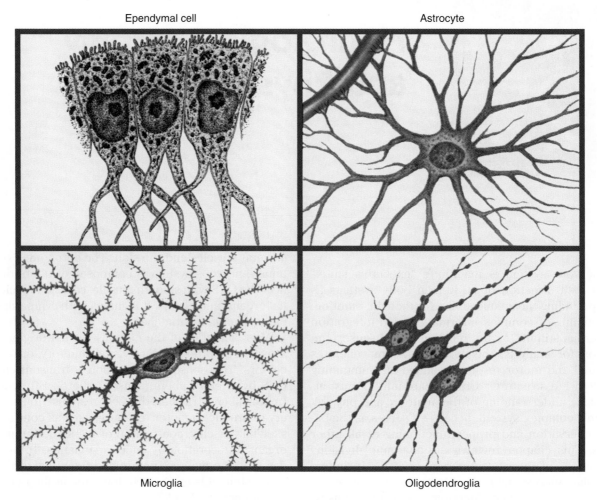

Ependymal cell

Astrocyte

Microglia

Oligodendroglia

Fig. 25-1   Types of neuroglial cells. (From Thompson JM et al: *Mosby's clinical nursing*, ed 5, St Louis, 2002, Mosby.)

Table 25-1	Types of Neuroglial Cells
Cell Type	**Function**
Astroglia (astrocyte)	Supplies nutrients to neuron structure and to support framework for neurons and capillaries; forms part of the blood-brain barrier
Oligodendroglia	Forms the myelin sheath in the central nervous system (CNS)
Ependyma	Lines the ventricular system; forms the choroid plexus, which produces cerebrospinal fluid (CSF)
Microglia	Occurs mainly in the white matter; phagocytizes waste products from injured neurons

NEURONS

Neurons are the basic unit of function within the CNS and are charged with the highly specialized task of data integration and signal transmission. The CNS is made up of more than 10 billion neurons.[1,3] The cellular appearance of neurons varies, but each cell contains three basic components: the cell body, dendrites, and an axon (Fig. 25-2). Neurons are structurally classified as unipolar, a cell body with one process that divides into a central branch (the axon) and a peripheral branch (the dendrite); as bipolar, a cell body with two processes (one axon and one dendrite); or multipolar, a cell body with one axon and several dendrites. The cell body (soma) controls the metabolic activity of the neuron and contains the organelles necessary for cellular metabolism and maintenance, such as the nucleus, mitochondria, endoplasmic reticulum, Golgi apparatus, and liposomes.

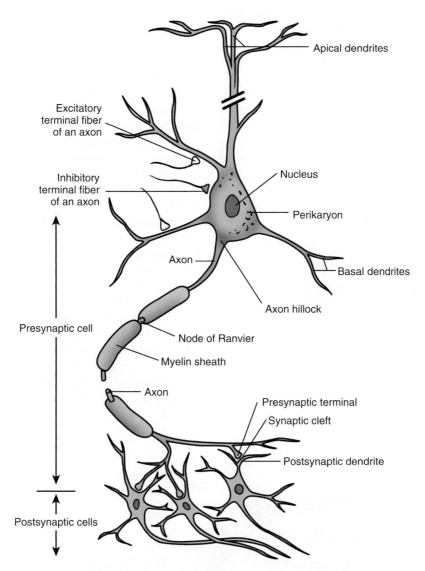

Fig. 25-2 Anatomy of a neuron. (From Layon AJ, Gabrielli A, Friedman WA: *Textbook of neurointensive care,* Philadelphia, 2004, Saunders.)

Compared to other body cells, the neuron's protein-embedded membrane with its phospholipid bilayer is unique, consisting of specialized pores that work as ion-specific channels or pumps to promote passage of ions through an otherwise impermeable plasma membrane.[3]

The neuronal cell body is the life support unit of the neuron. The metabolic demands of these specialized units are significant, necessitating uninterrupted perfusion with glucose and oxygen to maintain neuronal life and optimal functioning. Until recently it was believed that CNS neuronal repair was not possible, but research has validated that neurons are more *plastic* than was previously thought, although rates of repair *(plasticity)* and/or restoration of neuronal function are driven by factors that still remain largely unknown at this time.[4-6] Within the brain and spinal cord, neuronal cell bodies make up regions of gray matter. Outside the CNS, *ganglia* are cell bodies within the PNS that work in close relation and proximity to CNS neurons.[1,3]

Dendrites form the receptive component of the neuron; they are branched fibers extending only a short distance from the cell body. Each neuron may have several dendrites, which function as impulse receivers for the cell body.[1,3,7] The axon is the part of the neuron concerned with transmission of impulses away from the cell body to other neurons, muscle cells, endocrine glands, or some other effector organ. Neurons contain only one axon, which may be microscopic in length or, in some cases, may extend up to 4 feet in length. Some axons are protected by a myelin sheath, a white phospholipid complex laid down by Schwann cells in the PNS and by oligodendroglia in the CNS. Myelin sheathes not only protect neuronal axons, but also act as insulation for the conduction of nerve impulses.[1,3,8] Fibers enclosed in the sheath are called *myelinated fibers;* those not enclosed are called *unmyelinated fibers.* The white matter of the CNS is composed of myelinated fiber tracts.

Myelinated fibers use a process called *saltatory* conduction to support rapid axonal transmission of nerve impulses.[1,8] Structurally, axons participating in this form of impulse transmission are laid out with a noncontinuous myelin cover, interrupted with 2-μm bare segments called the *nodes of Ranvier.* These nodes are packed with sodium channels, making them extremely sensitive to membrane depolarization. Because segments of the axon covered by myelin are impervious to sodium influx, impulse transmission is pulled down the length of the axon to the next node of Ranvier. Saltatory conduction increases transmission velocity up to 100-fold, allowing transmission at rates as high as 120 m/second.[8]

Neuronal function is driven by depolarization-repolarization cycles, similar to that described for cardiac physiology (see Chapter 15), but what makes the nervous system so exceptional is its ability to undergo the depolarization-repolarization cycle up to 1000 times per second to ensure optimal receipt, integration, and transmission of information throughout the body.[3] The movement of ions across the neuronal membrane generates electrical action potentials (Figs. 25-3 and 25-4). Neuronal resting membrane potential (RMP) is −65 mV, approximating the equilibrium potential for potassium; upon depolarization, sodium channels open, shifting the equilibrium potential in a positive direction.[1,3,8] To better understand neuronal mechanisms for ionic movement,

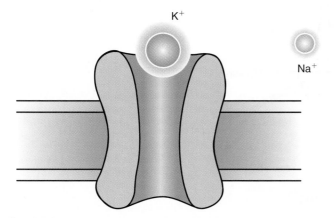

Fig. 25-3 Neuronal voltage-gated channel selectivity. (From Layon AJ, Gabrielli A, Friedman WA: *Textbook of neurointensive care,* Philadelphia, 2004, Saunders.)

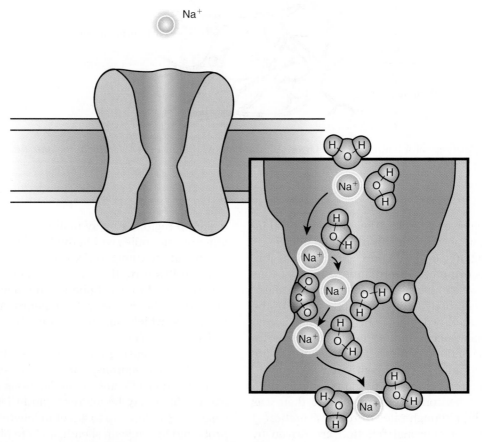

Fig. 25-4 Selectivity filter of voltage-gated channels. (From Layon AJ, Gabrielli A, Friedman WA: *Textbook of neurointensive care,* Philadelphia, 2004, Saunders.)

two classifications of neuronal channels will be discussed, *voltage-gated* and *ligand-gated*. Many pharmaceutical and therapeutic agents in use today or currently undergoing testing manipulate these ionic transport mechanisms.

Voltage-gated channels become activated with changes in transmembrane electrical potential, promoting sodium and calcium influx and potassium efflux. These channels are the primary drivers of cellular action potentials.[1,2,6] Ligand-gated channels are primarily concerned with mitigating the response of a postsynaptic neuron to synapse and will later be discussed in more detail.[2,3,9]

Action potentials begin with influx of sodium, producing a focal zone of membrane depolarization somewhere between −55 mV to −35 mV. Once this critical threshold is reached, a large number of sodium channels open, resulting in fast and massive localized depolarization of the plasma membrane. Rapid sodium influx (upstroke phase) increases the membrane potential to between 70 mV and 90 mV. As the membrane potential changes locally, it stimulates adjoining regions in the neuron to begin depolarization in a self-propagating fashion until depolarization is complete. Within a millisecond of opening, sodium channels close and become inactive.[1,2,6]

Depolarization causes potassium channels to open, allowing this ion to flow out into the extracellular space and thereby promoting the onset of repolarization. Potassium efflux triggers the cell membrane to return to a potassium equilibrium potential of approximately −75 mV, allowing potassium to reenter the cell but maintaining greater polarity than RMP to hold the cell refractory to another depolarization stimulus. Cellular pumps dependent on a steady supply of adenosine triphosphate (ATP) are also activated to remove sodium and restore the −65 mV RMP, allowing the cycle to begin anew.[1,6]

Once an action potential reaches the axon terminal it initiates a cascade of events that promote interneuronal communication, or *synapse*. Two types of synapse exist: electrical synapse and chemical synapse. In an electrical synapse, gap junctions made up of narrow (3.5 nm) bridges allow cytoplasm and intracellular metabolites to pass in an essentially continuous fashion between neurons, facilitating impulse conduction from one neuron to the next.[1,9] In chemical synapse, which comprises the majority of synaptic events, no physical bridge exists between neurons. Instead a large synaptic cleft measuring between 20 and 40 nm is present, preventing direct action potential transmission from one neuron to another (see Fig. 25-2).[9] When the wave of depolarization reaches the presynaptic terminal it signals the release of neurotransmitters into the synaptic cleft.

There are two classifications of neurotransmitters: small-molecule transmitters and neuroactive peptides.[9] Examples of small-molecule transmitters include acetylcholine, dopamine, norepinephrine, epinephrine, serotonin, histamine, gamma-aminobutyric acid (GABA), glycine, and glutamate. Neuroactive peptides include such substances as pituitary peptides, hypothalamic-releasing hormones and neurohypophyseal hormones. This text is primarily concerned with the small-molecule transmitters, which are stored in vesicles within the axon terminal and released into the synapse through a process called *exocytosis*. Exocytosis is stimulated by arrival of the action potential in the axon terminal and results in release of neurotransmitter into the synaptic cleft, where these molecules rapidly diffuse to interact with postsynaptic receptors.[8,9]

Ligand-gated channels are activated by ligand agonists' binding to receptors on the postsynaptic neuron.[1,9] Ions passing through ligand-gated channels promote either an excitatory or inhibitory response within postsynaptic neurons. Examples of excitatory ligand-gated channel receptors include the ionotropic glutamate receptors (N-methyl-D-aspartate [NMDA], alpha-amino-3-hydroxyl-5-methyl-4-isoxazolepropionic acid [AMPA], and kainite) which are primarily concerned with gating sodium, potassium, and calcium ions. Examples of inhibitory ligand-gated channel receptors include GABA receptors, glycine receptors, and nicotinic acetylcholine receptors. GABA receptors are primarily specific to the brain, where GABA serves as the primary inhibitory neurotransmitter, whereas glycine serves as the spinal cord's primary postsynaptic inhibitory neurotransmitter. GABA and glycine channels gate chloride ions, which inhibit by promoting repolarization to the chloride equilibrium potential (–60 mV), and by short-circuiting incoming excitatory potentials by gating anions and clamping the membrane shut to excitatory cations (shunting).[9] In other words, when inhibitor neurotransmitters are released, the neuron's internal charge becomes more negative, and the resistance to depolarization is increased.

Metabotropic receptors also contribute to impulse transmission, promoting sustained effects of postsynaptic excitation or inhibition. Examples of metabotropic receptors include catecholamine receptors, neuropeptide receptors and muscarinic receptors.[9]

Termination of synapse is most commonly accomplished through reuptake, where transporter proteins embedded in neuron and glial cell membranes direct neurotransmitter molecules within the cleft to move back to the intracellular compartment for vesicle repackaging. Neurotransmitter may also go through enzyme degradation, with their component parts taken up for further neurotransmitter synthesis and storage.[1,9] Ultimately, remaining neurotransmitter diffuses away from the synaptic cleft.

As noted, the response in the postsynaptic neuron to synapse is either an excitatory or inhibitory potential. Membrane potentials are not strong enough by themselves to generate a complete action potential within the postsynaptic neuron, but instead are summarized or integrated by the neuronal cell body in the process of information transmission.[9] When the postsynaptic neuron is bombarded with excitatory potentials, they may combine *(summation)* to become capable of stimulating an action potential.

APPLICATION OF NEURONAL ANATOMY AND PHYSIOLOGY TO THE PATHOPHYSIOLOGY OF NEURONAL INJURY

Fig. 25-5 provides examples of disease- or chemically-induced mechanisms that alter neuronal transmission. Two stages of CNS neuronal injury have been identified: *primary* and *secondary*. Primary injury occurs immediately and is typified by neuronal cell membrane dysfunction, local inflammation, cellular edema, and necrosis.[6,10] Disruption of normal vascular supply mechanisms devastates production of ATP, leading to ionic pump failure and massive neuronal depolarization, called *anoxic depolarization*.[4-6,10,11] The onset of depolarization promotes influx of sodium, calcium, chloride, and water into cells, as well as potassium efflux. Loss of ionic pump function aggravates neuronal edema. Within axon terminals, voltage-gated calcium channels open in response to depolarization, triggering a massive release of glutamate into the extracellular space.[4-6, 10-14] Glutamate release promotes excitotoxicity; peak glutamate levels can be measured within 5 minutes of injury, and the magnitude of these levels directly correlates with the severity of neuronal injury sustained.[10,12]

Glutamate facilitates neuronal injury by promoting calcium influx through receptor pores and voltage-gated channels. Calcium is also able to enter the depolarized neuron through sodium-calcium antiporters, pump systems that normally are charged with removal of both sodium and calcium. Activation of metabotropic glutamate receptors induces release of calcium from intracellular stores, causing free calcium ion concentrations to increase rapidly. Unchecked quantities of intracellular calcium ultimately destroy the neuron from the inside out, by activating phospholipase A_2 and phospholipase C, which digest the plasma membrane and linings of organelles.[12,13] Calcium-activated proteases such as calpains, as well as nucleases, further the destruction. Nucleases cause breaks in deoxyribonucleic acid (DNA) strands, and elevated intracellular calcium concentrations stimulate the arachidonic acid cascade (activation of 5-lipoxygenase, prostaglandin synthase and neuronal nitric oxide synthase), resulting in generation of free radicals with further internal cellular destruction.[5,6] Damage to the mitochondria liberates cytochrome C, activating proteases such as caspases shown to be associated with later stages of cell death.[14]

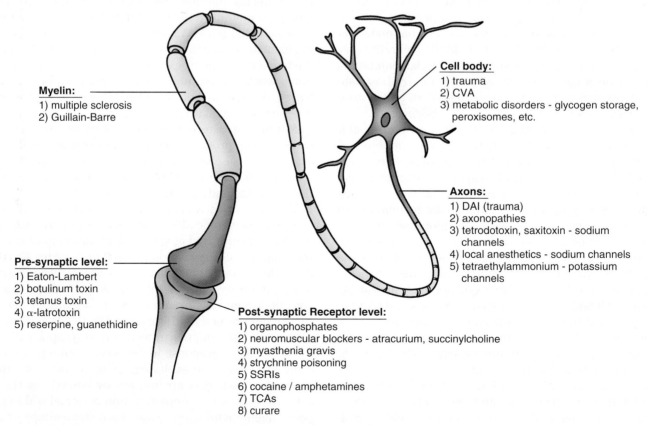

Myelin:
1) multiple sclerosis
2) Guillain-Barre

Cell body:
1) trauma
2) CVA
3) metabolic disorders - glycogen storage, peroxisomes, etc.

Axons:
1) DAI (trauma)
2) axonopathies
3) tetrodotoxin, saxitoxin - sodium channels
4) local anesthetics - sodium channels
5) tetraethylammonium - potassium channels

Pre-synaptic level:
1) Eaton-Lambert
2) botulinum toxin
3) tetanus toxin
4) α-latrotoxin
5) reserpine, guanethidine

Post-synaptic Receptor level:
1) organophosphates
2) neuromuscular blockers - atracurium, succinylcholine
3) myasthenia gravis
4) strychnine poisoning
5) SSRIs
6) cocaine / amphetamines
7) TCAs
8) curare

Fig. 25-5   Neuronal pathophysiology. (From Layon AJ, Gabrielli A, Friedman, WA: *Textbook of neurointensive care*, Philadelphia, 2004, Saunders.)

Knowledge of the intracellular processes associated with cell death continues to evolve, and many other substances are likely to contribute to cell necrosis or programmed cell death known as *apoptosis*. Inflammatory processes are also being examined to further the understanding of how they contribute to cell death following trauma or ischemic injury. Substances such as tumor necrosis factor-α and interleukin-1β, well known for their association with inflammatory injury, have been identified as potential contributors to cell death through aggravation of increased intracellular water concentrations, generation of free radicals, and destruction of the blood-brain barrier. Microvascular obstruction by a massive influx of neutrophils, macrophages, and monocytes furthers ischemia.[4-6,10-14]

Secondary injury occurs hours to weeks after the primary injury is sustained, affecting areas that neighbor the initial site of injury, called the *penumbra*. Apoptosis of penumbral cells may be triggered by the death of cells at the site of the primary insult and results in a characteristic pattern of degenerative changes that culminate in cell death.[12-14] Scientists continue to explore the mechanisms for apoptosis and necrosis to further discovery of agents that may alter the course of cell death following trauma or ischemia.

CENTRAL NERVOUS SYSTEM

The CNS consists of the brain and spinal cord. Serving as the control unit for all body systems, the CNS is remarkably delicate, requiring significant protection to preserve normal function. This section addresses the anatomy and physiology of the brain and spinal cord, supporting the critical care nurse's understanding of pathophysiologic changes that contribute to clinical examination findings.

CRANIAL PROTECTIVE MECHANISMS

Bony Structures. The outermost protective measures underneath the integument are the bony structures that encase the CNS. The skull, or cranium, surrounds the brain and is composed of eight flat, irregular bones fused at sutures during early childhood (Fig. 25-6).[1] The skull protects the brain from direct force and superficial trauma, although excessive force may fracture the skull, destroying this protective mechanism and driving bony fragments into fragile brain tissue.

Viewing the skull from the inside, the superior surfaces form a smooth inner wall, whereas the basilar skull contains ridges and folds with sharp edges (Fig. 25-7).[1] Traumatic impact to the head often results in fracture of the basilar skull as a result of gravitational forces that displace energy in a downward fashion toward the skull base.

The cranium is a solid, nonexpanding bony vault with only one large opening at the base called the *foramen magnum*, through which the brainstem projects and connects to the spinal cord. Several other very small openings in the base of the skull allow entrance and exit of blood vessels and nerve fibers.

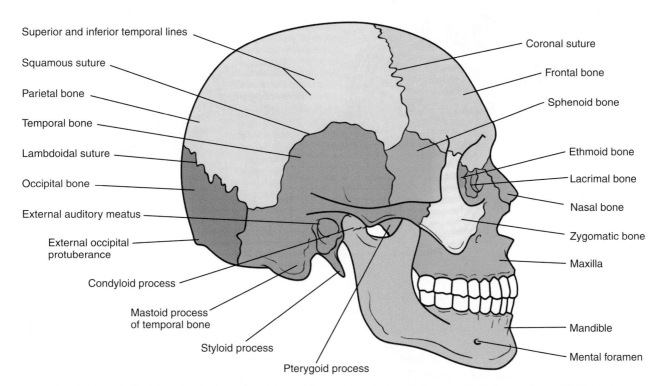

Fig. 25-6 Skull. (From Thibodeau GF, Patton KT: *Anatomy & physiology*, ed 5, Philadelphia, 2003, Mosby.)

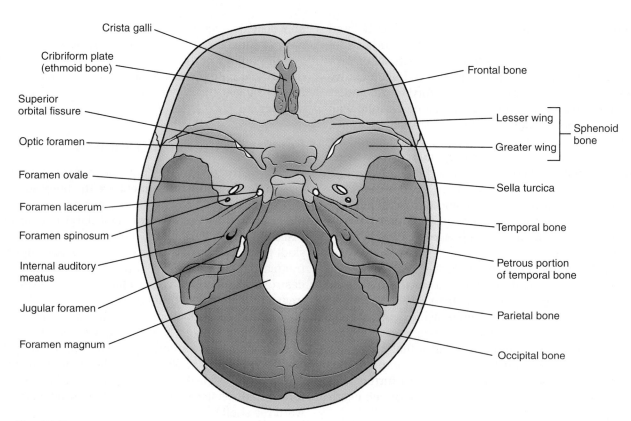

Fig. 25-7   Basilar skull. (From Thibodeau GF, Patton KT: *Anatomy & physiology,* ed 5, Philadelphia, 2003, Mosby.)

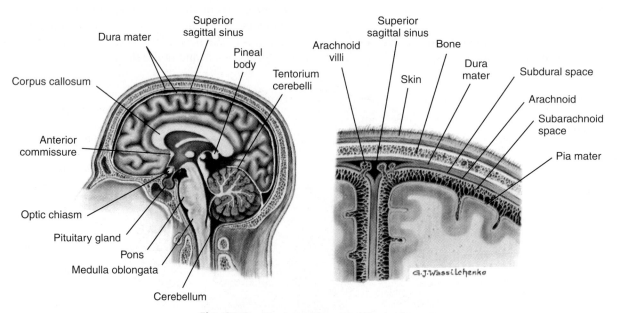

Fig. 25-8   Meningeal layers of the brain.

Meninges.   Directly beneath the skull lie the meninges, which form another source of protection for the CNS. The meninges consist of three layers, namely the *dura mater,* the *arachnoid mater,* and the *pia mater* (Fig. 25-8).

Dura Mater.   The outermost layer of meninges directly beneath the skull is the dura mater. *Dura* is the Latin term for tough, and true to its name, this layer is made up of fibrous tissue that is double-folded to support the CNS, nerves, and vascular structures.[1,3] Within the dura mater's double layers lie venous sinuses that collect blood from intracranial and meningeal veins for drainage into the internal jugular veins.

Four extensions of the dura mater directly support and separate specific areas of the brain, namely the falx cerebri, the tentorium cerebelli, the falx cerebelli, and the diaphragma sellae. The falx cerebri divides the right and left hemispheres of the brain vertically through the longitudinal fissures extending from the frontal lobe to the occipital lobe. The tentorium cerebelli forms a tent between the occipital lobes and the cerebellum and separates the cerebral hemispheres from the brainstem and cerebellum. Structures within the brain that are located above the tentorium are often referred to as *supratentorial*, while those located below the tentorium are referred to as *infratentorial* and make up the region of the brain referred to as the *posterior fossa*. The falx cerebelli forms the division between the two lateral lobes of the cerebellum, and the diaphragma sellae forms a roof over the sella turcica, which houses the pituitary gland.[1,3]

The main blood supply for the dura mater is the middle meningeal artery. This artery lies on the surface of the dura in the epidural space, within grooves formed on the inside of the parietal bone.[1] Traumatic disruption of the parietal bone may result in tearing of the middle meningeal artery and development of an epidural hematoma.

A potential space exists between the dura mater and the arachnoid mater. This area contains a large number of unsupported small veins that may become disrupted and torn when traumatic head injury occurs, leading to development of a subdural hematoma.[3]

Arachnoid Mater. The arachnoid membrane is a delicate, fragile membrane that loosely surrounds the brain. Fine threads of elastic tissue called *trabeculae* connect the arachnoid to the pia mater, creating a spongy, weblike structure called the *subarachnoid space*. Cerebrospinal fluid (CSF) circulates freely in the subarachnoid space, which also contains the origins of the brain's large arteries where they enter the skull and differentiate into anterior and posterior circulatory branches.[1,3,15,16] Rupture of an artery within the subarachnoid space allows for blood to mix with CSF, producing a *subarachnoid hemorrhage.*

At the base of the brain, widened areas of subarachnoid space form cisterns, or spaces filled with CSF. The largest of these cisterns, the cisterna magna, lies between the medulla and the cerebellum and communicates with the fourth ventricle.[1]

Tufts of arachnoid membrane, called *arachnoid villi*, or granulations, project into the superior sagittal and transverse venous sinuses. Absorption of CSF by arachnoid villi allows for removal by the venous drainage system. The delicate structure of the arachnoid villi places them at risk for obstruction by blood in subarachnoid hemorrhage, resulting in *communicating hydrocephalus.*[2,3,15]

Pia Mater. The pia mater adheres directly to brain tissue. Rich in small blood vessels that supply a large volume of arterial blood to the CNS, this membrane closely follows all folds and convolutions of the brain's surface.

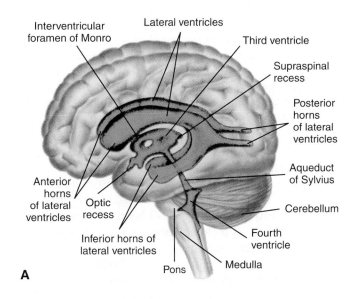

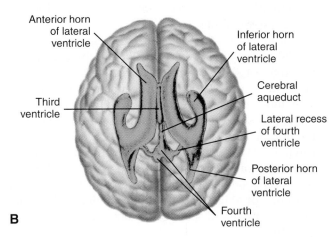

Fig. 25-9   Ventricular system. **A,** Lateral view. **B,** Superior view. (From Thompson JM et al: *Mosby's clinical nursing,* ed 5, St Louis, 2002, Mosby.)

Tufts or folds of the pia mater in the lateral, third, and fourth ventricles form a portion of the choroid plexus that is responsible for the production of CSF.[1,3]

Ventricular System. The *ventricular system* consists of four CSF-filled canals lined with ependymal cells, a type of neuroglial cell (Fig. 25-9). This system is made up of two large *lateral ventricles* that each lie within a hemisphere of the cerebral cortex. Extending from the frontal lobes to the occipital lobe, the lateral ventricles consist of a body, an atrium, and frontal, temporal, and occipital horns.[1,17] When cannulation of the ventricular system is required for intracranial pressure monitoring, CSF drainage, or placement of a CSF shunt, the frontal horn of the lateral ventricle on the nondominant side of the brain is most often selected.

The foramen of Monro connects the two lateral ventricles with a central cavity, the *third ventricle*. Located directly above the midbrain, the walls of the third ventricle are formed by the thalami. The *cerebral aqueduct (aqueduct of Sylvius)* is the canal between the third and *fourth ventricle*, which lies between the brainstem and the cerebellum. At the base of the fourth ventricle, two openings—the *foramen of Luschka* and the *foramen of Magendie*—open into the subarachnoid space.[1,3] Blockage of CSF flow occurring within the ventricular system obstructs the normal circulation of CSF, causing dilation of the ventricles, and is termed *noncommunicating hydrocephalus.*[2,3]

Cerebrospinal Fluid. CSF fills the ventricular system and surrounds the brain and spinal cord in the subarachnoid space. Protection of the CNS is further provided by CSF, which acts as a "shock absorber" when energy is displaced in traumatic injury.

CSF is normally clear, colorless, and odorless. It is secreted by the choroid plexuses of the ventricular system, although small amounts are also synthesized by capillaries of the pia mater. Believed to be a filtrate of blood, CSF contains some unique properties that make its synthesis a mystery (Table 25-2).[1,3]

The production of CSF occurs at a rate of approximately 20 ml/hour, or 500 ml/day. With a circulating volume of 135 to 150 ml, CSF must be regularly resorbed to prevent development of hydrocephalus. Resorption through intact arachnoid villi is favored by increased hydrostatic pressure mechanics that maintain CSF volume within normal limits.[1]

The flow of CSF is from the lateral ventricles, through the Foramina of Monro into the third ventricle, through the cerebral aqueduct into the fourth ventricle, and out the foramen of Magendie and the Foramina of Luschka into the subarachnoid space of the brain and spinal cord (Fig. 25-10).

Blood-Brain Barrier. The blood-brain barrier is a physiologic mechanism that helps maintain the delicate metabolic balance in the CNS. The blood-brain barrier regulates the transport of nutrients, ions, water, and waste products through selective permeability.[3]

Stabilization of the physical and chemical environment surrounding the neurons of the CNS is the task of the blood-brain barrier. Many substances, such as metabolites or toxic compounds, cannot cross the blood-brain barrier. Other substances, such as antibiotics, cross slowly, resulting in lower concentrations of them in the brain than in other areas of the body.

The blood-brain barrier operates on the concept of "tight junctions" between adjacent cells and actually consists of three separate barriers.[1,3] The vascular endothelial barrier is formed by tight junctions between the endothelial cells of cerebral blood vessels. The blood-CSF barrier consists of tight junctions between the epithelial cells of the choroid plexus. The arachnoid barrier is created by tight junctions between the cells that form the outermost layer of the arachnoid mater. The selective permeability of the blood-brain barrier keeps out toxic or harmful compounds and protects neuronal function.

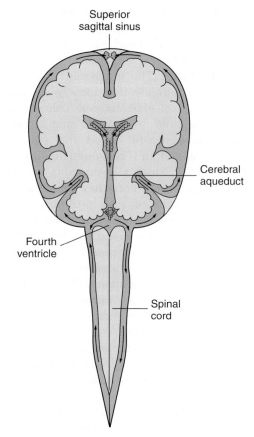

Fig. 25-10 Path of circulation of cerebrospinal fluid from its formation in the ventricles to its absorption into the superior sagittal sinus. (From Waxman SG, deGroot J: *Correlative neuroanatomy,* ed 23, Norwalk, Connecticut, 1996, Appleton & Lange. Reproduced with permission of the McGraw-Hill Companies.)

Table 25-2	Normal CSF Profile Values
Property	**Values**
pH	7.35-7.45
Specific gravity	1.007
Appearance	Clear and colorless
Cells	0 white blood cells (WBCs)
	0 red blood cells (RBCs)
	0-10 lymphocytes
Glucose	50-75 mg/dl (two thirds of blood sugar value)
Protein	5-25 mg/dl
Volume	135-150 ml
Pressure	70-200 mm H_2O (lumbar puncture)
	3-15 mm Hg (ventricular)

CSF, Cerebrospinal fluid.

Passage of substances across the blood-brain barrier is a function of particle size, lipid solubility, and protein-binding potential.[1,3] Most drugs or compounds that are lipid soluble and stable at body pH rapidly cross the blood-brain barrier. The blood-brain barrier is also very permeable to water, oxygen, carbon dioxide, and glucose.

The blood-brain barrier exists only in certain areas of the CNS. The areas in which it does not exist—the pineal region, the basal hypothalamus, and the floor of the fourth ventricle—require contact with plasma to sense changes in concentration of glucose and carbon dioxide, as well as changes in serum osmolality.[1] Initiation of feedback mechanisms by the hypothalamus in response to these changes regulates the internal environment of the rest of the body.

Of clinical significance, disruption or alteration of blood-brain barrier permeability occurs with injury to brain tissue from causes including trauma, toxic insults, and ischemic injury. Brain irradiation also may alter the permeability of the blood-brain barrier, although intravenously administered chemotherapeutic agents have been shown to have little effect on blood-brain barrier permeability.

CEREBRUM

The cerebrum is the largest portion of the brain, comprising 80% of its weight. It is composed of two cerebral hemispheres (right and left), separated by the longitudinal fissure and connected at the base by the *corpus callosum.*

The outermost aspect of the cerebrum is called the *cerebral cortex* and is made up of *gray matter,* consisting of neuronal cell bodies. Directly below the cerebral cortex lies *white matter,* consisting of myelinated axons, which communicate impulses from the cerebral cortex to other areas of the brain. White matter tracts consist of three types of fibers: *commissural* (transverse), *projection,* and *association.*[1,3] Commissural fibers are tracts that communicate between the two cerebral hemispheres, and the corpus callosum is the largest commissural tract. Projection fibers communicate between the cerebral cortex and lower regions of the brain and spinal cord. Association fibers communicate between various regions of the same hemisphere.

The cerebral hemispheres are divided into the *frontal, parietal, temporal,* and *occipital* lobes (Fig. 25-11). The *rhinencephalon* is often labeled as a fifth lobe of the cerebral cortex. Lying deep inside the cerebrum and anatomically associated with the temporal lobe, the rhinencephalon is also sometimes referred to as the *limbic lobe.*[1,18]

The primary functions of the cerebral cortex include sensory, motor, and intellectual (cognitive) functions, making this area of the brain vital to normal human functioning and providing capabilities that make humans unique as a species.[1] Brodmann's classification of cerebral cortical cytoarchitecture identifies more than 100 unique areas and provides a useful way to localize specific cortical functions within the brain (Fig. 25-12). This section will cover those areas within Brodmann's classification that are commonly assessed in relation to the development of specific neurologic pathology.

Frontal Lobe. The frontal lobe lies underneath the frontal bone of the skull and is separated posteriorly from the parietal lobe by the central sulcus (fissure of Rolando) and inferiorly from the temporal lobe by the lateral fissure (Sylvian fissure). The major functions of the frontal lobe are voluntary motor function, cognitive function (orientation, memory, insight, judgment, arithmetic, and abstraction), and expressive language (verbal and written).[1,3]

The prefrontal areas (Brodmann's areas 9 to 12), located just behind the frontal bone's distribution over the forehead, are concerned with cognition.[1-3,11] These areas work in concert with other areas of the brain to intellectually appraise and respond to environmental information or stimuli. They augment intellect with socially trained emotional responses learned over the course of childhood and young adulthood, and participate in triggering autonomic nervous system responses such as tachycardia, in relation to situational needs. The location of the prefrontal cortex makes it vulnerable to traumatic injury, often resulting in profound changes in cognitive capacity and social responses to environmental stimuli following brain injury.[10]

The motor strip of the frontal cortex is represented by Brodmann's area 4 and consists of cell bodies for neurons associated with *voluntary (pyramidal) motor* functions. It is important to remember that since most voluntary motor tracts cross over to the opposite side as they descend through the brainstem, the right motor strip represents voluntary motor function for the left side of the body and vice versa.[1-3] The motor *homunculus* (Fig. 25-13, *A*) is a graphic representation of the distribution of voluntary motor function throughout area 4. Appearing as an upside-down man, the foot of the homunculus is illustrated on the superior medial aspects of the frontal lobes, with the knees, hips, trunk, and shoulders extending along the lateral surfaces, and the hands, thumb, head, face, and tongue represented in a lateral inferior distribution extending to the Sylvian fissure. The homunculus demonstrates larger body part size to denote those areas with greater representation because of the amount of dexterity associated with the part's function. Therefore the large surface area of the trunk occupies a relatively small part of the motor strip, whereas smaller body areas, such as the thumb or tongue that involve a great deal of dexterity and fine motor movement, occupy a larger area of the motor strip. Damage to the motor strip results in compromise of motor function on the opposite side of the body.

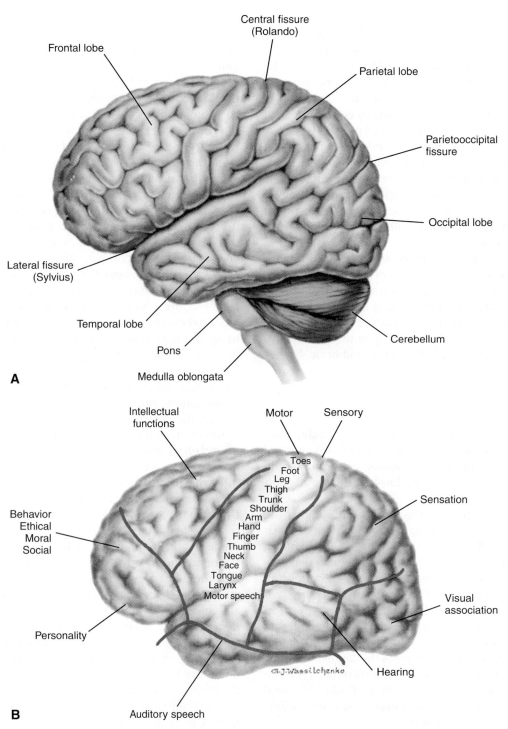

Fig. 25-11 **A,** Lateral view of the cerebral hemispheres (showing lobes and principal fissures), cerebellum, pons, and medulla oblongata. **B,** Principal functional subdivisions of cerebral hemisphere.

Broca's area (area 44) is located at the inferior frontal gyrus in close proximity to the motor strip's facial distribution (see Fig. 25-12). Most commonly, Broca's area is located on the left side of the frontal lobe, although it may on occasion be located in the right frontal hemisphere. Broca's area is responsible for expressive language and is used in the formation of both verbal and written communication.[1] Damage occurring to this area results in disability ranging from word-finding difficulties to an expressive or nonfluent aphasia, where verbal and written communication are significantly compromised, although verbal language reception and comprehension may remain intact.[3,11,15]

Parietal Lobe. The parietal lobe lies directly behind the frontal lobe on the opposite side of the central sulcus. The posterior border of the parietal lobe is the pari-

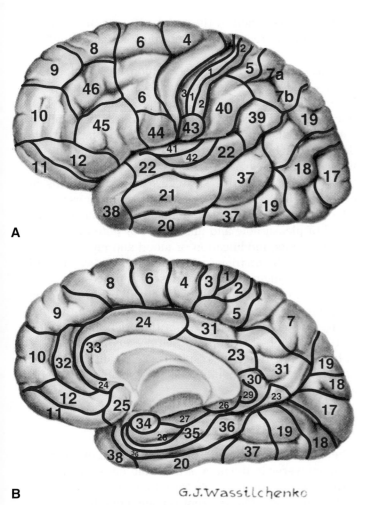

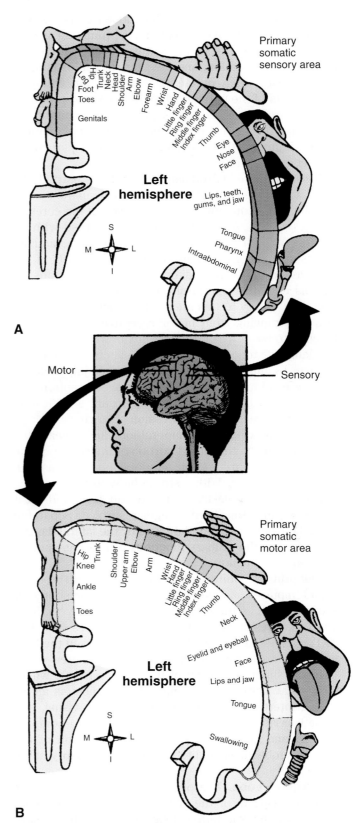

Fig. 25-12 Cytoarchitectural map of the lateral and medial surface of the human cortex according to Brodmann's primary somatic sensory **(A)** and motor **(B)** areas of the cortex. (From Thibodeau GA, Patton KT: *Anatomy & physiology,* ed 5, St Louis, 2003, Mosby.)

etooccipital fissure, which separates it from the occipital lobe. The parietal lobes are primarily concerned with sensory functions including integration of sensory information; awareness of body parts; interpretation of touch, pressure, and pain; and recognition of object size, shape, and texture.[1]

The parietal lobe contains a sensory strip (areas 1, 2, and 3) that lies opposite the motor strip of the frontal lobe (see Fig. 25-12). Similar to the homunculus of the motor strip, a sensory homunculus recreates a caricature of an upside-down man (Fig. 25-13, *B*) representing those areas that account for receipt and initial analyses of sensory information from different areas of the body. Areas of the body with greater sensory needs occupy larger areas on the sensory strip, which is concerned with both deep or internal sensations, as well as cutaneous sensations such as touch, pressure, position, and vibration. Injury to these areas may result in tactile sensory loss on the opposite side of the body.

Fig. 25-13 Primary somatic sensory **(A)** and motor **(B)** areas of the cortex. (From Thibodeau GA, Patton KT: *Anatomy & physiology,* ed 5, St Louis, 2003, Mosby.)

Associative areas of the parietal lobe (areas 5 and 7) further assessment of sensory stimuli, promoting an ability to determine size, shape, texture, locality of stimuli, temperature, vibration, and precise purpose of familiar objects based solely on tactile discrimination. Interpretive aspects of the parietal lobe's response to stimuli include awareness of body parts, perceptual orientation in space, and recognition of environmental spatial relationships.[1] Injury to these areas may result in perceptual neglect or inattention.[11,15]

Wernicke's area (Brodmann's area 22) is partially located within the parietal lobe and partially in the temporal lobe, most commonly on the left side of the cerebral cortex (see Fig. 25-12). This area is concerned with reception of both written and verbal language, and includes many intricate connections to other parts of the brain associated with auditory and visual functions, as well as cognitive appraisal and ultimately, expressive language.[1] Injury to this area of the brain may result in disability ranging from minor receptive language dysfunction to *receptive* or *fluent aphasia*, whereby expressive language function remains but is illogical in content or a *word salad*. In instances where brain injury includes those areas important to both language reception and expression, a *global aphasia* may result, significantly limiting both receipt and expression of language.[11,15]

Temporal Lobe. The temporal lobe lies beneath the temporal bone in the lateral portion of the cranium. The anterior, lower border of the temporal lobe is encased in the sphenoid wing. With a strong blow to the head the temporal lobe is easily contused and lacerated as it moves against this hard, irregular surface. Separated from the frontal and parietal lobes by the lateral fissure, this lobe has the primary functions of hearing, speech, behavior, and memory.[1,3]

The primary auditory areas (areas 41 and 42) receive sound impulses and assist in determining the source of sound as well as the meaning of sound. Injury to these areas may result in auditory perceptual loss (see Fig. 25-12). As noted previously, auditory centers in the temporal lobe are closely linked with Wernicke's area.

In the superior portion of the temporal lobe, where the frontal, parietal, and temporal lobes meet, is an essential interpretive area in which auditory, visual, and somatic association areas are integrated into complex thought and memory.[1,3] Seizures in this region of the temporal lobe cause auditory, visual, and sensory hallucinations.[2]

Occipital Lobe. The occipital lobe forms the most posterior aspects of the cerebral cortex and are concerned with interpretation of visual stimuli. The primary visual cortex (area 17) receives impulses from projections of the optic nerve (cranial nerve II). These impulses are then referred to the visual associative areas (areas 18 and 19) for interpretation and integration (see Fig. 25-12). Injury to the occipital lobes may result in cor-

tical blindness, whereby the eye structures remain intact but ability to receive and interpret visual stimuli is lost.[11,15]

Limbic Lobe. The rhinencephalon, or limbic lobe, lies medially along the inner aspects of the temporal lobe. The core of the limbic system consists of the hippocampus and the amygdaloid nucleus.[1,18] In comparison to animals living in the wild, the limbic lobe is poorly developed in humans as a result of the sophisticated cognitive capabilities of the frontal lobe, which mediate many of the protective strategies used by humans in everyday life. The limbic lobe's primary functions are related to self-preservation and include such functions as recall of pleasurable and unpleasant or potentially dangerous events, modification of mood and emotional responses in relation to perceived events, interpretation of smell, and augmentation of visceral processes (e.g., heart rate, respirations) associated with emotion. When the prefrontal cortex is injured resulting in cognitive disability, this controversial area of the brain may take on increased control to support self-preservation needs;[18] unfortunately, this may result in significantly aberrant behavior that is frequently judged as socially unacceptable in today's world.

INTERNAL CAPSULE

Fiber tracts from many portions of each half of the cerebrum converge in the area of the brain known as the internal capsule, as they progress toward the brainstem and spinal cord. The internal capsule contains both afferent and efferent fibers (Fig. 25-14). Afferent (sensory) impulses destined for the cortex travel through the internal capsule in the following succession: brainstem to thalamus, to internal capsule, to cerebral cortex. Efferent (motor) fibers leaving the cortex also pass through

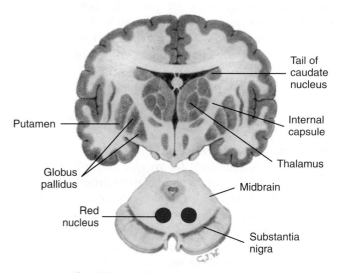

Fig. 25-14 Coronal section of brain.

Tail of caudate nucleus

Internal capsule

Thalamus

Midbrain

Substantia nigra

Red nucleus

Globus pallidus

Putamen

the internal capsule.[1] Injury to a portion of the internal capsule may result in pure sensory and/or motor loss on the opposite side of the body with preservation of cortical function.[11]

BASAL GANGLIA

The basal ganglia participate in regulating extrapyramidal (involuntary) motor function.[1-3] Located deep within the white matter of the cerebral hemispheres, the basal ganglia consist of four nuclei including the corpus striatum (caudate nucleus, putamen, and nucleus accumbens); the globus pallidus; the substantia nigra; and the subthalamic nucleus[1] (see Fig. 25-14). The basal ganglia are considered a telencephalic, or cerebral, structure and are embryologically separate from the thalamus, which is considered a diencephalic structure.[1,2]

Although the basal ganglia play a major role in regulating voluntary motor function, they do not provide direct input to motor tracts via the spinal cord. Instead, input from the cerebral cortex stimulates basal ganglia output, which is sent to the brainstem and the thalamus for relay back to the frontal cortex.[1] Ultimately, the basal ganglia integrate associated movements and postural adjustments with voluntary motor movement, suppressing skeletal muscle tone as needed to provide fluid, smooth

motor function. Dysfunction of the basal ganglia may result in tremor or other involuntary movements, rigid, nonfluid muscle tone, and slowness of movement without paralysis.[2]

DIENCEPHALON

The diencephalon lies below the cerebral cortex and consists of two structures, the thalamus and the hypothalamus (Fig. 25-15). Although structurally wedded to the hypothalamus, the pituitary gland is considered an endocrine organ, and is not a part of the CNS;[1-3] a complete discussion of pituitary gland anatomy and physiology is found in Chapter 34.

Thalamus. The thalamus consists of two connected ovoid masses of gray matter and forms the lateral walls of the third ventricle (see Figs. 25-14 and 25-15). The two thalami serve as a relay station and gatekeeper for both motor and sensory stimuli, preventing or enhancing transmission of impulses based on the behavioral needs of the person. More than 50 nuclei support thalamic function and are divided into specific, relay nuclei and nonspecific, diffusely projecting nuclei.[1] Relay nuclei have a specific relationship or trajectory within the cerebral cortex, while diffusely projecting nuclei are thought to mediate cortical arousal. Thalamic injury may result

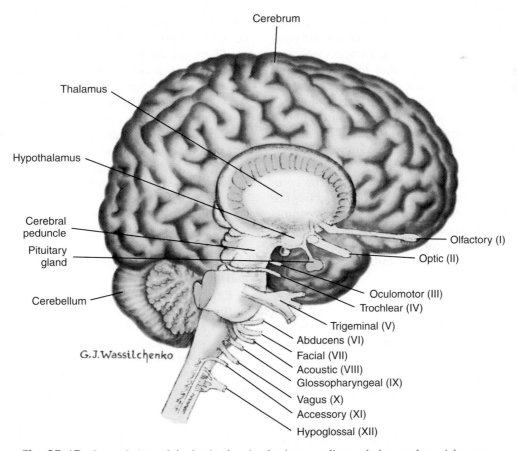

Fig. 25-15   Lateral view of the brain showing brainstem, diencephalon, and cranial nerves.

in sensory and/or motor dysfunction as normal impulse pathways are interrupted.[2,11]

Hypothalamus. The hypothalamus is located below the thalamus and is connected to the pituitary gland by the hypothalamic or pituitary stalk (see Fig. 25-15). Neural control of emotion involves many regions of the brain, including the amygdala and limbic associations with the prefrontal cortex, but to ensure homeostasis these systems all work through the hypothalamus to coordinate the body's behavioral responses to emotion. The hypothalamus maintains internal homeostasis through its ability to stimulate autonomic nervous system response and endocrine system function in relation to body needs, giving the hypothalamus a role in temperature regulation, regulation of food and water intake, control of pituitary hormone release, and augmentation of overall autonomic nervous system output to either a sympathetic or parasympathetic state.[1]

CEREBELLUM

The cerebellum (see Fig. 25-15), or "hind brain," is separated from the cerebrum by the dural fold named the *tentorium cerebelli.* Accounting for one fifth of the brain's size, the cerebellum consists of two lateral hemispheres connected by the *vermis.* The cerebellum is composed of an outer layer of gray matter, or cortex, with a core of white matter tracts lying beneath.[1,3]

Cerebellar impulses are communicated to descending motor pathways to integrate spatial orientation and equilibrium with posture and muscle tone, ensuring synchronized adjustments in movement that maintain overall balance and motor coordination.[1,2] Cerebellar monitoring and adjustment of motor activity occurs simultaneously with movement, enabling significant control of fine motor function. The cerebellum is literally bombarded with information related to the goals of movement and disparities between actual and intended movements. There are 40 times more axons projecting into the cerebellum, compared to the number of axons leaving the cerebellum, to ensure adequate receipt of motor information.[2] Injury to the cerebellum produces *ataxia,* defined as preservation of motor strength with lack of control (coordination) over fine motor function.[2,11]

BRAINSTEM

The brainstem consists of three major divisions—the midbrain, the pons, and the medulla oblongata—and is packed with sensory and motor pathways traveling between the spinal cord and the brain, as well as a number of centers that regulate vital mechanisms throughout the body (see Fig. 25-15).

Midbrain. The midbrain forms the junction between the pons and the diencephalon. The cell bodies of cranial nerves III and IV originate in the midbrain (Table 25-3).

The midbrain is divided by a sagittal plane into the two cerebral peduncles, and anatomically it constitutes the location of the aqueduct of Sylvius (see Fig. 25-15). The major function of the midbrain is to relay stimuli to and from the brain through ascending sensory tracts and descending motor pathways.[1,2]

Pons. Located above the medulla, the pons also relays information to and from the brain through sensory and motor pathways. The posterior aspects of the pons make up the upper surface of the fourth ventricle (see Fig. 25-15). Two respiratory control centers are located in the pons, namely the apneustic and pneumotaxic centers. The apneustic center controls the length of inspiration and expiration, whereas the pneumotaxic center controls respiratory rate.[1-3]

The cell bodies of cranial nerves V (trigeminal), VI (abducens), VII (facial), and VIII (acoustic) are located in the pons (see Table 25-3).[1] The medial longitudinal fasciculus (MLF) is an important fiber tract in the pons that connects cranial nerves III, IV, and VI with the vestibular portion of the acoustic nerve and pontine paramedian reticular formation, allowing coordinated and appropriate movements of the eyes in response to noise, motion, position, and arousal. The structural integrity of the brainstem may be assessed through clinical stimulation of the MLF in caloric testing.[2]

Medulla Oblongata. The medulla oblongata forms the last section of the brainstem, situated between the pons and the spinal cord (see Fig. 25-15). In the pyramids of the medulla, decussation (crossing) of voluntary motor fibers occurs, lending the name *pyramidal* to voluntary motor function. Below the point of decussation, stimuli from the right side of the brain control movement for the left side of the body and vice versa.[1]

Centers for control of involuntary functions such as swallowing, vomiting, hiccoughing, coughing, heart rate, arterial vasoconstriction, and respiration are located within the medulla oblongata. The medullary respiratory center works in conjunction with the apneustic and pneumotaxic centers in the pons to control respiratory function and is responsible for the rhythm of respiration. The cell bodies of cranial nerves IX (glossopharyngeal), X (vagus), XI (spinal accessory), and XII (hypoglossal) are also located in the medulla oblongata (see Fig. 25-15 and Table 25-3).[1,2]

Reticular Formation. The reticular formation (RF) of the brainstem is located at the core of the brainstem and is active in modulating sensation, movement, consciousness, reflexive behaviors, and the activities of the cranial nerves arising from the brainstem (III-XII). The RF extends from the upper pons to the diencephalon.[1] The ascending RF is referred to as the reticular activating system (RAS) and is responsible for increasing wakefulness, vigilance, and responsiveness of cortical and thalamic neurons to sensory stimuli. In the thalamus, the RAS activates both relay and diffuse projection nuclei to

Table 25-3	Cranial Nerves, Origins, Course, and Functions	
Cranial Nerve	**Origin and Course**	**Function**
I OLFACTORY Sensory	Mucosa of nasal cavity; only cranial nerves with cell body located in peripheral structure (nasal mucosa). Pass through cribriform plate of ethmoid bone and go on to olfactory bulbs at floor of frontal lobe. Final interpretation is in temporal lobe.	Smell. However, system is more than receptor/interpreter for odors; perception of smell also sensitizes other body systems and responses, such as salivation, peristalsis, and even sexual stimulus. Loss of sense of smell is termed *anosmia*.
II OPTIC Sensory	Ganglion cells of retina converge to the optic disc and form optic nerve. Nerve fibers pass to optic chiasm, which is above pituitary gland. Some fibers decussate; others do not. The two tracts then go to the lateral geniculate body near the thalamus and then on to the end station for interpretation in the occipital lobe.	Vision

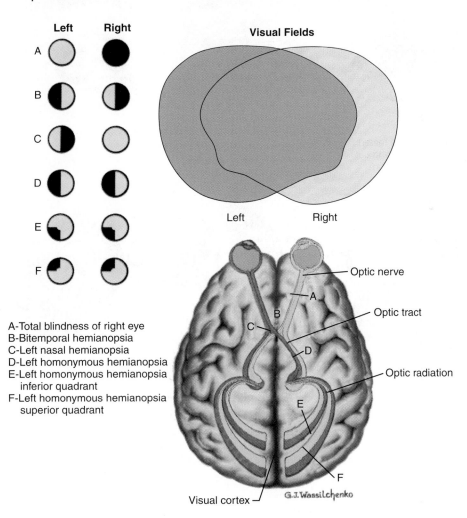

A-Total blindness of right eye
B-Bitemporal hemianopsia
C-Left nasal hemianopsia
D-Left homonymous hemianopsia
E-Left homonymous hemianopsia inferior quadrant
F-Left homonymous hemianopsia superior quadrant

Continued

Table 25-3	Cranial Nerves, Origins, Course, and Functions—cont'd	
Cranial Nerve	**Origin and Course**	**Function**
III OCULOMOTOR	Originates in midbrain and emerges from brainstem at upper pons.	Extraocular movement of eyes (see Fig. 23-10).
Motor	Motor fibers to superior, medial, inferior recti, and inferior oblique for eye movement; levator muscle of the eyelid.	Raise eyelid.
Parasympathetic	Parasympathetic fibers to ciliary muscles and iris of eye.	Constrict pupil; change shape of lens.

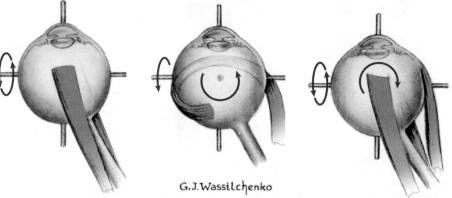

A
Superior rectus tested by gaze up and out

B
Inferior oblique tested by gaze up and in

C
Medial rectus tested by gaze directed in toward nose (medial)

Inferior rectus tested by gaze down and out

G.J.Wassilchenko

Table 25-3	Cranial Nerves, Origins, Course, and Functions—cont'd	
Cranial Nerve	**Origin and Course**	**Function**

IV TROCHLEAR

Motor — Midbrain origin near oculomotor, emerges at upper pons near cerebral peduncle. Motor fibers to superior oblique muscle of eyeball. | Extraocular movement of eyes.

Superior oblique tested
by gaze down and in

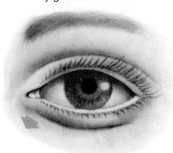 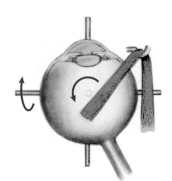 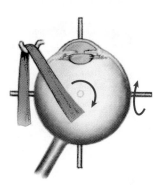

G.J.Wassilchenko

V TRIGEMINAL

Sensory — Originates in fourth ventricle and emerges at lateral parts of pons. Has three branches to face; ophthalmic, maxillary, and mandibular.

Ophthalmic branch: Sensation to cornea, ciliary body, iris, lacrimal gland, conjunctiva, nasal mucosal membranes, eyelids, eyebrows, forehead, and nose.
Maxillary branch: Sensation to skin of cheek, lower lid, side of nose and upper jaw, teeth, mucosa of mouth, sphenopolative-pterygoid region, and maxillary sinus.
Mandibular branch: Sensation to skin of lower lip, chin, ear, mucous membrane, teeth of lower jaw, and tongue.

Motor — Goes to temporalis, masseter, pterygoid gland, anterior part of digastric muscles (all for mastication), and the tensor tympani and tensor veli palatine muscles (clench jaw). — Muscles of chewing and mastication and opening jaw.

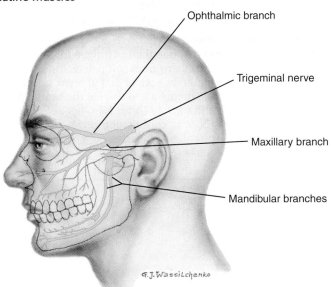

Ophthalmic branch

Trigeminal nerve

Maxillary branch

Mandibular branches

G.J.Wassilchenko

Continued

Table 25-3	Cranial Nerves, Origins, Course, and Functions—cont'd	
Cranial Nerve	**Origin and Course**	**Function**

VI ABDUCENS

Motor — Posterior part of pons goes to lateral rectus muscle for eye movement. — Extraocular eye movement; rotates eyeball outward.

Lateral rectus tested by gaze directed outward away from nose (lateral)

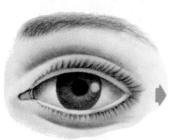
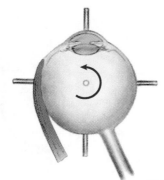
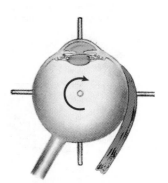

G.J.Wassilchenko

VII FACIAL

Sensory	Lower portion of pons goes to anterior two thirds of tongue and soft palate.	Taste in anterior two thirds of tongue. Sensation to soft palate.
Motor	Pons to muscles of forehead, eyelids, checks, lips, ears, nose, and neck.	Movement of facial muscles to produce facial expressions, close eyes.
Parasympathetic	Pons to salivary gland and lacrimal glands.	Secretory for salivation and tears.

VII ACOUSTIC

Sensory	Two divisions:	
	Cochlear division: Originates in spinal ganglia of the cochlea, with peripheral fibers to the organ of Corti in the internal ear. Goes to pons, and impulses transmitted to the temporal lobe.	Hearing.
	Vestibular division: Originates in otolith organs of the semicircular canals in the inner ear and in the vestibular ganglion. Terminates in pons, with some fibers continuing to cerebellum. The only cranial nerve that originates wholly within a bone, the petrous portion of the temporal bone.	Equilibrium.

IX GLOSSOPHARYNGEAL

Sensory	Posterior one third of tongue for taste sensation and sensations from soft palate, tonsils, and opening to mouth in back of oral pharynx (fauces). Fibers go to the medulla and then to the temporal lobe for taste and sensory cortex for other sensations.	Taste in posterior one third of tongue. Sensation in back of throat; stimulation elicits a gag reflex.
Motor	Medulla to constrictor muscles of pharynx and stylopharyngeal muscles.	Voluntary muscles for swallowing and phonation.
Parasympathetic	Medulla to parotid salivary gland via otic ganglia.	Secretory, salivary glands. Carotid reflex.

Table 25-3	Cranial Nerves, Origins, Course, and Functions—cont'd	
Cranial Nerve	**Origin and Course**	**Function**
X VAGUS		
Sensory	Sensory fibers in back of ear and posterior wall of external ear go to medulla oblongata and on to sensory cortex.	Sensation behind ear and part of external ear meatus.
Motor	Fibers go from medulla oblongata through jugular foramen with glossopharyngeal nerve and on to pharynx, larynx, esophagus, bronchi, lungs, heart, stomach, small intestine, liver, pancreas, and kidneys.	Voluntary muscles for phonation and swallowing. Involuntary activity of visceral muscles of heart, lungs, and digestive tract.
Parasympathetic	Medulla oblongata to larynx, trachea, lungs, aorta, esophagus, stomach, small intestines, and gallbladder.	Carotid reflex. Autonomic activity of respiratory tract and digestive tract, including peristalsis and secretion from organs.
XI SPINAL ACCESSORY		
Motor	This nerve has two roots, cranial and spinal. Cranial portion arises at several rootlets at side of medulla, runs below vagus, and is joined by spinal portion from motor cells in cervical cord. Some fibers go along with vagus nerve to supply motor impulse to pharynx, larynx, uvula, and palate. Major portion to sternomastoid and trapezius muscles, branches to cervical spinal nerves C2-C4.	Some fibers for swallowing and phonation. Turn head and shrug shoulders.
XII HYPOGLOSSAL		
Motor	Arises in medulla oblongata and goes to muscles of tongue.	Movement of tongue necessary for swallowing and phonation.

increase distribution of sensory stimuli throughout the cerebral cortex.[1,2] The RAS also works through activation of the hypothalamus, which results in diffuse cortical stimulation as well as autonomic stimulation.[1] Damage to either the thalamic or hypothalamic RAS pathways results in impaired consciousness.[19]

ARTERIAL CIRCULATION

The brain constitutes 2% of the body's weight but uses 20% of the body's total resting cardiac output.[1,15] It requires approximately 750 ml of blood flow per minute and can extract as much as 45% of arterial oxygen to meet normal metabolic needs.[1,15,16] It has no reserve of either oxygen or glucose, making reductions of these substances critical to the disruption of normal cellular function. Two pairs of arteries, the internal carotids and the vertebral arteries, provide blood to the brain and are anatomically separated into the anterior and posterior circulations that connect at the base of the brain to form the circle of Willis (Fig. 25-16).[1,16] Knowledge of the brain's arterial supply as it correlates to neurologic function is an essential aspect of neuroscience critical care nursing, especially in the care of stroke patients. Arterial distribution for the cerebral cortex is illustrated in Fig. 25-17.

Anterior Circulation. The anterior circulation of the brain is supplied by the right and left internal carotid arteries and their branches. Originating as the common carotids, the left common carotid takes off from the arch of the aorta, whereas the right common carotid originates from the innominate artery. At the level of the crycothyroid junction, the common carotid splits to form the external and internal carotid arteries. The external carotid feeds the face, the scalp, and the skull and includes the branch called the *middle meningeal artery*, which lies between the skull and the dura.[1]

The internal carotid artery continues upward through the carotid siphon and enters the base of the skull through an opening in the petrous bone. At the base of the brain the internal carotid gives off the right and left middle cerebral arteries (MCAs), the right and left anterior cerebral arteries (ACAs) which are connected by the anterior communicating artery (AcoA), and the two posterior communicating arteries (PcoAs).[16] The anterior circulation provides 80% of the blood flow to the cerebral hemispheres, covering the needs of the frontal lobes and most of the parietal and temporal lobes as well as the subcortical structures residing above the brainstem.[1,11,16]

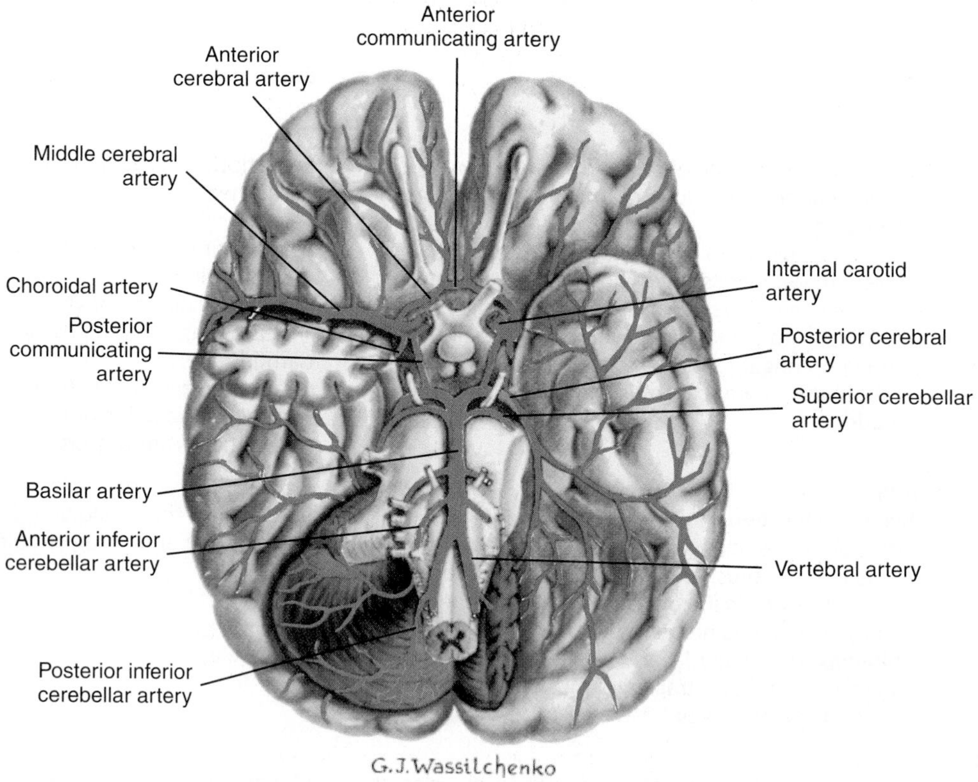

G. J. Wassilchenko

Fig. 25-16 Blood supply of the brain.

The internal carotid artery also gives rise to the ophthalmic artery at the siphon, before bifurcating into the anterior cerebral and middle cerebral arteries. The ophthalmic artery supplies blood to the optic nerve and eye, and may reverse its course to supplement the anterior circulation's arterial blood volume in the case of internal carotid artery occlusion.[16]

Posterior Circulation. The posterior circulation begins with the two vertebral arteries, which originate from the subclavian arteries and travel posteriorly through small openings in the lateral spinous processes of the cervical spine. They enter the skull through the foramen magnum, and at the level of the pons the two vertebral arteries fuse to form the basilar artery.[1] The terminal portion of the vertebral arteries gives rise to two important arterial branches prior to basilar artery fusion, namely, the posterior inferior cerebellar arteries (PICA).[11,16] Two major infratentorial branches of the basilar artery include the anterior inferior cerebellar arteries (AICA) and superior cerebellar arteries (SCA), which together with the PICA supply the cerebellum.[11] The distal basilar artery gives rise to the two posterior cerebral arteries (PCAs), which emerge in the supratentorial region to supply the posterior aspects of the cerebral cortex.[1,11,16]

Circle of Willis. The circle of Willis is a vascular supply system unique to the brain's circulation (see Fig. 25-16). Located above the optic chiasm in the subarach-

noid space, the circle is fed by branches of the internal carotid and basilar arteries. The anterior circulation is connected between the two ACAs by the AcoA, and to the posterior circulation by the two PcoAs.[1] Approximately 50% of the population has a complete or "ideal" circle of Willis. Most commonly, atretic (small and nonfunctional or hypoplastic) segments are often found in the A1 branch of the ACAs, the P1 branch of the PCAs, and the PcoAs.[16] When complete, the circle of Willis is capable of supporting some degree of collateral blood flow in the case of arterial occlusion, although a sufficient arterial supply in the face of arterial obstruction is not guaranteed.

Venous Circulation. Venous drainage occurs through venous sinuses, many of which are housed in the double-folded membrane of the dura mater. Capillaries drain into venules, which then flow into cerebral veins, ultimately emptying into sinuses located throughout the cranium. Blood from these sinuses empties into the internal jugular vein, which in turn empties into the superior vena cava (Fig. 25-18). Cerebral veins have thinner walls relative to veins in the general circulation and lack a muscular layer or valves.[1,2,15]

SPINAL CORD

The spinal cord makes up the last division of the CNS and extends from the medulla below the foramen mag-

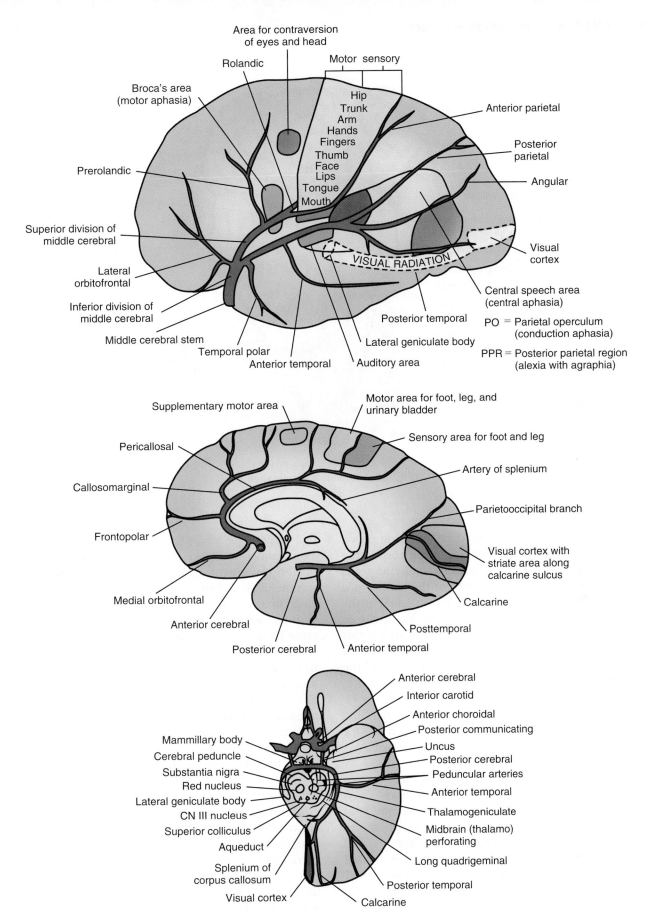

Fig. 25-17 Arterial distribution. (Modified from Adams RD, Victor M: *Principles of neurology,* ed 6, New York, 1997, McGraw-Hill.)

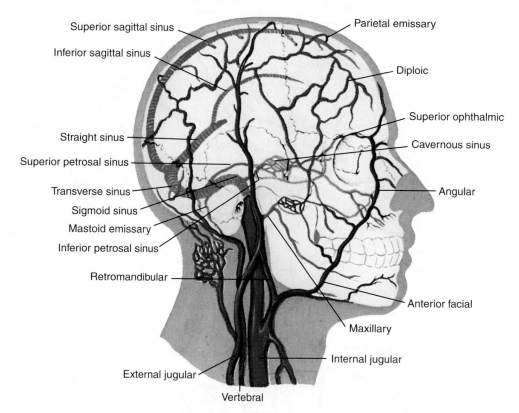

Fig. 25-18 Venous circulation.

num.[1,3] Similar to the brain, the spinal cord is composed of both gray and white matter, although the cord's gray matter is located internally whereas the white matter is located on its surface. The distal end of the spinal cord tapers to the *conus medullaris*, which is situated at the level of the first or second lumbar vertebra. Exiting from the spinal cord are 31 pairs of spinal nerves, which exit through intervertebral foramina. Because the spinal cord ends at L1 and the final nerve roots do not exit until the coccyx, long lengths of nerves, called the *cauda equina*, extend below the conus medullaris toward their associated intervertebral foramina to exit the spinal canal (Fig. 25-19). Similar protective mechanisms to those listed for the brain also provide protection to the spinal cord.[1]

Protective Mechanisms

Bony Structures. The bony structure that encases the spinal cord is the vertebral column. Comprising 33 vertebrae and 24 intervertebral disks, this column, held together by ligaments and tendons, provides support and protection for the spinal cord as well as structure and flexibility for body movement. The vertebrae are divided into sections in relation to their appearance. There are 7 cervical vertebrae, 12 thoracic vertebrae, 5 lumbar vertebrae, 5 sacral vertebrae (fused together as one), and 4 coccygeal vertebrae (fused together as one).[1]

Although differences in vertebral appearance exist, the basic structure includes a vertebral body connected by two pedicles to the transverse processes (Fig. 25-20). Two laminae connect the transverse processes to the posterior segment of the vertebra, the spinous process, forming a ring. The center of the spinal foramen is the canal housing the spinal cord.

Intervertebral Disk. Vertebral bodies are separated by an intervertebral disk. These fibrocartilaginous structures lie between each vertebral body, extending from the cervical vertebra to the beginning of the sacrum. Intervertebral disks are composed of two layers. The inner core, called the nucleus pulposus, is a soft, gelatinous material that assists in shock absorbency. Surrounding the nucleus pulposus is the annulus fibrosus, a thick, tough outer layer.[1] The diagnosis of herniated disk refers to dislocation of the normal anatomic position of an intervertebral disk in such a way as to compromise or put pressure on a spinal nerve.

Meninges. The meninges of the spinal cord are similar to those in the cranium (Fig. 25-21). The dura is a continuation of the intracranial dura mater and encases the cord, the nerve roots, and the spinal nerves until they exit from the vertebral column. The dura extends to the level of the second sacral vertebra, even though the spinal cord itself ends at the L1 or L2 level.[1]

The arachnoid mater provides the same weblike, delicate structure as in the cranium, with CSF flow within the subarachnoid space.[1] Because the spinal cord termi-

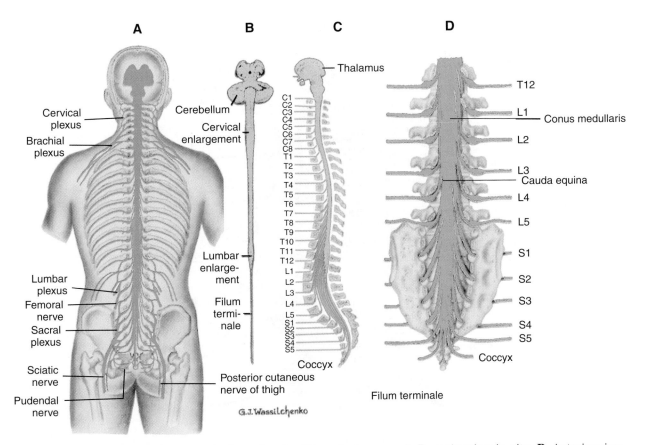

Fig. 25-19 Spinal cord within vertebral canal and exiting spinal nerves. **A,** Posterior view *in situ.* **B,** Anterior view. **C,** Lateral view. **D,** Cauda equina.

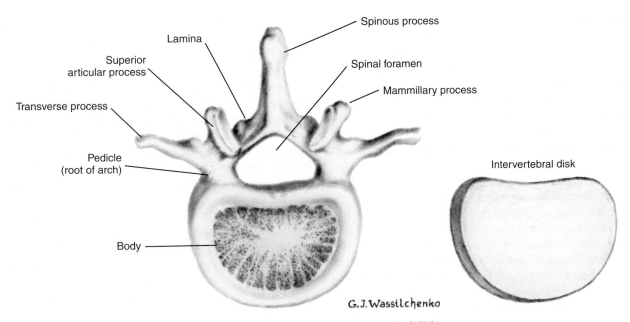

Fig. 25-20 Vertebra and intervertebral disk.

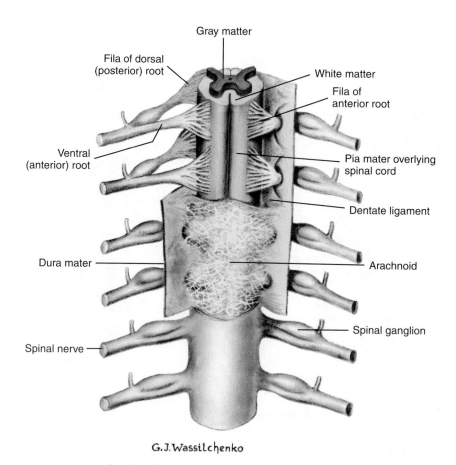

Gray matter

Fila of dorsal
(posterior) root

White matter

Fila of
anterior root

Ventral
(anterior) root

Pia mater overlying
spinal cord

Dentate ligament

Dura mater

Arachnoid

Spinal ganglion

Spinal nerve

G.J.Wassilchenko

Fig. 25-21   Meningeal layers of the spinal cord.

nates at L2 and the meninges continue to S2, a volume of CSF is contained in the lumbar cistern, and constitutes the site targeted for a lumbar puncture.[2,20] The pia mater of the spinal cord is a thicker, firmer, less vascular membrane than that in the cranium.[1]

Spinal Nerves. There are 31 pairs of spinal nerves: 8 cervical, 12 thoracic, 5 lumbar, 5 sacral, and 1 coccygeal (see Fig. 25-19).[1] In the cervical region, the first seven pairs of nerves exit the cord above the corresponding vertebrae. The C8 nerve pair exits the spinal cord below the C7 vertebra. From this point on, all thoracic, lumbar, and sacral nerves exit below the corresponding vertebrae. In other words, spinal cord segments associated with each spinal nerve, and the corresponding vertebra do not directly line up.

The spinal nerve has two roots: the dorsal root and the ventral root. The dorsal root is an afferent pathway and carries sensory impulses from the body into the spinal cord. The ventral root is an efferent pathway and carries motor information from the spinal cord to the body. The dorsal and ventral roots join together as they exit the spinal foramen and become a spinal nerve (see Fig. 25-21).[1] Distribution of the sensory components of each spinal nerve are illustrated as dermatomes. Der-

matome diagrams facilitate identification of sensory innervation throughout the body (Fig. 25-22).

Cross Section of the Spinal Cord. The spinal cord is composed of both gray matter and white matter. The central gray matter, which appears in the shape of an H, consists of cell bodies, small projection fibers, and glial support cells. The gray matter of the spinal cord has been divided into areas based on cell body type and location. The three basic divisions are the anterior horn, the lateral horn, and the posterior horn. The anterior horn contains motor neurons and is the final junction for motor information before it exits the CNS. The lateral horn contains preganglionic fibers of the autonomic nervous system: sympathetic fibers T1 to L2 and parasympathetic fibers S2 to S4. The posterior horn contains sensory neurons and becomes the entry point for afferent impulses to the CNS.[1,3]

The white matter, which surrounds the gray matter, contains the myelinated ascending and descending tracts, which carry information to and from the brain (Fig. 25-23). Spinal tracts are named so that the prefix denotes the origin of the tract and the suffix is the destination, promoting easy identification of sensory or motor tracts. Sensory tracts begin with the prefix *spino,*

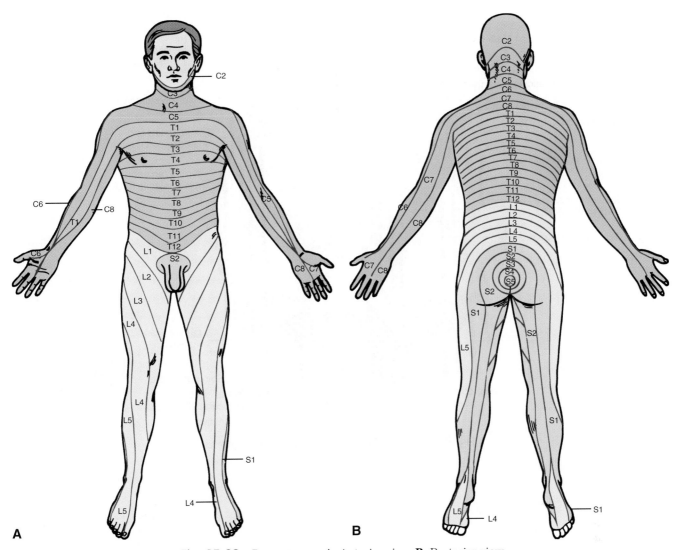

Fig. 25-22 Dermatomes. **A,** Anterior view. **B,** Posterior view.

---

and motor tracts end with the suffix *spinal* (Box 25-1). The complexity of spinal cord tracts is beyond the scope of this text, which is limited to those tracts that are most clinically significant and easily tested.

Vascular Supply. Arterial blood supply to the spinal cord is supplied by branches of the vertebral arteries and small radicular arteries that enter through intervertebral foramina. They combine to form the anterior spinal and two posterior spinal arteries. These three arteries, along with some additional radicular arterial flow from cervical, intercostal, lumbar, and sacral arteries, feed the entire length of the spinal cord (Fig. 25-24).

Arterial supply to the spinal cord is segmented at best, making portions of the spinal cord that receive blood supply from two separate sources vulnerable to low flow states. The most vulnerable of these areas are C2 to C3, T1 to T4, and L1 to L2. Evidence of this tenuous blood supply is occasionally evident following surgical proce-

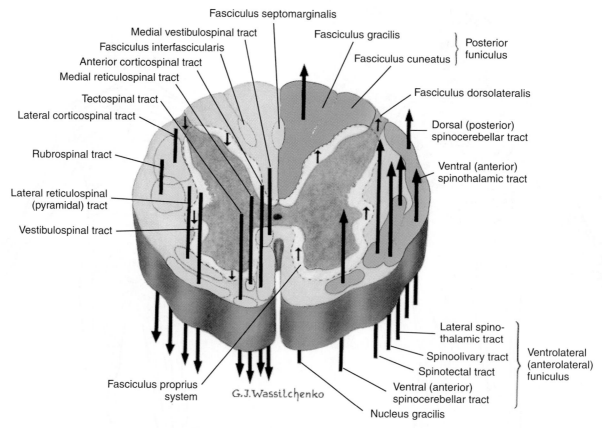

Fig. 25-23 Spinal cord tracts of the white matter.

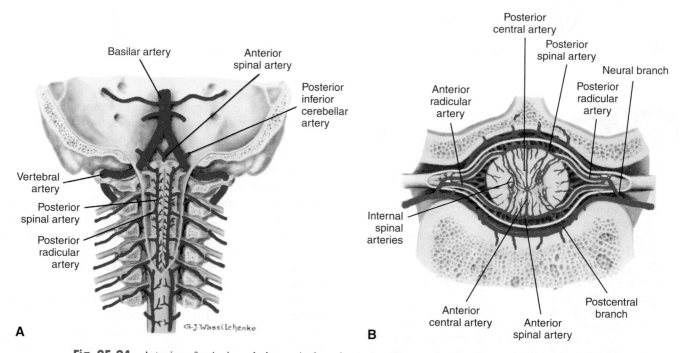

Fig. 25-24 Arteries of spinal cord. **A,** cervical cord arteries. **B,** vascular distribution in the spinal cord.

dures that involve cross-clamping of the aorta, resulting in spinal cord infarction.

REFERENCES

1. Williams PL: *Gray's anatomy,* ed 38, London, 1995, Churchill Livingstone.
2. Kandel ER, Schwartz JH, Jessel TM: *Principles of neuroscience,* ed 4, New York, 2000, McGraw Hill.
3. Waxman SG: *Correlative neuroanatomy,* ed 24, New York, 2000, Lange.
4. Dirnagl U, Iadecola C, Moskowitz MA: Pathobiology of ischaemic stroke: an integrated view, *Trends Neurosci* 22: 391, 1999.
5. Lee JM, Zipfel GJ, Choi DW: The changing landscape of ischaemic brain injury mechanisms, *Nature* 399:A7, 1999.
6. Povlishock JT: Pathophysiology of neural injury: therapeutic opportunities and challenges, *Clin Neurosurg* 46:113, 2000.
7. Stuart G, Spruston N, Hausser M: *Dendrites,* Oxford, 1999, Oxford University Press.
8. Waxman SG, Kocsys JD, Stys PK: *The axon,* Oxford, 1995, Oxford University Press.
9. Cowan WM, Sudhof TC, Stevens CF: *Synapses,* Baltimore, 2001, Johns Hopkins University Press.
10. Narayan RK, Wilberger JE, Povlishock JT: *Neurotrauma,* New York, 1996, McGraw-Hill.
11. Barnett HJM et al, editors: *Stroke: pathophysiology, diagnosis, and management,* ed 2, New York, 1998, Churchill Livingstone.
12. Zipfel GJ et al: Neuronal apoptosis after CNS injury: the roles of glutamate and calcium, *J Neurotrauma* 17:857, 2000.
13. Zipfel GJ, Lee JM, Choi DW: Reducing calcium overload in the ischemic brain, *N Engl J Med* 341:1543, 1999.
14. Green DR, Reed JC: Mitochondria and apoptosis, *Science* 281:1309, 1998.
15. Wojner AW: Neurovascular disorders. In Dunbar S et al, editors: *AACN clinical reference guide to critical care nursing,* ed 4, St Louis, 1998, Mosby.
16. Alexandrov AV: *Cerebrovascular ultrasound in stroke prevention and treatment,* Armonk, NY, 2003, Blackwell-Futura.
17. Frackowiak RSD, Gadian DG, Mazziotta JC: Functional neuroimaging. In Bradley WG et al, editors: *Neurology in clinical practice,* ed 3, Boston, 2000, Butterworth Heinemann.
18. Gloor P: *The temporal lobe and limbic system,* New York, 1997, Oxford University Press.
19. Bleck TP: Levels of consciousness and attention. In Goetz CG, Pappert EJ, editors: *Textbook of clinical neurology,* Philadelphia, 1999, Saunders.
20. Wojner AW, Malkoff M: Performing a lumbar puncture. In Lynn-McHale DJ, Carlson, KK, editors: *AACN's procedure manual for critical care nursing,* ed 4, Philadelphia, 2001, Saunders.

CHAPTER 26

Neurologic Clinical Assessment and Diagnostic Procedures

*A*ssessment of the critically ill patient with neurologic dysfunction includes a review of the patient's health history, a thorough physical examination, and an analysis of the patient's laboratory data. Numerous invasive and noninvasive diagnostic procedures may also be performed to assist in the identification of the patient's disorder. This chapter focuses on clinical assessments, laboratory studies, and diagnostic procedures for the critically ill patient with a neurologic dysfunction.

CLINICAL ASSESSMENT

A thorough clinical assessment of the patient with neurologic dysfunction is imperative for the early identification and treatment of neurologic disorders. Once completed, the assessment serves as the foundation for developing the management plan for the patient. The assessment process can be brief or can involve a detailed history and examination, depending on the nature and immediacy of the patient's situation.

HISTORY

Neurologic assessment encompasses a wide variety of applications and a multitude of techniques. This chapter focuses on the type of assessment performed in a critical care environment. The one factor common to all neurologic assessments is the need to obtain a comprehensive history of events preceding hospitalization. An adequate neurologic history includes information about clinical manifestations, associated complaints, precipitating factors, progression, and familial occurrences (see the Data Collection feature on Neurologic History). If the patient is incapable of providing this information, family members or significant others should be contacted as soon as possible. When someone other than the patient is the source of the history, it should be an individual who was in contact with the patient on a daily basis. Frequently, valuable information is gained that directs the caregiver

to focus on certain aspects of the patient's clinical assessment.[1]

PHYSICAL EXAMINATION

Five major components make up the neurologic examination of the critically ill patient: evaluation of (1) level of consciousness, (2) motor function, (3) pupillary function, (4) respiratory function, and (5) vital signs. Until all five components have been assessed, a complete neurologic examination has not been performed.[1]

Level of Consciousness. Assessment of the level of consciousness is the most important aspect of the neurologic examination. In most situations, a patient's level of consciousness deteriorates before any other neurologic changes are noted. These deteriorations often are subtle and must be monitored carefully. Assessment of level of consciousness focuses on two areas: (1) evaluation of arousal or alertness and (2) appraisal of content of consciousness or awareness.[1] Although universally accepted definitions for various levels of consciousness do not exist, the categories outlined in Box 26-1 are often used to describe the patient's level of consciousness.[1-4]

Evaluation of Arousal. Assessment of the arousal component of consciousness is an evaluation of the reticular activating system and its connection with the thalamus and the cerebral cortex. Arousal is the lowest level of consciousness, and observation centers on the patient's ability to respond to verbal or noxious stimuli in an appropriate manner. To stimulate the patient, the nurse should begin with verbal stimuli in a normal tone. If the patient does not respond, the nurse should increase the stimuli by shouting at the patient. If the patient still does not respond, the nurse should further increase the stimuli by shaking the patient. Noxious stimuli should follow if previous attempts to arouse the patient are unsuccessful. To assess arousal, central stimulation should be used (Box 26-2).

Appraisal of Awareness. Content of consciousness is a higher level function and is concerned with assessment of the patient's orientation to person, place,

DATA COLLECTION
Neurologic History

COMMON NEUROLOGIC SYMPTOMS
- Fainting
- Dizziness
- Blackouts
- Seizures
- Headache
- Memory loss
- Weakness
- Paralysis
- Tremors or other involuntary movements
- Pain
- Numbness
- Tingling
- Speech disturbances
- Vision disturbances

EVENTS PRECEDING ONSET OF SYMPTOMS
- Travel
- Animal contact
- Falls
- Infection
- Dental problems or procedures
- Sinus or middle ear infections
- Prodromal symptoms
- Food or drugs ingested

PROGRESSION OF SYMPTOMS
- Initial onset
- Evolution
- Frequency
- Severity
- Duration
- Associated activities/aggravating factors

FAMILY HISTORY
- Stroke (arteriovenous malformation, aneurysm)
- Diabetes mellitus
- Hypertension
- Seizures
- Tumors
- Headaches
- Emotional problems or depression

MEDICAL HISTORY
Child
- Birth injuries, congenital defects, encephalitis, meningitis, bedwetting, fainting, seizures, trauma

Adult
- Diabetes; hypertension; cardiovascular, pulmonary, kidney, liver, or endocrine disease; tuberculosis, tropical infection, sinusitis, visual problems, tumors, psychiatric disorders

SURGICAL HISTORY
- Neurologic, ear-nose-throat, dental, eye

TRAUMATIC HISTORY
- Motor vehicle accidents, falls, blows to the head, neck or back, being knocked out

ALLERGIES
- Drug, food, environment

PATIENT PROFILE
- Personal habits
  Use of alcohol, recreational drugs, over-the-counter medications, smoking, dietary habits, sleeping patterns, elimination patterns, exercise habits
- Recent life changes
- Living conditions
- Working conditions
  Exposure to toxins, chemicals, fumes; occupational duties
- General temperament

CURRENT MEDICATIONS USAGE
- Sedatives, tranquilizers
- Anticonvulsants
- Psychotropics
- Anticoagulants
- Antibiotics
- Calcium channel blockers
- Beta-blockers
- Nitrates
- Oral contraceptives

and time. Assessment of content of consciousness requires the patient to give appropriate answers to a variety of questions. Changes in the patient's answers that indicate increasing degrees of confusion and disorientation may be the first sign of neurologic deterioration.[1,3-4]

Glasgow Coma Scale. The most widely recognized level of consciousness assessment tool is the Glasgow Coma Scale (GCS).[5] This scored scale is based on evaluation of three categories: eye opening, verbal response, and best motor response (Table 26-1). The best possible score on the GCS is 15, and the lowest score is 3. Generally a score of 7 or less on the GCS in-

dicates coma. Originally the scoring system was developed to assist in general communication concerning the severity of neurologic injury. Recent testing of the GCS revealed a moderate to high agreement rating among both physicians and nurses.[6,7] Several points should be kept in mind when the GCS is used for serial assessment. It provides data about level of consciousness only and never should be considered a complete neurologic examination. It is not a sensitive tool for evaluation of an altered sensorium, nor does it account for possible aphasia. The GCS is also a poor indicator of lateralization of neurologic deterioration.[7] Lateralization involves

Table 26-1 Glasgow Coma Scale

Category	Score	Response
Eye opening	4	Spontaneous—eyes open spontaneously without stimulation
	3	To speech—eyes open with verbal stimulation but not necessarily to command
	2	To pain—eyes open with noxious stimuli
	1	None—no eye opening regardless of stimulation
Verbal response	5	Oriented—accurate information about person, place, time, reason for hospitalization, and personal data
	4	Confused—answers not appropriate to question, but use of language is correct
	3	Inappropriate words—disorganized, random speech, no sustained conversation
	2	Incomprehensible sounds—moans, groans, and incomprehensible mumbles
	1	None—no verbalization despite stimulation
Best motor response	6	Obeys commands—performs simple tasks on command; able to repeat performance
	5	Localizes to pain—organized attempt to localize and remove painful stimuli
	4	Withdraws from pain—withdraws extremity from source of painful stimuli
	3	Abnormal flexion—decorticate posturing spontaneously or in response to noxious stimuli
	2	Extension—decerebrate posturing spontaneously or in response to noxious stimuli
	1	None—no response to noxious stimuli; flaccid

Box 26-1

CATEGORIES OF CONSCIOUSNESS

Alert	Patient responds immediately to minimal external stimuli.
Confused	Patient is disoriented to time or place but usually oriented to person, with impaired judgment and decision making and decreased attention span.
Delirious	Patient is disoriented to time, place, and person with loss of contact with reality and often has auditory or visual hallucinations.
Lethargic	Patient displays a state of drowsiness or inaction in which the patient needs an increased stimulus to be awakened.
Obtunded	Patient displays dull indifference to external stimuli, and response is minimally maintained. Questions are answered with a minimal response.
Stuporous	Patient can be aroused only by vigorous and continuous external stimuli. Motor response is often withdrawal or localizing to stimulus.
Comatose	Vigorous stimulation fails to produce any voluntary neural response.

From Barker E: *Neuroscience nursing: a spectrum of care,* ed 2, St Louis, 2002, Mosby.

Box 26-2

STIMULATION TECHNIQUES IN PATIENT AROUSAL

CENTRAL STIMULATION
- *Trapezius pinch:* Squeeze trapezius muscle between thumb and first two fingers.
- *Sternal rub:* Apply firm pressure to sternum with knuckles, using a rubbing motion.

PERIPHERAL STIMULATION
- *Nailbed pressure:* Apply firm pressure, using object such as a pen, to nailbed.
- *Pinching of inner aspect of arm/leg:* Firmly pinch small portion of patient's tissue on sensitive inner aspect of arm or leg.

Evaluation of Muscle Size and Tone. Initially the muscles should be inspected for size and shape. The presence of atrophy or hypertrophy is noted. Muscle tone is assessed by evaluating the opposition to passive movement. The patient is instructed to relax the extremity while the nurse performs passive range of motion movements and evaluates the degree of resistance. Muscle tone is appraised for signs of flaccidity (no resistance), hypotonia (little resistance), hypertonia (increased resistance), spasticity, or rigidity.[8]

Estimation of Muscle Strength. Having the patient perform a number of movements against resistance assesses muscle strength. The strength of the movement is then graded on a six-point scale (Box 26-3). Asking the patient to grasp, squeeze, and release the nurse's index and middle fingers tests the upper extremities. If asymmetric weakness is suspected, the patient is instructed

decreasing motor response on one side or unilateral changes in pupillary reaction.

Motor Function. Assessment of motor function focuses on two areas: (1) evaluation of muscle size and tone and (2) estimation of muscle strength. Each side should be assessed individually and then compared against the other.[1,8]

Box 26-3

MUSCLE STRENGTH GRADING SCALE

0—No movement or muscle contraction
1—Trace contraction
2—Active movement with gravity eliminated
3—Active movement against gravity
4—Active movement with some resistance
5—Active movement with full resistance

Box 26-4

CLASSIFICATION OF ABNORMAL MOTOR FUNCTION

Spontaneous	Occurs without regard to external stimuli and may not occur by request
Localization	Occurs when the extremity opposite the extremity receiving pain crosses midline of the body in an attempt to remove the noxious stimulus from the affected limb
Withdrawal	Occurs when the extremity receiving the painful stimulus flexes normally in an attempt to avoid the noxious stimulus
Decortication	Abnormal flexion response that may occur spontaneously or in response to noxious stimuli (see Fig. 26-1, *A* and *C*)
Decerebration	Abnormal extension response that may occur spontaneously or in response to noxious stimuli (see Fig. 26-1, *B* and *C*)
Flaccid	No response to painful stimuli

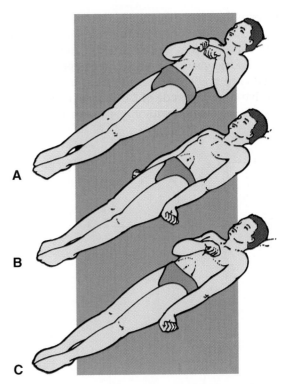

Fig. 26-1   Abnormal motor responses. **A,** Decorticate posturing. **B,** Decerebrate posturing. **C,** Decorticate posturing on right side and decerebrate posturing on left side of body.

to extend both arms with the palms turned upward and holds that position with the eyes closed. If the patient has a weaker side, that arm will drift downward and pronate. The lower extremities are tested by asking the patient to push and pull the feet against resistance.[9]

Abnormal Motor Responses. If the patient is incapable of comprehending and following a simple command, noxious stimuli are necessary to determine motor responses. The stimulus is applied to each extremity separately to allow evaluation of individual extremity function. Peripheral stimulation is used to assess motor function (see Box 26-2).[1,2] Motor responses elicited by noxious stimuli are interpreted differently than those elicited by voluntary demonstration. These responses may be classified into the categories as listed in Box 26-4.[8]

Abnormal flexion also is known as *decorticate posturing* (Fig. 26-1, *A*). In response to painful stimuli, the upper extremities exhibit flexion of the arm, wrist, and fingers with adduction of the limb. The lower extremity exhibits extension, internal rotation, and plantar flexion. Abnormal flexion occurs with lesions above the midbrain, in the region of the thalamus or cerebral hemispheres. Abnormal extension also is known as *decerebrate rigidity*, or *posturing* (Fig. 26-1, *B*). When the patient is stimulated, teeth clench and the arms are stiffly extended, adducted, and hyperpronated. The legs are stiffly extended with plantar flexion of the feet. Abnormal extension occurs with lesions in the area of the brainstem. Because abnormal flexion and extension appear similar in the lower extremities, the upper extremities are used to determine the presence of these abnormal movements. It is possible for the patient to exhibit abnormal flexion on one side of the body and extension on the other (Fig. 26-1, *C*).[1-3] Outcome studies indicate that abnormal flexion or decorticate posturing has a less serious prognosis than does extension, or decerebrate posturing. Onset of posturing or a change from abnormal flexion to abnormal extension requires immediate physician notification.[3]

Evaluation of Reflexes. Deep tendon reflexes (DTRs) are usually evaluated by a physician when a complete neurologic evaluation is performed. DTRs are tested by tapping the appropriate tendon using a reflex or percussion hammer. The muscle needs to be relaxed and the joint at midposition for reflex testing to be accurate. The four reflexes tested are the Achilles (ankle jerk), the quadriceps (knee jerk), the biceps, and the triceps. DTRs are graded on a scale from 0 (absent) to 4 (hyperactive). A DTR grade of 2 is normal (Fig 26-2). Hyperreflexia is associated with upper motor neuron inter-

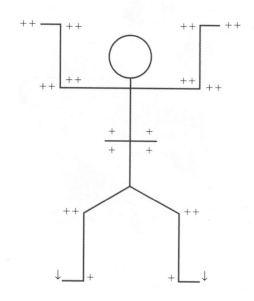

Scoring Deep Tendon Reflexes

Grade	Deep Tendon Reflex Response
0	No response
1+	Sluggish or diminished
2+	Active or expected response
3+	More brisk than expected, slightly hyperactive
4+	Brisk, hyperactive, with intermittent or transient clonus

Fig. 26-2 The patient's reflex scores are recorded by entering the correct scores at the correct location on the stick figure. (From Barker E: *Neuroscience nursing: a spectrum of care*, ed 2, St Louis, 2002, Mosby.)

ruption, and areflexia is associated with lesions of the lower motor neurons.[2]

Superficial reflexes are normal if present and abnormal if absent. Superficial reflexes are tested by stimulating cutaneous receptors of the skin, cornea, or mucous membrane. Stroking, scratching, or touching can be used as the stimulus (Table 26-2). The corneal reflex is present if the eyelids quickly close when the cornea is lightly stroked with a wisp of cotton. An alternative approach is to drop a small amount of water or saline onto the cornea.[1] The pathway for the corneal reflex is formed by the trigeminal cranial nerve (CN) V and facial (CN VII) nerves and the pons. The pharyngeal reflex is present if retching or gagging occurs with stimulation of the back of the pharynx.[1-3] The gag reflex is often stimulated during routine oral and pulmonary hygiene in the critical care environment. The presence of these reflexes should be noted and documented during completion of these activities.

The presence of pathologic reflexes is an abnormal neurologic finding. The grasp reflex is present when tactile stimulation of the palm of the hand produces a grasp response that is not a conscious voluntary act. The grasp reflex is a primitive reflex that normally disappears with maturational development. Presence of the grasp reflex in the adult indicates cortical damage. Babinski's reflex is a pathologic sign in any individual over 2 years of age. The presence of this reflex is tested by slow, deliberate stroking of the lateral half of the sole of the foot. Sustained extensor response of the big toe is indicative of a positive Babinski's reflex. This response is sometimes accompanied by the fanning out of the other four toes. Flexor response of all the toes in response to the same stimuli is a normal finding and indicates absence of Babinski's reflex (Fig. 26-3). Babinski's reflex is an extremely important neurologic finding, significantly indicative of an upper motor neuron lesion in the brain, brainstem, or spinal cord. The disease may be degenera-

Table 26-2	Superficial Reflexes	
Reflex	**Nerve(s) Involved**	**Normal Reaction**
Corneal	CN V and VII	Prompt closure of both eyelids when cornea touched with wisp of cotton
Pharyngeal	CN IX and X	Gagging response to pharyngeal stimulation
Abdominal	Epigastric (T6-T9); midabdominal (T9-T11); hypogastric (T11-L1)	Contraction of abdominal muscle when stroked, so that there is a brief, brisk movement of umbilicus toward stimulus
Cremasteric	L1, L2	Elevation of testicle when inner aspect of thigh stroked
Anal		Contraction of anal ring as perineum is stroked or scratched
Bulbocutaneous	S4, S5	
Anocutaneous	S5	
Plantar	L5, S1	Flexion of toes from stimulation of sole of foot

From Barker E: *Neuroscience nursing: a spectrum of care*, ed 2, St Louis, 2002, Mosby.

tive, neoplastic, inflammatory, vascular, or posttraumatic. Babinski's reflex may also become positive during transtentorial herniation.

Pupillary Function. Assessment of pupillary function focuses on three areas: (1) estimation of pupil size and shape, (2) evaluation of pupillary reaction to light, and (3) assessment of eye movements. Pupillary function is an extension of the autonomic nervous system. Parasympathetic control of the pupil occurs through innervation of the oculomotor nerve (CN III), which exits from the brainstem in the midbrain area. When the parasympathetic fibers are stimulated, the pupil constricts. Sympathetic control originates in the hypothalamus and travels down the entire length of the brainstem. When the sympathetic fibers are stimulated, the pupil dilates. Pupillary changes provide a valuable tool to assessment because of pathway location. The oculomotor nerve lies at the junction of the midbrain and the tentorial notch. Any increase of pressure that exerts force down through the tentorial notch compresses the oculomotor nerve. Oculomotor nerve compression results in a dilated, nonreactive pupil. Sympathetic pathway disruption occurs with involvement in the brainstem. Loss of sympathetic control leads to pinpoint, nonreactive pupils. Control of eye movements occurs with interaction of three cranial nerves: oculomotor (CN III), trochlear (CN IV), and abducens (CN VI). The pathways for these cranial nerves provide integrated function through the internuclear pathway of the medial longitudinal fasciculus (MLF) located in the brainstem. The MLF provides coordination of eye movements with the vestibular nerve (CN VIII) and the reticular formation.[3]

Estimation of Pupil Size and Shape. Pupil size should be documented in millimeters with the use of a pupil gauge to reduce the subjectivity of description. Although most people have pupils of equal size, a discrepancy up to 1 mm between the two pupils is normal. Inequality of pupils is known as anisocoria and occurs in 16% to 17% of the human population.[10] Change or inequality in pupil size, especially in patients who previously have not shown this discrepancy, is a significant neurologic sign. It may indicate impending danger of herniation and should be reported immediately. With the location of the oculomotor nerve (CN III) at the notch of the tentorium, pupil size and reactivity play a key role in the physical assessment of intracranial pressure changes and herniation syndromes. In addition to CN III compression, changes in pupil size occur for other reasons. Large pupils can result from the instillation of cycloplegic agents, such as atropine or scopolamine, or can indicate extreme stress. Extremely small pupils can indicate narcotic overdose, lower brainstem compression, or bilateral damage to the pons.[10,11]

Pupil shape is also noted in the assessment of pupils. Although the pupil is normally round, an irregularly shaped or oval pupil may be noted in patients with elevated intracranial pressure. An oval pupil can indicate the initial stages of CN III compression.[1] It has been observed that an oval pupil is almost always associated with an elevated intracranial pressure (ICP) between 18 and 35 mm Hg.[12]

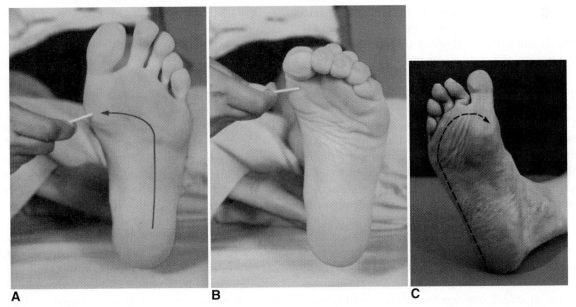

A   **B**   **C**

Fig. 26-3 Elicitation of the plantar reflex. **A,** A hard object is applied to the lateral surface of the sole, starting at the heel and going over the ball of the foot, ending beneath the great toe. **B,** Normal response to plantar stimulation: flexion of all toes. **C,** Babinski's sign: dorsiflexion of the great toe and fanning of the other toes. (**A** and **B** from Barkauskas VH, Baumann LC, Darling-Fisher CS: *Health & physical assessment,* ed 3, St Louis, 2002, Mosby. **C** from Seidel HM, Ball JW, Dains JE: *Mosby's guide to physical examination,* ed 5, St Louis, 2003, Mosby.)

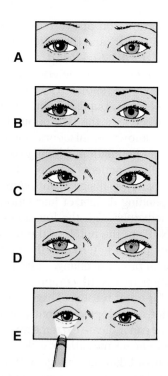

Fig. 26-4 Abnormal pupillary responses. **A,** Oculomotor nerve compression. **B,** Bilateral diencephalon damage. **C,** Midbrain damage. **D,** Pontine damage. **E,** Dilated, nonreactive pupils.

Evaluation of Pupillary Reaction to Light. The pupillary light reflex depends on both optic nerve (CN II) and oculomotor nerve (CN III) function (Fig. 26-4).[3] The technique for evaluation of the pupillary light response involves use of a narrow-beamed bright light shined into the pupil from the outer canthus of the eye. If the light is shined directly onto the pupil, glare or reflection of the light may prevent the assessor's proper visualization. Pupillary reaction to light is identified as brisk, sluggish, or nonreactive or fixed.[1] Each pupil should be evaluated both for direct light response and for consensual response. The consensual pupillary response is constriction in response to a light shined into the opposite eye. This reflex occurs as a result of the crossing of nerve fibers at the optic chiasm.[1] Evaluation of consensual response is necessary to rule out optic nerve dysfunction as a cause for lack of a direct light reflex. Because the optic nerve is the afferent pathway for the light reflex, shining a light into a blind eye will produce neither a direct light response in that eye nor a consensual response in the opposite eye. A consensual response in the blind eye produced by shining a light into the opposite eye demonstrates an intact oculomotor nerve. Oculomotor compression associated with transtentorial herniation will affect both the direct light response and the consensual response in the affected pupil.[1,2,10,11]

Assessment of Eye Movement. In the conscious patient, the function of the three cranial nerves of the eye and their MLF innervation can be assessed by asking the patient to follow a finger through the full range of eye motion. If the eyes move together into all six fields, extraocular movements are intact (Fig 26-5).[1]

In the unconscious patient, assessment of ocular function and innervation of the MLF is performed by eliciting the doll's eyes reflex. If the patient is unconscious as a result of trauma, the nurse must ascertain the absence of cervical injury before performing this examination. To assess the oculocephalic reflex, the nurse holds the patient's eyelids open and briskly turns the head to one side while observing the eye movements, then briskly turns the head to the other side and observes. If the eyes deviate to the opposite direction in which the head is turned, doll's eyes are present and the oculocephalic reflex arc is intact (Fig. 26-6, *A*). If the oculocephalic reflex arc is not intact, the reflex is absent. This lack of response, in which the eyes remain midline and move with the head, indicates significant brainstem injury (Fig. 26-6, *C*). The reflex may also be absent in severe metabolic coma. An abnormal oculocephalic reflex is present when the eyes rove or move in opposite directions from each other (Fig. 26-6, *B*). Abnormal oculocephalic reflex indicates some degree of brainstem injury.[1-3]

The oculovestibular reflex is performed by a physician, often as one of the final clinical assessments of brainstem function. Following confirmation that the tympanic membrane is intact, the head is raised to a 30-degree angle. Then 20 to 100 ml of ice water is injected into the external auditory canal. The normal eye movement response is a conjugate, slow, tonic, nystagmus deviating toward the irrigated ear and lasting 30 to 120 seconds. This response indicates brainstem integrity. Rapid nystagmus returns the eyes back to the midline only in the conscious patient with cortical functioning (Fig. 26-7).[1] An abnormal response is dysconjugate eye movement, which indicates a brainstem lesion, or no response, which indicates little to no brainstem function. The oculovestibular reflex may also be temporarily absent in reversible metabolic encephalopathy.[3] This test is an extremely noxious stimulation and may produce a decorticate or decerebrate posturing response in the comatose patient. In the conscious patient, this procedure may produce nausea, vomiting, or dizziness.[1,10,11]

Respiratory Function. Assessment of respiratory function focuses on two areas: (1) observation of respiratory pattern and (2) evaluation of airway status. The activity of respiration is a highly integrated function that receives input from the cerebrum, brainstem, and metabolic mechanisms. A close correlation exists in clinical assessment among altered levels of consciousness, the level of brain or brainstem injury, and the respiratory pattern noted. Under the influence of the cerebral cortex and the diencephalon, three brainstem centers control respirations. The lowest center, the medullary respira-

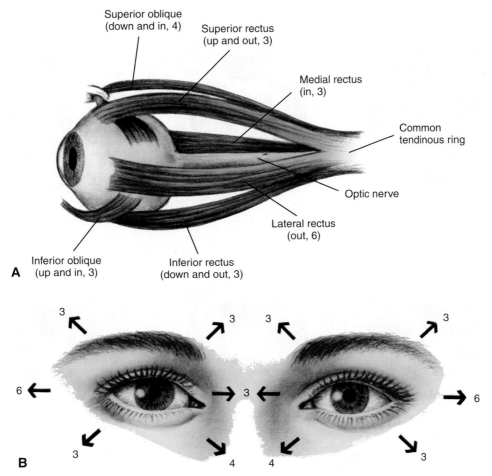

Fig. 26-5 Extraocular eye movements. **A,** Extraocular muscles. **B,** The six cardinal directions of gaze with each associated cranial nerve supply.

tory center, sends impulses through the vagus nerve to innervate muscles of inspiration and expiration. The apneustic and pneumotaxic centers of the pons are responsible for the length of inspiration and expiration and the underlying respiratory rate.[1-3]

Observation of Respiratory Pattern. Changes in respiratory patterns assist in identifying the level of brainstem dysfunction or injury (Fig. 26-8 and Table 26-3). Evaluation of respiratory pattern must also include evaluation of the effectiveness of gas exchange in maintaining adequate oxygen and carbon dioxide levels. Hypoventilation is not uncommon in the patient with an altered level of consciousness. Alterations in oxygenation or carbon dioxide levels can result in further neurologic dysfunction. ICP increases with hypoxemia or hypercapnia.[1-3]

Evaluation of Airway Status. Finally, assessment of the respiratory function in a patient with neurologic deficit must include assessment of airway maintenance and secretion control. Cough, gag, and swallow reflexes responsible for protection of the airway may be absent or diminished.[13]

Vital Signs. Assessment of vital signs focuses on two areas: (1) evaluation of blood pressure and (2) observation of heart rate and rhythm. As a result of the brain and brainstem influences on cardiac, respiratory, and body temperature functions, changes in vital signs can indicate deterioration in neurologic status.

Evaluation of Blood Pressure. A common manifestation of intracranial injury is systemic hypertension. Cerebral autoregulation, responsible for the control of cerebral blood flow, frequently is lost with any type of intracranial injury. After cerebral injury, the body often is in a hyperdynamic state (increased heart rate, blood pressure, and cardiac output) as part of a compensatory response. With the loss of autoregulation as blood pressure increases, cerebral blood flow and cerebral blood volume increase and, therefore, ICP increases. Control of systemic hypertension is necessary to stop this cycle. However, caution must be exercised. The mean arterial pressure must be maintained at a level sufficient to produce adequate cerebral blood flow in the presence of elevated ICP. Attention must also be paid to the pulse pressure because widening of this value may occur in the late stages of intracranial hypertension.[13]

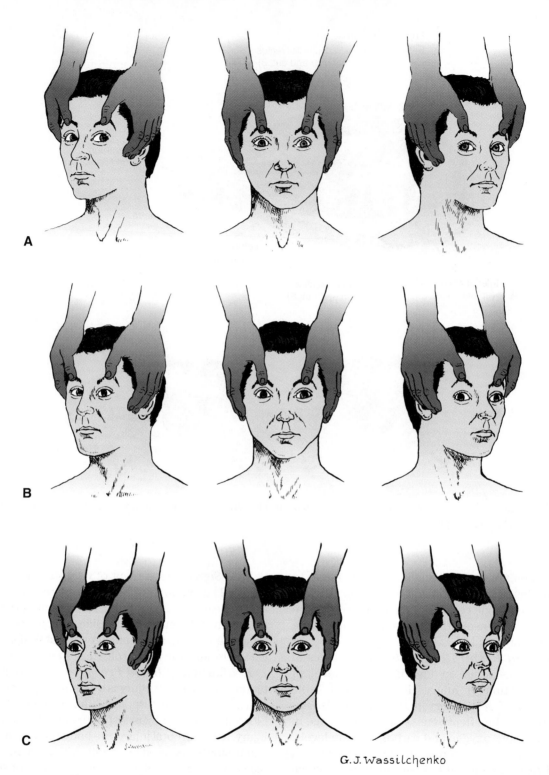

G. J. Wassilchenko

Fig. 26-6   Oculocephalic reflex (doll's eyes). **A,** Normal. **B,** Abnormal. **C,** Absent.

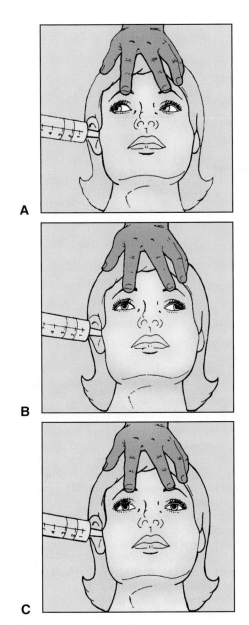

Fig. 26-7 Oculovestibular reflex (cold caloric test). **A,** Normal. **B,** Abnormal. **C,** Absent.

Observation of Heart Rate and Rhythm. The medulla and the vagus nerve provide parasympathetic control to the heart. When stimulated, this lower brainstem system produces bradycardia. Sympathetic stimulation increases the rate and contractility. Various intracranial pathologies and abrupt ICP changes can produce cardiac dysrhythmias, such as bradycardia, premature ventricular contractions (PVCs), atrioventricular block, or ventricular fibrillation and myocardial damage.[14]

Cushing's Triad. Cushing's triad is a set of three clinical manifestations (bradycardia, systolic hypertension, and widening pulse pressure) related to pressure on the medullary area of the brainstem. These signs often occur in response to intracranial hypertension or a herniation syndrome. The appearance of Cushing's triad is a late finding that may be absent in neurologic deterioration. Attention should be paid to alteration in each component of the triad and intervention initiated accordingly.[3]

RAPID NEUROLOGIC EXAMINATION

An adequate neurologic examination should focus on covering all major areas of neurologic control. Any abnormalities identified can then be further evaluated and investigated. Findings should always be evaluated in light of those of previous examinations. A neurologic examination should be organized, thorough, and simple so that it can be performed accurately and easily at each assessment point.[1]

The Conscious Patient. An example of a rapid neurologic examination that can be performed in the critical care unit on a conscious patient with known or potential neurologic deficit is outlined in Box 26-5. This examination, which usually takes less than 4 minutes, is meant to provide a starting point. If any neurologic deficit is identified that is new or different from that of the last assessment, attention must be focused in more detail on that abnormality.[1]

Table 26-3	Respiratory Patterns	
Pattern of Respiration	**Description of Pattern**	**Significance**
Cheyne-Stokes	Rhythmic crescendo and decrescendo of rate and depth of respiration; includes brief periods of apnea	Usually seen with bilateral deep cerebral lesions or some cerebellar lesions
Central neurogenic hyperventilation	Very deep, very rapid respirations with no apneic periods	Usually seen with lesions of the midbrain and upper pons
Apneustic	Prolonged inspiratory and/or expiratory pause of 2-3 sec	Usually seen in lesions of the mid to lower pons
Cluster breathing	Clusters of irregular, gasping respirations separated by long periods of apnea	Usually seen in lesions of the lower pons or upper medulla
Ataxic respirations	Irregular, random pattern of deep and shallow respirations with irregular apneic periods	Usually seen in lesions of the medulla

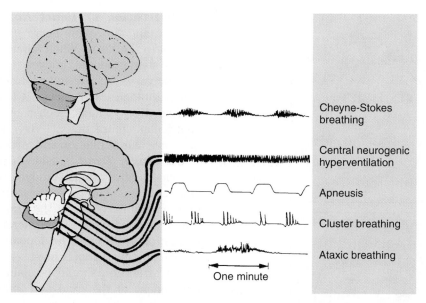

Fig. 26-8 Abnormal respiratory patterns with corresponding level of central nervous system activity.

Cheyne-Stokes breathing

Central neurogenic hyperventilation

Apneusis

Cluster breathing

Ataxic breathing

One minute

Box 26-5

RAPID NEUROLOGIC ASSESSMENT OF THE CONSCIOUS PATIENT

1. **Level of consciousness:** Address the patient and ask a variety of orientation questions; avoid the obvious, overused questions about name, date, and place, and focus on questions about recent and past events from the patient's experiences, such as spouse's name, home address, what was eaten at the previous meal; be sure that, as examiner, you are aware of the correct answers to all questions asked.
2. **Facial movements:** During assessment of level of consciousness, observe the patient's facial movements for symmetry; listen to speech patterns for evidence of slurred speech.
3. **Pupillary function and eye movements:** Perform pupil check and assess extraocular eye movements.
4. **Motor assessment:** Assess upper and lower extremity movement and strength.
5. **Sensory:** With a finger, stroke the patient bilaterally on the face, upper aspect of the arm, hand, leg, and foot; ask the patient to identify what is touched and whether there is any difference in sensation between the two sides.
6. **Vital signs:** Note any alterations in blood pressure, heart rate or rhythm, respiratory pattern, or temperature.
7. **Change in status:** Ask the patient if he or she feels any differences between this and the previous examination.

Box 26-6

RAPID NEUROLOGIC ASSESSMENT OF THE UNCONSCIOUS PATIENT

1. **Level of consciousness:** Perform the Glasgow Coma Scale assessment.
2. **Pupillary assessment:** Perform pupillary assessment with special attention to size, reactivity, and shape of pupil in comparison with the opposite eye.
3. **Motor examination:** Assess each extremity individually by means of a predetermined coding score of motor movement.
4. **Respiratory pattern:** If the patient is not receiving mechanical ventilation, observe respiratory patterns for evidence of deteriorating level of function.
5. **Vital signs:** Include comparison of preassessment vital signs with postassessment vital signs, paying special attention to arterial blood pressure and intracranial pressure (ICP) if these parameters are being monitored.

---

the patient has been stimulated, the examiner can proceed with the neurologic examination. As in the assessment of the conscious patient, if any abnormalities or changes from previous assessment are noted, further investigation must occur. This assessment takes 3 to 4 minutes.[1]

NEUROLOGIC CHANGES ASSOCIATED WITH INTRACRANIAL HYPERTENSION

Assessment of the patient for signs of increasing intracranial pressure is an important responsibility of the critical care nurse. Increasing ICP can be identified by changes in level of consciousness, pupillary reaction, motor response, vital signs, and respiratory patterns (Fig. 26-9).

The Unconscious Patient. In the assessment of the unconscious patient (Box 26-6), initial efforts are directed at achieving maximal arousal of the patient. Calling the patient's name, patting him or her on the chest, or shaking his or her shoulder accomplishes this task. Once

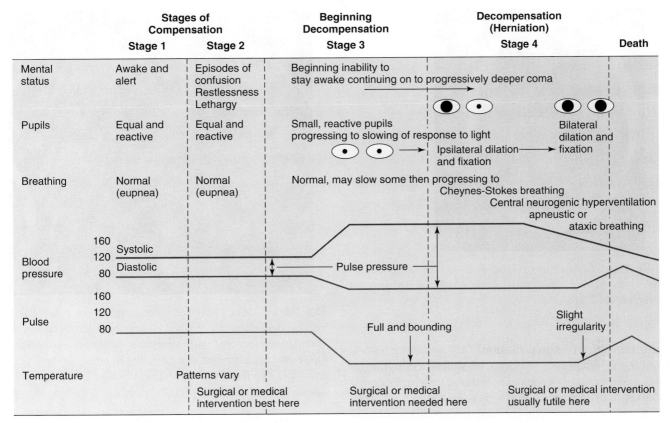

Fig. 26-9   Clinical correlates of compensated and decompensated phases of intracranial hypertension.   (From Beare PG, Myers JL: *Principles and practice of adult health nursing,* ed 3, St Louis, 1998, Mosby.)

DIAGNOSTIC PROCEDURES

RADIOLOGIC PROCEDURES

The following discussion focuses on the more commonly performed radiologic procedures that are used in diagnosis of the critically ill patient with neurologic dysfunction.

Skull and Spine Films. The purpose of radiographs of the skull or spine is to identify fractures, anomalies, or possible tumors. The role of skull radiographs in trauma has diminished with the advent of computed axial tomography (CT). If the patient is to undergo a CT scan during the initial assessment process, a skull radiograph may not be necessary.[15]

The procedure for obtaining skull and spine radiographs is relatively painless In many situations a single lateral view of the skull is adequate, but in some situations a full skull series is required. A skull series consists of four different views: lateral, posteroanterior, half-axial (Towne's), and submentovertical (base).[15] A cervical spine series consists of four views: atlas and axial, anteroposterior, lateral, and oblique. Thoracic and lumbar spine series consists of two views: anteroposterior and lateral.[15]

Proper patient positioning is essential, especially for spine radiographs. Spinal precautions (i.e., cervical col-

lar and strict maintenance of head alignment) must be maintained until lateral films confirm integrity of the cervical structures. Nursing care involves positioning the patient to obtain adequate films. In any situation in which traumatic injury, especially head injury, is the cause of the patient's admission to the critical care unit, the cervical spine must be treated as unstable until proven otherwise.[2]

Computed Tomography. Computed tomographic (CT) scanning provides the clinician with a mathematically reconstructed view of multiple sections of the head and body. This is accomplished by passage of intersecting x-ray beams through the examined area and measurement of the density of substances through which the x-ray beams pass. The denser the substance through which an x-ray beam passes, the whiter it appears on the finished film. The less dense a substance, the blacker it appears. Therefore with normal findings in a CT scan of the head, bone appears white, blood appears off-white, brain tissue appears shaded gray, cerebrospinal fluid (CSF) appears off-black, and air appears black (Fig. 26-10).[15]

CT scanning offers rapid, noninvasive visualization of structures and is the diagnostic study of choice to identify the presence of surgical lesions in acute head injury. Serial evaluations may be necessary to identify evolution

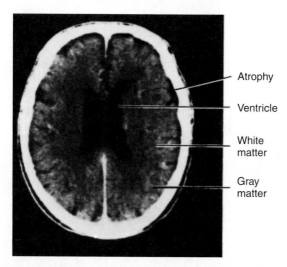

Fig. 26-10 CT scan image. (From Ballinger PW: *Merrill's atlas of radiographic positions and radiologic procedures,* ed 7, St Louis, 1991, Mosby.)

Labels on figure:
- Atrophy
- Ventricle
- White matter
- Gray matter

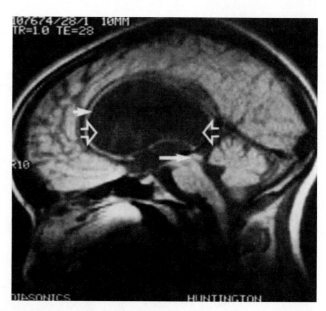

Fig. 26-11 Magnetic resonance image of the brain. Sagittal section demonstrating marked enlargement of the lateral ventricle *(open arrow)* with stretching of the corpus callosum *(arrowhead)* as a result of aqueductal stenosis *(arrow).* (From Stark DD, Bradley WG: *Magnetic resonance imaging,* ed 2, St Louis, 1992, Mosby.)

of diffuse injury to a mass lesion.[16] CT scanning also is used in the diagnostic workup of space-occupying lesions, hemorrhage, or vascular lesions; cerebral edema; seizures; hydrocephalus; and severe headache. CT scan is the preferred method for diagnosing subarachnoid hemorrhage and for differentiating intracranial hemorrhage and infarction.[17]

CT scans can be conducted with and without the use of a contrast medium. The noncontrast scan is noninvasive, requires no premedication of the patient, and is good for analysis and location of normal brain structures. A noncontrast CT scan of the head is appropriate in trauma patients in whom the goal is to view the intracranial area for evidence of intracranial hemorrhage, cerebral edema, or shift of structures. Noncontrast CT scan also is appropriate in the diagnosis of hydrocephalus.[18] A contrast CT scan involves the use of an intravenously injected contrast medium. The use of contrast enhances the vascular areas and allows for detection of vascular lesions or the further definition of lesions noted on a noncontrast scan. The letter **C** will be evident on the film when contrast has been used.[17]

Nursing management of the patient receiving a CT scan can be divided into two areas of focus: observation of patient tolerance of the procedure and observation of patient reaction to the dye in contrast scanning. Because of the associated activity and positioning, transporting and scanning of a critically ill patient with known or suspected intracranial hypertension can cause deterioration in the patient's condition. The nurse must always remain with the patient during the CT scan and closely observe the neurologic status, vital signs, and, if monitored, ICP.

If the patient is to receive a contrast CT scan, questions about possible sensitivity to iodine-based dye must

be asked beforehand if at all possible. During the infusion of the dye and for ten to thirty minutes afterward, the patient is to be observed closely for anaphylactic reaction. Of all patients receiving contrast CT scans, fewer than 1% per year have severe anaphylactic reactions, shock, or cardiac arrest. Another potential complication of the dye is acute tubular necrosis (ATN). Two measures reported to reduce the incidence and severity of ATN after contrast CT are antihistamine administration and adequate hydration before and after the study.[17]

Magnetic Resonance Imaging. Magnetic resonance imaging (MRI) has replaced CT as the diagnostic study of choice for many conditions. MRI produces images with greater detail than CT scanning and provides views of several planes (sagittal, coronal, axial, and oblique) not possible with CT scanning.[17] For MRI, the patient is placed in a large magnetic field that stimulates the nuclei of the atoms of the body. Introduction of radiofrequency waves causes resonance of the nuclei, which is emitted as the nuclei relax. A computer then constructs an image of the tissue (Fig. 26-11). Intravenous administration of a non–iodine-based contrast medium enhances the images by influencing the magnetic environment and signal intensity.[18]

With MRI, small tumors, whose tissue densities differ from those of the surrounding cells, can be identified before they would be visible by any other radiographic test. MRI also can identify small hemorrhages deep in the brain that are invisible on CT scan. And finally, MRI can

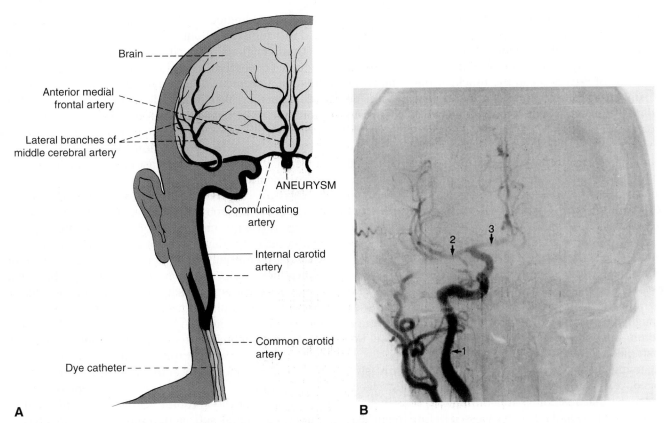

Fig. 26-12   Cerebral angiography. **A,** Insertion of contrast through a catheter in the common carotid. **B,** View of the vessels. *1,* Internal carotid artery. *2,* Middle cerebral artery. *3,* Middle meningeal artery. (From Black JM, Hawks JH: *Medical-surgical nursing: clinical management for positive outcomes,* ed 7, Philadelphia, 2005, Saunders.)

detect areas of cerebral infarct within a few hours of the incident, as well as small areas of plaque in patients with multiple sclerosis. MRI with contrast is the preferred study for detection of infectious and inflammatory processes of the central nervous system, malignancy, and metastatic lesions; cervical spine imaging; and post-operative evaluation of tumor recurrence.[17] MRI is the diagnostic study of choice in the evaluation of spinal cord injury.[19] Recent studies favor the use of MRI to determine prognosis after acute head injury and to diagnose cerebral fat embolism.[20,21]

Nursing management for the patient undergoing MRI is focused on patient tolerance of the procedure. Concerns related to transport of the neurologic patient for MRI are identical to those discussed for CT. Patient teaching and preparation are essential for successful MRI. The procedure is lengthy and requires the patient to lie motionless in a tight, enclosed space. Many patients experience anxiety, panic, and an acute sense of claustrophobia. Mild sedation or a blindfold, or both, may be necessary. The neurologically impaired patient may not be able to comprehend the instructions, and sedation, possibly combined with neuromuscular blockade, will be required. Removal of all metal from the patient's body and clothing is essential because the basis of MRI is a magnetic field. In the past it was believed that

any metal material, such as dental filling, prostheses, or internal clips or staples, would prevent scanning. Further study and changes in the type of metals used for many procedures have made the test safer. Any questions about specific devices or metals must be directed to the neuroradiologist before testing. The test is considered relatively safe and noninvasive, but all risks have not yet been identified in this procedure.[1]

Cerebral Angiography

Conventional Angiography. Conventional angiography involves the injection of radiopaque contrast medium into the intracranial or extracranial vasculature (Fig. 26-12).[22] With the use of serial radiologic filming, an angiogram traces the flow of blood from the arterial circulation through the capillary bed to the venous circulation. Cerebral angiography allows visualization of the lumen of vessels to provide information about patency, size (narrowing or dilation), any irregularities, or occlusion. Angiography is used in the diagnosis of cerebral aneurysm, vasospasm, arteriovenous (AV) malformation, carotid artery disease, and some vascular tumors. Angiography also is used to evaluate cerebral vasculature in the stroke patient. Information obtained from the angiogram guides the surgeon in choosing the operative approach or provides information on which to make medical management decisions other than surgery.[1]

The procedure involves placement of a catheter in the femoral artery and threading it up the aorta and into the origin of the cerebral circulation. Other injection sites include direct carotid or vertebral artery puncture or placement of a catheter in the brachial, the axillary, or the subclavian artery. Several views of vessels can be studied by means of angiogram. A four-vessel angiogram involves injections into the right and left internal carotid arteries and the right and left vertebral arteries. If the area of suspected disease already has been identified, a single vessel study may be all that is required. This is particularly true when angiography is used as a follow-up in the evaluation of intracranial vascular surgery. Also, if carotid artery disease is a working diagnosis, the angiogram may include views of the arch of the aorta, plus the external and internal carotid arteries.[22]

Once the catheter is appropriately placed, the contrast medium is injected. Then a rapid succession of radiographs is taken as the contrast medium progresses through the cerebral circulation. Separate contrast medium injections are administered for each vessel being studied.[2]

Nursing management associated with this invasive procedure is comprehensive. Renal insufficiency, bleeding, and cardiac instability are contraindications to cerebral angiography and must be assessed before the procedure.[2] As with contrast CT, the nurse must assess the patient for possible sensitivity to iodine-based contrast medium. Instruction and education of the patient are essential to patient preparation. The patient's complete understanding of the role this procedure plays in diagnosis, as well as the process itself, relieves anxiety about the unknown and also ensures cooperation in what is commonly an uncomfortable procedure.[1]

Before the procedure the patient is kept on nothing-by-mouth (NPO) status for at least 4 hours. Sedation is administered immediately before the procedure. Discomforts during the procedure include the need to lie still on a cold, hard table and the possibility of pain during preparation and insertion of the groin catheter. The patient often experiences a hot, burning sensation when the contrast medium is injected, especially if it is injected into the external carotid system. Preparation of patients for this burning sensation assures them that it is not an abnormal occurrence.[1]

And finally, the patient must be made aware of the postprocedure assessment. After the procedure, adequate hydration is necessary to assist the kidneys in clearing the heavy dye load. Inadequate hydration may lead to ATN and renal shutdown. If the patient cannot tolerate oral fluids, an intravenous line is placed before the procedure is begun. Postprocedure assessment involves vital signs' measurement, neurologic evaluation, observation of the puncture site, and assessment of neurovascular integrity distal to the puncture site every 15 minutes for the first hour. Any abnormalities noted must be reported immediately. The patient should be kept on bed rest for 8 to 12 hours.[1]

Complications associated with cerebral angiography include (1) cerebral embolus caused by the catheter dislodging a segment of atherosclerotic plaque in the vessel, (2) hemorrhage or hematoma formation at the insertion site, (3) vasospasm of a vessel caused by the irritation of catheter placement, (4) thrombosis of the extremity distal to the injection site, and (5) allergic or adverse reaction to the contrast medium, including renal impairment.[2]

Digital Subtraction Angiography. Digital subtraction angiography is a newer method of visualizing the arteriovenous circulation of the intracranial space. It can be used to identify tumors, AV malformations, and vascular abnormalities. Radiographic dye is injected into either the venous or the arterial circulation, but significantly less dye is necessary for this procedure than for arterial angiography. Films taken before and after dye injection are superimposed on each other, and all matching images are subtracted. Thus only the dye-enhanced cerebral vessels are left for study and evaluation. Digital subtraction angiography eliminates the shadows and distortions of bone or other material that sometimes block the viewing of the cerebral vessels.[23] The major disadvantage of digital subtraction angiography involves the patient's ability to remain motionless during the entire procedure. Even swallowing interferes significantly with the imaging process. Complications and nursing management are similar to those described for cerebral angiography. The risk of embolism is decreased with the intravenous route.[1]

Magnetic Resonance Angiography. Magnetic resonance angiography (MRA) is a technique that offers noninvasive visualization of the cerebrovascular system.[24] It uses MRI technology to evaluate cerebral blood flow and provide details about cerebral vessels. MRA of the carotid arteries has become an established complement to preoperative ultrasound evaluation.[17] MRA is also being used to identify intracranial aneurysms, AV malformations, and vasospasm.[18] A contrast-enhanced MRA (CEMRA) may be performed to improve image resolution and reduce artifact. The most commonly used agent is gadolinium, a nonnephrotoxic contrast medium, which is injected intravenously.[23]

Computed Tomography Angiography. Computed tomography angiography (CTA) is a technique that uses high-speed helical CT technology with the administration of contrast media to visualize the cerebrovascular system. It is used to assess the carotid arteries for stenosis and to evaluate cerebral aneurysms. Currently CTA is becoming a well-accepted substitute for conventional cerebral angiography.[24] The downside to this procedure is that it requires large doses of contrast and radiation.[23] CTA has also been used in determining prognosis in intracerebral hemorrhage.[25]

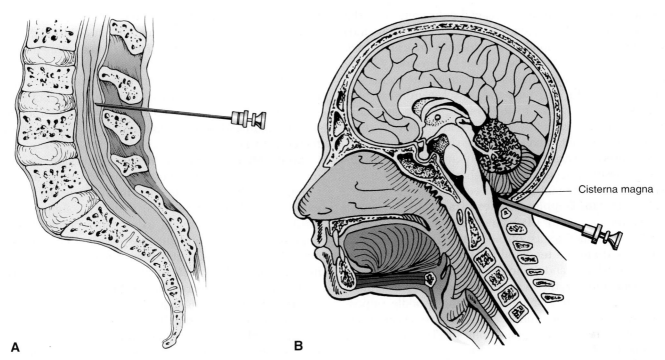

Fig. 26-13 **A,** Lumbar puncture. **B,** Cisternal puncture. (Modified from Phipps WJ et al: *Medical-surgical nursing: health and illness perspectives,* ed 7, St Louis, 2003, Mosby.)

Myelography. Myelography is radiographic examination of the spinal cord and vertebral column after injection of a contrast material into the subarachnoid space via the lumbar region of the spine between L2-L3 or L3-L4 or cisternal puncture.[4] Myelography allows visualization of the spinal canal, the subarachnoid space around the spinal cord, and the spinal nerve roots (Fig. 26-13). MRI has replaced myelography in most cases, but myelography may be necessary in postoperative patients with multiple clips or metallic hardware. Myelography is superior to MRI in identifying nerve root avulsions and dural tears.[26] Possible risks involved with the use of myelography include injection of the dye outside the subarachnoid space, arachnoiditis as a result of irritation of the arachnoid membranes from a foreign material, and allergic reaction. Other adverse reactions include confusion, hallucinations, headache, grand mal seizure, chest pain, and dysrhythmias.[26] Postprocedure care includes keeping the patient's head elevated 45 degrees for 8 hours, monitoring neurologic status, and encouraging oral fluids.[1]

CEREBRAL BLOOD FLOW STUDIES

The following discussion focuses on the more commonly performed cerebral blood studies that are used in diagnosis of the critically ill patient with neurologic dysfunction.

Perfusion Computed Tomography. Perfusion CT is a relatively new technique that allows rapid evaluation of cerebral perfusion. A perfusion CT scan is made by passing x-rays through the brain, just like a regular CT scan, but in addition to revealing the structure of brain tissue, it also measures cerebral blood flow (CBF), cerebral blood volume, and mean transit time. This is done by scanning the patient several times every few seconds before, during, and after the intravenous delivery of an iodine-containing contrast agent that absorbs the x-rays. Perfusion CT has been found to be useful for diagnosis of cerebral ischemia and infarction associated with stroke and for evaluation of cerebral ischemia associated with vasospasm after subarachnoid hemorrhage.[27,28]

Xenon Computed Tomography. Xenon CT is used to study regional CBF. The scan is a computerized x-ray study of the brain that is performed while the patient breathes a carefully regulated flow of xenon (a colorless, odorless gas). It has been demonstrated to have higher resolution in blood flow measurements than other techniques such as positron emission tomography (PET). A xenon CT scan has been used in the evaluation of a wide variety of disorders and has been most useful in the evaluation of cerebrovascular disease and brain metabolism. Xenon CT studies are occasionally used to determine brain death.[28]

Carotid Duplex Sonography. Ultrasound technology, although not an absolute measure of cerebral blood flow, uses a noninvasive technique to provide information about the flow velocity of blood through carotid vessels. Carotid duplex studies are used as a routine screening procedure for intraluminal narrowing of the common and internal carotid arteries as a result of atherosclerotic plaques. A Doppler probe is placed externally over the vessel, where high frequency sound waves (ultrasound) are generated and blood flow velocities are calculated. As the diameter of the vessel changes, the velocity of the flow of blood through the vessel changes; the higher the flow velocity, the narrower the vessel. Carotid duplex studies are noninvasive, relatively inexpensive, and painless. When changes in flow velocities are noted that may indicate significant occlusion of the vessel, CTA or MRA can be used to verify the degree of severity of the narrowed vessel. If necessary, a cerebral angiogram is performed to confirm ambiguous or equivocal findings.[1,15]

Transcranial Doppler Studies. Transcranial Doppler (TCD) studies monitor CBF velocity through cranial "windows," or thinned areas, of the skull. Three areas commonly used are the temporal bone (transtemporal), the eye (transorbital), and the foramen magnum (transoccipital). Depending on the angle of the Doppler probe, flow velocities can be measured in the anterior, middle, or posterior cerebral arteries and the vertebral and basilar arteries. Numerous clinical applications for TCD have been identified.[29]

TCD studies often are used in critical care for postintracranial aneurysm rupture in which concern about vasospasm development is a factor. The noninvasive technique and portability of the equipment allow for frequent bedside monitoring of flow velocity and therefore vascular diameter. Use of serial transcranial Doppler studies for the detection of cerebral vasospasm greatly reduces the need for cerebral angiograms to verify and follow postsubarachnoid hemorrhage vasospasm.[30]

Additional uses of TCD include identification of intracranial lesions in the stroke patient, evaluation of flow-velocity changes during carotid endarterectomy, and detection of cerebral blood flow changes associated with increased ICP. TCD has also been used to detect cerebral circulatory arrest in brain death determination but must be accompanied by clinical evaluation and additional diagnostic tests, because intracranial circulation may be preserved in brain-dead patients.[30]

Limitations of the TCD study must be understood. Accuracy of the TCD study is operator-dependent. Correct location and angle of the probe are essential. A small percentage of patients have temporal bones too thick for ultrasound penetration. And finally, a normal TCD study does not completely rule out the presence of vasospasm, because vasospasm may not be evident in the particular vessel examined. TCD results are always evaluated in conjunction with clinical assessment findings.[30]

During the TCD study, the patient will experience only mild pressure at the transducer site. No pain is involved. The patient must remain still during the study, which lasts 15 to 90 minutes.[1]

Transcranial Color-Coded Duplex Sonography. Transcranial color-coded duplex sonography (TCCS) is a new and noninvasive ultrasound study that enables the visualization of the intracranial structures and basal cerebral arteries and the measurement of blood flow velocities through the arteries. The color component of the study allows for more reliable data than the traditional TCD. TCCS is becoming a reliable tool for detecting the narrowing or occlusion of cerebral arteries, screening for vasospasm, and monitoring changes in intracranial dynamics. In addition, AV malformations can also be detected with TCCS.[31]

Emission Tomography. Positron emission tomography (PET) and single photon emission computed tomography (SPECT) are nuclear medicine scans used to calculate global and regional CBF. The ability of the SPECT and PET scanners to measure cerebral metabolic use of oxygen and glucose permits them to distinguish between brain tumor recurrence and brain or tumor necrosis. The PET scan uses positron-emitting radionucleotides, whereas the SPECT scan uses gamma emitters. PET scanning can quantify blood flow and can be used to evaluate the fraction of oxygen extracted from arterial blood by the cerebral tissue. Clinical use of PET is extremely limited because of the significant cost, lack of portability, and unavailability of the technology at many hospitals. SPECT is less expensive and more available in clinical practice. SPECT offers a qualitative, rather than an absolute, measure of cerebral blood flow. Results are described simply as normal, hypoperfused, or hyperperfused.[3,32] Nursing management of the patient undergoing PET or SPECT involves transportation of the patient to the scanning area and observation during the procedure.

Regional Cerebral Blood Flow Study. Regional cerebral blood flow studies used to be the gold standard for clinical bedside evaluation of CBF. Xenon-133 is administered by inhalation or injection into a peripheral vein. Scintillation detectors, or probes, placed on the outside of the skull monitor the uptake and clearance, or washout, of the xenon from the cerebral circulation. Information from the probes is then passed to a computer that calculates global or regional cerebral blood. One difficulty with this method is that all body tissues take up xenon and then clear it, including the skin and muscles of the scalp under detectors. Although mathematic calculations are factored in, cerebral blood flow results are an estimated value at best.[1]

ELECTROPHYSIOLOGY STUDIES

The following discussion focuses on the more commonly performed electrophysiology studies that are used in diagnosis of the critically ill patient with neurologic dysfunction.

Electroencephalography. Electroencephalography (EEG) is the recording of electrical impulses, commonly called *brain waves*, generated by the brain. This test has been in existence for many years and is well known to the general public. It is important for the nurse caring for a patient with a neurologic dysfunction to be aware of both the appropriate indications for use and the limitations of this diagnostic procedure. The purpose of EEG is to detect and localize abnormal electrical activity. This abnormal activity can be defined as *slowing*, which occurs in areas of injury or infarct, or as the *spikes* and *waves* seen in irritated tissue. Indications for the use of EEG include suspected seizure activity, cerebral infarct, metabolic encephalopathies, altered consciousness, infectious disease, some head injuries, and confirmation of brain death.[18,33]

Noninvasive electrodes are placed on the head, and the electrical impulses detected are transferred to a central recording device that records the information in wave form. Six types of waves or rhythms may be present (Table 26-4). Intermittent slowing with triphasic wave morphology is associated with metabolic encephalopathy. Continuous generalized slowing in the delta or theta range is associated with anoxic damage. The combination of alpha waves that do not change with stimulation and a coma state is termed *alpha coma* and is associated with a poor prognosis.[18]

Other EEG abnormalities associated with poor prognosis are *burst suppression* (occasional generalized bursts of activity with intervening inactivity or severe voltage depression) and *periodic patterns* (generalized spikes at fixed intervals of one to two per second).[18] Absence of electrical activity on EEG, *electrocerebral silence*, can occur transiently in the period immediately following cardiopulmonary resuscitation, severe hypothermia, and CNS depressant overdose.[18] Enduring electrocerebral silence provides evidence for the clinical determination of brain death.

The limitations of EEG are noteworthy. Only electrical activity involving large areas of cortex is recorded on EEG.[18] Accuracy of EEG varies depending on the location of electrophysiologic activity. Abnormal EEG findings are not cause-specific.[18] Similar EEG changes occur with a variety of conditions. And finally, it is important to note that the EEG can be normal even when significant pathology is present.[2,18]

In preparing the patient for an EEG, the nurse must stress the noninvasive aspects of this procedure. The awake patient may be asked to perform certain simple tasks during the procedure, such as blinking, closing the eye, or swallowing. Occasionally, testing must be performed during sleep or after a period of sleep deprivation.[1]

Evoked Potentials. Evoked potentials (EPs) are cerebral electrical impulses generated in response to a sensory stimulus.[18] Impulses are recorded as they travel through the brainstem and into the cerebral cortex. Measuring EPs is a sophisticated way of observing the status of sensory pathways as they enter the central nervous system, travel through the brainstem, and reach the cerebral cortex. EP studies are used in the determination of prognosis in coma and the existence and extent of brainstem or spinal cord injury in the traumatically injured patient. Evaluation of EPs is valuable during therapeutically-induced comas, such as barbiturate coma, inasmuch as these sensory pathways are unaffected by the depressive activity of such drugs.[18] Monitoring of EPs is also used intraoperatively during spinal surgery and cerebral tumor dissection.[34]

The four types of evoked potential tests are (1) visual evoked responses (VER), (2) brainstem auditory evoked responses (BAER), (3) somatosensory evoked responses (SSER), and (4) motor evoked potentials (MEP). VER involves monitoring of the visual pathways through the brainstem and cortex in response to the patient's viewing a shifting geometric pattern on a screen or a flashing light stimulus emitted from a mask placed over the eye. BAER involves monitoring the auditory pathway through the brainstem and cortex in response to a rhythmic clicking sound sent through earphones placed over the patient's ears. BAERs are useful in assessing brainstem integrity in the critical care unit when cranial nerve testing cannot be performed or is inconclusive. SSER involves monitoring of sensory pathways from the extremities ascending the spinal cord through the brainstem and into the cortex. This is performed by administering a small electrical shock to a nerve root in the periphery, such as the ulnar or radial nerve.[18] SSER can be used to evaluate cortical

Table 26-4	Types of Electrical Brain Waves	
Wave	**Duration**	**Description**
Delta	1-4 cycles/sec	Normal; seen in stages 3 and 4 of sleep
Alpha	8-13 cycles/sec	Normal; relaxed state with eyes closed, seen often in occipital leads
Theta	4-7 cycles/sec	Less common in adults than in children; characteristic of coma in brain injury
Beta	12-40 cycles/sec	Fast waves indicating mental or physical activity
Sleep spindles	12-14 cycles/sec	Seen in stage 2 sleep, not REM
Spike and slow waves	Variable	Seen in irritable brain tissue (such as seizure)

REM, Rapid eye movement.

functioning after cardiac arrest or head trauma.[35] SSER also is used routinely during spinal surgery.[34] MEPs assess the functional integrity of descending motor pathways. The motor cortex is stimulated via direct high-voltage electrical stimulation through the scalp or use of a magnetic field to induce an electrical current within the brain.[36] Electrical stimulation is a painful procedure and must be reserved for anesthetized patients. Magnetic stimulation is painless.

NURSING MANAGEMENT

The nursing management of a patient undergoing a diagnostic procedure involves a variety of interventions. Nursing activities are directed toward preparing the patient psychologically and physically for the procedure, monitoring the patient's responses to the procedure, and assessing the patient after the procedure. Preparing the patient includes teaching the patient about the procedure, answering any questions, and transporting and/or positioning the patient for the procedure. Monitoring the patient's responses to the procedure includes observing the patient for signs of pain, anxiety, or hemorrhage and monitoring vital signs. Assessing the patient after the procedure includes observing for complications of the procedure and medicating the patient for any postprocedure discomfort. Any evidence of increasing ICP should be immediately reported to the physician, and emergency measures to maintain circulation must be initiated.

LABORATORY STUDIES

The major laboratory study performed in the patient with neurologic dysfunction is CSF analysis obtained via a lumbar puncture or a ventriculostomy.[1-3]

LUMBAR PUNCTURE

The main purpose of lumbar puncture (LP) is to obtain CSF for analysis. CSF opening pressure may also be obtained. CSF samples are evaluated for the presence of subarachnoid blood or infection or are sent for laboratory analysis (Table 26-5).

An LP involves the introduction of a 20- to 22-gauge hollow needle into the subarachnoid space at L3-L4 or L4-L5, below the end of the spinal cord, which usually is at L1-L2 (Fig. 26-13, A). The patient can be placed either in the lateral decubitus position with the knees and head tightly tucked or in the sitting position leaning over a bedside table or some other support. Prior to initiating the procedure the patient's coagulation profile should be checked for any abnormalities.[3]

Two life-threatening risks associated with LP include possible brainstem herniation, if ICP is elevated, and res-

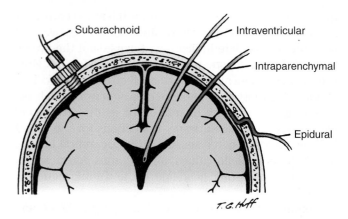

Fig. 26-14 Intracranial pressure monitoring sites. (From Lee KR, Hoff JT: *Youman's neurological surgery,* ed 4, Philadelphia, 1996, Saunders.)

piratory arrest associated with neurologic deterioration. During the procedure the nurse must monitor the patient's neurologic and respiratory status. Also, if the patient is not fully alert and cooperative, the nurse may need to assist the patient in maintaining the position necessary for performance of the LP.[1] The long-standing routine of keeping the patient flat in bed for several hours after a LP to prevent a headache has been refuted by scientific study.[37]

Cisternal puncture, which is the introduction of a needle into the cisterna magna at the C1-2 level (Fig. 26-13, B), is another method for obtaining access to the subarachnoid space. Risks of cisternal puncture are slightly higher than those associated with an LP, but cisternal puncture is necessary if the lumbar space cannot be entered because of scar tissue or some other physical barrier or if the CSF pathway is totally blocked somewhere along the spinal column.[3]

BEDSIDE MONITORING

INTRACRANIAL PRESSURE MONITORING

In the patient with suspected intracranial hypertension, a monitoring device may be placed within the cranium to quantify ICP. Under normal physiologic conditions, ICP is maintained below 15 mm Hg mean pressure. It is used to monitor serial intracranial pressures and assist with the management of intracranial hypertension. An increase in ICP can cause a decrease in blood flow to the brain, causing brain damage. It can also provide a sterile access for draining excess CSF.

Monitoring Sites. The four sites for monitoring ICP are the intraventricular space, the subarachnoid space, the epidural space, and the parenchyma (Fig. 26-14). Each site has advantages and disadvantages for monitoring ICP (Table 26-6). The type of monitor chosen de-

Table 26-5	Analysis of Cerebrospinal Fluid		
Characteristic	**Normal Findings**	**Abnormal Findings**	**Possible Causes/Comments**
Pressure	Less than 200 cm H_2O	<60 mm	Faulty needle placement Dehydration Spinal block along subarachnoid space Block of foramen magnum Hydrocephalus
		>200 mm	Muscle tension Abdominal compression Brain tumor Subdural hematoma Brain abscess Brain cyst Cerebral edema (any cause)
Color	Clear, colorless	Cloudy/turbid	Cloudy as a result of microorganisms (e.g., WBCs) Turbid as a result of increased cell count
		Yellow (xanthrochromic)	Breakdown of RBCs with RBC pigments, high protein count
		Smoky	RBCs
Blood	None	Red blood cells: blood tinged	Traumatic tap—bloody in first sample
		Grossly bloody	Traumatic tap—bloody in all samples
Volume	150 ml	Increase	Hydrocephalus
Specific gravity	1.007	Increase	Infection, presence of cells or protein
White blood cells (WBCs)	0-5 mm^3	<500 mm^3	Bacterial or viral infections of meninges, neurosyphilis, subarachnoid hemorrhage, infarction, abscess, tuberculous meningitis, metastatic lesions
		>500 mm^3	Purulent infection
Glucose	50-75 mg/dl or 60%-70% of blood glucose	<40 mg/dl	Meningitis: bacterial, tuberculosis, parasitic, fungal carcinomatous, subarachnoid hemorrhage
		>80 mg/dl	May not be of neurologic significance
Chloride	700-750 mg/dl	Decreased (<625 mg/dl)	Meningeal infection, tuberculosis meningitis, hypochloremia
		Increased (>800 mg/dl)	May not be of neurologic significance; correlated with blood levels of chloride and not routine—done only on request
Culture and sensitivity	No organisms present	*Neisseria* or *Streptococcus*	Identify organisms to begin therapy; Gram stain for some cultures may take several weeks
Serology for syphilis	Negative	Positive	Syphilis
Protein (If CSF contains blood, this will raise the protein level)	15-50 mg/dl	Increased (>60 mg/dl)	Bacterial meningitis, brain tumors (both benign and malignant), complete spinal block, ALS, Guillain-Barré syndrome, subarachnoid hemorrhage, infarction, CNS trauma, CNS degenerative diseases, herniated disk, DM with polyneuropathy
		Decreased (<10 mg/dl)	May not be of neurologic significance
Osmolality	295 Osm/L	Increased	Protein, WBCs, microorganisms, RBCs
Lactate	10-20 mg/dl	Increased	Bacterial, seizure activity, fungal meningitis, CNS trauma, coma related to toxic or metabolic causes

From Barker E: *Neuroscience nursing; a spectrum of care,* ed 2, St Louis, 2002, Mosby.
WBC, White blood cell; *RBC,* red blood cell; *CSF,* cerebrospinal fluid; *ALS,* amyotrophic lateral sclerosis; *CNS,* central nervous system; *DM,* diabetes mellitus.

Table 26-6	Advantages, Disadvantages, and Nursing Considerations of ICP Monitoring Techniques		
Monitoring Device	**Advantages**	**Disadvantages**	**Nursing Considerations**
Intraventricular catheter (ventriculostomy)	Allows accurate ICP measurement Provides access to CSF for drainage or sampling Provides access for instillation of contrast media Allows reliable evaluation of intracranial compliances (volume-pressure relationships)	Provides an additional site for infection Is most invasive ICP monitoring technique Requires frequent transducer balancing or recalibration Catheter may become occluded by blood clot or tissue debris Insertion is difficult if ventricles are small, compressed, or displaced Is associated with risk for CSF leakage around insertion site Is associated with increased risk for infection	Provide appropriate sedatives or analgesics during catheter insertion Do baseline and serial neurologic assessments Measure patient's temperature at least every 4 hours Note character, amount, and turbidity of CSF drainage Document ICP/CPP measurements, response to stimulation, nursing care activities per hospital/unit protocol Monitor quality of ICP waveform Monitor system/tubing for air bubbles, and flush or purge system as appropriate Drain CSF as indicated for treatment of ICP elevation Notify physician if CSF drainage is not within prescribed parameters Monitor insertion site for bleeding, drainage, swelling, CSF leakage Zero or calibrate device per hospital/unit protocol Level transducer at the foramen of Monro; external landmarks include the tragus of the patient's ear and the external auditory canal, among others; all ICP measurements should be made with the transducer at a consistent level relative to external landmarks Administer sedatives or analgesics as appropriate to decrease risk of catheter being dislodged by patient's movements Educate patient's family as indicated Notify physician if ICP/CPP not within specified parameters
Subarachnoid bolt or screw	Is associated with lower infection rates than is ventriculostomy Is quickly and easily placed Can be used with small or collapsed ventricles Requires no penetration of brain tissue	Has potential for dampened waveform (cerebral edema, blood or tissue debris) Is less accurate at high ICP elevations Requires frequent balancing/recalibration (and with position changes) Provides no access for CSF sampling	Administer appropriate sedatives or analgesics during insertion Do baseline and serial neurologic assessments Measure patient's temperature at least every 4 hours Monitor insertion site for bleeding, drainage, swelling, CSF leakage Monitor quality of ICP waveform Document ICP/CPP measurements, response to stimulation per hospital/unit protocol Administer sedatives or analgesics as appropriate to decrease risk of catheter being dislodged by patient's movements Zero or calibrate device per hospital/unit protocol Level transducer at the foramen of Monro; external landmarks include the tragus of the patient's ear and the external auditory canal, among others; all ICP measurements should be made with the transducer at a consistent level relative to external landmarks Educate patient's family as indicated Notify physician if ICP/CPP is not within specified parameters

From Arbour R: Intracranial hypertension: monitoring and nursing assessment, *Crit Care Nurse* 24(5):19, 2004.

Table 26-6	Advantages, Disadvantages, and Nursing Considerations of ICP Monitoring Techniques—cont'd		
Monitoring Device	Advantages	Disadvantages	Nursing Considerations*
Subdural or epidural catheter or sensor	Is least invasive Is associated with decreased risk of infection Is easily and quickly placed	Increase in baseline drift over time means possible loss of reliability or accuracy Provides no access for CSF drainage/sampling	Administer appropriate sedatives or analgesics during insertion Do baseline and serial neurologic assessments Measure patient's temperature at least every 4 hours Monitor insertion site for bleeding, drainage, swelling Monitor quality of ICP waveform, drift over time Document ICP/CPP measurements, response to stimulation per hospital/unit protocol Administer sedatives or analgesics as appropriate to decrease risk of catheter being dislodged or damaged by patient's movements Educate patient's family as indicated Notify physician if ICP/CPP is not within specified parameters
Fiberoptic transducer-tipped catheter	Can be placed in subdural or subarachnoid space, in a ventricle, or directly within brain tissue Is easily transported Requires zeroing only once (during insertion) Has baseline drift of up to 1 mm Hg per day Is associated with decreased risk for infection when brain tissue is not penetrated Provides good-quality ICP waveforms (less artifact than with other devices) Requires no adjustment in level of transducer with patient's change of position	Provides no access for CSF sampling/drainage Cannot be recalibrated after placement Requires periodic replacement of probe Is easily damaged	Administer appropriate sedatives or analgesics during insertion Do baseline and serial neurologic assessments Measure patient's temperature at lest every 4 hours Monitor insertion site for bleeding, drainage, swelling, CSF leakage Monitor quality of ICP waveform, drift over time Document ICP/CPP measurements, response to stimulation per hospital/unit protocol Administer sedatives or analgesics as appropriate to decrease risk of catheter being dislodged or damaged by patient's movements Educate patient's family as indicated Notify physician if ICP/CPP is not within specified parameters

pends on both the suspected pathologic condition and physician's preferences.[38,39] Nursing considerations for each type of device are also discussed in Table 26-6.

Intraventricular. ICP monitoring is accomplished by placing a small catheter into the ventricular system; this procedure is known as a *ventriculostomy.* The catheter is inserted through a burr hole with the patient under local anesthesia and usually is placed in the anterior horn of the lateral ventricle. If at all possible, the side chosen for placement of the ventriculostomy is the nondominant hemisphere.[38,39]

Subarachnoid Space. ICP monitoring is accomplished by placing a small hollow bolt or screw into the subarachnoid space. It is inserted though a burr hole,

usually located in the front of the skull behind the hairline, with the patient under local anesthesia. Inserting this device is easier than inserting the ventriculostomy catheter.[38,39]

Epidural Space. ICP monitoring is accomplished by placing a small fiberoptic sensor into the epidural space. It is also inserted through a burr hole while the patient is under local anesthesia. The physician strips the dura away from the inner table of the skull before inserting the epidural monitor.[38,39]

Intraparenchymal. ICP monitoring is accomplished by placing a small fiberoptic catheter into the parenchymal tissue. After placing a subarachnoid bolt (as just described), a hole is punched in the dura and the

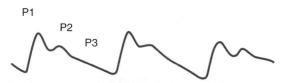

Fig. 26-15 Normal ICP waveform. (From Bader MK, Little-johns LR: *AANN core curriculum for neuroscience nursing,* ed 4, St Louis, 2004, Elsevier.)

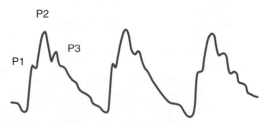

Fig. 26-16 Abnormal ICP waveform. (From Bader MK, Little-johns LR: *AANN core curriculum for neuroscience nursing,* ed 4, St Louis, 2004, Elsevier.)

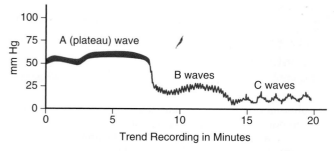

Fig 26-17 Intracranial pressure waves. Composite diagram of *A* (plateau) waves, *B* (sawtooth) waves, and *C* (small rhythmic) waves. (From Barker E: *Neuroscience nursing: a spectrum of care,* ed 2, St Louis, 2002, Mosby.)

catheter is inserted approximately 1 cm into the brain's white matter.[38,39]

Intracranial Pressure Waves. The ICP pulse waveform is observed on a continuous, real-time pressure display and corresponds to each heartbeat. The waveform arises primarily from pulsations of the major intracranial arteries, receiving retrograde venous pulsations as well.[38,39]

Normal ICP Waveform. The normal ICP wave has three or more defined peaks (Fig. 26-15). The first peak, or P1, is called the *percussion wave.* Originating from the pulsations of the choroid plexus, it has a sharp peak and is fairly consistent in its amplitude. The second peak, or P2, is called the *tidal wave.* The tidal wave is more variable in shape and amplitude, ending on the dicrotic notch. The P2 portion of the pulse waveform has been most directly linked to the state of decreased compliance. When the P2 component is equal to or higher than P1, decreased compliance occurs (Fig. 26-16). Immediately after the dicrotic notch is the third wave, P3, which is called the *dicrotic wave.* After the dicrotic wave, the pressure usually tapers down to the diastolic position, unless retrograde venous pulsations add a few more peaks.[39-41]

A, B, and C pressure waves are not true waveforms (Fig. 26-17). Rather, they are the graphically displayed trend data of intracranial pressure over time. These waves reflect spontaneous alterations in ICP associated with respiration, systemic blood pressure, and deteriorating neurologic status.

A Waves. Also called *plateau waves* because of their distinctive shape, A waves are the most clinically significant of the three types. They usually occur in an already elevated baseline ICP (greater than 20 mm Hg) and are characterized by sharp increases in ICP of 30 to 69 mm Hg, which plateau for 2 to 20 minutes and then return to baseline. The actual cause of A waves is unknown, but they may result from vasodilation and increased CBF, decreased venous outflow (and therefore increased cerebral blood volume), fluctuations in $PaCO_2$ (and therefore changes in cerebral blood volume), or decreased CSF absorption. B waves often precede A waves. Plateau waves are considered significant because of the reduced cerebral perfusion pressure associated with ICP in the 50 to 100 mm Hg range. Transient signs of intracranial hypertension such as a decreased level of consciousness, bradycardia, pupillary changes, or respiratory changes may accompany these waves. Some research suggests that prolonged increases in ICP associated with plateau waves could result in transient as well as permanent cell damage from ischemia.[2,39]

B Waves. B waves are sharp, rhythmic oscillations with a sawtooth appearance that occur every 30 seconds to 2 minutes and can raise the ICP from 5 to 70 mm Hg. They are a normal physiologic phenomenon that can occur in any patient, but they are amplified in states of low intracranial compliance. B waves appear to reflect fluctuations in cerebral blood volume. Decompensation of normal intracranial volume compensatory capacity is indicated by B waves with a high amplitude (greater than 15 mm Hg pressure change from peak to trough of wave).[2,39]

C Waves. C waves are smaller, rhythmic waves that occur every 4 to 8 minutes at normal levels of ICP. They are related to normal fluctuations in respiration and systemic arterial pressure. C waves are considered clinically insignificant.[2,39]

Cerebral Perfusion Pressure. Measuring CBF in the clinical setting is difficult, but at the bedside an estimated pressure of cerebral perfusion can be derived. Cerebral perfusion pressure (CPP) is the blood pressure gradient across the brain and is calculated as the difference between the incoming mean arterial pressure (MAP) and the opposing ICP on the arteries:

$$CPP = MAP - ICP$$

The CPP in the average adult is approximately 80 to 100 mm Hg, with a range of 60 to 150 mm Hg. The CPP must be maintained near 80 mm Hg to provide adequate blood supply to the brain. If the CPP drops below this point, ischemia may develop. A sustained CPP of 30 mm Hg or less usually results in neuronal hypoxia and cell death. When the mean systemic arterial pressure equals the ICP, CBF may cease.[1-3]

CEREBRAL OXYGENATION MONITORING

Cerebral Metabolism. The measurements of CBF and CPP do not address the brain's metabolic need for oxygen. Active neurons require greater amounts of oxygen than those which are inactive. The determination that CBF matches the brain's metabolic needs is expressed as *cerebral metabolic rate (CMRo$_2$)*, the normal value of which is 3.4 ml per 100 g of brain tissue per minute. Neuronal demand for oxygen is governed by their metabolic rate. This value is not easily attained for technical reasons, although it can be calculated. It is the product of the measured CBF and calculated arteriojugular oxygen difference (Ajdo$_2$):[42]

$$CMRo_2 = CBF \times Ajdo_2$$

CBF can be measured using a variety of complex techniques (e.g., PET and SPECT scans). Most recently, continuous bedside monitoring of regional cerebrocortical blood flow has become available.[8] Arteriojugular oxygen difference is the amount of oxygen extracted by the brain and is reflected in the difference between the arterial oxygen content and the jugular venous oxygen content. The normal value is 5.0 to 7.5 vol%.[42]

Jugular Venous Oxygen Saturation (Sjvo$_2$). One method of measuring CBF allows continuous measurement of oxygenation within the jugular venous system through the use of the jugular bulb monitor. Sjvo$_2$ can be used to reflect cerebral oxygen supply-and-demand balance. Any disorder that increases CMRo$_2$ or decreases oxygen delivery may decrease Sjvo$_2$, and conversely any disorder that that decreases CMRo$_2$ or increases oxygen delivery may increase Sjvo$_2$.[42,43]

To measure Sjvo$_2$ a fiberoptic catheter is placed retrograde through the internal jugular vein into the jugular bulb and attached to a bedside monitor. The normal value is 60% to 80%. Patients with values less than 50% and 55% are either hypoxemic or oligemic (low cerebral blood flow as compared with metabolic rate). Oligemia occurs as a result of decreased blood flow due to hypotension, vasospasm, or intracranial hypertension or as a result of increased brain metabolic requirements due to fever or seizures.[42,43] Sjvo$_2$ values below 45% are indicative of severe cerebral hypoxia.[42] Patients with values above 75% to 80% are considered hyperemic (CBF high compared with metabolic need). Sjvo$_2$ will also rise if the brain is so severely injured the neurons are unable to extract oxygen.[42,43]

There are a number of limitations to Sjvo$_2$ monitoring. Sjvo$_2$ is a global measure of cerebral oxygenation and thus a normal Sjvo$_2$ does not mean that there are not localized areas of cerebral ischemia.[42,43] Readings are affected by the movement of the patient's head.[43] Up to 50% of low Sjvo$_2$ readings are false and may be due to technical issues with the catheter, particularly catheter migration.[44] For accurate reading, the tip of the catheter must be within 1 cm of the jugular bulb.[43]

Brain Tissue Oxygen Pressure (Pbto$_2$). Over the last few years a new device has become available to measure the partial pressure of oxygen within brain tissue (Pbto$_2$). The device consists of a monitoring probe on the end of a catheter, which is inserted into the brain parenchyma and attached to a bedside monitor. The probe may be inserted into the damaged portion of the brain to measure regional oxygenation or inserted into the undamaged portion of the brain to measure global oxygenation. One risk associated with insertion of the catheter is bleeding with hematoma formation.[45] While there is no consensus on normal values because they vary from device to device, it has been concluded that the probability of death increases with prolonged periods of a Pbto$_2$ less than 15 mm Hg and any episode of a Pbto$_2$ less than 6 mm Hg.[45]

In the head-injured patient the goal of treatment is to maintain the Pbto$_2$ greater than 20 mm Hg. Factors that decrease Pbto$_2$ include tissue hypoxia, hypocapnia, hypovolemia, decreased blood pressure, low hemoglobin, intracranial hypertension, and hyperthermia.[46] Treatment is directed at the underlying cause.

REFERENCES

1. Barker E: *Neuroscience nursing: a spectrum of care*, ed 2, St Louis, 2002, Mosby.
2. Bader MK, Littlejohns LR: *AANN core curriculum for neuroscience nursing*, ed 4, St Louis, 2004, Elsevier.
3. Goetz CG: *Textbook of clinical neurology*, ed 2, St Louis, 2003, Elsevier.
4. Haymore J: A neuron in a haystack: advanced neurologic assessment, *AACN Clin Issues* 15:568, 2002.
5. Teasdale G, Jennett W: Assessment of coma and impaired consciousness—a practical scale, *Lancet* 2:81, 1974.
6. Juarez VJ, Lyons M: Interrater reliability of the Glasgow Coma Scale, *J Neurosci Nurs* 27:283, 1995.
7. Fischer J, Mathieson C: The history of the Glasgow Coma Scale: implications for practice, *Crit Care Nurs Q* 23(4):52, 2001.
8. Barnwell P: Assessing motor and sensory function—a focused survey, *Aust Emerg Nurs J* 2(3):16, 1999.
9. O'Hanlon-Nichols T: Neurologic assessment, *Am J Nurs* 99(6):44, 1999.
10. Bishop BS: Pathologic pupillary signs: self-learning module. Part 1, *Crit Care Nurs* 11(6):58, 1991.
11. Bishop BS: Pathologic pupillary signs: self-learning module. Part II, *Crit Care Nurs* 11(7):58, 1991.
12. Marshall LF et al: The oval pupil: clinical significance and relationship to intracranial hypertension, *J Neurosurg* 58:566, 1983.

13. Chesnut RM: Management of brain and spine injuries, *Crit Care Clin* 20:25, 2005.
14. Keller C, Williams A: Cardiac dysrhythmias associated with central nervous system dysfunction, *J Neurosci Nurs* 25:349, 1993.
15. Grainger RG et al: *Grainger & Allison's diagnostic radiology: a textbook of medical imaging,* ed 4, London, 2001, Churchill Livingstone.
16. Servadei F et al: The value of the "worst" computed tomographic scan in clinical studies of moderate and severe head injury, *Neurosurgery* 46:70, 2000.
17. Shpritz DW: Neurodiagnostic studies, *Nurs Clin North Am* 34:593, 1999.
18. Bradley WG et al: *Neurology in clinical practice,* ed 4, St Louis, 2003, Elsevier.
19. Selden NR et al: Emergency magnetic resonance imaging of cervical spinal cord injuries: clinical correlation and prognosis, *Neurosurgery* 44:785, 1999.
20. Wedekind C et al: Comparative use of magnetic resonance imaging and electrophysiologic investigation for the prognosis of head injury, *J Trauma* 74:44, 1999.
21. Takahashi M et al: Magnetic resonance imaging findings in cerebral fat embolism: correlation with clinical manifestations, *J Trauma* 46:324, 1999.
22. Fink JN, Caplan LR: Cerebrovascular cases, *Med Clin North Am* 87:755, 2003.
23. Rowe VL, Tucker SW: Advances in vascular imaging, *Surg Clin North Am* 84:1189, 2004.
24. Phillips CD, Bubash LA: CT angiography and MR angiography in the evaluation of extracranial carotid vascular disease, *Radiol Clin North Am* 40:783, 2002.
25. Becker KJ et al: Extravasation of radiographic contrast is an independent predictor of death in primary intracerebral hemorrhage, *Stroke* 30:2025, 1999.
26. Humphreys SC, Eck JC, Hodges SD: Neuroimaging in low back pain, *Am Fam Physician* 65:2299, 2002.
27. Hoeffner EG et al: Cerebral perfusion CT: technique and clinical applications, *Radiology* 231:632, 2004.
28. Perez-Arjona EA et al: New techniques in cerebral imaging, *Neurol Res* 24(Suppl 1):S17, 2002.
29. Miller RD: *Miller's anesthesia,* ed 6, St Louis, 2005, Elsevier.
30. Sloan MA et al: Assessment: transcranial Doppler ultrasonography: report of the Therapeutics and Technology Assessment Subcommittee of the American Academy of Neurology, *Neurology* 62:1468, 2004.
31. Krejza J: Clinical applications of transcranial color-coded duplex sonography, *J Neuroimaging* 14:215, 2004.
32. Alavi A et al: PET: a revolution in medical imaging, *Radiol Clin North Am* 42:983, 2004.
33. Cascino GD: Use of routine and video electroencephalography *Neurol Clin* 19:271, 2001.
34. Soriano SG, McCann ME, Laussen PC: Neuroanesthesia. Innovative techniques and monitoring, *Anesthesiol Clin North Am* 20:137, 2002.
35. Robinson LR et al: Predictive value of somatosensory evoked potentials for awakening from coma, *Crit Care Med* 31:960, 2003.
36. Papworth D: Intraoperative monitoring during vascular surgery, *Anesthesiol Clin North Am* 22:223, 2004.
37. Thoennissen J et al: Does bed rest after cervical or lumbar puncture prevent headache? A systematic review and meta-analysis, *CMAJ* 165:1311, 2001.
38. American Association of Neuroscience Nurses: *Clinical guideline series: intracranial pressure monitoring,* Chicago, 1997, The Association.
39. Arbour R: Intracranial hypertension: monitoring and nursing assessment, *Crit Care Nurse* 24(5):19, 2004.
40. March K: Intracranial pressure monitoring and assessing intracranial compliance in brain injury, *Crit Care Nurs Clin North Am* 12:429, 2000.
41. Kirkness CJ et al: Intracranial pressure waveform analysis: clinical and research implications, *J Neurosci Nurs* 32:271, 2000.
42. Smythe PR, Samra SK: Monitors of cerebral oxygenation, *Anesthesiol Clin North Am* 20:293, 2002.
43. Kidd JC, Criddle L: Using jugular venous catheters in patients with traumatic brain injury, *Crit Care Nurse* 21(6):16, 2001.
44. Coplin WM et al: Accuracy of continuous jugular bulb oximetry in the intensive care unit, *Neurosurgery* 42:533, 1998.
45. Littlejohn LR, Bader MK, March K: Brain tissue oxygen monitoring in severe brain injury, I: research and usefulness in critical care, *Crit Care Nurse* 23(4):17, 2003.
46. Littlejohn LR, Bader MK, March K: Brain tissue oxygen monitoring in severe brain injury, II: implications for critical care teams and case study, *Crit Care Nurse* 23(4):19, 2003.

CHAPTER 27

Neurologic Disorders and Therapeutic Management

*A*n understanding of the pathology of a disease or condition, the areas of assessment on which to focus, and the usual medical management allows the critical care nurse to more accurately anticipate and plan nursing interventions. Although a wide array of neurologic disorders exists, only a few routinely require care in the critical care environment.

COMA

Description. Normal consciousness requires both awareness and arousal. Awareness is the combination of cognition (mental and intellectual) and affect (mood) that can be construed based on the patient's interaction with the environment. Thus, alterations of consciousness may be the result of deficits in awareness, arousal, or both.[1] Box 27-1 lists the descending states of consciousness.

Coma is the deepest state of unconsciousness; both arousal and awareness are lacking.[1,2] The patient can neither be aroused nor demonstrates any purposeful response to the surrounding environment. Coma is actually a symptom, rather than a disease, and it occurs as a result of some underlying process.[1] The incidence of coma is difficult to ascertain because a wide variety of conditions can induce coma.[2] This state of unconsciousness is unfortunately very common in critical care and will be the focus of the following discussion.

Etiology. The causes of coma can be divided into two general categories: structural or surgical and metabolic or medical. Structural causes of coma include ischemic stroke, intracerebral hemorrhage, trauma, and brain tumors.[3] Metabolic causes of coma include drug overdose, infectious diseases, endocrine disorders, and poisonings.[3] Approximately 85% of coma is caused by metabolic disorders and 15% by structural disorders.[4] Table 27-1 provides a brief list of the possible causes of coma.

Pathophysiology. Consciousness involves both arousal, or wakefulness, and awareness. Neither of these functions is present in the patient in coma. Ascending fibers of the reticular activating system (ARAS) in the pons, hypothalamus, and thalamus maintain arousal as an autonomic function. Neurons in the cerebral cortex are responsible for awareness. Diffuse dysfunction of both cerebral hemispheres and/or diffuse or focal dysfunction of the reticular activating system will produce coma.[5,6] Structural etiologies usually cause compression or dysfunction in the area of the ARAS, whereas most medical etiologies lead to general dysfunction of both cerebral hemispheres.[7] Diffuse brain dysfunction can be due to neuronal damage caused by deprivation of oxygen, glucose, or metabolic factors, endogenous and exogenous toxins, endocrine and electrolyte disorders, intracranial hypertension, central nervous system infections, neuronal disorders, disorders of temperature regulation, and seizures.[4] Dysfunction of the ARAS can be due to hemorrhage, infarction, tumors, and abscesses.[4]

Assessment and Diagnosis. Diagnosis of the coma state is a clinical one, readily established by assessment of the level of consciousness. However, determining the full nature and cause of coma requires a thorough history and physical examination. A past medical history is essential, because events immediately preceding the change in level of consciousness can often provide valuable clues as to the origin of the coma. When limited information is available and the coma is profound, the response of the patient to emergency treatment may provide clues to the underlying diagnosis; for example, the patient who becomes responsive with the administration of naloxone can be presumed to have ingested some type of opiate.[6]

Detailed serial neurologic examinations are essential for all patients in coma. Assessment of pupillary size and reaction to light (normal, sluggish, or fixed), extraocular eye movements (normal, asymmetric, or absent), motor response to pain (normal, decorticate, decerebrate, or flaccid), and breathing pattern yields important clues to determining whether the etiology of the coma is structural or metabolic.[3,5]

The areas of the brainstem that control consciousness and pupillary responses are anatomically adjacent. The sympathetic and parasympathetic nervous systems control pupillary dilation and constriction, respectively.

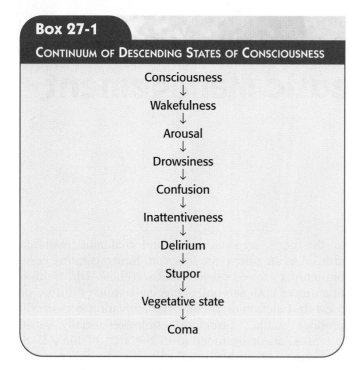

Box 27-1

Continuum of Descending States of Consciousness

Consciousness
↓
Wakefulness
↓
Arousal
↓
Drowsiness
↓
Confusion
↓
Inattentiveness
↓
Delirium
↓
Stupor
↓
Vegetative state
↓
Coma

Table 27-1   Etiologies of Coma

Structural/ Surgical Coma	Metabolic/ Medical Coma
Trauma	Infection
Epidural hematoma	Meningitis
Subdural hematoma	Encephalitis
	Metabolic
Diffuse axonal injury	Metabolic conditions
	Hypoglycemia
Brain contusion	Hyperglycemia
Intracerebral hemorrhage	Hyperosmolar
	Uremia
Subarachnoid hemorrhage	Hepatic encephalopathy
	Hypertensive encephalopathy
Posterior fossa hemorrhage	Hypoxic encephalopathy
	Hyponatremia
Supratentorial hemorrhage	Hypercalcemia
	Myxedema
Hydrocephalus	Intoxication
Ischemic stroke	Narcotic overdose
Tumor	Alcohol
Other	Poisonings
	Psychogenic

The anatomic directions of these pathways are known, and thus changes in pupillary responses can help identify where a lesion may be located (Fig. 27-1). For example, if damage occurs in the midbrain region, pupils will be slightly enlarged and unresponsive to light. Lesions that compress the third nerve result in a fixed and dilated pupil on the same side as the insult. Pupillary responses are usually preserved when the etiology of the coma is metabolic in origin. Pupillary light responses are often the key to differentiating between structural and metabolic causes of coma.[3,5,8]

Areas of the brainstem adjacent to those responsible for consciousness also control the oculomotor eye movement. The ability to maintain conjugate gaze requires preservation of the internuclear connections of cranial nerves III, VI, and VIII via the medial longitudinal fasciculus (MLF).[6,8] As with pupillary responses, structural lesions that impinge on these pathways will cause oculomotor dysfunction such as a disconjugate gaze. Thus deficits in extraocular eye movements usually accompany a structural etiology.[3,5,8]

Focal or asymmetric motor deficits usually also indicate structural lesions.[3,5] Abnormal motor movements may also help pinpoint the location of a lesion. Decorticate posturing (abnormal flexion) can be seen with damage to the diencephalon. Decerebrate posturing (abnormal extension) can be seen with damage to the midbrain and pons. Flaccid posturing is an ominous sign and can be seen with damage to the medulla.[8]

Abnormal breathing patterns may also assist in differentiating structural from metabolic etiologies of coma. Cheyne-Stokes respirations are seen in patients with cerebral hemispheric dysfunction and metabolic conditions. Central neurogenic hyperventilation occurs with damage to the midbrain and upper pons. Apneustic breathing may occur with damage to the pons, hypoglycemia, and anoxia. Ataxic breathing occurs with damage to the medulla. Agonal breathing occurs with failure of the respiratory centers in the medulla.[8]

In addition to physical assessment, laboratory studies and diagnostic procedures are done. Structural causes of coma are usually readily apparent with computed tomography (CT) or magnetic resonance imaging (MRI). Laboratory studies are also used to identify metabolic or endocrine abnormalities.[6] Occasionally the cause of coma is never clearly determined.

Medical Management. The goal of medical management of the patient in a coma is identification and treatment of the underlying cause of the condition. Initial medical management includes emergency measures to support vital functions and prevent further neurologic deterioration. Protection of the airway and ventilatory assistance are often needed. Administration of thiamine (at least 100 mg), glucose, and a narcotic antagonist is suggested whenever the cause of coma is not immediately known.[1,4-6] Thiamine is administered before glucose since the coma produced by thiamine deficiency, Wernicke's encephalopathy, can be precipitated by a glucose load.[5] The cervical neck is stabilized until traumatic injury is ruled out.[4]

The patient who remains in coma after emergency treatment requires supportive measures to maintain

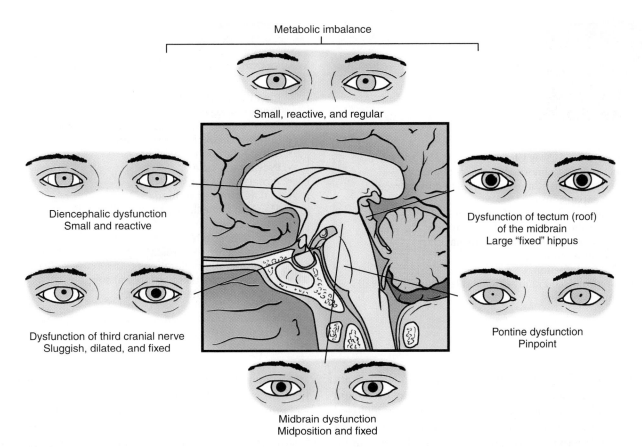

Metabolic imbalance

Small, reactive, and regular

Diencephalic dysfunction
Small and reactive

Dysfunction of tectum (roof)
of the midbrain
Large "fixed" hippus

Dysfunction of third cranial nerve
Sluggish, dilated, and fixed

Pontine dysfunction
Pinpoint

Midbrain dysfunction
Midposition and fixed

Fig 27-1   Pupils at different levels of consciousness. (From McCance KL, Huether SE: *Pathophysiology: the biologic basis for disease in adults and children,* ed 4, St Louis, 2002, Mosby.)

physiologic body functions and prevent complications. Continued airway protection and nutritional support are essential. Fluid and electrolyte management is often complex because of alterations in the neurohormonal system. Anticonvulsant therapy may be necessary to prevent further ischemic damage to the brain.[5,9]

The health care team and the patient's family make decisions jointly regarding the level of medical management to be provided. Family members require informational support in terms of probable cause of the coma and prognosis for recovery of both consciousness and function. Prognosis depends on the cause of the coma and the length of time unconsciousness persists. Sixty percent of patients in nontraumatic coma persisting for 6 or more hours die; 12% remain in a vegetative state.[10] The recovery rate for patients who are in coma for more than 1 week is only 3%.[10] As a general rule, metabolic coma has a better prognosis than coma caused by a structural lesion, and traumatic coma generally has a better outcome than nontraumatic.[6]

Much research has been directed toward identifying prognostic indicators for the patient in a coma after a cardiopulmonary arrest. As with all types of coma, the best prognosis is associated with early arousal. There is a 20% to 30% chance of survival with a good outcome in the comatose patient who responds to pain with reflex

posturing (decorticate or decerebrate) within 1 to 3 hours after an arrest. In one study the presence of speech at 24 hours after arrest predicted complete neurologic recovery.[11] Survival is unlikely in the coma patient who has absent pupillary light reflexes for more than 6 hours after cardiopulmonary resuscitation.[11] These statistics are helpful in guiding decision making. However, it must always be remembered that regardless of the cause or duration of coma, outcome for an individual cannot be predicted with 100% accuracy.[5]

Nursing Management. Nursing management of the patient in a coma incorporates a variety of nursing diagnoses (see the Nursing Diagnoses feature on Coma) and is directed by the specific etiology of the coma, although some common interventions are used. One of the most important things to remember is that the patient in a coma is totally dependent on the health care team. Nursing interventions are directed toward assessing for changes in neurologic status and clues to the origin of the coma, supporting all body functions, maintaining surveillance for complications, providing comfort and emotional support, and initiating rehabilitation measures.[5]

Measures to support body functions include promoting pulmonary hygiene, maintaining skin integrity, initiating range of motion exercises, and ensuring adequate nutritional support.[5]

NURSING DIAGNOSES — Coma

- Ineffective Airway Clearance related to excessive secretions or abnormal viscosity of mucus
- Ineffective Breathing Pattern related to decreased lung expansion
- Imbalanced Nutrition: Less Than Body Requirements related to lack of exogenous nutrients or increased metabolic demand
- Risk for Aspiration
- Risk for Infection
- Compromised Family Coping related to critically ill family member

Box 27-2

COLLABORATIVE MANAGEMENT

COMA
- Identify and treat underlying cause
- Protect airway
- Provide ventilatory assistance as required
- Support circulation as required
- Initiate nutritional support
- Provide eye care
- Protect skin integrity
- Initiate range of motion
- Maintain surveillance for complications
  - Infections
  - Metabolic alterations
  - Cardiac dysrhythmias
  - Temperature alterations
- Provide comfort and emotional support
- Plan for rehabilitation program

Eye Care. The blink reflex is often diminished or absent in the comatose patient. The eyelids may be flaccid and dependent on body positioning to remain in a closed position, and edema may prevent complete closure. Loss of these protective mechanisms results in drying and ulceration of the cornea, which can lead to permanent scarring and blindness.[5]

Two interventions that are commonly used to protect the eyes are instilling saline or methylcellulose lubricating drops and taping the eyelids in the shut position. There is evidence suggesting that an alternative technique may be more effective in preventing corneal epithelial breakdown. In addition to instilling saline drops every 2 hours, a polyethylene film is taped over the eyes, extending beyond the orbits and eyebrows. The film creates a moisture chamber around the cornea and assists in keeping the eyes moist and in the closed position.[12] This technique also prevents damage to the eyes that results from tape or gauze being placed directly on the delicate skin of the eyelids.[12]

Collaborative management of the patient in a coma is outlined in Box 27-2.

STROKE

Stroke is a descriptive term for the onset of acute neurologic deficit persisting for more than 24 hours and caused by the interruption of blood flow to the brain. Stroke is the third leading cause of death in the United States, preceded by heart disease and cancer, and the leading cause of adult disability.[13] Approximately 700,000 people experience a stroke each year, with 500,000 of these as first attacks and 200,000 as recurrent attacks.[13]

Strokes are generally classified as either ischemic or hemorrhagic. While approximately 80% of all strokes are ischemic, hemorrhagic strokes have a higher mortality rate. Approximately 8% to 12% of ischemic strokes and 37% to 38% of hemorrhagic strokes result in death within 30 days.[13] Hemorrhagic strokes can be further categorized as subarachnoid hemorrhages (SAHs) or intracerebral hemorrhages (ICHs). In 2005 the estimated annual cost for care and loss of productivity reached $56.8 billion.[13]

The national concern for the incidence and effects of stroke is illustrated by the inclusion of emergent stroke care in the American Heart Association guidelines for basic and advanced life support. Major public education programs, stroke appraisal screening programs, development of stroke centers, and algorithms for stroke management are based on the success these same approaches have had with coronary artery disease.

ISCHEMIC STROKE

Description. Ischemic stroke results from low cerebral blood flow, usually because of occlusion of a blood vessel. The occlusion can be either thrombotic or embolic in nature. Hypoperfusion resulting from hypotension also produces ischemic stroke. Eighty to eighty-five percent of all strokes are ischemic in nature.[14,15]

Strokes are preventable. Most thrombotic strokes are the result of the accumulation of atherosclerotic plaque in the vessel lumen, especially at bifurcations, or curves, of the vessel. The pathogenesis of cerebrovascular disease is identical to that of coronary vasculature. The greatest risk factor for ischemic stroke is hypertension (HTN).[6,14] Other risk factors are diabetes, elevated blood lipids, carotid artery disease, alcohol consumption, and smoking.[16] Common sites of atherosclerotic plaque are the bifurcation of the common carotid artery, the origins of the middle and anterior cerebral arteries, and the origins of the vertebral arteries.[6] Ischemic strokes secondary to vertebral artery dissection have been reported after chiropractic manipulation of the cervical spine.[17]

Etiology. An embolic stroke occurs when an embolus from the heart or lower circulation travels distally and lodges in a small vessel, resulting in loss of blood supply. At least 30% of ischemic strokes are attributed to a cardioembolic phenomenon.[6] The presence of valvular heart disease triples the risk for stroke.[18] Other risk factors include atrial fibrillation, myocardial infarction, ventricular aneurysm, and cardiomyopathy. Embolic strokes also arise from atherosclerosis of the ascending aorta.[19] Recent research has linked chronic inflammation, evidenced by elevated serum C-reactive protein,[16,20] and chronic periodontitis with significantly increased risk for stroke.[21]

Pathophysiology. Ischemic stroke is a cerebral hemodynamic insult. When cerebral blood flow is reduced to a level insufficient to maintain neuronal viability, ischemic injury occurs. In focal stroke, an area of marginally perfused tissue, the ischemic penumbra, surrounds a core of ischemic cells.[6] Sustained anoxic insult initiates a chain of events producing brain infarction. Irreversible neuronal injury soon follows. If infarction occurs, the affected brain tissue eventually softens and liquefies.[14]

The phenomenon of a focal ischemic stroke is identical to that associated with myocardial infarction, hence the term "brain attack" being used in public education strategies. Often a history of transient ischemic attacks (TIAs), brief episodes of neurologic symptoms, or reversible ischemic neurologic deficit (RIND), which last less than 24 hours, offers a warning that stroke is likely to occur. Sudden onset indicates embolism as the final insult to flow.[6,14] The size of the stroke depends on the size and location of the occluded vessel and the availability of collateral blood flow. Global ischemia results when severe hypotension or cardiopulmonary arrest provokes a transient drop in blood flow to all areas of the brain.[22,23]

Cerebral edema sufficient to produce clinical deterioration develops in 10% to 20% of patients with ischemic stroke and can result in intracranial hypertension. The edema results from a loss of normal metabolic function of the cells and peaks at 3 to 5 days. This process is commonly the cause of death during the first week after a stroke.[23] Secondary hemorrhage at the site of the stroke lesion, known as *hemorrhagic conversion*, and seizures are the two other major acute neurologic complications of ischemic stroke.[6] Mortality rates in the first 20 days after ischemic stroke range from 8% to 30%.

Assessment and Diagnosis. The characteristic sign of an ischemic stroke is the sudden onset of focal neurologic signs persisting for more than 24 hours. These

---

Box 27-3

NEUROLOGIC ABNORMALITIES IN ACUTE ISCHEMIC STROKES

LEFT (DOMINANT) HEMISPHERE
Aphasia; right hemiparesis; right-sided sensory loss; right visual field defect; poor right conjugate gaze; dysarthria; difficulty in reading, writing, or calculating

RIGHT (NONDOMINANT) HEMISPHERE
Neglect of the left visual space; left visual field defect, left hemiparesis, left-sided sensory loss, poor left conjugate gaze, extinction of left-sided stimuli; dysarthria; spatial disorientation

BRAINSTEM/CEREBELLUM/POSTERIOR HEMISPHERE
Motor or sensory loss in all four limbs, crossed signs, limb or gait ataxia, dysarthria, dysconjugate gaze, nystagmus, amnesia, bilateral visual field defects

SMALL SUBCORTICAL HEMISPHERE OR BRAIN STEM (PURE MOTOR STROKE)
Weakness of face and limbs on one side of the body without abnormalities of higher brain function, sensation, or vision

SMALL SUBCORTICAL HEMISPHERE OR BRAIN STEM (PURE SENSORY STROKE)
Decreased sensation of face and limbs on one side of the body without abnormalities of higher brain function, motor function, or vision

From Adams HP et al: *Circulation* 90(3):1588, 1994.

---

signs usually occur in combination. Box 27-3 lists common patterns of neurologic symptoms associated with an ischemic stroke. Hemiparesis, aphasia, and hemianopia are common. Changes in level of consciousness usually occur only with brainstem or cerebellar involvement, seizure, hypoxia, hemorrhage, or elevated intracranial pressure (ICP). These changes may be exhibited as stupor, coma, confusion, and agitation.[5] The reported frequency of seizures in patients with ischemic stroke is variable, ranging from 5% to 20%. If seizures occur, they are usually seen within 24 hours of insult.[24]

The National Institutes of Health Stroke Scale (NIHSS) is often used as the basis of the focused neurologic examination (Table 27-2). The scale has six major categories: (1) overall level of consciousness, (2) visual function, (3) motor skills, (4) sensation and inattention, (5) language, and 6) cerebellar integrity. The score ranges from 0 to 42 points: the higher the score, the more neurologically impaired the patient.[14,15]

Confirmation of the diagnosis of ischemic stroke is the first step in the emergent evaluation of these patients. Differentiation from intracranial hemorrhage is vital. Noncontrast CT scanning is the method of choice for this purpose and is considered the most important initial diagnostic study. In addition to excluding intracra-

Table 27-2	National Institutes of Health Stroke Scale

Administer stroke scale items in the order listed. Record performance in each category after each subscale examination. Do not go back and change scores. Follow directions provided for each examination technique. Scores should reflect what the patient does, not what the clinician thinks the patient can do. The clinician should record answers while administering the examination and work quickly. Except where indicated, the patient should not be coached (i.e., repeated requests to patient to make a special effort).

If any item is left untested, a detailed explanation must be clearly written on the form. All untested items will be reviewed by the medical monitor and discussed with the examiner by telephone.

Instructions	Scale Definition	Score

1A. LEVEL OF CONSCIOUSNESS

The investigator must choose a response, even if a full evaluation is prevented by such obstacles as an endotracheal tube, language barrier, orotracheal trauma/bandages. A 3 is scored only if the patient makes no movement (other than reflexive posturing) in response to noxious stimulation.

0 = Alert; keenly responsive.
1 = Not alert, but arousable by minor stimulation to obey, answer, or respond.
2 = Not alert, requires repeated stimulation to attend, or is obtunded and requires strong or painful stimulation to make movements (not stereotyped).
3 = Responds only with reflex motor or autonomic effects or totally unresponsive, flaccid, areflexic.

1B. LOC QUESTIONS

The patient is asked the month and his/her age. The answer must be correct—there is no partial credit for being close. Aphasic and stuporous patients who do not comprehend the questions will score 2. Patients unable to speak because of endotracheal intubation, orotracheal trauma, severe dysarthria from any cause, language barrier, or any other problem not secondary to aphasia are given a 1. It is important that only the initial answer be graded and that the examiner not "help" the patient with verbal or nonverbal cues.

0 = Answers both questions correctly.
1 = Answers one question correctly.
2 = Answers neither question correctly.

1C. LOC COMMANDS

The patient is asked to open and close the eyes and then to grip and release the nonparetic hand. Substitute another one-step command if the hands cannot be used. Credit is given if an unequivocal attempt is made but not completed due to weakness. If the patient does not respond to command, the task should be demonstrated to them (pantomime) and score the result (i.e., follows none, one, or two commands). Patients with trauma, amputation, or other physical impediments should be given suitable one-step commands. Only the first attempt is scored.

0 = Performs both tasks correctly.
1 = Performs one task correctly.
2 = Performs neither task correctly.

Table 27-2	National Institutes of Health Stroke Scale—cont'd	
Instructions	**Scale Definition**	**Score**

2. BEST GAZE

Only horizontal eye movements will be tested. Voluntary or reflexive (oculocephalic) eye movements will be scored but caloric testing is not done. If the patient has a conjugate deviation of the eyes that can be overcome by voluntary or reflexive activity, the score will be 1. If a patient has an isolated peripheral nerve paresis (CN III, IV, or VI), score a 1. Gaze is testable in all aphasic patients. Patients with ocular trauma, bandages, preexisting blindness, or other disorder of visual acuity or fields should be tested with reflexive movements and a choice made by the investigator. Establishing eye contact and then moving about the patient from side to side will occasionally clarify the presence of a partial gaze palsy.

0 = Normal.
1 = Partial gaze palsy. This score is given when gaze is abnormal in one or both eyes, but where forced deviation or total gaze paresis are not present.
2 = Forced deviation, or total gaze paresis not overcome by the oculocephalic maneuver.

3. VISUAL

Visual fields (upper and lower quadrants) are tested by confrontation, using finger counting or visual threat as appropriate. Patient must be encouraged, but if they look at the side of the moving fingers appropriately, this can be scored as normal. If there is unilateral blindness or enucleation, visual fields in the remaining eye are scored. Score 1 only if a clear-cut asymmetry, including quadrantanopia is found. If patient is blind from any cause, score 3. Double simultaneous stimulation is performed at this point. If there is extinction, patient receives a 1 and the results are used to answer question 11.

0 = No visual loss.
1 = Partial hemianopia.
2 = Complete hemianopia.
3 = Bilateral hemianopia (blind including cortical blindness).

4. FACIAL PALSY

Ask for or use pantomime to encourage the patient to show teeth or raise eyebrows and close eyes. Score symmetry of grimace in response to noxious stimuli in the poorly responsive or noncomprehending patient. If facial trauma/bandages, orotracheal tube, tape, or other physical barrier obscures the face, these should be removed to the extent possible.

0 = Normal symmetric movement.
1 = Minor paralysis (flattened nasolabial fold, asymmetry on smiling).
2 = Partial paralysis (total or near total paralysis of lower face).
3 = Complete paralysis of one or both sides (absence of facial movement in the upper and lower face).

Continued

Table 27-2	**National Institutes of Health Stroke Scale—cont'd**	
Instructions	**Scale Definition**	**Score**

5 AND 6. MOTOR ARM AND LEG

The limb is placed in the appropriate position: extend the arms (palms down) 90 degrees (if sitting) or 45 degrees (if supine) and the leg 30 degrees (always tested supine). Drift is scored if the arm falls before 10 seconds or the leg before 5 seconds. The aphasic patient is encouraged using urgency in the voice and pantomime but not noxious stimulation. Each limb is tested in turn, beginning with the nonparetic arm. Only in the case of amputation or joint fusion at the shoulder or hip may the score be "9," and the examiner must clearly write the explanation for scoring as a "9."

0 = No drift, limb holds 90 (or 45) degrees for full 10 seconds.
1 = Drift, limb holds 90 (or 45) degrees, but drifts down before full 10 seconds; does not hit bed or other support.
2 = Some effort against gravity, limb cannot get to or maintain (if cued) 90 (or 45) degrees, drifts down to bed, but has some effort against gravity.
3 = No effort against gravity, limb falls.
4 = No movement.
9 = Amputation, joint fusion; explain:

5A. LEFT ARM
5B. RIGHT ARM

0 = No drift, leg holds 30 degrees position for full 5 seconds.
1 = Drift, leg falls by the end of the 5 second period but does not hit bed.
2 = Some effort against gravity; leg falls to bed by 5 seconds, but has some effort against gravity.
3 = No effort against gravity, leg falls to bed immediately.
4 = No movement.
9 = Amputation, joint fusion; explain:

6A. LEFT LEG
6B. RIGHT LEG

0 = Absent.
1 = Present in one limb.
2 = Present in two limbs.

7. LIMB ATAXIA

This item is aimed at finding evidence of a unilateral cerebellar lesion. Test with eyes open. In case of visual defect, ensure that testing is done in intact visual field. The finger-nose-finger and heel-shin tests are performed on both sides, and ataxia is scored only if present out of proportion to weakness. Ataxia is absent in the patient who cannot understand or is paralyzed. Only in the case of amputation or joint fusion may the item be scored "9," and the examiner must clearly write the explanation for not scoring. In case of blindness, test by touching nose from extended arm position.

If present, is ataxia in?
Right arm: 1 = Yes, 2 = No, 9 = amputation or joint fusion; explain:
Left arm: 1 = Yes, 2 = No, 9 = amputation or joint fusion; explain:
Right leg: 1 = Yes, 2 = No, 9 = amputation or joint fusion; explain:
Left leg: 1 = Yes, 2 = No, 9 = amputation or joint fusion; explain:

Table 27-2	National Institutes of Health Stroke Scale—cont'd

Instructions	Scale Definition	Score

8. SENSORY

Sensation or grimace to pin prick when tested, or withdrawal from noxious stimulus in the obtunded or aphasic patient. Only sensory loss attributed to stroke is scored as abnormal, and the examiner should test as many body areas (arms [not hands], legs, trunk, face) as needed to accurately check for hemisensory loss. A score of 2, "severe or total," should only be given when a severe or total loss of sensation can be clearly demonstrated. Stuporous and aphasic patients will therefore probably score 1 or 0. The patient with brainstem stroke who has bilateral loss of sensation is scored 2. If the patient does not respond and is quadriplegic, score 2. Patients in coma (item 1a = 3) are arbitrarily given a 2 on this item.

0 = Normal; no sensory loss.
1 = Mild to moderate sensory loss; patient feels pinprick is less sharp or is dull on the affected side; or there is a loss of superficial pain with pinprick but patient is aware he/she is being touched.
2 = Severe to total sensory loss; patient is not aware of being touched in the face, arm, and leg.

9. BEST LANGUAGE

A great deal of information about comprehension will be obtained during the preceding sections of the examination. The patient is asked to describe what is happening in the attached picture, to name the items on the attached naming sheet, and to read from the attached list of sentences. Comprehension is judged from responses here as well as to all of the commands in the preceding general neurologic examination. If visual loss interferes with the tests, ask the patient to identify objects placed in the hand, repeat, and produce speech. The intubated patient should be asked to write. The patient in coma (question 1a = 3) will arbitrarily score 3 on this item. The examiner must choose a score in the patient with stupor or limited cooperation, but a score of 3 should be used only if the patient is mute and follows no one-step commands.

0 = No aphasia, normal.
1 = Mild to moderate aphasia; some obvious loss of fluency or facility of comprehension, without significant limitation on ideas expressed or form of expression. Reduction of speech and/or comprehension, however, makes conversation about provided material difficult or impossible. For example, in conversation about provided materials examiner can identify picture or naming card from patient's response.
2 = Severe aphasia; all communication is through fragmentary expression; great need for inference, questioning, and guessing by the listener. Range of information that can be exchanged is limited; listener carries burden of communication. Examiner cannot identify materials provided from patient response.
3 = Mute, global aphasia; no usable speech or auditory comprehension.

10. DYSARTHRIA

If patient is thought to be normal an adequate sample of speech must be obtained by asking patient to read or repeat words from the attached list. If the patient has severe aphasia, the clarity of articulation of spontaneous speech can be rated. Only if the patient is intubated or has other physical barrier to producing speech, may the item be scored "9," and the examiner must clearly write an explanation for not scoring. Do not tell the patient why he/she is being tested.

0 = Normal.
1 = Mild to moderate; patient slurs at least some words and, at worst, can be understood with some difficulty.
2 = Severe; patient's speech is so slurred as to be unintelligible in the absence of or out of proportion to any dysphasia, or is mute/anarthric.
9 = Intubated or other physical barrier; explain:

From the National Institutes of Health Stroke Scale (NIHSS).   *Continued*

Table 27-2	National Institutes of Health Stroke Scale—cont'd	
Instructions	**Scale Definition**	**Score**

11. EXTINCTION AND INATTENTION (FORMERLY NEGLECT)

Sufficient information to identify neglect may be obtained during the prior testing. If the patient has a severe visual loss preventing visual double simultaneous stimulation, and the cutaneous stimuli are normal, the score is normal. If the patient has aphasia but does appear to attend to both sides, the score is normal. The presence of visual spatial neglect or anosognosia may also be taken as evidence of abnormality. Since the abnormality is scored only if present, the item is never untestable.

0 = No abnormality.
1 = Visual, tactile, auditory, spatial, or personal inattention or extinction to bilateral simultaneous stimulation in one of the sensory modalities.
2 = Profound hemiinattention or hemiinattention to more than one modality. Does not recognize own hand or orients to only one side of space.

ADDITIONAL ITEM, NOT A PART OF THE NIH STROKE SCALE SCORE
A. DISTAL MOTOR FUNCTION

The patient's hand is held up at the forearm by the examiner and patient is asked to extend his/her fingers as much as possible. If the patient can't or doesn't extend the fingers the examiner places the fingers in full extension and observes for any flexion movement for 5 seconds. The patient's first attempts only are graded. Repetition of the instructions or of the testing is prohibited.

0 = Normal (no flexion after 5 seconds).
1 = At least some extension after 5 seconds, but not fully extended. Any movement of the fingers which is not command is not scored.
2 = No voluntary extension after 5 seconds. Movements of the fingers at another time are not scored.

A. LEFT ARM
B. RIGHT ARM

---

nial hemorrhage, CT can also assist in identifying early neurologic complications and the etiology of the insult.[15] An MRI will demonstrate actual infarction of cerebral tissue earlier than a CT but is less useful in the emergent differential diagnosis. Because of the strong correlation between acute ischemic stroke and heart disease, 12-lead electrocardiography, chest x-ray, and continuous cardiac monitoring are suggested to detect a cardiac etiology or coexisting condition. Echocardiography is valuable in identifying a cardioembolic phenomenon when a sufficient index of suspicion warrants its use.[25] Laboratory evaluation of hematologic function, electrolyte and glucose levels, and renal and hepatic function is also recommended. Arterial blood gas analysis is performed if hypoxia is suspected, and an electroencephalogram is obtained if seizures are suspected. Lumbar puncture is performed only if subarachnoid hemorrhage is suspected and the CT is normal.[26]

Medical Management. Major changes have taken place in the medical management of ischemic stroke since 1996. Based on results of the National Institute of Neurologic Disorders and Stroke (NINDS) rt-PA Stroke Study, thrombolytic therapy with intravenous rt-PA is now recommended within 3 hours of onset of ischemic stroke.[27,28] Indications and contraindications to thrombolysis are listed in Box 27-4.[28] Confirmation of diagnosis with CT must be accomplished before rt-PA administration. The recommended dose of rt-PA is 0.9 mg/kg up to a maximum dose of 90 mg. Ten percent of the total dose is administered as an initial intravenous bolus over 1 minute, and the remaining 90% is administered by intravenous infusion over 60 minutes.[29]

The desired result of thrombolytic therapy is to dissolve the clot and reperfuse the ischemic brain. The goal is to reverse or minimize the effects of stroke. The major risk and complication of rt-PA therapy is bleeding, especially intracranial hemorrhage. Unlike thrombolytic protocols for acute myocardial infarction, subsequent therapy with anticoagulant or antiplatelet agents is *not* recommended after rt-PA administration in ischemic stroke. Persons receiving thrombolytic therapy for stroke should not receive aspirin, heparin, warfarin, ticlopidine, or any other antithrombotic or antiplatelet drugs for at least 24 hours after treatment.[30]

Recent studies have demonstrated that these guidelines are safe for use in routine clinical practice.[31] The major barrier to effective application of thrombolytic therapy for ischemic stroke is prehospital and inhospital delays. This therapeutic breakthrough dictates that all those involved in the acute care of the ischemic

---

Box 27-4

INDICATIONS AND CONTRAINDICATIONS TO THROMBOLYTIC THERAPY IN ACUTE ISCHEMIC STROKE

INDICATIONS

Acute ischemic stroke within 3 hours from symptom onset

Age greater than 18 years old (rt-PA has not been studied in pediatric stroke)

CONTRAINDICATIONS

Evidence of intracranial hemorrhage on pretreatment evaluation

Suspicion of subarachnoid hemorrhage

Recent stroke, intracranial or intraspinal surgery, or serious head trauma in the past 3 months

Major surgery or serious trauma in the previous 14 days*

Arterial puncture at a noncompressible site or lumbar puncture in the last 7 days

Major symptoms that are rapidly improving or only minor stroke symptoms (NIHSS <4)*

History of intracranial hemorrhage

Uncontrolled hypertension at the time of treatment

Seizure at the stroke onset

Active internal bleeding

Intracranial neoplasm, arteriovenous malformation, or aneurysm

Known bleeding diathesis including but not limited to:

Current use of anticoagulants or an international normalized ratio (INR) >1.7 or a prothrombin time (PT >15 seconds)

Administration of heparin within 48 hours preceding the onset of stroke and an elevated activated partial thromboplastin time at presentation

Platelet count <100,000 mm^3

From Thurman RJ, Jauch EC: Acute ischemic stroke: emergent evaluation and management, *Emerg Med Clin North Am* 20:609, 2002.

*In the NINDS trial, not present in current package insert.

NIHSS, National Institutes of Health Stroke Scale.

---

patient must be prepared for rapid evaluation of the stroke patient and for rapid, knowledgeable institution of guideline protocols.[32]

Other emergent care of the patient with ischemic stroke must include airway protection and ventilatory assistance to maintain adequate tissue oxygenation.[15] Hypertension is often present in the early period as a compensatory response, and in most cases blood pressure (BP) must not be lowered (Table 27-3). For the patient who has not received thrombolytic therapy, antihypertensive therapy is considered only if the diastolic BP is greater than 120 mm Hg or the systolic BP is greater than 220 mm Hg.[33] Criteria differ for the patient who has received rt-PA. The BP for these patients is kept below 180/105 mm Hg to prevent intracranial hemorrhage. Intravenous labetalol or sodium nitroprusside is used to achieve BP control.[33] Body temperature and glucose levels also must be normalized.[23]

Medical management must also include the identification and treatment of acute complications such as cerebral edema or seizure activity. Prophylaxis for these complications is not recommended. Surgical decompression is recommended if a large cerebellar infarction compresses the brainstem.[34]

A number of additional therapies, both preventive and therapeutic, are under investigation. These include emergent carotid endarterectomy, embolectomy or angioplasty, hemodilution of the blood, and the administration of cytoprotective agents such as steroids, barbiturates, nimodipine, naloxone, glutamate antagonists, and monoclonal antibodies. These therapies are not recommended at this time for routine use because of insufficient evidence.[22,35]

SUBARACHNOID HEMORRHAGE

Description. Subarachnoid hemorrhage (SAH) is bleeding into the subarachnoid space, usually caused by rupture of a cerebral aneurysm or arteriovenous malformation (AVM). Subarachnoid hemorrhage accounts for 4.5% to 13% of all strokes[14]—with nontraumatic SAH affecting more than 30,000 Americans each year.[36] The incidence of SAH is greater in women and increases with age. The overall mortality rate is 25%, with most patients dying on the first day after insult.[36] The rate of significant morbidity approximates 50% to 60% of all survivors.[14] Unfortunately, no appreciable decrease in the incidence of SAH has occurred over time. Approximately 6% of the general population is believed to have an unruptured cerebral aneurysm,[37] the congenital anomaly responsible for most cases of SAH. The risk for rupture is 1% to 2% annually. The known risk factors for SAH include HTN, smoking, alcohol use, and stimulant use. As in ischemic stroke, the single most important risk factor is HTN.

Etiology. Cerebral aneurysm rupture accounts for approximately 85% of all cases of spontaneous SAH.[6] An aneurysm is an outpouching of the wall of a blood vessel that results from weakening of the wall of the vessel (Table 27-4). Ninety percent of aneurysms are congenital—the cause of which is unknown. The other 10% can be the result of traumatic injury (that stretches and tears the muscular middle layer of the arterial vessel) or infectious material (most often from infectious vegetation on valves of the left side of the heart after bacterial endocarditis) that lodges against a vessel wall and erodes the muscular layer, or are of undetermined cause.[5] Multiple aneurysms occur in 20% to 25% of the cases and often are bilateral, occurring in the same location on both sides of the cerebral vascular system.[6] It is possible for an individual to live a full life span with an unruptured cerebral aneurysm. Aneurysm rupture usually occurs during the fifth and sixth decades of life.[37]

Table 27-3	Blood Pressure Management for Stroke (American Stroke Association Guidelines)
Blood Pressure*	**Treatment**

NONTHROMBOLYTIC CANDIDATES

DBP > 140 mm Hg	Sodium nitroprusside (0.5 mcg/kg/min); aim for 10%-20% reduction in DBP
SBP > 220 mm Hg, DBP 121-140 mm Hg, or MAP† >130 mm Hg	10-20 mg labetalol‡ IV push over 1-2 min; may repeat or double labetalol every 20 min to a maximum dose of 300 mg
SBP < 220 mm Hg, DBP = 120 mm Hg, or MAP† <130 mm Hg	Emergency antihypertensive therapy is deferred in the absence of aortic dissection, acute myocardial infarction, severe congestive heart failure, or hypertensive encephalopathy

THROMBOLYTIC CANDIDATES
PRETREATMENT

SBP > 185 mm Hg or DBP > 110 mm Hg	1-2 inches of nitroglycerine paste (Nitropaste) or 1-2 doses of 10-20 mg labetalol‡ IV push; if BP is not reduced and maintained to <185/110 mm Hg, the patient should not be treated with TPA

DURING AND AFTER TREATMENT

Monitor BP	BP is monitored every 15 min for 2 hr, then every 30 min for 6 hr, and then hourly for 16 hr
DBP > 140 mm Hg	Sodium nitroprusside (0.5 mcg/kg/min)
SBP > 230 mm Hg or DBP 121-140 mm Hg	10 mg labetalol‡ IVP over 1-2 min; may repeat or double labetalol every 10 min to a maximum dose of 300 mg or give initial labetalol bolus and then start a labetalol drip at 2-8 mg/min If BP not controlled by labetalol, consider sodium nitroprusside
SBP 180-230 mm Hg or DBP 105-120 mm Hg	10 mg labetalol‡ IVP; may repeat or double labetalol every 10-20 min to a maximum dose of 300 mg or give initial labetalol bolus and then start a labetalol drip at 2-8 mg/min

From Bader MK, Littlejohns LR: *AANN core curriculum for neuroscience nursing,* ed 4, St Louis, 2004, Elsevier.
BP, Blood pressure; *DBP,* diastolic blood pressure; *MAP,* mean arterial pressure; *SBP,* systolic blood pressure; *TPA,* tissue plasminogen activator.
*All initial blood pressures should be verified before treatment by repeating reading in 5 minutes.
†As estimated by one third the sum of systolic and double diastolic pressure.
‡Labetalol should be avoided in patients with asthma, cardiac failure, or severe abnormalities in cardiac conduction. For refractory hypertension, alternative therapy maybe considered with sodium nitroprusside or enalapril.

Arteriovenous malformation rupture is responsible for less than 10% of all SAHs.[6] An AVM is a tangled mass of arterial and venous blood vessels that shunt blood directly from the arterial side into the venous side, bypassing the capillary system. They may be small, focal lesions or large, diffuse lesions that occupy almost an entire hemisphere. AVMs are always congenital, though the exact embryonic cause for these malformations is unknown. They also occur in the spinal cord and the renal, gastrointestinal, and integumentary systems. Small superficial AVMs are seen as port-wine stains of the skin. In contrast to the middle-aged population with SAH from aneurysm, SAH from an AVM usually occurs in the second to fourth decades of life.[6]

Pathophysiology. The pathophysiology of the two most common causes of SAH is distinctly different.

Cerebral Aneurysm. As the individual with a congenital cerebral aneurysm matures, blood pressure rises and more stress is placed on the poorly developed and thin vessel wall. Ballooning out of the vessel occurs, giv-

ing the aneurysm a berrylike appearance. Most cerebral aneurysms are saccular or berrylike with a stem or neck. Aneurysms are usually small, 2 to 7 mm in diameter, and often occur at the base of the brain on the circle of Willis. Fig. 27-2 illustrates the usual distribution between the vessels. Most cerebral aneurysms occur at the bifurcation of blood vessels.[5,6]

The aneurysm becomes clinically significant when the vessel wall becomes so thin that it ruptures, sending arterial blood at a high pressure into the subarachnoid space. For a brief moment after the aneurysm ruptures, intracranial pressure is believed to approach mean arterial pressure and cerebral perfusion falls. In other situations, the unruptured aneurysm expands and places pressure on surrounding structures. This is particularly true with posterior communicating artery aneurysms, because they put pressure on the oculomotor nerve (CN III), causing ipsilateral pupil dilation and ptosis.[5,6]

Arteriovenous Malformation. The pathophysiologic features of an AVM are related to the size and loca-

Table 27-4	Aneurysm Classification According to Type, Shape, Location, and Common Characteristics

Types of Aneurysms	Characteristics
Berry or saccular 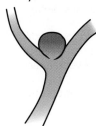	Most common type, usually congenital; appears at a bifurcation in the anterior circulation, primarily at the base of the brain or the circle of Willis and its branches; grows from the base of the arterial wall with a neck or stem; contains blood; thinned dome is usually the site of rupture
Giant or fusiform 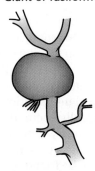	Can be irregular in shape and larger than 2.5 cm and atherosclerotic; involves mainly the internal carotid or vertebrobasilar artery; rarely ruptures; has no stem; can act like a space-occupying lesion in the brain; and is difficult to manage
Mycotic 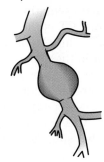	Rare form; usually occurs from septic emboli, usually secondary to bacterial infection, which weaken the vessel wall, causing dilation involving the distal branches of the middle cerebral arteries
Dissecting 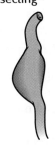	May occur during angiography, secondary to trauma, syphilis, or arteriosclerosis, or when blood is forced between layers of the arterial wall; the intima is pulled away from the medial layer, allowing blood to enter
Traumatic Charcot-Bouchard	Sometimes called a "pseudoaneurysm," which may resolve following trauma Small aneurysm that can be seen in the area of the basal ganglia and/or the brainstem in individuals with a history of hypertension; chronic hypertension causes fibrinoid necrosis in the penetrating and subcortical arteries, weakening the arterial walls and causing formation of small aneurismal outpouching[16]

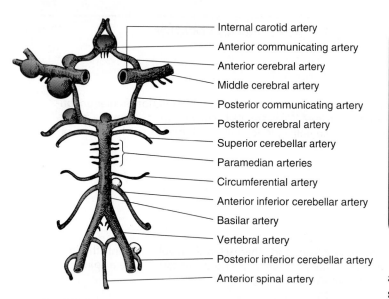

Internal carotid artery
Anterior communicating artery
Anterior cerebral artery
Middle cerebral artery
Posterior communicating artery
Posterior cerebral artery
Superior cerebellar artery
Paramedian arteries
Circumferential artery
Anterior inferior cerebellar artery
Basilar artery
Vertebral artery
Posterior inferior cerebellar artery
Anterior spinal artery

Fig. 27-2   Common sites of berry aneurysms. *Note:* The size of the aneurysm in the drawing is proportional to the frequency of occurrence at the various sites. (From Goldman L, Ausiello D, editors: *Cecil's textbook of medicine,* ed 22, Philadelphia, 2004, Saunders.)

Box 27-5

CLASSIFICATION OF SUBARACHNOID HEMORRHAGE

Grade I: asymptomatic or minimal headache and slight nuchal rigidity

Grade II: moderate to severe headache, nuchal rigidity, no neurologic deficit other than cranial nerve palsy

Grade III: drowsiness, confusion, or mild focal deficit

Grade IV: stupor, moderate to severe hemiparesis, possible early decerebrate rigidity, and vegetative disturbances

Grade V: deep coma, decerebrate rigidity, moribund appearance

---

tion of the malformation. One or more cerebral arteries, also known as *feeders,* feed an AVM. These feeder arteries tend to enlarge over time and increase the volume of blood shunted through the malformation, as well as increase the overall mass effect. Large, dilated, tortuous draining veins also develop as a result of increasing arterial blood flow being delivered at a higher than normal pressure. Normal vascular flow has a mean arterial pressure of 70 to 80 mm Hg, a mean arteriole pressure of 35 to 45 mm Hg, and a mean capillary pressure that drops from 35 to 10 mm Hg as it connects with the venous side. Lack of this capillary bridge allows blood with a mean pressure of 35 to 45 mm Hg to flow into the venous system. Because a vein has no muscular layer as does an artery, the veins become extremely engorged and rupture easily. Cerebral atrophy is also present sometimes in the patient with an AVM. It is the result of chronic ischemia because of the shunting of blood through the AVM and away from normal cerebral circulation.[5,6]

Assessment and Diagnosis. The patient with an SAH characteristically has an abrupt onset of pain, described as the "worst headache of my life." A brief loss of consciousness, nausea, vomiting, focal neurologic deficits, and a stiff neck may accompany the headache.[34] The SAH may result in coma or death.

Patient history may reveal one or more incidences of sudden onset of headache with vomiting in the weeks preceding a major SAH. These are "warning leaks" of an aneurysm in which small amounts of blood ooze from the aneurysm into the subarachnoid space. The presence of blood is an irritant to the meninges, particularly the

arachnoid membrane. This irritation causes headache, stiff neck, and photophobia. These small "warning leaks" seldom are detected because the condition is not severe enough for the patient to seek medical attention. If a neurologic deficit, such as third cranial nerve palsy, develops before aneurysm rupture, medical intervention is sought and the aneurysm may be surgically secured before the devastation of a rupture can occur. Symptoms of unruptured AVM—headaches with dizziness or syncope or fleeting neurologic deficits—also may be found in the history.[6]

Diagnosis of SAH is based on clinical presentation, CT scan, and lumbar puncture. Noncontrast CT is the cornerstone of definitive SAH diagnosis.[38-40] In 92% of the cases, CT scan can demonstrate a clot in the subarachnoid space, if performed within 24 hours of the onset of the hemorrhage. On the basis of the appearance and the location of the SAH, diagnosis of cause—aneurysm or AVM—may be made from the CT scan. MRI is relatively insensitive for detecting blood in the subarachnoid space.

If the initial CT scan is negative, a lumbar puncture is performed to obtain CSF for analysis. CSF after SAH is bloody in appearance with a red blood cell count greater than 1000/mm^3. If the lumbar puncture is performed more than 5 days after the SAH, CSF fluid is xanthochromic (dark amber), because the blood products have broken down.[38] Cloudy CSF usually indicates some type of infectious process, such as bacterial meningitis, not a subarachnoid hemorrhage.[6]

Once the SAH has been documented, cerebral angiography is necessary to identify the exact cause of the SAH (Fig. 27-3). If a cerebral aneurysm rupture is the cause, angiography is also essential for identifying the exact location of the aneurysm in preparation for surgery.[38-40] Once the aneurysm has been located, it is graded using the Hunt and Hess classification scale. This scale categorizes the patient based on the severity of the neurologic deficits associated with the hemorrhage (Box 27-5).[41] If AVM rupture is the cause, angiography is necessary to

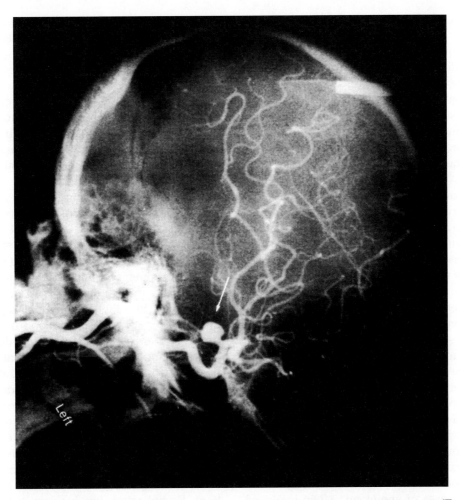

Fig. 27-3 Cerebral angiography showing location of aneurysm at posterior communicating artery. (From Tortorici M: *Fundamentals of angiography,* St Louis, 1982, Mosby.)

identify the feeding arteries and draining veins of the malformation.

Medical Management. SAH is a medical emergency, and time is of the essence. Preservation of neurologic function is the goal. Initial treatment must always support vital functions. Airway management and ventilatory assistance may be necessary. Early diagnosis is also essential. A ventriculostomy is performed to control ICP if the patient's level of consciousness is depressed.[38]

Evidence suggests that only 19% of the deaths attributable to aneurysmal SAH are related to the direct effects of the initial hemorrhage.[42] Research has shown that rebleeding accounts for 22% of deaths from aneurysmal SAH, cerebral vasospasm for 23%, and nonneurologic medical complications for 23%.[42] Principal nonneurologic causes of death are systemic inflammatory response syndrome (SIRS) and secondary organ dysfunction.[43] Once initial intervention has provided necessary support for vital physiologic functions, medical management of acute SAH is aimed primarily toward the prevention and treatment of the complications of SAH that can produce further neurologic damage and death.

Rebleeding. Rebleeding is the occurrence of a second SAH in an unsecured aneurysm or, less commonly, an AVM.[6] The incidence of rebleeding during the first 24 hours following the first bleed is 4%, with a 1% to 2% chance per day for the following month. Mortality with aneurysmal rebleeding is approximately 70%.[36]

Historically, conservative measures to prevent rebleeding have included BP control and SAH precautions (see section later in this chapter on nursing management of intracerebral hemorrhage). An elevation in BP is a normal compensatory response to maintain adequate cerebral perfusion after a neurologic insult. In the belief that hypertension contributes to rebleeding, nitroprusside, metoprolol, or hydralazine has been commonly used to maintain a systolic BP no greater than 150 mm Hg.[44] Individualized guidelines must be determined based on clinical condition and preexisting values of the patient. Evidence suggests that rebleeding has more to do with variations in BP than it does with absolute values and that BP control does not lower the incidence of rebleeding.[39] Prophylactic anticonvulsant therapy is recommended to prevent seizures.[36,39]

Surgical Aneurysm Clipping. Definitive treatment for the prevention of rebleeding is surgical clipping with complete obliteration of the aneurysm. Timing of the surgery is a key medical management issue. Since the introduction of microsurgery and improved surgical techniques, patients commonly are taken to the operating room within the first 48 hours after rupture. This early surgical intervention to secure the aneurysm eliminates the risk of rebleeding and allows more aggressive therapy to be used in the postoperative period for the treatment of vasospasm.[38] Early surgery also allows the neurosurgeon to flush out the excess blood and clots from the basal cisterns (reservoir of CSF around the base of the brain and circle of Willis) to reduce the risk of vasospasm.[45] Early surgery is recommended for patients with a grade I or grade II SAH and some patients with a grade III. In patients with a grade III SAH, the initial hemorrhage did not produce significant neurologic deficit, but the risk of rebleeding with a tragically high incidence of mortality is present until the aneurysm is secured. Because of the patient's clinical condition and the technical difficulty of the surgery, early surgical repair of the aneurysm is not always possible. Early surgery continues to be controversial for patients with grade IV or grade V SAH and those demonstrating vasospasm. However, recent studies have not supported the fear of worse ischemic sequelae with early surgery in these patients.[46] Careful consideration of the patient's clinical situation is necessary in determining the optimal time for surgery.

The surgical procedure involves a craniotomy to expose and isolate the area of aneurysm. A clip is placed over the neck of the aneurysm to eliminate the area of weakness (Fig. 27-4). This is a technically difficult procedure that requires the skill of an experienced neurosurgeon. It is not uncommon, particularly in early surgery, for the clot to break away from the aneurysm as it is surgically exposed. Extensive hemorrhage into the craniotomy site results, and cessation of the hemorrhage often causes increased neurologic deficits. Deficits also may occur as a result of surgical manipulation to gain access to the site of the aneurysm.[5]

Surgical AVM Excision. Management of AVM has traditionally involved surgical excision or conservative management of such symptoms as seizures and headache. The decision for surgical excision depends on the location and size of the AVM. Some malformations are located so deep in the cerebral structures (the thalamus or midbrain) that attempts to remove the AVM would cause severe neurologic deficits. History of a previous hemorrhage and the patient's age and overall condition are also taken into account when making the decision regarding surgical intervention.

Surgical excision of large AVMs includes the risk of reperfusion bleeding. As feeding arteries of the AVM are clamped off, the arterial blood that usually flowed into the AVM is now diverted into the surrounding circulation. In many cases the surrounding tissue has been in a state of chronic ischemia and the arterial vessels feeding these areas are maximally dilated. As arterial blood begins to flow at a higher volume and pressure into these dilated arteries, seeping of blood from the vessels may occur. Evidence of reperfusion bleeding in the operating room is an indication that no more arterial blood can be diverted from the AVM without risk of serious intracerebral hemorrhage. In the postoperative phase, a low blood pressure is maintained to prevent further reperfusion bleeding. In large AVMs, two to four stages of surgery may be required over 6 to 12 months.[6]

Embolization. Embolization is used to secure a cerebral aneurysm or AVM that is surgically inaccessible because of size, location, or medical instability of the patient. Embolization involves several new interventional neuroradiology techniques. All of the techniques use a percutaneous transfemoral approach in a manner similar to an angiogram. Under fluoroscopy, the catheter is threaded up to the internal carotid artery. Specially developed microcatheters are then manipulated into the area of the vascular anomaly, and embolic materials are placed endovascularly. Three different embolization techniques are used, depending on the underlying pathologic derangement.[6]

The first type of embolization is used to embolize an AVM. Small silastic beads or glue are slowly introduced into the vessels feeding the AVM. Blood flow then carries the material to the site, and embolization is achieved. This procedure may be used in combination with surgery. One to three sessions of embolization of the feeding vessels are performed to reduce the size of the lesion before a craniotomy is performed for total excision. The primary risk of this procedure is lodging of the embolic substance in a vessel that feeds normal tissue. This occurrence creates an embolic stroke with the immediate onset of neurologic symptoms.[5,6]

The second type of embolization involves placement of one or more detachable balloons into an aneurysmal sac or AVM. A liquid polymerizing agent is used to inflate the balloon. The material then solidifies. The third technique involves placement of one or more detachable

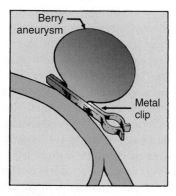

Fig. 27-4 Clipping of aneurysm. (From Chippo EM, Clonin NJ, Campbell UG: *Neurologic disorders,* St Louis, 1982, Mosby.)

platinum coils into an aneurysm to produce an endovascular thrombus. The advantage of this technique is that an electrical current creates positive charging of the coil, which induces electrothrombosis. The most common complication of these two techniques is the development of distal ischemia resulting from emboli. Again, the onset of neurologic symptoms is immediate. Other risks include subtotal occlusion and intraprocedural rupture of the vasculature and death.[5,6]

Cerebral Vasospasm. The presence or absence of cerebral vasospasm significantly affects the outcome of aneurysmal SAH. This complication does not occur with SAH resulting from AVM rupture. Cerebral vasospasm is a narrowing of the lumen of the cerebral arteries, possibly in response to subarachnoid blood clots coating the outer surface of the blood vessels. Inasmuch as aneurysms occur at the circle of Willis, the major vessels responsible for feeding the cerebral circulation are affected by vasospasm. Depending on the arterial vessels involved in the vasospasm reaction, decreased arterial flow occurs in large areas of the cerebral hemispheres.[6]

It is estimated that 70% of all SAH patients develop vasospasm, which is demonstrable by angiography.[46] Thirty-two percent of these patients develop symptomatic vasospasm, resulting in ischemic stroke and/or death for 15% to 20% of them despite the use of maximal therapy. The onset of vasospasm is usually 4 to 12 days after the initial hemorrhage.[47]

A variety of therapies have been evaluated in an attempt to reverse or overcome cerebral vasospasm. Research centers are evaluating such diverse therapies as barbiturate coma[48] and intraventricular sodium nitroprusside.[49] To date, three treatments are commonly used: induced hypertensive, hypervolemic, hemodilution therapy; oral nimodipine; and transluminal cerebral angioplasty.

Hypertensive, Hypervolemic, Hemodilution Therapy. Hypertensive, hypervolemic, hemodilution (HHH) therapy involves increasing the patient's blood pressure and cardiac output with vasoactive medications and diluting the patient's blood with fluid and volume expanders. Systolic BP is maintained between 150 and 160 mm Hg. The increase in volume and pressure forces blood through the vasospastic area at higher pressures. Hemodilution facilitates flow through the area by reducing blood viscosity. Many anecdotal reports exist of patients' neurologic deficits improving as systolic pressure increases from 130 mm Hg to between 150 and 160 mm Hg.[50] The Stroke Council of the American Heart Association (AHA) has recommended this therapy for prevention and treatment of vasospasm.[39]

The obvious deterrent to use of induced hypertension is the risk of rebleeding in an unsecured aneurysm. Surgical clipping of the aneurysm before HHH therapy is preferred. Cerebral edema, elevated intracranial pressure, cardiac failure, and electrolyte imbalance are also risks of HHH therapy. Careful monitoring of the patient's neurologic status, hemodynamic parameters, ICP, and serum electrolytes is necessary.[50]

Nimodipine. Nimodipine is strongly recommended to reduce the poor outcomes associated with vasospasm. The exact nature of the effect of nimodipine is not clear, but use of the drug has demonstrated consistently positive effects on outcome without any demonstrable effect on the incidence or severity of vasospasm.[49] Sixty milligrams of nimodipine is given orally every four hours for 21 days.[50] Nimodipine may produce hypotension, especially when administered concurrently with other antihypertensive agents.

Cerebral Angioplasty. Cerebral angioplasty is used when pharmacologic management of cerebral vasospasm has failed.[51] It is performed only when CT or MRI provides evidence that infarction has not yet occurred. An interventional neuroradiologist performs the procedure, and the patient is under local, general, or neuroleptic analgesia. The technique of cerebral angioplasty is very similar to that used in the coronary vasculature. Risks include intimal perforation or rupture, cerebral artery thrombosis or embolism, recurrence of stenosis, and severe diffuse vasospasm unresponsive to therapy. Hemorrhage at the femoral site also may occur. This procedure is recommended when conventional therapy is unsuccessful.[39,49,51]

Hyponatremia. Hyponatremia develops in 10% to 43% of patients with SAH as the result of a central salt-wasting syndrome. It usually occurs in around the same time frame as vasospasm, several days after initial hemorrhage.[36] There is strong evidence that the use of fluid restriction to treat hyponatremia is associated with poor outcome in the SAH patient. The AHA Stroke Council has strongly recommended that fluid restriction not be used in this instance and instead recommends sodium replenishment with isotonic fluids.[39]

Hydrocephalus. Hydrocephalus is a late complication that occurs in approximately 25% of patients after SAH.[39] Blood that has circulated in the subarachnoid space and has been absorbed by the arachnoid villi may obstruct the villi and reduce the rate of CSF absorption. Over time, increasing volumes of CSF in the intracranial space produce communicating hydrocephalus. Treatment consists of placing a drain to remove CSF. This can be accomplished temporarily by inserting a ventriculostomy or permanently by placing a ventriculoperitoneal shunt.[39]

INTRACEREBRAL HEMORRHAGE

Description. Intracerebral hemorrhage (ICH) is bleeding directly into cerebral tissue. ICH destroys cerebral tissue, causes cerebral edema, and increases ICP. The source of intracerebral bleeding is usually a small artery, but it can result also from rupture of an AVM or aneurysm. The most important cause of spontaneous ICH is hypertension, so this section concentrates on spontaneous hypertensive ICH.[52]

Spontaneous ICH is more than twice as common as SAH. The likeliness of death or disability is higher with ICH than with either ischemic stroke or SAH.[52-54] The mortality rate for hemorrhagic stroke is 35% to 52% within 1 month. Half of these deaths occur within the first 48 hours.[53] The key risk factors for ICH are age and hypertension. ICH occurs more often in men than in women and more often in nonwhite populations.[52,53]

Etiology. Intracerebral hemorrhage is most often caused by hypertensive rupture of a cerebral vessel, resulting from a long-standing history of hypertension (HTN). Other possible causes of spontaneous ICH are anticoagulation or thrombolytic therapy, coagulation disorders, drug abuse, and hemorrhage into cerebral infarct or brain tumors.[53,54] Many patients develop headache and neurologic symptoms after straining to have a bowel movement. Often on questioning, the patient with a hypertensive hemorrhage admits to having discontinued antihypertensive medication 2 to 3 weeks before the hemorrhage.

Pathophysiology. The pathophysiology of intracerebral hemorrhage is caused by continued elevated blood pressure exerting force against smaller arterial vessels that have become damaged from arteriosclerotic changes. Eventually these arteries break, and blood bursts from the vessels into the surrounding cerebral tissue, creating a hematoma. ICP rises precipitously in response to the increase in overall intracranial volume.[5,6]

Assessment and Diagnosis. Initial assessment usually reveals a critically ill patient who often is unconscious and requires ventilatory support. History from a relative or significant other describes a sudden onset of focal deficit often accompanied by severe headache, nausea, vomiting, and rapid neurologic deterioration. Approximately 50% of patients sustain early loss of consciousness, a key differential feature from ischemic stroke.[52,53] More than half of the patients with ICH present with a smooth progression of neurologic symptoms, an uncommon finding in either ischemic stroke or SAH.[53] One third of the patients have maximal symptoms at onset. Assessment of vital signs usually reveals a severely elevated BP (200/100 to 250/150 mm Hg). Signs of increased ICP are often present by the time the patient arrives in the emergency department. Diagnosis is established easily with CT. Angiography is recommended only in patients considered surgical candidates without a clear cause of hemorrhage.[52-54]

Medical Management. ICH is a medical emergency. Initial management requires attention to airway, breathing, and circulation. Intubation is usually necessary. Blood pressure management must be based on individual factors. Reduction in BP is usually necessary to decrease ongoing bleeding, but lowering BP too much or too rapidly may compromise cerebral perfusion pressure (CPP), especially in the patient with elevated ICP. National guidelines recommend keeping the *mean* arterial BP below 130 mm Hg in patients with a history of HTN and below 110 mm Hg after surgical treatment for ICH.[53] Va-

sopressor therapy, following fluid replenishment, is recommended if systolic BP falls below 90 mm Hg.[52-54]

Increased ICP is common with ICH and is a major contributor to mortality. Recommended management includes mannitol when indicated, hyperventilation, and neuromuscular blockade with sedation. Steroids are avoided. CPP must be kept greater than 70 mm Hg.[52-54]

The goal for fluid management is euvolemia with a recommended pulmonary artery occlusion pressure (PAOP) of 10 to 14 mm Hg. Body temperature is kept at less than 38.5° C using acetaminophen or cooling blankets. Use of short-acting benzodiazepines or propofol is recommended to treat agitation or hyperactivity. Pneumatic compression devices are used to decrease risk of pulmonary embolism. Prophylactic anticonvulsant therapy is sometimes used.[52-54]

The benefit of surgical treatment of spontaneous ICH is unclear. Recommendations for surgical removal of the clot depend on the size and location of the hematoma, the patient's ICP, and other neurologic symptoms. Medical treatment is recommended if the hemorrhage is small (less than 10 cm) or neurologic deficit is minimal.[52,53] Likewise, surgery offers no improvement in outcome for patients with a Glasgow Coma Scale (GCS) score of 4 or less. Surgical evacuation of the clot is recommended for patients with cerebellar hemorrhage greater than 3 cm with neurologic deterioration or hydrocephalus with brainstem compression, as well as for young patients with moderate or large lobar hemorrhage with clinical deterioration.[52,53] Numerous techniques are being investigated to lessen the risk of brain damage associated with craniotomy for ICH.

NURSING MANAGEMENT

Nursing management of the patient with stroke incorporates a variety of nursing diagnoses (see the Nursing Diagnoses feature on Stroke). Nursing interventions are directed toward performing frequent neurologic and hemodynamic assessments and maintaining surveillance for complications.

Performing Frequent Assessments. The goal of frequent assessments is early recognition of neurologic and/or hemodynamic deterioration. Close monitoring of the patient's neurologic signs and vital signs is essential and requires almost continuous observation. Automatic noninvasive devices such as a blood pressure cuff and a pulse oximeter are helpful. Seizure activity must be identified and treated immediately. It is essential that all personnel working with the patient be aware of the desired hemodynamic and neurologic parameters set by the physician and that the physician be notified at the first sign of any changes.

Maintaining Surveillance for Complications. The patient with stroke should be monitored closely for signs of bleeding, vasospasm, and increased ICP. Other complications of stroke include aspiration, malnutrition, pneumonia, deep vein thrombosis, pulmonary embolism, pressure

NURSING DIAGNOSES   Stroke

- Ineffective Cerebral Tissue Perfusion related to decreased cerebral blood flow
- Ineffective Cerebral Tissue Perfusion related to hemorrhage
- Acute Pain related to transmission and perception of cutaneous, visceral, muscular, or ischemic impulses
- Unilateral Neglect related to perceptual disruption
- Impaired Verbal Communication related to cerebral speech center injury
- Impaired Swallowing related to neuromuscular impairment, fatigue, and limited awareness
- Risk for Aspiration
- Risk for Infection
- Anxiety related to threat of biologic, psychologic, or social integrity
- Disturbed Body Image related to actual change in body structure, function, or appearance
- Compromised Family Coping related to critically ill family member
- Deficient Knowledge: Discharge Regimen related to lack of previous exposure to information (see Patient Education feature on Stroke)

ulcers, contractures, and joint abnormalities.[5] Nursing measures to prevent these complications are well known.

Additional complications that may be seen in the patient with stroke are related to the area of the brain that has been damaged. Damage to the temporoparietal area can create a variety of disturbances that affect the patient's ability to interpret sensory information. Damage to the dominant hemisphere (usually left) produces problems with speech and language and abstract and analytical skills. Damage to the nondominant hemisphere (usually right) produces problems with spatial relationships. The resulting deficits include agnosia, apraxia, and visual field defects. Perceptual deficits are not as readily noticeable as are motor deficits, but they may be more debilitating and can lead to the inability to perform skilled or purposeful tasks. In addition, the patient may develop impaired swallowing.[5]

Bleeding and Vasospasm. In the patient with a cerebral aneurysm, sudden onset of or an increase in headache and nausea and vomiting, increased BP, and changes in respiration herald the onset of rebleeding. The first indication of vasospasm is usually the appearance of new focal or global neurologic deficits. SAH precautions must be implemented to prevent any stress or straining that could potentially precipitate rebleeding. Precautions include BP control; bed rest; a dark, quiet environment; and stool softeners. Short-acting analgesics and sedatives

are used to relieve pain and anxiety. The patient must be kept calm. Limb restraints cause straining and must be avoided. The head of the bed should be elevated to 35 to 45 degrees at all times. The patient is taught to avoid any activities that correspond to performance of the Valsalva maneuver, such as pushing with the legs to move up in bed, straining for a bowel movement, or holding his or her breath during procedures or discomfort. Deep vein thrombosis precautions are routinely implemented. Collaboration with the patient and family is used to establish a visitation plan to meet patient and family needs. Often, family members at the bedside can assist the patient to remain calm.[5,14]

Increased Intracranial Pressure. Numerous signs and symptoms of increased ICP can be noted. A change in level of consciousness is the most sensitive indicator. Others include unequal pupil size, decreased pupillary response to light, headache, projectile vomiting, altered breathing patterns, Cushing's triad (bradycardia, systolic hypertension, and bradypnea), diminished brainstem reflexes, papilledema, and abnormal extension (decerebrate posturing) or flexion (decorticate posturing).[5,14]

Damage to Nondominant Hemisphere. Patients with nondominant hemispheric pathologic conditions may exhibit emotional lability, with periods of euphoria, impulsiveness, and inattention. A short attention span, lack of insight, and poor judgment may lead to injuries as the patient attempts to perform activities beyond his or her capabilities. In addition, these patients may suffer from agnosia, visual field defects, and apraxia.

Agnosia. Agnosia is a disturbance in the perception of familiar sensory (verbal, tactile, visual) information. Unilateral neglect is a form of agnosia characterized by an unawareness or denial of the affected half of the body. This denial may range from inattention to refusing to acknowledge a paralysis by neglecting the involved side of the body or by denying ownership of the side, attributing the paralyzed arm or leg to someone else. This neglect also may extend to extrapersonal space. This defect most often results from right hemispheric brain damage that causes left hemiplegia.

A variety of other types of agnosia exist in addition to unilateral neglect. Some patients are unable to recognize objects visually (visual object agnosia), whereas others cannot recognize faces (prosopagnosia) and may have to rely on the voice or characteristic mannerisms of a familiar person to identify that person. Tactile agnosia is a perceptual disorder in which a patient is unable to recognize by touch alone an object that has been placed in his or her hand. This may occur even in the presence of an intact sense of touch. If allowed to see or hear the object, the patient usually recognizes it.

Spatial orientation is also affected, resulting in interference with the patient's ability to judge position, distance, movement, form, and the relationship of his or her body parts to surrounding objects. Patients may confuse concepts such as up and down and forward and backward. They may have difficulty following a route from one place to another and may even get lost in areas that were once familiar. Stroke patients may also experience reading and writing problems related to visual perception and visuospatial deficits. One type of spatial dyslexia is related to unilateral spatial neglect. The patient may not look at the beginning of a line of written material that appears on the left. Instead, the patient fixes attention on a point to the right of the beginning of the line and reads to the end of the line. If asked to draw a design, the person completes only half a design or drawing.

Visual Field Defects. Visual field defects may accompany agnosia, although they do not cause it. A hemispheric lesion can interrupt the visual pathways, with the resulting visual defect dependent on the location and extent of the lesion. At the optic chiasm, nerve fibers coming from the nasal half of each retina cross to the opposite side, whereas fibers coming from the temporal half of each retina do not cross. This partial crossing allows binocular vision. In the optic chiasm, fibers from the nasal half of each retina join the uncrossed fibers from the temporal half of the retina to form the optic tract. Impulses conducted to the right hemisphere by the right optic tract represent the left field of vision, and those conducted to the left hemisphere by the left optic tract represent the right field of vision. Optic radiations extend back to the occipital lobes. Visual defects restricted to a single field, right or left, are termed *homonymous hemianopsia.*

The nurse may be the first person to detect that the patient has this defect. The patient with hemianopsia may neglect all sensory input from the affected side and initially may appear unresponsive if approached from the affected side. If the nurse approaches the patient from the healthy side, the patient actually may be quite alert. Another clue to hemianopsia is observing that the patient eats food only from one half of the tray. Hemianopsia may recede gradually with time. Many patients can learn to scan their environment visually to compensate for the defect, although in the acute stage of stroke the patient may be too lethargic to follow instructions in methods of visual scanning. This visual defect can lead to fear and confusion and can present a risk to the patient's safety.

Apraxia. Lesions in the parietal lobe, as well as in other cortical structures, can result in apraxia, an inability to perform a learned movement voluntarily. Even though the patient may understand the task to be performed and may have intact motor ability, he or she cannot perform the task and often fumbles and makes mistakes. The patient suffering from dressing apraxia, for example, may not be able to orient clothing in space, becoming tangled in his or her clothes when attempting to dress.

Damage to Dominant Hemisphere. Damage to the dominant hemisphere produces problems with speech and language. Impaired communication is a condition that results from a patient's difficulty in express-

ing and exchanging thoughts, ideas, or desires. The posterior temporoparietal area contains the receptive speech center known as *Wernicke's area.* The center for the perception of written language lies anterior to the visuoreceptive areas. Located at the base of the frontal lobe's motor strip and slightly anterior to it is Broca's area, also known as the *motor speech center.* These sensory and motor areas are connected by a large bundle of nerve fibers. Rather than receptive and motor language functions being entirely within discrete areas, it is believed that language is an integrated sensorimotor process, control of which is roughly located in these areas in the dominant cerebral hemisphere. It also is recognized that the elaborately complex functions of speech and language depend on other associative areas of the cerebrum and their thalamic connections. Consequently, much inconsistency exists in the degree of communication impairment among patients with lesions located in the same area of the brain.

Aphasia is a loss of language abilities caused by brain injury, usually to the dominant hemisphere. It involves more than just understanding speech or expressing oneself through verbal means. Language is a much broader term, referring to what the individual is attempting to interpret or convey through listening, speaking, reading, writing, and gesturing. Most cases of aphasia are partial, rather than complete. The severity of the disorder depends on the area and the extent of the cerebral damage.

Receptive Aphasia. Receptive aphasia, also referred to as *sensory, Wernicke's,* or *fluent aphasia,* occurs when the connection between the primary auditory cortex in the temporal lobe and the angular gyrus in the parietal lobe is destroyed. The patient's comprehension of speech is impaired, but he or she can still talk if the motor area for speech, Broca's area, is intact. The patient may in fact talk excessively, with many errors in the use of words. The patient can hear the examiner but cannot comprehend what is being said and cannot repeat the examiner's words. Such patients may talk nonsense, with rambling speech that gives little information. Patients with receptive aphasia also cannot read words, although they can see them.

Expressive Aphasia. Expressive aphasia, also known as *motor, Broca's,* or *nonfluent aphasia,* is primarily a deficit in language output or speech production. Depending on the lesion's size and exact location, a wide variation in the motor deficit can result. Expressive aphasia can range from a mild dysarthria (imperfect articulation as a result of weakness or lack of coordination of speech musculature) to incorrect intonation and phrasing and, in its most severe form, to complete loss of ability to communicate through verbal and written means. In this severe form of aphasia, the patient also has a loss of ability to communicate through conventional gestures, such as nodding or shaking the head for "yes" or "no." In most cases of expressive aphasia, the muscles of articulation are intact. If speech is possible at all, occasionally the

PATIENT EDUCATION   Stroke

- Pathophysiology of disease
- Specific etiology
- Risk factor modification
- Importance of taking medications
- Activities of daily living
- Measures to prevent injuries of impaired limbs
- Measures to compensate for residual deficits
- Basic rehabilitation techniques
- Importance of participating in neurologic rehabilitation program and/or support group

Box 27-6

COLLABORATIVE MANAGEMENT

STROKE
- Differentiate the cause of the stroke
  - Ischemic
  - Subarachnoid hemorrhage
  - Cerebral aneurysm
  - Arteriovenous malformation (AVM)
  - Intracerebral bleed
- Implement treatment according to cause of bleed
  - Ischemic
    Thrombolytic therapy
    Blood pressure control
  - Subarachnoid hemorrhage
    Surgical aneurysm clipping or AVM excision
    Embolization
  - Intracerebral bleed
    Blood pressure control
- Protect patient's airway
- Provide ventilatory assistance as required
- Perform frequent neurologic assessments
- Maintain surveillance for complications
  - Cerebral edema
  - Cerebral ischemia/vasospasm
  - Rebleeding
  - Impaired swallowing
  - Neurologic deficits
- Provide comfort and emotional support
- Design and implement appropriate rehabilitation program
- Educate patient and family

word "yes" or "no" is uttered, sometimes appropriately. In some cases the words of well-known songs may be sung. Other patients, when excited or angered, may utter expletives. Some patients with expressive aphasia struggle or hesitate in trying to express words. They struggle to form words while using motor musculature (verbal apraxia), an articulatory disorder that is a feature of some expressive types of aphasia. All these difficulties lead to exasperation and despair for the patient. Most patients with expressive aphasia also have severely impaired writing ability. Even though penmanship may be intact, they are unable to express themselves through writing—a deficit termed *agraphia*. If the right hand is paralyzed, as is often the case, the patient still cannot write or print with the left hand. In the recovery phase of severe expressive aphasia, patients become able to speak aloud to some degree, although words are uttered slowly and laboriously. Many patients, however, are able to learn to communicate ideas to some extent.

Global Aphasia. Global aphasia results when a massive lesion affects both the motor and sensory speech areas. The patient cannot transform sounds into words and cannot comprehend spoken words. All language modalities are affected, and impairment may be so severe that the patient may be unable to communicate on any level. These patients generally have severe hemiplegia and also homonymous hemianopsia. In these patients, language function rarely recovers to a significant degree unless the lesion is caused by some transient disorder, such as cerebral edema or a metabolic derangement.

Impaired Swallowing. Normal swallowing occurs in four phases that are controlled by the cranial nerves. Damage to the brain, brainstem, or cranial nerves can result in a variety of swallowing deficits that can place the patient at risk for aspiration. The stroke patient is observed for signs of dysphagia including drooling; difficulty handling oral secretions; absence of gag, cough, or swallowing reflexes; moist, gurgling voice quality; decreased mouth and tongue movements; and the presence of dysarthria. A speech therapy consult is initiated if any of these signs are present, and the patient must not be orally fed. In the absence of these warning signs, the patient may be fed, as ordered by the physician, though he or she must be continually monitored for signs of aspiration.[6]

Patient Education. Rehabilitation starts in the critical care area, with a multidisciplinary team designing and implementing an individualized plan for maximizing the patient's potential for neurologic rehabilitation. Early in the patient's hospital stay, the patient and family must be taught about stroke, its etiologies, and its treatment (see the Patient Education feature on Stroke). As the patient moves toward discharge, teaching focuses on the interventions necessary for preventing the reoccurrence of the event and on maximizing the patient's rehabilitation potential. The patient's family must be encouraged to participate in the patient's care; learn how to feed, dress, and bathe the patient; and learn some basic rehabilitation techniques. In addition, the importance of participating in a neurologic rehabilitation program and/or a support group must be stressed.

Collaborative management of the patient with a stroke is outlined in Box 27-6.

GUILLAIN-BARRÉ SYNDROME

Description. Guillain-Barré syndrome (GBS), once thought to be a single entity characterized by inflammatory peripheral neuropathy, is now understood to be a combination of clinical features with varying forms of presentation and multiple pathologic processes. A full discussion of the current understanding of this complex condition is beyond the scope of this text. Most cases of GBS do not require admission to a critical care unit. However, the prototype of GBS, known as *acute inflammatory demyelinating polyradiculoneuropathy (AIDP)*, involves a rapidly progressive, ascending peripheral nerve dysfunction leading to paralysis that may produce respiratory failure. Because of the need for ventilatory support, AIDP is one of the few peripheral neurologic diseases that necessitates care in a critical care environment.[55] For the sake of this discussion, all references to GBS will pertain to the AIDP prototype.

The annual incidence of GBS is 1.8 per 100,000 persons.[55] It occurs more often in males and is the most commonly acquired demyelinating neuropathy.[56] Occasionally clusters of cases are reported, such as occurred following the 1977 swine flu vaccinations.[57]

Etiology. The precise cause of GBS remains unknown, but the syndrome involves an immune-mediated response involving both cell-mediated immunity and development of IgG antibodies. Most patients report a viral infection 1 to 3 weeks before the onset of clinical manifestations, usually involving the upper respiratory tract.[55]

Numerous antecedent causes, or triggering events, have now been associated with GBS. These include viral infections (influenza; cytomegalovirus; hepatitis A, B, or C; Epstein-Barr; human immunodeficiency virus), bacterial infections (gastrointestinal *Campylobacter jejuni* and *Mycoplasma pneumoniae*), vaccines (rabies, tetanus, influenza), lymphoma, surgery, and trauma.[55,56]

Pathophysiology. This disease affects the motor and sensory pathways of the peripheral nervous system, as well as the autonomic nervous system functions of the cranial nerves. The major finding in GBS (AIDP type) is a segmental demyelination process of the peripheral nerves. GBS is believed to be an autoimmune response to antibodies formed in response to a recent physiologic event. T cells migrate to the peripheral nerves, resulting in edema and inflammation. Macrophages then invade the area and break down the myelin. Inflammation around this demyelinated area causes further dysfunction. Some axonal damage also occurs.[55,56]

The myelin sheath of the peripheral nerves is generated by Schwann's cells and acts as an insulator for the peripheral nerve. Myelin promotes rapid conduction of nerve impulses by allowing the impulses to jump along the nerve via nodes of Ranvier. Disruption of the myelin fiber slows and may eventually stop the conduction of impulses along the peripheral nerves. In GBS, the more thickly myelinated fibers of motor pathways and the cranial nerves are more severely affected than are the thinly myelinated sensory fibers of cutaneous pain, touch, and temperature.[6]

Once the temporary inflammatory reaction stops, myelin-producing cells begin the process of reinsulating the demyelinated portions of the peripheral nervous system. When remyelination occurs, normal neurologic function should return. In some instances the axon may be damaged during the inflammatory process. The degree of axonal damage is responsible for the degree of neurologic dysfunction that persists after recovery.[55]

Assessment and Diagnosis. Symptoms of GBS include motor weakness; paresthesias and other sensory changes; cranial nerve dysfunction (especially oculomotor, facial, glossopharyngeal, vagal, spinal accessory, and hypoglossal); and some autonomic dysfunction. The usual course of GBS begins with an abrupt onset of lower extremity weakness that progresses to flaccidity and ascends over a period of hours to days. Motor loss usually is symmetric, bilateral, and ascending. In the most severe cases, complete flaccidity of all peripheral nerves, including spinal and cranial nerves, occurs.[6]

The patient is admitted to the hospital when lower extremity weakness prevents mobility. Admission to the critical care unit is necessary when progression of the weakness threatens respiratory muscles. As the patient's weakness progresses, close observation is essential. Frequent assessment of the respiratory system, including ventilatory parameters such as inspiratory force and tidal volume, is necessary. The most common cause of death in patients with GBS is from respiratory arrest. As the disease progresses and respiratory effort weakens, intubation and mechanical ventilation are necessary. Continued, frequent assessment of neurologic deterioration is required until the patient reaches the peak of the disease and plateau occurs.[58]

The diagnosis of GBS is based on clinical findings plus CSF analysis and nerve conduction studies. The diagnostic finding is elevated CSF protein with normal cell count.[58] The increased protein count is usually present after the first week but does not occur in approximately 10% of all cases. Nerve conduction studies that test the velocity at which nerve impulses are conducted show significant reduction, as the demyelinating process of the disease suggests.

Medical Management. With no curative treatment available, the medical management of GBS is limited. The disease must simply run its course, which is characterized by ascending paralysis that advances over 1 to 3 weeks and then remains at a plateau for 2 to 4 weeks.[58] The plateau stage is followed by descending paralysis and return to normal or near-normal function. The main focus of medical management is the support of bodily functions and the prevention of complications.

Both plasmapheresis and intravenous immune globulin (IVIg) are used to treat GBS.[55,56,58] They have been shown to be equally effective.[59] Plasmapheresis involves the removal of venous blood via a catheter, separation of plasma from blood cells, and reinfusion of the cells plus autologous plasma or another replacement solution. Though the number of exchanges may vary, usually four to six exchanges are performed over a 5- to 8-day period.[55]

Nursing Management. The nursing management of the patient with GBS incorporates a variety of nursing diagnoses and interventions (see the Nursing Diagnoses feature on Guillain-Barré syndrome). The goal of nursing management is to support all normal body functions until the patient can do so on his or her own. Although the condition is reversible, the patient with GBS requires extensive long-term care, because recovery can be a long process. Nursing priorities are directed toward maintaining surveillance for complications, initiating rehabilitation, facilitating nutritional support, and providing comfort and emotional support.

Maintaining Surveillance for Complications. Continuous assessment of the progressive paralysis associated with GBS is essential to timely intervention and the prevention of respiratory arrest and further neurologic insult. Once the patient is intubated and placed on mechanical ventilation, close observation for pulmonary complications, such as atelectasis, pneumonia, and pneumothorax, is necessary. Autonomic dysfunction, dysautonomia, in the GBS patient can procuce variations in heart rate and blood pressure that can reach extreme values.[60,61] Hypertension and tachycardia may require beta-blocker therapy. All GBS patients must be observed for this phenomenon.

Initiating Rehabilitation. In patients with GBS, immobility may last for months. The usual course of GBS involves an average of 10 days of symptom progression and 10 days of maximal level of dysfunction, followed by 2 to 48 weeks of recovery. Although GBS is usually completely reversible, the patient will require physical and occupational rehabilitation because of the problems of long-term immobility. Rehabilitation starts in the critical care area, with a multidisciplinary team designing and implementing an individualized plan for maximizing the patient's potential for rehabilitation.

Facilitating Nutritional Support. Nutritional support is implemented early in the course of the disease. Because GBS recovery is a long process, adequate nutritional support will be a problem for an extended period. Nutritional support usually is accomplished through the use of enteral feeding.

Providing Comfort and Emotional Support. Pain control is another important component in the care of the patient with GBS. Although patients may have minimal to no motor function, most sensory functions remain, causing patients considerable muscle aching and pain. Because of the length of this illness, a safe, effective, long-term solution to pain management must be identified. These patients also require extensive psychologic support. Although the illness is almost 100% reversible, lack of control over the situation, constant pain or discomfort, and the long-term nature of the disorder create coping difficulties for the patient. GBS does not affect the level of consciousness or cerebral function. Patient interaction and communication are essential elements of the nursing management plan.

Patient Education. Early in the patient's hospital stay, the patient and family must be taught about GBS and its different treatments (see the Patient Education feature on Guillain-Barré syndrome). As the patient moves toward discharge, teaching focuses on the interventions to maximize the patient's rehabilitation potential. The patient's family must be encouraged to participate in the patient's care and to learn some basic rehabilitation techniques. In addition, the importance of participating in a neurologic rehabilitation program (if necessary) must be stressed.

Collaborative management of the patient with Guillain-Barre syndrome is outlined in Box 27-7.

NURSING DIAGNOSES | Guillain-Barré Syndrome

- Ineffective Breathing Pattern related to musculoskeletal fatigue or neuromuscular impairment
- Acute Pain related to transmission and perception of cutaneous, visceral, muscular, or ischemic impulses
- Activity Intolerance related to prolonged immobility or deconditioning
- Risk for Aspiration
- Imbalanced Nutrition: Less Than Body Requirements related to lack of exogenous nutrients or increased metabolic demand
- Risk for Infection
- Anxiety related to threat of biologic, psychologic, or social integrity
- Powerlessness related to lack of control over current situation and/or disease progression
- Ineffective Coping related to situational crisis and personal vulnerability
- Compromised Family Coping related to critically ill family member
- Deficient Knowledge: Discharge Regimen related to lack of previous exposure to information (see Patient Education feature on Guillain-Barré Syndrome)

Guillain-Barré Syndrome

- Pathophysiology of disease
- Importance of taking medications
- Measures to compensate for residual deficits
- Basic rehabilitation techniques
- Importance of participating in neurologic rehabilitation program (if necessary)

Box 27-8

OPERATIVE TERMS

Burr hole: hole made into the cranium using a special drill
Craniotomy: surgical opening of the skull
Craniectomy: removal of a portion of the skull without replacing it
Cranioplasty: plastic repair of the skull
Supratentorial: above the tentorium, separating the cerebrum from the cerebellum
Infratentorial: below the tentorium; includes the brainstem and the cerebellum; an infratentorial surgical approach may be used for temporal or occipital lesions

Box 27-7

COLLABORATIVE MANAGEMENT

GUILLAIN-BARRÉ SYNDROME
- Support bodily functions
  - Protect airway
  - Provide ventilatory assistance as required
- Initiate treatments to limit duration of the syndrome
  - Plasmapheresis
  - Intravenous immunoglobulin
- Initiate nutritional support
- Maintain surveillance for complications
  - Infections
  - Cardiac dysrhythmias
  - Blood pressure alterations
  - Temperature alterations
- Provide comfort and emotional support
- Design and implement appropriate rehabilitation program
- Educate patient and family

CRANIOTOMY

Types of Surgery. A craniotomy is performed to gain access to portions of the CNS inside the cranium, usually to allow removal of a space-occupying lesion such as a brain tumor (Table 27-5). Common procedures include tumor resection or removal, cerebral decompression, evacuation of hematoma or abscess, and clipping or removal of an aneurysm or arteriovenous malformation. Most patients who undergo craniotomy for tumor resection or removal do not require care in a critical care unit. Those patients who do usually need intensive monitoring or are at greater risk of complications because of underlying cardiopulmonary dysfunction or the surgical approach used. Box 27-8 provides definitions of common neurosurgical terms.[62] This section provides a generalized discussion of craniotomy care.

Preoperative Care. Protection of the integrity of the CNS is a major priority of care for the patient awaiting a craniotomy. Optimal arterial oxygenation, hemodynamic stability, and cerebral perfusion are essential to maintaining adequate cerebral oxygenation. Management of seizure activity is essential to controlling metabolic needs.

Detailed assessment and documentation of the patient's preoperative neurologic status are imperative for accurate postoperative evaluation. Specific attention is placed on identifying and describing the nature and extent of any preoperative neurologic deficits. When pituitary surgery is planned, thorough evaluation of endocrine function is necessary to prevent major intraoperative and postoperative complications.[63]

Current trends in health care demand judicious use of routine preoperative studies. Depending on the type of surgery to be performed and the general health of the patient, preoperative screening may include a complete blood count (CBC), blood urea nitrogen (BUN), creatinine, fasting blood sugar (FBS), chest x-ray, and electrocardiogram. A type and crossmatch for blood may also be ordered.[62]

Preoperative teaching is necessary to prepare both the patient and family for what to expect in the postoperative period. A description of the intravascular lines and intracranial catheters used during the postoperative period allows the family to focus on the patient, rather than be overwhelmed by masses of tubing. Some or all of the patient's hair is shaved off in the operating room, and a large, bulky, turbanlike craniotomy dressing is applied. Most patients experience some degree of postoperative eye or facial swelling and periorbital ecchymosis. An explanation of these temporary changes in appearance helps alleviate the shock and fear many patients and families experience in the immediate postoperative period.

All craniotomy patients require instruction to avoid activities known to provoke sudden changes in intracranial pressure. These activities include bending, lifting, straining, and the Valsalva maneuver. Patients com-

Table 27-5 Tumor Types and Characteristics

Tumor	Clinical Features	Treatment/Prognosis
Glioblastoma multiforme (GM)	Often presents with nonspecific complaints and increased ICP As tumor grows, focal deficits develop	Rapidly progressive course, with poor prognosis Total surgical removal usually not possible; response to radiation poor
Astrocytoma	Presentation similar to GM, but course more protracted, often over several years; cerebellar astrocytoma, especially in children, may have more benign course	Variable prognosis By diagnosis, total excision usually impossible; tumor often not radiosensitive In cerebellar astrocytoma, total excision often possible
Medulloblastoma	Glioma most often seen in children Generally arises from roof of fourth ventricle and leads to increased ICP, with brain stem and cerebellar signs; may seed subarachnoid space	Treatment consists of surgery with radiation therapy and chemotherapy
Ependymoma	Glioma arising from ependyma of ventricle, especially fourth; leads early to signs of increased ICP; arises also from central canal of spinal cord	Tumor not radiosensitive and best treated surgically, if possible
Oligodendroglioma	Slow-growing glioma, usually arises in cerebral hemisphere in adults Calcification may be visible on radiograph	Treatment is surgical and usually successful
Brainstem glioma	Presents in childhood with cranial nerve palsies, then long-tract signs in limbs; signs of increased ICP occur late in course	Tumor is inoperable Treatment with irradiation and shunt for increased ICP
Cerebellar hemangioblastoma	Presents with disequilibrium, ataxia of trunk or limbs, and signs of increased ICP; at times familiar; may be associated with retinal and spinal lesions; polycythema, and hypernephroma	Treatment is surgical
Pineal tumor	Presents with increased ICP, at times associated with impaired upward gaze (Parinaud's syndrome) and other deficits indicating midbrain lesion	Ventricular decompression by shunting, followed by surgical approach to tumor Irradiation if tumor malignant Prognosis depends on histopathologic findings and tumor extent
Craniopharyngioma	Originates from remnants of Rathke's pouch above sella turcica, depressing optic chiasm May present at any age but usually in childhood with endocrine dysfunction and bitemporal field deficits	Treatment is surgical, but total removal may not be possible
Acoustic neuroma	Most common initial symptom is ipsilateral hearing loss; subsequent symptoms may include tinnitus, headache, vertigo, facial weakness or numbness, and long-tract signs May be familial and bilateral when related to neurofibromatosis Most sensitive screening tests are MRI and brainstem AEP	Treatment is by excision by translabyrinthine approach, craniectomy, or combination Prognosis usually good
Meningioma	Originates from dura mater or arachnoid; compresses rather than invades adjacent neural structures Increasingly common with advancing age Tumor size varies greatly; symptoms vary with tumor site* Tumor usually benign; readily detected by CT; may lead to calcification and bone erosion visible on plain skull radiographs	Treatment is surgical Tumor may recur if removal is incomplete; patient may receive radiation with incomplete excision to decrease risk of recurrence
Primary central lymphoma	Associated with AIDS and other immunodeficiency states Presentation may be with focal deficits or disturbances of cognition and consciousness; may be indistinguishable from cerebral toxoplasmosis	Treatment is by whole-brain irradiation Chemotherapy may have adjunctive role Prognosis depends on CD4 cell count at diagnosis

From Gawlinski A, Hamwi D, editors: *Acute care nurse practitioner: clinical curriculum and certification review*, Philadelphia, 1999, Saunders.
*For example, unilateral exophthalmos (sphenoidal ridge), anosmia and optic nerve compression (olfactory groove).
AEP, Auditory-evoked potential; *AIDS*, acquired immunodeficiency syndrome; *CT*, computed tomography; *ICP*, intracranial pressure; *MRI*, magnetic resonance imaging.

monly elicit the Valsalva maneuver during repositioning in bed by holding their breath and straining with a closed epiglottis. Teaching the patient to continue to breathe deeply through the mouth during all position changes is an effective deterrent.

The patient undergoing transsphenoidal surgery requires preparation for the sensations associated with nasal packing. The patient often awakens with alarm because of the inability to breathe through the nose. Preoperative instruction in mouth breathing and avoidance of coughing, sneezing, or blowing of the nose facilitates postoperative cooperation.

The psychosocial issues associated with the prospect of neurosurgery cannot be overemphasized. Few procedures are as threatening as those involving the brain or spinal cord. For some patients the fear of permanent neurologic impairment may be as or more ominous than the fear of death. Steps to meet the needs of the patient, as well as the family, include collaboration with clergy and social services personnel, patient-controlled visitation, and provision of as much privacy as the patient's condition permits. Both the patient and the family must be provided with the opportunity to express their fears and concerns apart from each other as well as jointly.[62]

Surgical Considerations. Whereas the emphasis in surgical approach for most other types of surgery is to gain adequate exposure of the surgical site, the neurosurgeon must select a route that also produces the least amount of disruption to the intracranial contents. Neural tissue is unforgiving. A significant portion of neurologic trauma and postoperative deficits is related to the surgical pathway through the brain tissue, rather than to the procedure performed at the site of pathology. Depending on the location of the lesion and the surgical route decided on, either a transcranial or a transsphenoidal approach is used to open the skull.

Transcranial. In the transcranial approach, a scalp incision is made and a series of burr holes is drilled into the skull to form an outline of the area to be opened (Fig. 27-5). A special saw is then used to cut between the holes. In most cases the bone flap is left attached to the muscle to create a hinge effect. In some cases the bone flap is removed completely and either placed in the abdomen for later retrieval and implantation or discarded

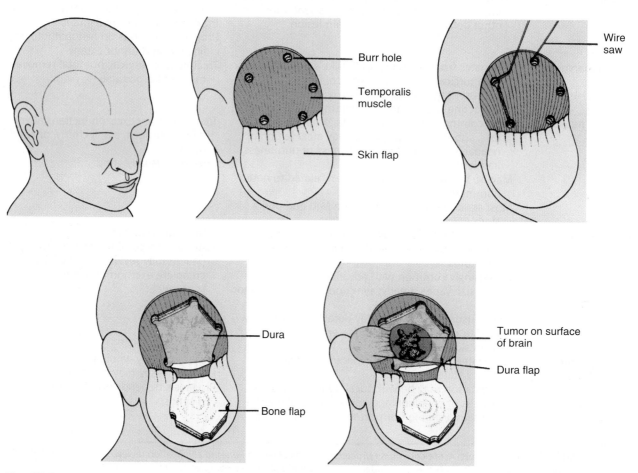

Fig. 27-5 Craniotomy. (From Beare PG, Myers JL: *Principles and practice of adult health nursing,* ed 2, St Louis, 1994, Mosby.)

and replaced with synthetic material. Next the dura is opened and retracted. After the intracranial procedure, the dura and the bone flap are closed, the muscles and scalp are sutured, and a turbanlike dressing is applied.[62]

Transsphenoidal. The transsphenoidal approach is the technique of choice for removal of a pituitary tumor without extension into the intracranial vault (Fig 27-6).[63] This approach involves making a microsurgical entrance into the cranial vault via the nasal cavity. The sphenoid sinus is entered to reach the anterior wall of the sella turcica. The sphenoid bone and the dura are then opened to gain intracranial access. After removal of the tumor, the surgical bed is packed with a small section of adipose tissue grafted from the patient's abdomen or thigh. After closure of the intranasal structures, nasal splints and soft packing or nasal tampons impregnated with antibiotic ointment are placed in the nasal cavities. Occasionally, epistaxis balloons are used instead. A nasal drip pad or mustache-type dressing is placed at the base of the nose to catch surgical drainage.[62]

The patient may be placed in a supine, prone, or even sitting position for a craniotomy procedure. A skull clamp connected to skull pins is used to position and secure the patient's head throughout the surgery. During a transsphenoidal approach or a transcranial approach into the infratentorial area, the patient's head is elevated during the surgery. This position places the patient at risk for an air embolism. Air can enter the vascular system either through the edges of the dura or a venous opening. Continuous monitoring of the patient's heart sounds by Doppler signal allows immediate recognition of this complication. If it occurs, an attempt may be made to withdraw the embolus from the right atrium through a central line. Flooding the surgical field with irrigation fluid and placing a moistened sterile surgical sponge over the surgical site creates an immediate barrier to any further air entrance.[62]

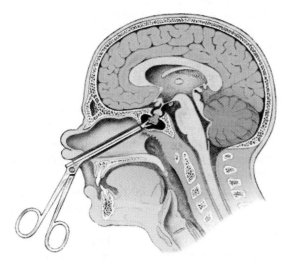

Fig. 27-6 Transsphenoidal hypophysectomy.

Postoperative Medical Management. Definitive management of the postoperative neurosurgical patient varies, depending on the underlying reason for the craniotomy. During the initial postoperative period, management is usually directed toward the prevention of complications. Complications associated with a craniotomy include intracranial hypertension, surgical hemorrhage, fluid imbalance, CSF leak, and deep vein thrombosis.

Intracranial Hypertension. Postoperative cerebral edema is expected to peak 48 to 72 hours after surgery. If the bone flap is not replaced at the time of surgery, intracranial hypertension will produce bulging at the surgical site. Close monitoring of the surgical site is important so that integrity of the incision can be maintained. Postcraniotomy management of intracranial hypertension is usually accomplished through CSF drainage, patient positioning, and steroid administration.[5]

Surgical Hemorrhage. Surgical hemorrhage after a transcranial procedure can occur in the intracranial vault and is manifested by signs and symptoms of increasing ICP. Hemorrhage after a transsphenoidal craniotomy may be evident from external drainage, patient complaint of persistent postnasal drip, or excessive swallowing. Loss of vision after pituitary surgery is also indicative of evolving hemorrhage. Postoperative hemorrhage requires surgical reexploration.[63]

Fluid Imbalance. Fluid imbalance in the postcraniotomy patient usually results from a disturbance in production or secretion of antidiuretic hormone (ADH). ADH is secreted by the posterior pituitary (neurohypophysis) gland. It stimulates the renal tubules and collecting ducts to retain water in response to low circulating blood volume or increased serum osmolality. Inoperative trauma or postoperative edema of the pituitary gland or hypothalamus can result in insufficient ADH secretion. The outcome is unabated renal water loss even when blood volume is low and serum osmolality is high. This condition is known as *diabetes insipidus (DI).* The polyuria associated with DI is often greater than 200 ml/hour. Urine specific gravity of 1.005 or less and elevated serum osmolality provide evidence of insufficient ADH. The loss of volume may provoke hypotension and inadequate cerebral perfusion. DI is usually self-limiting, with fluid replacement being the only necessary therapy. In some cases, however, it may be necessary to administer vasopressin intravenously to control the loss of fluid.[5]

The syndrome of inappropriate antidiuretic hormone (SIADH) commonly occurs with neurologic insult and results from excessive ADH secretion. SIADH is manifested by inappropriate water retention with hyponatremia in the presence of normal renal function. Urine specific gravity is elevated and urine osmolality is greater than serum osmolality. The dangers associated with SIADH include circulating volume overload and electrolyte imbalance, both of which may impair neurologic functioning. SIADH is usually self-limiting, with the mainstay of treatment being fluid restriction.[5]

CSF Leak. Leakage of CSF fluid results from an opening in the subarachnoid space, as evidenced by clear fluid draining from the surgical site. When this complication occurs after transsphenoidal surgery, it is evidenced by excessive, clear drainage from the nose or persistent postnasal drip. To differentiate CSF drainage from postoperative serous drainage, a specimen is tested for glucose content. A CSF leak is confirmed by glucose values of 30 mg/dl or greater. Management of the patient with a CSF leak includes bed rest and head elevation. Lumbar puncture or placement of a lumbar subarachnoid catheter may be used to reduce CSF pressure until the dura heals. The risk of meningitis associated with CSF leak often necessitates surgical repair to reseal the opening.[5,63]

Deep Vein Thrombosis. Deep vein thrombosis (DVT) has been reported to occur in 29% to 46% of all neurosurgical patients, as compared with a 25% incidence in general surgical patients. Early research demonstrated a greater risk after removal of a supratentorial tumor and a twofold risk in patients whose surgery lasted for more than 4 hours.[64] Recent research has demonstrated numerous additional risk factors significantly associated with DVT development: preoperative leg weakness, longer preoperative critical care unit stay, longer recovery room time, longer postoperative critical care unit stay, more days on bed rest, and delay of postoperative mobility and activity.[65] Clinical manifestations of DVT include leg or calf pain, edema, localized tenderness, and pain with dorsiflexion or plantar flexion (Homans' sign). Unfortunately, the patient with a DVT is often asymptomatic, and the diagnosis is not made until the patient experiences a pulmonary embolus.

The primary treatment for DVT is prophylaxis. In the neurosurgery patient, sequential (intermittent) pneumatic compression boots or stockings have been demonstrated to be effective in reducing the incidence of DVT. Effectiveness is enhanced when these devices are initiated in the preoperative period. Low-dose unfractionated heparin or low–molecular-weight heparin may also be used prophylactically in high-risk patients.[44]

Postoperative Nursing Management. The nursing management of the neurosurgical patient incorporates a variety of nursing diagnoses (see the Nursing Diagnoses feature on Craniotomy). As in preoperative care, the primary goal of postcraniotomy nursing management is protection of the integrity of the CNS. Nursing interventions are directed toward preserving adequate CPP, promoting arterial oxygenation, providing comfort and emotional support, maintaining surveillance for complications, and initiating early rehabilitation. Frequent neurologic assessment is necessary to evaluate accomplishment of these objectives and to identify and quickly intervene if complications do arise. Often a ventriculostomy is placed to facilitate ICP monitoring and/or CSF drainage.

NURSING DIAGNOSES   Craniotomy

- Decreased Intracranial Adaptive Capacity related to failure of normal intracranial compensatory mechanisms
- Ineffective Cerebral Tissue Perfusion related to decreased blood flow
- Ineffective Cerebral Tissue Perfusion related to hemorrhage
- Acute Pain related to transmission and perception of cutaneous, visceral, muscular, or ischemic impulses
- Disturbed Body Image related to actual change in body structure, function, or appearance
- Deficient Knowledge: Discharge Regimen related to lack of previous exposure to information (see Patient Education feature on Craniotomy)

Preserving Adequate Cerebral Perfusion. Nursing interventions to preserve cerebral perfusion include patient positioning, fluid management, and avoidance of postoperative vomiting and fever.

Positioning. Patient positioning is an important component of care for the craniotomy patient. The head of the bed should be elevated 30 to 45 degrees at all times to reduce the incidence of hemorrhage, facilitate venous drainage, and control ICP. Other positioning measures to control ICP include maintaining the patient's head in a neutral position at all times and avoiding neck or hip flexion. It is vital to adhere to these rules of positioning throughout all nursing activities, including linen changes and transporting the patient for diagnostic evaluation. Most craniotomy patients can still be turned from side to side within these restrictions, using pillows for support, except in some cases of extensive tumor removal, cranioplasty, and when the bone flap is not replaced. Specific orders from the surgeon must be obtained in these instances. The patient with an infratentorial incision may be restricted to only a very small pillow under the head to prevent strain on the incision. Avoidance of anterior or lateral neck flexion also protects the integrity of this type of incision.

Fluid Management. Fluid management is another important component of postcraniotomy care. Hourly monitoring of fluid intake and output facilitates early identification of fluid imbalance. Urine specific gravity must be measured if DI is suspected. Fluid restriction may be ordered as a routine measure to lessen the severity of cerebral edema or as treatment for the fluid and electrolyte imbalances associated with SIADH.

Vomiting and Fever. Postoperative vomiting must be avoided to prevent sharp spikes in ICP and possibly surgical hemorrhage. Antiemetics are administered as soon as nausea is apparent. Early nutrition in the neurosurgical patient is beneficial. If the patient is unable to eat, enteral hyperalimentation via feeding tube is the preferred method of nutritional support and can be initiated as early as 24 hours after surgery.[62] Postoperative fever may also adversely affect ICP and increase the metabolic needs of the brain. Acetaminophen is administered orally, rectally, or via a feeding tube. External cooling measures, such as a hypothermia blanket, may also be necessary.

Promoting Arterial Oxygenation. Routine pulmonary care is used to maintain airway clearance and prevent pulmonary complications. To prevent dangerous elevations in ICP, this care must be performed using proper technique and at time intervals that are adequately spaced from other patient care activities. If pulmonary complications do arise, consideration must be given to maintaining adequate oxygenation during repositioning. It may be necessary to restrict turning to only the side that places the good lung down.

Providing Comfort and Emotional Support. Pain management in the postcraniotomy patient primarily involves control of headache. Small doses of intravenous morphine are used in the critical care setting. As soon as oral analgesics can be tolerated, acetaminophen with codeine is used. Both of these analgesics cause constipation. Administration of stool softeners and initiation of a bowel program are important components of postcraniotomy care. Constipation is hazardous, because straining to have a bowel movement can create significant elevations in blood pressure and ICP.

Maintaining Surveillance for Complications. The postoperative neurosurgical patient is at risk for infection, corneal abrasions, and injury from falls or seizures.

Infection. Care of the incision and surgical dressings is institution- and physician-specific. The rule of thumb for a craniotomy dressing is to reinforce it as needed and change it only with a physician's order. Often a drain is left in place to facilitate decompression of the surgical site. If a ventriculostomy is present, it is treated as a component of the surgical site. All drainage devices must be secured to the dressing to prevent unintentional displacement with patient movement. Sterile technique is required to prevent infection and resultant meningitis.

Corneal Abrasions. Routine eye care may be necessary to prevent corneal drying and ulceration. Periorbital edema interferes with normal blinking and eyelid closure, which are essential to adequate corneal lubrication. Saline drops are instilled every 2 hours. If the patient remains in a coma state, covering the eyes with a

---

PATIENT EDUCATION — Craniotomy

Before Surgery
- Pathophysiology and expected outcome of underlying disease
- Need for intensive care management after surgery
- Routine postoperative surgical care

After Surgery
- Routine postoperative surgical care
- Discharge medications—purpose, dose, and side effects
- Incisional care
- Signs and symptoms of infection
- Signs and symptoms of increased intracranial pressure
- Measures to compensate for residual deficits
- Basic rehabilitation techniques
- Importance of participating in neurologic rehabilitation program

---

polyethylene film extending over the orbits and eyebrows may be beneficial.[12]

Injury. The postcraniotomy patient may also experience periods of altered mentation. Protection from injury may require use of restraint devices. The side rails of the bed must also be padded to protect the patient from injury. Having a family member stay at the bedside and/or use of music therapy is often helpful to keep the patient calm during periods of restlessness. In rare circumstances, neuromuscular blockade and sedation may be necessary to control patient activity and metabolic needs on a short-term basis.

Initiating Early Rehabilitation. Increased patient activity, including ambulation, is begun as soon as tolerated in the postoperative period. Rehabilitation measures and discharge planning may begin in the critical care unit but are beyond the scope of this text. Transfer to a general care or rehabilitation unit is usually accomplished as soon as the patient is considered to be stable and free of complications.

Patient Education. Preoperatively the patient and family should be taught about the precipitating event necessitating the need for the craniotomy and its expected outcome (see the Patient Education feature on Craniotomy). The severity of the disease and the need for critical care management postoperatively must be stressed. As the patient moves toward discharge, teaching focuses on medication instructions, incisional care including the signs of infection, and the signs and symptoms of increased ICP. If the patient has neurologic deficits, teaching focuses on the interventions to maximize the patient's rehabilitation potential, and the patient's family must be encouraged to participate in the patient's care and to learn some basic rehabilitation techniques. In addition, the importance of participating in a neurologic rehabilitation program must be stressed.

INTRACRANIAL HYPERTENSION

Pathophysiology. The intracranial space comprises three components: brain substance (80%), CSF (10%), and blood (10%). Under normal physiologic conditions, the ICP is maintained below 15 mm Hg mean pressure.[8] Essential to understanding the pathophysiology of ICP, the Monro-Kellie hypothesis proposes that an increase in volume of one intracranial component must be compensated by a decrease in one or more of the other components so that total volume remains fixed. This compensation, although limited, includes displacing CSF from the intracranial vault to the lumbar cistern, increasing CSF absorption, and compressing the low-pressure venous system.[66] Pathophysiologic alterations that can elevate ICP are outlined in Table 27-6.

Volume-Pressure Curve. When capable of compliance, the brain can tolerate significant increases in in-

tracranial volume without much increase in ICP. The amount of intracranial compliance, however, does have a limit. Once this limit has been reached, a state of decompensation with increased ICP results. As the ICP rises, the relationship between volume and pressure changes, and small increases in volume may cause major elevations in ICP (Fig. 27-7).[67] The exact configuration of the volume-pressure curve and the point at which the steep rise in pressure occurs vary among patients. The configuration of this curve is also influenced by the cause and the rate of volume increases within the intracranial vault; for example, neurologic deterioration occurs more rapidly in a patient with an acute epidural hematoma than in a patient with a meningioma of the same size.[5] Regardless of how fast the pressure increases, intracranial hypertension occurs when ICP is greater than 20 mm Hg.[67]

Cerebral Blood Flow and Autoregulation. Cerebral blood flow (CBF) corresponds to the metabolic demands of the brain and is normally 50 ml/100 g of brain tissue/min. Although the brain makes up only 2% of body weight, it requires 15% to 20% of the resting cardiac output and 15% of the body's oxygen demands. The normal brain has a complex capacity to maintain constant CBF, despite wide ranges in systemic arterial pressure—an effect known as *autoregulation.* Mean arterial pressure (MAP) of 50 to 150 mm Hg does not alter CBF when au-

Table 27-6	Mechanisms of Intracranial Pressure Elevation	
Pathophysiology	**Example**	**Treatment**
DISORDERS OF CSF SPACE		
Overproduction of CSF	Choroid plexus papilloma	Diuretics, surgical removal
Communicating hydrocephalus from obstructed arachnoid	Old subarachnoid hemorrhage	Surgical drainage from lumbar drain
Noncommunicative hydrocephalus	Posterior fossa tumor obstructing aqueduct	Surgical drainage by ventricular drain
Interstitial edema	Any of above	Surgical drainage of CSF
DISORDERS OF INTRACRANIAL BLOOD		
Intracranial hemorrhage causing increased ICP	Epidural hematoma	Surgical drainage
Vasospasm	Subarachnoid hemorrhage	Hypervolemia and hypertensive therapy
Vasodilation	Elevated $Paco_2$	Hyperventilation
Increasing cerebral blood volume and ICP	Hypoxia	Adequate oxygenation
DISORDERS OF BRAIN SUBSTANCE		
Expanding mass lesion with local vasogenic edema causing increased ICP	Brain tumor	Steroids Surgical removal
Ischemic brain injury with cytotoxic edema increasing ICP	Anoxic brain injury from cardiac or respiratory arrest	Resistant to therapy
Increased cerebral metabolic rate increasing cerebral blood flow and ICP	Seizures, hyperthermia	Anticonvulsant medications to control fever

Modified from Helfaer MA, Kirsch JR: *Crit Care Rep* 1:12, 1989.
CSF, Cerebrospinal fluid; *ICP,* intracranial pressure.

toregulation is present. Outside the limits of this autoregulation, CBF becomes passively dependent on the perfusion pressure.[6]

Factors other than arterial blood pressure that affect CBF are conditions that result in acidosis, alkalosis, and changes in metabolic rate. Conditions that cause acidosis (e.g., hypoxia, hypercapnia, and ischemia) result in cerebrovascular dilation. Conditions causing alkalosis (e.g., hypocapnia) result in cerebrovascular constriction. Normally, a reduction in metabolic rate (e.g., from hypothermia or barbiturates) decreases CBF, and increases in metabolic rate (e.g., from hyperthermia) increase CBF.[68,69]

Arterial blood gases exert a profound effect on CBF. Carbon dioxide, which affects the pH of the blood, is a potent vasoactive substance. Carbon dioxide retention (hypercapnia) leads to cerebral vasodilation, with increased cerebral blood volume, whereas hypocapnia leads to cerebral vasoconstriction and a reduction in cerebral blood volume. Prolonged hypocapnia, however, especially at an arterial partial pressure of carbon dioxide ($PaCO_2$) level lower than 20 mm Hg, can lead to cerebral ischemia. Low arterial partial pressure of oxygen (PaO_2) levels, especially below 40 mm Hg, lead to cerebral vasodilation, which increases the intracranial blood volume and can contribute to increased ICP. High PaO_2 levels have not been shown to affect CBF in either direction.[6,69]

Metabolic activity in the brain significantly influences CBF. Normally, when cerebral metabolic activity increases, CBF also increases to meet the demand. Any pathologic process that decreases CBF could lead to a mismatch between metabolic demand and blood supply, resulting in cerebral ischemia.[68]

Assessment and Diagnosis. The numerous signs and symptoms of increased ICP include decreased level of consciousness, Cushing's triad (bradycardia, systolic hypertension, and bradypnea), diminished brainstem reflexes, papilledema, decerebrate posturing (abnormal extension), decorticate posturing (abnormal flexion), unequal pupil size, projectile vomiting, decreased pupillary reaction to light, altered breathing patterns, and headache.[70] Patients may exhibit one or all of these symptoms, depending on the underlying cause of the elevation in ICP. One of the earliest and most important signs of increased ICP is a decrease in level of consciousness. This change must be reported immediately to the physician.[67]

In the patient with suspected intracranial hypertension, a monitoring device may be placed within the cranium to quantify ICP. Under normal physiologic conditions, ICP is maintained below 15 mm Hg mean pressure. The device is used to monitor serial intracranial pressures and assist with the management of intracranial hypertension. An increase in intracranial pressure can cause a decrease in blood flow to the brain, causing brain damage. The monitoring device can also provide a sterile access for draining excess CSF. The four sites for monitoring ICP are the intraventricular space, the subarachnoid space, the epidural space, and the parenchyma. Each site has advantages and disadvantages for monitoring ICP. The type of monitor chosen depends on both the suspected pathologic condition and physician's preferences.[67,71] See Chapter 26 for further discussion of ICP monitoring.

Medical and Nursing Management. Once intracranial hypertension is documented, therapy must be prompt to prevent secondary insults. Although the exact pressure level denoting intracranial hypertension remains uncertain, most current evidence suggests that ICP generally must be treated when it exceeds 20 mm Hg.[68] All therapies are directed toward reducing the volume of one or more of the components (blood, brain, CSF) that lie within the intracranial vault. A major goal of therapy is to determine the cause of the elevated pressure and, if possible, to remove the cause.[68] In the absence of a surgically treatable mass lesion, intracranial hypertension is treated medically. Nurses play an important role in rapid assessment and implementation of appropriate therapies for reducing ICP (see the Nursing Interventions Classification features on Cerebral Perfusion Promotion and Cerebral Edema Management).

Positioning and Other Nursing Activities. Positioning of the patient is a significant factor in the prevention and treatment of intracranial hypertension. Head elevation has long been advocated as a conventional nursing intervention to control ICP, presumably by in-

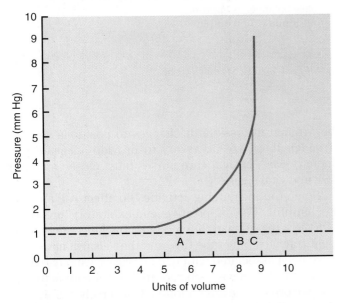

Fig. 27-7 Intracranial volume-pressure curve. *A,* Pressure is normal, and increases in intracranial volume are tolerated without increases in intracranial pressure. *B,* Increases in volume may cause increases in pressure. *C,* Small increases in volume may cause larger increases in pressure.

NIC Cerebral Perfusion Promotion

Definition: Promotion of adequate perfusion and limitation of complications for a patient experiencing or at risk for inadequate cerebral perfusion

Activities

Consult with physician to determine hemodynamic parameters, and maintain hemodynamic parameters within this range

Induce hypertension with volume expansion or intropic or vasoconstrictive agents, as ordered, to maintain hemodynamic parameters and maintain/optimize cerebral perfusion pressure (CPP)

Administer and titrate vasoactive drugs, as ordered, to maintain hemodynamic parameters

Administer agents to expand intravascular volume, as appropriate (e.g., colloid, blood products, and crystalloid)

Administer volume expanders to maintain hemodynamic parameters, as ordered

Monitor prothrombin time (PT) and partial thromboplastin time (PTT), if using hetastarch as a volume expander

Administer rheologic agents (e.g., low-dose mannitol or low–molecular-weight dextrans [LMDs]), as ordered

Keep hematocrit level around 33% for hypervolemic hemodilution therapy

Maintain serum glucose level within normal range

Consult with physician to determine optimal head of bed (HOB) placement (e.g., 0, 15, or 30 degrees) and monitor patient's responses to head positioning

Avoid neck flexion or extreme hip/knee flexion

Keep P_{CO_2} level at 25 mm Hg or greater

Administer calcium channel blockers, as ordered

Administer vasopressin, as ordered

Administer and monitor effects of osmotic and loop-active diuretics and corticosteroids

Administer pain medication, as appropriate

Administer anticoagulant medication, as ordered

Administer antiplatelet medications, as ordered

Administer thrombolytic mediations, as ordered

Monitor patient's prothrombin time (PT) and partial thromboplastin time (PTT) to keep 1 to 2 times normal, as appropriate

Monitor for anticoagulant therapy side effects

Monitor for signs of bleeding (e.g., test stool and nasogastric tube drainage for blood)

Monitor neurologic status

Calculate and monitor cerebral perfusion pressure (CPP)

Monitor patient's ICP and neurologic responses to care activities

Monitor mean arterial pressure (MAP)

Monitor CVP

Monitor pulmonary artery occlusion pressure (PAOP) and pulmonary artery pressure (PAP)

Monitor respiratory status (e.g., rate, rhythm, and depth of respirations; P_{O_2}, P_{CO_2}, pH, and bicarbonate levels)

Auscultate lung sounds for crackles or other adventitious sounds

Monitor for signs of fluid overload (e.g., rhonchi, jugular venous distention [JVD], edema, and increase in pulmonary secretions)

Monitor determinants of tissue oxygen delivery (e.g., Pa_{CO_2}, Sa_{O_2}, and hemoglobin levels and cardiac output), if available

Monitor lab values for changes in oxygenation or acid-base balance, as appropriate

Monitor intake and output

From Dochterman JM, Bulechek GM: *Nursing interventions classification (NIC),* ed 4, 2004, St Louis, Mosby.

creasing venous return. One recent study found that elevation of the bed at least 30 degrees did result in improvement in both ICP and CPP.[72] Other studies have suggested that while elevating the head of the bed does decrease ICP it can also decrease MAP and thus have an overall negative effect on CPP. Therefore the recent trend is to customize the head position to maximize CPP and minimize ICP measurements.[73]

Positions that impede venous return from the brain cause elevations in ICP. Obstruction of jugular veins or an increase in intrathoracic or intraabdominal pressure is communicated as increased pressure throughout the open venous system, thereby impeding drainage from the brain and increasing ICP. Positions that decrease venous return from the head (e.g., Trendelenburg, prone, extreme flexion of the hips, angulation of the neck) must

be avoided if possible. If changes to positions such as Trendelenburg are necessary to provide adequate pulmonary care, critical care nurses must closely monitor ICP and vital signs.[5,14]

Some routine nursing activities do affect ICP and can be harmful. Use of positive end-expiratory pressures (PEEP) greater than 20 cm H_2O, coughing, suctioning, tight tracheostomy tube ties, and the Valsalva maneuver have been associated with ICP increases. Cumulative increases in ICP have been reported when care activities are performed one after another. Conversely, family contact and gentle touch have been associated with decreases in ICP.[5,73,74]

Hyperventilation. Controlled hyperventilation has been an important adjunct of therapy for the patient with increased ICP. The rationale employed in hyperventila-

NIC Cerebral Edema Management

Definition: Limitation of secondary cerebral injury resulting from swelling of brain tissue

Activities

Monitor for confusion, changes in mentation, complaints of dizziness, syncope

Monitor neurologic status closely, and compare with baseline

Monitor vital signs

Monitor CSF drainage characteristics: color, clarity, consistency

Record CSF drainage

Monitor CVP, PAWP, and PAP, as appropriate

Monitor ICP and CPP

Analyze ICP waveform

Monitor respiratory status: rate, rhythm, depth of respirations; PaO_2, PCO_2, pH, bicarbonate levels

Allow ICP to return to baseline between nursing activities

Monitor patient's ICP and neurologic responses to care activities

Decrease stimuli in patient's environment

Plan nursing care to provide rest periods

Give sedation, as needed

Note patient's change in response to stimuli

Screen conversation within patient's hearing

Administer anticonvulsants, as appropriate

Avoid neck flexion or extreme hip/knee flexion

Avoid Valsalva maneuver

Administer stool softeners

Position with head of bed up 30 degrees or greater

Avoid use of PEEP

Administer paralyzing agent, as appropriate

Encourage family/significant other to talk to patient

Restrict fluids

Avoid use of hypotonic IV fluids

Adjust ventilator settings to keep $PaCO_2$ at prescribed level

Limit suction passes to less than 15 seconds

Monitor lab values: serum and urine osmolality, sodium, potassium

Monitor volume pressure indices

Perform passive range of motion exercises

Monitor intake and output

Maintain normothermia

Administer loop-active or osmotic diuretics

Implement seizure precautions

Titrate barbiturate to achieve suppression or burst-suppression of EEG as ordered

Establish means of communication: ask yes or no questions, provides magic slate, paper and pencil, picture board, flashcards, VOCAID device

From Dochterman JM, Bulechek GM: *Nursing interventions classification (NIC)*, ed 4, 2004, St Louis, Mosby.
CPP, Cerebral perfusion pressure; *CSF,* cerebrospinal fluid; *CVP,* central venous pressure; *EEG,* electroencephalogram; *ICP,* intracranial pressure; *IV,* intravenous; *PAP,* pulmonary artery pressure; *PAWP,* pulmonary artery wedge pressure; PEEP, positive end-expiratory pressure.

---

tion is that if the $PaCO_2$ can be reduced from its normal level of 35 to 40 mm Hg to a range of 25 to 30 mm Hg in the patient with intracranial hypertension, vasoconstriction of cerebral arteries, reduction of cerebral blood flow, and increased venous return will result. This practice is currently being reexamined. More and more research has indicated that severe or prolonged hyperventilation can actually reduce cerebral perfusion and lead to cerebral ischemia and infarction. Rather, the trend now is to maintain $PaCO_2$ levels on the lower side of normal (35 ± 2 mm Hg) by carefully monitoring arterial blood gas measurements and by adjusting ventilator settings.[66,75,76]

Although hypoxemia must obviously be avoided, excessively high levels of oxygen offer no benefits. In fact, increasing inspired oxygen concentrations above 60% may lead to toxic changes in lung tissue. The use of pulse oximetry has led to greater awareness of the circumstances, such as pain and anxiety, which can cause oxygen desaturation and therefore elevate ICP.[14,77]

Temperature Control. Directly proportional to body temperature, cerebral metabolic rate increases 7% per degree centigrade of increase in body temperature.[76]

This fact is significant because as the cerebral metabolic rate increases, blood flow to the brain must increase to meet the tissue demands. To avoid the increase in blood volume associated with an increased cerebral metabolic rate, nurses must prevent hyperthermia in the patient with a brain injury. Antipyretics and cooling devices must be used when appropriate while the source of the fever is being determined.[14,76,77]

Conversely, hypothermia reduces cerebral metabolic rate. Research done in patients with severe head injury who were unresponsive to barbiturate therapy for control of intractable intracranial hypertension demonstrated a significant decrease in ICP when subjected to mild hypothermia between 32° C and 35° C.[76]

Blood Pressure Control. Maintenance of arterial blood pressure in the high normal range is essential in the brain-injured patient. Inadequate perfusion pressure decreases the supply of nutrients and oxygen requirements for cerebral metabolic needs. On the other hand, a blood pressure too high increases cerebral blood volume and may increase ICP.[14,76] Fig. 27-8 shows the relationship between blood pressure and ICP.

Control of systemic hypertension may require nothing more than the administration of a sedative agent. Small, frequent doses may be sufficient to blunt noxious stimuli and prevent them from triggering rises in blood pressure. When sedation proves inadequate in controlling systemic arterial hypertension, antihypertensive agents are used. Care must be taken in choosing these agents because many of the peripheral vasodilators (e.g., nitroprusside and nitroglycerin) also are cerebral vasodilators. Still, all antihypertensives are believed to cause some degree of cerebral vasodilation. To reduce this va-

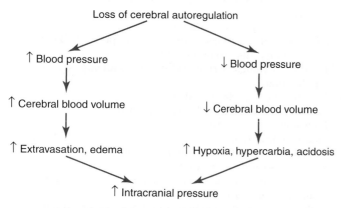

Fig. 27-8 Loss of pressure autoregulation.

sodilating effect, cotreatment with beta-blockers (e.g., metoprolol and labetalol) may be beneficial.[5]

Systemic hypotension should be treated aggressively with fluids to maintain a systolic blood pressure greater than 90 mm Hg.[5] Crystalloids, colloids, and blood products can be used depending on the patient's condition.[74] Recent studies have demonstrated a positive effect on ICP and CPP with hypertonic saline.[78] If fluids fail to adequately elevate the patient's blood pressure, the use of inotropic agents may be necessary[76] (see the Clinical Application feature on Neurologic Concepts for further discussion).

Seizure Control. The incidence of posttraumatic seizures in the head-injured population has been estimated at 5%. Because of the risk of a secondary ischemic insult associated with seizures, many physicians prescribe anticonvulsant medications prophylactically. Seizures cause metabolic requirements to increase, which results in elevation of CBF, cerebral blood volume, and ICP, even in paralyzed patients. If blood flow cannot match demand, ischemia develops, cerebral energy stores are depleted, and irreversible neuronal destruction occurs. The usual anticonvulsant regimen for seizure control includes phenytoin or phenobarbital, or both, in therapeutic doses.[77] Fast-acting, short-duration agents such as lorazepam may be indicated for break-

---

CLINICAL APPLICATION

Neurologic Concepts

Mrs. T is a 66-year-old woman with a medical history of hypertension controlled by diet and medication. While leaving the grocery store, Mrs. T complained of severe headache and collapsed to the floor. An ambulance transported her to the hospital. In the emergency room her initial vital signs are blood pressure (BP) 210/124; heart rate (HR) 98 (normal sinus rhythm with occasional premature ventricular contractions [PVCs]); and respiratory rate (RR) 24 (rhythm regular). Her Glasgow Coma Scale (GCS) score is as follows: Eye Opening, 4; Best Verbal, 4; and Best Motor, 6. Her pupils are round and equal and react briskly to light. No nuchal rigidity is evident, and the motor examination is symmetric. Mrs. T is admitted with the diagnosis of r/o cerebrovascular accident (CVA).

1. Which of Mrs. T's symptoms support the diagnosis of CVA? What are her risk factors?
2. What is the purpose of rating this patient using the GCS? What are the limitations?
3. What is the most likely diagnostic study to be ordered given this patient's presentation and why?
4. Should this patient's blood pressure be treated at this time? Why?

Labetalol 10 mg is administered intravenously as Mrs. T is prepared for an emergency computerized tomography (CT) scan of her head. Her neurologic status rapidly deteriorates, she becomes stuporous and difficult to arouse, and her respirations become irregular. Her pupils are midposition and sluggish in reaction to light. Intubation, oxygenation, and manual hyperventilation are carried out, and she is transported to the CT scanner. The CT scan reveals a subarachnoid hemorrhage (SAH) extending into the ventricles, complicated by acute obstructive hydrocephalus. Mrs. T is immediately transported to the operating room for placement of a ventriculostomy. At the end of the procedure she is transported to the critical care unit. Her GCS is 14.

5. Why was Mrs. T hyperventilated?
6. Based on Mrs. T's CT scan results, what is the advantage of placing a ventriculostomy rather than another type of ICP monitor?
7. What nursing precautions should be part of Mrs. T's plan of care?

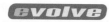 For the discussion and continuation of this Clinical Application, see the Evolve website.

through seizures until therapeutic drug levels can be achieved.

Lidocaine. Various forms of sensory stimulation (e.g., tracheal intubation and endotracheal suctioning) may provoke marked increases in ICP and MAP. One therapy used to prevent cerebral ischemia and acute intracranial hypertension has been the administration of lidocaine through an endotracheal tube or through intravenous infusion before nasotracheal suctioning.[79] Lidocaine is believed to be effective in blunting ICP spikes secondary to tracheal stimulation. Studies have found that peak lidocaine concentrations are linearly related to the administered dose and that the rate of absorption depends on the vascularity of the site of administration.[79] It also has been documented that lidocaine is initially distributed to the lungs, then to the heart and kidneys, and then to muscle and adipose tissue.

Prophylactic administration of lidocaine before endotracheal suctioning is widely practiced. Lidocaine protects the patient from the associated increases in ICP that occur with suctioning. To prevent hypoxemia, suctioning should only be performed if necessary. Suctioning should be preceded with hyperventilation using 100% oxygen, followed by a 10-second pass, and limited to no more than two passes.[80]

Cerebrospinal Fluid Drainage. Cerebrospinal fluid drainage for intracranial hypertension may be used with other treatment modalities. CSF drainage is accomplished by the insertion of a pliable catheter into the anterior horn of the lateral ventricle (ventriculostomy), preferably on the nondominant side. Such drainage can

help support the patient through periods of cerebral edema by controlling spikes in ICP. One of the major advantages of the ventriculostomy is its dual role as both a monitoring device and a treatment modality. Because CSF provides a favorable medium for the development of infection, flawless aseptic technique must be followed during insertion and maintenance of the system. The ventricular system is connected to a drainage bag and is then maintained as a closed system for the period the ventriculostomy remains in place—usually 3 to 5 days (Figs. 27-9 and 27-10).[81]

Diuretics

Osmotic Agents. Clinicians have known for decades that osmotic agents effectively reduce ICP. The mechanism by which these diuretics reduce ICP continues to be a subject of investigational interest. One theory is that these agents act by remaining relatively impermeable to the blood-brain barrier, thereby drawing water from normal brain tissue to plasma. The direction of flow is from the hypoconcentrated tissue to the hyperconcentrated cerebral vasculature. If the situation becomes reversed and the tissue becomes hyperconcentrated in relation to the cerebral vasculature, a rebound phenomenon could

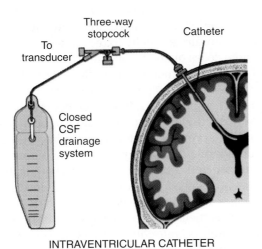

INTRAVENTRICULAR CATHETER

Fig. 27-9 Intermittent drainage system. Intermittent drainage involves draining cerebrospinal fluid (CSF) via a ventriculostomy when intracranial pressure (ICP) exceeds the upper pressure parameter set by the physician. Intermittent drainage involves opening the three-way stopcock to allow CSF to flow into the drainage bag for brief periods (30 to 120 seconds) until the pressure is below the upper pressure parameter. (From Barker E: *Neuroscience nursing*, ed 2, St Louis, 2002, Mosby.)

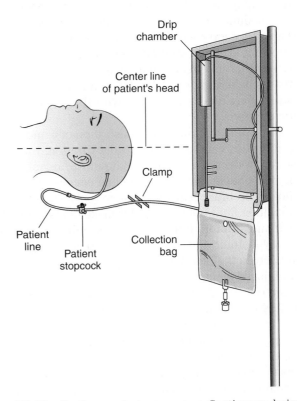

Fig. 27-10 Continuous drainage system. Continuous drainage involves placing the drip chamber of the drainage system at a specified level above the foramen of Monro (usually 15 cm). The system is left open to allow continuous drainage of cerebrospinal fluid (CSF) into the chamber (which drains into a collection bag) against a pressure gradient that prevents excessive drainage and ventricular collapse. (Courtesy Codman/Johnson & Johnson Professional, Inc., Raynham, Mass.)

occur. These agents have little direct effect on edematous cerebral tissue situated in an area of defective blood-brain barrier; instead, they require an intact blood-brain barrier for osmosis to occur.[66,82]

The most widely used osmotic diuretic is mannitol, a large molecule that is retained almost entirely in the extracellular compartment and has little to none of the rebound effect noted with other osmotic diuretics. Mannitol may improve perfusion to ischemic areas of the brain, producing cerebral vasoconstriction and resulting in a reduction of ICP.[66,82]

Perhaps the most common difficulty associated with the use of osmotic agents is the provocation of electrolyte disturbances. Careful attention must be paid to body weight and fluid and electrolyte stability. Serum osmolality must be kept between 300 and 320 mOsm/L. Hypernatremia and hypokalemia often are associated with repeated administration of osmotic agents. Central venous pressure readings must be monitored to prevent hypovolemia. Smaller doses of mannitol simplify fluid and electrolyte management, and their use is encouraged whenever possible.[77,82]

Nonosmotic Agents. Loop diuretics have also been used to decrease ICP. Furosemide, one such nonosmotic diuretic, may act differently from osmotic agents by pulling sodium and water from edematous areas and, perhaps, by decreasing CSF production. One advantage of furosemide administration over the use of osmotic diuretics is that its effect is not generally associated with increases in serum osmolality. Therefore electrolyte imbalances may not be as severe with the use of nonosmotic diuretics.[14,77]

Volume Maintenance. Administration of osmotic and loop diuretics can contribute to dehydration, thus precipitating a decrease in CPP. In the most favorable scenario, the patient is maintained in an euvolemic state to optimize cerebral perfusion. Volume replacement strategies include fluid boluses, fluid replacements, and albumin administration. Intravenous fluids administered are typically isotonic and low in glucose to prevent gradient shifts across the blood-brain barrier in the traumatically brain-injured patient.[74]

Control of Metabolic Demand. Any treatment modality that increases the incidence of noxious stimulation to the patient carries with it the potential for increasing ICP. Such noxious stimuli include pain, the presence of an endotracheal tube, coughing, suctioning, repositioning, bathing, and many other routine nursing interventions. Agents used to reduce metabolic demands include the use of benzodiazepines such as midazolam and lorazepam, intravenous sedative-hypnotics such as propofol, opioid narcotics such as fentanyl and morphine, and neuromuscular blocking agents such as vecuronium and atracurium. These agents may be administered separately or in combination, via continuous drip or as an intravenous bolus on an as-needed basis. The preferred treatment regimen begins with the administration of benzodiazepines for sedation and narcotics for analgesia. If these agents fail to blunt the patient's response to noxious stimuli, propofol and/or a neuromuscular blocking agent is added. The use of these medications is recommended only in patients who have an ICP monitor in place, because sedatives, narcotics, and neuromuscular blocking agents affect the reliability of neurologic assessment. The use of neuromuscular blocking agents without sedation is not recommended because these agents can cause skeletal muscle paralysis and thus have no analgesic effect and do not adequately protect the patient from pain and the physiologic responses that can occur from pain-producing procedures.[74,77] If these agents fail to control the patient's ICP, barbiturate therapy is considered.

Barbiturate Therapy. Barbiturate therapy is a treatment protocol developed for the management of uncontrolled intracranial hypertension that has not responded to the conventional treatments previously described.[66] The two most commonly used drugs in high-dose barbiturate therapy are pentobarbital and thiopental. The goal with either of these drugs is a reduction of ICP to 15 to 20 mm Hg while a MAP of 70 to 80 mm Hg is maintained. Patients are maintained on high-dose barbiturate therapy until ICP has been controlled within the normal range for 24 hours. Barbiturates must never be stopped abruptly but are tapered slowly over approximately 4 days.[5]

Complications of high-dose barbiturate therapy can be disastrous unless a specific and organized approach is used. The most common complications are hypotension, hypothermia, and myocardial depression. If any complications occur and are allowed to persist unchecked, they may cause secondary insults to an already damaged brain. Hypotension, the most common complication, results from peripheral vasodilation and can be compounded in an already dehydrated patient who has received large doses of an osmotic diuretic in an attempt to control ICP. Careful monitoring of fluid status by central venous pressure or a pulmonary artery catheter can help prevent this complication. Myocardial depression results from cardiac muscle suppression and can be avoided by frequent monitoring of fluid status, cardiac output, and serum drug levels. If an adequate cardiac output cannot be maintained in the presence of normothermia, barbiturates must be reduced, regardless of serum levels.[5,66]

The major unresolved issue in the use of high-dose barbiturates is their effect on outcome after head injury. Several laboratory and clinical trials have been undertaken to address this issue. Results of a multicenter randomized trial of barbiturates found that most elevations of ICP could be controlled with aggressive use of standard therapies of ICP management. For the small subset of patients in whom standard therapy fails to achieve ICP control, judicious, carefully monitored and administered high-dose barbiturate therapy is beneficial.[83]

Collaborative management of the patient intracranial hypertension is outlined in Box 27-9.

Box 27-9

COLLABORATIVE MANAGEMENT PRIORITIES

INTRACRANIAL HYPERTENSION
- ✔ Position patient to achieve maximal ICP reduction
- ✔ Reduce environmental stimulation
- ✔ Maintain normothermia
- ✔ Control ventilation to ensure a normal Paco₂ level (35 ± 2 mm Hg)
- ✔ Administer diuretic agents, anticonvulsants, sedation, analgesia, paralytic agents, and vasoactive medications to ensure CPP > 70 mm Hg
- ✔ Drain cerebrospinal fluid for ICP > 20 mm Hg

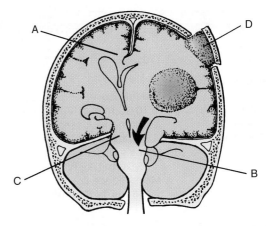

Fig. 27-11 Supratentorial herniation. *A*, Cingulate. *B*, Uncal. *C*, Central. *D*, Transcalvarial.

Herniation Syndromes. The goal of neurologic evaluation, ICP monitoring, and treatment of increased ICP is to prevent herniation. Herniation of intracerebral contents results in the shifting of tissue from one compartment of the brain to another and places pressure on cerebral vessels and vital function centers of the brain. If unchecked, herniation rapidly causes death as a result of the cessation of cerebral blood flow and respirations.

Supratentorial Herniation. The four types of supratentorial herniation syndrome are uncal; central, or transtentorial; cingulate; and transcalvarial (Fig. 27-11).

Uncal Herniation. Uncal herniation is the most often noted herniation syndrome. In uncal herniation, a unilateral, expanding mass lesion, usually of the temporal lobe, increases ICP, causing lateral displacement of the tip of the temporal lobe (uncus). Lateral displacement pushes the uncus over the edge of the tentorium, puts pressure on the oculomotor nerve (cranial nerve III) and the posterior cerebral artery ipsilateral to the lesion, and flattens the midbrain against the opposite side. Clinical manifestations of uncal herniation include ipsilateral pupil dilation, decreased level of consciousness, respiratory pattern changes leading to respiratory arrest, and contralateral hemiplegia leading to decorticate or decerebrate posturing. If no intervention occurs, uncal herniation results in fixed and dilated pupils, flaccidity, and respiratory arrest.[5,84]

Central Herniation. In central, or transtentorial, herniation an expanding mass lesion of the midline, frontal, parietal, or occipital lobes results in downward displacement of the hemispheres, basal ganglia, and diencephalon through the tentorial notch. Central herniation often is preceded by uncal and cingulate herniation. Clinical manifestations of central herniation include loss of consciousness; small, reactive pupils progressing to fixed, dilated pupils; respiratory changes leading to respiratory arrest; and decorticate posturing progressing to flaccidity. In the late stages, uncal and central herniation syndromes affect the brainstem similarly.[5,84]

Cingulate Herniation. Cingulate herniation occurs when an expanding lesion of one hemisphere shifts laterally and forces the cingulate gyrus under the falx cerebri. Cingulate herniation occurs often. Whenever a lateral shift is noted on CT scan, cingulate herniation has occurred. Little is known about the effects of cingulate herniation, and there are no accompanying clinical manifestations that assist in its diagnosis. Cingulate herniation is not in itself life-threatening, but if the expanding mass lesion that caused cingulate herniation is not controlled, uncal or central herniation will follow.[5,84]

Transcalvarial Herniation. Transcalvarial herniation is the extrusion of cerebral tissue through the cranium. In the presence of severe cerebral edema, transcalvarial herniation occurs through an opening from a skull fracture or craniotomy site.[5]

Infratentorial Herniation. The two infratentorial herniation syndromes are upward transtentorial herniation and downward cerebellar herniation.

Upward Transtentorial Herniation. Upward transtentorial herniation occurs when an expanding mass lesion of the cerebellum causes protrusion of the vermis (central area) of the cerebellum and the midbrain upward through the tentorial notch. Compression of the third cranial nerve and diencephalon occurs. Blockage of the central aqueduct and distortion of the third ventricle obstruct CSF flow. Deterioration progresses rapidly.[5,84]

Downward Cerebellar Herniation. Downward cerebellar herniation occurs when an expanding lesion of the cerebellum exerts pressure downward, sending the cerebellar tonsils through the foramen magnum. Compression and displacement of the medulla oblongata occur, rapidly resulting in respiratory and cardiac arrest.[5,84]

PHARMACOLOGIC AGENTS

A number of pharmacologic agents are used in the care of patients with neurologic disorders. The Pharmacologic Management table on Neurologic Disorders reviews the various agents used and any special considerations necessary for administering them.[85,86]

Pharmacologic Management: Neurologic Disorders

DRUG	DOSAGE	ACTIONS	SPECIAL CONSIDERATIONS
Anticonvulsants Phenytoin (Dilantin) Fosphenytoin (Cerebyx)	Loading dose: 10-20 mg/kg IV Maintenance dose: 100 mg q6-8h IV Loading dose: 15-20 mg/kg IV Maintenance dose: 4-6 mg/kg/24h IV	Used to prevent the influx of sodium at the cell membrane	Monitor serum levels closely; therapeutic level is 5-20 mcg/ml **Phenytoin** Infuse no faster than 50 mg/min; administer Dilantin with normal saline only because it precipitates with other solutions **Fosphenytoin** Dosage, concentration, and infusion rate of fosphenytoin is expressed as phenytoin sodium equivalents (FE)
Barbiturates Phenobarbital	Loading dose: 6-8 mg/kg IV Maintenance dose: 1-3 mg/kg/24h IV	Used to produce CNS depression and reduce the spread of an epileptic focus	May depress cardiac and respiratory function **Phenobarbital** Administer at a rate of 60 mg/min; monitor serum level closely; therapeutic level is 20-40 mcg/ml
Pentobarbital	Loading dose: 3-10 mg/kg over 30 min Maintenance dose: 0.5-3 mg/kg/hr IV	Used to induce barbiturate coma	**Pentobarbital** Monitor serum level closely; therapeutic level for coma is 20-40 mcg/ml
Osmotic Diuretics Mannitol	1-2 g/kg IV	Used to treat cerebral edema by pulling fluid from the extravascular space into the intravascular space; requires intact blood-brain barrier	Side effects include hypovolemia and increased serum osmolality Monitor serum osmolality and notify the physician if >310 mOsm/L Warm and shake before administering to ensure crystals are dissolved
Loop Diuretics Furosemide	0.1-2 mg/kg IV	Used to decrease sodium transport within the brain and thereby reduce cerebral edema; may inhibit CSF production	Side effects include hypovolemia and hypokalemia
Calcium Channel Blockers Nimodipine (Nimotop)	60 mg q4h NG or PO for 21 days	Used to decrease cerebral vasospasm	Side effects include hypotension, palpitations, headache, and dizziness Monitor blood pressure frequently when implementing therapy
Local Anesthetics Lidocaine	50-100 mg IV or 2 ml of 4% solution	Used to blunt the effects of tracheal stimulation on intracranial pressure	Must be administered not longer than 5 minutes before suctioning
Thrombolytics Tissue plasminogen activator (tPA)	0.9 mg/kg total with 10% of the dose administered as IV bolus over 1 min and 90% of the dose administered continuous IV infusion over 1 hr	Used to convert plasminogen to plasmin to dissolve clot	Treatment must start within 3 hr of the onset of the symptoms Do not exceed 90 mg Do not use anticoagulants during the first 24 hr Monitor patient for bleeding

CSF, Cerebrospinal fluid; *CNS*, central nervous system; *IV*, intravenous; *NG*, nasogastric; *PO*, by mouth.

REFERENCES

1. Wijdicks EFM: Coma in the critically ill, part 1: causes in medical and surgical patients, *J Crit Illness* 15:603, 2000.
2. Laureys S, Owen AM, Schiff ND: Brain function in coma, vegetative state, and related disorders, *Lancet Neurol* 3:537, 2004.
3. Malik K, Hess DC: Evaluating the comatose patient. Rapid neurologic assessment is key to appropriate management, *Postgrad Med* 111(2):38, 2002.
4. Marx JA et al: *Rosen's emergency medicine: concepts and clinical practice*, ed 5, St Louis, 2002, Mosby.
5. Barker E: *Neuroscience nursing: a spectrum of care*, ed 2, St Louis, 2002, Mosby.
6. Goetz CG: *Textbook of clinical neurology*, ed 2, St Louis, 2003, Elsevier.
7. Berger JR: Clinical approach to stupor and coma. In Bradley WG et al, editors: *Neurology in clinical practice*, ed 3, Boston, 2000, Butterworth Heinemann.
8. McCance KL, Huether SE: *Pathophysiology: the biologic basis for disease in adults and children*, ed 4, St Louis, 2002, Mosby.
9. Wijdicks EFM: Coma in the critically ill, part 2: the transplant patient; management overview, *J Crit Illness* 15:646, 2000.
10. Stubgen JP, Plum F: Evaluation of coma. In Grenvik A et al, editors: *Textbook of critical care*, ed 4, Philadelphia, 2000, Saunders.
11. Jorgensen EO, Holm S: Prediction of neurological outcome after cardiopulmonary resuscitation, *Resuscitation* 41:145, 1999.
12. Cortese D, Capp L, McKinley S: Moisture chamber versus lubrication for the prevention of corneal epithelial breakdown, *Am J Crit Care* 4:425, 1995.
13. American Heart Association: *Heart disease and stroke statistics—2005 update*, Dallas, 2005, The Association.
14. Bader MK, Littlejohns LR: *AANN core curriculum for neuroscience nursing*, ed 4, St Louis, 2004, Elsevier.
15. Thurman RJ, Jauch EC: Acute ischemic stroke: emergent evaluation and management, *Emerg Med Clin North Am* 20:609, 2002.
16. Sacco RL: Newer risk factors for stroke, *Neurology* 57:S31, 2001.
17. Hufnagel A et al: Stroke following chiropractic manipulation of the cervical spine, *J Neurol* 246:683, 1999.
18. Petty GW et al: Rates and predictors of cerebrovascular events among patients with valvular heart disease: a population-based study, *Stroke* 31:279A, 2000.
19. D'avila-Rom'an VG et al: Atherosclerosis of the ascending aorta is an independent predictor of long-term neurologic events and mortality, *J Am Coll Cardiol* 33:1308, 1999.
20. O'Rourke F et al: Current and future concepts in stroke prevention, *CMAJ* 170:1123, 2004.
21. Grau AJ et al: Periodontitis as a risk factor for cerebral ischemia, *Stroke* 31:317A, 2000.
22. Hock NH: Brain attack: the stroke continuum, *Nurs Clin North Am* 34:689, 1999.
23. Samples SD, Krieger DW: Acute ischemic stroke, *Curr Opin Crit Care* 6:77, 2000.
24. Silverman IE, Restrepo L, Mathews G: Poststroke seizures, *Arch Neurol* 59:195, 2002.
25. Wityk RJ, Beauchamp NJ: Diagnostic evaluation of stroke, *Neurol Clin* 18:357, 2000.
26. Becker K: Intensive care unit management of the stroke patient, *Neurol Clin* 18:439, 2000.
27. Adams JP et al: Guidelines for thrombolytic therapy for acute stroke: a supplement to the guidelines for the management of patients with acute ischemic stroke, *Circulation* 94:1167, 1996.
28. Baker WF: Thrombolytic therapy: clinical applications, *Hematol Oncol Clin North Am* 17:283, 2003.
29. Albers GW et al: Antithrombotic and thrombolytic therapy for ischemic stroke: the Seventh ACCP Conference on Antithrombotic and Thrombolytic Therapy, *Chest* 126:483S, 2004.
30. Adams HP: Emergent use of anticoagulation for treatment of patients with ischemic stroke, *Stroke* 33:856, 2002.
31. Hanson SK et al: Should use of tPA for ischemic stroke be restricted to specialized stroke centers? *Stroke* 31:313A, 2000.
32. Mohr JP: Thrombolytic therapy for ischemic stroke: from clinical trials to clinical practice, *JAMA* 283:1189, 2000.
33. Adams HP et al: Guidelines for the early management of patients with acute ischemic stroke. A statement from the Stroke Council of the American Stroke Association, *Stroke* 34:1056, 2003.
34. Swadron SP et al: The acute cerebrovascular event: surgical and other interventional therapies, *Emerg Med Clin North Am* 21:847, 2003.
35. Hickenbottom SL, Barson WG: Acute ischemic stroke therapy, *Neurol Clin* 18:379, 2000.
36. Fahy BG, Sivaraman V: Current concepts in neurocritical care, *Anesthesiol Clin North Am* 20:441, 2002.
37. Vega C, Kwoon JV, Lavine SD: Intracranial aneurysms: current evidence and clinical practice, *Am Fam Physician* 66:601, 2002.
38. Manno EM: Subarachnoid hemorrhage, *Neurol Clin* 22:347, 2004.
39. Mayberg MR et al: Guidelines for the management of aneurysmal subarachnoid hemorrhage: a statement for healthcare professionals from a special writing group of the Stroke Council, American Heart Association, *Circulation* 25:2315, 1994.
40. Shpritz DW: Neurodiagnostic studies, *Nurs Clin North Am* 34:593, 1999.
41. Hunt WE, Hess RM: Surgical risks as related to time of intervention in the repair of intracranial aneurysms, *J Neurosurg* 28:14, 1968.
42. Solenski NJ et al: Medical complications of aneurysmal subarachnoid hemorrhage: a report of the multicenter, cooperative aneurysm study, *Crit Care Med* 23:1007, 1995.
43. Classen J et al: Effect of acute physiologic derangements on outcome after subarachnoid hemorrhage, *Crit Care Med* 32:832, 2004.
44. Lefevre F, Woolger JM: Surgery in the patient with neurologic disease, *Med Clin North Am* 87:257, 2003.
45. Oyama K, Criddle L: Vasospasm after aneurysmal subarachnoid hemorrhage, *Crit Care Nurse* 24(5):58, 2004.
46. Bendo AA: Intracranial vascular surgery, *Anesthesiol Clin North Am* 20:377, 2002.
47. Treggiari-Venzi MM, Suter PM, Romand JA: Review of medical prevention of vasospasm after aneurysmal subarachnoid hemorrhage: a problem of neurointensive care, *Neurosurgery* 48:249, 2001.
48. Finfer SR, Ferch R, Morgan MK: Barbiturate coma for severe, refractory vasospasm following subarachnoid hemorrhage, *Intensive Care Med* 25:406, 1999.
49. Thomas JE, Rosenwasser RH: Reversal of severe cerebral vasospasm in three patients after aneurysmal subarachnoid hemorrhage: initial observations regarding the use of intraventricular sodium nitroprusside in humans, *Neurosurgery* 44:48, 1999.
50. Sen J et al: Triple-H therapy in the management of aneurysmal subarachnoid haemorrhage, *Lancet Neurol* 2:614, 2003.

51. Fahy BG, Sivaraman V: Current concepts in neurocritical care, *Anesthesiol Clin North Am* 20:441, 2002.

52. Gebel JM, Broderick JP: Intracerebral hemorrhage, *Neurol Clin* 18:419, 2000.

53. Broderick JP et al: Guidelines for the management of spontaneous intracerebral hemorrhage, *Stroke* 30:905, 1999.

54. Panagos PD, Jauch EC, Broderick JP: Intracerebral hemorrhage, *Emerg Med Clin North Am* 20:631, 2002.

55. Chitnis T, Khoury SJ: Immunologic neuromuscular disorders, *J Allergy Clin Immunol* 111:S659, 2003.

56. Newswanger DL, Warren CR: Guillain-Barré syndrome, *Am Fam Physician* 69:2405, 2004.

57. Keenlyside R, Brezman D: Fatal Guillain-Barré syndrome after the national influenza immunization program, *Neurology* 30:929, 1980.

58. Marinelli WA, Leatherman JW: Neuromuscular disorders in the intensive care unit, *Crit Care Clin* 18:915, 2002.

59. Hughes RA et al: Intravenous immunoglobulin for Guillain-Barré syndrome, *Cochrane Database Syst Rev* CD002063, 2004.

60. Kihara M et al: A dysautonomia case of Guillain-Barré syndrome with recovery: monitored by composite autonomic scoring scale, *J Auton Nerv Syst* 73:186, 1998.

61. Pfeiffer G et al: Indicators of dysautonomia in severe Guillain-Barré syndrome, *J Neurol* 246:1015, 1999.

62. Rothrock JC: *Alexander's care of the patient in surgery,* ed 12, St Louis, 2003, Mosby.

63. Vance ML: Perioperative management of patients undergoing pituitary surgery, *Endocrinol Metab Clin North Am* 32:355, 2003.

64. Valladeres JB, Hankinson J: Incidence of lower extremity deep vein thrombosis in neurosurgical patients, *Neurosurgery* 6:138, 1980.

65. Warbel A, Lewicki L, Lupica K: Venous thromboembolism: risk factors in the craniotomy patient population, *J Neurosci Nurs* 31:180, 1999.

66. Allen CH, Ward JD: An evidenced-based approach to management of increased intracranial pressure, *Crit Care Clin* 14:485, 1998.

67. Arbour R: Intracranial hypertension: monitoring and nursing assessment, *Crit Care Nurse* 24(5):19, 2004.

68. Cunning S, Houdek L: Preventing secondary brain injuries, *Dimen Crit Care Nurs* 18(5):20, 1999.

69. Vavilala MS, Lee LA, Lam AM: Cerebral blood flow and vascular physiology, *Anesthesiol Clin North Am* 20:247, 2002.

70. Wall BM, Philips JP, Howard JC: Validation of increased intracranial pressure and high risk for increased intracranial pressure, *Nurs Diag* 5:74, 1994.

71. American Association of Neuroscience Nurses: *Clinical guideline series: intracranial pressure monitoring,* Chicago, 1997, The Association.

72. Winkleman C: Effect of backrest position on intracranial and cerebral perfusion pressures in traumatically brain-injured adults, *Am J Crit Care* 9:373, 2000.

73. Simmons BJ: Management of intracranial hemodynamics in the adult: a research analysis of head positioning and recommendations for clinical practice and future research, *J Neurosci Nurs* 29:44, 1997.

74. Bader MK, Palmer S: Keeping the brain in the zone: applying the severe head injury guidelines to practice, *Crit Care Nurs Clin North Am* 12:413, 2000.

75. Coles JP et al: Effect of hyperventilation on cerebral blood flow in traumatic head injury: clinical relevance and monitoring correlates, *Crit Care Med* 30:1950, 2002.

76. Wong FWH: Prevention of secondary brain injury, *Crit Care Nurse* 20(5):18, 2000.

77. Arbour R: Aggressive management of intracranial dynamics, *Crit Care Nurse* 18(3):30, 1998.

78. Qureshi AI, Suarez JI: Use of hypertonic saline solutions in treatment of cerebral edema and intracranial hypertension, *Crit Care Med* 28:3301, 2000.

79. Brucia JJ, Owen DC, Rudy EB: The effects of lidocaine on intracranial hypertension, *J Neurosci Nurs* 24:205, 1992.

80. Kerr M et al: Head-injured adults: recommendations for endotracheal suctioning, *J Neurosci Nurs* 25:86, 1993.

81. Cummings R: Understanding ventricular drainage, *J Neurosci Nurs* 24:84, 1992.

82. Paczynski RP: Osmotherapy: basic concepts and controversies, *Crit Care Clin* 13:105, 1997.

83. Lee M et al: The efficacy of barbiturate coma in the management of uncontrolled intracranial hypertension following neurosurgical trauma, *J Neurotrauma* 11(3):325, 1994.

84. Morrison CAM: Brain herniation syndromes, *Crit Care Nurs* 7(5):34, 1987.

85. Gahart BL, Nazareno AR: *2005 Intravenous medications,* ed 21, St Louis, 2005, Mosby.

86. Stewart-Amidel C: Pharmacology advances in the neuroscience intensive care unit, *Crit Care Nurs Clin North Am* 14:31, 2002.

RENAL
ALTERATIONS

CHAPTER
28

Renal Anatomy and Physiology

The kidneys are complex organs responsible for numerous functions and substances necessary to maintain homeostasis. The primary roles of the kidneys are to remove metabolic wastes, maintain fluid and electrolyte balance, and help achieve acid-base balance. However, the kidneys also have an important role in blood pressure control, red blood cell synthesis, and bone metabolism. Without adequate kidney function, balance in all of these functions and therefore homeostasis is affected.

The purpose of this chapter is to provide an overview of the anatomy and physiologic processes of the kidneys. An understanding of normal kidney function is essential to understanding the pathophysiology, symptoms, and therapeutic management of kidney disease and failure.

MACROSCOPIC ANATOMY

The kidneys are paired organs located retroperitoneally, one on each side of the vertebral column between T12 and L3, with the right kidney slightly lower than the left because of the presence of the liver. The kidneys measure approximately 12 cm long, 6 cm wide, and 2.5 cm thick in the adult and weigh about 120 grams.[1] The kidneys are protected anteriorly and posteriorly by the rib cage and by a tough fibrous capsule that encloses each kidney. Additional protection is provided by a cushion of perirenal fat and the support of the renal fascia.[1]

Internally the kidneys are made up of two distinct areas: the cortex and the medulla. The cortex is the outer layer and contains the glomeruli, the proximal tubules, the cortical portions of the loops of Henle, the distal tubules, and the cortical collecting ducts.[2,3] The medulla is the inner layer, made up of the renal pyramids, which contain the medullary portions of the loops of Henle, the vasa recta, and the medullary portions of the collecting ducts. Numerous pyramids taper and join to form a minor calyx; several minor calyces join to form a major calyx. The major calyces then join and enter the funnel-shaped renal pelvis, a 5- to 10-ml conduit that directs urine into the ureter (Fig. 28-1).[1-3]

The renal system also includes the urinary drainage system—the ureters, bladder, and urethra (Fig. 28-2). The ureters are fibromuscular tubes that exit the central part of the renal pelvis and enter the urinary bladder at an oblique angle. As urine is formed by the kidneys, the urine flows through the ureters by peristalsis. The peristaltic action of the ureters and the angle at which the ureters enter the bladder help prevent reflux of urine from the bladder back up into the kidneys. The bladder is a muscular sac within the pelvis and has a capacity of 280 to 500 ml.[1] Urine leaves the bladder through the urethral orifice and is excreted from the body via the urethra. In the male the urethra is about 20 cm long; in the female the urethra is 3 to 5 cm long.[3]

VASCULAR ANATOMY

The kidneys are highly vascular and receive 20% to 25% of the cardiac output—about 1200 ml/minute. Blood enters the kidneys through the renal arteries, which branch bilaterally from the abdominal aorta. The renal artery divides into arterial branches that become progressively smaller vessels, eventually ending with the afferent arterioles.[1,3] A single afferent arteriole supplies blood to each glomerulus, a tuft of capillaries that is the first structure of the nephron, the functional unit of the kidneys.

Blood exits the glomerulus by the efferent arteriole, which divides into the vasa recta and the peritubular capillaries. The vasa recta extends into the medulla to supply the long medullary loops of Henle; the peritubular capillaries provide blood to the cortical portions of the nephron tubules. The intricate capillary network maintains the intracapillary pressure that allows water and solutes to move between the tubules and the capillaries for urine formation and the concentration and dilution of urine.[1] The capillaries then rejoin the gradually enlarging venous vessels until the blood finally leaves each kidney through the renal vein and returns to the general circulation by the inferior vena cava.

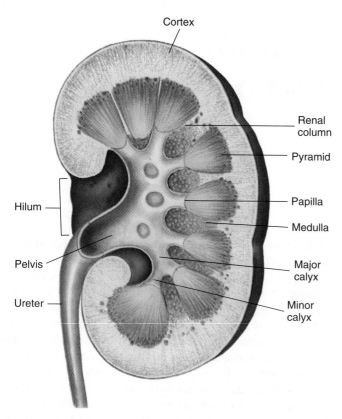

Fig. 28-1   Cross-section of the kidney. (From Thompson JM et al: *Mosby's clinical nursing,* ed 5, St Louis, 2002, Mosby.)

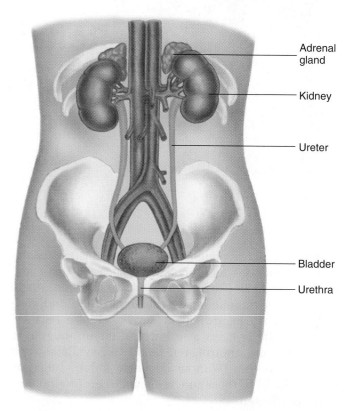

Fig. 28-2   Structures of the urinary system. (From Thompson JM et al: *Mosby's clinical nursing,* ed 5, St Louis, 2002, Mosby.)

MICROSCOPIC STRUCTURE AND FUNCTION

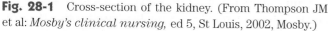

Each kidney is made up of about one million nephrons, the functional units of the kidneys. Due to the vast number of nephrons, the kidneys can continue to function even when several thousand nephrons are damaged or destroyed by disease or injury. Each nephron has the ability to perform all of the individual functions of the kidneys. The nephron is made up of several distinct structures: the glomerulus, Bowman's capsule, the proximal convoluted tubule, the loop of Henle, the distal convoluted tubule, and the collecting duct (Fig. 28-3).

Two types of nephrons make up each kidney: the cortical nephrons and the juxtamedullary nephrons.[1,3,4] Approximately 85% of the nephrons are cortical nephrons, and are either superficial or midcortical nephrons.[1] The superficial cortical nephrons have glomeruli located in the outer cortex and have short loops of Henle. The midcortical nephrons are located lower in the cortex and have loops of Henle that may be short or long. Both types of cortical nephrons perform excretory and regulatory functions. The remaining 15% of the nephrons are juxtamedullary nephrons with glomeruli located deep in the cortex and extending into the medullary layer of the kidney. The juxtamedullary nephrons have long loops of Henle that have an important role in the concentration and dilution of urine.[1,3,4] The vasa recta structures of the juxtamedullary nephrons maintain the concentration gradient that concentrates the urine.

GLOMERULUS

The first structure of each nephron is the glomerulus, a high-pressure capillary bed that serves as the filtering point for the blood. Positive filtration pressure in the glomerulus is achieved as a result of the high arterial pressure as the blood enters the afferent arteriole and the resistance created by the smaller efferent arteriole as the blood exits the glomerulus. As a result of the positive-pressure gradient, fluid and solutes are filtered through the glomerular capillary walls. The glomerulus has 3 layers: the endothelium, the basement membrane, and the epithelium.[1] The inner endothelial layer lines the glomerulus and contains numerous pores that allow filtration of fluid and small solutes from the blood. The middle basement membrane layer also controls filtration according to the size, the electrical charge, the protein-binding capability, and the shape of the molecules.[1] Large molecules such as albumin and red blood cells are prevented from entering the filtrate. The presence of large molecules in the urine is a signal that the glomeru-

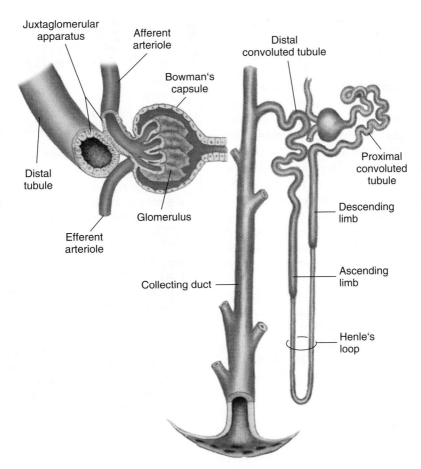

Fig. 28-3   Components of the nephron. (From Thompson JM et al: *Mosby's clinical nursing*, ed 5, St Louis, 2002, Mosby.)

lar membrane is damaged or affected by disease. Finally, the outer epithelium layer contains pores that allow the filtered blood, or filtrate, into Bowman's space.

BOWMAN'S CAPSULE

The filtrate (often called the *ultrafiltrate*) enters Bowman's space, which is surrounded by Bowman's capsule, a tough, membranous layer of epithelial cells that completely surrounds the glomerular capillary bed. Bowman's space is located between the capillary walls of the glomerulus and the inner layer of Bowman's capsule and is a small holding area for the initial filtrate from the blood. Fluid, solutes, and other substances filtered by the glomerulus collect in the space. The holding space connects with the first portion of the nephron's tubular system—the proximal convoluted tubule.[1]

PROXIMAL CONVOLUTED TUBULE

The proximal convoluted tubule is located in the cortex of the kidney and has a large surface area available for solute and fluid transportation.[1,3] The proximal tubule resorbs most of the filtered water and sodium and many

of the solutes the body does not routinely excrete in the urine. Solutes that are usually resorbed include all of the glucose and amino acids, some of the water-soluble vitamins, the majority of phosphate and bicarbonate, and much of the potassium, chloride, and calcium that is filtered by the glomerulus. Creatinine is not resorbed and is thus excreted in the urine. In addition to a major role in resorbing water and solutes from the filtrate, the proximal convoluted tubule also secretes organic anions and cations into the tubular lumen. Due to the presence of the large amount of solutes in the filtrate created by the glomerulus, the fluid that enters the proximal tubule is hyperosmotic. When the filtrate leaves the proximal tubule and enters the loop of Henle, it is isosmotic (equivalent to plasma) as a result of the resorption of both solutes and water.[1]

LOOP OF HENLE

After selective resorption in the proximal convoluted tubule, the isosmotic filtrate enters the loop of Henle. The loop of Henle consists of a thin descending limb, a thin ascending limb, and a thick ascending limb.[1,3] As noted previously, there are two types of nephrons: the cortical nephrons with short loops of Henle and the juxtamedullary nephrons with long loops of Henle. The nephrons with short loops of Henle do not have a thin ascending limb.[1] As a result, the cortical nephrons perform excretory and regulatory functions but play a minor role in the concentration or dilution of urine. The juxtamedullary nephrons have glomeruli that are next to (juxtaposed to) the medulla near where the cortex and medulla sections of the kidney join and contain a thin ascending limb.[1] As a result, these nephrons are critical for concentrating and diluting the urine by means of the countercurrent mechanism. The thin descending limb is very permeable to water but fairly impermeable to urea, sodium, and other solutes. As a result, water is resorbed back into the general circulation and a more concentrated filtrate is produced. The filtrate then moves up the thin ascending limb, which is impermeable to water but allows movement of sodium, chloride, and urea. Finally, the thick ascending limb is also impermeable to water but allows resorption of sodium, chloride, potassium, calcium, and bicarbonate. Due to the low water and high solute resorption in the loop of Henle, the filtrate leaves the ascending limb hypoosmotic (more dilute than plasma).[1]

DISTAL CONVOLUTED TUBULE

The hypoosmotic filtrate enters the distal convoluted tubule located in the cortex of the kidney. The first portion of the distal tubule contains the cells of the macula densa—specialized cells that are a component of the juxtaglomerular apparatus important in blood pressure control. The first section of the distal tubule is impermeable to water and transports solutes such as sodium, bicarbonate, calcium, and potassium.[1,3] The later section of the distal tubule further regulates sodium, bicarbonate, potassium, and calcium according to hormonal influences and acid-base and electrolyte balance needs of the body. The permeability of the late distal tubule is influenced by antidiuretic hormone (ADH). In the presence of ADH the late distal tubule is impermeable to water but resorbs some solutes, and the filtrate remains hypoosmotic. In the absence of ADH, the late distal tubule is more permeable to water, and the filtrate may become isosmotic.

COLLECTING DUCT

Several distal tubules join to form a collecting duct that begins in the cortex and extends through the medulla to empty into the papilla.[1] The final composition of the urine occurs in the collecting duct, primarily because of the transport of potassium, sodium, and water. Water permeability is again determined by the absence or presence of ADH.[3] In the absence of or with small amounts of ADH, the urine will be dilute, whereas larger amounts

---

Box 28-1

TUBULAR RESORPTION AND SECRETION

GLOMERULUS
- Filters fluid and solutes from blood

PROXIMAL CONVOLUTED TUBULE
- Resorbs Na^+, K^+, Cl^-, HCO_3^-, urea, glucose, amino acids
- Filtrate leaves isosmotic

LOOP OF HENLE
- Resorbs Na^+, K^+, CL^-
- Blocks resorption of H_2O from ascending limb
- Countercurrent mechanism dilutes/concentrates urine
- Filtrate leaves hypoosmotic

DISTAL TUBULE
- Na^+, K^+, Ca^{++}, PO_4 selectively resorbed
- H_2O resorbed in presence of ADH
- Na^+ resorbed in presence of aldosterone
- Filtrate leaves hypoosmotic

COLLECTING DUCT
- Resorption similar to that in distal tubule
- H_2O resorbed in presence of ADH
- HCO_3^- and H^+ resorbed/secreted to acidify urine
- Filtrate leaves hyperosmotic or hypoosmotic, depending on body needs

---

of ADH will result in a concentrated urine. The filtrate is generally more concentrated when it leaves the collecting duct than it was when it entered. Acidification of the urine is accomplished by the transport of bicarbonate and hydrogen in the collecting duct. Several collecting ducts then combine to form the pyramids. After the urine leaves the collecting ducts, no change in the composition of the filtrate occurs. Box 28-1 summarizes tubular resorption and secretion in the various structures of the nephron.[1,3]

NERVOUS SYSTEM INNERVATION

The autonomic nervous system provides the primary innervation to the kidneys and the urinary drainage system. The kidneys receive messages from the lowest splanchnic and inferior splanchnic nerves, which form the renal plexus. The inferior mesenteric plexus, the hypogastric plexus, and the pudic nerve from the sacral region serve the urinary bladder, the ureters, and the urethra.[5]

Nervous system control in the urinary tract is reflected in the process of micturition, or the release of urine. Bladder fullness stimulates stretch receptors in the bladder wall and a portion of the urethra. Signals are carried through nerves in the sacral area and return as parasympathetic messages to contract the detrusor muscle of the bladder. With a full bladder, contractions usually are powerful enough to relax the external sphincter. Sympathetic stimulation returns the external sphincter to contraction after the urine is released. The cerebral cortex and brain stem portions of the central nervous system also exert control over the urinary bladder. The central nervous system regulates the micturition reflex, frequency, and external sphincter tone and allows conscious control over release of urine from the bladder.[5]

PROCESSES OF URINE FORMATION

The nephrons are responsible for removing unwanted metabolic substances and wastes from the blood and retaining essential electrolytes and water as needed by the body. The entire blood volume of an individual is filtered by the kidneys 60 to 70 times each day, resulting in about 180 L of filtrate.[1] The glomerular filtration rate (GFR), or the amount of filtrate formed in the nephrons, is therefore about 125 ml/minute. The kidneys must reduce the 180 L of filtrate to an average of 1 to 2 L of urine per day. Thus, although 180 L of filtrate is formed, 99% of it is resorbed and only 1% is excreted as urine. The three processes necessary for changing the 180 L of filtrate into 1 to 2 L of urine are glomerular filtration, tubular resorption, and tubular secretion.[1,3,4]

GLOMERULAR FILTRATION

The first process in urine formation, glomerular filtration, depends on glomerular blood flow, the pressure in Bowman's space, and plasma oncotic pressure.[3,4,6] Glomerular blood flow is the most important of these three factors and is maintained through an intrarenal autoregulatory mechanism.[7] The autoregulatory mechanism (ARM) maintains a consistent renal blood flow and perfusion at a constant level as long as the mean arterial pressure remains between 80 and 100 mm Hg. The ARM is maintained by the afferent and efferent arterioles of the glomeruli, which have the ability to increase or decrease the glomerular blood flow rate through selective dilation and/or constriction.[7] When the mean arterial blood pressure is decreased, the afferent arteriole dilates and the efferent arteriole constricts to maintain a higher pressure in the glomerular capillary bed and maintain the GFR at 125 ml/minute. The ability of the kidneys to autoregulate blood flow fails when the mean arterial blood pressure is less than 80 mm Hg or greater than 180 mm Hg.[4,7]

The second factor that influences the GFR is the pressure in Bowman's space. An increase in pressure in this space will decrease filtration because the increased pressure resists the movement of solutes and water from the capillaries into the space. For example, if the tubules of the nephrons are blocked by cellular debris, backward pressure is exerted on Bowman's space, the

GFR drops below 125 ml/minute, and a decreased urine output results.

The final factor that influences GFR is plasma oncotic pressure. When the oncotic pressure in the blood is decreased (as in disease states that result in low plasma protein levels), pressure in the glomerular capillary bed is decreased. Therefore, although the mean arterial pressure in the glomerulus favors filtration, decreased amounts of fluid and solutes will leave the capillaries and enter Bowman's space because the oncotic pressure gradient in the plasma that encourages movement of fluid and solutes out of the plasma is less favorable. Filtration will still occur, but it is decreased from the normal 125 ml/minute, resulting in a decrease in the amount of filtrate and therefore urine.

The status of the glomerular filtration system is assessed by measuring the GFR. Creatinine is used as a measure of the GFR because it is a waste product produced at a fairly constant rate by the muscles, is freely filtered by the glomerulus, and is not resorbed or secreted by the tubules.[8] Therefore most of the creatinine produced by the body is excreted by the kidneys, making the creatinine clearance a good screening and follow-up test for estimating the GFR. In general, the creatinine clearance mirrors the GFR, so that a normal creatinine clearance is approximately 125 ml/minute. A creatinine clearance less than 100 ml/minute reflects a GFR of less than 100 ml/minute and is a signal of decreased kidney function. A creatinine clearance (and GFR) less than 20 ml/minute results in symptoms of kidney failure.[8]

TUBULAR RESORPTION

The second process in the formation of urine is tubular resorption—the movement of a substance from the tubular lumen (filtrate) into the peritubular capillaries (blood).[1] Tubular resorption allows the 180 L of solutes and water filtered by the glomerulus to be taken back into the circulation, decreasing the 180 L of filtrate to 1 to 2 L of urine per day. The majority of tubular resorption takes place in the proximal convoluted tubule and occurs by both passive and active transport processes.[1,3,4]

Passive Transport. Passive transport of substances in the tubule depends on changes in concentration gradients and does not require energy. Diffusion and osmosis are the primary passive transport processes in the nephrons.[1] Diffusion is the spontaneous movement of molecules/solutes from an area of higher concentration to an area of lower concentration across a semipermeable membrane ("semi" permeable because not all substances will cross, primarily because of the large size of a molecule). For example, when water is reabsorbed by the tubules, the concentration of urea in the tubules is increased. Urea then diffuses across the semipermeable membrane of the tubule and reenters the plasma to achieve balance in the concentration gradient.

Osmosis is the movement of water from an area of lower solute concentration to an area of higher solute concentration. Osmosis occurs any time the concentration of solutes on one side of a semipermeable membrane is greater than the concentration of solutes on the other side of the membrane. For example, when the concentration of sodium is greater in the peritubular capillaries than in the tubules, water passively moves from the tubules into the capillaries to balance the concentration gradient.

Active Transport. Active transport of substances into or out of the tubules requires substances to move against an electro-chemical gradient and takes energy in the form of adenosine triphosphate (ATP).[1,3] In active transport the substance combines with a carrier and then diffuses across the semipermeable tubular membrane. Substances that are actively resorbed include glucose, amino acids, calcium, potassium, and sodium. The rate at which substances can be actively resorbed depends on the availability of the carriers, saturation of the carriers, and availability of energy. The transport maximum refers to the maximum rate at which substances can be resorbed and varies according to each individual substance.[3]

The threshold concentration of a substance is also important in active transport. The threshold of a substance is the plasma level of a substance at which none of the substance appears in the urine.[3] When the threshold of a substance in the plasma is exceeded, progressively larger amounts of the substance appear in the urine because the large amounts cannot be resorbed. For example, the threshold concentration for glucose is about 180 mg/dl. At or below a plasma glucose concentration of 180 mg/dl, all glucose is actively resorbed from the tubules back into the circulation and none is excreted in the urine. When the plasma glucose concentration is above 180 mg/dl, the threshold concentration is exceeded, and some of the glucose cannot be resorbed from the tubules and is excreted in the urine.[9]

TUBULAR SECRETION

The third process in urine formation is tubular secretion, the transport of substances from the peritubular capillaries into the lumen of the tubules.[1] Tubular secretion allows the body to remove excess substances; it occurs by both diffusion and active transport and depends on the needs of the body. For example, potassium, hydrogen, and drugs/drug metabolites are secreted into the tubules to decrease their concentration in the body. Tubular secretion plays a lesser role than tubular resorption in changing the filtrate into urine.

FUNCTIONS OF THE KIDNEYS

The formation of urine through the processes just described is a major function of the kidneys. The kidneys are also responsible for a number of other functions essential to maintaining homeostasis. These additional functions include the elimination of metabolic wastes, blood pressure regulation, the regulation of erythrocyte production, the activation of vitamin D, prostaglandin synthesis, acid-base balance, and fluid-electrolyte balance.[2,3]

ELIMINATION OF METABOLIC WASTES

Metabolic processes in the body produce waste products that are selectively filtered out of the circulation by the kidneys. Urea, uric acid, and creatinine are by-products of protein metabolism that the kidneys filter out of the circulation and excrete in the urine. In addition, metabolic acids (e.g., ammonia), bilirubin, and drug metabolites are also eliminated as waste products.[3]

Urea. Urea and creatinine are the primary waste products that are measured in determining kidney function. Urea is measured as blood urea nitrogen (BUN) and is the end product of protein metabolism and results from the breakdown of ammonia in the liver. The level of urea in the blood is influenced by protein breakdown, the amount of protein in the diet, fluid volume, and excretion from the kidneys.[8] The body forms approximately 25 to 28 g of urea per day.[2] More urea is formed if protein intake is high or if the individual is in a catabolic state and is breaking down body protein stores. Urea is primarily excreted in the urine and will therefore accumulate if the glomerulus is unable to filter it from the blood.

Creatinine. Creatinine is an end product of protein metabolism produced by the muscles. Creatinine is normally completely filtered by the kidneys and excreted in the urine. As a result, the level of creatinine in the blood provides an indicator of kidney function.

BLOOD PRESSURE REGULATION

The kidneys regulate arterial blood pressure by maintaining the circulating blood volume by means of fluid balance and by altering peripheral vascular resistance via the renin-angiotensin-aldosterone system. Regulation by the renin-angiotensin-aldosterone system occurs in the juxtaglomerular apparatus (JGA), a group of specialized cells located around the afferent arteriole where the distal convoluted tubule and afferent arteriole make contact (see Fig. 28-3). This group of specialized cells is called the *macula densa* and provides a feedback message system from the distal tubule to control blood flow through the afferent arteriole.[3,7] An increase in tubular filtrate in the macula densa causes the afferent arteriole to constrict and therefore decrease the GFR and the amount of filtrate. Conversely, a decrease in the amount of tubular filtrate results in afferent arteriole dilation, an increased GFR, and an increased amount of filtrate.

The JGA synthesizes, stores, and releases renin.[3] Renin is released in response to reduced pressure in the glomerulus, sympathetic stimulation of the kidneys, and a decrease in the amount of sodium in the distal convoluted tubule.[7] Renin enters the lumen of the afferent arteriole and is released into the general circulation. Renin is then converted to angiotensin I, which is further converted to angiotensin II as the blood circulates through the lungs. Angiotensin II is an active compound that causes both afferent and efferent arteriole vasoconstriction, resulting in an increased vascular resistance, and therefore maintains hydrostatic pressure within the kidneys.[7] A powerful vasoconstrictor, angiotensin II also causes increased systemic vascular resistance and therefore increased arterial blood pressure.

Angiotensin II also stimulates the release of aldosterone by the adrenal cortex. Aldosterone acts on the distal tubule to facilitate sodium and water resorption, resulting in an expanded circulating blood volume and increased blood pressure. When the arterial blood pressure increases, the JGA stops releasing renin and the renin-angiotensin-aldosterone system (RAAS) is no longer in effect. Fig. 28-4 summarizes the major aspects of the renin-angiotensin-aldosterone mechanism.

ERYTHROCYTE PRODUCTION

The kidneys secrete erythropoietin, the hormone that controls erythrocyte (red blood cell) production in the bone marrow. Erythropoietin is released in response to a decrease in the amount of oxygen delivered to the kidneys, such as in anemia or prolonged hypoxia.[10] The hormone remains active for about 24 hours after release and stimulates the bone marrow to increase the production of erythrocytes. The absence of erythropoietin, which occurs in individuals with kidney failure, results in a profound anemia that is treated by administering synthetic erythropoietin or by blood transfusion therapy.

VITAMIN D ACTIVATION

The kidneys convert vitamin D from food sources into an active form for use by the body. Active vitamin D stimulates the absorption of calcium by the intestine and resorption of calcium by the tubules so that calcium is available for bone and tooth metabolism and blood clotting functions.[10] When the kidneys fail, the body is unable to convert dietary vitamin D to its active form, calcium is poorly absorbed, and bone disease results.

PROSTAGLANDIN SYNTHESIS

Prostaglandins are vasoactive substances that dilate or constrict the arteries. The kidney produces two vasodilatory protaglandins (PGs): E and I. These are typically abbreviated PGE_1 and PGI_2. The prostaglandins produced by the kidneys produce only local renal blood flow effects and have minimal, if any, systemic effects.[7,10] The primary prostaglandins produced by the kidneys are the vasodilators PGE_1 and PGI_2, which act on the afferent arteriole to maintain blood flow and glomerular perfusion and filtration. The vasodilating effects of the prostaglandins also counteract the effects of angiotensin II and the sympathetic nervous system on the kidneys and maintain renal blood flow despite systemic vasoconstriction.[7] Other prostagladins that may impact kidney function include PGF_2, which contributes to vasoconstriction in times of volume depletion. See Box 28-2 for the effects of prostaglandins.

ACID-BASE BALANCE

The kidneys are actively involved in acid-base regulation by resorbing or excreting acids and bases in the kidney

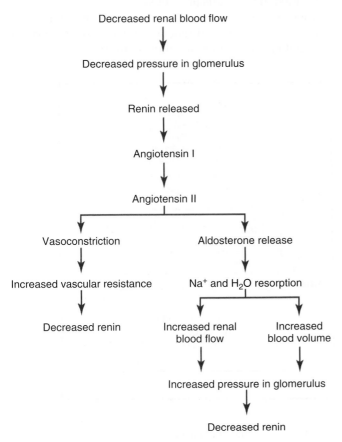

Fig. 28-4 Renin-angiotensin-aldosterone system.

Box 28-2

EFFECTS OF PROSTAGLANDINS

PROSTAGLANDINS E_1 AND I_2
- Vasodilation
- Increased sodium and water excretion
- Stimulation of renin release

PROSTAGLANDIN F_2
- Bronchoconstriction
- Vasoconstriction (PGF_2 in volume depletion)

tubules.[1,3] For example, bicarbonate, the principal blood buffer, is resorbed from the tubules, and hydrogen, a potent organic acid, is secreted into the tubules. However, the tubules do not function as rapidly in altering acid-base concentrations as do the lungs; therefore the kidneys regulate the day-to-day balance rather than coping with emergencies requiring quick response.

FLUID BALANCE

Regulation of the total amount of water in the body is vital for homeostasis and is one of the most important functions of the kidneys. In the absence of effective kidney function, fluid volume overload occurs and threatens homeostasis. Similarly, if the kidneys are unable to preserve adequate amounts of fluid, a severe volume deficit occurs that also disrupts homeostasis.

FLUID COMPARTMENTS

The fluid of the body is present in distinct internal spaces or compartments. The compartments are separated from each other by semipermeable membranes with openings (pores) that allow molecules of specific size and molecular weight to pass through while preventing larger, heavier molecules from doing so. As a result of the semipermeable membrane, fluid movement between the compartments is dynamic and constant.

The body has two basic fluid compartments: intracellular and extracellular.[5,10] The intracellular compartment is the fluid inside each of the body's cells and accounts for 40% of a person's total body weight and thus the majority of the water in the body. The remaining fluid is outside the body's cells and makes up the *extracellular compartment*. The extracellular compartment is made up of two distinct subcompartments: intravascular and interstitial. The intravascular compartment, the fluid within the blood vessels, accounts for 5% of the body's weight. The interstitial compartment corresponds to the fluid in the tissue spaces outside of both the body cells and the blood vessels and accounts for 15% of the body weight. Approximate amounts of fluid contained in each compartment are shown in Fig. 28-5, *A.*

The percentage of a person's total body weight that is made up of water varies slightly from individual to individual according to gender, age, and body fat content. An adult male has approximately a 60% body water content, whereas an adult female has closer to 50%. Infants have a body fluid content estimated at 77%, whereas body fluids may represent only 46% to 52% of body weight in elderly persons.[9] Also, with an increase in body fat, the body fluid percentage decreases because fat contains a smaller and less significant amount of water than muscle.

COMPOSITION

Any information about body fluids must also include a description of the substances contained within the fluids. When fluids move within the body, the substances contained in the fluids also move.

Electrolytes are elements or compounds that, when dissolved in water, dissociate into ions, electrically charged particles. Ions in solution in the fluid allow the

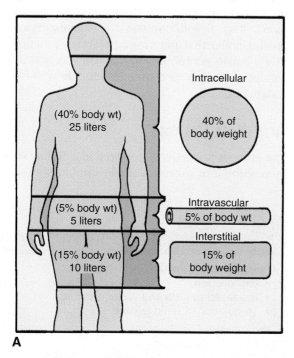

A

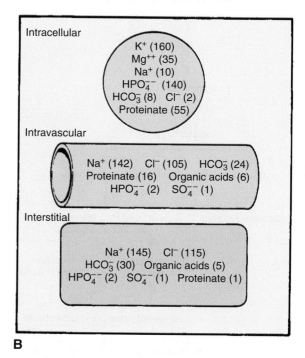

B

Fig. 28-5 **A,** Fluid compartments. **B,** Electrolytes by fluid compartment.

fluid to conduct an electrical current. A balance exists between cations (positively charged ions), anions (negatively charged ions), and other substances in the fluid compartments. Maintaining this balance is important to the normal function of all body systems. Electrolytes exist in differing amounts in each of the fluid compartments.[9] The primary electrolytes and other substances of importance in fluid and electrolyte balance are shown by fluid compartment in Fig. 28-5, *B*.

FLUID PHYSIOLOGY

An overall understanding is needed of both the structures containing or balancing fluids and electrolytes and the physiologic forces that govern movement and balance. In addition, knowledge of factors that inhibit or enhance the transfer of fluids and electrolytes is needed.

Tonicity. The terms *isotonic, hypotonic,* and *hypertonic* all refer to tonicity, or the osmolality of body fluids.[3] Osmolality is a measure of the number of particles in a solution and is stated in milliosmoles. The normal osmolality of body fluids is 275 to 295 mOsm/kg of body weight.[9] Different hospital laboratories may use slightly different numbers, but all fall within a range of 270 and 300 mOsm/kg.

Fig. 28-6 *A, B,* and *C* illustrates the effects of the tonicity of fluid in the body. An isotonic solution has roughly the same concentration of particles as the blood plasma; therefore cells within an isotonic solution maintain consistency and do not lose or gain fluid to their surroundings. A hypertonic solution contains a greater concentration of particles than that inside the cell and causes fluid to be drawn out of the cells. Used inappropriately, too much fluid may be withdrawn, causing a withering of the cell (crenation). A hypotonic solution contains a lesser concentration of particles than that inside the cell and causes fluid to be drawn into the cells. If used incorrectly, a hypotonic solution can cause too much fluid to enter the cell, causing the cells to swell and burst (hemolysis).

Hydrostatic Pressure. The force of left ventricular contraction of the heart propels the blood through the circulatory system, causing the blood to exert pressure against the vessel walls. This hydrostatic pressure creates the tendency for fluids and dissolved substances to move into the interstitial spaces via filtration (movement of fluid and substances from an area of high pressure to one of low pressure). Without opposing forces counteracting the hydrostatic pressure, fluid would leave the intravascular space until the space was depleted. However, whereas hydrostatic pressure favors fluid and electrolyte movement out of the intravascular compartment, the colloid osmotic pressure of the plasma holds the fluid and substances in the intravascular space.[4]

Osmotic Pressure. Osmotic pressure is created by solutes and other substances (albumin, globulin, fibrinogen) suspended in fluid. Colloid osmotic pressure is created primarily by the presence of plasma proteins in the intravascular space. Plasma proteins exert a pull on water molecules and therefore produce osmotic pressure, which retains fluid within the intravascular compartment. This force is maintained because proteins are large and cannot move or be transported across the semipermeable membrane unless the permeability of the membrane is changed by disease or other assaults on the body (e.g., burns, infections). Similarly, the solute and protein content of the interstitium results in interstitial colloid osmotic pressure. A decrease in serum protein lessens the osmotic pressure in the intravascular space so that the interstitial oncotic pressure is greater in relation to the intravascular pressure and pulls fluid from the vascular space into the interstitial space, causing edema.

Diffusion, Osmosis, and Active Transport. Fluid balance within the compartments is also achieved through the processes of diffusion, osmosis, and active transport. Just as in the kidney tubule cells, these three processes are constantly at work in other parts of the body to facilitate the movement of water and solutes to maintain homeostasis between the intracellular and extracellular compartments.

Movement of Water. The forces generated by left ventricular contraction, the colloid osmotic pressure in the intravascular space, and the solute content of both the extracellular fluid (ECF) and the intracellular fluid (ICF) result in the constant movement and balance of fluid throughout the fluid compartments. An increase in plasma volume results in increased capillary hydrostatic pressure, forcing fluid into the interstitial space and creating edema. Conversely, a decrease in plasma volume causes the movement of fluid from the intersti-

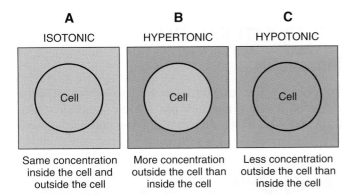

A	B	C
ISOTONIC	**HYPERTONIC**	**HYPOTONIC**
Cell	Cell	Cell
Same concentration inside the cell and outside the cell	More concentration outside the cell than inside the cell	Less concentration outside the cell than inside the cell

Fig. 28-6 **A,** Isotonic solution. The extracellular solution concentration is the same as the intracellular concentration, with no movement of water into or out of the cell. **B,** Hypertonic solution. The extracellular solution concentration is greater than the intracellular concentration. Water moves from the cell into the extracellular compartment. **C,** Hypotonic solution. The extracellular solution concentration is less than the intracellular concentration. Water moves from the extracellular compartment into the cell.

tium into the vascular space because the interstitial hydrostatic pressure is greater than the capillary hydrostatic pressure.

FACTORS CONTROLLING FLUID BALANCE

ANTIDIURETIC HORMONE

ADH is secreted by the posterior pituitary gland and functions as the primary controller of ECF volume.[11] Messages for release of ADH are sent by the osmoreceptors located in the hypothalamus and liver.[4,12] As serum osmolality rises above 285 mOsm/kg (normal, 275 to 295 mOsm/kg), ADH is released and carried through the circulation to the nephrons. ADH acts on the late distal convoluted tubule and the collecting ducts to resorb water.[12] In the presence of ADH, water is resorbed and the ECF volume remains high; in the absence of ADH, water resorption does not occur and the ECF volume is diminished.[3] ADH can sustain the effect on the renal tubules to a urinary osmolality of 1200 to 1400 mOsm/kg (normal, 500 to 800 mOsm/kg).[9] Box 28-3 identifies several additional mechanisms that stimulate the release of ADH. In addition to the usual stimuli, the presence of severe stress, either emotional or physical, can initiate ADH release through the limbic system that surrounds the hypothalamus.

ALDOSTERONE

As noted in Box 28-4, several factors stimulate the release of aldosterone. The relationship between sodium and water plays an important role in the influence of the renin-angiotensin-aldosterone system on body water regulation (see Fig. 28-4). A reduction in vascular volume stimulates the release of renin. Renin converts to angiotensin I, which converts to the powerful vasoconstrictor angiotensin II. In turn, angiotensin II stimulates the adrenal glands to secrete aldosterone, which acts on the distal tubules to resorb sodium from the tubular lumen into the circulation. When sodium is retained, so is water. Angiotensin II also constricts the renal vasculature, reducing renal blood flow and available glomerular filtrate, thus sending a signal to the posterior pituitary to release ADH. In this way the two systems intertwine, not only to maintain fluid balance but also to maintain electrolyte balance.[5,12]

ATRIAL NATRIURETIC PEPTIDE

An additional influence on fluid and electrolyte regulation comes from the synthesis of atrial natriuretic peptide (ANP).[3,12] This hormone is secreted from cells in the atria of the heart in response to hypernatremia, stimulation of stretch receptors as a result of increased volume, and increased pressure in the heart (Box 28-5).[12] ANP affects sodium and water balance by blocking aldosterone and ADH production, initiating vasodilation, and stimulating increased sodium and water excretion by the collecting ducts of the kidneys. Thus the physiologic effects of ANP include a reduction in fluid overload through diuresis, decreased cardiac workload, and reduction in cardiac preload and afterload.

ELECTROLYTE BALANCE

POTASSIUM

Potassium is the primary intracellular electrolyte and is responsible for numerous physiologic functions (Box 28-6). As with many solutes, diffusion and active trans-

---

Box 28-3

FACTORS STIMULATING RELEASE OF ANTIDIURETIC HORMONE

- Hyperosmolality of extracellular fluid (ECF)
- Hypovolemia
- Increased body temperature
- Medications
  - Opiods
  - Antineoplastics
  - Oral hypoglycemics
  - Beta-adrenergics
- Severe emotional or physical stress

Box 28-4

FACTORS STIMULATING RELEASE OF ALDOSTERONE

- Hypovolemia
- Hyponatremia
- Hyperkalemia
- Stress—emotional, physical

Box 28-5

FACTORS STIMULATING RELEASE OF ATRIAL NATRIURETIC PEPTIDE (ANP)

- Hypernatremia
- Hypervolemia
- Vasoconstriction
- Decreased cardiac output
- Increased cardiac preload and afterload
- Increased systemic vascular resistance

port across the cell membrane maintain potassium balance. Potassium leaves the cell by diffusion, moving toward the area of lesser concentration outside the cell, but it must be actively transported back into the cell to maintain cellular stability. One of the most important potassium functions in the body—that of aiding nervous impulse conduction and muscle contraction—is accomplished with the movement of potassium across the cell membrane.[10,13]

The gastrointestinal (GI) tract and skin excrete small amounts of potassium, but the major controllers of potassium stores are the kidneys. Potassium is resorbed by the proximal tubules and secreted into the distal tubules as needed to maintain balance. Resorption and secretion of potassium are influenced by many factors, which are presented in Box 28-7. Of the estimated 60 to 100 mEq/day ingested by an individual, 90% of the potassium is resorbed before arriving at the distal convoluted tubule, where the remainder is usually excreted.[13]

Potassium and sodium are in a constant state of competition within the body despite the need for electrolytes and their differing functions. Because both of these electrolytes are cations, one intracellular and one extracellular, potassium and sodium must remain in balance to preserve electrical neutrality at the cell membrane. As a result, when the sodium level is elevated, the potassium level will decrease and vice versa. In the presence of aldosterone, potassium is excreted by the tubules whereas sodium is retained. Therefore potassium wasting may occur despite the body's need for potassium. If potassium stores are low within the cell, the other intracellular electrolytes (magnesium and phosphorus) are often similarly depleted.[14]

SODIUM

Sodium is the most abundant extracellular electrolyte in the body and is primarily responsible for shifts in body water and the amount of water retained or excreted by the kidneys. In addition to water regulation, sodium plays a role in the transmission of nerve impulses through the "sodium pump," or active transport mechanism at the cellular level. Like potassium, sodium is key to a number of physiologic functions (Box 28-8).[9]

The body contains a complex system of safeguards and feedback mechanisms to protect the level of sodium in the ECF. Sodium balance is regulated by the kidneys, the adrenal glands (aldosterone secretion), and the posterior pituitary gland (ADH secretion). Most sodium resorption occurs in the proximal tubule under the influence of aldosterone. Because of the extremely sensitive mechanism for retaining sodium, ingestion of large amounts of sodium is not necessary.

CALCIUM

Calcium is the electrolyte of greatest quantity in the body, with stores estimated at 1200 g.[5] Of the total body calcium, 99% is contained in the bones.[15] The remaining 1% is contained primarily in the ECF in the vascular space. The calcium contained within bone is in an inactive form that maintains bone strength and is a ready storehouse for mobilization of calcium to the serum in cases of depletion. In addition to bone metabolism, cal-

---

Box 28-6

FUNCTIONS OF POTASSIUM

NORMAL SERUM VALUE
3.5-4.5 mEq/L

FUNCTIONS
Transmission of nerve impulses
Intracellular osmolality
Enzymatic reactions
Acid-base balance
Myocardial, skeletal, and smooth muscle contractility

Box 28-7

FACTORS AFFECTING RESORPTION AND SECRETION OF POTASSIUM

- Sodium balance—sodium deficit results in potassium loss
- Acid-base balance—acidosis moves hydrogen into the cell and potassium out, with potassium being excreted in the urine
- Diuretics—increased loss of potassium in distal tubule
- Gastrointestinal (GI) losses—vomiting and GI suction remove potassium
- Insulin—promotes movement of potassium into the cell
- Epinephrine—enhances potassium resorption from distal tubule

---

Box 28-8

FUNCTIONS OF SODIUM

NORMAL SERUM VALUE
135-145 mEq/L

FUNCTIONS
Body fluid movement and retention
Extracellular osmolality
Active transport mechanism (with potassium)
Neuromuscular activity
Enzyme activities
Acid-base balance

Box 28-9

FUNCTIONS OF CALCIUM

NORMAL SERUM VALUE
8.5-10.5 mg/dl

FUNCTIONS
Hardness of bone and teeth
Skeletal muscle contraction
Blood coagulation
Cellular permeability
Heart muscle contraction

Box 28-10

FUNCTIONS OF PHOSPHORUS

NORMAL SERUM VALUE
2.5-4.5 mg/dl

FUNCTIONS
Intracellular energy production (ATP)
Bone hardness
Structure of cellular membrane
Oxygen delivery to tissues
Enzyme regulation (ATPase)

---

cium is responsible for numerous other important functions including myocardial contractility, coagulation, and neuromuscular activity (Box 28-9).[15]

The mobilization of calcium from bone stores is accomplished through the influence of parathyroid hormone (PTH). The calcium in the intravascular space, the plasma calcium, exists in three general forms: ionized, protein-bound, or complexed.[15] Ionized calcium is the active form and functions in cell membrane stability and blood clotting. Protein-bound calcium, ionizes more quickly than the calcium in the bone, is readily put to use during immediate crisis. Complexed calcium is combined with other anions such as chloride, citrate, and/or phosphate and is available for filtration by the glomerulus for potential removal in the urine. Ionized calcium not needed for physiologic functions is returned to the bone under the influence of the hormone *calcitonin*.

In the ionized (active) form, calcium plays an important role in maintaining the internal integrity of the cell. The amount of ionized calcium in the serum depends on changes in serum pH and on the availability of plasma protein, primarily albumin. Because changes in pH and albumin levels occur with relative frequency, the measurement of total serum calcium alone can be deceptive. It is now clear that, to accurately determine the ionized calcium, it is necessary to measure it with a laboratory test because the results of calculated values are unreliable. Estimation of ionized calcium levels—calculated from the serum albumin and total serum calcium—were inaccurate 38% of the time in one study of critically ill patients.[16] Often both the total serum calcium and the ionized calcium values are measured. Increasingly the ionized calcium is the value that is used to accurately guide calcium management in critically ill patients.[16]

Calcium levels are highly dependent on individual dietary intake and on a variety of physiologic mechanisms related to absorption.[14,15] The uptake of calcium is influenced by the amount of phosphorus, magnesium, vitamin D and its breakdown products, PTH, and calcitonin.

PHOSPHORUS

As with calcium and magnesium, the serum values of phosphorus represent a minute portion of the actual body stores.[9] Approximately 75% of the phosphorus is found in the bones, and part of the remaining amount is intracellular, making it difficult to measure. The primary function of phosphorus is the formation of ATP, which provides intracellular energy for active transport mechanisms across the cell membrane. Additional functions of phosphorus include cell membrane structure, acid-base balance, oxygen delivery to the tissues, cellular immunity, and bone strength (Box 28-10).[17]

Absorption of phosphorus takes place in the GI tract, and serum phosphorus levels change frequently and dramatically, particularly in response to the ingestion of phosphate-rich foods such as milk, red meats, poultry, and fish. Excretion, for the most part, occurs in the kidneys. Over 90% of the phosphorus in the plasma is filtered by the glomerulus, and about 80% is resorbed by the proximal convoluted tubules. Resorption by the kidneys is increased when body stores are low and is combined with sodium and excess hydrogen ions to maintain acid-base balance.[3,17]

Phosphorus abnormalities are evident early in the course of kidney failure. The Third National Health and Nutrition Examination Survey (NHANES III, 1988-1994, which included 14,722 adults), revealed that people with mild-to-moderate kidney dysfunction—defined as a urinary creatinine clearance (CrCl) between 50 and 60 ml/min—already have elevations of serum phosphorus and potassium.[14] In contrast, serum ionized calcium remains relatively unchanged until the creatinine clearance is extremely low (CrCl less than 20 ml/min) and kidney failure is advanced.[14] In kidney failure hyper-

Box 28-11

FUNCTIONS OF MAGNESIUM

NORMAL SERUM VALUE
1.3-2.1 mEq/L

FUNCTIONS
Neuromuscular transmission
Contraction of heart muscle
Activation of enzymes for cellular metabolism
Active transport at cellular level
Transmission of hereditary information

Box 28-12

FUNCTIONS OF CHLORIDE

NORMAL SERUM VALUE
97-110 mEq/L

FUNCTIONS
Body fluid osmolality (with sodium)
Body water balance (with sodium)
Acid-base balance
Acidity of body fluids—specially gastric secretions
Red blood cell oxygenation, carbon dioxide transport

phosphatemia may contribute to lower serum calcium levels because both phosphate and calcium are deposited in bone and soft tissues.[17]

MAGNESIUM

Magnesium is the second most important and abundant intracellular electrolyte; about 60% of it is located in the bone.[9,17] The ECF contains only about 1% of the body's magnesium, and the remaining amount resides in the ICF. The levels of other intracellular electrolytes, such as calcium and potassium, are affected by the level of magnesium. For example, calcium and magnesium compete for absorption in the GI tract. If the dietary intake of calcium is higher than that of magnesium, calcium will be preferentially resorbed, and vice versa. The most important functions of magnesium are ensuring the transport of sodium and potassium across the cell membrane and as a cofactor in many intracellular enzyme reactions.[17] A depletion of magnesium liberates potassium to the ECF, which causes an increase in the renal excretion of potassium and hypokalemia. In addition, magnesium plays a role in transmitting central nervous system messages, maintaining neuromuscular activity, protein synthesis, and intracellular energy production (Box 28-11).[17]

CHLORIDE

Chloride is rarely found in the body unless in combination with one of the major cations, especially sodium. Therefore changes in serum chloride levels usually indicate changes in the other electrolytes or in acid-base balance. Because of its frequent combination with sodium, chloride plays a major role in maintaining serum osmolality, water balance, and acid-base balance because of competition with bicarbonate for combination with sodium. Additional functions of chloride are noted in Box 28-12.

Chloride is usually ingested with sodium in the form of salt and is resorbed or excreted in the proximal tubules of the kidney. Chloride is actively transported out of the tubules into the interstitium, again with sodium, to help maintain the high tubular interstitial osmolality and the mechanism for concentrating the urine.[3]

BICARBONATE

Bicarbonate (HCO_3^-) is an anion in the ECF and performs the essential function of maintaining acid-base balance. Although bicarbonate is not solely responsible for acid-base balance, it is the major ECF buffer. Bicarbonate levels in the body are in balance with carbonic acid (H_2CO_3) levels. The ratio between the two must remain proportional at 1 mEq of carbonic acid to 20 mEq of bicarbonate, or acid-base disturbances will result. When the carbonic acid level is elevated, acidosis results. When the bicarbonate level is high, alkalosis results.

The amount of bicarbonate available in the ECF is regulated by the kidneys.[3] Resorption of bicarbonate occurs primarily from the proximal tubule into the peritubular capillaries. Bicarbonate is also produced in the distal tubule and resorbed into the blood in response to acid-base balance and body requirements. In addition, the kidneys either resorb or excrete bicarbonate in response to the number of hydrogen ions present as part of the body buffer system. More bicarbonate will be resorbed when a large number of hydrogen ions are present, and more will be excreted when few hydrogen ions are present.

As described in this chapter, the kidneys carry out many functions that assist in the maintenance of homeostasis. Although fluid balance is one of the most important functions that the kidney provides, an understanding of the numerous other roles the kidneys play provides clues to total body function.

REFERENCES

1. Chmielewski C: Renal anatomy and overview of nephron function, *Nephrol Nurs J* 28(2):185, 2003.
2. Brundage D: *Renal disorders,* St Louis, 1992, Mosby.

3. Lancaster L: Renal anatomy and physiology. In Lancaster L, editor: *Core curriculum for nephrology nursing,* ed 4, Pitman, NJ, 2001, American Nephrology Nurses Association.
4. Peschman P: Renal physiology. In Clohesy J et al: *Critical care nursing,* ed 2, Philadelphia, 1996, Saunders.
5. Guyton A, Hall J: *Textbook of medical physiology,* ed 9, Philadelphia, 1996, Saunders.
6. Holechek M: Glomerular filtration: an overview, *Nephrol Nurs J* 28(3):285, 2003.
7. Holechek M: Renal hemodynamics: an overview, *Nephrol Nurs J* 28(4):441, 2003.
8. Richard D: Assessment of renal structure and function. In Lancaster L, editor: *Core curriculum for nephrology nursing,* ed 4, Pitman, NJ, 2001, American Nephrology Nurses Association.
9. Metheny N: *Fluid and electrolyte balance: nursing considerations,* ed 4, Philadelphia, 2000, Lippincott.
10. Lancaster L: Systemic manifestations of renal failure. In Lancaster L, editor: *Core curriculum for nephrology nursing,* ed 4, Pitman, NJ, 2001, American Nephrology Nurses Association.
11. Guthrie D, Yucha C: Urinary concentration and dilution, *Nephrol Nurs J* 31(3):297-301, 2004.
12. Candela L, Yucha C: Renal regulation of extracellular fluid volume and osmolality, *Nephrol Nurs J* 31(4):397, 2004.
13. Ludlow M: Renal handling of potassium, *Nephrol Nurs J* 28(5):493, 2003.
14. Hsu CY, Chertow GM: Elevations of serum phosphorous and potassium in mild-to-moderate chronic renal insufficiency, *Nephrol Dial Transplant* 17(8):1419-1425, 2002.
15. Yucha C, Guthrie D: Renal homeostasis of calcium, *Nephrol Nurs J* 28(6):621, 2003.
16. Brynes MC et al: A comparison of corrected serum calcium levels to ionized calcium levels among critically ill surgical patients, *Am J Surg* 189(3):310-314, 2005.
17. Yucha C, Dungan, J: Renal handling of phosphorus and magnesium, *Nephrol Nurs J,* 31(1):33, 2004.

CHAPTER 29

Renal Clinical Assessment and Diagnostic Procedures

*U*nderstanding the anatomic structures and physiologic workings of the renal system provides the basis for understanding the clinical manifestations that signal kidney/renal system dysfunction. The body presents a variety of clinical signs and symptoms that indicate kidney disorders. However, signs and symptoms of kidney dysfunction are often subtle and are exhibited in other body systems. A detailed history and careful physical examination provide data that help pinpoint the problem and often the cause of the problem.

HISTORY

A renal history begins with a description of the chief complaint, stated in the patient's own words. A description of the chief complaint includes the onset, location, duration, and factors or strategies that lessen or aggravate the problem.[1] The individual should be encouraged to describe the effects of any treatment for the problem thus far, medications taken to alleviate symptoms (both prescription and nonprescription), efforts taken to determine the cause of the problem, and/or procedures performed to improve the problem. A careful history that explores symptoms fully is an essential component of the clinical assessment.

Predisposing factors for acute kidney dysfunction are also elicited during the history, including the use of over-the-counter medicines, recent infections requiring antibiotic therapy, antihypertensive medicines, and any diagnostic procedures performed using radiopaque contrast media.[2] Nonsteroidal antiinflammatory drugs (such as ibuprofen), antibiotics (especially aminoglycosides), antihypertensives (especially medicines that block angiotensin), and iodine-based dyes may cause an acute or chronic decline in kidney function. A history of recent onset of nausea and vomiting or appetite loss caused by taste changes (uremia often causes a metallic taste) may also provide clues to the rapid onset of kidney problems.[2] And finally, symptoms that indicate rapid fluid volume gains are explored. For example, weight gains of more than 2 pounds per day, sleeping on additional pillows, and sitting in a chair to sleep are signals of volume overload and potential kidney dysfunction.

In addition to outlining the current reason for admission to the critical care unit, compiling a complete medical and social history is important. Similar symptoms, problems, or treatment for complaints in the past may help establish the cause of the current problem or provide clues for treatment. For example, a history of obstructive urology problems, frequent kidney infections, or previous acute renal failure may be significant in determining risk factors for current kidney problems. The patient and/or family or significant other must provide as much detail as possible during the history.

The family history also may provide important information that will aid in identifying the patient's disorder. For example, the patient may reveal that one or two close family members have always had swelling of the extremities or high blood pressure. These symptoms should lead to questions about any history of kidney problems in the family. The Data Collection feature summarizes the information gained from a renal history.

PHYSICAL EXAMINATION

In the critical care area, nursing assessment does not routinely include a full physical examination of the kidneys and renal system. However, many of the assessment parameters for the renal system provide information related to the volume status of the individual and are helpful in a large number of patients regardless of kidney function or status. Although not often performed in the depth described in the following sections, the critical care nurse must be aware of how to perform a thorough renal assessment in stable patients and as needed in patients with kidney dysfunction.

INSPECTION

Bleeding. Visual inspection related to the kidneys generally focuses on the flank and abdomen. Kidney trauma is suspected if a purplish discoloration is present

801

DATA COLLECTION

Renal History

COMMON KIDNEY-RELATED SYMPTOMS
- Dyspnea
- Peripheral dependent edema
- Nocturia
- Nausea
- Metallic taste in mouth
- Loss of appetite
- Headache
- Rapid weight gain
- Itching
- Dry, scaly skin
- Weakness, fatigue

PATIENT PROFILE
- Personal habits
- Use of over-the-counter drugs, herbs, vitamins, and dietary supplements
- Illicit drug use
- Change in employment caused by illness
- Financial problems resulting from illness—e.g., cost, time off work
- Sexual function—decreased libido, amenorrhea

RISK FACTORS
- Family history
- Hypertension
- Diabetes mellitus
- Previous acute renal failure

FAMILY HISTORY
- Hypertension
- Diabetes mellitus

- Polycystic kidney disease
- Kidney disease
- Chronically swollen extremities

RENAL STUDIES IN PAST
- Urinalysis with proteinuria
- Creatinine clearance
- Kidney-ureter-bladder (KUB) x-ray
- Intravenous pyelogram
- Renal ultrasound
- Renal arteriography
- Kidney biopsy

MEDICAL HISTORY

Childhood
- Nephrotic syndrome, streptococcal infection, hypoplastic kidneys, obstructive uropathy

Adult
- Frequent urinary tract infections
- Calculi
- Use of iodine-based radiographic contrast media
- Use of nonsteroidal antiinflammatory drugs

CURRENT MEDICATION USAGE
- Nonsteroidal antiinflammatory drugs
- Antibiotics
- Antihypertensives
- Diuretics

on the flank (Grey-Turner's sign) or near the posterior eleventh or twelfth ribs.[1] Bruising, abdominal distention, and abdominal guarding may also signal renal trauma or a hematoma around a kidney.

Volume. Inspection is especially helpful in looking for signs of volume depletion or overload that might signal kidney problems. Fluid volume assessment begins with an inspection of the patient's neck veins. The supine position facilitates normal venous distention. An absence of distention (or flat neck veins) indicates hypovolemia. Assessment continues with the head of the bed elevated 45 to 90 degrees.[1] If the neck veins remain distended more than 2 cm above the sternal notch when the bed is at 45 degrees, fluid overload may be present.[3]

Hand vein inspection may be helpful in assessing volume status and is performed by observing for venous distention when the hand is held in the dependent position. Venous filling that takes longer than 5 seconds suggests hypovolemia. When the hand is elevated, the dis-

tention should disappear within 5 seconds. If distention does not disappear within 5 seconds after the hand is elevated, fluid overload is suspected.

Assessment of skin turgor provides additional data for identifying fluid-related problems. To assess turgor, the skin over the forearm is picked up and released. Normal elasticity and fluid status allow an almost immediate return to shape once the skin is released. In fluid volume deficit, however, the skin remains raised and does not return to its normal position for several seconds. Because of the loss of skin elasticity in elderly persons, skin turgor assessment is not an accurate fluid assessment for this age-group.

Finally, inspection of the oral cavity provides clues to fluid volume status. When a fluid volume deficit exists, the mucous membranes of the mouth become dry. However, mouth breathing and some medicines (such as antihistamines) can also dry the mucous membranes temporarily. Therefore a more accurate way to

Table 29-1	Pitting Edema Scale
Rating	**Approximate Equivalent**
+1	2-mm depth
+2	4-mm depth (lasting up to 15 sec)
+3	6-mm depth (lasting up to 60 sec)
+4	8-mm depth (lasting longer than 60 sec)

assess the oral cavity is to inspect the mouth using a tongue blade. Dryness of the oral cavity is more indicative of fluid volume deficit than are complaints of a dry mouth.[3]

Edema. Edema is the presence of excess fluid in the interstitial space and can be a sign of volume overload. In the presence of volume excess, edema may be present in dependent areas of the body, such as the feet and legs of an ambulatory person or the sacrum of an individual confined to bed. The presence of edema, however, does not always indicate fluid volume overload. A loss of albumin from the vascular space can cause peripheral edema in the presence of hypovolemia or normal fluid states. A critically ill patient may have a low serum albumin level (hypoalbuminemia) because of inadequate nutrition after surgery, a burn, or a head injury and may exhibit edema as a result of the loss of plasma oncotic pressure and not as a result of volume overload. In addition, edema may signal circulatory difficulties. An individual who is fluid-balanced but who has poor venous return may experience pedal edema after prolonged sitting in a chair with the feet dependent. Similarly, an individual with heart failure may experience edema because the left ventricle is unable to pump blood effectively through the vessels. A key feature that distinguishes edema due to excess volume or hypoalbuminemia from circulatory compromise is that the edema does not reverse with elevation of the extremity.

Edema can be assessed by applying fingertip pressure on the skin over a bony prominence, such as the ankles, pretibial areas (shins), and sacrum. If the indentation made by the fingertip does not disappear within 15 seconds, "pitting" edema is present. Pitting edema indicates increased interstitial volume and is generally not evident until a weight gain of approximately 10% has occurred.[4] Edema also may appear in the hands and feet, around the eyes, and in the cheeks. Dependent areas, such as the feet and sacrum, are the areas most likely to demonstrate edema in patients confined to a wheelchair or bed. One way of measuring the extent of edema is by using a subjective scale of 1 to 4, with 1 indicating only minimal pitting and 4 indicating severe pitting (Table 29-1).[1] Other scales for assessing and measuring edema are used as well (see Table 16-3).

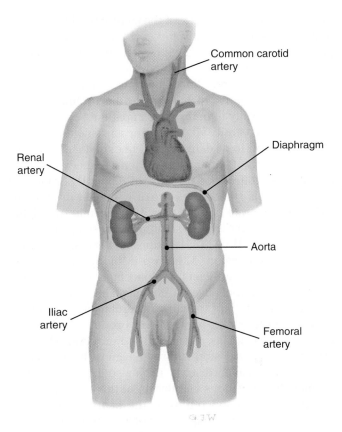

Fig. 29-1 Sites for auscultation of bruits.

AUSCULTATION

Auscultation of the kidneys yields virtually no useful information. However, the renal arteries are auscultated for a bruit, a blowing or swishing sound that resembles a cardiac murmur (Fig. 29-1). The examiner listens for bruits above and to the left and right of the umbilicus.[1] A renal artery bruit generally indicates stenosis, which may lead to acute or chronic kidney dysfunction due to compromised blood flow to the kidney(s). A bruit over the upper portion of the abdominal aorta may indicate an aneurysm or a stenotic area and could decrease blood flow to the kidneys.

Auscultation is especially helpful in providing information about extracellular fluid (ECF) volume status. Listening for specific sounds in the heart and lungs provides information about the presence or absence of increased fluid in the interstitium or vascular space.

Heart. Auscultation of the heart requires not only assessing rate and rhythm but also listening for extra sounds. Fluid overload is often accompanied by a third or fourth heart sound, which may be heard with the bell of the stethoscope.[1] Increased heart rate alone provides little information about fluid volume, but combined with a low blood pressure it may indicate hypovolemia.

The heart also is auscultated for the presence of a pericardial friction rub. A rub can best be heard at the third intercostal space to the left of the sternal border, with the individual leaning slightly forward.[1] The presence of a pericardial friction rub indicates pericarditis and may result from uremia in a patient with kidney failure.

Blood Pressure. Blood pressure and heart rate changes are very useful in assessing fluid volume deficit. In stable critically ill patients or in patients on a telemetry unit, orthostatic vital sign measurements provide clues to blood loss, dehydration, unexplained syncope, and the effects of some antihypertensive medications.[5,6] A drop in systolic blood pressure of 20 mm Hg or more, a drop in diastolic blood pressure of 10 mm Hg or more, or a rise in pulse rate of more than 15 beats/min from lying to sitting or from sitting to standing represents orthostatic hypotension. Box 29-1 describes how to assess for orthostatic hypotension. The drop in blood pressure occurs because a sufficient preload is not immediately available after the position change. The heart rate increases in an attempt to maintain cardiac output and circulation. Orthostatic hypotension produces subjective feelings of weakness, dizziness, or faintness. Although orthostatic hypotension is often a sign of hypovolemia, peripheral vascular disease may also be responsible. Damage to the venous circulation of the lower extremities decreases blood return to the heart, leading to a blood pressure drop in a normovolemic individual.

Lungs. Lung assessment also is extremely important in gauging fluid status. Crackles indicate fluid overload. Dyspnea with mild exertion, dyspnea at night that prevents sleeping in a supine position (orthopnea), or dyspnea that awakens the individual from sleep (paroxysmal nocturnal dyspnea) may indicate pooling of fluid in the lungs. Shallow, gasping breaths with periods of apnea reflect severe acid-base imbalances.

PALPATION

Although rarely performed in critically ill patients, palpation of the kidneys in stable patients provides information about the kidneys' size and shape. Palpation of the kidneys is achieved through the bimanual capturing approach. Capturing is accomplished by placing one hand posteriorly under the flank of the supine patient with fingers pointing to the midline, while placing the opposite hand just below the rib cage anteriorly.[1,4] The patient is asked to inhale deeply while pressure is exerted to bring the hands together (Fig. 29-2). As the patient exhales, the examiner may feel the kidney between the hands. After each kidney is palpated in this manner, the two should be compared for size and shape. Each kidney should be firm, smooth, and of equal size. The examiner is usually unable to palpate a normal left kidney. The right kidney is more easily palpated because of its lower position, being displaced downward by the liver. Problems should be suspected if a mass (cancer) or an irregular surface (polycystic kidneys) is palpated, a size difference is detected, the kidney extends significantly lower than the rib cage on either side, or there is evidence of recent blunt trauma.[1,7]

PERCUSSION

Percussion is performed to detect pain in the area of a kidney or to determine excess accumulation of air, fluid, or solids around the kidneys. Percussion of the kidneys also provides information about kidney location, size, and possible problems. Like palpation, percussion of the kidneys is not a routine part of a nursing assessment in critical care. However, the information gained through percussion can provide important patient care data.

Kidneys. Percussion of a kidney is performed with the patient in a side-lying or sitting position, with the examiner's hand placed over the costovertebral angle (lower border of the rib cage on the flank).[1] Striking the back of the hand with the opposite fist produces a dull

---

Box 29-1

ORTHOSTATIC HYPOTENSION ASSESSMENT

1. Take BP and HR with patient lying down
2. Assist patient to sitting position
   Monitor patient for complaints of dizziness, imbalance
   Take BP and HR immediately and record
   Take BP and HR after 3 minutes and record
3. Assist patient to standing position (if patient not dizzy, imbalanced)
   Assess as above

BP, Blood pressure; *HR,* heart rate.

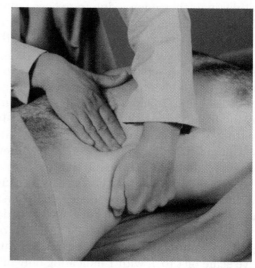

Fig. 29-2 Palpation of the kidney. (From Barkauskas V, Baumann V, Darling-Fisher C: *Health & physical assessment,* ed 3, St Louis, 2002, Mosby.)

thud, which is normal. Pain may indicate infection (such as a urinary tract infection that has extended into the kidneys) or injury resulting from trauma. Traumatic injury to the kidneys should be assessed in the presence of a penetrating abdominal wound, with blunt abdominal trauma, or with a fractured pelvis or ribs.[7,8]

Abdomen. Observation and percussion of the abdomen are of value in assessing fluid status. Percussing the abdomen with the patient in the supine position generally yields a dull sound (solid bowel contents or fluid) or a hollow sound (gaseous bowel).[1]

Ascites, or severe fluid distention of the abdominal cavity, is an important observation in determining fluid overload. Differentiating ascites from distortion caused by solid bowel contents is accomplished by producing a fluid wave. A fluid wave is elicited by exerting pressure to the abdominal midline while one hand is placed on the right or left flank.[1,4] Tapping the opposite flank produces a wave in the accumulated fluid that can be felt under the hands (Fig. 29-3). Other signs of ascites include a protuberant, rounded abdomen and abdominal striae.[1]

Individuals with kidney failure may have ascites caused by volume overload, which forces fluid into the abdomen because of increased capillary hydrostatic pressures. However, ascites may or may not represent fluid volume excess. Severe ascites in persons with compromised hepatic function may result from decreased plasma proteins. The ascites occurs because the increased vascular pressure associated with hepatic dysfunction forces fluid and plasma proteins from the vascular space into the interstitial space and abdominal cavity. Thus although the individual may exhibit marked edema, the intravascular space is volume-depleted and the patient is hypovolemic.

ADDITIONAL ASSESSMENT PARAMETERS

WEIGHT

One of the most important assessments of kidney and fluid status is the patient's weight. In the critical care unit, weight is monitored on every patient every day and is an important vital signs measurement. Significant fluctuations in body weight over a 1- to 2-day period indicate fluid gains and losses. Rapid weight gains or losses of greater than 2 pounds per day generally indicate fluid rather than nutritional factors. One liter of fluid equals 1 kg, or approximately 2.2 pounds.

Whenever possible, the patient is weighed during admission to the critical care unit. It is important to note whether the current weight differs significantly from the weight 1 to 2 weeks before admission. The patient is weighed daily for comparison with the previous day's weight. The weight is obtained at the same time each day, with the patient wearing the same amount of clothing.

The individual's weight is of critical importance to the dialysis nurse caring for a patient with acute or chronic kidney failure. The differences in weight from day to day are used to calculate the amount of fluid to remove during a dialysis treatment.[9]

INTAKE AND OUTPUT

Like patient weight, intake and output are monitored on all patients in the critical care unit. Intake and output can be compared with the patient's weight to more accurately evaluate fluid gains or losses. Urinary output plus insensible fluid losses (perspiration, stool, and water vapor from the lungs) can vary from 750 to 2400 ml/day. When intake exceeds output (excessive intravenous fluid, decreased urine output), a positive fluid balance exists. In impaired kidney function, the positive fluid balance results in fluid volume overload. Conversely, if output exceeds intake (fever, increased respiration, profuse sweating, vomiting, diarrhea, gastric suction, diuretic therapy), a negative fluid balance exists and volume deficit results. During a 24-hour period, fever can increase skin and respiratory losses by as much as 75 ml per degree of Fahrenheit temperature rise.

Individuals with acute renal failure (ARF) often exhibit a decrease in urine output, or oliguria (less than 30 ml/hour or 400 ml/day in adults; less than 1ml/kg/hour in infants and young children). However, there may be a fairly normal or only slightly decreased urine output that reflects water removal without solute removal in the

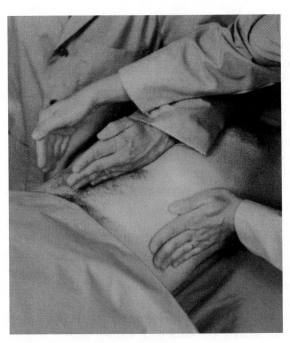

Fig. 29-3 Test for the presence of a fluid wave. (From Barkauskas V, Baumann V, Darling-Fisher C: *Health & physical assessment*, ed 3, St Louis, 2002, Mosby.)

Table 29-2	Hemodynamic Assessment of Fluid Status	
Measurement	**Volume Depletion**	**Volume Overload**
CVP	<2 mm Hg	>5 mm Hg
PAOP	<5 mm Hg	>12 mm Hg
CI	<2.2 L/min/m²	>4 L/min/m²
MAP	Decreased	Increased

CVP, Central venous pressure; *PAOP*, pulmonary artery occlusion pressure; *CI*, cardiac index; *MAP*, mean arterial pressure.

early phases of ARF. Therefore kidney function cannot be accurately determined by urine output alone.

Abnormal output of body fluids creates not only fluid imbalances but also electrolyte and acid-base disturbances. For example, gastrointestinal suction or loss by diarrhea can result in fluid deficit, sodium and potassium deficits, and metabolic acidosis from excessive loss of bicarbonate.

In maintaining daily records of intake and output, all gains or losses must be recorded. A standard list of the fluid volume held in various containers (e.g., milk cartons, juice containers) expedites this process. Discussions about the importance of accurate intake and output with the patient and family or friends are necessary and can improve the accuracy of intake and output volumes assessment.

Hemodynamic Monitoring. Body fluid status is accurately reflected in measurements of cardiovascular hemodynamics. Measurements such as central venous pressure (CVP), pulmonary artery occlusion pressure (PAOP), cardiac index (CI), and mean arterial pressure (MAP) provide a clear picture of the increases or decreases in vascular volume returning to and being ejected from the heart.[10] Indeed, both volume depletion and overload are easily detected by use of central venous or arterial catheters from which pressure measurements can be obtained (Table 29-2).

A central venous catheter is often inserted to evaluate fluid volume status and to measure the CVP. The CVP represents the filling pressure of the right atrium and is a measurement of right ventricular preload. The CVP will change with fluctuations in volume status. A normal CVP is 2 to 5 mm Hg. In volume depletion the CVP is less than 2 mm Hg, whereas volume overload is reflected by readings of more than 5 mm Hg (see "Hemodynamic Monitoring" in Chapter 17 for more information on CVP interpretation).

If the patient has coexisting cardiopulmonary disease or if more information about hemodynamic function is required, a pulmonary artery catheter may be inserted.

This catheter provides information about left ventricular filling pressures and cardiac output. The PAOP represents the left atrial pressure required to fill the left ventricle. When the left ventricle is full at the end of diastole, this represents the volume of blood available for ejection. It is also known as left ventricular preload and is measured by the PAOP. The normal PAOP is 5 to 12 mm Hg. In fluid volume excess, PAOP rises. In fluid volume deficit, PAOP is low.[10]

The CI demonstrates the cardiac output, or ejection volume, of the left ventricle over 1 minute, standardized for body size. The normal CI is 2.2 to 4 L/min/m². Compensatory mechanisms in early hypovolemic shock maintain the CI at or near normal. With prolonged fluid loss, however, the CI falls. Fluid volume overload increases heart rate, which in turn increases cardiac output, but only to a point. Pump failure may result from massive volume overload, such as with acute heart failure secondary to kidney failure, in which case the CI falls. The most frequent cause of acute renal failure that regains hemodynamic monitoring is severe sepsis.[10]

MAP is regulated by systemic vascular resistance (SVR) and the cardiac output and represents an average of blood pressure within the arterial system. Changes in SVR or cardiac output inevitably result in corresponding MAP changes. For example, an increase in SVR during the early stages of hypovolemic shock leads to elevation of the MAP. Ongoing fluid losses eventually lead to a decreased cardiac output, which leads to a reduction in MAP. The net effect of a decreased MAP to the kidneys is a reduction in blood flow, which may lead to ARF.

OTHER OBSERVATIONS

Kidney system dysfunction often leads to fluid and electrolyte imbalances and the retention of nitrogenous waste products. Some of the disturbances in fluid, electrolyte, and waste product levels are accompanied by clinical manifestations less observable or measurable than those previously mentioned but that indicate a change from normal function. Box 29-2 summarizes additional important aspects to consider during kidney and fluid and electrolyte assessment.

Sudden or slowly developing changes in mental status also must be investigated. For example, acidosis often results in disorientation. Lethargy, coma, and confusion may result from sodium, calcium, or magnesium excess or deficit or retained waste products. Apprehension or anxiety may be secondary to sodium deficit, a shift of fluid from the plasma to the interstitium, or respiratory changes caused by fluid volume overload.

Apathy and withdrawal may also accompany hypovolemic states. Patients with kidney failure and the accompanying systemic increases in electrolytes, fluids, and nitrogenous waste products often exhibit apathy, restlessness, confusion, and withdrawal.[2] The speed of

Box 29-2

FLUID AND ELECTROLYTE ASSESSMENT

FLUID STATUS
Skin turgor
Mucous membranes
Intake and output
Presence of edema/ascites
Neck and hand vein engorgement
Lung sounds—crackles
Dyspnea
Central venous pressure (CVP) <2 mm Hg, >5 mm Hg
Pulmonary artery occlusive pressure (PAOP) <5 mm Hg, >12 mm Hg
Tachycardia
Hypertension, hypotension
Cardiac index (CI) <2.2 $L/min/m^2$
S_3, S_4 heart sounds
Headache
Blurred vision
Vertigo on rising

Papilledema
Mental changes
Serum osmolality

ELECTROLYTE AND WASTE PRODUCT STATUS
Complete blood count (CBC)
Serum electrolyte levels, nitrogen waste products (BUN)
Electrocardiogram tracings (potassium, calcium, magnesium levels)
Behavioral and/or mental changes (sodium, BUN levels)
Chvostek's and Trousseau's signs (calcium levels)
Changes in peripheral sensation (numbness, tremor—sodium, potassium, calcium levels)
Muscle strength (potassium, BUN)
Gastrointestinal (GI) changes (nausea and vomiting—BUN)
Itching (calcium, phosphorus, BUN)
Therapies that can alter electrolyte status (GI suction, diuretics, antihypertensives, calcium channel blockers)

---

onset will vary according to how rapidly (or slowly) the kidney failure progresses and alters homeostasis. In some patients it may be difficult to separate the emotional component of critical illness from the physiologic mechanism; therefore both mechanisms are considered by the critical care nurse.

LABORATORY ASSESSMENT

SERUM

Blood Urea Nitrogen. In addition to history and physical examination, laboratory data are extremely helpful in the diagnosis, management, and ongoing evaluation of kidney system dysfunction. Blood urea nitrogen (BUN) is a by-product of protein and amino acid metabolism.[11] The normal value for BUN is 5 to 25 mg/dl and is increased when kidney function deteriorates.[12] With kidney dysfunction, the BUN is elevated because of a decrease in the glomerular filtration rate (GFR) and therefore a fall in urea excretion. Elevations in the BUN can be correlated with the clinical manifestations of uremia; as the BUN rises, symptoms of uremia become more pronounced.[2] However, a drop in the GFR and therefore an increase in the BUN also may be caused by hypovolemia and dehydration,[13] nephrotoxic drugs, or a sudden hypotensive episode. In these cases the rise in BUN is caused by a decreased GFR in the presence of normal kidney function.[13] BUN is also increased by changes in the rate of protein metabolism such as excessive protein intake and catabolism.[11] A catabolic state may occur with starvation (or chronic poor nutrition in a critically ill patient), severe infection, surgery, or trauma.

The BUN also may be elevated as the result of hematoma resorption, GI bleeding, excessive licorice ingestion, or steroid or tetracycline therapy. A decrease in the BUN may indicate volume overload, liver damage, severe malnutrition (as a result of depleted protein stores), use of phenothiazines, or pregnancy.[12]

Creatinine. Creatinine is a by-product of muscle and normal cell metabolism and appears in serum in amounts proportional to the body muscle mass. Although slightly higher in males than females, the normal serum creatinine level is about 0.5 to 1.5 mg/dl.[12] Creatinine is easily excreted by the renal tubules and is not resorbed or secreted in the tubules.[2] Measuring the creatinine clearance—the amount of creatinine in the excreted urine and the amount of creatinine in the blood over 24 hours—provides a reliable and accurate estimate of glomerular filtration and therefore of kidney function.[2] The normal value for creatinine clearance is 110 to 120 ml/minute; values less than 50 ml/minute indicate significant kidney dysfunction. The creatinine clearance is measured using a 12- or 24-hour urine collection and blood sample. The creatinine clearance can also be estimated from the serum creatinine (Box 29-3).[14,15] As kidney function decreases, creatinine clearance decreases and is useful in monitoring the severity, progression, and recovery of kidney function. The estimated/calculated creatinine clearance is widely used to determine changes in drug dosing with kidney dysfunction because many drugs are excreted by the kidneys.[15]

Creatinine levels are fairly constant and are affected by fewer factors than BUN. As a result, the serum creatinine level is a more sensitive and specific indicator of kidney function than BUN. Creatinine excess occurs most often in persons with kidney failure resulting from impaired excretion. Elevations in creatinine may occur in muscle growth disorders such as acromegaly or with skeletal muscle injury (such as may be found in a trauma patient) in the absence of kidney dysfunction. Also, malnutrition can result in transient increases in creatinine levels as the rapid muscle catabolism associated with malnutrition causes "dumping" of increased amounts of creatinine into the circulation. Decreased levels of creatinine are rare and may be associated with muscular dystrophy.

Another useful diagnostic parameter in kidney disease is the ratio of serum urea nitrogen to creatinine. In general, the ratio of BUN to creatinine is 10:1. A change in the ratio generally indicates kidney dysfunction and is often very useful in identifying the etiology of the acute kidney dysfunction.[12,15] For example, if both BUN and creatinine are elevated and maintain an approximate 10:1 ratio, the disorder is intrarenal, or affecting the tubules of the kidneys. If the ratio of BUN to creatinine is greater than 10:1, the etiology is most likely prerenal (such as hypovolemia).[11,13] In prerenal kidney failure the creatinine is excreted by functioning tubules but the urea nitrogen is retained because of the poor GFR and hemoconcentration, leading to the increased ratio.[11] Thus, in the diagnosis of prerenal failure, the ratio is a more useful indicator of kidney function than the separate tests of BUN and creatinine.

Osmolality. The serum osmolality reflects the concentration or dilution of vascular fluid and measures the dissolved particles in the serum. The normal serum osmolality is 275 to 295 mOsm/L.[3] An elevated osmolality indicates hemoconcentration or dehydration, while a decreased osmolality indicates hemodilution or volume overload. When the serum osmolality level increases, antidiuretic hormone (ADH) is released from the posterior pituitary gland and stimulates increased water resorption in the kidney tubules. This expands the vascular space, brings the serum osmolality back to normal, and results in more concentrated urine (and thus an elevated urine osmolality). The opposite occurs with a decreased serum osmolality level, which inhibits the production of ADH. The decreased ADH results in increased excretion of water in the tubules, producing dilute urine with a low osmolality, and brings the serum osmolality back to normal. Sodium accounts for 85% to 95% of the serum osmolality, therefore doubling the serum sodium gives an estimate of the serum osmolality.[12] A more precise value of the serum osmolality can be calculated from the following formula:

$$2 \times Na + BUN/3 + Glucose/18$$

Measurement of serum osmolality is a useful parameter in determining fluid balance and fluid replacement therapy in critically ill patients. Serum osmolality is also a useful parameter in determining disorders of ADH secretion that may occur in critically ill individuals. A decreased serum osmolality may indicate syndrome of inappropriate ADH secretion (SIADH), or too much ADH, whereas an elevation of serum osmolality may indicate diabetes insipidus (DI), or too little ADH.

Anion Gap. The anion gap is a calculation of the difference between the measurable cations (sodium and potassium) and the measurable anions (chloride and bicarbonate).[3] The value represents the remaining unmeasurable ions present in the extracellular fluid (phosphates, sulfates, ketones, lactate). The formula generally used in the calculation of the anion gap is as follows:

$$Na^+ - (Cl^- + HCO_3^-)$$

A normal anion gap is 1 to 12 mEq/L and should not exceed 14 mEq/L. An increased anion gap level reflects overproduction or decreased excretion of acid products and indicates metabolic acidosis; a decreased anion gap indicates metabolic alkalosis.

Acute and chronic kidney failure can increase the anion gap because of retention of acids and altered bicarbonate resorption. The anion gap is also increased in diabetic ketoacidosis caused by ketone production. The measurement of the anion gap is a rapid method for identifying acid-base imbalance but cannot be used to pinpoint the source of the acid-base disturbance specifically.

Hemoglobin and Hematocrit. The hemoglobin (Hgb) and hematocrit (Hct) levels can indicate increases or decreases in intravascular fluid volume.[11] Both Hgb and Hct vary between genders, with the Hgb in males normally 13.5 to 17.5 g/dl and in females 12 to 16 g/dl. The Hct ranges from 40% to 54% in males and 37% to 47% in females. Hct values are higher in newborns (up to 65%) and decrease to adult ranges between the ages of 4 and

10 years.[12] Hgb transports oxygen and carbon dioxide and is important in maintaining cellular metabolism and acid-base balance.[3]

The Hct is the proportion or concentration of red blood cells (RBCs) in a volume of whole blood and is expressed as a percentage.[12] Hematocrit is approximate three times the Hgb if the individual is in a normal fluid balance. An increase in the Hct often indicates a fluid volume deficit, which results in hemoconcentration. Although rare, true disorders of RBC production, such as polycythemia, also can result in an increased Hct.

Conversely, a decreased Hct can indicate fluid volume excess because of the dilutional effect of the extra fluid load. Decreases, however, also can result from anemias, blood loss, liver damage, or hemolytic reactions.[12] In individuals with acute kidney failure, anemia may occur early in the disease, so that a decreased Hct either may indicate the anemia of kidney failure or may reflect fluid volume overload. If the Hct is dropping but the Hgb remains constant, the cause is fluid volume overload. If both the Hct and the Hgb are decreased, this indicates a true loss of RBCs. The history and bedside assessment, including hemodynamic monitoring data, aid in determining whether fluid imbalances or disease states, or both, are responsible for changes in Hct in the critically ill patient.

Albumin. Slightly more than 50% of the total plasma protein is serum albumin. It is manufactured in the liver, with a normal blood level of 3.5 to 5 g/dl.[12] Albumin is primarily responsible for the maintenance of colloid osmotic pressure, which functions to hold fluid in the vascular space. The blood vessel walls, because of their impermeability to plasma proteins, prevent albumin from leaving the vascular space. However, in some disease states such as severe burns (cell membrane destruction) or ARF resulting from the nephrotic syndrome (increased glomerular capillary permeability to protein), albumin is lost from the vascular space.

Decreased albumin levels in the vascular space result in a plasma-to-interstitium fluid shift, creating peripheral edema. A decreased albumin level can occur as a result of protein-calorie malnutrition, which occurs in many critically ill patients in whom available stores of albumin are depleted. A decrease in the plasma oncotic pressure results, and fluid shifts from the vascular space to the interstitial space. Liver disease or severe injury to the liver also causes a fall in albumin levels as the diseased liver fails to synthesize sufficient albumin. Furthermore, severe portal hypertension can force albumin and other plasma proteins into the abdominal cavity, resulting in ascites.

Increased albumin levels are rare. The body uses a fixed amount of protein for energy and body cell replacement and converts excess protein into stored fat. If all plasma protein levels are elevated, fluid volume deficit (hemoconcentration) is suspected.

URINE ANALYSIS

Analysis of the urine provides excellent information about the patient's kidney function and condition relative to fluids and electrolytes. Specific tests and abnormal indications are presented in Table 29-3.[12,16,17] In many cases, urinalysis in the critically ill patient aids in locating the site of kidney damage or disease and therefore guides therapeutic management of the patient's care.

Appearance. Physical examination of the urine focuses on a general inspection of the urine's color, clarity, and odor.[17] Normal urine is pale yellow, but may vary due to food intake (carrots, beets, rhubarb), drugs (phenytoin, nitrofurantoin, phenazopyridine), and/or metabolic by-products (bilirubin, methemoglobin).[12] Clarity of the urine may be affected by bacteria, white blood cells, pus, or urates. Normal urine has minimal odor; therefore a strong odor may be due to concentrated urine (as in dehydrated states), infection, medicines (especially vitamins), or foods (broccoli, asparagus).

Urine pH. Urine pH indicates the acidity or alkalinity of the urine. The normal urinary pH is acidic, but with a range from 4.5 to 8.0.[12] The kidneys regulate acid-base balance; therefore more hydrogen ions are excreted than bicarbonate ions, causing the acidity of the urine. Changes in kidney function produce changes in urinary pH.

An increase in urinary acidity (decreased pH) indicates retention of sodium and acids by the body, which would be present in intrarenal ARF. Conversely, a decrease in urinary acidity (increased pH or more alkaline) means the body is retaining bicarbonate. In the presence of normal renal function, urinary pH levels are greatly affected by diet and medications. Certain food groups, such as citrus fruits and vegetables, lead to an alkaline urine, whereas a diet high in protein can produce an acid urine. In the critical care unit, patients receiving total parenteral nutrition or a high-protein tube-feeding formula may have an acidic urine because of a high protein intake.

Specific Gravity. Specific gravity measures the density or weight of urine compared with that of distilled water. The normal urinary specific gravity is 1.005 to 1.030 as compared with the normal specific gravity of distilled water at 1.000.[12] Because urine is composed of many solutes and substances suspended in water, the specific gravity should always be higher than that of water.

The specific gravity measures hydration status and indicates the ability of the kidneys to dilute or concentrate the urine.[17] Decreases in specific gravity reflect the inability of the kidneys to excrete the usual solute load into the urine (less dense with fewer solutes). Increases in specific gravity (a more concentrated urine) occur with fluid volume deficit as the result of fever, vomiting, or diarrhea. An increased specific gravity can also occur with diabetes or glomerular membrane disease, both of which allow glucose and protein to pass into the urine,

Table 29-3	Urinalysis Results		
Test	Normal	Possible Causes for Increased Values	Possible Causes for Decreased Values
pH	4.5-8.0	Alkalosis	Acidosis Intrarenal ARF
Specific gravity	1.003-1.030	Volume deficit Glycosuria Proteinuria Prerenal ARF (>1.020)	Volume overload Intrarenal ARF
Osmolality	300-1200 mOsm/kg	Volume deficit Prerenal ARF (urine > serum osmolality)	Volume excess Intrarenal ARF (urine < serum osmolality)
Protein	30-150 mg/24 hr	Trauma Infection Intrarenal ARF Transient with exercise Glomerulonephritis	
Sodium	40-220 mEq/24 hr	High-sodium diet Intrarenal ARF	Prerenal ARF
Creatinine	1-2 g/24 hr		Intrarenal ARF Chronic kidney failure
Urea	6-17 g/24 hr		Intrarenal ARF Chronic kidney failure
Myoglobin	Absent	Crush injury Rhabdomyolysis	
RBCs	0-5	Trauma Intrarenal ARF Infection Strenuous exercise Renal artery thrombus	
WBCs	0-5	Infection	
Bacteria	None-few	Infection	
Casts	None-few	RBC: glomerular disease WBC: pyelonephritis Glomerular disease Nephrotic syndrome Epithelial: glomerular disease	

ARF, Acute renal failure; *RBCs,* red blood cells; *WBCs,* white blood cells.

thereby increasing urine density. A fixed specific gravity (does not vary with fluid intake) suggests early kidney dysfunction as the kidneys are unable to excrete and/or resorb water and solutes.

Osmolality. The urine osmolality more accurately pinpoints fluid balance than does the urine specific gravity or the serum osmolality value. The serum osmolality reflects serum sodium concentration and therefore is subject to more influences than the urine osmolality. The simultaneous measurement of both the serum and urine osmolality levels provides an accurate assessment of fluid status. Normal urine osmolality is 500 to 1200 mOsm/kg and depends on resorption or excretion of water in the kidney tubules.[12,17] The urine osmolality level increases (and urine output decreases) during fluid volume deficit because of the retention of fluid by the body. Conversely, the urine osmolality level decreases (and

urine output increases) during volume excess because fluid is excreted by the kidneys. However, in intrarenal ARF the urine osmolality value and urine output are both decreased because solutes and fluids are being retained.[2]

Glucose. Glucose normally is completely resorbed by the renal tubules; therefore the urine should be free of glucose. The appearance of glucose in the urine may be transient, brought on by ingestion of a heavy carbohydrate load (as in patients on total parenteral nutrition), stress (trauma, surgery), or the renal changes that accompany pregnancy.

Consistent glycosuria occurs during hyperglycemic episodes of diabetes when the renal threshold for glucose is exceeded and the excess glucose spills into the urine. Glucose is generally present in the urine when serum glucose exceeds 180 mg/dl.[16,17] In the presence of acute or chronic kidney failure, glycosuria is not a reliable indicator of the level of hyperglycemia because of the erratic excretion of glucose by the damaged nephrons.

Protein. Protein, like glucose, normally is absent from urine because the large protein molecules are not filtered across the intact glomerular capillary membrane. Thus consistent appearance of protein in urine in amounts greater than 150 mg/day suggests compromise of the glomerular membrane and possible intrinsic kidney damage and requires further evaluation.[18] The amount of protein in the urine is often directly correlated with the severity of the damage and may exceed 4 g/day.

Transient appearance of protein in the urine can occur as the result of efferent arteriole constriction caused by extreme exercise but should decrease within 24 hours. Also, transient proteinuria can occur after ingestion of a high-protein meal or can accompany the renal changes associated with pregnancy.

Electrolytes. With the exception of sodium, levels of electrolytes in the urine are not measured as often as are levels in serum, but they too can yield information about kidney function. To measure urinary electrolyte levels, a 24-hour urine sample may be needed, although potassium and sodium are frequently measured in a randomly collected specimen. Urine electrolyte levels are highly variable, and the electrolytes depend on the kidneys for adequate excretion. Consequently, changes in urinary electrolyte levels are highly suggestive of kidney failure and generally indicate intrarenal ARF.

The most commonly measured electrolyte in the urine is sodium. Urinary sodium is a reflection of the action of aldosterone and subsequent retention or excretion of sodium by the kidney tubules to maintain fluid balance. In the presence of hypovolemia the tubules retain sodium (and therefore water), and the amount of sodium in the urine and the fractional excretion of sodium will be very low.[10] The opposite is true with volume overload and with kidney diseases that cause sodium wasting.

Sediment. The presence of sediment such as epithelial cells and casts aids in identifying problems related to the kidneys. In addition, the presence or absence of urine sediment can be helpful in identifying the etiology of ARF.[16] In prerenal ARF the kidneys are not damaged and urinary sediment is absent, which is normal. However, in intrarenal ARF the kidney glomeruli or tubules are damaged and urine sediment is abnormal, with the presence of casts and epithelial cells. Casts are shells or clumps of cellular breakdown or protein materials that form in the renal tubular system and are washed out in the urinary flow. Casts differ in composition and size and correlate with the severity and type of renal damage. White blood cell (WBC) casts indicate pyelonephritis or may occur during acute glomerulonephritis. RBC casts indicate glomerulonephritis, whereas hyaline casts are associated with renal parenchymal disease and glomerular capillary membrane inflammation. Consistent appearance of epithelial cells shed by the lining of the nephron may indicate nephritis. Although small numbers of epithelial cells normally appear in the urine and an occasional cast may be found, their consistent appearance is abnormal.[16,17]

Hematuria. Both obvious and microscopic hematuria may signal kidney damage. Although a few RBCs in the urine are normal, apparently bloody urine usually indicates bleeding within the urinary tract or renal trauma.[8] Microscopic hematuria may occur normally after strenuous exercise or the insertion of a retention catheter but should disappear within 48 hours.

The presence of myoglobin can also make the urine appear red. However, microscopic examination of the urine fails to reveal RBCs, with myoglobin being present instead.[19] Myoglobin in the urine may be present as a result of skeletal muscle damage (traumatic crush injury) or rhabdomyolysis. Rhabdomyolysis may develop in patients admitted to a critical care unit for a wide variety of reasons including cocaine abuse, status epilepticus, and heat prostration or collapse during intense physical exercise (such as running a marathon race on a hot day). Myoglobin is released by the muscle cells and blocks the tubules, resulting in intrarenal ARF.[19]

RADIOLOGIC ASSESSMENT

Although laboratory assessment is used most often in diagnosing kidney problems in the critically ill patient, radiologic assessment can confirm or clarify causes of particular disorders. Radiologic assessment ranges from basic to more complex (Table 29-4) and provides information about abnormal masses, abnormal fluid collection, obstructions, vascular supply alterations, and other disorders of the kidneys and urinary tract.[2,20,21]

Some of the radiologic studies require the use of contrast medium or injection of a radiopaque dye. Many of the dyes used in radiology are potentially nephrotoxic. Therefore dyes must be used carefully in patients with ARF or chronic kidney disease. For example, an individual with ARF undergoing a test using contrast medium may experience a further worsening of kidney function caused by the dye. In general, to prevent nephrotoxicity, adequate hydration before and after the test and careful monitoring of renal status are indicated any time a contrast medium is used.

KIDNEY BIOPSY

Kidney biopsy is the definitive tool for diagnosing disease processes of the kidney. Two methods are used: closed biopsy and open biopsy. Percutaneous needle biopsy (closed method) involves inserting a needle via the flank to obtain a specimen of cortical and medullary kidney tissue. An open biopsy is a surgical procedure

Table 29-4	Renal Imaging Tests
Test	**Comments**
Kidney-ureter-bladder (KUB)	Flat plate x-ray of abdomen; determines position, size, and structure of kidneys and urinary tract, and pelvis; useful to evaluate presence of calculi and masses Usually followed by additional tests
Intravenous pyelogram (IVP)	Intravenous (IV) injection of contrast medium with x-ray; allows visualization of internal kidney tissues
Renal angiography	Injection of contrast medium into arterial blood perfusing the kidneys; allows visualization of renal blood flow May also visualize stenosis, cysts, clots, trauma, and infarctions
Renal computed tomography (CT)	Radioisotope administered by IV route and absorbed by kidneys; scintillation photography is then performed in several planes; spiral or helical CT allows rapid imaging Density of the image helps evaluate kidney vessels, perfusion, tumors, cysts, hemorrhage, necrosis, and trauma
Renal ultrasound	High-frequency sound waves are transmitted to the kidneys and urinary tract, and image is viewed on an oscilloscope; noninvasive Identifies fluid accumulation or obstruction, cysts, and masses Useful to evaluate kidney before biopsy
Magnetic resonance imaging (MRI)	A scanner produces three-dimensional images in response to the application of high-energy radiofrequency waves to the tissues Produces clear images; the density of the image may indicate trauma, cysts, masses, malformation of the vessels or tubules, and necrosis

and is rarely done in critically ill patients. In either case, biopsy is often the last choice for diagnostic assessment in the critically ill patient because of the postprocedural risks of bleeding, hematoma formation, and infection.

REFERENCES

1. Seidel HM et al: *Mosby's guide to physical examination,* ed 5, St Louis, 2003, Mosby.
2. Richard C: Assessment of renal structure and function. In Lancaster L, editor: *Core curriculum for nephrology nursing,* ed 4, Pitman, NJ, 2001, American Nephrology Nurses Association.
3. Metheny NM: *Fluid and electrolyte balance—nursing considerations,* ed 4, Philadelphia, 2000, Lippincott.
4. Malasanos L, Barkauskas V, Stoltenberg-Allen K: *Health assessment,* ed 4, St Louis, 1990, Mosby.
5. Ejaz AA et al: Characteristics of 100 consecutive patients presenting with orthostatic hypotension, *Mayo Clin Proc* 79(7):890-894, 2004.
6. Irvin D: The importance of accurately assessing orthostatic hypotension, *Geriatr Nurs* 25(2):99, 2004.
7. Bozeman C et al: Selective operative management of major blunt renal trauma, *J Trauma* 57(2):305-309, 2004.
8. Knudson MM et al: Outcome after major renovascular injuries: a Western trauma association multicenter report, *J Trauma* 49(6):1116-1122, 2000.
9. Purcell W et al: Accurate dry weight assessment: reducing the incidence of hypertension and cardiac disease in patients on hemodialysis, *Nephrol Nurs J* 31(6):631-636, 2004.
10. Subramanian S, Ziedalski TM: Oliguria, volume overload, Na$^+$ balance, and diuretics, *Crit Care Clin* 21(20):291-303, 2005.
11. Robinson BE, Weber H: Dehydration despite drinking: beyond the BUN/creatinine ratio, *J Am Med Dir Assoc* 5(2 suppl):S67-S71, 2004.
12. Kee J: *Handbook of laboratory & diagnostic tests with nursing implications,* ed 5, Upper Saddle River, NJ, 2005, Pearson Prentice-Hall.
13. Thomas DR et al: Physician misdiagnosis of dehydration in older adults, *J Am Med Dir Assoc* 5(2 suppl):S30-S34, 2004.
14. Miller D et al: Challenges for nephrology nurses in the management of children with chronic kidney disease, *Neph Nurs J,* 31(3):287, 2004.
15. Simonson M: Measurement of glomerular filtration rate. In Hricik et al, editors: *Nephrology secrets,* ed. 2, Philadelphia, 2003, Hanley & Belfus.
16. Ganz M: Urinalysis. In Hricik et al, editors: *Nephrology secrets,* ed. 2, Philadelphia, 2003, Hanley & Belfus.
17. Hanson K: Laboratory studies in the evaluation of urologic disease: Part I, *Urol Nurs* 23(6):400, 2004.
18. Simonson M: Measurement of urinary protein. In Hricik et al, editors: *Nephrology secrets,* ed. 2, Philadelphia, 2003, Hanley & Belfus.
19. Russell T: Acute renal failure related to rhabdomyolysis: pathophysiology, diagnosis, and collaborative management, *Neph Nurs J* 27(5):567, 2000.
20. Hanson K: Diagnostic tests and tools in the evaluation of urologic disease: Part II, *Urol Nurs* 23(6):405, 2004.
21. Elashi E et al: Renal imaging techniques. In Hricik et al, editors: *Nephrology secrets,* ed 2, Philadelphia, 2003, Hanley & Belfus.

CHAPTER 30

Renal Disorders and Therapeutic Management

ACUTE RENAL FAILURE

Acute renal failure (ARF) is characterized by a sudden decline in glomerular filtration rate (GFR), with subsequent retention of products in the blood that are normally excreted by the kidneys; this disrupts electrolyte balance, acid-base homeostasis, and fluid volume equilibrium.

CRITICAL ILLNESS AND ARF

Once ARF has occurred in the critically ill patient, the risk of death rises dramatically.[1] Mortality ranges from 38% to 80%.[2] One of the reasons for the high mortality is that critical care patients often have coexisting nonrenal health problems that increase their susceptibility to the development of ARF. High-risk conditions include heart failure, shock, respiratory failure and sepsis.[1,2] The increasing number of comorbid conditions found in critically ill patients is changing the spectrum of acute renal failure. A recent observational study that examined the incidence and course of ARF in six academic medical centers in the United States found that acute renal failure was accompanied by extrarenal organ failure in most patients, even those who did not require dialysis.[1] In this study of 618 patients with ARF, 64% of patients required dialysis, the in-hospital mortality was 37%, and the rate of nonrecovery of the kidney and/or death was 50%.[1] The clinicians' conclusion is that mortality in the critically ill patient with ARF is related to the severity of the extrarenal disease.[1] Mortality rates exceeded 50% when four or more systems had failed.[1]

The high mortality related to ARF has not changed for over 4 decades in spite of increasingly complex technologies to treat acute renal failure.[1] One could argue that today patients with acute renal failure often have associated multiple organ dysfunction syndrome (MODS) and have more complex illnesses and comorbidities compared with patients 40 years ago. More critical care patients are receiving dialysis therapies in the critical care unit.[1]

Typically a patient is not admitted to the critical care unit with a diagnosis of acute renal failure alone; there is always coexisting hemodynamic, cardiac, pulmonary, or neurologic compromise. Many individuals come into the hospital with preexisting renal insufficiency (elevated serum creatinine), although they may be nonsymptomatic and unaware of their renal compromise.[3] This lack of renal reserve places them at increased risk of acute renal failure should complications occur in any of the other major organ systems. As a result, the picture of acute renal failure in the modern critical care unit has changed to encompass patients with renal failure who also have multisystem nonrenal diseases that complicate their clinical course.[1]

DEFINITION OF ARF

At this time there is no standardized definition of acute renal failure that may be applied to the critically ill.[4] Some researchers suggest that ARF be described according to whether it was community- or hospital-acquired, or by the speed of the rise of the serum creatinine level.[2] Others focus on the etiology of the acute renal failure.[1] For the purposes of understanding the etiology of acute renal dysfunction in this chapter, ARF is classified into three categories according to location of the insult relative to the kidney: prerenal, intrarenal, and postrenal (Box 30-1).

PRERENAL ARF

Any condition that decreases blood flow, blood pressure (BP), or renal perfusion before arterial blood reaches the kidney can cause prerenal failure. When renal hypoperfusion due to low cardiac output, hemorrhage, vasodilation, thrombosis, or other cause reduces the blood flow to the kidney, glomerular filtration decreases and consequently urine output decreases (see Box 30-1). This is a major reason that the critical care nurse monitors the urine output on an hourly basis. Initially, in prerenal states the integrity of the kidney's nephron structure and function is preserved. If normal perfusion and cardiac output are restored quickly, the kidney will not suffer any permanent injury. However, if the prerenal in-

---

Box 30-1

ETIOLOGIES OF ACUTE RENAL FAILURE

PRERENAL
Prolonged hypotension (sepsis, vasodilation)
Prolonged low cardiac output (heart failure, cardiogenic shock)
Prolonged volume depletion (dehydration, hemorrhage)
Renovascular thrombosis (thromboemboli)

INTRARENAL
Renal ischemia (advanced stage of prerenal failure)
Endogenous toxins (rhabdomyolysis, tumor lysis syndrome)
Exogenous toxins: (radiocontrast dye, nephrotoxic drugs)
Infection (acute glomerulonephritis, interstitial nephritis)

POSTRENAL
Obstruction (urethra/prostate/bladder)
Rare to be cause of ARF in critical care

---

sult is not corrected, the GFR will decline, the BUN will rise, and the patient will develop oliguria and risk significant kidney damage. *Oliguria*, or a urine output less than 400 ml/day, is a classic finding in ARF.[2] Prerenal ARF is seen frequently in the critically ill. In a study of hospitalized elderly patients with renal failure, prerenal ARF occurred in 58% of the patients.[2] This compares with 34% intrarenal and 8% postrenal causes in the same study.[2]

INTRARENAL ARF

Any condition that produces an ischemic or toxic insult directly at the site of the nephron places the patient at risk for development of intrarenal failure (see Box 30-1). Ischemic damage may be caused by prolonged hypotension or low cardiac output. Toxic injury reaction may occur in response to substances that damage the renal tubular endothelium such as some antimicrobial drugs and the contrast dye used in radiology diagnostic studies. The insult may involve both the glomeruli and the tubular epithelium. When the internal filtering structures are affected, this is known as *acute tubular necrosis*.

POSTRENAL ARF

Any obstruction that hinders the flow of urine from beyond the kidney through the remainder of the urinary tract may lead to postrenal failure. This is not a frequent cause of kidney failure in the critically ill. When monitoring of the urine output reveals a sudden decrease in the patient's urine output from the urinary catheter, a blockage may be responsible. Sudden development of *anuria* (urine output below 100 ml/24 hours) should prompt verification that the urinary catheter is not occluded.

AZOTEMIA

The term *azotemia* is used to describe an acute rise in blood urea nitrogen (BUN). *Uremia* is another term used to describe an elevated BUN.

ACUTE TUBULAR NECROSIS

Acute tubular necrosis (ATN) results from either nephrotoxic or ischemic injury that damages the renal tubular epithelium and, in severe cases, extends to the basement membrane. Injury that is limited to the epithelial layer recovers sooner than injury that also involves the basement membrane.

EPIDEMIOLOGY AND ETIOLOGY

Damage to the cells in the glomerular and tubular structures prevents normal concentration of urine, filtration of wastes, and regulation of acid-base, electrolyte, and water balance. The renal tubular cells are constantly at risk for damage because of their normally high blood flows, high oxygen requirements, and the constant resorption and secretion of metabolites. A number of disorders can result in ATN, and several contributing factors often work together to bring about tubular damage. Common causes of ATN are divided into two categories: ischemic injury and nephrotoxic injury (Box 30-2).

Ischemic Acute Tubular Necrosis. Ischemic damage secondary to inadequate perfusion impairs tubular endothelial function, causing nonuniform patchy areas of tubular cell damage and cast formation. Ischemic necrosis occurs as a result of vasodilation associated with sepsis and when hypotension or a low-cardiac-output episode is prolonged; it is worsened by renal hypoperfusion or dehydration. In other words, prerenal low perfusion can develop into intrarenal ischemic ATN (see Box 30-2). In the multicenter study of critical care patients with ARF by Mehta and colleagues, 50% of the patients had ischemic ATN, which was largely precipitated by hypotension (20%), and sepsis (19%).[1]

Toxic Acute Tubular Necrosis. Nephrotoxic damage results from damage by drugs and chemical agents. A common cause of toxic ATN is the radiopaque (contrast) dye administered during an interventional or diagnostic radiologic study. Complications from the contrast will cause ARF in 9% to 14% of patients.[1,5,6] In affected patients, the serum creatinine levels typically begin to rise 48 to 72 hours after the study, peak at 3 to 5 days, and return to baseline within another 3 to 5 days.[5] The renal dysfunction can persist up to 3 weeks after the procedure.[6] Although patients with normal renal function are not considered to be at risk, those with elevated serum creatinine levels, diabetes, or microvascular disease are highly vulnerable.[5,6]

Box 30-2

ISCHEMIC VS. NEPHROTOXIC ACUTE TUBULAR NECROSIS

ISCHEMIC INJURY
Advanced stage of prerenal injury
  Massive hemorrhage
  Severe volume loss
  Severe dehydration
  Severe, prolonged hypotension
  Shock: cardiogenic, hypovolemic, septic
  Sepsis
  Anaphylaxis

NEPHROTOXIC INJURY
Endogenous Toxins*
Rhabdomyolysis
Tumor lysis syndrome

Exogenous Toxins*
Radiocontrast dye

Nephrotoxic Antimicrobials
Aminoglycosides: gentamicin, tobramycin
Cephalosporins: cefazolin
Antifungals: amphotericin B
Antivirals: acyclovir

Nephrotoxic Immunosuppressants
Cyclosporin; tacrolimus (FK506)

Nephrotoxic Chemotherapeutics
5-Azacitidine; cisplatin; methotrexate

Nephrotoxic Street Drugs
Heroin; amphetamines; phencyclidine (PCP)

Nephrotoxic Analgesics:
Nonsteroidal antiinflammatory drugs (NSAIDs)

*Only represents a partial list of potential nephrotoxic medications.

Toxic damage causes uniform, widespread injury to the renal endothelium. Because the basement membrane is not injured as severely as with ischemic ATN, the healing is more rapid, the layer of the membrane can regenerate, and full recovery from ATN and resumption of renal function is more likely (see Box 30-2).

PATHOPHYSIOLOGY

The mechanisms responsible for tubular dysfunction in ischemic ATN are multifactorial. When "cellular debris" accumulates in the nephron tubular lumen, an obstruction will occur if there is not adequate flow of filtrate through the nephron. The obstruction is made up of casts and sloughing tissue and is exacerbated by interstitial edema. Filtration ceases when tubular hydrostatic pressure rises to match GFR. This decreases the formation of urine because of the lack of filtrate to process. The result is more tubular cell swelling, obstruction, decreased capillary blood flow, and finally, further ischemia and cell injury. The clinical course of ATN progresses through four phases.

PHASES OF ACUTE TUBULAR NECROSIS

Onset Phase. The onset (initiating) phase is the period from when an insult occurs until cell injury. Ischemic injury is evolving during this time. The GFR is decreased because of impaired renal blood flow and decreased glomerular ultrafiltration pressure. This disrupts the integrity of the tubular epithelium, which back-leaks the glomerular filtrate. This phase lasts from hours to days, depending on the cause, with toxic factors causing the phase to last longer. If treatment is initiated during this time, irreversible damage can be alleviated. A longer course of recovery reflects the presence of more extensive tubular injury.

Oliguric/Anuric Phase. The oliguric/anuric phase, the second phase of ATN, lasts 5 to 8 days in the nonoliguric patient and 10 to 16 days in the oliguric patient.[7] The accumulation of necrotic cellular debris in the tubular space blocks the flow of urine and causes damage to the tubular wall and basement membranes. Also, a back-leak phenomenon occurs because damage in the tubular wall causes the glomerular filtrate to flow passively into the renal tissue rather than be passed out as urine through the ureters and bladder. Oliguria is encountered more often in ischemic damage and is a sign that the damage is more extensive and severe. During the oliguric/anuric phase, GFR is greatly reduced, which leads to increased levels of BUN (azotemia), elevated serum creatinine levels, electrolyte abnormalities (hyperkalemia, hyperphosphatemia, hypocalcemia), and metabolic acidosis.

Diuretic Phase. The third phase, the diuretic phase, lasts 7 to 14 days and is characterized by an increase in GFR and sometimes polyuria with a urine output as high as 2 to 4 L/day. If the patient is receiving hemodialysis during this phase, the polyuria will not be evident because excess volume will be removed by dialysis. During the diuretic phase the tubular obstruction has passed, but edema and scarring are present. In this situation, the GFR returns before the ability of the tubules to function normally. The kidneys can clear volume but not solutes, which, with a large diuresis, can lead to volume depletion.

Recovery Phase. The last phase of ATN is the recovery, or convalescent, phase. Both oliguric and nonoliguric patients will demonstrate increased urine output if they enter the recovery stage. During this stage, renal function slowly returns to normal or near normal, with a GFR that is 70% to 80% of normal within 1 to 2 years.[8] However, if significant renal parenchymal damage has occurred, BUN and creatinine levels may never return to normal. For patients surviving ATN, approximately 62% will recover normal renal function, 33% will be left with residual renal insufficiency, and at least 5% will require long-term hemodialysis.[8]

Table 30-1	Initial Urine Laboratory Analysis Findings in Acute Renal Failure*		
	Prerenal†	**Intrarenal‡**	**Postrenal§**
Urine Volume	Normal	Oliguria or nonoliguria	Oliguria to anuria
Urine Specific Gravity	>1.020	1.010	1.000-1.010
Urine Osmolality (mOsm/kg)	>350	~300	300-400
Urine sodium (mEq/L)	<20	>30	20-40
FENa (%)	<1%	>2-3%	1%-3%
BUN/Cr ratio	20:1	Ischemic: 20:1	10:1
		Toxic: 10:1	
Urine microscopy (sediment)	Normal	ATN: dark granular casts, hyaline casts, renal epithelial cells	Normal

*Results of urine laboratory tests are only valid in the absence of diuretics.
†Urine in prerenal failure is concentrated, with low sodium.
‡Urine in intrarenal failure shows kidney damage because the nephron cannot concentrate urine or conserve sodium, and evidence of renal damage (casts) is seen.
§Urine test results in postrenal failure are variable, because initially the findings depend on the hydration status of the patient rather than the status of the kidney.
~ Approximately; *Cr,* creatinine; *BUN,* blood urea nitrogen; *anuria,* urine volume less than 100 ml/24 hr; *oliguria,* urine volume 100-400 ml/24 hr; *polyuria,* urine volume excessive over 24 hours; *mEq/L,* milliequivalents per liter; *mOsm/kg,* milliosmoles per kilogram; *FENa,* fractional excretion of sodium; *ATN,* acute tubular necrosis.

Table 30-2	Normal Serum Electrolyte Values
Electrolyte	**Normal Value**
Sodium	135-145 mEq/L
Potassium	3.5-4.5 mEq/L
Chloride	98-108 mEq/L
Calcium	8.5-10.5 mg/dl *or* 4.5-5.8 mEq/L
Phosphorus	2.7-4.5 mg/dl
Magnesium	1.5-2.5 mEq/L
Bicarbonate	24-28 mEq/L

ASSESSMENT AND DIAGNOSIS

LABORATORY ASSESSMENT

Once acute renal disease is suspected, the presence or degree or renal dysfunction is assessed using both urine and blood analysis. Table 30-1 lists the initial urine analysis findings in ARF. Most serum electrolytes will become increasingly elevated as ARF develops (Table 30-2). Clinical findings associated with acute renal failure are listed in Table 30-3. Normal and abnormal urinalysis findings and significance are summarized in Chapter 29.

Acidosis. Acidosis (pH below 7.5) is one of the trademarks of acute renal failure.[9] Metabolic acidosis occurs as a result of the accumulation of unexcreted waste products. The acid waste products consist of strong negative ions (anions), elevated serum phosphorus (hyperphosphatemia), and other normally "unmeasured ions" (sulfate, urate, lactate, and others) that decrease the serum pH.[9] A low serum albumin, often present in ARF, has a slight alkalinizing effect, but not enough to offset the metabolic acidosis.[9] Even though respiratory compensation may be present, or the patient may receive mechanical ventilatory support, this is rarely sufficient to reverse the metabolic acidosis. Acidosis in acute renal failure is complex, as evidenced by the fact that many ARF patients maintain a normal anion gap.[9] The reasons for this remain unknown.[9] Information on acidosis and arterial blood gas interpretation is found in Chapter 22. Anion gap measurement is discussed in Chapter 29.

Blood Urea Nitrogen. BUN is not a reliable indicator of kidney damage.[10] Although it reflects cellular damage, BUN is easily changed by protein intake, blood in the gastrointestinal (GI) tract, and cell catabolism and is diluted by fluid administration. A BUN-creatinine ratio may be calculated to determine the cause of the acute renal dysfunction (see Table 30-1). The BUN-creatinine ratio is most useful in diagnosing prerenal failure (often described as prerenal azotemia) where the BUN level is greatly elevated relative to the serum creatinine value.

Serum Creatinine. Creatinine is a by-product of muscle metabolism that is formed from nonenzymatic dehydration of creatine in the liver;[10] 98% of creatine is in the muscles[10] and it is almost totally excreted by the renal tubules. Thus, if the kidneys are not working the creatinine level will rise in the serum. When the serum creatinine doubles (for example from 0.75 to 1.5 mg/dl), this reflects a decrease of approximately 50% in the GFR.[10] Serum creatinine level is assessed daily to follow the trend of renal function and answer the question, is kidney function stable, getting better, or getting worse?[10]

Table 30-3	Serum Electrolytes in Acute Renal Failure	
Electrolyte Disturbance	**Serum Value**	**Clinical Findings**
POTASSIUM		
Hypokalemia	<3.5 mEq/L	Muscular weakness
		Cardiac irregularities on ECG
		Abdominal distention and flatulence
		Paresthesia
		Decreased reflexes
		Anorexia
		Dizziness, confusion
		Increased sensitivity to digitalis
Hyperkalemia	>4.5 mEq/L	Irritability and restlessness
		Anxiety
		Nausea and vomiting
		Abdominal cramps
		Weakness
		Numbness and tingling (fingertips and circumoral)
		Cardiac irregularities on ECG
SODIUM		
Hyponatremia	<135 mEq/L	Disorientation
		Muscle twitching
		Nausea/vomiting, abdominal cramps
		Headaches, dizziness
		Seizures, postural hypotension
		Cold, clammy skin
		Decreased skin turgor
		Tachycardia
		Oliguria
Hypernatremia	>145 mEq/L	Extreme thirst
		Dry, sticky mucous membranes
		Altered mentation
		Seizures (later stages)
CALCIUM		
Hypocalcemia	<8.5 mg/dl *or* <4.5 mEq/L	Irritability
		Muscular tetany, muscle cramps
		Decreased cardiac output (decreased contractions)
		Bleeding (decreased ability to coagulate)
		ECG changes
		Positive Chvostek's/Trousseau's signs
Hypercalcemia	>10.5 mg/dl *or* >5.8 mEq/L	Deep bone pain
		Excessive thirst
		Anorexia
		Lethargy, weakened muscles
MAGNESIUM		
Hypomagnesemia	<1.4 mEq/L	Choroid/athetoid muscle activity
		Facial tics, spasticity
		Cardiac dysrhythmias
Hypermagnesemia	>2.5 mEq/L	CNS depression
		Respiratory depression
		Lethargy
		Coma
		Bradycardia
		ECG changes
PHOSPHATE		
Hypophosphatemia	<3.0 mg/dl	Hemolytic anemias
		Depressed white cell function
		Bleeding (decreased platelet aggregation)
		Nausea/vomiting
		Anorexia

Continued

Table 30-3	Serum Electrolytes in Acute Renal Failure—cont'd	
Electrolyte Disturbance	**Serum Value**	**Clinical Findings**
PHOSPHATE—CONT'D		
Hyperphosphatemia	>4.5 mg/dl	Tachycardia
		Nausea, diarrhea, abdominal cramps
		Muscle weakness, flaccid paralysis
		Increased reflexes
CHLORIDE		
Hypochloremia	<98 mEq/L	Hyperirritability
		Tetany or muscular excitability
		Slow respirations
Hyperchloremia	>108 mEq/L	Weakness, lethargy
		Deep, rapid breathing
		Possible unconsciousness (later stages)
ALBUMIN		
Hypoalbuminemia	<3.8 g/dl	Muscle wasting
		Peripheral edema (fluid shift)
		Decreased resistance to infection
		Poorly healing wounds

ECG, Electrocardiogram; *CNS,* central nervous system.

Creatinine Clearance. If the patient is making sufficient urine, the urinary creatinine clearance can be measured. A normal urine creatinine clearance is 120 ml/min, but this value decreases with renal failure. Critical care patients in ARF are oliguric, and the urine creatinine clearance is infrequently measured.

Fractional Excretion of Sodium. The fractional excretion of sodium (FENa) in the urine is measured early in the ARF course to differentiate between a prerenal condition and ATN (intrarenal). A FENa value below 1% (in the absence of diuretics) suggests prerenal compromise, because resorption of almost all the filtered sodium is an appropriate response to decreased renal perfusion. If diuretics are administered, the test is meaningless. A FENa value above 2% implies the kidney cannot concentrate the sodium and that the damage is intrarenal (ATN).

Urinary sodium is measured in mEq/L (milliequivalents per liter). The interpretation of results is similar to the FENa. Urinary sodium less than 10 mEq/L (low) indicates a prerenal condition. Urinary sodium greater than 40 mEq/L suggests an intrarenal cause (see Table 30-1). As with other urinalysis tests, the use of diuretics invalidates any results. This is because the diuretics alter resorption of water and produce dilute urine and the test result will not reflect actual kidney function.

Radiologic Findings. A computed tomography (CT) scan of the abdomen is useful to evaluate the anatomic status of the kidney in the critically ill. Angiography is used more cautiously because of the association between use of contrast media and nephrotoxic renal failure.[6]

"AT RISK" DISEASE STATES AND ACUTE RENAL FAILURE

Many patients come into the critical care unit with disease states that predispose them to the development of acute renal failure. There are also many individuals who already have kidney damage but are unaware of this condition.[3]

UNDERLYING CHRONIC KIDNEY DISEASE

The incidence of chronic kidney disease (CKD) in United States is estimated to be 11% (19.2 million adults).[11] Recent clinical practice guidelines for management of end-stage kidney disease (ESKD) have classified renal dysfunction into five stages.[12] Because of the large numbers of adults with renal dysfunction (diagnosed or not), kidney function must be assessed on all critically ill patients at risk for fluid and electrolyte imbalance. The glomerular filtration rate associated with each stage and the numeric population estimates in each stage of kidney dysfunction are shown in Table 30-4.

Most people in the early stages of renal disease are unaware of their condition.[3] A national health survey queried individuals whether they had ever been told by their physician that they had "weak or failing kidneys." The answer to this question was then correlated with the individual's GFR and the presence of albuminuria by urine test to stratify them according to the five stages of kidney failure (see Table 30-4). The results showed that

Table 30-4	Decreased Kidney Function by Stage in Adult U.S. Population		
Stage*	Population Affected*	GFR‡ and Diagnosis*	Percent Who Know They Have Kidney Dysfunction (%)†
1	9 million (3.3%)	Normal; persistent albuminuria	40.5
2	5.3 million (3.0%)	60 to 89; persistent albuminuria	29.3
3	7.6 million (4.3%)	30 to 59	22.0
4	400,000 (0.2%)	15 to 29	44.5
5	300,000 (0.2%)	Below 15: End stage kidney disease	100

*Data from Coresh J et al: *Am J Kidney Dis* 41(1):1-12, 2003.
† Data from Nickolas TL et al: *Am J Kidney Dis* 44(2):185-197, 2004.
‡Glomerular filtration rate (GFR) in ml/min /1.73 m^2 body surface area.

Table 30-5	RIFLE Criteria for Acute Renal Dysfunction	
RIFLE	Serum Cr/GFR Criteria	Urine Output Criteria
Risk	Serum Cr increased 1.5 times above normal **or** GFR decreased more than 25%	<0.5 ml/kg/hr for 6 hours
Injury	Serum Cr increased 2 times above normal **or** GFR decreased more than 50%	<0.5 ml/kg/hr for 12 hours
Failure hours	Serum Cr increased 3 times above normal **or**	<0.3 ml/kg/hr for 24 hours **or** anuria for 12
	GFR decreased more than 75% **or** Serum Cr ≥ 4mg/dl **or** Serum Cr acute rise ≥ 0.5 mg/dl	
Loss	Persistent acute renal failure (ARF); complete loss of kidney function for more than 4 weeks	
ESKD	End-stage kidney disease for >3 months	

Data from Bellomo R et al. Acute renal failure: definition, outcome measures, animal models, fluid therapy and information technology needs: the Second International Consensus Conference of the Acute Dialysis Quality Initiative (ADQI) Group, *Crit Care* 8(4):R204-212, 2004.

over half the respondents were unaware that they had renal dysfunction until they reached stage 5 or end-stage kidney disease when they would become dialysis dependent.[3] The results categorized by stage of kidney failure are listed in Table 30-4.

RISK OF ACUTE RENAL FAILURE

A classification to determine risk of developing acute renal failure in critically ill patients has been proposed by a multinational group of nephrologists.[13] The classification uses the acronym *RIFLE:* *r*isk, *i*njury, *f*ailure, *l*oss, and *E*SKD (end-stage kidney disease).[13] The RIFLE system classifies patients into categories of risk, based on GFR criteria, urine output, or previous loss of renal function[13] (Table 30-5). If acute renal failure is superimposed on a kidney that is already compromised, the researchers recommend adding the term chronic to the RIFLE criteria to denote an "acute-on-chronic" renal failure etiology.[13]

OLDER AGE AND ARF

Older age appears to be a risk factor for development of chronic kidney disease, because 11% of individuals older than 65 years *without* hypertension or diabetes have stage 3 or worse CKD.[11] In the presence of diabetes or hypertension, the risk of developing chronic kidney disease increases substantially (see following section, as well as the Clinical Application feature on Renal Concepts).

HEART FAILURE AND ARF

There is a strong association between kidney failure and cardiovascular disease. In studies of critically ill patients with acute renal failure, 54%[1] to 63%[2] have both

CLINICAL APPLICATION

Renal Concepts

JT is a 55-year-old male who was diagnosed with severe hypertension 3½ years ago. His medication regimen includes at least two antihypertensive drugs, as well as furosemide (Lasix) and a potassium supplement. He states he has frequent omissions of his medications because of a hectic work schedule. Per paramedic report, JT presents to the hospital with a complaint of sudden, intense midabdominal to lower abdominal pain. He began to feel faint and nauseated but was unable to summon help. The paramedics arrived to find JT alert but ashen, and dyspneic. He complained of accelerating midabdominal pain radiating to his thoracic spine. The paramedics noted the following: blood pressure (BP), 88/40; heart rate (R), 126; respiratory rate (RR), 32; oxygen saturation (SpO_2), 94% (despite receiving 6 L O_2); and tense, distended abdomen without bowel sounds. En route to the hospital, JT's systolic BP fell to 74 mm Hg despite rapid IV infusion of lactated Ringer's solution. Before surgery JT received 1200 ml of intravenous (IV) fluids.

JT is diagnosed with an abdominal aortic aneurysm.

1. Which of JT's symptoms support the diagnosis of abdominal aortic aneurysm?
2. What is the most probable cause of JT's changes in blood pressure?
3. Given JT's medical diagnosis, what nursing diagnoses must be addressed?

During surgery, JT lost approximately 9 L of blood, which was replaced with lactated Ringer's (LR), Plasmanate, and packed red blood cells (PRBCs). He returned to the critical care unit in stable condition with the following assessment:

He has no neurologic deficits except that he is lethargic. His RR is 26/min. He has decreased excursion and diminished breath sounds throughout lung bases. His ABG values on oxygen at 4L/min per nasal cannula are PaO_2, 90; $PaCO_2$ 40; pH, 7.40; O_2 saturation, 96%. His BP is 118/60; HR, 98; mean arterial pressure (MAP), 80; right atrial pressure (RAP), 4 mm Hg; cardiac output (CO), 6 L/min; pulmonary artery occlusion pressure (PAOP), 8 mm Hg; systemic vascular resistance (SVR), 1014 dynes/sec/cm^{-5}. Regular heart rate with no extra heart sounds or murmurs. Peripheral pulses at 1+. His skin is cool and mottled over extremities, but upper body is warm and dry. Nasogastric (NG) tube per his right naris is draining pink-tinged fluid. Abdomen is soft and nondistended. Bowel sounds are absent. Bulky dressing at midabdomen is clean, dry, and intact. His urinary catheter is in place, draining clear, amber urine at 100-120 ml/hour. Approximately 500 ml of urine is in the bag. Hematocrit (Hct) is 28%; hemoglobin (Hgb), 8.4; Na^+, 136; K^+, 3.8; Cl^-, 108.

4. Interpret JT's hemodynamic values and fluid status.
5. What medical treatments would you anticipate to treat these values?
6. What medical treatments would you expect to treat the Hgb and Hct values and electrolytes?
7. Why would you expect hypothermia to be present in this patient?
8. Interpret JT's current acid-base status.
9. What other nursing diagnoses could you anticipate for this patient?

On the third postoperative day, JT was transferred to the medical/surgical unit. On day 4 he began to experience decreased urine output of 50 ml/hr. Output continued to drop to 30 ml/day. By day 5 his weight had increased 8 kg; 3+ edema was present in both lower extremities. JT complained of mild dyspnea and nausea. Despite furosemide (Lasix) administration, his renal output had not increased.

Laboratory values on day 5 were as follows: K^+, 6.4; Na^+, 138; Cl^-, 110; serum creatinine, 7.0; blood urea nitrogen (BUN), 73. ECG shows peaked T waves.

10. What do these findings show?
11. How would you treat these findings?
12. What other therapeutic measures may need to be initiated to treat this patient's low urine output?
13. As part of the patient's ongoing assessment, what things must the nurse monitor and address?

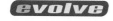 For the discussion of this Clinical Application and for additional clinical applications on renal concepts, see the Evolve website.

---

acute renal failure and heart failure. Hypertension, a major contributor to the development of heart failure, is also a major risk factor for the development of CKD.[14] Unfortunately the presence of hypertension and diabetes predisposes an individual to development of chronic kidney disease and exposes him or her to a higher risk of death.[11,15-17] As the patient's GFR declines, the risks of cardiovascular disease, myocardial infarction, and death increase, especially for patients with stage 3 or worse CKD.[18,19]

RESPIRATORY FAILURE AND ARF

There is a significant association between respiratory failure and kidney failure. In studies of critically ill patients with renal failure, 54% to 88% have respiratory failure.[1-2] The range in values is due to how the renal failure was classified. For example, in one study 57% have respiratory and renal failure but were not treated with dialysis;[1] and 88% have respiratory and renal failure and were given dialysis treatment with continuous renal replacement therapy (CRRT).[2] See later section for a detailed description of CRRT.

The process of mechanical ventilation also affects the kidney, although it is not known if this is deleterious.[20] Positive pressure ventilation reduces renal blood flow (RBF), lowers GFR, and decreases urine output.[20] These effects are intensified with the addition of positive end-expiratory pressure (PEEP).[20] Prolonged mechanical ventilation in critically ill patients is associated with an increased incidence of acute renal failure and dialysis.[20] It is likely that the real problem is respiratory failure and that mechanical ventilation is just a marker for the increased severity of illness.

SEPSIS AND ARF

Sepsis and septic shock create hemodynamic instability and decrease renal perfusion.[21,22] The mechanism is presumed to be prerenal. Sepsis caused 19% or ARF in one study,[1] and 55% of ARF in a population of elderly hospitalized patients.[2] Clinical guidelines for hemodynamic support in sepsis emphasize the need for adequate fluid resuscitation; since in 40% to 50% of cases, reversal of hypotension and restoration of hemodynamic stability can be achieved with fluids alone.[22] Unfortunately, in severely septic patients, inflammation increases vascular permeability and much of this fluid may move into the third space (interstitial space).[22] If the BP remains low, the use of vasopressors is recommended to raise refractory low BP. Vasopressors raise BP, increase systemic vascular resistance (SVR), and presumably also increase intrarenal vascular resistance. Other practices aimed at reversing the deleterious effects of sepsis include maintaining the patient's hemoglobin level over 8 mg/dl and achieving a pulmonary artery occlusion pressure (PAOP), or wedge pressure, between 12 and 15 mm Hg.[22]

TRAUMA AND ARF

Trauma patients with major crush injuries have an elevated risk of kidney failure because of the release of creatine and myoglobin from damaged muscle cells.[23] Myoglobin in large quantities is toxic to the kidney. Overall survival from rhabdomyolysis is 77%.[23]

Creatine kinase (CK), a marker of systemic muscle damage, will rise with rhabdomyolysis. One trauma service reported that out of 2,083 critical care trauma admissions, 85% had elevated CK levels and 10% developed acute renal failure secondary to rhabdomyolysis.[24] A CK level of 5000 units/L was the lowest abnormal value present in patients who developed ARF associated with rhabdomyolysis.[24]

Volume resuscitation is the primary treatment to preserve adequate kidney function and prevent development of acute renal failure. In many hospitals the intravenous (IV) fluids are alkalinized by the addition of sodium bicarbonate, and the urine output is increased by IV administration of the diuretic mannitol.[23] A bicarbonate/mannitol regimen is utilized to try to prevent acidosis and hyperkalemia, both frequent complications of rhabdomyolysis. Close attention is paid to urine output, CK, any rise in serum creatinine, and any signs of compartment syndrome in all patients admitted with this diagnosis.

CONTRAST-INDUCED NEPHROTOXIC INJURY AND ARF

Over 1 million studies or procedures that involve use of IV radiocontrast are performed every year.[5] Approximately 1% of those patients will require dialysis as a result of contrast-induced nephrotoxicity, with prolongation of the hospital stay to an average of 17 days.[5] Patients at risk are those with a baseline serum creatinine over 1.5 mg/dl, known diabetes, heart failure, or volume depletion.[25] A clinical definition of contrast-induced nephrotoxicity is a rise in serum creatinine of 0.5 mg/dl or more, or a 25% rise from the patient's baseline, within 48 to 72 hours of contrast medium exposure.[5,25] High–molecular-weight contrast medium is a potential cause of nephrotoxicity.[5,26] One strategy to prevent contrast-induced nephrotoxicity involves use of a lower quantity of contrast per study, and use of nonionic, low-osmolar or isoosmolar (iohexol) contrast media that are less nephrotoxic.[26] Research studies are still needed to determine how to avoid this complication. The best method of prevention is aggressive hydration with IV normal saline both during and after the procedure. Research results are mixed on the use of the oral drug N-acetylcysteine (NAC),[27-29] and IV infusion of fenoldopan.[5,6] Some studies report that these drugs are helpful,[6,28] and others report them as neutral, neither beneficial nor harmful.[5,27] Patients undergoing radiology studies with contrast represent a major at-risk population, and more research on the optimal treatment strategy is required to prevent contrast-induced nephrotoxicity.

HEMODYNAMIC MONITORING AND FLUID BALANCE

Hemodynamic monitoring is important for the analysis of fluid volume status in the critically ill patient with ARF.

Hemodynamic Monitoring. Hemodynamic monitoring includes surveillance of central venous pressure (CVP), pulmonary artery occlusion pressure (PAOP), cardiac output (CO), and cardiac index (CI).

Daily Weight. Less "high-tech" but also important is a daily weight and focused physical assessment.[30] The "daily weight," combined with accurate "intake and output" monitoring, is a powerful indicator of fluid gains or losses over 24 hours. A 1-kg weight gain over 24 hours represents 1000 ml of additional fluid retention.

Physical Assessment. Physical assessment signs and symptoms are used to assess fluid balance. Signs that suggest extracellular fluid (ECF) depletion include thirst, decreased skin turgor, and lethargy. Signs that imply intravascular fluid volume overload include pulmonary congestion, increasing heart failure, and rising blood pressure. The patient with untreated ARF is edematous. Several factors contribute to this state:

1. Fluid retention because of the inadequate urine output.
2. Low serum albumin creates a lower oncotic pressure in the vasculature, and more fluid seeps out into the interstitial spaces as peripheral edema.
3. Inflammation associated with ARF or a coexisting nonrenal disease increases vascular permeability to the movement of water into the tissues.

In critical illness, even though there is peripheral edema, and the patient may have gained 8 L over his or her "dry-weight" baseline, the patient may remain "intravascularly dry" and hemodynamically unstable. This is because the retained fluid is not inside a vascular compartment and thus cannot contribute to maintenance of hemodynamic stability. The patient in ARF is assessed frequently for pitting edema over bony prominences and in dependent body areas.

ELECTROLYTE BALANCE

Potassium. Electrolyte levels require frequent observation, especially in the critical phases of renal failure (see Table 30-3). Potassium may quickly reach levels of 6.0 milliequivalents per liter (mEq/L) and above. Specific ECG changes are associated with hyperkalemia, specifically peaked T waves, a widening of the QRS interval, and ultimately, ventricular tachycardia or fibrillation. If hyperkalemia is present, all potassium supplements are stopped.[31] If the patient is producing urine, IV diuretics can be administered. Acute hyperkalemia can be treated temporarily by IV administration of insulin and glucose. An infusion of 50 ml of 50% dextrose accompanied by 10 units of regular insulin forces potassium out of the serum and into the cells.

Finally, sodium polystyrene sulfonate (Kayexalate), a cation-exchange resin, is mixed in water and sorbitol and given orally, rectally, or through a nasogastric (NG) tube. The resin binds potassium in the bowel, which eliminates it in the feces. Kayexalate and dialysis are the only permanent methods of potassium removal.[31]

Sodium. Dilutional hyponatremia, associated with renal failure, is an expected finding (see Table 30-3). It can be corrected over a few days with fluid restriction. More rapidly, sodium levels may be raised during dialysis by changing the amount of sodium in the dialysate bath.

Calcium and Phosphorus. Serum calcium levels are reduced (*hypocalcemia*) in renal failure (see Table 30-3). This reduction results from multiple factors, in-

cluding *hyperphosphatemia*. Chronically elevated serum phosphorus levels (greater than 5.5 to 6.5 mEq/L) are associated with higher mortality in renal failure.[12,32] At the renal level, calcium and phosphorus are regulated in part by parathyroid hormone (PTH). Normally, PTH helps calcium be resorbed back into the bloodstream at the proximal tubule and distal nephron, and promotes excretion of phosphorus by the kidney to maintain homeostasis. In renal failure this mechanism is nonfunctional; thus the serum phosphorus level rises in the bloodstream, and the serum calcium level falls.

Calcium Replacement. Most calcium in the bloodstream is bound to protein. This can be measured as a total serum calcium level. The metabolically active, non–protein-bound portion is known as the *ionized calcium*. Without adequate levels of serum calcium, a compensatory mechanism "steals" calcium from the bones, making the patient with kidney failure more vulnerable to fractures.[33] Maintaining adequate calcium stores in the body is important and is achieved by administration of calcium supplements, vitamin D preparations, and synthetic calcitriol.

Dietary-Phosphorus Binding Drugs. A second method used in tandem with calcium supplements to achieve normal calcium levels is to lower the level of phosphorus in the bloodstream. Phosphorus occurs in many foods, and to eliminate all phosphorus containing foods from the diet would make it unpalatable.[34] Foods that contain particularly high levels of phosphorus include dairy products, processed meats, some carbonated drinks and nuts.[34] Unfortunately, once eaten, free phosphorus passes from the GI tract into the bloodstream and raises the serum level. Medications that bind dietary phosphorus in the GI tract are administered orally or via NG tube. The binding agent must be taken at the same time as a meal.[34] Once the dietary-phosphorus is bound to the binding substance in the bowel, it is eliminated from the intestine with stool. This lowers the serum phosphorus level.

The types of dietary-phosphorus binders used have changed over the years. The original binders were aluminum salts (aluminum hydroxide) that bound dietary phosphorus effectively in the GI tract, but conferred aluminum toxicity because some of the aluminum metal was also absorbed.[34] For this reason, aluminum binders have largely been abandoned.[34]

The second generation of dietary-phosphorus binding agents that are most widely prescribed use calcium salts (calcium carbonate; calcium acetate [PhosLo]) to bind dietary phosphorus in the GI tract. Calcium-based drugs are safer, but elevated serum calcium levels and calcium deposits in other areas of the body (extraosseous calcification) are a problem.[34]

A third generation of dietary-phosphorus binding medications has recently become available. These medications are non–aluminum-, non–calcium-based. They include sevelamer hydrochloride (RenaGel) and lanthanum carbonate (Fosrenol).[34]

MEDICAL MANAGEMENT

Treatment goals for patients experiencing ARF focus on prevention, compensation for the deterioration of renal function, and regeneration of the remaining kidney functional capacity. Over the past 4 decades, mortality from acute renal failure has remained at more than 50%.[1,2] Key areas that are evaluated include prevention strategies, fluid balance, anemia, medications, and electrolyte imbalance.

Prevention. The only truly effective remedy for ARF is prevention. For effective prevention the patient's risk for development of ARF must be assessed. Knowledge of the most frequent causes of ARF in the critically ill is essential if prevention strategies are to be enacted. The critical care team collaborates closely with the clinical pharmacist to avoid drugs with nephrotoxic side effects in patients with renal insufficiency or chronic kidney disease.[11,12] Nonsteroidal antiinflammatory drugs (NSAIDs) for pain relief are avoided in patients with elevated creatinine, those taking antibiotics, or those recovering from major surgery.[35] The use of intravascular contrast dye is delayed until the patient is fully rehydrated.[5,6]

Fluid Resuscitation. Prerenal failure is caused by decreased perfusion and flow to the kidney. It is often associated with trauma, hemorrhage, hypotension, and major fluid losses. If contrast dye is used, aggressive fluid resuscitation with either 0.9 normal saline (NaCl)[5] or 0.45 normal saline (NaCl)[6] is recommended.[6] Fluid replacement is the only treatment shown to prevent renal tubular injury.[36] The objectives of volume replacement are to replace fluid and electrolyte losses and to prevent ongoing loss. Maintenance IV fluid therapy is initiated when oral (PO) fluid intake is inadvisable. Maintenance fluids are calculated with consideration for individual body surface area. Adults require approximately 1500 ml/m^2/24 hr; fever, burns, and trauma significantly increase fluid requirements. Other important criteria when calculating fluid volume replacement include baseline metabolism, environmental temperature, and humidity. The rate of replacement depends on cardiopulmonary reserve, adequacy of renal function, urine output, fluid balance, ongoing loss, and type of fluid replaced.

Crystalloids and Colloids. Crystalloids and colloids refer to two different types of IV fluids used for volume management in critically ill patients. These IV solutions are used on all types of patients, not just those with acute renal failure. Adequacy of IV fluid replacement depends on strict, ongoing evaluation and frequent adjustment. Frequent monitoring of serum electrolyte levels is required, and strictly regulated intake and output are correlated with daily weight records. In septic shock, hemodynamic readings are frequently undertaken. Following a fluid challenge, a merely minimal increase in CVP implies that additional fluid replacement is required. Continued decreases in CVP, PAOP, and CI indicate ongoing volume losses. Which IV fluid to select to most successfully resuscitate hemodynamically unstable patients has been a controversial topic in critical care. The major debate centers on the differences between crystalloid versus colloid solutions.

Crystalloids. Crystalloid solutions, which are balanced salt solutions, are in widespread use for both maintenance infusion and replacement therapy. Crystalloid fluids include normal saline solution (0.9 NaCl), half-strength saline solution (0.45 NaCl), and lactated Ringer's (LR) solution (Table 30-6). LR solution is generally avoided in patients with renal failure, because it contains potassium. A noncrystalloid solution that may be infused is dextrose (5% or 10%) in water (D_5W, $D_{10}W$).

Colloids. Colloids are solutions containing oncotically active particles that are used to expand intravascular volume to achieve and maintain hemodynamic stability. Albumin (5% and 25%) and hetastarch are colloid solutions (see Table 30-6). Colloids expand intravascular volume, and the effect can last as long as 24 hours. The goal is to optimize PAOP or "wedge" pressure, raise mean arterial pressure (MAP), and increase CO and the CI to a therapeutic level.

The controversy over resuscitation fluids is not fully resolved, and some recent research study results have reopened the debate. The SAFE study was a randomized, prospective, double-blind trial that examined whether the selection of resuscitation fluid in the critical care unit affected survival at 28 days. SAFE stands for *s*aline vs. *a*lbumin *f*luid *e*valuation.[37] This was a huge study, with almost 7000 critical care patients randomized into two similar groups. One group received 4% albumin, and the other group received 0.9 normal saline (NaCl) for fluid resuscitation.[37] The patients in both groups were very similar in terms of organ dysfunction, mechanical ventilator support (64% of patients), and renal replacement therapy (1% of patients). The SAFE results showed that there was that there was no difference in mortality (death rate), time in the critical care unit, ventilator days, or renal replacement therapy days.[37] The researchers conclude that albumin and saline should be considered clinically equivalent treatments for intravascular volume expansion in critically ill patients.[37]

The findings of the SAFE study investigators have been validated by a meta-analysis of 71 studies that compared albumin with other IV solutions for fluid volume resuscitation.[38] These authors went further and declared that albumin reduces morbidity (complications) in acutely ill hospitalized patients.[38] The authors state that many of the previous studies were flawed because albumin was administered to both the investigational and the control group, thus invalidating many studies.[38] The authors are careful to point out that every patient is an in-

Table 30-6		Frequently Used Intravenous Solutions	
Solution		**Electrolytes**	**Indications**
CRYSTALLOIDS*			
Dextrose in water (D₅W)—isotonic		None	Maintain volume Replace mild loss Provide minimal calories
Normal saline solution (0.9% NaCl)		Sodium 154 mEq/L Chloride 154 mEq/L Osmolality 308 mEq/L	Maintain volume Replace mild loss Correct mild hyponatremia
Half-strength saline solution (0.45% NaCl)		Sodium 77 mEq/L Chloride 77 mEq/L	Free water replacement Correct mild hyponatremia Free water/electrolyte replacement (fluid/electrolyte-restricted conditions)
Lactated Ringer's solution		Sodium 130 mEq/L Potassium 4 mEq/L Calcium 2.7 mEq/L Chloride 107 mEq/L Lactate 27 mEq/L pH 6.5	Fluid and electrolyte replacement (contraindicated for patients with renal or liver disease or in lactic acidosis)
COLLOIDS			
5% Albumin (Albumisol)		Albumin 50 g/L Sodium 130-160 mEq/L Potassium 1 mEq/L Osmolality 300 mOsm/L Osmotic pressure 20 mm Hg pH 6.4 to 7.4	Volume expansion Moderate protein replacement Achievement of hemodynamic stability in shock states
25% Albumin (salt-poor)		Albumin 240 g/L Globulins 10 g/L Sodium 130-160 mEq/L Osmolality 1500 mOsm/L pH 6.4 to 7.4	Concentrated form of albumin sometimes used with diuretics to move fluid from tissues into the vascular space for diuresis
Hetastarch		Sodium 154 mEq/L Chloride 154 mEq/L Osmolality 310 mOsm/L Colloid osmotic pressure 30-35 mm Hg	Synthetic polymer (6% solution) used for volume expansion Hemodynamic volume replacement after cardiac surgery, burns, sepsis
Low–molecular-weight dextran (LMWD)		Glucose polysaccharide molecules with average molecular weight of 40,000; no electrolytes	Volume expansion and support (contraindi- cated for patients with bleeding disorders)
High–molecular-weight dextran (HMWD)		Glucose polysaccharide molecules with average molecular weight of 70,000; no electrolytes	Used prophylactically in some cases to pre- vent platelet aggregation; available in either saline or glucose solutions

*For the crystalloid solutions that contain electrolytes, specific concentrations of electrolytes and pH will vary according to the manufacturer.

dividual, that clinical situations are often unique, and that their findings would not necessarily apply to every clinical situation.[38] Nonetheless, these studies are certain to make clinicians reevaluate the use of albumin and normal saline as resuscitation fluids for the critically ill patient. If the outcomes are equal, the additional cost of albumin may not be justified for many patients.

Fluid Restriction. Fluid restriction constitutes a large part of the medical treatment for acute renal failure. Fluid restriction is used to prevent circulatory overload and the development of interstitial edema when the kidneys cannot remove excess volume. The fluid require-

ments are calculated on the basis of daily urine volumes and insensible losses. Obtaining daily weight measurements and keeping accurate intake and output records is essential. Renal failure patients are usually restricted to 1 L of fluid per 24 hours if urine output is 500 ml or less. Insensible losses range from 500 to 750 ml/day.

Fluid Removal. Acute renal failure promotes increased amounts of water, solutes, and potential toxins into the circulation; thus prompt measures are needed to decrease their levels. Diuretics are used to stimulate the urine output. However, renal replacement therapies (RRT), either hemodialysis or hemofiltration, are the

Pharmacologic Management: Renal Drugs

DRUG	DOSAGE	ACTIONS	SPECIAL CONSIDERATIONS
Diuretics			
Loop Diuretics			
Furosemide (Lasix)	20-80 mg/day (Lasix) 0.5-2 mg/day (Bumex)	Acts on loop of Henle to inhibit sodium and chloride	Ototoxicity if administered too rapidly or with other ototoxic drugs Monitor intake/output, hydration, watch for hypotension
Thiazide Diuretics			
Chlorothiazide (Diuril)	500 mg-2 g/day	Inhibit sodium, chloride resorption in distal tubule	Enhanced with low-sodium diet Synergistic effect with loop diuretics
Potassium-Sparing Diuretics			
Aldactone	100 mg/day for 5 days	Exert effects on collecting tubule; reduce potassium, hydrogen and increase sodium	Weak diuretic effect, so given with other diuretics Potassium supplements not required; monitor for hyperkalemia Used as an "aldosterone blocker" to treat heart failure
Osmotic Diuretics			
Mannitol	0.25-2.0 g/kg IV infusion as a 15%-20% solution over 30-90 min	Increases urine output because of increased plasma osmolality, increasing flow of water from tissues Increases sodium, potassium	Often used in head injury to decrease cerebral edema Can be used to promote urinary secretion of toxic substances Use in-line 5 micron IV filter with >20% solutions

GI, Gastrointestinal; *IV*, intravenous; *PO*, by mouth; *ECG*, electrocardiogram; *BP*, blood pressure.

treatment of choice, particularly if volume overload exacerbates pulmonary and heart failure.

PHARMACOLOGIC MANAGEMENT

The first step is to eliminate any nephrotoxic medications. Second, if drugs are eliminated through the kidneys, it is important to decrease the frequency of administration (e.g., from every 6 hours to every 12 hours) or to decrease the dose and to monitor the serum concentration by measuring serum drug levels.[35]

Diuretics. Diuretics are used to stimulate urinary output in the fluid overloaded patient with functioning kidneys. Care must be taken in their use to avoid the creation of secondary electrolyte abnormalities (see the Pharmacologic Management Table on Diuretic Drugs). Diuretics are used in many patient populations, not only those with incipient renal failure.

Loop Diuretics. The loop diuretic *furosemide* (Lasix) is the most frequently used diuretic in critical care patients. It may be prescribed as a bolus dose or as a continuous infusion. Electrolytic abnormalities are frequently encountered. Close monitoring of serum potassium, magnesium, and sodium is essential. Concurrent use of furosemide preceded by a synergistic thiazide diuretic is also seen.

Thiazide Diuretics. Diuretics may be prescribed in combination. A thiazide diuretic such as chlorothiazide (Diuril), or metolazone (Zaroxolyn) may be administered followed by a loop diuretic, to take advantage of the fact that these drugs work on different parts of the nephron.

Osmotic Diuretics. Osmotic diuretics (mannitol) are also prescribed to decrease fluid overload and improve urine output. It is important to use an in-line 5-micron filter when administering this drug. Mannitol is frequently prescribed for patients with brain injury and increased intracranial pressure (ICP). More information on the use of mannitol in this population can be found in Chapter 27.

Heart Failure. In patients with heart failure the natriuretic peptides (ANP and BNP) may be prescribed. These drugs work by stimulating natriuretic receptors in the atrium (ANP) and ventricular myocardium (BNP). The potassium-sparing diuretic Aldactone is also used in heart failure as an "aldosterone agonist," not as a diuretic. Most heart failure patients also require significant dosages of loop diuretics. One method of diuresis is to administer 50 ml of IV 25% albumin followed by a loop diuretic. The rationale is that the albumin will pull fluid from the tissues into the bloodstream and the diuretic will increase the water excretion. For more information on the use of diuretics in heart failure management, see Chapter 18.

Controversies. The use of diuretics continues to be controversial in the critically ill. This is a topic that is under active investigation. Mehta and colleagues published an observational study that showed that once ARF with oliguria was present, loop diuretics increased mortality and delayed kidney recovery in critically ill patients with established ARF.[39] A subsequent study found that furosemide helped maintain urine output, but had no more impact on survival and renal recovery than a placebo.[40] Finally, a third research trial found that furosemide (Lasix) neither helped nor worsened ARF in the critically ill.[41] Undoubtedly, the debate and the research studies will continue, but for now it appears that loop diuretics increase the urine output, which makes clinicians feel better, but have no impact on the outcome of established oliguric ARF.

Dopamine. Low-dose dopamine (2 to 3 mcg/kg/min), also known as "renal-dose dopamine," is frequently infused to stimulate renal blood flow. Dopamine is effective in increasing urine output in the short term, but dopamine-renal-receptor tolerance to the drug is theorized to develop in the critically ill patients who are most at risk for development of ARF.[42] A meta-analysis of related research studies determined that renal-dose dopamine did not prevent onset of ARF and did not decrease the need for dialysis or reduce mortality.[43] At this point the support for routine use of low-dose dopamine for the prevention of renal failure remains anecdotal only.[44]

Acetylcysteine. N-Acetylcysteine (Mucomyst, Mucosil) is a N-acetyl derivative of the amino acid L-cysteine.[6] It has been used for many years as a mucolytic agent to assist with expectoration of thick pulmonary secretions. It is now frequently prescribed for patients with mildly elevated serum creatinine before a radiology study using contrast dye.[6] Acetylcysteine is believed to work directly in the kidney to both vasodilate the tubule and "scavenge" oxygen free radicals. Research studies have shown a decreased incidence of contrast-induced nephrotoxicity when acetylcysteine was used.[6] The recommended dosage is 600 mg orally twice a day (morning and evening), on the day before and the day of any procedure that involves administration of IV radiopaque contrast.[6]

Fenoldopan. Fenoldopan mesylate (Corlopam) is a dopamine-1 (DA-1) receptor agonist similar in structure to dopamine and dobutamine. It is used to lower blood pressure and to prevent contrast-induced nephrotoxicity.[6] Fenoldopan dilates both renal afferent and efferent arterioles, increases blood flow to both the renal cortex and medulla, and is thought to improve the nephron's ability to remove the contrast dye.[6]

Other pharmacologic interventions that are recommended to reduce the impact of contrast dye on the kidney include stopping all diuretics on the day of the procedure to prevent volume depletion;[5] stopping administration of the hypoglycemic drug metformin (Glucophage) because of its association with nephrotoxicity and lactic acidosis on rare occasions;[6] limiting the quantity of contrast dye administered;[45] and providing adequate rehydration after the procedure.[5]

Dietary-Phosphorus Binders. Many patients with renal failure will be prescribed a dietary-phosphorus binding medication (see earlier section on calcium/phosphorus).[34] There are many dietary-phosphorus binding drugs available; some important issues concern all of them. The dietary-phosphorus binder must be taken at the time of the meal. If it is taken 2 hours later, it will only increase the level of the binding substance (such as calcium) in the bloodstream, and will not lower the serum phosphorus level. Other related issues such as the quantity of phosphorus in the diet should be discussed with a clinical nutritionist (dietitian).

NUTRITION

The diet for the patient with renal problems restricts the electrolytes potassium, sodium, and phosphorus. It also limits protein intake to control azotemia (increased BUN). Fluids are limited. By contrast, carbohydrates are encouraged, to provide energy for metabolism and healing.[46]

NURSING MANAGEMENT

Nursing management of acute renal failure patients involves a variety of nursing diagnoses (see the Nursing Diagnoses feature on Acute Renal Failure). "Prevention is the best cure" is an old saying that captures the role of the critical care nurse, who evaluates all patients for level of kidney function, risk of infection, fluid imbalance, electrolyte disturbances, anemia, readiness to learn, and need for education.

Risk Factors for ARF. Some individuals have an increased risk of developing ARF as a complication during their hospitalization, and the alert critical care nurse recognizes potential risk factors and acts as a patient advocate.[11,12] Patients at risk include elderly persons because their GFR may be decreased,[2] dehydrated patients because hypoperfusion of the kidneys may lead to ischemic ATN, patients with increased creatinine levels before their hospitalization,[13] and patients undergoing a radiology procedure involving contrast dye.[5,6]

Infectious Complications. The critical care patient with ARF is at risk for infectious complications. Signs of infection such as increased white blood cell (WBC)

NURSING DIAGNOSES — Acute Renal Failure

- Excess Fluid Volume related to renal dysfunction
- Ineffective Renal Tissue Perfusion related to decreased renal blood flow
- Anxiety related to threat to biologic, psychologic, and/or social integrity
- Decreased Cardiac Output related to decrease in preload
- Risk for Infection risk factors: protein-calorie malnourishment, invasive monitoring devices
- Disturbed Body Image related to functional dependence on life-sustaining technology
- Ineffective Coping related to situational crisis and personal vulnerability
- Disturbed Sleep Pattern related to fragmented sleep
- Deficient Knowledge: Fluid Restriction, Reportable Symptoms, and Medications related to lack of previous exposure to information

count, redness at a wound or IV site, or increased temperature are always a cause for concern. A urinary catheter is inserted to facilitate accurate urine measurement and patient comfort. However, any indwelling catheter is a potential source for infection. Therefore, when the patient no longer makes large quantities of urine, the catheter is removed and a scheduled "straight catheterization" is performed to minimize the risk of infection from an indwelling catheter and drainage system. This method allows the patient's bladder to be emptied, but the catheter does not remain in place. Pulmonary hygiene is maintained by asking the patient to cough and deep-breathe frequently if he or she is awake and alert. If the patient is intubated and ventilated, frequent turning, endotracheal suctioning, and frequent mouth care become mandatory. If the patient is immobile, changes of position and observation of potential sites for skin breakdown help avoid creating sites for infection.

Fluid Balance. Intravascular fluid balance is often assessed on an hourly basis for the critically ill patient who has hemodynamic lines inserted. Hemodynamic values (HR, BP, CVP, PAOP, CO, and CI) and daily weight measurements are correlated with the intake and output. Urine output is measured hourly, via a urinary catheter and drainage bag, throughout all phases of ARF, particularly in response to diuretics. Any fluid removed with dialysis is recorded in the fluid balance section of the nursing flowsheet. Recognition of the clinical signs and symptoms of fluid overload is important. Excess fluid

will move from the vascular system into the peripheral tissues (dependent edema), abdomen (ascites), the lungs (crackles, pulmonary edema and pulmonary effusions), around the heart (pericardial effusions), and into the brain (increased intracranial swelling).

Electrolyte Imbalance. Hyperkalemia, hypocalcemia, hyponatremia, hyperphosphatemia, and acid-base imbalances all occur during ARF (see Table 30-3). Clinical manifestations of these electrolyte imbalances must be prevented and their associated side effects controlled. The potential imbalances that are the most likely are hyperkalemia and hypocalcemia, which can result in life-threatening cardiac dysrhythmias. Dilutional hyponatremia may develop as fluid overload worsens in the patient with oliguria. Monitoring the serum sodium level is important to prevent this complication. Hyperphosphatemia results in severe pruritis. Nursing care is directed at soothing the itching by performing frequent skin care with emollients, discouraging scratching, and administering phosphate-binding medications.[34] The acid-base imbalances that occur with renal failure are monitored by arterial blood gas (ABG) analysis. The goal of treatment is to maintain the pH within the normal range.

Preventing Anemia. Anemia is an expected side effect of renal failure that occurs because the kidney no longer produces the hormone *erythropoietin.*[33] Thus the bone marrow is not stimulated to produce red blood cells (RBCs). Care is taken to prevent blood loss in the patient with ARF, and blood withdrawal is minimized as much as possible. Irritation of the GI tract from metabolic waste accumulation is expected, and GI bleeding is a possibility. Stool, NG drainage, and emesis are routinely tested for occult blood. Anemia is treated pharmacologically by the administration of recombinant human erythropoietin (rHuEPO), epoetin alfa (Procrit, Epogen), to stimulate erythrocyte production by the bone marrow, and if required by RBC transfusion.[33,47] Treatment of anemia early in the course of ARF (predialysis) appears to slow the progression of the renal failure and delays the initiation or renal replacement therapies.[33,48] Even in anemic critically ill patients without renal failure, administration of rHuEPO weekly significantly decreases the number of blood transfusions.[49]

PATIENT EDUCATION

It is vital to provide accurate and uncomplicated information to the patient and family about ARF, including its prognosis, treatment, and possible complications.[3] Education of the patient can be challenging because elevations of BUN and creatinine can negatively affect level of consciousness. Also, sleep-rest disorders and emotional upset often occur as complications of ARF and can disrupt short-term memory. Encouraging the patient and family to voice concerns, frustrations, or fears and allowing the patient to control some aspects of the acute

- Explain pathophysiology:
  "ARF is a sudden, severe impairment of renal function, causing an acute buildup of toxins in the blood."
- Explain etiology:
  Prerenal (before the kidney)
  Intrarenal (within the kidneys)
  Postrenal (past the kidneys)
- Identify predisposing factors; explain the level of renal function after the acute phase is over.
- Explain diet and fluid restrictions.
- Demonstrate how to check blood pressure, pulse, respirations, and weight.
- Discuss good hygiene and how to avoid infections.
- Emphasize need for exercise and rest.
- Describe medications and adverse effects.
- Explain need for ongoing follow-up with health care professional.
- Explain purpose of dialysis and importance of regular treatments.

Box 30-3

COLLABORATIVE MANAGEMENT

ACUTE RENAL FAILURE (ARF)
1. **Assess risk of renal failure.**
   - Assess baseline renal function on all patients at risk for development of ARF.
2. **Protect the kidneys.**
   - If patient has preexisting renal dysfunction, avoid nephrotoxic drugs, limit exposure to radiologic contrast dye, and prevent both hypotension and hypovolemia.
3. **Monitor urine output.**
   - Intervene for low urine output before patient is oliguric or anuric for several hours (see Table 30-1).
4. **Supply nutrition.**
   - Oral, enteral, or parenteral nutrition is needed to combat catabolism in critically ill patient with renal dysfunction.
5. **Provide renal replacement.**
   - If patient has lost renal function during acute illness, replace kidney function with intermittent hemodialysis or CRRT as indicated.

Box 30-4

INDICATIONS AND CONTRAINDICATIONS FOR HEMODIALYSIS

INDICATIONS
Blood urea nitrogen (BUN) exceeds 90 mg/dl
Serum creatinine 9 mg/dl
Hyperkalemia
Drug toxicity
Intravascular and extravascular fluid overload
Metabolic acidosis
Symptoms of uremia
- Pericarditis
- Gastrointestinal bleeding
Changes in mentation
Contraindications to other forms of dialysis

CONTRAINDICATIONS
Hemodynamic instability
Inability to anticoagulate
Lack of access to circulation

---

care environment and treatment also are essential (see the Patient Education feature on Acute Renal Failure).

COLLABORATIVE MANAGEMENT

Management of the patient with acute renal dysfunction is complex and requires the expertise of many different health care clinicians (Box 30-3). Recently developed clinical guidelines[12,13] can be used to guide the health care team in determining priority interventions for this high-risk group of patients.

RENAL REPLACEMENT THERAPY—DIALYSIS

A range of renal replacement therapies (RRT) is available for the treatment of ARF. These include intermittent hemodialysis (IHD) therapy and continuous renal replacement therapy (CRRT), and peritoneal dialysis (PD).

HEMODIALYSIS

Hemodialysis roughly translates as "separating from the blood." Indications and contraindications for hemodialysis are listed in Box 30-4. As a treatment, hemodialysis literally separates and removes from the blood the excess electrolytes, fluids, and toxins by use of a hemodia-

lyzer (Fig. 30-1). Although hemodialysis is efficient in removing solutes, it does not remove all metabolites. Furthermore, electrolytes, toxins, and fluids increase between treatments, necessitating hemodialysis on a regular basis. Hemodialysis therapy is always intermittent; each dialysis treatment takes 3 to 4 hours. In the acute phases of renal failure, dialysis is performed daily.[50] The dialysis frequency gradually decreases to three times per week as the patient moves into a more chronic phase of kidney failure.

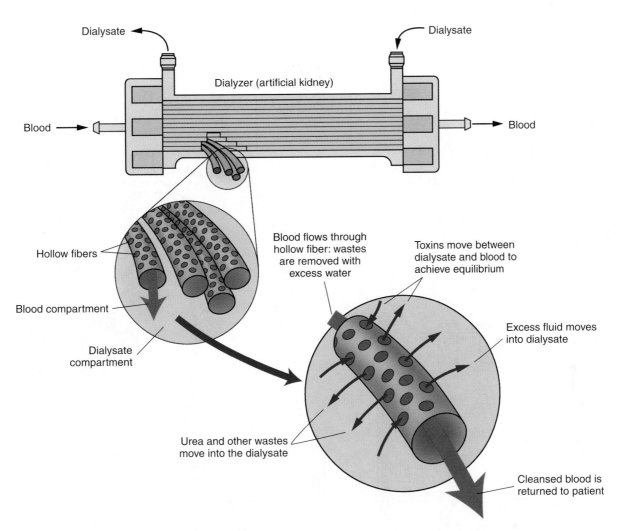

Fig. 30-1 Hemodialyzer.

Hemodialyzer. Hemodialysis works by circulating blood outside the body through synthetic tubing to a dialyzer, which consists of hollow-fiber tubes. The dialyzer is sometimes described as an "artificial kidney" (Fig. 30-2). While the blood flows through the membranes, which are semipermeable, a fluid "dialysate bath" bathes the membranes and, through osmosis and diffusion, performs exchanges of fluid, electrolytes, and toxins from the blood to the bath, where toxins and dialysate then pass out of the artificial kidney. The blood and the dialysate bath are shunted in opposite directions (countercurrent flow) through the dialyzer to match the osmotic and chemical gradients at the most efficient level for effective dialysis.

Ultrafiltration. To remove fluid, a positive hydrostatic pressure is applied to the blood and a negative hydrostatic pressure is applied to the dialysate bath. The two forces together, called *transmembrane pressure*, pull and squeeze the excess fluid from the blood. The difference between the two values (expressed in millimeters of mercury (mm Hg) represents the transmembrane pressure and results in fluid extraction, known as *ultrafiltration*, from the vascular space.

Anticoagulation. Either heparin or sodium citrate is added to the system just before the blood enters the dialyzer to anticoagulate the blood within the dialysis tubing. Without an anticoagulant the blood will clot because its passage through the foreign tubular substances of the dialysis machine activates the clotting mechanism. Heparin can be administered either by bolus injection or intermittent infusion. It has a short half-life, and its effects subside within 2 to 4 hours. If necessary, the effects of heparin are easily reversed with the antidote protamine sulfate. When there is concern about the development of heparin-induced thrombocytopenia (HIT),[51] alternative anticoagulants can be used. Citrate (trisodium citrate) can also be infused as an anticoagulant via intermittent bolus or continuous infusion.[52]

Vascular Access. Hemodialysis requires access to the bloodstream. Various types of temporary and permanent devices are in clinical use. It is important for patient safety to be able to recognize these different vascular access devices and to properly care for them. The following section discusses temporary vascular access catheters used in the acute care hospital environment and permanent methods used for long-term hemodialysis.

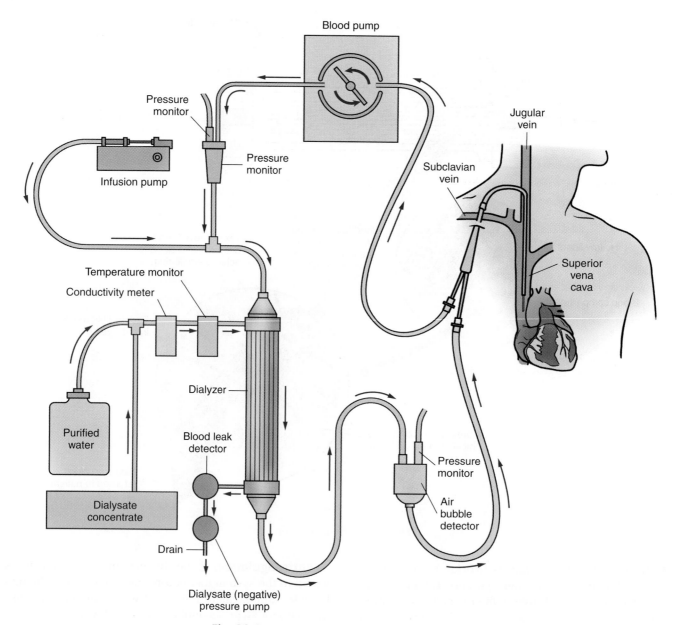

Fig. 30-2 Components of a hemodialysis system.

Temporary Acute Access. *Subclavian* and *femoral* veins are catheterized when short-term access is required or when vascular access is nonfunctional in a patient requiring immediate hemodialysis. Both subclavian and femoral catheters are routinely inserted at the bedside. Most temporary catheters are venous only. Blood flows out towards the dialyzer and flows back to the patient via the same vein. A dual-lumen venous catheter is the most commonly seen. It has a central partition running the length of the catheter. The outflow catheter section pulls the blood flow through openings that are proximal to the inflow openings on the opposite side (Fig. 30-3). This design helps prevent dialyzing the same blood just returned to the area (recirculation), which would severely reduce the procedure's efficiency. A silicone rub-

ber, dual-lumen catheter with a polyester cuff designed to decrease catheter-related infections is also available.

Permanent Vascular Access. The common denominator in permanent vascular access devices is a connection to the arterial circulation and a return conduit to the venous circulation.

Arteriovenous Fistula. The arteriovenous (AV) fistula is created by surgically exposing a peripheral artery and vein, creating a side-by-side opening in the artery and the vein, and joining the two vessels together. The high arterial flow creates a swelling of the vein, or a pseudoaneurysm, at which point (when healed) a large-bore needle can be inserted to obtain arterial outflow to the dialyzer. Inflow is accomplished through a second large-bore needle inserted into a peripheral vein distal to the fistula (Fig. 30-4,

Double Lumen Catheter

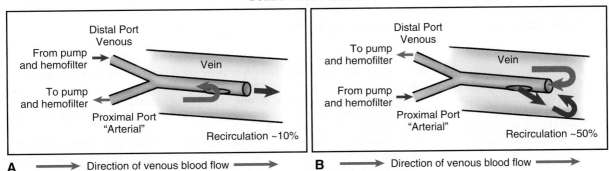

A   → Direction of venous blood flow →

B   → Direction of venous blood flow →

Fig. 30-3 Temporary dialysis venous access catheter.

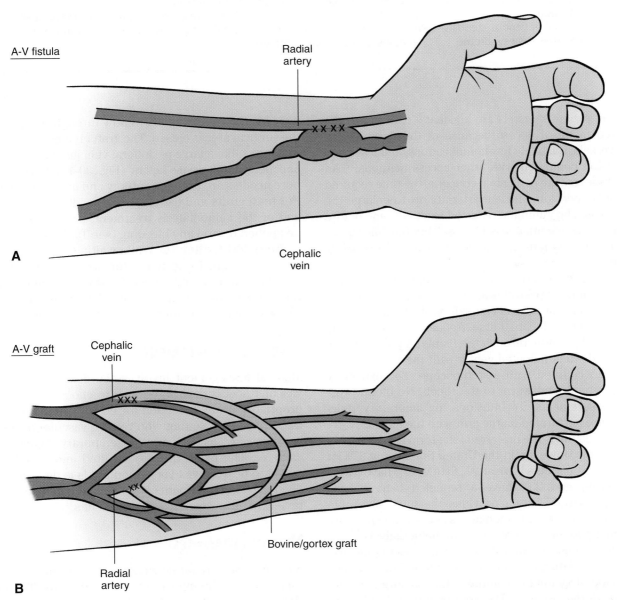

Fig. 30-4 Methods of vascular access for hemodialysis. **A,** Arteriovenous fistula between vein and artery. **B,** Internal synthetic graft corrects artery and vein.

Table 30-7 — Complications and Nursing Management of Arteriovenous Fistula/Graft

Type	Complications	Nursing Management
Fistula	Thrombosis Infection Pseudoaneurysm Vascular steal syndrome Venous hypertension Carpal tunnel syndrome Inadequate blood flow	Teach patients to avoid wearing constrictive clothing on limbs containing access. Teach patients to avoid sleeping on or bending accessed limb for prolonged periods. Use aseptic technique when cannulating access. Avoid repetitious cannulation of one segment of access. Offer comfort measures, such as warm compresses and ordered analgesics, to lessen pain of vascular steal. Teach patients to develop blood flow in the fistulas through exercises (squeezing a rubber ball) while applying mild impedance to flow just distal to the access (at least once per day for 10-15 minutes). Avoid too-early cannulation of new access.
Graft	Bleeding Thrombosis False aneurysm formation Infection Arterial or venous stenosis Vascular steal syndrome	Teach patients to avoid wearing constrictive clothing on accessed limbs. Avoid repeated cannulation of one segment of access. Use aseptic technique when cannulating access. Monitor for changes in arterial or venous pressure while patients are on dialysis. Provide comfort measures to reduce pain of vascular steal (e.g., warm compresses, analgesics as ordered).

A). If the patient's vessels are adequate, fistulas are the preferred mode of access because of the durability of blood vessels, relatively few complications, and less need for revision compared with other access methods.[12] An initial disadvantage of a fistula concerns the time required for development of sufficient arterial flow to enlarge the new access. The minimum reported length of time before a fistula can be cannulated is 14 days,[53] but the time lag for many patients is longer, as much as weeks to possibly months.[54]

In caring for a patient with a fistula, there are some important nursing priorities to ensure the ongoing viability of the vascular access and safety of the limb (Table 30-7). The critical care nurse frequently assesses the quality of blood flow through the fistula. A patent fistula has a thrill when palpated gently with the fingers and a bruit if auscultated with a stethoscope. The extremity should be pink and warm to the touch. No blood pressure measurements, IV infusions, or laboratory phlebotomy are performed on the arm with the fistula.

The AV fistula is the preferred long-term access for hemodialysis.[12] However, in the United States only 27% of hemodialysis patients have an AV fistula; 47% have a synthetic graft; and 23% have a tunneled hemodialysis catheter.[55] An AV fistula provides the most favorable long-term patency for hemodialysis access and is recommended if patients require long-term hemodialysis.[12]

Arteriovenous Grafts. AV grafts are vascular access devices for treating chronic kidney failure. The graft is a tube made of synthetic material, which is surgically implanted inside the limb. The area is surgically opened, and an artery and a vein are located. A tunnel is created in the tissue where the graft is placed. Anastomoses are made with the graft ends connected to the artery and

vein. The blood is allowed to flow through the graft, and the surgical area is closed. The graft creates a raised area that looks like a large peripheral vein just under the skin and peripheral tissue layers (Fig. 30-4, B). Two large-bore needles are used for outflow and inflow to the graft. For both grafts and fistulas, after needle removal at the end of the hemodialysis treatment, firm pressure must be applied to stop any bleeding (see Table 30-7).

Tunneled Catheters. While waiting for the fistula or graft to mature to be ready for access, some patients may have a long-term silastic catheter tunneled under the skin and inserted into the jugular or subclavian vein. These catheters are not common in critical care.

MEDICAL MANAGEMENT

Medical management involves the decision to place a vascular access device and then to choose the most appropriate type and location for each patient. Patients in the critical care setting who require vascular access for hemodialysis usually use a temporary hemodialysis catheter. The exact quantity of fluid and/or solute removal to be achieved via hemodialysis is determined individually for each patient by clinical examination and review of all relevant laboratory results.

NURSING MANAGEMENT

A noncritical care nurse who is specially trained in dialysis manages the intermittent hemodialysis. The dialysis nurse typically comes to the patient's bedside with the hemodialysis machine. During the acute phase of treatment, hemodialysis occurs daily. The frequency is reduced to 3 days a week as the patient becomes hemo-

NIC Hemodialysis Therapy

Definition: Management of extracorporeal passage of the patient's blood through a dialyzer

Activities

Draw blood sample and review blood chemistries (e.g., BUN, serum creatinine, serum sodium, potassium, and PO$_4$ levels) before treatment

Record baseline vital signs: weight, temperature, pulse, respirations, and blood pressure

Explain hemodialysis procedure and its purpose

Check equipment and solutions, according to protocol

Use sterile technique to initiate hemodialysis and for needle insertions and catheter connections

Use gloves, eyeshield, and clothing to prevent direct contact with blood

Initiate hemodialysis, according to protocol

Anchor connections and tubing securely

Check system monitors (e.g., flow rate, pressure, temperature, pH level, conductivity, clots, air detector, negative pressure for ultrafiltration, and blood sensor) to ensure patient safety

Monitor blood pressure, pulse, respirations, temperature, and patient response during dialysis

Administer heparin, according to protocol

Monitor clotting times and adjust heparin administration appropriately

Adjust filtration pressures to remove an appropriate amount of fluid

Institute appropriate protocol, if patient becomes hypotensive

Discontinue hemodialysis according to protocol

Compare postdialysis vital signs and blood chemistries with predialysis values

Avoid taking blood pressure or doing intravenous punctures in arm with fistula

Provide catheter or fistula care, according to protocol

Work collaboratively with patient to adjust diet regulations, fluid limitations, and medications to regulate fluid and electrolyte shifts between treatments

Teach patient to self-monitor signs and symptoms that indicate need for medical treatment (e.g., fever, bleeding, clotted fistula, thrombophlebitis, and irregular pulse)

Work collaboratively with patient to relieve discomfort from side effects of the disease and treatment (e.g., cramping, fatigue, headaches, itching, anemia, bone demineralization, body image changes, and role disruption)

Work collaboratively with patient to adjust length of dialysis, diet regulations, and pain and diversion needs to achieve optimal benefit of the treatment

From McCloskey JD, Bulechek GM: *Nursing interventions classification (NIC)*, ed 4, 2004, St Louis, Mosby.

---

dynamically stable. The essential nursing elements to manage a patient on hemodialysis are listed in the Nursing Interventions Classification feature on Hemodialysis Therapy. The essential role of the critical care nurse during dialysis is to monitor the patient's hemodynamic stability. The ARF patient on hemodialysis is dependent on a viable venous access catheter. When not in use the catheter is "heparin-locked" to preserve patency. The critical care nurse provides education about the disease process and treatment plan to patient and family.

CONTINUOUS RENAL REPLACEMENT THERAPY

Continuous renal replacement therapy (CRRT) is a newer mode of dialysis that has many similarities to traditional hemodialysis. CRRT has the advantage of being a continuous therapy, lasting 12 hours to several days, where the venous blood is circulated through a highly porous hemofilter.[56,57] As with traditional hemodialysis, it is rare to use an artery-to-vein setup; both access and return of blood are through a large venous catheter (venovenous) as shown in Fig. 30-3. The advantage of the

CRRT system is the continuous removal of fluid from the plasma. The fluid removal rate ranges from 5 to 45 ml/min, depending on the particular CRRT system used, plus removal of solutes (urea, creatinine, and electrolytes) as listed in Table 30-8. The removed fluid is described as *ultrafiltrate*. In an ideal situation the hydrostatic pressure exerted by a MAP greater than 70 mm Hg would propel a continuous flow of blood through the hemofilter to remove fluid and solute. However, because many critically ill patients are hypotensive and cannot provide adequate flow through the hemofilter, an electric roller pump "milks" the tubing to augment flow. If large amounts of fluid are to be removed, IV replacement solutions are infused. Indications and contraindications for CRRT are described in Box 30-5.

Because controlled removal and replacement of fluid is possible over many hours or days with CRRT, hemodynamic stability is maintained. This makes CRRT highly advantageous for use in the patient with multisystem problems. There are several CRRT methods used in critical care units:

1. Slow continuous ultrafiltration (SCUF).
2. Continuous venovenous hemofiltration (CVVH).

Table 30-8	Comparison of Continuous Renal Replacement Therapy Methods			
Type	**Ultrafiltration Rate**	**Fluid Replacement**	**Method of Solute Removal**	**Indication**
SCUF	100-300 ml/hr	None	None	Fluid removal
CVVH	500-800 ml/hr	Predilution or postdilution, calculating hourly net loss	Convection	Fluid removal, moderate solute removal
CVVHD	500-800 ml/hr	Predilution or postdilution, subtracting dialysate, then calculating hourly net loss	Diffusion	Fluid removal, maximum solute removal
CVVHDF		Predilution or postdilution, subtracting dialysate, then calculating hourly net loss	Convection and diffusion	Maximal fluid removal, maximum solute removal

CVVH, Continuous venovenous hemofiltration; *CVVHD,* continuous venovenous hemodialysis; *CVVHDF,* continuous venovenous hemodiafiltration; *SCUF,* slow continuous ultrafiltration.

Box 30-5	
INDICATIONS AND CONTRAINDICATIONS FOR CRRT	

INDICATIONS
Need for large fluid volume removal in hemodynamically unstable patient
Hypervolemic or edematous patients unresponsive to diuretic therapy
Patients with multiple organ dysfunction syndrome
Ease of fluid management in patients requiring large daily fluid volume
  • Replacement for oliguria
  • TPN administration
Contraindication to hemodialysis and peritoneal dialysis
Inability to be anticoagulated

CONTRAINDICATIONS
Hematocrit > 45%
Terminal illness

CRRT, Continuous renal replacement therapy; *TPN,* total parenteral nutrition; >, greater than.

3. Continuous venovenous hemodialysis (CVVHD).
4. Continuous venovenous hemodiafiltration (CVVHDF).

The decision as to which type of therapy to initiate is based on myriad factors including clinical assessment, metabolic status, severity of uremia, and whether a particular treatment modality is available at that institution.

CRRT Terminology. In CRRT, solutes are removed from the blood by *diffusion* or *convection.* Both processes remove fluid, and they remove molecules of different sizes depending on the method chosen.

Diffusion. Diffusion describes the movement of solutes along a *concentration gradient* from "high" concentration to a "low" concentration across a semipermeable membrane. This is the main mechanism used in hemodialysis. Solutes such as creatinine and urea cross the dialysis membrane from the blood to the dialysis fluid compartment.

Convection. Convection occurs when a pressure gradient is set up so that the water is pushed or pumped across the dialysis filter and carries the solutes from the bloodstream with it. This method of solute removal is known as *"solvent drag"* and is commonly employed in CRRT.

Absorption. The filter attracts solute, and molecules attach (absorb) to the dialysis filter.

The size of solute molecules is measured in *daltons.* The different sizes of molecules that can be removed by convection or diffusion methods are shown in Table 30-9. Very tiny molecules such as urea and creatinine are removed by both diffusion and convection (all methods). As the molecular size increases (above 500 daltons), convection is the more efficient method.

Ultrafiltrate volume. The fluid that is removed each hour is not called *urine;* it is known as *ultrafiltrate.*

Replacement fluid. Typically some of the ultrafiltrate is replaced via the CRRT circuit by a sterile "replacement fluid." This replacement fluid can be added before the filter (pre–filter dilution) or after the filter (post–filter dilution). The purpose is to increase the volume of fluid passing through the hemofilter and improve convection of solute.

Anticoagulation. Because the blood outside the body is in contact with artificial tubing and filters, the coagulation cascade and complement cascades are activated. To prevent the hemofilter from becoming obstructed by clotting, or clotting off, low-dose anticoagulation must be used. The dose should be low enough to have no effect on patient anticoagulation parameters. Systemic anticoagulation is not the goal. Typical anticoagulant choices include unfractionated heparin (UFH) and sodium citrate.

Table 30-9	Size of Molecules Cleared by CRRT		
Type of Molecule	**Size of Molecule**	**Solutes**	**Solute Removal Method**
Small	Below 500 daltons	Urea, creatinine	Convection, diffusion
Middle	500-5000 daltons	Vancomycin	Convection better than diffusion
Low–molecular-weight (small) proteins	5000-50,000 daltons	Cytokines, complement	Convection or absorption onto hemofilter
Large proteins	Over 50,000 daltons	Albumin	Minimal removal

CRRT, Continuous renal replacement therapy.

Because of the design of the CRRT machine it is not possible to look at the outside and follow the flow of blood and, if used, dialysate. The following section describes each of the CRRT methods and uses diagrams to clearly show the mechanism of CRRT that is used.

Slow Continuous Ultrafiltration. Slow continuous ultrafiltration (SCUF), as the name implies, slowly removes fluid, 100 to 300 ml/hour, through a process of ultrafiltration (Fig. 30-5, *A*). This consists of a movement of fluid, across a semipermeable membrane. SCUF has minimal impact on solute removal. Because small amounts of fluid are removed via this process, it was initially hoped it would be a suitable choice for edematous patients with acute heart failure and diminished renal perfusion who were unresponsive to diuretics. In reality, SCUF is an infrequent clinical choice because it requires both arterial and venous access for effective functioning. In addition, the SCUF system is more likely to thrombose (clot off) than other CRRT methods that use higher flows.

Continuous Venovenous Hemofiltration. Continuous venovenous hemofiltration (CVVH) is indicated when the patient's clinical condition warrants removal of significant volumes of fluid and solutes. Fluid is removed by ultrafiltration in volumes of 5 to 20 ml/min or up to 7 to 30 L/24 hr. Removal of solutes such as urea, creatinine, and other small non–protein-bound toxins is accomplished by convection. The replacement fluid rate of flow through the CRRT circuit can be altered to achieve desired fluid and solute removal without causing hemodynamic instability. Replacement fluid can be added via the addition of a prehemofilter replacement fluid (Fig. 30-5, *B*) or post–hemofilter replacement fluid.

As with other CRRT systems, the blood outside the body is anticoagulated and the ultrafiltrate is drained off either by gravity or by the addition of negative-pressure suction into a large drainage bag. Because large volumes of fluid may be removed in CVVH, some of the removed ultrafiltrate volume must be replaced hourly with a continuous infusion (replacement fluid) to avoid intravascular dehydration. Replacement fluids may consist of standard solutions of bicarbonate, potassium-free LR solution, acetate, or dextrose. Electrolytes such as potassium, sodium, calcium chloride, magnesium sulfate, and sodium bicarbonate also may be added. The formula used to calculate the volume removed from the patient follows with an example:

$$\text{Ultrafiltrate in bag} + \text{other output} -$$
$$(\text{CVVH replacement fluid} + \text{IV/oral/NG intake}) = \text{Output}$$
$$1000 \text{ ml} - 800 \text{ ml} = 200 \text{ ml/hr output}$$

Continuous Venovenous Hemodialysis. Continuous venovenous hemodialysis (CVVHD) is technically more like traditional hemodialysis and removes solute via diffusion because of a slow (15 to 30 ml/min) countercurrent drainage flow on the membrane side of the hemofilter (Fig. 30-5, *C*). Countercurrent flow is through the hemofilter. *Countercurrent* means the blood flows in one direction and the dialysate flows in the opposite direction. As with other types of CRRT and hemodialysis, while arterial access is always possible, venovenous vascular access is the most common choice today.

CVVHD is indicated for patients who require large-volume removal for severe uremia or critical acid-base imbalances or for those who are diuretic-resistant. A MAP of at least 70 mm Hg is desirable for effective volume removal and dialysis, and it is most effective when used over days, not hours. The use of replacement fluid is optional and depends on the patient's clinical condition and plan of care. The critical care nurse is responsible for calculating the hourly intake and output, noting fluid trends, and replacing excessive losses. This therapy is ideal for hemodynamically unstable patients in the critical care setting because they do not experience the abrupt fluid and solute changes that can accompany standard hemodialysis treatments.

Continuous Venovenous Hemodiafiltration. Another CRRT option is continuous venovenous hemodiafiltration (CVVHDF). CVVHDF combines two of the previously described methods (CVVH + CVVHD) to achieve maximal fluid and solute removal. A strong transmembrane pressure is applied to the hemofilter to push water across the filter, and a negative pressure is applied at the other side to pull fluid across the membrane and produce large volumes of ultrafiltrate, and also create a "solvent drag" (CVVH method). In addition, the blood and

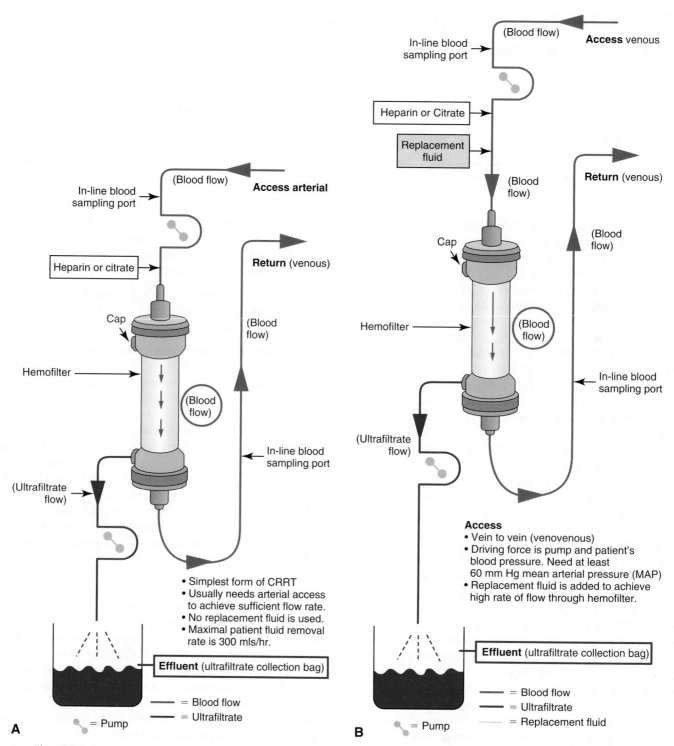

Fig. 30-5 Continuous renal replacement therapy (CRRT) systems. **A,** Slow, continuous ultrafiltration (SCUF). **B,** Continuous venovenous hemofiltration (CVVH).

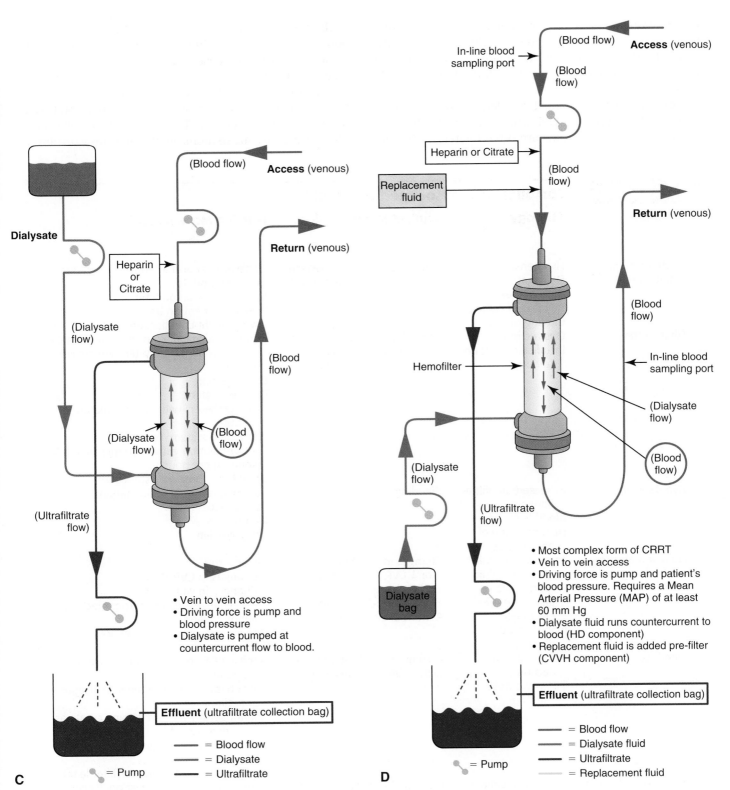

Dialysate

(Blood flow)   **Access** (venous)

Return (venous)

Heparin or Citrate

(Dialysate flow)

(Blood flow)

(Dialysate flow)   (Blood flow)

(Ultrafiltrate flow)

- Vein to vein access
- Driving force is pump and blood pressure
- Dialysate is pumped at countercurrent flow to blood.

Effluent (ultrafiltrate collection bag)

—— = Blood flow
—— = Dialysate
—— = Ultrafiltrate

= Pump

C

In-line blood sampling port   (Blood flow)   **Access** (venous)

(Blood flow)

Heparin or Citrate

Replacement fluid   (Blood flow)

Return (venous)

(Blood flow)

In-line blood sampling port

Hemofilter

(Dialysate flow)

(Blood flow)

(Dialysate flow)

(Ultrafiltrate flow)

Dialysate bag

- Most complex form of CRRT
- Vein to vein access
- Driving force is pump and patient's blood pressure. Requires a Mean Arterial Pressure (MAP) of at least 60 mm Hg
- Dialysate fluid runs countercurrent to blood (HD component)
- Replacement fluid is added pre-filter (CVVH component)

Effluent (ultrafiltrate collection bag)

—— = Blood flow
—— = Dialysate fluid
—— = Ultrafiltrate
—— = Replacement fluid

= Pump

D

Fig. 30-5, cont'd   C, Continuous venovenous hemofiltration dialysis (CVVHD). **D,** Continuous venovenous hemodiafiltration (CVVHDF).

the dialysate are circulated in a countercurrent flow pattern to remove fluid and solutes by diffusion (hemodialysis method). Thus CVVHDF can remove large volumes of fluid and solute because it employs both diffusion gradients and convection.

Complications. Potential problems associated with CRRT and appropriate nursing interventions are listed in Table 30-10. Complications are often related to the rate of flow through the system. If the patient becomes hypotensive, or the access lines remain kinked, the ultrafiltration rate will decrease. This in turn can lead to increased clot formation within the hemofilter. As the surface of the hemofilter becomes more clotted, it will not provide effective fluid or solute clearance and CRRT will be stopped; a new CRRT circuit must then be set up. The critical care nurse monitors the pressures displayed

Table 30-10	Complications Associated with CRRT		
Problem	**Etiology**	**Clinical Manifestations**	**Nursing Management**
Decreased ultrafiltration rate	Hypotension Dehydration Kinked lines Bending of catheters Clotting of filter	Ultrafiltration rate decreased Minimal flow through blood lines	Observe filter and arteriovenous system Control blood flow Control coagulation time Position patient on back Lower height of collection container
Filter clotting	Obstruction Insufficient heparinization	Ultrafiltration rate decreased, despite height of collection container being lower	Control anticoagulation (heparin/citrate) Maintain continuous system anticoagulation Call physician Remove system Prime catheters with anticoagulated solution Prime new system; connect it Start predilution with 1000 ml saline 0.9% solution per hour Do not use three-way stopcocks
Hypotension	Increased ultrafiltration rate Blood leak Disconnection of one of lines	Bleeding	Control amount of ultrafiltration Control access sites Clamp lines Call physician
Fluid and electrolyte changes	To much/too little removal of fluid Inappropriate replacement of electrolytes Inappropriate dialysate	Changes in mentation ↑ or ↓ CVP, ↑ or ↓ PAOP, ECG change ↑ or ↓ BP and heart rate Abnormal electrolyte levels	Observe for: • Changes in CVP/PAOP • Changes in vital signs • ECG changes resulting from electrolyte abnormalities Monitor output values every hour Control ultrafiltration
Bleeding	System disconnection ↑ Heparin dose	Oozing from catheter insertion site or connection	Monitor ACT no less than once every hour (heparin) Adjust heparin dose within specifications to maintain ACT Monitor serum calcium if using citrate as an anticoagulant Observe dressing on vascular access for blood loss Observe for blood in filtrate (filter leak)
Access dislodgement or infection	Catheter or connections not secured Break in sterile technique Excessive patient movement	Bleeding from catheter site or connections Inappropriate flow/infusion Fever Drainage at catheter site	Observe access site at least once every 2 hours Ensure that clamps are available within easy reach at all times Observe strict sterile technique when dressing vascular access

CRRT, Continuous renal replacement therapy; *CVP,* central venous pressure; *PAOP,* pulmonary artery occlusion pressure or "wedge" pressure; *BP,* blood pressure; *ECG,* electrocardiogram; *ACT,* activated coagulation time.

on the CRRT machine screen to monitor the positive pressure of fluid going into the hemofilter (inflow) and the pressures coming out of the hemofilter to ensure that resistance to the negative pressure "pull" of the fluid across the hemofilter membrane has not developed. Other patient-related complications include fluid and electrolyte alterations, bleeding secondary to anticoagulation, or problems with the access site such as dislodgement or infection.

Medical Management. The choice of the method of blood purification to use to treat ARF is a medical decision. There is no clear clinical or research consensus as to whether intermittent or continuous renal replacement therapy is the most beneficial.[56] Age, gender, and preexisting chronic conditions are of little help in determining the need for hemofiltration or hemodialysis. Often the acute clinical diagnosis, physician preference, availability of the CRRT machine, and knowledgeable physicians and nurses at the hospital are the deciding factors. Infectious complications are associated with a grave prognosis. Dialysis is prescribed for almost anyone who develops severe ARF, unless the patient is clearly dying.

Intermittent hemodialysis or CCRT is usually begun before the BUN level exceeds 90 mg/dl or the creatinine exceeds 9 mg/dl. In many hospitals the threshold to begin is considerably lower. Whether daily treatment is more effective than treatment every other day is controversial. The patient's serum creatinine, BUN, and fluid volume status are the deciding factors. CCRT is often prescribed when the BUN level is approximately 60 mg/dl. CRRT is more effective in the early stages of ARF. If severe electrolyte imbalance or fluid overload is present, even earlier intervention may be required.

Nursing Management. Critical care nurses play a vital role in monitoring the patient receiving CRRT. In many critical care units, the CRRT system is set up by the dialysis staff but is run on a 24-hour basis by critical care nurses with additional training. Complications can occur related to the CRRT circuit, the CRRT pump, or to the patient, as listed in Box 30-6. The critical care nurse monitors fluid intake and output, prevents and detects potential complications (e.g., bleeding, hypotension), trends electrolyte laboratory values, supervises safe operation of the CRRT equipment, and provides patient and family education about the patient's condition inclusive of CRRT.

PERITONEAL DIALYSIS

Peritoneal dialysis (PD) is a modality used in patients with chronic kidney disease.[58] Only 8.4% of patients with end-stage kidney disease (ESKD) are treated with PD.[59] When a PD-dependent patient is admitted to the critical care unit with a nonrenal acute illness, peritoneal dialysis may be continued. Peritoneal dialysis involves the introduction of sterile dialyzing fluid through an implanted catheter into the abdominal cavity. The dialysate bathes the peritoneal membrane, which covers the abdominal organs and overlies the capillary beds that support the organs.[58] By the processes of osmosis, diffusion, and active transport, excess fluid and solutes travel from the peritoneal capillary fluid through the capillary walls, through the peritoneal membrane, and into the dialyzing fluid. After a selected period the fluid is drained out of the abdomen by gravity (Fig. 30-6). The process is then repeated at regular prescribed intervals.[60]

Indications for peritoneal dialysis include renal failure, volume overload, electrolyte imbalances, hemodynamic instability, lack of access to circulation, and removal of high–molecular-weight toxins. In the critical care unit, patients who have PD at home may be admitted with a nonrenal critical illness but will continue to receive PD for chronic kidney failure in the hospital (Box 30-7).

The peritoneal membrane's structure and capillary blood flow to the peritoneum account for the relatively slow nature of PD. The small capillary pores, the capillary membrane, the interstitium, the mesothelium of the

---

Box 30-6
COMPLICATIONS OF CRRT

THE CIRCUIT
Air embolism
Clotted hemofilter
Poor ultrafiltration
Blood leaks
Broken filter
Recirculation/disconnection
Access failure
Catheter dislodgment

THE PUMP
Circuit pressure alarm
  Decreased inflow pressure
  Decreased outflow pressure
  Increased outflow resistance
Air bubble detector alarm
Power failure
Mechanical dysfunction

THE PATIENT
Code/emergency situation
Dehydration
Hypotension
Electrolyte imbalances
Acid-base imbalances
Blood loss/hemorrhage
Hypothermia
Infection
Blood transfusion reaction

From Headrick CL: *Nurse Clin North Am* 10(2):197-207, 1998.
CRRT: Continuous renal replacement therapy.

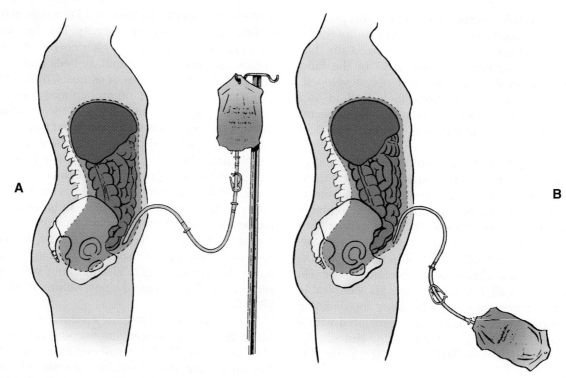

Fig. 30-6 Peritoneal dialysis. **A,** Inflow. **B,** Outflow (drains by gravity). (From Thompson JM et al: *Mosby's clinical nursing,* ed 5, St Louis, 2002, Mosby.)

Box 30-7

INDICATIONS AND CONTRAINDICATIONS FOR PERITONEAL DIALYSIS

INDICATIONS
Uremia
Volume overload
Electrolyte imbalances
Hemodynamic instability
Lack of access to circulation
Removal of high–molecular-weight toxins
Patients with nonrenal critical illness receiving peritoneal dialysis for chronic kidney failure
Severe cardiovascular disease
Inability to anticoagulate
Contraindication to hemodialysis

CONTRAINDICATIONS
Recent abdominal surgery
History of abdominal surgeries with adhesions and scarring
Significant pulmonary disease
Need for rapid fluid removal
Peritonitis

---

peritoneum, and the fluid film layers in the capillary and the peritoneal cavity provide formidable barriers to fluid and solute passage. If needed a "peritoneal equilibration test" can be performed to determine the level of solute clearance for a specific patient.[58]

The volume of dialysate instilled into the abdomen affects the clearance. Normally the PD-dependent patients are well versed in the amount, type, and frequency of dialysate to be infused into their abdomen, with subsequent drainage by gravity into a "waste" bag. The primary nursing consideration is to avoid contamination of the access point and monitor the patient's vital signs during this process. The dialysate should be instilled at body temperature to be comfortable, provide some vasodilation, and provide increased solute transport in the peritoneum. The length of time the solution remains in the peritoneal cavity *(dwell time)* and the solution composition affect the outcome. The dwell time affects the amount of fluid removed from the peritoneal capillaries, although a longer dwell time will not remove proportionately more fluid because of osmotic equilibration across the membranes. The various glucose concentrations of the dialysate provide for different rates of fluid removal.[58,61]

Catheter Placement. Most catheters have four segments: an external segment outside the abdomen, a tunnel segment that passes through subcutaneous tissue and muscle, a cuff for stabilization at the peritoneal membrane, and an internal segment with numerous holes for fast delivery and drainage of dialysate (Fig. 30-7). The infusion and removal of the dialysate fluid are sterile procedures.

Infection. The most significant risk to the patient with peritoneal dialysis is development of peritonitis

NIC Peritoneal Dialysis Therapy

Definition: Administration and monitoring of dialysis solution into and out of the peritoneal cavity.

Activities

Explain the selected peritoneal dialysis procedure and purpose

Warm the dialysis fluid before instillation

Assess patency of catheter, noting difficulty in inflow/outflow

Maintain record of inflow/outflow volumes and individual/cumulative fluid balance

Have patient empty bladder before peritoneal catheter insertion

Avoid excess mechanical stress on peritoneal dialysis catheters (e.g., coughing, dressing change, infusing large volumes)

Monitor blood pressure, pulse, respirations, temperature, and patient response during dialysis

Ensure aseptic handling of peritoneal catheter and connections

Draw blood samples and review blood chemistries (e.g., BUN; serum Cr; and serum sodium, potassium, and PO_4 levels)

Obtain cell count cultures of peritoneal effluent, if indicated

Record baseline vital signs: weight, temperature, pulse, respirations, and blood pressure

Measure and record abdominal girth

Measure and record daily weight

Anchor connections and tubing securely

Check equipment and solutions, according to protocol

Administer dialysis exchanges (inflow, dwell, and outflow), according to protocol

Monitor for signs of infection (e.g., peritonitis and exit-site inflammation/drainage)

Monitor for signs of respiratory distress

Monitor for bowel perforation or fluid leaks

Work collaboratively with patient to adjust length of dialysis, diet regulations, and pain and diversion needs to achieve optimal benefit of the treatment

Teach patient to monitor self for signs and symptoms that indicate need for medical treatment (e.g., fever, bleeding, respiratory distress, irregular pulse, cloudy outflow, and abdominal pain)

Teach procedure to patient requiring home dialysis

From McCloskey JD, Bulechek GM: *Nursing interventions classification (NIC)*, ed 4, 2004, St Louis, Mosby.

secondary to catheter contamination and infection. Infection accounts for about two thirds of all PD catheter losses.[58] PD catheter infection results in peritonitis in 25% to 50% of cases.[58] Serious infection is also a reason a patient who uses PD would be admitted to the hospital.[58] The critical care nurse must be acutely aware of the signs and symptoms of systemic infection, such as a sudden rise in the WBC count, increased temperature, and malaise. At the same time, clinicians remain vigilant for signs of localized catheter or abdominal infection manifested by catheter site redness, site swelling, cloudy dialysis effluent following the dwell time, and abdominal tenderness or pain which is present 75% of the time when infection is present.[58]

Medical Management. PD is used for long-term end-stage kidney failure. It is never used as a first-line acute care intervention. If a patient uses PD at home, PD will continue during the acute care hospitalization, provided the condition precipitating the admission is unrelated to the kidneys or abdomen.

Nursing Management. Nursing management of the patient receiving peritoneal dialysis is complex. A comprehensive list of nursing interventions while caring for the patients with PD is provided in the Nursing Interventions Classification feature on Peritoneal Dialysis Therapy. Nurses are vigilant about prevention and detection

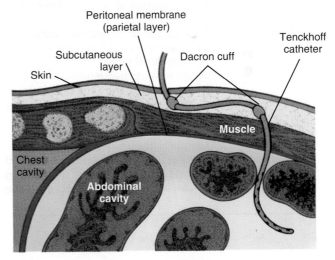

Fig. 30-7 Tenckhoff catheter used in peritoneal dialysis. (From Lewis SM, Heitkemper MM, Dirksen SR: *Medical-surgical nursing assessment and management of clinical problems*, ed 6, St Louis, 2004, Mosby.)

of complications related to PD (Table 30-11). The critical care nurse observes for signs and symptoms of infection, monitors fluid volume status, infuses the dialysate fluid, observes drainage of the ultrafiltrate fluid, prevents complications associated with the PD catheter, and provides

Table 30-11	Complications Associated With Peritoneal Dialysis
Complication	**Nursing Management**
Peritonitis	Assess for signs and symptoms: cloudy effluent, abdominal pain, rebound tenderness, nausea and vomiting, fever. Obtain effluent sample for culture. Administer antibiotics as ordered. Teach patient/family signs and symptoms and prevention.
Exit site infection	Monitor site daily for signs and symptoms of infection: induration, erythema, purulence, hyperthermia. Increase daily cleaning of site. Apply topical antibiotics as ordered (controversial). Teach patient/family to avoid agents such as creams and lotions around exit site.
Catheter-tunnel infection	Assess for signs and symptoms of infection: pain along tunnel, induration for several centimeters away from catheter, erythema leading away from exit site, drainage at exit site or as tunnel is "milked" toward exit site. Teach patient/family signs and symptoms of infection. Teach patient/family to avoid pulls or tugs on catheter or trauma to exit site. Emphasize need to maintain cleansing regimen at exit site.
Fluid obstruction	Change position of patient (standing, lying, side-lying, knee-chest). Relieve patient's constipation. Irrigate the catheter. Ensure that sufficient fluid is in abdomen (sometimes requires a residual reservoir of approximately 50 ml).
Rectal pain	Ensure a sufficient reservoir of fluid. Use slow infusion rate.
Shoulder pain	Ensure that all air is primed from infusion tubing. Attempt draining the effluent with patients in knee-chest position. Administer mild analgesics as ordered.
Hernia	Monitor for increase in size of or pain in area of hernia. Decrease volume of exchanges as ordered. Dialyze with patients in the supine position. Use abdominal binder or support for patients (as long as not binding on catheter exit site). Avoid initiation of peritoneal dialysis until exit site healing has taken place (approximately 1 to 2 weeks) if possible.
Fluid overload	Increase use of hypertonic solutions. Decrease oral (PO) fluid intake. Shorten dwell times. Weigh patients frequently. Monitor lung sounds and peripheral edema.
Dehydration	Assess patients for decreased skin turgor, muscle cramps, hypotension, tachycardia, and dizziness. Discontinue hypertonic solutions. Increase oral fluid intake. Lengthen dwell times.
Blood-tinged effluent	Monitor for change in effluent color (clear yellow to pink or rusty). Administer heparin, as ordered, to prevent fibrin formation. Obtain patient history about catheter trauma and patient activity before appearance of complication.

patient and family education. Patients who use PD are partners in the maintenance of their health because of the huge commitment they make in self-management of their peritoneal dialysis care.[59-62]

SUMMARY

Many critically ill patients have acute renal failure as a complication of their illness. The initial reason for ad-mission to the critical care unit may have been sepsis, hypovolemic shock, or trauma or may occur following major surgery; however, if acute renal failure develops, mortality increases. Because of the mortality and mor-bidity risks associated with ARF, prevention is always a top priority. Once a diagnosis of ARF is made, the critical care nurse must be knowledgeable about effective inter-ventions and provide patient comfort measures to ame-liorate symptoms experienced by the patient with acute renal failure.

REFERENCES

1. Mehta RL et al: Spectrum of acute renal failure in the intensive care unit: the PICARD experience, *Kidney Int* 66(4):1613-1621, 2004.
2. Sesso R et al: Prognosis of ARF in hospitalized elderly patients, *Am J Kidney Dis* 44(3):410-419, 2004.
3. Nickolas TL et al: Awareness of kidney disease in the U.S. population: findings from the National Health and Nutrition Examination Survey (NHANES) 1999 to 2000, *Am J Kidney Dis* 44(2):185-197, 2004.
4. Kellum JA et al: Developing a consensus classification system for acute renal failure, *Curr Opin Crit Care* 8(6):509-514, 2002.
5. Asif A, Epstein M: Prevention of radiocontrast-induced nephropathy, *Am J Kidney Dis* 44(1):12-24, 2004.
6. Thompson EJ, King SL: Acetylcysteine and fenoldopam. Promising new approaches for preventing effects of contrast nephrotoxicity, *Crit Care Nurse* 23(3):39-46, 2003.
7. Sheridan AM, Bonventre JV: Cell biology and molecular mechanisms of injury in ischemic acute renal failure, *Curr Opin Nephrol Hypertens* 9(4):427-434, 2000.
8. Liano F et al: The spectrum of acute renal failure in the intensive care unit compared with that seen in other settings. The Madrid Acute Renal Failure Study Group, *Kidney Int Suppl* 66:S16-24, 1998.
9. Rocktaeschel J et al: Acid-base status of critically ill patients with acute renal failure: analysis based on Stewart-Figge methodology, *Crit Care* 7(4):R60-66, 2003.
10. Bellomo R, Kellum JA, Ronco C: Defining acute renal failure: physiological principles, *Intensive Care Med* 30(1):33-37, 2004.
11. Coresh J et al: Prevalence of chronic kidney disease and decreased kidney function in the adult U.S. population: Third National Health and Nutrition Examination Survey, *Am J Kidney Dis* 41(1):1-12, 2003.
12. K/DOQI clinical practice guidelines for chronic kidney disease: evaluation, classification, and stratification, *Am J Kidney Dis* 39(2 Suppl 1):S1-266, 2002.
13. Bellomo R et al: Acute renal failure—definition, outcome measures, animal models, fluid therapy and information technology needs: the Second International Consensus Conference of the Acute Dialysis Quality Initiative (ADQI) Group, *Crit Care* 8(4):R204-212, 2004.
14. Warnock DG, Textor SC: Hypertension, *Am J Kidney Dis* 44(2):369-375, 2004.
15. K/DOQI clinical practice guidelines on hypertension and antihypertensive agents in chronic kidney disease, *Am J Kidney Dis* 43(5 Suppl 1):S1-290, 2004.
16. Mitch WE et al: Detecting and managing patients with type 2 diabetic kidney disease: proteinuria and cardiovascular disease, *Kidney Int Suppl* 92:S97-98, 2004.
17. Keith DS et al: Longitudinal follow-up and outcomes among a population with chronic kidney disease in a large managed care organization, *Arch Intern Med* 164(6):659-663, 2004.
18. Go AS et al: Chronic kidney disease and the risks of death, cardiovascular events, and hospitalization, *N Engl J Med* 351(13):1296-1305, 2004.
19. Anavekar NS et al: Relation between renal dysfunction and cardiovascular outcomes after myocardial infarction, *N Engl J Med* 351(13):1285-1295, 2004.
20. Pannu N, Mehta RL: Mechanical ventilation and renal function: an area for concern? *Am J Kidney Dis* 39(3):616-624, 2002.
21. Dellinger RP et al: Surviving Sepsis Campaign guidelines for management of severe sepsis and septic shock, *Crit Care Med* 32(3):858-873, 2004.
22. Hollenberg SM et al: Practice parameters for hemodynamic support of sepsis in adult patients: 2004 update, *Crit Care Med* 32(9):1928-1948, 2004.
23. Criddle LM: Rhabdomyolysis. Pathophysiology, recognition, and management, *Crit Care Nurse* 23(6):14-28, 2003.
24. Brown CV et al: Preventing renal failure in patients with rhabdomyolysis: do bicarbonate and mannitol make a difference? *J Trauma* 56(6):1191-1196, 2004.
25. Kandzari DE et al: Contrast nephropathy: an evidence-based approach to prevention, *Am J Cardiovasc Drugs* 3(6):395-405, 2003.
26. Aspelin P et al: Nephrotoxic effects in high-risk patients undergoing angiography, *N Engl J Med* 348(6):491-499, 2003.
27. Durham JD et al: A randomized controlled trial of N-acetylcysteine to prevent contrast nephropathy in cardiac angiography, *Kidney Int* 62(6):2202-2207, 2002.
28. Guru V, Fremes SE: The role of N-acetylcysteine in preventing radiographic contrast-induced nephropathy, *Clin Nephrol* 62(2):77-83, 2004.
29. Kshirsagar AV et al: N-acetylcysteine for the prevention of radiocontrast induced nephropathy: a meta-analysis of prospective controlled trials, *J Am Soc Nephrol* 15(3):761-769, 2004.
30. El-Shahawy MA, Agbing LU, Badillo E: Severity of illness scores and the outcome of acute tubular necrosis, *Int Urol Nephrol* 32(2):185-191, 2000.
31. Ahee P, Crowe AV: The management of hyperkalemia in the emergency department, *J Accid Emerg Med* 17(3):188-191, 2000.
32. Levey AS et al: National Kidney Foundation practice guidelines for chronic kidney disease: evaluation, classification, and stratification, *Ann Intern Med* 139(2):137-147, 2003.
33. Leavey SF, Weitzel WF: Endocrine abnormalities in chronic renal failure, *Endocrinol Metab Clin North Am* 31(1):107-119, 2002.
34. Emmett M: A comparison of clinically useful phosphorus binders for patients with chronic kidney failure, *Kidney Int Suppl* 90:S25-32, 2004.
35. Haney SL: Drug use in renal failure, *Crit Care Nurs Clin North Am* 14(1):77-80, 2002.
36. Mehta RL, Clark WC, Schetz M: Techniques for assessing and achieving fluid balance in acute renal failure, *Curr Opin Crit Care* 8(6):535-543, 2002.
37. Finfer S et al: A comparison of albumin and saline for fluid resuscitation in the intensive care unit, *N Engl J Med* 350(22):2247-2256, 2004.
38. Vincent JL, Navickis RJ, Wilkes MM: Morbidity in hospitalized patients receiving human albumin: a meta-analysis of randomized, controlled trials, *Crit Care Med* 32(10):2029-2038, 2004.
39. Mehta RL et al: Diuretics, mortality, and nonrecovery of renal function in acute renal failure, *JAMA* 288(20):2547-2553, 2002.
40. Cantarovich F et al: High-dose furosemide for established ARF: a prospective, randomized, double-blind, placebo-controlled, multicenter trial, *Am J Kidney Dis* 44(3):402-409, 2004.
41. Uchino S et al: Diuretics and mortality in acute renal failure, *Crit Care Med* 32(8):1669-1677, 2004.
42. Ichai C et al: Prolonged low-dose dopamine infusion induces a transient improvement in renal function in hemodynamically stable, critically ill patients: a single-blind, prospective, controlled study, *Crit Care Med* 28(5):1329-1335, 2000.

43. Kellum JA: Use of dopamine in acute renal failure: a meta-analysis, *Crit Care Med* 29(8):1526-1531, 2001.

44. Bellomo R et al: Low-dose dopamine in patients with early renal dysfunction: a placebo-controlled randomised trial. Australian and New Zealand Intensive Care Society (ANZICS) Clinical Trials Group, *Lancet* 356(9248):2139-2143, 2000.

45. Freeman RV et al: Nephropathy requiring dialysis after percutaneous coronary intervention and the critical role of an adjusted contrast dose, *Am J Cardiol* 90(10):1068-1073, 2002.

46. Druml W: Nutritional management of acute renal failure, *Am J Kidney Dis* 37(1 Suppl 2):S89-94, 2001.

47. Pearl RG, Pohlman A: Understanding and managing anemia in critically ill patients, *Crit Care Nurse* Suppl:1-12, 2002.

48. Gouva C et al: Treating anemia early in renal failure patients slows the decline of renal function: a randomized controlled trial, *Kidney Int* 66(2):753-760, 2004.

49. Corwin HL et al: Efficacy of recombinant human erythropoietin in critically ill patients: a randomized controlled trial, *JAMA* 288(22):2827-2835, 2002.

50. Schiffl H, Lang SM, Fischer R: Daily hemodialysis and the outcome of acute renal failure, *N Engl J Med* 346(5):305-310, 2002.

51. Warkentin TE, Greinacher A: Heparin-induced thrombocytopenia: recognition, treatment, and prevention: the Seventh ACCP Conference on Antithrombotic and Thrombolytic Therapy, *Chest* 126(3 Suppl):311S-337S, 2004.

52. Monchi M et al: Citrate vs. heparin for anticoagulation in continuous venovenous hemofiltration: a prospective randomized study, *Intensive Care Med* 30(2):260-265, 2004.

53. Rayner HC et al: Creation, cannulation and survival of arteriovenous fistulae: data from the Dialysis Outcomes and Practice Patterns Study, *Kidney Int* 63(1):323-330, 2003.

54. Beathard GA et al: Aggressive treatment of early fistula failure, *Kidney Int* 64(4):1487-1494, 2003.

55. Asif A et al: Arteriovenous fistula creation: should US nephrologists get involved? *Am J Kidney Dis* 42(6):1293-1300, 2003.

56. Kellum JA et al: Continuous versus intermittent renal replacement therapy: a meta-analysis, *Intensive Care Med* 28(1):29-37, 2002.

57. Rempher KJ: Continuous renal replacement therapy for management of overhydration in heart failure, *AACN Clin Issues* 14(4):512-519, 2003.

58. Teitelbaum I, Burkart J: Peritoneal dialysis, *Am J Kidney Dis* 42(5):1082-1096, 2003.

59. Curtin RB, Johnson HK, Schatell D: The peritoneal dialysis experience: insights from long-term patients, *Nephrol Nurs J* 31(6):615-624, 2004.

60. Kelley KT: How peritoneal dialysis works, *Nephrol Nurs J* 31(5):481-482, 488-489, 2004.

61. Crawford-Bonadio TL, Diaz-Buxo JA: Comparison of peritoneal dialysis solutions, *Nephrol Nurs J* 31(5):499-507, 520, 2004.

62. Maaz DE: Troubleshooting non-infectious peritoneal dialysis issues, *Nephrol Nurs J* 31(5):521-532, 2004.

GASTROINTESTINAL ALTERATIONS

CHAPTER 31

Gastrointestinal Anatomy and Physiology

*T*he major function of the gastrointestinal (GI) tract is digestion—that is, to convert ingested nutrients into simpler forms that can be transported from the tract's lumen to the portal circulation and then used in metabolic processes. The GI system also plays a vital role in detoxification and elimination of bacteria, viruses, chemical toxins, and drugs. Disturbances of the GI system itself or of the complex hormonal and neural controls that regulate it can severely upset homeostasis and compromise the overall nutritional status of the patient. Furthermore, any circumvention of the normal feeding mechanism can alter digestive processes or contribute to malabsorption.[1] Thus it is vital for the critical care nurse to have a comprehensive knowledge of the normal function of the GI tract to facilitate assessment, diagnosis, and intervention in patients with GI dysfunction.

The GI tract consists of the mouth, the esophagus, the stomach, the small intestine, and the large intestine (Fig. 31-1).

MOUTH

The mouth and accessory organs, which include the lips, cheeks, gums, tongue, palate, and salivary glands, perform the initial phases of digestion, which are ingestion, mastication, and salivation.[1]

INGESTION AND MASTICATION

The mouth is the beginning of the alimentary canal (see Fig. 31-1), and is the means for ingestion and entry of nutrients. The teeth cut, grind, and mix food, transforming it into a form suitable for swallowing and increasing the surface area of food available to mix with salivary secretions. Healthy dentition is vital for this process. Mucous glands located behind the tip of the tongue and serous glands located at the back of the tongue aid in the lubrication of food and in its distribution over the taste buds.[2]

SALIVATION

Salivation has an important role in the first stage of digestion because saliva lubricates the mouth, facilitates the movement of the lips and the tongue during swallowing, and washes away bacteria. Saliva consists of approximately 99.5% water[3] that contains a large amount of ions such as potassium, chloride, bicarbonate,[1] thiocyanate, and hydrogen,[3] as well as immunoglobulin A, which is vital for destroying oral bacteria,[1] and mucus. Approximately 1000 to 1500 ml of saliva is produced each day by three pairs of major salivary glands: the submandibular glands, the sublingual glands, and the parotid glands. Parotid gland secretions are enzymatic, containing amylase (ptyalin), which begins the chemical breakdown of large polysaccharides into dextrins and sugars. The mouth and pharynx also are lined with minor salivary glands that provide additional lubrication.[3]

The salivary glands are regulated by the autonomic nervous system, with parasympathetic effects predominating. Increased parasympathetic stimulation results in profuse secretions of watery saliva, whereas decreased parasympathetic stimulation results in inhibition of salivation.[1,3]

ESOPHAGUS

The esophagus is a hollow muscular tube that lacks cartilage. In adults it is 23 to 25 cm (9 to 10 inches) long and 2 to 3 cm (1 inch) wide. It is the narrowest part of the digestive tube and lies posterior to the trachea and heart, with attachments at the hypopharynx and at the cardiac portion of the stomach below the diaphragm. It begins at the level of the C6 to T1 vertebrae and extends vertically through the mediastinum and diaphragm to the level of T11.[4]

The esophagus has two sphincters, the upper esophageal (also known as *hypopharyngeal*) and the lower esophageal (also known as *cardioesophageal* or *gastroesophageal*).[5] The upper esophageal sphincter in-

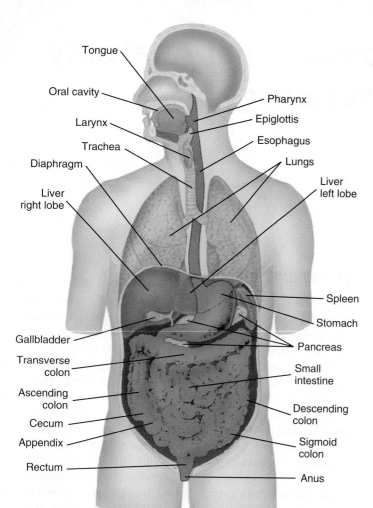

Fig. 31-1 Anatomy of the gastrointestinal system. (From Thompson JM et al: *Mosby's clinical nursing,* ed 5, St Louis, 2002, Mosby.)

hibits air from entering the esophagus during respiration.[1] The lower esophageal sphincter controls the passage of food into the stomach[5] and prevents reflux of gastric contents.[1]

SWALLOWING

The functions of the esophagus are to accept a bolus of food from the oropharynx, to transport the bolus through the esophageal body by gravity and peristalsis, and to release the bolus into the stomach through the lower esophageal sphincter. This process is known as *swallowing.*[6] Peristalsis consists of waves of circular muscle contractions and relaxations. Peristalsis that is initiated by swallowing is known as *primary peristalsis,* whereas peristalsis that is initiated by esophageal distention is known as *secondary peristalsis.*[1,5] Peristaltic waves begin in the pharynx and move distally at a rate of 2 to 6 cm per second.[1]

STOMACH

The stomach is an elongated pouch approximately 25 to 30 cm (10 to 12 inches) long and 10 to 15 cm (4 to 6 inches) wide at the maximal transverse diameter. It lies obliquely beneath the cardiac sphincter at the esophagogastric junction and above the pyloric sphincter, next to the small intestine. The anatomic divisions of the stomach are the cardia (proximal end), the fundus (portion above and to the left of the cardiac sphincter), the body (middle portion), the antrum (elongated, constricted portion), and the pylorus (distal end connecting the antrum to the duodenum) (Fig. 31-2). The greater curvature, which begins at the cardiac orifice and arches backward and upward around the fundus, is in contact with the transverse colon and the pancreas at the posterior edge. The lesser curvature extends from the cardia to the pylorus. Two sphincters control the rate of food passage: the lower esophageal at the esophagogastric junction and the pyloric at the gastroduodenal junction.[5]

The stomach wall has four layers (Fig. 31-3). The outermost layer, the serous layer (serosa), consists of squamous epithelial tissue and continues as a double fold from the lower edge of the stomach to cover the intestine. The second layer, the muscular layer (muscularis), extends from the fundus to the antrum and consists of three smooth muscle layers, which are the longitudinal layer, the circular layer, and the oblique layer. The third layer, the submucous layer (submucosa), consists of connective tissue that contains blood vessels, lymphatics, and nerve plexuses. The innermost layer, the mucous layer (mucosa), consists of a muscular layer that is arranged in longitudinal folds, or rugae, that can expand as the stomach fills.[5] This layer also contains glands that secrete up to 3000 ml of gastric juice per day.[7]

The celiac artery provides the blood supply required for the motor and secretory activity of the stomach. The splenic vein provides venous drainage for the right side of the stomach, and the gastric vein provides it for the left.[1] Numerous lymphatic channels arise in the submucosa and terminate in the thoracic duct. The stomach is innervated by the autonomic nervous system. Sympathetic fibers arise from the celiac plexus; parasympathetic fibers arise from the gastric branch of the vagus nerve.[5]

The epithelial cells of the gastric mucosa are packed very close together and serve as a protective barrier, preventing diffusion of hydrogen ions into the mucosa. The surface epithelial cells produce alkaline mucus and secrete a bicarbonate-laden fluid. The mucus further protects the gastric mucosa by delaying back-diffusion of hydrogen ions and trapping them for neutralization by the secreted bicarbonate.[8] In addition, gastric mucosal cells can compensate for cell destruction. Epithelial cells are in a constant state of growth, migration, and desquamation and are shed at a rate of one-half million cells per minute. The gastric mucosa also has the ability to in-

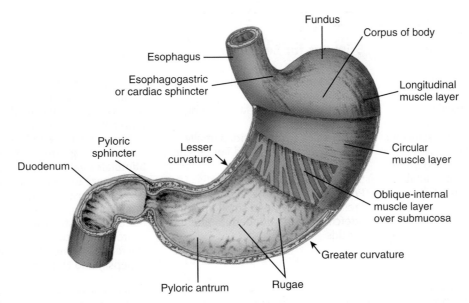

Fig. 31-2   Gross anatomy of the stomach. (From Thompson JM et al: *Mosby's clinical nursing,* ed 5, St Louis, 2002, Mosby.)

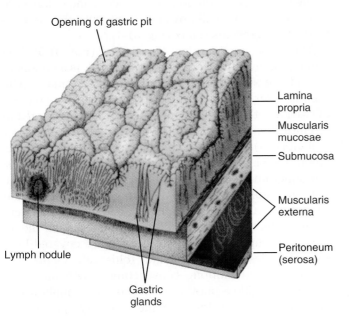

Fig. 31-3   Structure of the gastric mucosa. (From Berne RM, et al: *Physiology,* ed 5, St Louis, 2005, Mosby.)

crease blood flow, providing an additional buffer for acid neutralization and aiding in the removal of toxic metabolites and chloride ions from injured mucosa. Finally, the gastric mucosal cells synthesize a family of unsaturated fatty acids known as *prostaglandins*. Prostaglandins facilitate mucosal bicarbonate secretion and inhibit acid secretion by preventing the activation of parietal cells by histamine (a local biochemical mediator). Certain lipid-soluble substances, such as alcohol, aspirin and other nonsteroidal antiinflammatory drugs, regurgitated bile, and uremic toxins, can break through the mucosal bar-

rier and penetrate the cells, causing their destruction, edema, and eventual bleeding.[8]

GASTRIC SECRETION

The stomach has three different types of glands—cardiac, oxyntic, and pyloric—that contain cells of various types that secrete 1500 to 3000 ml of gastric juice into the lumen per day, depending on the diet and other stimuli.[7] Gastric juice is composed of hydrochloric acid (HCl), pepsin, (necessary for the breakdown of protein), mucus, intrinsic factor (necessary for vitamin B_{12} absorption), sodium, and potassium. Pepsinogen, secreted by the chief cells of the stomach lining, is converted to its active form, pepsin, in the acidic environment of the stomach.[1] The cardiac glands secrete mucus and pepsinogen. The oxyntic glands contain parietal cells, which secrete HCl and intrinsic factor, and chief cells, which secrete pepsinogen. Pyloric glands contain mucus cells, which secrete mucus and pepsinogen, and G cells, which secrete gastrin (Table 31-1).[5] Gastric glands are stimulated by the parasympathetic stimulation and gastrin and inhibited by gastric-inhibitory peptide and enterogastrone. Histamine and entero-oxyntin also stimulate the parietal cells to produce acid, and secretin also stimulates the chief cells to produce pepsinogen.[1]

The pH of gastric juice is 1.0, but when mixed with food, it rises to 2.0 to 3.0. Gastric juice dissolves soluble foods and has bacteriostatic action against swallowed microorganisms. The composition of gastric secretions will vary depending on a variety of factors including flow rate, volume, and the time of day. In addition, pain, fear, or rage will inhibit gastric secretion, whereas aggression or hostility will stimulate it.[1]

Table 31-1	Digestive Hormones		
Source	**Hormone**	**Stimulus for Secretion**	**Action**
Mucosa of the stomach	Gastrin	Presence of partially digested proteins in the stomach	Stimulates gastric glands to secrete hydrochloric acid and pepsinogen
Mucosa of the small intestines	Motilin	Presence of acid and fat in the duodenum	Increases gastrointestinal motility
	Secretion	Presence of chyme (acid, partially digested proteins, and fats) in the duodenum	Stimulates pancreas to secrete alkaline pancreatic juice and liver to secrete bile; decreases gastrointestinal motility
	Cholecystokinin	Same as for secretin	Stimulates gallbladder to eject bile and pancreas to secrete alkaline fluid; decreases gastric motility
	Enterogastrone	Presence of fat in the duodenum	Inhibits gastric secretion and motility
	Entero-oxyntin	Presence of chyme in small intestine	Stimulates gastric glands to secrete hydrochloric acid
	Gastric-inhibitory peptide	Stretching of the duodenum and fatty acids	Decreases gastric motility and secretion of pepsin and HCl

From McCance KL, Huether SE, editors: *Pathophysiology: the biologic basis for disease in adults and children,* ed 4, St Louis, 2002, Mosby.

GASTRIC MOTILITY

The functions of the stomach include food storage, digestion, and emptying. The stomach receives food through the lower esophageal sphincter, stores it for a period of time, and mixes it with gastric secretions. The food is then ground into a semifluid consistency called *chyme*, which is delivered via the pylorus to the duodenum. Gastric motility is regulated by the autonomic nervous system, digestive hormones, and neural reflexes. Gastrin, motilin (see Table 31-1), and parasympathetic stimulation increase gastric motility, whereas secretin, cholecystokinin, enterogastrone, gastric-inhibitory peptide (see Table 31-1), and sympathetic stimulation decrease it. The ileogastric reflex inhibits gastric motility when the ileum is distended.[9]

SMALL INTESTINE

The small intestine, a coiled, folded tube approximately 7 m (22 to 23 feet) long, extends from the pyloric sphincter to the cecum and fills most of the abdominal cavity. It has three anatomic divisions: duodenum, jejunum, and ileum. The duodenum, shaped like the letter C, begins at the pyloric sphincter of the stomach and ends at the ligament of Treitz. It is 30 cm (12 inches) long and 4 cm (1 to 1.5 inches) wide.[10] The jejunum, which is 250 cm (8 to 9 feet) long and 4 cm (1 to 1.5 inches) wide, lies in the left iliac and umbilical regions. The ileum, which is 375 cm (12 feet) long and 2.5 cm (1 inch) wide, lies in the hypogastric, right iliac, and pelvic regions. Although the demarcating line between the jejunum and the ileum is somewhat arbitrary, the ileum is narrower than the jejunum. The ileocecal valve, located at the terminal end of the ileum at the junction of the cecum and colon, controls the flow of small bowel contents into the large intestine and prevents reflux (Fig. 31-4).[1]

The small intestine has four layers (Fig. 31-5). The outermost layer, the serous layer (serosa), is a continuation of the serous coat surrounding the stomach. The second layer, the muscular layer (muscularis), consists of two smooth muscle layers called the *longitudinal* and *circular layers.* The third layer, the submucous layer (submucosa), consists of connective tissue that contains blood vessels, lymphatics, glands, and nerve plexuses. The innermost layer, the mucous layer (mucosa), consists of simple columnar epithlelium.[5] The mucosa and submucosa are arranged in circular folds (plicae circulares),[5] which are largest and most numerous in the jejunum and upper ileum.[1] These folds are covered by a second series of projectile-like folds called *villi* that are in constant motion—constricting, lengthening, and shortening (villous movement). The 4 to 5 million villi (see Fig. 31-4) give the intestine a velvety appearance; they are more numerous and larger in the jejunum than in the ileum. Villi contain a network of capillaries and blind lymphatic vessels called *lacteals.* The outer layer of the villus is composed of microvilli. The circular folds of the small intestine, along with the villi and microvilli, increase the digestive-absorptive surface of the small intestine 600 times.[5,10]

The gastroduodenal artery provides the blood supply for the duodenum, and branches of the superior mesenteric artery provide for the jejunum and the ileum. The superior mesenteric vein provides for venous drainage of the small intestine.[11] Numerous lymphatic channels arise in the submucosa and terminate in the thoracic duct. The small intestine is extrinsically innervated by the autonomic nervous system. Sympathetic fibers arise

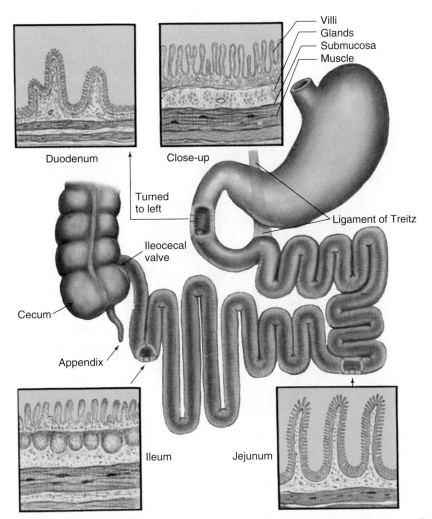

Fig. 31-4   Clinical anatomy of the small intestine. (From Thompson JM et al: *Mosby's clinical nursing,* ed 5, St Louis, 2002, Mosby.)

from the celiac plexus, whereas parasympathetic fibers arise from the gastric branch of the vagus nerve. Intrinsic innervation, which initiates motor functions, is provided by two plexuses (Auerbach's and Meissner's) located in the intestinal wall.[1]

INTESTINAL SECRETION

The small intestine has two major types of glands, Brunner's glands and intestinal glands. Brunner's glands lie in the mucosa of the duodenum and secrete mucus, an alkaline fluid (pH of 9) that neutralizes chyme and protects the mucosa.[5] Intestinal glands are found in pits of the submucosa and are called the *crypts of Lieberkühn.* These crypts secrete 2 to 3 L per day of yellow fluid containing enzymes that assist in nutrient digestion.[7]

INTESTINAL MOTILITY

Intestinal motility consists of two separate motions: peristalsis and haustral segmentation. Peristalsis is se-

quential contraction and relaxation of short segments of the small intestine that facilitate digestion and absorption. Haustral segmentation is rhythmic contractions that facilitate the mixing and forward movement of chyme. It is controlled by Auerbach's plexus. Intestinal motility is also affected by neural reflexes located along the length of the small intestine. Motility is inhibited by the intestinointestinal reflex, which is activated by distention of the small intestine, and stimulated by the gastroileal reflux, which is initiated by an increase in gastric motility.[9]

DIGESTION AND ABSORPTION

The functions of the small intestine include digestion and absorption. Digestion, which involves breaking down large molecules into small ones, is essential for nutrient absorption from the small intestine. Maintenance of pH and osmolality is crucial for digestion in the small intestine. The entry of chyme into the duodenum stimulates the production of secretin, which in turn stimulates

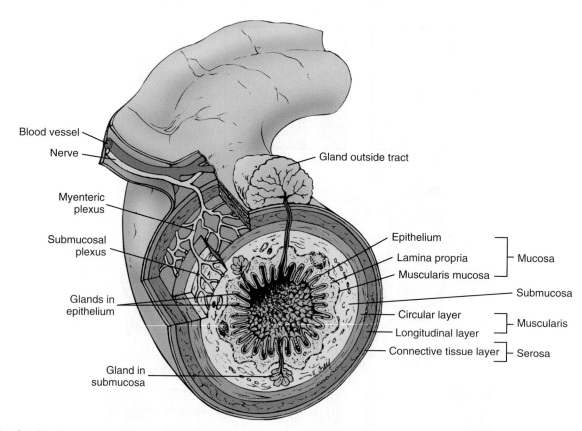

Fig. 31-5   Cross section of the small intestine. (From Moffett DF, Moffett SB, Schauff CL: *Human physiology: foundations and frontiers*, ed 2, St Louis, 1993, Mosby.)

the pancreas to secrete a highly alkaline fluid into the duodenum. Once in the small intestine, the chyme mixes with pancreatic enzymes, intestinal enzymes, and bile from the liver and gallbladder and is then reduced to absorbable elements of proteins, fats, and carbohydrates. The nutrients are absorbed through the villi and transported to the liver via the portal system for further processing (Table 31-2). The small intestine absorbs up to 8 L of fluid per day, passing only a small part of this fluid into the large intestine. In addition to the nutrients, electrolytes, water, components of saliva, gastric juice, and bile, intestinal and pancreatic secretions are also absorbed.[1]

LARGE INTESTINE

The large intestine, which extends from the ileocecal valve to the anus, is approximately 90 to 150 cm (4 to 5 feet) long and 4 to 6 cm (2 inches) in diameter. It is divided into the ascending colon, the hepatic flexure, the transverse colon, the splenic flexure, the descending colon, the sigmoid colon, the rectum, and the anal canal.[5]

The colon has four layers. The outermost layer, the serous layer (serosa), is formed from the visceral peritoneum and covers most of the large intestine, with the exclusion of the sigmoid colon. The second layer, the muscular layer (muscularis), consists of two smooth muscle layers: the longitudinal and the circular. These muscles work together to propel fecal matter through the colon and to "knead" the stool into a compact bolus. The longitudinal muscle consists of three muscular bands that stretch from the cecum to the distal sigmoid colon. These muscular bands create sacculations of haustra, important clinical features that normally are apparent on a barium enema radiograph. Haustra aid segmentation so that absorption of fluid from the fecal bolus is achieved. The third layer, the submucous layer (submucosa), consists of connective tissue that contains blood vessels, lymphatics, glands, and nerve plexuses. The innermost layer, the mucous layer (mucosa), is lined with simple columnar epithelial cells and contains deep crypts of Lieberkühn that are lined with mucus-producing goblet cells. Mucus is produced that eases the passage of the fecal material and protects the mucosal surface from trauma.[5]

The rectum begins midsacrum, is 12 to 15 cm (5 inches) long, and is quite angulated. These angles, also known as *Houston's valves*, are important in the defecation process because they tend to slow the passage of fecal material in the rectal vault, thus assisting the continence mechanism.

Arterial blood is supplied to the colon from branches of the superior and inferior mesenteric arteries. Venous drainage occurs via the branches of the superior and in-

Table 31-2	Nutrient Digestion and Absorption	
Digestive Enzymes	**Site of Action/Absorption**
CARBOHYDRATES	
Amylase	Produced in mouth (salivary glands)
	Absorbed in stomach (limited)
	Produced in small intestine (pancreas)
	Absorbed in small intestine
Disaccharidases (sucrase, maltase isomaltase, lactase)	Produced in small intestine (brush border)
	Absorbed in small intestine
Pepsin	Produced in stomach (chief cells)
	Absorbed in small intestine
PROTEINS	
Trypsin, chymotrypsin	Produced in small intestine (pancreas)
	Absorbed in small intestine
Carboxypeptidase	Produced in small intestine (brush border)
Peptidases	Absorbed in small intestine
Bile (not enzyme)	Produced in liver and delivered to duodenum
	Absorbed in small intestine
LIPIDS	
Lipase	Produced in small intestine (pancreas, brush border)
	Absorbed in small intestine
Esterase	Produced in small intestine (pancreas)
	Absorbed in small intestine

From Doughty DB, Jackson DB: *Gastrointestinal disorders,* St Louis, 1993, Mosby.

ferior mesenteric veins into the portal system. The colon is intrinsically innervated by Auerbach's plexus, which controls secretion and motility, and extrinsically innervated by the autonomic nervous system. Both the sympathetic and parasympathetic branches of the autonomic system innervate the colon, regulating motility. Sympathetic stimulation inhibits colonic activity and constricts the anal sphincters, whereas parasympathetic stimulation increases colonic activity and secretion and relaxes the anal sphincters.[10]

COLONIC MOTILITY

Colonic motility consists of both haustral shuttling and peristalsis. Haustral shuttling, a variation of haustral segmentation, consists of the contraction and relaxation of the circular muscle. It moves the contents of the colon back and forth to facilitate the grinding of food masses and fluid absorption. Peristalsis is produced primarily by the longitudinal muscles and propels the fecal bolus forward. Mass peristalsis is a strong, slow contraction in which the distal left colon contracts en masse to move the fecal bolus into the rectum.[12]

RESORPTION

The major functions of the colon are resorption of water, sodium, chloride, glucose, and urea; dehydration of undigested residue; putrefaction of contents by bacteria; movement of the fecal bolus through the colon; and elimination of the fecal mass. The colon receives approximately 1000 to 2000 ml of chyme per day, with all but 50 to 250 ml of it absorbed in the ascending and transverse colon.[5]

The colon contains billions of anaerobic bacteria that serve to putrefy remaining proteins and indigestible residue; synthesize folic acid, vitamin K, nicotinic acid, riboflavin, and some B vitamins; and convert urea salts to ammonium salts and ammonia for absorption into the portal circulation.[1] Common colonic bacteria include *Bacteroides, Lactobacillus,* and *Clostridium.*[5]

ACCESSORY ORGANS

The accessory organs of digestion are the liver, the biliary system, and the pancreas (Fig. 31-6).

LIVER

The liver is the largest internal organ in the body. Weighing 1200 to 1600 g (3 to 4 lb), it is friable, dark red, and of a soft-solid consistency. Located in the right upper abdominal quadrant, it fits snugly against the right interior diaphragm. The liver is surrounded by connective tissue known as *Glisson's capsule*, which is covered by serosa

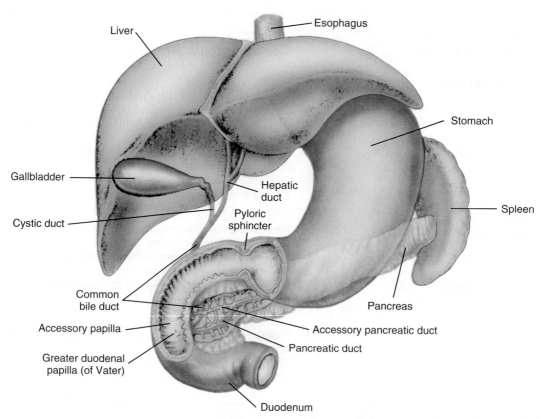

Fig. 31-6   Liver, gallbladder, and pancreas. (From Thompson JM et al: *Mosby's clinical nursing,* ed 5, St Louis, 2002, Mosby.)

and contains blood vessels and lymphatics. The peritoneum covering the liver forms the falciform ligament, which attaches the liver to the anterior portion of the abdomen between the diaphragm and umbilicus and divides the liver into two main lobes, right and left (Fig. 31-6). The right lobe, which is six times larger than the left, has three sections: the right lobe proper, the caudate lobe, and the quadrate lobe. The left lobe is divided into two sections. Each lobe is divided into numerous lobules.[5,13]

The liver receives one third of the total cardiac output from two major sources: the hepatic artery, which provides oxygenated blood; and the portal vein, which is supplied with nutrient-rich blood from the gut, pancreas, spleen, and stomach (Fig. 31-7). The portal vein, which accounts for 75% of the total liver blood flow, branches into sinusoids to transport blood to each lobule. Unlike capillaries, sinusoids lack a definite cell wall but contain a lining of phagocytic (Kupffer's) cells and some non-phagocytic cells of modified epithelium. Sinusoids empty blood into an intralobular vein in the center of the lobule. Intralobular veins empty into larger veins and finally into the hepatic vein, which empties on the posterior surface of the liver and eventually into the vena cava. The hepatic artery also divides and subdivides between the lobules, supplying sinusoids with oxygenated blood before emptying into the hepatic vein. Lymphatic spaces are be-

tween liver cells. Lymph drains into lymphatic vessels that surround the hepatic vein and bile ducts.[14]

Nutrient Metabolism. The liver plays a key role in metabolizing and storing carbohydrates, fats, proteins, and vitamins. Glycogen, the stored form of glucose, can be synthesized from glucose or from protein, fat, or lactic acid. Glycogen is broken down to glucose by the liver to maintain normal blood glucose levels. The liver also has a vital role in amino acid metabolism and can synthesize amino acids from metabolites of carbohydrates and fats or can deaminate amino acids to produce ketoacids and ammonia, from which urea is formed. In fat metabolism the liver hydrolyzes triglycerides to glycerol and fatty acids in the process of ketogenesis and synthesizes phospholipids, cholesterol, and lipoproteins.[5]

Hematologic Function. The liver synthesizes plasma proteins, such as globulins and albumin, which are important in maintaining the normal osmotic balance of blood. It also synthesizes a number of clotting factors including fibrinogen and prothrombin. Kupffer's cells destroy worn red blood cells, and hepatocytes conjugate bilirubin (by-product of red cell destruction) for excretion.[5]

Detoxification and Storage. Steroid hormones are conjugated, and polypeptide hormones are inactivated by the liver. In addition, the liver stores fat-soluble vitamins, vitamin B$_{12}$, and the minerals *iron* and *copper*. And

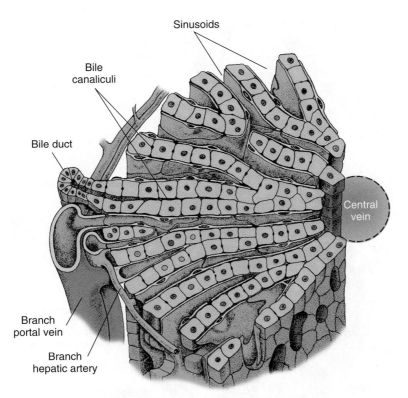

Fig. 31-7   Cross section of a liver lobule. (From Berne RM, Levy MN: *Principles of physiology,* ed 3, St Louis, 1993, Mosby.)

finally, detoxification of drugs and toxins occurs in Kupffer's cells.[5]

Bile. The production of bile makes the liver a vital organ in digestion and absorption. The major components of bile are bile pigments, bile salts, cholesterol, neutral fats, phospholipids, inorganic salts, fatty acids, mucin, conjugated bilirubin, lecithin, and water. Traces of albumin, gamma globulin, urea, nitrogen, and glucose are also present in bile. The principal electrolytes of bile are sodium, chloride, and bicarbonate.[15]

Bile functions to emulsify fat globules and absorb fat-soluble vitamins. Bile salts also serve as an excretion route for bilirubin, cholesterol, and various hormones. Approximately 80% of bile salts are actively resorbed in the distal ileum and are recycled to the liver through the enterohepatic circulation; only 20% are lost in the feces.[1]

Bilirubin. The primary bile pigment, bilirubin, is formed from the heme portion of hemoglobin during the degradation of red blood cells by Kupffer's cells. When released into the blood stream, bilirubin binds to albumin as fat-soluble, unconjugated bilirubin. Taken up by liver hepatocytes, unconjugated bilirubin is conjugated with glucuronic acid to form water-soluble, conjugated bilirubin, which is then excreted through hepatic ducts into the large intestine. If the amount of bilirubin sent to the liver is in excess, the ability of the liver to conjugate the bilirubin may be taxed; thus free, unconjugated indirect bilirubin will appear in the blood. High levels of un-

conjugated bilirubin in the blood suggest hepatocellular dysfunction, whereas high levels of conjugated bilirubin suggest biliary tract obstruction.[1]

BILIARY SYSTEM

The biliary system (Fig. 31-8) consists of the gallbladder and its related ductal system, including the hepatic, cystic, and common bile ducts. The hepatic duct, from the liver, joins the cystic duct, from the gallbladder, to form the common bile duct, which empties into the duodenum. The common bile duct is surrounded by Oddi's sphincter, which pierces the wall of the duodenum and controls the flow of bile into the duodenum. The gallbladder is a pear-shaped organ that is 7 to 10 cm (3 to 4 inches) long and 2.5 to 3.5 cm (approximately 1 inch) wide, lying on the underside of the liver (see Fig. 31-6). It is attached to the liver by connective tissue, peritoneum, and blood vessels.[5,16]

Bile. The main functions of the gallbladder are to collect, concentrate, acidify, and store bile. Bile is continuously formed in the liver and excreted into the hepatic duct for transport to the gallbladder via the cystic duct. The gallbladder can store up to 90 ml of bile and concentrate it approximately 15 to 29 times by removing approximately 90% of the water. Cholesterol and pigment are likewise concentrated. Bile, which is golden or orange-yellow in the liver, becomes dark brown when

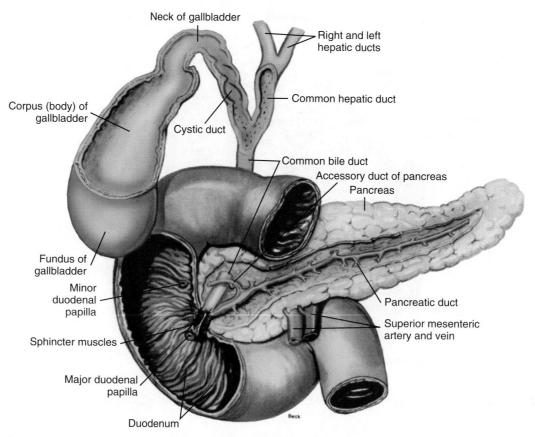

Fig. 31-8   Gallbladder and pancreas. (From McCance KL, Huether SE, editors: *Pathophysiology: the biologic basis for disease in adults and children,* ed 4, St Louis, 2002, Mosby.)

concentrated in the gallbladder. By altering its shape and volume, the gallbladder regulates pressure within the biliary system. Relaxation of the sphincter of Oddi is coordinated with gallbladder contraction through the regulatory action of cholecystokinin. Factors such as sight, smell, and taste can stimulate gallbladder contraction, whereas fear or excitement can decrease contraction. After a meal the amount of bile entering the duodenum increases as a result of enhanced liver secretion and gallbladder contraction. Intestinal secretion of cholecystokinin and secretin, high levels of bile salts in the blood, and vagal stimulation increase biliary secretion.[15]

PANCREAS

The pancreas is a soft, lobulated, fish-shaped gland (see Fig. 31-8) lying beneath the duodenum and the spleen (see Fig. 31-6). It is a pinkish-yellow color, 15 to 20 cm (6 to 8 inches) long, and 5 cm (1 to 1.5 inches) wide. Its anatomic divisions include the head, which lies in the C-shaped curve of the duodenum to which it is attached; the body, the main part of the gland, which extends horizontally across the abdomen and is largely hidden behind the stomach; and the tail, a thin, narrow portion in contact with the spleen. The main pancreatic duct, called the

duct of Wirsung, traverses the entire length of the organ. Wirsung's duct empties exocrine secretions into the ampulla of Vater, which is the same lumen draining the common bile duct, at the entrance to the duodenum.[5]

The internal structural unit of the pancreas is the lobule, consisting of numerous small ducts with secretory cells called *tubuloacinar* cells. Each acinus has a small duct that empties into lobular ducts. Lobules are joined by connective tissue into lobes, which unite to form the gland. The ducts from each lobule empty into the duct of Wirsung.[5]

Arterial blood supply to the pancreas is provided by branches of the superior mesenteric artery and celiac arteries. Venous drainage of the head of the pancreas is via the portal vein, and drainage of the body and tail is via the splenic vein. The pancreas is innervated by the autonomic nervous system. Sympathetic stimulation decreases pancreatic secretion, and parasympathetic stimulation increases it.[5]

Exocrine Functions.   Exocrine functions of the pancreas are limited to digestion. Acinar cells secrete pancreatic juice, which consists of water, sodium bicarbonate, and electrolytes at a highly alkaline pH. Enzymes produced in the pancreas include trypsin, chymotrypsin, carboxypeptidase, amylase, and lipase. The pancreas also produces a trypsin inhibitor that prevents activation of trypsinogen (inactive form of trypsin), which inhibits autodigestion. Autodigestion is the underlying cause of acute pancreatitis. Pancreatic exocrine function is regulated by digestive hormones. Signals provided primarily by the intestinal hormones *secretin* and *cholecystokinin* stimulate the pancreas to secrete pancreatic juice. The two hormones potentiate each other's effects on the pancreas.[17]

Endocrine Functions. Endocrine tissue in the pancreas consists of spherical islets called *islets of Langerhans*, which are embedded within the lobules of acinar tissue throughout the pancreas, especially in the distal body and tail. Endocrine products include insulin, which is produced in beta cells; glucagon, which is produced in alpha cells; and gastrin. All of these hormones are secreted directly into the blood stream.[17]

REFERENCES

1. Huether SE: Structure and function of the digestive system. In McCance KL, Huether SE, editors: *Pathophysiology: the biologic basis for disease in adults and children,* ed 4, St Louis, 2002, Mosby.
2. Staff D, Shaker R: Aging in the gastrointestinal tract, *Dis Mon* 47:72, 2001.
3. Silvers AR, Som PM: Salivary glands, *Radiol Clin North Am* 36:941, 1998.
4. Johnson MC: The esophagus, *Prim Care* 28:459, 2001.
5. Society of Gastroenterology Nurses and Associates Core Curriculum Committee: *Gastroenterology nursing: a core curriculum,* ed 3, St Louis, 2003, Mosby.
6. Lind CD: Dysphagia: evaluation and treatment, *Gastroenterol Clin North Am* 32:553, 2003.
7. Guyton AC: *Textbook of medical physiology,* ed 10, Philadelphia, 2000, Saunders.
8. Cryer B: Mucosal defense and repair. Role of prostaglandins in the stomach and duodenum, *Gastroenterol Clin North Am* 30:877, 2001.
9. Quigley EMM: Gastric and small intestinal motility in health and disease, *Gastroenterol Clin North Am* 25:113, 1996.
10. Androulakis J et al: Embryologic and anatomic basis of duodenal surgery, *Surg Clin North Am* 80:171, 2000.
11. Lin PH, Chaikof EL: Embryology, anatomy, and surgical exposure of the great abdominal vessels, *Surg Clin North Am* 80:417, 2000.
12. O'Brien MD: Colonic motility in health and disease, *Gastroenterol Clin North Am* 25:147, 1996.
13. Vauthey JN, Rousseau DL: Liver imaging. A surgeon's perspective, *Clin Liver Dis* 6:271, 2002.
14. Delattre JF, Avisse C, Flament JB: Anatomic basis of hepatic surgery, *Surg Clin North Am* 80:345, 2000.
15. Tomer G, Shneider BL: Disorders of bile formation and biliary transport, *Gastroenterol Clin North Am* 32:839, 2003.
16. Adkins RB, Chapman WC, Reddy VS: Embryology, anatomy, and surgical applications of the extrahepatic biliary system, *Surg Clin North Am* 80:363, 2000.
17. Kang SY, Go VLW: Pancreatic exocrine-endocrine interrelationships: clinical implication, *Gastroenterol Clin North Am* 28:551, 1999.

CHAPTER 32

Gastrointestinal Clinical Assessment and Diagnostic Procedures

Assessment of the critically ill patient with gastrointestinal (GI) dysfunction includes a review of the patient's history, a thorough physical examination, and analysis of the patient's laboratory data. Numerous invasive and noninvasive diagnostic procedures may also be performed to help identify the disorder.

CLINICAL ASSESSMENT

A thorough clinical assessment of the patient with GI dysfunction is imperative for the early identification and treatment of GI disorders. Once completed, the assessment serves as the foundation for developing the management plan for the patient. The assessment process can be brief or can involve a detailed history and examination, depending on the nature and immediacy of the patient's situation.[1]

HISTORY

Taking a thorough and accurate history is extremely important to the assessment process. The patient's history provides the foundation and direction for the rest of the assessment. The overall goal of the patient interview is to expose key clinical manifestations that will facilitate the identification of the underlying cause of the illness. This information will then assist in the development of an appropriate management plan.[2]

The initial presentation of the patient determines the rapidity and direction of the interview. For a patient in acute distress, the history should be curtailed to just a few questions about the patient's chief complaint and the precipitating events. For a patient in no obvious distress, the history should focus on current symptoms, patient medical history, and family history. Specific items regarding each of these areas are outlined in the Data Collection feature on Gastrointestinal History.[3,4]

PHYSICAL EXAMINATION

The physical examination helps establish baseline data about the physical dimensions of the patient's situation.[3] The abdomen is divided into four quadrants (left upper, right upper, left lower, and right lower), with the umbilicus as the middle point, to help specify the location of examination findings (Fig. 32-1 and Box 32-1). The assessment should proceed when the patient is as comfortable as possible and in the supine position; however, the position may need readjustment if it elicits pain. To prevent stimulation of GI activity, the order for the assessment should be changed to inspection, auscultation, percussion, and palpation.[4]

INSPECTION

Inspection should be performed in a warm, well-lighted environment with the patient in a comfortable position and with the abdomen exposed. Although assessment of the GI system classically begins with inspection of the abdomen, the patient's oral cavity also must be inspected to determine any unusual findings. Abnormal findings of the mouth include joint tenderness, inflammation of the gums, missing teeth, dental caries, ill-fitting dentures, and mouth odor.[5]

Observe the skin for pigmentation, lesions, striae, scars, petechiae, signs of dehydration, and venous pattern. Pigmentation may vary considerably and still be within normal limits because of race and ethnic background, although the abdomen is generally lighter in color than other exposed areas of the skin. Abnormal findings include jaundice, skin lesions, and a tense and glistening appearance of the skin. Old striae (stretch marks) are generally silver in color, whereas pinkish-purple striae may be indicative of Cushing's syndrome.[4] A bluish discoloration of the umbilicus (Cullen's sign) or of the flank (Grey Turner's sign) indicates intraperitoneal bleeding.[1]

Observe the abdomen for contour, noting whether it is flat, slightly concave, or slightly round; observe for sym-

DATA COLLECTION
Gastrointestinal History

DEMOGRAPHIC DATA
- Name, address, phone number, birth date, sex, race, marital status, occupation, education, religious preference

CHIEF COMPLAINT/REASON FOR VISIT
- In patient's own words

PRESENT PROBLEM/CURRENT HEALTH STATUS
- Description to include onset, duration, severity, associated factors, associated symptoms, exacerbating or relieving factors, patient's concerns

MEDICAL HISTORY
- Chronic illnesses
- Previous weight gain or loss
- Tooth extractions or orthodontic work
- Gastrointestinal (GI) disorders (e.g., peptic ulcer, inflammatory bowel disease, polyps, cholelithiasis, diverticular disease, pancreatitis, intestinal obstruction)
- Hepatitis or cirrhosis
- Abdominal surgery
- Abdominal trauma
- Cancer affecting GI system
- Spinal cord injury
- Women: episiotomy or fourth-degree laceration during delivery

FAMILY HISTORY
- Investigate for history of following disorders, and document (+ or −) responses
- Hirschsprung's disease
- Obesity
- Metabolic disorders
- Inflammatory disorders
- Malabsorption syndromes
- Familial Mediterranean fever
- Rectal polyps
- Polyposis syndromes
- Cancer of the GI tract

PERSONAL AND SOCIAL HISTORY
- Dietary habits
  Usual number of meals or snacks per day
  Usual fluid intake per day
- Exercise patterns
- Oral care patterns
  Frequency of toothbrushing/denture care
  Frequency of flossing
- Alcohol intake (frequency and usual amounts)

REVIEW OF GI SYSTEM
General Data
- Usual height and weight
- Nutrient intake
  Types of food usually eaten at each meal or snack
  Food likes and dislikes
  Religious or medical food restrictions
  Food intolerances
  Patient's perceptions and concerns about adequacy of diet and appropriateness of weight
  Effects of lifestyle on food intake, weight gain or loss
  Vitamins or nutritional supplements (type, amount, frequency)
- Oral hygiene
  Last visit to dentist
  Presence of braces, dentures, bridges, or crowns
- Bowel elimination
  Usual frequency of bowel movements
  Usual consistency and color of stool
  Ability to control elimination of gas and stool
  Any changes in bowel elimination patterns
  Use of enemas or laxatives (reason for use, frequency, type, response)
- Medications (e.g., laxatives, stool softeners, antiemetics, antidiarrheals, antacids, frequent or high doses of aspirin, acetaminophen, corticosteroids)

Specific Data
- Oral lesions
- Appetite
- Digestion or indigestion (heartburn)
- Dysphagia
- Nausea
- Vomiting
- Hematemesis
- Change in stool color or contents (clay-colored, tarry, fresh blood, mucus, undigested food)
- Constipation
- Diarrhea
- Flatulence
- Hemorrhoids
- Abdominal pain
- Hepatitis
- Jaundice
- Ulcers
- Gallstones
- Polyps
- Tumors
- Anal discomfort
- Fecal incontinence
- Exposure to infectious agents (e.g., foreign travel, water source, other exposure)

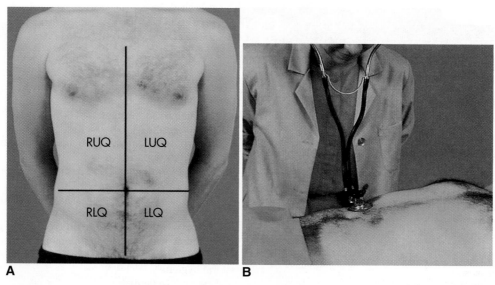

Fig. 32-1   **A,** Anatomic mapping of the four quadrants of the abdomen. **B,** Auscultation for bowel sounds. (From Barkauskas V et al: *Health & physical assessment,* ed 3, St Louis, 2002, Mosby.)

Box 32-1

ANATOMIC CORRELATES OF THE FOUR QUADRANTS OF THE ABDOMEN

RIGHT UPPER QUADRANT
Liver and gallbladder
Pylorus
Duodenum
Head of pancreas
Right adrenal gland
Portion of right kidney
Hepatic flexure of colon
Portion of ascending and transverse colon

RIGHT LOWER QUADRANT
Lower pole of right kidney
Cecum and appendix
Portion of ascending colon
Bladder (if distended)
Ovary and salpinx
Uterus (if enlarged)
Right spermatic cord
Right ureter

LEFT UPPER QUADRANT
Left lobe of liver
Spleen
Stomach
Body of pancreas
Left adrenal gland
Portion of left kidney
Splenic flexure of colon
Portions of transverse and descending colon

LEFT LOWER QUADRANT
Lower pole of left kidney
Sigmoid colon
Portion of descending colon
Bladder (if distended)
Ovary and salpinx
Uterus (if distended)
Left spermatic cord
Left ureter

Barkauskas V et al: *Health & physical assessment,* ed 3, St Louis, 2002, Mosby.

---

metry and for movement. Marked distention is an abnormal finding. In particular, ascites may cause generalized distention and bulging flanks. Asymmetric distention may indicate organ enlargement or a mass. Peristaltic waves should not be visible except in very thin patients. In the case of intestinal obstruction, hyperactive peristaltic waves may be noted. Pulsation in the epigastric area is often a normal finding, but increased pulsation may indicate an aortic aneurysm. Symmetric movement of the abdomen with respirations is usually seen in men.[4,5]

AUSCULTATION

Auscultation of the abdomen provides clinical data regarding the status of the bowel's motility. Initially, listen with the diaphragm of the stethoscope below and to the right of the umbilicus. Proceed methodically through all four quadrants, lifting and then replacing the diaphragm of the stethoscope lightly against the abdomen (Fig. 32-1). Normal bowel sounds include high-pitched, gurgling sounds that occur approximately every 5 to 15 sec-

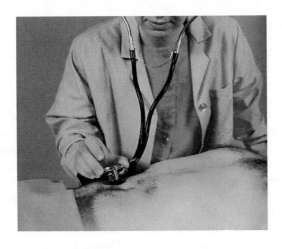

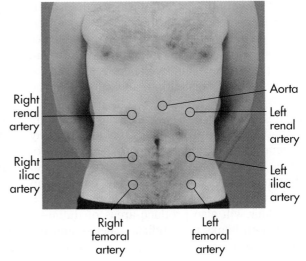

Right renal artery

Right iliac artery

Aorta

Left renal artery

Left iliac artery

Right femoral artery

Left femoral artery

Fig. 32-2   Auscultation for bruits. Note that the left illustration shows correct placement of the stethoscope. (From Barkauskas V et al: *Health & physical assessment,* ed 3, St Louis, 2002, Mosby.)

Table 32-1	Abnormal Abdominal Sounds
Sound	**Cause**
Hyperactive bowel sounds (borborygmi), loud and prolonged	Hunger, gastroenteritis, or early intestinal obstruction
High-pitched, tinkling sounds	Intestinal air and fluid under pressure; characteristic of early intestinal obstruction
Decreased (hypoactive) bowel sounds	Possible peritonitis or ileus
Infrequent and abnormally faint	
Absence of bowel sounds (confirmed only after auscultation of all four quadrants and continuous auscultation for 5 min)	Temporary loss of intestinal motility, as occurs with complete ileus
Friction rubs	Pathologic conditions such as tumors or infection that cause inflammation of organ's peritoneal covering
High-pitched sounds heard over liver and spleen (RUQ and LUQ), synchronous with respiration	
Bruits	Abnormality of blood flow (requires additional evaluation to determine specific disorder)
Audible swishing sounds that may be heard over aortic, iliac, renal, and femoral arteries	
Venous hum	Increased collateral circulation between portal and systemic venous systems
Low-pitched, continuous sound	

From Doughty DB, Jackson DB: *Gastrointestinal disorders,* St Louis, 1993, Mosby.
RUQ, Right upper quadrant; *LUQ,* left upper quadrant.

onds or at a rate of 5 to 34 times per minute. Colonic sounds are low-pitched and have a rumbling quality. A venous hum also may be audible at times.[6] See Table 32-1 for a list of abnormal abdominal sounds.

Abnormal findings include the absence of bowel sounds throughout a 5-minute period, extremely soft and widely separated sounds, and increased sounds with a high-pitched, loud rushing sound (peristaltic rush). Absent bowel sounds may occur as a result of inflammation, ileus, electrolyte disturbances, and ischemia. Bowels sounds may be increased with diarrhea and early intestinal obstruction.[6]

The abdomen also should be auscultated for the presence of bruits, using the bell of the stethoscope (Fig. 32-2). Bruits are created by turbulent flow over a partially obstructed artery and are always considered an abnormal finding. The aorta, the right and left renal arteries, and the iliac arteries should be auscultated.[5,6]

PERCUSSION

Percussion is used to elicit information about deep organs, such as the liver, spleen, and pancreas (Fig. 32-3). Because the abdomen is a sensitive area, muscle tension may interfere with this part of the assessment. Percussion often helps relax tense muscles, so it is performed before palpation. Percussion, in the absence of disease, is most helpful in delineating the position and size of the liver and spleen, and it also assists in the detection of fluid, gaseous distention, and masses in the abdomen.[5]

Percussion should proceed systematically and lightly in all four quadrants. Normal findings include tympany over the stomach when empty, tympany or hyperresonance over the intestine, and dullness over the liver and spleen. Abnormal areas of dullness may indicate an underlying mass. Solid masses, enlarged organs, and a distended bladder will also produce areas of dullness. Dullness over both flanks may indicate ascites and necessitates further assessment.[6]

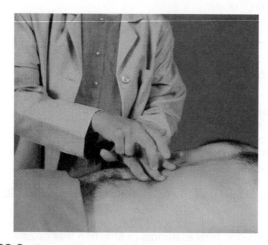

Fig. 32-3   Percussion of the abdomen. (From Barkauskas V et al: *Health & physical assessment*, ed 3, St Louis, 2002, Mosby.)

PALPATION

Palpation is the assessment technique most useful in detecting abdominal pathologic conditions. Both light and deep palpation of each organ and quadrant should be completed. Light palpation, which has a palpation depth of approximately 1 cm, assesses to the depth of the skin and fascia (Fig. 32-4, *A*). Deep palpation assesses the rectus abdominis muscle and is performed bimanually to a depth of 4 to 5 cm (Fig. 32-4, *B*). Deep palpation is most helpful in detecting abdominal masses. Areas in which the patient complains of tenderness should be palpated last.[6]

Normal findings include no areas of tenderness or pain, no masses, and no hardened areas. Persistent involuntary guarding may indicate peritoneal inflammation, particularly if it continues even after relaxation techniques are used. Rebound tenderness, in which pain increases with quick release of a palpated area, is indicative of an inflamed peritoneum.[4]

ASSESSMENT FINDINGS OF COMMON DISORDERS

Table 32-2 presents a variety of common gastrointestinal disorders and their associated assessment findings.

LABORATORY STUDIES

The value of various laboratory studies used to diagnose and treat diseases of the GI system has been emphasized often. However, no single study provides an overall picture of the various organs' functional state. Also, no single value is predictive by itself. Laboratory studies used in the assessment of GI function, liver function, and pan-

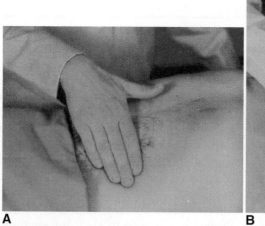
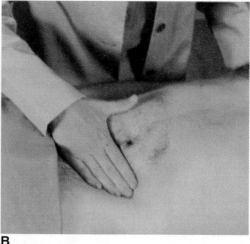

A   **B**

Fig. 32-4   Palpation of the abdomen. **A,** Light. **B,** Deep. (From Barkauskas V et al: *Health & physical assessment*, ed 3, St Louis, 2002, Mosby.)

Table 32-2	Assessment Findings of Common Gastrointestinal Disorders		
Condition	**History**	**Symptoms**	**Signs**

RIGHT LOWER QUADRANT (RLQ) OF THE ABDOMEN

Condition	History	Symptoms	Signs
Appendicitis	Children (except infants) and young adults	Anorexia Nausea Pain: early vague epigastric, periumbilical, or generalized pain after 12-24 hours; RLQ at McBurney's point	Signs may be absent early Vomiting Localized RLQ guarding and tenderness after 12-24 hours Rovsing's sign: pain in RLQ with application of pressure, iliopsoas sign Obturator sign White blood cell count 10,000/mm^3 or shift to left Low-grade fever Cutaneous hyperesthesia in RLQ Signs highly variable
Perforated duodenal ulcer	Prior history	Abrupt onset pain in epigastric area or RLQ	Tenderness in epigastric area or RLQ Signs of peritoneal irritation Hem-positive stool Increased white blood cell count
Cecal volvulus	Seen most often in the elderly	Abrupt severe abdominal pain	Distention Localized tenderness Tympany
Strangulated hernia	Any age Women: femoral Men: inguinal	Severe localized pain If bowel obstructed, generalized pain	If bowel obstructed, distention

RIGHT UPPER QUADRANT (RUQ) OF THE ABDOMEN

Condition	History	Symptoms	Signs
Liver hepatitis	Any age, often young blood product user Drug addict	Fatigue Malaise Anorexia Pain in RUQ Low-grade fever May have severe fulminating disease with liver failure	Hepatic tenderness Hepatomegaly Bilirubin elevated Jaundice Lymphocytosis in one third of cases Liver enzymes elevated Hepatitis A or B or antibodies to the viruses may be found
Acute hepatic congestion	Usually elderly with acute heart failure Pericardial disease Pulmonary embolism	Symptoms of acute heart failure	Hepatomegaly Acute heart failure
Biliary stones, colic	"Fair, fat, forty" (90%) but can be 30 to 80 years of age	Anorexia Nausea Pain severe in RUQ or epigastric area Episodes lasting 15 minutes to hours	Tenderness in RUQ Jaundice
Acute cholecystitis	"Fair, fat, forty" (90%) but may be 30 to 80 years of age	Severe RUQ or epigastric pain Episodes prolonged up to 6 hours	Vomiting Tenderness in RUQ Peritoneal irritation signs Increased white blood cell count
Perforated peptic ulcer	Any age	Abrupt RUQ pain	Tenderness in epigastrum and/or right quadrant Peritoneal irritation signs Free air in abdomen

LEFT UPPER QUADRANT (LUQ) OF THE ABDOMEN

Condition	History	Symptoms	Signs
Splenic trauma	Blunt trauma to LUQ of abdomen	Pain: LUQ pain of the abdomen often referred to the left shoulder (Kehr's sign)	Hypotension Syncope Increased dyspnea X-ray studies show enlarged spleen

Continued

Table 32-2	Assessment Findings of Common Gastrointestinal Disorders—cont'd		
Condition	**History**	**Symptoms**	**Signs**
LEFT UPPER QUADRANT (LUQ) OF THE ABDOMEN—CONT'D			
Pancreatitis	Alcohol abuse Pancreatic duct Obstruction Infection Cholecystitis	Pain in LUQ or epigastric region radiating to the back or chest	Fever Rigidity Rebound tenderness Nausea Vomiting Jaundice Cullen's sign Grey Turner's sign Abdominal distention Diminished bowel sounds
Pyloric obstruction	Duodenal ulcer	Weight loss Gastric upset Vomiting	Increasing dullness in LUQ Visible peristaltic waves in epigastric region
LEFT LOWER QUADRANT (LLQ) OF THE ABDOMEN			
Ulcerative colitis	Family history Jewish ancestry	Chronic, watery diarrhea with bloody mucus Anorexia Weight loss Fatigue	Fever Cachexia Anemia Leukocytosis
Colonic diverticulitis	Over age 39 Low-residue diet	Pain that recurs in LUQ	Fever Vomiting Chills Diarrhea Tenderness over descending colon

Modified from Barkauskas V et al: *Health & physical assessment,* ed 3, St Louis, 2002, Mosby.

creatic function are found in Tables 32-3 to 32-5, respectively.

DIAGNOSTIC PROCEDURES

To complete the assessment of the critically ill patient with GI dysfunction, the patient's diagnostic tests are reviewed. Although many procedures exist for diagnosing GI disease, their application in the critically ill patient is limited. Only those procedures that are currently used in the critical care setting are presented here.

The nursing management of a patient undergoing a diagnostic procedure involves a variety of interventions. Nursing actions include preparing the patient psychologically and physically for the procedure, monitoring the patient's responses to the procedure, and assessing the patient after the procedure. Preparing the patient includes teaching the patient about the procedure, answering any questions, and transporting and/or positioning the patient for the procedure. Monitoring the patient's responses to the procedure includes observing the patient for signs of pain, anxiety, or hemorrhage and monitoring vital signs. Assessing the patient after the proce-

dure includes observing for complications of the procedure and medicating the patient for any postprocedural discomfort. Any evidence of GI bleeding should be immediately reported to the physician, and emergency measures to maintain circulation must be initiated.

ENDOSCOPY

Available in several forms, fiberoptic endoscopy is a diagnostic procedure for the direct visualization and evaluation of the GI tract. An endoscopy can provide information regarding lesions, mucosal changes, obstructions, and motility dysfunction. A biopsy can also be obtained during the procedure. The main difference between the various diagnostic forms is the length of the anatomic area that can be examined. An esophagogastroduodenoscopy (EGD) permits viewing of the upper GI tract from esophagus to the upper duodenum and is used to evaluate sources of upper GI bleeding. A colonoscopy permits viewing of the lower GI tract from the rectum to the distal ileum and is used to evaluate sources of lower GI bleeding. An enteroscopy permits viewing of the small bowel beyond the ligament of Treitz and is used to evaluate sources of GI bleeding that have not been iden-

Table 32-3	Selected Laboratory Studies of Gastrointestinal Function	
Test	**Normal Findings**	**Clinical Significance of Abnormal Findings**
Stool studies	Resident microorganisms: clostridia, enterococci, *Pseudomonas,* a few yeasts Fat: 2-6 g/24 hr Pus: none Occult blood: none (Ortho-Tolidin or guaiac test) Ova and parasites: none	Detection of *Salmonella typhi* (typhoid fever), *Shigella* (dysentery), *Vibrio cholerae* (cholera), *Yersinia* (enterocolitis), *Escherichia coli* (gastroenteritis), *Staphylococcus aureus* (food poisoning), *Clostridium botulinum* (food poisoning), *Clostridium perfringens* (food poisoning), *Aeromonas* (gastroenteritis) Steatorrhea (increased values) can result from intestinal malabsorption or pancreatic insufficiency Large amounts of pus are associated with chronic ulcerative colitis, abscesses, and anorectal fistula Positive tests associated with bleeding Detection of *Entamoeba histolytica* (amebiasis), *Giardia lamblia* (giardiasis), and worms
D-Xylose absorption	5-hr urinary excretion: 4.5 g/L Peak blood level: >30 mg/dl	Differentiation of pancreatic steatorrhea (normal D-xylose absorption) from intestinal steatorrhea (impaired D-xylose absorption)
Gastric acid stimulation	11-20 mEq/hr after stimulation	Detection of duodenal ulcers, Zollinger-Ellison syndrome (increased values), gastric atrophy, gastric carcinoma (decreased values)
Manometry (use of water-filled catheters connected to pressure transducers passed into the esophagus, stomach, colon, or rectum to evaluate contractility)	Values vary at different levels of the intestine	Inadequate swallowing, motility, sphincter function
Culture and sensitivity of duodenal contents	No pathogens	Detection of *Salmonella typhi* (typhoid fever)

From McCance KL, Huether SE, editors: *Pathophysiology: the biologic basis for disease in adults and children,* ed 4, St Louis, 2002, Mosby.

tified previously with an EGD or colonoscopy. An endoscopic retrograde cholangiopancreatography (ERCP) enables viewing of the biliary and pancreatic ducts and is used in evaluation of pancreatitis. During this procedure, contrast is injected into the ducts via the endoscope and x-rays films are taken.[7] In addition, endoscopy provides therapeutic benefits for a variety of conditions including the treatment of GI bleeding.[8]

Nursing Management. The patient should take nothing by mouth (NPO) for 6 to 12 hours before an endoscopy of the upper GI tract. The patient should receive a bowel preparation before an endoscopy of the lower GI tract.[7] In some cases the procedure is performed at the patient's bedside, particularly if the patient is actively bleeding and too unstable to be moved to the GI suite. Fiberoptic endoscopy may present risks for the patient. Although rare, potential complications include perforation of the GI tract, hemorrhage, aspiration, vasovagal stimulation, and oversedation.[7] Signs of perforation include abdominal pain and distention, GI bleeding, and fever.[9]

ANGIOGRAPHY

Angiography is used as both a diagnostic and a therapeutic procedure. Diagnostically it is used to evaluate the status of the GI circulation (Fig. 32-5).[7] Therapeutically it is used to achieve transcatheter control of GI bleeding.[8] Angiography is used in the diagnosis of upper gastrointestinal (UGI) bleeding only when endoscopy fails, and it is used to treat those patients (approximately 15%) whose GI bleeding is not stopped with medical measures or endoscopic treatment.[8] In addition, angiography also is used to evaluate cirrhosis, portal hypertension, intestinal ischemia, and other vascular abnormalities.[7]

The radiologist cannulates the femoral artery with a needle and passes a guidewire through it into the aorta. The needle is removed, and an angiographic catheter is inserted over the guidewire. The catheter is advanced into the vessel supplying the portion of the GI tract that is being studied. Once the catheter is in place, contrast medium is injected and serial x-rays are taken. If the procedure is undertaken to control bleeding, vasopressin

Table 32-4	Common Laboratory Studies of Liver Function	
Test	**Normal Value**	**Interpretation**
SERUM ENZYMES		
Alkaline phosphatase	13-39 units/ml	Increases with biliary obstruction and cholestatic hepatitis
Aspartate amino transferase (AST; previously serum glutamate oxaloacetate transaminase [SGOT])	5-40 units/ml	Increases with hepatocellular injury
Alanine amino transferase (ALT; previously serum glutamate pyruvate transaminase [SGPT])	5-35 units/ml	Increases with hepatocellular injury
Lactate dehydrogenase (LDH)	200-500 units/ml	Isoenzyme LD_5 is elevated with hypoxic and primary liver injury
5'-Nucleotidase	2-11 units/ml	Increases with increase in alkaline phosphatase and cholestatic disorders
BILIRUBIN METABOLISM		
Serum bilirubin		
Indirect (unconjugated)	<0.8 mg/dl	Increases with hemolysis (lysis of red blood cells)
Direct (conjugated)	0.2-0.4 mg/dl	Increases with hepatocellular injury or obstruction
Total	<1.0 mg/dl	Increases with biliary obstruction
Urine bilirubin	0	Decreases with biliary obstruction
Urine urobilinogen	0-4 mg/24 hr	Increases with hemolysis or shunting or portal blood flow
SERUM PROTEINS		
Albumin	3.3-5.5 g/dl	Reduced with hepatocellular injury
Globulin	2.5-3.5 g/dl	Increases with hepatitis
Total	6-7 g/dl	
Albumin/globulin (A/G) ratio	1.5:2.5:1	Ratio reverses with chronic hepatitis or other chronic liver disease
Transferrin	250-300 mcg/dl	Liver damage with decreased values, iron deficiency with increased values
Alpha-fetoprotein	6-20 ng/ml	Elevated values in primary hepatocellular carcinoma
BLOOD CLOTTING FUNCTIONS		
Prothrombin time	11.5-14 sec or 90%-100% of control	Increases with chronic liver disease (cirrhosis) or vitamin K deficiency
Partial thromboplastin time	25-40 sec	Increases with severe liver disease or heparin therapy
Bromsulphalein (BSP) excretion	<6% retention in 45 min	Increased retention with hepatocellular injury

From McCance KL, Huether SE, editors: *Pathophysiology: the biologic basis for disease in adults and children,* ed 4, St Louis, 2002, Mosby.

(Pitressin Synthetic) or embolic material (Gelfoam) is injected once the site of the bleeding is located.[8]

Nursing Management. Complications include overt and covert bleeding at the femoral puncture site, neurovascular compromise of the affected leg, and sensitivity to the contrast medium. Before the procedure the patient should be asked about any sensitivities to contrast. Postprocedural assessment involves monitoring vital signs, observing the injection site for bleeding, and assessing neurovascular integrity distal to the injection site every 15 minutes for the first 1 to 2 hours. Depending on how the puncture site is stabilized after the procedure, the patient may have to remain flat in bed for a specified length of time. Any evidence of bleeding or neurovascular impairment must be immediately reported to the physician.[10]

PLAIN ABDOMINAL SERIES

Although numerous radiologic studies are available to investigate GI dysfunction further, many of these studies are not performed on the critically ill patient. The radiologic study that is performed most often is the plain abdominal series (Fig. 32-6). An abdominal film is useful in the diagnosis of a bowel obstruction and perforation.[11,12]

Air in the bowel serves as a contrast medium to aid in the visualization of the bowel. Gas patterns (the presence of gas inside or outside the bowel lumen and the distribution of gas in dilated and nondilated bowel) are best revealed by plain films. Common radiologic signs of free air in the abdomen include the presence of air on both sides of the bowel wall and the presence of air in the right upper quadrant anterior to the liver.[11,12] Table

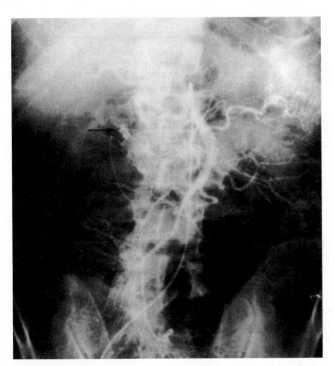

Fig. 32-5 Arteriogram of superior mesenteric artery showing diverticular bleeding. Note area of contrast extravasation. (From Doughty DB, Jackson DB: *Gastrointestinal disorders*, St Louis, 1993, Mosby.)

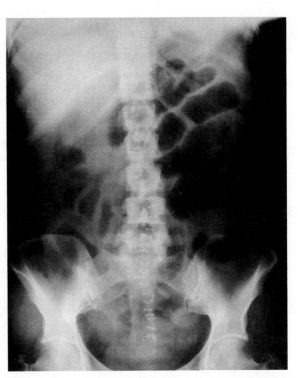

Fig. 32-6 Abdominal flat plate x-ray. Note the dilated loops of small bowel consistent with a postoperative ileus. (From Doughty DB, Jackson DB: *Gastrointestinal disorders*, St Louis, 1993, Mosby.)

Table 32-5	Common Laboratory Studies of Pancreatic Function	
Test	**Normal Value**	**Clinical Significance**
Serum amylase	60-180 Somogyi units/ml	Elevated levels with pancreatic inflammation
Serum lipase	1.5 Somogyi units/ml	Elevated levels with pancreatic inflammation (may be elevated with other conditions; differentiates with amylase, isoenzyme study)
Urine amylase	35-260 Somogyi units/hr	Elevated levels with pancreatic inflammation
Secretin test	Volume 1.8 ml/kg/hr Bicarbonate concentration: >80 mEq/L Bicarbonate output: >10 mEq/L/30 sec	Decreased volume with pancreatic disease because secretin stimulates pancreatic secretion
Stool fat	2-5 g/25 hr	Measures fatty acids: decreased pancreatic lipase increases stool fat

From McCance KL, Huether SE, editors: *Pathophysiology: the biologic basis for disease in adults and children,* ed 4, St Louis, 2002, Mosby.

32-6 lists common radiologic findings. In addition, the abdominal films are used to verify nasogastric or feeding tube placement.

Nursing Management. An abdominal series can be obtained at the patient's bedside using a portable x-ray machine. The series includes two views of the abdomen: one in the supine and one in the upright position. In patients unable to sit upright, a lateral decubitus film with the left side down may be done instead. No special interventions are required before or after the procedure.[10]

ABDOMINAL ULTRASOUND

Abdominal ultrasound is useful in evaluating the status of the gallbladder and biliary system, the liver, the spleen, and the pancreas. It plays a key role in the diagnosis of many acute abdominal conditions, such as acute cholecystitis and biliary obstructions, because it is sensitive in detecting obstructive lesions, as well as ascites. Ultrasound is used to identify gallstones and hepatic abscesses, candidiasis, and hematomas. Intestinal gas, as-

Table 32-6	Plain Film Findings	
Finding	**Appearance**	**Associations**
Pneumoperitoneum	Air seen under diaphragm on upright chest or overlying right lobe of liver on left lateral decubitus films	Most commonly associated with bowel perforation, although other causes exist
Peritoneal fluid	Medial displacement of colon separated from flank stripes by fluid density on flat plate	Ascites or hemorrhage
Adynamic ileus	Dilatation of entire intestinal tract including stomach	Multiple causes including trauma, infection (intraabdominal and extraabdominal), metabolic disease, and medications (e.g., narcotics)
Sentinel loop	Single distended loop of small bowel containing an air-fluid level	Represents localized ileus associated with localized inflammatory process such as cholecystitis, appendicitis, or pancreatitis
Small bowel obstruction	Dilated loops of small bowel (distinguished by valvulae conniventes, thin, transverse linear densities that extend completely across diameter of bowel) with air-fluid levels	Can be associated with other serious pathology such as incarcerated hernia, appendicitis, or mesenteric ischemia
Large bowel obstruction	Dilated loops, usually more peripheral in the abdomen (distinguished by haustra—short, thick indentations that do not completely cross bowel and are less frequently spaced than valvulae conniventes)	Can be associated with diverticulitis and malignancy
Cecal volvulus	Usually found in middle or upper abdomen to the left; often kidney-shaped	
Sigmoid volvulus	Dilated loop of colon arising from left side of pelvis and projecting obliquely upward toward right side of abdomen	
Early ischemic bowel findings	Might resemble mechanical obstruction with dilated loops and air-fluid levels	
Later ischemic bowel findings	Might resemble adynamic ileus; thumbprinting (edema of bowel wall with convex indentations of lumen) and pneumatosis intestinalis (linear or mottled gas pattern in bowel wall)	
Gallbladder emergency findings	Ring of air outlining gallbladder	Emphysematous cholecystitis
	Air in biliary tree combined with signs of small bowel obstruction, possibly with visible calculus in pelvis	Gallstone ileus
Abdominal aortic aneurysm (AAA)	Usually appears left of midline on supine film and anterior to spine in lateral projection; calcification in wall of aneurysm is variable	Ruptured or leaking AAA might reveal loss of psoas shadows or large soft tissue mass

From Hendrickson M, Naparst TR: Abdominal surgical emergencies in the elderly, *Emerg Med Clin North Am* 21:937, 2003.

cites, and extreme obesity can interfere with transmission of the sound waves and thus limit the usefulness of the procedure.[13]

The procedure uses sound waves to produce echoes that are converted into electrical energy and transferred to a screen for viewing. A transducer, which emits and receives sound waves, is moved slowly over the area of the abdomen being studied. Tissues of varying densities produce different echoes, which then translate into the different structures on the viewing screen.[13]

Nursing Management. An ultrasound can be obtained at the patient's bedside using a portable scanning unit. Ultrasound is easily performed, noninvasive, and well tolerated by critically ill patients. The procedure re-

quires only that the patient lie still for 20 to 30 minutes. No special interventions are required before or after the procedure.[10]

COMPUTED TOMOGRAPHY OF THE ABDOMEN

Computed tomography (CT) scan is a radiographic examination that provides cross-sectional images of internal anatomy. It may be used to evaluate abdominal vasculature and identify focal points found on nuclear scans as solid, cystic, inflammatory, or vascular. CT detects mass lesions more than 2 cm in diameter and allows visualization and evaluation of many different aspects of GI disease. It is particularly useful in identifying pancreatic pseudocysts, abdominal abscesses, biliary obstructions, and a variety of GI neoplastic lesions.[14]

The procedure involves taking the patient to the CT scanner, placing the patient on the table, and inserting the area to be studied into the opening of the scanner. Multiple x-rays are then taken at a variety of angles. Next, a computer synthesizes images of the structures being studied. Intravenous or GI contrast also may be used to facilitate the imaging of the blood vessels or the GI tract, respectively.[14]

Nursing Management. Before the procedure the patient should be asked about any sensitivities to contrast. The procedure usually takes 30 minutes without contrast and 60 minutes with contrast, during which time the patient must lie very still. No special interventions are required before or after the procedure.[10]

HEPATOBILIARY SCINTIGRAPHY

A hepatobiliary scan is a nuclear scan that is used to assess the status of the liver and the biliary system. It is valuable in detecting various abnormalities such as acute and chronic cholecystitis, biliary obstruction, and bile leaks and yields additional information regarding organ size.[15]

The scan involves injecting an intravenous technetium-99m–([99m]Tc-) labeled iminodiacetic agent (radiotracer), such as disofenin (DISIDA) or mebrofenin (TMBIDA). Serial images are then obtained using a gamma (scintillation) camera.[13] The liver cells take up 80% to 90% of the radiotracer, which is then secreted into the bile and transported throughout the biliary system, allowing visualization of the biliary tract, the gallbladder, and the duodenum.[7] Pooling of the iminodiacetic agent around the liver indicates poor uptake and hepatocellular dysfunction.[15]

Nursing Management. The scan is relatively noninvasive and safe, although the patient must be transported to the nuclear medicine department. In addition, the patient may need to maintain NPO status for 2 to 4 hours before the procedure. Sedation is usually not required, but the patient must be able to lie flat and still for 60 minutes during the scanning procedure. No special interventions are required after the procedure.[10]

GASTROINTESTINAL BLEEDING SCAN

A GI bleeding scan is used to evaluate the presence of an active GI bleed, to identify the site of the bleed, and to assess the need for an arteriogram.[15] The GI bleeding scan is sensitive to low rates of bleeding (0.1 to 0.35 mg/min)[15] but is reliable only when the patient is actively bleeding.[7]

The scan is usually performed with intravenous ^{99m}Tc-labeled sulfur colloid or ^{99m}Tc-labeled red blood cells (radiotracers). To tag the red blood cells, a blood sample is taken from the patient. The red blood cells are separated, tagged with ^{99m}Tc, and then returned to the patient. Serial images are obtained using a gamma (scintillation) camera. Extravasation and accumulation or pooling of radiotracers in the bowel lumen indicates active bleeding is occurring and facilitates identification of the site.[7,15]

Nursing Management. The scan is relatively noninvasive and safe, although the patient must be transported to the nuclear medicine department. Sedation usually is not required, but the patient must be able to lie flat and still for 60 minutes during the scanning procedure. No special interventions are required after the procedure.[10]

MAGNETIC RESONANCE IMAGING

Magnetic resonance imaging (MRI) is used to identify tumors, abscesses, hemorrhages, and vascular abnormalities. Small tumors, whose tissue densities differ from those of the surrounding cells, can be identified before they would be made visible by any other radiographic test.[7] Magnetic resonance angiography is a form of MRI that is used to assess blood vessels and blood flow.[16] Magnetic resonance cholangiopancreatography (MRCP) is a new form of MRI used to evaluate the biliary and pancreatic ducts.[17]

During the MRI the patient is placed in a large magnetic field that stimulates the protons of the body. Introduction of radiofrequency waves causes resonance of these protons, which then emit an image that a computer is able to reconstruct for viewing. Intravenous administration of a non–iodine-based contrast medium enhances the image by influencing the magnetic environment and signal intensity.[18]

Nursing Management. The procedure is lengthy and requires that the patient be transported to the scanner. The patient must lie motionless in a tight, enclosed space; thus sedation is usually necessary. Removal of all metal from the patient's body is essential because the basis of MRI is a magnetic field. Patients with implanted metal objects are not candidates for the procedure. No special interventions are required after the procedure.[10]

PERCUTANEOUS LIVER BIOPSY

Liver biopsy is a diagnostic procedure that is used to evaluate liver disease. Morphologic, biochemical, bacteriologic, and immunologic studies are performed on the tissue sample to diagnose a variety of liver disorders such as cirrhosis, hepatitis, infections, or cancer. The biopsy can also yield information about the progression of the patient's disease and response to therapy.[7,19]

Percutaneous liver biopsy can be performed at the bedside or in the imaging department using an imaging guided-needle approach. Before the test the patient should maintain NPO status for 6 hours and have coagulation studies drawn. The procedure is performed by anesthetizing the pericapsular tissue, inserting either a coring or suction needle between the eighth and ninth intercostal space into the liver while the patient holds his or her breath on exhalation, withdrawing the needle with the sample, and applying pressure to stop any bleeding.[7]

Nursing Management. During the procedure the patient may experience a deep pressure sensation or dull pain that radiates to the right shoulder. Afterwards the patient is positioned on the right side for 2 hours and kept on complete bed rest for the next 6 to 8 hours.[7,19] Hemorrhage is the major complication associated with a liver biopsy, although it occurs in fewer than 1% of patients. Other complications include damage to neighboring organs (kidney, lung, colon, gallbladder), bile peritonitis, hemothorax, and infection at the needle site. Puncturing the gallbladder can cause leakage of the bile into the abdominal cavity, resulting in peritonitis.[19]

REFERENCES

1. O'Toole MT: Advanced assessment of the abdomen and gastrointestinal problems, *Nurs Clin North Am* 24:771, 1990.
2. Gehring PE: Physical assessment begins with a history, *RN* 54(11):26, 1991.
3. Seidel HM et al: *Mosby's guide to physical examination,* ed 5, St Louis, 2003, Mosby.
4. Barkauskas V et al: *Health & physical assessment,* ed 3, St Louis, 2002, Mosby.
5. Thompson JM et al: *Mosby's clinical nursing,* ed 5, St Louis, 2002, Mosby.
6. O'Hanlon-Nicholas T: Basic assessment series: gastrointestinal system, *Am J Nurs* 98(4):48, 1998.
7. Society of Gastroenterology Nurses and Associates Core Curriculum Committee: *Gastroenterology nursing: a core curriculum,* ed 3, St Louis, 2003, Mosby.
8. Lefkovitz Z et al: Radiologic diagnosis and treatment of gastrointestinal hemorrhage and ischemia, *Med Clin North Am* 86:1357, 2002.
9. Putcha RV, Burdick JS: Management of iatrogenic perforation, *Gastroenterol Clin North Am* 32:1289, 2003.
10. Pangana KD, Pangana TJ: *Mosby's diagnostic and laboratory test reference,* ed 6, St Louis, 2002, Mosby.
11. Hendrickson M, Naparst TR: Abdominal surgical emergencies in the elderly, *Emerg Med Clin North Am* 21:937, 2003.
12. Rubesin SE, Levine MS: Radiologic diagnosis of gastrointestinal perforation, *Radiol Clin North Am* 41:1095, 2003.
13. Puylaert JB: Ultrasonography of the acute abdomen: gastrointestinal conditions, *Radiol Clin North Am* 41:1227, 2003.
14. Kundra V, Silverman PM: Impact of multislice CT on imaging of acute abdominal disease, *Radiol Clin North Am* 41:1083, 2003.
15. Zuckier LS, Freeman LM: Selective role of nuclear medicine in evaluating the acute abdomen, *Radiol Clin North Am* 41:1275, 2003.
16. Anderson CM: GI magnetic resonance angiography, *Gastrointest Endosc* 55:S42, 2002.
17. Fulcher AS, Turner MA: MR cholangiopancreatography, *Radiol Clin North Am* 40:1363, 2002.
18. Pedrosa I, Rofsky NM: MR imaging in abdominal emergencies, *Radiol Clin North Am* 41:1243, 2003.
19. Shankar S, van Sonnenberg E, Silverman SG, Tuncali K: Interventional radiology procedures in the liver. Biopsy, drainage, and ablation, *Clin Liver Dis* 6:91, 2002.

CHAPTER 33

Gastrointestinal Disorders and Therapeutic Management

*U*nderstanding the pathology of a disease, the areas of assessment on which to focus, and the usual medical management allows the critical care nurse to more accurately anticipate and plan nursing interventions. This chapter focuses on gastrointestinal disorders commonly seen in the critical care environment.

ACUTE GASTROINTESTINAL HEMORRHAGE

DESCRIPTION

Gastrointestinal (GI) hemorrhage is a medical emergency that remains a very common complication of critical illness[1] and results in almost 300,000 hospital admissions yearly.[2] Despite advances in medical knowledge and nursing care, the mortality rate for patients with acute GI bleeding has not changed in more than 50 years; it remains between 7% and 10%.[2,3]

ETIOLOGY

GI hemorrhage occurs from bleeding in the upper or lower GI tract. The ligament of Treitz is the anatomic division used to differentiate between the two areas. Thus bleeding proximal to the ligament is considered to be upper GI in origin, and bleeding distal to the ligament is considered to be lower GI in origin.[4] The various etiologies of acute GI hemorrhage are listed in Box 33-1.[1,5] Only the three main causes of GI hemorrhage commonly seen in the intensive care unit are discussed further.

Peptic Ulcer Disease. Peptic ulcer disease (gastric and duodenal ulcers), resulting from the breakdown of the gastromuscosal lining, is the leading cause of upper GI hemorrhage, accounting for 50% to 70% of cases.[5,6] Normally protection of the gastric mucosa from the digestive effects of gastric secretions is accomplished in several ways. First, the gastroduodenal mucosa is coated by a glycoprotein mucus barrier that protects the surface of the epithelium from hydrogen ions and other noxious substances present in the gut lumen.[7] Adequate gastric mucosal blood flow is necessary to maintain this mucosal barrier function. Second, gastroduodenal epithelial cells are protected structurally against damage from acid and pepsin because they are connected by tight junctions that help prevent acid penetration. Third, prostaglandins and nitric oxide protect the mucosal barrier by stimulating mucus and bicarbonate secretion and inhibiting the secretion of acid.[8]

Peptic ulceration occurs when these protective mechanisms cease to function, thus allowing gastroduodenal mucosal breakdown. Once the mucosal lining is penetrated, gastric secretions autodigest the layers of the stomach or duodenum, leading to injury of the mucosal and submucosal layers. This results in damaged blood vessels and subsequent hemorrhage. The two main causes of disruption of gastroduodenal mucosal resistance are nonsteroidal antiinflammatory drugs and the bacterial action of *Helicobacter pylori*.[3,9,10]

Stress-Related Erosive Syndrome. Stress-related erosive syndrome (SRES), also known as a *stress ulcer* or *hemorrhagic gastritis*, is a term used to describe the gastric mucosal abnormalities often found in the critically ill patient.[4] These abnormalities develop rapidly within hours of admission. They range from superficial mucosal erosions to deep ulcers and are usually limited to the stomach.[7] SRES occurs via the same pathophysiologic mechanisms as peptic ulcer disease, but the main cause of disruption of gastric mucosal resistance is increased acid production and decreased mucosal blood flow resulting in ischemia and degeneration of the mucosal lining.[4,7] Patients at risk include those in high physiologic stress situations, such as occur with mechanical ventilation, extensive burns, severe trauma, major surgery, shock, or acute neurologic disease.[3] GI hemorrhage is estimated to occur in 1% to 30% of patients who develop SRES, with an associated mortality of 30% to 80%.[3] SRES is the second leading cause of upper GI hemorrhage, accounting for approximately 20% of cases.[4,7]

Esophagogastric Varices. Esophagogastric varices are engorged and distended blood vessels of the esophagus and proximal stomach that develop as a result of portal hypertension secondary to hepatic cirrhosis, a chronic disease of the liver that results in damage to the liver sinusoids (Fig. 33-1). Without adequate sinusoid function, resistance to portal blood flow is increased and pressures within the liver are elevated. This leads to a rise in portal venous pressure (portal hypertension),

causing collateral circulation to divert portal blood from areas of high pressure within the liver to adjacent areas of low pressure outside the liver, such as into the veins of the esophagus, the spleen, the intestines, and the stomach. The tiny, thin-walled vessels of the esophagus and proximal stomach that receive this diverted blood lack sturdy mucosal protection. The vessels become engorged and dilated, forming esophagogastric varices that are vulnerable to damage from gastric secretions and may result in subsequent rupture and massive hemorrhage.[11,12] The risk of variceal bleeding increases with disease severity and variceal size, but overall, bleeding occurs in 19% to 50% of patients with varices and has an associated mortality of 40% to 70%.[2,11,13]

PATHOPHYSIOLOGY

GI hemorrhage is a life-threatening disorder that is characterized by acute, massive GI bleeding. Regardless of the etiology, acute GI hemorrhage results in hypovolemic shock, initiation of the shock response, and the development of multiple organ dysfunction syndrome if left untreated (Fig. 33-2).[8] However, the most common cause of death in GI hemorrhage is exacerbation of the underlying disease, not intractable hypovolemic shock.

ASSESSMENT AND DIAGNOSIS

The initial clinical presentation of the patient with acute GI hemorrhage is that of a patient in hypovolemic shock;

Box 33-1

ETIOLOGIES OF ACUTE GASTROINTESTINAL (GI) HEMORRHAGE

UPPER GI
Peptic ulcer disease
Stress-related erosive syndrome
Esophagogastric varices
Mallory-Weiss tear
Esophagitis
Neoplasm
Aortoenteric fistula
Angiodysplasia

LOWER GI
Diverticulosis
Angiodysplasia
Neoplasm
Inflammatory bowel disease
Trauma
Infectious colitis
Radiation colitis
Ischemia
Aortoenteric fistula
Hemorrhoids

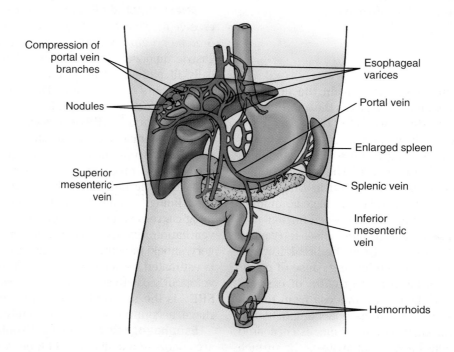

Fig. 33-1 Esophageal varices caused by cirrhosis. (Modified from Powell LW, Piper DW: *Fundamentals of gastroenterology*, Sydney, 1991, McGraw-Hill. Reproduced with permission of the McGraw-Hill Companies.)

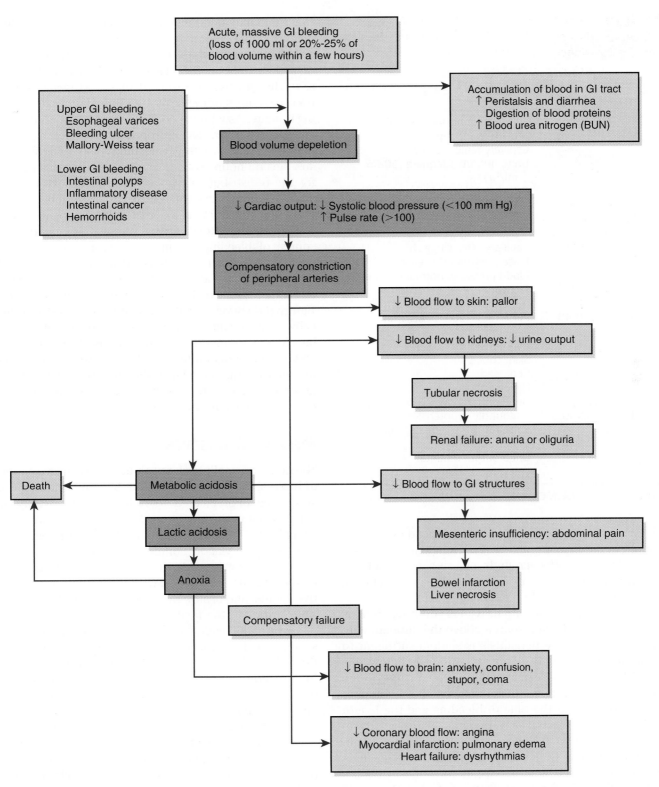

Fig. 33-2 Pathophysiology of acute gastrointestinal hemorrhage. (From Huether SE, McCance KL, Tarmina MS: Alterations of digestive function. In McCance KL, Huether SE, editors: *Pathophysiology: the biologic basis for disease in adults and children,* ed 4, St Louis, 2002, Mosby.)

Table 33-1		Clinical Classification of Hemorrhage
Class	**Blood Loss (%)**	**Clinical Signs/Symptoms**
1	≤15	Pulse rate: normal or <100 beats/min (supine) Capillary refill: <3 sec Urine output: adequate (30-35 ml/hr) Orthostatic hypotension Apprehensive
2	15-30	Pulse rate: increased (>100 beats/min) Capillary refill: sluggish Pulse pressure: decreased Blood pressure: normal (supine) Tachypnea Urine output: low (25-30 ml/hr)
3	30-40	Pulse rate: 120+ beats/min (supine) Hypotension Skin: cool, pale Confused Hyperventilating Urine output: low (5-15 ml/hr)
4	≥40	Profoundly hypotensive Pulse rate: 140+ beats/min Confused, lethargic Urine output minimal

From Klein DG: *AACN Clin Issues Crit Care Nurs* 1:508, 1990.

the clinical presentation will vary depending on the amount of blood lost (Table 33-1).[8] Hematemesis (bright red or brown, coffee grounds emesis), hematochezia (bright red stools), and melena (black, tarry, or dark red stools) are the hallmarks of GI hemorrhage.[4,8]

Hematemesis. The patient who is vomiting blood is usually bleeding from a source above the duodenojejunal junction; reverse peristalsis is seldom sufficient to cause hematemesis if the bleeding point is below this area. The hematemesis may be bright red or like coffee grounds in appearance, depending on the amount of gastric contents at the time of bleeding and the length of time the blood has been in contact with gastric secretions. Gastric acid converts bright red hemoglobin to brown hematin, accounting for the coffee grounds appearance of the emesis. Bright red emesis results from profuse bleeding with little contact with gastric secretions.[4]

Hematochezia and Melena. The presence of blood in the GI tract results in increased peristalsis and diarrhea. Hematochezia (bright red stool) occurs from massive lower GI hemorrhage and, if rapid enough, upper GI hemorrhage. Melena (black, tarry, or dark red stool) occurs from digestion of blood from an upper GI hemor-

rhage and may take several days to clear after the bleeding has stopped.[4]

Laboratory Studies. Laboratory tests can help determine the extent of bleeding, although it is important to realize that the patient's hemoglobin and hematocrit are poor indicators of the severity of blood loss if the bleeding is acute. As whole blood is lost, plasma and red blood cells are lost in the same proportion; thus if the patient's hematocrit is 45% before a bleeding episode, it will still be 45% several hours later.[8] It may take as long as 72 hours for the redistribution of plasma from the extravascular space to the intravascular space to occur and cause the patient's hemoglobin and hematocrit to drop.[2,14]

Diagnostic Procedures. To isolate and treat the source of bleeding, an urgent fiberoptic endoscopy is usually undertaken. If performed within 12 hours of the bleeding event, endoscopy therapy has a 90% effectiveness rate in achieving hemostasis and reduces mortality.[1] Before the endoscopy, the patient must be hemodynamically stabilized and the area that is to be visualized must be cleared of blood.[2,15] A tagged red blood cell scan and/or an angiogram may be done to assist with localizing and treating a bleeding lesion in the GI tract when it is impossible to clearly view the GI tract because of continued active bleeding.[14]

MEDICAL MANAGEMENT

To reduce mortality related to GI hemorrhage, patients at risk should be identified early and interventions should be implemented to reduce gastric acidity and support the gastric mucosal defense mechanisms. Management of the patient at risk for GI hemorrhage should include prophylactic administration of pharmacologic agents for gastric acid neutralization. These agents include antacids, histamine-2 (H_2) antagonists, cytoprotective agents, and proton-pump inhibitors (PPIs).[2,4]

Priorities in the medical management of the patient with GI hemorrhage include airway protection, fluid resuscitation to achieve hemodynamic stability, correction of comorbid conditions (coagulopathy), therapeutic procedures to control and/or stop bleeding, and diagnostic procedures to determine the exact etiology of the bleeding.[1,5]

Stabilization. The initial treatment priority is the restoration of adequate circulating blood volume to treat or prevent shock. This is accomplished with the administration of intravenous infusions of crystalloids, blood, and blood products.[2,6] A central venous catheter[5] or pulmonary artery catheter[2] may be necessary to guide fluid replacement therapy, particularly in those patients at risk for developing cardiac failure. Supplemental oxygen therapy is initiated to increase oxygen delivery and improve tissue perfusion.[2,5] Intubation may be necessary in the patient at risk for aspiration or to facilitate gastric lavage.[1] A large nasogastric (NG) tube may be inserted to confirm the diagnosis of active bleeding and to prepare the esophagus, stomach, and proximal duodenum for endoscopic evaluation.[5] A urinary drainage catheter should be inserted to monitor urine output.[2]

Control Bleeding. Interventions to control bleeding are the second priority for the patient with GI hemorrhage.

Peptic Ulcer Disease. In the patient with GI hemorrhage related to peptic ulcer disease, bleeding hemostasis may be accomplished via endoscopic thermal therapy or endoscopic injection therapy. Endoscopic thermal therapy uses heat to cauterize the bleeding vessel, whereas endoscopic injection therapy uses a variety of agents such as hypertonic saline, epinephrine, ethanol, and sclerosants to induce localized vasoconstriction of the bleeding vessel.[1,3] Intraarterial infusion of vasopressin into the gastric artery or intraarterial injection of an embolizing agent (Gelfoam pledgets, stainless steel coils, platinum microcoils, and polyvinyl alcohol particles) can also be performed during arteriography to control bleeding once the site has been identified.[4,16] Intraarterial administration of vasopressin is less effective for duodenal lesions because of the dual blood supply of the duodenum.[2]

SRES. In the patient with GI hemorrhage caused by SRES, bleeding hemostasis may be accomplished via intraarterial infusion of vasopressin and intraarterial embolization. Endoscopic therapies have been shown to be of minimal benefit because of the diffuse nature of the disease.[4]

Esophagogastric Varices. In acute variceal hemorrhage, control of bleeding may be initially accomplished through the use of pharmacologic agents and endoscopic therapies. Intravenous vasopressin, somatostatin, and octreotide have been shown to reduce portal venous pressure and slow variceal hemorrhaging by constricting the splanchnic arteriolar bed.[11,12] Two commonly used endoscopic therapies are injection therapy and variceal ligation. Endoscopic injection therapy (also referred to as sclerotherapy) controls bleeding via the injection of a sclerosing agent in or around the varices. This creates an inflammatory reaction that induces vasoconstriction and results in the formation of a venous thrombosis. During endoscopic variceal band ligation, bands are placed around the varices to create an obstruction to stop the bleeding.[11,12]

If these initial therapies fail, esophagogastric balloon tamponade or transjugular intrahepatic portosystemic shunting (TIPS) may be necessary. Balloon tamponade tubes (Sengstaken-Blakemore, Linton, and Minnesota tubes) stop hemorrhaging by applying direct pressure against bleeding vessels while decompressing the stomach.[11,12] In a TIPS procedure, a channel between the systemic and portal venous systems is created to redirect portal blood, thereby reducing portal hypertension and decompressing the varices to control bleeding (Fig. 33-3).[12,17]

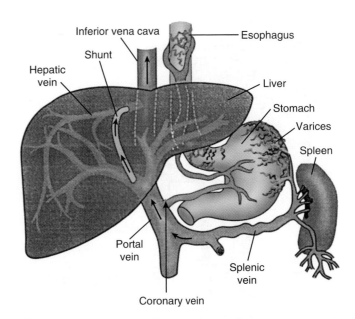

Fig. 33-3 Anatomic location of the transjugular intrahepatic portosystemic shunt (TIPS). (From Vargas HE, Gerber D, Abu-Elmagd K: *Surg Clin North Am* 79:1, 1999.)

Surgical Intervention. The patient who remains hemodynamically unstable despite volume replacement may need urgent surgery.

Peptic Ulcer Disease. The operative procedure of choice to control bleeding from peptic ulcer disease is a vagotomy and pyloroplasty. During this procedure the vagus nerve to the stomach is severed, thus eliminating the autonomic stimulus to the gastric cells and reducing hydrochloric acid production. Because the vagus nerve also stimulates motility, a pyloroplasty is performed to provide for gastric emptying.[16]

SRES. There are several operative procedures to control bleeding from SRES. A total gastrectomy is performed when bleeding is generalized. An oversew of the ulcers is performed when bleeding is localized. A total gastrectomy involves the complete removal of the stomach with anastomosis of the esophagus to the jejunum. During an oversew of the ulcers, the bleeding vessel is ligated and the ulcer crater is closed.[16]

Esophagogastric Varices. Operative procedures to control bleeding gastroesophageal varices include portacaval shunt, mesocaval shunt, and splenorenal shunt (Fig. 33-4).[17] These shunt procedures are also referred to as decompression procedures, since they result in the diversion of portal blood flow away from the liver and decompression of the portal system. The portacaval shunt procedure has two variations. An end-to-side portacaval shunt procedure involves the ligation of the hepatic end of the portal vein with subsequent anastomosis to the vena cava. During a side-to-side portacaval shunt procedure, the side of the portal vein is anastomosed to the side of the vena cava. A mesocaval shunt procedure involves the

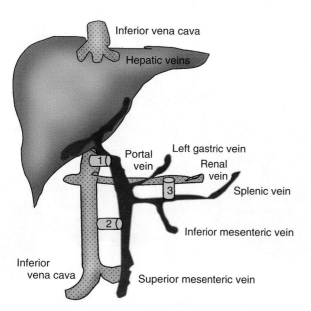

Fig. 33-4 The anatomy of the portal venous system and the sites in which surgical anastomoses are made to shunt blood from the portal *(dark)* to the systemic *(light)* venous circulation. Sites used for surgical portal decompression: (1) portacaval shunt; (2) mesocaval shunt; (3) splenorenal shunt. (From Luketic VA, Sanyal AJ: *Gastroenterol Clin North Am* 29:387, 2000.)

NURSING DIAGNOSES	Acute Gastrointestinal Hemorrhage

- Deficient Fluid Volume related to absolute loss
- Decreased Cardiac Output related to alterations in preload
- Risk for Aspiration
- Imbalanced Nutrition: Less Than Body Requirements related to lack of exogenous nutrients and increased metabolic demand
- Risk for Infection
- Powerlessness related to health care environment or illness-related regimen
- Compromised Family Coping related to critically ill family member
- Deficient Knowledge: Discharge Regimen related to lack of previous exposure to information (see the Patient Education feature on Acute Gastrointestinal Hemorrhage)

---

insertion of a graft between the superior mesenteric artery and the vena cava. Lastly, during a distal splenorenal shunt procedure, the splenic vein is detached from the portal vein and anastomosed to the left renal vein.[16,17]

NURSING MANAGEMENT

All critically ill patients should be considered at risk for stress ulcers and therefore GI hemorrhage. Routine assessments should include gastric fluid pH monitoring with a goal of keeping the pH greater than 4.[4,7] Gastric pH measurements, either via litmus paper or direct NG tube probes, may be used to assess gastric fluid pH and the effectiveness or need for prophylactic agents. In addition, patients at risk should be assessed for the presence of bright red or coffee grounds emesis, bloody NG aspirate, and bright red, black, or dark red stools.[1] Any signs of bleeding should be promptly reported to the physician.

Nursing management of a patient experiencing acute GI hemorrhage incorporates a variety of nursing diagnoses (see the Nursing Diagnoses feature on Acute Gastrointestinal Hemorrhage). Nursing priorities are directed toward administering volume replacement, controlling the bleeding, providing comfort and emotional support, maintaining surveillance for complications, and educating the patient and family.

Administering Volume Replacement. Measures to facilitate volume replacement include obtaining intravenous access and administering prescribed fluids and blood products. Two large-diameter peripheral intra-

venous (IV) catheters should be inserted to facilitate the rapid administration of prescribed fluids.[1,2]

Controlling the Bleeding. One measure to control active bleeding is gastric lavage. It is used to decrease gastric mucosal blood flow and evacuate blood from the stomach. Gastric lavage is performed by inserting a large-bore NG tube into the stomach and irrigating it with normal saline or water until the returned solution is clear. It is important to keep accurate records of the amount of fluid instilled and aspirated to ascertain the true amount of bleeding. Historically iced saline was favored as a lavage irrigant. Research has shown, however, that low-temperature fluids shift the oxyhemoglobin dissociation curve to the left, decrease oxygen delivery to vital organs, and prolong bleeding time and prothrombin time. Iced saline also may further aggravate bleeding; therefore room-temperature water or saline is the currently preferred irrigant for use in gastric lavage.[5]

Maintaining Surveillance for Complications. The patient should also be continuously observed for signs of gastric perforation. Although a rare complication, gastric perforation constitutes a surgical emergency. Signs and symptoms include sudden, severe, generalized abdominal pain with significant rebound tenderness and rigidity. Perforation should be suspected when fever, leukocytosis, and tachycardia persist despite adequate volume replacement.[5]

Patient Education. Early in the hospital stay, the patient and family should be taught about acute GI hemorrhage and its causes and treatments. As the patient moves toward discharge, teaching should focus on the interven-

PATIENT EDUCATION

Acute Gastrointestinal Hemorrhage

- GI hemorrhage
- Specific etiology
- Precipitating factor modification
- Interventions to reduce further bleeding episodes
- Importance of taking medications
- Lifestyle changes
- Stress management
- Diet modifications
- Alcohol cessation
- Smoking cessation

Box 33-2

COLLABORATIVE MANAGEMENT

ACUTE GASTROINTESTINAL HEMORRHAGE

Initiate fluid resuscitation to achieve hemodynamic
   stability
   Crystalloids
   Colloids
   Blood and blood products
Determine the etiology of the bleeding
   Gastric lavage
Control bleeding
   Endoscopic interventions
   Vasopressin, somatostatin, octreotide
   Esophagogastric balloon tube
   Transjugular intrahepatic portosystemic shunting
   Surgery
Provide comfort and emotional support
Maintain surveillance for complications
   Hypovolemic shock
   Gastric perforation

Box 33-3

RANSON'S CRITERIA FOR ESTIMATING THE SEVERITY OF ACUTE PANCREATITIS

AT ADMISSION
Age >55 years
Hypotension
Abnormal pulmonary findings
Abdominal mass
Hemorrhagic or discolored peritoneal fluid
Increased serum LDH levels (>350 units/L)
AST >250 units/L
Leukocytosis (>16,000/mm^3)
Hyperglycemia (>200 mg/dl; no diabetic history)
Neurologic deficit (confusion, localizing signs)

DURING INITIAL 48 HOURS OF HOSPITALIZATION
Fall in hematocrit >10% with hydration or hematocrit
   <30%
Necessity for massive fluid and colloid replacement
Hypocalcemia (<8 mg/dl)
Arterial Po$_2$ <60 mm Hg with or without acute respira-
   tory distress syndrome
Hypoalbuminemia (<3.2 mg/dl)
Base deficit >4 mEq/L
Azotemia

From Latifi R, McIntosh JK, Dudrick SJ: *Surg Clin North Am*
71:583, 1991.
LDH, Lactate dehydrogenase: *AST,* aspartate aminotransferase;
Po$_2$, partial pressure of oxygen.

---

tions necessary for preventing the recurrence of the precipitating disorder. If an alcohol abuser, the patient should be encouraged to stop drinking and be referred to an alcohol cessation program (see the Patient Education feature on Acute Gastrointestinal Hemorrhage).

Collaborative management of the patient with acute GI hemorrhage is outlined in Box 33-2.

ACUTE PANCREATITIS

DESCRIPTION

Acute pancreatitis is an inflammation of the pancreas that produces exocrine and endocrine dysfunction that may also involve surrounding tissues and/or remote or-

gan systems. The clinical course can range from a mild, self-limiting disease to a systemic process characterized by organ failure, sepsis, and death. In approximately 80% of patients it takes the milder form of *edematous interstitial pancreatitis*, whereas the other 20% develop severe *acute necrotizing pancreatitis*.[7] Reported mortality rates for acute pancreatitis vary, but range from 2% to 15% overall and from 20% to 50% in patients with severe disease.[18-20] Several prognostic scoring systems have been developed to predict the severity of acute pancreatitis. One of the most commonly used is Ranson's Criteria (Box 33-3). If the patient has 0 to 2 factors present, predicted mortality is 2%; with 3 to 4 factors, 15% mortality; with 5 to 6 factors, 40% mortality; and with 7 to 8 factors, predicted mortality is 100%.[18,21]

ETIOLOGY

The two most common causes of acute pancreatitis are gallstones and alcoholism. Together they account for approximately 80% of cases. Other less common causes are quite diverse and include surgical trauma, hypercalcemia, various toxins, ischemia, infections, and the use of certain drugs (Box 33-4). In 10% to 20% of patients with acute pancreatitis, no etiologic factor can be determined.[21,22]

Box 33-4

ETIOLOGIES OF ACUTE PANCREATITIS

- Toxins—ethyl alcohol, methyl alcohol, scorpion, venom, parathion
- Biliary disease—stones, sludge, common bile duct obstruction
- Drugs—sulfonamides, thiazide diuretics, furosemide, estrogens, tetracycline, pentamidine, procainamide, salicylates, steroids, cyclosporine, amphetamines, nonsteroidal antiinflammatory agents, valpoic acid, azathioprine, allopurinol
- Hypercalcemia—hyperparathyroidism
- Hyperlipidemia
- Tumors
- Infections—bacterial, viral, parasitic
- Trauma—abdominal, surgical, endoscopic
- Ischemia
- Transplant
- Vasculitis
- Pregnancy
- Hypothermia
- Sphincter of Oddi dysfunction
- Systemic lupus erythematosus
- Ampullary stenosis
- Idiopathic

Data from Steer ML: Acute pancreatitis. In Taylor MB, editor: *Gastrointestinal emergencies,* Baltimore, 1992, Williams & Wilkins.

Box 33-5

PRESENTING CLINICAL MANIFESTATIONS OF ACUTE PANCREATITIS

- Pain
- Vomiting
- Nausea
- Fever
- Abdominal distention
- Abdominal guarding
- Abdominal tympany
- Hypoactive/absent bowel sounds
- Severe disease
  Peritoneal signs
  Ascites
  Jaundice
  Palpable abdominal mass
  Grey Turner's sign
  Cullen's sign
  Signs of hypovolemic shock

From Krumberger JM: *Crit Care Nurs Clin North Am* 5:185, 1993.

PATHOPHYSIOLOGY

In acute pancreatitis the normally inactive digestive enzymes become prematurely activated within the pancreas itself, leading to autodigestion of pancreatic tissue. The enzymes become activated through various mechanisms, including obstruction of or damage to the pancreatic duct system, alterations in the secretory processes of the acinar cells, infection, ischemia, and/or other unknown factors.[8,19]

Trypsin is the enzyme that becomes activated first and initiates the autodigestion process by triggering the secretion of proteolytic enzymes such as kallikrein, chymotrypsin, elastase, phospholipase A, and lipase. Release of kallikrein and chymotrypsin results in increased capillary membrane permeability, leading to leakage of fluid into the interstitium and the development of edema and relative hypovolemia. Elastase is the most harmful enzyme in terms of direct cell damage. It causes dissolution of the elastic fibers of blood vessels and ducts, leading to hemorrhage. Phospholipase A, in the presence of bile, destroys the phospholipids of cell membranes, causing severe pancreatic and adipose tissue necrosis. Lipase flows into the damaged tissue and is absorbed into the systemic circulation, resulting in fat necrosis of the pancreas and surrounding tissues.[22]

The extent of injury to the pancreatic cells determines which form of acute pancreatitis will develop. If injury to the pancreatic cells is mild and without necrosis, edematous pancreatitis develops. The acinar cells appear structurally intact and blood flow is maintained through small capillaries and venules. This form of acute pancreatitis is self-limiting. If injury to the pancreatic cells is severe, acute necrotizing pancreatitis develops.[23] Cellular destruction in pancreatic injury results in the release of toxic enzymes and inflammatory mediators into the systemic circulation and causes injury to vessels and other organs distant from the pancreas; this may result in systemic inflammatory response syndrome (SIRS), multiorgan failure, and/or death.[18,22,23] Local tissue injury results in infection, abscess and pseudocyst formation, disruption of the pancreatic duct, and severe hemorrhage with shock.[18]

ASSESSMENT AND DIAGNOSIS

The clinical manifestations of acute pancreatitis range from mild to severe and often mimic those of other disorders (Box 33-5). Epigastric to midabdominal pain may vary from mild and tolerable to severe and incapacitating. Many patients report a twisting or knifelike sensation that radiates to the low dorsal region of the back. Nausea and vomiting is present in more than 80% of patients.[19,24] The patient may obtain some comfort by leaning forward or assuming a semifetal position. Other clinical findings include fever, diaphoresis, weakness, tachypnea, hypotension, and tachycardia. Depending on the extent of fluid loss and hemorrhage, the patient may exhibit signs of hypovolemic shock.[19,23,25]

Table 33-2	Laboratory Tests and Diagnostic Procedures in Acute Pancreatitis
Study	**Finding in Pancreatitis**

LABORATORY

Serum amylase	Elevated
Serum isoamylase	Elevated
Urine amylase	Elevated
Serum lipase (if available)	Elevated
Serum triglycerides	Elevated
Glucose	Elevated
Calcium	Decreased
Magnesium	Decreased
Potassium	Decreased
Albumin	Decreased or increased
White blood cell count	Elevated
Bilirubin	May be elevated
Liver enzymes	May be elevated
Prothrombin time	Prolonged
Arterial blood gases	Hypoxemia, metabolic acidosis

RADIOGRAPHIC
Abdominal
Ultrasonography
Magnetic resonance imaging
ERCP
Abdominal films (flat plate and upright or decubitus)
Chest films (posteroanterior and lateral)

From Krumberger JM: *Crit Care Nurs Clin North Am* 5:185, 1993.
ERCP, Endoscopic retrograde cholangiopancreatograph.

Physical Examination. The results of physical assessment usually reveal hypoactive bowel sounds and abdominal tenderness, guarding, distention, and tympany. Findings that could indicate pancreatic hemorrhage include Grey Turner's sign (gray-blue discoloration of the flank) and Cullen's sign (discoloration of the umbilical region), however, they are rare and would generally be seen several days into the illness.[24,26] A palpable abdominal mass indicates the presence of a pseudocyst or abscess.[25,27]

Laboratory Studies. Assessment of laboratory data usually demonstrates elevated levels of serum amylase and lipase. Serum lipase is more pancreas-specific than amylase and a more accurate marker for acute pancreatitis. Amylase is present in other body tissues, and other disorders (intraabdominal emergencies, renal insufficiency, salivary gland trauma, liver disease) may contribute to an elevated level. Unlike other serum enzymes, however, amylase is excreted in urine, and this clearance increases with acute pancreatitis. Measurement of urinary versus serum amylase should be considered in light of the patient's creatinine clearance. In addition, serum amylase may be elevated for only 3 to 5 days; if the patient delays seeking treatment, a normal level (false negative) may be noted. Leukocytosis, hypocalcemia, hyperglycemia, hyperbilirubinemia, and hypoalbuminemia may also be present (Table 33-2).[8,24]

Diagnostic Procedures. An abdominal ultrasound is obtained as part of the diagnostic evaluation to determine the presence of biliary stones. A contrast-enhanced computed tomography (CT) scan is considered the gold standard for diagnosing pancreatitis as well as for ascertaining the overall degree of pancreatic inflammation and necrosis.[20,24]

MEDICAL MANAGEMENT

Initial management of the patient with severe acute pancreatitis includes ensuring adequate fluid and electrolyte replacement, providing nutritional support, and correcting metabolic alterations. In addition, careful monitoring for systemic and local complications is critical.[24]

Fluid Management. Because pancreatitis if often associated with massive fluid shifts, intravenous crystalloids and colloids are administered immediately to prevent hypovolemic shock and maintain hemodynamic stability. In severe forms of acute pancreatitis, the use of a pulmonary artery catheter may be used to guide ongoing fluid management.[20,26] Electrolytes are monitored closely; and abnormalities such as hypocalcemia, hypokalemia, and hypomagnesemia are corrected.[26] If hyperglycemia develops, exogenous insulin may be required.[24]

Nutritional Support. Until recently, conventional nutritional management was to place the patient on a nothing by mouth (NPO) regimen and institute intravenous hydration. The rationale was to rest the inflamed pancreas and prevent enzyme release. Oral feeding was only initiated when the attack had subsided and enzymes had normalized. Total parenteral nutrition (TPN) was started on patients anticipated to have oral feedings held for greater than 5 days. Although this practice is still followed in many hospitals, recent randomized clinical trials have demonstrated that enteral feeding (gastric or jejunal) is safe and cost-effective, and that it is associated with fewer septic and metabolic complications and should be considered. However, TPN still has a role in the critically ill patient with acute pancreatitis, especially in the presence of paralytic ileus or duodenal obstruction.[18,20] In the past, nasogastric suction was also recommended, but this intervention has not been shown to be of benefit and should only be instituted if the patient has persistent vomiting, obstruction, or gastric distention.[21,24]

Systemic Complications. Acute pancreatitis can affect every organ system, and recognition and treatment of systemic complications is crucial to management of the patient (Box 33-6). The most serious complications are hypovolemic shock, acute lung injury (ALI), acute renal failure (ARF), and GI hemorrhage. Hypovolemic shock is the result of relative hypovolemia resulting from third spacing of intravascular volume and vasodilation caused by the release of inflammatory immune mediators. These mediators also contribute to the development of ALI and ARF. Other possible pulmonary complications include pleural effusions, atelectasis, and pneumonia. Stress ulcers and bleeding gastroesophageal varices (in the alcoholic patient) can precipitate the development of GI hemorrhage.[24]

Local Complications. Local complications include the development of infected pancreatic necrosis and pancreatic pseudocyst.[18] The necrotic areas of the pancreas can lead to the development of a widespread pancreatic infection (infected pancreatic necrosis) which significantly increases the risk of death.[20] Prophylactic antibiotics have been shown to reduce sepsis and mortality and are initiated in patients suspected of having necrotizing pancreatitis.[18,20] Once the patient develops

infected necrosis, however, surgical debridement is necessary.[20] The procedure of choice is a necrosectomy, which entails careful debridement of the necrotic tissue in and around the pancreas. It often requires postoperative lavage and multiple reexplorations with further debridement to remove all the necrotic tissue.[20,28] A pancreatic pseudocyst is a collection of pancreatic fluid enclosed by a nonepithelialized wall. Cyst formation may result from liquefaction of a pancreatic fluid collection or from direct obstruction in the main pancreatic duct.[18] A pancreatic pseudocyst may (1) resolve spontaneously; (2) rupture, resulting in peritonitis; (3) erode a major blood vessel, resulting in hemorrhage; (4) become infected, resulting in abscess; or (5) invade surrounding structures, resulting in obstruction.[18] Treatment involves drainage of the pseudocyst either surgically,[28] endoscopically,[29] or percutaneously.[30]

NURSING MANAGEMENT

Nursing management of the patient with pancreatitis incorporates a variety of nursing diagnoses (see the Nursing Diagnoses feature on Acute Pancreatitis). Nursing priorities are directed toward providing pain relief and emotional support, maintaining surveillance for complications, and educating the patient and family.

Providing Comfort and Emotional Support. Pain management is a major priority in acute pancreatitis. Ad-

---

Box 33-6

COMPLICATIONS OF ACUTE PANCREATITIS

RESPIRATORY
Early hypoxemia
Pleural effusion
Atelectasis
Pulmonary infiltration
ALI
Mediastinal abscess

CARDIOVASCULAR
Hypotension
Pericardial effusion
ST-T changes

RENAL
Acute tubular necrosis
Oliguria
Renal artery or vein
  thrombosis

HEMATOLOGIC
DIC
Thrombocytosis
Hyperfibrinogenemia

ENDOCRINE
Hypocalcemia
Hypertriglyceridemia
Hyperglycemia

NEUROLOGIC
Fat emboli
Psychosis
Encephalopathy

OPHTHALMIC
Purtscher's retinopathy—
  sudden blindness

DERMATOLOGIC
Subcutaneous fat necrosis

GI/HEPATIC
Hepatic dysfunction
Obstructive jaundice
Erosive gastritis
Paralytic ileus
Duodenal obstruction
Pancreatic
  Pseudocyst
  Phlegmon
  Abscess
  Ascites
Bowel infarction
Massive intraperitoneal
  bleed
Perforation
  Stomach
  Duodenum
  Small bowel
  Colon

From Ranson JHC: Complication of pancreatitis. In Taylor MB, editor: *Gastrointestinal emergencies,* Baltimore, 1992, Williams & Wilkins.
ALI, Acute lung injury; *DIC,* disseminated intravascular coagulation; *GI,* gastrointestinal.

NURSING DIAGNOSES | **Acute Pancreatitis**

- Acute Pain related to transmission and perception of cutaneous, visceral, muscular, ischemia impulses
- Deficient Fluid Volume related to relative fluid loss
- Decreased Cardiac Output related to alterations in preload
- Ineffective Breathing Pattern related to decreased lung expansion
- Imbalanced Nutrition: Less Than Body Requirements related to lack of exogenous nutrients or increased metabolic demand
- Anxiety related to threat to biologic, psychologic, and/or social integrity
- Compromised Family Coping related to critically ill family member
- Deficient Knowledge: Discharge Regimen related to lack of previous exposure to information (see the Patient Education feature on Acute Pancreatitis)

ministration of analgesics to achieve pain relief is essential. For years, meperidine (Demerol) was considered to be the preferred agent in the patient with acute pancreatitis because morphine produced spasms at the sphincter of Oddi. Recent studies, however, have demonstrated that all opioids have a spasmogenic effect on the sphincter of Oddi. Therefore there is no evidence to indicate that morphine is contraindicated for use in acute pancreatitis, and it may provide more effective analgesia with fewer side effects than meperidine.[31] Relaxation techniques and positioning the patient in the knee-chest position can also assist in pain control.

Maintaining Surveillance for Complications. The patient must be routinely monitored for signs of local or systemic complications (see Box 33-6). Intensive monitoring of each of the organ systems is imperative, since organ failure is a major indicator of the severity of the disease.[20,24] In addition, the patient must be closely monitored for signs and symptoms of pancreatic infection, which include increased abdominal pain and tenderness, fever, and increased white blood cell count (Box 33-7).[19]

Patient Education. Early in the patient's hospital stay, the patient and family should be taught about acute pancreatitis and its causes and treatment. As the patient moves toward discharge, teaching should focus on the interventions necessary for preventing the recurrence of the precipitating disorder. If the patient has sustained permanent damage to the pancreas, the patient will re-quire teaching specific to diet modification and supplemental pancreatic enzymes. Diabetes education may also be necessary. If an alcohol abuser, the patient should be encouraged to stop drinking and be referred to an alcohol cessation program (see the Patient Education feature on Acute Pancreatitis and the Clinical Application feature on Gastrointestinal Concepts).[19]

Collaborative management of the patient with pancreatitis is outlined in Box 33-8.

FULMINANT HEPATIC FAILURE

DESCRIPTION

Fulminant hepatic failure (FHF) is a life-threatening condition characterized by severe and sudden liver cell dysfunction, coagulopathy, and hepatic encephalopathy.[32] Although uncommon, FHF is associated with a mortality rate as high as 80% and generally occurs in patients without preexisting liver disease.[33] Because liver transplantation is one of the few definitive treatments for FHF, the

---

Box 33-7

SIGNS AND SYMPTOMS OF PANCREATIC INFECTION

SYMPTOMS
Persistent abdominal pain
Abdominal tenderness

SIGNS
Prolonged fever
Abdominal distention
Palpable abdominal mass
Vomiting

DIAGNOSTICS
Laboratory
    Increased white blood cell count
    Persistent elevation of serum amylase
    Hyperbilirubinemia
    Elevated alkaline phosphatase
    Positive culture and Gram's stain
Radiography/CT
    Pancreatic inflammation or enlargement
    Necrosis
    Cystic or mass lesions
    Fluid accumulations
    Pseudocyst abscess

From Krumberger JM: *Crit Care Nurs Clin North Am* 5:185, 1993. *CT,* Computed tomography.

PATIENT EDUCATION | **Acute Pancreatitis**

- Pancreatitis
- Specific etiology
- Precipitating factor modification
- Interventions to reduce further episodes
- Importance of taking medications
- Lifestyle changes
- Diet modification
- Stress management
- Alcohol cessation
- Diabetes management (if present)

Box 33-8

COLLABORATIVE MANAGEMENT

ACUTE PANCREATITIS
Ensure adequate circulating volume
Provide nutritional support
Correct metabolic alterations
Minimize pancreatic stimulation
Provide comfort and emotional support
Maintain surveillance for complications
    Multiple organ dysfunction syndrome

CLINICAL APPLICATION

Gastrointestinal Concepts

Mr. P is a 43-year-old man admitted with complaints of severe epigastric pain and intractable nausea and vomiting after a weekend of heavy drinking. He has a history of alcohol abuse with previous admissions for GI bleeding. Mr. P's initial vital signs are temperature, 100° F (37.8° C); heart rate (HR), 102; respiratory rate (RR), 24; and blood pressure (BP), 92/54. His initial laboratory studies reveal serum amylase, 320 units/L; serum lipase, 770 units/L; white blood cell (WBC) count, 17,000 mm³; lactate dehydrogenase (LDH), 365 units/L; aspartate aminotransferase (AST), 90 units/L; and serum glucose, 350 mg/dl. An ultrasound examination reveals an enlarged, edematous pancreas but shows no gallstones. A diagnosis of acute pancreatitis is made.

On admission to the unit, Mr. P is oriented to person and place, and is anxious and uncooperative. His temperature is 101.5° F. He is tachycardic, diaphoretic, and tachypneic. Auscultation of the chest reveals clear breath sounds bilaterally. His abdomen is distended without bowel sounds, and guarding is noted on palpation. A urinary drainage catheter is placed with an output of 45 ml of dark, amber urine. A central line is placed, and a central venous pressure (CVP) of 1 mm Hg is obtained.

1. What is the most likely precipitating factor for Mr. P's acute pancreatitis?
2. Is serum amylase or serum lipase a better indicator of acute pancreatitis? Why?
3. What intervention would you anticipate being initiated FIRST for Mr. P?
4. Mr. P continues to complain of severe abdominal pain. What is the drug of choice in treating pain in acute pancreatitis? Why?
5. The following day Mr. P's vital signs become unstable, and you notice a bluish discoloration of the periumbilical and flank areas. What do you suspect has happened to Mr. P?
6. What are your nursing priorities for Mr. P?

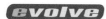 For the discussion of this Clinical Application, see the Evolve website.

---

patient with FHF should be transferred to a critical care unit and strongly considered for referral to a major medical center where transplant services are available.[33,34]

ETIOLOGY

The etiologies of FHF include infections, drugs, toxins, hypoperfusion, metabolic disorders, and surgery (Box 33-9); however, viral hepatitis and drug-induced liver damage are the predominant etiologies in North America. Patients are usually healthy before the onset of symptoms because FHF tends to occur in patients with no known liver history. Therefore a thorough medication and health history is imperative to determine a possible etiology. The patient should be questioned about exposure to environmental toxins, hepatitis, intravenous drug use, and sexual history. Viral hepatitis, drug toxicity, poisoning, and metabolic disorders such as Reye's syndrome and Wilson's disease should be considered.[35]

PATHOPHYSIOLOGY

FHF is a syndrome characterized by the development of acute liver failure over 1 to 3 weeks, followed by the development of hepatic encephalopathy within 8 weeks, in a patient with a previously healthy liver. Generally the interval between the actual failure of the liver and the onset of hepatic encephalopathy is less than 2 weeks. The underlying cause is massive necrosis of the hepatocytes.[33-35]

Acute liver failure results in a number of derangements including impaired bilirubin conjugation, decreased production of clotting factors, depressed glucose synthesis, and decreased lactate clearance. This results in jaundice, coagulopathies, hypoglycemia, and metabolic acidosis. Other effects of acute liver failure include increased risk of infection and altered carbohydrate, protein, and glucose metabolism. Hypoalbuminemia, fluid and electrolyte imbalances, and acute portal hypertension contribute to the development of ascites.[33,34] Hepatic encephalopathy is thought to result from failure of the liver to detoxify various substances in the bloodstream and may be worsened by metabolic and electrolyte imbalances.[36]

The patient may also experience a variety of other complications including cerebral edema, cardiac dysrhythmias, acute respiratory failure, sepsis, and acute renal failure. Cerebral edema and increased intracranial pressure (ICP) develops as a result of breakdown of the blood-brain barrier and astrocyte swelling. Circulatory failure that mimics sepsis is common in FHF and may exacerbate low cerebral perfusion pressure (CPP). Hypoxemia, acidosis, electrolyte imbalances, and/or cerebral edema can precipitate the development of cardiac dysrhythmias. Acute respiratory failure, progressing to ALI, can result from pulmonary edema, aspiration pneumonia, and atelectasis. Acute renal failure may be caused by acute tubular necrosis, hypotension, or hemorrhage.[33,34]

Box 33-9

ETIOLOGIES OF FULMINANT HEPATIC FAILURE

INFECTIONS
Hepatitis A, B, C, D, E, non-A, non-B, non-C
Herpes simplex virus (types 1 and 2)
Epstein-Barr virus
Varicella zoster
Dengue fever virus
Rift Valley fever virus

DRUGS/TOXINS
Industrial substances (chlorinated hydrocarbons, phosphorus)
Amanita phalloids (mushrooms)
Aflatoxin (herb)
Medications (isoniazid, rifampin, halothane, methyldopa, tetracycline, valproic acid, monoamine oxidase inhibitors, phenytoin, nicotinic acid, tricyclic antidepressants, isoflurane, ketoconazole, trimethoprim-sulfamethoxazole, sulfasalazine, pyrimethamine, octreotide)
Acetaminophen toxicity
Cocaine

HYPOPERFUSION
Venous obstructions
Budd-Chiari syndrome
Veno-occlusive disease
Ischemia

METABOLIC DISORDERS
Wilson's disease
Tyrosinemia
Heat stroke
Galactosemia

SURGERY
Jejunoileal bypass
Partial hepatectomy
Liver transplant failure

OTHER
Reye's syndrome
Acute fatty liver of pregnancy
Massive malignant infiltration
Autoimmune hepatitis

ASSESSMENT AND DIAGNOSIS

Early recognition of FHF is extremely important. The diagnosis should include potentially reversible conditions (e.g., autoimmune hepatitis) and should differentiate FHF from decompensating chronic liver disease. Prognostic indicators such as coma grade, serum bilirubin, prothrombin time (PT), coagulation factors, and pH should be noted, and potential etiologies investigated.[33]

Signs and symptoms of FHF include headache, hyperventilation, jaundice, mental status changes, palmar erythema, spider nevi, bruises, and edema. The patient should be evaluated for the presence of asterixis or "liver flap," best described as the inability to voluntarily sustain a fixed position of the extremities. Asterixis is best demonstrated by having the patient extend the arms and dorsiflex the wrists, resulting in downward flapping of the hands. Hepatic encephalopathy is assessed using a grading system that stages the encephalopathy according to the patient's clinical manifestations (Box 33-10).[35,36] Diagnostic findings include elevated serum bilirubin, aspartate aminotransferase (AST), alkaline phosphatase, and serum ammonia, and decreased serum albumin. Arterial blood gases (ABGs) reveal respiratory alkalosis and/or metabolic acidosis. Hypoglycemia, hypokalemia, and hyponatremia also may be present.[33,35]

Factors I (fibrinogen), II (prothrombin), V, VII, IX, and X are produced exclusively by the liver. Prothrombin time may be the most useful of tests of these in the evaluation of acute FHF because levels may be 40 to 80 seconds above control values. Decreased levels of plasmin and plasminogen and increased levels of fibrin and

---

Box 33-10

STAGING OF HEPATIC ENCEPHALOPATHY

I   Euphoria or depression, mild confusion, slurred speech, disordered sleep rhythm; slight asterixis and normal EEG
II   Lethargy, moderate confusion; marked asterixis and abnormal EEG
III Marked confusion, incoherent speech, sleeping but arousable; asterixis present and abnormal EEG
IV   Coma; initially responsive to noxious stimuli, later unresponsive; asterixis absent and abnormal EEG

EEG, Electroencephalogram.

---

fibrin-split products also are noted. Platelet counts may be decreased to 80,000/mm^3 or less.[33]

MEDICAL MANAGEMENT

Medical interventions are directed toward management of the multiple system impact of FHF.

Ammonia Levels. Neomycin or lactulose is administered to remove or decrease production of nitrogenous wastes in the large intestine. Neomycin, given orally or rectally, reduces bacterial flora of the colon. This aids in decreasing ammonia formation by decreasing bacterial action on protein in the feces. Side effects include renal toxicity and hearing impairment. Lactulose, a synthetic ketoanalog of lactose split into lactic acid and acetic acid in the intestine, is given orally, via NG tube, or as a retention enema. The result is the creation of an acidic environment that decreases bacterial growth. Lactulose also traps ammonia and has a laxative effect that promotes expulsion.[36] Various experimental therapies such as exchange transfusion, charcoal hemoperfusion, and plasmapheresis have been used to lower ammonia levels, but have not improved survival.[35]

Complications. Bleeding is best controlled through prevention. Because these patients are at risk for acute GI hemorrhage, stress ulcer prophylaxis is essential.[35] If an invasive procedure (central line placement, ICP monitor) will be performed or the patient develops active bleeding, vitamin K, fresh-frozen plasma (to maintain reasonable prothrombin time), and platelet transfusions are necessary.[37] Metabolic disturbances such as hypoglycemia, metabolic acidosis, hypokalemia, and hyponatremia should be monitored and treated appropriately. Prophylactic antibiotic administration may be initiated because the patient is at high risk for an infection.[33,34]

The development of cerebral edema necessitates intracranial pressure (ICP) monitoring. Mannitol is the only treatment shown to be of benefit in managing increased ICP in the patient with FHF, but must be used with caution in patients with renal failure.[35,37] Other interventions to control intracranial hypertension include elevating the head of the bed (HOB) to 20 to 30 degrees, treating fever and hypertension, minimizing noxious stimulation, and correcting hypercapnia and hypoxemia.[38] If renal failure develops, continuous renal replacement therapy (CRRT) should be initiated.[34] Intubation and mechanical ventilation may be necessary as hypoxemia develops.[38] Hemodynamic instability is a common complication necessitating fluid administration and vasoactive medications to prevent prolonged episodes of hypotension. A pulmonary artery catheter may be used to guide clinical management.[33,34]

If FHF continues and the patient shows no immediate signs of improvement or reversal, the patient should be considered for a liver transplant. Prompt referral to a transplant center should be a high priority for patients experiencing fulminant hepatic failure.[34]

NURSING MANAGEMENT

Nursing management of the patient with FHF incorporates a variety of nursing diagnoses (see the Nursing Diagnoses feature on Fulminant Hepatic Failure). Nursing priorities are directed toward protecting the patient from injury, providing comfort and emotional support, maintaining surveillance for complications, and educating the patient and family.

Protecting the Patient from Injury. Use of benzodiazepines and other sedatives is discouraged in the FHF patient because of the "masking" of pertinent neurologic changes and further potentiation of hepatic encephalopathy.[35] These patients are often very difficult to manage because they may be extremely agitated and combative.

NURSING DIAGNOSES Fulminant Hepatic Failure

- Ineffective Breathing Pattern related to decreased lung expansion
- Impaired Gas Exchange related to ventilation/perfusion mismatching or intrapulmonary shunting
- Decreased Cardiac Output related to alterations in preload
- Decreased Cardiac Output related to alterations in heart rate
- Decreased Intracranial Adaptive Capacity related to failure of normal compensatory mechanisms
- Ineffective Renal Tissue Perfusion related to decreased renal blood flow
- Risk for Infection
- Imbalanced Nutrition: Less Than Body Requirements related to lack of exogenous nutrients or increased metabolic demand
- Disturbed Body Image related to actual change in body structure, function, or appearance
- Compromised Family Coping related to critically ill family member
- Deficient Knowledge: Discharge Regimen related to lack of previous exposure to information (see the Patient Education feature on Fulminant Hepatic Failure)

Physical restraint is generally required to prevent patient injury.

Maintaining Surveillance for Complications. As the neurologic condition worsens, respiratory depression and arrest can occur quickly. Continuous pulse oximetry monitoring and ABG analysis are helpful in assessing adequacy of respiratory efforts. A thorough neurologic assessment should be performed at least every hour.

Educating Patient and Family. Early in the patient's hospital stay, the patient and family should be taught about fulminant hepatic failure and its causes and treatment. As the patient moves toward discharge, teaching should focus on the interventions necessary for preventing the recurrence of the precipitating etiology. If the patient is considered a liver transplant candidate, the patient and family will need specific information regarding the procedure and care. Liver transplant evaluation may include screening for medical contraindications, human immunodeficiency virus (HIV) serology, anticipated compliance, and assessment of the social support system. Psychiatric and other specialty team consults are necessary for a thorough evaluation of the patient's suitability for a transplant (see the Patient Education feature on Fulminant Hepatic Failure).

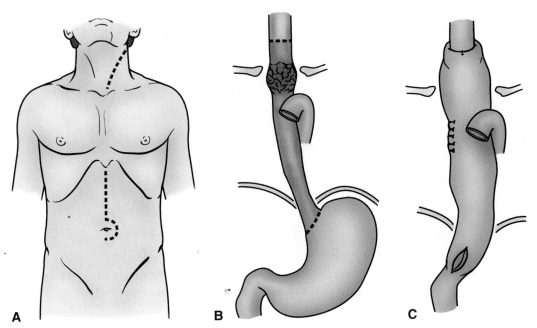

Fig. 33-5   **A** to **C**, Overview of transhiatal esophagectomy with gastric mobilization and gastric pull-up for cervical-esophagogastric anastomosis. (**A** to **C** adapted from Ellis F: Esophagogastrectomy for carcinoma: technical considerations based on anatomic location of lesion, *Surg Clin North Am* 60:275, 1980.)

PATIENT EDUCATION

Fulminant Hepatic Failure

- Specific etiology
- Precipitating factor modification
- Interventions to reduce further episodes
- Importance of taking medications
- Lifestyle changes
- Diet modification
- Alcohol cessation

Box 33-11

COLLABORATIVE MANAGEMENT

FULMINANT HEPATIC FAILURE
- Decrease ammonia levels
- Control bleeding
- Correct metabolic alterations
- Prevent infection
- Prepare patient for liver transplantation if necessary
- Protect patient from injury
- Provide comfort and emotional support
- Maintain surveillance for complications
    - Cerebral edema
    - Renal failure

Collaborative management of the patient with fulminant hepatic failure is outlined in Box 33-11.

GASTROINTESTINAL SURGERY

TYPES OF SURGERY

Gastrointestinal surgery refers to a wide variety of surgical procedures that involve the esophagus, the stomach, the intestine, the liver, the pancreas, or the biliary tract. Indications for gastrointestinal surgery are numerous and include bleeding or perforation from peptic ulcer disease, obstruction, trauma, inflammatory bowel disease, and malignancy. Patients may be admitted to the critical care unit for monitoring after GI surgery as a result of their underlying medical condition; however, this portion of the chapter will focus only on several surgical procedures that commonly require postoperative critical care.

Esophagectomy. Esophagectomy is usually performed for cancer of the distal esophagus and gastroesophageal junction. The procedure involves the removal of part or the entire esophagus, part of the stomach, and lymph nodes in the surrounding area. The stomach is then pulled up into the chest and connected to the remaining part of the esophagus. If the entire esophagus and stomach must be removed, part of the bowel may be used to form the esophageal replacement (Figs. 33-5 and 33-6).[39,40]

Pancreaticoduodenectomy. The standard operation for pancreatic cancer is a pancreaticoduodenectomy, or "Whipple procedure." In the Whipple procedure the pan-

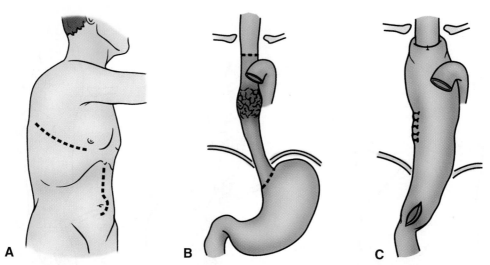

Fig. 33-6 Overview of right thoracotomy **(A)** with esophageal resection, gastric mobilization **(B),** and intrathoracic anastomosis **(C)** for midesophageal tumor. (**A** to **C** adapted from Ellis FH: Esophagogastrectomy for carcinoma: technical considerations based on anatomic location of lesion, *Surg Clin North Am* 60:273, 1980.)

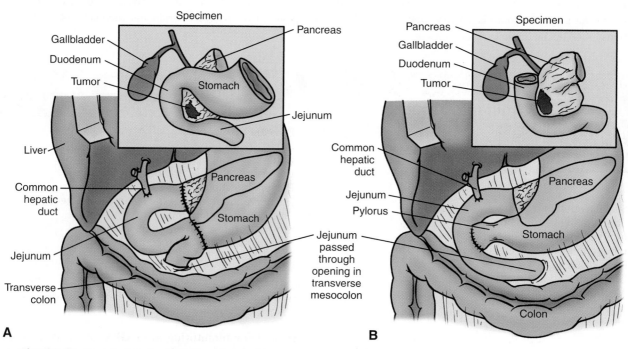

Fig. 33-7 Standard and pylorus-preserving Whipple procedure. **A,** The "standard Whipple" involves resection of the gastric antrum, head of pancreas, distal bile duct, and entire duodenum with reconstruction as shown. **B,** The "pylorus-preserving Whipple" does not include resection of the distal stomach, pylorus, or proximal duodenum. (From Cameron JL: Current status of the Whipple operation for periampullary carcinoma, *Surg Rounds* 77-87, 1998.)

creatic head, the duodenum, part of the jejunum, the common bile duct, the gallbladder, and part of the stomach are removed. The continuity of the GI tract is restored by anastomosing the remaining portion of the pancreas, the bile duct, and the stomach to the jejunum (Fig. 33-7).[40]

Bariatric Surgery. Bariatric surgery refers to surgical procedures of the GI tract that are performed to induce weight loss. Bariatric procedures are divided into two broad types: restrictive and malabsorptive. Restrictive procedures such as vertical banded gastroplasty (VBG) (Fig. 33-8, *A*) and gastric banding (Fig. 33-8, *B*) reduce the capacity of the stomach and limit the amount of food that can be consumed. Malabsorptive procedures such as the biliopancreatic diversion (BPD) (Fig. 33-8, *C*) alter the GI tract to limit the digestion and absorption of food.

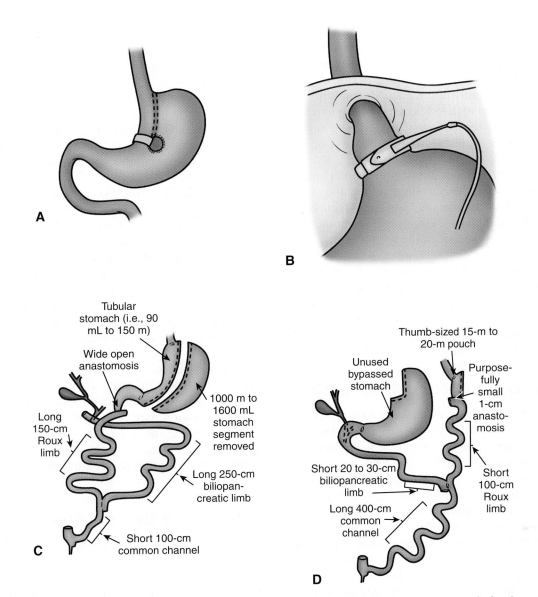

Fig. 33-8   Bariatric surgical procedures. **A,** Vertical banded gastroplasty creates a tubular stomach that is restrictive. **B,** Gastric banding systems are adjustable and reversible and can be placed laparoscopically. **C,** Biliopancreatic diversion with duodenal switch and vertical gastroplasty/sleeve gastrectomy. **D,** Roux-en-Y proximal gastric bypass. (From Association of Perioperative Registered Nurses: Standards, recommended practices, and guidelines, 2005 edition.)

The Roux-en-Y gastric bypass (RYGBP) (Fig. 33-8, *D*) combines both strategies by creating a small gastric pouch and anastomosing the jejunum to the pouch. Food then bypasses the lower stomach and duodenum, resulting in decreased absorption of digestive materials.[41,42]

PREOPERATIVE CARE

A thorough preoperative evaluation should be conducted to evaluate the patient's physical status and identify risk factors that may affect the postoperative course. Since obesity is associated with a higher incidence of comorbidities such as cardiovascular disease, hypertension, diabetes, gastroesophageal reflux, obstructive sleep apnea, and heart failure, an extensive workup may be required for the bariatric patient.[43] Before esophagectomy or pancreaticoduodenectomy, the patient may undergo multiple diagnostic tests such as CT, positron emission tomography (PET), and endoscopic ultrasound (EUS), to determine the invasiveness of the tumor.[39]

SURGICAL CONSIDERATIONS

Two approaches may be used for esophageal resection, transhiatal or transthoracic (see Figs. 33-5 and 33-6). In both approaches, the stomach is mobilized through an abdominal incision then transposed into the chest. The anastomosis of the stomach to the esophagus is then performed either in the chest (transthoracic) or in the neck (transhiatal). The approach selected depends upon the location of the tumor, the patient's overall health and pulmonary function, and the experience of the surgeon. After surgery the patient will have an NG tube in place that should not be manipulated because of the potential to cause damage to the anastomosis. Those who undergo transthoracic esophagectomy will have one or more chest tubes.[39,40]

Most bariatric procedures can be performed using either an open or laparoscopic surgical technique. Although laparoscopic approaches are more technically difficult to perform, they have largely replaced open procedures because they are associated with decreased pulmonary complications, less postoperative pain, reduced length of hospital stay, fewer wound infections, and an earlier return to full activity.[44,45] Open procedures are performed on patients who have had prior upper abdominal surgery, are morbidly obese, or who may not be able to tolerate the increased abdominal pressure associated with laparoscopic procedures.[40]

COMPLICATIONS AND MEDICAL MANAGEMENT

A number of complications are associated with GI surgery. They include, but are not limited to, respiratory failure, atelectasis, pneumonia, anastomotic leak, deep vein thrombosis, pulmonary embolus, and bleeding. It is important to note that the morbidly obese patient is at even greater risk for many postoperative complications.[44]

Pulmonary Complications. The risk for pulmonary complications is substantial after GI surgery, and adverse respiratory events such as atelectasis and pneumonia are twice as likely to occur in the obese patient.[46] Aggressive pulmonary toilet should be initiated in the immediate postoperative period. Early ambulation and adequate pain control will assist in reducing the risk of atelectasis development. Suctioning, chest physiotherapy, or bronchodilators may be needed to optimize pulmonary function. Patients should be closely monitored for the development of oxygenation problems. Treatment should be aimed at supporting adequate ventilation and gas exchange. Mechanical ventilation may be required in the event of respiratory failure.

Anastomotic Leak. An anastomotic leak is a severe complication of GI surgery. It occurs when there is a breakdown of the suture line in a surgical anastomosis and results in leakage of gastric or intestinal contents into the abdomen or mediastinum (transthoracic esophagectomy).[39,47] The clinical signs and symptoms of a leak can be very subtle and often go unrecognized. They include tachycardia, tachypnea, fever, abdominal pain, anxiety, and restlessness.[42] In the patient with an esophagectomy, a leak of the esophageal anastomosis may manifest itself as subcutaneous emphysema in the chest and neck.[39] If undetected, a leak can result in sepsis,

multiorgan failure, and death. Patients with progressive tachycardia and tachypnea should have a radiologic study (upper GI or CT scan) with contrast to rule out an anastomotic leak.[42,46] The type of treatment is dependent upon the severity of the leak. If the leak is small and well contained, it may be managed conservatively by making the patient NPO, administering antibiotics, and draining the fluid percutaneously. If the patient is deteriorating rapidly, an urgent laparotomy is indicated in order to repair the defect.[46,47]

Deep Vein Thrombosis/Pulmonary Embolism. Pulmonary embolism (PE) is a very serious complication of any surgical procedure. Deep vein thrombosis (DVT) prophylaxis should be initiated before surgery and continue until the patient is fully ambulatory to reduce the risk of clot development. Typically a combination of sequential compression devices and subcutaneous unfractionated heparin or low–molecular-weight heparin is used. Patients determined to be at high risk for PE may benefit from prophylactic inferior vena cava filter placement.[39,46]

Bleeding. Upper GI bleeding is an uncommon, but life-threatening complication of GI surgery. Early bleeding generally occurs at the site of the anastomosis and can usually be treated through endoscopic intervention. Surgical revision may be needed for persistent, uncontrolled bleeding. Late bleeding is usually a result of ulcer development. Medical therapy is aimed at the prevention of this complication through administration of H_2 antagonists or PPIs.[39,42]

POSTOPERATIVE NURSING MANAGEMENT

Nursing care of the patient who has had GI surgery incorporates a number of nursing diagnoses (see the Nursing Diagnoses feature on Gastrointestinal Surgery). Nursing management involves interventions aimed at optimizing oxygenation and ventilation, preventing atelectasis, providing comfort and emotional support, and maintaining surveillance for complications.

Pulmonary Management. Nursing interventions in the postoperative period are focused on promoting ventilation and adequate oxygenation and preventing complications such as atelectasis and pneumonia. After the patient is extubated, deep-breathing exercises and incentive spirometry should be initiated and then performed regularly. Early ambulation is encouraged to promote maximal lung inflation and thereby reduce the risk of pulmonary complications, as well as reduce the potential for pulmonary embolus.

Pain Management. It is imperative to appropriately manage the patient's pain after GI surgery. Adequate analgesia is necessary to promote mobility of the patient and decrease pulmonary complications. Initial pain management may be accomplished by IV opioid (morphine, Dilaudid) administration via a patient-controlled analgesia (PCA) pump or through continuous epidural infusion

NURSING DIAGNOSES

Gastrointestinal Surgery

- Ineffective Breathing Pattern related to decreased lung expansion
- Impaired Gas Exchange related to alveolar hypoventilation
- Decreased Cardiac Output related to alterations in preload
- Acute Pain related to transmission and perception of cutaneous, visceral, muscular, or ischemic impulses
- Anxiety related to threat to biologic, psychologic, and/or social integrity
- Disturbed Body Image related to actual change in body structure, function, or appearance
- Deficient Knowledge related to cognitive/perceptual learning limitations

of an opioid and local anesthetic (bupivacaine).[40,43] Oral pain medications can be started after an anastomosis leak is ruled out. Nonpharmacologic interventions such as positioning, application of heat or cold, and distraction may also be used. If the patient's pain is not being sufficiently relieved, the pain management service should be consulted.[39]

THERAPEUTIC MANAGEMENT

GASTROINTESTINAL INTUBATION

Because GI intubation is used so often in critical care units, it is important for nurses to know the clinical indications and responsibilities inherent in tube use. The four categories of GI tubes are based on function: NG suction tubes, long intestinal tubes, feeding tubes, and esophagogastric balloon tamponade tubes.

Nasogastric Suction Tubes. NG tubes remove fluid regurgitated into the stomach, prevent accumulation of swallowed air, may partially decompress the bowel, and reduce the patient's risk for aspiration. NG tubes also can be used for collecting specimens, assessing for the presence of blood, and administering tube feedings. The most common NG tubes are the single-lumen Levin tube and the double-lumen Salem sump. The Salem sump has one lumen that is used for suction and drainage, and another that allows air to enter the patient's stomach and prevents the tube from adhering to the gastric wall and damaging the mucosa. The tube is passed through the nose into the nasopharynx and then down through the pharynx into the esophagus and stomach. The length of time the NG tube remains in place depends on its use. The tube is then placed to gravity, low intermittent suction, or low continuous suction, or in rare instances is clamped.[48]

Nursing management is focused on preventing complications common to this therapy, such as ulceration and necrosis of the nares, esophageal reflux, esophagitis, esophageal erosion and stricture, gastric erosion, and dry mouth and parotitis from mouth breathing. In addition, interference with ventilation and coughing, aspiration, and loss of fluid and electrolytes can be critical problems. Interventions include irrigating the tube every 4 hours with normal saline, ensuring the blue air vent of the Salem sump is patent and maintained above the level of the patient's stomach, and providing frequent mouth and nares care. The Nursing Interventions Classification feature on Tube Care: Gastrointestinal, outlines the nursing activities for managing a patient with a GI tube.[49]

Long Intestinal Tubes. Miller-Abbott, Cantor, and Anderson tubes are examples of long, weighted-tip intestinal tubes that are placed either preoperatively or intraoperatively. The long length allows removal of contents from the intestine to treat an obstruction that cannot be managed by an NG tube. These tubes can decompress the small bowel and can splint the small bowel intraoperatively or postoperatively. Because progression of the tubes depends on bowel peristalsis, their use is contraindicated in patients with paralytic ileus and severe mechanical bowel obstructions. Older tubes like the Cantor and Miller-Abbott are rarely used today because the balloon and the distal end is filled with mercury; the newer Anderson tube has a weighted tungsten tip and is a safer option.[48]

Interventions used in the care of the patient with a long intestinal tube are similar to those with an NG tube. The patient should be observed for (1) gaseous distention of the balloon section, which makes removal difficult; (2) rupture of the balloon or spillage of mercury into the intestine; (3) overinflation of the balloon, which can lead to intestinal rupture; and (4) reverse intussusception if the tube is removed rapidly. Intestinal tubes should be removed slowly; usually 6 inches of the tube is withdrawn every hour.

Feeding Tubes. Small-diameter (8 Fr to 12 Fr) flexible feeding tubes, such as Dobhoff tubes, are commonly placed at the bedside for patients who can't take nourishment by mouth. The feeding tube may be inserted orally or nasally so that the tip ends up in either the stomach or duodenum. To facilitate passage into the gastrointestinal tract, these tubes generally have a weighted tungsten tip, and a guidewire is needed to prevent them from curling up in the back of the patient's throat. An x-ray film must be obtained to verify correct placement of the tube before initiating feeding. The tube should also be marked with indelible ink where it exits the

NIC	Tube Care: Gastrointestinal

Definition: Management of a patient with a gastrointestinal tube

Activities

Monitor for correct placement of the tube, per agency protocol

Verify placement with x-ray exam, per agency protocol

Connect tube to suction, if indicated

Secure tube to appropriate body part, with consideration for patient comfort and skin integrity

Irrigate tube, per agency protocol

Monitor for sensations of fullness, nausea, and vomiting

Monitor bowel sounds

Monitor for diarrhea

Monitor fluid and electrolyte status

Monitor amount, color, and consistency of nasogastric output

Replace the amount of gastrointestinal output with the appropriate intravenous (IV) solution, as ordered

Provide nose and mouth care 3 to 4 times daily or as needed

Provide hard candy or chewing gum to moisten mouth, as appropriate

Initiate and monitor delivery of enteral tube feedings, per agency protocol, as appropriate

Teach patient and family how to care for tube, when indicated

Provide skin care around tube insertion site

Remove tube when indicated

From Dochterman JM, Bulechek GM: *Nursing intervention classification (NIC),* ed 4, St Louis, 2004, Mosby.

mouth or nares so that the nurse can later verify that the tube has not been dislodged.[48]

Nursing management of the patient with a feeding tube includes prevention of complications and monitoring the tolerance of feeding. Before administering medications or feedings, it is important to make sure that the tube is in the patient's stomach or duodenum. Assessing the exit point marked on the tube helps to determine if the tube has maintained the same position. Looking for coiling in the mouth or throat can help detect upward displacement that may have occurred as a result of vomiting. The traditional practice of confirming placement by ascultating air inserted through the tube over the epigastrum is not reliable and is not recommended. If there is any doubt as to the tube's position, a repeat x-ray film should be obtained. During feedings, the HOB should be elevated 30 to 45 degrees to minimize the risk of aspiration, and gastric residuals should be checked at least every 8 hours. Increased residuals (greater than 150 ml), cramping, and abdominal distention may indicate intolerance of feeding, and the physician should be notified. Other interventions include nares and oral care and flushing the tube with normal saline or water to maintain patency.[49]

Esophagogastric Balloon Tamponade Tubes. Tamponading tubes may be used to stop bleeding in patients when endoscopic therapy fails or while waiting for surgical intervention. Although effective in 80% to 90% of patients, they are only a temporizing measure until definitive treatment can occur, and over 50% of patients will rebleed when the balloon is deflated.[13,50] Currently, three different types of balloon tamponade tubes are available. The Sengstaken-Blakemore tube has three lumens: one for the gastric balloon, one for the esophageal balloon, and one for the gastric suction (Fig. 33-9, *A*). The Linton-Nachlas tube also has three lumens: for the gastric balloon, gastric suction, and esophageal suction (Fig. 33-9, *B*). The Minnesota tube has four lumens: for the gastric balloon, the esophageal balloon, gastric suction, and esophageal suction (Fig. 33-9, *C*). The Sengstaken-Blakemore and Minnesota tubes are considered the standard for tamponade therapy; however, the Minnesota tube is preferable because it offers both a gastric and an esophageal balloon and allows suction to be applied both above and below the balloons (in the stomach and in the esophagus).[51]

Balloon tamponade tubes are inserted by the physician. Once the tube is passed into the stomach and placement is confirmed by gastric aspirate, the gastric balloon is slowly inflated to a total contents of 500 ml of air (or as specified by the tube manufacturer). After radiographic confirmation of placement, the tube is secured and placed under tension so that the gastric balloon places pressure on the gastroesophageal junction. Usually 1 to 3 pounds of tension are applied using a helmet with a constant-traction spring device. If bleeding continues, the esophageal balloon is inflated to a pressure of 25 to 45 mm Hg. Low intermittent suction is applied to both the gastric and esophageal ports. Typically balloons are deflated after 24 hours to prevent tissue necrosis; however, the gastric balloon may be inflated for up to 72 hours if needed. When discontinuing tamponade ther-

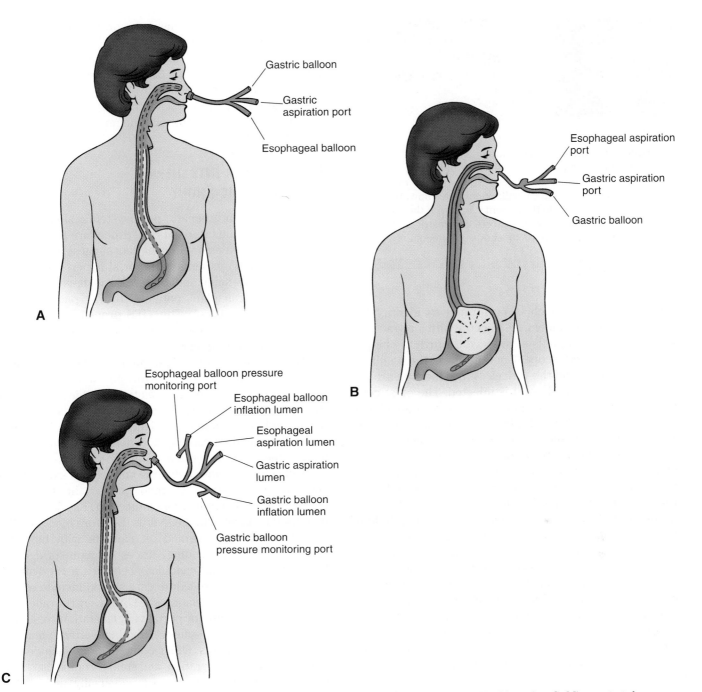

Fig. 33-9   Esophageal tamponade tubes. **A,** Sengstaken-Blakemore tube. **B,** Linton-Nachlas tube. **C,** Minnesota tube.

apy, the esophageal balloon pressure should be gradually decreased and the patient observed for evidence of bleeding. If no bleeding is noted, the gastric balloon may be deflated. If no further bleeding occurs, the tube is removed 4 hours later.[51]

Nursing management of the patient with a balloon tamponade tube includes monitoring for rebleeding and observing for complications of the tube. The most common complication is pulmonary aspiration, which can be limited by emptying the stomach and placing an endotracheal tube before passing the balloon tamponade tube.

Additional complications include esophageal erosion and rupture, balloon migration, and nasal necrosis (see the Patient Safety feature on Esophagogastric Balloon Tamponade Tubes).[37]

ENDOSCOPIC INJECTION THERAPY

Endoscopic injection therapy is used to control bleeding of varices and ulcers. It may be performed emergently, electively, or prophylactically. An endoscope is introduced through the patient's mouth, and endoscopy of the

PATIENT SAFETY ALERT

Esophagogastric Balloon Tamponade Tubes

Balloon migration can be a potentially life-threatening complication of this type of therapy. If the gastric balloon is allowed to slowly deflate or ruptures, the esophageal balloon migrates upward where it can occlude the patient's airway. If the patient develops respiratory distress, the gastric and esophageal balloon ports must be cut immediately.

esophagus and stomach is performed to identify the bleeding varices or ulcers. An injector with a retractable 23- to 25-gauge needle is introduced through the biopsy channel of the endoscope. Once in place, the needle is inserted in or around the varices or into the area around the ulcer, and a liquid agent is injected. The most commonly used agent is epinephrine, which results in localized vasoconstriction and enhanced platelet aggregation. Sclerosing agents such as ethanolamine, alcohol, and polidocanol also may be used. These agents cause an inflammatory reaction in the vessel that results in thrombosis and eventually a fibrous band. Repeated sclerotherapy results in the development of supportive scar tissue around the varices. Other agents used include fibrinogen and thrombin, which when injected together react to form an active fibrin clot, and cyanoacrylate glue, which is used as a sealant to stop the bleeding.[52,53]

Endoscopic injection therapy controls acute variceal bleeding in as many as 70% to 90% of patients.[52] Complications can vary from mild to severe and include esophageal perforation, extravasation of the injection agent, and strictures of the esophagus.[52] This procedure is contraindicated in patients with severe coagulopathies.[53]

ENDOSCOPIC VARICEAL LIGATION

Endoscopic variceal ligation involves applying bands or metal clips around the circumference of the bleeding varices to induce venous obstruction and control bleeding. One or two days after the procedure, necrosis and scar formation promote band and tissue sloughing. Fibrinous deposits within the healing ulcer potentiate vessel obliteration. Band ligation is accomplished via endoscopy, with 5 to 10 bands placed initially. The procedure may be repeated on an inpatient or outpatient basis over 1 to 4 weeks until all the varices are obliterated.[53]

Endoscopic variceal ligation controls bleeding approximately 86% of the time.[52] This procedure is reported to require fewer endoscopic treatment sessions and has a lower rebleeding rate and fewer complications than endoscopic sclerotherapy.[2,13] The most common complication of endoscopic variceal ligation is the development of superficial mucosal ulcers. Systemic complications are very rare.[9]

TRANSJUGULAR INTRAHEPATIC PORTOSYSTEMIC SHUNT

A transjugular intrahepatic portosystemic shunt (TIPS) is an angiographic interventional procedure for decreasing portal hypertension. Recent data suggest that TIPS is advocated in (1) patients with portal hypertension who are also experiencing active bleeding or have poor liver reserve, (2) transplant patients, or (3) patients with other operative risks.[16] The TIPS procedure is usually performed by a gastroenterologist, vascular surgeon, or interventional radiologist.

Portal hypertension is first confirmed via direct measurement of the pressure in the portal vein (gradient greater than 10 mm Hg). Cannulation is achieved through the internal jugular vein, and an angiographic catheter is advanced into the middle or right hepatic vein. The mid-hepatic vein is then catheterized, and a new route is created connecting the portal and hepatic veins, using a needle and guidewire with a dilating balloon. An expandable stainless steel stent is then placed in the liver parenchyma to maintain that connection (Fig. 33-10). The increased resistance in the liver is therefore bypassed.[53]

TIPS may be performed on patients with bleeding varices, refractory bleeding varices, or as a "bridge" to liver transplant if the candidate becomes hemodynamically unstable. Postprocedure care should include observation for overt (cannulation site) or covert (intrahepatic site) bleeding, hepatic or portal vein laceration (resulting in rapid loss of blood volume), and inadvertent puncture of surrounding organs. Other complications include bile duct trauma, stent migration, and stent thrombosis.[53] Portal hypertension recurs almost universally after TIPS, whereas stent stenosis occurs in 3% to 10% of patients.[16,53]

GASTRIC TONOMETRY

Gastric tonometry is an indirect means of assessing regional perfusion of the gut by measuring the CO_2 of the gastric mucosa. Because the gut is extremely sensitive to decreased oxygen delivery and decreased blood flow results in increased hydrogen ion production, lactate formation, and CO_2 accumulation, measurement of the partial pressure of CO_2 in the stomach may allow for early identification of hypoperfusion. This information provides the clinician with an enhanced clinical picture and

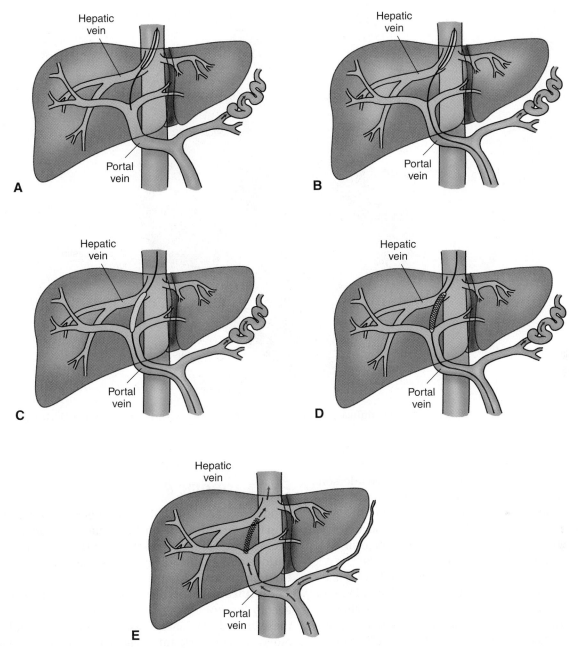

Fig. 33-10 Transjugular intrahepatic portosystemic shunt (TIPS). **A,** Needle directed though liver parenchyma to portal vein. **B,** Needle and guidewire passed down to midportal vein. **C,** Balloon dilation. **D,** Deployment of stent. **E,** Intrahepatic shunt from portal to hepatic vein. (From Zemel G et al: *JAMA* 266:391, 1991. ©1991 American Medical Association.)

assists with recognition and treatment of shock. This relatively noninvasive measurement is obtained via a modified nasogastric tube that has been combined with a gas-permeable silicone balloon system.[54]

There are two types of tonometry methods that are currently available: saline tonometry and air tonometry. In saline tonometry, the nasogastric tonometer (NGT) is primed to clear all air and then is inserted as a normal nasogastric tube (Fig. 33-11). Once inserted, the balloon lies in close proximity to the gastric mucosa. The balloon is then infused with anaerobic saline. The balloon is semipermeable to CO_2, which is produced by cells during the normal metabolic process. The level of CO_2 in the saline in the balloon equilibrates with the level of CO_2 in the gastric mucosal cells after 30 to 60 minutes. A sample of the saline is then withdrawn anaerobically and sent along with an arterial blood gas sample to the blood gas laboratory. The CO_2 from the saline and the HCO_3 from the arterial

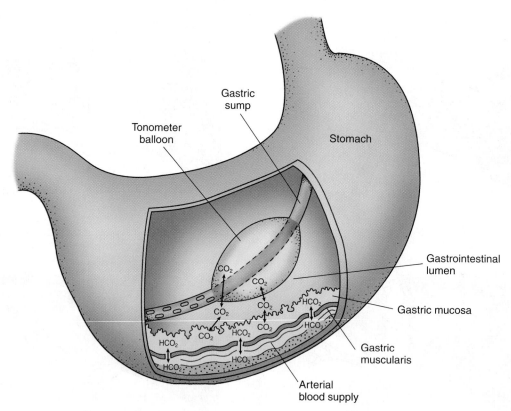

Fig. 33-11 Principles of $Paco_2$ and HCO_3^- diffusion in gastric tonometry. (From Clark CH, Gutierrez G: *Am J Crit Care* 1:53, 1992.)

blood gas sample are then correlated in the Henderson-Hasselbalch equation to determine the intramucosal pH (pHi). Air tonometry is a newer technique in which air from the balloon is automatically withdrawn and analyzed by an infrared sensor; the pHi and gut mucosal CO_2 ($PgCO_2$) are then displayed at 10-minute intervals.[54,55]

A normal pH is 7.35 to 7.45 and a normal $PgCO_2$ is 35 mm Hg to 45 mm Hg, the same as an arterial blood gas. In the presence of decreased gastric/splanchnic perfusion, such as occurs in shock, the $PgCO_2$ increases and pHi decreases as a result of anaerobic metabolism. The PCO_2 gap is the difference between the mucosal and the arterial CO_2 and has been proposed as a better indicator of gastrointestinal mucosal perfusion. A normal gap is less than 10 mm Hg. A widening gap indicates compromised blood flow to the splanchnic bed.[54,55]

Nursing considerations with the use of gastric tonometry monitoring include accurate user sampling procedures if using saline tonometry. Mistakes in sample drawing or timing may produce a measurement that misdirects therapy. Enteral feedings and an acidic gastric environment can also affect readings. If feedings are not distal to the pyloric valve, they should be discontinued at least 1 hour before measurement in order to avoid obtaining a falsely lowered pHi. Because accuracy is improved with a gastric pH of 4.0, patients monitored by tonometry should be on H_2 antagonists.[54,55]

PHARMACOLOGIC AGENTS

A number of pharmacologic agents are used in the care of patients with GI disorders. The Pharmacologic Management table on Gastrointestinal Disorders reviews the various agents and any special considerations necessary for administering them.

Antiulcer Agents. A number of different antiulcer agents are commonly used in the critical care setting; these include H_2 antagonists, gastric PPIs, and gastric mucosal agents. H_2 antagonists are used to decrease the volume and concentration of gastric secretions and control gastric pH, thus decreasing the incidence of stress-related upper GI bleeding. These agents work by blocking histamine stimulation of the H_2 receptors on the gastric parietal cells, thus reducing acid production. Although these drugs may be administered orally (PO), intramuscularly (IM), or by IV, they are generally given IV in the critical care setting.[56,57]

Proton-pump inhibitors decrease gastric acid secretion by binding to the proton pump, thus blocking the release of acid from the gastric parietal cells. PPIs are potent acid inhibitors and have greater suppressive ability than the H_2 agonists.[57] Five PPIs are currently available in the United States; however, pantoprazole is the only PPI available for intravenous administration. The oral PPIs are formulated as enteric coated tablets or as delayed-

Pharmacologic Management: Gastrointestinal Disorders

MEDICATION	DOSAGE	ACTIONS	SPECIAL CONSIDERATIONS
Antacids	30-90 ml q1-2 hr PO or NG; possibly titrated to NG pH	Used to buffer stomach acid and raise gastric pH	Can cause diarrhea or constipation and electrolyte disturbances Irrigate NG tube with water after administration because antacids can clog tube
Histamine-2 Antagonists Cimetidine (Tagamet) Ranitidine (Zantac) Famotidine (Pepcid)	300 mg q6h IV or PO 150 mg q12h PO or 50 mg q8h IV 40 mg daily PO or 20 mg q12h IV	Used to reduce volume and concentration of gastric secretions	Side effects include CNS toxicity (confusion or delirium) and thrombocytopenia Separate administration of antacids and histamine blocking agents by 1 hour
Gastric Mucosal Agents Sucralfate (Carafate)	1 g q6h NG or PO	Forms an ulcer-adherent complex with proteinaceous exudates Covers the ulcer and protects against acid, pepsin, and bile salts	Requires an acid medium for activation; do not administer within 30 minutes of an antacid May cause severe constipation May cause decreased absorption of certain drugs
Gastric Proton-Pump Inhibitors Omeprazole (Prilosec) Lansoprazole (Prevacid) Rabeprazole (Acipnex) Esomeprazole (Nexium) Pantoprazole (Protonix)	20-40 mg q12h PO 15-30 mg q24h PO 20 mg q24PO 20-40 mg q24h PO 40mg q12-24h PO 80 mg IV bolus followed by 8 mg/hr × 72° IV infusion	Inactivates acid, or hydrogen, acid pump, thus blocking secretion of hydrochloric acid by gastric parietal cells	Capsules should be swallowed intact May increase levels of phenytoin, diazepam, warfarin May administer concomitantly with antacids
Vasopressin (Pitressin Synthetic)	Loading dose of 20 units over 20 min IV followed by 0.2-0.6 units/min IV infusion	Decreases splanchnic blood flow, thus reducing portal pressure	Side effects include coronary, mesenteric, and peripheral vasoconstriction May be administered concurrently with nitroglycerin to minimize side effects
Octreotide (Sandostatin)	Loading dose of 50-100 mcg IV followed by 25-50 mcg/hr IV infusion	Decreases splanchnic blood flow, thus reducing portal pressure	May cause hyperglycemia or hypoglycemia when initiating the drip and changing dosages

PO, By mouth; *NG,* nasogastric; *IV,* intravenous; *CNS,* central nervous system.

release capsules containing enteric coated granules. Absorption occurs in an alkaline environment and thus begins only after the granules leave the stomach and enter the duodenum.[58,59] To administer via an NG or gastrostomy tube, the capsule can be opened and the granules either mixed with 8.4% sodium bicarbonate to form a suspension or mixed with 40 ml of apple juice. If administered in juice, the tube must be flushed with additional juice to ensure that all the granules have been cleared.[58]

Unlike H_2 antagonists or gastric PPIs, sucralfate does not affect gastric acid concentration but rather exerts its action locally. Sucralfate reacts with hydrochloric acid to form a sticky, pastelike substance that adheres to the surface of the ulcer and shields it from pepsin, acid, and bile. Sucralfate predominantly binds to damaged GI mucosa, with minimal adherence to normal tissue. It is administered orally or via a gastric tube. Sucralfate should not be crushed but may be dissolved in 10 ml of water to form a slurry. It is also available as a suspension.[56,57]

Vasopressin. As discussed earlier, vasopressin is a treatment modality used to control gastric ulcer and variceal bleeding. It is administered intraarterially, through a catheter inserted into the right or left gastric artery (via the femoral artery, aorta, and celiac trunk), or intravenously. It causes splanchnic and systemic vasoconstriction, subsequently reducing portal blood flow and pressure.[53]

A major side effect of the drug is systemic vasoconstriction, which can result in cardiac ischemia and chest pain, hypertension, acute heart failure, dysrhythmias, phlebitis, bowel ischemia, and cerebrovascular accident. These side effects can be offset with concurrent administration of nitroglycerin. Other complications include bradycardia and fluid retention. Nursing responsibilities with the use of this therapy include maintenance of a patent infusion line and continuous monitoring for vasoconstrictive complications of therapy.[54]

Somatostatin and Octreotide. Somatostatin is a peptide that is administered parenterally in the acutely bleeding cirrhotic patient. It reduces splanchnic vasodilation and portal pressure through the inhibition of secretion of various vasodilator hormones, and is as effective as vasopressin in treating variceal bleeding with minimal side effects. Octreotide is a commonly used long-acting synthetic analog of somatostatin.[53]

REFERENCES

1. Conrad SA: Acute upper gastrointestinal bleeding in critically ill patients: causes and treatment modalities, *Crit Care Med* 30:S365, 2002.
2. Kupfer Y, Cappell MS, Tessler S: Acute gastrointestinal bleeding in the intensive care unit: the intensivist's perspective, *Gastroenterol Clin North Am* 29:275, 2000.
3. Huang CS, Lichtenstein DR: Nonvariceal upper gastrointestinal bleeding, *Gastroenterol Clin North Am* 32:1053, 2003.
4. Beejay U, Wolfe MM: Acute gastrointestinal bleeding in the intensive care unit: the gastroenterologist's perspective, *Gastroenterol Clin North Am* 29:309, 2000.
5. Zuckerman GR, Prakash C: Acute lower intestinal bleeding. Part II. Etiology, therapy, and outcomes, *Gastrointest Endosc* 49:228, 1999.
6. Fallah MA, Prakash C, Edmundowics S: Acute gastrointestinal bleeding, *Med Clin North Am* 84:1183, 2000.
7. Fennerty MB: Pathophysiology of the upper gastrointestinal tract in the critically ill patient: rationale for the therapeutic benefits of acid suppression, *Crit Care Med* 30:S351, 2002.
8. McCance KL, Huether SE: *Pathophysiology: the biologic basis for disease in adults and children,* ed 4, St Louis, 2002, Mosby.
9. Smoot DT, Go MF, Cryer B: Peptic ulcer disease, *Prim Care* 28:487, 2001.
10. Moss SF, Sood S: *Helicobacter pylori, Curr Opin Infect Dis* 16:445, 2002.
11. Luketic VA, Sanyal AJ: Esophageal varices. I. Clinical presentation, medical therapy, and endoscopic therapy, *Gastroenterol Clin North Am* 29:337, 2000.
12. Sharara AI, Rockey DC: Medical progress: gastroesophageal variceal hemorrhage, *N Engl J Med* 345:669, 2001.
13. Harry R, Wendon J: Management of variceal bleeding, *Curr Opin Crit Care* 8:164, 2002.
14. Velayos F: Upper and lower gastrointestinal bleeding in the critically ill patient. In Parsons PE, Wiener-Kronish JP, editors: *Critical care secrets: questions and answers reveal the secrets to effective critical care,* ed 3, Philadelphia, 2003, Hanley & Belfus.
15. Barkun A et al: Consensus recommendations for managing patients with nonvariceal upper gastrointestinal bleeding, *Ann Intern Med* 139:843, 2003.
16. Stabile BE, Stamos MJ: Surgical management of gastrointestinal bleeding, *Gastroenterol Clin North Am* 29:189, 2000.
17. Luketic VA, Sanyal AJ: Esophageal varices. II. TIPS (transjugular intrahepatic portosystemic shunt) and surgical therapy, *Gastroenterol Clin North Am* 29:387, 2000.
18. Bank S et al: Evaluation of factors that have reduced mortality from acute pancreatitis over the past 20 years, *J Clin Gastroenterol* 35:50, 2002.
19. Hughes E: Understanding the care of patients with acute pancreatitis, *Nursing Standard* 18:45, 2003.
20. Yousaf M, McCallion K, Diamond T: Management of severe acute pancreatitis, *Br J Surg* 90:407, 2003.
21. Hale AS, Moseley MJ, Warner SC: Treating pancreatitis in the acute care setting, *Dimens Crit Care Nurs* 19(4):15, 2000.
22. Sakorafas GH, Tsioyou AG: Etiology and pathogenesis of acute pancreatitis: current concepts, *J Clin Gastroenterol* 30:343, 2000.
23. Bentrem DJ, Joehl RJ: Pancreas: healing response in critical illness, *Crit Care Med* 31:S582, 2003.
24. Faigel DO, Metz DC: Acute pancreatitis. In Hanson CW, Manaker SM, editors: *The intensive care unit manual,* Philadelphia, 2001, Saunders.
25. Wrobleski DM, Barth MM, Oyen LJ: Necrotizing pancreatitis: pathophysiology, diagnosis, and acute care management, *AACN Clin Issues* 10:464, 1999.
26. Bowyer MW: Acute pancreatitis. In Parsons PE, Wiener-Kronish JP, editors: *Critical care secrets: questions and answers reveal the secrets to effective critical care,* ed 3, Philadelphia, 2003, Hanley & Belfus.
27. Cothren C, Burch JM: Acute pancreatitis. In Harken AH, Moore EE, editors: *Abernathy's surgical secrets: questions and answers reveal the secrets to successful surgery,* ed 5, Philadelphia, 2004, Hanley & Belfus.
28. Cooperman AM: Surgical treatment of pancreatic pseudocysts, *Surg Clin North Am* 81:411, 2001.
29. Venu RP et al: Endoscopic transpapillary drainage of pancreatic abscess: technique and results, *Gastrointest Endosc* 51:391, 2000.
30. Neff R: Pancreatic pseudocysts and fluid collections: percutaneous approach, *Surg Clin North Am* 81:399, 2001.
31. Thompson DR: Narcotic analgesic effects on the sphincter of Oddi: a review of the data and therapeutic implications in treating pancreatitis, *Am J Gastroenterol* 96:1266, 2001.
32. Farmer DG et al: Liver transplantation for fulminant hepatic failure: experience with more than 200 patients over a 17-year period, *Ann Surg* 237:666, 2003.
33. Gill RQ, Sterling RK: Acute liver failure, *J Clin Gastroenterol* 33:191, 2001.
34. Riordan SM, Williams R: Fulminant hepatic failure, *Clin Liver Dis* 4:25, 2000.
35. Riaz Q, Sterking RK: Acute liver failure, *J Clin Gastroenterol* 33:191, 2001.
36. Jones EA: Pathogenesis of hepatic encephalopathy, *Clin Liver Dis* 4:467, 2000.

37. Lucey MR: Acute liver failure. In Hanson CW, Manaker SM, editors: *The intensive care unit manual,* Philapelphia, 2001, Saunders.

38. Sass DA, Shakil AO: Fulminant hepatic failure. *Gastroenterol Clin North Am* 32:1195, 2003.

39. Mackenzie DJ, Popplewell PK, Billingsley KG: Care of patients after esophagectomy, *Crit Care Nurse* 24:16, 2004.

40. Jaffe RA, Samuels SI: *Anesthesiologist's manual of surgical procedures,* ed 3, Philadelphia, 2004, Lippincott Williams & Wilkins.

41. Association of Perioperative Registered Nurses: AORN bariatric surgery guideline, *AORN J* 79:1026, 2004.

42. Ukleja A, Stone RL: Medical and gastroenterologic management of the post-bariatric patient, *J Clin Gastroenterol* 38:312, 2004.

43. Abir F, Bell, R: Assessment and management of the obese patient, *Crit Care Med* 32:S87, 2004.

44. Miller TA, Savas JF: Gastric surgery, *Curr Opin Gastroenterol* 17:533, 2001.

45. Brolin RE: Bariatric surgery and long-term control of morbid obesity, *JAMA* 288:2793, 2002.

46. Levi D et al: Critical care of the obese and bariatric surgery patient, *Crit Care Clin* 19:11, 2003.

47. Rubesin SE, Levine MS: Radiologic diagnosis of gastrointestinal perforation, *Radiol Clin North Am* 41:1095, 2003.

48. Noble KA: Name that tube, *Nursing* 33:56, 2003.

49. Kowalak JP, Hughes AS, Mills JE: *Best practices: A guide to excellence in nursing care,* Philadelphia, 2003, Lippincott Williams & Wilkins.

50. Stotland BR, Ginsberg GG: Upper gastrointestinal bleeding. In Hanson CW, Manaker SM, editors: *The intensive care unit manual,* Philapelphia, 2001, Saunders.

51. Day MW: Esophagogastric tamponade tube. In Lynn-McHale DJ, Carlson KK, editors: *The AACN procedure manual for critical care,* ed 4, Philapelphia, 2001, Saunders.

52. Savides TJ, Jensen DM: Therapeutic endoscopy for nonvariceal gastrointestinal bleeding, *Gastroenterol Clin North Am* 29:465, 2000.

53. Comar KM, Sanyal AJ: Portal hypertensive bleeding, *Gastroenterol Clin North Am* 32:1079, 2003.

54. Ruffolo DC, Headley JM: Regional carbon dioxide monitoring: a different look at tissue perfusion, *AACN Clin Issues* 14:168, 2003.

55. Heard SO: Gastric tonometry: the hemodynamic monitor of choice, *Chest* 123:469S, 2003.

56. McKenry LM, Salerno E: *Pharmacology in nursing,* ed 21, St Louis, 2003, Mosby.

57. Katzung BG: *Basic and clinical pharmacology,* ed 8, New York, 2002, Lange Medical Books/McGraw-Hill.

58. Der G: An overview of proton pump inhibitors, *Gastroenterol Nurs* 26:182, 2003.

59. Welage LS: Pharmacologic features of proton pump inhibitors and their potential relevance to clinical practice, *Gastroenterol Clin North Am* 32:S25, 2003.

UNIT

VIII

ENDOCRINE
ALTERATIONS

Endocrine Anatomy and Physiology

*M*aintaining dynamic equilibrium among the various cells, tissues, organs, and systems of the human body is a highly complex and specialized process. Two systems regulate these critical relationships: the nervous system and the endocrine system. The nervous system communicates by nerve impulses that control skeletal muscle, smooth muscle tissue, and cardiac muscle tissue. The endocrine system controls and communicates by distributing potent hormones throughout the body. (Fig. 34-1 lists the endocrine glands and their hormones, target tissues, and actions.) When stimulated, the endocrine glands secrete hormones into surrounding body fluids. Once in circulation, these hormones travel to specific target tissues, where they exert a pronounced effect. Receptors found on or within these specialized target tissue cells are equipped with molecules that recognize the hormone and bind it to the cell, producing a specific response.

PANCREAS

ANATOMY

The pancreas is a long, triangular organ. It is clinically described as consisting of a *head*, *body*, and *tail*. The "head" end of the organ lies in the C-shaped curvature of the duodenum, and the "tail" extends behind and below the stomach toward the spleen. It is approximately 15 cm (6 inches) long and 4 cm (1 to 2 inches) wide. The pancreas receives arterial blood supply from the pancreaticoduodenal arteries that branch from the superior mesenteric artery. Venous drainage is via the pancreaticoduodenal veins that ultimately empty into the portal vein. The pancreas has two major and different functions, one digestive and one hormonal.

Exocrine. Specialized exocrine cells within the pancreas secrete digestive enzymes into a duct that is 3 millimeter (mm) wide that transverses the length of the pancreas and empties into the duodenum. Pancreas exocrine anatomy is illustrated in Fig. 31-8, and pancreatic digestive juices are discussed as part of the physiology

of the gastrointestinal system. Most pancreatic tissue is devoted to production of exocrine digestive juices.

Endocrine. The pancreas also contains specialized endocrine cells that secrete hormones directly into the bloodstream. The endocrine tissue is less than 5% of the total volume of the pancreas. The function of the endocrine hormones is the focus of the following discussion.

PHYSIOLOGY

Clusters of cells that appear to form tiny islands among the exocrine cells accomplish the endocrine functions of the pancreas. These "islands" are known as the *islets of Langerhans* and are composed of four distinct cell types. The cells are known as *alpha*, *beta*, *delta*, and *PP* cells. The location of the cells that produce these hormones is shown in Fig. 34-2. Alpha cells secrete glucagon, beta cells secrete insulin, delta cells secrete somatostatin, and PP cells secrete pancreatic polypeptide hormone. Glucagon, insulin, somatostatin, and polypeptide hormones are released into the surrounding capillaries to empty into the portal vein, where they are distributed to target cells in the liver. They then go into general circulation to reach other target cells.

Insulin. Insulin is a potent anabolic hormone whose production is stimulated by the presence of glucose. Insulin is produced by the beta cells of the pancreas. It is the only hormone produced in the body that directly lowers glucose levels in the bloodstream. Insulin is responsible for the storage of carbohydrate, protein, and fat nutrients.[1] Insulin also augments the transport of potassium into the cells, decreases the mobilization of fats, and stimulates protein synthesis (Table 34-1). Box 34-1 defines terms commonly used when discussing glucose/insulin balance. The major stimulant for insulin secretion is an elevation of serum glucose. The greater the rise in blood glucose, the more insulin the normal pancreas will produce. Other hormones inhibit the release of insulin, as listed in Box 34-2.

In patients with symptoms of diabetes, beta cell destruction has already occurred. In type 1 diabetes all of

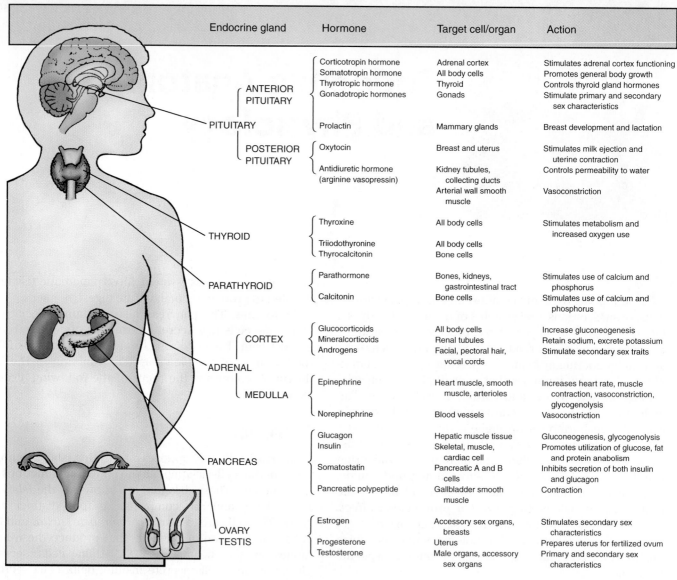

Endocrine gland		Hormone	Target cell/organ	Action
PITUITARY	ANTERIOR PITUITARY	Corticotropin hormone	Adrenal cortex	Stimulates adrenal cortex functioning
		Somatotropin hormone	All body cells	Promotes general body growth
		Thyrotropic hormone	Thyroid	Controls thyroid gland hormones
		Gonadotropic hormones	Gonads	Stimulate primary and secondary sex characteristics
		Prolactin	Mammary glands	Breast development and lactation
	POSTERIOR PITUITARY	Oxytocin	Breast and uterus	Stimulates milk ejection and uterine contraction
		Antidiuretic hormone (arginine vasopressin)	Kidney tubules, collecting ducts	Controls permeability to water
			Arterial wall smooth muscle	Vasoconstriction
THYROID		Thyroxine	All body cells	Stimulates metabolism and increased oxygen use
		Triiodothyronine	All body cells	
		Thyrocalcitonin	Bone cells	
PARATHYROID		Parathormone	Bones, kidneys, gastrointestinal tract	Stimulates use of calcium and phosphorus
		Calcitonin	Bone cells	Stimulates use of calcium and phosphorus
ADRENAL	CORTEX	Glucocorticoids	All body cells	Increase gluconeogenesis
		Mineralcorticoids	Renal tubules	Retain sodium, excrete potassium
		Androgens	Facial, pectoral hair, vocal cords	Stimulate secondary sex traits
	MEDULLA	Epinephrine	Heart muscle, smooth muscle, arterioles	Increases heart rate, muscle contraction, vasoconstriction, glycogenolysis
		Norepinephrine	Blood vessels	Vasoconstriction
PANCREAS		Glucagon	Hepatic muscle tissue	Gluconeogenesis, glycogenolysis
		Insulin	Skeletal, muscle, cardiac cell	Promotes utilization of glucose, fat and protein anabolism
		Somatostatin	Pancreatic A and B cells	Inhibits secretion of both insulin and glucagon
		Pancreatic polypeptide	Gallbladder smooth muscle	Contraction
OVARY		Estrogen	Accessory sex organs, breasts	Stimulates secondary sex characteristics
TESTIS		Progesterone	Uterus	Prepares uterus for fertilized ovum
		Testosterone	Male organs, accessory sex organs	Primary and secondary sex characteristics

Fig. 34-1 Location of endocrine glands with hormones, target cell/organ, and hormone action.

Table 34-1 — Pancreatic Endocrine Cells, Hormones, Stimulant Release Factor, Target Tissue, and Response/Action

Cell	Hormone	Stimulant Release Factor	Target Tissue	Response/Action
Alpha	Glucagons	↓Glucose Exercise ↑Amino acids SNS stimulation	Hepatocyte Myocyte	↑Glucose in bloodstream ↑Gluconeogenesis ↑Glycogenolysis Fat mobilization Protein mobilization
Beta	Insulin	Glucose	Skeletal cells Muscle cells Cardiac cells	↓Blood glucose ↓Fat mobilization ↑Fat storage ↓Protein mobilization ↑Protein synthesis ↑Glucogenesis
Delta	Somatostatin	Hyperglycemia	A cells B cells	↓Blood glucose ↓Glycogen secretion ↓Insulin secretion
PP	Pancreatic polypeptide	Acute hypoglycemia	Gallbladder Smooth muscle	↑Gallbladder contraction ↓Pancreatic enzyme

SNS, Sympathetic nervous system.

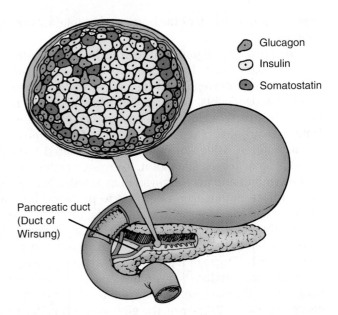

Glucagon

Insulin

Somatostatin

Pancreatic duct (Duct of Wirsung)

Fig. 34-2 Macroscopic and microscopic structure of the islets of Langerhans and of the pancreas.

Box 34-2

AGENTS THAT RELEASE OR INHIBIT INSULIN

INSULIN RELEASE (MAJOR STIMULANT: ELEVATED BLOOD GLUCOSE LEVEL)	INSULIN INHIBITION (MAJOR INHIBITOR: LOW BLOOD GLUCOSE LEVEL)
Hormones	
Glucagons	Somatostatin
Corticotropic hormone	Norepinephrine
Thyrotropin	Epinephrine
Somatotropin	
Glucocorticoids	
Secretin	
Gastrin	
Drugs	
β-adrenergic stimulators	β-adrenergic blocking
Sulfonylurea	agents
Theophylline	Diazoxide
Acetylcholine	Phenytoin
	Thiazide/sulfonamide
	diuretics

the beta cells are nonfunctional. In type 2 diabetes, about 50% of the beta cells are destroyed by the time the patient exhibits signs and symptoms of diabetes.[2]

Carbohydrate Anabolism. Glucose is admitted to the skeletal, cardiac, and adipose cells for use as energy in the presence of effective insulin. The movement of glucose from the circulation into the intracellular compartment reduces the presence of glucose in the bloodstream and helps preserve the blood's osmolality. Simultaneously, glucose is available to the cell as its main energy source. Excess glucose, in the form of glycogen, is stored in the hepatic and muscle cells for use as fuel at a later time.

The central nervous system (CNS) is freely permeable to glucose and does not rely on insulin for the transport of glucose across the cell membrane. The CNS cells require glucose and are unable to use the end product of gluconeogenesis for energy. Hyperglycemia from decreased insulin levels does not damage brain cells; however, these cells cannot survive the glucose deficiency (hypoglycemia) that occurs from hypersecretion of insulin. Brain cells store only a minimum of glycogen for energy release.

Fat Anabolism. Adequate, effective insulin levels also affect fat metabolism. In the presence of insulin, fat is stored in connective tissues, thereby reducing fat mobilization and fat catabolism. Dyslipidemias are strongly associated with type 2 diabetes.[3] Disorders of carbohydrate and fat metabolism are also associated with the metabolic syndrome, a precursor to diabetes and cardiovascular disease.[4]

Protein Sparing. Insulin facilitates the transfer of glucose across the cell wall to the cell receptor site. By having glucose (carbohydrate) available as the body's fuel source, protein is spared from use as energy. Protein is then available for critical protein synthesis, for amino acid active transport into the cells, for construction of blood proteins, and for the conversion of ribonucleic acid (RNA) into new protein. Thus protein metabolism also benefits from an adequate insulin supply. Only in acute hyperglycemia of diabetic ketoacidosis (DKA) or in starvation states does the body use protein for energy sources.[5]

Glucagon. Glucagon, synthesized by alpha cells in the pancreas, has the opposite effect of insulin. Glucagon counterregulates insulin levels and raises blood glucose levels. It is a potent gluconeogenic hormone. By means of gluconeogenesis, it can form glucose from noncarbohydrate sources such as fat and protein when required. Glucagon release is stimulated by low blood glucose levels, starvation, exercise, or stimulation of the sympathetic nervous system as listed in Box 34-3. The purpose of glucagon release is to protect the body from the consequences of hypoglycemia.

Initially glucagon stimulates the release of glycogen stored in the liver and muscle cells to meet short-term energy needs. Through a process called *glycogenolysis*, the glycogen stored in the liver and muscles is converted back into a glucose form to be used by the cells. If the energy needs are long-term, the glucagon stimulates glucose release through the more complex process of *gluconeogenesis*. In gluconeogenesis, fat and protein nutrients are rapidly broken down into end products that are then changed into glucose.

A normal blood glucose level is maintained in the healthy body by the insulin/glucagon ratio. When the blood glucose level is high, insulin is released and glucagon is inhibited. When blood glucose levels are low, glucagon rather than insulin is released in order to raise blood glucose (see Box 34-3).

Somatostatin. Somatostatin is a hormone that is produced in the pancreatic delta cells. It inhibits the release of both insulin and glucagon. Somatostatin de-creases glucagon secretion, and in high quantities it decreases insulin release (see Table 34-1). Hyperglycemia stimulates the activity of the delta cells. It is theorized that the release of insulin enables somatostatin to control beta cell activity. Somatostatin may be involved in the regulation of the postprandial influx of glucose into cells. Somatostatin-analog drugs are now commercially available after ingestion of a meal; however, the clinical role of these agents is still being researched.[6]

Pancreatic Polypeptide. The role of pancreatic polypeptide, synthesized by the PP cells within the islets of Langerhans, is not yet completely understood. Pancreatic polypeptide release can be stimulated by acute hypoglycemia or by an intake that is high in protein and low in carbohydrate. The effect of hypersecretion versus hyposecretion of this hormone is not yet been identified. The hormone represses pancreatic enzyme secretion and relaxes the smooth muscle tissue of the gallbladder.

PITUITARY GLAND AND HYPOTHALAMUS

ANATOMY

The hypothalamus is linked to the pituitary gland in two distinct ways: a vascular network connects the anterior portion of the pituitary with the hypothalamus, whereas a separate pathway of nerve fibers connects the posterior pituitary with the hypothalamus. Understanding the proximity of the hypothalamus and the pituitary gland is necessary to appreciate the correlation that exists between these organs.

The hypothalamus lies in the base of the brain, superior to the pituitary gland. It is composed of specialized nervous tissue responsible for the integrated functioning of the nervous system and endocrine system, which is termed *neuroendocrine control*. The hypothalamus weighs approximately 4 g and forms the walls and lower portion of the third ventricle of the brain. The area composing the floor of the ventricle thickens in the center and elongates. It is from this funnel-shaped portion, called the *infundibular stalk* (or *stem*), that the pituitary gland is suspended as illustrated in Fig. 34-3. The infundibular stalk contains a rich vascular supply and a network of communicating neurons that travel from the hypothalamus to the pituitary. The vascular network and neural pathways transport chemical and neural signals and maintain constant communication between the nervous system and the endocrine system.

The pituitary gland is also called the *hypophysis*. It is attached below the hypothalamus and is found recessed in the base of the cranial cavity in a hollow depression of the sphenoid bone known as the *sella turcica*. Secured in such a protected environment, the pituitary is one of the most inaccessible endocrine glands in humans. Yet it is because of this very location that the pituitary gland is

---

Box 34-3

INSULIN/GLUCAGON RATIO AND ITS EFFECT ON CARBOHYDRATE, FAT, AND PROTEIN METABOLISM

BALANCED INSULIN/GLUCAGON	DECREASED INSULIN/ INCREASED GLUCAGON
↑Use of glucose by cells	↓Use of glucose by cells
↑Movement of potassium intracellularly	↓Movement of potassium intracellullarly
↑Carbohydrate metabolism	↑Blood glucose
↓Gluconeogenesis	↑Gluconeogenesis
↑Glycogen storage	↓Glycogen storage
↓Glycogenolysis	↑Glycogenolysis
↓Lipolysis	↑Lipolysis
↓Fat mobilization	↑Fat mobilization
↑Fat storage	↓Fat stores
↓Protein mobilization	↑Hepatic metabolism fats
↑Protein synthesis	↑Ketogenesis
	↑Mobilization of protein
	↑Proteolysis
	↑Lipoprotein

susceptible to injury from surgical and accidental trauma to the face and head.[7] The pituitary is composed of the anterior lobe and the posterior lobe (see Fig. 34-3). Each component within the pituitary has its own origin, morphology, and function.

Anterior Pituitary. The anterior lobe of the pituitary, also called the *adenohypophysis*, is the largest portion of the gland. It communicates with the hypothalamus by means of a vascular network. The glandular tissue of the anterior pituitary produces several hormones including adrenocorticotropic hormone (ACTH), thyroid-stimulating hormone (TSH), follicle-stimulating hormone (FSH), luteinizing hormone (LH), growth hormone, and prolactin. Information about all the hormones, their target tissue, and their action is found in Fig. 34-1.

Posterior Pituitary. The posterior lobe of the pituitary gland is also known as the *neurohypophysis*. It retains its continuity with the hypothalamus by means of neural fibers running through the infundibular stalk. The neurohypophysis has no glandular properties but functions as an extension of the hypothalamus. It collects, stores, and later releases hormones that are produced in the hypothalamus. Oxytocin and antidiuretic hormone (ADH) are both manufactured in the hypothalamus and stored in the posterior pituitary.

PHYSIOLOGY

The hypothalamus gland is known as the master gland because of the major influence it has over all areas of body functioning. The hypothalamus controls pituitary gland action and response by secreting substances termed *release-inhibiting factors*. These factors then control the release or inhibition of hormones. Thyrotropin-releasing hormone (TRH) is an example of a release-inhibiting factor. Virtually every function necessary to maintaining the human body in a state of dynamic equilibrium is regulated in this manner. One of the most important hormones to understand in caring for the critically ill patient is ADH.[8]

Antidiuretic Hormone. ADH, known also as *arginine vasopressin*, is an important hormone responsible for regulating fluid balance within the body. ADH acts via specialized vasopressin receptors (V receptors) in specific target tissue[9]:

V_1 receptors—in arterial wall

V_2 receptors—in renal tissue

V_3 receptors—in pituitary tissue

ADH (vasopressin) has two functions. Via the V_1 receptors it constricts smooth muscles within the arterial wall; via V_2 receptors it regulates fluid balance by altering the permeability of the kidney tubule to water.[9] ADH also contributes to control of the sodium level in the extracellular fluid by control of plasma osmolality. The sodium ion concentration in the plasma largely determines plasma osmolality.[10] Osmoreceptors, believed to be sodium receptors, are located in the hypothalamus and are sensitive to changes in the circulating plasma osmolality. A low sodium level is associated with a low serum osmolality.[10] When sodium levels rise, plasma osmolality increases. ADH is then released to stimulate water resorption at the nephron to maintain sodium balance. This process decreases water loss from the body and subsequently concentrates and reduces urine volume. Fluid conserved in this manner is returned to the circulating plasma, where it dilutes the concentration (osmolality) of plasma, as shown in Fig. 34-4.

The release of ADH increases with hypovolemia. Primarily, the plasma osmotic pressure and the volume of circulating blood regulate the release of ADH. Stretch receptors located in the left atrium are sensitive to volume changes in the plasma that may be caused by vomiting, diarrhea, or blood loss. Hemorrhage, sufficient to lower the blood pressure, or emesis, sufficient to reduce fluid volume, will stimulate the release of ADH. Other factors capable of influencing ADH secretion are pain, stress, malignant disease, surgical intervention, alcohol, and drugs.[7-9,11] See Box 34-4 for additional factors that affect ADH (vasopressin) levels.

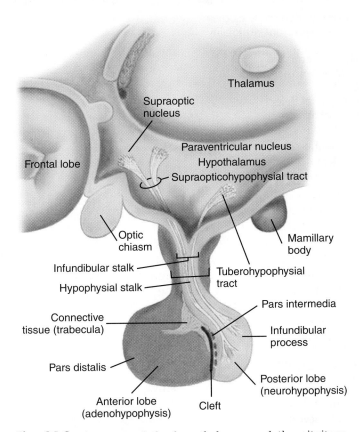

Fig. 34-3 Anatomy of the hypothalamus and the pituitary gland and their location in the skull. (From Thompson JM et al: *Mosby's clinical nursing*, ed 5, St Louis, 2002, Mosby.)

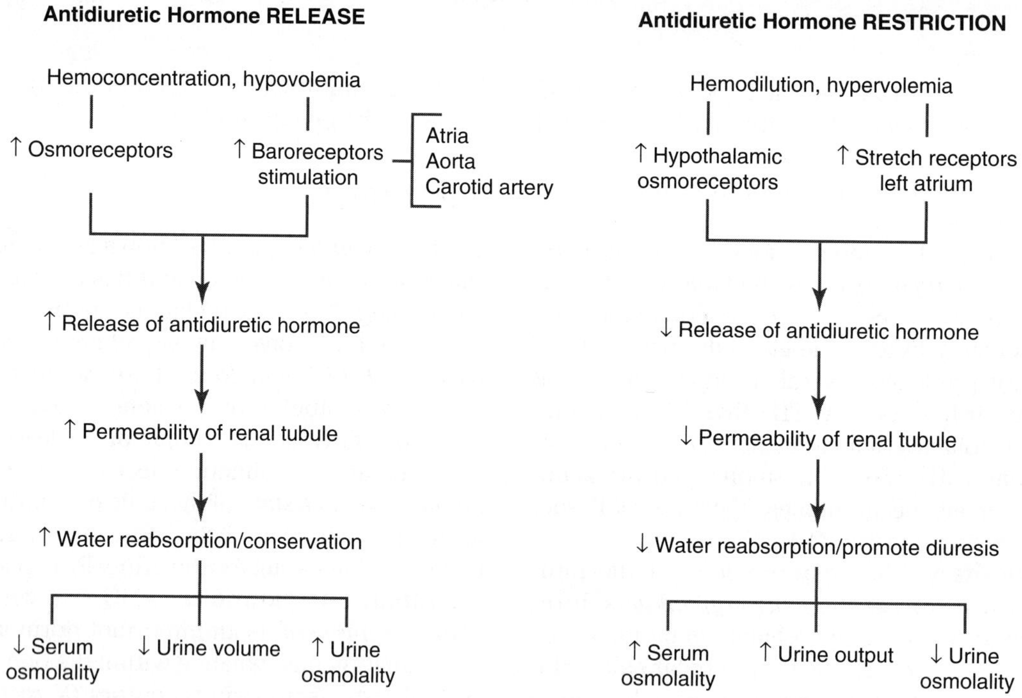

Antidiuretic Hormone RELEASE

Hemoconcentration, hypovolemia

↑ Osmoreceptors   ↑ Baroreceptors stimulation — Atria, Aorta, Carotid artery

↓

↑ Release of antidiuretic hormone

↓

↑ Permeability of renal tubule

↓

↑ Water reabsorption/conservation

↓ Serum osmolality   ↓ Urine volume   ↑ Urine osmolality

Antidiuretic Hormone RESTRICTION

Hemodilution, hypervolemia

↑ Hypothalamic osmoreceptors   ↑ Stretch receptors left atrium

↓

↓ Release of antidiuretic hormone

↓

↓ Permeability of renal tubule

↓

↓ Water reabsorption/promote diuresis

↑ Serum osmolality   ↑ Urine output   ↓ Urine osmolality

Fig. 34-4 Physiology of the release and restriction of antidiuretic hormone.

Box 34-4

FACTORS AFFECTING ANTIDIURETIC HORMONE

ANTIDIURETIC HORMONE STIMULATION
Increased serum osmolality
  Emesis
Hypovolemia
  Hemorrhage
Pain

Trauma to Hypothalamic-Hypophyseal System
  Accidental
  Surgical
  Pathologic
Stress
  Physical
  Emotional
Acute infections
Malignancies
Nonmalignant pulmonary disorders
Stimulated pulmonary baroreceptors
Nocturnal sleep

Drugs
  Nicotine
  Barbiturates
  Oxytocin
  Glucocorticoids
  Anesthetics
  Acetaminophen
  Amitriptyline
  Carbamazepine
  Cyclophosphamide
  Chlorpropamide
  K^+-depleting diuretics
  Vincristine
  Isoproterenol

ANTIDIURETIC HORMONE RESTRICTION
Decreased serum osmolality

Hypervolemia
  Water intoxication
Cold
Congenital defect
CO_2 inhalation

Accidental
Surgical
Pathologic

  Phenytoin
  Chlorpromazine
  Reserpine
  Norepinephrine
  Ethanol
  Opioids
  Lithium
  Demeclocycline
  Tolazamide

THYROID GLAND

ANATOMY

The thyroid gland weighs from 15 to 20 g in the adult human.[12] There is variation in the size of the adult gland according to the availability of dietary iodine in different parts of the world. The gland partially encases the trachea, is wrapped around the second to fourth tracheal rings anteriorly and laterally, and is located at the level of the sixth and seventh cervical vertebrae posteriorly. The thyroid gland lies below the thyroid cartilage and the articulating surface of the cricoid cartilage.

This bow tie–shaped gland has two lateral lobes that are partially covered by the sternohyoid and sternothyroid muscles. The thyroid isthmus, the band of narrow thyroid tissue that connects the lateral lobes, lies directly below the cricoid cartilage, as shown in Fig. 34-5. The richly vascularized thyroid tissue receives about 5 ml of blood per gram of thyroid tissue per minute. The basic functional units of the thyroid gland are spherical cells called *follicles*. Follicles are filled with a protein named *thyroglobulin*.

PHYSIOLOGY

The functioning of the thyroid gland depends upon multiple factors that respond to a delicate hormonal interplay: hypothalamus, anterior pituitary, dietary intake of iodine, and circulating protein bodies in the blood all affect thyroid gland function.

Pituitary gland and TSH. The anterior lobe of the pituitary gland secretes thyroid-stimulating hormone (TSH), also known as thyrotropin. TSH then stimulates the thyroid gland to produce thyroid hormone (T_4 and T_3).[13]

Iodine and Iodide. Through a complex process, dietary iodine is absorbed and concentrated in the thyroid follicles. About 100 mcg of iodide is needed on a daily basis to generate sufficient quantities of thyroid hormone.[12] In the U.S. dietary ingestion of iodide ranges from 200 to 500 mcg per day.[12] The iodine is oxidized to iodide by the enzyme thyroid perioxidase.[12] Then through active transport, the amino acid tyrosine binds the iodide to thyroglobulin, eventually yielding triiodothyronine (T_3) and thyroxine (T_4). More than 99% of T_3 and T_4 circulates in the bloodstream bound to transport proteins: thyroxin-binding globulin, prealbumin,

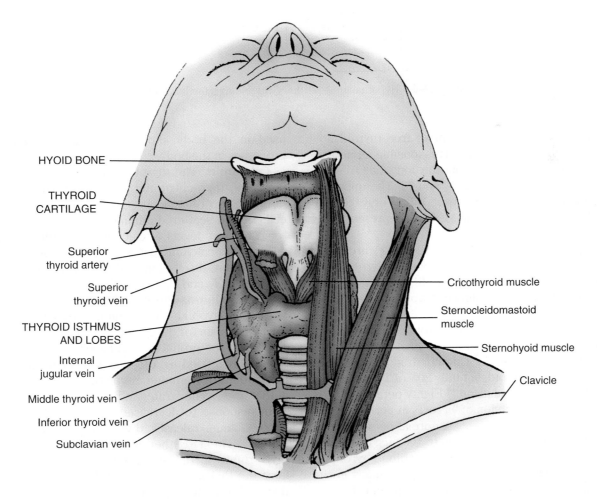

Fig. 34-5 Gross anatomy of the human thyroid.

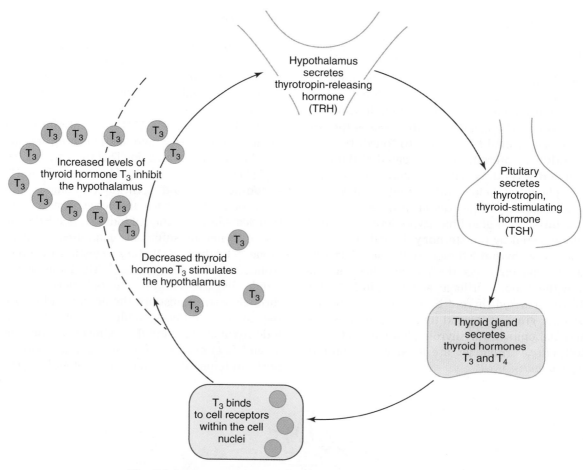

Fig. 34-6 Hypothalamus-pituitary-thyroid axis feedback loop.

and albumin. The minute amount of free thyroid hormone that is not protein-bound is responsible for activating thyroid responses throughout the body. The free thyroid hormone is measured as T_3 and T_4. The unbound, physiologically active, free fraction of T_4 is only 0.02% of the total T_4 in the bloodstream. Free T_3 represents only 0.03% of the total serum level.[14]

Thyroglobulin. Thyroglobulin (Tg) is a key precursor in the biosynthesis of thyroid hormone. Thyroglobulin is stored in the thyroid follicles until needed. TSH release stimulates thyroglobulin secretion into the bloodstream.[15]

T_3 and T_4. TSH prompts the thyroid cells to produce thyroid hormone (T_4 and T_3) in the presence of iodine from food that is ingested.[12] One hundred percent of T_4 is produced in the thyroid, but only 20% of T_3 is secreted directly from the thyroid gland.[12] Eighty percent of T_3 is the result of the conversion of T_4 to T_3 in peripheral tissues of the liver and kidneys.[12] A normal person with a healthy thyroid gland produces 90 to 100 mcg of T_4 (thyroxine) per day and 30-35 mcg of T_3 (triiodothyronine) per day.[12] T_3 acts more rapidly on target tissues in the body than does T_4 and is more actively potent than T_4. Both thyroid hormones affect the rate at which oxygen is

used in the body and therefore affect all metabolic processes in the body.

Calcitonin. The thyroid gland also produces a third hormone, thyrocalcitonin, also called *calcitonin*. This hormone is produced by the parafollicular cells, or C cells, found scattered among the follicular cells. Calcitonin reduces levels of calcium in the blood stream by augmenting calcium absorption in the bone.[16] Throughout this unit, discussion of thyroid hormone refers collectively to T_3 and T_4, not calcitonin.

Hypothalamus-Pituitary-Thyroid Axis Feedback Loop. The hypothalamic-pituitary-thyroid axis regulates the mechanism for the synthesis and secretion of thyroid hormone. The production and secretion of thyroid hormone is regulated by a feedback mechanism that limits the amount of hormone circulating to the cellular need at that time, as illustrated in Fig. 34-6.

In response to decreased circulating T_3 and T_4, the hypothalamus releases thyrotropin-releasing hormone (TRH).[12] The TRH then activates TSH (also known as thyrotropin) in the anterior pituitary. TSH then stimulates the thyroid gland to manufacture and release the thyroid hormones T_3 and T_4 in the presence of iodine.[12] When serum blood levels of T_3 and T_4 become high, the

Box 34-5

MAJOR FUNCTIONS OF THYROID HORMONES

- Interact with growth hormone
  Maturation of skeletal system
  Development of central nervous system
- Stimulate carbohydrate metabolism
  Increase the rate of glucose absorption from the gastrointestinal tract
  Increase the rate of glucose use by the cells
- Accelerate the rate of fat metabolism
  Increase cholesterol degradation in the liver
  Decrease serum cholesterol levels
- Increase protein anabolism and catabolism
  Mobilize protein and release amino acids into circulation
  Increase energy from protein nutrients through gluconeogenesis
- Increase body's demand for vitamins
- Increase oxygen consumption and use
- Increase basal metabolic rate
- Have marked chronotropic and inotropic effects on heart
- Increase cardiac output
- Stimulate contractility and excitability of myocardium
- Increase blood volume
- Expand respiratory rate and depth necessary for normal hypoxic and hypercapnic drive
- Promote sympathetic overactivity
- Boost erythropoiesis
- Increase metabolism and clearance of various hormones and pharmacologic agents
- Stimulate bone resorption

Box 34-5 lists the major functions of thyroid hormone in more detail.

REFERENCES

1. Standards of medical care in diabetes, *Diabetes Care* 27(Suppl 1):S15-35, 2004.
2. Rolla A: The pathophysiological basis for intensive insulin replacement, *Int J Obes Relat Metab Disord* 28(Suppl 2): S3-7, 2004.
3. Krauss RM, Siri PW: Dyslipidemia in type 2 diabetes, *Med Clin North Am* 88(4):897-909, 2004.
4. Grundy SM et al: Clinical management of metabolic syndrome: report of the American Heart Association/National Heart, Lung, and Blood Institute/American Diabetes Association conference on scientific issues related to management, *Circulation* 109(4):551-556, 2004.
5. Kitabchi AE et al: Hyperglycemic crises in diabetes, *Diabetes Care* 27(Suppl 1):S94-102, 2004.
6. Boehm BO: The therapeutic potential of somatostatin receptor ligands in the treatment of obesity and diabetes, *Expert Opin Investig Drugs* 12(9):1501-1509, 2003.
7. Vance ML: Perioperative management of patients undergoing pituitary surgery, *Endocrinol Metab Clin North Am* 32(2):355-365, 2003.
8. Verbalis JG: Disorders of body water homeostasis, *Best Pract Res Clin Endocrinol Metab* 17(4):471-503, 2003.
9. Holmes CL, Landry DW, Granton JT: Science review: vasopressin and the cardiovascular system, part 1—receptor physiology, *Crit Care* 7(6):427-434, 2003.
10. Janicic N, Verbalis JG: Evaluation and management of hypoosmolality in hospitalized patients, *Endocrinol Metab Clin North Am* 32(2):459-481, 2003.
11. Verbalis JG: Management of disorders of water metabolism in patients with pituitary tumors, *Pituitary* 5(2):119-132, 2002.
12. Demers LM: Thyroid disease: pathophysiology and diagnosis, *Clin Lab Med* 24(1):19-28, 2004.
13. Ross DS: Serum thyroid-stimulating hormone measurement for assessment of thyroid function and disease, *Endocrinol Metab Clin North Am* 30(2):245-264, 2001.
14. Langton JE, Brent GA: Nonthyroidal illness syndrome: evaluation of thyroid function in sick patients, *Endocrinol Metab Clin North Am* 31(1):159-172, 2002.
15. Torrens JI, Burch H.B. Serum thyroglobulin measurement. Utility in clinical practice, *Endocrinol Metab Clin North Am* 30(2):429-467, 2001.
16. Baloch Z et al: Laboratory medicine practice guidelines. Laboratory support for the diagnosis and monitoring of thyroid disease, *Thyroid* 13(1):3-126, 2003.

pituitary inhibits the production of additional TSH. When levels of T_3 and T_4 become too low, the pituitary is stimulated to secrete additional TSH.

Thyroxine (T_4) prompts the activation of β-adrenergic receptors in widespread areas of the body. These receptors trigger a sympathetic nervous system response and release norepinephrine at sympathetic nerve endings. The effect is stimulation of the cardiac tissue, nervous tissue, and smooth muscle tissue, as well as an increase in metabolism and thermogenesis (increased body heat).

Endocrine Assessment and Diagnostic Procedures

*A*ssessment of the patient with endocrine dysfunction is a systematic process that incorporates both the history and the physical examination. Most of the endocrine glands are deeply encased in the human body. Although the placement of the glands provides security for the glandular functions, their resulting inaccessibility limits clinical examination. Nevertheless, the endocrine glands can be assessed indirectly. The critical care nurse who understands the metabolic actions of the hormones produced by endocrine glands assesses the physiology of the gland by monitoring that gland's target tissue as listed in Fig. 34-1. This chapter describes clinical and diagnostic evaluation of the pancreas, the posterior pituitary, and the thyroid gland.

HISTORY

The initial presentation of the patient determines the rapidity and direction of the interview. For a patient in acute distress the history is curtailed to only a few questions about the patient's chief complaint and precipitating events. For the patient without obvious distress the endocrine history focuses on four areas: (1) current health status, (2) history of present illness, (3) past history and general endocrine status, and (4) family history. Data collection in the endocrine history for diabetes complications is outlined in the Data Collection feature on Diabetic Complications.

PANCREAS

PHYSICAL ASSESSMENT

Insulin, which is produced by the pancreas, is responsible for glucose metabolism. The clinical assessment provides information about pancreatic functioning. Clinical manifestations of abnormal glucose metabolism often manifest as hyperglycemia, which is the initial assessment priority for the patient with pancreatic dysfunction.[1-4] Patients with hyperglycemia may ultimately be diagnosed with either type 1 or type 2 diabetes[4] or be hyperglycemic in association with a severe critical illness.[1,5] All of these conditions have specific identifying features. More information on the specific pathophysiology related to each condition is discussed in Chapter 36.

Hyperglycemia. Because severe hyperglycemia affects a variety of body systems, all systems are assessed. The patient may complain of blurred vision, headache, weakness, fatigue, drowsiness, anorexia, nausea, and abdominal pain. On *inspection* the patient has flushed skin, polyuria, polydipsia, vomiting, and evidence of dehydration. Progressive deterioration in the level of consciousness, from alert to lethargic or comatose, is observed as the hyperglycemia exacerbates. If ketoacidosis occurs the patient's breathing becomes deep and rapid (Kussmaul respirations), and the breath may have a fruity odor. *Auscultation* of the abdomen reveals hypoactive bowel sounds. *Palpation* elicits abdominal tenderness. *Percussion* reveals diminished deep tendon reflexes. Because hyperglycemia results in osmotic diuresis, the patient's fluid volume status is assessed. Signs of dehydration include tachycardia, orthostatic hypotension, and poor skin turgor. The key laboratory tests that assist in assessment are discussed below.

LABORATORY STUDIES

Pertinent laboratory tests for pancreatic function measure the short and long-term blood glucose levels, which can identify and diagnose diabetes. Laboratory studies can also measure the amount of insulin produced by the pancreatic beta cells and the effectiveness of insulin in transporting glucose from the bloodstream into the cell, although this is not a common test in clinical practice.

Blood Glucose. Fasting plasma glucose (FPG) is assessed by a simple blood test when the person has not eaten for 8 hours. A normal FPG is between 70 and110 mg/dl. A fasting glucose between 110 and 126 mg/dl identifies a person with *impaired glucose tolerance*, that is, one who is *prediabetic*. Even prediabetic individuals are at increased risk to develop complications of diabetes such as coronary heart disease and stroke. A FPG level

DATA COLLECTION
Diabetic Complications

CURRENT HEALTH STATUS
- The body may not be able to adjust to increased insulin needs resulting from sudden physiologic changes such as infection, injury, or surgery, among others. The nurse would assess whether the patient had a severe infection, surgical wound, or traumatic injury.
- Recent/current signs and symptoms
  Unexplained changes in weight, thirst, hunger
  Headache, blurred vision
  Long-standing, unhealed infection
  Vaginitis, pruritus
  Leg pain, numbness
- Unexplained change in urinary patterns (i.e., daytime and night time, frequency, and volume)
  Energy/stamina changes
  Endurance level
  Weakness
  Unexplained, excessive fatigue
- Behavior/mental changes (also ask family member or significant other for input)
  Memory loss
  Orientation

HISTORY OF PRESENT ILLNESS—ONSET, CHARACTERISTICS, COURSE
- Chronic illness—physiologic or psychologic stress could increase endogenous glucose

- Recent treatments that could be a source of exogenous glucose
  Hyperalimentation
  Peritoneal dialysis
  Hemodialysis
- Medications—prescription and over-the-counter preparations (Pharmacologic agents can alter pancreatic function by either increasing or decreasing release of the endocrine hormones. Drugs also may interfere with hormonal action at the receptor site on the target cell.)

Past History
- Previous pancreatic surgery?
- Ever been told any of the following applied to you:
  Too much sugar in the urine?
  Too much sugar in the blood?
  Would probably develop too much sugar later in life?
- If "yes" answer to any of the above, what treatment, if any, was prescribed?
- Are you currently following such a treatment?

Family History
- Has a family member ever been diagnosed with diabetes/sugar in the blood?
- If so, how did he or she treat the condition?

---

of greater than 126 mg/dl (7 mmol/L) is diagnostic of diabetes (Table 35-1). In nonurgent settings the test is repeated on another day to make sure the result is accurate. Following a meal the level glucose rises in the bloodstream. It is recommended that postprandial glucose levels do not exceed 180 mg/dl (10 mmol/L).[6]

All hospitalized patients must have their blood glucose level monitored frequently while in the hospital.[1] Clinical practice recommendations emphasize maintaining blood glucose as close to normal as possible for all critically ill patients, whether or not they have a diagnosis of diabetes. If a continuous insulin drip is infused to normalize blood glucose levels, point-of-care blood glucose testing is performed hourly by the critical care nurse, until the blood glucose is within the target range.[1,5]

Before discharge home, diabetic patients should be taught to self-monitor their own blood glucose levels.[6] Maintaining blood glucose within the normal range is associated with fewer diabetes-related complications and a lower rate of complications of diabetes.[4] Laboratory tests or point-of-care or self-monitoring of blood glucose represent the standard of care for management of diabetes at this time. Unfortunately, home monitoring of

Table 35-1	Blood Glucose Levels	
Patient Status	**(mg/dl)**	**mmol/L**
Hypoglycemia	<60	
Normal FPG	70-110	>1-6.1
Impaired FPG	110-126	6.1-7.0
Fasting FPG diagnostic of diabetes	>126	>7.0
Non-FPG diagnostic of diabetes	>200	>11.1

Data from *Diabetes Care* 27 (suppl 1), 2004.
FPG, Fasting plasma glucose.

blood glucose is not the norm, in spite of research evidence that maintaining blood glucose levels as close to normal as possible prolongs life and reduces complications. Only 40% of patients with type 1 diabetes, and 26% of patients with type 2 diabetes, monitor their blood glucose at least once a day.[6]

Urine Glucose. Testing the urine for glucose is not recommended for diabetic patients because there is too much variation in the renal threshold for glucose when kidney damage secondary to diabetes has occurred.[6]

Urine glucose measurements are affected by variation in fluid intake, reflect an average glucose and not a specific point in time, and are altered by some drugs.[6] The other limitation of urine glucose testing is that it does not offer any help in the identification of hypoglycemia.[6] For all of these reasons urine testing is not recommended.

Glycated Hemoglobin. Blood testing of glucose is useful for daily management of diabetes. However, a different blood test is used to achieve an objective measure of blood glucose over an extended period of time. The glycated hemoglobin test (also known as the glycosylated hemoglobin, or HbA_{1C} or A_{1C}), provides information about the average amount of glucose that has been present in the patient's bloodstream over the previous 3 to 4 months.[6] During the 120-day life span of red blood cells (erythrocytes), the hemoglobin within each cell binds to the available blood glucose through a process known as *glycosylation*. Typically 4% to 6% of hemoglobin contains the glucose group hemoglobin A_{1C}. A normal hemoglobin A_{1C} level is 4% to 6%, with an acceptable target level for diabetic patients below 7%.[4] The hemoglobin A_{1C} value correlates with specific blood glucose levels as shown in Table 35-2. Not all clinical laboratories use the same analytical techniques to measure the glycated hemoglobin A_{1C}, and methods to standardize the reporting of results worldwide are underway.[6,7]

Glycated Serum Proteins. Serum fructosamine level, a newer and less frequently used test, measures the glycosylation of the serum protein albumin.[6] Albumin has a half-life of about 14 days, compared with approximately 120 days for hemoglobin; thus glycemic levels reflect a shorter period covering the preceding 2 to 4 weeks. This test is a useful measure for patients who have a hemoglobin abnormality such as hemolytic anemia. Normal serum fructosamine levels are 1.5 to 2.4 mmol/L when serum albumin level is 5 g/dl. At the present time the glycated serum proteins (albumin) do not have widespread clinical utility.[6]

Table 35-2	Correlation between Hemoglobin (HbA$_{1c}$) and Blood (Plasma) Glucose	
HbA$_{1c}$ (%)	**Mean Plasma Glucose (mg/dl)**	**(mmol/L)**
6	135	7.5
7	170	9.5
8	205	11.5
9	240	13.5
10	275	15.5
11	310	17.5
12	345	19.5

From *Diabetes Care*, 27(7):1761-1773, 2004.

Blood Ketones. In a serum blood test, normal ketone level is 2 to 4 mg/dl of blood, and normal acetone 0.3 to 2.0 mg/dl of blood. Ketones are by-products of fat metabolism. In most cases, when the body uses carbohydrate as its main source of energy, the liver completes fat metabolism and minimal or no ketones are found in the blood. Elevated blood ketones (ketonemia) are also detected by a fruity, sweet-smelling odor on the exhaled breath. This odor is the result of the body's attempt to keep the pH within the normal range. A sweet-smelling breath occurs when the patient exhales in an attempt to decrease the accumulated acids.

Urine Ketones. Urine ketone monitoring is important, particularly in patients with type 1 diabetes.[6] The presence of ketones may signify impending or established ketoacidosis. In diabetic ketoacidosis (DKA), fat breakdown (lipolysis) occurs so rapidly that fat metabolism is incomplete, and ketone bodies (acetone, β-hydroxybutyric acid, and acetoacetic acid) accumulate in the blood *(ketonemia)* and are excreted in the urine *(ketonuria)*. It is recommended that all diabetic patients self-test, or have their urine tested for the presence of ketones during any acute illness or stress, with a blood glucose greater than 300 mg/dl (16.7 mmol/L), with symptoms of nausea, vomiting, or abdominal pain, and for women during pregnancy.[6]

Normally, in healthy nonfasting individuals only minute quantities of ketones are present in the urine, and the levels are so low they are below the threshold of detectability with routine testing methods.[6] In fasting and starvation states, ketones may be present in the urnie.[6]

PITUITARY GLAND

The pituitary gland, recessed in the base of the cranium, is not accessible to physical assessment. The critical care nurse must therefore be aware of the systemic effects of a normally functioning pituitary to be able to identify dysfunction. One essential hormone formed in the hypothalamus but secreted through the posterior pituitary gland is *antidiuretic hormone* (ADH), also known as *vasopressin*.

PHYSICAL ASSESSMENT

ADH controls the amount of fluid lost and retained within the body. Acute dysfunction of the posterior pituitary or the hypothalamus can result in insufficient or excessive ADH production. Thus the clinical signs of posterior pituitary dysfunction often manifest as fluid volume deficit (insufficient ADH production) or fluid volume excess (excessive ADH production).

Hydration Status. The nurse determines the effectiveness of ADH production by conducting a hydration assessment. A hydration assessment includes observations of skin integrity, skin turgor, and buccal membrane moisture. Moist, shiny buccal membranes indicate satisfactory fluid balance. Skin turgor that is resilient and returns to its original position in less than 3 seconds after being pinched or lifted indicates adequate skin elasticity. Skin over the forehead, clavicle, and sternum is the most reliable for testing tissue turgor because it is less affected by aging and thus more easily assessed for changes related to fluid balance. A well-hydrated patient has skin in the groin and axilla that is slightly moist to touch. In elderly patients these "typical" assessment findings may be absent. Elderly persons, especially women, experience a as much as a 50% decreases in total body water content by age 75.[8]

Other indicators that the patient's hydration status is adequate for metabolic demands include a balanced intake and output and absence of thirst. Absence of thirst, however, is not a reliable indicator of dehydration in those with decreased thirst mechanisms, such as the elderly or critically ill patients. Absence of abrupt changes in mental status may also indicate normal hydration. Other indicators of normal hydration include absence of edema, stable weight, and urine specific gravity that falls within the normal range (1.005 to 1.030).

Vital Signs. Changes in heart rate, blood pressure (BP), and central venous pressure (when available) are useful to determine fluid volume status. BP and pulse are monitored frequently. Decreased BP with increased pulse is characteristic of hypovolemia, whereas elevated blood pressure and a rapid, bounding pulse may indicate hypervolemia. In contrast, orthostatic hypotension, which occurs when intravascular fluid volume decreases, is identified by a drop in systolic BP of 20 millimeters of mercury (mm Hg) or a drop in diastolic BP of 10 mm Hg when the patient changes position from lying to standing.

Weight and Intake/Output. Daily weight changes coincide with fluid retention and fluid loss. Sudden changes in weight could result from a change in fluid balance; 1 L of fluid lost or retained is equal to approximately 2.2 pounds, or 1 kg, of weight gained or lost. To use weight as a true determinant of the fluid balance, all extraneous variables are eliminated, and the same scale is used at the same time each day. Precise measurement and notation of intake and output are used as criteria for fluid replacement therapy.

LABORATORY ASSESSMENT

No single diagnostic test identifies dysfunction of the posterior pituitary gland. Diagnosis usually is made through an array of laboratory tests combined with the clinical profile of the patient.

Serum Antidiuretic Hormone. The result of a blood test for normal levels of serum ADH is 1 to 5 pg/ml (picogram per milliliter).[8] To prepare the patient for the test, all drugs that may alter the release of ADH are withheld for a minimum of 8 hours. Common medications that affect ADH levels include morphine sulfate, lithium carbonate, chlorothiazide, carbamazepine, oxytocin, and certain neoplastic and anesthetic agents. Nicotine, alcohol, both positive-pressure and negative-pressure ventilation, and emotional stress also influence ADH levels and must be considered in the interpretation of values.

The test, read by comparing serum ADH levels with the blood and urine osmolality, is helpful in differentiating the *syndrome of inappropriate antidiuretic hormone* (SIADH) from central *diabetes insipidus* (DI). The presence of increased ADH in the bloodstream compared with a low serum osmolality and elevated urine osmolality confirms the diagnosis of SIADH. Reduced levels of serum ADH in a patient with high serum osmolality, hypernatremia, and reduced urine concentration signal central DI.

Urine and Serum Osmolality. Values for serum osmolality in the bloodstream range from 275 to 295 mOsm/kg H_2O (milliosmoles per kilogram of water). *Osmolality* measurements determine the concentration of dissolved particles in a solution. In a healthy person a change in the concentration of solutes triggers a chain of events to maintain adequate serum dilution. Urine osmolality in the person with normal kidneys is highly dependent on fluid intake. With high fluid intake, particle dilution is low but will increase if fluids are restricted, and therefore the expected range for urine osmolality is wide, ranging from 50 to 1400 mOsm/kg.

Increased serum osmolality stimulates the release of ADH, which in turn reduces the amount of water lost through the kidney. Body fluid thereby is retained to dilute the particle concentration in the bloodstream. Decreased serum osmolality inhibits the release of ADH, the kidney tubules increase their permeability, and fluid is eliminated from the body in an attempt to regain normal concentration of particles in the bloodstream. The most accurate measures of the body's fluid balance are obtained when urine and blood samples are collected simultaneously.

ADH Test. The ADH test is used to differentiate between *neurogenic* DI (central) and *nephrogenic* (kidney) DI. The patient is challenged with 0.05 to 1.0 ml intranasally administered ADH in the form of desmopressin or DDAVP.[9] An IV is inserted before the ADH; urine volume and osmolality are measured every 30 minutes for 2 hours before and after the ADH challenge. The patient with normal posterior pituitary functioning responds to the exogenous ADH by resorbing water at the renal tubule and raising the urine osmolality slightly. In severe central DI, where the pituitary is affected, the urine osmolality shows a significant rise (becomes more concentrated), which indicates that the cell receptor sites on the renal tubules are responsive to vasopressin. Test results in which urine osmolality remains unchanged indicate nephrogenic DI, suggesting renal dysfunction because the kidneys are no longer responsive to ADH. This test is rarely performed in the critical care unit because of the unstable hemodynamic and volume status of most patients.[9]

DIAGNOSTIC PROCEDURES

In addition to laboratory tests, radiographic examination, computed tomography (CT), and magnetic resonance imaging (MRI) are used to diagnose structural lesions such as cranial bone fractures, tumors, or blood clots in the region of the pituitary. Although these procedures do not diagnose DI or SIADH, they are useful in uncovering the likely underlying cause.[8]

Radiographic Examination. A basic x-ray examination of the inferior skull views the sella turcica and surrounding bone formation. Bone fractures or tissue swelling at the base of the brain, which are apparent on a radiograph, suggest interference with the vascular supply and nerve impulses to the hypothalamic-pituitary system. Dysfunction can occur if the hypothalamus, infundibular stalk, or pituitary is impaired.

Computed Tomography. CT scan of the base of the skull identifies pituitary tumors, blood clots, cysts, nodules, or other soft tissue masses. This rapid procedure causes no discomfort except that it requires the patient to lie perfectly still. CT studies can be performed with radiopaque contrast (sodium iodine solution) or "without contrast." The contrast dye is given intravenously to highlight the hypothalamus, infundibular stalk, and pituitary gland. This dye may cause allergic reactions in iodine-sensitive persons, and the patient must be carefully questioned about iodine allergy before the test. Size and shape of sella turcica and position of hypothalamus, infundibular stalk, and pituitary are identified.

Magnetic Resonance Imaging. MRI enables the radiologist to visualize internal organs and cellular characteristics of specific tissue. MRI uses a magnetic field rather than radiation to produce high-resolution cross-sectional images. The soft brain tissue and surrounding cerebrospinal fluid (CSF) make the brain especially suited to MRI scanning. Although not a definitive diagnostic test for posterior pituitary hormonal imbalance, MRI may identify anatomic disruption of the gland and the surrounding area to uncover a primary cause of DI or SIADH.

THYROID GLAND

CLINICAL ASSESSMENT

History. The history of a patient in the critical care area should be as detailed as possible. Information regarding the clinical manifestations of either hypothyroidism or hyperthyroidism must be obtained from the patient, family, or others with knowledge about the patient. Sample questions considered pertinent to detection of thyroid disease are presented in the Data Collection feature on Thyrotoxicosis (Hyperthyroidism) and Myxedema (Hypothyroidism).

Physical Examination. The thyroid is palpated for tenderness, nodules, and enlargement and auscultated for bruits. The normal-size thyroid gland is generally not visible or palpable in the anterior neck. Palpation may be from an anterior or posterior approach. Auscultation of the thyroid is accomplished by use of the bell portion of the stethoscope to identify a bruit or blowing noise from the circulation through the thyroid gland. The presence of a bruit indicates enlargement of the thyroid as evidenced by increased blood flow through the glandular tissue.

LABORATORY STUDIES

There is controversy about "routine" measurement of thyroid function in adults without clinical symptoms. The American Thyroid Association recommends thyroid function measurement in all adults beginning at age 35 years and every 5 years thereafter; more frequent screening is recommended in high-risk or symptomatic individuals.[10] More recently, the U.S. Preventive Services Task Force (USPSTF) found the research evidence insufficient to either recommend or recommend against routine screening for thyroid disease in asymptomatic adults.[11] At this time there are no specific recommendations related to thyroid function screening for critically ill patients.

Thyroid hormone blood tests measure the levels of circulating thyroid hormone and thus assess the integrity of the hormonal negative feedback response within the hypothalamic-pituitary axis. Laboratory diagnosis of hyperthyroidism and hypothyroidism usually is based on the value of thyroid-stimulating hormone (TSH) and measurement of free T_4.[12,13] Laboratory tests developed to analyze TSH have become much more sensitive over the last decade, allowing more accurate measurement of low levels of thyroid hormone.[13] Thyroid hormone reference ranges in adults are listed in Table 35-3.[12,14] Serum values vary slightly between laboratory methods, so it is imperative to know the normal reference values used by the hospital laboratory.[14,15]

The upper limit "normal" for some of these values is currently under scrutiny. This is because a U.S. national survey found the average level of TSH in the population in all ages to be only 1.49 milli-International Units/L, considerably lower than most cited laboratory norms.[12] In addition, the serum level of TSH increases as people grow older, which may signal declining thyroid function as more stimulation of the thyroid gland is required.[12]

The average TSH level is:
- 1.60 milli-International Units/L after age 50
- 1.79 milli-International Units/L after age 60

DATA COLLECTION

Thyrotoxicosis (Hyperthyroidism) and Myxedema (Hypothyroidism)

NOTE: The patient would be the best from whom to obtain the following information. However, if the patient is unable to respond, the following questions are directed to family, friends, significant other, and/or those involved in admission of the patient to the intensive care unit.

- Have you ever been diagnosed with overactive thyroid, increased metabolism, or hyperthyroidism? What about underactive thyroid, slowed metabolism, or hypothyroidism?
- Have you ever been treated for hyperthyroidism or hypothyroidism?
- Have you ever had an operation for thyroid disease?
- Have you ever received radioactive iodine for thyroid disease?
- Were you taking any medicine for thyroid disease? If so, what is the name of the medicine, dose, frequency?
- When did you first notice the constant restlessness and/or extreme fatigue?
- Has your weight been the same or changed over the last year?
- Has your appetite changed over the last 6 months?
- Have you lost weight even though your appetite has increased? (May indicate hyperthyroidism)
- Have you gained weight or stayed at the same weight even though you haven't felt like eating over the last 6 months? (May indicate hypothyroidism)

- Are you always feeling warm? (May indicate hyperthyroidism)
- Do you open windows in house, even in winter months?
- Do you wear lightweight clothing, even when everyone around is wearing layers of heavier clothing?
- Are you always feeling cold? (May indicate hypothyroidism)
- Do you wear multiple layers of clothing despite warm weather or the use of a heater/furnace?
- Do you use several blankets with closed windows, even in warm weather?
- Does patient complain of never being able to "warm-up"?
- Over the last 6 months to 1 year, have you developed any of the following?

INDICATORS FOR HYPOTHYROIDISM	INDICATORS FOR HYPERTHYROIDISM
Hair thinning	Tremors
Facial puffiness	Insomnia
Decreased appetite	Increased appetite
Severe constipation	Diarrhea
Pain when moving hands, wrist, feet	Muscle weakness/wasting
Change in menstruation	Change in menstruation

Table 35-3	Thyroid Tests			
Name of Test		**Abbreviation**	**Reference Value***	**Reference Value***
Total serum thyroxine		TT_4	58-160 nmol/L	4.5 – 12.6 mcg/dl
Free thyroxine		T_4	9-23 pmol/L	0.7-1.8 ng/dl
Total serum triiodothyronine		TT_3	1.2-2.7 nmol/L	80-180 ng/dl
Free triiodothyronine		T_3	3.5-7.7 pmol/L	0.2-0.5 ng/dl
Thyroid-stimulating hormone (thyrotropin)		TSH	0.4-4.0 milli-International Units/L	
Thyroglobulin†		Tg	3.0-40 mcg/L	

Reference values from Demers LM et al: Laboratory medicine practice guidelines. Laboratory support for the diagnosis and monitoring of thyroid disease, *Thyroid* 13(1):3-126, 2003.
*Some tests are reported with more than one reference value because different laboratories report results in several reference scales.
†Thyroglobulin (Tg) reference values should be determined locally because serum Tg concentrations are influenced by iodide intake.

- 1.98 milli-International Units/L after age 70
- 2.08 milli-International Units/L for those older than 80[12]

However, because this age adjusted rise is predictable, it is not recommended that laboratories use age-adjusted reference values when assessing thyroid function.[14] Most asymptomatic people with a normal thyroid gland have a TSH level below 2.5 milli-International Units/L.[12,14]

Thyroid Tests in the Critically Ill. Thyroid hormone testing in patients with nonthyroidal critical illness is often inconclusive because of the hormonal disruption caused by the illness.[14-16]

Drugs and Thyroid Testing. Additional measurement difficulties involve concomitant use of certain drugs that interfere with thyroid function.[12] Glucocorticoids in large doses can lower the serum T_3 and inhibit

<table>
<tr><td colspan="2">

Box 35-1

DRUGS THAT INFLUENCE DIAGNOSTIC THYROID LEVELS

</td></tr>
<tr><td>

TRIIODOTHYRONINE (T_3)
Increase
Methadone
Estrogens
Progestins
Amiodarone

THYROXINE (T_4)
Increase
Oral contraceptives
Heparin
Aspirin
Furosemide
Clofibrate
Phenylbutazone
Some nonsteroidal antiinflam-
   matory drugs (NSAIDs)
Propranolol
Corticosteroids
Amiodarone

THYROID-STIMULATING HORMONE (TH)

Increase TSH
Metocloproamide
Iodides
Lithium
Potassium iodide
Morphine sulfate

THYROXINE-BINDING GLOBULIN (TBG)
Increase
Opiates
Oral contraceptives
Estrogens
Clofibrate
5-Fluorouracil (5-FU)
Perphenazine

</td><td>

Decrease
Anabolic steroid
Androgens
Salicylates
Phenytoin
Lithium
Reserpine
Propranolol
Sulfonamides
Propylthiouracil
Methylthiouracil

Decrease
Phenytoin
Steroids
Diphenylhydantoin
Chlorpromazine
Lithium
Sulfonylurea
Sulfonamides
Reserpine
Chlordiazepoxide

Decrease TSH and TSH
Response to TRH
Glucocorticoids
Dopamine
Heparin
Aspirin
Carbamazepine

Decrease
Androgen therapy
L-Asparaginase

</td></tr>
</table>

TSH secretion.[14] Dopamine directly inhibits TSH stimulation and consequently lowers serum levels.[13] Dobutamine infusions decrease serum TSH by 10% to 15%.[13] The antidysrhythmic drug amiodarone inhibits conversion of T_3 to T_4 and thus decreases serum T_4 levels.[13] Several drugs increase the serum level of T_4 by displacing protein-bound T_4.[17] Drugs that displace T_4, including heparin (both unfractionated and low–molecular-weight heparins), cause an increase in serum T_4 levels.[17] Salicylates (aspirin) and furosemide (Lasix) also raise T_4 serum levels by the same mechanism.[17] A more complete list of drugs that alter thyroid hormone serum levels are

listed in Box 35-1. How, or if, it is necessary to adjust management of the critically ill patient in response to these laboratory findings is not yet clear.

Serum TSH/T_4 Relationship. There is an inverse, linear relationship between thyroid-stimulating hormone and T_4.[14] When the hypothalamic-pituitary axis is normal, TSH production is inhibited by the presence of normal thyroid hormone.[14] It is more common to come across misleading serum T_4 results than to encounter misleading TSH results.[14] High TSH and low T_4 is characteristic of hypothyroidism.[14] Conversely, low TSH and high serum T_4 is indicative of hyperthyroidism.[14] According to clinical practice guidelines on thyroid laboratory measurement, the sensitivity and specificity of TSH assays have improved so much that the indirect measurement of thyroid function (TSH measurement) offers better diagnostic sensitivity than does direct T_4 measurement.[14,15]

Thyrotoxicosis, the precursor of thyrotoxic crisis, is diagnosed in part by elevated T_4 and T_3 serum levels. Laboratory levels of TSH and thyrotropin-releasing hormone (TRH) are measured to confirm thyrotoxicosis, as well as to identify the cause as intrinsically thyroid, a thyroid malignancy, or perhaps related to pituitary dysfunction.

DIAGNOSTIC PROCEDURES

Thyroid scanning involves the use of oral radioactive iodine. The preferred isotope to use in a scan to determine the cause of the hyperthyroidism is ^{123}I.[15] It is low-energy, with a short half-life to minimize the patient's exposure to radioactive material. The thyroid-scanning procedure is useful in detecting the presence of ectopic thyroid tissue and thyroid carcinomas. Thyroid scans also identify the presence and amount of viable thyroid glandular tissue after irradiation treatment.

REFERENCES

1. Clement S et al: Management of diabetes and hyperglycemia in hospitals, *Diabetes Care* 27(2):553-591, 2004.
2. Clement S et al: Diagnosis and classification of diabetes mellitus, *Diabetes Care* 27(Suppl 1):S5-S10, 2004.
3. Clement S et al: Screening for type 2 diabetes, *Diabetes Care* 27(Suppl 1):S11-S14, 2004.
4. Clement S et al: Standards of medical care in diabetes, *Diabetes Care* 27(Suppl 1):S15-S35, 2004.
5. Van Den Berghe G et al: Intensive insulin therapy in the critically ill patients, *N Engl J Med* 345(19):1359-1367, 2001.
6. Goldstein DE et al: Tests of glycemia in diabetes, *Diabetes Care* 27(7):1761-1773, 2004.
7. Jeffcoate SL: Diabetes control and complications: the role of glycated haemoglobin, 25 years on, *Diabet Med* 21(7): 657-665, 2004.
8. Janicic N, Verbalis JG: Evaluation and management of hypo-osmolality in hospitalized patients, *Endocrinol Metab Clin North Am* 32(2):459-481, 2003.

9. Holcomb S: Diabetes insipidus, *DCCN* 21(3):94-97, 2002.

10. Ladenson PW et al: American Thyroid Association guidelines for detection of thyroid dysfunction, *Arch Intern Med* 160(11):1573-1575, 2000.

11. US Preventive Services Task Force (USPSTF): Screening for thyroid disease, retrieved from the World Wide Web at www.AHRQ.gov, 2004.

12. Demers LM: Thyroid disease: pathophysiology and diagnosis, *Clin Lab Med* 24(1):19-28, 2004.

13. Ross DS: Serum thyroid-stimulating hormone measurement for assessment of thyroid function and disease, *Endocrinol Metab Clin North Am* 30(2):245-264, 2001.

14. Demers LM et al: Laboratory medicine practice guidelines. Laboratory support for the diagnosis and monitoring of thyroid disease, *Thyroid* 13(1):3-126, 2003.

15. American Association of Clinical Endocrinologists medical guidelines for clinical practice for the evaluation and treatment of hyperthyroidism and hypothyroidism, *Endocr Pract* 8(6):458-469, 2002.

16. Langton JE, Brent GA: Nonthyroidal illness syndrome: evaluation of thyroid function in sick patients, *Endocrinol Metab Clin North Am* 31(1):159-172, 2002.

17. Stockigt JR: Free thyroid hormone measurement. A critical appraisal, *Endocrinol Metab Clin North Am* 30(2):265-289, 2001.

CHAPTER 36

Endocrine Disorders and Therapeutic Management

The endocrine system is almost invisible when it functions well and causes widespread upset whenever an organ is suppressed, hyperstimulated or under physiologic stress. This results in a wide spectrum of possible disorders; some are rare, whereas others are frequently encountered in the critical care unit. This chapter focuses initially on the neuroendocrine stress associated with critical illness and disorders of three major endocrine glands: the pancreas, the thyroid gland, and the posterior pituitary gland.

NEUROENDOCRINOLOGY OF STRESS AND CRITICAL ILLNESS

Major neurologic and endocrine changes occur when an individual is confronted with physiologic stress caused by critical illness,[1] trauma,[2] sepsis,[3] burns,[4] major surgery,[5] stroke,[6] cardiovascular disease,[7] or cardiac arrest.[8] The normal "fight or flight" response that is initiated in times of physiologic or physiologic stress is exacerbated in critical illness through activation of the neuroendocrine system, specifically the hypothalamic-pituitary-adrenal axis (HPA),[3,8] thyroid[9] and pancreas.[1] HPA influence on the course of critical illness is just beginning to be understood. Hormonal neuroendocrine output is very active at the beginning of a critical insult but greatly diminishes if the critical illness is prolonged.[10-11] All endocrine organs are affected by acute critical illness, as shown in Table 36-1. How much influence hormonal fluctuations have on morbidity and mortality remains the focus of ongoing research.

ACUTE NEUROENDOCRINE RESPONSE TO CRITICAL ILLNESS

The initial "fight or flight" acute response to physiologic threat is a rapid discharge of the catecholamines *norepinephrine* and *epinephrine* into the bloodstream.[8] Norepinephrine is released from the nerve endings of the sympathetic nervous system (SNS).[8]

Hypothalamic-Pituitary-Adrenal Axis in Acute Stress. Epinephrine, also known as *adrenaline*, is released from the medulla of the adrenal glands. Epinephrine increases cerebral blood flow and cerebral oxygen consumption and may be the trigger for recruitment of the hypothalamic-pituitary axis.[8]

The pituitary gland has two parts (anterior and posterior) that function under control of the hypothalamus, as described in Chapter 34. As a response to stress the *posterior pituitary gland* releases antidiuretic hormone (ADH) also known as *vasopressin* (pitressin). This hormone is an antidiuretic with a powerful vasoconstrictive effect on blood vessels.[8] The combination of epinephrine and vasopressin raises blood pressure quickly, and also decreases gastric motility.[8] Epinephrine increases heart rate, causes ventricular dysrhythmias in susceptible patients, and provides some analgesia or lack of pain awareness during acute physical stress.[8]

The *anterior pituitary gland* is also under the control of the hypothalamus (see Chapter 34). In acute physiologic stress, "pulses" of growth hormone (GH) are released from the anterior pituitary gland to boost serum GH levels.[11] In critical illness the anterior pituitary actively secretes hormone, but the quantity may be insufficient for extreme physiologic needs. A different problem is that peripheral tissues may be "resistant" and unable to use the anabolic (tissue building) growth hormone.[12] The anterior pituitary gland also produces *corticotrophin*, which stimulates release of *cortisol* from the adrenal cortex.[13]

Cortisol release is an important protective response to stress, and serum levels will increase sixfold with normal adrenal function.[13] High cortisol levels alter carbohydrate, fat, and protein metabolism so that energy is immediately and selectively available to vital organs such as the brain.[11]

Liver and Pancreas in Acute Stress. The liver releases the hormone *glucagon* to stimulate the liver to pour additional glucose into the bloodstream. This greatly raises blood glucose levels.[3] Paradoxically the pancreas does not produce more insulin. Serum insulin levels remain normal, even with the increased metabolic

Table 36-1		Endocrine Responses to Stress
Gland/Organ	**Hormone**	**Response/Physical Examination**
Adrenal cortex	Cortisol	↑ Insulin resistance → ↑ glycogenolysis → ↑ glucose circulation
		↑ Hepatic gluconeogenesis → ↑ glucose available
		↑ Lipolysis
		↑ Protein catabolism
		↑ Sodium → ↑ water retention to maintain plasma osmolality by movement of extravascular fluid to intravascular space
		↓ Connective tissue fibroblasts → poor wound healing
	Glucocorticoid	↓ Histamine release → suppresses immune system
		↓ Lymphocytes, monocytes, eosinophils, basophils
		↑ Polymorphonuclear leukocytes → ↑ infection risk
		↑ Glucose
		↓ Gastric acid secretion
	Mineralocorticoids	↑ Aldosterone → ↓ sodium excretion → ↓ water excretion → ↑ intravascular volume
		↑ Potassium excretion → hypokalemia →
		↑ Hydrogen ion excretion → metabolic acidosis
Adrenal medulla	Epinephrine	↑ Endorphins → ↓ pain
	Norepinephrine, epinephrine	↑ Metabolic rate to accommodate stress response
		↑ Live glycogenolysis → ↑ glucose
		↑ Insulin (cells are insulin resistant)
		↑ Cardiac contractility
		↑ Cardiac output
		↑ Dilation of coronary arteries
		↑ Blood pressure
		↑ Heart rate
		↑ Bronchodilation → ↑ respirations
		↑ Perfusion to heart, brain, lungs, liver, and muscle
		↓ Perfusion to periphery of body
		↓ Peristalsis
	Norepinephrine	↑ Peripheral vasoconstriction
		↑ Blood pressure
		↑ Sodium retention
		↑ Potassium excretion
Pituitary	All hormones	↑ Endogenous opioids → ↓ pain
Anterior pituitary	Adrenocorticotropic hormone	↑ Aldosterone → ↓ sodium excretion → ↓ water excretion → ↑ intravascular volume
		↑ Cortisol to ↑ blood volume
	Growth hormones	↑ Protein anabolism of amino acids to protein
		↑ Lipolysis → ↑ gluconeogenesis
Posterior pituitary	Antidiuretic hormone	↑ Vasoconstriction
		↑ Water retention → restoration of circulating blood volume
		↓ Urine output
		↑ Hypoosmolality
Pancreas	Insulin	Insulin resistance → hyperglycemia
	Glucagon	Directly opposes action of insulin → ↑ glycolysis
		↑ Glucose for fuel
		↑ Glycogenolysis
		↑ Gluconeogenesis
		↑ Lipolysis
Thyroid	Thyroxine	↓ Routine metabolic demands during stress
Gonads	Sex hormones	Energy and oxygen supply diverted to brain, heart, muscles, and liver

↑, Increased; →, causes; ↓, decreased.

demand associated with critical illness or sepsis. Cells become *insulin-resistant.*[3] In other words the tissues are unable to use the available insulin to transport glucose inside the cells for normal metabolism. This raises blood glucose levels, causing persistent hyperglycemia. Continuous infusion of insulin to return and maintain blood glucose levels within the normal range significantly reduces morbidity and mortality.[1] Management of hyperglycemia for the nondiabetic critically ill patient is discussed in detail in a later section.

Thyroid Gland in Acute Stress. Within 2 hours of trauma or surgery serum levels of T_3 decrease.[11] The greater the decrease of T_3 in the first 24 hours the more severe the critical illness. Thyroid-stimulating hormone (TSH) and T_4 briefly increase and then return to normal levels. In the acute phase of critical illness a high serum cortisol or a low serum T_3 are associated with a poor prognosis.[11]

Systemic illnesses that do not directly involve the thyroid gland, but alter thyroid gland metabolism, are referred to as a *nonthyroidal illness syndrome*, or *sick euthyroid syndrome.*[9] The significance of altered thyroid function in critical illness is unknown at this time.[9]

PROLONGED NEUROENDOCRINE RESPONSE TO CRITICAL ILLNESS

If critical illness is prolonged the neuroendocrine response changes dramatically. The initially high hormonal levels are greatly reduced and output is decreased from all the major endocrine glands.

Hypothalamic-Pituitary-Adrenal Axis in Prolonged Stress. When critical illness is prolonged over 7 to 10 days the production of hormones from the pituitary gland is significantly lessened.

Normally the posterior pituitary gland produces ADH, or vasopressin. The impact of prolonged critical illness on vasopressin production has not been reported.

Growth hormone (GH) from the anterior pituitary is greatly decreased and lacks the "pulses" or bolus doses delivered during the initial acute phase.[11] Growth hormone levels are low when compared with the high levels seen as part of the initial stress response (see preceding paragraphs).[11] Unexpectedly, when critically ill patients were given high-dose GH as part of a large multicenter study, the morbidity increased and the mortality doubled.[11] Because of this finding, exogenous administration of growth hormone is not recommended.

Adrenal dysfunction is common in prolonged critical illness that lasts more than 7 to 10 days.[11] Serum adrenal corticotropin hormone level (ACTH) decreases, whereas the cortisol level remains high.[11] The reason for this paradoxical effect is unknown. Some researchers believe that an alternative metabolic pathway, as yet unidentified, may be stimulating the adrenal cortex to produce cortisol outside of the normal channels.[11] With time, all pathways fail as indicated by a twentyfold increase in adrenal failure seen in critically ill patients over 50 years of age who spend more than 14 days in a critical care unit.[11] If the critical illness is prolonged and the patient remains hypotensive, vasopressor-dependent, and mechanically ventilated, adequacy of adrenal function must be evaluated. Even if a corticotropin test was performed earlier in the hospitalization, it is important to repeat the test since the adrenal gland may have been initially normal, but has since failed due to the stress of the critical illness.[13] Older patients are particularly susceptible to adrenal failure.[11,13,14]

Liver-Pancreas in Prolonged Stress. Hyperglycemia is often persistent. Gluconeogenesis (the metabolism of glucose from fat or protein) and proteolysis (protein breakdown) continue throughout the catabolic phase of critical illness.[12] Critically ill patients can lose up to 10% of their lean body mass per week.[12] The addition of adequate supplemental nutrition is recommended, in addition to an IV insulin infusion, to reduce hyperglycemia and provide additional substrate other than the patient's own body tissues.[1] Insulin is an anabolic hormone and can improve protein synthesis and reduce protein breakdown.[12] While the critical illness is ongoing, nutrition and insulin seem to limit rather than stop the loss of lean body mass.

Thyroid Gland in Prolonged Stress. The thyroid gland appears to follow a similar pattern to the pituitary gland when critical illness is prolonged. The serum levels of T_3, T_4 and TSH are greatly reduced.[11] Also, the normal pulses of TSH are flattened.[11] The significance of this is unknown, and investigation of the impact of thyroid hormone infusions is underway.[11]

Gonads in Prolonged Stress. If critical illness is prolonged, hypogonadism develops. This is measured as a low serum testosterone in men.[11] Testosterone is an endogenous anabolic steroid (builds muscle) and the level is decreased in catabolic states such as starvation, acute myocardial infarction, burns, and prolonged critical illness.[11] Again, the significance of this finding is unknown.

When critical illness is prolonged beyond 7 to 10 days there is profound suppression of pituitary, thyroid, adrenal, and gonadal gland function. This finding is in addition to the initial clinical problem and to any other organ dysfunction that may be present. Research is ongoing to understand the neuroendocrine pathways in both acute and prolonged critical illness with a view to blocking counterproductive metabolic pathways. The critical care nurse who understands the pathophysiology of the stress response in critical illness will be in a better position to recognize the neuroendocrine symptoms and collaborate with the multidisciplinary team to return the patient to physiologic normalcy.

ADRENAL DYSFUNCTION IN CRITICAL ILLNESS

Diminished adrenal gland function may result from one or more causes during critical illness:

- *Primary hypoadrenalism* describes an intrinsic failure of the adrenal gland to produce normal endogenous glucocorticosteroid hormones such as cortisol. Absolute adrenal failure is rare and occurs in 0.01% to 3% of critically ill patients.[15,16]
- *Secondary hypoadrenalism* occurs as a result of the administration of therapeutic steroids. In response to exogenous glucocorticosteroids the adrenal glands stop production of intrinsic hormones. Patients who have taken steroids before their admission to the hospital will need their dosage increased. One recommendation is to double the dose for a febrile illness.[13]
- *Relative adrenal insufficiency* describes a situation where the adrenal gland produces glucocorticosteroids but the quantity is insufficient for the disease process. Estimates of the frequency of adrenal insufficiency in critical illness range from 0% to 77% but are as high as 50% to 75% in septic shock.[15]
- *Peripheral adrenal resistance* is thought to occur in severe sepsis and septic shock.[15] In septic patients, inflammatory cytokines induce cellular resistance to cortisol; low-dose, short-term replacement corticosteroids may be required.[13,15]

Assessment of Adrenal Function. Clinical assessment of adrenal dysfunction is difficult in the critically ill, and a specialized laboratory assay is necessary for an accurate diagnosis. First, a baseline serum cortisol level is obtained. Adrenal failure is likely if the cortisol level is below 15 mcg/dl, and suspected if the level is above 15 but below 34 mcg/dl.[13]

Further confirmation may be obtained by performance of a corticotropin stimulation test *(cosyntropin test)*.[13,15] Cosyntropin is a medication made from the first 24 amino acids of corticotropin.[13] In the test, 250 mcg Cosyntropin is administered by intravenous (IV) route, and serum blood levels are measured 30 and 60 minutes later. If the serum cortisol rise from baseline is less than 9 mcg/dl after 30 to 60 minutes, this denotes inability of the adrenal gland to respond to a stress stimulus (nonresponder).[13,15] When the cortisol rise is greater than 18 mcg/dl in response to corticotropin stimulation, this indicates normally functioning adrenal glands (responder).[16] Corticosteroids are only given to nonresponders.[16]

The combination of a low baseline cortisol value (below 15 mcg/dl) with minimal or no rise in cortisol level (below 9 mcg/dl) after the cosyntropin test is firm evidence of adrenal failure.[13] The cosyntropin test is particularly helpful to determine level of adrenal dysfunction in patients whose serum cortisol level falls between 15 and 34 mcg/dl. One study demonstrated that after surgery, older patients with cortisol levels below 30 mcg/dl and who were vasopressor-dependent were successfully weaned off the vasopressor drips following cortisol replacement (hydrocortisone).[14] Further clinical trials will be required to fully explore the role of short-term corticosteroids in critical illness.

Corticosteroid Replacement. Clinical guideline recommendations promote short-term provision of low-dose hydrocortisone for patients with depleted cortisol levels who do not demonstrate a rise in cortisol level following corticotropin stimulation, and have a diagnosis of septic shock.[11,13,15] Hydrocortisone is the recommended replacement because it is the pharmacologic steroid that most resembles endogenous cortisol.[15] One suggested replacement regimen is 50 mg of hydrocortisone (glucocorticoid) every 6 hours (200 mg per day total), plus an optional 50 mg of fludrocortisone (mineralocorticoid) via a nasogastric tube (NG) once per day.[13,15] Fludrocortisone can only be taken by mouth or via a feeding tube.[15] Steroid replenishment is recommended as early as possible once septic shock with depleted cortisol levels is identified, but only if the septic patient is vasopressor-dependent.[15] High-dose steroid replacement is never recommended in management of sepsis.[15]

The role of corticosteroid replacement with other diagnoses is less well defined, but the current trend is to supplement low cortisol levels in critically ill patients. Corticosteroids are never discontinued abruptly and must be tapered gradually over several days.

HYPERGLYCEMIA IN CRITICAL ILLNESS

When hyperglycemia is actively managed with an insulin drip and blood glucose is maintained within the normal range, clinical outcomes are better both for diabetic and nondiabetic patients. Plasma blood glucose in the normal range (below 110 mg/dl) is associated with a lower morbidity and mortality.[1,17] The landmark study of "tight glucose control" by van den Berghe and colleagues found that for every 20 mg/dl serum glucose was elevated above normal (100 mg/dl), mortality rose 30%.[1,17]

Hospitalized Patients Who Are Diabetic. Not all patients who are hyperglycemic in the critical care unit have a previous diagnosis of diabetes. Estimates of the number of in-hospital patients who are diabetic ranges from 12% to 25%.[17] This wide range is due to the different methodologies used to define diabetes in hospitalized patients—sometimes by the serum glucose and sometimes by discharge diagnosis.[17] The range is also an indication that no one is really tracking how many hospitalized patients have diabetes as a primary or secondary diagnosis.

Hyperglycemia and the Cardiovascular System. Many patients who are admitted to the hospital with acute complications of cardiovascular disease are also diabetic.

The connection between acute cardiovascular events and diabetes is perhaps due to inflammatory changes in the vessel wall that are driven by hyperglycemia.[17] Phagocytic white blood cells (WBC) that are exposed to high serum glucose produce inflammatory mediators—tumor necrosis factor (TNF) and interleukin-6 (IL-6)—that are known to be damaging to endothelial tissue.[17] It has been suggested that elevated blood glucose contributes to acute cardiovascular events because hyperglycemia inhibits vasodilation by blocking the action of nitric oxide (NO) a vasodilator normally released by the vascular endothelium.[17]

Hyperglycemia and the Neurologic System. Acute hyperglycemia is associated with increased neuron damage following brain ischemia or ischemic stroke.[6,17] Most at risk is the *penumbra*—the potentially viable area of brain tissue around the ischemic core. More than one third of patients admitted with acute stroke are hyperglycemic when they arrive at the hospital.[18] Hyperglycemia decreases cerebral blood flow and increases brain lactate production.[19] If the hyperglycemia is not controlled after the stroke, the potentially viable penumbra (ischemic brain tissue) is more likely to progress to infarction.[20] Thus, the area of brain tissue affected is larger in patients with acute hyperglycemia at the time of an ischemic stroke.[18,20]

Hyperglycemia and Infection. Elevated serum blood glucose is associated with an increased incidence of infection and sepsis.[1,17] In cardiac surgery patients, many of whom are diabetic, hyperglycemia increases the incidence of deep sternal wound infections[21] and increases mortality.[17]

INSULIN MANAGEMENT IN THE CRITICALLY ILL

A profound shift in the management of the hyperglycemic critically ill ventilated patient has recently taken place.[17] As a result of the research that has highlighted the deleterious effects of hyperglycemia in critical illness, most hospitals have developed an institution-specific "tight glucose control" algorithm to lower blood glucose into the normal range. Many of these protocols are now published to enable others to use and adapt the developed algorithims.[21,22] The vigilance of the critical care nurse is pivotal to the success of any intervention to lower blood glucose using a continuous insulin infusion.

Some clinical interventions increase the likelihood that the patient will receive exogenous insulin. Infusion of total parental nutrition (TPN) typically requires a continuous insulin infusion to normalize blood glucose. In a study of critically ill surgical patients with preexisting type 2 diabetes who did not previously require insulin, 77% of patients needed insulin to control the blood sugar while receiving TPN.[17] Some enteral nutrition formulas are high in carbohydrates and will increase blood sugar in the same way. In this situation, either the composition

of the enteral feeding is altered or the insulin dosage is increased to achieve normal blood glucose levels. It is important to provide nutrition, and insulin can be a powerful adjunct to nutritional support.

Frequent Blood Glucose Checks. Monitoring the blood glucose using a point-of-care glucometer is the basis of targeted glucose control. As part of the comprehensive initial assessment the blood sugar is measured either by a standard laboratory sample or by a "fingerstick" capillary blood sample. In many institutions, if the blood sugar is greater than 130 mg/dl (although the initial value will vary between hospitals) the patient is started on a continuous IV insulin infusion. In critically ill catabolic patients the initial blood glucose can be well above 200 mg/dl. While the glucose is elevated, blood sample measurements are generally tested hourly to allow titration of the insulin drip to lower blood glucose. Once the patient is stable, blood glucose measurements can be spaced every 2 hours, although the actual time intervals will vary based on individual hospital protocols.

Several different blood-sampling methods are available. A capillary finger-stick is perhaps the easiest initial option, although the fingers can become noticeably marked if there are numerous sticks over several days. Trauma to the fingers is also exacerbated if there is diminished peripheral perfusion. If a central venous catheter (CVC) or an arterial line with a blood conservation system attached is in place, this can be a highly efficient system because there is no blood wastage. If there is not a blood conservation set-up attached, the venous/arterial catheter access method is unacceptable because of the amount of waste-blood that would be discarded.

Continuous Insulin Infusion. Many hospitals use insulin infusion protocols for management of stress-induced hyperglycemia that are implemented by the critical care nurse.[1,7] Effective glucose protocols gauge the insulin infusion rate based on two parameters:

1. The immediate blood glucose result;
2. The rate of change in the blood glucose since the last hourly measurement.

The following three examples illustrate this concept:

- Patient A receives 3 units of continuous IV regular insulin per hour and has a blood glucose measurement of 110 mg/dl, but 1 hour ago it was 190 mg/dl; so the insulin rate must be decreased to avoid sudden hypoglycemia.
- Patient B receives 3 units of continuous IV regular insulin per hour and has a blood glucose measurement of 110 mg/dl, but an hour before it was 112 mg/dl; in this situation, no change is made in the insulin infusion rate.
- Patient C receives 3 units of continuous IV regular insulin per hour and has a blood glucose measurement of 190 mg/dl, and one hour ago it was 197

mg/dl; in this situation, the insulin rate must be increased to more rapidly move the patient's blood sugar toward normoglycemia.

The important point to emphasize is that the *rate of change* of the blood glucose is as important as the *most recent* blood glucose measurement. Each of the patients described may have the same insulin infusion rate, depending on their catabolic state, but individualization between different patients with different diagnoses can be safely achieved as long as the rate of change is also considered. A person's insulin requirement often fluctuates over the course of their illness. This occurs in response to changes in the clinical condition such as development of an infection; caloric alterations caused by stopping or starting enteral nutrition or TPN; administration of therapeutic steroids; or because the person is less catabolic.[17] A method to allow for corrective incremental changes (up or down) to adapt to the reality of clinical developments and maintain the glucose within the target range is essential.[17] Some protocols alter only the infusion rates, and others incorporate bolus insulin doses when the glucose is above a preestablished threshold such as 180 mg/dl. Typically, when the blood glucose has remained within target range for a number of hours (varies with hospital protocol from 4 to 12 hours) the time interval between blood glucose monitoring is extended to every 2 hours.

Transition from Continuous to Intermittent Insulin Coverage. The transition from a continuous insulin infusion to intermittent insulin coverage must be handled with care to avoid large fluctuations in blood glucose. Before the conversion the regular insulin infusion should be at a stable and preferably low rate and the patient's blood glucose maintained consistently within the target range. Even after the IV infusion has been turned off the insulin effect in the tissues extends for at least 30 minutes beyond circulating plasma insulin levels.[23] Recommended methods to facilitate the transition from IV to subcutaneous (SQ) insulin administration include the following[17,23]:

- Administer short-acting insulin SQ 1 to 2 hours before discontinuation of the continuous IV infusion. Example: regular insulin.
- Administer intermediate-acting insulin SQ 2 to 4 hours before stopping the continuous IV infusion. Example: NPH and Lente insulin.
- Administer long-acting insulin SQ 4 to 6 hours before stopping the continuous IV infusion. Example: Lantus (glargine) insulin.

Clinicians use various methods to calculate the quantity of insulin to prescribe during the transition to maintain stable blood glucose levels. Fig. 36-1 depicts hypothetical examples of how a combination of basal and bolus insulin regimens (prandial insulin) can work in clinical practice. One method is described below for Al-ice Smith, a 67-year-old patient recovering from critical illness and recently extubated.

1. Mrs. Smith is in stable condition on a regular insulin drip at 1 unit per hour. She is ready to be transitioned to SQ insulin. Mrs. Smith is now going to be taking food and liquids by mouth. Her total insulin over the previous 24 hours was 24 units. Mrs. Smith will require both *basal* coverage (provided by SQ intermediate or long-acting insulin) and *nutritional* coverage for mealtimes (provided by short-acting SQ insulin).

2. The 24 units of insulin infused during the previous 24 hours is her required insulin dose. Half of this (12 units) will be administered SQ as intermediate or long-acting insulin; the other half will be administered as short-acting insulin to coincide with meals (4 units insulin SQ with each meal—12 units total).

3. Insulin administration options:
   - Basal insulin: 12 units once a day (*or* 6 units twice a day) of Neutral Protamine Hagedorn (NPH) SQ; *or* glargine 12 units once a day.[21]
   - Prandial/nutritional insulin: 4 units regular insulin SQ before each meal (short-acting), *or* 4 units Lispro or Aspart SQ with meals (ultra–short-acting insulin).[21]
   - Supplemental correction dosages: A sliding insulin scale can be used to cover any hyperglycemia above target, combined with scheduled blood glucose measurement.[21,23]

Subsequently the SQ insulin dosage is adjusted to the individual patient's needs. In a stable *insulin-sensitive* patient 1 unit of short-acting insulin will lower the blood glucose by 50 to 100 mg/dl.[17] In critical care patients, more insulin is typically required to reduce blood glucose levels, because of the stress of the critical illness.[21] See the Pharmacologic Management Table on Insulin for a description of the different types of insulin available for use. These include ultra–short-acting, short-acting, intermediate-acting, long-acting, and combination insulin replacement options. Even after the transition to SQ insulin, blood glucose is monitored frequently to maintain blood glucose within the target range, and detect hyperglycemia or hypoglycemia.

Intermittent Insulin Coverage. As the critical illness resolves and the glucose levels become more predictable and stable, the patient can be transitioned to intermittent insulin using a "sliding scale." These scales can be either IV or SQ. The intermittent scales are generally not as proactive as the continuous IV infusion method and should be reserved for the stable patient. A frequent criticism of "sliding scale" therapy is that the dosages are rarely reevaluated or adjusted once established.[17] A second criticism is that the scales treat hyperglycemia only after it has occurred. They are not proactive in the manner of continuous insulin infusions.[17]

A. Intermediate-acting insulin (NPH) every 12 hours with short-acting (regular) insulin to cover meals.

B. Intermediate-acting insulin (NPH) every 12 hours with rapid acting insulin (Lispro or Aspart) with meals.

C. Intermediate-acting insulin (NPH) every 12 hours with short acting insulin (regular) to cover meals.

D. Long-acting insulin (glargine) one a day, with rapid-acting insulin (Lispro, Aspart) at mealtimes.

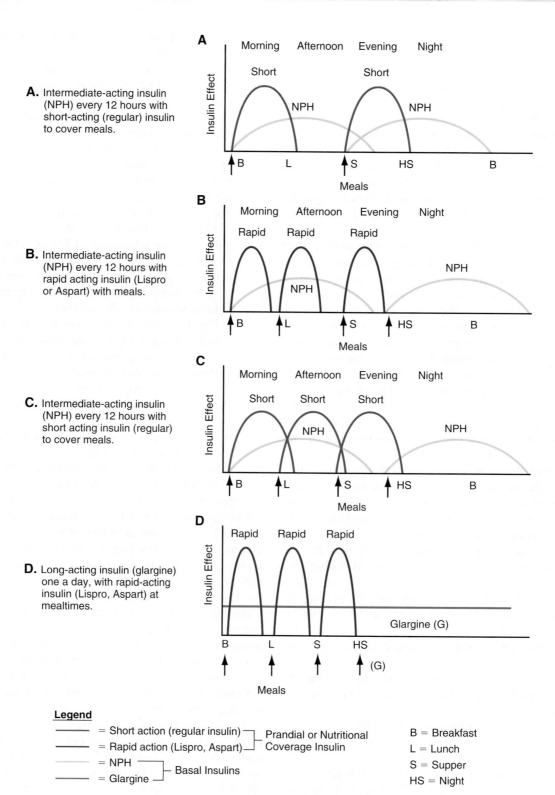

Fig. 36-1 Basal-nutritional bolus insulin combinations.

Pharmacologic Management: Insulin

INSULIN	ROUTE	ACTION	ONSET/PEAK/ DURATION	SPECIAL CONSIDERATIONS
Ultra–Short-Acting Insulins				
Lispro (Humalog)	SQ*	Insulin replacement, rapid onset	10-15 min/0.5-2.5hr/3-6.5 hr	First available synthetic insulin (analog), almost *immediately* absorbed **Must be taken with food** Shorter duration of action than regular insulin; should be used with basal longer-acting insulin See Fig. 36-1
Aspart (NovoLog)	SQ*	Insulin replacement, rapid onset	10-20 min/1–3 hr/3-5 hr	Insulin analog almost *immediately* absorbed **Must be taken with food** Insulin appearance should be clear Must be used in combination with intermediate acting or long-acting basal insulin regimen See Fig. 36-1
Short-Acting Insulin				
Regular	IV or SQ	Insulin replacement therapy	IV: Under 15 minutes SQ: In under 1 hr/2-4 hr/ 5-8 hr	Only type of insulin suitable for IV continuous infusion or bolus administration
Intermediate-Acting Insulins				
Neutral Protamine Hagedorn (NPH)	SQ*	Insulin replacement Intermediate action	3-4 hr/6-12 hr/ 18-28 hr	
Zinc suspension (Ultralente)	SQ*	Insulin replacement Extended action	4-6 hr/18-24 hr/ 36 hr	Also available as extended insulin zinc, human
Long-Acting Insulins				
Glargine (Lantus)	SQ*	Long-acting basal insulin analog Longer-acting than NPH or Ultralente	Does not produce peak concentrations; relatively constant concentrations over 24 hr	Synthetic insulin (analog), differs from human insulin by three amino acids, slowing release over 24 hours No peak Decrease dose by 20% if switching from NPH to glargine Must not be diluted or mixed with other insulins See Fig. 36-1
Combination (Premixed) Insulins				
Various	SQ*	Rapid plus intermediate or long-acting insulin combination		Varies according to combination used, and many other combinations exist **Long-acting component/short-acting component** —70% NPH with 30% Regular (70/30 regular) —70% aspart-protamine suspension with 30% aspart (NovoLog mix 70/30) —75% lispro-protamanine suspension with 25% lispro (Humalog mix 75/25)

Dosages are individualized according to patient's age and size.
*Not for IV use.
IV, Intravenous; *SQ*, subcutaneous.

HYPOGLYCEMIA MANAGEMENT

It is important to have a protocol for the management of hypoglycemia. The major drawback to use of intensive insulin protocols, as described above, is the potential for hypoglycemia. Whenever hypoglycemia is detected it is important to *stop* any continuous infusion of insulin. An example of one protocol to reverse hypoglycemia is described below:

- Blood glucose below 40 mg/dl: administer an IV bolus of 50 ml dextrose 50% in water ($D_{50}W$).
- Blood glucose 40 to 60 mg/dl: administer an IV bolus of 25 ml $D_{50}W$.
- Blood glucose 60 to 80 mg/dl: supplementary bolus glucose is not generally required.

In all cases of hypoglycemia the blood glucose is monitored every 15 to 20 minutes until the blood sugar has risen into a safe range. Some protocols use the patient's level of consciousness as a guide to glucose replacement with hypoglycemia. A different protocol suggests the following for a blood glucose below 60 mg/dl[21]:

- Blood glucose below 60 mg/dl and patient is awake and responsive: administer IV push 25 ml $D_{50}W$.
- Blood glucose below 60 mg/dl and patient is unresponsive: administer IV push 50 ml $D_{50}W$.

NURSING MANAGEMENT

Nursing management of the patient with neuroendocrine stress secondary to critical illness incorporates a variety of nursing diagnoses (see the Nursing Diagnosis feature on Stress of Critical Illness). The goals of nursing management are to monitor the glycemic side-effects of vasopressor therapy, Administer prescribed corticosteroids, monitor blood glucose and insulin effectiveness, provide nutrition, maintain surveillance for complications; and provide education to the patient's family and supportive others (see the Patient Education feature on Stress of Critical Illness).

Monitor Glycemic Side Effects of Vasopressor Therapy. Two vasopressors frequently used as continuous infusions to counteract hypotension in the critically ill also raise blood glucose. Epinephrine and, to a lesser extent, norepinephrine stimulate an increase in gluconeogenesis (creation of new glucose), an increase of skeletal muscle and hepatic glycogenolysis (increased glucose production), an increase in lipolysis (increased fat breakdown), direct suppression of insulin secretion, and an increase in peripheral insulin resistance.[24] All of these actions serve to raise the serum glucose level in the bloodstream. If hyperglycemia develops while a patient is receiving vasopressor therapy, IV insulin and a dextrose infusion should be instituted.[1,17]

Administer Prescribed Corticosteroids. Critically ill patients with below normal cortisol levels may be prescribed IV hydrocortisone. Therapeutic steroids raise

blood glucose levels and make glycemic control more difficult. Frequent monitoring of the blood glucose is necessary to guide treatment of hyperglycemia in the patient receiving IV corticosteroids. Ongoing monitoring for presence of new infection is mandatory, although short-term use of therapeutic steroids does confer greater benefit than harm in the septic patient population.[13]

Monitor Blood Glucose and Insulin Effectiveness. Hyperglycemia is associated with an increase in both morbidity and mortality in the critically ill patient.[1,7,17] The critical care nurse is responsible for the hourly monitoring of blood glucose and titration of the insulin infu-

EVIDENCE-BASED COLLABORATIVE PRACTICE
Stress of Critical Illness

Summary of evidence and evidence-based recommendations for controlling symptoms related to physiologic stress of critical illness

Strong Evidence to Support:
Maintenance of normal blood glucose levels
    Maintaining blood glucose levels between 80–110 mg/dl reduces patient morbidity and mortality.
    For patients who are eating, maintain preprandial blood glucose below 110 mg/dl; maintain peak postprandial blood glucose below 180 mg/dl.

Use of continuous IV insulin to control hyperglycemia is safe for critical care patients who have tight monitoring of their blood glucose.
Use of a multidisciplinary team approach
    Use of a multidisciplinary team that implements institutional guidelines, protocols, and standardized order-sets for the hospital results in fewer hypoglycemic and hyperglycemic events.

Moderate Evidence to Support:
Maintenance of normal cortisol levels
    In septic patients with depleted cortisol levels, hydrocortisone IV is administered short-term.

From Garber AJ et al: American College of Endocrinology position statement on inpatient diabetes and metabolic control, *Endocr Pract* 10(suppl 2):4-9, 2004; Clement S et al: Management of diabetes and hyperglycemia in hospitals, *Diabetes Care* 27(2):553-591, 2004; and Keh D, Sprung CL: Use of corticosteroid therapy in patients with sepsis and septic shock: an evidence-based review, *Crit Care Med* 32(11):S527-S533, 2004.

sion according to the hospital's established protocol while the patient is hyperglycemic. The use of standardized protocols makes possible a systematic approach to the control of blood glucose. This results in improved glycemic control and lower rates of hypoglycemia.[7] It is essential and recommended that nurses receive effective and ongoing education about the anabolic impact of insulin therapy in critical illness.[7]

Provide Nutrition. When an insulin infusion is started to lower blood glucose, it may be necessary to add a 10% dextrose infusion if the patient is not receiving other nutritional support (enteral or TPN).[23] While the 10% dextrose will further increase the blood glucose and the need for insulin, it offers the advantage of carbohydrate calories for metabolism, limits fluctuations in the blood sugar, and reduces the risk of hypoglycemia. Once the patient's metabolic condition is stable, introduction of non–glucose nutrition (protein and fat) is highly desirable.

PATIENT EDUCATION

When the patient is acutely ill the majority of the educational interventions are directed to the family at the bedside. Numerous explications are required to describe the IV medications, the nutritional needs, the purpose of insulin, the role of steroids (if applicable), the ongoing nursing care, prevention of complications, risk of multiorgan system dysfunction (MODS) and management of the underlying disease process. Educational issues that may be discussed are listed in the Patient Education feature on Stress of Critical Illness.

COLLABORATIVE MANAGEMENT

It is well established that standardized protocols designed to manage the complications of critical illness result in a lower morbidity and mortality for the patients.[7] Optimally, all disciplines concerned with the endocrine status of the patient have participated in design of these guidelines in each critical care area. The guideline that will apply to most patients is the use of tight glucose control. Many professional organizations endorse the importance of normalizing blood glucose in the hospitalized patient as described in the Evidence-Based Collaborative Practice feature on Stress of Critical Illness.

DIABETES MELLITUS

Diabetes mellitus is a progressive endocrinopathy associated with carbohydrate intolerance and insulin dysregulation.[5]

Morbidity and Mortality Associated with Diabetes Mellitus. Diabetes is the sixth most common cause of death in U.S. adults as reported by the U.S. Centers for Disease Control and Prevention (CDC).[25] Heart disease and stroke are the first and third leading causes of death among U.S. adults.[25] This data must be interpreted in light of the knowledge that adults with diabetes have a risk for dying from cardiovascular diseases that is two to four times greater than adults without diabetes.[26] Although the annual incidence of deaths attributed to cardiovascular diseases has decreased substantially, the decline is less among those with diabetes.[26] Age-adjusted prevalence of heart disease and stroke is approximately two to three times greater among adults with diabetes than among those without.[26] Diabetes is also associated with an increased risk of cancer. Malignant neoplasms are the second leading cause of death in the United States.[25] The CDC reports that diabetes is also an independent predictor of mortality from cancer of the colon, the pancreas, the female breast, and, in men, of the liver and the bladder.[27] Annual cost for hospital care per capita for persons with diabetes is $6,309, compared with $2,971 for persons without diabetes.[17] This represents a cost ratio of 2:1.[17]

Diagnosis of Diabetes. Diabetes mellitus is diagnosed by measurement of the fasting plasma glucose (FPG), also known as a fasting blood glucose (FBG) or fasting blood sugar (FBS).[28] The benchmarks for "normal" FPG have been progressively lowered in recent years as more knowledge has been gained about the benefits of maintaining the plasma glucose as close to normal as possible.

The current values endorsed by the American Diabetes Society are listed below[28]:

- FPG below 100 mg/dl (5.6 mmol/l) signifies normal fasting glucose.
- FPG between 100 and 125 mg/dl (5.6 and 6.9 mmol/L) implies impaired fasting glucose (IFG).
- FPG above 126 mg/dl (7 mmol/L) provides a diagnosis of diabetes (result is verified by testing more than once).

Two fasting blood glucose values of 126 mg/dl or higher confirm the diagnosis of diabetes.[28] For the acutely ill patient, hyperglycemia is actively treated with insulin to lower the blood sugar to within the normal range.[1] There are differences in the values of plasma versus whole blood glucose measurements. Plasma glucose values are 10% to 15% higher than whole blood glucose values, and it is essential that health care clinicians and people with diabetes know whether their monitor and strips provide whole blood or plasma results, especially when results from more than one setting (laboratory or monitor) are being compared.[29] Although most laboratories measure plasma glucose levels, most home-monitoring units and point-of-care units measure glucose using whole blood from a finger-stick.[30]

The benefit and importance of maintaining blood glucose at levels as close to normal as possible was conclusively demonstrated in patients with both type 1 and type 2 diabetes.[30] The Diabetes Control and Complications Trial (DCCT) of 1995 on type 1 diabetes and the United Kingdom Prospective Diabetes Study (UKPDS), published in 1998 on type 2 diabetes, demonstrated that lifestyle changes and use of medications that lead to consistently normal glucose levels reduce microvascular diabetes-related complications and decrease mortality.[30]

Types of Diabetes. There are two distinct types of diabetes that will be discussed in this chapter[31]:

- Type 1 diabetes results from beta-cell destruction, usually leading to absolute insulin deficiency.
- Type 2 diabetes results from a progressive insulin secretory defect in addition to insulin resistance.

The two diseases are different in nature, etiology, treatment, and prognosis.[28] A further category of *prediabetes* has recently been added to describe patients with impaired fasting glucose (FPG between 100 and 125 mg/dl) who are likely to develop diabetes at some time in the future and are also at increased risk for coronary artery disease and stroike.[28,31] Other conditions such as gestational diabetes are not discussed in this chapter.

Glycated Hemoglobin. For individuals with diabetes, maintenance of blood glucose within a tight normal range is fundamental to avoid development of microvascular and neuropathic secondary conditions. Although the fasting plasma glucose produces a "snapshot" of the blood glucose at a single point in time, the *glycated hemoglobin* (hemoglobin A_{1C}), also known as a *glycosylated hemoglobin*, identifies a percentage of glucose that the red cells have absorbed from the plasma over the previous 3- to 4-month period. A normal hemoglobin A_{1C} falls between 4% and 6%.[31] The target for diabetic patients is an A_{1C} value below 7%.[31] Long-term studies have shown that for every 1% increase in the hemoglobin A_{1C} there is an approximate 30% increase in microvascular complications.[32] A clinical study is underway to determine if a more stringent A_{1C} target of less than 6% will reduce complications even further for those with diabetes.[31] Additional information about the glycosylated hemoglobin and the correlation with the plasma glucose is shown in Table 35-2. Currently the hemoglobin A_{1C} is not recommended as a diagnostic tool for new diabetics, but only for those with known diabetes as a means to track their degree of glycemic control.[31] However, it is obvious that in the newly admitted critical care patient with an elevated hemoglobin A_{1C} that the hyperglycemia has been present prior to admission.[21] This situation offers an opportunity to reevaluate and manage the ongoing hyperglycemia.

TYPE 1 DIABETES

Type 1 diabetes mellitus accounts for only about 5% to 10% of the diabetic population.[28] Older names for this condition include insulin-dependent diabetes (IDDM) and juvenile diabetes. Type 1 diabetes is a cellular-mediated autoimmune disease that causes progressive destruction of the beta cells of the islets of Langerhans in the pancreas. Autoantibodies that falsely identify "self" as a foreign invader to be destroyed can now be identified by laboratory analysis. There are multiple responsible autoantibodies that contribute to pancreatic destruction; these include autoantibodies to the islet cell, to insulin, to glutamic acid decarboxylase (GAD65), and to the tyrosine phosphatases IA-2 and IA-2β.[28] One or more of these autoantibodies are present in 85% to 90% of individuals when fasting hyperglycemia is initially detected.[28] Over time the autoantibodies render the pancreatic beta cells incapable of secreting insulin and regulating intracellular glucose. In type 1 diabetes, the rate of beta-cell destruction is highly variable. It occurs rapidly in some individuals (mainly infants and children) and slowly in others (mainly adults). Some patients, particularly children and adolescents, may be seen with ketoacidosis as the first manifestation of their disease.

Genetic predisposition and as yet unknown environmental factors are also believed to play an important role.[28] Patients with type 1 diabetes are prone to development of other autoimmune disorders such as Graves' disease (hyperthyroidism), Hashimoto's thyroiditis, Addison's disease, autoimmune hepatitis, myasthenia gravis, and pernicious anemia.[28] Lack of insulin impairs carbohydrate, protein, and fat metabolism.

Management of Type 1 Diabetes. Patients with type 1 diabetes must receive IV or subcutaneous (SQ) insulin therapy. Treatment with exogenous insulin replacement restores normal entry of glucose into the cells. The range of insulin replacements available is expanding, and it is essential that critical care nurses are knowledgeable about this class of medications (see the Pharmacologic Management Table on Insulin). Insulin is manufactured using human-based recombinant DNA technology.[33] Without insulin, the rapid breakdown of noncarbohydrate substrate, particularly fat, leads to ketonemia, ketonuria, and diabetic ketoacidosis (DKA), a life-threatening complication associated with type 1 diabetes (see also the Clinical Application feature on Endocrine Concepts).

TYPE 2 DIABETES

The estimated prevalence of type 2 diabetes among adults in the United States was 8.7% in 2002.[34] Almost 90% to 95% of those with diabetes have type 2 diabetes.[28] Most patients with this type of diabetes are older and obese, and many also have a condition known as *metabolic syndrome*.[28] Up to one third of people who have diabetes are undiagnosed. Patients at high risk of developing type 2 diabetes include those who meet the following criteria[34]:

- A family history of type 2 diabetes in first- and second-degree relatives.[34]
- Member of racial or ethnic groups known to be at greater risk of developing type 2 diabetes: Native Americans, African-Americans, Hispanic Americans, Asians/South Pacific Islanders.[34]
- Have signs of *insulin resistance syndrome* or conditions associated with insulin resistance such as hypertension, dyslipidemia, polycystic ovary syndrome, or metabolic syndrome.[34,35]

In type 2 diabetes, pancreatic beta cells are present and functioning but the amount of insulin they produce is highly variable in different patients as described in the following paragraphs:

- In some patients the pancreatic beta cells do not produce sufficient insulin to meet the metabolic need. In these patients there is evidence that the beta cells may be in decline for years before the appearance of clinical symptoms. This is termed an *inadequate insulin response.*

CLINICAL APPLICATION

Endocrine Concepts

Mr. E is a 45-year-old accountant with a history of type 1 diabetes that has been treated for 30 years. He was found sitting at his desk in a stuporous state on April 16. Family members report Mr. E is normally very careful about his diet and medications, but he has been working very late for the last 2 weeks. His initial assessment reveals warm, dry, flushed skin; poor skin turgor; rapid, deep respirations; and a fruity odor to his breath. Finger-stick blood glucose performed at the bedside was 764 mg/dl. Vital signs are as follows: heart rate (HR), 140; respiratory rate (RR), 40; and blood pressure (BP), 80/60 mm Hg.

1. What complication of diabetes do you suspect Mr. E has developed? What probably precipitated this event?

2. Is Mr. E acidotic? Why or why not?
3. Is Mr. E dehydrated? Why or why not?
4. What is the first goal of medical therapy for Mr. E?
5. Mr. E is placed on an insulin drip. The physician tells you that Mr. E's blood glucose should drop by no more than 75 to 100 mg/dl/hour. Why?
6. The physician orders state to change Mr. E's intravenous fluids from 0.45% normal saline to 5% dextrose in 0.45% normal saline when his blood sugar decreases to 250 mg/dl. Would you question this order? Why or why not?
7. Identify five complications that Mr. E should be closely monitored for while you are caring for him.

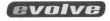 For the discussion of this Clinical Application and for additional clinical applications on endocrine concepts, see the Evolve website.

- In other individuals the pancreas may produce sufficient insulin, or even more than is needed (hyperinsulinemia) but the tissues are resistant to the effects of the insulin. This is known as *insulin resistance syndrome.*[35]
- Some patients may have a combination of the above, a lower than normal level of insulin production and a heightened insulin resistance at the cellular level.

Insulin resistance describes a complex metabolic situation where organ and tissue cells deny entry to insulin and glucose. This creates the clinical paradox in which elevated serum insulin levels and hyperglycemia are present at the same time. Abdominal obesity increases insulin resistance.[28] Insulin resistance has a strong association with type 2 diabetes. Until researchers clarify the exact nature of insulin resistance, many labels are used to describe similar clusters of symptoms, including insulin resistance syndrome and metabolic syndrome.[35-37]

Metabolic Syndrome. The major known stimuli for development of metabolic syndrome are obesity and disorders of insulin resistance.[37] Specific measurable factors are diagnostic of metabolic syndrome. These include abdominal adiposity as demonstrated by a waist measurement greater than 40 inches in men and over 35 inches in women; triglyceride levels higher than 150 mg/dl; high-density lipoprotein (HDL) cholesterol levels below 40 mg/dl in men and below 35 mg/dl in women; a blood pressure higher than 130/85 mg Hg; and a fasting plasma glucose higher than 100 mg/dl. The American Diabetes Association (ADA) uses the fasting plasma glucose cut-off point of 100 mg/dl in order to identify individuals who are prediabetic.[37] Metabolic syndrome is strongly associated with the development of heart disease and is also discussed in Chapter 18.

Screening for Type 2 Diabetes. The ADA recommends screening individuals at risk for type 2 diabetes at 3-year intervals beginning at age 45, particularly in those who are overweight or obese (body mass index [BMI] of 25 kg/m^2 or greater).[34] With the rise of obesity in the United States the incidence of type 2 diabetes in children and adolescents has also increased dramatically in the last decade.[31] Consistent with screening recommendations for adults, only children and youth at increased risk for the presence or the development of type 2 diabetes should be tested outside the hospital setting.[31]

Lifestyle Management with Type 2 Diabetes. The majority of adults with type 2 diabetes are overweight or obese as demonstrated by a BMI that exceeds 25 kg/m^2 (overweight) or 30 kg/m^2 (obese). Most patients with type 2 diabetes are recommended a program of weight reduction, increased physical exercise, and a change in diet pattern. Diets that contain large quantities of carbohydrate are discouraged.[37] The diet should contain less than 30% calories from fat, reduced sugar intake, low levels of saturated and trans fats, and an increased quantity of whole grains, vegetables, and fruits. "Crash diets" are not recommended, and a gradual program of weight loss, if needed, is preferred.[37] The exercise program is tailored to the individual but might start with 30 minutes of brisk walking each day if the person was previously sedentary.

Pharmacologic Management of Type 2 Diabetes. If lifestyle changes are unsuccessful in reversing the pattern of type 2 diabetes, oral antihyperglycemic medications are prescribed (see the Pharmacologic Management Table on Oral Medications for Type 2 Diabetes).[32] These drugs are not oral forms of insulin, because insulin would be destroyed by gastric juices. There are six major classes of oral agents (sulfonylureas, meglitinides, phenylalanine derivatives, biguanides, thiazolidinediones, and alpha-glucosidase inhibitors). These medications can also be classified according to their mechanism of action to lower plasma glucose levels. The oral drugs work in several different ways[32] (Box 36-1).

Insulin secretagogues stimulate pancreatic secretion of insulin and decrease hyperglycemia. Three classes of drugs have this action: the sulfonylureas (glyburide, glypizide, and glimepiride), the meglitinides (repaglinide), and phenylalanine derivatives (nateglinide).[32] The sulfonylurea drugs are taken once or twice a day, lower hyperglycemia, and have a long duration of action but little effect on postprandial hyperglycemia. Both of the other drugs are taken with meals, lower hyperglycemia, and also lower postprandial blood glucose levels.[32]

Insulin sensitizers work at two locations in the body. The drugs increase insulin sensitivity in the liver, increasing the ability of insulin to suppress endogenous glucose production, and also increase insulin sensitivity at the peripheral cellular level, allowing an increased uptake of glucose.[38] This class of drugs is considered first-line therapy for patients with type 2 diabetes. Two separate drug classes work in different ways to increase insulin sensitivity. The biguanide drugs (metformin) increase insulin sensitivity in the liver and have only a

---

Box 36-1

ORAL ANTIHYPERGLYCEMIC DRUG ACTIONS

Drugs that stimulate the pancreas to make more insulin (insulin secretagogues)
    Sulfonylureas
    Meglitinides
    Phenylalanine derivatives
Drugs that sensitize the body to insulin (insulin sensitizers)
    Thiazolidinediones
    Biguanides
Drugs that delay carbohydrate absorption
    Alpha-glucosidase inhibitors

Pharmacologic Management: Oral Medications for Type 2 Diabetes

Drug	Dosage	Action	Onset/Peak/Duration	Special Consideration
Insulin Secretalogues				
First-Generation Antihyperglycemics				
Tolbutamide (Orinase)	0.5-2.0 g bid-tid	Stimulates release of insulin	Rapid absorption 30 min-1 hr/ 3-5 hr/6-12 hr	Metabolized in liver; excreted in kidneys; Renal insufficiency: start with lower dose; observe for signs of hypoglycemia; Contraindicated in pregnancy; Numerous drug interactions
Tolazamide (Tolinase)	0.1-1.0 g single dose or bid	Stimulates release of insulin	4 hr/4 hr/10 hr	
Chlorpropamide (Diabinese)	0.1-0.5 g single dose	Stimulates release of insulin; Antidiuretic	1 hr/2-4 hr/48 hr	Frequent monitoring for patients with fluid retention or cardiac dysfunction
Second-Generation Antihyperglycemics				
Glipizide (Glucotrol, Glucotrol XL)	5-10 mg bid; 5-20 mg bid	Stimulates release of insulin	1 hr/1-3 hr/ 12-24 hr	
Glyburide (Micronase, Diabeta, Glynase Prestab)	5 mg single dose or bid; 3-6 mg daily	Stimulates release of insulin	1 hr/4 hr/ 18-24 hr	
Glimepiride (Amaryl)	1-4 mg daily	Stimulates release of insulin	Duration 24 hr	
Phenylalanine Derivatives				
Nateglinide (Starlix)	120 mg tid (1-30 minutes before meals)	Stimulates release of insulin	Peak < 1 hr	*Contraindications:* • Pregnancy, breast-feeding • Children • Hepatic disorders Dose may need to be adjusted with increased glucose during times of stress (infection, surgery, trauma)
Meglitinides				
Repaglinide (Prandin)	0.5-4.0 mg before meals	Binds to potassium on pancreatic beta cells; increases insulin secretion		Useful in patients with sulfa allergies

Second-generation hypoglycemics in this table are considered second-generation *oral* hypoglycemics and are more potent. Dosage is lower than for the first-generation drugs, but fewer side effects are associated with the second-generation agents.

bid, Twice daily; *tid,* three times daily; *BP,* blood pressure; *LDL,* low-density lipoprotein.

Continued

Pharmacologic Management: Oral Medications for Type 2 Diabetes—cont'd

Drug	Dosage	Action	Onset/Peak/ Duration	Special Consideration
Insulin Sensitizers *Biguanide* Metformin (Glucophage)	Max: 500-2550 mg divided dose	Sensitizer Antihyperglycemic Suppresses hepatic glucose production	1-3 hr/24 hr/ 24-48 hr	Lowers serum glucose by reducing hepatic glucose output. Decreases peripheral insulin resistance Temporarily withhold if patient having contrast radiography Adverse effects: lactic acidosis, GI upset Promotes weight loss *Contraindications:* • Pregnancy • Renal insufficiency • Acute/chronic acidosis • Diabetic ketoacidosis • Hepatic dysfunction • Excessive alcohol intake
Thiazolidinediones Pioglitazone (Actos)	15-45 mg	Enhances insulin action by increasing cell receptors to exogenous and endogenous insulin	Peak 2-3 hr	Decreases insulin resistance and decreases hepatic glucose production Take with meals to increase absorption
Rosiglitazone (Avandia)	4-8 mg			Reduces BP and triglycerides Administration with oral contraceptives reduces efficacy of both drugs by 30%
Carbohydrate Inhibitors *Alpha-Glucosidase Inhibitors* Acarbose (Precose)	100 mg tid with meals	Inhibits activity of intestinal enzymes that metabolize carbohydrate Reduces postprandial glucose mobilization	Peak 2-3 hr	With "first bite" each meal First drug to reduce effectively postprandial glucose Delays carbohydrate digestion by blocking absorption of complete carbohydrates in small intestine Does not promote weight loss; carbohydrate absorbed in distal small intestine and perhaps colon

Miglitol (Glyset)	50-100 mg tid	No apparent effect on lactose absorption, so lactose (not sucrose) substances should be used to treat hypoglycemia
		Side effects: flatulence, abdominal pain, diarrhea; minimized with slow titration
		Not recommended in severe renal impairment; safety in pregnancy not established
	Peak 2-3 hr	Same as for acarbose
		Administration with digoxin reduces average plasma concentration of digoxin
		Administration with propranolol or ranitidine greatly reduces bioavailability of these two drugs
		Do not take concomitantly with digestive enzymes (e.g., amylase, pancreatin)
Combination	Initial 25 mg daily, adjust bi-weekly per GI tolerance	
Glyburide and metformin (Glucovance)	1.25 mg/250 mg	Initial or second-line therapy
	2.5 mg/500 mg	Glyburide stimulates insulin secretion
	5.0 mg/500 mg	Metformin decreases glucose production and absorption
		See glyburide and metformin
		Common side effects: diarrhea, nausea, upset stomach

minor effect on skeletal muscle. In contrast, the thiazo-lidinedione drugs (pioglitazone and rosiglitazone) are about 70% more effective at increasing peripheral insulin sensitivity compared with metformin.[32] Both of these drug classes have rare but significant side effects that must be recognized if they occur. Metformin is associated with a risk of metabolic acidosis, especially for patients with elevated creatinine clearance.[39,40] The thiazo-lidinediones cause fluid gain and pedal edema in 3% to 5% of patients and heart failure in under 1%.[41] Of greater concern is when the thiazolidinedione drugs are combined with insulin therapy, the incidence of heart failure rises to between 2% and 3%.[41] The reasons for this occurrence are not yet known.

The third group of drugs slows digestion of ingested carbohydrates, delays glucose absorption, and reduces postprandial (after meals) hyperglycemia.[32] These are the *alpha-glucosidase inhibitors.* The drugs in this class are acarbose and miglitol.[32] A review of the physiology of carbohydrate digestion is helpful to understand how these drugs work. Carbohydrates are broken down to absorbable components in the duodenum and upper jejunum. The carbohydrates are digested to *oligosaccharides* in the small intestine by pancreatic lipase; then, the oligosaccharides are cleaved to *monosaccharides* by the *alpha-glucosidase* group of enzymes. The *monosaccharides* are then available to be absorbed from the intestine into the bloodstream. The alpha-glucosidase inhibitor drugs work by decreasing the conversion of carbohydrates from oligosaccharides to monosaccharides, thus limiting the glucose blood rise that occurs after eating. The most frequently prescribed drug in this class is acarbose, which is nonabsorbable.[32]

Combination therapy, either by prescription of drugs from more than one class, or use of a drug that combines two different methods of action, is the treatment of choice in most patients with type 2 diabetes.[32] The number of oral antihyperglycemic agents is increasing rapidly, and the critical care nurse must be familiar with these categories of drugs. See the Pharmacologic Management Table on Oral Medications for Type 2 Diabetes for more specific details related to the oral antihyperglycemic drugs. Pancreatic beta cell decline occurs as type 2 diabetes progresses and eventually, in many patients, oral agents alone will fail to control hyperglycemia. Insulin may be added to the drug regimen to maintain normal blood sugar levels.[32,42] At this stage, many patients with type 2 diabetes take oral medications and receive SQ insulin.[32] Some patients convert entirely to type 1 diabetes.[42] When a patient with type 2 diabetes is admitted to the critical care unit, he or she is often switched to either SQ or IV insulin and the oral medications are temporarily stopped.[43]

Patients who have type 2 diabetes are prone to a wide range of other complications that increase morbidity and mortality. Thus, in addition to antihyperglycemic drugs, patients with type 2 diabetes often require medications to lower their blood pressure,[44] lower their cholesterol and triglyceride levels,[45] treat ischemic heart disease,[46] and manage symptoms of heart failure.[47]

A serious complication of type 2 diabetes that, if present, mandates admission to a critical care unit, is hyperglycemic hyperosmolar syndrome (HHS). This severe, sustained elevation of glucose levels leads to a serum hyperosmolality and, if left untreated, progresses toward cellular dehydration, coma, and death. HHS is discussed in a later section.

DIABETIC KETOACIDOSIS

EPIDEMIOLOGY AND ETIOLOGY

Diabetic ketoacidosis (DKA) is a life-threatening complication of diabetes mellitus. Type 1 diabetics who are dependent on insulin are typically affected.[48] Some elderly patients with type 2 diabetes can develop DKA, but this is not as frequently encountered.[49,50]

The clinical diagnostic criteria for DKA are a blood glucose greater than 250 mg/dl; an arterial pH below 7.3; serum bicarbonate below 15 mEq/L; and moderate or severe ketonemia or ketouria.[29,48-50]

The annual incidence of DKA ranges from 4.6 to 8 episodes per 1,000 patients with diabetes.[48] Annual hospital costs for patients with DKA exceed $1 billion per year.[48] Infection is the major reason that diabetic patients develop and progress to DKA. Symptoms of fatigue and polyuria may precede the development of full-blown DKA, which can develop in under 24 hours, in a person with type 1 diabetes.[48] In an undiagnosed diabetic patient, it is unknown how long it may take to develop as the pancreatic beta cells gradually fail. About 20% of hospital admissions for DKA are related to diagnosis of new-onset type 1 diabetes.[50] Mortality in DKA is below 5% in patients with type 1 diabetes, when patients are managed by clinicians experienced in treatment of this disorder.[48]

Changes in the type of insulin, change in dosage, or increased metabolic demand can precipitate DKA in individuals with type 1 diabetes.[48] Life cycle changes, such as growth spurts in the adolescent, require an increase in insulin intake, as do surgery, infection, and trauma. In young persons with diabetes, psychologic problems combined with eating disorders may be a contributing factor in up to 20% of recurrent ketoacidosis.[48]

Ketoacidosis also occurs with acute pancreatitis. In addition to elevated glucose and acidosis, the serum amylase and lipase are abnormally high, which helps to establish the diagnosis as separate from type 1 diabetes.[50] Other nondiabetes causes of ketoacidosis are *starvation ketoacidosis* and *alcoholic ketoacidosis.* Both of these are distinguished from classical DKA by clinical history and usually, by a plasma glucose level below 250 mg/dl.[48]

PATHOPHYSIOLOGY

Insulin Deficiency. Insulin is the metabolic key to the transfer of glucose from the bloodstream into the cell, where it can be used immediately for energy or stored for use at a later time. Without insulin, glucose remains in the bloodstream, and cells are deprived of their energy source. A complex pathophysiologic chain of events fol-

lows (Fig. 36-2). The release of glucagon from the liver is stimulated when insulin is ineffective in providing the cells with glucose for energy. Glucagon increases the amount of glucose in the bloodstream by breaking down stored glucose (glycogenolysis). In addition, noncarbohydrates (fat and protein) are converted into glucose (gluconeogenesis). Blood glucose levels for the patient in DKA typically range from 300 to 800 mg/dl of blood. The

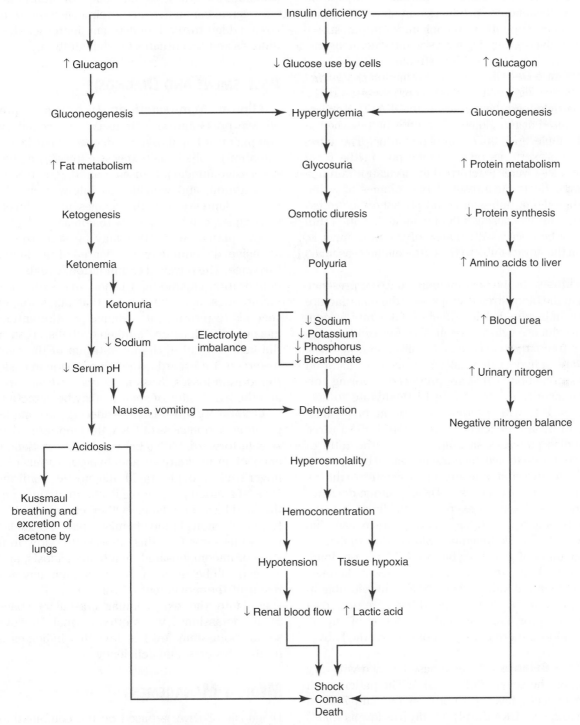

Fig. 36-2 Pathophysiology of diabetic ketoacidosis (DKA).

reason the plasma glucose is not higher is because of the short time period in which DKA develops. Elevated serum glucose levels alone do not define DKA; the major determining factor is the presence of ketoacidosis.

Hyperglycemia. Hyperglycemia increases the plasma osmolality, and blood volume becomes hyperosmolar. Cellular dehydration occurs as the hyperosmolar extracellular fluid draws the more dilute intracellular and interstitial fluid into the vascular space in an attempt to return the plasma osmolality to normal. Dehydration stimulates catecholamine production in an effort to provide emergency support. Catecholamine output stimulates further glycogenolysis, lipolysis, and gluconeogenesis, pouring glucose into the bloodstream.

Fluid Volume Deficit. Excessive urination *(polyuria)* and *glycosuria* (sugar in the urine) occur as a result of the osmotic particle load that occurs with DKA. The excess glucose, filtered at the glomeruli, cannot be resorbed at the renal tubule and "spills" into the urine. The unresorbed solute exerts its own osmotic pull in the renal tubules, and less water is returned to circulation through the collecting ducts. As a result, large volumes of water, along with sodium, potassium, and phosphorus, are excreted in the urine, causing a fluid volume deficit. Serum sodium may be decreased because of the movement of water from the intracellular to the extracellular (vascular) space.[48]

Ketoacidosis. In the healthy individual, the presence of insulin in the bloodstream suppresses the manufacture of ketones. In insulin deficiency states, fat is rapidly converted into glucose (gluconeogenesis). Ketoacidosis occurs when free fatty acids are metabolized into ketones: acetoacetate, β-hydroxybutyrate, and acetone make up the three ketone bodies that are produced.[49] During normal metabolism the ratio of β-hydroxybutyrate to acetoacetate is 1:1, with acetone present in only small amounts. In insulin deficiency the quantity of all three ketone bodies increases substantially, and the ratio of β-hydroxybutyrate to acetoacetate increases by as much as 10:1.[49] β-hydroxybutyrate and acetoacetate are the ketones responsible for acidosis in DKA. Acetone does not cause acidosis and is safely excreted in the lungs, causing the characteristic "fruity" odor.[49] Ketones are measurable in the bloodstream (ketonemia). Blood tests that measure the quantity of β-hydroxybutyric acid, the predominant ketone body, are the most useful.[29] Because ketones are excreted via the kidney they are also measurable in the urine *(ketonuria).* Ketone blood tests are preferred over urine tests for diagnosis and monitoring of DKA.[29] When the blood and urine are clear of ketones the DKA is resolved.

Acid-Base Balance. The acid-base balance will vary depending on the severity of the DKA. The patient with mild DKA typically has a pH between 7.25 and 7.30. In moderate to severe DKA the pH will drop as low as 7.00.[48] Acid ketones dissociate and yield hydrogen ions (H^+) that accumulate and precipitate a fall in serum pH. The level of serum bicarbonate also decreases consistent with a diagnosis of metabolic acidosis. Breathing becomes deep and rapid (Kussmaul respirations) to release carbonic acid in the form of carbon dioxide. Acetone is exhaled, giving the breath its characteristic "fruity" odor.

Gluconeogenesis. Gluconeogenesis is the process of breaking down fat or protein to make new glucose. Fat is metabolized to ketones as described above. Protein used for gluconeogenesis leaves no reserve protein available for synthesis and repair of vital body tissues. Nitrogen accumulates as protein is metabolized to urea. Urea, added to the bloodstream, increases the osmotic diuresis and accentuates the dehydration.

ASSESSMENT AND DIAGNOSIS

Clinical Manifestations. DKA has a predictable clinical presentation. It is usually preceded by patient complaints of malaise, headache, polyuria (excessive urination), polydipsia (excessive thirst), and polyphagia (excessive hunger). Nausea, vomiting, extreme fatigue, dehydration, and weight loss follow. Central nervous system depression, with changes in the level of consciousness, can lead quickly to coma.[48,49,51]

The patient with DKA may be stuporous or unresponsive, depending on the degree of fluid-balance disturbance. The physical examination reveals evidence of dehydration, including flushed dry skin, dry buccal membranes, and skin turgor that takes longer than 3 seconds to return to its original position after the skin has been lifted. Often, "sunken eyeballs," resulting from the lack of fluid in the interstitium of the eyeball, are observed. Tachycardia and hypotension may signal profound fluid losses. *Kussmaul respirations* are present and the fruity odor of acetone may be detected.

Laboratory Studies. Considering the complexity and potential seriousness of DKA, the laboratory diagnosis is straightforward. With a known diabetic patient, the presence of urine ketones and hyperglycemia on bedside finger-stick provide rapid diagnostic confirmation of DKA. If a blood gas sample is obtained, this can confirm the acid-base imbalance. Other clues may be gleaned from the venous blood chemistry panel. If the laboratory panel measures CO_2 this value will be low in the presence of uncompensated metabolic acidosis, and the anion gap will be elevated. Serum sodium may be low as a result of the movement of water from the intracellular space into the extracellular (vascular) space.[48] The serum potassium level is often normal. However, if the serum potassium level is low this indicates a severe total-body potassium deficiency.[48]

MEDICAL MANAGEMENT

Diagnosis of DKA is based on the combination of presenting symptoms, patient history, medical history (type 1 diabetes), precipitating factors if known, and results of

Management of Adult Patients with DKA

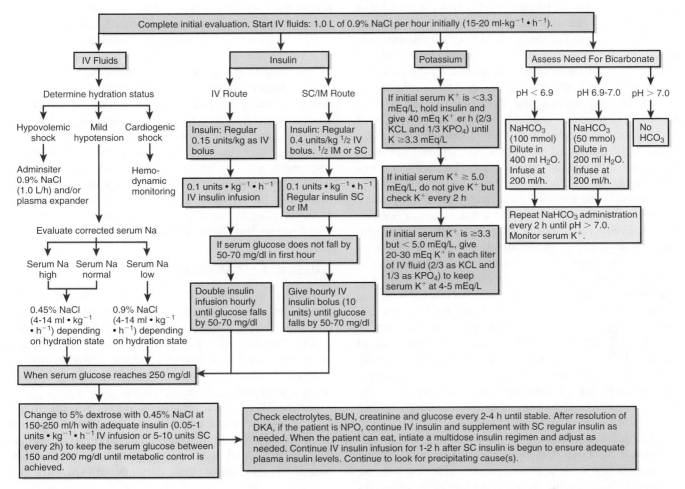

Fig. 36-3 Protocol for the management of adult patients with DKA. (From Kitabchi AE et al: *Diabetes Care*, 27(Suppl 1):S94-S102, 2004.)

serum glucose and urine ketone testing. Once diagnosed, DKA requires aggressive clinical management to prevent progressive decompensation. The goals of treatment are the following:

- Reverse dehydration
- Replace insulin
- Reverse ketoacidosis
- Replenish electrolytes

Reverse Hydration. The patient with DKA is dehydrated and may have lost 5% to 10% of body weight in fluids. A fluid deficit up to 6 L can exist in severe dehydration.[48] Aggressive fluid replacement is provided to rehydrate both the intracellular and the extracellular compartments and prevent circulatory collapse as detailed in Fig. 36-3.[48] An assessment of hydration is an important first step. Isotonic normal saline (0.9% NaCl) IV is infused to replenish the vascular deficit and to reverse hypotension. For the severely dehydrated patient, 1 to 1.5 L of normal saline is infused immediately.[48] Laboratory assessment of the serum osmolality and of serum sodium can help guide the subsequent interventions. If the serum osmolality is elevated and serum

sodium is high (hypernatremia), infusions of hypotonic sodium chloride (0.45% to 0.75%) will follow the initial saline replacement. The replacement infusion typically includes 20 to 30 mEq potassium per liter to restore the intracellular potassium debt, provided kidney function is normal.[48] Fluid replacement should correct intravascular volume deficits within 24 hours, with the caveat that the hourly changed in serum osmolality should not exceed 3 mOsm per kg H_2O each hour.[48] In patients without normally functioning kidneys, or with cardiopulmonary disease, very careful attention must be paid to the volume of fluid replacement to avoid fluid overload.

Once the serum glucose level decreases to between 150 and 250 mg/dl, the infusing solution is changed again to a 50/50 mix of isotonic or hypotonic saline and 5% dextrose.[48] Dextrose is added to replenish depleted cellular glucose as the circulating serum glucose level falls. Dextrose infusion will also prevent unexpected hypoglycemia when the insulin drip is continued, but before the patient can take in sufficient carbohydrate from an oral diet.

Replace Insulin. In moderate to severe DKA, an initial IV bolus of regular insulin at 0.15 units for each kg of body weight is administered.[48] Subsequently, a continuous infusion of regular insulin is infused simultaneously with IV fluids.[48] The amount of insulin can be calculated by multiplying 0.1 unit of regular insulin by the patient's body weight. Typically this represents 5 to 7 units of regular insulin per hour in adults. If the plasma glucose does not fall by 50 mg/dl in the first hour of treatment, recheck the glucose measurement and reevaluate the hydration status of the patient. If the plasma glucose is decreasing as expected, the insulin infusion may be doubled every hour until a steady glucose decline between 50-75 mg/dl is achieved.[48] See Fig. 36-3 for a diagrammatic representation of both IV and SQ insulin administration options in DKA. Frequent assessment of the patient's blood glucose is mandatory in moderate to severe DKA. Initially blood glucose tests are performed hourly; frequency decreases to every 2 to 4 hours as the patient's blood glucose levels stabilize and approach normal. Once the blood glucose has decreased to between 150 and 250 mg/dl, acidosis is corrected and dehydration is achieved, it will be possible to decrease the insulin infusion rate to 0.05 to 0.1 unit per kg body weight, hourly. This usually represents 3 to 6 units per hour in an adult receiving a continuous IV insulin infusion.[48] It is advised to verify that the serum potassium is not below 3.3 mEq/L, and to replace the serum potassium if necessary, before administering the initial insulin bolus.[48]

Reverse Ketoacidosis. Replacement of fluid volume and insulin will interrupt the ketotic cycle and reverse the metabolic acidosis. In the presence of insulin, glucose will enter the cells, and the body will cease to convert fats into glucose. The ketoacidotic cycle is broken by the provision of fluid volume and insulin replacement.

Adequate hydration and insulin replacement will usually correct the acidosis and is sufficient treatment for many patients with DKA. As shown in Fig. 36-3, replacement of bicarbonate is no longer routine except for the severely acidotic patient with a serum pH below 7.0.[48] An indwelling arterial line provides access for hourly sampling of arterial blood gases (ABGs) to evaluate pH, bicarbonate, and other laboratory values in the patient with severe DKA. If an arterial line is not available the pH can be assessed using the venous pH.[48]

Hyperglycemia generally resolves before ketoacidemia. In one clinical report, patients with previously diagnosed type 1 diabetes in DKA took an average of 21 hours after being started on an IV insulin protocol to clear ketones from the urine; the IV insulin infusion was continued for 36 hours until the patients could tolerate an oral diet, and the patients received a total of 9.5 liters of normal saline for rehydration.[50] It is important to be aware that patients who are newly diagnosed type 1 diabetics take longer to clear their urine ketones and require more insulin to achieve normal glycemic control.[50]

Replenish Electrolytes. Low serum potassium (hypokalemia) will occur as insulin promotes the return of potassium into the cell and metabolic acidosis is reversed. Replacement of potassium using potassium chloride (KCl) begins as soon as the serum potassium falls below normal. Frequent verification of the serum potassium level is required for the DKA patient receiving fluid resuscitation and insulin therapy. The serum phosphate level is sometimes low (hypophosphatemia) in DKA. Insulin treatment may make this more obvious as phosphate is returned to the interior of the cell. If the serum phosphate level is below 1 mg/dl, phosphate replacement is recommended.[48] Some of the potassium replacement may be provided in the form of potassium phosphate (KPO_4).[48] See Fig. 36-3 for further information about potassium replacement options.

NURSING MANAGEMENT

Nursing management of the patient with diabetic ketoacidosis incorporates a variety of nursing diagnoses (see the Nursing Diagnoses feature on Diabetic Ketoacidosis). The goals of nursing management are to administer prescribed fluids, insulin, and electrolytes; monitor response to therapy; maintain surveillance for complications; and provide patient education.

Administer Fluids, Insulin, and Electrolytes. Rapid IV fluid replacement requires the use of a volumetric pump. Insulin is administered IV to patients who are severely dehydrated or have poor peripheral perfusion to ensure effective absorption. Patients with DKA are kept

---

NURSING DIAGNOSES **Diabetic Ketoacidosis**

- Decreased Cardiac Output related to alterations in preload
- Deficient Fluid Volume related to absolute loss
- Anxiety relate to threat to biologic, psychologic, and/or social integrity
- Disturbed Body Image related to functional dependence on life-sustaining technology
- Ineffective Coping related to situational crisis and personal vulnerability
- Powerlessness related to lack of control over current situation and/or disease progression
- Deficient Knowledge: Discharge Regimen related to lack of previous exposure to information (see Patient Education feature on Diabetic Ketoacidosis)

on NPO status (nothing by mouth) until the hyperglycemia is under control. Throughout the insulin therapy, both patient response and laboratory data are assessed for changes relating to blood glucose levels. The critical care nurse is responsible for monitoring the rate of plasma glucose decline in response to insulin. The goal is to achieve a fall in glucose levels of approximately 50 to 75 mg/dl each hour.[48] The coordination involved in monitoring blood glucose, potassium and often blood gases on an hourly basis is considerable. When the blood glucose level falls to between 150 and 250 mg/dl, a 5% or 10% dextrose solution is infused to prevent hypoglycemia.[48] At this time, it is likely the insulin dose per hour will also be decreased. The regular insulin drip is not discontinued until the ketoacidosis subsides, as identified by a normal pH on an arterial or venous blood gas.[48] Insulin is given subcutaneously when glucose levels, dehydration, hypotension and acid-base balance are normalized and the patient is in stable condition and taking an oral diet.

Monitor Response to Therapy. Accurate intake and output (I&O) measurements must be maintained to monitor reversal of dehydration. Measuring hourly urine output is an indicator of renal function and provides information to prevent overhydration or underhydration. Vital signs, especially heart rate (HR), hemodynamic values, and BP, are continuously monitored to assess response to the fluid replacement. Evidence that fluid replacement is effective includes normal central venous pressure (CVP), decreased HR, and normal BP. Box 36-2 lists the standard features to be included in an assessment of hydration status. More invasive hemodynamic monitoring, such as a pulmonary artery catheter, is rarely needed. Further evidence of hydration improvement includes a change from a previously weak, thready pulse to a pulse that is strong and full, and a change from hypotension to a gradual elevation of systolic BP. Respirations are assessed frequently for changes in rate, depth, and presence of the fruity acetone odor.

Blood glucose is measured each hour in the initial period. Sometimes potassium is measured just as frequently. Serum osmolality and serum sodium are evaluated, and blood urea nitrogen (BUN) and creatinine levels are assessed for possible renal impairment related to decreased kidney perfusion. The purpose of these frequent assessments is to determine that the patient's clinical status is improving. Once the patient has stable laboratory indicators and is awake and alert, the transition to SQ insulin and an oral diet can be made. Hypoglycemia is a risk during the transition period. For example, in anticipation of discontinuing the insulin and IV dextrose infusion, a patient would receive a SQ dose of insulin and would be expected to eat a meal. However, if the patient is then unable to eat an adequate amount, hypoglycemia results secondary to the SQ insulin without adequate glucose.[50]

The markers for resolution of DKA include a blood glucose below 200 mg/dl, serum bicarbonate above 18 mEq/L, and a venous pH greater than 7.3.[48]

Survey for Complications. The patient in DKA can experience a variety of complications, including risk for fluid volume overload, hypoglycemia, hypokalemia or hyperkalemia, hyponatremia, cerebral edema, and infection.

Fluid Volume Overload. Fluid overload from rapid volume infusion is a serious complication that can occur in the patient with a compromised cardiopulmonary system, renal system, or both. Neck vein engorgement, dyspnea without exertion, and pulmonary crackles on auscultation signal circulatory overload. Reduction in the rate and volume of infusion, elevation of the head of the bed, and provision of oxygen may be required to manage the increased intravascular volume. Hourly urine measurement is mandatory to assess renal output and adequacy of fluid replacement.

Hypoglycemia. Hypoglycemia is defined as serum glucose level below 60 mg/dl. Most acute care hospitals have specific procedures for management of the hypoglycemic patient (see the Nursing Intervention Classification feature on Hypoglycemia Management). For example, if hypoglycemia is detected by finger-stick point-of-care testing at the bedside, a blood sample is sent to the laboratory for a verification, the physician is notified immediately, and replacement glucose is given either IV or by mouth. The route of administration is based on the patient's clinical condition, diagnosis, and level of consciousness.

Unexpected behavior change or decreased level of consciousness, diaphoresis, and tremors are physical warning signs that the patient has become hypoglycemic. These symptoms are especially important to recognize if the frequency of glucose testing has lengthened to 2- to 4-hour intervals. A comparison between the physical symptoms expected with hypoglycemia versus hyperglycemia is provided in Box 36-3.

Box 36-2

HYDRATION ASSESSMENT

Hourly intake
Blood pressure changes
  Orthostatic hypotension
  Pulse pressure
  Pulse rate, character, rhythm
Neck vein filling
Skin turgor
Skin moisture
Body weight
Central venous pressure
Pulmonary arterial occlusion pressure
Hourly output
Complaints of thirst

NIC   Hypoglycemia Management

Definition: Preventing and treating low blood glucose levels

Activities

Identify patient at risk for hypoglycemia

Determine recognition of hypoglycemia signs and symptoms

Monitor blood glucose levels, as indicated

Monitor for signs and symptoms of hypoglycemia (e.g., shakiness, tremor, sweating, nervousness, anxiety, irritability, impatience, tachycardia, palpitation, chills, clamminess, lightheadedness, pallor, hunger, nausea, headache, tiredness, drowsiness, weakness, warmth, dizziness, faintness blurred vision, nightmares, crying out in sleep, paresthesias, difficulty concentrating, difficulty speaking, incoordination, behavior change, confusion, coma, seizure)

Provide simple carbohydrate, as indicated

Provide complex carbohydrate and protein, as indicated

Administer glucagons, as indicated

Contact emergency medical services, as necessary

Administer intravenous glucose, as indicated

Maintain IV access, as appropriate

Maintain patent airway, as necessary

Protect from injury, as necessary

Review events prior to hypoglycemia to determine probable cause

Provide feedback regarding appropriateness of self-management of hypoglycemia

Instruct patient and significant others on signs and symptoms, risk factors, and treatment of hypoglycemia

Instruct patient to have simple carbohydrates available at all times

Instruct patient to obtain and carry/wear appropriate emergency identification

Instruct significant others on the use and administration of glucagons, as appropriate

Instruct on interaction of diet, insulin/oral agents, and exercise

Provide assistance in making self-care decisions to prevent hypoglycemia (e.g., reducing insulin/oral agents and/or increasing food intake for exercise)

Encourage self-monitoring of blood glucose levels

Encourage ongoing telephone contact with diabetes care team for consultation regarding adjustments in treatment regimen

Collaborate with patient and diabetes care team to make changes in insulin regimen (e.g., multiple daily injections), as indicated

Modify blood glucose goals to prevent hypoglycemia in the absence of hypoglycemia symptoms

Inform patient of increased risk of hypoglycemia with intensive therapy and normalization of blood glucose levels

Instruct patient regarding probable changes in hypoglycemia symptoms with intensive therapy and normalization of blood glucose levels

From Dochterman JM, Bulechek GM: *Nursing interventions classification, (NIC),* ed 4, St Louis, 2004, Mosby.

Hypokalemia/Hyperkalemia. Hypokalemia can occur within the first 4 hours of rehydration and insulin treatment. Continuous cardiac monitoring is required because low serum potassium (hypokalemia) can cause ventricular dysrhythmias. Hyperkalemia occurs with acidosis or with overaggressive administration of potassium replacement in patients with renal insufficiency. Severe hyperkalemia is noted on the cardiac monitor by a large, peaked T wave, flattened P wave, and widened QRS complex. Ventricular fibrillation can follow.

Hyponatremia. Sodium is eliminated from the body as a result of the osmotic diuresis and compounded by the vomiting and diarrhea that occur during DKA. Clinical manifestations of hyponatremia include abdominal cramping, apprehension, postural hypotension, and unexpected behavioral changes. Sodium chloride is infused as the initial IV solution. Maintenance of the saline infusion depends on clinical manifestations of sodium imbalance plus serum laboratory values.

Risk for Cerebral Edema. Changes in the patient's neurologic status may be insidious. Alterations in level of consciousness, pupil reaction, and motor function may be the result of fluctuating glucose levels and cerebral fluid shifts. Confusion and sudden complaints of headache are ominous signs that may signal cerebral edema. These observations require immediate action to prevent neurologic damage. Neurologic assessments are performed every hour or as needed during the acute phase of hyperglycemia and rehydration. Assessment of level of consciousness serves as the cerebral index of the patient's response to the rehydration therapy.

Risk for Infection. Skin care takes on new dimensions for the patient with DKA. Dehydration, hypovolemia, and hypophosphatemia interfere with oxygen delivery at the cell site and contribute to inadequate perfusion and tissue breakdown. Patients must be repositioned frequently to relieve capillary pressure and promote adequate perfusion to body tissues. The typical

Box 36-3

CLINICAL MANIFESTATIONS OF HYPOGLYCEMIA AND HYPERGLYCEMIA

HYPOGLYCEMIA	HYPERGLYCEMIA
Restlessness	Excessive thirst
Apprehension	Excessive urination
Irritability	Hunger
Trembling	Weakness
Weakness	Listlessness
Diaphoresis	Mental fatigue
Pallor	Flushed, dry skin
Paresthesia	Itching
Pallor	Headache
Headache	Nausea
Hunger	Vomiting
Difficulty thinking	Abdominal cramps
Loss of coordination	Dehydration
Difficulty walking	Weak, rapid pulse
Difficulty talking	Postural hypotension
Visual disturbances	Hypotension
Blurred vision	Acetone breath odor
Double vision	Kussmaul respirations
Tachycardia	Rapid breathing
Shallow respirations	Changes in level of con-
Hypertension	sciousness
Changes in level of con-	Stupor
sciousness	Coma
Seizures	
Coma	

PATIENT EDUCATION — Diabetic Ketoacidosis

- Acute phase
  Explain rationale for critical care unit admission
  Reduce anxiety associated with critical care unit
- Predischarge
  Assess knowledge level
  Assess compliance history
  Diabetes disease process
  Target glucose levels
  Causes of DKA
  Pathophysiology of DKA
  Self-care monitoring blood glucose
  Insulin regimen
  Sick-day management
  Universal precautions for caregivers
  Signs and symptoms to report to health care practitioner

patient with type 1 diabetes is either of normal weight or underweight. Bony prominences must be assessed for tissue breakdown and the patient's body weight repositioned every 1 to 2 hours. Irritation of skin from adhesive tape, shearing force, and detergents should be avoided. Maintenance of skin integrity will prevent unwanted portals of entry for microorganisms.

Oral care, including tooth brushing and lip balm, helps keep lips supple and prevents cracking. Prepared sponge sticks or moist gauze pads can be used to moisten oral membranes of the unconscious patient. Swabbing the mouth moistens the tissue and displaces the bacteria that collect when saliva, which has a bacteriostatic action, is curtailed by dehydration. The conscious patient removes bacteria and provides oral comfort with frequent tooth brushing and oral rinsing.

Strict sterile technique is used to maintain all IV systems. All venipuncture sites are checked every 4 hours for signs of inflammation, phlebitis, or infiltration. Strict surgical asepsis is used for all invasive procedures. Sterile technique is used if urinary catheterization is necessary to obtain urine samples for testing. Urinary catheter care is provided every 8 hours.

PATIENT EDUCATION

It is important to be aware of the knowledge level and compliance history of patients with previously diagnosed diabetes to formulate an appropriate teaching plan. Learning objectives include a discussion of target glucose levels, definition of hyperglycemia and its causes, harmful effects, and symptoms and how to manage insulin and diet when one is unwell and unable to eat.[50] Additional objectives include a definition of DKA and its causes, symptoms, and harmful consequences. The patient and family are also expected to learn the principles of diabetes management. Universal precautions must be emphasized for all family caregivers.[17] The patient and family must also learn the warning signs to report to the attention of a health care practitioner. Education of the patient, family, or other support persons to achieve knowledge-based, independent self-management of blood glucose level and avoidance of diabetes-related complications are the ultimate goals of the teaching process (see the Patient Education feature on Diabetic Ketoacidosis).

COLLABORATIVE MANAGEMENT

In all aspects of patient care management, health care professionals work as a team, with the major collaborative goal of providing the best possible outcome for each

EVIDENCE-BASED COLLABORATIVE PRACTICE
Diabetic Ketoacidosis

Summary of evidence and evidence based recommendations for controlling symptoms related to diabetic ketoacidosis (DKA):

Strong Evidence to Support:
Unless the DKA is mild, regular insulin by continuous infusion is recommended.

Replace serum phosphate if level is below 1.0 mg/dl.

Very Little Evidence to Support:
No support for use of routine bicarbonate to correct low serum pH. May be considered if pH is below 7.0.

From Kitabchi AE et al: *Diabetes Care* 27 (suppl 1):S94-S102, 2004.

---

patient. Current guidelines related to collaborative management of patients with hyperglycemia crisis are listed in the Evidence-Based Collaborative Practice feature on Diabetic Ketoacidosis (DKA).

HYPERGLYCEMIC HYPEROSMOLAR STATE

EPIDEMIOLOGY AND ETIOLOGY

Hyperglycemic hyperosmolar state (HHS) is a potentially lethal complication of type 2 diabetes. The hallmarks of HHS are extremely high levels of plasma glucose with resultant elevation in hyperosmolality causing osmotic diuresis. Ketosis is absent or mild.[48] Inability to replace fluids lost through diuresis leads to profound dehydration and changes in level of consciousness. Overall mortality from HHS is 15%.[48] However, because patients with HHS have type 2 diabetes as an underlying disorder, they are older and have associated illnesses, which will increase their mortality risk.[49,50] When the mortality for diabetic patients is stratified by age there is no difference in death rates based on the underlying hyperglycemic crisis (HHS or DKA).[49] For HHS patients less than 75 years of age, mortality is 10%; for patients aged 75-84, mortality is 19%; and for those older than 85 years, mortality is 35%.[49]

The diagnostic criteria for HHS include blood glucose above 600 mg/dl, arterial pH above 7.3, bicarbonate greater than 15 mEq/L, and serum osmolality greater than 320 mOsm/kg H_2O (320 mmol/kg).[29] Most patients with this level of metabolic disruption will also experience visual changes, mental status changes, and potentially hypovolemic shock.

HHS occurs when the pancreas produces a relatively insufficient amount of insulin for the high levels of glucose that flood the bloodstream. HHS primarily affects older obese persons with underlying cardiovascular conditions. Infection is the primary reason that type 2 diabetics develop HHS. The patient may have type 2 diabetes treated with diet and oral hypoglycemic agents that is destabilized by an infection. The most common infections are pneumonia and urinary tract infections. Other precipitating causes of HHS include stroke, myocardial infarction, trauma, burns, or the stress of a major illness. Many classes of medications have been associated with the development of HHS including corticosteroids, phenytoin, thiazide diuretics, beta-blockers, dobutamine, trebutaline, and antipsychotics.[48,49]

Differences between HHS and DKA. Clinically HHS is distinguished from DKA by the presence of extremely elevated serum glucose, more profound dehydration, and minimal or absent ketosis (Table 36-2). There is another major difference between HHS and DKA. In HHS, protein and fats are not used to create new supplies of glucose as in DKA, and the ketotic cycle is either never started, or does not occur until the glucose level is extremely elevated. Patients with type 1 diabetes do not develop HHS. Some patients with type 2 diabetes do develop DKA.[49,50]

PATHOPHYSIOLOGY

HHS represents a deficit of insulin and an excess of glucagons (Fig. 36-4). Reduced insulin levels prevent the movement of glucose into the cells, thus allowing glucose to accumulate in the plasma. The decreased insulin triggers glucagon release from the liver, and hepatic glucose is poured into the circulation. As the number of glucose particles increases in the blood, serum hyperosmolality increases. In an effort to decrease the serum osmolality, fluid is drawn from the intracellular compartment (inside the cells) into the vascular bed. Profound intracellular volume depletion occurs if the patient's thirst sensation is absent or decreased. HHS may evolve over days or even weeks.[48]

Hemoconcentration persists despite removal of large amounts of glucose in the urine (glycosuria). The glomerular filtration and elimination of glucose by the

Table 36-2	Comparison of Diabetic Ketoacidosis (DKA) and Hyperglycemic Hyperosmolar Syndrome (HHS)	
	DKA	**HHS**
Cause	Insufficient exogenous glucose for glucose needs	Insufficient exogenous/endogenous insulin for glucose needs
Onset	Sudden (hours)	Slow, insidious (days, weeks)
Precipitating factors	Noncompliance with type 1 diabetes, illness, surgery, decreased activity	Elderly patients with recent acute illness; therapeutic procedures
Mortality	9%-14%	10%-50%
Population affected	Type 1 diabetes	Type 2 diabetes
Clinical manifestations	Dry mouth, polydipsia, polyuria, polyphagia, mental confusion, tachycardia, changes in level of consciousness	dehydration, dry skin, hypotension, weakness,
	Ketoacidosis; air hunger, acetone breath odor, respirations deep and rapid, nausea, vomiting	No ketosis, no breath odor, respirations rapid and shallow, usually mild nausea/vomiting
LABORATORY TESTS		
Glucose	300-800 mg/dl	600-2000 mg/dl
Ketones	Strongly positive	Normal or mildly elevated
pH	<7.3	Normal*
Osmolality	<350 mOsm/L	>350 mOsm/L
Sodium	Normal or low	Normal or elevated
Potassium (K^+)	Normal, low, or elevated (total body K^+ depleted)	Low, normal, or elevated
Bicarbonate	<15 mEq/L	Normal
Phosphorus	Low, normal, or elevated (may decrease after insulin therapy)	Low, normal, or elevated (may decrease after insulin therapy)
Urine acetone	Strong	Absent or mild

*Except if lactic acidosis develops. With severe HHS, lactic acidosis may result from dehydration and severe tissue hypoperfusion and ischemia.

kidney tubules is ineffective in reducing the serum glucose level sufficiently to maintain normal glucose levels. The hyperosmolality and reduced blood volume stimulate release of ADH to increase the tubular resorption of water. ADH, however, is powerless in overcoming the osmotic pull exerted by the glucose load. Excessive fluid volume is lost at the kidney tubule with simultaneous loss of potassium, sodium, and phosphate in the urine. This chain of events results in progressively worsening hypovolemia.

Hypovolemia reduces renal circulation, and oliguria develops. Although this process conserves water and preserves the blood volume, it prevents further glucose loss, and hyperosmolality increases. Ketosis is absent or mild in HHS. However, the patient with HHS with an extremely elevated serum glucose (greater than 1000 mg/dl) can develop a metabolic acidosis secondary to dehydration, poor tissue perfusion, and lactic acid accumulation.

The sympathetic nervous system reacts to the body's stress response to try to restore homeostasis. Epinephrine, a potent stimulus for gluconeogenesis, is released, and additional glucose is added to the bloodstream. Unless the glycemic diuresis cycle is broken by aggressive fluid replacement and insulin, intracellular dehydration negatively affects fluid and oxygen transport to the brain

cells. Central nervous system dysfunction may result and lead to coma. Hemoconcentration increases the blood viscosity, which may result in clot formation, thromboemboli, and cerebral, cardiac, and pleural infarcts.

ASSESSMENT AND DIAGNOSIS

Clinical Manifestations. HHS has a slow, subtle onset and develops over several days. Initially the symptoms may be nonspecific and may be ignored or attributed to the patient's concurrent disease processes. History reveals malaise, blurred vision, polyuria, polydipsia (depending on patient's thirst sensation), weight loss and advancing weakness.[49] Medical attention may not be obtained for these nonspecific, nonacute symptoms until the patient is unable to take sufficient fluids to offset the fluid losses. Progressive dehydration follows and leads to mental confusion, convulsions, and eventually coma, especially in the elderly.

The physical examination may reveal a profound fluid deficit. Signs of severe dehydration include longitudinal wrinkles in the tongue, decreased salivation, and decreased CVP, with increases in HR and rapid respirations (Kussmaul air hunger is not present). In elderly patients, assessment of clinical signs of dehydration is challeng-

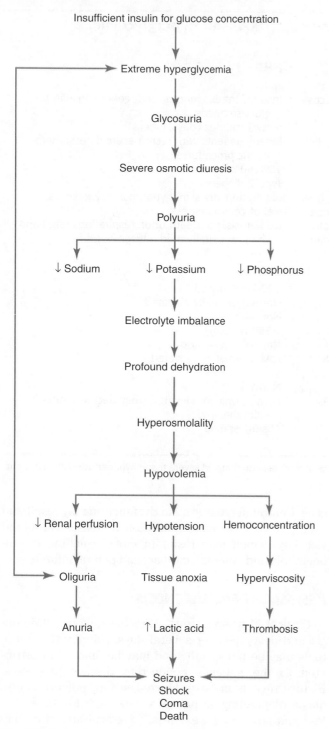

Fig. 36-4   Pathophysiology of hyperglycemic hyperosmoloar nonketotic syndrome (HHS).

ing. Neurologic status is affected as the serum glucose climbs, especially above 1500 mg/dl. Without intervention, obtundation and coma will occur.

Laboratory Studies. Laboratory findings are used to establish the definitive diagnosis of HHS. Plasma glucose levels are strikingly elevated with blood glucose above 600 mg/dl. Serum osmolality is above 320 mOsm/kg. Acidosis is absent with an arterial pH above 7.3, a serum bi-

carbonate greater than 15 mEq/L, and absent or mild ketonuria.[48-50] Elevated hematocrit and depleted potassium and phosphorus levels may also be noted.

Point-of-care finger-stick or arterial-line testing of glucose at the bedside is the usual method for frequent monitoring of the serum blood glucose. Insulin replacement is then prescribed according to the blood glucose result. Some electrolytes also can be tested at the bedside (potassium, sodium, ionized calcium) but generally require an arterial line for frequent blood access. If point-of-care testing is not available, traditional serial laboratory tests keep the clinician apprised of the fluctuating serum electrolyte levels and provide the basis for electrolyte replacement. Intracellular potassium and phosphate levels usually are depleted as a result of dehydration.[48]

Elevated BUN and creatinine levels suggest kidney impairment as a result of the severe reduction in renal circulation. Metabolic acidosis usually is absent at lower glucose levels. Acidosis may result from starvation ketosis or an increase in lactic acid production secondary to poor tissue perfusion.

MEDICAL MANAGEMENT

The goals of medical management are rapid rehydration, insulin replacement, and correction of electrolyte abnormalities, specifically potassium replacement. The underlying stimulus of HHS must be discovered and treated. The same basic principles used to treat DKA are used for the patient with HHS.

Rapid Rehydration. The primary intervention for HHS is rapid rehydration to restore intravascular volume. The fluid deficit may be as much as 150 ml/kg of body weight. The average 150-pound adult can lose more than 7 to 10 L of fluid and perhaps 5 to 10 mEq/kg of sodium a day.[52] Physiologic normal saline solution (0.9%) is infused for the first 1 L, especially for the patient in hypovolemic shock.[48] The patient may need replacement of 6 to 10 L of fluid in the first 10 hours to achieve a BP and CVP within normal range.

Serum sodium is the parameter that is monitored to determine when to change from isotonic (0.9%) to hypotonic (0.45%) saline. For example, patients with sodium levels equal to or less than 140 mEq/L receive 0.9% normal saline solution. Patients with levels greater than 140 mEq/L receive 0.45% saline solution as shown in Fig. 36-5. In reality it is difficult to assess serum sodium in the presence of hemoconcentration. Another recommendation is to calculate a *corrected sodium value.* This involves adding 1.6 mEq to the sodium laboratory value for each 100 mg/dl plasma glucose above normal.[48,49] Sodium input should not exceed the amount required to replace the losses. Careful monitoring of serum sodium is recommended to avoid a sodium-water imbalance and hemolysis as the hemoconcentration is reduced.[52]

To prevent hypoglycemia, when the serum glucose falls to the 250 to 300 mg/dl range, the hydrating solution

Management of Adult Patients with HHS

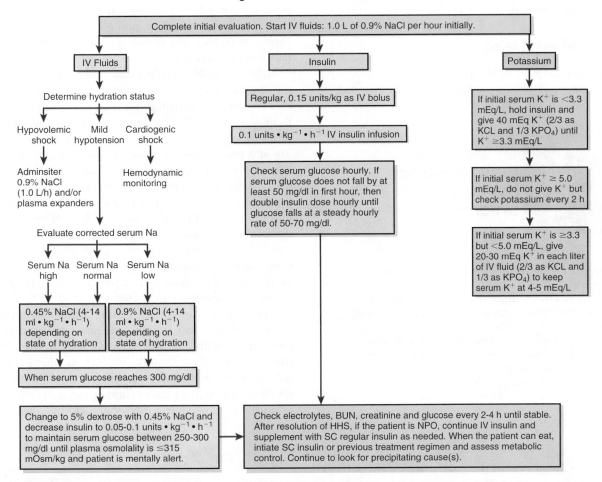

Fig. 36-5 Protocol for the management of adult patients with HHS. (From Kitabchi AE et al: *Diabetes Care* 27(Suppl 1):S94-S102, 2004.)

is changed to 5% dextrose in water, in 0.45% saline solution (D5% and 0.45%NS).[48]

Insulin Administration. Volume resuscitation will lower serum glucose levels and improve symptoms even without insulin.[49] However, insulin replacement is recommended to treat HHS because of clinical reports that acidosis can develop when insulin is withheld.[49] Insulin is given to facilitate the cellular use of glucose.

Methods to lower the glucose level vary. One method is initially to administer an IV bolus of regular insulin (0.15 unit per kg body weight), followed by a continuous insulin drip. Regular insulin infusing at an initial rate calculated as 0.1 unit per kg hourly (7 units/hour for a person weighing 70 kg) should lower the plasma glucose by 50 mg/dl in the first hour of treatment.[48] If the measured glucose does not decrease by this amount, the insulin infusion rate may be doubled until the blood glucose is declining at a rate of 50 to 75 mg/dl per hour.[48]

Insulin Resistance. Patients with HHS have underlying type 2 diabetes; many will have metabolic syndrome and exhibit signs of *insulin resistance.*[37] In critical illness the presence of *counterregulatory hormones,* also known as *stress hormones* (cortisol, glucagon, growth hormone,

epinephrine) will both increase glucose production and induce insulin resistance.[49] Patients with HHS may require supraphysiologic doses of insulin initially to overcome the hyperglycemia and insulin resistance.[49] Hourly serial monitoring of the blood glucose will permit safe glycemic management and avoid the most common complication, which is hypoglycemia caused by overzealous insulin administration.[48] Once the patient is over the hyperglycemic crisis and the insulin is discontinued, oral agents designed to decrease insulin resistance in type 2 diabetics will be prescribed (see the Pharmacologic Management Table on Oral Medications for Type 2 Diabetes).

Electrolyte Replacement. Increasing the circulating levels of insulin with therapeutic doses of IV insulin will promote the rapid return of potassium and phosphorus into the cell. Serial laboratory tests keep the clinician apprised of the serum electrolyte levels and provide the basis for electrolyte replacement. Potassium is typically added to the IV infusion as shown in Fig. 36-5. If the serum potassium is below 3.3 mEq/L it is wise to replenish the serum potassium before giving insulin.[48] Many hospitals also have potassium replacement algorithms that are used to treat hypokalemia. Phosphate levels are carefully monitored and replaced if the serum phosphate level is below 1.0 mg/dl.[48]

NURSING MANAGEMENT

Nursing management of the patient with HHS incorporates a variety of nursing diagnoses (see the Nursing Diagnoses feature on Hyperglycemic Hyperosmotic Syndrome). Nursing management goals are similar to that outlined for DKA. The critical care nurse administers prescribed fluids, insulin, and electrolytes; monitors the response to therapy; maintains surveillance for complications; and provides patient education.

Administer Fluids, Insulin, and Electrolytes. Rigorous fluid replacement and continuous IV insulin replacement must be controlled with an electronic volumetric pump. Accurate I&O measurements are maintained to monitor fluid balance. I&O includes the total of all IV fluids and hourly losses, typically urine output and sometimes emesis. Hemodynamic monitoring may include an arterial line and CVP if the patient manifests signs of hypovolemic shock. Arterial line access is very helpful to monitor serial blood glucose and electrolyte values. The use of a blood conservation system on the arterial line is essential to avoid iatrogenic exsanguination of the patient. Most critical care units have developed protocols or guidelines to ensure that patients in hyperglycemic crisis are managed safely (see Fig. 36-3). The major responsibility for delivery of insulin, hourly monitoring of blood glucose, and infusion of appropriate crystalloid solutions is with the critical care nurse (see the Nursing Interventions Classification on Hyperglycemia Management). Many hospitals mandate a "double check" for medications such as insulin and potassium that have the potential to cause harm if wrongly administered.

NURSING DIAGNOSES Hyperglycemic Hyperosmolar Syndrome

- Decreased Cardiac Output related to alterations in preload
- Deficient Fluid Volume related to absolute loss
- Anxiety related to threat to biologic, psychologic, and/or social integrity
- Deficient Knowledge: Discharge Regimen related to previous lack of exposure to information (see Patient Education feature on Hyperglycemic Hyperosmotic Syndrome)

NIC Hyperglycemia Management

Definition: Preventing and treating above-normal blood glucose levels

Activities

Monitor blood glucose levels, as indicated
Monitor for signs and symptoms of hyperglycemia: polyuria, polydipsia, polyphagia, weakness, lethargy, malaise, blurring of vision, or headache
Monitor urine ketones, as indicated
Monitor ABG, electrolyte, and beta-hydroxybutyrate levels, as available
Monitor orthostatic blood pressure and pulse, as indicated
Administer insulin, as prescribed
Encourage oral fluid intake
Monitor fluid status (including intake and output)
Maintain IV access, as appropriate
Administer IV fluids, as needed
Administer potassium, as prescribed
Consult physician if signs and symptoms of hyperglycemia persist or worsen
Assist with ambulation if orthostatic hypotension is present
Provide oral hygiene, if necessary
Identify possible causes of hyperglycemia
Anticipate situations in which insulin requirements will increase (e.g., intercurrent illness)

Restrict exercise when blood glucose levels are greater than 250 mg/dl, especially if urine ketones are present
Instruct patient and significant others on prevention, recognition, and management of hyperglycemia
Encourage self-monitoring of blood glucose levels
Instruct on urine ketone testing, as appropriate
Instruct on indications for, and significance of, urine ketone testing, if appropriate
Instruct patient to report moderate or high urine ketone levels to the health professional
Instruct patient and significant others on diabetes management during illness, including use of insulin and/or oral agents, monitoring fluid intake; carbohydrate replacement; and when to seek health professional assistance, as appropriate
Provide assistance in adjusting regimen to prevent and treat hyperglycemia (e.g., increasing insulin or oral agent), as indicated
Facilitate adherence to diet and exercise regimen
Test blood glucose levels of family members

From Dochterman JM, Bulechek GM: *Nursing interventions classification, (NIC),* ed 4, St Louis, 2004, Mosby.

Monitor Response to Therapy. The BP, HR, and CVP are monitored to evaluate the degree of dehydration, the effectiveness of hydration therapy, and the patient's fluid tolerance. Because patients with HHS have underlying type 2 diabetes, many have preexisting illnesses such as heart failure and renal failure. Thus, it is important to monitor for symptoms of circulatory overload in susceptible individuals. Symptoms to anticipate include elevated CVP, tachycardia, bounding pulse, dyspnea, tachypnea, lung crackles, and engorged neck veins. The astute critical care nurse is aware of the clinical manifestations of fluid overload and observes for potential complications when rehydrating the patient with HHS and cardiac, pulmonary, or renal disease.

The serum glucose should decrease by 50-75 mg/dl per hour with insulin administration.[48] This is monitored by hourly blood glucose determinations. Based upon the glucose result the critical care nurse can alter the infusion of insulin based upon hospital protocol (see Fig. 36-5).

Surveillance for Complications. The potential complications are similar in HHS to those described in the previous section on DKA: hypoglycemia, hypokalemia or hyperkalemia, and infection. In addition, the patient with HHS is at risk for other complications specific to associated disease entities. A history of cardiovascular, pulmonary or kidney disease, whether known or latent, creates a high risk of complications for HHS patients.

Patient Education

As the patient's condition improves and demonstrates readiness to learn, education about type 2 diabetes and voiding a recurrence of HHS becomes a priority (see the Patient Education feature on Hyperglycemic Hyperosmotic Syndrome). Most teaching will occur after the patient has left the critical care unit. Teaching topics include a description of type 2 diabetes and how it relates to HHS, dietary restrictions, exercise requirements, medication protocols, home testing of blood glucose, signs and symptoms of hyperglycemia and hypoglycemia, foot care, and lifestyle modifications if cardiovascular disease is present.

Collaborative Management

Because HHS is an acute condition superimposed upon the chronic health problem of type 2 diabetes, many health professionals provide care and work collaboratively to restore homeostasis for each patient (see the Evidence-Based Collaborative Practice feature on Hyperglycemic Hyperosmolar Syndrome).

PATIENT EDUCATION

Hyperglycemic Hyperosmolar Syndrome

- Acute phase
  Explain rationale for critical care unit admission
- Predischarge
  Assess knowledge level
  Assess compliance history
  Diabetes disease process
  Definitions of hyperglycemic hyperosmotic syndrome (HHS)
  Causes of HHS
  Self-care diabetes
  Signs and symptoms to report to health care practitioner

EVIDENCE-BASED COLLABORATIVE PRACTICE

Hyperglycemic Hyperosmolar Syndrome

Summary of evidence and evidence based recommendations for controlling symptoms related to hyperglycemic hyperosmolar syndrome (HHS)

Strong Evidence to Support:
Regular insulin by continuous infusion is recommended to normalize blood glucose to 80-110 mg/dl (euglycemic levels).
Replace serum phosphate if level is below 1 mg/dl.

A multidisciplinary team approach to care reduces length of stay and improves clinical outcomes.
Close follow-up after discharge is recommended to maintain hemoglobin A_{1C} below 7% and prevent diabetes-related complications.

Weak Evidence to Support:
Use of a "sliding insulin scale" alone is discouraged because it is associated with both hyperglycemia and hypoglycemia in hospitalized patients.

From Kitabchi AE et al: *Diabetes Care* 27(suppl 1):S94-S102, 2004; Garber AJ, et al: American College of Endocrinology position statement on inpatient diabetes and metabolic control, *Endocr Pract* 10(suppl 2):4-9, 2004; and Clement S et al: Management of diabetes and hyperglycemia in hospitals, *Diabetes Care* 27(2):553-591, 2004.

DIABETES INSIPIDUS

Diabetes insipidus (DI) is recognized by the vast quantities of very dilute urine that are produced in susceptible patients. In the critically ill patient the extreme diuresis is most likely to be due to a lack of antidiuretic hormone (ADH). Any patient with head trauma or those after neurosurgery have an increased risk of developing DI. Normally ADH is produced in the hypothalamus and is stored in the posterior pituitary gland, as described in Chapter 34. Physiologically ADH is primarily released in response to even small elevations in serum osmolality and secondarily in reaction to hypovolemia or hypotension.[53] ADH is also known by the name *vasopressin*.[54] DI can occur at any one of the physiologic steps listed below[54]:

- The hypothalamus produces insufficient ADH.
- The posterior pituitary fails to release ADH.
- The kidney nephron is resistant (unresponsive) to ADH.

ETIOLOGY

DI is categorized into three types according to cause: central, nephrogenic, and psychogenic (Box 36-4). Only central DI, also known as neurogenic DI because of the association with the brain, is encountered with any frequency in the critical care unit.

Central Diabetes Insipidus. In central diabetes insipidus, there is an inability to secrete an adequate amount of vasopressin in response to osmotic or nonosmotic stimuli, resulting in inappropriately dilute urine.[55] Either the synthesis of ADH is incomplete in the hypothalamus, or the release of ADH from the pituitary is interrupted. Central DI can be congenital or idiopathic, but this is not typically seen in critical care. The most likely acute cause of central DI is secondary to neurosurgery, traumatic head injury,[56] tumors,[57] increased intracranial pressure (ICP), brain death, and infections such as encephalitis or meningitis.[55] In patients undergoing surgery on the pituitary gland, DI occurs in approximately 12% of patients and is permanent in 3%.[58] The degree of hormone replacement required following surgery is dependent on the quantity of pituitary tissue that is removed.[58] One clinical study reported the incidence of central DI to be almost 3% in patients with traumatic brain injury (TBI).[56]

Nephrogenic Diabetes Insipidus. Nephrogenic DI results from the inability of the kidney nephrons to respond to circulating ADH.[59] Nephrogenic DI is a rare disorder that occurs in the setting of kidney disease when V_2 receptors on the kidney tubule become nonresponsive to the action of ADH. Some drugs cause nephrogenic DI by decreasing the responsiveness of the kidney tubules to ADH. Long-term use of lithium carbonate, prescribed for bipolar disorder, is a frequent culprit.[59,60]

Psychogenic DI. Psychogenic DI is a rare form of the disease that occurs with compulsive drinking of more than 5 L of water a day. Long-standing psychogenic DI closely mimics nephrogenic DI because the kidney tubules become less responsive to ADH as a result of prolonged conditioning to hypotonic urine. This is uncommon to see in the critical care unit.

PATHOPHYSIOLOGY

The purpose of ADH is to maintain normal serum osmolality and circulating blood volume. Normally ADH binds to the V_2 receptors on the kidney collecting tubules, causing insertion of water channels known as *aquaporins*, along the luminal surface.[53] Even small (1% to 2%) increases in plasma osmolality are sufficient to stimulate ADH release.[53] Although there are several types of DI, this discussion focuses on neurogenic central DI, the condition encountered in the critical care unit following neurosurgery or head injury[56] (Fig. 36-6).

In DI, as free water is eliminated the urine osmolality and specific gravity decrease (dilute urine). By contrast, in the bloodstream, serum sodium and serum osmolality rise.[54] Normally, when the serum osmolality rises above 290 mOsm per kg H_2O (290 mmol/L) this triggers the syn-

---

Box 36-4

ETIOLOGY OF DIABETES INSIPIDUS

CENTRAL DI
Primary (Rare in Critical Care)
ADH deficiency from hypothalamic-hypophyseal malformation
    Congenital defect
    Idiopathic

Secondary (Most Common in Critical Care)
ADH deficiency from damage to the hypothalamic-hypophyseal system
    Trauma
    Infection
    Surgery
    Primary neoplasms
    Metastatic malignancies

NEPHROGENIC DI
Inability of kidney tubules to respond to circulating ADH
    Decrease or absence of ADH receptors
    Cellular damage to nephron, especially loop of Henle
    Kidney damage (e.g., hydronephrosis, pyelonephritis, polycystic kidney)
    Untoward response to drug therapy (e.g., lithium carbonate, demeclocyline)

PSYCHOGENIC DI
Rare form of water intoxication
    Compulsive water drinking

ADH, Antidiuretic hormone; *DI,* diabetes insipidus.

thesis and release of ADH.[53] At 295 mOsm per kg H_2O the thirst sensors are activated in the hypothalamus.[53] In central DI, however, no ADH is released, or the ADH released is insufficient. Without ADH, the kidney collecting tubules are incapable of concentrating urine and retaining water.

As the extracellular dehydration ensues, hypotension and hypovolemic shock occur. If the person is alert, extreme thirst will permit the individual to replace lost fluids by drinking lots of water. This excessive intake of water reduces the serum osmolality to a more normal level and prevents dehydration. In the person with decreased level of consciousness, the polyuria leads to severe hypernatremia, dehydration, decreased cerebral perfusion, seizures, loss of consciousness, and death.

ASSESSMENT AND DIAGNOSIS

Clinical Manifestations. The clinical diagnosis is made by the dramatic increase in dilute urine output in the absence of diuretics, a fluid challenge, or hyperglycemia. Central DI is anticipated in conditions where the underlying disease process is likely to disrupt pituitary function. If central DI occurs because of increasing ICP, this is life-threatening. It is imperative that the underlying condition be recognized and treated appropriately. In this situation medications that treat DI are not sufficient.

Laboratory Studies. The core diagnostic tests used to establish the presence of DI that evaluate the body's ability to balance fluid and electrolytes are not specific

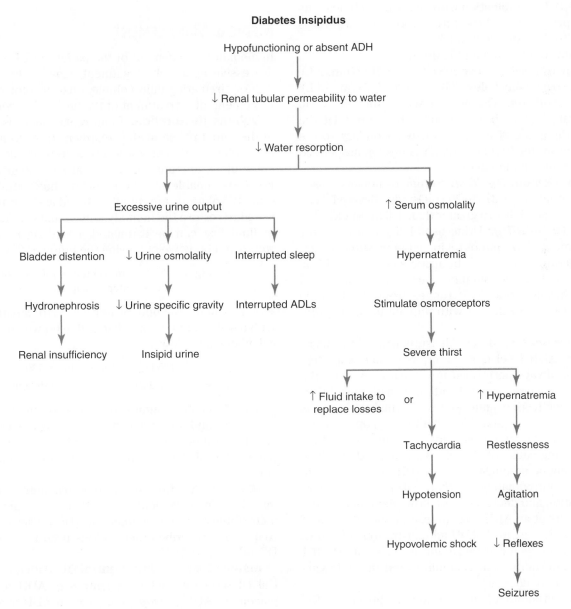

Fig. 36-6   Pathophysiology of diabetes insipidus (DI). *ADH,* Antidiuretic hormone; *ADLs,* activities of daily living.

Table 36-3	Laboratory Values for Patients With DI and SIADH		
Value	**Normal**	**DI**	**SIADH**
Serum ADH	1-5 pg/ml	*Central DI:* decreased serum ADH level.	Elevated ADH level
Serum osmolality	275-295 mOsm/L*	>295 mOsm/L*	<270 mOsm/L
Serum sodium	135-145 mEq/L	>145 mEq/L	<120 mEq/L
Urine osmolality	300-1400 mOsm/L	<300 mOsm/L	Increased
Urine specific gravity	1.005-1.030	<1.005	>1.030
Urine output	1.0-1.5 L per day	1.0-1.5 L per hour	Below normal

* Some hospitals use 280-300 mOsm/L as their normal reference value.
DI, Diabetes insipidus; *SIADH,* syndrome of inappropriate antidiuretic hormone; *ADH,* antidiuretic hormone.

to the endocrine system. The most common tests are serum sodium, serum osmolality, and urine osmolality (Table 36-3). In combination with an obvious clinical picture the presence of these three laboratory criteria is sufficient to diagnose central DI:

- Serum sodium above 145 mEq/L.
- Serum osmolality above 295 mOsm/kg H$_2$O (mmol/L).
- Urine osmolality below 300 mOsm/kg H$_2$O (mmol/L).

Serum Sodium. The normal serum sodium is 140 mEq/L (range (135 to 145 mEq/L). In central DI the serum sodium can rise precipitously secondary to the loss of free water. Hypernatremia is always associated with serum hyperosmolality.[61]

Serum Osmolality Test. Serum osmolality has a narrow normal range, 275 to 295 mOsm/kg. Severe DI can raise serum osmolality to greater than 320 mOsm/kg.[53]

Urine Osmolality. Urine osmolality is low, below 300 mOsm/kg H$_2$O (mmol/L) in patients with central DI. For greatest accuracy the urine sample should be collected and tested simultaneously with the blood sample. Normal urine ADH ranges from 500 to 1400 mOsm/L H$_2$O, and will vary with fluid intake and hydration status.

Measurement of ADH. Measurement of the baseline serum ADH level is an additional diagnostic step. This is not always performed in critical care when the clinical circumstances (e.g., head injury with raised ICP) make further testing unnecessary. Normal ADH levels range from 1 to 5 pg/ml. Most hydrated people have a morning fasting serum level below 4 pg/ml.[62] To test for the underlying cause of the DI, exogenous ADH (vasopressin) may be administered. An ADH plasma concentration of approximately 1 pg/ml will increase urinary concentration and decrease urine flow. Maximum antidiuresis occurs at an ADH (vasopressin) concentration of approximately 5 pg/ml.[55] ADH administration is used to distinguish between central DI and nephrogenic DI. If 1 mcg SQ of desmopressin is administered the following responses are diagnostic[61]:

- Urine output greatly decreased in response to ADH administration diagnoses central DI.

- Urine output unchanged in response to ADH administration suggests nephrogenic DI.

MEDICAL MANAGEMENT

Immediate management of the patient in DI requires an aggressive approach. Treatment goals include restoration of circulating fluid volume, pharmacologic ADH replacement, plus treatment of the underlying condition.

Volume Restoration. Fluid replacement is provided in the initial phase of the treatment to prevent circulatory collapse. Patients who are able to drink are given voluminous amounts of fluid orally to balance output. For those unable to take sufficient fluids orally, hypotonic IV solutions are rapidly infused and carefully monitored to restore the hemodynamic balance. The amount of fluid lost can be estimated, based on normal fluid stores and body weight, using the following formula:

$$(0.6 \{kg\ wt\}) \times (\text{Serum sodium} - 140) \div 140 = \text{Body water deficit (L)}$$

For example the body water deficit for a patient in DI with a serum sodium of 160 mEq/L who weighs 135 kg is calculated as follows:

$$(0.6 \times 135\ kg) \times (160 - 140) \div 140 =$$
$$81 \times 20 \div 140 = 11.57\ L\ \text{water deficit}$$

The formula assumes that 60% of an individual's weight is fluid, although this is not always exact. The calculated liters of body water deficit can be used for planning replacement fluids to restore hemodynamic stability.

Medications. Central DI requires immediate pharmacologic management.[54] The Pharmacologic Management Table on Diabetes Insipidus [DI] presents the most frequently prescribed medications used to treat central DI and replace ADH.

Medications Used for Central DI. Patients with central DI who are unable to synthesize ADH require replacement ADH *(vasopressin)*, or an ADH analog. The most commonly prescribed drug is the synthetic analog

Pharmacologic Management: Diabetes Insipidus

DRUG	DOSAGE	ACTIONS	SPECIAL CONSIDERATIONS
Central Diabetes Insipidus			
Desmopressin acetate (DDAVP) available IV, as nasal spray, Rhinal tube, Rhinyle drops, Stimate)	Nasal: 10-40 mcg at bedtime or in divided doses Parenteral: 2-4 mcg twice daily	*Central diabetes insipidus (DI)* Antidiuretic Increases water resorption in nephron Prevents and controls polydipsia, polyuria	Few side effects Observe for nasal congestion, upper respiratory infection, allergic rhinitis Monitor intake/output, urine osmolality, serum sodium
Vasopressin (Pitressin Synthetic, Pressyn)	Intramuscular, intravenous, subcutaneous, intraarterial Topical: nasal mucosa	*Central DI* Antidiuretic Promotes resorption of water at kidney tubule Decreases urine output Increases urine osmolality Diagnostic aid Increases gastrointestinal peristalsis	Monitor fluid volume often, especially in elderly patients Assess cardiac status May precipitate angina, hypertension, or myocardial infarction if increased dose given to patient with cardiac history Parenteral extravasation may cause skin necrosis
Lypressin (Diapid)	Intranasal: 1-2 sprays (7-14 mcg) each nostril four times daily	*Central DI* Synthetic antidiuretic hormone Increases resorption of sodium and water in nephron	Proper instillation important for absorption and action Patient sits upright while holding bottle upright for administration Repeat sprays (>2-3) ineffective, wasteful; if dose increased to 2-3 sprays, shorten time between dosing Cough, chest tightness, shortness of breath
Nephrogenic Diabetes Insipidus			
Thiazide diuretics	Varies according to diuretic chosen, patient's size and age	*Nephrogenic DI* Leads to mild fluid depletion Increased water/sodium resorbed in proximal nephron; less fluid travels to distal nephron, excreting less water	Varies according to diuretic chosen
Psychogenic Diabetes Insipidus			
Anti–compulsive disorder drugs, anxiolytics, psychopharmacologic agents; dosage varies		*Psychogenic DI*	Varies according to medication chosen

Parenteral, indicates intravenous or subcutaneous.

of ADH, *desmopressin* (DDAVP). It is preferred over vasopressin (Pitressin) because it has a stronger antidiuretic action with little effect on blood pressure. DDAVP can be given IV, SQ, or as a nasal spray. A typical DDAVP dose is 1 to 2 mcg IV or SQ every 12 hours.[63] Sometimes only 0.5 mcg IV is used. The dosage is subsequently titrated according to the patient's antidiuretic response to the drug. In order to avoid a medication error it is important to be aware that DDAVP is also used to control hemorrhage caused by platelet disorders and that the dose ranges for all of these conditions are different.[63]

Vasopressin (Pitressin) 5 to 10 units intramuscularly (IM) every 3 to 4 hours will produce a reduction in urine output.[63] Vasopressin acts on the V_1 receptors in vascular smooth muscle and can elevate systemic blood pressure. Water intoxication also can occur if the dosage is higher than the therapeutic level. Because of the risk of hypertension this is not typically the first drug of choice for treating central DI. Clinicians must be aware that vasopressin can also prescribed in septic shock states as an IV infusion, and in cardiac arrest IV push.[64,65] Dosages for these conditions are very different from the dosage used to treat central DI. Extreme care must be taken to ensure that all drug dosages are accurate for each specific diagnosis.

Medications Used for Nephrogenic DI. The mainstay of therapy is to stop any medications that are inducing the ADH resistance. Nephrogenic DI is treated with hydrochlorothiazide 12.5-25 mg administered 1 or 2 times/day. The dosage is titrated according to the patient's antidiuretic response.

Nursing Management

Nursing management of the patient with diabetes insipidus incorporates a variety of nursing diagnoses (see the Nursing Diagnoses feature on Diabetes Insipidus). Nursing management is directed toward administration of prescribed fluids and medications, evaluation of response to therapy, surveillance for complications, and provision of patient education.

Administration of Fluids and Medications. Rapid IV fluid replacement requires the use of a volumetric pump. Initially a hypotonic IV solution is used to replace fluids lost and lower the serum hyperosmolality. ADH replacement is accomplished with extreme caution in the patient with a history of cardiac disease because ADH may cause hypertension and overhydration. At the first signs of cardiovascular impairment, the drug is discontinued and fluid intake restricted until urine specific gravity is less than 1.015 and polyuria resumes.

Evaluation of Response to Therapy. Critical assessment and management of the fluid status are the most important initial concerns for the patient with DI. Monitoring of HR, BP, CVP, and pulmonary artery (PA) pressures (if PA catheter in place) provide early indications of response to fluid volume replacement. I&O measurement, condition of buccal membranes, skin turgor, daily weight measurements, presence of thirst, and temperature provide a basic assessment list that is vital for the patient unable to regulate fluid needs and losses. Placement of a urinary catheter is essential to accurately monitor the urinary output. Simultaneous urine and blood specimens for osmolality, sodium, and potassium levels are collected and results relayed to the physician as necessary. The patient who is unable to satisfy sensations of thirst or to complete any task or self-care activity without the need to urinate may be confused and frightened. For patients who are able to verbalize their fears, having a caring nurse who is interested and nonjudgmental will help reduce the emotional turmoil associated with their condition.

Surveillance for Complications. The most dangerous potential complication is hypertension and vasospasm of cardiac cerebral or mesenteric arterial vessels secondary to vasopressin (Pitressin) replacement. In most cases, DDAVP will be the ADH replacement selected to avoid this complication. A less serious complication from DI is constipation from fluid loss, treated with dietary fiber, stool softeners, or both. Conversely, diarrhea, abdominal cramping, and intestinal hyperactivity may accompany vasopressin therapy. Untoward effects can be mitigated by modification of the vasopressin dose.

Patient Education

Educating the patient and the family about the disease process and how it affects thirst, urination, and fluid balance will encourage patients to participate in their care and reduce the feelings of hopelessness (see the Patient Education feature on Diabetes Insipidus). For most critical care patients central DI is a temporary condition that

---

NURSING DIAGNOSES | **Diabetes Insipidus**

- Deficient Fluid Volume related to compromised regulatory mechanism
- Decreased Cardiac Output related to alterations in preload
- Anxiety related to threat to biologic, psychologic, and/or social integrity
- Deficient Knowledge: Discharge Regimen related to lack of previous exposure to information (see Patient Education feature on Diabetes Insipidus)

PATIENT EDUCATION | **Diabetes Insipidus**

- Acute phase
  Explain rationale for critical care unit admission
- Predischarge
  Assess knowledge base
  Measurement of fluid intake and output
  Urine specific gravity
  Causes of Diabetes insipidus
  Disease process of Diabetes insipidus
  Nutritional information to prevent constipation and diarrhea
  Medications: explain purpose, side effects, dosage, and how often to use
  Signs and symptoms to report to health care professional

resolves as their underlying medical condition (e.g., brain injury) improves. Patients who are discharged with DI are taught, along with their families, the signs and symptoms of dehydration and overhydration, and procedures for accurate daily weight and urine specific gravity measurement. Printed information pertaining to drug actions, side effects, dosages, and timetable is provided, as well as an outline of factors that must be reported to the physician.

COLLABORATIVE MANAGEMENT

Central DI is a life-threatening condition. The collaborative assessment and clinical skills of all health care professionals with a clear plan of care is essential to achieve optimal outcomes for each patient.

SYNDROME OF INAPPROPRIATE SECRETION OF ANTIDIURETIC HORMONE

The opposing syndrome to DI is the syndrome of inappropriate secretion of antidiuretic hormone (SIADH). The patient with SIADH has an excess of antidiuretic hormone (ADH) secreted into the bloodstream, more than the amount needed to maintain normal blood volume and serum osmolality. Excessive water is resorbed at the kidney tubule, leading to dilutional hyponatremia.

ETIOLOGY

Numerous causes of SIADH are observed in patients who are critically ill (Box 36-5). Central nervous system

---

Box 36-5

ETIOLOGY OF SYNDROME OF INAPPROPRIATE SECRETION OF ANTIDIURETIC HORMONE (SIADH)

- *Malignant disease* associated with autonomous production of ADH
  Bronchogenic small cell carcinoma
  Pancreatic adenocarcinoma
  Duodenal, bladder, ureter, prostatic carcinomas
  Lymphosarcoma, Ewing's sarcoma
  Acute leukemia, Hodgkin's disease
  Cerebral neoplasm, thymoma
- *Central nervous system diseases* that interfere with the hypothalamic-hypophyseal system and increase the production and/or release of ADH
  Head injury
  Brain abscess
  Hydrocephalus
  Pituitary adenoma
  Subdural hematoma
  Subarachnoid hemorrhage
  Cerebral atrophy
  Guillain-Barré syndrome
- *Neurogenic stimuli* capable of increasing ADH
  Decreased glomerular filtration rate
  Physical and/or emotional stress
    Pain
    Fear
    Trauma
    Surgery
    Myocardial infarction
    Acute infection
    Hypotension
    Hemorrhage
    Hypovolemia
- *Pulmonary diseases* believed to stimulate the baroreceptors and increase ADH
  Pulmonary tuberculosis
  Viral and bacterial pneumonia
  Empyema

Lung abscess
Chronic obstructive lung disease
Status asthmaticus
Cystic fibrosis
- *Endocrine disturbances* that hormonally influence ADH
  Myxedema
  Hypothyroidism
  Hypopituitarism
  Adrenal insufficiency—Addison's disease
- *Medications* that mimic, increase the release of, or potentiate ADH
  Hypoglycemics
    Insulin
    Tolbutamide
    Chlorpropamide
  Potassium-depleting thiazide diuretics
  Tricyclic antidepressants
    Imipramine
    Amitriptyline
  Phenothiazine
    Fluphenazine
    Thioridazine
  Thioxanthenes
    Thiothixene
    Chlorprothixene
  Chemotherapeutic agents
    Vincristine
    Cyclophosphamide
  Opiates
  Carbamazepine
  Clofibrate
  Acetaminophen
  Nicotine
  Oxytocin
  Vasopressin
  Anesthetics

ADH, Antidiuretic hormone.

injury, tumors or diseases interfering with the normal functioning of the hypothalamic-pituitary system can cause SIADH. A common cause is malignant bronchogenic small cell carcinoma (also known as oat cell carcinoma). This type of malignant cell is capable of synthesizing and releasing ADH regardless of the body's needs.[53,66] With much less frequency, other cancers that involve the brain, head and neck, gastroenteral, gynecologic, and hematologic systems are capable of autonomous production of ADH.[53] Levels of ADH rise with use of positive-pressure ventilators that decrease venous return to the thorax, simultaneously stimulating pulmonary baroreceptors to release and increase levels of circulating ADH.

PATHOPHYSIOLOGY

ADH (vasopressin) is a powerful, complex polypeptide compound. When released into the circulation by the posterior pituitary gland, ADH regulates water and electrolyte balance in the body. In SIADH, profound fluid and

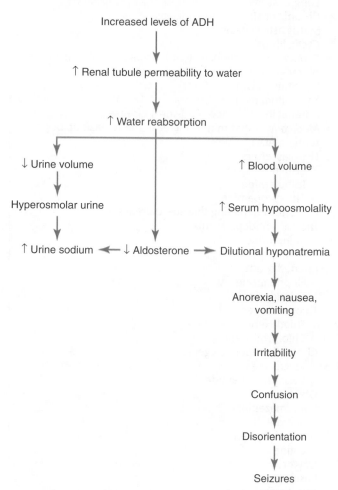

Fig. 36-7 Pathophysiology of syndrome of inappropriate secretion of antidiuretic hormone (SIADH). *ADH,* Antidiuretic hormone.

electrolyte disturbances result from the unsolicited, continuous release of the hormone into the bloodstream (Fig. 36-7). Excessive ADH stimulates the kidney tubules to retain fluid regardless of need. This results in severe overhydration.

Excessive ADH dramatically alters the sodium balance in the extracellular vascular compartment. The overhydration causes a dilutional hyponatremia and reduces the sodium concentration to critically low levels. In the healthy adult, hyponatremia inhibits the release of ADH; however, in SIADH the increased levels of circulating ADH are unrelated to the serum sodium. Aldosterone production from the adrenal glands is also suppressed. Serum hypoosmolality leads to a shift of fluid from the extracellular fluid space into the intracellular fluid compartment (inside the cells) in an attempt to equalize osmotic pressure. Because minimal sodium is present in this fluid, edema usually does not result. Without ADH and aldosterone, water is retained, urine output is diminished, and further sodium is excreted in the urine. The urine has an increased osmolality from the decreased water excretion. Urinary concentration is also elevated by excess sodium in the urine. It is believed that despite the serum hyponatremia, the increased release of ADH promotes sodium loss through the kidneys into the urine.

ASSESSMENT AND DIAGNOSIS

Clinical Manifestations. The clinical manifestations of SIADH relate to the excess fluids in the extracellular compartment and the proportionate dilution of the circulating sodium. Edema usually is not present;[67] slight weight gain may occur from the expanded extracellular fluid volume. Early clinical manifestations of dilutional hyponatremia include lethargy, anorexia, nausea, and vomiting. Severe neurologic symptoms generally do not develop until the serum sodium drops below 120 mEq/L.[61,67] Progressively deteriorating neurologic signs of hyponatremia then predominate, and the patient is admitted to the critical care unit. Symptoms of severe hyponatremia include inability to concentrate, mental confusion, apprehension, seizures, decreased level of consciousness, coma, and death.

Laboratory Values. SIADH presents with very dilute serum and very concentrated urine output. Laboratory values confirm this clinical picture. In SIADH the serum is hypoosmolar (less than 275 mOsm/kg H$_2$O) with low serum sodium and a urine osmolality greater than would be expected of such hypotonic blood.[61] A serum sodium below 125 mEq/L (some cite below 120 mEq/L) is associated with increasing severity of neurologic symptoms.[61,67] An elevated urine sodium, greater than 30 mEq/L, is congruent with the concentrated urine output of SIADH.[61,67] Use of diuretics negates the reliability of the urine sodium and urine osmolality levels.[67] A comparison of the typical laboratory values associated with SIADH versus those in DI is presented in Table 36-3.

MEDICAL MANAGEMENT

In the critical care unit, SIADH often occurs as a secondary disease. Ideally, recognition and treatment of the primary disease will reduce the production of ADH. If the patient is receiving any of the medications suspected of causing the disease, discontinuing the drug may return ADH levels to normal. Several drugs that alter ADH levels are listed in Box 36-5.

Fluid Restriction. The medical therapy that is the most successful (along with treatment of the primary disease) is simple reduction of fluid intake.[61] This is achieved most successfully for the patient with a moderate increase in body fluid volume with hyponatremia. Although fluid restrictions are calculated on the basis of individual needs and losses, a general criterion is to restrict fluids to 500 ml less than average daily output.[53]

Sodium Replacement. Patients with severe hyponatremia (less than 125 mEq/L serum sodium) experience severe neurologic symptoms, even seizures. How rapidly the sodium should be corrected and which sodium concentration to use remains controversial.[68] One recommended regimen is an IV rate that provides sufficient sodium to raise serum sodium levels by up to 12 mEq/day for the first 24 hours, with a total rise of 18 mEq/L in the initial 48 hours.[61] There are other regimens that are more aggressive[61] and others that are less so.[69] Another option is to add furosemide (Lasix) to increase the diuresis of free water.

An infusion of 3% hypertonic saline solution may be used to replenish the serum sodium without adding extra volume when hyponatremia is severe (below 120 mEq/L). It is imperative that clinicians are aware that hypertonic saline solution is dangerous if administered too quickly, and calculation of the quantity of sodium that will be administered is advised. An example of one sodium replacement regimen is an infusion of 3% saline infusion at 35 ml/hour in a 70-kg patient, which will increase the serum sodium by approximately 0.5 mEq/L per hour (12 mEq/day).[61] Suggested end-points at which to stop the acute sodium repletion include the following[61]:

- The patient's symptoms are abolished.
- A safe serum sodium level is achieved, generally greater than 120 mEq/L.
- A total correction of 20 mEq/L is achieved.

Too-rapid serum sodium correction must be avoided to reduce the risk of *osmotic demyelination*, previously known as *central pontine myelinolysis*.[69] The demyelination occurs in the pons and in other areas of the brain's white matter.[53] The lesions may be detected on imaging studies (CT and MRI), and severe neurologic damage or even death can result.[53] Patients with a baseline serum

sodium below 120 mEq/L are most at risk.[53] Serum sodium levels must be evaluated at least every 4 hours during the acute phase of sodium replacement.[61]

Medications. Medications are only prescribed if water restriction is ineffective in correcting the SIADH. Certain drugs decrease the output of ADH from the pituitary gland, and other medications increase the action of ADH on the V_2 tubule receptors so that more water is excreted.

Medications That Increase Renal Water Excretion. The preferred agent to treat SIADH is demeclocycline, a derivative of tetracycline.[61] The required dosage range is from 600-1200 mg per day, and several days of therapy are necessary to achieve maximal effects.[61] Thus, it is advisable to wait several days before changing the initial dose regimen.[61]

NURSING MANAGEMENT

Nursing management of the patient with SIADH incorporates a variety of nursing diagnoses (see the Nursing Diagnoses feature on Syndrome of Inappropriate Secretion of Antidiuretic Hormone). Nursing management is directed toward restriction of fluids, surveillance for complications, and provision of patient education.

Restriction of Fluids. Thorough, astute nursing assessments are required for care of the patient with SIADH, while an attempt is made to correct the fluid and sodium imbalance; the systemic effects of hyponatremia occur rapidly and can be lethal. Frequent assessment of the patient's hydration status is accomplished with serial measurements of urine output, serum sodium levels, and serum osmolality. Accurate measurement of I&O is required to calculate fluid replacement for the patient with SIADH. All fluids are restricted. Intake that equals urine output may be given until serum sodium level returns to

NURSING DIAGNOSES

Syndrome of Inappropriate Secretion of Antidiuretic Hormone

- Excess Fluid Volume related to comprised regulation mechanism
- Anxiety related to lack of control over current situation or disease progression
- Deficient Knowledge: Discharge Regimen related to lack of previous exposure to information (see Patient Education feature on Syndrome of Inappropriate Secretion of Antidiuretic Hormone)

normal. Frequent mouth care through moistening the buccal membrane may give comfort during the period of fluid restriction. The patient is weighed daily to gauge fluid retention or loss. Weight gain signifies continual fluid retention, whereas weight loss indicates loss of body fluid.

Constipation is a frequent complication of decreased fluid intake. Cathartics or low-volume hypertonic enemas may be given to stimulate peristalsis. Tap water or hypotonic enemas should never be given because the water in the enema solution may be absorbed through the bowel and potentiate water intoxication.

Surveillance for Complications. The patient's neurologic status, especially level of consciousness, should be evaluated on an hourly basis if the serum sodium is critically low, below 125 mEq/L. Seizure precautions for the patient with SIADH are provided regardless of the degree of hyponatremia. Serum sodium levels may fluctuate rapidly, and neurologic impairment may occur with no apparent warning. The patient's altered neurologic response also may be influenced by the acuity of the primary disease (central nervous system disease) and not solely by the result of low sodium levels. Seizure precautions include nursing actions to protect the patient from injury (padded side rails, bed in low position when patient is unattended) and to provide an open airway (oral airway, head turned to side without forcibly restraining the patient, suction apparatus). Oxygen may be required to maintain a saturation level greater than 92% if there is pulmonary congestion or edema than interferes with alveolar gas exchange.

PATIENT EDUCATION

Rapidly occurring changes in the patient's neurologic status may frighten visiting family members. Sensitivity to the family's unspoken fears can be shown by words that express empathy and by providing time for the patient and family to communicate their feelings. The nurse may discuss the course of SIADH, its effect on water balance, and the reasons for fluid restrictions (see the Patient Education feature on Syndrome of Inappropriate Secretion of Antidiuretic Hormone).

COLLABORATIVE MANAGEMENT

At this time there are no published guidelines that discuss acute collaborative care management of the patient with SIADH. This is a complex condition, and effective clinical management requires the skills of many health care professionals working as a team with goals that are clearly communicated to all team members.

THYROID STORM

DESCRIPTION

Thyroid storm always occurs as a complication of preexisting hyperthyroidism. Hyperthyroidism, also called *thyrotoxicosis*, occurs when the thyroid gland produces thyroid hormone in excess of the body's need.[70] The most common cause of primary hyperthyroidism is *Graves' disease*, an autoimmune disease that affects 0.4% of the U.S. population with a 5:1 ratio favoring women to men.[71] The antidysrhythmic drug amiodarone (Cordarone) causes thyroid dysfunction in 14% to 18% of patients.[70] Hyperthyroid conditions also may result from ingestion of excessive thyroid replacement drugs. Conditions associated with hyperthyroidism are presented in Box 36-6.[70]

Thyroid storm, also called *thyroid crisis*, is a critical stage of hyperthyroidism. It is a rare and life-threatening condition. The pathophysiology underlying the transition from hyperthyroidism to thyroid storm is not fully understood. Activation of the sympathetic nervous system (SNS) and enhanced sensitivity to the effects of thyroid hormone are apparent.[72] Major stressors, such as infection,[72] surgery,[73] trauma,[74] pregnancy,[75] or critical illness can precipitate thyroid storm in the hyperthyroid patient.

ETIOLOGY

In hyperthyroidism, excessive thyroid hormone causes increased metabolic activity and stimulates the β-adrenergic receptors, which results in a heightened SNS response. There is hyperactivity of cardiac tissue,

Box 36-6

CONDITIONS ASSOCIATED WITH HYPERTHYROIDISM

- Iodine-induced hyperthyroidism (e.g., related to amiodarone therapy)
- Excessive pituitary TSH or trophoblastic disease
- Excessive ingestion of thyroid hormone
- Toxic diffuse goiter (Graves' disease)
- Toxic adenoma
- Toxic multinodular goiter (Plummer's disease)
- Painful subacute thryoiditis
- Silent thyroiditis, including lymphocytic and postpartum variations

TSH, Thyroid-stimulating hormone.

nervous tissue, and smooth muscle tissue and tremendous heat production.[72]

PATHOPHYSIOLOGY

Thyroid hormone increases cellular oxygen consumption in almost all metabolically active cells. Energy in the form of heat is lost rather than used by the cell. Excess metabolism generates heat, and the body temperature may rise to as high as 41° C (105.8° F). Cellular oxygen demands are dramatically increased. The cardiac response is to increase the cardiac output and pump more blood more rapidly to deliver oxygen and to expel carbon dioxide. Hypertension and tachycardia follow. The oxygen demands in the hypermetabolic state are so great that the cardiac system cannot compensate adequately. Tremors, fatigue, and tachydysrhythmias follow.[72] A critically high fever is typically present.[76]

Increased metabolic rate requires increased oxygen and sufficient energy sources. Catabolism and a negative nitrogen balance occur. Metabolic acidosis is a potential problem. Intestinal peristalsis increases, often resulting in diarrhea, nausea, and vomiting. These symptoms all lead to dehydration and compound the problem of malnutrition and weight loss. Muscular contraction and relaxation increase more rapidly and are referred to as the *hyperreflexia of hyperthyroidism.* Muscular weakness occurs and is compounded by the excessive protein breakdown.

Hypersensitivity to the increased adrenergic-binding sites potentiates the cardiovascular and nervous system responses to the hypermetabolic state. Atrial fibrillation or flutter is reported in 8.3% of patients with hyperthyroidism.[77] Tachydysrhythmias are to be anticipated in thyroid storm.[72-73] Pulmonary edema and acute heart failure also can occur. Increased β-adrenergic activity manifests in emotional lability, fine muscular tremors, agitation and even delirium. Clinical manifestations of thyroid storm are listed in Box 36-7.

ASSESSMENT AND DIAGNOSIS

Thyroid storm is a potentially lethal complication of thyrotoxicosis. Early symptoms may be missed and insidious, creating a paradoxically abrupt presentation of a cluster of symptoms. Thyroid storm lacks a "textbook" profile to signal its presence. The presenting symptoms and severity of the disease differ from one patient to another and change during the course of the disease, posing a profound threat to the patient's survival. It is the patient who is hospitalized for a major illness—the person with either undiagnosed or previously controlled thyrotoxicosis—who is at high risk of experiencing thyroid storm. No diagnostic test is available to differentiate thyroid storm from its predecessor, thyrotoxicosis. The condition, therefore, is identified by a combination of past medical history and current clinical manifestations.[71]

MEDICAL MANAGEMENT

The goal of acute medical management of thyroid storm is to reduce the clinical effects of thyroid hormone as rapidly as possible. During this time the goal is to prevent cardiac decompensation, reduce hyperthermia, reverse dehydration as a result of pyrexia or GI loses.

Prevent Cardiovascular Collapse. The body's heightened sensitivity to the increased adrenergic and catecholamine receptors must be suppressed. Cardiac irregularities need to be controlled and progression of heart failure halted. Beta-blockers are the mainstay of therapy for cardiac protection.[72,73]

Reduce Hyperthermia. Pyrexia is treated with hypothermia measures such as a cooling blanket and acetaminophen. Reduction in body temperature is managed by use of a cooling blanket and the antipyretic agent acetaminophen. Salicylates (aspirin) are contraindicated because they prevent protein binding of T_3 to T_4, increasing the free, metabolically active, thyroid hormone.[76]

Reverse Dehydration. Vigorous fluid replacement must be instituted to treat or prevent dehydration. Antibiotic therapy may be warranted in the presence of systemic infection. Other existing pathologic conditions have to be treated appropriately. When dehydration and metabolic acidosis are present, they are treated with large volumes of glucose and sodium solutions to replace circulating fluid and sodium losses caused by hypermetabolism.

PHARMACOLOGIC MANAGEMENT

Pharmacologic treatment is essential in treatment of thyroid storm. Drug administration is divided into three phases[72]:

1. Initially prescribed are drugs that block the synthesis and release of thyroid hormone into circulation.

Box 36-7

CLINICAL MANIFESTATIONS OF THYROID STORM

CARDIOVASCULAR SYSTEM
Prompted by Increased Affinity of β-Adrenergic Receptors in the Heart
    Tachycardia
    Systolic murmur
    Increased stroke volume
    Increased cardiac output
    Increased systolic blood pressure
    Decreased diastolic blood pressure
    Extra systoles
    Paroxysmal atrial tachycardia
    Premature ventricular contraction
    Palpitations
    Chest pain
    Increased cardiac contractility
    Congestive heart failure
    Pulmonary edema
    Cardiogenic shock

CENTRAL NERVOUS SYSTEM
Resulting From an Increased Catecholamine Response
    Hyperkinesis
    Nervousness
    Muscle weakness
    Confusion
    Convulsions
    Heat intolerance
    Fine tremor
    Emotional lability
    Frank psychosis
    Apathy
    Stupor
    Diaphoresis

GASTROINTESTINAL SYSTEM
    Nausea
    Vomiting
    Diarrhea
    Liver enlargement
    Abdominal pain
    Weight loss
    Increased appetite

INTEGUMENTARY SYSTEM
    Pruritus
    Hyperpigmentation of skin
    Fine, straight hair
    Alopecia

THERMOREGULATORY SYSTEM
    Hyperthermia
    Heat dissipation
    Diaphoresis

SERUM/URINE
    Hypercalcemia
    Hyperglycemia
    Hypoalbuminemia
    Hypoprothrombinemia
    Hypocholesterolemia
    Creatinuria

2. Second, drugs that block and inhibit the conversion of T_4 to T_3 are given.
3. Third, drugs to decrease the peripheral cellular sensitivity to catecholamines are used.

Drugs That Block Thyroid Synthesis. The synthesis of new thyroid hormone is blocked by the administration of *antithyroid drugs* in the *thiouricil class*.[72] Two drugs are frequently used: propylthiouracil (PTU) and methimazole (MMI).[76] Neither drug is available in parenteral form and must be given by mouth or via a nasogastric tube. PTU is especially therapeutic because it also blocks the conversion of T_4 to T_3. Methimazole has a slower action rate, but it is more potent than PTU. Both drugs act within about 1 to 2 hours following absorption from the GI tract. These drugs have no impact on previously released thyroid hormone.

Drugs That Block Release of Thyroid Hormone. The administration of inorganic iodine will block the release of any "preformed" thyroxine already in the thyroid gland but not yet released.[72] It is essential that iodine therapy not be administered until adequate inhibition of new hormone synthesis has occurred. The iodide preparations are rapid-acting with a short duration. They are given approximately 1 hour after the administration of the antithyroid drugs (see above) to prevent the iodide from being used for thyroid hormone and possibly worsening the clinical state. Oral (or NG) *iodides* are given in large amounts to decrease thyroid hormone production.[76] The iodides maintain and increase the levels of protein-bound thyroid hormone, thereby decreasing the levels of free active thyroid. The iodide most commonly used for thyroid storm is sodium iodide. Potassium iodide, saturated solution of potassium iodide, or strong iodide solution also may be used.

Drugs That Block Catecholamine Effect. To decrease the catecholamine effects of excessive thyroid hormone, β-adrenergic blocking agents are used. Propranolol is the most frequently used drug.[72] Beta-blockers have no effect on thyroid hormone but reduce the exaggerated myocardial stimulation and contractile force, and slow atrioventricular (AV) conduction rate. Therapeutic doses vary from patient to patient, but typically higher doses (60 to 80 mg every 6 hours orally) are required to effectively control the symptoms.[72] Esmolol, a short-acting beta-blocker, administered via IV infusion, can also be used.[72] Calcium channel blockers are effective in controlling heart rate in patients for whom beta-blockers are contraindicated.[76]

Some patients with thyroid storm have concomitant adrenal insufficiency, and they may be prescribed dexamethasone, or hydrocortisone, during the initial stages of thyroid storm management.[72] The Pharmacologic Management Table on Thyrotoxic Crisis lists the most commonly used medications and their nursing implications for the patient in thyroid storm.

NURSING MANAGEMENT

Nursing management of the patient with thyroid storm incorporates a variety of nursing diagnoses (see the Nursing Diagnoses feature on Thyroid Storm). Nursing interventions are directed toward safe administration and monitoring of the effects of prescribed medications, normalizing body temperature, rehydration with correction of other metabolic derangements, and provision of patient education.

Medication Administration. The timely and ordered sequence of medication administration is essential in the management of thyroid storm (see previous sections on pharmacologic management). The patient in thyroid storm is agitated, anxious, and unable to rest and benefits from an environment that is calm. Gradually, the effects of the antithyroid medications, iodides, and β-adrenergic blocking drugs will decrease the neurologic symptoms related to the catecholamine sensitivity. Heart rate should decrease following beta-blockade. The patient and family needs to be reassured that this extreme agitation is the result of the disease process and that the medications will help control the nonstop fidgeting and tremors. Frequent reassurance and clear, simple explanations of the patient's condition help decrease the fear brought on by the onset thyroid storm.

Normalize Body Temperature. In thyroid storm the patient has hyperthermia related to a hypermetabolic state, as evidenced by critically high body temperature; diaphoresis; hot, flushed skin; intolerance to heat; tachycardia; and tachypnea. Temperature is assessed frequently until safe levels are attained. Nursing measures to provide comfort while the patient is intolerant to heat include a room with a cool environment and a fan to circulate air, lightweight bed coverings, and comfortable, nonrestrictive bedclothes. A tepid sponge bath helps to reduce heat by evaporation, and cold-pack application to the groin and axilla increase heat loss at major blood vessels. If antipyretic drugs are required, acetaminophen is the agent of choice to avoid the use of salicylates.[72]

NURSING DIAGNOSES | Thyroid Storm

- Hyperthermia related to increased metabolic rate
- Imbalanced Nutrition: Less Than Body Requirements related to lack of exogenous nutrients or increased metabolic demand
- Decreased Cardiac Output related to alterations in heart rate
- Anxiety related to threat to biologic, psychologic, and/or social integrity
- Disturbed Sleep Pattern related to fragmented sleep
- Deficient Knowledge: Discharge Regimen related to lack of previous exposure to information (see Patient Education feature on Thyroid Storm)

Rehydration and Correction of Metabolic Derangements. Hyperthermia, tachypnea, diaphoresis, vomiting, and diarrhea predispose the patient to a fluid volume deficit. Fluids and electrolytes are as vigorously replaced as the decompensated cardiovascular system can tolerate. Glucose solutions are given to replace glycogen stores, which are depleted. Insulin is administered to treat the hyperglycemia that results from mobilization of nutrients and glucocorticoids. Point-of-care (bedside) blood glucose measurements are performed frequently to use as a reference point for insulin dose. Hyponatremia from active loss, such as vomiting, is monitored by means of laboratory serum values. Hyponatremia is prevented and/or treated with isotonic IV fluid replacement. Additional nursing measures focus on frequent hydration assessments (see Box 36-2). I&O includes estimating diaphoretic fluid loss through the number of gown and linen changes, checking buccal membranes for moisture, and recording the patient's weight daily.

PATIENT EDUCATION

During the critical events surrounding the thyroid storm, the patient and family are given information according to their emotional state and cognitive level of understanding. The cause of the high fever, anxiety, and cardiac dysrhythmias is explained in understandable terms (see the Patient Education feature on Thyroid Storm). Often the patient and family are relieved to know that the agitation and nervousness result from circulating chemicals that may be decreased by taking daily medications. Side effects of drug therapy are taught before discharge. Patients treated with beta-blockers or are taught to report

Pharmacologic Management: Thyrotoxic Crisis

DRUG	DOSAGE	ACTIONS	SPECIAL CONSIDERATIONS
Blocks Synthesis of Thyroid Hormone			
Prophylthiouracil	Loading dose: 800-1200 mg Maintenance dose: 100-400 mg q4-6hr PO or gavage	Blocks synthesis of thyroid hormone Blocks conversion of T_3 to T_4	Monitor thyrotoxic response (i.e., heart rate, nervousness, fever, diarrhea, diaphoresis) Observe for sudden conversion to hypothyroidism: headache, sluggish responses Assess for skin rash Administer with meals to reduce gastrointestinal (GI) effects May cause rash, nausea, vomiting, agranulocytosis, skin hyperpigmentation, prothrombin deficiency
Methimazole	10-20 mg q 6-8 hr PO or gavage	Blocks synthesis of thyroid hormone	More toxic than propylthiouracil Presence of rash may be reason to discontinue drug Monitor signs listed for propylthiouracil May cause rash, agranulocytosis
Suppresses Release of Thyroid Hormone			
Sodium iodide	1 g/L q12hr IV	Suppresses releases of thyroid hormone	Give iodide 1 hr after propylthiouracil or methimazole Toxic iodinism poisoning: edema, mucosal stomatitis, hemorrhage, metallic taste, skin lesions, severe GI upset
Potassium iodide	2-5 gtts q8hr PO	Suppresses release of thyroid hormone	Discontinue if rash appears Signs of toxic iodinism as above
Saturated solution of potassium iodide (SSKI)	10 gtt q8hr PO	Suppresses release of thyroid hormone	Give through a straw to prevent teeth discoloration Mix with juice or milk to lessen GI upset Signs of toxic iodinism as above
Dexamethasone	2 mg q6hr, variable, IV	Suppresses thyroid hormone release Blocks conversion of T_4 to T_3	Monitor intake and output; monitor serum glucose levels May cause hypertension, nausea, vomiting, anorexia, increased susceptibility to infection
Beta-Blockers			
Propranolol	1-3 mg q1-4hr IV 40-80 mg q4-6hr PO	β-adrenergic blocking agent to counter sympathetic activity	Monitor cardiac activity, CVP, PAOP, bradycardia, hypotension, pending CHF Hold if heart rate <50 beats/min Have atropine available, may cause GI upset, weakness, fatigue
Esmolol	500 mcg/kg/min for first minute, then 50 mcg/kg/min for 4 minutes IV	β-adrenergic blocker	Monitor for bradycardia, orthostatic hypotension, dysrhythmia Measure intake and output May cause edema, diarrhea, diaphoresis, vertigo
Alpha-Blockers			
Reserpine	1-2.5 mg q24hr PO	Depletes stores of catecholamine in sympathetic nerve endings	Monitor BP, heart rate changes in hyperthyroid conditions May cause bradycardia, drowsiness, GI bleeding, diarrhea
Guanethidine sulfate	50-150 mg q24hr PO	Antiadrenergic Inhibits norepinephrine release in response to sympathetic nerve stimulation	Monitor orthostatic hypotension Measure and record intake and output Monitor diarrhea May cause GI upset, edema, fatigue, drowsiness

PO, By mouth; *gtts*, drops; *IV*, intravenous; *CVP*, central venous pressure; *PAOP*, pulmonary artery occlusion pressure; *CHF*, congestive heart failure; *BP*, blood pressure.

PATIENT EDUCATION

Thyroid Storm

- Acute phase
  Explain reasons for critical care unit admission
  Explain reasons for extreme hypermetabolism
- Predischarge
  Assess knowledge level
  Disease process of thyrotoxicosis
  Causes of thyrotoxic crisis
  Medications: explain purpose, side effects, dosage, and how often to use
  Signs and symptoms to report to health care professional

signs of bradycardia, unexplained fatigue, and orthostatic hypotension, among other untoward effects. Patients discharged with antithyroid drugs are alerted to the main side effect: agranulocytosis. Symptoms of agranulocytosis include sudden cough, fever, rash, and inflammation. These symptoms must be brought to the attention of the primary care provider. Patients are instructed to use acetaminophen rather than salicylates, since the salicylate increases the free thyroid hormone in circulation.

COLLABORATIVE MANAGEMENT

There are no published guidelines that discuss acute collaborative care management of the patient with thyroid storm. Guidelines do exist for nonacute care of the patient with hyperthyroidism.[70] The patient with thyroid storm requires interventions by many health care professionals with clearly communicated goals to facilitate rapid recovery.

MYXEDEMA COMA

DESCRIPTION

A severe deficiency or absence of thyroid hormone produces hypothyroidism. Hypothyroidism as defined by laboratory tests and clinical symptoms ranges from mild to severe. Mild hypothyroidism has no symptoms.[78] Severe hypothyroidism leads to a comatose state called *myxedema coma*, which can be fatal.[79] Discussion of myxedema coma necessitates frequent reference to its precursor state, hypothyroidism. The term *myxedema* is used only referring to myxedema coma, as a description of the progressive worsening or terminal stage of hypothyroidism.

ETIOLOGY

Hypothyroidism is caused by a deficiency of circulating thyroid hormone. Lack or insufficient thyroid hormone affects all body cells and organs, and slows metabolic rate and response time in every system.[71] Subclinical hypothyroidism is underdiagnosed and is present in up to 20% of the adult U.S. population over 60 years of age.[70] Myxedema coma is rare, afflicts the elderly more commonly, and affects more women than men.[79] Early recognition of the symptoms and prompt treatment will decrease mortality rate, although it remains high compared with many other diseases—35% in one clinical report.[79] Myxedema coma is rarely seen as a single disease entity in the critical care unit. Its underlying presence often is revealed by an acute primary disease, surgery, or as a consequence of increased metabolic demands. Cardiopulmonary disease, systemic infection, and exposure to extreme cold are a few of the physiologic stressors that increase metabolic demand.[80]

PATHOPHYSIOLOGY

The effects of hypothyroidism are widespread and varied. When the basal metabolic rate of oxygen consumption is reduced, the cell is unable to maintain the processes necessary to sustain life. Without thyroid hormone, protein synthesis is severely curtailed and amino acid production, manufacture of blood proteins, and repair of tissues are halted. Metabolism of carbohydrate and fat is incomplete, and gluconeogenesis cannot supply additional sources of glucose. Lipolysis is ineffective, and cholesterol collects in the blood stream. All systems are affected as described below.

Skin. The composition of the skin changes as *hyaluronic acid* deposits (gel-like substance capable of holding large amounts of fluid) accumulate in the interstitial spaces, giving rise to a full, puffy appearance of face, hands, and feet. The facial expression is dull and mask-like. The skin is pale, with an overall yellowish appearance resulting from the increase of carotene deposits. The nails and hair are thin and brittle. Absence of thyroid hormone also leads to decreased or absent sweat production. The hyaluronic acid deposits are evident in cardiac muscle tissue, skeletal muscles, and muscles of the tongue, pharynx, and proximal esophagus. These striated muscular changes of the tongue, pharynx, and esophagus most probably contribute to the hoarse, husky voice and dull facial expression of hypothyroid patients.

Cardiopulmonary System. Interstitial edema impairs cardiac myocytes, resulting in bradycardia and diminished cardiac output. The heart appears to be enlarged, but its size may be exaggerated by serous fluid accumulation in the pericardial sac. Cardiac output decreases by 30% to 50% in severe hypothyroidism.[80] A decreased sensitivity to catecholamines is present even though serum catecholamine levels are elevated.[80] Resting heart rate and stroke volume are reduced. The force of myocardial contraction is weakened, with a decrease in the systolic blood pressure and an increase in diastolic pressure, causing a narrowed pulse pressure. Electrocardiogram typically reveals low-voltage QRS complexes and nonspecific ST segment changes.[80]

Pulmonary System. Pleural effusions and muscular changes affect gas exchange. The basal rate of oxygen consumption decreases, with a resulting insensitivity to CO_2. Hypoventilation increases the CO_2 serum content, which increases cerebral hypoxia. Both hypoxic and hypercapneic ventilatory drive are severely impaired.[80] Respiratory acidosis can occur.[81] Pleural effusion, reduced vital capacity, and shallow respirations occur with any exertion. Respiratory muscle weakness, sleep apnea, and upper airway obstruction all may be present. Patients with myxedema are a high-risk category for any surgical procedure or critical care admission due to their limited ventilatory capacity.[80]

Kidneys and Fluid and Electrolyte Balance. Renal blood flow is reduced with decreased glomerular filtration rate (GFR), decreased urine specific gravity, and decreased urine osmolality. ADH level is increased (fluid retention), and sodium is decreased. Urea production is diminished. Elimination of drugs via the kidneys is severely slowed in hypothyroidism.[80] Coexisting adrenal insufficiency should also be considered.[81]

Nutrition and Elimination. Decreased gastric motility or even ileus is an expected complication for the patient with severe hypothyroidism.[80] Food utilization and nutrient mobilization decrease with insufficient thyroid hormone. Intestinal hypomotility and abdominal distention prevent absorption of food nutrients in the small intestine. Lipolysis decreases, and serum cholesterol increases. Abdominal distention, decreased intestinal peristalsis, and eventual paralytic ileus lead to extreme constipation. These finding make provision of enteral nutrition a challenge. Understandably, in the more alert patient, a lack of appetite and inability to eat coexist.

Thermoregulation. Heat production decreases as a result of insufficient energy for the base metabolic rate within the cells. The inability to maintain body heat is further restricted by the hypoglycemia. Sweating and insensible water loss diminish.

Anemia. Anemia is a common problem that is present in 25% to 50% of patients with hypothyroidism.[80] Symptoms of fatigue and depression are associated. Erythropoiesis (red cell production) is impaired and inadequate. Coagulation abnormalities may coexist.[80]

ASSESSMENT AND DIAGNOSIS

The diagnosis of myxedema coma is based on the clinical manifestations of end-stage hypothyroidism. A comparison of the difference between severe hyper- (thyroid

storm) and hypothyroidism (myxedema) is provided in Box 36-8.

Clinical Presentation. The diagnosis of end-stage hypothyroidism is based on the clinical presentation of the patient. Increasing signs of somnolence, depression, and

---

Box 36-8

CLINICAL MANIFESTATIONS OF HYPERTHYROIDISM (THYROID STORM) AS COMPARED WITH HYPOTHYROIDISM (MYXEDEMA COMA)

HYPERTHYROIDISM (THYROTOXICOSIS) Thyroid Crisis	HYPOTHYROIDISM (MYXEDEMA) Myxedema Coma
Elevated T_4, T_3	Decreased T_4, T_3
Decreased TSH	Elevated TSH
Hypercalcemia	Hyponatremia
Hyperglycemia	Hypoglycemia
Metabolic acidosis	Respiratory acidosis
	Metabolic acidosis
	Hypercholesterolemia
	Anemia
Tachycardia	Bradycardia
Angina	Enlarged heart
Palpitations	Decreased stroke volume
Atrial fibrillation	Decreased cardiac output
ST wave changes	Flattened, inverted T waves
Shortened QT	Prolonged QT and PR intervals
Hypertension	Increased total body fluid with
AV block	decreased effective arterial
Hypovolemia	blood volume
Angina	Peripheral vasoconstriction
Acute heart failure	Pericardial effusion
Tachypnea	Hypoventilation
SOB	Possible CO_2 retention
Hypermetabolism	Depressed metabolism
Polyphagia	Decreased lipolysis
	Increased cholesterol
Weight loss	Weight gain
Nausea, vomiting	Constipation
Increased peristalsis	
Tremor	Depression
Extreme restlessness	Seizures
Insomnia	Slowness
Anxiety	Hypothermia
Uneasiness	Impaired short-term memory
Emotional instability	Slow, deliberate speech
Despondency	Thickened tongue
Diaphoresis	Coarse, dry, scaly, edematous skin
Heat intolerance	Frank delirium (myxedema madness)
	Lethargy → stupor → coma (myxedema coma)
Increased deep tendon reflexes (DTRs)	Diminished DTRs
Muscle weakness/muscle wasting	Paresthesia of hands
Oligoamenorrhea	Menorrhagia

TSH, Thyroid-stimulating hormone; *SOB*, shortness of breath; *AV*, atrioventricular.

diminished mental acuity signal diminished cellular functioning. Interstitial edema collects in almost all tissues. Organs become infiltrated with the mucoidal-rich substrate, mucopolysaccharides, which compromises organ functioning. Patients manifest cardiovascular collapse, hypothermia, decreased renal functioning, fluid excess, hypoventilation, and severe metabolic disorders.

Weight gain is attributed to the collection of mucopolysaccharides in the interstitium, increase in fluid retention, and decrease in metabolism. Paresthesia of hands and feet is caused by the hyaluronic acid accumulation in the synovial sacs, which leads to the compression of nerves and carpal tunnel syndrome. The compression of nerves interferes with the simplest hand grasp and the ability to raise one's hands. Reflexes contract briskly but take extended seconds to relax.

Hypothermia is a very distressing symptom. The patient is unable to keep the body warm. Temperatures have been reported to fall below 35° C (95.9° F).[81] Most cases of myxedema are diagnosed in the winter months.[81] The myxedematous patient has hypotension, reduced total blood volume, decreased cardiac output, and bradycardia—all related to a decrease in the β-adrenergic stimulation. Neuropsychiatric symptoms of depression, confusion, and decreased mental acuity may degenerate to a psychosis aptly termed "myxedema madness."

Laboratory Studies. Laboratory test results do not differentiate between hypothyroidism and myxedema coma. The blood test results simply confirm the clinical diagnosis. Typically patients with myxedema have primary hypothyroidism with a low T_4 level, a low T_3 level, and a high TSH level.[81] If the TSH level is normal or low, other causes of the hypothyroidism must be investigated.[81] TSH is released by the pituitary gland (see Chapter 34); endocrine studies to evaluate the level of pituitary function should be undertaken.

MEDICAL MANAGEMENT

The patient's primary admitting diagnosis may mask an underlying hypothyroidism. However, clinical manifestations can trigger the alert clinician to suspect a hypofunctioning thyroid. Both the primary disease condition and the myxedema coma must be treated immediately to improve the patient's chances for recovery. A complete blood count and differential are evaluated to establish the presence of infection. Hypothyroidism produces a characteristically low white blood cell count. A normal white blood cell count and a differential with elevated and immature neutrophils indicate an ongoing acute infection. Severe systemic infection, often a precipitating factor for the myxedema coma, must be treated to decrease the stress on the thyroid-pituitary axis. Empiric antibiotic therapy may be required.

The goal for the treatment of end-stage or decompensated hypothyroid condition is to restore the patient to an euthyroid (normal thyroid function) condition. This is accomplished with thyroid hormone replacement and support measures for the multisystem involvement.

PHARMACOLOGIC MANAGEMENT

Methods of treating end-stage hypothyroidism with medications vary among practitioners. A common method is to replete T_4 levels with an initial dose of levothyroxine 100 to 500 mcg IV to saturate the previously empty T_4 binding sites.[81] The thyroid-binding globulin must be saturated before any free thyroxine can circulate. The loading dose is followed by daily administration of 75 to 100 mcg of levothyroxine.[81] If an elderly patient with concurrent heart disease is treated with replacement hormones, it is necessary to start the treatment slowly so as not to precipitate heart failure or angina.

Glucocorticoids may be necessary to assist the patient to respond to the stress state of hypothyroidism until a coexisting adrenal insufficiency is ruled out.

NURSING MANAGEMENT

Nursing care of the patient with myxedema coma focuses on management of the precipitating disease as well as the severe hypothyroid impact on multiple organ systems. Many nursing diagnoses are associated with management of myxedema coma and are listed in the Nursing Diagnoses feature on Myxedema Coma.

Pulmonary Care. The patient with myxedema coma who is admitted to the critical care unit may require intubation and mechanical ventilatory support. Individuals who are not intubated are monitored for development of respiratory failure. Arterial blood gas measurements are evaluated to monitor for CO_2 retention and respiratory acidosis.

NURSING DIAGNOSES   Myxedema Coma

- Hypothermia related to decreased metabolic rate
- Impaired Spontaneous Ventilation related to respiratory fatigue or metabolic factors
- Activity Intolerance related to prolonged immobility or deconditioning
- Disturbed Body Image related to functional dependence on life-sustaining technology
- Deficient Knowledge: Discharge Regimen related to lack of previous exposure to information (see Patient Education feature on Myxedema Coma)

Cardiac Concerns. Dysrhythmias are common in the myxedematous patient with impaired myocardial contraction and can quickly be identified by continuous electrocardiogram (ECG) monitoring. Expected signs of myxedema, such as flattened or inverted T waves or prolonged QT and PR intervals, resolve in a positive response to thyroxine replacement therapy. Hypotension management requires cautious fluid replacement of 5% to 10% glucose in 0.45% sodium chloride or 0.9% sodium chloride, depending on serum sodium levels.

Thermoregulation. Hypothermia will gradually improve as the patient is treated with thyroid hormone. Several warm blankets comfortably wrapped around the patient (with mild hypothermia) may be sufficient to help raise the body temperature to normal. Active warming devices are also used. Continuous assessments are important to avoid too-rapid heating and vasodilation. Temperature is measured with electronic devices that can measure accurately at the extreme lower range of body temperatures.

Thyroid Replacement Therapy. Elderly patients or those with a cardiac history receive IV thyroxine with due precautions. Thyroxine can precipitate angina and dysrhythmias. Hemodynamic monitoring includes HR, BP, ECG, CVP, and in rare situations information from a PA catheter. Improvement in the patient's cardiopulmonary and neurologic status, plus change in T_4 and TSH laboratory values, are used to gauge success of the thyroid hormone replacement therapy.

Skin Care. Patients with myxedema coma have rough, dry skin. Measures are taken to avoid skin breakdown related to decreased circulation and widespread edema. Soap is used sparingly, followed by an emollient. Frequent positioning minimizes pressure against capillary beds over bony prominences.

Elimination. Constipation is managed on a daily basis to avoid impaction. Use of fiber-enriched enteral nutrition may be helpful. When eating, food choices include sources of increased fiber, such as fresh fruits and vegetables. Fluids are encouraged as the hypovolemia is corrected and blood pressure stabilizes. Increased fiber is preferable to use of enemas. Enemas are to be avoided, because insertion of the rectal tube may stimulate the vagal nerve.

PATIENT EDUCATION

Patients with myxedema coma have decreased comprehension and mental acuity. All instructions, procedures, and activities are to be explained slowly, and provided in written form. Family members, as well as the patient experiencing myxedema coma, may go through myriad emotions with one constant: fear of the unknown. Before any teaching, the nurse is to evaluate the family's ability to accept the patient's slowed thinking and slowed response time. The family may benefit from a referral to the

---

PATIENT EDUCATION | **Myxedema Coma**

- Acute phase
  Explain reasons for critical care unit admission
  Explain reasons for extreme hypermetabolism
- Predischarge
  Assess knowledge level
  Disease process of thyrotoxicosis
  Causes of thyrotoxic crisis
  Medications: explain purpose, side effects, dosage, and how often to use
  Signs and symptoms to report to health care professional

---

hospital's social service department for assistance in dealing with the patient's neuropsychiatric symptoms.

All instructions given to the patient and/or family are to be given both verbally and in writing. In addition, a written copy of all schedules is given as a reference for home care before discharge. The nurse is to discuss the medication schedule and the frequency of the drug doses with the patient and family. Side effects of each drug are to be included. The patient and family are to know the side effects of drugs so that they can deal with them at home, as well as know which signs or symptoms are to be reported to the health care provider. Over-the-counter medications are not to be taken unless the physician approves of the drug and the dose (see the Patient Education feature on Myxedema Coma).

COLLABORATIVE MANAGEMENT

There are no published guidelines that discuss acute collaborative care management of the patient with myxedema coma. Guidelines do exist for nonacute care of the patient with hypothyroidism.[70] Collaborative management is required to decrease mortality in myxedema coma. Early recognition of symptoms and a willingness to request laboratory tests to confirm the diagnosis will allow therapy to be instituted as early as possible by the clinical team.

SUMMARY

The endocrine system is complex, and assessment relies heavily on laboratory tests for confirmation of disease processes. As clinicians gain a more comprehensive understanding of the role of the endocrine system critical illness, the tests of endocrine organ function will be more frequently requested as part of a complete critical care evaluation. Hormone deficiencies will be replenished if this practice is supported by adequate research. To fully participate in the care of these complex patients it is imperative that critical care nurses are familiar with the intricacies of the endocrine system.

REFERENCES

1. Van Den Berghe G et al: Intensive insulin therapy in the critically ill patients, *N Engl J Med* 345(19):1359-1367, 2001.
2. Laird AM et al: Relationship of early hyperglycemia to mortality in trauma patients, *J Trauma* 56(5):1058-1062, 2004.
3. Marik PE, Raghavan M: Stress-hyperglycemia, insulin and immunomodulation in sepsis, *Intensive Care Med* 30(5): 748-756, 2004.
4. Holm C et al: Acute hyperglycaemia following thermal injury: friend or foe? *Resuscitation* 60(1):71-77, 2004.
5. Coursin DB, Connery LE, Ketzler JT: Perioperative diabetic and hyperglycemic management issues, *Crit Care Med* 32(4 Suppl):S116-S125, 2004.
6. Capes SE et al: Stress hyperglycemia and prognosis of stroke in nondiabetic and diabetic patients: a systematic overview, *Stroke* 32(10):2426-2432, 2001.
7. Garber AJ et al: American College of Endocrinology position statement on inpatient diabetes and metabolic control, *Endocr Pract* 10(Suppl 2):4-9, 2004.
8. Wortsman J: Role of epinephrine in acute stress, *Endocrinol Metab Clin North Am* 31(1):79-106, 2002.
9. Langton JE, Brent GA: Nonthyroidal illness syndrome: evaluation of thyroid function in sick patients, *Endocrinol Metab Clin North Am* 31(1):159-172, 2002.
10. Van Den Berghe G: Neuroendocrine pathobiology of chronic critical illness, *Crit Care Clin* 18(3):509-528, 2002.
11. Van Den Berghe G: Endocrine evaluation of patients with critical illness, *Endocrinol Metab Clin North Am* 32(2): 385-410, 2003.
12. Weekers F, Van Den Berghe G: Endocrine modifications and interventions during critical illness, *Proc Nutr Soc* 63(3): 443-450, 2004.
13. Cooper MS, Stewart PM: Corticosteroid insufficiency in acutely ill patients, *N Engl J Med* 348(8):727-734, 2003.
14. Rivers EP et al: Adrenal insufficiency in high-risk surgical ICU patients, *Chest* 119(3):889-896, 2001.
15. Keh D, Sprung CL: Use of corticosteroid therapy in patients with sepsis and septic shock: an evidence-based review, *Crit Care Med* 32(11):S527, 2004.
16. Axelrod L: Perioperative management of patients treated with glucocorticoids, *Endocrinol Metab Clin North Am* 32(2):367-383, 2003.
17. Clement S et al: Management of diabetes and hyperglycemia in hospitals, *Diabetes Care* 27(2):553-591, 2004.
18. Baird TA et al: The influence of diabetes mellitus and hyperglycaemia on stroke incidence and outcome, *J Clin Neurosci* 9(6):618-626, 2002.
19. Parsons MW et al: Acute hyperglycemia adversely affects stroke outcome: a magnetic resonance imaging and spectroscopy study, *Ann Neurol* 52(1):20-28, 2002.
20. Baird TA et al: Persistent poststroke hyperglycemia is independently associated with infarct expansion and worse clinical outcome, *Stroke* 34(9):2208-2214, 2003.
21. Moghissi E: Hospital management of diabetes: beyond the sliding scale, *Cleve Clin J Med* 71(10):801-808, 2004.
22. Robinson LE, Van Soeren MH: Insulin resistance and hyperglycemia in critical illness: role of insulin in glycemic control, *AACN Clin Issues* 15(1):45-62, 2004.
23. Dinardo MM, Korytkowski MT, Siminerio LS: The importance of normoglycemia in critically ill patients, *Crit Care Nurs Q* 27(2):126-134, 2004.
24. Langdon CD, Shriver RL: Clinical issues in the care of critically ill diabetic patients, *Crit Care Nurs Q* 27(2):162-171, 2004.
25. Anderson RN, Smith BL: Deaths: leading causes for 2001, *Natl Vital Stat Rep* 52(9):1-85, 2003.
26. Self-reported heart disease and stroke among adults with and without diabetes—United States, 1999-2001, *MMWR Morb Mortal Wkly Rep* 52(44):1065-1070, 2003.
27. Coughlin SS et al: Diabetes mellitus as a predictor of cancer mortality in a large cohort of U.S. adults, *Am J Epidemiol* 159(12):1160-1167, 2004.
28. Diagnosis and classification of diabetes mellitus, *Diabetes Care* 27(Suppl 1):S5-S10, 2004.
29. Goldstein DE et al: Tests of glycemia in diabetes, *Diabetes Care* 27(Suppl 1):S91-S93, 2004.
30. Blake DR, Nathan DM: Point-of-care testing for diabetes, *Crit Care Nurs Q* 27(2):150-161, 2004.
31. Standards of medical care in diabetes, *Diabetes Care* 27(Suppl 1):S15-S35, 2004.
32. Lebovitz HE: Oral antidiabetic agents: 2004, *Med Clin North Am* 88(4):847-863, 2004.
33. Richter B, Neises G, Bergerhoff K: Human versus animal insulin in people with diabetes mellitus. A systematic review, *Endocrinol Metab Clin North Am* 31(3):723-749, 2002.
34. Screening for type 2 diabetes, *Diabetes Care* 27(Suppl 1): S11-S14, 2004.
35. American Association of Clinical Endocrinologists: Position statement on the insulin resistance syndrome, *Endocr Pract* 9(S2):5-21, 2003.
36. Fletcher B, Lamendola C: Insulin resistance syndrome, *J Cardiovasc Nurs* 19(5):339-345, 2004.
37. Grundy SM et al: Clinical management of metabolic syndrome: report of the American Heart Association/National Heart, Lung, and Blood Institute/American Diabetes Association conference on scientific issues related to management, *Circulation* 109(4):551-556, 2004.
38. Yki-Jarvinen H: Thiazolidinediones, *N Engl J Med* 351(11): 1106-1118, 2004.
39. Kruse JA: Metformin-associated lactic acidosis, *J Emerg Med* 20(3):267-272, 2001.
40. Khan JK et al: Lactic acidemia associated with metformin, *Ann Pharmacother* 37(1):66-69, 2003.
41. Nesto RW et al: Thiazolidinedione use, fluid retention, and congestive heart failure: a consensus statement from the American Heart Association and American Diabetes Association, *Circulation* 108(23):2941-2948, 2003.
42. Davis T, Edelman SV: Insulin therapy in type 2 diabetes, *Med Clin North Am* 88(4):865-895, 2004.
43. Lien LF, Angelyn Bethel M, Feinglos MN: In-hospital management of type 2 diabetes mellitus, *Med Clin North Am* 88(4):1085-1105, 2004.
44. Toto RD: Lessons learned from recent clinical trials in hypertensive diabetics: what's good for the kidney is good for the heart and brain, *Am J Hypertens* 17(11 Suppl):S7-S10, 2004.
45. Krauss RM: Lipids and lipoproteins in patients with type 2 diabetes, *Diabetes Care* 27(6):1496-1504, 2004.
46. Wilson Tang WH, Maroo A, Young JB: Ischemic heart disease and congestive heart failure in diabetic patients, *Med Clin North Am* 88(4):1037-1061, 2004.

47. Langford M: Type 2 diabetes and chronic systolic heart failure: clinical implications, *J Cardiovasc Nurs* 19(6s):S35-S44, 2004.

48. Kitabchi AE et al: Hyperglycemic crises in diabetes, *Diabetes Care* 27(Suppl 1):S94-S102, 2004.

49. Gaglia JL, Wyckoff J, Abrahamson MJ: Acute hyperglycemic crisis in the elderly, *Med Clin North Am* 88(4):1063-1084, 2004.

50. Newton CA, Raskin P: Diabetic ketoacidosis in type 1 and type 2 diabetes mellitus: clinical and biochemical differences, *Arch Intern Med* 164(17):1925-1931, 2004.

51. Magee MF, Bhatt BA: Management of decompensated diabetes. Diabetic ketoacidosis and hyperglycemic hyperosmolar syndrome, *Crit Care Clin* 17(1):75-106, 2001.

52. Unger RH, Foster DW: Diabetes mellitus. In Williams RH et al, editors: *Williams textbook of endocrinology,* ed 10, Philadelphia, 2002, Saunders.

53. Janicic N, Verbalis JG: Evaluation and management of hypo-osmolality in hospitalized patients, *Endocrinol Metab Clin North Am* 32(2):459-481, 2003.

54. Holcomb S: Diabetes insipidus, *DCCN* 21(3):94-97, 2002.

55. Wong LL, Verbalis JG: Systemic diseases associated with disorders of water homeostasis, *Endocrinol Metab Clin North Am* 31(1):121-140, 2002.

56. Boughey JC, Yost MJ, Bynoe RP: Diabetes insipidus in the head-injured patient, *Am Surg* 70(6):500-503, 2004.

57. Verbalis JG: Management of disorders of water metabolism in patients with pituitary tumors, *Pituitary* 5(2):119-132, 2002.

58. Vance ML: Perioperative management of patients undergoing pituitary surgery, *Endocrinol Metab Clin North Am* 32(2):355-365, 2003.

59. Innis J: Treating nephrogenic diabetes insipidus: a case study, *DCCN* 21(3):98-99, 2002.

60. Olson DM, Meek LG, Lynch JR: Accurate patient history contributes to differentiating diabetes insipidus: a case study, *J Neurosci Nurs* 36(4):228-230, 2004.

61. Verbalis JG: Disorders of body water homeostasis, *Best Pract Res Clin Endocrinol Metab* 17(4):471-503, 2003.

62. Holmes CL et al: Physiology of vasopressin relevant to management of septic shock, *Chest* 120(3):989-1002, 2001.

63. *Mosby's Drug Consult,* St. Louis, 2004, Mosby.

64. Holmes CL, Landry DW, Granton JT: Science review: vasopressin and the cardiovascular system part 1—receptor physiology, *Crit Care* 7(6):427-434, 2003.

65. Holmes CL, Landry DW, Granton JT: Science review: vasopressin and the cardiovascular system part 2—clinical physiology, *Crit Care* 8(1):15-23, 2004.

66. Seute T et al: Neurologic disorders in 432 consecutive patients with small cell lung carcinoma, *Cancer* 100(4):801-806, 2004.

67. Freda BJ, Davidson MB, Hall PM: Evaluation of hyponatremia: a little physiology goes a long way, *Cleve Clin J Med* 71(8):639-650, 2004.

68. Johnson AL, Criddle LM: Pass the salt: indications for and implications of using hypertonic saline, *Crit Care Nurse* 24(5):36-48, 2004.

69. Rabinstein AA, Wijdicks EF: Hyponatremia in critically ill neurological patients, *Neurologist* 9(6):290-300, 2003.

70. American Association of Clinical Endocrinologists: Medical guidelines for clinical practice for the evaluation and treatment of hyperthyroidism and hypothyroidism, *Endocr Pract* 8(6):458-469, 2002.

71. Demers LM: Thyroid disease: pathophysiology and diagnosis, *Clin Lab Med* 24(1):19-28, 2004.

72. Wald DA, Silver A: Cardiovascular manifestations of thyroid storm: a case report, *J Emerg Med* 25(1):23-28, 2003.

73. Grimes CM et al: Intraoperative thyroid storm: a case report, *AANA J* 72(1):53-55, 2004.

74. Vora NM, Fedok F, Stack BC Jr: Report of a rare case of trauma-induced thyroid storm, *Ear Nose Throat J* 81(8):570-572, 574, 2002.

75. Waltman PA, Brewer JM, Lobert S: Thyroid storm during pregnancy. A medical emergency, *Crit Care Nurse* 24(2):74-79, 2004.

76. Holcomb SS: Thyroid diseases: a primer for the critical care nurse, *Dimens Crit Care Nurs* 21(4):127-133, 2002.

77. Frost L, Vestergaard P, Mosekilde L: Hyperthyroidism and risk of atrial fibrillation or flutter: a population-based study, *Arch Intern Med* 164(15):1675-1678, 2004.

78. Surks MI et al: Subclinical thyroid disease: scientific review and guidelines for diagnosis and management, *JAMA* 291(2):228-238, 2004.

79. Rodriguez I et al: Factors associated with mortality of patients with myxoedema coma: prospective study in 11 cases treated in a single institution, *J Endocrinol* 180(2):347-350, 2004.

80. Stathatos N, Wartofsky L: Perioperative management of patients with hypothyroidism, *Endocrinol Metab Clin North Am* 32(2):503-518, 2003.

81. Wall CR: Myxedema coma: diagnosis and treatment, *Am Fam Physician* 62(11):2485-2490, 2000.

UNIT

IX

MULTISYSTEM ALTERATIONS

CHAPTER 37

Trauma

Trauma is the leading cause of death for all age-groups under the age of 44. Injury costs the United States hundreds of billions of dollars annually. It is one of the most pressing health problems in the United States today. However, the problem continues to go largely unrecognized.

Injury as a result of trauma is no longer considered to be an "accident." The term *motor vehicle accident (MVA)* has been replaced with *motor vehicle crash (MVC)*, and the term *accident* has been replaced with *unintentional injury.* Unintentional injury is no accident. Accident traditionally has implied an act of God or an unpredictable accident. Domestic violence and alcohol-related issues are priority prevention areas with which health care providers must be actively involved.

Domestic violence constitutes a major public health issue in the United States. It is unrecognized and underreported.[1] Domestic violence is the leading cause of injury to women in the United States, and it has been estimated that one million women every year are severely beaten or assaulted with weapons by male partners.[2] Domestic violence and alcohol abuse have a high prevalence among female trauma patients admitted to trauma centers.[1,3] Health care providers should consider routinely inquiring about domestic violence as part of the history, at a minimum for all female adolescents and adult patients.[4] Key points in prevention, recognition, and treatment of domestic violence summarized by Sisley et al (1999) are listed in Box 37-1.[5]

An alcohol-related motor vehicle crash kills someone every 30 minutes and nonfatally injures someone every 2 minutes.[6] Each year, alcohol-related crashed in the United States cost about $51 billion.[7] To decrease the incidence of alcohol-related crashes, communities need to implement and enforce strategies that are known to be effective such as sobriety checkpoints, regulations limiting driving to those whose blood alcohol levels are below 0.08%, minimum legal drinking age laws, and "zero tolerance" for young drivers.[8,9] Alcohol screening and intervention have been recommended as routine compo-

nents of trauma care.[10] CAGE, a screening questionnaire, has been recommended (Box 37-2).[11]

Over the past few decades, major advances have been made in the management of patients with traumatic injuries, and significant improvements have been made in their care in both prehospital and emergency department settings. These improvements have affected critical care in that patients with complex, multisystem trauma are admitted to critical care units. These patients require complex nursing care. This chapter reviews nursing management of patients with traumatic injuries, particularly in the critical care setting.

MECHANISMS OF INJURY

Trauma occurs when an external force of energy impacts the body and causes structural or physiologic alterations, or "injuries." External forces can be radiation, electrical, thermal, chemical, or mechanical forms of energy. This chapter focuses on trauma from mechanical energy. Mechanical energy can produce either blunt or penetrating traumatic injuries. Knowledge of the mechanism of injury helps health care providers anticipate and predict potential internal injuries.

BLUNT TRAUMA

Blunt trauma is seen most often with MVCs, contact sports, blunt force injuries (e.g., trauma caused by a baseball bat), or falls. Injuries occur because of the forces sustained during a rapid change in velocity (deceleration). To estimate the amount of force a person would sustain in an MVC, multiply the person's weight by miles per hour of speed the vehicle was traveling. A 130-pound woman in a vehicle traveling at 60 miles per hour that hits a brick wall, for example, would sustain 7800 pounds of force within milliseconds. As the body stops suddenly, tissues and organs continue to move forward. This sudden change in velocity causes injuries that result in lacerations or crush injuries of internal body structures.

PENETRATING TRAUMA

Penetrating injuries occur with stabbings, firearms, or accidents resulting in impalement—injuries that penetrate the skin and result in damage to internal structures. Damage occurs along the path of penetration. Penetrating injuries can be misleading inasmuch as the condition of the outside of the wound does not determine the extent of internal injury. Bullets can create internal cavities 5 to 30 times larger than the diameter of the bullet.[12]

Several factors determine the extent of damage sustained as a result of penetrating trauma. Different weapons cause different types of injuries. The severity of a gunshot wound depends on the type of gun, type of ammunition used, and the distance and angle from which the gun was fired. Pellets from a shotgun blast expand on impact and cause multiple injuries to internal structures. Handgun bullets, on the other hand, usually damage what is directly in the bullet's path. Once inside the body, the bullet can ricochet off bone and create fur-

ther damage along its pathway. With penetrating stab wounds, factors that determine the extent of injury include the type and length of object used, as well as the angle of insertion.

PHASES OF TRAUMA CARE

Care of trauma victims during wartime enhanced principles of triage and rapid transport of the injured to medical facilities. The military experience has demonstrated that more lives can be saved by decreasing the time from injury to definitive care. It also has enhanced incentives and models for improvements in civilian trauma care, such as emergency medical service (EMS) systems and trauma care centers.

Statistics demonstrate that deaths as a result of trauma occur in a trimodal distribution (Fig. 37-1).[12] The first peak includes victims who die before medical attention can be provided. The second peak occurs within a few hours after injury. It is this peak that commonly is referred to as the *golden hour* for those critically injured. The golden hour is a 60-minute time frame that incorporates activation of the EMS system, stabilization in the prehospital setting, transportation to a medical facility, rapid resuscitation on arrival in the emergency department, and provision of definitive care. In the critically injured patient, the primary goal is to minimize the time from injury to definitive care and to optimize prehospital care so that the patient arrives at the hospital alive. The third death peak occurs days to weeks after injury as a result of complications, including infection or multiple organ dysfunction syndrome. It is a nursing challenge to influence the quality of care the trauma patient receives in an attempt to "beat" the trimodal distribution of trauma deaths.

Nursing management of the patient with traumatic injuries begins the moment a call for help is received, and continues until the patient's death or return to residential rehabilitation.[13] Care of the trauma patient is seen as a continuum that includes six phases: prehospital resuscitation, hospital resuscitation, definitive care and operative phase, critical care, intermediate care, and rehabilitation.

PREHOSPITAL RESUSCITATION

The goal of prehospital care is immediate stabilization and transportation. This is achieved through airway maintenance, control of external bleeding and shock, immobilization of the patient, and immediate transport (ground or air) to the closest appropriate medical facility.[12] Personnel providing prehospital care should also communicate information needed for triage at the hospital. Advance planning for the injured patient is essential.

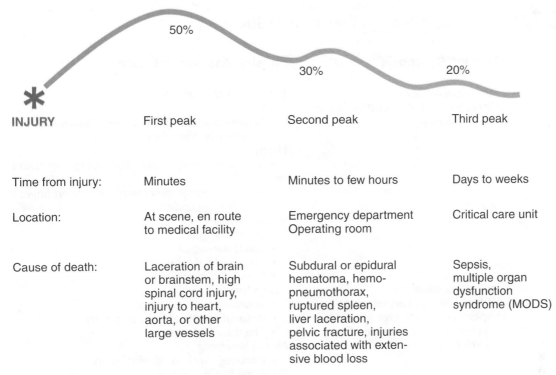

	First peak	Second peak	Third peak
	50%	30%	20%
INJURY			
Time from injury:	Minutes	Minutes to few hours	Days to weeks
Location:	At scene, en route to medical facility	Emergency department Operating room	Critical care unit
Cause of death:	Laceration of brain or brainstem, high spinal cord injury, injury to heart, aorta, or other large vessels	Subdural or epidural hematoma, hemo-pneumothorax, ruptured spleen, liver laceration, pelvic fracture, injuries associated with extensive blood loss	Sepsis, multiple organ dysfunction syndrome (MODS)

Fig. 37-1   Trimodal distribution of trauma deaths.

EMERGENCY DEPARTMENT RESUSCITATION

The American College of Surgeons developed guidelines (Advanced Trauma Life Support [ATLS]) for rapid assessment, resuscitation, and definitive care for trauma patients in the emergency department.[12] These guidelines delineate a systematic approach to care of the trauma patient: rapid primary survey, resuscitation of vital functions, more detailed secondary survey, and initiation of definitive care. This process constitutes the ABCDEs of trauma care described in the following section and assists in identifying injuries.

Primary Survey. On arrival of the trauma patient in the emergency department, the primary survey is initiated. During this assessment, life-threatening injuries are discovered and treated. The five steps in the primary survey comprise the ABCDEs: *A*irway maintenance with cervical spine protection; *B*reathing and ventilation; *C*irculation with hemorrhage control; *D*isability and neurologic status; and *E*xposure/environmental control (Table 37-1).

Airway. The patient's airway is assessed for ineffective airway clearance and airway obstruction. The trauma patient is at risk for ineffective airway clearance, especially in the presence of altered consciousness, drugs and alcohol, and maxillofacial or thoracic injuries. Airway obstruction can be caused by foreign bodies, blood clots, or broken teeth. Airway patency should be assessed by inspecting the oropharynx for foreign body obstruction, listening for air movement at the patient's nose and mouth, and auscultating lung fields. Airway assessment must incorporate cervical spine immobilization. The patient's head should not be rotated, hyperflexed, or hyperextended to establish and maintain an airway. The cervical spine must be immobilized in all trauma patients until a cervical spinal cord injury has been definitively ruled out. If the patient can communicate verbally, it is likely that the airway is patent. Patients who display nonpurposeful motor movements or who have a Glasgow Coma Scale score of 8 or less usually require the placement of a definitive airway.[12]

Breathing. The patient is assessed for ineffective breathing patterns and impaired gas exchange. It is crucial to remember that an open, clear airway does not ensure adequate ventilation and gas exchange. Assessment includes chest wall integrity and respiratory rate, depth, and symmetry. Auscultation is performed to assess gas flow in the lungs. Air or blood in the chest may be identified by percussion. Decreased breath sounds or alteration in chest wall integrity necessitate chest tube placement. Endotracheal intubation may be required for patients who have compromised airways caused by mechanical factors, who are unconscious, or who have ventilatory problems.[12] Supplemental oxygen is administered to all injured patients.[12]

Circulation. The next step is to assess for decreased cardiac output, impaired tissue perfusion, and deficient fluid volume. External exsanguination is identified and controlled by direct manual pressure on the wound. Rapid assessment of the circulatory status includes as-

Table 37-1	Primary Survey of the Trauma Patient	
Survey Component	Nursing Diagnosis	Nursing Assessment. Care
Airway	Ineffective Airway Clearance related to obstruction or actual injury	Immobilize cervical spine Look • Is there obvious airway trauma, tachypnea, accessory muscle use, tracheal shift? Listen • Stridor, hyperresonance, dullness to percussion? Feel • For air exchange over the mouth; insert finger sweep to clear foreign bodies Secure airway • Oropharyngeal • Nasopharyngeal • Endotracheal tube • Cricothyrotomy
Breathing	Ineffective Breathing Pattern related to actual injury Impaired Gas Exchange related to actual injury or disrupted tissue perfusion	Assess for • Spontaneous breathing • Respiratory rate, depth, symmetry • Chest wall integrity Absent breathing • Intubate, mechanical ventilation Breathing but ineffective • Assess life-threatening conditions (e.g., tension pneumothorax, flail chest) Administer supplemental oxygen Initiate pulse oximetry
Circulation	Decreased Cardiac Output related to actual injury Alteration in Tissue Perfusion related to actual injury or shock Deficient Fluid Volume related to actual loss of circulating volume	Assess pulse quality/rate ECG monitoring No pulse • Initiate ACLS Pulse but ineffective • Assess and treat life-threatening conditions (uncontrolled bleeding, shock) Initiate two large-bore IVs or central catheter; obtain serum samples for laboratory tests Fluid replacement
Disability	Ineffective Cerebral Tissue Perfusion Risk for Injury related to actual injury of brain or spinal cord	Assess Glasgow Coma Scale Assess pupil size and reactivity
Exposure/ environmental control	Risk for Imbalanced Body Temperature	Remove all clothing to inspect all body regions Prevent hypothermia

ECG, Electrocardiogram; *ACLS,* advanced cardiac life support; *IV,* intravenous line.

sessment of level of consciousness, skin color, and pulse.[12] Level of consciousness provides data on cerebral perfusion. Ashen, gray facial skin color or white, pale extremities may be ominous signs of hypovolemia.[12] Central pulses (femoral or carotid artery) should be assessed bilaterally for rate, regularity, and quality. If a pulse is not present, advanced cardiac life support (ACLS) protocols are instituted. Cardiac monitoring should be initiated to assess for rhythm disturbances. Life-threatening dysrhythmias are treated according to ACLS protocols.

Disability. A rapid neurologic assessment is performed next. During this step the nurse assesses the potential for injury by completing a brief neurologic assessment to establish the patient's level of consciousness and pupillary size and reaction. The AVPU method can be used to quickly describe the patient's level of consciousness: *A,* alert; *V,* responds to verbal stimuli; *P,* responds to painful stimuli; and *U,* unresponsive. The patient's Glasgow Coma Scale (GCS) can be assessed if time allows (see Chapter 26).

Box 37-3

SERUM SAMPLES TO OBTAIN WITH INTRAVENOUS PLACEMENT

- Complete blood cell (CBC) count
- Electrolyte profile (Na^+, K^+, Cl^-, CO_2, glucose, blood urea nitrogen [BUN] creatinine [Cr])
- Coagulation parameters: prothrombin time (PT); partial thromboplastin time (PTT)
- Type and screen (ABO compatibility)
- Amylase
- Toxicology screens
- Liver function studies
- Pregnancy test (for females of childbearing age)
- Lactate

Box 37-4

HISTORY OF MECHANISM OF INJURY

PENETRATING TRAUMA
Weapon used (handgun, shotgun, rifle, knife)
Caliber of weapon
Number of shots fired
Gender of assailant
Position of victim and assailant when injury occurred

BLUNT TRAUMA
Height of fall
Motor vehicle crash (MVC) extrication time
Ejection
Steering wheel deformation
Location in automobile (passenger, driver, front seat, back seat)
Restraint status (lap belt, shoulder harness, or combination; unrestrained)
Speed of automobile(s)/direction of impact
Occupants (number and morbidity status)

Exposure. The final step in the primary survey is exposure and environmental control. All clothing is removed to facilitate a thorough examination of all body surfaces for the presence of injury. After all clothing is removed, it is imperative to protect the patient from hypothermia. This can be accomplished through external blankets, warm ambient room temperature, and warmed IV fluids.

Resuscitation Phase. After the primary survey the resuscitation phase begins. Hypovolemic shock is the most common type of shock that occurs in trauma patients.[12] Hemorrhage must be identified and treated rapidly. Two large-bore peripheral intravenous (IV) catheters (14- to 16-gauge) or a central venous catheter is inserted. During the initiation of IV lines, blood samples are drawn (Box 37-3). Intravenous therapy with Ringer's lactate solution should be administered rapidly. High-flow fluid warmers may be used to deliver warmed IV solutions at rates greater than 1000 ml/minute. If the patient remains unresponsive to bolus intravenous therapy, O-negative blood or type-specific blood may be administered.[12] Transfusion of autologous salvaged blood (autotransfusion) also may be used to replace intravascular volume and to provide oxygen-carrying capacity.

Placement of urinary and gastric catheters is part of the resuscitation phase. An indwelling urinary catheter can help evaluate urine output as an indicator of volume status and renal perfusion. A gastric tube is inserted to reduce gastric distention and assist in reducing the risk of aspiration.[12]

The resuscitation phase begins in the emergency department and may continue well into the critical care phase. Resuscitation is aimed at ensuring adequate perfusion of tissues with oxygen and nutrients to support cellular function. The patient's response to resuscitation efforts is a priority nursing assessment because the patient's response to these efforts is key to determining subsequent therapy. Resuscitation endpoints (i.e., variables or parameters) must be viewed across the continuum of resuscitation from shock. During resuscitation from traumatic hemorrhagic shock, normalization of standard clinical parameters such as blood pressure, heart rate, and urine output are not adequate.[14] The optimal resuscitation endpoint is a major focus of recent research in trauma care. Current guidelines recommend that during resuscitation, attempts should be made to improve oxygen delivery to normalize base deficit, lactate or gastric pH_i during the first 24 hours after injury.[14]

Optimizing hemodynamic variables including cardiac index, oxygen delivery, and oxygen consumption may be beneficial, especially when initiated as soon as possible during resuscitation.[15] Central venous pressure and pulmonary artery pressures are useful, but have limitations due to changes in ventricular compliance and intrathoracic pressures.[14] Given these limitations, some trauma centers use the right ventricular end-diastolic volume index using a right ventricular ejection fraction/oximetry volumetric catheter to more accurately reflect preload.

Secondary Survey. The secondary survey begins when the primary survey is completed, resuscitation is well established, and the patient is demonstrating normalization of vital signs. During the secondary survey, a head-to-toe approach is used to thoroughly examine each body region. The history is one of the most important aspects of the secondary survey. Often head injury, shock, or the use of drugs or alcohol may preclude taking a good history, so the history must be pieced together from other sources. The prehospital care providers (paramedics, emergency medical technicians) usually can provide most of the vital information pertaining to the accident. Specific information that must be elicited pertaining to the mechanism of injury is summarized in Box 37-4. This information can help predict internal in-

Table 37-2	Effects of Trauma Resuscitation
Aspect of Injury/Resuscitation	**Effect on ICU Course**
Prolonged extrication time	Gives an indication of length of time patient may have been hypotensive and/or hypothermic before medical care
Period of respiratory or cardiac arrest	Effects of loss of perfusion to brain (anoxic injury), kidneys, and other vital organs
Time on backboard	Potentiates risk of sacral or occipital breakdown
Number of units of blood; whether any were not fully cross-matched; packed cells versus whole blood used	Potentiates risk of ARDS, MODS

ICU, Intensive care unit; *ARDS,* acute respiratory distress syndrome; *MODS,* multiple organ dysfunction syndrome.

juries and facilitate rapid intervention. The patient's pertinent past history can be assessed by use of the mnemonic AMPLE: *A*llergies, *M*edications currently used, *P*ast medical illnesses/pregnancy, *L*ast meal, and *E*vents/environment related to the injury.

During the secondary survey the nurse ensures the completion of special procedures, such as an electrocardiogram (ECG); radiographic studies (chest, cervical spine, thorax, and pelvis); diagnostic peritoneal lavage; and ultrasonography. Throughout this survey the nurse continuously monitors the patient's vital signs and response to medical therapies. Emotional support to the patient and family also is imperative.

DEFINITIVE CARE/OPERATIVE PHASE

Once the secondary survey has been completed, specific injuries usually have been diagnosed. Definitive care related to specific injuries is described throughout this chapter. Trauma is often referred to as a "surgical disease" because the nature and extent of injuries usually requires operative management. After surgery, depending on the patient's status, a transfer to the intensive care unit may be indicated.

CRITICAL CARE PHASE

Critically ill trauma patients are admitted into the intensive care unit (ICU) as direct transfers from the emergency department (ED) or operating room (OR). Information the ICU nurse must obtain from the ED or OR nurse, or both, is summarized in Box 37-5. This information must be obtained before patient admission to the ICU to ensure availability of needed personnel, equipment, and supplies. This information also helps the ICU nurse to assess the impact of trauma resuscitation on the patient's ICU presentation and course. Table 37-2 summarizes the prehospital, ED, and OR resuscitative measures that can affect the trauma patient's care in the ICU.

On the patient's arrival to the ICU, the nurse, using the primary and secondary surveys and resuscitative mea-

---

Box 37-5

NURSING REPORT FROM REFERRING AREA

- Mechanism of injury/injuries sustained
- Diagnostic tests completed and results
- Medications administered (particularly narcotics, sedatives, neuromuscular blocking agents)
- Diagnostic/therapeutic procedures performed (diagnostic peritoneal lavage [DPL], chest tube insertion, intravenous [IV] access)
- Vital signs
- Established airway/mechanical ventilation settings/O_2 flow devices
- Any loss of consciousness and its duration
- Current Glasgow Coma Scale score
- Fluid replacement (colloid and crystalloid)
- Fluid loss (urine output, chest tube drainage, estimated intraoperative blood loss)
- Laboratory tests (including blood alcohol and toxicology screen)
- Past medical/surgical history (including medications taken at home, allergies)
- Family members present (assessment of coping and current knowledge of nature and extent of injuries and treatment plan)

Modified from Johnson KL: Critical care of the trauma patient. In Neff JA, Kidd PS, editors: *Trauma nursing: the art and science,* St Louis, 1993, Mosby.

---

sures in accordance with ATLS guidelines, assesses the trauma patient's status. Priority nursing care during the critical care phase includes ongoing physical assessments and monitoring the patient's response to medical therapies. The ICU nurse constantly is aware that the third peak of the trimodal distribution of trauma deaths occurs in the ICU setting as a result of complications, including acute respiratory distress syndrome (ARDS), sepsis, prolonged shock states, and multiple organ dysfunction syndrome (MODS). Ongoing nursing assessments are imperative for early detection and treatment of complications.

Table 37-3	Factors Predisposing the Trauma Patient to Impaired Oxygenation	
Factor	**Impairment**
Impaired ventilation	Injury to airway structures, loss of CNS regulation of breathing, impaired level of consciousness
Impaired pulmonary gas diffusion	Pneumothorax, hemothorax, aspiration of gastric contents
	Shifts to the left of the oxyhemoglobin dissociation curve (can be secondary to infusion of large volumes of banked blood, hypocarbia or alkalosis, or hypothermia)
Decreased oxygen supply	Reduced hemoglobin (secondary to hemorrhage)
	Reduced cardiac output (cardiovascular injury, decreased preload)
Increased oxygen supply	Increased metabolic demands (associated with the stress response to injury)

CNS, Central nervous system.

One of the most important nursing roles is assessment of the balance between oxygen delivery and oxygen demand. Oxygen delivery must be optimized to prevent further system damage. Assessment of circulatory status includes the use of noninvasive and invasive techniques (see "Cardiovascular Clinical Assessment," Chapter 16). The trauma patient is at high risk for impaired oxygenation as a result of a variety of factors (Table 37-3). These risk factors must be promptly identified and treated to prevent life-threatening sequelae. Prevention and treatment of hypoxemia depend on accurate assessment of the adequacy of pulmonary gas exchange, oxygen delivery, and oxygen consumption.

Frequent and thorough nursing assessment of all body systems is important because these assessments are the cornerstone to the medical and nursing management of the critically ill trauma patient. The nurse can detect subtle changes and facilitate the implementation of timely therapeutic interventions to prevent complications often associated with trauma. The nurse must be knowledgeable about specific organ injuries, as well as their associated sequelae.

SPECIFIC TRAUMA INJURIES

TRAUMATIC BRAIN INJURIES

Over 1.5 million traumatic brain injuries (TBIs) occur annually in the United States,[16] with approximately 15% of those patients hospitalized as a result of their injury. Approximately 50,000 Americans die each year from TBI, which accounts for about one third of all trauma-related deaths.[16] Approximately 50% of all trauma deaths are associated with some type of head injury.[12] Of the patients with head trauma who are hospitalized, approximately 35% of the survivors will suffer long-term disability, posing a tremendous economic impact on society due to both health care costs as well as life years lost.[17]

Mechanism of Injury. TBIs occur when mechanical forces are transmitted to brain tissue. Mechanisms of injury include penetrating or blunt trauma to the head. Be-

fore 1990, the incidence of transportation-related TBI exceeded that of TBI related to firearm use. Since 1994 this has switched, with firearm-related TBIs exceeding injuries due to transportation, such as MVC.[16] Penetrating trauma can result from the penetration of a foreign object (e.g., a bullet) that causes direct damage to cerebral tissue. Blunt trauma can be the result of deceleration, acceleration, or rotational forces. Deceleration causes the brain to crash against the skull after it has hit something (e.g., the dashboard of a car). Acceleration injuries occur when the brain has been hit by something (e.g., a baseball bat). In many instances, TBIs can be caused by both acceleration and deceleration. Acceleration injuries occur when the skull is hit by a force that causes the brain to move forward to the point of impact; and then as the brain reverses direction and hits the other side of the skull, deceleration injuries occur.

Pathophysiology. The review of the pathophysiology of a TBI can be divided into two categories: primary injury and secondary injury. It is important that the critical care nurse understands this pathophysiology, because goals of ICU care include efforts to reduce morbidity and mortality from primary and secondary injuries.

Primary Injury. The primary injury occurs at the moment of impact as a result of mechanical forces to the head. The extent of and recovery from injury are related to whether the primary injury was localized to an area or whether it was diffuse or widespread throughout the brain. Primary injuries may occur as direct damage to the parenchyma or as injury to the vessels that causes hemorrhage, compressing nearby structures. Examples of primary injuries include contusion, laceration, shearing injuries, and hemorrhage. Primary injury may be mild, with little or no neurologic damage, or severe, with major tissue damage. Immediately after injury, a cascade of neural and vascular processes is activated.

Secondary Injury. Secondary injury is the biochemical and cellular response to the initial trauma that can exacerbate the primary injury and cause loss of brain tissue not originally damaged.[18] Secondary injury can be caused by ischemia, hypercapnia, hypotension, cerebral edema, sustained hypertension, calcium toxicity, or metabolic derangements. Hypoxia or hypotension, the best-known culprits for secondary injury, typically are the result of extracranial trauma.[18] A self-perpetuating cycle develops that may result in the expansion of a relatively focal primary injury into uncontrolled, refractory secondary injury.[12,18]

Tissue ischemia occurs in areas of poor cerebral perfusion as a result of hypotension and/or hypoxia. The cells in ischemic areas become edematous. Extreme vasodilation of the cerebral vasculature occurs in an attempt to supply oxygen to the cerebral tissue. This increase in blood volume increases intracranial volume and intracranial pressure (ICP).

Significant hypotension causes inadequate perfusion to neural tissue. It is important to note that hypotension rarely is associated with TBI. Hypotension typically is not caused by brain injury unless terminal medullary failure occurs.[18] If a trauma patient is unconscious and hypotensive, an aggressive assessment of the chest, abdomen, and pelvis is performed to rule out internal injuries.

Hypercapnia is a powerful vasodilator. Most often caused by hypoventilation in an unconscious patient, hypercapnia results in cerebral vasodilation and increased cerebral blood volume and ICP.

Cerebral edema occurs as a result of the changes in the cellular environment caused by contusion, loss of autoregulation, and increased permeability of the blood-brain barrier. Cerebral edema can be focal as it localizes around the area of contusion, or diffuse as a result of hypotension or hypoxia. The extent of cerebral edema can be minimized by controlling the other aspects of secondary injury, such as oxygenation, ventilation, and perfusion.

Initial hypertension in the patient with severe TBI is common. As a result of the loss of autoregulation, increased blood pressure results in increased intracranial blood volume and ICP. Every effort must be made to control hypertension to prevent the secondary injury caused by increased ICP (see "Intracranial Hypertension" in Chapter 27). The effects of increases in intracranial pressure may be varied. As pressure increases inside the enclosed vault of the skull, cerebral perfusion decreases, which leads to further compromise of the intracranial contents. The effects of increasing pressure and decreasing perfusion precipitate a downward spiral of events (see "Intracranial Hypertension" in Chapter 27).

Classification. Injuries of the brain are described by the functional changes or losses that occur. Some of the major functional abnormalities seen in head injury are described here.

Skull Fracture. Skull fractures are common, but they do not by themselves cause neurologic deficits. Skull fractures can be classified as open (dura is torn) or closed (dura is not torn), or they can be classified as those of the vault or those of the base. Common vault fractures occur in the parietal and temporal regions. Basilar skull fractures usually are not visible on conventional skull films, and a computerized tomography is typically required. Assessment findings may include cerebrospinal fluid otorrhea or rhinorrhea, Battle's sign (ecchymosis overlying the mastoid process), "raccoon eyes" (subconjunctival and periorbital ecchymosis), or palsy of the seventh cranial nerve.

The significance of a skull fracture is that it identifies the patient with a higher probability of having or developing an intracranial hematoma. Open skull fractures require surgical intervention to remove bony fragments and to close the dura. The major complications of basilar skull fractures are cranial nerve injury and leakage of cerebrospinal fluid (CSF). CSF leakage may result in a fistula, which increases the possibility of bacterial contamination and resultant meningitis. Because fistula formation may be delayed, patients with a basilar skull fracture are admitted to the hospital for observation and possible surgical intervention.

Concussion. A concussion is a brain injury accompanied by a brief loss of neurologic function, especially loss of consciousness.[17] If loss of consciousness occurs, it may last for seconds to an hour. The neurologic dysfunctions include confusion, disorientation, and sometimes a period of antegrade or retrograde amnesia. Other clinical manifestations that occur after concussion are headache, dizziness, nausea, irritability, inability to concentrate, impaired memory, and fatigue. The diagnosis of concussion is based on the loss of consciousness inasmuch as the brain remains structurally intact despite functional impairment.

Contusion. Contusion, or bruising of the brain, usually is related to acceleration-deceleration injuries, which result in hemorrhage into the superficial parenchyma, often the frontal and temporal lobes. Frontal or temporal contusions are most common and can be seen in a coup-contrecoup mechanism of injury (Fig. 37-2). Coup injury affects the cerebral tissue directly under the point of impact. Contrecoup injury occurs in a line directly opposite the point of impact.

The clinical manifestations of contusion are related to the location of the contusion, the degree of contusion, and the presence of associated lesions. Contusions can be small, in which localized areas of dysfunction result in a focal neurologic deficit. Larger contusions can evolve over several days after injury as a result of edema and further hemorrhaging. A large contusion can produce a mass effect that can cause a significant increase in ICP. Contusions are almost always associated with subdural hematoma.[12]

Contusions of the tips of the temporal lobe are a common occurrence and are of particular concern. Because the inner aspects of the temporal lobe surround the opening in the tentorium where the midbrain enters the cerebrum, edema in this area can cause rapid deteriora-

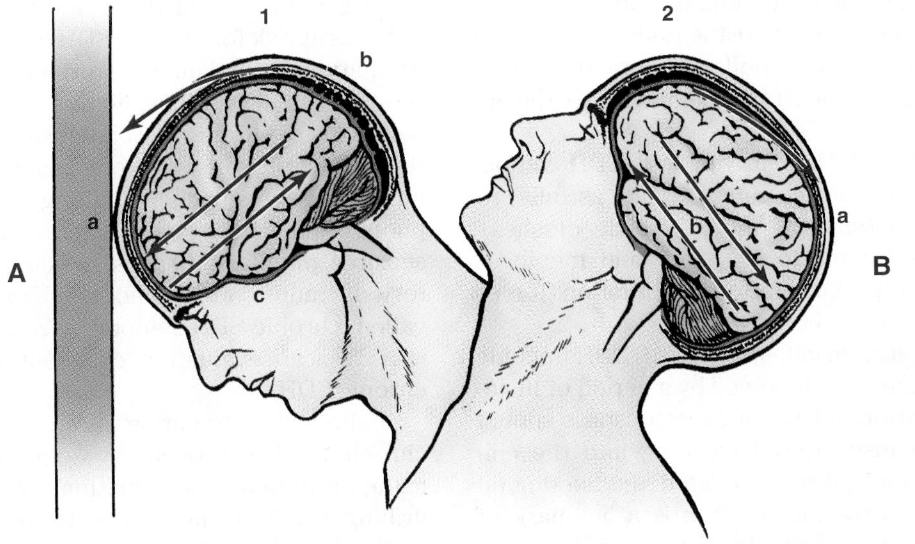

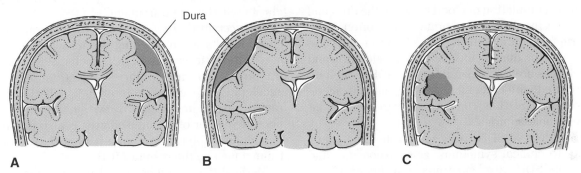

Fig. 37-2 Coup and contrecoup head injury after blunt trauma. **A,** Coup injury: impact against object. *a,* Site of impact and direct trauma to brain. *b,* Shearing of subdural veins. *c,* Trauma to base of brain. **B,** Contrecoup injury: impact within skull. *a,* Site of impact from brain hitting opposite side of skull. *b,* Shearing forces throughout brain. These injuries occur in one continuous motion—the head strikes the wall (coup), then rebounds (contrecoup).

Fig. 37-3 Types of hematomas. **A,** Subdural hematoma. **B,** Epidural hematoma. **C,** Intracerebral hematoma.

tion of the patient's condition and can lead to herniation. Because of the location, this deterioration can occur with little or no warning at a deceptively low ICP.

Diagnosis of contusion is made by computed tomography (CT) scan. If the CT scan indicates contusion, especially in the temporal area, the nurse must pay particular attention to neurologic assessments and look for subtle changes in pupillary signs or vital signs, irrespective of a stable ICP.

Medical management of cerebral contusions may consist of medical or surgical therapies. Because a contusion can progress over several days after injury, secondary injury may occur. If contusions are small, focal, or multiple, they are treated medically with serial neurologic assessments and possibly ICP monitoring. Larger contusions that produce considerable mass effect require surgical intervention to prevent the increased edema and intracranial pressure as the contusion ma-

tures. Outcome of cerebral contusion varies, depending on the location and the degree of contusion.

Hematomas. Extravasation of blood produces a space-occupying lesion on the brain and leads to increased ICP. Three types of hematomas are discussed here (Fig. 37-3). The first two hematomas, epidural and subdural, are extraparenchymal (outside of brain tissue) and produce injury by pressure effect and displacement of intracranial contents. The third type of hematoma, intracerebral, directly damages neural tissue and can produce further injury as a result of pressure and displacement of intracranial contents.

Epidural Hematoma. Epidural hematoma (EDH) is a collection of blood between the inner table of the skull and the outermost layer of the dura. EDHs are most often associated with patients with skull fractures and middle meningeal artery lacerations (two thirds of patients) or skull fractures with venous bleeding.[12] A blow to the head that causes a linear skull fracture on the lateral surface of the head may tear the middle meningeal artery. As the artery bleeds, it pulls the dura away from the skull, creating a pouch that expands into the intracranial space.

The incidence of EDH is relatively low. EDH can occur as a result of low-impact injuries (such as falls) or high-impact injuries (such as motor vehicle crashes). EDH occurs from trauma to the skull and meninges rather than from the acceleration-deceleration forces seen in other types of head trauma.

The classic clinical manifestations of EDH include brief loss of consciousness followed by a period of lucidity. Rapid deterioration in level of consciousness should be anticipated because arterial bleeding into the epidural space can occur quickly. A dilated and fixed pupil on the same side as the impact area is a hallmark of EDH.[12] The patient may complain of a severe, localized headache and may be sleepy. Diagnosis of EDH is based on clinical symptoms and evidence of a collection of epidural blood identified on CT scan. Treatment of EDH involves surgical intervention to remove the blood and to cauterize the bleeding vessels.

Subdural Hematoma. Subdural hematoma (SDH), which is the accumulation of blood between the dura and the underlying arachnoid membrane, most often is related to a rupture in the bridging veins between the cerebral cortex and the dura.[19] Acceleration-deceleration and rotational forces are the major causes of SDH, which often is associated with cerebral contusions and intracerebral hemorrhage. SDH is common, representing about 30% of severe head injuries.

The three types of SDH are based on the time frame from injury to clinical symptoms: acute, subacute, and chronic. Acute SDHs are hematomas that occur after a severe blow to the head. The clinical presentation of acute SDH is determined by the severity of injury to the underlying brain at the time of impact and the rate of blood accumulation in the subdural space. In other situations the patient has a lucid period before deterioration. Careful observation for deterioration in level of consciousness or lateralizing signs, such as inequality of pupils or motor movements, is essential. Rapid surgical intervention including craniectomy, craniotomy, or burr hole evacuation, and aggressive medical management can reduce mortality.

Subacute SDHs are hematomas that develop symptomatically 2 days to 2 weeks after trauma. In subacute hematomas the expansion of the hematoma occurs at a rate slower than that in acute SDH; therefore it takes longer for symptoms to become obvious. Clinical deterioration with subacute SDH usually is slower than that with acute SDH, but treatment by surgical intervention, when appropriate, is the same.

Chronic subdural hematoma is the term used when symptoms appear days or months after injury. Most patients with chronic SDH are elderly or in late middle age. Patients at risk for chronic SDH include patients with coordination or balance disturbances, the elderly, and those receiving anticoagulation therapy. Clinical manifestations of chronic SDH are insidious. The patient may report a variety of symptoms, such as lethargy, absent-mindedness, headache, vomiting, stiff neck, and photophobia, and may show signs of transient ischemic attack, seizures, pupillary changes, or hemiparesis. Because history of trauma often is not significant enough to be recalled, chronic SDH seldom is seen as an initial diagnosis. CT scan evaluation can confirm the diagnosis of chronic SDH.

If surgical intervention is required, evacuation of the chronic SDH may occur by craniotomy, burr holes, or catheter drainage. Evacuation by burr hole involves drilling a hole in the skull over the site of the chronic SDH and draining the fluid. Drains or catheters are left in place for at least 24 hours to facilitate total drainage. Outcome after chronic SDH evacuation is variable. Return of neurologic status often depends on the degree of neurologic dysfunction before removal. Because this condition is most common in the elderly or debilitated patient, recovery is a slow process. Recurrence of chronic SDH is not infrequent.

Intracerebral Hematoma. Intracerebral hematoma (ICH) results when bleeding occurs within cerebral tissue. Traumatic causes of ICH include depressed skull fractures, penetrating injuries (bullet, knife), or sudden acceleration/deceleration motion. The ICH can act as a rapidly expanding lesion; however, late ICH into the necrotic center of a contused area is also possible. Sudden clinical deterioration of a patient 6 to 10 days after trauma may be the result of ICH.

Medical management of ICH may include surgical or nonsurgical management. Generally it is believed that hemorrhages that do not cause significant ICP problems should be treated nonsurgically. Over time, the hemorrhage may be reabsorbed. If significant problems with ICP occur as a result of the ICH producing a mass effect, surgical removal is necessary. Outcome from ICH depends greatly on the location of the hemorrhage. Size, mass effect, and displacement of other intracranial structures also affect the outcome.

Missile Injuries. Missile injuries are caused by objects that penetrate the skull to produce a significant focal damage but little acceleration/deceleration or rotational injury. The injury may be depressed, penetrating, or perforating (Fig. 37-4). Depressed injuries are caused by fractures of the skull, with penetration of bone into cerebral tissue. Penetrating injury is caused by a missile that enters the cranial cavity but does not exit. A low-velocity penetrating injury (knife) may involve only focal damage and no loss of consciousness. A high-velocity missile (bullet) can produce shock waves that are transmitted throughout the brain, in addition to injury caused

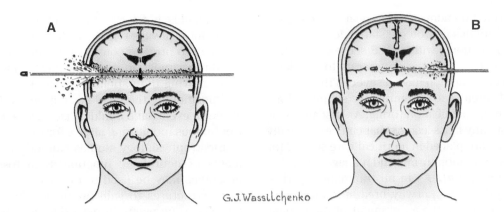

Fig. 37-4 Bullet wounds of the head. Bullet wound or other penetrating missile wounds cause an open (compound) skull fracture and damage to brain tissue. Shock wave effects are transmitted throughout the brain. **A,** Perforating injury. **B,** Penetrating injury.

by the bullet. Perforating injuries are missile injuries that enter and then exit the brain. Perforating injuries have much less ricochet effect but are still responsible for significant injury.

Risk of infection and cerebral abscess is a concern in missile injuries. If fragments of the missile are embedded within the brain, careful consideration of the location and risk of increasing neurologic deficit is weighed against the risk of abscess or infection. The outcome after missile injury is based on the degree of penetration and the location of the injury, as well as the velocity of the missile.

Diffuse Axonal Injury. Diffuse axonal injury (DAI) is a term used to describe prolonged posttraumatic coma that is not due to a mass lesion, although DAI with mass lesions has also been reported.[19] DAI covers a wide range of brain dysfunction typically caused by acceleration/deceleration and rotational forces. DAI occurs as a result of damage to the axons or disruption of axonal transmission of the neural impulses.

The pathophysiology of DAI is related to the stretching and tearing of axons as a result of movement of the brain inside the cranium at the time of impact. The stretching and tearing of axons result in microscopic lesions throughout the brain, but especially deep within cerebral tissue and the base of the cerebrum. Disruption of axonal transmission of impulses results in loss of consciousness. Unless surrounding tissue areas are significantly injured, causing small hemorrhages, DAI may not be visible on CT scan or magnetic resonance imaging (MRI). DAI can be classified into three grades based on the extent of lesions: mild, moderate, or severe. The patient with mild DAI may be in a coma for 24 hours and may exhibit periods of decorticate and decerebrate posturing. Patients with moderate DAI may be in a coma for longer than 24 hours and may exhibit periods of decorticate and decerebrate posturing. Severe DAI is usually manifested as a prolonged deep coma with periods of hypertension, hyper-

thermia, and excessive sweating. Treatment of DAI includes support of vital functions and maintenance of ICP within normal limits. The outcome after severe DAI is poor because of the extensive dysfunction of cerebral pathways.

Assessment. The neurologic assessment is the most important tool for evaluating the patient with a severe TBI, because it can indicate severity of injury, provide prognostic information, and dictate the speed with which further evaluation and treatment must proceed.[17] The cornerstone of the neurologic assessment is the Glasgow Coma Scale (GCS).[18] The GCS does not provide a complete neurologic examination, however. Pupillary and motor strength assessment must also be incorporated into the early and ongoing assessments. Once injuries are specifically identified, a more thorough, focused neurologic examination, extending for instance to the cranial nerves, is warranted. To assist with the initial assessment, TBIs are divided into three descriptive categories on the basis of the patient's GCS score and duration of the unconscious state.

Degree of Injury

Mild Injury. Mild TBI is described as a GCS score of 13 to 15, with a loss of consciousness that lasts up to 15 minutes. Patients with mild injury often are seen in the ED and discharged home with a family member who is instructed to evaluate the patient routinely and to bring the patient back to the hospital if any further neurologic symptoms appear.

Moderate Injury. Moderate TBI is described as a GCS score of 9 to 12, with a loss of consciousness for up to 6 hours. Patients with this type of TBI usually are hospitalized. They are at high risk for deterioration from increasing cerebral edema and ICP, and therefore serial clinical assessments are an important function of the nurse. Hemodynamic and ICP monitoring and ventilatory support often are not required in this group unless other systemic injuries make them necessary. A CT scan usually is performed on admission. Repeat CT scans are indicated if the patient's neurologic status deteriorates.

Severe Injury. Patients with a GCS score of 8 or less after resuscitation or those who deteriorate to that level within 48 hours of admission have a severe TBI. Patients with severe TBI often receive ventilatory support along with ICP and hemodynamic monitoring. A CT scan is performed to rule out any mass lesions that can be surgically removed. Patients are placed in a critical care setting for continual assessment, monitoring, and management.

Nursing Assessment. As in all traumatic injuries, the evaluation of the ABCs (airway, breathing, and circulation) is the first step in the assessment of the patient with TBI in the ICU. Patients with moderate primary injury may deteriorate as a result of diffuse swelling or bleeding.[17] A patient with severe TBI who is breathing spontaneously may require prophylactic endotracheal or nasotracheal intubation with mechanical ventilatory support to reduce the risk of hypoxia and hypercapnia. After stabilization of the ABCs is ensured, a neurologic assessment is performed.

Level of consciousness, motor movements, pupillary response, respiratory function, and vital signs are all part of a complete neurologic assessment in the patient with traumatic brain injury. Level of consciousness can be elicited to assess wakefulness. Consciousness is assessed by obtaining the patient's response to verbal and painful stimuli. Determination of orientation to person, place, and time is a means to assess mental alertness. Pupils are assessed for size, shape, equality, and reactivity. Asymmetry must be reported immediately. Pupils are also assessed for constriction to a light source (parasympathetic innervation) or dilation (sympathetic innervation). Because parasympathetic fibers are present in the brain stem, pupils that are slow to react to light may indicate a brain stem injury. A "blown" pupil can be caused by compression of the third ocular nerve or transtentorial herniation. Bilateral fixed pupils can indicate midbrain involvement (see Chapter 26).

Neurologic assessments are ongoing throughout the patient's critical care stay as part of the initial shift assessment and as part of ongoing assessments to detect subtle deterioration. Serial assessments include monitoring hemodynamic status and ICP. The use of muscle relaxants and sedation for ICP control may mask neurologic signs in the patient with severe head injury. In these situations, observations for changes in pupils and vital signs become extremely important. Newer, shorter-acting sedatives with a very short half life, such as propofol (Diprivan) can be discontinued and within minutes, a neurologic examination can be performed.

Diagnostic Procedures. The cornerstone of diagnostic procedures for evaluation of TBI is the CT scan.[18] The CT scan is a rapid, noninvasive procedure that can provide invaluable information about the presence of mass lesions and cerebral edema. Serial CT scans may be used over a period of several days to assess areas of con-

tusion and ischemia and to detect delayed hematomas. A nurse must always remain with a TBI patient during the CT scan to provide continued observation and monitoring during transport and scanning. Transporting the patient, moving the patient from the bed to the CT table, and positioning the head flat during the CT scan are all stressful events and could cause severe increases in ICP. Continuous monitoring allows for rapid intervention.

Electrophysiology studies can aid in ongoing assessments of neurologic function. Somatosensory evoked potentials may be used to evaluate injures deep in the brain structures to gain prognostic information.[18] MRI appears to be useful in detecting hematomas and cerebral edema (see Chapter 26).

Medical Management

Surgical Management. If a lesion, identified by CT scan, is causing a shift of intracranial contents or an increase in ICP, surgical intervention is necessary. A craniotomy is performed to remove the EDH, SDH, or large ICH. Occasionally, if an area of contusion is large, hemorrhagic, and associated with an elevated ICP, a craniotomy for removal of the contused area may be performed to relieve pressure and prevent herniation. Patients who have had surgery for penetrating head trauma have an increased incidence of posttraumatic seizures, and therefore these patients may receive anticonvulsants.

Nonsurgical Management. No longer is surgery the mainstay of treatment of traumatic brain injuries because approximately 95% of management occurs in the intensive care unit.[18] Nonsurgical management includes management of ICP, maintenance of adequate cerebral perfusion pressure and oxygenation, and treatment of any complications (e.g., pneumonia or infection). The decision of when to initiate intracranial pressure monitoring is critical. ICP monitoring may be required for patients with a GCS less than 8 and abnormal findings on a head CT scan[20] (see "Intracranial Hypertension" in Chapter 27).

Nursing Management. Nursing diagnoses for the patient with TBI are listed in the Nursing Diagnoses feature on Traumatic Brain Injury. Priority nursing goals include stabilization of vital signs, prevention of further injury, and reduction of increased ICP. Ongoing nursing assessments are the cornerstone of the care of patients with TBI. Such assessments are the primary mechanism for determining secondary brain injury from cerebral edema and increased ICP. If secondary injury is to be prevented, the ICU nurse must respond immediately to hypotensive events and, in collaboration with physicians, maximize cerebral perfusion pressure through reduction of ICP and restoration of mean arterial pressure[21] (see "Intracranial Hypertension" in Chapter 27).

All aspects of care, including hemodynamic management, pulmonary care, maintenance of body temperature, and control of the environment, can affect outcome after TBI.[20] Hemodynamic and fluid management are vital. Arterial blood pressure should be monitored because hypotension in a patient with TBI is rare and may indicate

NURSING DIAGNOSES

Traumatic Brain Injury

- Ineffective Breathing Pattern related to neuromuscular impairment, perceptual/cognitive impairment
- Risk for Aspiration risk factors: impaired laryngeal sensation or reflex; impaired pharyngeal peristalsis or tongue function; impaired laryngeal closure or elevation; increased gastric volume; decreased lower esophageal sphincter pressure
- Impaired Gas Exchange related to ventilation/perfusion mismatching
- Imbalanced Nutrition: Less Than Body Requirements related to lack of exogenous nutrients and increased metabolic demand
- Disturbed Sensory Perception related to altered sensory reception or transmission (neurologic trauma)
- Powerlessness related to lack of control over current situation
- Decreased Intracranial Adaptive Capacity related to failure of normal compensatory mechanisms
- Impaired Physical Mobility related to perceptual/cognitive impairment
- Ineffective Cerebral Tissue Perfusion related to hemorrhage, cerebral edema

Box 37-6

RECOMMENDATIONS FOR SUCTIONING PATIENTS WITH TRAUMATIC BRAIN INJURY

Pass the suction catheter for no longer than 10 seconds.
Limit the number of suction catheter passes, preferably to no more than 2 passes per suctioning episode.
Hyperoxygenate the patient before and after each passage of the suction catheter (e.g., deliver 4 ventilator breaths at 135% of the patient's tidal volume on 100% Fio_2, at a rate of 4 breaths in 20 seconds).
Minimize airway stimulation (i.e., stabilize endotracheal tube, avoid passing the suction catheter all the way to the carina).

From McQuillan KA, Mitchell P: Traumatic brain injuries. In McQuillan KA et al, editors: *Trauma nursing: from resuscitation through rehabilitation,* ed 3, Philadelphia, 2002, Saunders.

additional injuries. Cerebral perfusion pressure should be maintained at a minimum of 60 mm Hg.[21] In the absence of cerebral ischemia, aggressive attempts to keep cerebral perfusion pressure (CPP) >70 mm Hg with intravenous fluids and vasopressors should be avoided secondary to the risk of acute respiratory distress syndrome (ARDS)[21] (see "Intracranial Hypertension" in Chapter 27). Close monitoring of hemodynamic status is of paramount importance in patients with TBI because in addition to fluid management, changes in cardiovascular function and circulating catecholamines contribute to hemodynamic instability.[18] Pulmonary artery catheterization may be required to optimize fluid status and cardiac output. Capnography is suggested for monitoring patients to prevent inadvertent hypocapnia or hypercapnia.[18] Aggressive pulmonary care must be instituted. However, endotracheal suctioning can elevate ICP. Techniques to eliminate elevation in ICP with suctioning include are outlined in Box 37-6. Cerebral oxygen consumption is increased during periods of increased body temperature, and therefore euthermia may be a goal to be achieved with early workup and intervention in case of infection, and the use of antipyretics.

In the early postinjury phase, the patient's environment must be controlled. Stimuli that produce pain, agitation, or discomfort can increase intracranial pressure. Analgesics and sedatives should be administered. Patients should be given rest periods. After ICP stabilization, stimulation programs for patients in a coma may be used. These programs provide stimulation to the tactile, olfactory, gustatory, auditory, and visual senses. Several methods have been used to stimulate coma patients: (1) intense multisensory stimulation program defined as stimulatory cycles lasting approximately 15 to 20 minutes, repeated every hour for 12 to 14 hours per day, 6 days a week; (2) formalized not-intensive stimulation program, defined as cycles of stimulation 10 to 60 minutes twice a day, and (3) sensory regulation program, defined as single brief sessions of stimulation in a quiet environment completely free of noise.[22] Whatever program is used, a stimulation schedule should be established, and accurate documentation of the stimulus and response is essential. Coma stimulation programs should be individualized and family members encouraged to participate.

SPINAL CORD INJURIES

Approximately 10,000 new spinal cord injuries (SCIs) occur annually, with an overwhelming majority of injuries occurring in males between the ages of 16 and 30.[23] Of the new cases of SCI each year, about 4000 patients will die before arrival to the hospital and 1000 patients will die of complications of their SCI during the hospitalization.[23] The diagnosis of SCI begins with a detailed history of events surrounding the incident, precise evaluation of sensory and motor function, and radiographic studies of the spine.

Mechanism of Injury. The type of primary injury sustained depends on the mechanism of injury. Mechanisms of injury can include hyperflexion, hyperextension, rotation, axial loading (vertical compression), and missile or penetrating injuries.

Hyperflexion. Hyperflexion injury most often is seen in the cervical area, especially at the level of C5 to C6, because this is the most mobile portion of the cervical spine. This type of injury most often is caused by sudden deceleration motion, as in head-on collisions. Injury occurs from compression of the cord by fracture fragments or as a result of dislocation of the vertebral bodies. Instability of the spinal column occurs because of the rupture or tearing of the posterior muscles and ligaments.

Hyperextension. Hyperextension injuries involve backward and downward motion of the head. With this injury, often seen in rear-end collisions or diving accidents, the spinal cord itself is stretched and distorted. Neurologic deficits associated with this injury are often caused by contusion and ischemia of the cord without significant bony involvement. A mild form of hyperextension is the *whiplash* injury.

Rotation. Rotation injuries often occur in conjunction with a flexion or extension injury. Severe rotation of the neck or body results in tearing of the posterior ligaments and displacement (rotation) of the spinal column.

Axial Loading. Axial loading, or vertical compression, injuries occur from vertical force along the spinal cord. This is most commonly seen in a fall from a height in which the person lands on the feet or buttocks. Compression injuries cause burst fractures of the vertebral body that often send bony fragments into the spinal canal or directly into the spinal cord (Fig. 37-5).

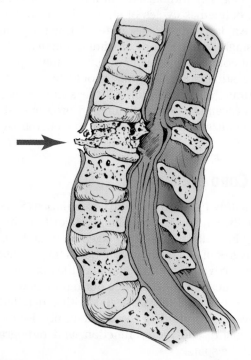

Fig. 37-5 Spinal cord compression burst fractures. Compression injuries cause burst fractures of the vertebral body that often send bony fragments into the spinal canal or directly into the spinal cord.

Penetrating Injuries. Penetrating injury to the spinal cord can be caused by a bullet, knife, or any other object that penetrates the cord. These types of injury cause permanent damage by anatomically transecting the spinal cord.

Pathophysiology. Spinal cord injuries are the result of a mechanical force that disrupts neurologic tissue or its vascular supply, or both. Much like the pathophysiology of TBI, the injury process includes both primary and secondary injury mechanisms. Primary injury is the neurologic damage that occurs at the moment of impact. Secondary injury refers to the complex biochemical processes affecting cellular function. Secondary injury can occur within minutes of injury and can last for days to weeks.[23]

Several events after a spinal cord injury can lead to spinal cord ischemia and loss of neurologic function. A cascade of events is initiated that includes systemic and local vascular changes, electrolyte and biochemical changes, neurotransmitter accumulation, and local edema (Box 37-7). Collectively, these pathophysiologic events result in worsening of the injury, potentially extending the level of functional deficit, and worsening long-term outcome.[23] Knowledge of the pathophysiology of secondary processes has led to the development of new drugs, which target the cellular changes contributing to injury.[23] Despite ongoing research efforts at repairing the primary injury, minimizing damage through reducing secondary injury has shown the most promise.

Functional Injury of the Spinal Cord. Functional injury of the spinal cord refers to the degree of disruption of normal spinal cord function. This depends on what specific sensory and motor structures within the cord are damaged. SCIs are classified as complete or incomplete (see the Nursing Diagnoses feature on Spinal Cord Injury). SCI cannot be classified until spinal shock has resolved.

Complete Injury. Complete SCI results in a total loss of sensory and motor function below the level of injury. Regardless of the mechanism of injury, the result is a complete dissection of the spinal cord and its neurochemical pathways, resulting in one of two conditions: quadriplegia or paraplegia.

Quadriplegia. With quadriplegia the injury occurs from the C1 to T1 level. Residual muscle function depends on the specific cervical segments involved. The potential functional status resulting from different neurologic levels of injury is described in Table 37-4.

Paraplegia. With paraplegia the injury occurs in the thoracolumbar region (T2 to L1). Patients with injuries in this area may have full use of the arms and may need a wheelchair, although some may have limited ability to ambulate short distances with crutches and orthoses. Thoracic L1 and L2 injuries produce paraplegia with variable innervation to intercostal and abdominal muscles.

Incomplete Injury. Incomplete SCI results in a mixed loss of voluntary motor activity and sensation below the level of the lesion. Incomplete SCI exists if any function remains below the level of injury. Incomplete injuries can result in one of a variety of syndromes, which are classified according to the degree of motor and sensory loss below the level of injury. Some of the more common syndromes are described here.

Brown-Séquard's Syndrome. Brown-Séquard's syndrome is associated with damage to only one side of the cord. This produces loss of voluntary motor movement on the same side as the injury, with loss of pain, temperature, and sensation on the opposite side. Functionally, the side of the body with the best motor control has little or no sensation, whereas the side of the body with sensation has little or no motor control.

Central Cord Syndrome. Central cord syndrome is associated with cervical hyperextension/flexion injury and hematoma formation in the center of the cervical cord. This injury produces a motor and sensory deficit more pronounced in the upper extremities than in the lower extremities. Varying degrees of bowel and bladder dysfunction may be present.

Anterior Cord Syndrome. The anterior cord syndrome is associated with injury to the anterior gray horn

Table 37-4	Quadriplegia Functional Status
Neurologic Level of Complete Injury (Vertebrae)	**Functional Ability**
C1-C4	Requires electric wheel chair with breath, head, or shoulder controls
C5	Needs electric wheelchair with hand control and/or manual wheel chair with rim projections; may require adaptive devices to assist with ADLs
C6	Independent in manual wheel chair on level surface; may need hand controls; adaptive devices may be needed for ADLs
C7	Requires manual wheel chair on most surfaces
C8-T1	May need adaptive devices

ADLs, Activities of daily living.

Box 37-7

PRIMARY AND SECONDARY MECHANISMS OF ACUTE SPINAL CORD INJURY

PRIMARY INJURY MECHANISMS
Acute compression
Impact
Missile
Distraction
Laceration
Shear

SECONDARY INJURY MECHANISMS
Systemic Effects
Heart rate: brief increase, then prolonged bradycardia
Blood pressure: brief hypertension, then prolonged hypotension
Decreased peripheral resistance
Decreased cardiac output
Increased catecholamines, then decreased
Hypoxia
Hyperthermia
Injudicious movement of the unstable spine leading to worsening compression
Local vascular changes
Loss of autoregulation
Systemic hypotension (neurogenic shock)
Hemorrhage (especially gray matter)
Loss of microcirculation

Reduction in blood flow
Vasospasm
Thrombosis
Electrolyte changes
Increased intracellular calcium
Increased intracellular sodium
Increased sodium permeability
Increased intracellular potassium

Biochemical Changes
Neurotransmitter accumulation
Catecholamines (e.g., norepinephrine, dopamine)
Excitotoxic amino acids (e.g., glutamate)
Arachidonic acid release
Free radicals production
Eicosanoid production
Prostaglandins
Lipid peroxidation
Endogenous opioids
Cytokines
Edema
Loss of energy metabolism
Decreased adenosine triphosphate production
Apoptosis

Adapted from Sekhon LHS, Fehlings MG: Epidemiology, demographics, and pathophysiology of acute spinal cord injury, *Spine* 26(24S):S2, 2001.

Spinal Cord Injury

- Decreased Cardiac Output related to lack of sympathetic innervation
- Risk for Autonomic Dysreflexia related to spinal cord injury above T8
- Impaired Gas Exchange related to alveolar hypoventilation
- Ineffective Breathing Pattern related to impairment of innervation of diaphragm (lesion above C5), complete or mixed loss of intercostal muscle function
- Impaired Physical Mobility related to neuromuscular impairment, immobilization by traction, paralysis
- Risk for Impaired Skin Integrity related to immobility, traction, tissue pressure, altered peripheral circulation, and sensation
- Bowel Incontinence related to disruption of innervation to bowel and rectum, perceptual impairment, altered fluid and food intake
- Constipation related to disruption of innervation to bowel and rectum, perceptual impairment, altered fluid and food intake
- Impaired Urinary Elimination related to disruption in bladder innervation, bladder atony
- Disturbed Body Image related to actual change in body structure, function, or appearance
- Ineffective Coping related to situational crisis and personal vulnerability

cells (motor), the spinothalamic tracts (pain), anterior spinothalamic tract (light touch), and the corticospinal tracts (temperature). The result is a loss of motor function, as well as loss of the sensations of pain and temperature below the level of injury. However, below the level of injury, position sense and sensations of pressure and vibrations remain intact. Anterior cord syndrome is commonly caused by flexion injuries or acute herniation of an intervertebral disk.

Posterior Cord Syndrome. Posterior cord syndrome is associated with cervical hyperextension injury, with damage to the posterior column. This results in the loss of position sense, pressure, and vibration below the level of injury. Motor function and sensation of pain and temperature remain intact. These patients may not be able to ambulate because the loss of position sense impairs spontaneous movement.

Spinal Shock. Spinal shock is a condition that can occur shortly after traumatic injury to the spinal cord. Spinal shock is the complete loss of all muscle tone and normal reflex activity below the level of injury.[12] Patients

with spinal shock may appear to be completely without function below the area of the injury, although all of the area may not necessarily be destroyed.

Neurogenic Shock. Neurogenic shock results from injury to the descending sympathetic pathways in the spinal cord. This results from loss of vasomotor tone and sympathetic innervation to the heart. A relative hypovolemia and hypovolemic shock ensues, causing hypotension and a decreased systemic vascular resistance. Patients with SCI at T6 or above may have profound neurogenic shock as a result of interruption of the sympathetic nervous system and loss of vasoconstrictor response below the level of the injury. Blood vessels cannot constrict and the heart rate is slow, which results in hypotension, venous pooling, and decreased cardiac output. Cellular oxygenation is threatened as cardiac output falls secondary to both a decrease in stroke volume (hypovolemia) and heart rate (bradycardia). The duration of this shock state can persist for up to 1 month after injury. Blood pressure support may be required with the use of sympathomimetic drugs. Because hypotension is a problem, the nurse must be cautious when adjusting backrest position or when repositioning a patient in bed, because orthostatic blood pressure changes can occur (see "Neurogenic Shock" in Chapter 38).

Autonomic Dysreflexia. Autonomic dysreflexia is a life-threatening complication that may occur with SCI. This condition is caused by a massive sympathetic response to a noxious stimulus (full bladder, line insertions, fecal impaction), which results in bradycardia, hypertension, facial flushing, and headache. Immediate intervention is needed to prevent cerebral hemorrhage, seizures, and acute pulmonary edema. Treatment is aimed at alleviating the noxious stimulus. A clinical algorithm for treatment of autonomic dysreflexia is provided in Box 37-8.[24] If symptoms persist, antihypertensive agents can be administered to reduce blood pressure. Prevention of autonomic dysreflexia is imperative and can be accomplished through the use of a good bowel and bladder program.

Assessment. On admission to the ICU, attention to the ABCs is imperative in the patient with known or suspected SCI. Stabilization of the spinal cord is mandatory to prevent further injury and spinal precautions are maintained until the spine is cleared of injury. Stabilization in the ICU may include the use of bed rest with logrolling maneuvers and a hard cervical collar until definitive stabilization is achieved.

Airway. Assessment of ABCs is essential to ensure optimal oxygenation and perfusion to all vital organs, including the spinal cord. Complete cardiovascular and respiratory assessments are essential to the patient's survival and prognosis. The primary assessment begins with an evaluation of airway clearance. In an unresponsive person, an oral airway is inserted while the patient's neck is maintained in a neutral position. The patient

Table 37-5	Effects of Spinal Cord Injury on Ventilatory Functions	
Neurologic Level of Complete Injury (Vertebrae)	**Respiratory Function**	**Comment**
C1-C2	Paralysis of diaphragm	Ventilator-dependent
C3-C5	Varying degrees of diaphragm paralysis	Some diaphragm control; may need ventilatory support; weaning depends on preinjury pulmonary status
C6-T11	Varying degrees of impaired intercostal muscles and abdominal muscles	Compromised respiratory function; reduced inspiratory ability; paradoxical breathing patterns; ineffective cough, sneeze

Modified from Moore EE et al: *Surg Clin North Am* 74:295, 1995.

Box 37-8

AUTONOMIC DYSREFLEXIA

- If patient is supine, immediately sit the patient up.
- Begin frequent vital sign monitoring: perform every 5 minutes.
- Survey for instigating causes: begin with urinary system.
- Loosen clothing, constrictive devices.
- If indwelling catheter is not present, catheterize the patient:
  - Lidocaine jelly may be instilled 5 minutes before catheter insertion.
- If indwelling catheter is present:
  - Check system for kinks, obstructions to flow.
  - Irrigate bladder with small amount of fluid.
  - If not draining, remove catheter and replace.
- If systolic blood pressure is greater than 150 mm Hg, consider rapid-onset, short-duration antihypertensive agent.
- If acute symptoms persist, suspect fecal impaction:
  - Instill lidocaine jelly into rectum; wait at least 5 minutes.
  - Perform digital examination to check for presence of stool; if present, gently remove. If signs of autonomic dysreflexia persist, stop exam; instill additional lidocaine jelly, and wait 20 minutes to reexamine.
  - If no stool found and abdominal distention noted, consider administration of laxative

---

must undergo intubation before severe hypoxia can occur, which could further damage the spinal cord.

Breathing. Assessment of breathing patterns and gas exchange is made after an airway has been secured. The level of injury dictates the degree of altered breathing patterns and gas exchange (Table 37-5). Because complete injuries above the C3 level result in paralysis of the diaphragm, patients with these injuries require ventilatory assistance.

Circulation. Assessment of cardiac output and tissue perfusion is imperative to detect life-threatening injuries and promote recovery of injured spinal cord tissue. The patient with SCI is at high risk for developing alterations in cardiac output and tissue perfusion because the cardiovascular system is subjected to a variety of serious and potential physiologic alterations, including dysrhythmias, cardiac arrest, orthostatic hypotension, emboli, and thrombophlebitis.

The patient with an SCI is assessed for adequate tissue perfusion by means of both invasive and noninvasive hemodynamic monitoring techniques. Cardiac monitoring is required to detect bradycardia and other dysrhythmias that occur in response to reflex vagus activity mediated by the dominant parasympathetic nervous system, as well as changes in cardiac rhythm that result from hypothermia or hypoxia.

Once the ABCs have been evaluated and interventions for life-threatening complications have been initiated, a full physical assessment is made to determine the extent of injury.

Neurologic. The initial neurologic assessment may not be an accurate indication of eventual motor and sensory loss. It focuses on the rapid and accurate identification of present, absent, or impaired functioning of the motor, sensory, and reflex systems that coordinate and regulate vital functions. A detailed motor and sensory examination includes the assessment of all 32 spinal nerves for evidence of dysfunction. Carefully mapped pathways for the sensory portion of the spinal nerves, termed *dermatomes*, can assist in localizing the functional sensory level of injury. Motor function may be graded on a 6-point scale (Box 37-9). Initial assessment must be performed correctly and findings thoroughly documented in detail so that subsequent serial assessments can rapidly identify deterioration. Ongoing spinal cord assessments must be documented during the critical care phase.

Diagnostic Procedures. Diagnostic radiographic evaluations can identify the severity of damage to the spinal cord. Initial evaluation includes anteroposterior and lateral views for all areas of the spinal cord. Films of all seven cervical vertebrae and the top of T1 must be obtained to rule out cervicothoracic junction injury. Flexion and extension views can identify subtle ligamentous injuries. CT scan, tomograms, myelography, and MRI also may be used in the diagnostic process (see Chapter 26).

Screening for Spinal Cord Injury. About 15% of trauma patients with injury will have a cervical spine injury.[18] Screening of the spinal cord for injury becomes an integral part of the assessment for all trauma patients. The degree of trauma, alteration in mentation, intoxication, or distracting injuries will dictate the type and extent of exam required to clear the cervical spine. The Eastern Association of Surgeons in Trauma developed guidelines for the clearance of the cervical spine (Table 37-6). On admission, the spine is palpated for obvious deformity and the patient is assessed for the subjective response of pain to palpation. If the patient has distracting injuries, such as rib fractures, is intoxicated, or has received analgesics, examination of the spinal cord may be deferred.[18] An MRI may be done to make a definitive diagnosis.

Medical Management. After assessment and diagnosis of the SCI, medical management begins. The primary treatment goal is to preserve remaining neurologic function. Medical interventions are divided into pharmacologic, surgical, and nonsurgical interventions.

Pharmacologic Management. Methylprednisolone has been shown to improve neurologic outcome after spinal cord injury. Patients with SCI should receive a methylprednisolone bolus followed by a continuous infusion for at least 24 hours, and preferably 48 hours, if their treatment began 3 to 8 hours after their injury.[25] Methylprednisolone directly affects the changes that occur within the spinal cord after injury, primarily by preventing posttraumatic spinal cord ischemia, improving energy metabolism, restoring extracellular calcium, and improving nerve impulse conduction.

Surgical Management. Surgical intervention provides spinal column stability in the presence of an unstable injury. Unstable injuries include disrupted ligaments and tendons, as well as a vertebral column that cannot maintain normal alignment. Identification and immobilization of unstable injuries is particularly important for the patient with incomplete neurologic deficit. Without adequate stabilization, movement and dislocation of the vertebral column could cause a complete neurologic deficit. A variety of surgical procedures may be performed to achieve decompression and stabilization. The question of when surgery should be performed remains controversial.

Laminectomy. The laminectomy procedure is the removal of the lamina of the vertebral ring to allow decom-

---

Box 37-9

MUSCLE STRENGTH SCALE

Active movement against maximal resistance
Active movement through range of motion against resistance
Active movement through range of motion against gravity
Active movement through range of motion with gravity eliminated
Flicker or trace of contraction
No contraction; total paralysis

Table 37-6	EAST Guidelines for Cervical Spine Clearance
Patient Population	**Recommendation**
Alert, awake, not intoxicated, neurologically normal, no complaints of neck pain	Neck is palpated in all directions for tenderness or pain If physical exam is negative for pain or tenderness, plain films are not necessary.
Awake, alert, not intoxicated, with complaints of neck pain	Cervical spine x-ray films are obtained. CT scan may be obtained through suspicious areas identified on 3-view cervical spine x-rays.
Neurologic deficits referable to a spine injury	Plain films and CT images with MRI of the cervical spine
Altered mental status and return of normal mental status not anticipated for 2 days or more (e.g., severe traumatic or hypoxic, ischemic brain injury)	Plain films and CT images Axial CT images at 3-mm intervals with sagittal reconstruction from the base of the occiput through C2. If plain films and CT are normal, flexion/extension lateral cervical spine fluoroscopy with static images obtained at extremes of flexion and extension.

EAST Guidelines: Determination of Cervical Spine Stability in Trauma Patients, 2000.
CT, Computed tomography; *MRI,* magnetic resonance imaging; *EAST,* Eastern Association for the Surgery of Trauma.

pression and removal of bony fragments or disk material from the spinal canal.

Spinal Fusion. Spinal fusion entails the surgical fusion of two to six vertebral elements to provide stability and to prevent motion. Fusion is accomplished through the use of bone parts or bone chips taken from the iliac crest or by use of wire or acrylic glue.

Rodding. The rodding procedure stabilizes and realigns larger segments of the spinal column by means of a variety of rodding materials such as Harrington rods. The rods are attached by screws and glue to the posterior elements of the spinal column. These types of procedures most often are performed to stabilize the thoracolumbar area.

Nonsurgical Management. If the injury to the spinal cord is stable, nonsurgical management is the treatment of choice. Nonsurgical management for cervical and thoracolumbar injuries is discussed here.

Cervical Injury. Management of cervical injuries involves the immobilization of the fracture site and realignment of any dislocation. This is accomplished through skeletal traction that involves the use of two-point tongs, which are inserted into the skull through shallow burr holes and are connected to traction weights. Several types of cervical tongs are used. Gardner-Wells and Crutchfield tongs are the most common. These tongs can be applied at the bedside with the use of a local anesthetic.

After the procedure the patient can be immobilized on a kinetic therapy bed or a regular bed. The kinetic therapy bed is the most popular method used for cervical immobilization because it maintains spinal column alignment while providing constant turning motion to reduce pulmonary and skin breakdown. Use of cervical skeletal traction on a regular bed makes it difficult to provide adequate care to the pulmonary system and skin because of the extensive degree of immobility.

After the spinal column has been adequately realigned by means of skeletal traction, a halo traction brace often is applied. The halo vest consists of a metal ring secured to the skull with two occipital and two temporal screws. Steel bars anchor the screws to the vest to provide cervical immobilization (Fig. 37-6). The halo traction brace immobilizes the cervical spine, which allows the patient to ambulate and participate in self-care.

Thoracolumbar Injury. Nonsurgical management of the patient with a thoracolumbar injury also involves immobilization. Skeletal traction may be used in high thoracic injury. For the most part, misalignment of the spinal canal does not occur in stable injuries of the thoracolumbar spine. Immobilization to allow fractures to heal is accomplished by bed rest (with bed flat) and the use of a plastic or fiberglass jacket, a body cast, or a brace.

Nursing Management. Nursing diagnoses and management for the patient with spinal cord injury are summarized in the Nursing Diagnoses feature on Spinal Cord Injury. The goal during the critical care phase is to prevent life-threatening complications while maximizing the function of all organ systems. Nursing interventions are aimed at preventing secondary damage to the spinal cord and managing the complications of the neurologic deficit. Because almost all body systems are affected by SCI, nursing management also must include interventions that optimize nutrition, elimination, skin integrity, and mobility. In addition, patients with SCI have complex psychosocial needs that necessitate a great deal of emotional support from the critical care nurse.

Cardiovascular. The risk for cardiovascular instability is especially profound in patients with SCI at the C3 to C5 levels, although cardiovascular alterations can occur with most injuries above T6. Alteration in tissue perfusion secondary to hypotension may require the administration of IV fluids. Astute assessment of fluid volume is required, however, because pulmonary edema is a threat to SCI patients. Pulmonary artery catheterization may be required to assess for this complication. Once fluid volume status has been optimized, inotropic or vasopressor support, or both, may be implemented.

Another consequence of sympathetic nervous system dysfunction is loss of thermoregulation (poikilothermy), in which body temperature is regulated by the external environment. Thus judicious use of heat or cold for therapeutic or comfort measures is required. Profound changes in body temperature must be avoided. Hypothermia can produce bradydysrhythmias and sinus ar-

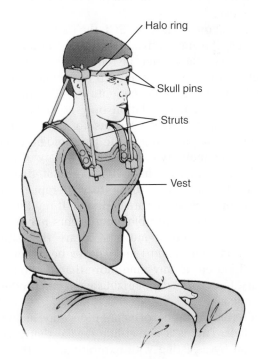

Fig. 37-6 Halo vest. The halo traction brace immobilizes the cervical spine, which allows the patient to ambulate and participate in self-care.

rest. Symptomatic bradydysrhythmias can be treated with inotropic drugs (isoproterenol), alone or in combination with a pacemaker (temporary transvenous or transcutaneous). Before antipyretics are given or a cooling blanket is used, the environment must be assessed for potential causes of hyperthermia/hypothermia.

After a prolonged period of bed rest, orthostatic hypotension may become a significant problem. It may be helpful when initially mobilizing the patient with an SCI to gradually elevate the head of bed and dangle the legs over the side of the bed. The incidence of orthostatic hypotension may be reduced by leg elevation or the use of antiembolic hose or an abdominal binder.[24] As with any immobilized patient, the risk for the development of deep vein thrombosis (DVT) is high. However, detection of DVT is difficult since pain, tenderness, and positive Homans' sign are not applicable to the patient with an SCI. Prevention of DVT is imperative and may include a combination of therapies such as low-dose heparin, low–molecular-weight heparin, sequential compression devices, and embolic hose.

Pulmonary. Pulmonary complications are the most common cause of mortality in SCI patients.[25] Initial and ongoing nursing assessments of respiratory status are imperative for identifying actual or potential impairment in ventilation. These include observation of respiratory rate and rhythm, observation of symmetry of chest expansion and use of accessory muscles, inspection of quantity and character of secretions, and auscultation of breath sounds. Judicious use of serial arterial blood gas (ABG) values provides information on the adequacy of gas exchange.

Depending on the level of SCI, the patient's breathing pattern may be ineffective (Box 37-5). Intubation and mechanical ventilation may be required. Patients with lesions at C3 to C5 may be able to be weaned from mechanical ventilation. Some patients with C3 injuries may require mechanical ventilation only at night. Weaning can be a complex process because of physical requirements of the diaphragm and the psychologic effects of the fear of the inability to breathe. A variety of weaning methods may be used, but a well-coordinated approach by the nurse, physician, respiratory therapist, and patient is required Setbacks are common. If reintubation is required, neuromuscular blocking agents may be used. The critical care nurse must be aware that succinylcholine (Suxamethonium) must never be administered to an SCI patient at any time more than 72 hours after the injury. Use of this depolarizing agent can produce hyperkalemic arrest.

An alternative mode of ventilation may include the pneumobelt. This is a corset-like device that produces ventilation by assisting with expiration. Another assistive device is the abdominal binder. This is thought to support the sagging diaphragm in higher SCI due to loss of abdominal muscle innervation.

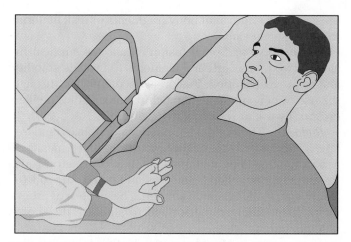

Fig. 37-7 Cough assistance. A hand or both hands are placed over the upper diaphragm. After the patient inhales, pressure is directed inward and upward as the patient attempts to cough.

Ineffective airway clearance is a particular problem for the SCI patient as a result of hypoventilation (paralysis of respiratory muscles), increased bronchial secretions, and atelectasis secondary to decreased cough. Frequent suctioning for airway clearance is required. Caution must be used with vigorous suctioning because the unopposed vagus nerve (which runs alongside the trachea), when stimulated, can cause profound bradycardia. Bradycardia exacerbated by hypoxia is likely to develop in patients with cervical SCI. Use of hyperventilation breaths with 100% oxygen before suctioning may help. Chest percussion and drainage facilitate removal of secretions. Kinetic therapy beds, which can rotate up to 60 degrees on each side, may provide continual postural drainage and mobilization of secretions. To further aid in mobilizing secretions in the presence of an ineffective cough, a technique of cough assistance can be used (Fig. 37-7). This procedure is similar to the Heimlich maneuver. Exact hand placement may vary, and it is important to assess which placement works best for the patient.

Impaired gas exchange can occur in the SCI patient as a result of hypoventilation (because of paralysis of respiratory muscles), increased bronchial secretions that interfere with adequate gas diffusion, shunting secondary to atelectasis and associated pulmonary injuries, and pulmonary complications (pulmonary embolism). Nursing interventions are directed at improving and maintaining adequate gas exchange.

Musculoskeletal. Immobilized patients are at high risk for developing contractures. When a muscle is denervated, as in the case of SCI, the muscle fibers shorten and produce a contracture. Irreversible contractures may result in skin breakdown, inability to perform activities of daily living, poor wheelchair posture, and inability to use adaptive devices.[24] Physical therapy and occupational therapy personnel should be consulted early in the patient's ICU course. Range of motion exercises are initiated as soon as the spine has been stabilized. Foot drop splints should be applied on admission to prevent contractures and prevent skin breakdown of the heels.[24] Hand splints should be applied for quadriplegics. Both hand and foot splints should be removed and reapplied every 2 hours. Nursing management of the patient in a halo vest includes inspection of pins and traction for security, correct positioning and turning (traction bars or the halo ring must never be used to lift or reposition the patient), placement of wrenches on the front of the vest in case of cardiac arrest, and maintenance of skin integrity inside the halo vest.

Integumentary. Patients with an SCI are at high risk for developing pressure ulcers because of the lack of motor control and sensation. Prevention is the best treatment; diligent assessments, meticulous skin care, and frequent position changes are required. It should not be assumed that specialty surfaces or low air loss beds may be necessary in the prevention of pressure ulcers in patients with an SCI.[24]

Elimination. Initially after SCI, bowel and bladder tone are flaccid. The degree of bladder and urinary sphincter dysfunction will depend on the location and completeness of the injury. Initially a Foley catheter is in place. This should be removed 3 to 4 days after admission, at which time the patient is placed on an intermittent catheterization schedule every 4 to 6 hours. It is not unusual for the male patient with an upper motor neuron injury to experience a reflexogenic erection when being catheterized.[24] An overdistended bladder in the patient with an injury at T6 or above may trigger autonomic dysreflexia. Abdominal distention, constipation, and fecal impaction are major problems encountered in care of the SCI patient. Innervation between the brain and defecation center in the sacral cord has been disrupted. A bowel program to prevent fecal impaction and encourage normal, regular bowel function must be instituted. The patient should not go longer than 3 to 4 days without a bowel movement. Laxatives and stool softeners may be needed, especially if the patient is receiving narcotics. Aspects of a successful bowel program include consistent timing of evacuation, proper positioning, physical activity, appropriate fluid intake, high-fiber diet, and reflex stimulation for those with upper motor neuron injuries.[24]

Maximizing Psychosocial Adaptation. Nursing management of the patient with SCI must include the provision of dedicated emotional support. In the critical care unit, the patient and family experience anxiety, grief, denial, anger, frustration, and hopelessness, because long-term neurologic deficits remain unknown.

Nursing interventions include the promotion of coping mechanisms, support systems, and adaptive skills. Simple, accurate, and consistent information can alleviate fear and anxiety. Feelings of powerlessness may be reduced by including the patient and family in care and decision making. Further psychosocial support can be given by social workers, occupational therapists, psychiatric clinical nurse specialists, and pastors.

MAXILLOFACIAL INJURIES

Trauma to the face results in complex physiologic and psychologic sequelae. Vital functions that depend on facial integrity include mastication; deglutination; perception of the environment (vision, hearing, speech, olfaction); and respiration. The face also represents a direct link to self and to expression by playing a major role in personal identity, appearance, and communication. Consequently, maxillofacial trauma and disfigurement has the potential to produce long-term sequelae, with emotional, psychologic, and sensory implications.

Mechanism of Injury. Maxillofacial injury results from blunt or penetrating trauma. Blunt trauma may occur from motor vehicle, industrial, or athletic injuries, violent blows to the head, or falls. The mechanism for this injury is exemplified by the unbelted driver or passenger who is thrown into the dashboard or windshield. Associated injuries may include concussion, skull fracture, rhinorrhea, spinal cord injury, and fractures of other bones. The facial skeleton serves as an energy-absorbing shield to protect the brain, spinal cord, eyes, and pharynx. Nasal bones, the zygoma, and the mandibular condyle are the most susceptible to fracture. Bullet wounds can be life-threatening because of hemorrhage and airway obstruction. Maxillofacial trauma can result in soft tissue injury ranging from abrasions to destruction of most of the face, as well as maxillofacial skeletal fractures. This section is limited to the discussion of maxillofacial skeletal injuries.

Maxillofacial Skeletal Injuries. Fractures of the maxilla are diagnosed according to Le Fort's classification. Le Fort's fractures are classified into three broad categories, depending on the level of the fracture (Fig. 37-8). The most common, Le Fort I, consists of horizontal fractures in which the entire maxillary arch moves separately from the upper facial skeleton. Le Fort II fractures are an extension of Le Fort I and involve the orbit, ethmoid, and nasal bones. Le Fort III fractures are associated with craniofacial disruption. Cerebrospinal fluid frequently leaks with Le Fort II and III fractures because there is frequently communication between the cranial base and the cribriform plate.[26]

Assessment. Patients with maxillofacial trauma are especially prone to ineffective airway clearance, deficient fluid volume related to hemorrhage, and risk for injury. Life-threatening complications associated with maxillofacial trauma include airway obstruction and head and/or cervical spine injury. Major or minor facial deformities should not distract the trauma team from the standard assessments and interventions needed to stabilize the airway, breathing, and circulation of the patient.

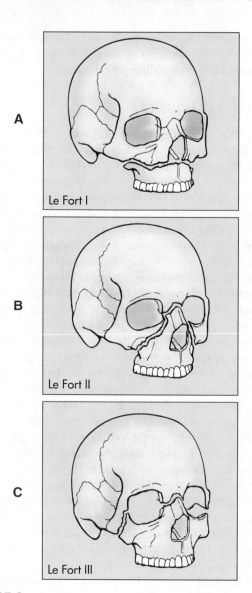

A, Le Fort I

B, Le Fort II

C, Le Fort III

Fig. 37-8   Fractures of the maxillae are diagnosed according to Lefort's classification, which consists of three broad categories based on the level of the fracture. **A,** Le Fort I. **B,** Le Fort II. **C,** Le Fort III.

Patients with maxillofacial trauma are at high risk for ineffective airway clearance. The tongue, edema, hemorrhage, foreign objects, vomit, broken teeth, or bone fragments can obstruct the airway. The look, listen, and feel methods (see Table 37-1). should be used to assess for airway obstruction. An artificial airway may be required. An oral endotracheal tube is used unless there is a laryngeal fracture. Nasotracheal (as well as nasogastric) intubation is contraindicated in the presence of unstable facial fractures, because if a fracture of the cribriform plate is present the tube could be inadvertently placed through the fractured base of the cranium and into the brain.[12] A tracheostomy may be required for patients with hypopharynx swelling or hemorrhage.

Patients with maxillofacial trauma are at risk for deficient fluid volume related to massive hemorrhage as a result of bleeding from the ethmoid or maxillary sinuses. Profuse bleeding through the nares may occur with nasal fractures, maxillary fractures, or cranial base fractures, and for these, nasal packing may be required to control the bleeding.[26] Fluids are given intravenously to correct the deficient fluid volume.

Once life-saving interventions are initiated, the comprehensive exam of facial structures is begun as part of the general head-to-toe sequence of assessment. Specifically, assessment of the face involves a careful inspection and palpation of the soft tissue. A small abrasion or contusion of the face may seem unobtrusive, but the impact to the underlying structures may have disrupted facial bone integrity, the parotid gland, or the facial nerve.[26] The mouth is inspected for traumatic tooth dislodgement, recognizing that some teeth may intrude into the underlying alveolar bone. The ear canal is inspected for occult lacerations of the tympanic membrane. Many of the facial structures enter from the cranium through the eye orbit; therefore careful inspection and palpation of the eye orbit is required.

Maxillofacial trauma often is associated with cervical spinal cord injury. An altered level of consciousness in the presence of maxillofacial fractures strongly suggests neurotrauma. Fractures involving the cranium and dura mater may enable oral bacterial flora to enter cerebrospinal fluid (CSF), placing the patient at risk for meningitis. Nasal and auditory canals must be inspected for discharge. The drainage also can be tested for glucose inasmuch as CSF has a high glucose content.

Diagnostic Procedures.   The location and displacement of fractures is determined by axonal and coronal CT scan.[12] When true coronal CT is unavailable, CT with facial reconstruction may be substituted.[26]

Medical Management.   Treatment of Le Fort fractures includes direct visualization and reduction of the fragments, and stabilization with plates and screws.[27]

Nursing Management.   Nursing diagnoses for the patient with maxillofacial trauma are listed in the Nursing Diagnoses feature on Maxillofacial Trauma. Nursing interventions are directed toward the nursing diagnoses for the patient with maxillofacial trauma. Nursing management of the patient with jaw wires requires interventions aimed at protecting the airway by reducing the risk of emesis and aspiration. Proper orogastric tube functioning must be ensured. Antiemetics may be administered. Unless contraindicated, the head of the bed is elevated 30 degrees. If vomiting occurs, the patient is placed in a side or forward position and oral/nasal suctioning is used. Wire cutters must be available at the bedside in case the vomit cannot clear the wires and occludes the airway. Although this seldom is necessary, the principle in cutting the wires is to cut the vertical attachments, not the horizontal ones.

NURSING DIAGNOSES — Maxillofacial Trauma

- Risk for Aspiration risk factors: impaired pharyngeal peristalsis or tongue function; impaired laryngeal sensation or reflex; impaired laryngeal closure or elevation
- Deficient Fluid Volume related to absolute loss
- Imbalanced Nutrition: Less Than Body Requirements related to lack of exogenous nutrients and increased metabolic demands
- Acute Pain related to transmission and perception of cutaneous, visceral, muscular, or ischemic impulses

THORACIC INJURIES

Thoracic injuries involve trauma to the chest wall, the lungs, the heart, the great vessels, and the esophagus. Thoracic trauma most commonly is the result of a violent crime or MVC.

Mechanism of Injury

Blunt Thoracic Trauma. Blunt trauma to the chest most often is caused by MVCs or falls. Second only to head and spinal cord injury, thoracic injuries account for 20% of trauma deaths. The underlying mechanism of injury tends to be a combination of acceleration/deceleration injury and direct transfer mechanics, such as in a crush injury. Varying mechanisms of blunt trauma are associated with specific injury patterns. After head-on collisions, drivers have a higher frequency of injury than do backseat passengers because the driver comes in contact with the steering assembly. Severe thoracic injuries often are seen in patients who are unrestrained. Falls from greater than 20 feet are associated with thoracic injury.

Penetrating Thoracic Injuries. The penetrating object involved determines the damage sustained from penetrating thoracic trauma. Low-velocity weapons (.22-caliber gun, knife) usually damage only what is in the weapon's direct path. Of particular concern, however, are stab wounds that involve the anterior chest wall between the midclavicular lines, Louis's angle, and the epigastric region because of the proximity of the heart and/or great vessels.

Specific Thoracic Traumatic Injuries

Chest Wall Injuries

Rib Fractures. Fractures of certain ribs or multiple rib fractures can be more serious. Fractures of certain ribs are associated with more underlying, life-threatening injuries. Fractures of the first and second ribs are associated with intrathoracic vascular injuries (brachial plexus, great vessels). Right-sided fractures at the eighth rib and below are associated with liver injury.[28] Left-sided fractures at the same level are associated with spleen injury.[28] Lack of bone calcification in the pediatric trauma patient results in more compliant chest walls. Thus, rib fractures not need be present for a tremendous amount of force to have been absorbed by the underlying structures.[29]

The pain associated with rib fractures can be aggravated by respiratory excursion. As a result, the patient often splints, takes shallow breaths, and refuses to cough, which can result in atelectasis and pneumonia. Localized pain that increases with respiration or that is elicited by rib compression may indicate rib fractures. Definitive diagnosis can be made with a chest film. Nursing diagnoses may include Pain, Ineffective Airway Clearance, Ineffective Breathing Pattern, and Impaired Gas Exchange. Interventions include aggressive pulmonary physiotherapy and pain control to improve chest expansion efforts and gas exchange. Pain management interventions must be tailored to the individual patient's response to therapy. The primary goal of pain management in patients with rib fractures is prevention of pulmonary complications and, of course, patient comfort. Nonsteroidal antiinflammatory agents (NSAIDs), intercostal nerve blocks, thoracic epidural analgesia, and narcotics may all come into consideration to assist with pain control.[28] Epidural analgesia has been shown to help increase the functional residual capacity, dynamic lung compliance, and vital capacity; decrease the airway resistance; and increase partial pressure of oxygen (PaO_2).[30] External splints are not recommended because they further limit chest wall expansion and may add to atelectasis.[30] The patient's preexisting pulmonary status and age may dictate the course of recovery.[29]

Flail Chest. Flail chest, caused by blunt trauma, disrupts the continuity of chest wall structures. A flail chest occurs when two or more ribs are fractured in two or more places and are no longer attached to the thoracic cage.[31] This results in a free-floating segment of the chest wall. This segment moves independently from the rest of the thorax and results in paradoxic chest wall movement during the respiratory cycle (Fig. 37-9). During inspiration the intact portion of the chest wall expands, while the injured part is sucked in. During expiration the chest wall moves in, and the flail segment moves out. The effects of impaired chest wall motion include decreased tidal volume and vital capacity and impaired cough, which lead to hypoventilation and atelectasis.

Inspection of the chest reveals paradoxic movement. Palpation of the chest may indicate crepitus and tenderness near fractured ribs. A chest x-ray that reveals multiple rib fractures and evidence of hypoxia demonstrated by an ABG measure aid in the diagnosis. Nursing diagnoses for the patient with a flail chest include Ineffective Breathing Patterns, Impaired Gas Exchange, and Pain.

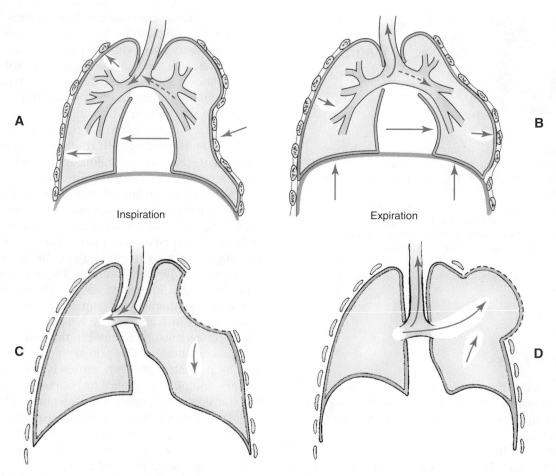

Fig. 37-9   Flail chest. **A,** Normal inspiration. **B,** Normal expiration. **C,** Inspiration: area of lung underlying unstable chest wall sucks in on inspiration. **D,** Same area balloons out on expiration. Note movement of mediastinum toward opposite lung on inspiration.

Interventions focus on ensuring adequate oxygenation, judicious administration of fluids, and analgesia to improve ventilation.[32] Intubation and mechanical ventilation may be required to prevent further hypoxia.

Ruptured Diaphragm. Diagnosis of a diaphragmatic rupture is often missed in trauma patients because of the subtle and nonspecific symptoms this injury produces. The mechanism of injury appears to be a rapid rise in intraabdominal pressure as a result of compression force applied to the lower part of the chest or upper region of the abdomen. This injury can occur when a person is thrown forward over the tip of the steering wheel in a high-speed deceleration accident. The force can cause the diaphragm, which offers little resistance, to rupture or tear. Abdominal viscera then can gradually enter the thoracic cavity, moving from the positive pressure of the abdomen to the negative pressure in the thorax. Diaphragmatic rupture can be life-threatening. Massive herniation of abdominal contents into the thoracic cavity can compress the lungs and mediastinum, which then hampers venous return and leads to decreased cardiac output. In addition, herniated bowel can become strangulated and perforate.

Diaphragmatic herniation may produce significant compromise and changes in respiratory effort. Auscultation of bowel sounds in the chest or unilateral breath sounds may indicate a ruptured diaphragm. The patient may complain of shoulder pain, shortness of breath, or abdominal tenderness. Thoracoscopy may be helpful in evaluating the diaphragm in indeterminate cases.[33] A chest film may reveal the tip of a nasogastric tube above the diaphragm, a unilaterally elevated hemidiaphragm, a hollow or solid mass above the diaphragm, and a shift of the mediastinum away from the affected side. Treatment of a ruptured diaphragm includes its immediate repair.

Pulmonary Injuries

Pulmonary Contusion. A pulmonary contusion is fundamentally a bruise of the lung. Pulmonary contusion often is associated with blunt trauma and other chest injuries, such as rib fractures and flail chest, and is the most common potentially lethal chest injury.[31] Pulmonary contusions can occur unilaterally or bilaterally. A contusion manifests initially as a hemorrhage followed by alveolar and interstitial edema. The edema can remain rather localized in the contused area or can spread to other lung areas. Inflammation affects alveolar-capillary units. As

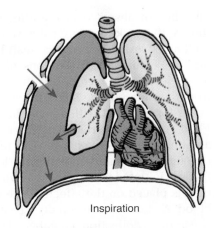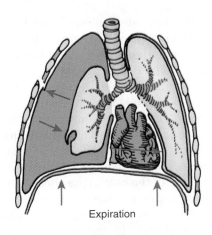

Inspiration   Expiration

Fig. 37-10 A tension pneumothorax usually is caused by an injury that perforates the chest wall or pleural space. Air flows into the pleural space with inspiration and becomes trapped. As pressure in the pleural space increases, the lung on the injured side collapses and causes the mediastinum to shift to the opposite side. (From Marx J et al: Rosen's *Emergency medicine: concepts and clinical practice,* ed 5, St Louis, 2002, Mosby.)

more units are affected by inflammation, further pathophysiologic events can occur, including decreased compliance, increased pulmonary vascular resistance, and decreased pulmonary blood flow. These processes result in a ventilation/perfusion imbalance, which results in hypoxemia and poor ventilation that progresses over a 24- to 48-hour period.

Clinical manifestations of pulmonary contusion may take up to 24 to 48 hours to develop. Inspections of the chest wall may reveal ecchymosis at the site of impact. Moist crackles may be noted in the contused lung. A cough may be present with blood-tinged sputum. Abnormal lung function can be detected by systemic arterial hypoxemia. The diagnosis is made primarily by chest x-ray studies consistent with pulmonary infiltrate corresponding to the area of external chest impact that is manifested within 12 to 24 hours of injury. Pulmonary contusions tend to worsen over a 24- to 48-hour period and then slowly resolve unless complications occur (infection, ARDS). Nursing diagnoses for the patient with pulmonary contusions may include Impaired Gas Exchange, Risk for Infection, Acute Pain, Ineffective Tissue Perfusion, and Ineffective Airway Clearance.

Aggressive respiratory care is the cornerstone for care of nonintubated patients with pulmonary contusion. Interventions include ambulation, deep-breathing exercises, turning, and incentive spirometry. Chest physiotherapy is not tolerated if there are coexisting rib fractures. Aggressive removal of airway secretions is important to avoid infection and to improve ventilation. Patients with unilateral contusions are placed with the injured side up and uninjured side down ("down with the good lung"). This positioning maximizes the match between pulmonary ventilation and perfusion. Patients with severe contusions may continue to show decompensation despite aggressive nursing management. Res-

piratory acidosis, increases in peak airway and plateau pressures, and increased work of breathing may require endotracheal intubation and mechanical ventilation with positive end-expiratory pressure (PEEP). Adequate pain control is accomplished with administration of NSAIDs, opiates, intercostal nerve blocks, or thoracic epidural analgesia. Complications resulting from pulmonary contusions include pneumonia, ARDS, lung abscesses, emphysema, and pulmonary embolism. Factors that contribute to mortality include shock, coexisting head injury, flail chest, falls from heights greater than 20 feet, advanced age, and preexisting disease (coronary artery disease, chronic obstructive pulmonary disease).

Tension Pneumothorax. A tension pneumothorax usually is caused by an injury that perforates the chest wall or pleural space. Air flows into the pleural space with inspiration and becomes trapped. As pressure in the pleural space increases, the lung on the injured side collapses and causes the mediastinum to shift to the opposite side (Fig. 37-10). As pressure continues to build, the shift exerts pressure on the heart and thoracic aorta, which results in decreased venous return and decreased cardiac output. Tissue perfusion with oxygenated blood is further hampered because the collapsed lung cannot participate in gas exchange.

Clinical manifestations of a tension pneumothorax include dyspnea, tachycardia, hypotension, or sudden chest pain extending to the shoulders. Tracheal deviation will be noted as the trachea shifts away from the injured side. On the injured side, breath sounds can be decreased or absent. Percussion of the chest reveals a hyperresonant sound over the affected side. Diagnosis of tension pneumothorax is made by clinical assessment. There is no time for a chest film inasmuch as this potentially lethal condition must be treated immediately.[12] A large-bore (14-gauge) needle or chest tube is inserted into the affected lung. This procedure allows immediate release of air from the pleural space. A hissing sound is heard as the tension pneumothorax is converted to a simple pneumothorax. Nursing diagnoses for a patient with a tension pneumothorax include Decreased Cardiac Output and Impaired Gas Exchange.

Open Pneumothorax. An open pneumothorax, or "sucking chest wound," usually is caused by penetrating trauma. Open communication between the atmosphere and intrathoracic pressure results in immediate lung deflation. Air moves in and out of the hole in the chest, producing a sucking sound heard on inspiration.

An open pneumothorax produces the same symptoms as does a tension pneumothorax. In addition, subcutaneous emphysema may be palpated around the wound. Initial management of an open pneumothorax is accomplished by promptly closing the wound at end expiration with a sterile occlusive dressing (plastic wrap or petroleum gauze) large enough to overlap the wound's edges.[32] This dressing should be taped securely on three sides. As the patient breathes in, the dressing gets sucked in to occlude the wound and prevent air from entering. A chest tube is placed as soon as possible. Surgical intervention may be required to close the wound.

Hemothorax. Blunt or penetrating thoracic trauma can cause bleeding into the pleural space, resulting in a hemothorax (Fig. 37-11). A massive hemothorax results from the accumulation of more than 1500 ml in the chest cavity.[32] The source of bleeding may be the intercostal or internal mammary arteries, the lungs, the heart, or the great vessels. Lacerations to the lung parenchyma are low-pressure bleeds, and therefore typically stop bleeding spontaneously.[31] Arterial bleeding from hilar vessels usually requires immediate surgical intervention.[12] In either case, increasing intrapleural pressure results in a decrease in vital capacity. Increasing vascular blood loss into the pleural space causes decreased venous return and decreased cardiac output.

Assessment findings for patients with a hemothorax include hypovolemic shock. Breath sounds may be diminished or absent over the affected lung. With hemothorax, the neck veins are collapsed and the trachea is at midline. Massive hemothorax can be diagnosed on the basis of clinical manifestations of hypotension associated with the absence of breath sounds and/or dullness to percussion on one side of the chest.[12] Nursing diagnoses for a patient with a hemothorax include Deficient Fluid Volume, with resulting Decreased Cardiac Output, and Impaired Gas Exchange. This life-threatening condition must be treated immediately. Resuscitation with IV fluids is initiated to treat the hypovolemic shock. A chest tube is placed on the affected side to allow drainage of blood. An autotransfusion device can be attached to the chest tube collection chamber. Thoracotomy may be necessary for patients who require persistent blood transfusions or who have significant bleeding (200 ml/hr for 2 to 4 hours) or when there are injuries to major cardiovascular structures.[34]

Cardiac and Vascular Injuries

Penetrating Cardiac Injuries. Penetrating cardiac trauma can occur from mechanical injuries as a result of bullets, knives, or impalements. The chest wall offers little protection to the heart from penetrating trauma. The most common site of injury is the right ventricle because of its anterior position. Mortality from penetrating trauma to the heart is high. Prehospital mortality for penetrating cardiac injuries is very high, and most deaths occur within minutes after injury as a result of exsanguination or tamponade.

Cardiac Tamponade. Cardiac tamponade is the progressive accumulation of blood in the pericardial sac (Fig. 37-12). With cardiac tamponade a progressive accumulation of blood, 120 to 150 ml, increases the intracardiac pressure and compresses the atria and ventricles.[32] An increase in intracardiac pressure leads to decreased venous return and decreased filling pressure, which leads to decreased cardiac output, myocardial hypoxia, cardiac failure, and cardiogenic shock.[32]

Classic assessment findings associated with cardiac tamponade are termed *Beck's triad*—presence of ele-

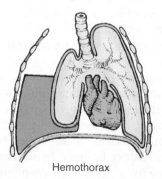

Hemothorax

Fig. 37-11 Blunt or penetrating thoracic trauma can cause bleeding into the pleural space to form a hemothorax.

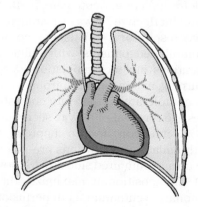

Fig. 37-12 Cardiac tamponade is the progressive accumulation of blood in the pericardial sac.

vated central venous pressure with neck vein distention, muffled heart sounds, and hypotension. Pulsus paradoxus may be present. Pulseless electrical activity (PEA) in the absence of hypovolemia and tension pneumothorax is suggestive of cardiac tamponade.[12] Ultrasonography in the emergency setting may be used in penetrating cardiac injuries to identify a hemopericardium.[35] The major nursing diagnosis for this injury is Decreased Cardiac Output. Immediate treatment is required to remove the accumulation of fluid in the pericardial sac. Pericardiocentesis involves the aspiration of fluid from the pericardium by use of a large-bore needle. The inherent risk in this procedure is potential laceration of the coronary artery. Other approaches include surgical procedures, such as thoracotomy or median sternotomy. The goal of these procedures is to locate and control the source of bleeding.

Blunt Cardiac Injuries. The most common causes of blunt cardiac trauma include high-speed MVCs, direct blows to the chest, and falls. The heart, because of its mobility and its location between the sternum and thoracic vertebrae, is susceptible to blunt traumatic injury. Sudden acceleration (as from contact with a steering wheel) can cause the heart to be thrown against the sternum (Fig. 37-13). Sudden deceleration can cause the heart to be thrown against the thoracic vertebrae by a direct blow to the chest (such as blows caused by a baseball, animal kick, or fall).

Blunt cardiac injury (BCI), formerly called *myocardial contusion*, covers the spectrum of myocardial contusion, concussion, and rupture. The most often injured chambers include the right atrium and ventricle because of their anterior position in the chest.[36]

Few clinical signs and symptoms are specific for BCI. Evidence of external chest trauma, such as steering wheel imprint or sternal fractures, should raise the suspicion for blunt cardiac injury. However, the presence of a sternal fracture does not predict the incidence of BCI. The patient may complain of chest pain that is similar to anginal pain. However, it is not typically relieved with nitroglycerin.[36] The chest pain is usually caused by associated injuries. The Eastern Association for the Surgery of Trauma (EAST) Guidelines for screening of BCI are listed in Box 37-10. An electrocardiogram (ECG) may reveal dysrhythmias, ST changes, heart block, or unexplained sinus tachycardia. Medical management is aimed at preventing and treating complications. This may include administration of antidysrhythmic medications, treatment of heart failure, or insertion of a temporary pacemaker to control conduction abnormalities. Assessment of fluid and electrolyte balance is imperative to ensure adequate cardiac output and myocardial conduction.

Aortic Injury. Blunt aortic injury is one of the most lethal blunt thoracic injuries. Disruption of the aorta in blunt chest trauma is a leading cause of immediate death in trauma patients: 22% die before reaching the ED, 37% die during initial resuscitation or in the operating room, and 14% die after surgery.[37] Of the survivors, 19% develop paraplegia or paresis.[37] Injuries associated with aortic injury include a first or second rib fracture, high sternal fracture, left-clavicular fracture at the level of the sternal margin, and massive hemothorax.[38] However, blunt aortic injury should be suspected in all victims of trauma with a rapid deceleration or acceleration mechanism of injury.[32]

The thoracic aorta is relatively mobile and tears at fixed anatomical points within the thorax. Sites of aortic disruption in order of frequency include the aortic isthmus, just distal to the subclavian artery (where the vessel is fixed to the chest by the ligamentum arteriosum); at the ascending aorta (where the aorta leaves the peri-

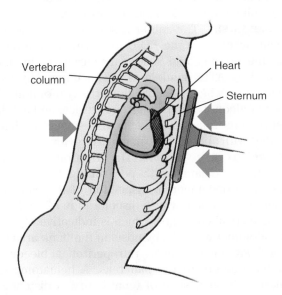

Fig. 37-13 Blunt cardiac trauma. Sudden acceleration (as from contact with the steering wheel) can cause the heart to be thrown against the sternum.

Vertebral column

Heart

Sternum

> ### Box 37-10
>
> **EAST GUIDELINES FOR SCREENING OF BLUNT CARDIAC INJURY (BCI)**
>
> - Admission ECG for all patients in whom there is suspected BCI.
> - If ECG is abnormal, the patient should be admitted for continuous ECG monitoring for 24 to 48 hours.
> - If the patient is hemodynamically unstable, an echocardiogram may be performed.
> - Cardiac enzymes and/or cardiac troponin T are not useful in predicting which patients will have complications related to BCI.

EAST, Eastern Association for the Surgery of Trauma; *ECG*, electrocardiogram.

cardial sac); at the descending aorta (where the aorta enters the diaphragm); and avulsion of the innominate artery from the aortic arch.[32]

The nurse assesses blood pressure bilaterally because a tear in the aortic arch may create a pressure gradient, resulting in blood pressures changes between upper extremities. If aortic disruption is suspected, blood pressure is also compared between upper and lower extremities. Baroreceptors are stimulated, resulting in upper extremity hypertension with relative lower extremity hypotension. Additional clinical assessment findings include a pulse deficit anywhere, unexplained hypotension, sternal pain, precordial systolic murmur, hoarseness, dyspnea, and lower extremity sensory deficits.

Initial radiograph is obtained in the upright position once it is considered safe to do so.[32] Radiograph findings suggestive of aortic injury include a widened mediastinum, obscured aortic knob, deviation of the left mainstem bronchus or nasogastric tube, and opacification of the aortopulmonary window.[38] A spiral or helical CT may be warranted if the initial radiograph is inconclusive, but definitive diagnosis is made by aortography in indeterminate cases.[38]

During the resuscitation phase for a patient with aortic disruption, blood pressure management is the primary goal to minimize injury. Patients with tears at the aortic isthmus are typically hypertensive, and minimizing stress on the vessel is achieved by maintaining the systolic blood pressure at less than 90 mm Hg by using antihypertensive agents such as sodium nitroprusside.[38] The nurse anticipates definitive surgical intervention early in the resuscitation. Surgical repair may be achieved by grafting, primary anastomosis, and bypassing.[38]

Postoperative care is directed toward BP stabilization with the goal of minimizing vessel stress while maintaining tissue perfusion, typically accomplished by use of sodium nitroprusside. Careful assessment of postoperative paraplegia is needed, since lack of blood flow to the spinal column may have occurred perioperatively. Paraplegia is closely related to duration of clamp time intraoperatively.[32] The critical care nurse monitors for signs of bowel ischemia (tube feeding intolerance, lactic acidosis) and renal failure (poor urinary output, rising creatinine) because mesenteric and renal blood flow may have been compromised as a result of the injury or aortic clamp time.

ABDOMINAL INJURIES

Abdominal injuries often are associated with multisystem trauma. Abdominal injuries are the third leading cause of traumatic death. Injuries to the abdomen are the result of blunt or penetrating trauma. Two major, life-threatening conditions that occur after abdominal trauma are hemorrhage and hollow viscus perforation with its associated peritonitis. Death occurring after 48

hours following injury is the result of sepsis and its complications. The critical care nurse must pay particular attention to complication prevention strategies throughout the trauma cycle.

Mechanism of Injury

Blunt Trauma. Blunt abdominal injuries are common. They result most often from MVCs, falls, and assaults. In MVCs, abdominal injury is more likely to occur when a vehicle is struck from the side. In the passenger position of the front seat, hepatic injury is likely when the point of impact is on the same side as the passenger. A driver is likely to sustain injury to the spleen when the impact is on the driver's side. Pedestrians hit by motor vehicles are at risk for serious abdominal injuries. Blunt trauma to the thorax can produce injuries to the liver, the spleen, and the diaphragm.[39] Deceleration and direct forces can produce retroperitoneal hematomas. Intestinal injuries are more common sources of injury when compared to penetrating trauma injuries.[39] Blunt abdominal injuries often are hidden, requiring careful assessment and reassessment. Unrecognized abdominal trauma is a frequent cause of preventable deaths, and blunt abdominal injury deaths are more likely to be fatal than are penetrating abdominal injuries.

Penetrating Trauma. Penetrating abdominal trauma is caused most often by knives or bullets. The danger of penetrating abdominal trauma is that the outside appearance of the wound does not reflect the extent of internal injury. Commonly injured organs from knife wounds are the colon, the liver, the spleen, and the diaphragm. Gunshot wounds to the abdomen usually are more serious than are stab wounds. A bullet destroys tissue along its path. Once inside the abdomen, a bullet can travel in erratic paths and ricochet off bone. Death from penetrating injuries depends on the injury to major vascular structures and resultant intraabdominal hemorrhage.

Assessment. The initial assessment of the trauma patient, whether in the ED or the critical care unit, follows the primary and secondary survey techniques as outlined by ATLS guidelines.[12] The initial physical assessment may be unreliable given the confounding influences of alcohol, illicit drugs, analgesics, and an altered level of consciousness. Specific assessment findings associated with abdominal trauma are reviewed here.

Physical Assessment. The location of entry and exit sites associated with penetrating trauma are assessed and documented. Inspection of the patient's abdomen may reveal purplish discoloration of the flanks or umbilicus (Cullen's sign), which is indicative of blood in the abdominal wall. Ecchymosis in the flank area (Grey-Turner's sign) may indicate retroperitoneal bleeding or a possible fracture of the pancreas. A hematoma in the flank area is suggestive of renal injury. A distended abdomen may indicate the accumulation of blood, fluid, or gas secondary to a perforated organ or ruptured blood vessel. Auscultation of the abdomen may reveal friction rubs over the liver or spleen and may indicate rupture. The abdomen is assessed for rebound tenderness and rigidity. Presence of these assessment findings indicates peritoneal inflammation. Referred pain to the left shoulder (Kehr's sign) may indicate a ruptured spleen or irritation of the diaphragm from bile or other material in the peritoneum. Subcutaneous emphysema palpated on the abdomen suggests free air as a result of a ruptured bowel.

Diagnostic Procedures. Insertion of a nasogastric tube and urinary catheter serves as a useful diagnostic and therapeutic aid. A nasogastric tube can decompress the stomach, and the contents can be checked for blood. Urine obtained from the urinary catheter can be tested for the presence of blood.

Serial laboratory test results may be nonspecific for the patient with abdominal trauma. A serum amylase determination can detect pancreatic injuries. Because of hemoconcentration, hemoglobin and hematocrit results may not reflect actual values. Serial values are more valuable in diagnosing abdominal injuries.

Diagnostic testing may occur simultaneously during the primary and secondary surveys. Tests may include the diagnostic peritoneal lavage (DPL), bedside ultrasound, and chest radiograph. DPL can exclude or confirm the presence of intraabdominal injury with a high accuracy rate. After the patient's bladder has been emptied, a small incision is made in the abdomen through the skin and into the peritoneum. A small catheter is inserted (Fig. 37-14). If frank blood is encountered, intraabdominal injury is obvious and the patient is taken immediately to the operating room (OR). If gross blood is not initially encountered, a liter of fluid (lactated Ringer's or 0.9% normal saline) is infused through the catheter into the abdomen. The IV bag is then placed in a dependent position, and abdominal fluid is allowed to drain into the IV bag. The drainage fluid is sent to the laboratory for analysis. Positive DPL results signal intraabdominal trauma and usually necessitate surgical intervention (Box 37-11). DPL is invasive, has been associated with complications, and cannot exclude retroperitoneal injuries.

Bedside ultrasonography has gained wide use in the United States for the detection of abdominal free fluid and hemoperitoneum. Focused Assessment with Sonography for Trauma (FAST) is noninvasive, does not involve potentially dangerous dyes, is convenient, and cost-effective. Typically four areas are examined: the right upper quadrant (RUQ) Morrison's pouch; the pericardial sac; the left upper quadrant (LUQ) splenorenal area; and the pelvis (Douglas' pouch).[40] The primary disadvantage of FAST is the need for free intraperitoneal fluid to cause a positive study.[41] An initial negative FAST may be followed with either serial ultrasound examinations, DPL, or abdominal CT.[42]

Although this test has been shown to have good sensitivity and specificity, it is not intended to replace DPL or CT. Obese abdomens and patients with ascites may have

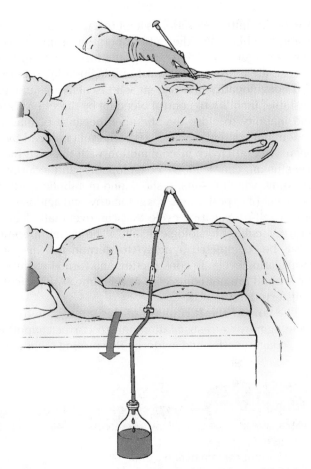

Fig. 37-14 Diagnostic peritoneal lavage (DPL) can exclude or confirm the presence of intraabdominal injury with a high accuracy rate.

Box 37-11

POSITIVE PERITONEAL LAVAGE RESULTS

- Red blood cell count: 100,000/mm^3
- White blood cell count: 500/mm^3
- Amylase: 175 units/dl
- Presence of blood, stool, bile, bacteria

---

erroneous results and further work-up for these patients is warranted.[40] Ultrasound is also limited in its ability to diagnose diaphragmatic, intestinal, or pancreas injuries.[41] Abdominal CT scanning is the mainstay of diagnostic evaluation in the hemodynamically stable trauma patient.[41] Abdominal CT provides information as to specific organ injury, pelvic injury, and retroperitoneal hemorrhage.

Combined Abdominal Organ Injuries. Patients with multivisceral injuries may require surgical intervention that uses somewhat nontraditional techniques, referred to as "damage control" surgery. The three phases to this treatment strategy are *initial operation, ICU resuscitation,* and *definitive reoperation* (Box 37-12).[43] The duration of this initial operation is kept to a minimum. The decision to abbreviate the initial operation is made early during surgery. Decisions that could lead the surgeon to choose an abbreviated laparotomy include hypothermia and coagulopathy in a patient who is hemodynamically unstable, inability to control bleeding by direct pressure, and inability to close the abdomen because of massive abdominal content edema.[43] Hypothermia induced by an open visceral cavity in conjunction with massive blood transfusion can lead to coagulopathy and continued bleeding, which results in shock and metabolic acidosis. The triad of hypothermia, coagulopathy, and acidosis creates a self-propagating cycle that can eventually lead to an irreversible physiologic insult.[43] The initial operation must be completed quickly to terminate this self-propagating cycle. Reconstruction and formal closure of the wound are not completed at this time. The patient is transferred to the ICU.

The goal of the ICU phase of this strategy is to continue aggressive resuscitation and to correct hypothermia, coagulopathy, and acidosis. Rewarming techniques, described in Table 37-7, are used to correct hypothermia. Coagulation factors and platelets may be given to correct coagulopathies. Serial lactate and base deficit measurements, as well as a mixed venous oxygen saturation (Svo_2) pulmonary artery catheter, may be used to guide fluid resuscitation, inotropic support, and oxygenation to prevent further development of acidosis.

The patient is assessed for additional complications, including ongoing hemorrhage, intraabdominal hypertension, and abdominal compartment syndrome. Abdominal compartment syndrome is defined as end-organ dysfunction secondary to intraabdominal hypertension.[43] The increased pressure can be caused by bleeding, ileus, visceral edema, or a noncompliant abdominal wall. Increased abdominal cavity pressure can impinge on diaphragmatic excursion and also can affect ventilation. Clinical manifestations of abdominal compartment syndrome include decreased cardiac output, increased pulmonary vascular resistance, increased peak pulmonary pressures, decreased urine output, and hypoxia.[44] (For additional information, see the Clinical Application feature on Trauma.)

Intraabdominal pressure can be measured through a bladder catheter after the injection of 50 to 100 ml of normal saline.[44] Serial monitoring of bladder pressures, about every 2 to 4 hours, is useful in detecting the onset of intraabdominal hypertension and the progression to abdominal compartment syndrome. Measurements may be graded: grade I (10 to 15 mm Hg), grade II (15 to 25 mm Hg), grade III (25 to 35 mm Hg), and grade IV (greater than 35 mm Hg).[44] Surgical decompression of the abdomen may be required for abdominal pressures greater than 20 to 25 mm Hg that are associated with other assessment findings such as decreased cardiac output, hypotension, elevated peak inspiratory pressures, and decreased urine output.[44] Surgical decompression involves opening the abdomen and then temporarily closing the abdomen with a sterile perforated plastic sheet, clips, vacuum-assisted techniques, as well as many other options.[43] The open abdomen is then cov-

---

Box 37-12

DAMAGE CONTROL SEQUENCE

1. Initial operation
   Control contamination
   Control hemorrhage
   Intraabdominal packing
   Temporary closure
2. Intensive care unit (ICU) resuscitation
   Correct coagulopathy
   Rewarming
   Maximize hemodynamics
   Ventilatory support
   Injury identification
3. Planned reoperation
   Pack removal
   Definitive repair

Table 37-7   Interventions for Rewarming the Trauma Patient

	External Rewarming Procedures	Internal Rewarming Procedures
Passive	Maintain a warm room temperature Remove all wet clothing and linen Cover the patient with blankets Avoid bathing patient until normothermia achieved	Administer warmed, humidified oxygen Administer warmed intravenous fluids
Active	Use radiant heat lamps, heating blankets/pads, hot water bottles	Perform GI irrigation with warmed solutions Perform extracorporeal rewarming for profound hypothermia Use esophageal rewarming tubes

Adapted from Morris J: Environmental emergencies. In Newberry L, editor: *Sheehy's emergency nursing: principles and practice*, ed 5, St Louis, 2003, Mosby.
GI, Gastrointestinal.

ered with towels or dressings, and closed suction drains are placed over the top and brought out through a plastic drape over the entire wound. The wound is closed permanently several weeks later, or it is allowed to heal by secondary intention and eventual skin grafting.

Once the patient is hemodynamically stable and the triangle of hypothermia, coagulopathy, and acidosis has been corrected, the patient is taken back to the OR for the definitive operation. This usually occurs within 48 to 72 hours of the initial operation.[43] It is during this phase that definitive repairs and wound closure are made. After surgery the patient is transported back to the ICU for continued care.

Specific Organ Injuries. Physical assessment findings, DPL, and CT scanning aid in making a diagnosis of specific abdominal organ injury. The medical and nursing management vary according to specific organ injuries. Liver, spleen, and bowel injuries, which are seen more commonly, are discussed here.

Liver Injuries. The liver is the primary organ injured in penetrating trauma and the second most often injured organ in blunt trauma. Abdominal CT is considered to be the most reliable diagnostic tool to identify and assess the severity of the injury to the liver.[45] The severity of liver injuries is graded to provide a mechanism for determining the amount of trauma sustained by that organ, the care needed, and possible outcomes (Table 37-8). Nonoperative management is considered the standard of care for hemodynamically stable patients with liver injury.[45] Patients are admitted to the ICU or a step-down unit and are monitored for signs of hemor-

rhage. Serial serum hematocrit and hemoglobin levels and vital signs are monitored over several days.

Patients with penetrating or blunt liver trauma who are hemodynamically unstable may require surgical intervention to correct the defect. Resection of the devitalized tissue is required for massive injuries. Hemorrhage is common with liver injuries, and ligation of the hepatic arteries or veins may be required to control hemorrhage. Drains may be placed intraoperatively to drain areas of blood and to prevent hematomas.

Care of the patient with severe liver injuries can be challenging for the critical care nurse. Lack of hemodynamic stability can result from hemorrhage and hypovolemic shock, leading to fluid volume deficit, decreased cardiac output, and decreased tissue perfusion. Combinations of crystalloid and colloid IV solutions may be used to correct hypovolemia. Fresh-frozen plasma, platelets, and cryoprecipitate may be administered to correct coagulopathies. A crucial nursing responsibility is to monitor the patient's response to medical therapies. Continued hemodynamic instability (hypotension, decreased cardiac output) in spite of aggressive medical intervention may indicate continued hemorrhage, in which case an exploratory laparotomy may be required to determine and correct the source of bleeding. The patient's postoperative ICU course may be complicated by coagulopathy, acidosis, and/or hypothermia. Jaundice may occur as a sign of hepatic dysfunction, but it may also be caused by resorption of hematomas or breakdown of transfused blood.

Spleen Injuries. The spleen is the organ most commonly injured by blunt abdominal trauma and is second

CLINICAL APPLICATION

Trauma

Mr. J is a 32-year-old man who was driving home from a Super Bowl party. He hit a patch of ice and lost control of his car, hitting a guard rail and a tree. He was not wearing a seat belt. The emergency medical technicians at the scene reported a prolonged extrication time of 45 minutes.

1. Mr. J is 45 minutes into the "golden hour." What is the golden hour?
2. What are the goals of prehospital care? How are these achieved?
3. Mr. J was involved in an MVC. What information is important to obtain from the paramedics regarding this mechanism of injury?
4. What aspects present at the scene will affect his ICU presentation and ICU course?

5. Mr. J is transported via helicopter to the emergency department. What systematic approach should be used to assess this patient? Why?
6. During the secondary survey a DPL is performed. The DPL is positive. What is a DPL and what is the significance of this positive result?
7. Mr. J is taken to the operating room. Intraoperatively he remains hypothermic and coagulopathic. He remains hypotensive despite a 12-L fluid resuscitation. A decision is made to institute "damage control" surgery. The operation is terminated, and he is brought to the ICU. What are the goals of the ICU phase of the damage control sequence? How will these be accomplished?
8. The patient is at high risk for developing abdominal compartment syndrome. What are the clinical manifestations of this complication?

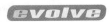 For the discussion of this Clinical Application and for an additional clinical application on trauma, see the Evolve website.

Table 37-8	Liver Injury Scale	
Grade*		**Injury Description**
I	Hematoma	Subcapsular, <10% surface area
	Laceration	Capsular tear, <1 cm parenchymal depth
II	Hematoma	Subcapsular, 10%-50% surface area; intraparenchymal <10 cm in diameter
	Laceration	Capsular tear, 1-3 cm parenchymal depth, <10 cm in length
III	Hematoma	Subcapsular, >50% surface area or expanding; ruptured subcapsular or parenchymal hematoma; intraparenchymal hematoma >10 cm or expanding
	Laceration	>3 cm parenchymal depth
IV	Laceration	Parenchymal disruption involving 25%-75% of hepatic lobe or 1-3 Couinaud's segments within a single lobe
V	Laceration	Parenchymal disruption involving >75% of hepatic lobe or >3 Couinaud's segments within a single lobe
	Vascular	Juxtahepatic venous injuries (i.e., retrohepatic vena cava/central major hepatic veins)
VI	Vascular	Hepatic avulsion

Modified from Trunkey DD: *Surg Clin North Am* 84:442, 2004.
*Advance one grade for multiple injuries up to grade II.

Table 37-9	Spleen Injury Scale	
Grade*		**Injury Description**
I	Hematoma	Subcapsular, <10% surface area
	Laceration	Capsular tear, <1 cm, parenchymal depth
II	Hematoma	Subcapsular, 10%-50% surface area; intraparenchymal <5 cm in diameter
	Laceration	Capsular tear: 1-3 cm parenchymal depth, which does not involve a trabecular vessel
III	Hematoma	Subcapsular, >50% surface area or expanding; ruptured subcapsular or parenchymal hematoma; intraparenchymal hematoma >5 cm or expanding
IV	Laceration	>3 cm parenchymal depth or involving trabecular vessels
	Laceration	Laceration involving segmental or hilar vessels producing major devascularization (>25% of spleen)
V	Laceration	Completely shattered spleen
	Vascular	Hilar vascular injury that devascularizes spleen

*Advance one grade for multiple injuries up to grade II.

to the liver as a source of life-threatening hemorrhage. Spleen injuries, like liver injuries, are graded for the purpose of determining the amount of trauma sustained, the care needed, and possible outcomes (Table 37-9). Hemodynamically stable patients may be monitored in the critical care unit by means of serial hematocrit values and vital signs. Progressive deterioration may indicate the need for operative management.[45]

Patients who exhibit hemodynamic instability require operative intervention with splenectomy, partial splenectomy, or splenorraphy. Patients who have had a splenectomy are at risk for the development of overwhelming postsplenectomy sepsis with streptococcal pneumonia. These patients require polyvalent pneumococcal vaccine (Pneumovax) to help promote immunity against most pneumococcal bacteria. Patients with isolated spleen injuries that necessitate surgical intervention rarely are ad-

mitted to the critical care unit. Complications after splenic trauma include wound infection; sepsis; subdiaphragmatic abscess; and fistulas of the colon, pancreas, and stomach.

Intestinal Injuries. Intestinal injuries can result from blunt or penetrating trauma. The diagnosis of small intestinal injuries is difficult. Surgical intervention is usually required in the presence of multiple findings on CT scan (unexplained free fluid, pneumoperitoneum, bowel wall thickening, mesenteric fat streaking, mesenteric hematoma, or IV contrast extravasation).[41] Regardless of the mechanism of injury, intestinal contents (bile, stool, enzymes, bacteria) leak into the peritoneum and cause peritonitis. Surgical resection and repair are required. The patient's postoperative course is dictated by the amount of spillage of intestinal contents. The patient is observed for signs of sepsis and abscess or fistula formation.

GENITOURINARY INJURIES

Trauma to the genitourinary (GU) tract seldom occurs as an isolated injury. A GU injury must be suspected in any patient with penetrating trauma to the torso; pelvic fracture; blunt trauma to the lower chest or flank; contusions, hematoma, tenderness over the flank, lower abdomen, or perineum; genital swelling or discoloration; blood at the urethral meatus; hematuria after Foley catheter placement; or difficulty with micturition.[12]

Mechanism of Injury. GU injuries, like all other traumatic injuries, can result from blunt or penetrating trauma.

Assessment. Evaluation of GU trauma begins after the primary survey has been conducted and immediately life-threatening conditions have been effectively managed. The conscious patient may complain of flank pain or colic pain. Rebound tenderness can be elicited if intraperitoneal extravasation of urine has occurred. Inspection may reveal blood at the urethral meatus. Bluish discoloration of the flanks may indicate retroperitoneal bleeding, whereas perineal discoloration may indicate a pelvic fracture and possible bladder or urethral injury. Hematuria is the most common assessment finding with GU trauma; however, the absence of gross or microscopic hematuria does not exclude a urinary tract injury.[12]

Specific Genitourinary Injuries

Renal Trauma. Most renal trauma is caused by blunt trauma, resulting in contusions or lacerations without urinary extravasation. Renal injury may be reflected by flank ecchymosis and fracture of inferior ribs or spinous processes. Gross or microscopic hematuria may be present; however, the extent of renal damage is often incongruous with the degree of hematuria.[46] Gross hematuria can be present with minor injuries and usually clears within a few hours. CT scan is the most accurate modality available for diagnosing renal injuries because it can assess the extent of parenchymal laceration, urine extravasation, surrounding hemorrhage, and the presence of vascular injury.[47] Contusions and minor lacerations can usually be treated with observation. The success of nonoperative management may be assisted and enhanced by using angiographic embolization. Nonoperative treatment of patients with major lacerations and vascular injuries may be achieved in patients who are hemodynamically stable.[47] Operative intervention may be performed in patients with renal injuries with a devascularized segment of the kidney. Postoperative and postinjury complications can include infection, hemorrhage, infarction, extravasation, calcification, acute tubular necrosis, and hypertension.

Bladder Trauma. A large percentage of bladder injuries result from pelvic fractures.[48] Physical findings may include lower abdominal bruising, distention, and pain. More definitive findings include difficulty in voiding or incomplete recovery of irrigation fluids from catheterized patients.[46] Definitive diagnosis is made by retrograde urethrogram. Bladder injuries are classified as contusions, extraperitoneal ruptures, intraperitoneal ruptures, or combined injuries. The type of injury depends on the location and strength of the blunt force and volume of urine in the bladder at the time of injury. Extraperitoneal rupture of the bladder may be managed conservatively with catheterization and antibiotics for 7 to 10 days.[47] Unresolved extravasation may require surgical intervention.

Nursing Management. Nursing diagnoses that can be applicable in caring for a patient with GU trauma include Ineffective Tissue Perfusion, Pain, Risk for Infection, and Risk for Deficient Fluid Volume.

After the patient is admitted to the critical care unit, the nurse makes an assessment according to ATLS guidelines. Once the patient's condition has stabilized, nursing management of postoperative renal trauma is similar to that for GU surgery. The primary nursing interventions include assessment for hemorrhage, maintenance of fluid and electrolyte balance, and maintenance of patency of drains and tubes. Measurement of urinary output includes drainage from the urinary catheter and the nephrostomy or suprapubic tubes. Drainage from these areas is recorded separately. Urine output is measured frequently until bloody drainage and clots have cleared. Gentle irrigation of drainage tubes may be required to clear clots and maintain the patency of the tubes.

PELVIC FRACTURES

More patients die from pelvic fractures than from any other skeletal injury, and survivors of this injury often suffer prolonged disability.[49] The pelvis is a ring-shaped structure composed of the hip bones, the sacrum, and the coccyx. Because the pelvis protects the lower urinary tract and major blood vessels and nerves of the lower extremities, pelvic trauma can result in life-threatening hemorrhage as well as urologic and neurologic dysfunction.

Mechanism of Injury. Blunt trauma to the pelvis can be caused by MVCs, falls, or a crushing accident. Pelvic injuries may be associated with damage to underlying tissues. Pelvic injuries often are associated with motorcycle crashes, pedestrian-vehicle collisions, direct crushing injury to the pelvis, and falls from heights greater than 12 feet.[50]

Assessment. Signs of pelvic fracture include perianal ecchymosis (scrotum or vulva) indicating extravasation of urine or blood, pain on palpation or "rocking" of the iliac crests, lower limb paresis or hypoesthesia, and hematuria. Lower extremity rotation or leg shortening is also cause for suspicion of a pelvic injury. Patients with a suspected pelvic injury should also have a rectal exam to assess for spinal cord injury or presence of occult or obvious rectal bleeding.

The diagnosis of pelvic fracture is made by an anteroposterior pelvic x-ray study with the patient in the supine position.[51] Further films may be required for definitive treatment, but the timing depends on the patient's hemodynamic stability.

Classification of Pelvic Fractures. Pelvic fractures constitute a spectrum of complexity ranging from a single, nondisplaced fracture of a pubic ramus to a life-threatening condition in which there are multiple fractures and crush injuries associated with significant hemorrhage and internal injuries. The three classifications of pelvic fractures follow.

Lateral Compression (LC). The lateral compression vector of pelvic injury is the most common.[50] This type of fracture produces a shortening of the pelvis diameter and typically does not involve ligamentous injury. While this type of fracture is forgiving to the pelvic ring vessels, localized bleeding may occur, particularly to the posterior pelvis. There are three types of LC fractures. Type I includes the posterior compression of the sacroiliac joint without ligament disruption or an oblique pubic ramus fracture. Type II includes rupture of the posterior sacroiliac ligament or internal rotation of the hemipelvis with a crush injury of the sacrum and an oblique pubic ramus fracture. Type III includes the findings of type II LC injury with additional evidence of AP compression to the contralateral hemipelvis.

Anterior-Posterior (AP) Compression. When force is applied in the anterior-posterior direction, the pelvic diameter widens. In this case, the injury can be completely ligamentous; it manifests as an open sacroiliac joint or open pubic symphasis.[50] This type of injury is also commonly associated with vascular injury. There are three types of AP compression fractures. Type I includes disruption of the pubic symphysis with less than 2.5 cm of diastasis with insignificant posterior pelvic involvement. Type II includes the disruption of the pubic symphysis of more than 2.5 cm with tearing of associated ligaments. Type III is a complete disruption of the pubic symphysis, posterior ligament complexes, and hemipelvic involvement.

Vertical Shear. A vertical shear pelvic injury includes a complete disruption of a hemipelvis associated with a hemipelvic displacement. This type of injury typically occurs in people who fall from a great height and land on one extremity.

Open Fractures. Open pelvic fractures involve an open wound with direct communication between the site of the fracture and a laceration involving the vagina, rectum, or perineum. Mortality from these injuries is high because, unlike closed pelvic fractures that bleed into the peritoneum, open pelvic fractures result in external exsanguination.[50]

Medical Management. The priority of the medical management of pelvic fractures is to prevent or to control life-threatening hemorrhage. External exsanguination is an immediate threat to patients with an open pelvic fracture. These patients are taken directly to the OR for aggressive resuscitation, ligation, and packing to control the exsanguination.[50] Patients with an open pelvic fracture may require an exploratory laparotomy to treat intraabdominal injuries. A diverting colostomy may be performed to prevent ongoing contamination of the pelvic wound from feces. If there are no obvious intraabdominal injuries, the pelvis is stabilized. After the initial operation, frequent operative débridement and pelvic wound irrigations are required for several days. Once the wound is clean and granulation tissue is present, definitive closure of the wound is done using a combination of techniques including free flap closure, split-thickness skin grafts, and rotation flaps.[49]

Patients who are hemodynamically stable and have stable closed pelvic fractures are usually treated conservatively with bed rest. These patients may receive elective orthopedic stabilization within 2 to 3 days after injury.[50] Patients who remain hemodynamically unstable may undergo temporary pelvic stabilization by wrapping the pelvis with a sheet between the greater trochanter and the iliac crests. Advantages of this technique are that it is quick, does not involve specialized training, allows continued access to the patient during the resuscitation, and does not require specialized equipment.[51] Temporary external fixation is performed concurrently with resuscitation in order to reduce further bleeding of the vessels in the pelvis. These patients require more drastic means to control hemorrhage including embolization by angiography and external pelvic fracture stabilization. Definitive management of pelvic fracture may include placement of internal or external fixation devices. Immediate external fixation is used as the primary method for controlling hemorrhage associated with closed pelvic fractures.[51] Angiography may be used to embolize bleeding vessels and achieve hemostasis in the hemodynamically unstable patient when other sources of bleeding have been excluded. Later, as the patient becomes more hemodynamically stable, internal fixation may be required.

Nursing Management. Initial assessment of the patient with a pelvic fracture in the critical care unit proceeds according to ATLS guidelines. Nursing diagnoses include Ineffective Tissue Perfusion, Pain, Risk for Infection, and Risk for Injury.

Massive blood loss contributes to alteration in tissue perfusion. On the patient's admission to the critical care unit, hemodynamic instability, with abnormal coagulation factors, may be present. Interventions include intravenously administered crystalloid and colloid fluids. The nurse must ensure that an appropriate amount of blood remains cross-matched and available if needed. Adequate oxygenation is assessed by means of pulse oximetry and SvO_2 and by monitoring serial hematocrit and hemoglobin levels.

The patient is at high risk for injury secondary to neurovascular compromise, development of abdominal compartment syndrome, fat embolism syndrome, and wound infection. These syndromes are discussed in further detail later in this chapter. Before the patient is moved, it is important that the nurse knows whether the physician has classified the closed pelvic fracture as *stable* or *unstable*. A stable pelvic injury implies that no further pathologic displacement of the pelvis can occur with physical turning or moving. An unstable pelvic fracture means that further pathologic displacement of the pelvis can occur with turning or moving.[49] Routine nursing assessments include neurovascular assessments of the lower extremities. Neurologic injury as a result of pelvic fracture may be transient and temporary. Open pelvic fractures may necessitate complex, time-consuming dressing changes. Aggressive pain management strategies should be employed during these dressing changes, because they can be quite painful.

Patients with open pelvic fractures usually have a prolonged critical care course, with varying degrees of complications. The patient with pelvic fractures is at risk for infection because of associated injuries and internal or external fixation devices. Nursing management of external fixation insertion sites is directed at preventing infection. Most institutions have protocols for pin care that require strict compliance.

COMPLICATIONS OF TRAUMA

In the trimodal distribution of trauma deaths, the third peak of death often occurs in the critical care unit as a result of complications days to weeks after the initial injury. Ongoing nursing assessments are imperative for early detection of complications often associated with traumatic injuries. A single complication can increase hospital length of stay, in addition to the associated costs of treating the complication.

HYPERMETABOLISM

Nutritional support is being recognized increasingly as an essential component in the care of critically ill trauma patients. Within 24 to 48 hours after traumatic injury, a predictable hypermetabolic response occurs. The metabolic response to injury mobilizes amino acids and accelerates protein synthesis to support wound healing and the immunologic response to invading organisms.[52] Stress hypermetabolism occurs after any major injury and is characterized by increases in metabolic rate and oxygen consumption. Energy requirements accelerate to promote immune function and tissue repair. The goal of early aggressive nutrition is to maintain host defenses by supporting this hypermetabolism and preserve lean body mass.[52] Most nutrition experts advocate beginning enteral nutrition. Current guidelines recommend enteral feedings be initiated within 72 hours for patients with blunt and penetrating abdominal injuries and those with severe head injuries.[52] Enteral feeding sites can include the gastric route or any site beyond the pylorus of the stomach, including the duodenum and jejunum. Prompt feeding tube placement by the critical care nurse must be a priority, unless contraindicated. Diminished or absent bowel sounds should not be interpreted to mean that the small bowel is not working. Small bowel function and the ability to absorb nutrients remains intact, despite the presence of gastroparesis and absent bowel sounds.[53] Because access to the stomach can be obtained more quickly and easily than to the duodenum, early gastric feeding is possible.[52] Patients at risk for pulmonary aspiration due to gastric retention or gastroesophageal reflex should receive enteral feedings into the jejunum.[52] If enteral feeding is not successful, parenteral nutrition should be initiated by day 7.[52]

INFECTION

Infection remains a major source of mortality and morbidity in critical care units. The trauma patient is at risk for infection because of contaminated wounds, invasive therapeutic and diagnostic catheters, intubation and mechanical ventilation, host susceptibility, and the critical care environment. Nursing management must include interventions to decrease and eliminate the trauma patient's risk of infection.

The patient with multiple trauma is at risk for infection because of host susceptibility (including preexisting medical conditions) and the adverse effect of trauma on the immune system (see "Systemic Inflammatory Response Syndrome" in Chapter 39).

Wound contamination poses an infection risk to the trauma patient, especially with injuries resulting from deep or penetrating trauma. Exogenous bacteria (from the external environment) can enter through open wounds. Exogenous bacteria can be introduced by dirt, grass, and debris inoculated into the wound at the time of injury, or they can be introduced by personnel during wound care. Endogenous bacteria (from the internal environment) can be released as a result of gastrointestinal or genitourinary perforation, which spills bacteria into the internal environment. Meticulous wound care is essential. The goals of wound care include minimizing infection risks, removing dead and devitalized tissue, allowing for wound drainage, and promoting wound epithelialization and contraction. Wound healing also is accomplished through interventions that promote tissue perfusion of well-oxygenated blood and that ensure adequate nutritional support for wound healing.

SEPSIS

The patient with multiple injuries is especially at risk for overwhelming infections and sepsis. The source of sepsis in the trauma patient can be invasive therapeutic and diagnostic catheters or wound contamination with exogenous or endogenous bacteria. The source of the septic nidus must be promptly evaluated. Gram's stain and cultures of blood, urine, sputum, invasive catheters, and wounds are obtained (see "Severe Sepsis and Septic Shock" in Chapter 38).

PULMONARY

Respiratory Failure. Posttraumatic respiratory failure often leads to the development of acute respiratory distress syndrome (ARDS). ARDS can be caused by direct injury to the lungs or indirect injury (see Chapter 23). The primary direct injuries in the trauma patient can include aspiration, inhalation, and pulmonary contusion.[54] The indirect injuries include sepsis, massive transfusion, fat emboli, and missed injury.[54] ARDS in the trauma patient can develop 24 to 72 hours after initial injury.

Fat Embolism Syndrome. Fat embolism syndrome (FES) can occur as a complication of orthopedic trauma. The clinical onset of FES ranges from 12 to 72 hours after injury, although 90% of patients with FES develop it within 24 hours after injury.[51] FES appears to develop as a result of fat droplets that leak from fractured bone and embolize to the lungs. The droplets are broken down into free fatty acids that are toxic to the pulmonary microvascular membranes. Pulmonary fat embolization alters pulmonary hemodynamics and pulmonary vascular permeability. The lung becomes highly edematous and hemorrhagic. The clinical presentation is almost indistinguishable from ARDS (see Chapter 23). Early stabilization of unstable extremity fractures may limit the seeding of fat droplets into the pulmonary system.[51]

PAIN

Pain in the ICU may come from many sources including surgery, procedures, and trauma. Trauma may contribute to cellular death and or inflammation that leads to pain.[55] Relief of pain is a major component in the care of trauma patients. An issue that often complicates pain management is the high incidence of substance abuse in patients who sustain traumatic injury. The Society of Critical Care Medicine (SCCM) proposed guidelines for the optimal use of sedatives and analgesics[56] (see Chapter 8).

RENAL COMPLICATIONS

Renal Failure. Assessment and ongoing monitoring of renal function are critical to the survival of the trauma patient. The etiology of posttraumatic renal failure is complex and may involve a variety of factors, as listed in Box 37-13.

Box 37-13

ETIOLOGIC FACTORS IN POSTTRAUMATIC RENAL FAILURE

- Preexisting disease
  Hypertension
  Diabetes
  Chronic renal insufficiency
  Chronic liver disease
- Prolonged shock states
- Profound acidosis
- SIRS/reperfusion injury
- Abdominal compartment syndrome
- Muscle ischemia; myoglobinuria
- Microemboli
- Nephrotoxic drugs
- Radiocontrast dye

SIRS, Systemic inflammatory response syndrome.

Prevention of renal failure is the best treatment and begins with ensuring adequate renal perfusion. Serial assessments of blood urea nitrogen (BUN) and creatinine levels are commonly used to evaluate renal function. Urine output as a measurement to determine renal function can be misleading because posttraumatic renal insufficiency can manifest as nonoliguric renal failure. Progressive renal failure requires prompt diagnosis and treatment (see "Acute Renal Failure" in Chapter 30).

Myoglobinuria. Patients with a crush injury are susceptible to the development of myoglobinuria, with subsequent secondary renal failure. Crush injuries can compromise blood flow. Loss of arterial blood flow, particularly to the extremities, results in the loss of oxygen transport to distal tissues and ischemia. This initiates a cascade of events that leads to the necrosis of skeletal muscle cells. As cells die, intracellular contents—particularly potassium and myoglobin—are released. Myoglobin (muscular pigment) is a large molecule. There are three mechanisms by which circulating myoglobin can lead to the development of renal failure: decreased renal perfusion, cast formation with tubular obstruction, and direct toxic effects of myoglobin in the renal tubuoles.[57]

Dark, tea-colored urine is suggestive of myoglobinuria. Testing for myoglobin in the urine can be done but may take several days, depending on laboratory resources available for this test. The most rapid screening test is a serum creatine kinase (CK) level. Urine output and serial CK levels should be monitored.

Once myoglobinuria is diagnosed, treatment is aimed at prevention of subsequent renal failure. Aggressive administration of intravenous fluids increases renal blood flow and decreases the concentration of nephrotoxic pigments. Continuous infusion of mannitol and sodium bicarbonate ($NaHCO_3$) may be used. Mannitol and $NaHCO_3$ are thought to alkalinize the urine and prevent myoglobin crystallization in the renal tubules. Acetazolamide (Diamox) may be given to prevent metabolic alkalosis that may be caused by the continuous $NaHCO_3$ infusion. Nursing management is directed toward achievement of fluid and electrolyte balance. The patient should be assessed for hypernatremia, hyperosmolality, and volume overload. Assessment parameters may include maintaining urine output greater than or equal to 200 ml/hr and maintaining urine pH 6.0 to 7.0 and serum pH < 7.5.[57]

VASCULAR COMPLICATIONS

Compartment Syndrome. Compartment syndrome is a condition in which increased pressure within a limited space compromises circulation, resulting in ischemia and necrosis of tissues within that space. Among those at high risk for the development of compartment syndrome are patients with lower extremity trauma including fractures, penetrating trauma, vascular ruptures, massive tissue injuries, or venous obstruction. Clinical manifestations of compartment syndrome include obvious swelling and tightness of an extremity, paresis, and pain of the affected extremity. Diminished pulses and decreased capillary refill do not reliably identify compartment syndrome because they may be intact until after irreversible changes have occurred. Elevated intracompartmental pressures confirm the diagnosis. The treatment can consist of simple interventions, such as removing an occlusive dressing, to more complex interventions, including a fasciotomy.

Deep Venous Thrombosis. Despite improvements in the care of the trauma patient, deep venous thrombosis (DVT) and the attendant risk of pulmonary embolism are important causes of morbidity and mortality in the trauma patient with multiple injuries. Major trauma patients have a DVT risk exceeding 50%.[58] The factors that are thought to form the basis of pathophysiology of DVT are stasis (reduction of blood flow in the veins), injury (to the intimal surface of the vessel), and hypercoagulopathy. Trauma patients are at risk for developing DVT because of endothelial injury, coagulopathy, immobility, and bed rest.

Trauma patients are at the greatest risk for developing thromboembolism early in their hospitalization. Prevention is key. The Eastern Association for the Surgery of Trauma developed practice guidelines for the prevention and management of DVT.[59] They recommended that trauma patients at high risk for DVT wear sequential compression devices for prophylaxis against DVT. High-risk patients include those with spinal cord injury, lower extremity or pelvic fractures, need for surgical procedure, increasing age, central venous catheters or venous injury, and prolonged immobility or hospital stay.[58] For patients in whom the lower leg is inaccessible, foot pumps may act as an effective alternative to lower the rate of DVT formation. Low–molecular-weight heparin

---

(e.g., enoxaparin) is recommended for DVT prophylaxis in trauma patients with the following injury patterns: (1) pelvic fractures requiring operative fixation or prolonged bed rest (>5 days), (2) complex lower extremity fractures requiring operative fixation or prolonged bed rest, and (3) SCI with complete or incomplete motor paralysis. The selection of DVT prophylaxis in trauma patients is often challenging because a balance between DVT risk and bleeding risk must be evaluated.

MISSED INJURY

Nursing assessment of the patient with multiple injuries in the critical care unit may reveal missed diseases or missed injuries. Missed "diseases" may include preexisting undiagnosed medical illnesses, such as endocrine disorders (diabetes, hypothyroidism); myocardial infarction; hypertension; respiratory insufficiency; renal insufficiency; or malnutrition.

Occasionally injuries may not be diagnosed in the precritical care phases. Missed injuries are commonly discovered in the first 24 to 48 hours of the hospital stay. Injuries are missed for a variety of reasons[60] as summarized in Box 37-14. In the critical care unit, a missed injury may be suspected if the patient fails to show appropriate response to medical or surgical intervention. Change in the character of drainage from wounds or catheters may represent biliary or duodenal injuries. Hypotension and a falling hematocrit level despite aggressive fluid administration may indicate an expanding hematoma. The critical care nurse must be alert to the possibility of a missed injury, especially when the patient does not appear to be responding appropriately to interventions. The physician must be notified immediately because potential complications of infection and hemorrhage may be life-threatening. Nurses play a key role in identifying missed injuries, particularly when patients regain consciousness and begin to increase their activity.

MULTIPLE ORGAN DYSFUNCTION SYNDROME

Multiple organ dysfunction syndrome (MODS) is a clinical syndrome of progressive dysfunction of organ systems. Trauma patients are at high risk for systemic inflammatory response syndrome (SIRS) and MODS. Organ dysfunction can be the result of "primary MODS," which is caused by direct traumatic injury such as that which occurs with acute lung dysfunction because of pulmonary contusion. Organ dysfunction that occurs latently in the trauma patient's ICU course, "secondary MODS," results from uncontrolled systemic inflammation with resultant organ dysfunction. Trauma patients may experience both primary and secondary MODS. Treatment is aimed at controlling or eliminating the source of inflammation, maintenance of oxygen delivery and consumption, and nutritional and metabolic support for individual organs (see Chapter 39).

SPECIAL CONSIDERATIONS

MEETING THE NEEDS OF FAMILY MEMBERS/SIGNIFICANT OTHERS

The impact of traumatic injury can be devastating not only for patients but also and especially for family members and significant others. "Trauma doesn't happen to an individual; it happens to a family."[61] They are faced with a crisis situation for which they have had little time to prepare. Trauma can precipitate a crisis within the family. Families may exhibit physical and sociocultural reactions as well as a combination of emotional reactions, including anger, fear, powerlessness, confusion, and mistrust. Recovery from traumatic injury can be long and frustrating for families. There may be many peaks and valleys of good days and bad days. During this time the family may exhaust its social and financial support systems. Nurses should recognize this and facilitate supportive relationships for families.

A valuable intervention is to bring families of trauma patients together in support group experiences. Trauma family support groups can offer sharing of experiences, the opportunity to express emotions, mutual support, sharing of coping strategies, and education about hospital and community services.

TRAUMA IN THE ELDERLY

Trauma is a disease that affects people of all ages. The elderly are predisposed to traumatic injuries because of the inevitable consequences of aging. The ability to react to or avoid environmental hazards is impaired because of age-related deterioration of the senses and changes in motor strength, postural stability, balance, and coordination.

The elderly experience the majority of all falls that result in injuries, and these falls are likely to occur from

---

Box 37-15

RISK FACTORS FOR FALLS IN THE ELDERLY

ACUTE ILLNESS
Cerebrovascular accidents
Dysrhythmias
Syncope
Diabetes

COGNITIVE IMPAIRMENT
Dementia

NEUROMUSCULAR DISORDERS
Arthritis
Lower extremity weakness
Unstable gait

MEDICATIONS
Antidepressants
Benzodiazepines
Diuretics
Phenothiazines

Box 37-16

FACTORS THAT PREDISPOSE THE ELDERLY TO MOTOR VEHICLE CRASHES

- Alterations in visual and auditory acuity
- Deterioration in strength and slower reaction times
- Diminution of cerebral skills
- Diminution of motor skills
- Exacerbation of acute or chronic medical conditions
- Medications that may interfere with safe driving

---

level surfaces or steps.[62] Factors that predispose the elderly to falls are summarized in Box 37-15.[63] Because many of the falls may be caused by an underlying medical condition (e.g., syncope, myocardial infarction, dysrhythmias), management of the elderly patient who has fallen must include an evaluation of events and conditions immediately preceding the fall. The exposure of the elderly to MVC trauma is a consequence of the increasing growth of the elderly population and the growing number of elderly drivers and occupants of motor vehicles. Factors that predispose the elderly to MVCs are summarized in Box 37-16.[63] A pedestrian struck by a motor vehicle receives some of the most devastating injuries. Many deaths that occur at crosswalks are of elderly individuals. Physiologic deterioration of cerebral and motor skills, and alterations in visual and auditory acuity cause elder pedestrians to walk directly into the path of oncoming vehicles.

Trauma in the elderly is associated with higher mortality even when the injuries are less severe. The elderly have a higher complications rate and a higher mortality rate, starting at 39 years of age, due to preexisting medical conditions, decreased physiologic reserves, and decreased ability to compensate for severe injury.[64] Elderly patients who do survive traumatic injury are often faced with changes in their preinjury functional status. Relatively minor trauma can be the event that changes the lifestyle of an elderly person from one of relative independence to one that requires prolonged rehabilitation or skilled nursing care. Discharge planning early in the patient's hospitalization is necessary.

The concept of "limited physiologic reserve" in the elderly trauma patient highlights the key difference between the average younger trauma patient with normal physiologic reserve and the elderly patient with underlying physiologic derangements.[65] Age-related changes that occur in virtually every organ system may not produce evidence of organ dysfunction in the resting state. However, the ability of organs to augment function in response to traumatic stress may be greatly compromised. Fluid resuscitation is an integral part of trauma resuscitation. Patients on chronic diuretic therapy may require more volume and potassium supplementation as a result of chronic volume and potassium depletion. The assessment and management of hypovolemic shock is more complex in the elderly trauma patient. The elderly have limited ability to increase their heart rate in response to blood loss, thus obscuring one of the earliest signs of hypovolemia—tachycardia.[12] Loss of physiologic reserve and the presence of preexisting medical conditions are likely to produce further conflicting hemodynamic data. The older patient's lack of physiologic reserve makes it imperative that early nutritional support is initiated.

Trauma protocols are well established for the management of young patients after injury. Clinicians increasingly are recognizing that these protocols must be individualized for the elderly trauma patient. The best outcomes in this trauma patient population have been achieved through early appropriate aggressive trauma care including early hemodynamic monitoring in high-risk elderly trauma patients (those with a high risk mechanism of injury, unknown cardiovascular status, or preexisting cardiac or renal disease).[66]

REFERENCES

1. Davis JW et al: Victims of domestic violence on the trauma service, *J Trauma* 54:352, 2003.
2. Guth AA, Pachter L: Domestic violence and the trauma surgeon, *Am J Surg* 179:134, 2000.
3. Melnick DM et al: Domestic violence and alcohol abuse in female trauma patients admitted to trauma centers, *J Trauma* 53:33, 2002.
4. Anglin D, Sachs C: Preventative care in the emergency department: screening for domestic violence in the ED, *Acad Emerg Med* 10:1118, 2003.
5. Sisley A, Jacobs LM, People G: Violence in America: a public health crisis—domestic violence, *J Trauma* 46:1105, 1999.
6. National Traffic Safety Association: *Traffic safety facts 2002: alcohol*, Washington, DC, 2003, NTSA.
7. Blincoe L et al: *The economical impact of motor vehicle crashes: 2000*. Washington, DC, 2002, Department of Transportation, NHTSA.
8. Shults RA et al: Reviews of evidence regarding mechanisms to reduce alcohol-impaired driving, *Am J Prev Med* 21(4S): 66, 2001.
9. Shults RA et al: Association between state level drinking and driving countermeasures and self-reported alcohol impaired driving, *Inj Prev* 8:106, 2002.
10. McCarthy MC: Trauma and critical care, *J Am Coll Surg* 190:232, 1999.
11. Nilssen O, Ries RK, Rivara FP: The CAGE questionnaire and the Michigan Alcohol Screening Test in trauma patients: comparisons of their correlations with biological markers, *J Trauma* 36:784, 1994.
12. American College of Surgeons: *Advanced trauma life support*, ed 6, Chicago, 1997, American College of Surgeons.
13. Cordonna V: *Trauma reference manual*, Baltimore, 1985, Brady Communications.
14. Eastern Association for the Surgery of Trauma: *Clinical practice guidelines: endpoints of resuscitation*, 2003, Eastern Association for the Surgery of Trauma, available on the Internet at http://www.east.org, 2003.
15. Kern JW, Shoemaker WC: Meta-analysis of hemodynamic optimization in high risk patients, *Crit Care Med* 30:1686, 2002.
16. Centers for Disease Control and Prevention: Traumatic brain injury in the United States: a report to Congress, September 23, 2003, accessed on the Internet at http://www.cdc.gov/doc.do/id/0900f3ec800101e6, June 29, 2004.
17. McQuillan KA, Mitchell PH: Traumatic brain injuries. In McQuillan KA et al, editors: *Trauma nursing: from resuscitation through rehabilitation*, ed 3, Philadelphia, 2002, WB Saunders.
18. Chestnut RM: Management of brain and spinal cord injuries, *Crit Care Clin* 20(1):25, 2004.
19. Valadka AB: Injury to the cranium. In Moore EE, Feliciano DV, Mattox KL: *Trauma*, ed 5, New York, 2004, McGraw Hill.
20. Brain Trauma Foundation: management and prognosis of severe traumatic brain injury, Part I: Guidelines for the management of severe traumatic brain injury. Available on the Internet at: http://www2.braintrauma.org/guidelines/downloads/btf_guidelines_management.pdf, 2000.
21. Brain Trauma Foundation: Guidelines for the management of severe traumatic brain injury.: Cerebral Perfusion Pressure. Available on the Internet at http://www2.braintrauma.org/guidelines/downloads/btf_guidelines_cpp_u1.pdf, 2003.
22. Lombardi F et al: Sensory stimulation for brain injured individuals in coma or vegetative state, *Cochrane Database of Systematic Reviews* 2: 2004.
23. Sekhon LHS, Fehlings MG: Epidemiology, demographics, and pathophysiology of acute spinal cord injury, *Spine* 26(24S):S2, 2001.
24. Russo-McCourt TA: Spinal cord injuries. In McQuillan KA et al, editors: *Trauma nursing: from resuscitation through rehabilitation*, ed 3, Philadelphia, 2002, WB Saunders.
25. Marion DW, Przybylski GJ: Injury to the vertebrae and spinal cord. In Mattox KL, Feliciano DV, Moore EE, editors: *Trauma*, ed 4, New York, 2004, McGraw Hill.
26. Robertson B, McQuillan KA: Maxillofacial injuries. In McQuillan KA et al, editors: *Trauma nursing: from resuscitation through rehabilitation*, ed 3, Philadelphia, 2002, WB Saunders.

27. Seyfer AE, Hansen JE: Facial trauma. In Moore EE, Feliciano DV, Mattox KL, editors: *Trauma,* ed 5, New York, 2004, McGraw Hill.
28. Easter A: Management of patients with multiple rib fractures, *Am J Crit Care* 10(5):320, 2001.
29. Holmes JF et al: A clinical decision rule for identifying children with thoracic injuries after blunt torso trauma, *Ann Emerg Med* 39(5):492, 2002.
30. Karmakar MK, Ho AM: Acute pain management of patients with multiple fractured ribs, *J Trauma* 54(3):615, 2003.
31. Keough V, Pudelek B: Blunt chest trauma: review of selected pulmonary injuries focusing on pulmonary contusion, *AACN Clin Issues* 12(2):270, 2001.
32. Sherwood S, Hartsock RL: Thoracic injuries. In McQuillan KA et al, editors: *Trauma nursing: from resuscitation through rehabilitation,* ed 3, Philadelphia, 2002, WB Saunders.
33. Asensio JA, Demetriades D, Rodriguez A: Injury to the diaphragm. In Mattox KL, Feliciano DV, Moore EE, editors: *Trauma,* ed 4, New York, 2004, McGraw Hill.
34. Wall MJ, Storey JH, Mattox KL: Indications for thoracotomy. In Mattox KL, Feliciano DV, Moore EE, editors: *Trauma,* ed 4, New York, 2004, McGraw Hill.
35. Ivatury RR: The injured heart. In Mattox KL, Feliciano DV, Moore EE, editors: *Trauma,* ed 4, New York, 2004, McGraw Hill.
36. Schultz JM, Trunkey DD: Blunt cardiac injury, *Crit Care Clin* 20(1):57, 2004.
37. Morgan PB, Buetchter KJ: Blunt thoracic aortic injuries: Initial evaluation and management, *South Med J* 93(2):173, 2000.
38. Eastern Association of Surgeons in Trauma: *Guidelines for the diagnosis and management of blunt aortic injury,* available on the Internet at http://www.east.org, 2000.
39. Fabian T, Crose N: Abdominal trauma, including indications for celiotomy. In Moore EE, Feliciano DV, Mattox KL, editors: *Trauma,* ed 5, New York, 2004, McGraw Hill.
40. Montonye J: Abdominal injuries. In McQuillan KA et al, editors: *Trauma nursing: from resuscitation through rehabilitation,* ed 3, Philadelphia, 2002, WB Saunders.
41. Todd SR: Critical concepts in abdominal injury, *Crit Care Clin* 20:119, 2004.
42. Eastern Association of Surgeons in Trauma: *Practice management guidelines for the evaluation of blunt abdominal trauma,* available on the Internet at http://www.east.org, 2001.
43. Schreiber MA: Damage control surgery, *Crit Care Clin* 20:119, 2004.
44. McNelis J, Marini CP, Simms HH: Abdominal compartment syndrome: clinical manifestations and predictive factors, *Curr Opin Crit Care* 9:133, 2003.
45. Eastern Association of Surgeons in Trauma: *Practice management guidelines for the nonoperative management of blunt injury to the liver and spleen,* 2003, Eastern Association for the Surgery of Trauma.
46. Peterson N: Genitourinary trauma. In Moore EE, Feliciano DV, Mattox KL, editors: *Trauma,* ed 5, New York, 2004, McGraw Hill.
47. Eastern Association of Surgeons in Trauma: *Practice management guidelines for the management of genitourinary trauma,* available on the Internet at http://www.east.org, 2003.
48. Nayduch DA: Genitourinary injuries and renal management. In McQuillan KA et al, editors: *Trauma nursing: from resuscitation through rehabilitation,* ed 3, Philadelphia, 2002, WB Saunders.
49. Walsh C: Musculoskeletal injuries. In McQuillan KA et al, editors: *Trauma nursing: from resuscitation through rehabilitation,* ed 3, Philadelphia, 2002, WB Saunders.
50. Scalea TM, Burgess AR: Pelvic fractures. In Moore EE, Feliciano DV, Mattox KL, editors: *Trauma,* ed 5, New York, 2004, McGraw Hill.
51. Mirza A, Ellis T: Initial management of pelvic and femoral fractures in the multiply injured patient, *Crit Care Clin* 20:159, 2004.
52. Eastern Association for the Surgery of Trauma: *Practice management guidelines for nutritional support of the trauma patient,* 2003, Eastern Association for the Surgery of Trauma.
53. Marik PE, Zaloga GP: Early enteral nutrition in acutely ill patients: a systematic review, *Crit Care Med* 29:2264, 2001.
54. Micheals AJ: Management of post-traumatic respiratory failure, *Crit Care Clin* 29:83, 2004.
55. Hall LG, Oyen LJ, Murray MJ: Analgesic agents: pharmacology and application in critical care, *Crit Care Clin* 17:899, 2001.
56. Jacobi F et al: Clinical practice guidelines for the sustained use of sedatives and analgesics in the critically ill adult, *Crit Care Med* 30:119, 2002.
57. Malinowski DJ, Slater MS, Mullins RJ: Crush injury and rhabdomyolysis, *Crit Care Clin* 20:171, 2004.
58. Geerts WH, Heit JA: Prevention of venous thromboembolism, *Chest* 119:1325, 2001.
59. Eastern Association for the Surgery of Trauma: *Practice management guidelines for the management of venous thromboembolism in trauma patients,* 1998, available on the Internet at www.east.org.
60. Sommers MS: Missed injuries: a case of trauma hide and seek, *AACN Clin Issues* 6:187, 1995.
61. Richmond TS: Trauma: beyond the hospital for patients and families, *Crit Care Nurse* 15(4):75, 1995.
62. Sterling DA, O'Connor JA, Bondies J: Geriatric falls: injury severity is high and disproportionate to mechanisms, *J Trauma* 50:116, 2001.
63. Johnson KL, Johnson SB: Geriatric trauma. In Fulmer T, Walker M, Foreman M, editors: *Critical care nursing of the elderly,* New York, 2001, Springer.
64. Victorino G, Chong TJ, Pal JD: Trauma in the elderly, *Arch Surg* 138:1093, 2003.
65. Jacobs DG: Special considerations in geriatric trauma, *Curr Opin Crit Care* 9:535, 2003.
66. Eastern Association for the Surgery of Trauma: *Practice management guidelines for geriatric trauma,* available from the Internet at www.east.org, 2001.

CHAPTER 38

Shock

Shock is an acute, widespread process of impaired tissue perfusion that results in cellular, metabolic, and hemodynamic alterations. Ineffective tissue perfusion occurs when an imbalance develops between cellular oxygen supply and cellular oxygen demand. This imbalance can occur for a variety of reasons and eventually results in cellular dysfunction and death. This chapter presents an overview of the general shock response, or shock syndrome, followed by a discussion of the different shock states.

SHOCK SYNDROME

DESCRIPTION

Shock is a complex pathophysiologic process that often results in multiple organ dysfunction syndrome (MODS) and death. All types of shock eventually result in ineffective tissue perfusion and the development of acute circulatory failure. The shock syndrome is a pathway involving a variety of pathologic processes that may be categorized into four stages: initial, compensatory, progressive, and refractory. Progression through each stage varies with the patient's prior condition, duration of initiating event, response to therapy, and correction of underlying cause.

ETIOLOGY

Shock can be classified as hypovolemic, cardiogenic, or distributive, depending on the pathophysiologic cause and hemodynamic profile. Hypovolemic shock results from a loss of circulating or intravascular volume. Cardiogenic shock results from the impaired ability of the heart to pump. Distributive shock results from maldistribution of circulating blood volume and can be further classified as septic, anaphylactic, or neurogenic. Septic shock is the result of microorganisms entering the body. Anaphylactic shock is the result of a severe antibody-antigen reaction. Neurogenic shock is the result of the loss of sympathetic tone.[1]

PATHOPHYSIOLOGY

During the initial stage, cardiac output (CO) is decreased and tissue perfusion is threatened. Almost immediately, the compensatory stage begins as the body's homeostatic mechanisms attempt to maintain CO, blood pressure (BP), and tissue perfusion. The compensatory mechanisms are mediated by the sympathetic nervous system (SNS) and consist of neural, hormonal, and chemical responses. The neural response includes an increase in heart rate (HR) and contractility, arterial and venous vasoconstriction, and shunting of blood to the vital organs. Hormonal compensation includes activation of the renin response and stimulation of the anterior pituitary and adrenal medulla. Activation of the renin response results in the production of angiotensin II, which causes vasoconstriction and the release of aldosterone and antidiuretic hormone (ADH), leading to sodium and water retention. Stimulation of the anterior pituitary results in the secretion of adrenocorticotropic hormone (ACTH), which in turn stimulates the adrenal cortex to produce glucocorticoids, causing a rise in blood glucose levels. Stimulation of the adrenal medulla causes the release of epinephrine and norepinephrine, which further enhance the compensatory mechanisms.

During the progressive stage, the compensatory mechanisms begin failing to meet tissue metabolic needs and the shock cycle is perpetuated. As tissue perfusion becomes ineffective, the cells switch from aerobic to anaerobic metabolism as a source of energy. Anaerobic metabolism produces small amounts of energy but large amounts of lactic acid, producing lactic acidemia. Increased vascular permeability from endothelial and epithelial hypoxia and inflammatory mediators results in intravascular hypovolemia, tissue edema, and further decline in tissue perfusion.[1,2] At the cellular level, the small amount of energy created by anaerobic metabolism is not enough to keep the cell functional and irreversible damage begins to occur. Some cells die as a result of apoptosis, an injury-activated preprogrammed cellular suicide.[3] Others die as the sodium-potassium pump in the cell membrane fails, causing the cell and its organelles to swell. Cellular energy production comes to a complete halt as the mitochondria swell and rupture. At this point the problem becomes one of oxygen utilization instead of oxygen delivery. Even if the cell were to receive more oxygen, it would be unable to use it because of damage to the mitochondria. The cell's digestive organelles swell, resulting in leakage of destructive enzymes into the cell, accelerating cell death.[1]

Every system in the body is affected by this process (Box 38-1). Cardiac dysfunction develops as a result of myocardial hypoperfusion and the release of myocardial depressant substances.[1,2] Ventricular failure eventually occurs, further perpetuating the entire process. Central nervous system (CNS) dysfunction develops as a result of cerebral hypoperfusion, leading to failure of the SNS, cardiac and respiratory depression, and thermoregulatory failure. Endothelial injury from hypoxia and inflammatory cytokines and impaired blood flow result in microvascular thrombosis. Hematologic dysfunction occurs as a result of consumption of clotting factors, release of inflammatory cytokines, and dilutional thrombocytopenia. Disseminated intravascular coagulation (DIC) may eventually develop. Pulmonary dysfunction occurs as a result of increased pulmonary capillary membrane permeability, pulmonary microemboli, and pulmonary vasoconstriction. Ventilatory failure and acute lung injury (ALI) eventually develop. Renal dysfunction develops as a result of renal vaso-

constriction and renal hypoperfusion, leading to acute tubular necrosis (ATN). Gastrointestinal dysfunction occurs as a result of splanchnic vasoconstriction and hypoperfusion and leads to failure of the gut organs. Disruption of the intestinal epithelium releases gram-negative bacteria into the system, which further perpetuates the entire shock syndrome.[3]

During the refractory stage, shock becomes unresponsive to therapy and is considered irreversible. As the individual organ systems die, MODS, defined as failure of two or more body systems, occurs (see Chapter 39). Death is the final outcome. Regardless of etiologic factors, death occurs from ineffective tissue perfusion because of the failure of the circulation to meet the oxygen needs of the cell.

ASSESSMENT AND DIAGNOSIS

The patient with a systolic blood pressure (SBP) less than 90 mm Hg and accompanied by tachycardia and altered mental status is considered to be in a shock state.[1] However, clinical manifestations will differ according to underlying cause and the stage of the shock, and are related to both the cause of and the patient's response to shock.[1,4]

Compensatory mechanisms may produce normal hemodynamic values even when tissue perfusion is compromised.[5,6] Global indicators of systemic perfusion and oxygenation include serum lactate and base deficit levels. Inadequate cellular oxygenation with anaerobic metabolism produces an elevated serum lactate. The level and duration of this hyperlactatemia are predictive of morbidity and mortality.[6,7] The base deficit derived from arterial blood gas (ABG) values also reflects global tissue acidosis and is frequently used to assess severity of shock.[6,7] (See individual sections on the different types of shock for a discussion of clinical assessment and diagnosis of the patient in shock.)

MEDICAL MANAGEMENT

The major focus of the treatment of shock is the improvement and preservation of tissue perfusion. Adequate tissue perfusion depends on an adequate supply of oxygen being transported to the tissues and the cell's ability to use it. Oxygen transport is influenced by pulmonary gas exchange, CO, and hemoglobin level. Oxygen use is influenced by the internal metabolic environment. Management of the patient in shock focuses on supporting oxygen transport and oxygen utilization.[1]

Adequate pulmonary gas exchange is critical to oxygen transport. Establishing and maintaining an adequate airway are the first steps in ensuring adequate oxygenation. Once the airway is patent, emphasis is placed on improving ventilation and oxygenation. Therapies in-

---

Box 38-1

CONSEQUENCES OF SHOCK

CARDIOVASCULAR
Ventricular failure
Microvascular thrombosis

NEUROLOGIC
Sympathetic nervous system dysfunction
Cardiac and respiratory depression
Thermoregulatory failure
Coma

PULMONARY
Acute respiratory failure
Acute lung injury (ALI)

RENAL
Acute tubular necrosis (ATN)

HEMATOLOGIC
Disseminated intravascular coagulation (DIC)

GASTROINTESTINAL
Gastrointestinal tract failure
Hepatic failure
Pancreatic failure

clude administration of supplemental oxygen and mechanical ventilatory support.

An adequate CO and hemoglobin level are crucial to oxygen transport. CO depends on HR, preload, afterload, and contractility. A variety of fluids and drugs are used to manipulate these parameters. The types of fluids used include both crystalloids and colloids. The categories of drugs used include vasoconstrictors, vasodilators, positive inotropes, and antidysrhythmics.

Indicated for decreased preload related to intravascular volume depletion, fluid administration can be accomplished by use of either a crystalloid or colloid solution, or both. Crystalloids are balanced electrolyte solutions that may be hypotonic, isotonic, or hypertonic. Examples of crystalloid solutions used in shock situations are normal saline and lactated Ringer's solution. Colloids are protein- or starch-containing solutions. Examples of colloid solutions are blood and blood components and pharmaceutical plasma expanders, such as hetastarch, dextran, and mannitol.

The choice of fluid is the subject of much debate and depends on the situation.[1,8-11] Advantages of colloids include faster restoration of intravascular volume and use of smaller amounts. Colloids are believed to stay in the intravascular space as opposed to crystalloids, which readily leak into the extravascular space. Disadvantages include expense, allergic reactions, and difficulties in typing and cross-matching blood. Colloids also can leak out of damaged capillaries and cause a variety of additional problems, particularly in the lungs. Blood should be used to augment oxygen transport if the patient's hemoglobin level is low, although controversy exists as to what threshold value should be used.[2,10]

Vasoconstrictor agents are used to increase afterload by increasing the systemic vascular resistance (SVR) and improving the patient's blood pressure level. Vasodilator agents are used to decrease preload or afterload, or both, by decreasing venous return and SVR. Positive inotropic agents are used to increase contractility. Antidysrhythmic agents are used to influence HR. Box 38-2 provides examples of each of these agents.

Sodium bicarbonate is no longer recommended in the treatment of shock-related lactic acidosis.[1,5,10,12] No overall benefit has been found and risks associated with its use are significant. These include shifting of the oxyhemoglobin dissociation curve to the left, rebound increase in lactic acid production, development of hyperosmolar state, fluid overload resulting from excessive sodium, and rapid cellular electrolyte shifts.[5,10,12]

The patient also should be started on a nutritional support therapy. The type of nutritional supplementation initiated varies according to the cause of shock and should be tailored to the individual patient's need, as indicated by the underlying condition and laboratory data. The enteral route is preferred over the parenteral.[13,14]

NURSING MANAGEMENT

The nursing management of a patient in shock is a complex and challenging responsibility. It requires an in-depth understanding of the pathophysiology of the disease and the anticipated effects of each intervention, as well as a solid understanding of the nursing process. (Individual shock sections contain separate discussions of specific interventions for the patient in shock.)

The psychosocial needs of the patient and family dealing with shock are extremely important. These needs, which differ with each patient and family, are based on situational, familial, and patient-centered variables. Nursing interventions for the psychosocial stress of critical illness include providing information on patient status, explaining procedures and routines, supporting the family, encouraging the expression of feelings, facilitating problem solving and decision making, involving the family in the patient's care, and establishing contacts with necessary resources.[15-17]

Collaborative management of the patient with shock is outlined in Box 38-3.

Box 38-2

AGENTS USED IN THE TREATMENT OF SHOCK

VASOCONSTRICTORS
Epinephrine (Adrenalin)
Norepinephrine (Levophed)
Alpha-range dopamine (Intropin)
Metaraminol (Aramine)
Phenylephrine (Neo-Synephrine)
Ephedrine
Vasopressin (Pitressin)

VASODILATORS
Nitroprusside (Nipride, Nitropress)
Nitroglycerin (Nitrol, Tridil)
Hydralazine (Apresoline)
Labetalol (Normodyne, Trandate)

INOTROPES
Beta-range dopamine (Intropin)
Dobutamine (Dobutrex)
Epinephrine (Adrenalin)
Isoproterenol (Isuprel)
Norepinephrine (Levophed)

ANTIDYSRHYTHMICS
Lidocaine (Xylocaine)
Adenosine (Adenocard)
Procainamide (Pronestyl)
Labetalol (Normodyne, Trandate)
Verapamil (Calan, Isoptin)
Esmolol (Brevibloc)
Diltiazem (Cardizem)
Amiodarone (Cordarone)

SHOCK
- Support oxygen transport
  - Establish a patent airway
  - Initiate mechanical ventilation
  - Administer oxygen
  - Administer fluids (crystalloids, colloids, blood and other blood products)
  - Administer vasoactive medications
  - Administer positive inotropic medications
  - Ensure sufficient hemoglobin and hematocrit
- Support oxygen use
  - Identify and correct cause of lactic acidosis
  - Ensure adequate organ and extremity perfusion
  - Initiate nutritional support therapy
- Identify underlying cause of shock and treat accordingly
- Maintain surveillance for complications
- Provide comfort and emotional support

ABSOLUTE
Loss of whole blood
  Trauma or surgery
  Gastrointestinal bleeding
Loss of plasma
  Thermal injuries
  Large lesions
Loss of other body fluids
  Severe vomiting or diarrhea
  Massive diuresis
Loss of intravascular integrity
  Ruptured spleen
  Long bone or pelvic fractures
  Hemorrhagic pancreatitis
  Hemothorax or hemoperitoneum
  Arterial dissection or rupture
RELATIVE
Vasodilation
  Sepsis
  Anaphylaxis
  Loss of sympathetic stimulation
Increased capillary membrane permeability
  Sepsis
  Anaphylaxis
  Thermal injuries
Decreased colloidal osmotic pressure
  Severe sodium depletion
  Hypopituitarism
  Cirrhosis
  Intestinal obstruction

HYPOVOLEMIC SHOCK

DESCRIPTION

Hypovolemic shock occurs from inadequate fluid volume in the intravascular space. The lack of adequate circulating volume leads to decreased tissue perfusion and initiation of the general shock response. Hypovolemic shock is the most commonly occurring form of shock.

ETIOLOGY

Hypovolemic shock can result from either absolute or relative hypovolemia. Absolute hypovolemia occurs when there is a loss of fluid from the intravascular space. This can result from an external loss of fluid from the body or when there is an internal shifting of fluid from the intravascular space to the extravascular space. Fluid shifts can result from loss in intravascular integrity, increased capillary membrane permeability, or decreased colloidal osmotic pressure. Relative hypovolemia occurs when vasodilation produces an increase in vascular capacitance relative to circulating volume (Box 38-4).

PATHOPHYSIOLOGY

Hypovolemia results in a loss of circulating fluid volume. A decrease in circulating volume leads to a decrease in venous return, which in turn results in a decrease in end-diastolic volume or preload. Preload is a major determinant of stroke volume (SV) and CO. A decrease in preload results in a decrease in SV and CO. The decrease in CO leads to inadequate cellular oxygen supply and ineffective tissue perfusion (Fig. 38-1).

ASSESSMENT AND DIAGNOSIS

The clinical manifestations of hypovolemic shock vary, depending on the severity of fluid loss and the patient's ability to compensate for it. Clinical classes have been developed by the American College of Surgeons to describe the levels of severity of hypovolemic shock. Class I indicates a fluid volume loss up to 15% or an actual volume loss up to 750 ml. Compensatory mechanisms maintain CO, and the patient appears free of symptoms other than slight anxiety.[2,18]

Class II hypovolemic shock occurs with a fluid volume loss of 15% to 30% or an actual volume loss of 750 to 1500 ml. Falling CO activates more intense compensatory responses. The HR increases to over 100/min in response to increased SNS stimulation. The pulse pressure (PP) narrows as the diastolic blood pressure increases because of vasoconstriction. Respiratory rate (RR) increases to 20 to 30/min, and respiratory depth increases in an attempt to improve oxygenation. ABG specimens drawn during this phase reveal respiratory alkalosis and hypoxemia, as evidenced by a low partial pressure of carbon dioxide ($Paco_2$) and a low partial pressure of

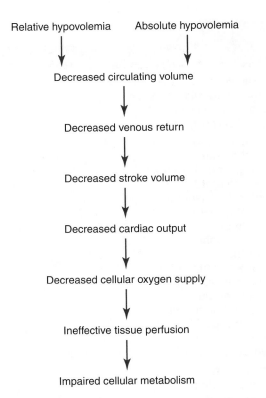

Relative hypovolemia   Absolute hypovolemia

↓   ↓

Decreased circulating volume

↓

Decreased venous return

↓

Decreased stroke volume

↓

Decreased cardiac output

↓

Decreased cellular oxygen supply

↓

Ineffective tissue perfusion

↓

Impaired cellular metabolism

Fig. 38-1 The pathophysiology of hypovolemic shock.

oxygen (PaO_2), respectively. Urine output (UO) starts to decline to 20-30 ml/hour as renal perfusion decreases. Urine sodium decreases, whereas urine osmolality and specific gravity increase as the kidneys start to conserve sodium and water. The patient's skin becomes pale and cool, with delayed capillary refill because of peripheral vasoconstriction. Jugular veins appear flat as a result of decreased venous return.[2,18]

Hypovolemic shock that is class III occurs with a fluid volume loss of 30% to 40% or an actual volume loss of 1500 to 2000 ml. This level of severity produces the progressive stage of shock as compensatory mechanisms become overwhelmed and ineffective tissue perfusion develops. Systolic BP decreases. The HR increases to over 120/min, and dysrhythmias develop as myocardial ischemia ensues. Respiratory distress occurs as the pulmonary system deteriorates. ABG values during this phase reveal respiratory and metabolic acidosis and hypoxemia, as evidenced by a high $PaCO_2$, low bicarbonate (HCO_3^-), and low PaO_2, respectively. Decreased renal perfusion results in the development of oliguria. Blood urea nitrogen (BUN) and serum creatinine levels start to rise as the kidneys begin to fail. The patient's skin becomes ashen, cold, and clammy, with marked delayed capillary refill. The patient appears confused as cerebral perfusion decreases and level of consciousness (LOC) deteriorates.[2,6,18]

Class IV hypovolemic shock is usually refractory in nature. It occurs with a fluid volume loss of greater than 40% or an actual volume loss of more than 2000 ml. The compensatory mechanisms of the body completely deteriorate, and organ failure occurs.[6] Severe tachycardia and hypotension ensue. Peripheral pulses are absent, and because of marked peripheral vasoconstriction, capillary refill does not occur. The skin appears cyanotic, mottled, and extremely diaphoretic. Urine output ceases. The patient becomes lethargic and unresponsive, and a variety of clinical manifestations associated with failure of the different body systems develop.[2,6,18]

Assessment of the hemodynamic parameters of a patient in hypovolemic shock varies by stage, but commonly reveals a decreased CO and cardiac index (CI). Loss of circulating volume leads to a decrease in venous return to the heart, which results in a decrease in the preload of the right and left ventricles. This is evidenced by a decline in the right atrial pressure (RAP) and pulmonary artery occlusion pressure (PAOP). Vasoconstriction of the arterial system results in an increase in the afterload of the heart as evidenced by an increase in the SVR. This vasoconstriction may produce a falsely elevated systolic BP when measured by arterial catheter. Mean arterial pressure (MAP) is more accurate in this low-flow state.[6]

MEDICAL MANAGEMENT

Treatment of the patient in hypovolemic shock requires an aggressive approach. The major goals of therapy are to correct the cause of the hypovolemia and to restore tissue perfusion. This approach includes identifying and stopping the source of fluid loss and vigorously administering fluid to replace circulating volume. Fluid administration can be accomplished with use of either a crystalloid or a colloid solution, or a combination of both. The type of solution used usually depends on the type of fluid lost, the degree of hypovolemia, and the severity of hypoperfusion.

Aggressive fluid resuscitation in the trauma patient with uncontrolled hemorrhage is a subject of debate. Research is evaluating the benefit of limited or hypotensive (SBP > 70) volume resuscitation, which is postulated to lessen bleeding and improve survival.[19-22]

NURSING MANAGEMENT

Prevention of hypovolemic shock is one of the primary responsibilities of the nurse in the critical care area. Preventive measures include the identification of patients at risk and frequent assessment of the patient's fluid balance. Accurate monitoring of intake and output and daily weights are essential components of preventive nursing care. Early identification and treatment result in decreased mortality.

Management of the patient in hypovolemic shock requires continuous evaluation of intravascular volume, tissue perfusion, and response to therapy. The patient in

NURSING DIAGNOSES | Hypovolemic Shock

- Deficient Fluid Volume related to active blood loss
- Deficient Fluid Volume related to interstitial fluid shift
- Decreased Cardiac Output related to alterations in preload
- Imbalanced Nutrition: Less Than Body Requirements related to increased metabolic demands or lack of exogenous nutrients
- Risk for Infection
- Anxiety related to threat to biologic, psychologic, and/or social integrity
- Compromised Family Coping related to critically ill family member

---

Box 38-5

ETIOLOGIC FACTORS IN CARDIOGENIC SHOCK

PRIMARY VENTRICULAR ISCHEMIA
Acute myocardial infarction
Cardiopulmonary arrest
Open heart surgery

STRUCTURAL PROBLEMS
Septal rupture
Papillary muscle rupture
Free wall rupture
Ventricular aneurysm
Cardiomyopathies
  Congestive
  Hypertrophic
  Restrictive
Intracardiac tumor
Pulmonary embolus
Atrial thrombus
Valvular dysfunction
Acute myocarditis
Cardiac tamponade
Myocardial contusion

DYSRHYTHMIAS
Bradydysrhythmias
Tachydysrhythmias

---

hypovolemic shock may have any number of nursing diagnoses, depending on the progression of the process (see the Nursing Diagnoses feature on Hypovolemic Shock). Nursing interventions also include minimizing fluid loss, administering volume replacement, and maintaining surveillance for complications.

Measures to minimize fluid loss include limiting blood sampling, observing lines for accidental disconnection, and applying direct pressure to bleeding sites. Measures to facilitate the administration of volume replacement include insertion of large-bore peripheral intravenous catheters, rapid administration of prescribed fluids, and positioning the patient with the legs elevated, trunk flat, and head and shoulders above the chest. In addition, monitoring the patient for clinical manifestations of fluid overload or complications related to blood product administration is critical to preventing further problems.

CARDIOGENIC SHOCK

DESCRIPTION

Cardiogenic shock is the result of failure of the heart to effectively pump blood forward. It can occur with dysfunction of either the right or the left ventricle, or both. The lack of adequate pumping function leads to decreased tissue perfusion and circulatory failure. It occurs in approximately 6% to 10% of the patients with an acute myocardial infarction (MI), and is the leading cause of death in patients hospitalized with MI.[23-25] The mortality rate for cardiogenic shock has decreased with the advent of early revascularization therapy and is currently around 50% to 60%.[23,26-27]

ETIOLOGY

Cardiogenic shock can result from primary ventricular ischemia, structural problems, and dysrhythmias.[1,23,25] The most common cause is acute MI resulting in the loss of 40% or more of the functional myocardium. The damage to the myocardium may occur after one massive MI (usually anterior wall), or it may be cumulative as a result of several smaller MIs or a small MI in a patient with preexisting ventricular dysfunction.[1,23] Structural problems of the cardiopulmonary system and dysrhythmias also may cause cardiogenic shock if they disrupt the forward motion of the blood through the heart (Box 38-5).[1,23,25]

PATHOPHYSIOLOGY

Cardiogenic shock results from the impaired ability of the ventricle to pump blood forward, which leads to a decrease in SV and an increase in the blood left in the ventricle at the end of systole. The decrease in SV results in a decrease in CO, which leads to decreased cellular oxygen supply and ineffective tissue perfusion. Typically myocardial performance spirals downward as compensatory vasoconstriction increases myocardial afterload and low blood pressure worsens myocardial ischemia. Recent research suggests that an alternate physiologic sequence may occur at some point in this process in a subset of patients. Evidence of a systemic inflammatory

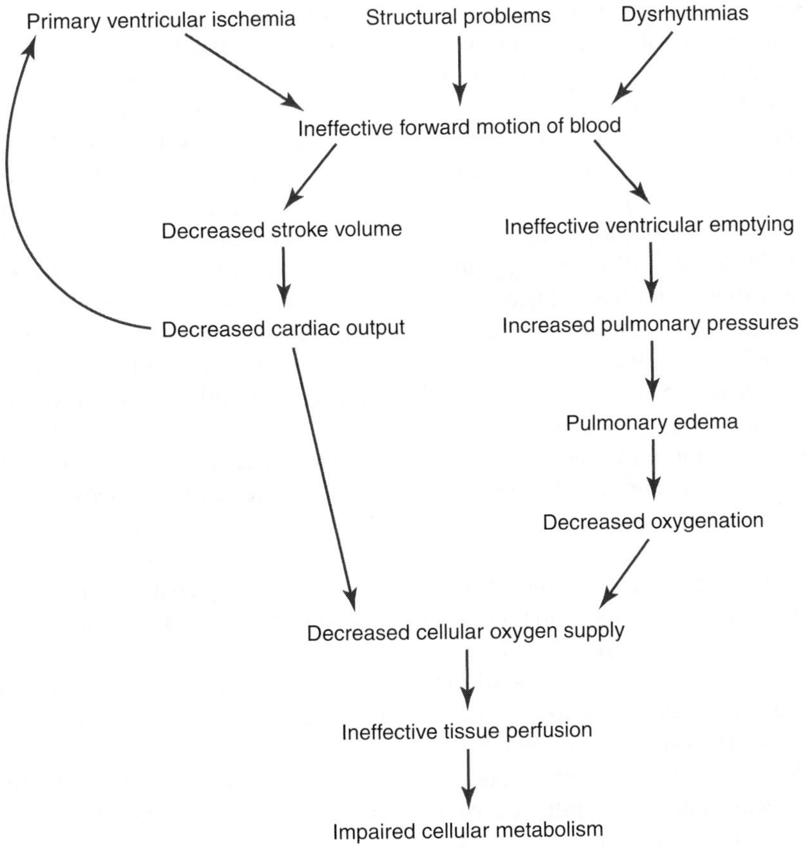

Fig. 38-2 The pathophysiology of cardiogenic shock.

response has been noted in a number of patients with cardiogenic shock.[26,28,29] Activation of inflammatory cytokines may induce systemic vasodilation, normalization of the CO, and defective cellular oxygen use. It is unknown whether this process contributes to the genesis or the outcome of cardiogenic shock.[26,29] As left ventricular contractility falls, an increase in end-systolic volume results in the back-up of blood into the pulmonary system and the subsequent development of pulmonary edema. Pulmonary edema causes impaired gas exchange and decreased oxygenation of the arterial blood, which further impair tissue perfusion (Fig. 38-2). Death due to cardiogenic shock may result from multiple organ failure or cardiopulmonary collapse.[25,26,28,29]

ASSESSMENT AND DIAGNOSIS

A variety of clinical manifestations occur in the patient in cardiogenic shock, depending on etiologic factors in pump failure, the patient's underlying medical status, and the severity of the shock state. Some clinical manifestations are caused by failure of the heart as a pump, whereas many relate to the overall shock response (Box 38-6).

Initially the clinical manifestations relate to the decline in CO. These signs and symptoms include SBP less

> **Box 38-6**
>
> **CLINICAL MANIFESTATIONS OF CARDIOGENIC SHOCK**
>
> - Systolic blood pressure <90 mm Hg
> - Heart rate >100 beats/min
> - Weak, thready pulse
> - Diminished heart sounds
> - Change in sensorium
> - Cool, pale, moist skin
> - Urine output <30 ml/hr
> - Chest pain
> - Dysrhythmias
> - Tachypnea
> - Crackles
> - Decreased cardiac output
> - Cardiac index <2.2 L/min/m^2
> - Increased pulmonary artery occlusion pressure
> - Increased right atrial pressure
> - Increased systemic vascular resistance

than 90 mm Hg; decreased sensorium; cool, pale, moist skin; and UO less than 30 ml/hr. The patient also may complain of chest pain. Tachycardia develops to compensate for the fall in CO. A weak, thready pulse develops, and heart sounds may reveal a diminished S_1 and S_2

as a result of the decrease in contractility. RR increases to improve oxygenation. ABG values at this time indicate respiratory alkalosis as evidenced by a decrease in $Paco_2$. Urinalysis findings demonstrate a decrease in urine sodium and an increase in urine osmolality and specific gravity as the kidneys start to conserve sodium and water. The patient also may experience a variety of dysrhythmias, depending on the underlying problem.[25]

As the left ventricle fails, auscultation of the lungs may disclose crackles and rhonchi, indicating the development of pulmonary edema. Hypoxemia occurs as evidenced by a fall in Pao_2 and Sao_2 as measured by ABG values. Heart sounds may reveal an S_3 and S_4. Jugular venous distention is evident with right-sided failure.

Assessment of the hemodynamic parameters of a patient in cardiogenic shock reveals a decreased CO with a CI less than 2.2 L/min/m^2 in the presence of elevated PAOP over 15 to18 mm Hg.[23,25] Increased filling pressures are necessary to rule out hypovolemia as the cause of circulatory failure. The increase in PAOP reflects an increase in the left ventricular end-diastolic pressure (LVEDP) and left ventricular end-diastolic volume (LVEDV) resulting from decreased SV. With right ventricular failure, the RAP also will increase. Compensatory vasoconstriction results in an increase in the afterload of the heart as evidenced by an increase in the SVR. Echocardiography confirms the diagnosis of cardiogenic shock and rules out other causes of circulatory failure.[23,25]

As compensatory mechanisms fail and ineffective tissue perfusion develops, a variety of other clinical manifestations appear. Myocardial ischemia progresses as evidenced by continued increases in HR, dysrhythmias, and chest pain. Pulmonary function deteriorates, which leads to respiratory distress. ABG values during this phase reveal respiratory and metabolic acidosis and hypoxemia as indicated by a high $Paco_2$, low HCO_3^-, and low Pao_2, respectively. Renal failure occurs as exhibited by the development of anuria and increases in BUN and serum creatinine levels. Cerebral hypoperfusion manifests as decreasing LOC.[25]

MEDICAL MANAGEMENT

Treatment of the patient in cardiogenic shock requires an aggressive approach. The major goals of therapy are to treat the underlying cause, enhance the effectiveness of the pump, and improve tissue perfusion. This approach includes identifying the etiologic factors of pump failure and administering pharmacologic agents to enhance CO. Inotropic agents are used to increase contractility and maintain adequate BP and tissue perfusion. Diuretics are used for preload reduction. Once blood pressure has been stabilized, vasodilating agents are used for preload and afterload reduction. Antidysrhythmic agents should be used to suppress or control dys-

rhythmias that can affect CO.[23,25] Intubation and mechanical ventilation may be necessary to support oxygenation.

Intraaortic balloon pump (IABP) support should be instituted if drug therapy does not quickly reverse the shock state.[26,27] The IABP is a temporary measure to decrease myocardial workload by improving myocardial supply and decreasing myocardial demand. It achieves this goal by improving coronary artery perfusion and reducing left ventricular afterload. See Chapter 19 for further discussion on IAPB therapy.

Once the cause of pump failure has been identified, measures should be taken to correct the problem if possible. If the problem is related to an acute MI, early revascularization by coronary angioplasty or coronary artery bypass surgery provides significant survival benefit.[23,26,27] Thrombolytic agents may be used in select patients. Therapies to decrease myocardial demand should include activity restrictions, analgesics, and sedatives.[25] When conventional therapies fail, extracorporeal membrane oxygenation (ECMO) and/or a ventricular assist device (VAD) may be used to support the patient in acute cardiogenic shock.[30-33] These mechanical circulatory assist devices provide an external means to sustain effective organ perfusion, allowing time for the patient's ventricle to heal or for cardiac transplantation to take place.

NURSING MANAGEMENT

Prevention of cardiogenic shock is one of the primary responsibilities of the nurse in the critical care area. Preventive measures include the identification of patients at risk and frequent assessment and management of the patient's cardiopulmonary status. Measures to limit myocardial oxygen demand include administering analgesics, sedatives, and agents to control afterload and dysrhythmias; positioning the patient for comfort; limiting activities; providing a calm and quiet environment and offering support to reduce anxiety; and teaching the patient about the condition. Measures to enhance myocardial oxygen supply include administering supplemental oxygen, monitoring the patient's respiratory status, and administering prescribed medications.

Effective nursing management of cardiogenic shock requires precise monitoring and management of HR, preload, afterload, and contractility. This is accomplished through accurate measurement of hemodynamic variables and controlled administration of fluids and inotropic and vasoactive agents. Close assessment and management of respiratory function is also essential to maintain adequate oxygenation.

Patients who require IABP therapy need to be observed frequently for complications. Complications include embolus formation, infection, rupture of the aorta, thrombocytopenia, improper balloon placement, bleed-

NURSING DIAGNOSES Cardiogenic Shock

- Ineffective Cardiopulmonary Tissue Perfusion related to acute myocardial ischemia
- Decreased Cardiac Output related to alterations in contractility
- Decreased Cardiac Output related to alterations in heart rate
- Imbalanced Nutrition: Less Than Body Requirements related to increased metabolic demands or lack of exogenous nutrients
- Risk for Infection
- Disturbed Body Image related to functional dependence on life-sustaining technology
- Compromised Family Coping related to critically ill family member

---

Box 38-7

ETIOLOGIC FACTORS IN ANAPHYLACTIC SHOCK

FOODS
Eggs and milk
Fish and shellfish
Nuts and seeds
Legumes and cereals
Citrus fruits
Chocolate
Strawberries
Tomatoes
Avocados
Bananas
Other

FOOD ADDITIVES
Food coloring
Preservatives

DIAGNOSTIC AGENTS
Iodinated contrast dye
Sulfobromophthalein (Bromsulphalein) (BSP)
Dehydrocholic acid (Decholin)
Iopanoic acid (Telepaque)

BIOLOGIC AGENTS
Blood and blood components
Insulin and other hormones

Gamma globulin
Seminal plasma
Enzymes
Vaccines and antitoxins

ENVIRONMENTAL AGENTS
Pollens, molds, and spores
Sunlight
Animal hair
Latex

DRUGS
Antibiotics
Aspirin
Narcotics
Dextran
Vitamins
Local anesthetic agents
Muscle relaxants
Barbiturates
Other

VENOMS
Bees and wasps
Snakes
Jellyfish
Spiders
Deer flies
Fire ants

---

ing, improper timing of the balloon, balloon rupture, and circulatory compromise of the cannulated extremity.

The patient in cardiogenic shock may have any number of nursing diagnoses, depending on the progression of the process (see the Nursing Diagnoses feature on Cardiogenic Shock). Nursing interventions include limiting myocardial oxygen demand, enhancing myocardial oxygen supply, and monitoring the patient's response to care.

ANAPHYLACTIC SHOCK

DESCRIPTION

Anaphylactic shock, a type of distributive shock, is the result of an immediate hypersensitivity reaction. It is a life-threatening event that requires prompt intervention. The severe antibody-antigen response leads to decreased tissue perfusion and initiation of the general shock response.[34-36]

ETIOLOGY

Anaphylactic shock is caused by an antibody-antigen response. Almost any substance can cause a hypersensitivity reaction. These substances, known as *antigens*, can be introduced by injection or ingestion or through the skin or respiratory tract. A number of antigens have been identified that can cause a reaction in a hypersensitive person. This list includes foods, food additives, diagnostic agents, biologic agents, environmental agents, drugs, and venoms (Box 38-7).[35,36] Latex allergies are discussed in Box 38-8.

Anaphylactic reactions can be either IgE-mediated or non–IgE-mediated responses. IgE is an antibody that is formed as part of the immune response. The first time an antigen enters the body, an antibody IgE, specific for the antigen, is formed. The antigen-specific IgE antibody is then stored by attachment to mast cells and basophils. This initial contact with the antigen is known as a *primary immune response*. The next time the antigen enters the body, the preformed IgE antibody reacts with it and a secondary immune response occurs. This reaction triggers the release of biochemical mediators from the mast cells and basophils and initiates the cascade of events that precipitates anaphylactic shock.[35-37] (For further discussion, see also the Clinical Application feature on Shock.)

Some anaphylactic reactions are non–IgE-mediated responses in that they occur in the absence of activation of IgE antibodies. These responses occur as a result of direct activation of the mast cells to release biochemical mediators. Direct activation of mast cells can be triggered by humoral mediators, such as the complement

Box 38-8

LATEX ALLERGIES

Latex is the milky sap of the rubber tree *Hevea brasilliensis.* It is treated with preservatives, accelerators, stabilizers, and antioxidants to make a more elastic, stable rubber. Reactions to products containing latex can be triggered by either the latex protein or by an additive used in the manufacturing process.

Latex reactions can be classified into three different categories: *irritation* (nonallergic inflammation occurring when the skin is abraded), *type IV delayed hypersensitivity* (non–IgE-mediated response to the chemical agents added during the manufacturing process), or *type I immediate sensitivity* (IgE-mediated response to latex proteins). Although the overall prevalence of latex allergy in the general population is only 1%, it is much higher (10% to 55%) in selected groups, such as patients with neural tube defects (spina bifida, myelomeningocele, lipomyelomeningocele) or congenital urologic disorders; those who have undergone multiple surgeries or who have a history of allergy to anesthetic drugs; and health care, rubber industry, or glove–manufacturing plant workers.

Five routes of exposure to latex proteins have resulted in systemic reactions: cutaneous (contact with moist skin); mucous membranes (mouth, vagina, urethra, or rectum); internal tissue (during surgery and other invasive procedures); intravascular; and inhalation (exposure to anesthesia equipment or endotracheal tubes or through the aerosolization of glove powder). It has been postulated that the latex allergen adheres to the cornstarch or powder and is released into the air with the manipulation of rubber gloves.

The American Academy of Allergy and Immunology has published guidelines for providing care to persons with latex allergy. All persons at risk for latex allergy should have a careful history and should complete a standardized latex allergy questionnaire. A history suggestive of reactivity to latex includes local swelling or itching after blowing up balloons, dental examinations, contact with rubber gloves, vaginal or rectal examinations, using condoms or diaphragms, and contact with other rubber products. Other historical information that may suggest increased risk of latex allergy includes hand eczema; previous, unexplained anaphylaxis; oral itching after eating bananas, chestnuts, kiwis, or avocados; and multiple surgical procedures in infancy. Patients at high risk should be offered clinical testing for latex allergy.

The patient with a latex allergy should be cared for in a latex-free environment; that is, an environment in which no latex gloves are used and there is no direct patient contact with other latex devices.

From Muller BA: *Postgraduate Medicine* 113:91, 2003; and Reed D: *AORN* 78:409, 2003.

system and the coagulation-fibrinolytic system. In addition, biochemical mediators can be released as a direct or indirect response to many drugs. This type of reaction is known as *anaphylactoid reaction.* Anaphylactoid reactions are produced in persons not previously sensitized and can occur with the first exposure to an antigen.[35-37]

PATHOPHYSIOLOGY

The antibody-antigen response (immunologic stimulation) or the direct triggering (nonimmunologic activation) of the mast cells results in the release of biochemical mediators. These mediators include histamine, eosinophil chemotactic factor of anaphylaxis (ECF-A), neutrophil chemotactic factor of anaphylaxis (NCF), platelet activating factor (PAF), proteinases, heparin, serotonin, leukotrienes (also known as *slow-reacting substance of anaphylaxis*), and prostaglandins. The activation of the biochemical mediators causes vasodilation, increased capillary permeability, bronchoconstriction, excessive mucus secretion, coronary vasoconstriction, inflammation, cutaneous reactions, and constriction of the smooth muscle in the intestinal wall, the bladder, and the uterus. Coronary vasoconstriction causes severe myocardial depression. Cutaneous reactions cause stimulation of nerve endings followed by itching and pain.[34-36]

ECF-A promotes chemotaxis of eosinophils, thus facilitating the movement of eosinophils into the area. During allergic reactions, eosinophils phagocytose the antibody-antigen complex and other inflammatory debris and release enzymes that inhibit vasoactive mediators, such as histamine and leukotrienes. In addition, secondary mediators are produced that either enhance or inhibit the already released biochemical mediators. For example, bradykinin, a secondary mediator, increases capillary permeability and facilitates vasodilation.[35]

Peripheral vasodilation results in relative hypovolemia and decreased venous return. Increased capillary membrane permeability results in the loss of intravascular volume, worsening the hypovolemic state. Decreased venous return results in decreased end-diastolic volume and SV. The decline in SV leads to a fall in CO and ineffective tissue perfusion. Death may result from airway obstruction or cardiovascular collapse, or both (Fig. 38-3).[34-37]

ASSESSMENT AND DIAGNOSIS

Anaphylactic shock is a severe systemic reaction that can affect any number of organ systems. A variety of clinical manifestations occur in the patient in anaphylactic shock, depending on the extent of multisystem involvement. The symptoms usually start to appear within

CLINICAL APPLICATION

Shock

Mr. H is a 27-year-old man born with a neural tube defect and a neurogenic bladder. Shortly after birth, he underwent a meningomyelocele repair with a ventriculoperitoneal (VP) shunt placement. During the following years, Mr. H underwent six major surgeries, all of which were fairly uneventful. However, when he was 17 years old, while undergoing a surgical release of his lower leg contractures, Mr. H suddenly became hypotensive and tachycardic and developed a lower extremity rash and wheezing. The anesthesiologist was able to reverse this episode with the administration of fluids and ephedrine. The reaction was attributed to an allergic reaction to cefazolin (Kefzol) because 500 mg IV had been administered 30 minutes before the event.

On this admission, Mr. H is taken to the operating room for an anterior spinal release. After 30 minutes of surgery, Mr. H develops generalized erythema, severe hypotension, tachycardia, wheezing, and hypoxemia, despite being ventilated with 100% oxygen. His jugular veins appear flat. Fluid resuscitation is initiated, epinephrine is administered, surgery is terminated, and Mr. H is transferred to the critical care unit on a ventilator. Upon arrival in the unit, Mr. H's vital signs are as follows: blood pressure (BP), 76/45; heart rate (HR), 145 (sinus tachycardia); temperature (T), 97° F; and urine output (UO), 35 ml/hr. Ventilation is continued at a rate of 8 (assist/control mode), tidal volume of 1000 ml, FiO_2 of 100%, and positive end-expiratory pressure (PEEP) of 5 cm H_2O. Breath sounds reveal wheezing over both lung fields. His arterial blood gas values are PaO_2, 70 mm Hg; $PaCO_2$, 37 mm Hg; pH, 7.30; HCO_3^-, 19 mEq/L; SaO_2, 92%.

1. What type of shock is Mr. H experiencing at this time?
2. Outline a brief plan of care for Mr. H.

Initially the cause of the anaphylactic reaction is unclear. Mr. H is given fluid boluses and started on a dopamine drip, which is titrated to 12 mcg/kg/min to keep his systolic BP greater than 90 mm Hg. A β_2-agonist aerosol, diphenhydramine (Benadryl), and a corticosteroid also are started. A pulmonary artery (PA) catheter is inserted, and Mr. H's hemodynamic values are right atrial pressure (RAP), 3 mm Hg; pulmonary artery occlusion pressure (PAOP), 5 mm Hg; cardiac output (CO), 3.4 L/min; cardiac index (CI), 1.8 L/min/m²; and systemic vascular resistance (SVR), 650. A dobutamine drip is initiated and titrated to 4.5 mcg/kg/min to maintain a CI greater than 2.0 L/min/m². Throughout the day Mr. H continues to have low filling pressures, persistent vasodilation, and wheezing despite the discontinuation of all suspected offending agents and the implementation of aggressive treatment. A thorough review of his history reveals Mr. H to be at high risk for an allergy to latex.

3. What are Mr. H's risk factors for developing a latex allergy?
4. How was Mr. H exposed to the latex allergen?
5. How would you modify Mr. H's environment to limit his exposure to latex while in the hospital?

All latex products are removed, and Mr. H is placed in a latex-free environment. Over the next 24 hours Mr. H becomes awake and alert, his vital signs stabilize, and his symptoms are quickly reversed. The remainder of Mr. H's stay in the critical care unit is uneventful. Weaning from the dopamine drip and mechanical ventilation is accomplished. Mr. H is transferred to the intermediate care unit, where discharge teaching regarding latex allergy is initiated. His surgery is rescheduled for 3 weeks later.

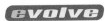 For the discussion of this Clinical Application, see the Evolve website.

---

minutes of exposure to the antigen, but they may not occur for up to 1 hour (Box 38-9).[34] Symptoms may also reappear following a 1- to 12-hour window of resolution. These late-phase reactions may be similar to the initial anaphylactic response, milder, or more severe.[34,35]

The cutaneous effects may appear first and include pruritus, generalized erythema, urticaria, and angioedema. Commonly seen on the face and in the oral cavity and lower pharynx, angioedema develops as a result of fluid leaking into the interstitial space. The patient may appear restless, uneasy, apprehensive, and anxious and may complain of being warm. Respiratory effects include the development of laryngeal edema, bronchoconstriction, and mucus plugs. Clinical manifestations of laryngeal edema include inspiratory stridor, hoarseness, a sensation of fullness or a lump in the throat, and dyspha-

gia. Bronchoconstriction causes dyspnea, wheezing, and chest tightness.[34-36] In addition, gastrointestinal and genitourinary manifestations may develop as a result of smooth muscle contraction. These include vomiting, diarrhea, cramping, and abdominal pain.

As the anaphylactic reaction progresses, hypotension and reflex tachycardia develop. This occurs in response to massive vasodilation and loss of circulating volume. Jugular veins appear flat as right ventricular end-diastolic volume is decreased. The eventual outcome is circulatory failure and ineffective tissue perfusion.[34-36] The patient's LOC may deteriorate to unresponsiveness.

Assessment of the hemodynamic parameters of a patient in anaphylactic shock reveals a decreased CO and CI. Venous vasodilation and massive volume loss lead to a decrease in preload, which results in a decline in the

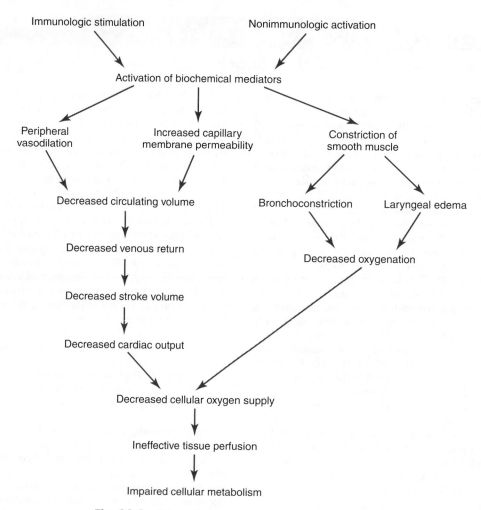

Fig. 38-3   The pathophysiology of anaphylactic shock.

RAP and PAOP. Vasodilation of the arterial system results in a decrease in the afterload of the heart, as evidenced by a decrease in the SVR.

MEDICAL MANAGEMENT

Treatment of anaphylactic shock requires an immediate and direct approach. The goals of therapy are to remove the offending antigen, reverse the effects of the biochemical mediators, and promote adequate tissue perfusion. When the hypersensitivity reaction occurs as a result of administration of medications, dye, blood, or blood products, the infusion should be immediately discontinued. Many times it is not possible to remove the antigen because it is unknown or has already entered the patient's system.

Reversal of the effects of the biochemical mediators involves the preservation and support of the patient's airway, ventilation, and circulation. This is accomplished through oxygen therapy, intubation, mechanical ventilation, and administration of drugs and fluids.

Epinephrine is given to promote bronchodilation and vasoconstriction and to inhibit further release of bio-

chemical mediators. In mild cases of anaphylaxis, 0.3 to 0.5 mg (0.3 to 0.5 ml) of a 1:1000 dilution of epinephrine is administered by either intramuscular or subcutaneous route and repeated every 5 to 15 minutes until anaphylaxis is resolved.[34-37] Evidence suggests that intramuscular administration into the lateral thigh achieves maximum absorption.[38] For anaphylactic shock with hypotension, epinephrine is administered intravenously. The IV dose is 0.3 to 0.5 mg (3 to 5 ml) of a 1:10,000 dilution administered over at least 3 to 10 minutes and repeated every 15 minutes if needed. If hypotension persists, a continuous infusion of epinephrine is recommended, administered at 1 mcg/min with titration up to 10 mcg/min as needed.[35,36] It must be noted that patients receiving beta-blockers may have a limited response to epinephrine. Intravenous glucagon administered at 5 to 15 mcg/min is recommended for inotropic and vasoactive support for these patients.[34,36]

Diphenhydramine (Benadryl), 1 to 2 mg/kg (maximum 50 mg) by intravenous (IV) route every 4 to 8 hours, is used to block the histamine response.[34-36] Corticosteroids also may be given with the goal of preventing a delayed reaction and stabilizing capillary membranes.[34-36]

Box 38-9

CLINICAL MANIFESTATIONS OF ANAPHYLACTIC SHOCK

CARDIOVASCULAR
Hypotension
Tachycardia

RESPIRATORY
Lump in throat
Dysphagia
Hoarseness
Stridor
Wheezing
Rales and rhonchi

CUTANEOUS
Pruritus
Erythema
Urticaria
Angioedema

NEUROLOGIC
Restlessness
Uneasiness
Apprehension
Anxiety
Decreased level of
   consciousness

GASTROINTESTINAL
Nausea
Vomiting
Diarrhea

GENITOURINARY
Incontinence
Vaginal bleeding

SUBJECTIVE COMPLAINTS
Sensation of warmth
Dyspnea
Abdominal cramping and pain
Itching

HEMODYNAMIC PARAMETERS
Decreased cardiac output
   (CO)
Decreased cardiac index (CI)
Decreased right atrial pressure
   (RAP)
Decreased pulmonary occlu-
   sion pressure (PAOP)
Decreased systemic vascular
   resistance (SVR)

NURSING DIAGNOSES — Anaphylactic Shock

- Deficient Fluid Volume related to relative loss
- Decreased Cardiac Output related to alterations in preload
- Decreased Cardiac Output related to alterations in afterload
- Ineffective Breathing Pattern related to decreased lung expansion
- Impaired Gas Exchange related to ventilation/perfusion mismatching or intrapulmonary shunting
- Imbalanced Nutrition: Less Than Body Requirements related to increased metabolic demands or lack of exogenous nutrients
- Risk for Infection
- Ineffective Coping related to situational crisis and personal vulnerability
- Compromised Family Coping related to critically ill family member

Fluid replacement is accomplished by use of either a crystalloid or colloid solution. In addition, positive inotropic agents and vasoconstrictor agents may be necessary to reverse the effects of myocardial depression and vasodilation.[34-36]

NURSING MANAGEMENT

Prevention of anaphylactic shock is one of the primary responsibilities of the nurse in the critical care area. Preventive measures include the identification of patients at risk and cautious assessment of the patient's response to the administration of drugs, blood, and blood products. A complete and accurate history of the patient's allergies is an essential component of preventive nursing care. In addition to a list of the allergies, a detailed description of the type of response for each one should be obtained.

The patient in anaphylactic shock may have any number of nursing diagnoses, depending on the progression of the process (see the Nursing Diagnoses feature on Anaphylactic Shock). Nursing interventions include facilitating ventilation, administering volume replacement, promoting comfort and emotional support, and maintaining surveillance for complications.

Measures to facilitate ventilation include positioning the patient to assist with breathing and instructing the patient to breathe slowly and deeply. Airway protection through prompt administration of prescribed medications is essential. Measures to facilitate the administra-

tion of volume replacement include inserting large-bore peripheral intravenous catheters, rapidly administering prescribed fluids, and positioning the patient with the legs elevated, trunk flat, and head and shoulders above the chest. Measures to promote comfort include administering medications to relieve itching, applying warm soaks to skin, and if necessary, covering the patient's hands to discourage scratching. In addition, observing the patient for clinical manifestations of a delayed reaction is critical to preventing further problems.

NEUROGENIC SHOCK

DESCRIPTION

Neurogenic shock, another type of distributive shock, is the result of the loss or suppression of sympathetic tone. The lack of sympathetic tone leads to decreased tissue perfusion and initiation of the general shock response. Neurogenic shock is the rarest form of shock.

ETIOLOGY

Neurogenic shock can be caused by anything that disrupts the SNS. The problem can occur as the result of interrupted impulse transmission or blockage of sympathetic outflow from the vasomotor center in the brain.[39,40] The most common cause is spinal cord injury. Neurogenic shock may mistakenly be referred to as *spinal shock.* The latter condition refers to loss of neurologic activity below the level of spinal cord injury, but does not necessarily involve ineffective tissue perfusion.[40]

PATHOPHYSIOLOGY

Loss of sympathetic tone results in massive peripheral vasodilation, inhibition of the baroreceptor response, and impaired thermoregulation. Arterial vasodilation leads to a decrease in SVR and a fall in blood pressure. Venous vasodilation leads to relative hypovolemia and pooling of blood in the venous circuit. The decreased venous return results in a decrease in end-diastolic volume or preload, causing a decrease in SV and CO. The fall in blood pressure and CO leads to inadequate or ineffective tissue perfusion. Loss of sympathetic tone and inhibition of the baroreceptor response result in bradycardia.[41] The slow HR worsens CO, which further compromises tissue perfusion. Impaired thermoregulation occurs because of loss of vasomotor tone in the cutaneous blood vessels that dilate and constrict to maintain body temperature. The patient becomes poikilothermic, or dependent on the environment for temperature regulation (Fig. 38-4).

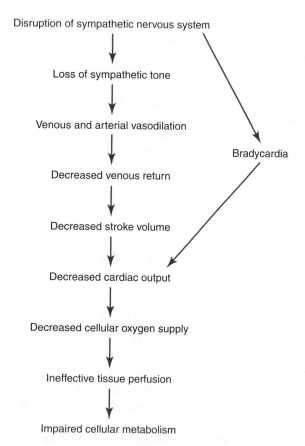

Fig. 38-4   The pathophysiology of neurogenic shock.

ASSESSMENT AND DIAGNOSIS

The patient in neurogenic shock characteristically presents with hypotension, bradycardia, and warm, dry skin.[40,41] The decreased blood pressure results from massive peripheral vasodilation. The decreased HR is caused by inhibition of the baroreceptor response and unopposed parasympathetic control of the heart.[41] Hypothermia develops from uncontrolled peripheral heat loss. The warm, dry skin occurs as a consequence of pooling of blood in the extremities and loss of vasomotor control in surface vessels of the skin that control heat loss.[39]

Assessment of the hemodynamic parameters of a patient in neurogenic shock reveals a decreased CO and CI. Venous vasodilation leads to a decrease in preload, which results in a decline in the RAP and PAOP. Vasodilation of the arterial system causes a decrease in the afterload of the heart as evidenced by a decrease in the SVR.[39]

MEDICAL MANAGEMENT

Treatment of neurogenic shock requires a careful approach. The goals of therapy are to treat or remove the cause, prevent cardiovascular instability, and promote optimal tissue perfusion. Cardiovascular instability can occur from hypovolemia, bradycardia, and hypothermia. Specific treatments are aimed at preventing or correcting these problems as they occur.

Hypovolemia is treated with careful fluid resuscitation. The minimal amount of fluid is administered to ensure adequate tissue perfusion. Volume replacement is initiated for SBP lower than 90 mm Hg, UO less than 30 ml/hr, or changes in mental status that indicate decreased cerebral tissue perfusion. The patient is carefully observed for evidence of fluid overload. Vasopressors are used as necessary to maintain blood pressure and organ perfusion.[39,40] Bradycardia should be treated with atropine when necessary.[40] Hypothermia is treated with warming measures and environmental temperature regulation.

NURSING MANAGEMENT

Prevention of neurogenic shock is one of the primary responsibilities of the nurse in the critical care area. This includes the identification of patients at risk and constant assessment of the neurologic status. Vigilant immobilization of spinal cord injuries and slight elevation of the head of the patient's bed after spinal anesthesia are essential components of preventive nursing care. Early identification allows for early treatment and decreased mortality.

The patient in neurogenic shock may have any number of nursing diagnoses, depending on the progression of the process (see the Nursing Diagnoses feature on Neurogenic Shock). Nursing interventions include treating hypovolemia, maintaining normothermia, and monitoring for dysrhythmias.

Venous pooling in the lower extremities promotes the formation of deep vein thrombosis (DVT), which can result in a pulmonary embolism. All patients at risk for DVT should be started on prophylaxis therapy. DVT-prophylactic measures include monitoring of calf and thigh measurements, passive range of motion exercises, application of antiembolic stockings and/or sequential pneumatic stockings, and administration of prescribed anticoagulation therapy.

SEVERE SEPSIS AND SEPTIC SHOCK

DESCRIPTION

Sepsis occurs when microorganisms invade the body and initiate a systemic inflammatory response. This host response often results in perfusion abnormalities with organ dysfunction (severe sepsis) and eventually hypotension (septic shock).[42] The primary mechanism of this type of shock is the maldistribution of blood flow to the tissues.[5,43,44] Severe sepsis is estimated to occur in 650,000 to 750,000 patients annually in the United States,[45,46] with an estimated mortality rate for septic shock at 45%.[5]

Specific terms are used to describe the continuum of conditions that the patient with an infection may experience. In 1991 at the American College of Chest Physicians/Society of Critical Care Medicine (ACCP/SCCM) Consensus Conference, definitions were developed to describe and differentiate these conditions (Box 38-10).[42] A second conference in 2001 reinforced and clarified these

---

NURSING DIAGNOSES — Neurogenic Shock

- Deficient Fluid Volume related to relative loss
- Decreased Cardiac Output related to sympathetic blockade
- Hypothermia related to exposure to cold environment, trauma, or damage to the hypothalamus
- Imbalanced Nutrition: Less Than Body Requirements related to increased metabolic demands or lack of exogenous nutrients
- Risk for Infection
- Anxiety related to threat to biologic, psychologic, or social integrity
- Compromised Family Coping related to critically ill family member

---

Box 38-10   DEFINITIONS FOR SEPSIS AND ORGAN FAILURE

Infection Microbial phenomenon characterized by an inflammatory response to the presence of microorganisms or the invasion of normally sterile host tissue by those organisms.

Bacteremia Presence of viable bacteria in the blood.

Systemic inflammatory response syndrome (SIRS) Systemic inflammatory response to a variety of severe clinical insults. The response is manifested by two or more of the following conditions: (1) temperature >38° C or <36° C; (2) heart rate >90 beats/min; (3) respiratory rate >20 breaths/min or $Paco_2$ <32 mm Hg; and (4) white blood cell count >12,000/mm^3, <4,000/mm^3, or >10% immature (band) forms.

Sepsis Systemic response to infection, manifested by two or more of the following conditions as a result of infection: (1) temperature >38° C or <36° C; (2) heart rate >90 beats/min; (3) respiratory rate >20 breaths/min or $Paco_2$ <32 mm Hg; and (4) white blood cell count >12,000/mm^3, <4,000/mm^3, or >10% immature (band) forms.

Severe sepsis Sepsis associated with organ dysfunction, hypoperfusion, or hypotension. Hypoperfusion and perfusion abnormalities may include, but are not limited to, lactic acidosis, oliguria, or an acute alteration in mental status.

Septic shock Sepsis-induced shock with hypotension despite adequate fluid resuscitation, along with the presence of perfusion abnormalities that may include, but are not limited to, lactic acidosis, oliguria, or an acute alteration in mental status. Patients who are receiving inotropic or vasopressor agents may not be hypotensive at the time that perfusion abnormalities are measured.

Sepsis-induced hypotension A systolic blood pressure <90 mm Hg or a reduction of ≥40 mm Hg from baseline in the absence of other causes for hypotension.

Mutliple organ dysfunction syndrome (MODS) Presence of altered organ function in an acutely ill patient such that homeostasis cannot be maintained without intervention.

From American College of Chest Physicians/Society of Critical Care Medicine Consensus Conference Committee: *Crit Care Med* 20:864, 1992.

Box 38-11

PRECIPITATING FACTORS ASSOCIATED WITH SEPTIC SHOCK

INTRINSIC FACTORS
Extreme of age
Coexisting diseases
   Malignancies
   Burns
   Acquired immunodeficiency syndrome (AIDS)
   Diabetes
   Substance abuse
   Dysfunction of one or more of the major body systems
Malnutrition

EXTRINSIC FACTORS
Invasive devices
Drug therapy
Fluid therapy
Surgical and traumatic wounds
Surgical and invasive diagnostic procedures
Immunosuppressive therapy

definitions.[47] This discussion focuses on severe sepsis and septic shock.

ETIOLOGY

Sepsis is caused by a wide variety of microorganisms including gram-negative and gram-positive aerobes, anaerobes, fungi, and viruses. The source of these microorganisms is varied. Exogenous sources include the hospital environment and members of the health care team. Endogenous sources include the patient's skin, gastrointestinal (GI) tract, respiratory tract, and genitourinary tract. In recent years, the incidence of chest-related infections has risen dramatically and the lungs have replaced the intraabdominal organs as the most common site of infection producing severe sepsis and septic shock.[48,49] Gram-negative bacteria are responsible for more than half of the cases of septic shock, though the proportionate incidence of gram-positive septicemia is rising dramatically.[49] Sepsis and septic shock are associated with a wide variety of intrinsic and extrinsic precipitating factors (Box 38-11). All of these factors interfere directly or indirectly with the body's anatomic and physiologic defense mechanisms. Several of the intrinsic factors are not modifiable or are very difficult to control. Several of the extrinsic factors may be required for diagnosis and management. All critically ill patients are therefore at risk for the development of septic shock.

PATHOPHYSIOLOGY

The syndrome encompassing severe sepsis and septic shock is a complex systemic response that is initiated when a microorganism enters the body and stimulates the inflammatory/immune system. Shed protein fragments and the release of toxins and other substances from the microorganism activate the plasma enzyme cascades (complement, kinin/kallikrein, coagulation, and fibrinolytic factors), as well as platelets, neutrophils, monocytes, and macrophages. Once activated, these systems and cells release a variety of mediators, or cytokines, that initiate a chain of complex interactions.[48,50-53] This host response is normally a protective mechanism controlled by feedback mechanisms. In severe sepsis and septic shock, the host response is altered and often exaggerated and uncontrolled.[51,54]

Once the mediators are activated, a variety of physiologic and pathophysiologic events occur that affect clotting, the distribution of blood flow to the tissues and organs, capillary membrane permeability, and the metabolic state of the body. Subsequently, a systemic imbalance between cellular oxygen supply and demand develops that results in cellular hypoxia, damage, and death (Fig. 38-5).[2]

Hallmarks of severe sepsis are endothelial damage and coagulation dysfunction.[50,54,55] Tissue factor is released from endothelial cells and monocytes in response to stimulation by the inflammatory cytokines.[48,50] Release of tissue factor initiates the coagulation cascade, producing widespread microvascular thrombosis and further stimulation of the systemic inflammatory pathways.[48] Diffuse endothelial damage impairs endogenous anticlotting mechanisms.[48,51] Mediator-induced suppression of fibrinolysis slows clot breakdown. Eventual consumption of coagulation factors may produce bleeding and hemorrhage.[55]

Significant alterations in cardiovascular hemodynamics are also caused by the activation of inflammatory cytokines and endothelial damage.[5,51,54] Massive peripheral vasodilation results in the development of relative hypovolemia. Increased capillary permeability produces loss of intravascular volume to the interstitium, which accentuates the reduction in preload and CO. These changes, coupled with the microvascular thrombosis, produce maldistribution of circulating blood volume, decreased tissue perfusion, and inadequate oxygen delivery to the cells. Impaired ventricular contractility results from cytokine activity and hypoxic myocyte dysfunction.[2,5]

Activation of the central nervous and endocrine systems also occurs as part of the response to invading microorganisms. This activation leads to stimulation of the SNS and the release of ACTH. These events trigger the release of epinephrine, norepinephrine, glucocorticoids, aldosterone, glucagon, and renin, resulting in the development of a hypermetabolic state and contributing to vasoconstriction of the renal, pulmonary, and splanchnic beds. Selective vasoconstriction in the splanchnic bed may contribute to hypoperfusion of the gastric mucosa. The resulting gut injury propagates the inflammatory response.[44,56] Activation of the CNS also causes the release

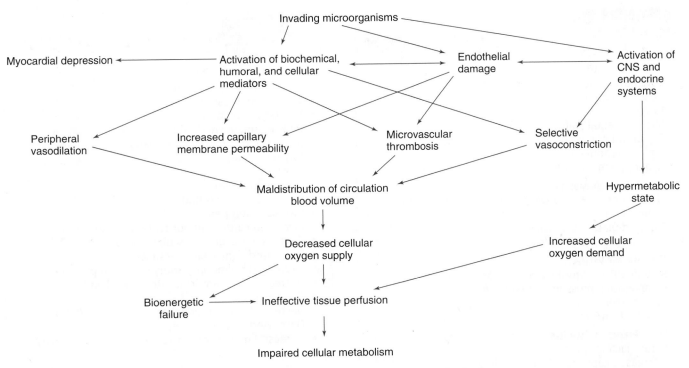

Fig. 38-5 The pathophysiology of septic shock.

of endogenous opiates that are believed to cause vasodilation and to further decrease myocardial contractility.[57]

A number of metabolic alterations occur as a result of CNS and endocrine system activation. The hypermetabolic state increases cellular oxygen demand and contributes to cellular hypoxia. Lactic acid is produced as a result of anaerobic metabolism. Glucocorticoids, ACTH, epinephrine, and glucagon are all catabolic hormones that are released as part of this response. These hormones favor the use of fats and proteins over glucose for energy production.[57]

The hypermetabolic state also increases the cellular metabolic needs. Increased glucose requirements in conjunction with the high level of catabolic hormones results in the limited ability of the cells to use glucose as a substrate for energy production. This causes glucose intolerance, hyperglycemia, relative insulin resistance, and the use of fat for energy (lipolysis).[43] The relative insulin resistance causes the body to produce more insulin, which inhibits the use of fat as an energy substrate. This promotes the use of protein as an energy substrate and catabolism of protein stores in the visceral organs and skeletal muscles.[57]

Metabolic derangements in severe sepsis and septic shock may also include an inability of the cells to use oxygen even if blood flow is adequate. Mitochondrial dysfunction is thought to be the underlying mechanism.[58] This bioenergetic failure may play an important role in the development of multiple organ dysfunction.[5,58] In addition, the exaggerated inflammatory response in severe sepsis also results in apoptosis, a programmed cell death or cellular suicide.[54]

These complex and interrelated pathophysiologic changes associated with severe sepsis and septic shock produce a pathologic imbalance between cellular oxygen demand and cellular oxygen supply/consumption. If unabated, this situation ultimately results in tissue ischemia, multiple organ dysfunction syndrome, and death.

ASSESSMENT AND DIAGNOSIS

Effective treatment of severe sepsis and septic shock is dependent on timely recognition. The diagnosis of severe sepsis is based on the identification of three conditions: known or suspected infection, two or more of the clinical indications of the systemic inflammatory response, and evidence of at least one organ dysfunction. Clinical indications of systemic inflammatory response and sepsis were included in the original ACCP/SCCM consensus definitions and are listed in Box 38-11. The second consensus conference expanded this list to facilitate prompt clinical recognition (Box 38-12).[47]

Signs of individual organ dysfunction are discussed in Chapter 39. The two most common organs to demonstrate dysfunction in severe sepsis are the cardiovascular system and the lungs. The patient with persistent hypotension requiring vasopressor therapy despite adequate volume resuscitation is demonstrating cardiovascular dysfunction. Pulmonary dysfunction is manifested by a Pao_2/Fio_2 (fraction of oxygen in inspired air) ratio

Box 38-12

EXPANDED LIST OF DIAGNOSTIC CRITERIA FOR SEPSIS

GENERAL VARIABLES
Core temperature >38.3° or <36 °C
Heart rate >90
Tachypnea
Altered mental status
Significant edema or positive fluid balance >20 ml/kg over 24 hours
Hyperglycemia (>120 mg/dl) in absence of diabetes

INFLAMMATORY VARIABLES
WBC count >12,000, <4,000 mm³, or >10% immature forms
Elevated plasma C-reactive protein
Elevated plasma procalcitonin

HEMODYNAMIC VARIABLES
Systolic BP <90 mm Hg or decrease >40 mm Hg
Mean arterial pressure <70 mm Hg
Svo_2 >70%
CI >3.5 L/m/m³

TISSUE PERFUSION VARIABLES
Serum lactate >1mmol/L
Decreased capillary refill or mottling

ORGAN DYSFUNCTION VARIABLES
Pao_2/Fio_2 <300
Urine output <0.5 ml/kg/hour
Creatinine increase >0.5 mg/dl
INR >1.5 or aPTT >60 sec
Ileus
Platelet count <100,000 mm³
Hyperbilirubinemia (plasma total bilirubin >4mg/dl

Modified from Levy MN et al: 2001 SCCM/ESICM/ACCP/ATS/SIS international sepsis definitions conference, *Crit Care Med* 31:1250, 2003.
aPTT, Activated partial thromboplastin time; *BP*, blood pressure; *CI*, cardiac index; *Fio₂*, fraction of oxygen in inspired air; *INR*, international normalized ratio; *Pao₂*, partial pressure of oxygen; *Svo₂*, mixed venous oxygen saturation; *WBC*, white blood cells.

Box 38-13

CLINICAL MANIFESTATIONS OF SEPTIC SHOCK

- Increased heart rate
- Decreased blood pressure
- Wide pulse pressure
- Full, bounding pulse
- Pink, warm, flushed skin
- Increased respiratory rate (early)/decreased respiratory rate (late)
- Crackles
- Change in sensorium
- Decreased urine output
- Increased temperature
- Increased cardiac output and cardiac index
- Decreased systemic vascular resistance
- Decreased right atrial pressure
- Decreased pulmonary artery occlusion pressure
- Decreased left ventricular stroke work index
- Decreased Pao_2
- Decreased $Paco_2$ (early)/increased $Paco_2$ (late)
- Decreased HCO_3^-
- Increased mixed venous oxygen saturation (Svo_2)

Paco₂, Partial pressure of carbon dioxide; *Pao₂*, partial pressure of oxygen; *Svo₂*, mixed venous oxygen saturation.

less than 300, indicative of acute lung injury.[50] Signs indicating septic shock are hypotension despite adequate fluid resuscitation and the presence of perfusion abnormalities such as lactic acidosis, oliguria, or acute change in mentation.

The patient in severe sepsis or septic shock may present with a variety of clinical manifestations that may change dynamically as the condition progresses (Box 38-13). During the initial stage, massive vasodilation occurs in both the venous and arterial beds. Dilation of the venous system leads to a decrease in venous return to the heart, which results in a decrease in the preload of the right and left ventricles. This is evidenced by a decline in the RAP and PAOP. Dilation of the arterial system results in a decrease in the afterload of the heart as evidenced by a decrease in the SVR. The patient's skin becomes pink, warm, and flushed as a result of the massive vasodilation. Myocardial contractility is decreased, as evidenced by a decline in the left ventricular stroke work index (LVSWI).

The HR rises in response to increased SNS, metabolic, and adrenal gland stimulation. If circulating volume and preload are adequate, this results in a normal-to-high CO and CI in spite of the impaired contractility. The PP widens as the diastolic blood pressure decreases because of the vasodilation, and the SBP increases because of the elevated CO. A full, bounding pulse develops. The net result of these changes is a relatively normal blood pressure in severe sepsis. However, as the reduction in preload and afterload becomes overwhelming and contractility fails, hypotension ensues resulting in septic shock.

In the lungs, ventilation/perfusion mismatching develops as a result of pulmonary vasoconstriction and the formation of pulmonary microemboli. Hypoxemia occurs, and the RR increases to compensate for the lack of oxygen. Crackles develop as increased pulmonary capillary membrane permeability leads to pulmonary edema.[43,59]

LOC starts to change as a result of decreased cerebral perfusion, immune mediator activation, hyperthermia, and lactic acidosis. This septic encephalopathy is demonstrated by acute onset of impaired cognitive functioning, or delirium, which may fluctuate during its course.[43] The patient may appear disoriented, confused, combative, or lethargic.

Arterial blood gas values initially reveal respiratory alkalosis, hypoxemia, and metabolic acidosis. This is demonstrated by a low PaO_2, low $PaCO_2$, and low HCO_3^-, respectively. The respiratory alkalosis is caused by the patient's increased RR. As pathologic pulmonary changes progress and the patient becomes fatigued, effectiveness of respirations decreases and the $PaCO_2$ increases, resulting in respiratory acidosis. The metabolic acidosis is the result of lack of oxygen to the cells and the development of lactic acidemia. Serum lactate levels rise over 2 mmol/L secondary to anaerobic metabolism. The mixed venous oxygen saturation (SvO_2) may increase because of maldistribution of the circulating blood volume and impaired cellular metabolism.[44] The white blood cell (WBC) count is elevated as part of the immune response to the invading microorganisms. In addition, the WBC differential reveals an increase in immature neutrophils (shift to the left). This occurs because the body has to mobilize increasing numbers of WBCs to fight the infection. Serum glucose also increases as part of the hypermetabolic response and the development of insulin resistance. The patient's temperature is elevated in response to pyrogens released from the invading microorganisms, immune mediator activation, and increased metabolic activity.[59] Urine output declines because of decreased perfusion of the kidneys. As impaired tissue perfusion develops, a variety of other clinical manifestations appear that indicate the development of MODS.

MEDICAL MANAGEMENT

Treatment of the patient in severe sepsis or septic shock requires a multifaceted approach. The goals of treatment are to reverse the pathophysiologic responses, control the infection, and promote metabolic support. This approach includes supporting the cardiovascular system and enhancing tissue perfusion, identifying and treating the infection, limiting the systemic inflammatory response, restoring metabolic balance, and initiating nutritional therapy. In addition, dysfunction of the individual organ systems must be prevented. Guidelines for the management of severe sepsis and septic shock have been developed under the auspices of the Surviving Sepsis Campaign (SSC), an international effort of 11 organizations to improve patient outcomes.[10]

The patient in severe sepsis or septic shock requires immediate resuscitation of the hypoperfused state. Specific interventions are aimed at increasing cellular oxygen supply and decreasing cellular oxygen demand. These treatments include administration of fluids, vasopressors, and positive inotropic agents. Early goal-directed therapy during the first 6 hours of resuscitation improves survival[60] and is recommended in the SSC guidelines.[10] This therapy includes aggressive fluid resuscitation to augment intravascular volume and increase preload until a central venous pressure (CVP) of 8 to 12

mm Hg (12 to 15 mm Hg in mechanically ventilated patients) is achieved. Crystalloids or colloids may be used. Administration of vasopressors, either norepinephrine or dopamine as first-choice agents, should be used as necessary to maintain a MAP of at least 65 mm Hg. These agents reverse the massive peripheral vasodilation and increase SVR. Vasopressin may be considered only for patients refractory to high doses of the first-choice agents.[10] Arterial line placement is recommended for any patient requiring vasopressor therapy. Intermittent or continuous monitoring of central venous or mixed venous oxygen saturation ($ScvO_2$ or SvO_2) allows evaluation of the effectiveness of oxygen delivery. If the $ScvO_2$ is less than 70%, administration of packed red cells is recommended to achieve a hematocrit of at least 30%.[60] Inotropic stimulation with dobutamine (administered to a maximum of 20 mcg/kg/min) is recommended as necessary to counteract myocardial depression and maintain adequate CO and $ScvO_2$ greater than 70%.[10,60] The dobutamine infusion should be reduced or discontinued if a tachycardia greater than 120 beats/min develops.[60]

Intubation and mechanical ventilatory support are also usually required to optimize oxygenation and ventilation for the patient in severe sepsis or septic shock. Ventilation with lower than traditional tidal volumes (6 ml/kg vs. 12 ml/kg) in patients with acute lung injury (ALI) and acute respiratory distress syndrome (ARDS) decreases mortality.[61] SSC guidelines recommend the goal of 6 ml/kg of predicted body weight for patients with severe sepsis or septic shock with ALI or ARDS.[10] Increased $PaCO_2$ may result from this therapy and is acceptable if tolerated as evidenced by hemodynamic stability. Ventilator settings should be adjusted to provide the patient with a PaO_2 greater than 70 mm Hg and a pH within the normal range. Patients receiving mechanical ventilation should be maintained in a semirecumbent position with the head of the bed raised to 45 degrees to decrease the incidence of ventilator-acquired pneumonia.[10] Prone positioning should be considered in the septic patient with ARDS requiring high levels of oxygen.[10] Sedation protocols using either intermittent bolus or continuous infusion using a standardized sedation scale and specific goals are recommended for all patients requiring mechanical ventilation. Daily interruption of sedative infusions to allow wakefulness and reevaluation of sedation needs reduces duration of mechanical ventilation and is recommended.[10,62] Neuromuscular blocking agents should be avoided, if possible, to prevent prolonged blockade following discontinuation.[10]

A key measure in the treatment of septic shock is finding and eradicating the cause of the infection. At least two blood cultures plus urine, sputum, and wound cultures should be obtained to find the location of the infection before antibiotic therapy is initiated.[10] Antibiotic therapy should be started within 1 hour of recognition of severe sepsis. If the microorganism is unknown, antiinfective therapy with one or more agents known to be effective against likely pathogens should be initiated. Once the microorganism is identified, an antibiotic more specific to the microorganism should be started.[10] Surgical intervention to debride infected or necrotic tissue or to drain abscesses also may be necessary to facilitate removal of the septic source.[10] Intravascular devices that might be the source of the infection should be removed following establishment of alternative vascular access.

Recombinant human activated protein C (rhAPC) administration has been demonstrated to improve survival in patients with severe sepsis.[10,48] Xigris, (drotrecogin alfa [activated]), is indicated for adult patients with severe sepsis who have a high risk of death. Patients with sepsis-induced ARDS or multiple organ failure or with septic shock meet these criteria.[10] Although its specific mechanisms for improving survival are not fully understood, drotrecogin alfa has anticoagulant, profibrinolytic, and antiinflammatory properties.[10,48] The proposed mechanisms of action of endogenous activated protein C are illustrated in Fig. 38-6. Guidelines for patient selection and appropriate administration of this agent must be strictly followed for safe and effective use. It is administered intravenously at an infusion rate of 24 mcg/kg/hr for a total infusion duration of 96 hours. Interruption of the infusion is necessary for invasive procedures. The most common serious side effect of drotrecogin alfa is bleeding. Contraindications for use include active internal bleeding, recent hemorrhagic stroke (within 3 months) or intracranial/intraspinal surgery (within 2 months); severe head trauma, trauma with

an increased risk of life-threatening bleeding, or presence of an epidural catheter; and intracranial neoplasm/mass lesion or evidence of cerebral herniation.[63] Studies of numerous other drugs believed to block or alter the effects of immune mediators have failed to demonstrate effectiveness or have been associated with unacceptable adverse effects.[55,64]

Intravenous corticosteroids reduce mortality in catecholamine-dependent septic shock patients with relative adrenal insufficiency.[65] The patient in septic shock who requires vasopressor therapy despite adequate fluid replacement should receive intravenous hydrocortisone at a stress dose of 200 to 300 mg/day in divided doses or continuous infusion for 7 days without waiting for ACTH stimulation results.[10] Doses greater than 300 mg/day may be harmful and should not be used.

Continuous infusion of insulin and glucose to maintain blood glucose less than 150 mg/dl improves outcomes[66] and is recommended by SSC guidelines following initial stabilization. Platelets should be administered when counts are less than 5000/mm^3.[10] Stress ulcer prophylaxis using histamine$_2$ (H$_2$-)-receptor blockers and DVT prophylaxis are recommended for all patients with severe sepsis or septic shock. Treatment of lactic acidemia with bicarbonate therapy is not beneficial and is not recommended if pH is equal to or greater than 7.15. Low-dose dopamine infusion for renal protection is not beneficial and should not be used either.[10,44]

The initiation of nutritional therapy is critical in the management of the patient in severe sepsis or septic shock. The goal is to improve the patient's overall nutritional status, enhance the immune system, and promote

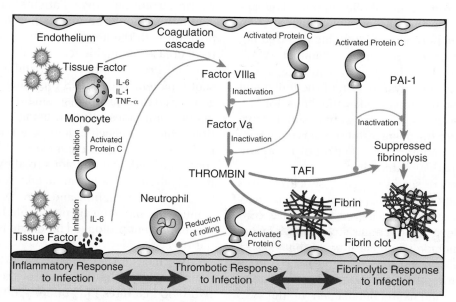

Fig. 38-6 Proposed mechanisms of action of endogenous activated protein C in severe sepsis. (From Eli Lilly and Company.)

wound healing. A daily caloric intake of 25 to 30 kcal/kg of usual body weight is recommended. The enteral route is preferred. The ideal nutritional supplement for the patient in septic shock should be high in protein because of the metabolic derangements that develop in the hypermetabolic state. The amount of protein calories given depends on the patient's nitrogen balance. In early sepsis, the mix of nonprotein calories may be divided evenly between carbohydrates and fats. In the later stages, significant alterations in fat metabolism occur and the lipid content should be limited to 10% to 15% of the total nonprotein calories. The lipid emulsion should contain long-chain fatty acid triglycerides for their protein-sparing effects.[57]

NURSING MANAGEMENT

Prevention of severe sepsis and septic shock is one of the primary responsibilities of the nurse in the critical care area. These measures include the identification of patients at risk and reduction of their exposure to invading microorganisms. Handwashing, aseptic technique,

and an understanding of how microorganisms can invade the body are essential components of preventive nursing care. Early identification allows for early treatment and decreases mortality.[43]

The patient in septic shock may have any number of nursing diagnoses, depending on the progression of the process (see the Nursing Diagnoses feature on Septic Shock). Nursing interventions include early identification of the sepsis syndrome; administering prescribed fluids, vasoactive agents, antibiotics, rhAPC, and other drugs; preventing complications of critical illness and therapeutic interventions; preventing the development of concomitant infections; observing for complications of all therapy; and monitoring the patient's response to care. Continual observation to detect subtle changes that indicate the progression of the septic process is also very important.

Evidence-based guidelines for the management of the patient with severe sepsis or septic shock are listed in the Evidence-Based Collaborative Practice feature on Severe Sepsis and Septic Shock Management Guidelines.

EVIDENCE-BASED COLLABORATIVE PRACTICE

Severe Sepsis and Septic Shock Management Guidelines

The following recommendations are supported by at least two large randomized trials with clear-cut results (grade A) or at least one large randomized trials with clear-cut results (grade B).

- Resuscitation should be initiated as soon as severe sepsis is recognized with the following goals as targets: CVP between 8 and 12 mm Hg; mean arterial pressure (MAP) of 65 mm Hg or greater; UO or 0.5 ml/kg/hr or greater; and ScvO$_2$ or SvO$_2$ of 70% or greater. (Grade B)
- If the above goals are not reached within the first 6 hours of resuscitation, then packed red blood cells should be transfused and/or dobutamine should be administered up to 20 mcg/kg/min. (Grade B)
- Low-dose dopamine for renal protection is not recommended. (Grade B)
- Increasing cardiac index to increase oxygen delivery to supranormal levels is not recommended. (Grade A)
- Corticosteroid doses greater than 300 mg a day are not recommended. (Grade A)
- Recombinant human activated protein C should be given to patients at high risk of death as long as no absolute contraindications to its use are present, and to patients with relative contraindications as long as the benefits of the drug outweigh the risks. (Grade B)

- Once tissue hypoperfusion has resolved, red blood cell transfusions should be used only when hemoglobin decreases below 7 g/dl or extenuating circumstances (e.g., acute hemorrhage) are present. (Grade B)
- Erythropoietin for anemia is not recommended unless another accepted reason for its administration is present. (Grade B)
- Antithrombin use is not recommended.
- Maintain tidal volume of 6 ml/kg and an end-inspiratory plateau pressure less than 30 cm H$_2$O while mechanically ventilated.
- Daily spontaneous breathing trials should be used to gauge the patient's readiness for extubation. (Grade A)
- A sedation protocol should be used to guide treatment of mechanically ventilated patients. (Grade B)
- The sedation protocol should include daily interruption or lightening of sedation. (Grade B)
- Continuous venovenous hemofiltration and intermittent hemodialysis are equally effective in the hemodynamically stable patient with acute renal failure. Continuous hemofiltration provides easier management of fluid balance in hemodynamically unstable patients. (Grade B)
- Deep vein thrombosis and stress ulcer prophylaxis should be given to patients with severe sepsis. (Grade A)

Data from Dellinger RP et al: Surviving Sepsis Campaign guidelines for management of severe sepsis and septic shock, *Crit Care Med* 32:858, 2004.

NURSING DIAGNOSES Septic Shock

- Deficient Fluid Volume related to relative loss
- Decreased Cardiac Output related to alterations in preload
- Decreased Cardiac Output related to alterations in afterload
- Decreased Cardiac Output related to alterations in contractility
- Impaired Gas Exchange related to ventilation/perfusion mismatching or intrapulmonary shunting
- Imbalanced Nutrition: Less Than Body Requirements related to increased metabolic demands or lack of exogenous nutrients
- Risk for Infection
- Anxiety related to threat to biologic, psychologic, or social integrity
- Compromised Family Coping related to critically ill family member

REFERENCES

1. Kumar A, Parrillo JE: Shock: classification, pathophysiology, and approach to management. In Parrillo JP, Dellinger RP, editors: *Critical care medicine: principles of diagnosis and management in the adult*, ed 2, St Louis, 2001, Mosby.
2. Hameed SM, Aird WC, Cohn SM: Oxygen delivery, *Crit Care Med* 31:S658, 2003.
3. Hotchkiss RS et al: Rapid onset of intestinal epithelial and lymphocyte apoptotic cell death in patients with trauma and shock, *Crit Care Med* 28:3207, 2000.
4. Kellum JA, Pinsky MR: Use of vasopressor agents in critically ill patients, *Curr Opin Crit Care* 8:236, 2002.
5. Dellinger RP: Cardiovascular management of septic shock, *Crit Care Med* 31:946, 2003.
6. Wilson M, Davis DP, Coimbra R: Diagnosis and monitoring of hemorrhagic shock during the initial resuscitation of multiple trauma patients: a review, *J Emerg Med* 24:413, 2003.
7. Chang MC: Monitoring of the critically injured patient, *New Horizons* 7:35, 1999.
8. Choi P et al: Crystalloids vs. colloids in fluid resuscitation: a systematic review, *Crit Care Med* 27:200, 1999.
9. Cook D, Guyatt G: Colloid use for fluid resuscitation: evidence and spin, *Ann Internal Med* 135:205, 2001.
10. Dellinger RP et al: Surviving Sepsis Campaign guidelines for management of severe sepsis and septic shock, *Crit Care Med* 32:858, 2004.
11. Wilkes MM, Navickis RJ: Patient survival after human albumin administration, *Ann Internal Med* 135:149, 2001.
12. Forsythe SM, Schmidt GA: Sodium bicarbonate for the treatment of lactic acidosis, *Chest* 117:260, 2000.
13. Cerra FB et al: Applied nutrition in ICU patients: a consensus statement of the American College of Chest Physicians, *Chest* 111:769, 1997.

14. Heys SD et al: Enteral nutritional supplementation with key nutrients in patients with critical illness and cancer: a meta-analysis of randomized controlled clinical trials, *Ann Surg* 222:467, 1999.
15. De Jong MJ: Family perceptions of support interventions in the intensive care unit, *Dimens Crit Care Nurs* 19(5):40, 2000.
16. Stein-Parbury J, McKinley S: Patients' experiences of being in an intensive care unit: a select literature review, *Am J Crit Care* 9:20-27, 2000.
17. Van Horn E, Tesh A: The effect of critical care hospitalization on family members: stress and responses, *Dimens Crit Care Nurs* 19(4):40, 2000.
18. Groeneveld ABJ: Hypovolemic shock. In Parrillo JP, Dellinger RP, editors: *Critical care medicine: principles of diagnosis and management in the adult*, ed 2, St Louis, 2001, Mosby.
19. Dutton RP, Mackenzie CF, Scalea TM: Hypotensive resuscitation during active hemorrhage: impact on in-hospital mortality, *J Trauma* 52:1141, 2002.
20. Revell M, Greaves I, Porter K: Endpoints for fluid resuscitation in hemorrhagic shock, *J Trauma* 54:S63, 2003.
21. Solomonov E et al: The effect of vigorous fluid resuscitation in uncontrolled hemorrhagic shock after massive splenic injury, *Crit Care Med* 28:749, 2000.
22. Stern SA: Low-volume fluid resuscitation for presumed hemorrhagic shock: helpful or harmful? *Curr Opin Crit Care* 7:422, 2001.
23. Ashby DT, Stone GW, Moses JW: Cardiogenic shock in acute myocardial infarction, *Catheter Cardiovasc Interv* 59:34, 2003.
24. Goldberg RJ et al: Recent magnitude of and temporal trends (1994-1997) in the incidence and hospital death rates of cardiogenic shock complicating acute myocardial infarction: the second National Registry of Myocardial Infarction, *Am Heart J* 141:65, 2001.
25. Hollenberg SM, Parrillo JP: Cardiogenic shock. In Parrillo JP, Dellinger RP, editors: *Critical care medicine: principles of diagnosis and management in the adult*, ed 2, St Louis, 2001, Mosby.
26. Hochman JS: Cardiogenic shock complicating acute myocardial infarction: expanding the paradigm, *Circulation* 107:2998, 2003.
27. Menon V, Fincke R: Cardiogenic shock: a summary of the randomized SHOCK trial, *Congest Heart Fail* 9:35, 2003.
28. Geppert A et al: Multiple organ failure in patients with cardiogenic shock is associated with high plasma levels of interleukin-6, *Crit Care Med* 30:1987, 2002.
29. Lim N et al: Do all nonsurvivors of cardiogenic shock die with a low cardiac index? *Chest* 124:1885, 2003.
30. Bowen FW et al: Application of "double bridge mechanical" resuscitation for profound cardiogenic shock leading to cardiac transplantation, *Ann Thorac Surg* 71:86, 2001.
31. Magliato KE et al: Biventricular support inpatient with profound cardiogenic shock: a single center experience, *ASAIO J* 49:475, 2003.
32. Meyns B et al: Initial experiences with the Impella device in patients with cardiogenic shock—Impella support for cardiogenic shock, *Thorac Cardiovasc Surg* 51:312, 2003.
33. Samuels LE et al: Management of acute cardiac failure with mechanical assist: experience with the ABIOMED BVS 5000, *Ann Thorac Surg* 71:S67, 2001.
34. Ellis AK, Day JH: Diagnosis and management of anaphylaxis, *CMAJ* 169:307, 2003.
35. Haupt MT: Anaphylaxis and anaphylactic shock. In Parrillo JP, Dellinger RP, editors: *Critical care medicine: principles of diagnosis and management in the adult*, ed 2, St Louis, 2001, Mosby.

36. Tang A: A practical guide to anaphylaxis, *Am Fam Physician* 38:1325, 2003.

37. McLean APC et al: Adrenaline in the treatment of anaphylaxis: what is the evidence? *BMJ* 327:1332, 2003.

38. Sicherer SH: Advances in anaphylaxis and hypersensitivity reactions to foods, drugs, and insect venom, *J Allergy Clin Immunol* 111:S829, 2003.

39. Frohna WJ: Emergency department evaluation and treatment of the neck and cervical spine injuries, *Emerg Med Clin North Am* 17:739, 1999.

40. Karlet MC: Acute management of the patient with spinal cord injury, *Int J Trauma Nurs* 7:43, 2001.

41. Bilello JF et al: Cervical spinal cord injury and the need for cardiovascular intervention, *Arch Surg* 138:1127, 2003.

42. American College of Chest Physicians/Society of Critical Care Medicine Consensus Conference Committee: Definitions for sepsis and organ failure and guidelines for the use of innovative therapies in sepsis, *Crit Care Med* 20:864, 1992.

43. Ely EW, Kleinpell RM, Goyette RE: Advances in the understanding of clinical manifestations and therapy of severe sepsis: an update for critical care nurses, *Am J Crit Care* 12:120, 2003.

44. Vincent JL: Hemodynamic support in septic shock, *Intensive Care Med* 27:S80, 2001.

45. Angus DC et al: Epidemiology of severe sepsis in the United States: analysis of incidence, outcome, and associated costs of care, *Crit Care Med* 29:1303, 2001.

46. Martin GS et al: The epidemiology of sepsis in the United States from 1979 through 2000, *N Engl J Med* 348:1546, 2003.

47. Levy MN et al: 2001 SCCM/ESICM/ACCP/ATS/SIS International sepsis definitions conference, *Crit Care Med* 31:1250, 2003.

48. Bernard GR et al: Efficacy and safety of recombinant human activated protein C for severe sepsis, *JAMA* 344:699, 2001.

49. Fish DN: Optimal antimicrobial therapy for sepsis, *Am J Health Syst Pharm* 59:S13, 2002.

50. Ahrens T, Vollman K: Severe sepsis management: are we doing enough? *Crit Care Nurs* 23(Suppl):2, 2003.

51. Dettenmeier P et al: Role of activated protein C in the pathophysiology of severe sepsis, *Am J Crit Care* 12:518, 2003.

52. Groeneveld AB et al: Circulating inflammatory mediators predict shock and mortality in febrile patients with microbial infection, *Clin Immunol* 106:106, 2003.

53. Russwurm S et al: Platelet and leukocyte activation correlate with severity of septic organ dysfunction, *Shock* 17:263, 2002.

54. Sharma S, Kumar A: Septic shock, multiple organ failure, and acute respiratory distress syndrome, *Curr Opin Pulm Med* 9:199, 2003.

55. Angus DC, Crowther MA: Unraveling severe sepsis: why did OPTIMIST fail and what's next? *JAMA* 290:256, 2003.

56. Tamion F et al: Gastric mucosal acidosis and cytokine release in patients with septic shock, *Crit Care Med* 31:2237, 2003.

57. Mizock BA: Metabolic derangements in sepsis and septic shock, *Crit Care Clin* 16:319, 2000.

58. Brealey D et al: Association between mitochondrial dysfunction and severity and outcome of septic shock, *Lancet* 360:219, 2002.

59. Balk RA: Severe sepsis and septic shock: definitions, epidemiology, and clinical manifestations, *Crit Care Clin* 16:179, 2000.

60. Rivers E et al: Early goal-directed therapy in the treatment of severe sepsis and septic shock, *N Engl J Med* 345:1368, 2001.

61. The ARDS Network: Ventilation with lower tidal volumes as compared with traditional tidal volumes for acute lung injury and the acute respiratory distress syndrome, *N Engl J Med* 342:1301, 2000.

62. Kress JP et al: Daily interruption of sedative infusions in critically ill patients undergoing mechanical ventilation, *N Engl J Med* 342:1471, 2000.

63. Powers J, Jacobi J: Treatment of severe sepsis with Xigris: implications for the clinical nurse specialist, *Clin Nurse Spec* 17:128, 2003.

64. Dellinger RP, Parrillo JE: Mediator modulation therapy of severe sepsis and septic shock: does it work? *Crit Care Med* 32:282, 2004.

65. Annane D et al: Effect of treatment with low doses of hydrocortisone and fludrocortisone on mortality in patients with septic shock, *JAMA* 288:862, 2002.

66. Van den Berghe G et al: Intensive insulin therapy in the critically ill patients, *N Engl J Med* 345:1359, 2001.

Systemic Inflammatory Response Syndrome and Multiple Organ Dysfunction Syndrome

*A*dvanced cardiopulmonary life support techniques and technology have allowed for the survival of some critically ill or injured patients who previously would have died of an initial insult such as trauma, infection, shock, or other acute process. However, continued patient survival and long-term quality of life are threatened by two clinical syndromes—systemic inflammatory response syndrome (SIRS) and multiple organ dysfunction syndrome (MODS)—that may result in death or profound disability. SIRS is characterized by generalized systemic inflammation in organs remote from an initial insult. MODS results from SIRS and pertains to progressive physiologic failure of several interdependent organ systems; it is the major cause of death of patients cared for in critical care units.[1-3]

In 1992 the American College of Chest Physicians and the Society of Critical Care Medicine adopted a framework that described the interrelationships among the systemic inflammatory response, sepsis, bacteremia, and infection (Fig. 39-1) and multiple organ dysfunction (see Fig. 39-2).[4] New terminology was proposed to describe the clinical manifestations of SIRS and its relationship to sepsis and MODS. Critical care professionals were urged to standardize terminology used in diagnosis, intervention, and research protocols.[4] In the past, terms such as *multiple systems organ failure, multiple organ failure syndrome*, and *progressive* or *sequential organ failure* were used to describe clinical syndromes of organ failure in critically ill patients. Because these terms imply organ failure rather than the dynamic process of organ dysfunction, the name of the syndrome was changed to *multiple organ dysfunction syndrome*.[4]

In 2001 the Society of Critical Care Medicine, the European Society of Intensive Care Medicine, the American College of Chest Physicians, the American Thoracic Society, and the Surgical Infection Society revisited the definitions for SIRS and sepsis, and attempted to identify methodologies for improving the accuracy and reliability in diagnosis. No changes to the proposed definitions from ten years earlier were made; however, an expansion of the list of signs and symptoms of sepsis based on experienced clinical observations was established.[5]

This chapter provides information regarding the pathogenesis of SIRS and MODS. Current clinical management, select investigational therapies, and appropriate nursing diagnoses are addressed.

THE INFLAMMATORY RESPONSE

Acute inflammation is a biochemical and cellular process that only occurs in vascularized tissue in response to an insult or invasion.[6] During inflammation the body creates a lethal microenvironment to localize the injury and kill microorganisms. Normally the inflammatory process is contained within a restricted environment. If it is not contained, a systemic widespread response (SIRS) occurs that is deleterious to organ function.[1,6,7] Fortunately, the body normally has a complex system of checks and balances to localize inflammation.

LOCAL INFLAMMATORY RESPONSE

The acute inflammatory response is a self-limiting (generally 8 to 10 days), nonspecific response that usually occurs in an identical manner regardless of the cause. The response generally starts within seconds of the insult. Cell injury or death initiates the acute inflammatory response. Cellular injury may result from trauma, hypoxia, or microorganisms.[6]

Mediators, facilitators of the local inflammatory response, are housed in the circulatory system and enhance the movement of plasma and blood cells from the circulation into the tissue around the injury. Mediators of the vascular response include leukocytes; plasma protein cascades (complement, coagulation, kinin/kallikrein); platelets; and other inflammatory biochemicals, such as arachidonic acid (AA) metabolites (e.g., prostaglandins [PGs], interleukins [ILs], and tumor necrosis factor [TNF]).[6]

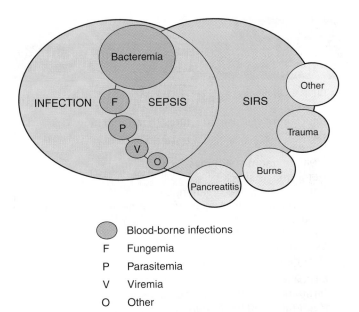

Fig. 39-1 Interrelationships among systemic inflammatory response syndrome (SIRS), sepsis, and infection. (From American College of Chest Physicians/Society of Critical Care Medicine Consensus Conference Committee: *Crit Care Med* 20:865, 1992.)

Blood-borne infections
F   Fungemia
P   Parasitemia
V   Viremia
O   Other

Vascular Response. The local vascular effects of inflammation start immediately and sustain increased vascular permeability that lasts through acute inflammation. Several mechanisms are operable. Arterioles near the injury constrict briefly and then dilate to increase blood flow to the injured area and allow exudation of plasma and cells into tissues. Exudation causes interstitial edema and slows the microcirculation, making it more viscous. Concurrently, mediators such as bradykinin stimulate capillary and venule endothelial cells to retract, creating spaces at junctions between cells. Endothelial cell retraction allows leukocytes to squeeze out of the cell. The net effect is the movement of blood cells and plasma proteins into the inflamed tissue.[6]

Neutrophil Response. Neutrophils engage in four functions related to inflammation: margination, diapedesis, chemotaxis, and phagocytosis. Many neutrophils normally adhere to the inside of blood vessel walls until needed (margination). On activation, neutrophils move to the area of injury by squeezing through the pores of blood vessels (diapedesis), are attracted to microbials or debris by chemical substances (chemotaxis), phagocytose bacteria or cellular debris, and then die. Monocytes and macrophages perform similar functions in a later stage of the inflammatory process.[6]

Plasma Protein Response. Three major plasma protein systems—the complement, kinin/kallikrein, and coagulation systems—participate in the acute inflammatory response.

Complement System. The complement system, a complex cascade of more than 20 serum proteins, is in-

volved in inflammatory and immune processes that destroy bacteria and contribute to vascular changes. Eleven principal proteins, labeled C1 through C9, have been identified. Activation of the complement cascade occurs through the classic pathway in response to an antigen/antibody complex or through an alternate pathway by exposure to polysaccharide from bacterial cell walls. The terminal pathway for both the classic and alternate pathways results in lysis of the target cell. The effects of complement during inflammation are outlined in Box 39-1.[6] With activation of complement proteins, stimulation of coagulation, mast cells, and platelets ensues.[8] Complement proteins are considered to be the most potent defenders against bacterial infection.[6]

Kinin/Kallikrein System. The kinin/kallikrein system controls vascular tone and permeability and is activated by stimulation of the plasma kinin cascade. Hageman factor (factor XII) of the coagulation cascade is also directly involved in kinin activation. Kinins are biochemicals that are controlled by kinases, enzymes present in the plasma and tissues. The end result of kinin activation is the production of bradykinin. Bradykinin has profound effects, including vasodilation at low doses, pain, extravascular smooth muscle contraction, increased vascular permeability, and leukocyte chemotaxis. Bradykinin facilitates endothelial retraction and increased vascular permeability, processes involved in acute inflammation.[6]

Coagulation System. The coagulation system traps bacteria in injured tissue to prevent the spread of infection and together with platelets functions to control excessive bleeding. The human body normally maintains a balance between clot formation (thrombosis), which is needed to minimize blood loss and to repair wounds, and clot lysis (fibrinolysis), which maintains the patency of blood vessels.[6] The coagulation system is a plasma protein system that, like the complement cascade, can be activated through two pathways. The intrinsic pathway is activated when damaged endothelial cells come into direct contact with circulating blood. In this contact phase, proteins activate additional coagulation factors

(XII, XI, IX, and VIII). The extrinsic pathway is activated by damaged tissue, which releases tissue factor and activates coagulation factor VII. Both pathways converge at factor X and proceed to fibrin polymerization and clot formation. Thirteen plasma proteins (factors I to XIII), produced primarily in the liver, participate in the coagulation cascade. The fibrinolytic system lyses fibrin clots through the actions of proteolytic and lysosomal enzymes. Plasmin splits fibrin and fibrinogen into fibrin degradation products; consequently, the clots dissolve. It is this delicate balance between thrombin and plasmin in the circulation that maintains normal coagulation and lysis during the inflammatory process. The end result of these complex interactions is a lesion that is ready to heal.[6,8,9] For further discussion of the coagulation system, see Chapter 42.

Platelets. Platelets normally circulate in the bloodstream until vascular injury occurs. Immediately after cellular injury, platelets work synergistically with the coagulation cascade to stop bleeding. Secondly, platelets degranulate and release biochemical mediators, which have profound vascular effects. Normally, complex systems work together to limit and localize the inflammatory response, thus limiting and confining the potentially destructive effects of uncontrolled mediator activity. Antiproteases, circulating albumin, vitamins C and E, red blood cells, and phagocytic cells limit the inflammatory response by inhibiting proteolytic enzyme activity, scavenging reactive oxygen metabolites, and removing the stimulus by phagocytosis.[6,8-10]

SYSTEMIC INFLAMMATORY RESPONSE

The systemic inflammatory response is an abnormal host response characterized by generalized inflammation in organs remote from the initial insult.[1] SIRS pertains to the widespread inflammation or clinical responses to inflammation occurring in patients suffering a variety of insults. Clinical conditions and manifestations associated with SIRS are listed in Box 39-2. These insults produce similar or identical systemic inflammatory responses, even in the absence of infection. SIRS is present when two or more of four clinical manifestations are present in the high-risk patient. Manifestations of SIRS must represent an acute alteration from the patient's normal baseline and must not be related to other causes (e.g., neutropenia from chemotherapy). Organ dysfunction or failure, such as acute lung injury, acute renal failure, and MODS, is a complication of SIRS.[1,2,4,5,7] The findings of a recent epidemiology study suggest that SIRS occurs in one third of all hospitalized patients, in more than 50% of all patients in critical care units, and in about 80% of all patients in surgical critical care units.[11]

When SIRS is a result of infection, the term *sepsis* is used. Severe sepsis is sepsis with either hypoperfusion or systemic manifestations of hypoperfusion. Septic shock is sepsis-induced hypotension despite fluid resuscitation.

Box 39-2

CLINICAL CONDITIONS AND MANIFESTATIONS ASSOCIATED WITH SIRS

CLINICAL CONDITIONS
Infection
Infection of vascular structures (heart and lungs)
Pancreatitis
Ischemia
Multiple trauma with massive tissue injury
Hemorrhagic shock
Immune-mediated organ injury
Exogenous administration of tumor necrosis factor or other cytokines
Aspiration of gastric contents
Massive transfusion
Host defense abnormalities

CLINICAL MANIFESTATIONS
Temperature >38° C or <36° C
Heart rate >90 beats/min
Respiratory rate >20 breaths/min or $Paco_2$ <32 mm Hg
WBC >12,000 cells/mm³ or <4000 cells/mm³ or >10% immature (band) forms

SIRS, Systemic inflammatory response syndrome.

Therefore SIRS, sepsis, severe sepsis, and septic shock represent a hierarchical continuum of the inflammatory response to infection.[12] Although infection and shock remain the most common precipitating factors, any disease that can induce a major inflammatory response is capable of initiating the events that lead to MODS.[2]

When SIRS is not contained, several consequences occur that lead to organ dysfunction including intense, uncontrolled activation of inflammatory cells; direct damage of vascular endothelium; disruption of immune cell function; persistent hypermetabolism; and maldistribution of circulatory volume to organ systems.[1-3] Consequently, inflammation becomes a systemic, self-perpetuating process that is inadequately controlled and results in organ dysfunction[2,6,13] (see the Clinical Application feature on Multiple Organ Dysfunction Syndrome, which discusses a patient who experiences SIRS).

However, not all patients develop MODS from SIRS. The development of MODS appears to be associated with failure to control the source of inflammation or infection, persistent hypoperfusion, flow-dependent oxygen consumption (Vo_2), and/or the continued presence of necrotic tissue.[2]

MULTIPLE ORGAN DYSFUNCTION SYNDROME

MODS results from progressive physiologic failure of two or more separate organ systems. It is defined as the "presence of altered organ function in an acutely ill pa-

CLINICAL APPLICATION

Multiple Organ Dysfunction Syndrome

Mr. H is a 38-year-old white, well-nourished construction worker who sustained abdominal injuries and a liver laceration that required surgical intervention (exploratory laparotomy, repair of liver laceration, splenectomy) after volume resuscitation in the field and emergency room. His previous medical history reveals no chronic health problems. However, he is a 20-pack/year smoker. During the immediate postoperative period (days 1 and 2), Mr. H was extubated. He was lethargic but oriented and hemodynamically stable, with mild volume depletion (as evidenced by measured and derived hemodynamic data from the pulmonary artery catheter). He required low-flow nasal oxygen (2 L/min) to maintain a PaO_2 of 75 mm Hg and an O_2 saturation above 95% (assessed continuously via pulse oximetry). Despite his relatively stable hemodynamic profile, he was tachycardic (sinus) and mildly tachypneic (respiratory rate, 26 breaths/min), with diminished breath sounds at both bases. He comprehended and was able to use patient-controlled analgesia (PCA) but frequently awakened anxious and in pain. Urine output was low but adequate for intravenous intake; skin and extremities were cool to the touch; and core temperature was 37° C. Mr. H's abdomen was distended, with absent bowel sounds. A nasogastric tube was draining small amounts of dark-green drainage. His surgical wound was well approximated, with no redness or drainage. Laboratory data revealed normochromic normocytic anemia (hemoglobin, 9.8 g/dl; hematocrit, 25%); leukocytosis (white blood cell [WBC] count, 13,000/mm^3); and an elevated serum lactate level. Arterial blood gas (ABG) values indicated a primary respiratory alkalosis and metabolic acidosis. Serum potassium levels were high; consequently no potassium was added to intravenous fluids.

1. You suspect Mr. H is experiencing systemic inflammatory response syndrome (SIRS). What signs and symptoms are evident to support your suspicions?
2. What are your nursing priorities for Mr. H at this time?
3. What additional interventions should you incorporate into your plan of care?

Despite his relatively stable clinical status during the first 2 postoperative days, on day 3 Mr. H was becoming progressively more tachycardic, tachypneic, and anxious. He required 100% oxygen via face mask. Chest film results demonstrated widespread alveolar opacification consistent with acute respiratory distress syndrome (ARDS). ABG values revealed refractory hypoxemia, with high anion gap primary metabolic and respiratory acidosis. Consequently, oral intubation and volume-cycled mechanical ventilation were used. Positive end-expiratory pressure (PEEP) at 10 cm H_2O was added incrementally to maximize oxygenation without compromising cardiac output and oxygen delivery.

Measures of static and dynamic lung compliance were consistent with decreasing lung compliance; oxygen indexes and derived shunt calculations demonstrated severe ventilation/perfusion mismatching and intrapulmonary shunting. Hemodynamic data continued to show a hyperdynamic cardiovascular profile. ABG values remained unchanged. Energy expenditure as measured with use of a metabolic cart demonstrated hypermetabolism, with increased oxygen consumption and carbon dioxide production. Enteral nutrition via a small-bore jejunal feeding tubing was attempted without success; consequently, total parenteral nutrition (TPN) was started at 25 to 30 kcal/kg/day via a newly placed internal jugular catheter. Appropriate fat supplementation also was provided.

4. Early nutritional support is important in preventing or limiting which complication of SIRS?

On days 6 and 7 Mr. H remained intubated and required 100% O_2 to maintain a PaO_2 of 70 mm Hg. Core temperature was 38.4° C and WBC count 18,000/mm^3 with a shift to the left. However, blood, urine, and wound cultures were negative. Despite the aggressive administration of diuretics, Mr. H was oliguric and azotemic, with renal indexes consistent with acute tubular necrosis. Serum creatinine and blood urea nitrogen (BUN) levels were approaching the need for hemodialysis. His level of consciousness was difficult to evaluate because paralytic agents and narcotics had been used to facilitate effective mechanical ventilation. Since admission, Mr. H had lost 8 pounds. His condition was highly catabolic, hyperglycemic, and in a negative nitrogen balance. Visceral protein (serum albumin, transferrin, prealbumin) levels were low despite nutritional and metabolic support. Hepatic function was altered as evidenced by elevated serum bilirubin, aspartate aminotransferase (AST), alanine aminotransferase (ALT), and lactate dehydrogenase (LDH) levels; clinical jaundice was evident. Mr. H's abdomen was distended, and bowel sounds were absent. He was unresponsive to all noxious stimuli and no longer required paralytics or narcotics for effective ventilation. Cardiovascular function was dependent on vasoactive drugs (dopamine at 10 mcg/kg/min) to maintain a subnormal cardiac output. Mr. H's family was notified of his grave prognosis. They were angry and grief-stricken.

5. Which of Mr. H's organs are failing? List the signs and symptoms to support your answer.
6. What treatments should you anticipate being initiated to support Mr. H's failing organs?
7. What are your nursing priorities for Mr. H at this time?
8. What are your nursing priorities for Mr. H's family at this time?

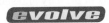 For the discussion of this Clinical Application and for an additional clinical application on MODS, see the Evolve website.

tient such that homeostasis cannot be maintained without intervention."[4] Dysfunction of one organ may amplify dysfunction in another. Organ dysfunction may be absolute or relative and is a leading cause of late mortality after trauma.[13-15]

INCIDENCE

Lack of consensus regarding definitions for organ dysfunction, the number of organs involved, and the duration of organ dysfunction have hampered an accurate account of organ dysfunction in critically ill patients. Failure of two or more organs is associated with an estimated 45% to 55% mortality. This may increase to 80% when three or more organ systems fail, and 100% if three or more organ systems fail for longer than 4 days.[3] Patient outcome is directly related to the number of organs that fail.

HIGH-RISK PATIENTS

Although various patient populations are at risk for organ dysfunction, trauma patients are particularly vulnerable because they often experience no–flow-reflow (or ischemia-reperfusion) events secondary to hemorrhage, blunt trauma, or sympathetic nervous system–induced vasoconstriction.[16] Other high-risk patients include those who have experienced infection, a shock episode, various ischemia-reperfusion events, acute pancreatitis, sepsis, burns, aspiration, multiple blood transfusions, or surgical complications.[17,18] Patients aged 65 years and older are at increased risk secondary to their decreased organ reserve and comorbidities.[19]

CLINICAL COURSE AND PROGRESSION

Organ dysfunction may be a direct consequence of the insult (primary MODS) or can manifest latently and involve organs not directly affected in the initial insult (secondary MODS) (Fig. 39-2). Patients can experience both primary and secondary MODS.

Primary MODS. Primary MODS "directly results from a well-defined insult in which organ dysfunction occurs early and is directly attributed to the insult itself"[4] and accounts for only a small fraction of MODS cases. Direct insults initially cause localized inflammatory responses. Examples of primary MODS include the immediate consequences of posttraumatic pulmonary failure, thermal injuries, acute tubular necrosis, or invasive infections.[2] These cellular or microcirculatory events may lead to a loss of critical organ function induced by failure of delivery of oxygen and substrates, coupled with the inability to remove end-products of metabolism.[2,14] Primary MODS generally results in one of three patient outcomes: recovery, a stable hypermetabolic state (limited SIRS), or death.[18]

Secondary MODS. Secondary MODS is a consequence of widespread systemic inflammation that results in dysfunction of organs not involved in the initial insult.[4-5] The focus of the following discussion pertains to the relationship between SIRS and secondary MODS.

Secondary MODS develops latently after an initial insult. The early impairment of organs normally involved in immunoregulatory function, such as the liver and the gastrointestinal (GI) tract, intensifies the host response to the insult. This intensified host response may be determined by factors such as age, comorbidities, gene transcription, and others.[20] It is postulated that the initial insult "primes" the inflammatory system in such a way that a mild second "hit" may perpetuate a hyperinflammatory response. SIRS/sepsis is a common initiating event in the development of secondary MODS. Severe sepsis appears to initiate a period of circulatory instability and relative physiologic shock that is perpetuated by a cascade of inflammatory mediators, endothelial injury, bacterial insult, and microcirculatory failure.[13] Noninfectious stimuli (inflammation, perfusion deficit, or dead tissue) also initiate similar cellular consequences. Interruption of tissue perfusion may ensue as a result of mismatched oxygen supply and demand, setting the stage for activation of SIRS and MODS.[18]

The definitive clinical course of secondary MODS has not been completely identified. One theory suggests that organ dysfunction may occur in a sequential or progressive pattern. This pattern generally begins with the lungs, the most commonly affected major organ, then goes on to involve the liver, the gut, and finally the kidneys. A late component is cardiac and, at times, bone marrow dysfunction. Neurologic and coagulopathic impairment may occur at any time during this progression.[21] Organs may fail simultaneously; for example, re-

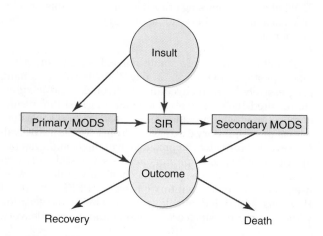

Fig. 39-2 Different causes and results of primary and secondary multiple organ dysfunction syndrome (MODS). *SIR,* Systemic inflammatory response. (From American College of Chest Physicians/ Society of Critical Care Medicine Consensus Conference Committee: *Crit Care Med* 20:868, 1992.)

nal dysfunction may occur concurrently with hepatic dysfunction. After the initial insult and resuscitation, patients develop persistent hypermetabolism, a metabolic consequence of sustained systemic inflammation and physiologic stress, followed closely by pulmonary dysfunction, manifested as acute lung injury (ALI).

Hypermetabolism accompanies SIRS but may not occur immediately after insult. Hypermetabolism generally lasts from 7 days to more than 3 weeks, and may be defined as resting energy expenditure greater than 115% of the predicted basal energy expenditure and oxygen consumption.[22] During hypermetabolism, changes occur in cellular anabolic and catabolic function, resulting in autocatabolism. Autocatabolism manifests as a severe decrease in lean body mass, severe weight loss, anergy, and increased cardiac output and Vo_2 secondary to profound alterations in carbohydrate, protein, and fat metabolism and production.[22] Concurrently, GI, hepatic, and immunologic dysfunction may occur, which intensifies the SIRS. Clinical consequences may affect gut function, wound healing, muscles wasting, host response, respiratory function, and continued promotion of the hypermetabolic response.[22]

A significant predictor of mortality in MODS is a change in organ system dysfunction over the initial 3 days. Worsening neurologic, renal, and hematologic function are specific to an increased mortality.[23] The development of renal and hepatic failure is a preterminal event in MODS, with death most common approximately 14 to 21 days after the initial insult.[18] Patients with decreased physiologic organ reserve may manifest signs and symptoms of organ dysfunction earlier than previously healthy patients.[1,13,19] Survivors may develop generalized polyneuropathy and a chronic form of pulmonary disease from ALI, complicating recovery. These patients often require prolonged, expensive rehabilitation.

PATHOPHYSIOLOGIC MECHANISMS

Secondary MODS results from altered regulation of the patient's acute immune and inflammatory responses. Dysregulation, or failure to control the host inflammatory response, leads to the excessive production of inflammatory cells and biochemical mediators that cause widespread damage to vascular endothelium and organ damage.[1,18,24] The critically ill patient's compromised immune state also fosters an environment conducive to organ failure.

The inflammatory and immune responses implicated in SIRS and MODS are evoked by certain cells and biochemicals that, in turn, affect cellular activity. As outlined in Box 39-3, mediators associated with SIRS and MODS can be classified as inflammatory cells, biochemical mediators, or plasma protein systems. Activation of one mediator often leads to activation of another. The biologic activity of inflammatory cells, biochemical media-

tors, and plasma protein systems and how they work in concert to cause SIRS and MODS has not yet been totally determined. The plasma protein systems were discussed earlier in the chapter in the local inflammatory response section.

Inflammatory Cells. Neutrophils, macrophages, monocytes, mast cells, platelets, and endothelial cells are inflammatory cells that mediate SIRS through their production of cytokines (biochemical mediators). Along with proinflammatory biochemicals released from damaged or necrotic tissue and circulating catecholamines (stress response), these inflammatory cells create a hypermetabolic state, cause maldistribution of circulatory volume, and alter inflammatory and immune function.[1,24]

Neutrophils. During SIRS and MODS, neutrophils overreact systemically and damage normal cells, in addition to killing bacteria. Specifically, neutrophils adhere to vascular endothelium and release cytotoxic biochemicals including platelet-activating factor (PAF), TNF, AA metabolites, and toxic oxygen metabolites.[1-3,7,8,11] These substances cause tissue damage, vascular injury, edema, thrombosis, and hemorrhage in multiple organ systems. During SIRS/sepsis, neutrophilic function also is modulated by other circulating mediators that intensify its inflammatory response.[24]

Box 39-3

INFLAMMATORY MEDIATORS ASSOCIATED WITH SIRS AND MODS

INFLAMMATORY CELLS
Neutrophils
Macrophages/monocytes
Mast
Lymphocytes
Endothelial

BIOCHEMICAL MEDIATORS
Reactive oxygen species
    Superoxide radical
    Hydroxyl radical
    Hydrogen peroxide
Tumor necrosis factor
Interleukins
Platelet activating factor
Arachidonic acid metabolites
    Prostaglandins
    Leukotrienes
    Thromboxanes
Proteases

PLASMA PROTEIN SYSTEMS
Complement
Kinin
Coagulation

SIRS, Systemic inflammatory response syndrome; *MODS,* multiple organ dysfunction syndrome.

Monocytes and Macrophages. Monocytes and macrophages normally perform three major functions relative to inflammation: antigen processing and presentation, bacterial phagocytosis, and mediator production. Monocytes and macrophages detect, process, and present antigen to lymphocytes for initiation of the humoral and cellular components of the lymphocytic immune response. Macrophages play a significant role in organ injury by producing oxygen metabolites, initiating procoagulant activity, and releasing IL-1 and TNF. Both TNF and IL-1 then stimulate neutrophils and lymphocytes to activate the AA cascade. AA metabolites are vasoactive and cause vascular instability and altered organ blood flow.[8,24,25]

In the lungs, alveolar macrophages produce toxic oxygen metabolites and proteolytic enzymes that destroy alveolar epithelial cells. The role of macrophages and monocytes in organ dysfunction is most directly linked to their production of TNF and IL-1.[1,6,8]

Mast Cells. Mast cells are found in all body tissues, especially those adjacent to blood vessels. As tissue-based cells, mast cells produce mediators that have both systemic and local effects. Endotoxin, direct cellular injury, complement proteins (C3a and C5a), and bradykinin stimulate the release of mast cell mediators. Mediators from mast cells include histamine, proteases, heparin, TNF, select AA metabolites, and PAF.[1,25]

Lymphocytes. Lymphocytes adhere to and are sequestered in the microvascular endothelium. Stimulated T and B lymphocytes produce cytokines such as IL-1 and IL-2, which in turn activate other inflammatory cells.[25]

Endothelial Cells. The endothelium is a unicellular layer that lines the entire vascular system. Normally little interaction occurs between the endothelium and leukocytes. However, during SIRS and MODS, endothelial cells not only become targets for leukocyte-derived mediators but also become dysfunctional and release prothrombotic, proinflammatory, and vasoactive mediators. Endothelial damage results in the production of procoagulants such as PAF, plasminogen-activating inhibitor, angiotensin II, and prostacyclin (AA metabolite), as well as in the development of a procoagulant state, leading to introduction of thrombin in the microvasculature.[16,24] In addition, endothelial cells manufacture chemotactic agents that attract neutrophils to areas of inflammation and endothelial injury. Collectively, these processes cause widespread endothelial destruction, intravascular coagulation, and vascular instability and permeability, key elements in SIRS/sepsis. Inflammatory mediators that cause endothelial damage include endotoxin, TNF, IL-1, and PAF. These mediators also recruit and activate neutrophils and activate complement and perpetuate destruction of the endothelium.[24] Endothelial cells also produce and maintain a physiologic equilibrium between endothelin (the most potent vasoconstrictor known) and endothelial-derived relaxant factor (ni-

tric oxide), a vasodilator. An alteration in this balance leads to vascular instability, vasodilation, and the perfusion abnormalities commonly seen in patients with SIRS/sepsis.[6,26]

Biochemical Mediators. Multiple biochemical inflammatory mediators play a role in SIRS and MODS, including proteases, TNF, interleukins, PAF, AA metabolites, and oxygen metabolites. TNF, IL-1, IL-6, and IL-8 appear to be the most important cytokines associated with SIRS and MODS.

Reactive Oxygen Species. Reactive oxygen species are produced in excessive amounts during critical illness and have been implicated in MODS. Oxygen metabolites are normally produced as the result of many physiologic processes. However, the body has numerous antioxidant and enzyme systems to convert free oxygen radicals to nontoxic substances to prevent tissue injury. Excessive oxygen metabolites cause lipid peroxidation and damage to the cell membrane, activate the complement and coagulation cascades, and cause deoxyribonucleic acid (DNA) damage.[10] Inflammatory neutrophils cause tissue injury by producing excessive numbers of reactive oxygen metabolites (ROM). For example, ROMs produced by neutrophils cause lung injury in ALI.[10,27] Reperfusion organ injury is partially attributed to excessive ROMs. During reperfusion, severe tissue injury follows the massive production of oxygen free radicals. The organs most susceptible to injury include the small intestines, the liver, the lungs, the muscles, the heart, the brain, the stomach, and the skin. In the future, antioxidant drug therapy may be effective in preventing organ dysfunction.[1,10,20,27]

Tumor Necrosis Factor-α. Tumor necrosis factor-α (TNF-α, also known as *cachectin*) is a polypeptide that is released from macrophages and lymphocytes in response to endotoxin, tissue injury, viral agents, and interleukins. When present in excessive amounts, TNF-α causes widespread destruction in most organ systems and is responsible for the pathophysiologic changes in SIRS/sepsis and gram-negative shock, including fever, hypotension, decreased organ perfusion, and increased capillary permeability.[13] TNF-α may precipitate organ injury by causing generalized endothelial injury, fibrin deposition, and a procoagulant state. TNF-α causes disseminated intravascular coagulopathy (DIC); interstitial pneumonitis; acute tubular necrosis (ATN); and necrosis of the GI tract, liver, and adrenal glands. TNF-α stimulates AA metabolism, the clotting cascade, and the production of PAF. Metabolically, excessive TNF-α causes hyperglycemia that progresses to hypoglycemia and hypertriglyceridemia. The destructive effects of TNF-α are exacerbated by AA metabolites and stress hormones.[13,15,20,22,24] Biologic effects of TNF-α are numerous and are outlined in Box 39-4.

Interleukins. The interleukins are a class of cytokines that have similar biologic responses to those of TNF-α, and both work similarly. At this time 14 interleukins have been identified. Interleukin-1 (IL-1) has two known forms that cause organ dysfunction synergistically. However, the effects of TNF-α are more destructive. Interleukins are produced primarily by monophagocytic and endothelial cells. Macrophages secrete substantial amounts of IL-1, whereas less is secreted by endothelial cells, epithelial cells, neutrophils, and B lymphocytes. IL-1 causes vascular congestion, capillary leakage, and increased coagulation, all of which are associated with SIRS/sepsis. Like TNF-α, IL-1 has profound vascular endothelial effects. IL-1 stimulates the production of procoagulants by endothelial cells, increases catabolism of muscle tissue, and causes neutrophilia. Cardiovascular and inflammatory effects commonly include hypotension, fever, tachycardia, diarrhea, ALI, leukopenia, platelet aggregation, and disseminated intravascular coagulation.[24] IL-1 and other immune cells enhance the production of IL-2, which amplifies the cardiovascular responses. IL-6 is a glycoprotein released by lymphocytes, macrophages, and fibroblasts; it mediates the acute phase response to injury and stimulates the proliferation of B cells.[27] IL-8 is a potent leukocyte activator, specifically for neutrophilic chemotactic recruitment.[28] Raised levels of IL-8 have been detected soon after IL-6 is identified after insult. The influences of IL-8 on leukocyte activities and attraction suggest that IL-8 is important in the development of MODS and acute lung injury.[15,28,29]

Platelet-Activating Factor. PAF is a lipid that attaches to cell membrane phospholipids and is released from inflammatory and immune cells in response to a multitude of factors or stimuli that also initiate AA metabolism. PAF is released by platelets, mast cells, monocytes, macrophages, neutrophils, and endothelial cells. PAF has widespread effects on the heart, the vascular system, coagulation, platelets, and the lungs. Effects of PAF include platelet aggregation, with resultant microvascular stasis and ischemia in the microvascular bed; platelet release of serotonin, which increases vascular permeability; and increased vasoconstriction from increased production of thromboxane A_2, an AA metabolite.[24,30]

Arachidonic Acid Metabolites. AA is a highly metabolic fatty acid that is a precursor of many biologically active substances known as *eicosanoids*. Select eicosanoids are implicated in the pathogenesis of SIRS and MODS. Eicosanoids contribute to organ failure by altering vascular reactivity and permeability and by fostering the accumulation and activation of inflammatory cells.[31] Activation of the AA cascade by hypoxia, ischemia, endotoxin, catecholamines, and tissue injury produces metabolites from both the cyclooxygenase and lipooxygenase pathways. AA metabolites produced via the cyclooxygenase pathway are called *prostaglandins* (PGs) and *thromboxanes* (Txs), whereas those from the lipooxygenase pathway are called *leukotrienes* (LTs). AA metabolites have profound effects on vasculature and cause vascular instability and maldistribution of blood flow. Eicosanoids (such as PGH_2 and PGF_2, TxA_2 and TxB_2) and leukotrienes LTD_4, LTC_4, and LTE_4 are vasoconstrictors. In contrast, some eicosanoids have vasodilatory properties. All leukotrienes and TxA_2 enhance capillary membrane permeability and increase vascular leakage. TxA_2, PGH_2, and PGF_2 are potent platelet aggregators.[31]

Proteases. Proteases are proteolytic (protein-digesting) enzymes released from inflammatory cells. Proteases digest tissue and can cause significant parenchymal damage. Neutrophils in the lung, for example, produce proteases that destroy lung tissue. In the GI tract, protease-induced mucosal injuries occur.[32]

ORGAN-SPECIFIC MANIFESTATIONS

Secondary MODS is a systemic disease with organ-specific manifestations. Organ dysfunction is influenced by numerous factors, including organ host defense function, response time to the injury, metabolic requirements, organ vasculature response to vasoactive drugs, and organ sensitivity to damage and physiologic reserve. The responses of the GI, hepatobiliary, cardiovascular, pulmonary, renal, and coagulation systems are discussed in the following text. Clinical manifestations of organ dysfunction are outlined in Box 39-5.

Gastrointestinal Dysfunction. The GI tract plays an important role in MODS. GI organs normally have immunoregulatory functions. The GI tract contains about 70% to 80% of the immunologic tissue of the entire body. Consequently, GI dysfunction amplifies SIRS and gut damage, which may lead to bacterial translocation and endogenous endotoxemia.[6,32-34]

Three specific mechanisms link the GI tract and latent organ dysfunction. First, hypoperfusion and/or shocklike states damage the normal GI mucosa barrier by decreasing mesenteric blood flow, leading to hypoperfusion of the villi, mucosal edema, ischemic necrosis, sloughing of the mucosa, and malabsorption. The GI tract is extremely vulnerable to oxygen metabolite–induced reperfusion injury. Endothelial injury and GI lesions occur in response to mediator-induced tissue damage. In addition, ischemic events and the absence of feedings can disrupt the normal metabolism of the gastric/intestinal lumen and the normal protective function of the gut barrier.[1,24,32-34]

Second, the translocation of normal GI bacteria via a "leaky gut" into the systemic circulation initiates and perpetuates an inflammatory focus in the critically ill

---

Box 39-5

CLINICAL MANIFESTATIONS OF ORGAN DYSFUNCTION

GASTROINTESTINAL
Abdominal distention
Intolerance to enteral feedings
Paralytic ileus
Upper/lower GI bleeding
Diarrhea
Ischemic colitis
Mucosal ulceration
Decreased bowel sounds
Bacterial overgrowth in stool

LIVER
Jaundice
Increased serum bilirubin (hyperbilirubinemia)
Increases serum ammonia
Decreased serum albumin
Decreased serum transferrin

GALLBLADDER
Right upper quadrant tenderness/pain
Abdominal distention
Unexplained fever
Decreased bowel sounds

METABOLIC/NUTRITIONAL
Decreased lean body mass
Muscle wasting
Severe weight loss
Negative nitrogen balance
Hyperglycemia
Hypertriglyceridemia
Increased serum lactate
Decreased serum albumin, serum transferrin, prealbumin
Decreased retinol-binding protein

IMMUNE
Infection
Decreased lymphocyte count
Anergy

PULMONARY
Tachypnea
ARDS pattern of respiratory failure (dyspnea, patchy infiltrates, refractory hypoxemia, respiratory acidosis, abnormal O_2 indexes)
Pulmonary hypertension

RENAL
Increased serum creatinine, BUN levels
Oliguria, anuria, or polyuria consistent with prerenal azotemia or acute tubular necrosis
Urinary indexes consistent with prerenal azotemia or acute tubular necrosis

CARDIOVASCULAR
Hyperdynamic
Decreased pulmonary capillary occlusion pressure
Decreased systemic vascular resistance
Decreased right atrial pressure
Decreased left ventricular stroke work index
Increased oxygen consumption
Increased cardiac output, cardiac index, heart rate

Hypodynamic
Increased systemic vascular resistance
Increased right atrial pressure
Increased left ventricular stroke work index
Decreased oxygen delivery and consumption
Decreased cardiac output and cardiac index

CENTRAL NERVOUS SYSTEM
Lethargy
Altered level of consciousness
Fever
Hepatic encephalopathy

COAGULATION/HEMATOLOGIC
Thrombocytopenia
DIC pattern

GI, Gastrointestinal; *AST,* aspartate aminotransferase (SGOT); *ALT,* alanine aminotransferase; *LDH,* lactic dehydrogenase; *ARDS,* acute respiratory distress syndrome; *BUN,* blood urea nitrogen; *DIC,* disseminated intravascular coagulation.

patient. The GI tract harbors organisms that present an inflammatory focus when translocated from the gut into the portal circulation and inadequately cleared by the liver. Hepatic macrophages respond to the presence of enteric organisms by producing tissue-damaging amounts of TNF. Bacterial translocation has been associated with paralytic ileus and drugs commonly used in the critically ill patient, including antibiotics, antacids, and histamine blockers.[18,20,32]

The third mechanism linking the GI tract and organ dysfunction is colonization. The oropharynx of the critically ill patient becomes colonized with potentially pathogenic organisms from the GI tract. Pulmonary aspiration of colonized sputum presents an inflammatory focus. Antacids, histamine blockers, and antibiotics also increase colonization of the upper GI tract.[1,11,18]

Hepatobiliary Dysfunction. The liver plays a vital role in host homeostasis related to the acute inflammatory response. In addition, the liver responds to SIRS by selectively changing carbohydrate (CHO), fat, and protein metabolism. Consequently, hepatic dysfunction after a critical insult threatens the patient's survival.[35]

The liver normally controls the inflammatory response by several mechanisms. Kupffer's cells, which are hepatic macrophages, detoxify substances that might normally induce systemic inflammation, as well as vasoactive substances that cause hemodynamic instability. Failure to detoxify gram-negative bacteria translocated from the GI tract causes endotoxemia, perpetuates SIRS, and may lead to MODS. In addition, the liver produces proteins and antiproteases to control the inflammatory response; however, hepatic dysfunction limits this response.[18,35]

The liver and gallbladder are extremely vulnerable to ischemic injury. Ischemic hepatitis occurs after a prolonged period of physiologic shock and is associated with centrilobular hepatocellular necrosis.[36] The degree of hepatic damage is related directly to the severity and duration of the shock episode. Terms such as *shock liver* and *posttraumatic hepatic insufficiency* have been used to describe ischemic hepatitis. Both anoxic and reperfusion injury damage hepatocytes and the vascular endothelium.[37] Patients at high risk for ischemic hepatitis after a hypotensive event include those with a history of cardiac failure and/or cardiac dysrhythmias. Clinical manifestations of hepatic insufficiency are evident 1 to 2 days after the insult. Jaundice and transient elevations in serum transaminase and bilirubin levels occur. Hyperbilirubinemia results from hepatocyte anoxic injury and an increased production of bilirubin from hemoglobin catabolism. Ischemic hepatitis may either resolve spontaneously or progress to fulminant hepatic failure. Although ischemic hepatitis is not a life-threatening complication, it can contribute to patient morbidity and mortality as a component of MODS.[37] Researchers have recently proposed that serum bilirubin is a valid indicator of hepatic dysfunction in MODS because it signifi-

cantly differentiates MODS survivors from nonsurvivors.[35,36,38] For further discussion on fulminant hepatic failure, see Chapter 33.

Acalculous cholecystitis manifests 3 to 4 weeks after an insult. Its pathogenesis is unclear but may be related to ischemic reperfusion injury, positive end-expiratory pressure (PEEP) greater than 5 cm H_2O, volume depletion, total parenteral nutrition, narcotics, and cystic duct obstruction as a result of hyperviscous bile.[39] Visceral hypotension and vasoactive medication use may decrease perfusion of the gallbladder mucosa contributing to ischemia. Bacterial invasion may stimulate activation of factor XII and initiate the coagulation pathway.[39] Clinical manifestations of acalculous cholecystitis may mimic acute cholecystitis with gallstones. However, patients may demonstrate vague symptoms including right upper quadrant pain and tenderness. Critical to the detection of acalculous cholecystitis is the recognition of abdominal distention, unexplained fever, loss of bowel sounds, and a sudden deterioration in the patient's condition. About 50% of patients with acalculous cholecystitis have gallbladder gangrene, and 10% have gallbladder perforation. Consequently, a cholecystectomy may be performed.[40]

Hypermetabolism accompanies SIRS and is commonly referred to as the "metabolic response to injury." During hypermetabolism and SIRS, the liver perpetuates select changes in metabolism including increased gluconeogenesis, glucogenesis, lipogenesis, and increased production of acute phase reactant proteins. Concurrently, the liver decreases synthesis of proteins, particularly albumin and transferrin. This metabolic response is partially mediated by IL-1, TNF, select AA metabolites, and the stress hormones.[18,35,41]

Pulmonary Dysfunction. The lungs, a frequent and early target organ for mediator-induced injury, are usually the first organs affected in secondary MODS. Acute pulmonary dysfunction in secondary MODS manifests as ALI. Patients who develop MODS generally develop ALI; however, not all patients with ALI develop secondary MODS. ALI patients who develop SIRS/sepsis concurrently with acute respiratory failure are at the greatest risk for MODS.[23]

ALI generally occurs 24 to 72 hours after the initial insult and manifests in four phases.[41] In summary, patients initially exhibit a low-grade fever, tachycardia, dyspnea, and mental confusion. As dyspnea, hypoxemia, and the work of breathing increase, intubation and mechanical ventilation are required. Pulmonary function is acutely disrupted, resulting in refractory hypoxemia secondary to intrapulmonary shunting, decreased pulmonary compliance, and altered airway mechanics, and there is generally radiographic evidence of noncardiogenic pulmonary edema.[1,22]

Mediators associated with ALI include inflammatory cells such as polymorphonuclear cells, macrophages, monocytes, endothelial cells, and mast cells; and biochemical mediators such as AA metabolites, toxic oxygen metabolites, proteases, TNF, PAF, and interleukins.[1] Intense mediator activity damages the pulmonary vascular endothelium and the alveolar epithelium, resulting in surfactant deficiency, mild pulmonary hypertension, and increased lung water (noncardiogenic pulmonary edema) resulting from increased pulmonary capillary permeability. Pulmonary hypertension and hypoxic pulmonary vasoconstriction occur secondary to loss of the vascular bed.[1,12,15,18] For further discussion on ALI, see Chapter 24.

Renal Dysfunction. Acute renal failure is a common manifestation of MODS. The kidney is highly vulnerable to reperfusion injury. Consequently, renal ischemic-reperfusion injury may be a major cause of renal dysfunction in MODS. The patient may demonstrate oliguria or anuria secondary to decreased renal perfusion and relative hypovolemia. The condition may become refractory to diuretics, fluid challenges, and dopamine. Additional signs and symptoms include azotemia, decreased creatinine clearance, abnormal renal indices, and fluid and electrolyte imbalances. Prerenal oliguria may progress to acute tubular necrosis, necessitating hemodialysis or other renal therapies.[22,42] The frequent use of nephrotoxic drugs during critical illness also intensifies the risk of renal failure. Researchers have proposed that the serum creatinine is a valid indicator of renal function because it significantly differentiates MODS survivors from nonsurvivors.[43] For further discussion of acute renal failure see Chapter 30.

Cardiovascular Dysfunction. The initial cardiovascular response in SIRS/sepsis is myocardial depression; decreased right atrial pressure and systemic vascular resistance (SVR); and increased venous capacitance, V_{O_2}, cardiac output (CO), and heart rate (HR). Despite an increased CO, myocardial depression occurs and is accompanied by decreased SVR, increased HR, and ventricular dilation. These compensatory mechanisms help maintain CO during the early phase of SIRS/sepsis. An inability to increase CO in response to a low SVR may indicate myocardial failure or inadequate fluid resuscitation and is associated with increased mortality. V_{O_2} may be twice that of normal and may be flow-dependent. Mediators implicated in the hyperdynamic response include bradykinin, select AA metabolites, PAF, endogenous opioids, and β-adrenergic stimulators.[3,16,21]

As MODS progresses, cardiac failure develops. Cardiac dysfunction is characterized by ventricular dilation, decreased diastolic compliance, and decreased systolic contractile function. Cardiovascular function becomes vasopressor-dependent. Cardiac failure may be caused by immune mediators, TNF, acidosis, or myocardial depressant factor (MDF), a substance secreted by the pancreas. TNF has a myocardial-depressant effect and is associated with myocardial depression during septic shock.[44] Myocardial depression is exacerbated by myocardial hypoperfusion from a low CO state and persistent lactic acidosis. Cardiogenic shock and biventricular failure occur and lead to death.[1,21] For further discussion of cardiac failure see Chapter 18, and for cardiogenic shock see Chapter 38.

Coagulation System Dysfunction. Anemia and coagulation abnormalities are common hematologic findings in the patient with SIRS/MODS.[21] Coagulation system dysfunction manifests as disseminated intravascular coagulation (DIC). DIC is a complex, consumptive coagulopathy that occurs in patients with a variety of disorders including sepsis, tissue injury, and shock; it is an overstimulation of the normal coagulation process. DIC results simultaneously in microvascular clotting and hemorrhage in organ systems, leading to thrombosis and fibrinolysis in life-threatening proportions. Clotting factor derangement leads to further inflammation and further thrombosis. Microvascular damage leads to further organ injury. Cell injury and damage to the endothelium activate the intrinsic or extrinsic coagulation pathways.[1,13] Low platelet counts and elevated D-dimer concentrations and fibrinogen degradation products are clinical indicators of DIC.[7] For further discussion of DIC see Chapter 42.

NURSING MANAGEMENT OF HIGH-RISK PATIENTS

Caring for the high-risk SIRS/MODS patient requires astute assessments to detect early organ manifestations of this syndrome. Patients who continue to experience sites of inflammation, septic foci, and inadequate tissue perfusion may be at higher risk. Nursing diagnoses applicable to this patient population are outlined in the Nursing Diagnoses feature on Multiple Organ Dysfunction Syndrome.

The patient with MODS requires interdisciplinary collaboration in clinical management, including fluid resuscitation and hemodynamic support (when appropriate), prevention and treatment of infection, maintenance of tissue oxygenation, nutritional/metabolic support, pain control, and support for individual organ function.[1,4,20] The use of investigational therapies may be part of the patient's clinical management.

PREVENTION, DETECTION, AND TREATMENT OF INFECTION

Identification and treatment of the underlying source of inflammation or infection are the most important aspects to reducing mortality. Medical and surgical intervention to remove sources of infection or contamination may limit the inflammatory response and improve chances of recovery.[1] Therefore surgical procedures such as early fracture stabilization, removal of infected organs or tissue, and burn excision are helpful. Appropriate antibiotics are needed if the focus cannot be removed surgically.[1,45] Other timely interventions, such as prevention of skin ulceration and early nutritional support, assist in improving outcomes.[1,13] Risk for Infection is a highly relevant nursing diagnosis during this time period. Nursing management includes strict adherence to standards of practice to prevent infection. Practices related to infection control with invasive hemodynamic monitoring, urinary catheters, mechanical ventilators, endotracheal tubes, intracranial pressure monitoring devices, total parenteral nutrition, and wound care must be stringent to prevent further infection. Prevention of ventilator-associated pneumonia and aspiration pneumonia is a priority.[1,46] Regardless of the identification of potential risk factors, clinical markers, bacterial contaminants, and investigative approaches for detection and prevention, treatment remains largely supportive and little improvement in the mortality rate has been appreciated.[45]

MAINTENANCE OF TISSUE OXYGENATION

Normally under steady state conditions, V_{O_2} is relatively constant and independent of oxygen delivery (D_{O_2}) unless delivery becomes severely impaired. The relationship is termed *supply-independent oxygen consumption* (V_{O_2} is about 25% of D_{O_2}). Consequently a percentage of oxygen is not used (physiologic reserve). Patients with SIRS/MODS often develop supply-dependent oxygen consumption in which V_{O_2} becomes dependent on D_{O_2}, rather than demand, at a normal or high D_{O_2}. When V_{O_2} does not equal demand, a tissue oxygen debt develops, subjecting organs to failure.[1,18]

Hypoperfusion and resultant organ hypoxemia often occur in patients at high risk for MODS, subjecting essential organs to failure. Therefore effective fluid resuscitation and early recognition of flow-dependent V_{O_2} is essential. Patients at risk for MODS require pulmonary artery catheterization, frequent measurements of D_{O_2} and V_{O_2}, and arterial lactate levels to guide therapy. Arterial lactate levels provide information regarding the severity of impaired perfusion and the presence of lactic acidosis[22] and differ significantly in MODS survivors and nonsurvivors. Failure to maintain adequate oxygenation to vital organs results in organ dysfunction. Despite adequate D_{O_2}, V_{O_2} may not meet the needs of the body during MODS.

Patients with ALI and sepsis frequently manifest supply-dependent oxygen consumption and are unable to use oxygen appropriately despite normal delivery.[1,18-19,48] Interventions that decrease oxygen demand and increase oxygen delivery are essential. Decreasing oxygen demand may be accomplished by sedation, mechanical ventilation, temperature and pain control, and rest. D_{O_2} may be increased by maintaining normal hematocrit and Pa_{O_2} levels, using PEEP, increasing preload or myocardial contractility to enhance CO, or reducing afterload to increase CO. Many critical care clinicians advocate the maintenance of a supranormal D_{O_2} to increase V_{O_2}; however, this therapeutic measure has not significantly improved survival, except in select groups of trauma patients.[14,48]

NUTRITIONAL/METABOLIC SUPPORT

Hypermetabolism in SIRS/MODS results in profound weight loss, cachexia, and loss of organ function. The goal of nutritional support is the preservation of organ structure and function. Although nutritional support may not alter the course of organ dysfunction, it prevents generalized nutritional deficiencies and preserves gut integrity. The enteral route is preferable to parenteral support.[1,49-53] Enteral feedings are given distal to the pylorus to prevent pulmonary aspiration. Enteral feedings may limit bacterial translocation. In addition to early nutritional support, the pharmacologic properties of enteral feeding formulas may limit SIRS for select critical care populations. Supplementation of enteral feedings with glutamine and arginine may be beneficial. Enteral feedings with omega-3 fatty acids may lessen the development of SIRS.[18,20,49-54] Guidelines for nutritional support during SIRS for trauma patients are outlined in the Evidence-Based Collaborative Practice feature on Nutritional Support During SIRS for Trauma Patients. For further discussion on nutritional support see Chapter 7.

EXPERIMENTAL APPROACHES IN SIRS AND MODS

Neither organ-specific nor pharmacologic interventions have been highly effective in improving survival in patients with MODS. At present the focus is on improving the host response to inflammation by targeting and controlling the effects of mediators that cause SIRS and MODS. Animal model studies continue to provide information regarding the efficacy of drugs that prevent organ dysfunction. Experimental treatments and drugs are being tested in human clinical trials. However, the initial enthusiasm about inflammatory therapies has been dampened, with many clinical trials reporting negative findings.[55]

The efficacy of continuous venovenous hemofiltration as a method of removing mediators that potentiate the inflammatory response has been researched numerous times with little success.[56,57] Although filtration of large leukocytes has been successful, the inflammatory response has not been halted. Therefore, hemofiltration will remain as an organ-specific therapy to improve survival for the MODS patient with acute renal failure.

Immunomodulatory strategies should prevent the conversion from SIRS to bacterial sepsis, septic shock, and MODS. Clinical trials with anti-TNF antibodies, IL-1 receptor antagonists, and antilipopolysaccharide mono-

clonal antibodies have been carried out, but no significant treatment effects were discerned.[1,58] Recent efforts have focused on the prophylactic effects of granulocyte/macrocyte colony-stimulating factor (GM-CSF) and attenuating the systemic inflammatory response via the use of xanthine derivatives such as pentoxifylline, which attenuates the formation of TNF.[59]

Pharmacologic approaches that inhibit neutrophil function may be beneficial in SIRS and are listed in Box 39-6. As immunomodulators, these drugs moderate neutrophil-induced injury in endothelial cells. Specifically, pentoxifylline reduces the adhesiveness of activated neutrophils to the endothelium and the release of toxic oxygen metabolites and lysosomal enzymes and inhibits neutrophil activation by endotoxin, TNF, and IL-1. Adenosine, another potential neutrophil inhibitor, reduces granulocyte adherence, inhibits superoxide ion formation, limits the effects of reperfusion injury, and protects endothelial cells.[55,60]

Naturally occurring substances, including some interleukins, inhibit the adherence of neutrophils to the endothelium. Monoclonal antibodies may be available to decrease the adhesion of neutrophils to the endothelium. Antioxidants, drugs that scavenge oxygen radicals or bind free oxygen radicals, and protease inhibitors may be effective in SIRS/sepsis.[1,55] There have been studies of attempts at decreasing the damage from the pro-oxidant activity of xanthine oxidase and radical oxygen species after ischemia-reperfusion using methylene blue, allopurinol, and mannitol. These studies have only been performed on animals in the laboratory but larger studies are being planned in the future.[16]

Eicosanoid modulation involves the use of pharmacologic agents to negate the destructive effects of AA metabolites. Agents that may inhibit the release or destructive activity of AA metabolites are listed in Box 39-6. The effectiveness of these agents in modulating the response to sepsis is under investigation. In contrast to

---

> ### Box 39-6
>
> #### EXPERIMENTAL PHARMACOLOGIC APPROACHES IN SIRS AND MODS
>
> - Neutrophil inhibitors (pentoxifylline, adenosine, aminophylline, terbutaline, dibutyl-cAMP, caffeine, forskolin)
> - WBC adherence inhibitors
> - Antioxidants/oxygen radical scavengers
> - Arachidonic acid metabolite modulators
>   Monoclonal antibodies to Phospholipase A_2
>   Cyclooxygenase inhibitors (ibuprofen, indomethacin)
>   Thromboxane synthetase inhibitors
>   Thromboxane receptor blockers
>   Lipooxygenase inhibitors
>   Leukotrienes antagonists
> - PAF inhibitors
> - Monoclonal antibodies to decrease adhesion of neutrophils to the endothelium
> - Protease inhibitors
> - Modulation of macrophage function (n-3 polyunsaturated fatty acids)
> - Stimulation of lymphocyte function (arginine, n-3 polyunsaturated fatty acids)
> - Antiendorphin therapy
> - Antihistamines
> - Glucocorticoids

SIRS, Systemic inflammatory response syndrome; *MODS,* multiple organ dysfunction syndrome; *WBC,* white blood cell; *PAF,* platelet-activating factor.

AA metabolites that have damaging effects, the administration of prostaglandin-1 may be effective in limiting the systemic inflammatory response because of its local vasodilatory effects and antiplatelet properties.[55]

Other therapies that have been investigated include antiendorphin therapy with SIRS/sepsis patients. No scientific evidence exists that endorphin neutralization with naloxone benefits patients with sepsis or multiple organ involvement.[58] Other investigational therapies that have demonstrated conflicting effects in limiting SIRS include those using corticosteroids.[60]

Recent investigational emphasis has been placed on anticytokine therapy in the treatment of SIRS and MODS. Several cytokines play an important role in uncontrolled inflammation, including TNF-α and IL-1. Therefore TNF-α inhibitors, anti–TNF-α antibody agents, and IL-1 receptor antagonists may demonstrate efficacy in the future.[1,55] It is highly likely that a combination of drugs will prove to be needed to suppress SIRS and to prevent MODS.

REFERENCES

1. Meeran H, Messent M: The systemic inflammatory response syndrome, *Trauma* 3:89, 2001.
2. Fry DE: Systemic inflammatory response and multiple organ dysfunction syndrome: biologic domino effect. In Baue AE, Faist E, Fry DE, editors: *Multiple organ failure: pathophysiology, prevention, and therapy,* New York, 2000, Springer-Verlag.
3. Baldwin KM, Morris SE: Shock, multiple organ dysfunction syndrome, and burns in adults. In McCance KL, Huether SE, editors: *Pathophysiology: the biologic basis for disease in adults and children,* ed 4, St Louis, 2002, Mosby.
4. American College of Chest Physicians/Society of Critical Care Medicine Consensus Conference Committee: Definitions for sepsis and organ failure and guidelines for the use of innovative therapies in sepsis, *Crit Care Med* 20:864, 1992.
5. Levy MM et al: 2001 SCCM/ESICM/ACCP/ATS/SIS International sepsis definitions conference, *Crit Car Med* 31:1250, 2003.
6. Rote NS: Inflammation. In McCance KL, Huether SE, editors: *Pathophysiology: the biologic basis for disease in adults and children,* ed 4, St Louis, 2002, Mosby.
7. Jacobi J: Pathophysiology of sepsis, *Am J Hlth Sys Pharm* 59:S3, 2002.
8. Fry DE: Microcirculatory arrest theory of SIRS and MODS. In Baue AE, Faist E, Fry DE, editors: *Multiple organ failure: pathophysiology, prevention, and therapy,* New York, 2000, Springer-Verlag.
9. Nimah M, Brilli RJ: Coagulation dysfunction in sepsis and multiple organ system failure, *Crit Care Clin* 19:441, 2003.
10. Nathan A, Singer M: Reactive oxygen species in clinical practice. In Baue AE, Faist E, Fry DE, editors: *Multiple organ failure: pathophysiology, prevention, and therapy,* New York, 2000, Springer-Verlag.
11. Brun-Breson C: The epidemiology of the systemic inflammatory response, *Intensive Care Med* 26:S64, 2000.
12. Khadaroo RG, Marshall JC: ARDS and the multiple organ dysfunction syndrome. Common mechanisms of a common systemic process, *Crit Care Clin* 18:127, 2002.
13. Ely EW, Kleinpell RM, Goyette RE: Advances in the understanding of clinical manifestations and therapy of severe sepsis: an update for critical care nurses, *Am J Crit Care* 12:120, 2003.
14. Lee CC et al: A current concept of trauma-induced multiorgan failure, *Ann Emerg Med* 38:170, 2001.
15. Zallen G et al: Circulating postinjury neutrophils are primed for the release of proinflammatory cytokines, *J Trauma* 46:42, 1999.
16. Weinbroum AA et al: Multiple organ dysfunction after remote circulatory arrest: common pathway of radical oxygen species? *J Trauma* 47:691, 1999.
17. Motoyama T et al: Possible role of increased oxidant stress in multiple organ failure after systemic inflammatory response syndrome, *Crit Care Med* 31:1048, 2003.
18. Kim PK, Deutschman CS: Inflammatory responses and mediators, *Surg Clin North Am* 80:885, 2000.
19. Epstein CD et al: Oxygen transport and organ dysfunction in the older trauma patient, *Heart Lung* 31:315, 2002.
20. Biffle WL, Moore EE: Role of the gut in multiple organ failure. In Grenvik A et al, editors: *Textbook of critical care,* ed 4, Philadelphia, 2000, Saunders.
21. Evans TW, Smithies M: ABC of intensive care: organ dysfunction, *Br Med J* 318:1606, 1999.
22. Majetschak M, Waydhas C: Infection, bacteremia, sepsis, and the sepsis syndrome: metabolic alterations, hypermetabolism, and cellular alterations. In Baue AE, Faist E, Fry DE, editors: *Multiple organ failure: pathophysiology, prevention, and therapy,* New York, 2000, Springer-Verlag.

23. Russell JA et al: Changing pattern of organ dysfunction in early human sepsis is related to mortality, *Crit Care Med* 28:3405, 2000.

24. Zimmerman JJ, Ringer TV: Inflammatory host responses in sepsis, *Crit Care Clin* 8:163, 1992.

25. Wort SJ, Evans TW: The role of the endothelium in modulating vascular control in sepsis and related conditions, *Br Med J* 55:30, 1999.

26. Kerr ME, Bender CM, Monti EJ: An introduction to oxygen free radicals, *Heart Lung* 25:200, 1996.

27. Rotstein OD: Oxidants and antioxidant therapy, *Crit Care Clin* 17:239, 2001.

28. Sablotzki A et al: The systemic inflammatory response syndrome following cardiac surgery: different expression of proinflammatory cytokines and procalcitonin in patients with and without multiorgan dysfunctions, *Perfusion* 17:103, 2002.

29. Rumalla V, Lowry SF: Counterregulation of severe inflammation: when more is too much and less is inadequate. In Baue AE, Faist E, Fry DE, editors: *Multiple organ failure: pathophysiology, prevention, and therapy,* New York, 2000, Springer-Verlag.

30. Zimmerman GA et al: The platelet-activating factor signaling system and its regulators in syndromes of inflammation and thrombosis, *Crit Care Med* 30:S294, 2002.

31. Manley FT, Vassar MJ, Holcroft JW: Eicosanoids. In Baue AE, Faist E, Fry DE, editors: *Multiple organ failure: pathophysiology, prevention, and therapy,* New York, 2000, Springer-Verlag.

32. Deitch EA: Gut failure: its role in the multiple organ failure syndrome. In Deitch EA, editor: *Multiple organ failure: pathophysiology and basic concepts of therapy,* New York, 1990, Thieme Medical.

33. Crouser ED: Gastrointestinal tract dysfunction in critical illness: pathophysiology and interaction with acute lung injury in adult respiratory distress syndrome/multiple organ dysfunction syndrome, *New Horizons* 2:476, 1994.

34. Cole L: Early enteral feeding after surgery, *Crit Care Nurs Clin North Am* 11:227, 1999.

35. Dhainaut JF et al: Hepatic response to sepsis: interaction between coagulation and inflammatory processes, *Crit Care Med* 29:S42, 2002.

36. Baue AE: Liver: multiple organ dysfunction and failure. In Baue AE, Faist E, Fry DE, editors: *Multiple organ failure: pathophysiology, prevention, and therapy,* New York, 2000, Springer-Verlag.

37. Wong F: Liver and kidney diseases, *Clin Liver Dis* 6:981, 2002.

38. Marshall JC et al: Multiple organs dysfunction score: a reliable descriptor of a complex clinical outcome, *Crit Care Med* 23:1638, 1995.

39. Puc MM et al: Ultrasound is not a useful screening tool for acute acalculous cholecystitis in critically ill trauma patients, *Am Surg* 68:65, 2002.

40. Proctor DD: Critical issues in digestive diseases, *Clin Chest Med* 24:623, 2003.

41. McMahon K: Multiple organ failure: the final complication of critical illness, *Crit Care Nurs* 15:23, 1995.

42. Huether S: Alterations of renal and urinary tract function. In McCance KL, Huether SE, editors: *Pathophysiology: the biologic basis for disease in adults and children,* ed 4, St Louis, 2002, Mosby.

43. Mullins RJ: Renal function and dysfunction in multiple organ failure. In Baue AE, Faist E, Fry DE, editors: *Multiple organ failure: pathophysiology, prevention, and therapy,* New York, 2000, Springer-Verlag.

44. Kumar A et al: Myocardial dysfunction in septic shock: part II. Role of cytokines and nitric oxide, *J Cardiothorac Vasc Anesth* 15:485, 2001.

45. Richards M, Thursky K, Buising K: Epidemiology, prevalence, and sites of infections in intensive care unit, *Semin Resp Crit Care Med* 24:3, 2003.

46. Grap MJ, Munro CL: Preventing ventilator-associated pneumonia: evidenced-based care, *Crit Care Nurs Clin North Am* 16:349, 2004.

47. Reference deleted in proofs.

48. Hauser CJ: Is supranormal oxygen delivery beneficial? pro. In Deitch EA, Vincent JL, Windsor ACJ, editors: *Sepsis and multiple organ dysfunction: a multiple disciplinary approach,* London, 2001, Harcourt International.

49. McQuiggan MM, Moore FA: Nutrition support in blunt and penetrating torso trauma. In Pichard C, Kudsk KA, editors: *From nutrition support to pharmacologic nutrition in the ICU,* Berlin, 2000, Springer-Verlag.

50. Fitzsimmons L, Hadley SA: Nutritional management of the metabolically stressed patient, *Crit Care Nurs Q* 17:1, 1994.

51. Cheever KH: Early enteral feeding of patients with multiple trauma, *Crit Care Nurse* 19:40, 1999.

52. McClave SA, Mallampalli A: Nutrition in the ICU, part1: enteral feeding—when and why? *J Crit Illness* 16:197, 2001.

53. Alexander JW: Is early enteral feeding of benefit? *Int Care Med* 25:129, 1999.

54. Epstein CD: Applications of indirect calorimetry, *Crit Care Nurs Clin North Am* 12:187, 2000.

55. Orr PA, Case KO, Stevenson JJ: Metabolic response and parenteral nutrition in trauma, sepsis, and burns, *J Infus Nurs* 25:45, 2002.

56. Ruffell AF: The utilization of continuous veno-venous haemofiltration for the removal of septic mediators in patients with systemic inflammatory response syndrome, *Int Crit Care Nurs* 19:207, 2003.

57. Treacher DF, Sabbato M, Brown KM: The effects of leucodepletion in patients who develop the systemic inflammatory response syndrome following cardiopulmonary bypass, *Perfusion* 16:S67, 2001.

58. Faist E, Kim C: Therapeutic immunomodulatory approaches for the control of systemic inflammatory response syndrome and the prevention of sepsis, *New Horizons* 6:S97, 1998.

59. Malham GM, Souter MJ: Systemic inflammatory response syndrome and acute neurological disease, *Br J Neurosurg* 15:381, 2001.

60. Kilger E et al: Stress doses of hydrocortisone reduce severe systemic inflammatory response syndrome and improve early outcome in a risk group of patients after cardiac surgery, *Crit Care Med* 31:1068, 2003.

CHAPTER 40

Burns

During the past two decades, trends of burn incidence, hospitalization, and death have all decreased. These decreases are attributed to fire and burn prevention education, management of burn patients in specialized burn centers, regulation of consumer products, and implementation of occupational safety standards.[1] The nurse, too, can play an active role in preventing fires and burns by promoting legislation and teaching safety practices. Many programs and organizations are dedicated to the prevention of burn injury. Societal changes involving decreased smoking and alcohol abuse, changes in home cooking practices, and reduced industrial employment also have contributed to the decline in burn incidence.[1]

Total burn injuries in America have decreased from estimates of 2.5 million to 1.25 million.[1] Approximately 100,000 thermally injured patients were hospitalized annually in the 1970s; this number has decreased to approximately 51,000 in the 1990s.[1] A shift in treatment from inpatient to outpatient settings has contributed as well to this decline in the hospitalization rate. In addition, deaths from burns and smoke inhalation have dramatically decreased from approximately 12,000 annually in the 1970s to 4000 deaths annually in the 1990s.[2]

Great advances have been made in the care of burn patients. A 30% total body surface area (TBSA) burn in an otherwise healthy adult 50 years ago was associated with a 50% mortality rate, whereas today an 80% TBSA burn carries the same mortality. The leading cause of in-hospital deaths 50 years ago was associated with burn shock. With improvements in fluid resuscitation, better critical care management, and the trend toward early excision and grafting, most in-hospital deaths are associated with late infectious complications.[3]

To provide comprehensive, holistic care for burn patients, close collaboration is required among members of the multidisciplinary team. The burn team comprises nurses, physicians, physical therapists, occupational therapists, recreational therapists, nutritionists, psychologists, social workers, family, and spiritual support staff members. The burn patient is characterized as the universal trauma model. The patient's response to a major burn injury is dramatic and involves multisystem alterations. Knowledge of local and systemic changes associated with patient needs is essential in providing care, which places extraordinary demands on the nurse in burn practice who must be both a specialist and a broadly based generalist.[4] The purpose of this chapter is to provide a basic understanding of the complexities of burn care and the patient's response to burn injury.

ANATOMY AND FUNCTIONS OF THE SKIN

The skin is the largest organ of the human body, ranging from 0.2 m^2 in the newborn to more than 2 m^2 in the adult. The integumentary system consists of two major layers: the epidermis and the dermis (Fig. 40-1).

The outermost layer of epidermis varies from 0.07 to 0.12 mm in thickness, with the deepest layer found on the soles of the feet and the palms of the hands. The epidermis is composed of dead, cornified cells that act as a tough protective barrier against the environment. From the surface inward its five layers are stratum corneum, stratum lucidum, stratum granulosum, stratum spinosum, and stratum germinativum. The deepest layer of epidermis contains fibronectin, which adheres the epidermis to the basement membrane. The epidermis regenerates every 2 to 3 weeks. The second, thicker layer, the dermis, ranges from 1 to 2 mm in thickness and lies below the epidermis and also continuously regenerates. The dermis is composed of two layers: the more superficial, papillary layer next to the stratum germinativum and the deeper, reticular layer. The dermis, composed primarily of connective tissue and collagenous fiber bundles made from fibroblasts, provides nutritional support to the epidermis. The dermis contains the blood vessels; sweat and sebaceous glands; hair follicles; nerves to the skin and capillaries that nourish the avascular epidermis; and sensory fibers for pain, touch, and temperature. Mast cells in the connective tissue perform the functions of secretion, phagocytosis, and production of fibroblasts. Beneath the dermis is the hypodermis, which con-

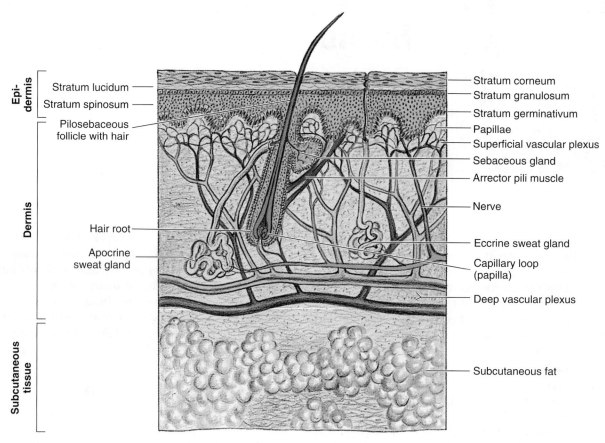

Fig. 40-1 Anatomy of the skin. (From Dains JE: Integumentary system. In Thompson JM et al: *Mosby's clinical nursing,* ed 5, St Louis, 2002, Mosby.)

tains the fat, smooth muscle, and areolar tissue. The hypodermis acts as a heat insulator, shock absorber, and nutritional depot.

The skin provides functions crucial to human survival. These functions include maintenance of body temperature; barrier to evaporative water loss; metabolic activity (vitamin D production); immunologic protection by preventing microbes from entering the body; protection against the environment through the sensations of touch, pressure, and pain; and overall cosmetic appearance.

PATHOPHYSIOLOGY AND ETIOLOGY OF BURN INJURY

A burn is an injury resulting in tissue loss or damage. Injury to tissue can be caused by exposure to thermal, electrical, chemical, and/or radiation sources. The temperature or causticity of the burning agent and duration of tissue contact with the source determine the extent of tissue injury. Tissue damage can occur at varying temperatures, usually between 40° and 44° C and above. The burn wound itself is responsible for both the local and systemic effects seen in the burned patient.[5] Tissue damage is caused by enzyme malfunction and denaturation

of proteins. Prolonged exposure or higher temperatures can lead to cell necrosis and a process known as *protein coagulation.* The areas extending outward from this central area of injury sustain varying degrees of damage and are identified by zones of injury.[5]

ZONES OF INJURY

Three concentric zones are present in burn injury. These include, from the center portion out, the zone of coagulation, the zone of stasis, and the zone of hyperemia. The central zone is the site of the most severe damage, the peripheral zone of the least. The central portion, the zone of coagulation, is usually the site of greatest heat transfer and where irreversible skin death occurs. This area is surrounded by the zone of stasis, which is characterized by impaired circulation that can lead to cessation of blood flow secondary to pronounced inflammatory reaction. This area is potentially salvageable; however, local or systemic factors can convert it into a full-thickness injury. Some of the factors that can lead to deeper wound conversion are toxic mediators of the inflammatory process, infection, inappropriate volume resuscitation, malnutrition, chronic illness, or the local wound care provided. It may take up to 48 hours to determine the full extent of

Box 40-1

BURN CENTER REFERRAL

Patients with the following burn injuries are best treated in a burn center:

- Partial thickness burns 10% or more of the TBSA
- Full-thickness burns in any age group
- Burns of face, hands, feet, genitalia, perineum, or major joints that may result in cosmetic or functional disability
- Electrical burns, including lightning injury
- Inhalation injury
- Chemical burns
- Burns in patients with preexisting disease that would increase the risk of dying (e.g., diabetes mellitus, symptomatic cardiopulmonary disease)
- Burn injury with concomitant trauma
- Burned children in hospitals without qualified personnel or equipment for the care of children
- Burn injury in patients who will require special social, emotional, or long-term rehabilitative intervention

TBSA, Total body surface area.
From the American Burn Association: website: www.ameriburn.org.

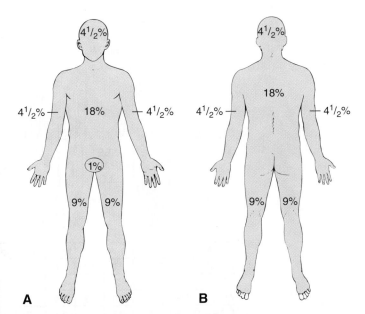

Fig. 40-2   Estimation of adult burn injury: rule of nines. **A,** Anterior view. **B,** Posterior view. (From Marx, J et al: *Rosen's Emergency medicine concepts and clinical practice,* ed 5, St Louis, 2002, Mosby.)

the injury in this area. The outermost area is the zone of hyperemia, where there is vasodilation and increased blood flow but minimal cell involvement. Early spontaneous recovery can occur in this area.[6]

CLASSIFICATION OF BURN INJURIES

Burns are classified primarily according to the size and depth of the injury. However, the type and location of the burn, as well as the patient's age and medical history, are also significant considerations. Recognition of the magnitude of burn injury, which is based on the depth and size of the burn and the previous health of the patient, is of crucial importance in the overall plan of care. Decisions concerning patient management and appropriate referral to a burn center are based on this assessment (Box 40-1).[2] Patient age and the burn size are the cardinal determinants of survival.[6-9]

SIZE OF INJURY

Several different methods can be used to estimate the size of the burn area. A quick and easy method is the *rule of nines,* which often is used in the prehospital setting for initial triage of the burn patient (Fig. 40-2). With this method the adult body is divided into surface areas of 9%. This method is modified in infants and very small children. In the adult the head and the anterior and pos-

terior surfaces of the trunk are each 18% of the TBSA, each arm is 9%, each leg is 18%, and the perineum is 1%. Another method uses the measure of the palmar surface of the victim's hand as a gauge for estimating burn area. The palmar surface, which represents 1% of the TBSA, also can be useful for making burn estimates in the prehospital setting or for estimating the percentage of involvement in small and scattered areas of burn.

In the hospital setting, the Lund and Browder method (Fig. 40-3) is the most accurate and accepted method for determining the percentage of burn. Surface area measurements are assigned to each body part in terms of the age of the patient. This method is highly recommended for use with children younger than 10 years because it corrects for smaller surface areas of the lower extremities. It is also recommended in adult burn victims because of its accuracy.

The Berkow method also can be used to estimate burn size for infants and children because it accounts for the proportionate growth. This method requires special charts provided by the National Burn Institute, which are not always available in local hospitals but may be at hand in a designated burn center.

DEPTH OF INJURY

Traditionally burn depth has been classified in degrees of injury based on the amount of injured epidermis or dermis, or both (i.e., first-, second-, or third-degree burns). However, these terms are not descriptive of the burn surface.

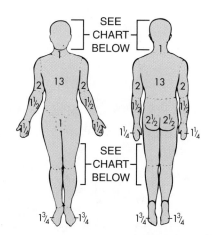

AREA	Inf.	1-4	5-9	10-14	15	Adult	Part.	Full	Total	Donor areas
HEAD	19	17	13	11	9	7				
NECK	2	2	2	2	2	2				
ANT. TRUNK	13	13	13	13	13	13				
POST. TRUNK	13	13	13	13	13	13				
R. BUTTOCK	$2\frac{1}{2}$	$2\frac{1}{2}$	$2\frac{1}{2}$	$2\frac{1}{2}$	$2\frac{1}{2}$	$2\frac{1}{2}$				
L. BUTTOCK	$2\frac{1}{2}$	$2\frac{1}{2}$	$2\frac{1}{2}$	$2\frac{1}{2}$	$2\frac{1}{2}$	$2\frac{1}{2}$				
GENITALIA	1	1	1	1	1	1				
R.U. ARM	4	4	4	4	4	4				
L.U. ARM	4	4	4	4	4	4				
R.L. ARM	3	3	3	3	3	3				
L.L. ARM	3	3	3	3	3	3				
R. HAND	$2\frac{1}{2}$	$2\frac{1}{2}$	$2\frac{1}{2}$	$2\frac{1}{2}$	$2\frac{1}{2}$	$2\frac{1}{2}$				
L. HAND	$2\frac{1}{2}$	$2\frac{1}{2}$	$2\frac{1}{2}$	$2\frac{1}{2}$	$2\frac{1}{2}$	$2\frac{1}{2}$				
R. THIGH	$5\frac{1}{2}$	$6\frac{1}{2}$	8	$8\frac{1}{2}$	9	$9\frac{1}{2}$				
L. THIGH	$5\frac{1}{2}$	$6\frac{1}{2}$	8	$8\frac{1}{2}$	9	$9\frac{1}{2}$				
R. LEG	5	5	$5\frac{1}{2}$	6	$6\frac{1}{2}$	7				
L. LEG	5	5	$5\frac{1}{2}$	6	$6\frac{1}{2}$	7				
R. FOOT	$3\frac{1}{2}$	$3\frac{1}{2}$	$3\frac{1}{2}$	$3\frac{1}{2}$	$3\frac{1}{2}$	$3\frac{1}{2}$				
L. FOOT	$3\frac{1}{2}$	$3\frac{1}{2}$	$3\frac{1}{2}$	$3\frac{1}{2}$	$3\frac{1}{2}$	$3\frac{1}{2}$				
						TOTAL				

Fig. 40-3   The Lund and Browder burn estimate diagram. (Modified from Cardona VD: *Trauma nursing from re-suscitation through rehabilitation,* Philadelphia, 1995, Mosby.)

Currently, burns are classified as *superficial, partial-thickness,* or *full-thickness.* These descriptions are based on the surface appearance of the wound. Superficial burns include first-degree burns. Partial-thickness wounds include varying stages of second-degree burns, and full-thickness burns include third-degree burns. Some authors further separate partial-thickness burns as being *superficial, mid-dermal* or *deep-dermal partial-thickness burns.* Wound assessment involves recognition of the depth of injury and the size of burn and can be challenging even for experienced caregivers. Because the management of burn wounds is closely tied to the correct assessment of wound severity, some newer strategies, other than observation, are being investigated. Some of these techniques include burn wound biopsy and tissue histology, ultrasound, use of the laser Doppler flowmeter, thermography, light reflectance, and

magnetic resonance imaging (MRI). Research with these techniques is ongoing, but they are currently limited by their clinical usefulness at the bedside.[5]

A *superficial burn (first-degree)* involves only the first two or three of the five layers of the epidermis. Erythema and mild discomfort characterize superficial partial-thickness wounds. Pain, the chief symptom, usually resolves in 48 to 72 hours. Common examples of these burn injuries are sunburns and minor steam burns such as those that may occur while a person is cooking. Generally, these wounds heal in 2 to 7 days and usually do not require medical intervention aside from pain relief and oral fluids.

A *partial-thickness* or *superficial dermal burn (second-degree)* involves the upper third of the dermis. These burns usually are caused by brief contact with flames, hot liquid, or exposure to dilute chemicals (Fig. 40-4). A light

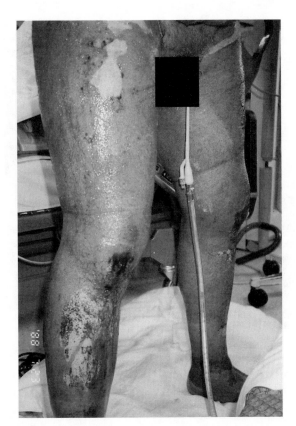

Fig. 40-4 Partial-thickness burn to lower extremities from hydrofluoric acid.

to bright red or mottled appearance characterizes superficial second-degree burns. These wounds may appear wet and weeping, may contain bullae, and are extremely painful and sensitive to air currents. The microvessels that perfuse this area are injured, and permeability is increased, resulting in the leakage of large amounts of plasma into the interstitium. This fluid, in turn, lifts off the thin damaged epidermis, causing blister formation. Despite the loss of the entire basal layer of the epidermis, a burn of this depth will heal in 7 to 21 days. Minimal scarring can be expected. Mid-dermal partial-thickness wounds commonly take 4 to 6 weeks to heal.

Deep-dermal partial-thickness burns (second-degree) involve the entire epidermal layer and part of the dermis. These burns often result from contact with hot liquids or solids or with intense radiant energy. A deep-dermal partial-thickness burn generally is not characterized by blister formation. Only a modest plasma surface leakage occurs because of severe impairment in blood supply. The wound surface usually is red with patchy white areas that blanch with pressure. The appearance of the deep-dermal wound changes over time. Dermal necrosis, along with surface coagulated protein, turns the wound from white to yellow. These wounds have a prolonged healing time. They can heal spontaneously as the epidermal elements germinate and migrate until the epidermal surface is restored, or they may require a skin substitute or surgical excision and grafting for wound closure. This process of healing by epithelialization can take up to 6 weeks. Left untreated, these wounds can heal primarily with unstable epithelium, late hypertrophic scarring, and marked contracture formation. Partial-thickness injuries can become full-thickness injuries if they become infected, if blood supply is diminished, or if further trauma occurs to the site. The treatment of choice is surgical excision and skin grafting.

A *full-thickness burn (third-degree)* involves destruction of all the layers of the skin down to and including the subcutaneous tissue. The subcutaneous tissue is composed of adipose tissue, includes the hair follicles and sweat glands, and is poorly vascularized. A full-thickness burn appears pale white or charred, red or brown, and leathery. The surface of the burn may be dry, and if the skin is broken, fat may be exposed. Full-thickness burns usually are painless and insensitive to palpation. All epithelial elements are destroyed; therefore the wound will not heal by reepitheliazation. Wound closure of small full-thickness burns (less than a 4 cm area) can be achieved with healing by contraction. All other full-thickness wounds require skin grafting for closure. Extensive full-thickness wounds leave the patient extremely susceptible to infections, fluid and electrolyte imbalances, alterations in thermoregulation, and metabolic disturbances.

The exact depth of many burn wounds cannot be clearly defined on the first inspection, and many burn wounds may contain both superficial, mid-dermal and deep-dermal wounds. A major difficulty is distinguishing deep-dermal partial-thickness from full-thickness injury. It is important to identify the depth of injury for appropriate treatment. Deep, partial-thickness wounds that will not heal within a relatively short time will be treated with wound excision and grafting. Burn wounds can evolve over time, and they require frequent reassessment. Special consideration must always be given to very young and elderly patients because of their thin dermal layer. Burn injuries in these age-groups may be more severe than they initially appear.[10]

At the same time that assessment for wound depth occurs, the total percentage, or TBSA, of the burn is calculated by means of either the rule of nines or the Lund and Browder chart. This calculation provides the basis for determining the amount of fluid required for treatment. All burn wound surface area percentages, except for superficial burns, are used to calculate the patient's fluid requirements.

TYPES OF INJURY

Thermal Burns. The most common type of burn is a thermal burn caused by steam, scalds, contact with heat, and fire injuries. The age-groups most often involved are toddlers (2 to 4 years), for whom the most common cause is scalds, and young adults (17 to 25 years, usually male), for whom the most common cause is flammable liquid. Structural fires account for fewer than 5% of hospital admissions but are responsible for more than 45% of burn-related deaths.[11]

Electrical Burns. Electrical and lightning injuries result in 1000 deaths per year in the United States.[12] Low-voltage (alternating) current or high-voltage (alternating or direct) current can cause electrical burns. Children have the highest incidence of electrical injury. These accidents occur as a result of insertion of an object into an outlet or by biting or sucking electrical cords. Common situations that may increase the risk for electrical injuries include occupational exposure and accidents involving household current. Lightning causes approximately 80 deaths a year in the United States; the incidence is seven times greater in men than women.[12]

Chemical Burns. Acids and alkalis cause chemical burns. Alkalis commonly result in more severe injuries than do acid burns. Acids and alkali agents are found in many household and industrial substances, such as liquid concrete. The concentration of the chemical agent and the duration of exposure are the key factors that determine the extent and depth of damage. Progression of injury from chemical burns to their complete depth may be delayed, and the full extent of the injury may not be apparent until up to 48 hours after injury. Time must not be wasted in looking for the specific neutralizing agents because the injury is related directly to the concentration of the chemical and the duration of the exposure; also, the heat of neutralization can extend the injury. Tar and asphalt burns are serious and rather common injuries (Fig. 40-5).[8] Approximately 70% of chemical burns occur to the hands.

Radiation Burns. Burns associated with radiation exposure are uncommon. Radiation burns usually are localized and indicate high radiation doses to the affected area. Radiation burns may appear identical to thermal burns. The major difference is the time between exposure and clinical manifestation; it can be days to weeks, depending on the level of the dose. Radiation injury can occur with exposure to industrial equipment, such as accelerators and cyclotrons, and equipment used for medical treatment.

Location of Injury

Location of injury can be a determining factor in differentiating the level of care required. According to triage criteria from the American College of Surgeons, burns on the face, hands, feet, genitalia, major joints, and perineum are best treated in a burn center. Such burns involve functional areas of the body and often require specialized intervention. Injuries to these areas can result in significant long-term morbidity, both from impaired function and altered appearance.

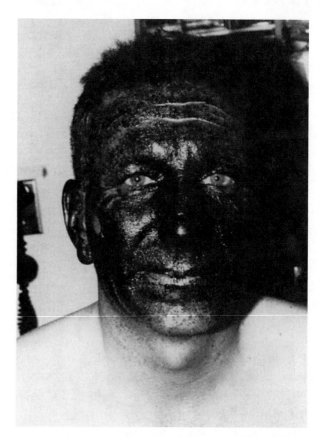

Fig. 40-5 Tar burn to the face.

Patient Age and History

Age and history are significant determinants of survival. Patients considered most at risk are those younger than 2 years and those older than 60 years. History of inhalation injury and electrical burns, and all burns complicated by trauma and fractures, considered major injuries, significantly increase mortality. Obtaining a past medical history is important, particularly a history relating to cardiac, pulmonary, and renal disorders, as well as diabetes and central nervous system disorders.

INITIAL EMERGENCY BURN MANAGEMENT

The goals of acute care of the patient with thermal injuries are to save life, minimize disability, and prepare the patient for definitive care. The burn injury may involve multiple organ systems, and the approach to the injured patient should be expeditious and methodical in identifying problems and establishing priorities of care.[13]

The resuscitation phase begins immediately after the burn insult has occurred; therefore the nurse is concerned with patient management at the scene until admission to an appropriate medical facility. As with any major trauma, the first hour after injury is crucial, but the first 24 to 36 hours after injury also are vitally important in burn patient management. Management during this time interval has a major impact on the patient's survival and ultimate rehabilitation.

Obtaining a history regarding the nature of the injury is important in the management of the burn patient. Water heater, propane gas, grain elevator, and other types of explosions often throw the patient some distance and may result in concomitant orthopedic, neurologic, and/or internal trauma. It is valuable to know the specific agents involved if the burns are chemical. It also helps to know what substance was burned or inhaled and how long the patient was exposed to smoke or superheated air. A detailed patient history should include the mechanism of injury, patient's age, location and size of burn, type and amount of fluid already administered, known allergies, status of tetanus immunization, and significant past medical history. All rings, watches, and jewelry are removed from injured limbs to avoid a tourniquet effect when edema occurs as a result of fluid shifts and fluid resuscitation.

AIRWAY MANAGEMENT

The first priority of emergency burn care is to secure and protect the airway. If there is any possibility of underlying cervical instability, cervical precautions must be initiated.[13] For patients with facial burns or exposure to fire in an enclosed space, or both, a high index of suspicion should exist for inhalation injury. Carbon monoxide (CO) poisoning is associated with high mortality. Carboxyhemoglobin levels are obtained, and oxygen therapy is initiated. All patients with major burns or suspected inhalation injury are initially administered 100% oxygen.[13] The nurse should continue to observe the patient for clinical manifestations of impaired oxygenation, such as tachypnea, agitation, anxiety, and upper airway obstruction (e.g., hoarseness, stridor, wheezing). Early intubation may save the life of the patient who has an inhalation injury, since it may be impossible to perform this procedure later, when edema has obstructed the larynx. The potential need for frequent blood sampling as well as the benefit of continuous blood pressure monitoring may necessitate an arterial line.

RESPIRATORY MANAGEMENT

Circumferential full-thickness burns to the chest wall can lead to restriction of chest wall expansion and decreased compliance. Decreased compliance requires higher ventilatory pressures to provide the patient with adequate tidal volumes. In the patient who has not undergone intubation, clinical manifestations of chest wall restriction include rapid, shallow respirations, poor chest wall excursion, and severe agitation. Arterial blood gas analysis will

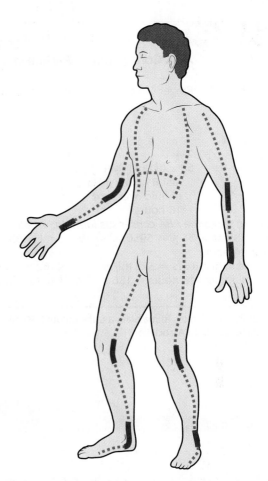

Fig. 40-6 Preferred sites of escharotomy incisions. (From Carrougher GJ: *Burn care and therapy*, St Louis, 1998, Mosby.)

reveal a decrease in oxygen tension and an increasing partial pressure of carbon dioxide ($Paco_2$) level. Patients receiving mechanical ventilation will demonstrate rising peak airway pressure.

Escharotomies, burn eschar incisions, may need to be performed immediately to increase compliance and thereby lead to improved ventilation. These incisions generally are made bilaterally along the anterior axillary lines and are connected by a transverse incision at the costal margin (Fig. 40-6).

CIRCULATORY MANAGEMENT

At this point, the extent and depth of the burn are assessed. The extent of TBSA of the burn is calculated for estimation of fluid resuscitation requirements (Table 40-1); the Parkland formula is the most widely used method of calculation. (For further discussion, see the Clinical Application feature on Burns.) Burn shock is caused by the loss of fluid from the vascular compartment into the area of injury, resulting in hypovolemia. Therefore the larger the percentage of burn area, the greater the potential for development of shock. Lactated

Table 40-1	Formulas for Fluid Replacement/Resuscitation in First 24 Hours				
	ABA Consensus	**Parkland**	**Modified Brooke**	**Brooke**	**Hypertonic**
ELECTROLYTE SOLUTION	Ringer's lactate	Ringer's lactate	Ringer's lactate	Ringer's lactate	Hypertonic lactated saline (sodium, 250 mEq/L)
ML/KG/% BURNED*	2-4 50% of fluid over first 8 hours; 50% of fluid over next 16 hours	4	2	1.5	Rate based on urine output of 30-50 ml/hr

Example using the ABA consensus formula: an 85-kg patient with 35% TBSA burn

2 ml × 85 kg × 35% = 5950 ml in first 24 hours	3 ml × 85 × 35% = 8925 ml	4 ml × 85 × 35% = 11,900 ml
2975 ml in first 8 hrs = 372 ml/hr	4462 ml in first 8 hours = 558 ml/hr	5950 ml in first 8 hours = 744 ml/hr
2975 ml in next 16 hours = 186 ml/hr	4462 ml in next 16 hours = 279 ml/hr	5950 ml in next 16 hours = 372 ml/hr

*Adjust the above rates to maintain a urine output >30 ml/hr in adults or 1 ml/kg/hr in children.
ABA, American Burn Association.

CLINICAL APPLICATION

Burns

Ms. G is a 23-year-old female victim of a house fire. The source of the blaze is undetermined. She is sent from the emergency department to your trauma unit. She arrives chemically sedated and intubated. She has partial-thickness burns to her face, ears, upper chest, and upper back. She has deep partial-thickness wounds to her bilateral arms circumferentially and a full-thickness burn to her forehead. She jumped out of a window approximately 10 feet off the ground to get out of the burning house. The paramedics reported she was alert and oriented but hysterical at the scene. She has a 4-year-old son who was rescued by firefighters and is not injured. Her carboxyhemoglobin level was 3.4 in the emergency department. She is allergic to penicillin but has no other past medical or surgical history.

1. What are your first priorities in the care of Ms. G?
2. After the airway is secure and breathing is resumed by a mechanical ventilator with 100% FiO_2, what are the next steps in Ms. G's care?

Ms. G has a carboxyhemoglobin level of 3.4 and arterial blood gas analysis of pH, 7.27; $PaCO_2$, 29; PaO_2, 313; and HCO_3^-, 14. Her weight is 52.16 kg. She has a triple-lumen catheter in her right femoral vein with good blood return to all ports. An endotracheal tube (ETT) is secure, and breath

sounds are present bilaterally but are coarse. Her sputum has dark carbon present.

3. What is her estimated TBSA burn?
4. What is her estimated fluid need using the Parkland formula?

After the initial assessment and interventions, it is necessary to rule out associated injury because other injuries may take precedence over the burn wounds. Ms. G jumped 10 feet and landed on her left hand. She has obvious swelling and grimaces to touching of her left fifth finger. She also has seven lacerations to her bilateral upper extremities that are bleeding and require sutures. X-ray film reveals a left fifth digit fracture of the proximal phalanx. Examination reveals no other associated injuries. Attention is turned to débriding Ms. G's wounds and applying dressings.

5. What route and type of medications will be used for Ms. G?
6. What would guide your selection of a topical antimicrobial cream?
7. After hemodynamic stability is achieved and the patient is not at risk for pulse loss in her extremities, what are your priorities?
8. What referrals would be necessary?

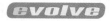 For the discussion of this Clinical Application and for an additional clinical application on burns, see the Evolve website.

Ringer's (LR) solution is infused via large-bore cannula (16-gauge or larger) in a peripheral vein. LR, an isotonic crystalloid, is the resuscitation fluid used most often. LR given in large amounts can restore cardiac output toward normal in most patients. It is preferred over normal saline because it most closely matches extracellular fluid. Because isotonic salt solutions generate no difference in osmotic pressure between plasma and interstitial space, the entire extracellular space must be expanded to replace intravascular losses. Diuretics should not be given during the resuscitative phase of burn care.

Per the Parkland formula, in the first 8 hours after injury, half the calculated amount of fluid is administered to the patient; 25% is given in the second 8 hours, and 25% in the third 8 hours. It is important to remember that calculated fluid requirements are guidelines. Fluid resuscitation is a dynamic process. The rate of fluid administration is adjusted according to the individual's response, which is determined by monitoring urine output, heart rate, blood pressure, and level of consciousness. Meticulous attention to the patient's intake and output is imperative to ensure that he or she is appropriately resuscitated. Underresuscitation may result in inadequate cardiac output leading to inadequate organ perfusion and the potential for wound conversion from partial- to full-thickness. Overresuscitation may lead to moderate to severe pulmonary edema; to excessive wound edema causing a decrease in perfusion of unburned tissue in the distal portions of the extremities; or to edema inhibiting perfusion of the zone of stasis, resulting in wound conversion.[9]

Continuous electrocardiogram (ECG) monitoring should be done on seriously burn-injured patients. In the presence of electrical injury, inhalation injury, or associated injury that can occur as a result of trauma, fluid requirements may be much higher than estimated using the Parkland formula. The recommendations for these situations are included later in this chapter.

PATHOPHYSIOLOGY OF BURN SHOCK

Burn injuries greater than 35% TBSA can result in burn shock.[7] Shock is defined as inadequate cellular perfusion. Significant burn injury results in hypovolemic shock and tissue trauma. Both of these cause the production and release of several local and systemic mediators. Burn shock can occur even when hypovolemia is corrected.

The first component of burn shock is hypovolemic shock. At the cellular level the burning agent produces a dilation of the capillaries and small vessels, thus increasing the capillary permeability. Plasma seeps out into the surrounding tissue, producing blisters and edema. The type, duration, and intensity of the burn all affect the amount and extent of fluid loss. This progressive fluid loss in extensive burns results in significant intravascular fluid volume deficit. The edema occurs locally in the burn wound and systemically in unburned tissues. Edema formation is unique to thermal injury.

Burn edema has been attributed to several factors. Barrier property changes of the capillary wall occur by direct injury and indirect mediator-modulated changes. Increases in permeability of both protein and water occur, resulting in edema. In most forms of shock, capillary pressure decreases as a result of arteriolar vasoconstriction. However, after burn injury, an increase in capillary pressure has been found in the burned tissue in the first minutes to hours after injury.[7] Coupled with this increase in capillary pressure is a negative interstitial hydrostatic pressure that occurs in the dermis layer of burned skin after thermal injury.[14] This negative interstitial hydrostatic pressure represents an edema-generating mechanism and occurs for approximately 2 hours after injury. In addition, plasma colloid osmotic pressure is decreased as a result of protein leakage into the extravascular space. Plasma is then further diluted with fluid resuscitation. Thus osmotic pressure is decreased and further fluid extravasation can occur.

In addition to the problem of leaking capillaries, local and systemic mediators cause edema and the cardiovascular problems seen in burn patients. Some of these mediators include histamine, prostaglandins, kinins, oxygen radicals, and others. These mediators increase arteriolar vasodilation. Manipulation of these mediators to stop the cascade of burn edema and burn shock is being researched.

The intravascular fluid changes combined with the action of inflammatory mediators and vasoconstricting mediators result in hemodynamic consequences in the burn patient. The hemodynamic alterations include decreased myocardial contractility and cardiac output despite adequate volume resuscitation, increased systemic vascular resistance (SVR), and increased pulmonary vascular resistance (PVR).[7] This increase in PVR can lead to pulmonary edema. Large but judicious volumes of resuscitation fluids, as previously discussed, are required to maintain the vascular volume during the first few hours after a large burn injury to provide optimal resuscitation. Early and full fluid resuscitation will prevent the complications of acute renal failure, cardiovascular collapse, and death from shock. However, overresuscitation will result in increased edema formation, which can further impair tissue oxygen diffusion. Therefore the nurse must assess the patient's fluid status and response to resuscitation to obtain the optimal response.

RENAL MANAGEMENT

If fluid resuscitation is inadequate, acute renal failure may occur. An indwelling urinary catheter is placed while the patient is in the emergency department to monitor urine output and the effectiveness of fluid resuscitation. The nurse measures urine output hourly. Adequate urine output for adults is 0.5 to 1 ml/kg/hr, or 30 to 50 ml/hr; for children it is 1 ml/kg/hr.[9,15]

GASTROINTESTINAL MANAGEMENT

Patients with burns of more than 20% TBSA are prone to gastric dilation as a result of paralytic ileus. Nasogastric or orogastric tubes are placed in these patients to prevent abdominal distention, emesis, and potential aspiration. This decrease in gastrointestinal (GI) function is caused by a combination of the effects of hypovolemia and the neurologic and endocrine response to injury. Gastrointestinal activity usually returns in 24 to 48 hours. Gastric prophylaxis with histamine$_2$ (H$_2$) blockers or sucralfate is initiated, since burn patients are prone to Curling stress ulcers.

PAIN MANAGEMENT

Burn injuries are very painful, so pain management must be addressed early and frequently reassessed to determine adequacy of interventions. Intravenous opiates, such as morphine sulfate, are indicated and are titrated to effect. The use of intravenous benzodiazepines for anxiolysis should also be administered and titrated to effect. Intramuscular or subcutaneous injections must not be administered, since absorption by these routes is unpredictable because of the fluid shifts that occur with burn injury.[16] The use of pain management guidelines for administration and monitoring of patients may be helpful and is recommended.[17]

EXTREMITY PULSE ASSESSMENT

Edema formation may cause neurovascular compromise to the extremities; frequent assessments are necessary to evaluate pulses, skin color, capillary refill, and sensation. Arterial circulation is at greatest risk with circumferential burns. If not corrected, reduced arterial flow will result in ischemia and necrosis. The Doppler flow probe is one of the best ways to evaluate arterial pulses. An escharotomy may be required to restore arterial circulation and to allow for further swelling. The escharotomy can be performed at the bedside with a sterile field and scalpel. Care must be taken to avoid major nerves, vessels, and tendons. The incision extends through the length of the eschar, over joints, and down to the subcutaneous fat. The incision is placed laterally or medially on the extremity. If a single incision does not restore circulation, bilateral incisions are required (see Fig. 40-6).[6,8] If escharotomy is required before the patient is transferred to a burn center, consultation with the receiving physician is advised.

LABORATORY ASSESSMENT

Initial laboratory studies are performed: hematocrit, electrolytes, blood urea nitrogen (BUN), urinalysis, and chest roentgenogram. Special situations, such as inhalation injury, warrant arterial blood gas, carboxyhemoglobin, and alcohol and drug screens. An ECG is obtained for all patients with electrical burns or preexisting cardiac problems.

WOUND CARE

After the wounds have been assessed, topical antimicrobial therapy is not a priority during emergency care. However, the wounds must be covered with clean, dry dressings or sheets. Every attempt must be made to keep the patient warm because of the high risk of hypothermia. The administration of tetanus prophylaxis is recommended for all burns >10% TBSA or for patients with a questionable immunization history.

BURN CENTER REFERRAL

After initial treatment and stabilization at an emergency department, referral to a burn center is considered (see Box 40-1). By definition, a burn center must be able to deliver all therapy required, including rehabilitation, and must perform personnel training and burn research.[11] Patients meeting the criteria for referral need the expertise of a multidisciplinary team. Referring hospitals must always contact the burn center in their region.[11]

SPECIAL MANAGEMENT CONSIDERATIONS

INHALATION INJURY

Inhalation injury can occur in either the presence or the absence of cutaneous injury. Inhalation injuries are strongly associated with burns sustained in a closed space. Inhalation injury is the leading cause of fire-related deaths.[18] For any given severity of skin burns, the addition of inhalation injury doubles the mortality rate.[19] Inhalation injury appears in three basic forms, alone or in combination: carbon monoxide poisoning, direct heat injury, and/or chemical damage. The three distinguishing types of inhalation injury are carbon monoxide poisoning, upper airway injury, and lower airway injury.

Immediate measures to save the life of the burn patient include management of the airway. The burn patient may exhibit few if any signs of airway distress; however, thermal injury to the airway must be anticipated if facial burns, singed eyebrows and nasal hair, carbon deposits in the oropharynx, or carbonaceous sputum is present, or if the history suggests confinement in a burning environment. Any of these findings indicates acute inhalation injury and requires immediate and definitive care. To prevent the necessity of tracheostomy or cricothyrotomy, the use of early intubation and respiratory support must be considered before tracheal edema occurs. Inhalation injury predisposes the patient to the development of pneumonia and acute lung injury (ALI).[18,19] Management of ALI necessitates mechanical ventilatory support and in extreme cases high-frequency oscillatory ventilation or extracorporeal membrane oxygenation. The occurrence of inhalation injury with cutaneous burns increases the fluid requirements during resuscitation to a higher level than would be predicted by the cutaneous burn alone.

Carbon Monoxide (CO) Poisoning. Persons found dead at the scene of a fire may have little or no cutaneous thermal injuries but will have died instead of CO poisoning. Carbon monoxide is a colorless, odorless, and tasteless gas. Inhalation of CO, a by-product of the incomplete combustion of carbon, results in its bonding to available hemoglobin, producing carboxyhemoglobin (HbCO), which effectively decreases oxygen saturation of hemoglobin. The affinity of hemoglobin molecules for carbon monoxide is approximately 200 times greater than that for oxygen.[22] Carboxyhemoglobin binds poorly with oxygen, reducing the oxygen-carrying capacity of blood and causing hypoxia. The shortage of oxygen at the tissue level is worsened by a shift to the left of the oxyhemoglobin dissociation curve so that the oxygen in the hemoglobin is not readily given up to the cells.

Arterial oxygen saturation measurement is of limited value because oxygen saturation may be quite high despite dangerously low levels of oxygen content. Remember that the pulse oximeter cannot distinguish between oxyhemoglobin and carboxyhemoglobin, thus making it unreliable during initial stages of CO poisoning. Arterial blood gas with oxygen saturation must be drawn to accurately assess hemoglobin oxygen saturation level. Normal HbCO levels are less than 2%. Carboxyhemoglobin levels of 40% to 60% often produce unresponsiveness or obtundation; levels of 15% to 40% may result in central nervous system dysfunction of varying degrees; and levels of 10% to 15%, which can be found in cigarette smokers, are rarely symptomatic but may cause a headache.

The major clinical manifestations of severe CO poisoning are related to the central nervous system and the heart. Symptoms associated with CO poisoning include headache, dizziness, nausea, vomiting, dyspnea, and confusion. In severe cases, CO poisoning may lead to myocardial ischemia and central nervous system complications caused by lowered oxygen delivery and the already compromised circulatory system. Early signs of CO poisoning may include tachycardia, tachypnea, confusion, and lightheadedness. As the CO level rises, the patients will exhibit a decreased level of responsiveness, which may progress to unresponsiveness and respiratory failure.

The treatment of choice for CO poisoning is high-flow oxygen administered at 100% through a tight-fitting nonrebreathing mask or endotracheal intubation. The half-life of CO in the body is 4 hours at room air (21% oxygen), 2 hours at 40% oxygen, and 40 to 60 minutes at 100% oxygen.[22] The half-life of CO is 30 minutes in a hyperbaric oxygen chamber at three times the atmospheric pressure. Currently the use of hyperbaric oxygen is of controversial benefit in the care of the burn patient. Because of the rapid removal of CO with the administration of 100% oxygen, the time required to transport a patient who has received oxygen in the field should always be considered to avoid possible underestimation of inhalation injury.

Upper Airway Injury. Burns of the upper respiratory tract include those involving the pharynx, larynx, glottis, trachea, and larger bronchi. Injuries are caused either by direct heat or by chemical inflammation and necrosis. Respiratory injury is most often confined to the upper airway. The heat exchange capability is so efficient that most heat absorption and damage occur in the pharynx and larynx above the true vocal cords.

Heat damage may be severe enough to cause upper airway obstruction at any time beginning from time of injury through the resuscitation period. Caution is taken for patients with severe hypovolemia, because supraglottic edema may be delayed until fluid resuscitation is under way. Patients must be monitored for hoarseness, stridor, audible airflow turbulence, and the production of carbonaceous sputum. Maximal edema occurs 24 hours after injury with upper airway injuries; therefore these patients should be observed in the intensive care unit for a minimum of 24 hours.[5]

The prediction of an upper airway obstruction is based on consideration of the following variables: extent of injury to the face and neck, the presence of blisters on or redness of the posterior pharynx, signs of singed nasal hair, increased HbCO levels, increased rate and decreased depth of breathing, hoarseness (which indicates a significant decrease in the diameter of the airway), increased amount of sputum, and the circumstances of the burn event (i.e., whether it occurred in an enclosed space and/or whether it involved superheated gases or steam). Steam has a heat-carrying capacity many times that of dry air and is capable of overwhelming the extremely efficient heat-dissipating capabilities of the upper airway.

Intubation is recommended when airway patency is questionable at any time, rather than delaying intubation until airway obstruction is so severe that intubation becomes very challenging. Once the airway is secure, priority is given to minimizing airway edema, maintaining pulmonary toilet, and treating bronchospasm. Elevating of the head of the bed to 30 degrees or higher decreases airway edema. Therapeutic deep breathing and coughing, early mobility, suctioning, and bronchodilators will assist in mobilizing and removing secretions. Fiberoptic bronchoscopy may be required to remove secretions in some patients. Mechanical ventilatory support is necessary when respiratory fatigue or failure occurs. When prolonged ventilatory failure is expected because of severe inhalation, a tracheostomy is performed.[5]

Lower Airway Injury. Heated air rarely causes lower airway injury. If it does, it usually is associated with death at the scene. Lower airway injuries also may be caused by chemical damage to mucosal surfaces. Tracheobronchitis with severe spasm and wheezing may occur in the first minutes to hours after injury. The most accurate method of documenting lower airway injury is the xenon-ventilation perfusion lung scan. Prolonged retention or symmetry of washout of the radioisotope indicates pulmonary parenchyma injury on the side of the retained emissions.

The fiberoptic bronchoscope is used by the physician both in the diagnosis and in the management of inhalation injury associated with complications.[23] The onset of symptoms is so unpredictable with possible smoke inhalation that patients at risk must be closely observed for at least 24 to 48 hours after injury. Research on the use of high-frequency ventilation early in the care of patients with inhalation injury has promising results.[20,24] Benefits include decreased rates of pneumonia and increased survival.[25] Treatment of lower airway injury is largely symptomatic. As with upper airway injury management, removal of secretions, ventilatory support, and tracheostomy may be required.

NONTHERMAL BURNS

Chemical Burns. Chemical burns can be caused by a variety of products. Acids, alkalis, and organic and inorganic compounds cause chemical burns. The acid or base quality determines the injurious nature of a product. The injury is caused by the pH of the product or by the concentration of the product. In the past, the irrigation of chemical burns with neutralizing solutions was recommended to limit the extent and depth of chemical burns. This practice is no longer advocated because neutralizing agents may cause reactions that are exothermic (i.e., produce heat), thereby increasing the extent and depth of the burn. It also is possible that the neutralizing agent is neither immediately known nor available. Therefore the use of large amounts of water to flush the area is recommended. Clothing and shoes should be removed if they have been in contact with the chemical. Alkali burns of the eyes require continuous irrigation for many hours after the injury. Removal of contact lenses is necessary before irrigation.

Treatments for chemical burns will vary. Phenol burns are first diluted, and then the skin is wiped quickly with polyethylene glycol or vegetable oil to decrease the severity of the burn. Areas exposed to hydrofluoric acid must also be copiously irrigated with water; the burned area then can be treated with 2.5% calcium gluconate gel. The patient may need calcium gluconate replacements because the fluoride ion precipitates serum calcium, causing hypocalcemia. White phosphorus can ignite if kept dry; therefore wounds must be covered with a moist dressing. After a tar or asphalt injury, the removal of tar or asphalt is best accomplished with the use of petroleum-containing distillates. One such product is Detachol (Ferndale Laboratories, Inc., Ferndale, Mich.). The solution can be placed directly on the wound and gently wiped off. Routine débridement of loose skin is initiated after tar removal. Topical antimicrobial therapy is then applied.

Electrical Burns. In electrical burns, the type and voltage of the circuit, resistance, pathway of transmission through the body, and duration of contact are considered in determining the amount of damage sustained. Often in these situations the rescuer also may be injured if he or she becomes part of the electrical circuit. The rescuer must disconnect the electrical source to break the circuit or must know how to avoid becoming part of the circuit. The use of appropriately insulated equipment that diverts the circuit elsewhere is essential. Extreme caution must be used in the rescue of victims.

Electricity always travels toward the ground. Current research proves that the body conducts electrical current as a whole, as opposed to the earlier belief that it traveled most quickly through the nerves and circulatory system.[25] Electrical burns often are much more serious than the surface appearance of the wound suggests. As the electrical current passes through the body, it damages the inner tissues and may leave little evidence of a burn on the skin surface (Fig. 40-7).

The electrical burn process can result in a profound alteration in acid-base balance and rhabdomyolysis resulting in myoglobinuria, which poses a serious threat to renal function. Myoglobin is a normal constituent of muscle. With extensive muscle destruction, it is released into the circulatory system and filtered by the kidneys. It can be highly toxic and can lead to intrinsic renal failure. Fluid resuscitation for the electrical burn patient does not correlate with the Parkland formula, and the fluid is adjusted according to the patient's urine output. If myoglobin is present in the urine, a urine output of 100 to 150 ml/hr in adults and 2 ml/kg/hr in children is established until the urine is clear of all gross pigment.

In the presence of hemoglobinuria, the clinician should assume that myoglobinuria and acidosis are present. Sodium bicarbonate may be administered to bring the pH level into normal range, to correct a documented acidosis, and/or to alkalize urine to promote myoglobin excretion. Diuretics also may be administered intravenously until myoglobinuria resolves. Sodium bicarbonate infusions and diuretic therapy are termed *forced alkaline diuresis*. Baseline ECG and cardiac enzyme levels are obtained while the patient is in the emergency department. The following are criteria for the cardiac monitoring of patients:

- A history of loss of consciousness or cardiac arrest
- Documentation of cardiac dysrhythmia at the scene of the accident or in the emergency department
- Abnormal ECG findings on admission

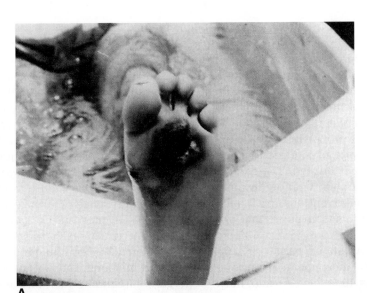

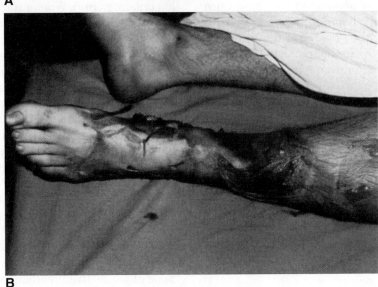

Fig. 40-7 **A,** Exit site of electrical burn on sole of foot. **B,** Same leg several days later, illustrating extension of tissue damage after the injury.

- TBSA burns of >20%
- Very young or elderly persons
- Previous cardiac history

Other burn patients may be admitted to nonmonitored settings and observed closely. Cardiac dysrhythmias must be treated promptly, and a protocol to rule out myocardial infarction must be followed.[26]

BURN NURSING DIAGNOSES AND MANAGEMENT

The clinical course of a burn injury comprises three phases: the resuscitative phase, the acute care phase, and the rehabilitative phase. Each phase is unique and has its own set of actual and potential problems. The resuscitative phase begins with the initial hemodynamic response to the injury and lasts until capillary integrity is restored and the repletion of plasma volume by fluid replacement occurs. Spontaneous diuresis is the hallmark that demonstrates that the capillaries have regained their integrity. The acute phase begins with the onset of diuresis of fluid mobilized from the interstitial space and ends with the closure of the burn wound. The major focus of the acute phase is wound healing, wound closure, and prevention of infection. The rehabilitative phase begins when the patient is admitted to the hospital, with correction of functional deficits and scar management being major considerations. The rehabilitative phase may last from months to years depending on the severity of injury. The rehabilitation phase focuses on support for adequate wound healing, prevention of scarring and contractures, and psychologic support of the patient and family.[27]

RESUSCITATION PHASE

Cardiopulmonary instability, life-threatening airway and breathing problems, and hypovolemia characterize the resuscitation phase, or shock phase. Every organ is involved in the physiologic response that occurs with thermal injury of greater than 20% TBSA. The magnitude of this pathophysiologic response is proportional to the extent of cutaneous injury. The response is maximal when approximately 60% of the TBSA is burned. The goal of the resuscitation phase is to maintain vital organ function and perfusion. Emergent interventions for inhalation injury, airway management, and hypovolemia are concurrently addressed.

Oxygenation Alterations. As stated earlier, inhalation injuries have emerged as the most common cause of death in burn patients, whereas 40 to 50 years ago, burn shock and then burn sepsis accounted for most burn deaths. Early diagnosis of inhalation injury is vital to minimize complications and to decrease the mortality rate. Three separate oxygenation complications are associated with smoke inhalation during the resuscitation phase: *CO poisoning, upper airway obstruction,* and *chemical pneumonitis.* The assessment of a patient for inhalation injury includes the following parameters: physical assessment (singed facial hairs, mucosal burns of nose or mouth, carbonaceous sputum); arterial blood gas analysis; HbCO levels; chest radiography; flexible fiberoptic bronchoscopy; xenon-133 lung scan; and pulmonary function tests.[18,19] Nursing actions include the following:

- Assess breath sounds, as well as the rate and quality of respirations, and document.
- Administer oxygen as prescribed.
- Monitor HbCO levels.
- Elevate the head of the bed.
- Assess and assist with pulmonary secretions removal, and document.
- Provide suction as needed.
- Observe for signs of airway obstruction (e.g., increased respiratory rate and heart rate, increased work of breathing, use of accessory muscles, stridor, wheezing, hoarseness, and crackles).
- Prepare for endotracheal intubation and mechanical ventilation.

Impaired Gas Exchange. As previously discussed, the most common pulmonary burn complication is CO poisoning. High-flow oxygen should be administered at 100% through a nonrebreathing mask or endotracheal intubation until the HbCO level is <10% to 15%.

Chemical pneumonitis is caused by inhalation of the by-products of combustion of substances such as those in burning cotton, aldehydes, oxides of sulfur, and nitrogen. Burning polyvinylchloride yields at least 75 potentially toxic compounds, including hydrochloric acid and CO. Within days after a burn, ARDS commonly develops in patients with chemical pneumonitis. The primary clinical manifestation of ARDS is hypoxemia refractory to oxygen therapy.[19] Early signs include increased pH, decreased $Paco_2$, and an increased respiratory rate. Ventilatory support with the use of positive end-expiratory pressure (PEEP) is the treatment of choice.

Ineffective Airway Clearance. Laryngeal swelling and upper airway obstruction may occur anytime in the first 24 hours after the burn injury. As previously stated, endotracheal intubation must be accomplished early because this simple procedure can become extremely difficult in the presence of laryngeal edema. Generally, however, time to intervene is available after obtaining the history and transporting the patient to the primary hospital. Edema may continue to develop for 72 hours after the burn incident. The patient who has not initially undergone intubation must be carefully monitored during this critical period. When prolonged ventilatory failure is expected as a result of severe inhalation, a tracheostomy is performed.[5]

Extubation should occur only if the patient can meet extubation criteria: level of consciousness assessed as "awake," intact cough and gag reflexes, inspiratory effort greater than −25 cm water in adults, vital capacity of 10 ml/kg, and decreased volume and tenacity of the sputum. Resolution of airway edema can be assessed by deflating the endotracheal cuff and observing the patient's ability to breathe around the endotracheal tube.

Laryngospasm is another complication that, although not commonly seen, must be addressed. It generally is brought on by airway irritation secondary to inhalation of noxious agents.

Ineffective Breathing Pattern. Circumferential full-thickness burns to the chest wall are the most common cause of ineffective breathing patterns. As previously discussed, escharotomies should be performed in this situation, which will lead to improved chest wall compliance and breathing efficiency.

Fluid Resuscitation. Current resuscitation protocols emphasize fluid delivery rates based on the extent of burn and the patient's weight. Therefore patient weight measured in kilograms must be obtained upon admission to the hospital. The extent of the burn is calculated by using one of the methods previously described. Several formulas are available to guide fluid resuscitation and should be used to assist in the management of fluid replacement (see Table 40-1). The formulas differ primarily in terms of administration, volume, and sodium content. The actual amount of fluid given to any patient must be based on that individual's response.

The type of fluid used in resuscitation and at what point one should switch to colloid solution are subjects of controversy. There are no clear-cut guidelines for resuscitation. The administration of crystalloid fluid, namely LR, for the first 24 to 36 hours after the burn is the most common practice. LR solution is the crystalloid solution of choice because of its physiologic similarity to the composition of extracellular fluid. Ideally the capillary leak seals approximately 24 hours after the injury and theoretically makes it possible to give colloid without leakage of protein into the interstitium. Colloid deficits are replaced in the next 24 hours with salt-free albumin or dextran at 0.3 to 1 ml/kg/% TBSA burn. In addition to colloid, maintenance fluids are given to replace evaporative losses, and the amount is adjusted according to the patient's serum electrolytes, urine output, weight, volume status, and clinical assessment.

The proposed benefit of colloid use is that less burn edema occurs and therefore increased hemodynamic stability results. Arguments have been made that colloid administration shows no more benefit than crystalloid and should be used judiciously because the cost is high. Hypertonic saline (LR with varying concentrations of sodium lactate) also is used. The controversial benefit of hypertonic saline is an overall decrease in total fluid requirements. Routine serum sodium levels should be monitored, and hypertonic saline should be stopped for sodium levels of 160 mEq/dl or greater.

Deficient Fluid Volume. The physiologic effects of the burn complicate tissue damage that occurs after the burn insult. Coagulation factors are affected, protein is denatured, and cellular content is ionized. These factors, coupled with the dilation of capillaries and small vessels, lead to increased capillary permeability and fluid shifts from the intravascular space to the interstitial space. The lymphatic system, which normally would carry away the increased interstitial fluid, may be damaged or overloaded and unable to function to its normal capacity.

In addition to the protein and electrolyte shift, an increased insensible water loss occurs. In the healthy adult this loss is estimated at 35 to 50 ml/hr. The burn patient's insensible water loss may be as much as 300 to 3000 ml per day. This increase may be related to temperature elevation, tracheostomy, and the size of the burn.

Burn shock is proportional to the extent and depth of injury. The loss of plasma begins almost immediately after the injury and reaches its peak within the first 48 hours. Desired clinical responses to fluid resuscitation include a urinary output of 0.5 to 1 ml/kg/hr; a pulse rate lower than 120 beats/min; blood pressure in normal to high ranges; a central venous pressure less than 12 cm H_2O or a pulmonary artery occlusion pressure less than 18 mm Hg; clear lung sounds; clear sensorium; and the absence of intestinal events, such as nausea and paralytic ileus. Heart rate, blood pressure, and central venous pressure values are not always accurate or reliable predictors of successful fluid resuscitation.

Potassium and sodium, the two electrolytes of concern during the resuscitation period, must be monitored carefully. *Hyperkalemia* can occur during this phase because of the release of potassium from damaged cells; because of metabolic acidosis; and/or because of im-

paired renal function secondary to hemoglobinuria, myoglobinuria, or decreased renal perfusion. The patient must be assessed for the clinical manifestations of hyperkalemia. Treatment includes correction of acidosis. During the resuscitation phase, using cation-exchange resins or intravenously administered insulin and hypertonic dextrose to transport potassium back into the cell is not recommended because of the unpredictable nature of fluid shifts that occur.

Hypokalemia also can occur during the resuscitation phase because of the massive loss of fluids and electrolytes through the burn wounds or because of hemodilution. During the acute phase it may be related to hemodilution; inadequate replacement; loss associated with diuresis, diarrhea, vomiting, nasogastric drainage, and long hydrotherapy sessions; and/or the shift of potassium from the intravascular space to the cell after the acidosis has been corrected. Nursing interventions include treating nausea and vomiting, limiting immersive hydrotherapy sessions to less than 30 minutes, preventing fluid volume excess, and judicious replacement of potassium.

Hyponatremia is not uncommon during the resuscitation phase because of the loss of sodium through the burn wound, the shift of fluid into the interstitial space, vomiting, nasogastric drainage, diarrhea, and/or the use of hypotonic salt solutions during the early phase of resuscitation. During this phase it may be necessary to monitor serum sodium levels every 4 to 8 hours. Hyponatremia also may occur during the acute phase because of hemodilution and loss through the wound, lengthy hydrotherapy sessions, and excessive diuresis resulting from the fluid shift back into the intravascular space. Interventions are followed for treating nausea and vomiting, hydrotherapy sessions are limited, and intravenous replacement of sodium is considered. During diuresis, which occurs during the acute phase, restricting free water intake usually is the only required intervention to increase the serum sodium.

Risk for Infection. Preventing infection in the burn patient is a true challenge and involves complex decision making. Infection leading to sepsis and multisystem organ failure is the most common cause of death after the initial resuscitation period.

There has been considerable discussion in recent years regarding the infection control precautions to use with burn patients. The burn wound is the most common source of infection in the burn patient. The loss of the protective mechanism of the skin and contamination from the patient's own bacterial flora can lead to bloodstream infections. Some centers advocate routine wound surveillance cultures and wound biopsy to identify infection early. Daily wound inspection for changes in appearance, such as an increase in exudate, odor, or color, is necessary to minimize the risk of bacteremia. Patients should not be treated with antibiotics prophylactically; rather, treatment should be tailored based on positive culture results.

Cross-contamination by direct contact is a significant source of infection and a subsequent cause of sepsis.[28] Proper hand-washing technique cannot be overemphasized. Nurses must wash their hands and change gloves when moving from area to area on the same patient. For example, after changing the chest dressing, which may be contaminated with sputum from the tracheostomy, hands must be washed and gloves changed before the nurse moves to the legs. Gowns, gloves, and masks should be worn whenever there is contact with body fluids. These garments also must be changed and hands washed before caring for a different patient. Maintaining patient-specific dressings and topical agents is recommended. Equipment such as thermometers, intravenous pumps, and stethoscopes should be designated for each patient or, when shared, should be cleaned with appropriate bactericidal cleansers between patients. Some centers advocate the practice of protective isolation for all burn patients.

Whichever precautions are used, it is vital that everyone coming in contact with the patient, including the family and visitors, is knowledgeable about the standard for infection control. These precautions should be strictly followed by all. Precautions should have sound rationale and should not increase the workload or the frustration of the burn team. Otherwise, compliance and consistent application of the standard will not occur, thus increasing the risk of infection and sepsis for the burn patient.

TISSUE PERFUSION

Ineffective Renal Tissue Perfusion. Urinalysis to determine the myoglobin level may be performed early after burn injury. Myoglobinuria can be detected grossly by a dark, port-wine color of the urine. Myoglobin is extremely toxic to the kidneys and can cause massive tubular destruction. It is best treated with rapid fluid administration and forced diuresis with diuretics such as mannitol, an osmotic diuretic. The goal is an hourly urine output that is at least double the general recommendations to flush the renal tubules. All other diuretics are avoided because they will deplete the already compromised intravascular volume. Sodium bicarbonate is sometimes given intravenously to alkalinize the urine and assist in the elimination of heme pigments.

Maintaining and monitoring the renal system is vital in burn patient management. Impairment of the renal system may be related to hemoglobinuria, myoglobinuria, hypoperfusion, and hypovolemia. Urinary output must be monitored every hour for the first 48 to 72 hours, and specific gravity values can be useful to determine adequacy of hydration status and renal competency. Urine glucose is monitored, as are urine sodium, creatinine, and BUN

levels. Use of an indwelling urinary catheter is appropriate for the first 48 to 72 hours. Because of the tremendous risk of infection related to indwelling catheters, they are removed as soon as possible. However, leaving the catheter in place may be necessary if perineal burns are involved. Oliguria is usually related to inadequate fluid resuscitation but may be associated with acute renal failure. Other signs of renal failure include increasing creatinine, BUN, phosphorus, and potassium levels; excessive weight gain; excessive edema; elevated blood pressure; lethargy; and confusion.

The presence of glucose in the urine causes osmotic diuresis. In this clinical situation, urine output will be an unreliable estimate of volume status. Because of the increased loss of fluid via the kidneys, glucosuria may actually suggest the need for additional fluid beyond the original estimates.

Ineffective Cerebral Tissue Perfusion. The patient's neurologic status is assessed frequently during the first few days. Changes may be related to an associated head injury that occurred at the time of burn injury, hypoperfusion related to hypovolemia, hypoxemia associated with inadequate ventilation, CO poisoning, and/or electrolyte imbalances. Patients with electrical burns or major thermal burns may have peripheral neurologic injuries, which may not become evident for several days after the injury. The neurologic assessment includes use of the Glasgow Coma Scale. It is not unusual for the patient to be agitated, restless, and extremely anxious during the resuscitation phase of burn injury as a result of hypovolemia, pain, and/or the fear of disfigurement or even death. However, the possibility of neurologic involvement must not be overlooked. Maintaining an adequate mean arterial pressure is essential to ensure adequate cerebral perfusion pressure.

Ineffective Peripheral Tissue Perfusion. Ineffective peripheral tissue perfusion results from third spacing of fluid during the resuscitation phase, which restricts blood flow to extremities. As hypovolemia ensues, vasoconstriction increases, which can be potentiated by the loss of body temperature. Peripheral tissue perfusion must be monitored carefully in all burn patients, as discussed earlier. Burned and unburned areas are carefully assessed for warmth, color, and peripheral pulses. Capillary refill time should be less than 2 seconds in unburned areas. Any clinical manifestation of diminished systemic tissue perfusion must be reported immediately. Nursing actions are taken to minimize any compromise of peripheral circulation. Close monitoring of appropriate fluid resuscitation and careful positioning of the patient are necessary to prevent compromised blood flow. Avoid such positions as crossed legs or dependent positions, and avoid pillows under knees. The limbs should be elevated above the heart to decrease peripheral edema and enhance venous return.[9] Assisted range of motion exercises also can help decrease edema.

Monitoring the peripheral circulation is crucial in the burn patient with circumferential full-thickness burns of the extremities. The resulting edema may severely compromise the venous system and then the arterial system. Neurovascular integrity of extremities with circumferential burns must be assessed every hour for the first 24 to 48 hours using the "six p's": *pulselessness, pallor, pain, paresthesia, paralysis,* and *poikilothermy.* Careful, ongoing assessment is necessary, especially in patients who are intubated and may not be able to communicate pain or paresthesia. The use of a Doppler flowmeter may be necessary. Loss of pulses is a late sign of compromised vascular flow. If any changes are noted, the physician must be notified immediately. Numbness and paresthesia may occur only 30 minutes before loss of pulses. Irreversible nerve ischemia resulting in loss of function may begin after 12 to 24 hours. An escharotomy may become necessary to allow the underlying tissue to expand. In deeper wounds, a fasciotomy, which involves incision into the fascia, may be necessary.

An unfortunate scenario results when the patient's reports of ischemic pain and paresthesia in a circumferentially burned extremity go unheeded and neurovascular compromise is allowed to persist. Sensory nerve fibers become damaged, and altered sensations cease, which may be misinterpreted as improvement in neurovascular status. Permanent disability and possible loss of limb are eventual outcomes.

Ineffective Gastrointestinal Tissue Perfusion. Paralytic ileus is a common GI complication that can occur during resuscitation or when sepsis develops. The abdomen and bowel sounds should be assessed every 2 hours during the initial phase and every 4 hours thereafter. If clinical manifestations of a paralytic ileus occur, oral intake is withheld and a nasogastric tube is inserted and placed on low to medium suction. A paralytic ileus can be related to hypokalemia, the sympathetic response to severe trauma, and/or decreased tissue perfusion related to hypovolemia.

A stress ulcer (Curling ulcer) may develop as a result of decreased tissue perfusion to the GI tract, a change in the quantity or quality of mucus (which has a pH of 1), and/or an increase in gastric acid secretion resulting from the stress response. Gastric acid should be maintained above a pH of 5 through the administration of antacids, H_2 blockers, or proton pump inhibitors to prevent the development of these ulcers. The patient should be carefully monitored for GI bleeding. All stools and gastric content are tested for occult blood. The patient should be observed for epigastric discomfort or fullness, decreased blood pressure, or increased pulse. Advances in burn care such as early fluid resuscitation, early gastric feeding, and antacid therapy have decreased the incidence of stress ulcers to a reported 2%.[29]

Invasive Monitoring. The decision to use invasive monitoring techniques requires careful consideration of the potential risk factors and how the data collected will influence the course of treatment. Invasive monitoring certainly should be considered if treatment seems ineffective or if complicating factors occur, such as severe respiratory involvement, major life-threatening injuries, head injuries, or pneumothorax. Patients with preexisting medical conditions such as chronic obstructive pulmonary disease (COPD), congestive heart failure, and renal failure also may require invasive monitoring.[30]

Invasive monitoring includes direct measurement of central venous pressure, pulmonary artery pressure, arterial pressure, core temperature, cardiac output, SVR, and PVR. The use of an arterial line is considered if serial and frequent arterial blood gas values are required for respiratory management or for hemodynamic instability requiring the titration of vasoactive drugs. Central venous catheters can be helpful in the early stages of fluid resuscitation to deliver the massive amount of fluids required. The physician selects the catheter insertion site based on burn location and the purpose of the catheter. It is preferable not to insert catheters through burned skin. It may be appropriate to use a multilumen catheter that can serve as a route for fluid resuscitation, maintenance fluids, antibiotic therapy, and vasoactive drugs. The risks involved include the increased chance of infection, potential for pneumothorax, and difficulty with insertion if hypovolemia is present.

Pulmonary artery catheters are placed only when necessary for optimal care. They may be absolutely essential to the survival of the septic patient despite the risks involved. Pulmonary artery catheters can provide data about pulmonary artery occlusion pressure (PAOP), cardiac output, stroke volume, systemic and pulmonary vascular resistance, core temperature, and mixed venous oxygen saturation levels.

Centrally placed intravascular catheters require meticulous care. Strict guidelines should be established and monitored. Catheters are inserted under sterile conditions, and the dressings are changed under the same conditions. Because infection is such a major concern, all invasive catheters are removed as early as possible.[28]

Hypothermia. Thermoregulation maintenance is a nursing challenge. The patient with extensive burn injury is at high risk for hypothermia. Hypothermia is especially problematic during initial treatment, during hydrotherapy, and immediately after surgery. Heat is lost through open burn wounds by means of evaporation and radiation. The patient's core temperature should be maintained at 99.6° to 101° F. Heat shields/lamps, hypothermia blankets, and fluid warmers can be individually or simultaneously used to maintain body temperature.

Laboratory Assessment. Laboratory assessment is another important aspect of burn care. Because of the invasive nature of drawing blood, it is done only if absolutely indicated. Consideration should be given to the age of the patient, the size of the burn, the time since injury, and any underlying disease process.

White blood cell (WBC) counts usually are monitored for elevation, a sign of sepsis. It is not unusual, however, for the WBC count to fall below 5000 mm^3 within 48 hours after injury. It may drop even lower—1500/mm^3 to 2000/mm^3—with the use of silver sulfadiazine. If the WBC count stays in this range for more than 12 hours, the use of a different topical agent is recommended. The WBC count will generally become normal again. At this point the use of silver sulfadiazine can be tested again by applying it to a small area. If the WBC count does not drop again within 12 hours, the use of silver sulfadiazine can be resumed. In practice, the need for discontinuation of silver sulfadiazine is not common but must be considered if the WBC count continues to fall.

Hemoglobin and hematocrit data can be useful in the resuscitative phase to guide fluid administration. If surgical débridement is required, monitoring blood counts in the postoperative period is important. Serum chemistry information is helpful for ongoing assessment of renal function and electrolyte balance. The myriad tests available should be used appropriately and as indicated by individual patient needs.

ACUTE CARE PHASE

The acute care phase of burn management begins after resuscitation and lasts until complete wound closure is achieved. The early postresuscitation phase is a period of transition from the shock phase to the hypermetabolic phase. Major cardiopulmonary and wound changes occur that substantially alter the manner of patient care from that given during resuscitation. In general, cardiopulmonary stability is optimal during this period because wound inflammation and infection have not developed. Hypermetabolic changes can be complicated with the onset of wound infection and sepsis. Early wound excision and skin grafting procedures, local wound care, nutritional support, and infection control characterize this phase.

Critical care nurses play a major role in promoting the healing process. Nurses, as skilled clinicians of the burn team, provide daily wound assessment, hydrotherapy, débridement, preoperative and postoperative management, and pain management. Appropriate treatment results in critical differences in patient care and outcomes.

Immediately after injury, the body responds by initiating a series of physiologic changes to restore skin integrity. These physiologic changes include the inflammatory phase, the proliferative phase, and the maturation phase.

The Inflammatory Phase. The inflammatory phase begins immediately after injury. Vascular changes and cellular activity characterize this period. Changes in the severed vessels occur in an attempt to wall off the wound from the external environment. Platelets, activated as a result of vessel wall injury, aggregate; blood coagulation

is initiated; and in larger vessels, smooth muscle tissue contraction occurs, resulting in reduction in the diameter of the vessel lumen. These brief but important compensatory mechanisms serve to protect the individual from excessive blood loss and increased exposure to bacterial contamination. As vasodilation occurs, vascular permeability and blood supply to the wound site increase. As extravascular volume increases, signs of erythema, edema, and tenderness become apparent. Granulocytes invade the wound within 24 hours and initiate the phagocytosis of necrotic tissue and bacteria. Fibroblasts migrate to the wound and multiply, producing a bed of collagen. This phase of healing lasts from the moment of injury to day 3 or 4 after the traumatic event.[31]

The Proliferative Phase. The proliferative phase of healing occurs approximately 4 to 20 days after injury. The key cell in this phase of healing, the fibroblast, rapidly synthesizes collagen. Collagen synthesis provides the needed strength for a healing wound. Epithelial cells migrate across the wound bed. Once these cells contact each other, the wound is covered. This process is known as *epithelialization*. Myofibroblasts also play a role in healing by pulling down the wound edge toward the center in an effort to close the wound; this process is known as *wound contraction*.

The Maturation Phase. The maturation phase of healing occurs from approximately 20 days after injury to longer than 1 year after injury. During this period the wound develops tensile strength as collagen deposits form scar tissue. Regardless of how well collagen realigns itself, the tissue of the wound will never regain the degree of strength or intactness inherent in uninjured tissue. Over time, scar tissue matures and becomes smaller and less bulky, and pigmentation returns.

IMPAIRED TISSUE INTEGRITY

Management of the burn wound is the top priority after the resuscitation phase. The depth of the burn wound is the principal determinant of wound management. Expedient closure of the wounds decreases the potential for multiple complications, such as fluid and electrolyte imbalances, loss of proteins and nitrogen, and infection. The major goal of burn wound care is wound closure. Initial débridement is done by removing blisters and loose skin. The assessment of wound depth by the clinician guides the treatment based on whether the wound will close in a reasonable time with daily dressings or will require surgical débridement. As previously mentioned, the assessment of wound depth can be a difficult challenge. There are many alternative dressing regimens for wound closure that are either temporary, semipermanent or permanent. These will be discussed in later sections. Several objectives must be met for optimal wound closure: to control infection through meticulous cleansing and débridement, to promote reepitheliazation, and to prepare the wound for grafting and closure. Other goals are to reduce scarring and contracture formation and to provide patient comfort with appropriate psychologic support and pharmacologic intervention.

Factors Affecting Healing of the Burn Wound. Prompt application of topical antimicrobial therapy is important to prevent bacterial contamination, and the agent is selected based on the depth and location of burn injury. The sources of contamination are many and include the patient's endogenous flora found on the skin, the upper respiratory tract, and the gastrointestinal tract. Exogenous flora found in the patient care setting include bacteria carried by staff members and the environment. Patient-specific factors that predispose the patient to infection include age, diabetes, steroid therapy, extreme obesity, severe malnutrition, and infections in remote sites. Because both wound healing and clinical infection are inflammatory responses, it is essential to differentiate between normal wound inflammation in the presence of colonization of microorganisms and that of invading organisms. In diagnosing infection, the importance of microbiologic results must be evaluated in conjunction with clinical findings such as excessive erythema, edema, pain, and purulence. Generally, clinical findings in conjunction with burn wound biopsy or culture results are the hallmark determinants of wound sepsis. Other factors that affect wound healing are tissue hypoxia from low blood flow to the burn wound, the presence of eschar that will require débridement, exudate on the wound that can be harmful to the granulating wound or consume oxygen in the wound, and trauma to the wound from daily dressing changes or lack of protection from the outside environment.

Wound Cleansing. A variety of equally appropriate methods can be used to cleanse burn wounds (e.g., sterile normal saline at the bedside or tap water in a hydrotherapy room). At some centers, a mild antimicrobial cleansing agent is used, such as chlorhexidine (Hibiclens). Wounds are gently cleansed with a gauze dressing or washcloth and patted dry before application of topical agents. Hydrotherapy facilitates the removal of debris and loose eschar. Denatured protein-rich pseudo eschar should be cleansed daily because it can slow healing and limit the innate ability of growth factors.[32] Daily cleansing and inspection of the wound and unburned skin are performed to assess for signs of healing and local infection. Generally this therapy is performed once or twice daily. The wound care exposure is limited in length as much as feasible to prevent hypothermia and decrease exposure to bacteria. Pain management and measures to reduce hypothermia are used. Patients must receive adequate premedication with analgesics, narcotics, and/or sedatives.[17] Morphine or other opioids are administered intravenously and titrated to effect. The patient's vital signs are carefully monitored during this time, especially body temperature and blood pressure.

Total immersion therapy has fallen out of favor recently because of the risk of infection. Currently, spray tables and specially designed upright and chair showers are used. The force of the spray assists in the removal of topical agents and débridement.[6,8]

Wound Care. Although many options for burn wound care are available, the basic principle of maintaining a moist wound environment while prevention burn wound infection is the standard of care. The universal belief that moist wound healing is advantageous is described by many authors.[32-34] Some of these benefits are preventing wound desiccation, optimal function of local wound growth factors and proteolytic enzymes to remove dead tissue, increased reepitheliazation and collagen synthesis and decreased wound fluid loss.[35-38] The most common regimen for burn wound care today continues to involve the application of a topical antimicrobial agent, followed by a primary gauze dressing to absorb burn wound drainage and an outer layer to provide increased absorption, compression, and occlusion. Daily wound care is managed in one of the following three methods: open, semiopen, or closed. The open method involves leaving the burn open with only a topical agent applied. Advantages to this method are (1) the wound can be easily assessed, (2) no dressings limit range of motion, and (3) the risk of diminishing circulation is decreased. Several disadvantages to the open method include (1) the need for strict isolation technique or increased risk of infection, (2) a possible increase in patient discomfort with this method because the wound is exposed to air currents and environmental temperatures, (3) increased risk of hypothermia, and (4) wound desiccation.

The semiopen method consists of covering the wound with a thin layer of gauze or nonadherent dressing that can be impregnated with petroleum product (e.g., Adaptic or Xeroform) with or without topical antimicrobial and netting material to keep the antimicrobial agent in place (BandNet). This method is useful for less acute wounds when the amount of drainage has decreased and wound closure has almost been achieved.

The closed method of management generally consists of the application of topical agents covered with gauze or a nonadherent dressing followed by a woven gauze dressing (e.g., Kerlix or Stockinette) to secure the dressing in place. Advantages to this method include (1) greater ease of patient mobility, (2) the decreased likelihood that the agent will be wiped off with movement, and (3) decreased risk of infection from outside contamination. Disadvantages of this method include (1) the significant amount of nursing time required to change these dressings, (2) the inability to assess the wound directly except during dressing change, (3) the increased risk of impaired peripheral circulation,[8] and (4) increased costs for dressings.

Topical Antibiotic Therapy. The decision to apply a topical antimicrobial is usually the presence of burn eschar. Burn injuries destroy the function of the skin's protective mechanism, including that of the sebaceous glands. Sebaceous glands normally secrete sebum, which contains fatty acids, including oleic acid. In addition to lubricating the skin, sebum is believed to help destroy some microorganisms, such as streptococci and some strains of staphylococci. In addition, serum is lost from damaged capillaries, providing a rich nutritional medium for bacterial colonization. Topical antibiotic agents are used to control this colonization. Effective antibacterial agents should control colonization so that specimens for wound biopsy reflect fewer than 10^{23} microorganisms per gram of tissue. More than 10^{23} microorganisms per gram of tissue make control of wound sepsis with topical antibiotics questionable. Parenteral therapy must then be considered. Topical antibiotics selected must meet the following criteria: side effects are minimal; resistant strains will not develop with use; application must be easy and rapid; and use must be relatively economical. Currently the most commonly used topical antibiotics are silver sulfadiazine (SSD), mafenide acetate cream (Sulfamylon), bacitracin ointment, and pure silver impregnated into the primary dressing (Acticoat and Aquacel Ag).[32,35,39] (See the Pharmacologic Management Table on Topical Antimicrobial Agents.) The use of pure silver is the current focus of much interest and research.

SSD is a broad-spectrum antimicrobial agent that has bactericidal action against many gram-negative and gram-positive bacteria. It does not penetrate eschar as readily as mafenide acetate. Its application is usually painless to the patient and requires only one dressing change daily. A common side effect of silver sulfadiazine is leukopenia secondary to bone marrow suppression,

which may develop 24 to 72 hours after application. SSD is indicated for use with partial- and full-thickness wounds and is the most popular topical antimicrobial agent used to treat burn wounds.

Mafenide acetate cream, Sulfamylon, penetrates through burn eschar and is bacteriostatic against many gram-negative and gram-positive organisms. Its use is limited because the application is generally uncomfortable for the patient and it is rapidly absorbed, thereby requiring twice-a-day dressing changes. It is used routinely for coverage of small wounds involving anatomic areas that contain cartilage, such as the ears and nose. Metabolic acidosis can result from the use of mafenide acetate. The patient must be observed closely for hyperventilation (see the Pharmacologic Management table on Topical Antimicrobial Agents).

A 5% mafenide acetate solution is less painful on application than cream and is isoosmolar and less desiccating to the burn wound. Gauze dressings are saturated with the solution and then applied over the burn wound and remoistened as needed. The eschar penetration of the solution and the antimicrobial benefits are superior to SSD, but it does not provide fungal coverage.

Bacitracin ointment is a topical agent applied to superficial burns and facial burns. Bacitracin is effective against gram-positive organisms but not gram-negative organisms or fungus. The open method of wound care is required with the use of bacitracin to prevent yeast overgrowth. A previously mentioned benefit of the open method is better visualization.

Pure silver has been shown to prevent the growth of and kills all organisms found on wounds more rapidly than traditionally used silver-containing compounds.[32,39]

Pharmacologic Management: Topical Antimicrobial Agents

AGENT	ADVANTAGES	DISADVANTAGES	IMPLICATIONS
Silver sulfadiazine	Painless application Broad spectrum Easy application Rare sensitivities	May produce transient leukopenia by bone marrow suppression Minimal eschar penetration Some gram-negative resistance	Monitor white cell count Observe wounds for tunneling and subeschar infection Monitor culture reports
Mafenide acetate cream	Broad-spectrum (esp. *Pseudomonas* coverage) Easy application Penetrates eschar	Painful application Rare acid-base imbalance Frequent sensitivities	Provide adequate analgesia Monitor arterial blood gases Observe for hyperventilation Observe for rashes
Bacitracin	Painless application Nonirritating Transparent Nontoxic	No eschar penetration No gram-negative or fungal coverage	
Pure silver	Painless application Broad spectrum, including fungus and resistant organisms Rare sensitivity Less frequent dressing changes	Keep moist with sterile water, not saline	Maintain dry linens No reported side effects

Silver works by interfering with bacterial enzyme systems, by binding to and destroying the bacterial cell membrane, and by interaction with bacterial DNA to inhibit cell division. Silver is harmless to normal skin, with no reports of toxicity. The Acticoat dressing is three-ply material with an polyester absorbent layer between two layers of silver-coated polyethylene (Westaim Biomedical, Exeter, New Hampshire). This dressing can be used on partial- and full-thickness wounds and recently received FDA approval for use on skin grafts. To provide antimicrobial benefit, the sustained release of silver is necessary. This is achieved with moisture, either by wound exudate or by the intermittent application of sterile water, not saline. Acticoat is cut to the size of the wound and then either applied directly to the wound surface or saturated before application and then placed next to the wound surface and held in place with gauze dressings (Fig. 40-8). The dressing is kept moist but not wet enough to traumatize the tissue. The dressing should be evaluated daily and changed as recommended by the manufacturer—at least every 3 days. Another dressing that utilizes topical silver is Aquacel Ag. This dressing is an absorbent hydrofiber dressing with 1.2% ionic silver distributed throughout the dressing.[40] This dressing is applied to clean partial-thickness or mid-dermal burns and held in place with gauze until it attaches to the wound bed. After the dressing adheres the gauze is removed and the Aquacel Ag stays intact to the wound. As the wound heals the dressing is trimmed to the size of open wound. The benefits of topical pure silver, which is only available in conjunction with dressings, include less pain to the patient, less frequent dressing changes, a decrease in burn wound sepsis, and a decrease in secondary bacteremia from burn wound infection.[40]

Wound Débridement. Mid-dermal and deep-dermal wounds require removal of eschar for wound healing and closure. *Eschar is* the nonviable tissue that forms after the burn injury. This tissue has no blood supply. Therefore polymorphonuclear leukocytes, antibodies, and systemic antibodies cannot reach these areas. Eschar provides an excellent medium for bacterial growth; thus it is vital that burn wounds be cleansed daily and loose eschar débrided as necessary. Débridement has two major aims: (1) removal of tissue contaminated by foreign bodies and bacteria, thus protecting patients from invasive infection, and (2) removal of devitalized tissue. The three types of débridement are as follows:

1. Mechanical
2. Enzymatic
3. Surgical

Mechanical débridement involves the use of scissors and forceps to gently lift and trim loose, necrotic tissue. Experienced professional nurses and physicians perform this procedure. Sterile gauze also may be used in the form of a wet-to-dry or wet-to-wet dressing to further débride the wound bed. Enzymatic débridement involves the topical application of proteolytic substances to the wound bed. These agents are useful in softening eschar and dissolving devitalized tissue. They promote the separation of eschar, which can lead to earlier wound closure. An experienced surgeon performs surgical débridement in the operating room. The goal of débridement is to remove nonviable tissue down to bleeding viable tissue with an electric dermatome or surgical knife.

Skin Substitutes. To assist in wound closure the use of many temporary and permanent skin substitute dressings has gained popularity throughout the United States during the past 10 years. A wide variety of products is currently available on the market. Each dressing has specific indications for use. Temporary substitutes are designed for placement on partial-thickness or clean excised wounds, and permanent substitutes are a permanent skin replacement. Skin substitutes must possess properties that mimic the native epidermis and dermis. This involves a bilayer that has a collagen network that adheres to the wound bed with a protective synthetic outer layer. They are made from a variety of synthetic materials such as nylon, polyurethane, or solid silicone polymers. Skin barrier substitutes must possess several properties to accomplish their desired effect as a temporary wound covering to protect the granulating tissue and/or to preserve a clean, viable wound surface for future autografting (Box 40-2). The most important property of these materials is adherence so that the skin substitute can simulate the function of the skin. Adherence must be uniform to prevent fluid accumulation beneath the surface of the substitute, which could lead to bacterial proliferation. For application of skin substitutes, the wound must be clean and ideally should have a bacterial count of less than 10^5 organisms per gram of tissue. The burn wound must be free from eschar, and hemostasis

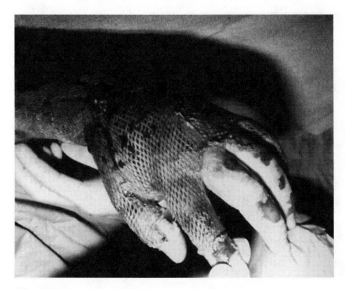

Fig. 40-8 Scarlet red applied to donor site on upper thigh.

must be present. Both eschar and blood provide an excellent medium for bacterial proliferation, and the presence of blood may interfere with adherence. The surface is cleaned and rinsed with saline solution, and the skin barrier substitutes must be applied according to established procedures by means of sterile techniques.[6]

Temporary Skin Substitutes

Polyurethane Film. Polyurethane film, such as Tegaderm, is a semiocclusive dressing that is impermeable to bacteria and liquid. Polyurethane film is used primarily in the coverage of donor sites, but some practitioners report using it over some partial-thickness burn wounds. To apply a polyurethane film dressing, a 2-inch margin of healthy tissue is required to obtain adequate adherence of the adhesive side of the dressing. It may take two persons to apply large pieces of polyurethane film because of its tendency to wrinkle and stick to itself. Polyurethane film dressings possess many of the properties of an ideal skin substitute. However, fluid can collect under the dressing

in large quantities. When fluid collects, it often leaks and decreases the adherence of the dressing. The fluid can be removed with a needle and syringe, but the needle puncture must be patched afterwards with a small piece of polyurethane film.

Biosynthetic Dressing. Biobrane and TransCyte are semipermeable, biosynthetic, temporary wound dressings. They are composed of nylon and Silastic membrane combined with a collagen derivative and can be used on several types of wounds, including partial-thickness burns and wounds, granulating wounds, and donor sites, and over split-thickness grafts. These wounds must be clean or débrided to healthy tissue before application.

Biosynthetic dressings have many of the properties of an ideal skin barrier substitute. These dressings have two advantages that other skin barrier substitutes do not share. A biosynthetic dressing has elasticity in all directions and conforms well to surfaces that are difficult to dress, such as the face, breasts, joints, and axilla. Also, because of its porosity, it allows the passage of some topical antibiotics to penetrate its membrane, reducing the bacterial count of the burn wound. A biosynthetic dressing may be applied after daily cleaning at the bedside or in the operating room. It is applied with the dull or nylon mesh side facing the wound. It can be held in place with a gauze dressing and the area is immobilized for 24 to 48 hours, depending on the site, until adherence occurs (Fig. 40-9). If fluid or air accumulates under the biosynthetic skin, it may be slit and the fluid expressed. If a large amount of fluid accumulates, the biosynthetic skin is removed and replaced. Biosynthetic skin initially adheres to the wound fibrin, which binds to the collagen and nylon backing of the material. Later the cells migrate into the nylon mesh and further bind to the wound. As the wound heals, the dressing will turn opaque and should be trimmed or peeled back. If bleeding occurs on

---

Box 40-2

IDEAL PROPERTIES OF SKIN SUBSTITUTES

- Adherence
- Decrease pain
- Easy application and removal
- Intact bacterial barrier
- Shelf storage capability
- Inexpensive in relation to alternatives
- Nonantigenic
- Similar to normal skin in transport of water vapor
- Elastic and durable
- Hemostatic
- Decreased protein and electrolyte loss
- Enhanced natural healing processes

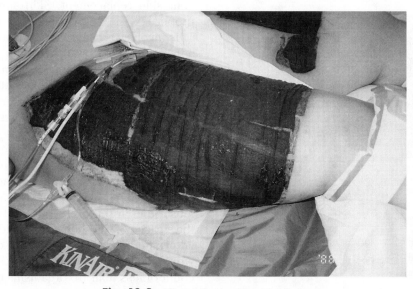

Fig. 40-9 Biosynthetic skin substitute.

removal, the dressing should be left in place and reevaluated for removal in a few days.

Hydrocolloidal Dressings. These are oxygen-impermeable, waterproof occlusive dressings that are composed of an outer layer of polyurethane foam and an inner layer of hydrocolloid polymer complex. Hydrocolloid dressings are indicated for use on partial-thickness wounds. The dressing does not adhere to the wound bed; therefore it does not damage new epithelium and decreases pain. Fear of bacterial proliferation limits the use of these dressings for burn wounds. To date, clinical investigations have revealed colonization but not clinical infection. The adhesive side is applied to the wound, allowing for an occlusive margin of intact skin. Disadvantages of using hydrocolloid dressings include large amounts of exudate, odor, and an inability to visualize the wound bed. Advantages include rapid healing times and decreased pain. A newer, highly absorbent hydrocolloidal dressing with fibers known as a hydrofiber is Aquacel. This product has recently been integrated with pure silver, Aquacel Ag, and can offer the benefits of adherence, decrease in pain, and ease of application while reducing the risk of infection.[41]

DEFINITIVE BURN WOUND CLOSURE

The primary goal of burn wound management is wound closure during the acute phase. It is now recommended that if a burn wound will not heal in 10 to 14 days, early excision should be undertaken to improve functional and cosmetic results, to decrease in-hospital time, and to reduce the cost of burn care.[6] Surgical débridement may begin as early as 3 to 5 days after the burn insult when hemodynamic stability has been achieved. Some physicians operate within 24 hours of admission if the patient is hemodynamically stable. Typically, excision procedures are limited to 20% of the body surface or 2 hours of operating time. In patients with massive burns, excision procedures are commonly staged, requiring the patient to return to the operating room every 2 to 3 days until all wounds have been excised. This technique helps avoid excessive transfusions and limits the physiologic stress.[6]

Autografting is the preferred choice for wound closure. However, with large TBSA burns, availability of donor sites can be problematic. When autograft is not available, many alternate methods are used to achieve this goal. Creative attempts have been initiated to establish a skin substitute that permanently closes the wound in a cosmetically and functionally acceptable fashion. Temporary skin substitutes may be used to provide permanent wound closure but the process is complex. These bilayer products, such as Integra, involve application to a clean, excised burn wound. After 14 to 21 days a neodermis is formed and a thin epidermal autograft is placed.[34] This is an area of evolving technology. These materials temporarily restore the protective barrier that the skin provides naturally. Skin substitutes can be used until the patient's own skin is available for harvesting. Previously used and healed donor sites can be used again in later return visits to the operating room. Table 40-2 reviews advantages and disadvantages of different graft types.

Autograft. An autograft is a skin graft harvested from a healthy, uninjured donor site on the burn patient and then placed over the patient's burn wound to provide permanent coverage of the wound. Autografts are the only grafts that provide permanent wound coverage. Preferred sites for obtaining these grafts are the thighs, back, and abdomen; however, grafts can be harvested from almost anywhere on the body.

Surgical excision is performed to mechanically remove necrotic tissue from the burn wound; it may be performed tangentially or fascially. Tangential excision involves sequentially excising the eschar down to bleed-

Table 40-2	Types of Grafts		
Graft	**Usage**	**Advantages**	**Disadvantages**
Autograft	Provides permanent coverage of burn wounds	Permanent coverage	Lack of available donor sites, which may delay wound coverage
		Nonantigenic	
		Least expensive	Donor sites are painful partial-thickness wounds
	Used in sheets or meshed form	Meshing allows a small amount of tissue to cover a large area	Must be done in surgical suite
Homograft (allograft)	Temporary wound coverage	Can be placed at bedside or in operating room	Possibility of disease transmission
			Antigenic; body rejects in approximately 2 weeks
		Allows for vascularization over deep wound	Not readily available to all burn centers
		Provides better control over bacterial growth than xenograft	Expensive
			Requires rigorous quality controls
Heterograph (xenograft)	Temporary wound coverage	Longer shelf life than allograft	Antigenic; body rejects in 3 to 4 days
		Can be meshed or comes in a variety of sizes	Potential for digestion by wound collagenase, thus leading to increased chance of infection

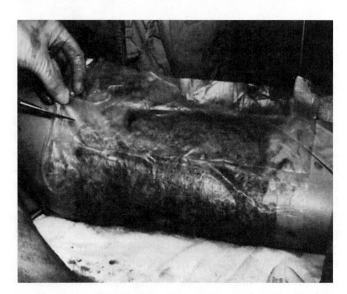

Fig. 40-10 Meshed autograft.

ing, viable tissue and then placing a split-thickness skin graft over the wound. Fascial excision is used when the wounds are deep and the fat does not appear viable. Surgical intervention with split-thickness skin grafts often yields a better cosmetic result than does the natural healing process in deep partial- and full-thickness injuries.

Sheets of the patient's epidermis and a partial layer of the dermis are harvested with use of a dermatome. These grafts are referred to as *split-thickness grafts* and can be applied to the wound bed as a sheet or in meshed form (Fig. 40-10). Split-thickness skin grafts are harvested at approximately twelve-thousandths of an inch in thickness. The split-thickness skin graft can be meshed 1½:1 to 4:1 in a mesher and then placed on the wounds.[6] The size of the mesh is based on the areas requiring grafting and the availability of donor skin. This meshing prevents serum accumulation under the graft and permits coverage of a surface area larger than its original surface. Grafts that are placed on the face, neck, lower portions of the arms, and hands generally are sheet grafts when possible. Grafts that are meshed can cover more area but may not produce the cosmetic appearance desired and therefore usually are placed on areas generally covered by clothing.

The grafts can be secured with sutures, fibrin glue, or staples. The choice of dressing that is placed over the graft varies widely based on physician and institution preference. One choice is fine mesh gauze impregnated with an emollient. It is placed over the graft, covered with a heavy gauze dressing, and secured to the patient with or without a splint, depending on the anatomic area of the graft. Great care must be taken not to disturb the graft. Trained nursing professionals or physicians remove the dressings on postoperative day 3 to 5 for assessment.[6] Graft adherence and survival can be assessed

in 48 to 72 hours. Autograft sites are assessed for adherence, presence of infection, and closure of interstices. Nurses, in collaboration with the multidisciplinary team, provide proper positioning, splinting, and pain management in the postoperative period.

Care of the donor site is equally important because it represents a wound similar to that of a partial-thickness injury. Donor sites can be covered with many different types of dressings. Fine mesh gauze, Tegaderm, Acticoat, or Xeroform can be applied. The gauze is then trimmed as it separates from the healing donor site over the next 10 days. Xeroform is a fine mesh gauze that contains 3% bismuth tribromophenate in a petrolatum blend. Xeroform has no major disadvantages and is trimmed away as the donor site heals. Application is easy, and it does not have the disadvantages of scarlet red. These dressings should not be removed forcibly, because this would interfere with the reepitheliazation process and cause considerable pain.

Biosynthetic Skin Substitutes. Skin substitutes include homograft (allograft) and heterograft (xenograft). *Homograft skin* can be obtained from live or deceased donors (cadaver skin). The homograft is harvested from cadaver skin and with advances in cryopreservation can be frozen and stored in a tissue bank. It is possible to transmit disease through the application of a homograft; therefore tissue banks must adhere to strict guidelines. Before application, homograft skin is tested for a variety of transmittable diseases, including the human immunodeficiency virus (HIV) and hepatitis B surface antigens. Homograft skin can be applied as a biologic dressing for débridement at the bedside or as a temporary wound coverage on excised burn wounds. The patient's wound readily accepts the homograft. Vascular ingrowth occurs, and the homograft seals the wound and protects it from bacterial invasion; however, it is rejected approximately 2 weeks after its application. Homografts must be handled and applied very carefully. They must be placed with the shiny surface down and must be wrinkle-free. They must neither overlap each other nor lap over infected areas or uninjured areas. The grafts can be dressed with a nonadherent agent that usually is not changed for 24 to 48 hours.

Disadvantages include the homograft antigenicity, lack of accessibility, difficulties with storage and quality control, expense of procurement, and possibility of disease transmission from the donor. The microbiologic cleanliness of the cadaver skin is of extreme concern because of the burn patient's debilitated immunologic condition. Homografts are harvested during the first 4 hours after death. They generally are taken from the abdomen, thighs, and back. Partial-thickness grafts are obtained, leaving the graft sites looking as if they were sunburned. Homografts usually are available only in centers in which the rigorous processing procedure can be achieved. These centers usually have skin and tissue bank facilities. Procurement of the allograft is much the same as for

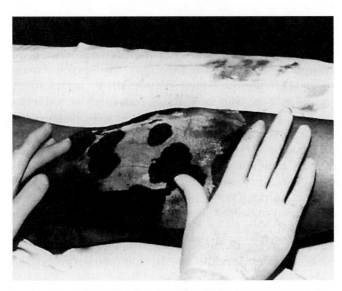

Fig. 40-11 Xenograft (pigskin).

any other donated organ. The public, however, is not as well educated about the need for this organ as it is about eyes, liver, lung, kidneys, and hearts.

The *xenograft*, or *heterograft*, is a graft transferred between two different species to provide temporary wound coverage. The most common and widely accepted xenograft is pigskin (porcine). Pigskin is available in frozen and shelf forms, with each type having a much longer storage life than the allograft. Depending on how the pigskin was prepared, it can have a shelf life of 1 month to 1 year. The pigskin is packaged in a variety of ways and in various sizes. It can be treated with silver sulfadiazine and can be meshed or nonmeshed. Pigskin can be used for temporary coverage of full- and partial-thickness wounds, burn wounds, and donor sites. It meets many of the ideal skin substitute properties mentioned previously. It has two disadvantages, however; it is antigenic, and it has the potential for being digested by the wound collagenase, possibly leading to infection.

Pigskin is applied in the same manner as homograft (Fig. 40-11). If the pigskin was frozen, it is thawed in a warm saline-solution bath. If it has been treated with silver sulfadiazine, it is thawed in water. The pigskin is placed on the wound with the dermal side down (the dermal side faces the center of the roll); it may be distinguished by its tendency to curl toward the dermal surface when held up at one end. Shelf-stored pigskin may be applied with either side to the wound. Once the pigskin is in place, it may be dressed with antibacterial-impregnated dressings or other forms of dressings. Pigskin usually is removed or dissolves because of lack of blood supply in 5 to 7 days. If sloughing or purulent drainage occurs, the xenograft is removed (see Table 40-2).

Synthetic Skin. The lack of available donor sites for major burn injury often delays wound closure. In an effort to minimize infection and to promote healing, many at-

tempts have been made to develop skin substitutes that will seal the wound in a functional and cosmetically acceptable fashion. Integra with a ultrathin layer of epidermal autograft has been used successfully.[42] A technique that involves the growth and subsequent graft placement of cultured epithelial autograft (CEA) has become an adjunct to treatment of burn wounds. A complex process that allows for separation of keratinocytes is performed. The CEA is grown over a period of 2 to 3 weeks to achieve a graft size of 25 cm^2. This represents an expansion of 50 to 70 times the original specimen. These confluent sheets of cultured epithelial cells are attached to a gauze backing and placed on the wound. The published results reveal that graft take is unpredictable because CEA lacks dermis. Even when grafts take initially, graft loss can still occur later. The CEA also is more fragile, and the technique is quite costly. This therapy is being recommended as an adjunct for traditional split-thickness skin graft (STSG) and continues to be investigated and combined with newer dermal skin substitutes.

Long-Term Postgraft Wound Care. A problem with the formation of tiny water blisters often occurs 2 to 6 weeks after wound closure. These blisters usually open and heal without incident in 3 to 5 days. These areas must be kept clean with mild soap and covered with a bland ointment. For 6 to 8 weeks, a mild nonalcohol-based skin cream is applied every 4 hours to these areas to lubricate the skin until natural lubrication occurs. Pruritus is common in the maturing burn wound. Patients can be relieved of this discomfort by the administration of an antipruritic agent, such as diphenhydramine hydrochloride or doxepin hydrochloride 5% and by the application of moisturizing creams.

Another concern in burn wound healing is the prevention or reduction of hypertrophic scarring. Its prevention or reduction depends on the timely application of uniform pressure. Hypertrophic scarring can be controlled with the use of tubular support bandages applied within 5 to 7 days after the graft. Bandages are available in a variety of sizes and have the advantage of applying pressure to selected body areas while allowing the remaining burned area to heal sufficiently. They also are readily available for immediate use during the wait for the commercial manufacture of the customized elastic pressure garment for long-term use, which can take up to 3 or 4 weeks.

Tubular support bandages apply tension in the medium range of 10 to 20 mm Hg. Tensions lower than this do not exert adequate pressure to control scarring, and higher tensions tend to cause edema in the distal parts of the extremities and may be too abrasive for newly grafted skin. Tension can be elevated if needed by placing silicone foam under the tubular support bandages over areas such as the axilla and knees.

Custom-made elastic pressure garments generally are worn for 6 months to 1 year after grafting. It is important to assess the patient for pressure points as weight is gained and as growth occurs in patients who are children. It is necessary to assess the garment for elasticity over time, because the elasticity will decrease with washing.

ACUTE PAIN

Pain is an individualized and subjective phenomenon. It comprises both physiologic and psychologic aspects. A guideline-based approach can be helpful in properly recognizing and treating the pain related to burn injury.[17] Pain after burn injury is complex and includes background pain, breakthrough pain, and procedural pain. Background pain is related to the physiologic changes associated with the burn injury and includes the damage or exposure of the nerve endings within partial-thickness burns and donor sites. Range of motion of the affected limbs and routine activities contribute to background pain. Breakthrough pain is described as episodes of pain more severe than background pain and is not relieved by routine pain medications. Procedural pain includes pain caused by interventions such as daily wound care, arterial punctures, chest physical therapy, and use of splints.[16]

Loss of control, forced dependence, loneliness, and separation from home and family all can contribute to anxiety, which heightens the patient's perception of pain. The patient's fears abound in thoughts of disfigurement and loss of love, function, and job. The psychologic experience or subjective component may be related to past experiences, anxiety, and altered coping mechanisms. Attention to the psychologic component of the patient's pain may lead to very useful strategies that decrease perceived pain. If possible, past experiences with pain, hospitalization, and successful coping strategies should be explored.

Patients with partial-thickness burns experience a great deal of discomfort. The slightest air current to the surface of the burn may stimulate pain. Covering wounds with topical agents, dressings, and linen significantly decreases the pain. The nerve endings that have been completely destroyed by full-thickness burns are initially insensate but do transmit pain sensation when they regenerate. It is a common misconception that these wounds are painless. Patients may experience deep somatic pain from ischemia or inflammation. It is unlikely that all wounds will be full-thickness. A combination of varying wound depths is more common. Wound edges, as they transition to less severely burned areas, will be hypersensitive.[16,31]

Pain continues even after healing; some patients describe the itching, tingling, and paresthesias as being as equally discomforting as the initial injury. Paresthesias can last 1 year or more after injury. It may be a false assumption to believe burn pain decreases over time.[31]

The burn patient confronts pain on a daily basis for many weeks. Pharmacotherapy is the mainstay for analgesia in burn patients. Inadequate pain management is a problem in many burn units because of the fear of opioid side effects and opioid addiction and the lack of pain evaluation and/or lack of treatment protocols. Initially after burn injury, narcotics are administered intravenously in small doses and titrated to effect. The constant background pain may be addressed with the use of a patient-controlled analgesia device. Once hemodynamic stability has occurred and GI function has returned, oral narcotics can be useful. Additional premedication and analgesics will be necessary during therapeutic procedures. The use of acetaminophen and nonsteroidal antiinflammatory drugs can be useful in patients who are not at risk for bleeding. Anxiolytics and antidepressants also should be considered and used appropriately. The nurse must be flexible with dosing and assess the effectiveness of medication by using a numerical or visual analog scale. The nurse should assure the patient that pain control issues will be continually addressed.

Nonpharmacologic techniques, such as imagery, hypnosis, distraction, and methods adapted from some of the popular childbirth techniques, can be effective in reducing anxiety and the pain experience. Giving the patient some management control also can reduce the anxiety and the pain experience. The perception of pain often is increased in the patient who is anxious and lacks control of the situation.[40]

Treatment strategies need to be individualized. Failure to adequately treat pain can increase burn hypermetabolism, result in loss of confidence between the burn team and patient, and lead to the development of psychiatric disorders. Assess and discuss on a regular basis the patient's psychologic status. Avoid using psychotropics for analgesia and narcotics for anxiety and depression.[40]

IMBALANCED NUTRITION: LESS THAN BODY REQUIREMENTS

The basal metabolic rate of a burn patient may be elevated 40% to 100% above the normal rate, depending on the amount of TBSA involved. The metabolic rate is influenced by the amount of protein and albumin lost through the wounds, the catabolic response associated with stress, associated injuries, fluid loss, fever, infection, immobility, gender, and the height and weight of the patient before the injury.[41] The goal in nutritional management of the burn patient is to provide adequate calories to prevent starvation and to enhance wound healing. To achieve this goal, nutritional support and the reduction of energy demand are imperative. Every effort should be made to reduce the release of catecholamines, which increase metabolic rate. Pain, fear, anxiety, and cold stimulate release of catecholamine stores. Appropriate interventions for each of these stimuli must be performed.

The use of enteral and oral routes is preferred in the management of burn patients. Because of the increased nutritional needs of the burn patient, oral feedings are usually inadequate and supplemental tube feedings are necessary. Caloric requirements are calculated on the basis of size of the burn; the age, height, and weight of the patient; and the stress factors. Protein and caloric requirements for the burn patient are elevated in light of a negative nitrogen balance. The daily protein requirement may increase to 2 to 4 times the normal 0.8 g/kg of body weight. Carbohydrates and fat are used for energy and to spare proteins required for wound healing. Daily caloric intake can be 2 to 20 times higher than normal. Vitamins and minerals generally are given in doses higher than normal also. Serum iron, zinc, calcium, phosphate, and potassium values are monitored and supplements given as indicated.[41]

REHABILITATION PHASE

The rehabilitation phase is one of recuperation and healing, both physically and emotionally. The patient is not acutely ill but may or may not be ready for discharge. This phase can last several years. The patient may require extensive reconstructive surgery. Psychologically the patient focuses on attaining specific personal goals related to achieving as much preburn function as possible.[27] Minor and major accomplishments must be praised. This phase is characterized by scar management techniques and by physical and occupational therapy. The burn team and the patient prepare for the transition to the outside world. The use of group therapy is a valuable tool used at many burn centers. Patients, family members, and health care providers express ideas and feelings. Many times burn patients establish priorities and make realistic decisions about their lives. Staff intervention during this phase is primarily one of support.

IMPAIRED PHYSICAL MOBILITY

Tremendous advances have been made during the past 10 to 15 years in the physical care of the burn patient. The survival rate of patients with full-thickness burns greater than 40% of TBSA has increased significantly. Currently, survival of patients with burns greater than 90% of TBSA is not impossible. As patients with larger and deeper burns survive, the challenge to maintain their optimal mobility and cosmetic appearance has been met with increased success. It is imperative that rehabilitation needs are addressed early in burn care. Nursing prescriptions for range of motion exercises, positioning, splinting, ambulation, and activities of daily living are initiated within the first 48 hours of hospitalization.

Despite the advances in other areas of burn care, contractures still develop after a burn injury. Contractures develop because of a variety of factors: the extent, depth, location, and configuration of the burn; the position of comfort the patient most frequently assumes; the relative underlying muscle strength; and the patient's motivation and compliance. Positioning the affected body parts in antideformity positions is vital. Frequent change of position also is important and may need to be performed as often as every hour. Burn patients are at greater risk for the development of pressure sores than the general hospital population, as well as the possible conversion of their partial-thickness burns to full-thickness burns.

Splints can be used to prevent and/or correct contracture or to immobilize joints after grafting. If splints are used, they must be checked daily for proper fit and effectiveness. Splints that are used to immobilize body parts after grafting must be left on at all times except to assess the graft site for pressure points every shift. Splints to correct severe contracture may be off for 2 hours per shift to allow burn care and range of motion exercises. Mild contracture may be kept in splints for 4 hours and out of splints for 4 hours to promote exercise and mobility.

Active exercise is encouraged and is preferred, although active-assisted or gentle-passive exercises also may be an important part of the rehabilitation program. Active exercise maintains muscle mass, aids in restoring protein structures within the muscle tissue, aids in venous and lymphatic return, and reduces the risk of pulmonary embolus and deep vein thrombosis. Patient tolerance must be carefully evaluated. The number of repetitions will be proportional to the degree of anticipated contracture and the patient's tolerance. Anticipation of the patient's pain also must be carefully considered. Before range of motion exercises and activities of daily living are performed, the need for pain medication must be assessed.[10] Nursing diagnoses for the burn patient are summarized in the Nursing Diagnoses feature on Burn Injury.

NURSING DIAGNOSES | **Burn Injury**

- Impaired Gas Exchange related to ventilation/perfusion mismatching
- Ineffective Airway Clearance related to excessive secretions or abnormal viscosity of mucus
- Deficient Fluid Volume related to relative loss
- Risk for Infection risk factors: invasive lines, immunodeficiencies
- Acute Confusion related to sensory overload, sensory deprivation, sleep pattern disturbance
- Disturbed Body Image related to actual change in body structure, function, or appearance
- Powerlessness related to physical deterioration despite compliance

OUTPATIENT BURN CARE

Outpatient burn care must be considered for minor burns. It is cost-effective and removes the potential for a wound infection from endemic, drug-resistant microorganisms within the hospital environment. The hospital environment also changes many of the self-care routines, such as diet, family contact, hygiene, and coping mechanisms. However, patients considered for outpatient burn care must be screened carefully. Nursing evaluation of the patient or family, or both, includes consideration of motivation, willingness to participate in care, ability to understand and perform the necessary procedures, potential aversions to wound care or dressing changes, and reliability of transportation. Medical considerations include hemodynamic stabilization, nutritional status, fluid and electrolyte balance, adequate pain control, and ruling out any complications.[42]

In general, small burns must be washed daily with a mild soap and water, and an appropriate ointment and/or synthetic antimicrobial agent can be applied and held in place with dressings. Initially these wounds must be monitored daily and then on a weekly basis until the wound begins to reepitheliaze. Home health nurses are helpful in monitoring these patients. Generally, if epithelialization of these wounds has not occurred in 2 to 3 weeks, use of primary excision and grafting must be considered.

To check for evidence of scarring, partial-thickness injuries must be monitored until the epithelialization has occurred. If scarring occurs, compression dressings must be fitted and worn until the wound becomes quiescent, which requires 12 to 18 months.

STRESSORS OF BURN NURSING

Burn units are fascinating environments in which to work. They offer the fast-paced, high-technology atmosphere of any critical care setting; the complexity of advanced nursing management; and the dynamics of an interdisciplinary, collaborative model of practice. However, all of these elements combined contribute to a potentially stressful work environment for the nurse. The physical environment can be a difficult one in which to work for a variety of reasons. The amount of equipment necessary to maintain the patient can be overwhelming and can limit the work space dramatically. The temperature of the room generally is kept at approximately 85° F and can get much warmer, depending on the amount of equipment in the room. Odors vary and can be very unpleasant. Noise levels within a unit also are distressing. These variables exact a physical toll on nursing staff members. The decision to specialize in burn nursing is a meaningful one, an important one; however, this decision also must be an informed one.

Self-care and care of other nurses are issues just as important as the care of the patient and his or her significant other.

In addition, there are patient care complexities unique to burn nursing. The daily dressing changes are extremely stressful for both the nurse and the patient. The nursing management of patients' pain is a complex issue in burn care and is one that contributes significantly to the stress level of nurses who specialize in burn injuries. The psychodynamics associated with the patient's burn injury experience are just that—dynamic—and require constant, high-level nursing assessment and intervention.

REFERENCES

1. Brigham PA, McLoughlin E: Burn incidence and medical care use in the United States: estimates, trends, and data sources, *J Burn Care Rehabil* 17:95, 1996.
2. American Burn Association: http//www.ameriburn.org.
3. Saffle JR, Davis B, Williams P: Recent outcomes in the treatment of burn injury in the United States: a report from the American Burn Association patient registry, *J Burn Care Rehabil* 16:219, 1995.
4. Demling RH: The advantage of the burn team approach, *J Burn Care Rehabil* 16:569, 1995.
5. Williams WG, Phillips LG: Pathophysiology of the burn wound. In Herndon DN, editor: *Total burn care*, ed 2, London, 2002, Saunders.
6. Pruitt BA: Burn wound. In Cameron JL, editor: *Current surgical therapy*, ed 5, St Louis, 1995, Mosby.
7. Kramer GC, Nguyen, TT: Pathophysiology of burn shock and burn edema. In Herndon DN, editor: *Total burn care*, ed 2, London, 2002, Saunders.
8. Still JM, Law EJ: Primary excision of the burn wound, *Clinic Plas Surg* 27(1):23, 2000.
9. Larson, K: Initial evaluation and management of the critically burned patient, *Mod Med* 100(6):582, 2003.
10. Cadier MA, Shakespeare PG: Burns in octogenarians, *Burns* 21:200, 1995.
11. Nebraska Burn Institute: Advanced burn life support (ABLS) course (first rev), Lincoln, 1990, The Institute.
12. Pruitt BA, Mason AD: Epidemiological, demographic and outcome characteristics of burn injury. In Herndon DN, editor: *Total burn care*, ed 2, London, 2002, Saunders.
13. Shaw A et al: Early management of large burns, *Br J Hos Med* 53(6):247, 1995.
14. Lund T: Edema generation following thermal injury: an update, *J Burn Care Rehabil* 20:445, 1999.
15. Goodwin CW: Fluid management and nutritional support of the burn patient. In Cameron JL, editor: *Current surgical therapy*, ed 5, St Louis, 1995, Mosby.
16. Laterjet J, Choinere M: Pain in burn patients, *Burns* 21:344, 1995.
17. Ulmer JF: Burn pain management: a guideline-based approach, *J Burn Care Rehabil* 19:151, 1998.
18. Flynn MB: Identifying and treating inhalation injuries in fire victims, *DCCN* 18(4):18, 1999.
19. Darling GE et al: Pulmonary complications in inhalation injuries with associated cutaneous burn, *J Trauma* 40:83, 1996.
20. Cartotto R, Ellis S, Smith T: Use of high-frequency oscillatory ventilation in burn patients, *Crit Care Med* 33(suppl 3): S175-181, 2005.

21. Thompson JT et al: Successful management of adult smoke inhalation with extracorporeal membrane oxygenation, *J Burn Care Rehabil* 26(1):62-66, 2005.

22. Traber DL et al: The pathophysiology of inhalation injury. In Herndon DN, editor: *Total burn care,* ed 2, London, 2002, Saunders.

23. Masanes MJ et al: Fiberoptic bronchoscopy for the early diagnosis of subglottal inhalation injury: comparative value in the assessment of prognosis, *J Trauma* 36:59, 1994.

24. Yowler CJ, Fratianne RB: Current status of burn resuscitation, *Clin Plast Surg* 27:1, 2000.

25. Luce EA: Electrical burns, *Clin Plast Surg* 27:133, 2000.

26. Carleton S: Cardiac problems associated with electrical injury, *Cardiol Clin* 13:263, 1995.

27. Partridge J, Robinson E: Psychological and social aspects of burns, *Burns* 21:453, 1995.

28. Weber J et al: Infection control in burn patients, *Burns* 30(8):A16-A24, 2004.

29. Robie DK, Herndon DN: Surgical management of complications of burn injury. In Herndon DN, editor: *Total burn care,* ed 2, London, 2002, Saunders.

30. Carleton S: Cardiac problems associated with burns, *Cardiol Clin* 13:257, 1995.

31. Arturson G: Pathophysiology of the burn wound pharmacological treatment, *Burns* 22:255, 1996.

32. Demling RH et al: Burn wound module, Part III: Managing the burn wound, available on the Internet at www.Burnsurgery.org.

33. Winter G: Formation of the scab and rate of epithelialization of superficial wound in the skin, *Nature* 193:293, 1962.

34. Vogt P et al: Dry, moist and wet skin wound repair, *Ann Plastic Surg* 34:493, 1995.

35. Tredget EE et al: A matched-pair, randomized study evaluating the efficacy and safety of Acticoat silver-coated dressing for the treatment of burn wounds, *J Burn Care Rehabil* 19:531, 1998.

36. Patterson DR: Non-opioid based approaches to burn pain, *J Burn Care Rehabil* 116:372, 1995.

37. Deitch E: Nutritional support of the burn patient, *Crit Care Clin* 11:735, 1995.

38. Bolinger B: Burn care in the home, *J Wound Ostomy Continence Nurs* 22(3):122, 1995.

39. Yin HQ, Langford R, Burrell R: Comparative evaluation of the antimicrobial activity of Acticoat antimicrobial barrier dressing, *J Burn Care Rehabil* 20:195-200, 1999.

40. Wright J et al: Wound management in an era of increasing bacterial antibiotic resistance: a role for topical silver treatment, *Am J Infect Control* 26:572, 1998.

41. Caruso D et al: Aquacel Ag in the management of partial-thickness burns: results in a clinical trial, *J Burn Care Rehabil* 25:89, 2004.

42. Heimbach D et al: Multicenter postapproval clinical trial of Integra dermal regeneration template for burn treatment, *J Burn Care Rehabil* 24:42, 2003.

Organ Donation and Transplantation

INTRODUCTION

Major advances in transplantation have been achieved since the first cadaver organ transplants in the 1960s. Today transplantation has become an accepted form of therapy for end-stage organ failure. The field of transplantation is highly specialized and requires expert teams of surgeons, immunologists, and medical and nurse specialists to achieve successful outcomes.

Many problems are yet to be solved in the field of transplantation. Organs remain a scarce commodity, and a lack of available organs restricts the availability of transplantation for many individuals. Safe and efficacious control of the immune system remains elusive. Rejection and infection as a result of immunosuppression persist as the major causes of death in recipients. Chronic rejection is still not well understood. This type of rejection results in eventual graft failure and limits long-term survival in many types of organ recipients.

This chapter gives an overview of the specialized areas of organ donation, the immune system, immunosuppressant medications used to prevent rejection, and solid organ transplantation.

ORGAN DONATION

The evolution of organ donation has moved in tandem with the development of transplantation since the 1950s. With the evolution of organ procurement organizations (OPO), organ donation has developed as a separate and distinct entity from the field of transplantation.

Animal research was used to establish renal transplantation procedures both for related and nonrelated donor organs. These investigational procedures led to the recovery of kidneys from donors before autopsy and led to the original source of organs for transplantation.

BRAIN DEATH

The first organ recovered for transplantation from a "dead" donor was in 1962. The recovery (procurement) of

organs from a "dead body" led to the evolution of the concept of brain death as distinguished from the cessation of the heart beating (death). Initially, the belief in medicine was that a person was alive until the heart stopped beating. Before the use or definition of brain death and the establishing of brain death criteria, patients with an "irreversible" head injury were used for the recovery of kidneys for transplantation. The ventilator was removed and the recovery procedure was initiated with the cessation of the heartbeat. In essence, the early donors were the same or similar to what is now referred to as the deceased after cardiac death (DCD) donor.

Criteria. The criteria for brain death were developed late in the 1960s,[1] soon after the proposal of a brain death standard of death. The debate began as to how much of the brain must be destroyed for a patient to be declared dead. As a result, a nonsurvivable injury was defined as a head injury resulting in an individual devoid of cerebral and brainstem function. This included the loss of cellular function, which is not congruent with the heart not beating. These decisions provided the basis for the conclusion that an individual was dead when the requirements were met and not when the heart stopped beating. This resulted in the passing of the Uniform Determination of Death Act of 1982.[2]

Source of Organ Donors. The current potential donor source that the critical care professional will work with is comprised of patients who are rapidly approaching death or have been declared brain-dead. However, there are multiple sources of donor organs for transplantation.

OPOs are responsible for the recovery of organs from deceased and DCD donors. Descriptions of the different categories of donors are listed in Table 41-1. The Transplant Center has predominantly living and unrelated living donors as a part of its program. In 2003 the United Network for Organ Sharing (UNOS) reported the following donor outcomes[3]:

Total donors	13,276
Deceased donors	6,457
Deceased after cardiac death (DCD) donor	264 (included in deceased donor total above)
Living donors	6,819

Table 41-1	Descriptions of the Different Categories of Donors
Donor	**Definition**
Deceased donor (cadaver donor)	A person who has been declared "brain-dead"
Deceased after cardiac death (DCD) donor	Donor whose death is determined by cessation of heart and respiratory functions (not brain death)
Living, related donor	A family member who donates a kidney, part of a lung, liver, or pancreas to another family member
Living, unrelated donor (benevolent)	A person who is not related by blood, who donates a kidney, part of a lung, liver, or pancreas to another person (such as a husband, wife, friend or in-law) Stranger-to-stranger, living, unrelated donations are included in this definition

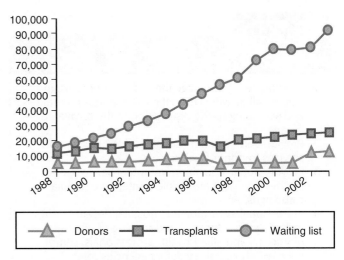

Fig. 41-1 Comparison of number of available donors, transplants performed, and waiting list for transplantation.

THE NEED

National Organ Transplant Act. With the passage of the National Organ Transplant Act (NOTA) in 1984,[4] the federal government began the process of establishing a comprehensive framework for the development and administration of a national transplant system. During the past 20 years, nearly 350,000 patients have received organ transplants and the national waiting list has grown from 8400 patients to more than 85,000.[3] More than 85,000 patients await an organ for transplantation, and approximately 50% will die while on the waiting list (Fig. 41-1).

Organ Donation and Recovery Improvement Act. The Organ Donation and Recovery Improvement Act (ODRIA) of 2004,[5] is the first federal legislation since 1990 amending the NOTA. The act focuses on strengthening efforts to increase organ donation rates. There are three important aspects of the legislation:

1. The federal government's role in educating the public about organ donation
2. The importance of discussing organ and tissue donation as a family
3. The contribution of living donors and the advancements in medical technology that make living donation possible

The key provisions of the act concern the following:

1. Assistance for living organ donation
2. Public awareness, studies, and demonstrations
3. Funds for states' efforts
4. Grants for hospital donor coordinators
5. Studies relating to organ donation and the recovery, preservation, and transplantation of organs
6. Organ procurement organizations (OPO)

The realization that organs from donors could be successfully transplanted into other individuals created the awareness that there was a need to develop a process to establish this organ source. The development of organ procurement organizations was a natural result of the increased demand for organs to transplant. This resulted in a slow evolution of the use of health care professionals to assist in the organ recovery process and the development of organ procurement as a function within the hospital.

National Transplant Act. The passage of the National Transplant Act resulted in the formation of the Organ Procurement and Transplant Network (OPTN),[6] which was to have oversight for transplantation and organ donation. The Health Care Financing Administration (HCFA) was given the authority under legislative provisions to certify organ procurement organizations.

Today there are 58 organ procurement organizations.[3] All organ procurement organizations are nonprofit corporations, serving organ donation needs in the United States, Puerto Rico, and Bermuda. Each OPO provides organ donation services to a designated service area. These service areas vary significantly according to populations served, geographic areas, transplant centers served, and the number of donor hospitals. The organ procurement organization is a complex health care business that is the frontline constituent for organ donation. Organ procurement organizations are central in bringing together the acquisition, placement, and transport of organs for transplantation. The organ procurement organization is responsible for numerous activities as listed in Box 41-1.

Box 41-1

ROLE OF THE ORGAN PROCUREMENT ORGANIZATION (OPO)

1. Coordinate and manage the donation process, including all activities from the initial donor referral and screening to the distribution of the recovered organs.
2. Provide bereavement care and additional support services to donor families.
3. Provide public education, volunteer services, and the development and implementation of media campaigns, etc.
4. Professional education and hospital development, including the education and training of nurses, physicians and allied health professionals, compliance with hospital regulatory agencies Joint Commission for Accreditation of Health Care Organizations (JCAHO) and Center for Medicare and Medicaid Services (CMS), implementation of donation policies and procedures, etc.
5. Manage and distribute data and information to various clients.
6. Manage of a publicly responsible financial program that provides the support to successfully provide various donation and donation related services.

Box 41-2

COLLABORATION BETWEEN ORGAN PROCUREMENT ORGANIZATION AND HOSPITALS

1. All hospitals must have an agreement with the designated organ procurement organization (OPO). This includes an agreement with at least one tissue bank and one eye bank.
2. The hospital will contact the OPO in a timely manner about individuals who die or whose death is imminent in the hospital.
3. The OPO will then determine the medical suitability for donation.
4. The hospital must ensure, in collaboration with the OPO, that every family of every potential donor is informed of its option to donate organs or tissues.
5. Hospitals must work with the OPO and at least one tissue bank and eye bank in educating staff on donation, reviewing death records to improve identification of potential donors, and maintaining physiologic organ/tissue function of donors.

ADDITIONAL FACTORS IN DONATION AND TRANSPLANTATION

Conditions of Participation. Today's regulatory environment for hospitals is the result of the promulgation of Conditions of Participation (COP).[7] On August 21, 1998, the Center for Medicare and Medicaid Services implemented Conditions of Participation (revised January 1, 2003). Conditions of Participation imposes requirements a hospital must meet that are designed to increase organ donation. These requirements are listed in Box 41-2.

Donation Outcomes. "Outcome is measured in terms of consent rate, conversion rate, and referral rate. It is not good enough for hospitals to point to an obligatory policy and procedure for donation. Critical care nurses are the key ingredients to a hospital's successful donation program. They must work closely, collaboratively, and effectively with OPO staff if the ever-widening gap between organ supply and organ demand is to be decreased."[8]

Informed Consent. The consent process for donation has changed since the early recovery of kidneys for transplantation. Adequate information and certain facts were rarely provided to families. With the advances and prevalence of donation and transplantation, the consent process has become more complex. Consent in the United States has now advanced to two processes:

1. Family consent for donation
2. Donor designation (donor consent for donation)

Informed consent is the process of reaching an agreement based on a full disclosure and full understanding of what will take place. Informed consent has components of disclosure, comprehension, competence, and voluntary response.[8] Consistent with other consent processes for medical procedures, there remains an ongoing debate as to how much information constitutes "informed consent." In 1998 Verble and Worth stated, "We believe that hospital personnel and procurement professionals would do well to adhere to what in legal circles is termed 'the minority point of view of disclosure'" (i.e., what a reasonable person would want to know).[9]

Presumed Consent. Presumed consent (opt-out system) is practiced in some other countries. Presumed consent provides every adult the opportunity to express his or her refusal to be a donor of solid organs and tissues, and to have this refusal recorded by publicly accountable authorities. A clinically and legally indicated candidate for deceased organ and tissue recovery is presumed to have consented to organ and tissue recovery if he or she had not registered a refusal.

Obtaining consent for donation has changed from a task predominantly for hospital personnel to one for OPO personnel and/or "a team approach." This practice uses organ procurement personnel in collaboration with hospital personnel such as the critical care nurse, hospital clergy, and physicians. This process has improved on the problem areas identified by Verble and Worth in 1998[9]:

- Lack of knowledge of what constitutes an adequate consent
- Providing inadequate information to provide an adequate basis for the donation decision
- Not adequately managing family anxieties

- Improper introduction of the donation subject. Questions asked without skill in the consent process often evoke negative responses.

Each consent for donation from the family has variables that are the results of a variety of factors, such as those listed below:

- The circumstances of the death of the potential donor
- Prior discussion regarding intent to donate
- The care provided and experienced by the family from hospital personnel
- Religious and/or cultural beliefs
- Misinformation and inadequate information
- Family members do not understand or accept the death, especially brain death
- The relationship or approach of the hospital personnel and OPO professionals

For both legal and ethical reasons, it is necessary that the public be properly informed regarding organ and tissue donation before individuals decide to become organ and/or tissue donors. An assurance that an informed consent process is in place strengthens the ability to use donor documentation as consent.

Medical Examiners and Coroners. Consistent and respectful working relationships between medical examiners and coroners and the organ and tissue donation agencies is essential in preventing the loss of organs and tissues for donation. In the United States there are three death investigation types: medical examiner, coroner, and a combination of both. The type of system varies from state to state. Each state and the District of Columbia have legislation outlining the death investigation system. In some instances, states have specific language regarding the investigational process for deceased potential donors.

Medical examiners and coroners play an integral role in organ and tissue donation. The majority of donation cases fall under their jurisdiction. Medical examiners and coroners are responsible for investigating and determining the cause of death in unexpected and violent circumstances. These deaths often engender organ and tissue donor candidates. The release of these patients' remains for donation is essential to a successful donation outcome.

Needs of Donor Families. The importance of the care provided to grieving families before and after organ and tissue donation should not be overlooked despite the clinical, technical, and legal focus within donation. These families have special needs that result from their life- (donation) and-death (loss of a loved one) decision.

The care of this family usually begins in an intensive care unit with the hospital and OPO professionals. "The influence of the nurse's sensitivity at the time of the family's agonizing decisions and emotional upheaval is critical to the family's long-term response to grief."[10]

The critical care nurse and the OPO professional establish a unique relationship with the grieving family. They are not only part of the donation process with the

---

Box 41-3

FAMILY SUPPORT DURING AND FOLLOWING ORGAN DONATION

- Follow-up by phone and letters
- Answering questions
- Providing basic information regarding the outcome for the organs and tissues transplanted
- Providing reference materials such as books, newsletters, and cards
- Providing keepsakes, such as a lock of hair or a handprint from the donor
- Presenting a donor medal

---

family, but they are entrusted to carry out the specific wishes of the deceased and/or the family. For this reason these professionals make a difference in the lives of the families at a time that makes an enduring impression.

Bereavement and/or family support mechanisms are an integral part of most OPOs. Trained personnel from the OPO provide support to families approached about donation, whether the donation becomes a reality or not. Trained family support personnel can also be used to assist with families during the actual donation process.

The support services provided are intended to assist the family through the early grieving period. This "support" is not directed at actual family counseling. If other sources of professional counseling are needed, families are provided with resource contacts. The services provided by the family support personnel are varied. Examples of support are listed in Box 41-3.

It is not infrequent that the family of the donor and the recipient of the organ(s) donated communicate with each other. Their interaction can be facilitated with mutual concurrence, including the support of the OPO and the transplant center. This interaction can range from an exchange of letters to actually meeting each other.

OPOs believe that providing donor families with personalized support is fundamental to their healing process. Various donor family surveys are conducted by OPOs; most frequently the surveys determine that families find that the ongoing support and follow-up by family support personnel facilitates their healing and helps reaffirm their lack of regret about the decision for donation. Giving compassionate and appropriate support to donor families assists them and in doing so, they become advocates for donation in the community.

Fears and Concerns About Donation. Fears and concerns about donation do affect the outcome for consent to donation. "Research into fears and concerns families have about donation and other issues at the time of donation spans a quarter of a century."[11] Examples of these fears and concerns follow:

- Disfigurement or mutilation of the donor
- Funeral for donor will not allow for an open casket

- Potential donor will be given inferior medical treatment
- Potential donor may not really be dead
- The family will have to pay for the donation process

Because of these fears and concerns, which do not change over time, and the numerous individualized variables affecting families of potential donors, there may be no "right way" to support and communicate with each family. These variables are not dissimilar from those that affect families of other critically ill patients in a critical care unit. Examples of these variables are the following:

- Timing (i.e., suddenness)
- Circumstances such as attempted suicide
- Child versus an adult
- Loss of control
- Unknown environment
- Feelings of blame or responsibility
- Disbelief

Studies by Verble and Worth indicate that strategies for communication and support can be taught and planned for by the OPO personnel in collaboration with the hospital staff.[11] Their research provides recommendations such as the use of gentle, probing questions. A question can led to the family's real concerns. Targeted strategies by trained requestors, who can provide immediate reassurance, may successfully address many fears and concerns.

Generally families in these circumstances need information to be provided many times. Assist the family by providing as much clarity as possible. Families need time, time to work their way through all that has happened, is happening, and is about to happen. They will need to have access to their loved one: easy access can be reassuring, and they need to say good-bye.

"Critical care nurses do make a difference in the lives of those entrusted to their care. Professionals in the field of transplantation emphasize the value of critical care nurses in determining which patients are potential donors and introducing the topic of donation."[10] The current strategies for these discussions are, as indicated previously, the result of the collaborative work provided by the critical care nurse and the OPO professional. This team approach offers the family the benefit of a process that includes the professionals who are trained to support them, and who have the collective ability to make the appropriate connection during times of significant grief and loss.

TISSUE DONATION

The critical care nurse is undoubtedly more aware of or familiar with organ donation than with tissue donation. It is important that the critical care nurse consider not only organ donor candidates for tissue donation, but also deceased patients who might contribute other tissues.

Organs donated save lives. It is important to know as well that tissue donation, although not specifically "life-saving," does improve the quality of life for multitudes of people. Organ transplants such as hearts, livers, and kidneys usually attract media attention because of the drama associated with life-saving operations. However, more than 1 million people benefit from tissue donation each year. One tissue donor can potentially benefit as many as 50 people. Tissue transplants make possible the following:

- Skin grafts and reconstructive therapy for thousands of critically burned patients
- Donated corneas that avert or correct blindness
- Cardiovascular tissues, including heart valves to help repair cardiac defects or damage, pericardium to repair damaged dura, and saphenous veins for vascular repair
- Bone, cartilage, and tendon grafts to help restore function in people who would otherwise be incapacitated or disabled

Each hospital is to have a formalized arrangement with one or more tissue banks for the referral of potential tissue donors. The standards and procedures have some similarities to organ donors (i.e., identification of a potential donor and referrals). The most significant difference is the status of the potential donor. As indicated previously, there are significant physiologic support factors to consider for organ donors, such as mechanical ventilation. Any deceased patient has the potential to be considered for tissue donation. The consent process for the deceased family is the same as for organ donors. There are different screening requirements for tissue donors, and each tissue bank provides these specific details.

CURRENT CHANGES IN ORGAN AND TISSUE DONATION

Donor Designation. Statistics for donation point to the reality that there continue to be barriers to higher donation rates. These include low rates of family consent to donation and missed opportunities to identify and refer all potential donors to OPOs so that families may be approached.

Multiple surveys spanning the last 20 years have indicated that a high percentage of Americans, 85%, support organ donation for transplants. The same studies indicate that only about 50% of families consent to donating a loved one's organs when presented with the opportunity. Most polls also indicate that knowledge of the decedent's wishes to donate would positively influence the family's decision to consent to donation. Moreover, potential organ donors in hospitals are not consistently identified and/or no request is made to the family.

Over the last 30 plus years, efforts to increase donation have included legislation, professional education and development, public education, training of donation requestors, media campaigns, and donor registries. Unfortunately, organ donor cards (or, similarly, the affirmative designation found on drivers' licenses) have not had a substantial effect on increasing donation. Although a donor card or donor designation on a drivers' license meets the legal requirement of an advance directive, health care personnel are reluctant to rely solely on the signed donor card for authorization to remove organs for transplantation purposes. Among the reasons commonly given for ignoring a valid donor document and seeking consent from the family are the following:

- Respect for the grieving family
- The need for a medical and social history
- Fear of bad publicity
- Fear of litigation
- Concern about whether the decision to sign a donor card is based on informed consent

As organ and tissue donation has evolved, the public has come to expect that the donor designation will be honored, and that family consent will be sought when there is no donor designation. Donor registries have resulted in many states. The primary issue for donor registries is the ability to demonstrate that the designated donor is adequately informed regarding the decision.

With "donor designation" for organ and tissue donation, the family is informed of the decedent's wishes rather than being asked to consent; OPO accepts a signed donor card or related document for donation, with or without a donor registry. This is changing the long-standing process for family consent and requires an even stronger and cohesive working relationship between the critical care nurse and OPO professionals.

The concept of a national donor registry system has been contemplated. However, in the absence of a national registry system and considering the ongoing need to increase organ and tissue donation, 33 states have currently implemented systems based on the concept of donor designation.[3] This number of state registries is projected to continue to increase. The majority of donor designation systems are tied to a donor registry.

Deceased After Cardiac Death (DCD) Donor. A DCD donor is determined by cessation of heart and respiratory functions (not brain death). DCD donors were previously termed *non–heart-beating* donors. The recovery and transplantation of organs from DCD donors represents both new practice and a return to a former practice in organ donation and transplantation; that is, the recovery of organs for transplantation from patients who are not brain dead.

In December 1997 the Institute of Medicine (IOM) published a report, "Non–Heart-Beating Organ Transplantation: Medical and Ethical Issues in Procurement."[12] The findings and recommendations of that study defined the ethical and scientific recommendations for non–heart-beating organ donation (NHBD) and transplantation. The IOM study concluded, "The recovery of organs from NHBDs is an important, medically effective, and ethically acceptable approach to reducing the gap between the demand for and the available supply of organs for transplantation."[12]

Following the 1997 study the Department of Health and Human Services (DHHS) requested a follow up study to promote DCD donation. The study promoted a patient- and family-centered approach to organ and tissue donation.[12]

The renewed interest in DCD donation comes from two central themes:

1. Patient and family interest in organ donation in cases where neurologic criteria for death cannot be met, but the decision has been made to withdraw life-sustaining treatment
2. The potential for increasing the supply of organs for transplantation[12]

Predominantly kidneys and liver are recovered from DCD donors. Overall the organs recovered per donor for transplantation are fewer for DCD donors. As technical expertise increases, the inclusion of other organs is expected to follow, but to what extent remains unknown at this point.

A patient can become a DCD donor when medical intervention is stopped, cardiac and respiratory functions cease, death is declared, and organs are removed. This process can occur in the critical care unit or the operating room (protocol-dependent) and must be carried out rapidly to remove organs before they become unsuitable for transplantation.

There are two types of DCD donors from whom organs can be recovered: "controlled" and "uncontrolled." In uncontrolled recovery, the organs are removed after the patient suffers a sudden cardiopulmonary arrest. In controlled recovery, a decision is made to discontinue life-sustaining medical intervention. Life-sustaining treatment is discontinued, although interventions to maintain the quality of the organs may be undertaken, such as cannulae placement, fluid administration, or medication. Death is declared when cardiopulmonary function ceases. Organs are removed after death has been declared.

The critical care nurse, in collaboration with the local OPO, plays a key role in DCD donation. The decision pathway involves both the patient care team and the OPO team. Each team has separate but intersecting responsibilities regarding medications, procedures, family support, withdrawing support, and declaring death. Each decision point involves cooperation between the OPO and the hospital representatives, generally the critical care nurse and the attending physician. Important features include the following:

- Family support and communication when the option is to withdraw life-sustaining treatment or stop cardiopulmonary resuscitation
- Assisting in establishing an environment of confidence with the family considering DCD donation by

assuring family members that the decision to stop aggressive treatment has been made based on appropriately communicated information
- Early notification of, referral to, and involvement of the local OPO
- Participating in the timing and the content of interactions between the OPO and the family

Barriers to DCD Organ Donation. As this addition for organ availability evolves there are issues or barriers that are prevalent (Table 41-2).[12] There were 264 DCD donors in the United States in 2003. The number of hospitals and OPOs participating in a DCD program was small, with approximately 80% of the DCD donors coming from five OPOs. The early results for 2004 indicated an increase in DCD donors and participating hospitals and OPOs. For January to June 2004 there were 180 DCD donors.

Although an increase in DCD donors will not "fix" the supply and demand gap, organs transplanted from DCD donors are positively affecting transplants. A concern that is beginning to surface is that with the changing hospital practices for treatment of devastating injuries to patients, with the public increased "ease" in making end-of-life decisions, and with hospital comfort care policies and procedures, there will be a natural decline in brain-dead donors and an increase in DCD donors. The probable outcome of this change is significant: whereas the number of donors may increase, the number of organs for transplantation will decrease, especially the availability of thoracic organs.

Table 41-2	Barriers to Organ Donation	
Issue Source	**Examples**	
Hospital factors	Lack of interest	
	Resistance	
	Failure to approve protocols	
	Rapid decisions to terminate life-sustaining medical interventions	
OPO factors	Limited resources	
	Resource skill for recovery process	
	Low priority	
	Resistance	
Organs	Unknown outcomes over time	
Adverse publicity	Media and public misunderstandings and anxiety	
Ethics	Resistance to discontinuing life-sustaining medical interventions	
	Perceived association with physician aid-in-dying	
	Medical interventions	
	Determinations of death	

OPO, Organ procurement organization.

DETERMINING BRAIN DEATH

Brain death is the term used to describe complete, irreversible cessation of function of the entire brain and brainstem. Spinal reflexes may continue to be present. At the point this occurs, the patient is dead, regardless of the presence of a heartbeat, maintenance of respiration via mechanical means, or functioning of other vital organs. The diagnosis of brain death is made by physical examination of the patient, usually by a neurologist. Absence of hypothermia and any central nervous system–depressant drugs in the blood is necessary to make the diagnosis of brain death. Several diagnostic procedures may be used to confirm the clinical diagnosis, although they are not mandatory in most cases. Transcranial Doppler, angiography, or positron emission tomography (PET) can confirm cessation of cerebral blood flow. Cessation of electrophysiologic function can be confirmed by electroencephalogram (EEG) or evoked potential testing.[1]

The following guidelines reflect generic, scientifically-based recommendations that may vary across practice settings and states according to variations in institutional policy and local legislation. Box 41-4 describes the initial requirements for clinical determination of brain death.[13] In addition; clinical determination of brain death includes coma or unresponsiveness, absence of cerebral motor responses to pain in all extremities, absence of brainstem reflexes, and apnea. In patients who are in a coma, the cause of the condition may determine what is visualized on neuroimaging studies. In most patients with brain death, the studies will show abnormalities that are consistent with loss of brain and brainstem function. However, occasionally patients will have normal neuroimaging results and have nonetheless sustained ischemic-anoxic cerebral injury.[13] In these patients the determination of brain death must be made through appropriate observation and application of the clinical criteria.

Cerebral Motor Responses. Cerebral motor responses to pain in all extremities are absent in brain death. These motor responses can be stimulated by the

---

Box 41-4

INITIAL REQUIREMENTS FOR CLINICAL DETERMINATION OF BRAIN DEATH

- Clinical or neuroimaging evidence of an acute catastrophic cerebral event consistent with the clinical diagnosis of brain death
- Exclusion of conditions that may confound clinical assessment of brain death (e.g., acute metabolic or endocrine derangements)
- Confirmation of the absence of drug intoxication or poisoning
- Core body temperature above 32° C (90° F)

application of pressure to the nailbeds as well as the supraorbital ridge. Some motor responses may occur spontaneously during apnea testing because of the presence of hypoxia or hypotension and are considered spinal cord reflexes. These may also be elicited in the presence of respiratory acidosis, and can include spontaneous flexion, and muscle stretch reflexes in arms and legs that can resemble grasping movements. It is important to determine if the patient has been given neuromuscular blocking agents that may induce pharmacologic motor weakness.

Brainstem reflexes that will be tested include pupillary signs, ocular movements, facial sensory and motor responses, and pharyngeal and tracheal reflexes.

Pupillary Signs. Pupillary signs are evaluated by the absence of the light reflex, which is consistent with brain death. Most often the pupils are round, oval, or irregularly shaped, although dilated pupils may remain even when brain death has occurred. This dilation may exist if the sympathetic cervical pathways to the pupillary dilator muscle are intact. Medications do not normally alter pupil response although the application of topical drugs as well as severe trauma to the eye may affect pupil reactivity.

Ocular Movements. Ocular movements also described as "doll's eyes" and vestibulo-ocular or "cold caloric" reflexes are not present in brain death. A description of the method of testing for each of these reflexes is included in Chapter 26. The so-called doll's eyes are elicited by the rapid turning of the head to 90 degrees laterally on both sides. The normal response is for the eyes to deviate to the opposite side of the head turning. In brain death, no eye movements occur in response to head movement (see Fig. 26-6).

The vestibulo-ocular reflex is elicited by elevating the patient's head 30 degrees and irrigating both tympanic membranes with 50 ml of iced saline or water (see Fig. 26-8). In brain death, no deviation of the eyes occurs in response to ear irrigation. It is recommended that the patient be observed for up to 1 minute after each ear irrigation; with a 5-minute wait between the testing of each ear. It is important to observe that several classes of drugs can influence the vestibulo-ocular reflex, including sedatives, aminoglycosides, tricyclic antidepressants, anticholinergics, and antiseizure medications.

Facial Sensory and Motor Responses. Facial sensory and motor responses are elicited by testing for corneal and jaw reflexes. Corneal reflexes can be tested using a cotton-tipped swab stroked across the cornea. Grimacing to pain can be demonstrated when deep pressure is applied to the nailbeds, the supraorbital ridge, or the temporomandibular joint. Severe trauma within these areas could inhibit interpretation of facial brainstem reflexes.

Pharyngeal and Tracheal Reflexes. Pharyngeal and tracheal reflexes are absent in patients with brain death.

The gag reflex can be evaluated by stimulating the posterior part of the pharynx with a tongue blade. The cough reflex can be tested using bronchial suctioning.

Apnea Testing. The loss of brainstem function results in the loss of centrally controlled breathing, causing apnea. The respiratory neurons are controlled by central chemoreceptors that sense changes in partial pressure of carbon dioxide ($PaCO_2$) and pH of the cerebrospinal fluid, which in turn accurately reflects changes in plasma $PaCO_2$. The exact level of $PaCO_2$ necessary to maximally stimulate the chemoreceptors of central respiratory centers remains unknown in conditions consistent with hyperoxygenation and brainstem destruction. Target $PaCO_2$ levels have been derived on the basis of both clinical observations and research involving apnea testing in brain death. Guidelines for determination of death based on these clinical and research data recommend achieving $PaCO_2$ levels greater than 60 mm Hg for maximal stimulation of brainstem respiratory centers.[13] Box 41-5 provides the procedure for apnea testing.

To avoid cardiac dysrhythmias and the systemic hypotension that may occur during the apnea test, clinicians should follow the precautions outlined in Box 41-6. Finally, the interpreted results of an apnea test are shown in Table 41-3. Apnea test results can be (1) posi-

---

Box 41-5

APNEA TESTING PROCEDURE

1. Disconnect the ventilator.
2. Deliver 100% oxygen at a rate of 6 L/min via the endotracheal tube. The oxygen cannula can be placed at the level of the carina.
3. Observe the patient closely for the respiratory movements (i.e., abdominal or chest excursions that produce adequate tidal volumes).
4. Measure PaO_2, $PaCO_2$, and pH after approximately 8 minutes and reconnect the ventilator.

Box 41-6

PRECAUTIONS TO OBSERVE DURING APNEA TESTING

- Maintain patient's core body temperature at ≥36.5° C.
- Maintain patient's systolic blood pressure at ≥90 mm Hg.
- Establish euvolemia (normal volume) in the patient.
- Establish eucapnia ($PaCO_2 \approx 40$ mm Hg) in the patient.

Maintain or achieve normal oxygen levels (option: $PaO_2 \approx 200$ mm Hg) in the patient.

Table 41-3	Apnea Test Results
Result	**Findings**
Positive	Respiratory movements are absent. Posttest arterial Pa_{CO_2} is ≥60 mm Hg. Result supports clinical determination of brain death.
Negative	Respiratory movements occur regardless of arterial Pa_{CO_2} level. Result does not support clinical determination of brain death. Apnea test can be repeated.
Occurrence of cardiovascular or pulmonary instability	Systolic blood pressure decreases to <90 mm Hg. Arterial oxygen desaturation occurs. Cardiac dysrhythmia occurs. The nurse should immediately obtain a blood sample for arterial blood gas analysis and reconnect the ventilator. Confirmatory test to finalize clinical determination of brain death may be performed at discretion of physician.
Inconclusive	No respiratory movements are observed. Posttest arterial Pa_{CO_2} is <60 mm Hg without marked cardiovascular instability.

Table 41-4	Confirmatory Tests of Brain Death
Test	**Results**
Cerebral angiography	No intracerebral filling at level of carotid bifurcation or circle of Willis. Patent external carotid circulation
Electroencephalography	No electrical activity during a period of a least 30 minutes of recording
Transcranial Doppler sonography	No diastolic or reverberating flow. Systole-only or retrograde diastolic flow. Small systolic peaks in early systole
Somatosensory and brainstem auditory evoked potentials testing	No responses
Technetium Tc 99m brain scan (cerebral blood flow scan)	No uptake of radionuclide in brain parenchyma ("hollow skull phenomenon")
Magnetic resonance imaging	Not yet determined

tive, (2) negative, (3) demonstrative of cardiovascular or pulmonary instability, or (4) inconclusive.

Although brain death policies vary by institution and may also be defined by statutes in each state, most experts recommend an arbitrary interval of 6 hours between initial and repeat examinations. In some patients, confirmatory tests are necessary to determine brain death. Table 41-4 provides a reference to the types of confirmatory testing most frequently used in declaring brain death. All clinical tests of cardinal findings are equally essential in declaring brain death.

Communication With Family. The nurse caring for a potential organ donor and the patient's family may find that confusion and misconceptions are often associated with brain death. Family members of patients who are being evaluated for brain death often think their loved one is being "kept alive" by the ventilator because the patient is warm, coloring indicates adequate perfusion to vital organs, and he or she appears to have respirations. It is important to establish with families that brain death is indeed irreversible, and it is not the same as a comatose state. The patient will not recover or get better through additional medical treatment or through a prolonged rehabilitation. Critical care nurses benefit from becoming familiar with the concept of brain death and its medical

and legal criteria, because they may need to explain brain death to families who are confused and in crisis.[13]

The use of terminology that is applied to cases in which patients are pronounced dead on the basis of neurologic criteria can be confusing for families. The term *brain death* can mean to some that only the brain is dead, and that other organs are alive. Similarly, the use of the term *life support* can imply that the patient is not truly dead, and the use of terms such as *artificial respiration* or *mechanical ventilation* may create less confusion. There may also be confusion about when death is to be recorded in a patient who is declared brain dead. When death is pronounced on the basis of neurologic criteria, the time of death is established as the time of brain death pronouncement as opposed to the time the patient is withdrawn from mechanical support.[14]

MANAGEMENT OF THE ORGAN DONOR

Once the potential organ donor has been officially declared brain dead by established confirmatory tests, the phase of management of the potential organ donor shifts to care of the patient that preserves and promotes organ function and viability. Referred to as donor management, this is a process that focuses on maintaining hemody-

Box 41-7

DONOR MANAGEMENT PLAN OF CARE

- Transfer care to (name of OPO).
- Discontinue all previous orders.
- Measure blood pressure, heart rate, temperature, urine output, central venous pressure (CVP; if central venous catheter is present), pulmonary artery occlusion pressure (PAOP; if pulmonary artery [PA] catheter is present) every hour.
- Reorder mechanical ventilator parameters as previously set.
- Maintain head of bed at 30 to 40 degrees of elevation.
- Continue routine pulmonary suctioning and side-to-side body positioning.
- Use warming blanket to maintain body temperature above 36.5° C.
- Maintain sequential compression devices.
- Continue chest tube suction or water seal (if present) as previously ordered.
- Set nasogastric (orogastric) tube (if present) to low intermittent suction.
- Administer intravenous (IV) fluid: 5% dextrose in 0.45% sodium chloride solution plus 20 mEq/L (mmol/L) potassium chloride at 75ml/hour
- Call the OPO coordinator when any of the following occur:
  - The mean arterial pressure (MAP) is less than 70 mm Hg
  - Systolic pressure is greater than 170 mm Hg
  - Heart rate is fewer than 60 or more than 130 beats/min
  - Temperature is less than 36.5° C or more than 37.8° C
  - Urine output is less than 75 or more than 250 ml/hour
  - CVP or PAOP is less than 8 or more than 18 mm Hg

- Administer pantoprazole 40 mg intravenously every 24 hours, first dose stat; give artificial tears every hour and as needed to prevent corneal drying.
- Administer albuterol and Atrovent unit dose per aerosol every 4 hours.
- Continue antibiotics previously ordered at same dose and frequency.
- Continue vasoactive drug infusions (e.g., dopamine, norepinephrine) at previously ordered concentrations and infusion rates.
- Review all medications previously ordered. Most medications (anticonvulsant agents, pain medications, laxatives, gastrointestinal [GI] motility agents, subcutaneous heparin, osmotic agents [mannitol], and diuretic agents) are unnecessary during donor care and will be discontinued automatically as the care is transferred to the OPO. Review any other medications in question with the physician.
- Send blood samples to the laboratory at once for measurement of electrolytes, magnesium, ionized calcium, complete blood cell count, platelets, glucose, blood urea nitrogen (BUN), creatinine, phosphorous, arterial blood gas values, prothrombin time (PT), and partial thromboplastin time (aPTT); and resample every 4 hours.
- Send blood for type and screen with the preceding blood sample (if not previously done).
- Obtain finger-stick glucose values every 2 hours—contact the OPO if the glucose level is less than 5.0 mmol/L (90 mg/dl) or greater than 10.0 mmol/L (180 mg/dl).
- Obtain an electrocardiogram (ECG) at initial donor evaluation.
- Add other orders for specific organ evaluation as indicated.

namic stability and normative laboratory parameters. The care of the donor in this phase may last for several hours, and is generally under the direction of the OPO professional working collaboratively with the attending physicians and critical care nursing staff. A standardized set of orders is most often used by the OPO professional to initiate treatment and provide a continuing evaluation tool that can be used to address management concerns as they arise. In addition, it serves as a baseline to indicate significant trends or shifts in the donor's status. These standardized orders should emphasize the following treatment guidelines:[15]

- Hypertension and hypotension
- Glucose management
- Temperature management
- Anemia
- Coagulopathy and thrombocytopenia
- Mechanical ventilation
- Fluid and electrolytes

- Polyuria
- Acid-base management

The clinical donor coordinator will normally be the person to write orders for the hospital chart to initiate standard donor care as listed in Box 41-7.

The OPO professional will also initiate a thorough physical examination of the patient and complete an extensive medical and social history. It is critical that events leading to the hospitalization, extent and duration of any cardiac arrest, cardiopulmonary resuscitation efforts, drugs administered, and signs of chest and abdominal trauma are identified. In addition to the treatment guidelines that are initiated, the OPO professional is responsible for ordering serologic testing that screens the patient for a variety of transmissible diseases including, but not limited to, human immunodeficiency virus (HIV), hepatitis, and other sexually transmitted diseases (STDs).

The medical social history is sensitive for determining high-risk social behavior of the donor, such as use of tobacco, alcohol, and drugs. The completion of these tests and the accompanying medical and social history are is necessary to determine the suitability of the donor and the subsequent allocation and recovery of the organs for transplantation.

NURSING MANAGEMENT

The primary goals of nursing management of the donor are to accomplish the following:
- Oxygenate the organs
- Maintain hemodynamic stability
- Maintain fluid and electrolyte balance
- Maintain temperature regulation

These goals can be accomplished by the use of treatment guidelines such as standard orders provided by the OPO, as well as the Critical Pathway for the Organ Donor (Table 41-5). This tool, developed by UNOS, is a multidisciplinary approach to identifying key events, processes, and timelines to anticipate in the care of an organ donor. It also promotes more efficient care of the donor by eliminating unnecessary and expensive tests, while adopting a standard of care that maximizes organ recovery and transplantation. Although hospitals and OPOs may vary in their standing orders or guidelines, the basic principles reflected in the pathway are universally recognized as effective donor care and management.

The role of the critical care nurse in continuing care of the donor is complex. The use of tools such as the standing orders provided by the OPO professional are focused on managing the circumstances a brain dead patient presents. However, it is important that physicians and other health care resources, such as respiratory therapists, also assist in the management of the potential donor. The nursing goals for care of the potential donor focus on maintaining the donor in a state of hemodynamic stability that supports organ function. The complications that arise from brain death lead to a lack of autoregulation of the brain and create intense vasodilation and potentially, cardiac dysrhythmias. In addition, the lack of blood flow in the brain forces a loss of temperature regulation, as well as a lack of antidiuretic hormone, causing diabetes insipidus and resultant fluid and electrolyte disorders.

RECOVERY OF ORGANS

The donor management phase continues into the operating room setting once the OPO professional has successfully identified potential recipients for the organs that have been donated. A time is set with the operating room, and the recovery and transplant teams are activated. The role of the OPO professional continues to ensure that the patient remains in a stable condition during transport to the operating room and through the recovery procedure. Donors are transferred to the operating room with ongoing monitoring of heart rate, blood pressure, and any intravenous medications. Ventilator support is continued, and a nurse anesthetist or anesthesiologist supports the patient management to ensure maximum stability. The OPO professional serves as a vital part of the recovery team and ensures that ongoing monitoring and documentation is completed. The OPO professional also provides communication back to the critical care staff and to the donor's family, once the case is completed and organs are recovered. At the completion of the donor case, the critical care nurse may still be providing support to the donor family in the critical care unit, or the family may have decided to leave the hospital and return home. The OPO professional will provide immediate feedback to the nursing and medical staff who have been an integral part of the donation process.

ROLE OF THE CRITICAL CARE NURSE IN ORGAN DONATION

The role of the critical care nurse in organ donation is one that is complex and challenging and contributes to saving lives. Critical care nurses provide the link to the OPO, donor families, and potential organ transplant recipients. As the health care provider responsible for the care of a critically ill patient, the nurse is also often in the role of providing support to the donor family. The nurse may be involved in helping the family to understand the diagnosis of brain death, as well as answering questions and concerns that arise. This unique role is instrumental in ensuring that a potential organ donor and his or her family is offered the opportunity to donate organs for transplantation. The nurse must be familiar with the criteria for brain death, as well as the protocols for their institutions, and may also be involved in obtaining consent for donation. In accordance with the federal government and the Health Care Financing Administration Conditions of Participation (COP), all patients who meet the criteria for brain death must be referred to the local organ procurement organization (OPO) and considered potential organ donors. The local OPO is consulted when it is believed that the patient's brain death is imminent.[16] This call sets into motion the referral process, and involves the nurse and the OPO working together while the patient is evaluated for medical suitability.

As the patient's condition is identified as meeting criteria for brain death, the focus of care the nurse has been providing shifts from that of saving the patient, to promoting optimal physiologic status to preserve organ function. The critical care nurse's efforts will be focused on the care and preservation of organ function; he or she works with the OPO professional to assume responsibility for the medical management of the donor. The OPO professional is generally not an employee of the hospital the donor is in and so depends upon the support and

Table 41-5   Critical Pathway for the Organ Donor

Patient name: _____

ID number: _____

Collaborative Practice	Phase I Referral	Phase II Declaration of Brain Death and Consent	Phase III Donor Evaluation	Phase IV Donor Management	Phase V Recovery Phase
The following professionals may be involved to enhance the donation process: Check all that apply Physician Critical Care RN **Organ procurement organization (OPO)** **Organ procurement coordinator (OPC)** Medical examiner (ME)/coroner Respiratory Laboratory Pharmacy Radiology Anesthesiology OR/Surgery staff Clergy Social worker	Notify physician regarding OPO referral Contact OPO ref: potential donor with severe brain insult **OPC on site and begins evaluation** **Time** _____ **Date** _____ **Ht** _____ **Wt** _____ **as documented** **ABO as documented** **Notify house supervisor/charge nurse of presence of OPC unit**	Brain death documented Time _____ Date _____ **Patient accepted as potential donor** MD notifies family of death Plan family approach with OPC Offer support services to family (clergy, etc.) **OPC/hospital staff talks to family about donation** Family accepts donation **OPC obtains signed consent and medical/social history** **Time** _____ **Date** _____ ME/coroner notified ME/coroner releases body for donation *Family/ME/coroner denies donation—stop pathway, initiate post mortem protocol, support family*	**Obtain pre/post transfusion blood for serology testing (HIV, hepatitis, VDRL, CMV)** **Obtain lymph nodes and/or blood for tissue typing** **Notify house supervisor of pending donation** Chest and abdominal circumference Lung measurements per CXR by OPC Cardiology consult as requested by OPC *Donor organs unsuitable for transplant—stop pathway, initiate post mortem protocol, support family*	**OPC writes orders** **Organ placement** **OPC sets tentative OR time** Insert arterial line/2 large-bore IVs Possibly insert central venous catheter	**Checklist for OR Supplies given to OR** Prepare patient for transport to OR IVs Pumps O₂ Ambu PEEP valve Transport to OR Date _____ Time _____ OR nurse Reviews consent form Reviews brain death documentation Checks patient's ID band

Table 41-5 Critical Pathway for the Organ Donor—con'td

Patient name: _____
ID number: _____

Collaborative Practice	Phase I Referral	Phase II Declaration of Brain Death and Consent	Phase III Donor Evaluation	Phase IV Donor Management	Phase V Recovery Phase
Labs/diagnostics		Review previous laboratory results Review previous hemodynamics	Blood and chemistry CBC = + diff UA C&S PT, PTT ABO A subtype Liver function test Blood culture × 2; 15 minutes to 1 hour apart Sputum Gram's stain and C&S Type and cross-match ____ # units PRBCs CXR ABGs ECG Echo **Consider cardiac death** Consider **bronchoscopy**	**Determine need for additional lab testing** CXR after line placement (if done) Serum electrolytes H&H after PRBC Rx PT, PTT BUN, serum, creatinine after correcting fluid deficit Notify OPC for ____ PT > 14 sec ____ aPTT < 28 sec ____ Urine output ____ <1 ml/kg/h ____ >3 ml/kg/h HCt ↓30 Hgb ↓10 Na ↑150 mmol/L	Samples for laboratory test obtained in OR as per surgeon or OPC request **Communicate with pathology: Bx liver and/or kidney as indicated**
Respiratory	Pt on ventilator Suction q 2 hr Reposition q 2 hr	Prep for apnea testing: set Fio2 at 1.00 and anticipate need to decrease rate if Pco2 ↓45 mm Hg	**Maximize ventilator settings to achieve Sao2 of 98%-99%** **PEEP = 5 cm H2O** **Challenge for lung placement: Fio2 at 1.00, PEEP at 5 cm H2O × 10 min** **ABGs as ordered** **VS q 1°**	Notify OPC for ____ BP < 90 mm Hg systolic ____ HR < 70 or > 120 beats/min ____ CVP < 4 or > 11 ____ Pao2 < 90 mm Hg or ____ Sao2 < 95%	Portable O2 at Fio2 of 1.00 for transport to OR Ambu bag and PEEP valve Move to OR
Treatments/ongoing care		Use warming/cooling blanket to maintain temperature at 36.5°C to 37.5°C NG to low intermittent suction	Check NG placement and output Obtain actual Ht ____ and Wt ____ if not previously obtained		Set OR temperature as directed by OPC Postmortem care at conclusion of case

Medications	The potential donor is identified and a referral is made to the OPO.	The family is offered the option of donation and their decision is supported.	Medication as requested by OPC	**Fluid resuscitation: consider crystalloids, colloids, blood products** **DC meds except vasopressors and antibiotics** **Broad-spectrum antibiotic if not previously ordered** **Vasopressor support to maintain BP >90 mm Hg systolic** **Electrolyte K, Ca^{++} PO$_4$, Mg^{++} replacement** **Hyperglycemia: consider insulin infusion** **Oliguria: consider diuretics** **Diabetes insipidus: consider antidiuretics** **Paralytic as indicated for spinal reflexes**	**DC antidiuretics** **Diuretics as needed** **Heparin, 350 units/kg or as directed by surgeon**
Optimal outcomes	The donor is evaluated and found to be a suitable candidate for donation.			Optimal organ function is maintained.	All potentially suitable organs for which consent obtained are recovered for transplantation.

Areas in bold indicate Organ Procurement Coordinator (OPC) activities. Reprinted with permission of the United Network for Organ Sharing.

ABGs, Arterial blood gases; *aPTT*, activated partial thromboplastin time; *BP*, blood pressure; *BUN*, blood urea nitrogen; *C&S*, culture and sensitivities; *CBC*, complete blood count; *CMV*, cytomegalovirus; *CVP*, central venous pressure; *CXR*, chest x-ray; *DC*, discontinue; *ECG*, electrocardiogram; *H&H*, hematocrit and hemoglobin; *Hct*, hematocrit; *Hgb*, hemoglobin; *HIV*, human immunodeficiency virus; *HR*, heart rate; *ID*, identification; *NG*, nasogastric; *OR*, operating room; *PaO$_2$*, partial pressure of oxygen; *PEEP*, positive end-expiratory pressure; *PRBC*, packed red blood cells; *PT*, prothrombin time; *PTT*, partial thromboplastin time; *Sa O$_2$*, oxygen saturation; *UA*, urinalysis; *VDRL*, Venereal Disease Research Laboratories; *VS*, vital signs.

involvement of the bedside nurse. Together, they will work to keep the patient hemodynamically stable while the various organs are evaluated for suitability for transplantation. The nurse will coordinate with the OPO professional, a variety of evaluative tests, such as electrocardiograms, chest x-rays, and echocardiograms, along with tests that determine the function of the liver, the kidney, and the pancreas. The use of standing orders that the OPO professional provides assist the critical care nurse in the management of the donor, a process that can be challenging and may last for several hours until the patient is taken to the operating room.

The role of the critical care nurse is vital to the successful recovery of transplantable organs. Research indicates that the attitude of health care professionals toward donation affects donation rates.[17] If a health care professional is not supportive of organ donation, the family is denied the autonomy to make its own decision and a potential transplant recipient is denied a chance at life.[17] Although the process is complex and challenging, it is also unique in that lives are saved as a result of a family's decision to donate and the care that is provided to the donor.

IMMUNOLOGY OF TRANSPLANT REJECTION

Organ transplantation has become a commonly practiced procedure for end-stage cardiac, pulmonary, liver, kidney, and pancreatic disease. Major advances have been made in organ procurement and preservation, surgical techniques, and identifying and treating rejection. The ultimate long-term success of any organ transplant depends on the immune system's tolerance of the transplanted graft. Virtually every body cell carries distinctive molecules that enable the immune system to distinguish self from non-self. A normally functioning immune system is designed to eliminate the foreign invader recognized as non-self. Tolerance of the transplanted organ can be achieved only by suppressing or regulating this normal immune response to the foreign organ. To understand the principles of immunosuppressive therapy, it is important to have some understanding of the cells of the immune system, the immune response, and the process of organ rejection.

IMMUNE MECHANISM

Whenever the body is confronted with any substance that is non-self, a primary immune response is elicited. There are three phases of any *primary immune response:*

1. Recognition of the substance as non-self
2. Proliferation of immunocompetent cells
3. Effector phase, or action against the foreign substance. During this primary response, immunologic

memory is established, and any subsequent encounter with the same substance will provide a more rapid and intense immune response. Subsequent encounters are termed *secondary immune responses.*

An antigen is a substance that is capable of eliciting an immune response. Each cell has antigens on its surface that are genetically predetermined by a series of linked genes known as the *major histocompatibility complex (MHC).* If tissue from one person is transplanted into a genetically different person, the antigens on the transplanted tissue cells are immediately recognized as non-self and rejection occurs. MHC determines the antigens to which the immune system should respond. The human MHC is called *human leukocyte antigen (HLA)* because these markers were first discovered on lymphocytes. The HLA gene complex is located on chromosome number 6. Each chromosome contains four loci: HLA-A, HLA-B, HLA-C, and HLA-D. More than 150 antigens have been recognized in the HLA system: 23 on the A locus, 52 on the B locus, 11 on the C locus, and 61 on the D locus.[18] Because a potential for millions of different arrangements of these antigens exists, the chances of finding a donor organ with the same histocompatibility genes as a recipient are virtually impossible unless donor and recipient are identical twins.

HLA antigens are divided into three classes of antigens. Class I antigens are present on almost all body cells and are thus the markers of self. The class II antigens are present on B lymphocytes, macrophages, and other cells responsible for presenting foreign antigen to the immune system and inducing the immune response. Class III antigens include some red blood cell antigens and complement.

CELLS OF THE IMMUNE SYSTEM

The immune system houses a vast number of cells responsible for general defense and very specific immune responses. Only a few cells of each specificity are stored. When a specific antigen appears, those few cells are stimulated to multiply and mount a response to the foreign antigen. Immune cells are originally produced in the bone marrow as stem cells. Their descendants become either lymphocytes or phagocytes (Fig. 41-2).

The two major classes of lymphocytes are B cells and T cells. B cells remain in the bone marrow to complete their maturation. The T cells migrate to the thymus gland, where they mature. In the thymus, T cells acquire the ability to distinguish self from non-self. Once mature, some B and T cells are housed in the lymph nodes, whereas others circulate in the blood and lymph system.

Humoral Immunity. Humoral immunity is mediated by B cells. They are responsible for the production of antibody or immunoglobulin. When a B cell encounters an antigen to which it is specifically coded to respond, the B

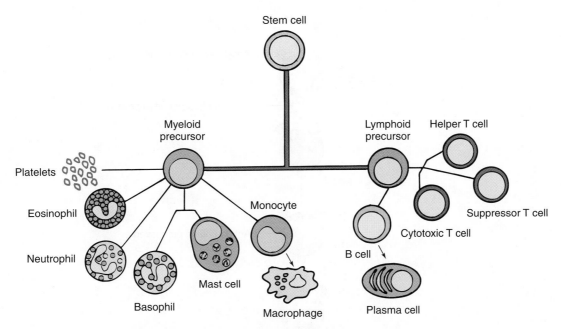

Fig. 41-2   All cells of the immune system originate from stem cells in the bone marrow. (From Schindler LW: *Understanding the immune system*, NIH Pub No. 90-529, Bethesda, Md, 1990, US Department of Health and Human Services.)

cell enlarges, divides, and differentiates into a plasma cell. It is the plasma cell that actually produces and secretes antigen-specific antibody (Fig. 41-3). Once exposed to an antigen, the immune system retains a memory of that antigen. Subsequent exposure stimulates the B cell memory cells, resulting in a rapid mobilization of antibody-secreting cells. Antibodies work in several ways, but their primary purpose is to mark an antigen for destruction by the immune system. Other antibodies are capable of neutralizing toxins produced by bacteria, or they can trigger the release of serum proteins known as *complement*.

Cell-Mediated Immunity. Cell-mediated immunity is determined by T cells that are specifically sensitized. Approximately 65% to 80% of all lymphocytes are T cells, of which there are three basic types: cytotoxic T cells, helper T cells, and suppressor T cells.

Cytotoxic T cells. Cytotoxic T cells are cells capable of killing invading cells. Their primary role is to rid the body of cells that have become infected; transformed by cancer; or are non-self, as in the case of transplanted tissue. They also are called *T8 or CD8 lymphocytes,* referring to a marker that distinguishes cytotoxic T cells from other T cells. Cytotoxic T cells are activated by macrophages that present the foreign antigen to immature cytotoxic T cells. With the assistance of the helper T cell and its release of chemical mediators, the cytotoxic T cell matures and kills foreign cells that carry that specific antigen (Fig. 41-4).

Helper T Cells. Helper T cells up-regulate the immune response by stimulating B cells to differentiate into plasma cells and begin antibody production, by activating cytotoxic T cells, and by stimulating natural killer cells and macrophages. Helper T cells are identified by their T4 or CD4 marker. Fig. 41-5 illustrates the process responsible for activating helper T cells. Macrophages are responsible for presenting processed antigen to the immature helper T cells. With the assistance of chemical mediators (interleukins) released by the macrophage, the helper T cell matures and begins to activate other cells of the immune system previously described.

Suppressor T Cells. A third type of T cell is the *suppressor T cell*. These cells suppress, or down-regulate, the immune response. They play an important role in keeping the immune response controlled and in turning off the response once the antigenic threat is no longer present.

Other Immune System Defenses. T and B cells work with other parts of the immune system, notably natural killer cells, phagocytic cells, and complement to enhance the immune response as described below.

Natural Killer Cells. Natural killer cells represent another type of lymphocyte. These cells are not targeted for any specific antigen but will attack and destroy any cell that is identified as non-self. Natural killer cells contain granules filled with potent chemicals that are released when the natural killer cell binds to the targeted non-self cell. These chemicals are capable of lysing the cell membrane and causing the cell's death.

Phagocytes. Phagocytes are a major category of immune cells capable of destroying alien cells. Critical phagocytes include monocytes, macrophages, neutrophils, eosinophils, and basophils. Table 41-6 outlines the primary function of these cells. Macrophages are vi-

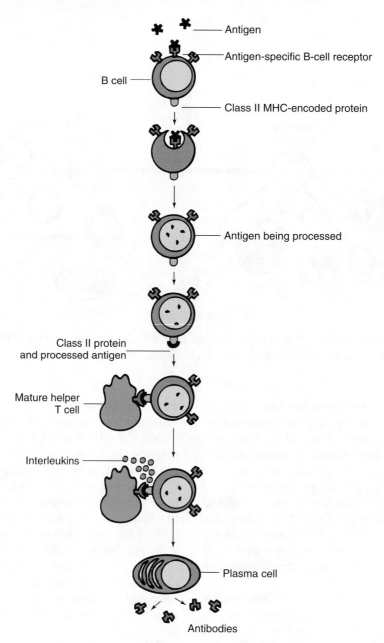

B cell — Antigen

Antigen-specific B-cell receptor

Class II MHC-encoded protein

Antigen being processed

Class II protein and processed antigen

Mature helper T cell

Interleukins

Plasma cell

Antibodies

Fig. 41-3   Foreign antigen is processed by the B cell and displayed with its MHC class II antigen (protein), which attracts helper T cells. The release of interleukins by the helper T cell stimulates differentiation of the B cell into a plasma cell, which begins to produce antibody. (From Schindler LW: *Understanding the immune system,* NIH Pub No. 90-629, Bethesda, Md, 1990, US Department of Health and Human Services.)

tally important to the immune response because of their role in "presenting" the antigen to the helper and cytotoxic T cells. This presentation alerts the T cells to the presence of antigen. Macrophages also produce chemical regulators, or interleukins, that stimulate the maturation of helper and cytotoxic T cells.

As just described, chemical substances are released by macrophages, helper T cells, and cytotoxic T cells, which allow these immune cells to communicate with each other. These substances provide a network of solu-ble, low–molecular-weight peptides called *cytokines,* or more specifically, *interleukins (ILs).*[19] Interleukins are capable of activating or suppressing the proliferation of lymphocyte subsets. Several different types of interleukins with specific functions have been identified, but researchers are just beginning to understand the role that interleukins play in modulating the immune response.

Complement. An important system in the immune response is complement. Complement consists of a

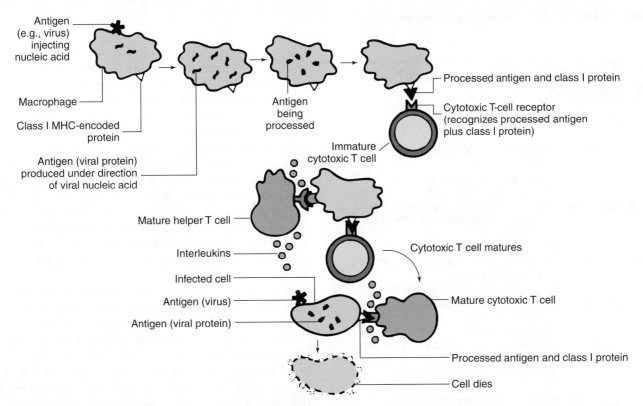

Fig. 41-4 The macrophage presents the processed antigen from the foreign organism on the major histocompatibility complex (MHC) class I protein to the cytotoxic and helper T cell. Aided by the release of interleukins from helper T cell, the cytotoxic T cell matures and kills the foreign cell. (From Schindler LW: *Understanding the immune system,* NIH Pub No. 90-629, Bethesda, Md, 1990, U.S. Department of Health and Human Services.)

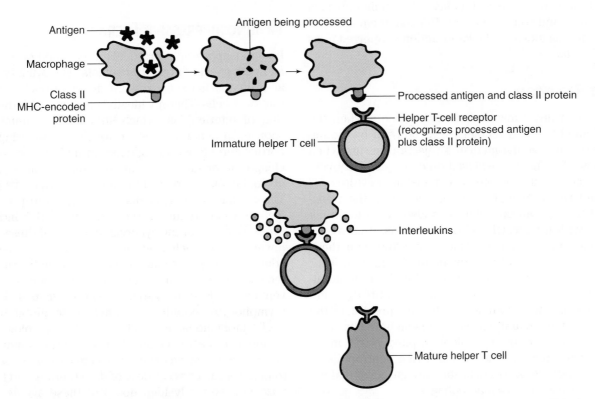

Fig. 41-5 The helper T cell is activated by the presence of processed antigen in combination with the class II antigen (protein) on the surface of a macrophage. It matures with the stimulus from interleukins. *MHC,* Major histocompatibility complex. (From Schindler LW: *Understanding the immune system,* NIH Pub No. 90-629, Bethesda, Md, 1990, U.S. Department of Health and Human Services.)

Table 41-6	Phagocytes and Their Functions
Phagocyte	**Function**
Monocytes	Migrate from blood tissues to become macrophages
	Scavenger cells in tissues
	Present antigen to T cells
Macrophages	Secrete enzymes, complement proteins, and immune regulatory factors (cytokines)
	Activated by lymphokines
Neutrophils	Contain granules capable of destroying alien organisms
	Key role in inflammatory reactions
Eosinophils	Contain granules capable of destroying alien organisms
	Weaker phagocyte
Basophils	Contain granules capable of destroying alien organisms
	Key role in allergic reaction

series of 25 proteins, which, when activated, develop into powerful enzymes capable of lysing alien cell walls. Complement is triggered by the presence of antibody bound to an alien cell or antigen (antigen-antibody complex). Complement also stimulates basophils, attracts neutrophils, and coats alien cells to make them more attractive to phagocytes. The latter action is referred to as *opsonization*.

GRAFT REJECTION

Rejection of any transplanted organ occurs when the transplanted tissue is recognized as non-self by the immune system. Cellular-mediated rejection occurs when HLA class II antigens, displayed on donor cells, activate helper T cells that promote the expansion of cytotoxic T cells and recruitment of macrophages into the transplanted tissue. Natural killer cells also begin to attack any cell with foreign HLA class I antigens. As a result, the transplanted organ becomes infiltrated with these cells, which proceed to destroy the foreign graft tissue.

At the same time, antibody-mediated or humoral-mediated rejection occurs as antigen-antibody complexes form. These complexes also are present in the transplanted organ and release complement that is capable of cell destruction. Complement plays a role in recruiting basophils and tissue-destroying neutrophils to the site. Antibody also coats the foreign cells, making them more attractive to macrophages.

Graft rejection can occur at different time intervals and has different injury patterns. The three different types of rejection patterns are hyperacute rejection, acute rejection, and chronic rejection.

Hyperacute rejection occurs within hours after transplantation and results in immediate graft failure. The primary mechanism triggering this response is activation of humoral-mediated rejection. Such an immediate response by the immune system is caused by the presence of preformed reactive antibodies resulting from previous exposure to antigens. Presensitization can be the result of previous blood transfusions, multiple pregnancies, or previous organ transplants.[20] Transplanting an organ from a donor with an incompatible blood type can have the same effect. Hyperacute rejection is prevented by testing for the presence of preformed antibodies in the recipient and by selecting donors with compatible blood types.

Acute rejection occurs weeks to months after transplantation. Class I or II antigens on the cells of the transplanted graft activate cellular-mediated rejection.

Chronic rejection occurs at varying times after transplantation and progresses for years until the ultimate deterioration of the transplanted organ. Chronic rejection is the result of both humoral-mediated and cellular-mediated immune responses. Chronic inflammation results in diffuse scarring of tissue and stenosis of the vasculature of the organ. Lack of blood supply leads to ischemia and necrosis of tissue. Chronic lung rejection results in small airway destruction, and chronic liver rejection causes diminution of bile ducts.

IMMUNOSUPPRESSIVE THERAPY

Immunosuppressive protocols vary among institutions and with specific organ transplants. The primary goal of all protocols is to suppress the activity of helper and cytotoxic T cells. Therapy ideally interferes with the secretion of interleukins, which stimulate the immune response. In general, most protocols combine high-dose corticosteroids with a calcineurin inhibitor such as cyclosporine or tacrolimus in addition to azathioprine or mycophenolate mofetil during the perioperative period. These triple drug regimens are designed to prevent rejection while reducing the toxicity of the individual drugs. Because of the synergistic nature of these agents, lower doses of each drug can almost always be used.[21] In addition to these primary agents, cytolytic therapy is often used in an attempt to induce graft tolerance and prevent early rejection episodes.[22] These agents include antilymphocyte globulins, antithymocyte globulins, and OKT3 monoclonal antibody. The Pharmacologic Management Table on Organ Transplantation summarizes immunosuppressive drugs. Absolute care must be taken to monitor the effectiveness of drug therapy and to minimize unnecessarily high doses of these agents, which could predispose patients to greater risks for infection, malignancy, or other toxic effects.

Corticosteroids. Corticosteroids (intravenous methylprednisolone [Solu-Medrol] and oral prednisone) have

Pharmacologic Management: Organ Transplantation

DRUG	DOSAGE*	ACTIONS	SPECIAL CONSIDERATIONS
Azathioprine	Titrate to WBC between 3000-6000 cells/mm^3	Inhibits purine synthesis	Monitor for bone marrow depression
Cyclosporine gelatin (Neoral)† Oral solution and capsules	Standard dose range (organ-specific): 14-18 mg/kg/day (liver transplant) 10-14 mg/kg/day (kidney transplant) Tapered to 5-10 mg/kg/day 4-6 mg/kg/day (heart transplant) Dosage split bid Therapeutic range: 100-400 ng/ml	Suppresses T lymphocytes	Hold for elevated levels Watch for nephrotoxicity, HTN, hepatotoxity, tremors, and seizures Watch for drugs that exhibit nephrotoxic synergy (i.e., gentamicin, tobramycin, vancomycin, amphotericin B, ketoconazole, cimetidine, and ranitidine)
Daclizumab (Zenapax)	1 mg/kg	Blocks interleukin-2 receptor sites	Used as induction therapy No pretreatment needed
Muromonab-CD3 (Orthoclone OKT3)	5 mg/day for 5-7 days (less in some centers)	Suppresses circulating T lymphocytes	Watch for reactions Pretreatment for initial doses with: Acetaminophen (Tylenol) Diphenhydramine (Benadryl) Hydrocortisone 50 mg
Mycophenolate mofetil (CellCept)	2-3 g/day split bid	Similar to azathioprine but less toxic to bone marrow	Increased blood level concentrations when used with other drugs excreted via the renal tubules
Prednisone	1 mg/kg/day Tapered to 0.3 mg/kg/day or off, if tolerated	Suppresses inflammatory response	Tapered to as low a dose as tolerated Dose is increased with rejection
Rabbit antithymocyte globulin (Thymoglobulin, RATG)	2.5 mg/kg for 1-7 days May be given daily initially then every other day	Suppresses circulating T lymphocytes	Used in lung transplants for induction therapy Used as rescue therapy for other transplants Watch for reactions Pretreatment may be used
Sirolimus (Rapamycin, Rapammune)	10 mg/day tapered to trough level of 12-20 mg/ml (depending of organ and center)	Blocks cytokines' ability to activate T and B lymphocytes	Synergistic effects when used with cyclosporine or tacrolimus Watch for thrombocytopenia Used in place of azathioprine or mycophenolate mofetil
Tacrolimus (Prograf, FK506)	0.1-0.3 mg/kg/day Dosage split bid Therapeutic range: 5-20 ng/ml	Inhibition of interleukin release	Nephrotoxicity with high doses Hyperkalemia

*These dosage ranges are general guidelines. Significant variations in dosages occur based on institutional practices, other drugs being used in combination, transplant type, and patient response to the drugs.
†Neoral and Sandimmune, although both cyclosporine preparations, are not bioequivalent and cannot be used interchangeably. Gengraf and Neoral are bioequivalent.
HTN, Hypertension.

complex and diverse effects on the immune system. They are used both for maintenance therapy and to treat acute rejection. The antiinflammatory actions of steroids provide important protection of the transplanted organ from permanent damage from the rejection process. As a maintenance therapy, steroids impair the sensitivity of T cells to antigen, decrease the proliferation of sensitized T cells, and impair the production of interleukins. Steroids also decrease macrophage mobility. Chronic steroid therapy is associated with numerous adverse effects and predisposes the patient to an increased risk of infection (see the Pharmacologic Management Table on

Organ Transplantation). A primary goal of therapy is to titrate the drug dose to as minimal a level as possible. An ideal therapeutic regimen would allow for the elimination of the drug altogether. Chronic use is associated with painful osteoporosis, avascular necrosis of joints, fragile skin that is easily traumatized, poor wound healing, susceptibility to skin cancers, steroid-induced acne, and problems with obesity. Eliminating these side effects would enhance the quality of life for many recipients.

Cyclosporine. Graft survival has improved dramatically since the introduction of cyclosporine. Its primary action seems to be inhibition of cytotoxic T cell generation.[23-25] It also interferes with the secretion of interleukins by helper T cells and the ability of cytotoxic T cells to respond to interleukins. Interleukin secretion by macrophages also is impaired. Because cyclosporine is specifically targeted for T cells, the patient's immune system is not totally impaired and some ability to protect the body from infection is preserved. T cells play a major role in providing protection from viral infections; thus cyclosporine's interference with T cell function prevents full immunologic competence against viral infection.[26]

Three preparations of cyclosporine are available. The first preparation to arrive on the market was Sandimmune (Novartis), followed by Neoral (Novartis). Neoral has demonstrated greater bioavailability and drug exposure when compared with Sandimmune, with no significantly greater adverse events.[27,28] Neoral is also associated with a decreased incidence of cytomegalic virus infection related to a decreased need to use supplemental antilymphocyte therapy as compared with Sandimmune after 1 year of therapy.[29] However, Neoral and Sandimmune are not bioequivalent and cannot be used interchangeably. Gengraf (Abbott Laboratories) is the latest form of cyclosporine to be introduced to the market. Unlike Sandimmune, Gengraf is bioequivalent to Neoral and since it is a generic formulation of cyclosporine, is also less costly. Gengraf is also generally better tolerated by patients who report that it is easier to swallow, tastes better, and has less impact on breath and body odor.[30]

Tacrolimus. Tacrolimus (Prograf, FK506) was first approved for use in clinical trials for liver transplant recipients in February 1989.[31] The immunologic action of tacrolimus is mediated through the inhibition of a specific type of interleukin release (interleukin-2).[32] Tacrolimus has been shown to have fewer side effects than cyclosporine and is used in place of cyclosporine in the immunosuppressive regimen of some transplant programs. Tacrolimus does not appear to be as nephrotoxic as cyclosporine, nor does it cause hypertension. Another benefit of tacrolimus is that unlike cyclosporine, it does not cause hypertrichosis, gingival hyperplasia, or facial dysmorphism.[32] In addition, patients receiving tacrolimus tend to require lower doses of azathioprine or mycophe-

nolate mofetil and corticosteroids long-term, factors that may improve the quality of life for transplant recipients. Unfortunately, tacrolimus is not free of side effects including nausea and vomiting.[32] These side effects are encountered most often with intravenous administration. Hyperkalemia associated with low aldosterone and renin levels has been reported and may require treatment with potassium-restricted diets. Other adverse effects of tacrolimus include neurotoxicity and glucose intolerance. When transitioning a patient from cyclosporine to tacrolimus, the cyclosporine should be discontinued for at least 24 hours before the administration of tacrolimus to prevent synergistic side effects including hypertension and body rash.[32] The dose is then adjusted according to the patient's liver chemistry findings, blood levels, and tolerance to the medication.

Azathioprine. Azathioprine (Imuran) is an antimetabolite that interferes with the purine synthesis necessary for the production of antibodies. Purine synthesis is also necessary for the synthesis of nucleic acids in rapidly proliferating cells, such as the cells of the immune system. Azathioprine is used as a maintenance drug to prevent the activation and rapid proliferation of T cells responding to an antigen. A common adverse effect is the suppression of other rapidly proliferating cells, resulting in leukopenia, thrombocytopenia, and anemia. The dose of the drug is adjusted to keep the white blood cell (WBC) count between 3000 and 5000 cells/mm^3, thus protecting the patient from an increased risk of infection. The actual minimum acceptable WBC count varies with institutional preferences and type of organ transplant.

Mycophenolate Mofetil. Mycophenolate mofetil (CellCept) is a derivative of mycophenolic acid. Mycophenolic acid is a fermentation product of several *Penicillium* species.[33] Mycophenolate mofetil inhibits inosine monophosphate dehydrogenase, which is a key enzyme in the *de novo* pathway of purine synthesis.[33,34] Therefore it is a potent inhibitor of the proliferative responses of T and B lymphocytes.[33] This inhibition also disrupts antibody formation and the generation of cytotoxic T cells. It effectively suppresses both cellular-mediated and humoral-mediated immunity. The mechanism of action is similar to that of azathioprine except that mycophenolate mofetil selectively inhibits T and B cells. Global bone marrow suppression is not seen with mycophenolate mofetil.[35] Clinical immunosuppression can thus be obtained without increased susceptibility to bacterial and fungal infections.[33]

In both animal studies and clinical trials, long-term heart transplant recipients had a lower incidence and severity of the proliferative arteriopathy seen with chronic rejection.[33,36,37] The drug may have an effect in reducing mechanisms that are thought to participate in the smooth muscle cell proliferation that causes concentric intimal thickening, resulting in obliterative arteriopathy of transplanted organs. Doses vary from 100 mg/day to 3500 mg/day, administered orally in conjunction with cyclosporine and corticosteroids.[33] Responses to the drug are dose-dependent. Preliminary data suggest that the fewest episodes of rejection occur in patients receiving doses of at least 200 mg/day. Doses of greater than 2000 mg/day are considered rescue doses. Side effects consist mainly of gastrointestinal symptoms such as nausea, vomiting, and diarrhea.[33,35] Ileus and gastritis are less common.[33,35] If the drug becomes intolerable because of side effects, the dose can be adjusted.

Many centers are now substituting azathioprine with mycophenolate mofetil to avoid the leukopenia, thrombocytopenia, and anemia associated with the bone marrow suppression that can occur with azathioprine. Mycophenolate mofetil has been shown to offer better protection against death from rejection, infection, and cardiovascular events in one large multicenter trial involving 26 centers and 650 patients.[38] Another study found lower levels of C-reactive protein, a marker of inflammation, in patients receiving mycophenolate mofetil compared to patients receiving azathioprine.[39] Elevated levels of C-reactive protein or CRP have been associated with cardiac allograft vasculopathy.[39,40] Furthermore, continuous therapy with mycophenolate mofetil has also been associated with protective effects against declining renal function and even improved renal function in kidney transplant recipients.[41]

Sirolimus. Sirolimus (Rapamycin, Rapamune) is a relatively new immunosuppressive agent that is also a macrolide antibiotic known for its powerful antifungal properties. Whereas cyclosporine and tacrolimus inhibit cytokine production, the mechanism of action of sirolimus is to block the effect of cytokines on the proliferation of lymphoid cells (T and B lymphocytes) by inhibiting a protein (mTOR) essential for cytokine-driven T cell proliferation.[42-44] Several large clinical trials of sirolimus in renal transplant recipients found fewer incidences of rejection in patients who received sirolimus compared to those who received azathioprine or placebo.[42] Studies have also shown that heart transplant recipients treated with sirolimus not only have lower rates of rejection but fewer episodes of rejection, all without increased rates of infection.[44]

Sirolimus also inhibits the proliferation of nonlymphoid cells like endothelial and smooth muscle cells, as well as fibroblasts.[44] The inhibition of these cells is especially promising in the prevention of allograft vasculopathy, a form of chronic rejection that will be discussed later in the chapter. Studies are beginning to show that sirolimus slows the progression of graft vasculopathy in heart transplant recipients.[45,46] Unfortunately, the fibroblasts and endothelial cells which are inhibited by sirolimus are also the cell types responsible for wound healing. Anecdotal reports and small studies are beginning to surface that report prolonged wound healing in transplant recipients receiving sirolimus. Other primary side effects of the drug include hyperlipidemia and myelosuppression.[47,48] Most of the myelosuppressive effect is directed at platelets, and severe thrombocytopenias can result, making it necessary to discontinue the drug.

Although dosages vary between institutions, several administer a loading dose followed by a maintenance dose to achieve serum levels between 5 to 15 nanograms per milliliter (ng/ml). Due to its prolonged half-life, sirolimus is only administered daily. Sirolimus also has been shown to have synergistic effects when combined with cyclosporine and tacrolimus, which can result in a lower dose requirement for these drugs. Because both cyclosporine and tacrolimus can be nephrotoxic, lower doses of the two medications can be advantageous.[43,47] A new form of sirolimus called *everolimus* is currently undergoing clinical trials. Everolimus is an analog of sirolimus with greater bioavailability and shorter half-life.[46,49]

INDUCTION THERAPY

Induction therapy involves the intraoperative and/or postoperative use of an immunosuppressive agent for a limited period of time. The purpose of induction therapy is to induce tolerance to the transplanted graft. It is used by some, but not all, transplant centers, since there is ongoing debate regarding the need for and effectiveness of induction therapy.

Antilymphocyte Preparations. Muromonab-CD3 (Orthoclone OKT3) was one of the first drugs introduced to target distinct subpopulations of T cells. The drug is a monoclonal antibody produced in mice to specifically target cells with the T3 surface antigen found on mature T cells. Orthoclone OKT3 removes these cells from circulation by forming antibody-antigen complexes. Orthoclone OKT3 also interferes with T cell recognition of foreign antigen, which renders the T cells incapable of responding.[24,35] The drug is used as induction therapy by some centers to eliminate T cell response for the first 2 weeks after transplantation. Other centers use it to treat and reverse a severe rejection episode. Because the drug is an animal protein, antibodies against it develop in some patients. For that reason, it cannot be used repeatedly in patients with sensitivity. Its initial adverse effects seem to be caused by the massive destruction of T cells, resulting in fever, general malaise, and rigors.[35] Reactions usually subside with subsequent doses. As the T cell population declines, the severity of the reaction diminishes. Orthoclone OKT3 usually is administered for 5 to 7 days and then stopped. The severity of reactions can be minimized with pretreatment of patients with acetaminophen and diphenhydramine for the initial doses. In addition, 50 mg of hydrocortisone is often given with the first dose of Orthoclone OKT3. A greater concern regarding the use of Orthoclone OKT3 is the increased incidence of lymphoma in patients who have received the drug.[22,50] Incidence varies from center to center, probably related to the length of therapy in any given protocol. It is expected that many newer, more specific, safer monoclonal antibodies will progress from laboratory testing to clinical settings.[51]

Antithymocyte Preparations. Antithymocyte preparations are made by injecting human thymocytes into an animal, usually a horse, rabbit, or goat. The animal produces antibody in response to the foreign human antigen. Antibody to human thymocytes can then be extracted from the serum of the animal. The same process can be used to obtain antilymphocyte preparations. Antibody preparations are made with serum or globulin. If globulin is produced, globulin molecules are extracted from the animal serum.[26] Many centers make their own preparations. A few preparations are commercially available, and they are made from horse and rabbit serum. Depending on the protocol of the institution and the type of organ transplant, antithymocyte or antilymphocyte preparations may be given as part of the induction therapy or may be used only to treat rejection. The duration of therapy is typically around 7 days but may be shorter or longer, depending on institutional preference. Administration of the drug depletes circulating T cells and reduces the proliferative function of the T cells. As with Orthoclone OKT3, patients are subject to reactions from the release of pyrogens during the massive T cell lysis, as well as to the foreign animal protein contained in the preparation.

Antilymphocyte and antithymocyte preparations are referred to as *cytolytic drugs.* Use of cytolytic drugs has been associated with an increased incidence of malignancy.[22,50] This increased incidence is most likely caused by the suppression of cytotoxic T cells, which play an important role in identifying and eliminating cancer cells. For that reason, many centers use these drugs only to reverse rejections that are unresponsive to conventional treatment with increased corticosteroids. However, a short 3-day course of antihuman thymocyte immunoglobulin has been successfully used for induction therapy, with a demonstrated lower rate of early rejection and an absence of a long-term cancer-promoting effect at 5 and 10 years of follow-up.[51]

Interleukin-2 Receptor Antagonists. There are currently two preparations of interleukin-2 receptor antagonist (IL-2Ra), daclizumab and basiliximab. Both are monoclonal antibodies; however, basiliximab is a combination of human and murine antibodies while daclizumab is 90% human.[52] IL-2Ra are antibodies to a receptor found on activated T lymphocytes. As discussed earlier, IL-2 mediates the activation of T-lymphocytes. IL-2Ra competitively antagonizes the IL-2–mediated activation of the T-lymphocytes.[53] Data from the kidney transplant studies have shown that patients who received daclizumab for induction therapy had the small-

est risk of posttransplant lymphoproliferative disease (PTLD) when compared to antithymocyte and antilymphocyte induction agents.[54] However, long-term studies on the impact of interleukin-2 receptor antagonists on posttransplant malignancies have yet to be released. IL-2Ra are generally better tolerated than other induction agents with fewer incidences of fever, leukopenia, thrombocytopenia, and other adverse reactions.[53]

HEART TRANSPLANTATION

The first human heart transplantation was performed at the University of Capetown in 1967 by Christian Barnard, with the patient surviving 18 days. In 1968 Shumway and colleagues performed the first transplant in the United States at Stanford University.[55] Heart transplant procedures grew dramatically in number for the first few years and then rapidly declined because of poor results. It was not until 1972 to 1974 that clinical survival improved and interest regenerated. The development of the endomyocardial biopsy in 1972 was a major milestone in the detection of allograft rejection. In addition, the introduction of T cell–specific agents, such as rabbit antithymocyte globulin, and the ability of laboratories to measure specific T cells (rosette counts) contributed to an increase in 1-year survival by approximately 20% of patients.[55] In 1981 the immunosuppressive drug *cyclosporine* was introduced in the clinical setting, improving survival by about 20% at 1 year. Once again the number of transplant procedures grew rapidly.[55]

INDICATIONS AND SELECTION

The general candidate criterion for heart transplantation is a life expectancy of only 6 to 12 months because of end-stage cardiac disease.[55] Common causes of such conditions are cardiomyopathy of various origins (idiopathic, viral, valvular) and coronary artery disease.[56] Other, less common etiologic factors include severe heart failure resulting from chemotherapy, radiation treatment, myocardial tumor, and complex congenital defects. Many centers grade the severity of heart failure by the New York Heart Association (NYHA) functional classification (Box 41-8), which is based on the amount of exertion required to cause symptoms. Although most patients fall into the category of NYHA class IV, the condition of some is graded class III because of recent recompensation.[56] The anticipated length of hospital stay is 13 days.

In addition to satisfying medical criteria, patients generally are evaluated for the presence of familial or social support; absence of chemical dependence; and commitment to adhering to a strict, lifelong medical regimen and follow-up.

Specific contraindications to cardiac transplantation are listed in Box 41-9. The age range in heart transplanta-

Box 41-8

NEW YORK HEART ASSOCIATION PHYSICAL MANIFESTATIONS OF HEART DISEASE

CLASS	PHYSICAL MANIFESTATION
I	No limitation of physical activity; no dyspnea, fatigue, or palpitations with ordinary activity.
II	Slight limitation of physical activity; patients have fatigue, palpitations, and dyspnea with ordinary physical activity but are comfortable at rest.
III	Marked limitation of activity; less than ordinary physical activity results in symptoms, but patients are comfortable at rest.
IV	Symptoms are present at rest, and any physical exertion exacerbates the symptoms.

Box 41-9

HEART TRANSPLANTATION CONTRAINDICATIONS

- Advanced age
- Significant systemic or multisystem disease
- Fixed severe pulmonary hypertension
- Active infection
- Recent pulmonary infarction
- Cachexia or obesity
- Psychiatric illness
- Drug or alcohol abuse

tion is from the neonatal period to approximately 65 years; upper age limits vary among transplant institutions. Preexisting malignancy has been an absolute contraindication because of the potential for recurring cancer or development of second cancers as a result of therapeutic immunosuppression. Some centers, however, consider cured, nonmetastatic malignancies as a relative contraindication.[57-59] Severe liver and kidney dysfunctions that are not reversible by an increase in cardiac output are contraindications for transplantation.[56] Diabetes mellitus (DM) was once an absolute contraindication because steroid administration can cause exacerbation of the condition. However, with good medical management, hyperglycemia can be controlled.

It also was believed that persons with diabetes would incur an increased risk for infectious complications. Currently, however, DM is considered a relative contraindication if the hyperglycemia is adequately treated, because it has been demonstrated that the early survival rates of patients with DM are equal to those without DM.[61-64] If patients have active infections, transplantation is delayed until the infections are cleared. Recent pulmonary infarctions increase the risk for postoperative infection and complicate oxygenation and ventila-

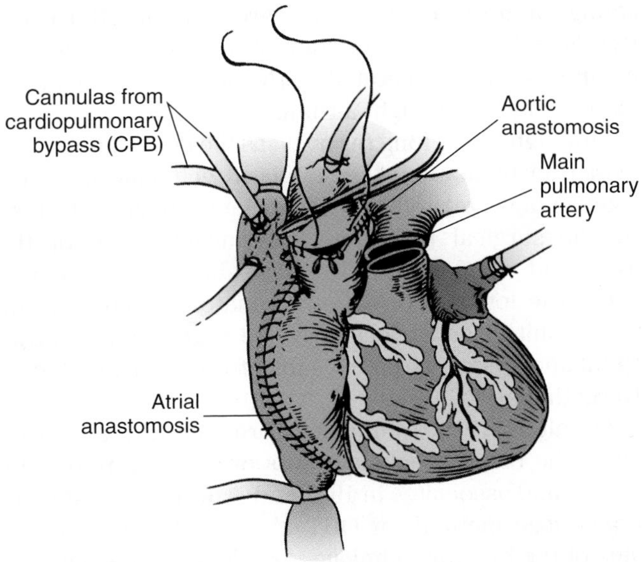

Fig. 41-6 Heart transplantation: surgical procedure. (Modified from Hurst JW et al: *The heart,* ed 7, New York, 1990, Mc-Graw-Hill.)

tion. Thus a recent history of infarction often precludes transplantation.

The active waiting list is prioritized by acuity, length of time on the list, ABO blood group, and weight. Distribution of organs is regulated by a regional, state, and national network organized and managed by UNOS, contracted by the federal government.[3] Acuity is determined by a patient's need for inotropic support or mechanical assist devices. Patients requiring this degree of assistance are listed as *status 1A* or *1B.* All other heart transplant candidates are listed as *status 2.*

HEART TRANSPLANT SURGICAL PROCEDURE

The standard surgical procedure for orthotopic heart transplantation (OHT) was originally developed by Lower and Shumway in 1960.[62] A standard median sternotomy is used, the great vessels are cannulated, and cardiopulmonary bypass (CPB) is instituted after anticoagulation and standard hypothermic technique. The donor heart is prepared by interconnecting the pulmonary veins to form a single left atrial cuff and by trimming the aorta and pulmonary artery to fit the recipient's anatomy. All of the recipient's heart is removed except the posterior walls of the atria that contain the orifices of the pulmonary veins and vena cava. Four major anastomoses are performed between the donor heart and recipient's native atrial remnant including those of the right and left atria, the aorta, and the pulmonary artery, in that order (Fig. 41-6).[63] The native atrial remnant remains innervated by the parasympathetic and sympathetic nerve fibers from the autonomic nervous system (ANS). The donor heart, however, is now denervated, resulting in a faster resting heart rate of 90 to 100 beats/min. The rate of the transplanted heart is the normal intrinsic rate generated by the donor sinoatrial (SA) node located in the right atrium.

Although it was long regarded as the gold standard for heart transplantation, the standard technique did have disadvantages related to anatomic abnormalities following the surgical procedure. The anastomosis of the donor and recipient atria left large abnormal atrial cavities.[64] The loss of normal atrial anatomy increases the risk of mitral and tricuspid valve regurgitation, atrial septal aneurysms, atrial thrombus formation, and tachy-dysrhythmias.[65,66]

An alternative to the standard surgical approach called the bicaval technique was originally reported by Sievers and associates in 1991 and is now the most commonly used method for OHT.[63,67] The five anastomotic sites of the bicaval technique include the left atrial cuff, which contains the pulmonary veins, superior and inferior vena cava, aorta, and the main pulmonary artery. This technique leaves the recipient with more anatomically normal atria. Benefits of the bicaval technique include preserved sinoatrial node function with decreased incidence of atrial dysrhythmias, and decreased incidences of mitral and tricuspid regurgitation.[68,69] Though fairly rare, superior vena caval stenosis is a complication that has been reported in the literature.[68]

POSTOPERATIVE MEDICAL AND NURSING MANAGEMENT

Immediate postoperative management of the transplant recipient is similar to that of patients undergoing other heart surgery procedures. Nursing care of the transplant recipient involves several nursing diagnoses, as listed in the Nursing Diagnoses feature on Heart Transplantation. The most frequently used diagnosis is Decreased Cardiac Output (CO). Possible causes for a decrease in CO are dysrhythmia, hypothermia, myocardial depression, tamponade, and rejection.

Variables that influence myocardial performance include prolonged ischemic times (time from excision of heart from the donor to removal of the aortic cross-clamp after the implant to the recipient); reperfusion injury; and hypothermia. Dysrhythmias may occur as a result of myocardial irritation, local ischemia, edema around the atrial suture line, and disruption of the SA nodal blood supply.[70]

An electrocardiogram abnormality unique to the transplanted heart is the presence of a second P wave, generated by the native SA node left in the atrial cuff. Because this impulse does not cross the suture line, it is capable of conducting only through the remnant of the native recipient atria. However, this is not seen in hearts transplanted using the bicaval technique since the native right atrium and therefore the SA node is removed.

NURSING DIAGNOSES   Heart Transplantation

- Decreased Cardiac Output related to alterations in preload
- Decreased Cardiac Output related to alterations in afterload
- Decreased Cardiac Output related to alterations in heart rate
- Risk for Infection risk factor: immunosuppressive drugs required to prevent rejection of transplanted organ
- Disturbed Body Image related to actual change in body structure, function, or appearance
- Anxiety related to threat to biologic, psychologic, and/or social integrity
- Readiness for Enhanced Knowledge: Posttransplant Self-Care Regimen, immunosuppressive drugs, cardiac drugs, diuretics, and clinical manifestations of infection.

Isoproterenol, a powerful β-adrenergic antagonist, is sometimes used in the postoperative period for chronotropic (heart rate) support. Its chronotropic and vasodilator properties effectively sustain heart rate, increase CO, and decrease pulmonary vascular resistance (PVR). PVR may be increased as a result of preexisting left ventricular failure and may be a cause of transient right ventricular dysfunction in the newly transplanted heart. Dopamine and epinephrine are often used for inotropic support in the postoperative period. However, the use of inotropic and chronotropic drugs are highly individualized based on institutional preference. Generally speaking, inotropic drugs are gradually discontinued over 24 to 48 hours as tolerated by the patient, and the need for isoproterenol decreases as the heart begins to maintain its normal intrinsic rate of 100 beats/min. Temporary pacing is required only occasionally, and fewer than 10% of transplant patients require a permanent pacemaker implant.[70]

Cardiac tamponade generally does not occur with greater frequency in transplantation than it does in other cardiac surgeries, but it may occur insidiously as a result of an enlarged pericardial sac from longstanding cardiomyopathy.[71] Patients who have had chronic right ventricular failure, subsequent liver enlargement, and abnormal coagulation studies may benefit from preoperative administration of fresh plasma or fresh-frozen plasma (FFP). Plasma contains most clotting factors and is indicated for liver dysfunction. Administration of plasma may decrease the risk of bleeding and tamponade.

Box 41-10

STANDARDIZED CARDIAC BIOPSY GRADING

GRADE	NOMENCLATURE
0	No evidence of acute rejection (NER)
1A	Focal, mild acute rejection (AR)
1B	Diffuse, mild AR
2	Focal, moderate AR
3A	Multifocal aggressive, low moderate AR
3B	Diffuse borderline, severe AR
4	Diffuse aggressive, severe AR

Rejection Surveillance. Rejection is the most common etiologic factor responsible for causing low CO for the first 3 months after transplantation.[71] Hyperacute rejection occurs only in the immediate postoperative period. It is a rare complication that necessitates retransplantation for survival. Acute rejection occurs most often in the first 3 to 6 months after transplantation.

Diagnosis of rejection is determined by endomyocardial biopsy. Biopsy specimens are obtained by inserting a bioptome percutaneously through the right internal jugular vein, and advancing it through the right atrium to the right ventricle with the aid of fluoroscopy or echocardiography. Four to five samples of myocardial tissue are obtained from the interventricular septum. The samples are microscopically evaluated for interstitial and perivascular infiltration. Cardiac biopsies are graded according to the severity of the interstitial infiltration of lymphocytes. This standardized cardiac biopsy grading scale ranges from 0 to 4 (Box 41-10).[72]

Surveillance for rejection is generally performed weekly for the first 4 to 6 weeks. The frequency of surveillance biopsies gradually decreases relative to the patient's rejection history and by institutional preference. A major but rare complication of biopsy is ventricular perforation, resulting in cardiac tamponade. This emergency situation may require open heart surgical repair. Pneumothorax may result from the perforation of the visceral pleura during cannulation of the jugular vein. Clinical manifestations are a sudden onset of sharp pain in the affected side and dyspnea. Many institutions require transplant patients to undergo biopsy monitoring for the rest of their lives.

Treatment of acute rejection episodes may require intravenously administered methylprednisolone (Solu-Medrol). Management of recurrent rejection is treated with various pharmacologic agents, depending on the clinical picture and institution. Strategies include augmenting current maintenance immunosuppression or switching to alternatives such as tacrolimus, mycophenolate mofetil, or Rapamycin. Orthoclone OKT3, a monoclonal antibody, is used for recurrent rejection. It is used also as an induction immunosuppressive agent for the first 7 to 14 days after surgery. If Orthoclone OKT3 is being used for a second time, the patient must be tested for the presence of antibodies. Antibodies may contraindicate use of Orthoclone OKT3. Other agents used for recurrent rejection are polyclonal antibodies, such as antilymphocyte globulin (ALG) or antithymocyte globulin (ATG).

Salvage therapy for persistent rejection that has not responded to conventional immunosuppression, multiple steroid boluses, or anti–T cell antibodies consists of total lymphoid irradiation (TLI). Low-dose ionizing radiation is used to treat the lymphoid tissue. Areas exposed to radiation are the axilla, the sternum, the clavicle, the para-aorta, the ilium, the inguinofemoral lymph nodes, and the spleen.[73]

Infection Surveillance. Infection surveillance is a high priority for the immunocompromised person. It is well known that immunosuppression predisposes the patient to infection by a multitude of opportunistic pathogens, which cannot easily be prevented with infection control. Development of infection is encountered most often in the early postoperative period when immunosuppression is maximized. Infection is the leading cause of death during this period (up to 2 years after surgery).[74] Great care must be taken to use aseptic technique for all intravenous line and dressing changes. Centers differ widely in protective practices regarding the transplant recipient. Some use reverse isolation, whereas others put transplant recipients in rooms with other patients and simply use Standard Precautions.

Development of fever is aggressively investigated, with systematic blood, wound, and respiratory tract cultures, chest x-ray films, and observation. Because steroids are known to suppress the body's inflammatory reaction, a temperature generally is considered significant at 38° C (100.4° F). Nurses must be suspicious of any new productive cough, dry cough, change in type of secretions, or change in chest roentgenogram findings.

Cytomegalovirus (CMV) is a particular threat to transplant recipients. CMV is a herpes virus that can produce latent infection that persists throughout life; approximately 50% of the general population is infected. The virus can be transmitted through organ and blood product donation; thus the transplantation from a CMV-seropositive donor to a CMV-seronegative recipient poses the highest risk to the recipient for acquiring a primary infection. An antiviral agent, ganciclovir, can inhibit viral replication and ameliorate symptoms and thus is used in the prophylaxis and treatment of CMV infections.[75,76] In addition, CMV immune globulin (CMVIG) is being used increasingly for the prevention of primary CMV disease and for treatment of CMV disease.[77-79]

PATIENT EDUCATION

As with all transplant patients, postoperative care includes educating the patient regarding compliance and record keeping. Education is provided on the immunosuppressive medication regimen, risks and signs and symptoms of infection, myocardial biopsy, and symptoms of heart failure. Patients may be required to check their blood glucose, blood pressure, and daily weight at home. At first, frequent clinic visits are needed to monitor progress and adjust medications. As the patient progresses, a schedule is established for routine laboratory tests and clinic visits to ensure long-term success of the transplant.

LONG-TERM CONSIDERATIONS

Chronic immunosuppression results in significant morbidity. Steroid administration can result in osteoporosis, avascular necrosis of joints, fragile skin, and obesity. Cyclosporine can induce renal insufficiency, excessive hair growth, gingival hyperplasia, tremor, and hypertension that necessitate pharmacologic control. Azathioprine can be hepatotoxic. Concomitant use of these immunosuppressants also leaves patients more susceptible to malignancies and late infections as listed in the Pharmacologic Management Table on Organ Transplantation.

Graft vasculopathy, or coronary artery disease in the transplanted heart, is a major cause of late morbidity and mortality.[80] Graft vasculopathy is a diffuse and rapidly progressive type of coronary artery disease that causes concentric narrowing of the coronary arteries. Because the lesions are not discrete, they are not amenable to angioplasty or bypass grafting.[80] The etiology of graft vasculopathy remains unclear, but chronic rejection likely plays a role.[81] Patients with denervated hearts usually cannot feel anginal pain, although recent literature reports evidence of reinnervation and subsequent chest pain.[82] More often, their symptoms are ischemic injury, heart failure, or sudden death. The disease is recognized initially by angiographic screening and, later in the course of the disease, by the presence of silent infarctions on electrocardiogram. Many patients may have the disease and demonstrate no clinical sequelae.[80] The only therapy for advanced graft vasculopathy is retransplantation.

In general, heart transplant recipients report being highly satisfied with their quality of life.[83-85] Fewer than 35% return to full-time employment, but many who are able to work cannot find suitable employment because of employers' concerns about liability, lack of health insurance, and the need to qualify for medical disability.[86,87]

In 2003, 2057 heart transplants were performed in the United States. On May 28, 2004 there were 3520 people registered on waiting lists to receive a heart transplant.[3] The number of heart transplants performed is greatly influenced by the limited donor pool. Current 1-year survival for heart transplant recipients, as reported by the UNOS Scientific Registry, is 85.1%.[3]

HEART-LUNG TRANSPLANTATION

Combined heart-lung transplantation research has been built on the foundation established by heart transplantation through years of laboratory investigation. Interest in the procedure gained momentum with the introduction of cyclosporine, because it permitted the delay of high-dose steroid therapy (whose use impaired bronchial healing and favored early postoperative infections). In 1981 at Stanford University, Reitz and colleagues performed the first heart-lung transplant resulting in long-term survival; the patient lived for more than 5 years.[55]

Heart-lung transplantation, now in its third decade, currently is the therapy of choice for some cardiac and cardiopulmonary diseases. Research and laboratory investigations continue in the development of new immunosuppressants, preservation solutions, and techniques. Recent advances have led to single-lung and double-lung transplantation, lobar lung transplantation, and single-lung transplantation with cardiac repair.

INDICATIONS AND SELECTION

Heart-lung transplantation (HLT) is an established treatment for selected patients with irreversible, progressively disabling end-stage cardiopulmonary and pulmonary disease.[88-90] Transplantation is usually offered to patients as an option when life expectancy is limited to 15 to 24 months.[88,89] Patients are evaluated and listed earlier than are heart transplant recipients because of the paucity of heart-lung donors and the inevitably long wait for transplantation.

Specific etiologic factors in pulmonary disease can be grouped according to the type of lung abnormality. Categories are pulmonary vascular disease, obstructive lung disease, and restrictive lung disease.[88,89] Box 41-11 lists indications for heart-lung transplantation. Optional lung transplantation, such as single- or bilateral- or double-lung transplantation are discussed in a later section.

HLT is the operation of choice for patients whose pulmonary disease process has irreversibly disabled the heart. HLT is considered the preferential procedure because transplantation of the entire heart-lung block eliminates having to separate the pulmonary artery and veins, avoiding subsequent reanastomoses and thus decreasing bleeding complications. However, in the case of disease processes in which the heart is judged to be only temporarily dysfunctional and can be expected to regain adequate function after the transplantation of a healthy lung or lungs, the native heart may be left in place,[89,90] and a single- or double-lung transplant performed. Another option is to transplant the heart-lung block into such an individual and then donate the native heart to another recipient, which is referred to as the *domino procedure.*[91]

The evaluation of HLT candidates is similar to that for heart transplant recipients with respect to patient com-

Box 41-11

SINGLE-LUNG, DOUBLE-LUNG, AND HEART-LUNG TRANSPLANTATION INDICATIONS

PULMONARY VASCULAR DISEASE
Primary pulmonary hypertension
Pulmonary hypertension due to secondary thromboembolic disease
Eisenmenger's syndrome
Cardiomyopathy with pulmonary hypertension

OBSTRUCTIVE LUNG DISEASE
Emphysema
Alpha-1 antitrypsin deficiency
Cystic fibrosis
Bronchiectasis
Bronchopulmonary dysplasia
Idiopathic or posttransplant obliterative bronchiolitis
Lymphangioleiomyomatosis

RESTRICTIVE LUNG DISEASE
Idiopathic pulmonary fibrosis
Sarcoidosis
Asbestosis
Histiocytosis X
BOOP: bronchiolitis obliterans organizing pneumonia
Desquamative interstitial pneumonitis

Box 41-12

SINGLE-LUNG, DOUBLE-LUNG, AND HEART-LUNG TRANSPLANTATION CONTRAINDICATIONS

ABSOLUTE CONTRAINDICATIONS
Significant systemic or multisystem disease
Active intrapulmonary or extrapulmonary infection
Cachexia or obesity
Current cigarette smoking
Psychiatric illness
Drug or alcohol abuse
Symptomatic osteoporosis
Severe chest wall deformity
Hepatitis B
Malignancy precluding long-term survival

RELATIVE CONTRAINDICATIONS
Corticosteroid therapy
Previous cardiothoracic surgery
Age (transplant program–specific)
Kidney disease
Liver disease
Previous cardiothoracic surgery

mitment to compliance with a strict, lifelong medical regimen. Contraindications to HLT are listed in Box 41-12. Systematic disease, active extrapulmonary infection, and other organ diseases are absolute contraindications. Cachexia and obesity are obstacles that can be eliminated by nutritional support and weight reduction.

Truncal obesity is especially undesirable because it significantly decreases diaphragmatic excursion, hinders postoperative mobilization, and may complicate recovery.[88] Preoperative use of corticosteroids has been implicated as a cause of tracheal and bronchial dehiscence in the early postoperative period.[88,89] Previous cardiothoracic surgery is a relative contraindication because of the risk of bleeding associated with the presence of pleural adhesions.[88] Removal of the native lung may precipitate pleural bleeding in the posterior pleural space, which can be particularly difficult to control because of location.[92]

HEART-LUNG TRANSPLANT SURGICAL PROCEDURE

Success of HLT depends in part on selection and procurement of suitable donor organs. The lungs are particularly difficult to procure because they are vulnerable to complications related to brain death. Prolonged mechanical ventilation is required, which increases the risk of infection. Any infection generally precludes donation. Neurogenic pulmonary edema also may damage the lungs, making their donation impossible. Lungs have a limited ischemic time of about 4 hours, which limits the geographic area for donor procurement.[92] Lung preservation has improved, and distant procurement with 2 to 3 hours transport time has increased the donor pool.[93]

Before the removal of the heart-lung block, alprostadil (prostaglandin E_1 [PGE_1]) is administered gradually until a systemic effect is achieved. PGE_1 is used to ensure complete pulmonary vasodilation for uniform cooling and distribution of pulmonoplegia.[93,94]

The operative procedure for the recipient is through a median sternotomy or a bilateral thoracosternotomy (clamshell) incision. The patient is heparinized and placed on cardiopulmonary bypass, and the heart is excised.[95] Care is used to ensure the preservation of the recipient's phrenic, vagus, and laryngeal nerves. The lungs are removed separately to decrease the risk of nerve damage. A left pneumonectomy is usually performed first since it is technically easier. The pulmonary artery, veins, and mainstem bronchus are isolated and excised in that order.[96] The donor heart and lungs are then implanted as a block. The heart is put into the orthotopic position and anastomosed to the native aorta and remnant recipient atria. The tracheal anastomosis in HLT is performed just above the level of the carina, as illustrated in Fig. 41-7.[94]

POSTOPERATIVE MEDICAL AND NURSING MANAGEMENT

Immediate postoperative care of the heart-lung transplant recipient is similar to that used for the heart transplant recipient. Several nursing diagnoses are associated with care of the heart-lung transplant recipient, as listed

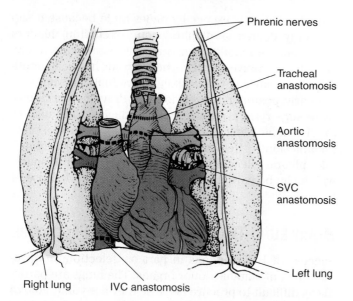

Fig. 41-7 Heart-lung transplantation: surgical procedure. *IVC,* Inferior vena cava; *SVC,* superior vena cava. (Modified from Reitz BA et al: Heart and lung transplantation, *J Thorac Cardiovasc Surg* 80(3):360, 1980.)

in the Nursing Diagnoses feature on Heart-Lung Transplantation. The most common complication is bleeding. Patients who have been cyanotic often have large bronchial vessels that cross behind the trachea and tend to be a source of bleeding. Control of bleeding at this site is difficult because of the location. Patients who have had previous thoracic surgery require more surgical dissection because of scarring and therefore achieve hemostasis with more difficulty.

Careful monitoring of bleeding and maintenance of the patency and function of mediastinal and pleural chest tubes are essential. Bleeding of greater than 100 to 200 ml/hour for more than 3 hours with normal coagulation studies is cause for concern about a surgical bleed. If bleeding of this nature persists, reexploration of the chest usually is indicated. The transplanted lung is susceptible to fluid overload because of the disruption of pulmonary lymphatics and the increase in extravascular lung water that is common after lung transplantation.[89] Replacement of blood loss with crystalloid or colloid therapy must be used carefully to minimize the risk of fluid overload of the transplanted lungs and the development of acute lung injury (ALI) (see "ALI," Chapter 23).

Patients are maintained on mechanical ventilation to support oxygenation for 12 to 48 hours. At least 5 mm Hg of positive end-expiratory pressure (PEEP) is used routinely to prevent atelectasis. Endotracheal tube (ETT) placement is monitored by auscultation and chest x-ray evaluation. The ETT must be well secured and movement minimized to protect the tracheal anastomosis. In addition, suctioning must be gentle, and to avoid disrup-

tion of the suture line, the suction catheter is not advanced beyond the end of the tube. Small amounts of bloody secretions can be expected with suctioning, but overt hemoptysis can be a sign of dehiscence, which requires immediate attention. Patients are weaned from ventilatory support as soon as possible. The longer the period of intubation, the higher the risk of pneumonia.[89] After extubation, patients are encouraged to cough, deep-breathe, and ambulate at the bedside.

Pharmacologic support is similar to that used for heart transplantation. Isoproterenol is given to augment heart rate, and dopamine is used for inotropic support and renal vasodilation. Additional inotropic support is achieved with epinephrine if necessary. PGE_1 is administered primarily for pulmonary vasodilation, and sodium nitroprusside is given for its systemic vasodilative properties (see "Vasodilators Drugs," p. 558).

Immunosuppression. Initial immunosuppression usually does not include the use of methylprednisolone for the HLT recipient. A single dose of methylprednisolone is usually given in the operating room, and maintenance dosing begins within the first 2 weeks. The use of methylprednisolone in the immediate postoperative period varies with institution. Daily steroid use is

Table 41-7	Standardized Pulmonary Biopsy Grading
Nomenclature	**Grade**
A. Acute rejection	0 - none 1 - minimal 2 - mild 3 - moderate 4 - severe
B. Airway inflammation—lymphocytic bronchitis/bronchiolitis	0 - none 1 - minimal 2 - mild 3 - moderate 4 - severe X - ungradable
C. Chronic airway rejection—bronchiolitis obliterans	a. active b. inactive
D. Chronic vascular rejection-accelerated graft vascular sclerosis	

Adapted from Yousem SA et al: Revision of the working formulation for the classification of pulmonary allograft rejection: Lung Rejection Study Group, *J Heart Lung Transplant* 15:1, 1996.

generally avoided for the first 2 weeks because of the deleterious effects on wound healing, in this case of the tracheal anastomosis.

Infection Surveillance. Surveillance for infection and rejection in the HLT recipient is accomplished by bronchoscopy. This is performed initially at clinically determined or set intervals to monitor the tracheal anastomosis for evidence of healing, to obtain bronchoalveolar lavage washings for appropriate cultures, and to take biopsy specimens for the diagnosis of rejection. Bronchoscopic examination provides visual evidence of tracheal anastomosis healing, which can determine the introduction of maintenance corticosteroids to the immunosuppressive regimen.[97]

As in the heart transplant recipient, presence of fever is an indication for aggressive evaluation. Serial chest x-ray films are used to monitor for infiltrate. However, it is difficult to distinguish infection from rejection by means of chest x-ray films. Radiographic changes are used with other clinical evidence, including the partial pressure of oxygen (PaO_2) level, O_2 saturation, presence or absence of fever, and culture reports, to determine the course of action. Documented infections are treated with appropriate antibiotics.

Rejection Surveillance. Rejection, which can be definitively diagnosed only by transbronchial biopsy, is graded by histologic findings of acute and chronic lung rejection (Table 41-7).[98] Procedural complications after bronchoscopic examination are a transient fever, fall in the PaO_2 level, infection, and pneumothorax. Chest x-ray examination must follow each bronchoscopy to rule out pneumothorax.

Pulmonary rejection is treated either by augmentation of maintenance immunosuppression, pulses of intravenously administered corticosteroid, or switching to alternative immunosuppressants. Augmentation may be in the form of increasing the cyclosporine or tacrolimus dose to achieve a higher drug level, and/or increasing azathioprine or mycophenolate mofetil, and/or increasing the maintenance prednisone dose. Pulsing is the method of administering large doses of corticosteroids over a relatively short period of time. A common pulse of steroid is 1 g of Solu-Medrol every day for 3 consecutive days. Quick resolution of radiographic changes after the administration of steroid pulses provides a retrospective confirmation of the diagnosis of rejection. Monoclonal and polyclonal antibodies also can be used to treat acute intractable rejection in similar fashion to the treatment of recurrent heart rejection.

Pulmonary function testing is a noninvasive method of assessing lung function and the presence of rejection. Lung denervation does not adversely affect the control of ventilation, at rest or during exercise.[99] Pulmonary function testing uses a wide range of parameters to measure the function of the lung at rest and during exercise. The functions are measured in percentages based on weight, gender, and age. The focus is usually on forced expiratory volume in 1 second (FEV_1), forced vital capacity (FVC), forced expiratory flow rate between 25% and 75% of FVC (FEF 25% to 75%), and the measurement of arterial blood gases. These functions are sensitive to slight changes in oxygenation and ventilation caused by infection or rejection. Acute changes in pulmonary function test (PFT) results and in PaO_2 are indications for transbronchial biopsy.[97]

Heart rejection occurs less often in the HLT recipient. Thus endomyocardial biopsy is performed less often;[100] when required, the procedure is similar to that in the heart transplant recipient.

PATIENT EDUCATION

It is important that patient education is provided to cover all aspects of the immunosuppressive medication regimen, signs and symptoms of infection, role of pulmonary function tests, myocardial biopsy, transbronchial biopsy and clinical signs of cardiac and pulmonary failure. In addition, a discussion of lifestyle adjustments, long-term considerations, and follow-up visits is always included.

LONG-TERM CONSIDERATIONS

Chronic immunosuppression in the HLT patient carries the same consequences as it does in the heart transplant recipient. Accelerated graft atherosclerosis can be a late complication in HLT patients and follows a course similar to that in the heart recipient. A major long-term complication in the pulmonary transplant patient is oblitera-

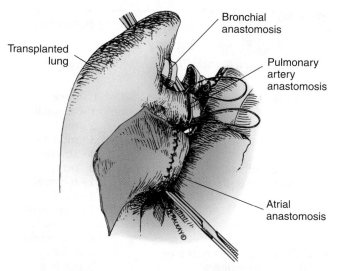

Fig. 41-8   Single-lung transplant: surgical procedure. (Modified from Baumgartner WA et al: *Heart and heart-lung transplantation,* ed 2, Philadelphia, 2002, Saunders.)

tive bronchiolitis (OB). Obliterative bronchiolitis is an inflammatory disorder of the small airways, which leads to obstruction and destruction of pulmonary bronchioles.[101] Features of obliterative bronchiolitis are listed in Box 41-13. OB may represent a manifestation of chronic pulmonary allograft rejection.[102] The only treatment for end-stage obliterative bronchiolitis is retransplantation. Retransplantation in the HLT group carries a high risk for complications related to infection, delayed healing as a result of steroids, renal insufficiency related to chronic cyclosporine use, and bleeding from scarring from the previous surgery.

CMV is also a significant threat to the lung transplant recipient. Prophylaxis and treatment of CMV disease are similar to those for heart recipients; however, institutions vary regarding the anti-CMV agents used and duration of prophylaxis and treatment.[75-78]

Heart-lung transplantation has increased annually for the past 10 years. Between 2002-2003, 62 heart-lung transplants were performed in the United States. The number of patients listed as candidates by UNOS in that same year was cited as 194.[3] The national 1-year survival rate for patients receiving HLT was 61.8%.[3] The limited donor pool remains the major factor limiting the number of heart-lung transplants performed.

SINGLE-LUNG AND DOUBLE-LUNG TRANSPLANTATIONS

SINGLE-LUNG TRANSPLANTS

Transplant teams have explored, modified, and successfully pursued the development of pulmonary transplantation, building upon the knowledge gained from heart-lung transplantation. Considerations in choosing lung transplantation include the specific disease process, the need for cardiac repair, and donor availability. Single-lung transplantation (SLT) is an alternative to HLT in a select group of patients. Generally speaking, SLT is most appropriate for patients with restrictive lung diseases such as idiopathic pulmonary fibrosis (IPF) and sarcoidosis or noninfectious obstructive lung diseases such as emphysema in the absence of significant cardiac dysfunction.

SINGLE-LUNG TRANSPLANT SURGICAL PROCEDURE

Transplantation contralateral (opposite side) to a previous thoracotomy is preferable in order to avoid adhesions that require further surgical dissection.[88] The left lung is sometimes preferred because it is easier to expose and has a longer left main bronchus. The longer bronchus gives the surgeon more flexibility in trimming the suture site as needed for anastomosis (Fig. 41-8).[103] If there is a significant disproportion of ventilation and perfusion to one side, transplantation of the worse side may be the preferred option.[89] With SLT the remaining native lung, which has either restrictive or obstructive pathophysiology, will have a higher vascular resistance than the transplanted lung. The blood flow is then automatically directed toward the new lung. Advantages to SLT are better use of donor resources, decreased operative risks, and decreased short-term and fewer long-term complications, as listed in Box 41-14. Contraindications to SLT are similar to those listed for the HLT candidate.

DOUBLE-LUNG OR BILATERAL-LUNG TRANSPLANTS

Pulmonary diseases that typically are associated with chronic lung infections, such as cystic fibrosis and bronchiectasis, require transplantation of both lungs because of the risk of cross-infection from the native lung into the transplanted lung.

DOUBLE LUNG TRANSPLANT SURGICAL PROCEDURE

Use of CPB is becoming less and less common during lung transplantation. However, patients with moderate to severe pulmonary hypertension generally require CPB because clamping of the pulmonary artery necessary for removal of the diseased lung may cause sudden right heart failure.[97] Inability to maintain adequate oxygenation and ventilation with a single lung, sudden increases in pulmonary artery pressure, poor right ventricular function, and hemodynamic compromise indicate the need for CPB.[104]

The surgical procedure for both single and double lung transplantation (DLT) is similar, with a few exceptions. In fact, a DLT is performed as a bilateral, sequential SLT. The surgical incision for an SLT can either be through an anteriolateral or posteriolateral thoracotomy at the level of the fourth or fifth intercostal space. A DLT is performed through bilateral anterior thoracosternotomies extending from the midaxillary line and across the sternum at the fourth intercostal space.[96] This approach is also known as a *clamshell incision*. The clamshell incision is exquisitely painful for the majority of patients, necessitating frequent pain assessment and intervention by the nurse. A median sternotomy or bilateral anterior thoracotomies are alternative surgical approaches.

The anastomotic sites for DLT include the back wall of the atria (containing the four pulmonary vein orifices), the bronchus, and the main pulmonary artery as illustrated in Fig. 41-9.[96] Donor and recipient arteries are trimmed to suitable lengths, and an end-to-end anastomosis is performed. Bronchial anastomosis is performed with a running suture. After the atrial clamp is slowly removed, the patient is assessed for bleeding.[89,103] In some transplant centers the omentum is brought through the diaphragm from the abdomen and is wrapped around the bronchus for added stability of the anastomosis and increased vascular supply. Disadvantages of this maneuver include a larger incision and involvement of the abdominal cavity.[89]

Lung Volume Reduction Surgery. Lung volume reduction is a surgical procedure that may be an option for lung transplant candidates. Although the procedure does not result in better lung function than does transplantation, it does avoid immunosuppression-related and transplant-related complications. It may be an early option for patients who may require lung transplant in the future.[103,105]

Living Donor Lung Transplantation. Another alternative to traditional lung transplantation is living donor lung transplantation. In living donor transplantation the lungs are harvested not from a brain-dead donor but from two living donors who provide either a right or left lower lobe to the recipient. The two donated lobes essentially function as new lungs. Recipients of this type of transplant tend to be patients with cystic fibrosis or other patients who are smaller in size. Smaller recipients increase the likelihood that two lobes are able to provide adequate pulmonary function.[106] Living donor lung transplantation is still fairly specialized and is therefore not as commonly practiced as cadaveric lung transplantation. Large studies comparing the risk and benefit as well as the rates of survival between traditional lung transplant versus living donor lung transplant have yet to be released.

POSTOPERATIVE MEDICAL AND NURSING MANAGEMENT

Postoperative care of single-lung and double-lung transplant recipients is similar to that for HLT patients, as described in the previous discussion. Several nursing diagnoses are associated with care of single-lung and double-lung transplant patients, as listed in the Nursing Diagnoses feature on Single-Lung and Double-Lung Transplantation. SLT patients generally require mechanical ventilation for a shorter duration. Less bleeding can be anticipated because of the brevity of the surgical procedure. A single pleural chest tube usually is sufficient for drainage. A pulmonary artery catheter may be used to measure right ventricular response when significant

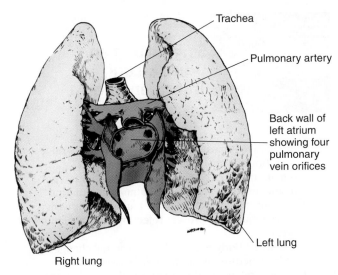

Fig. 41-9 Double-lung transplant graft before implantation into a recipient. (Modified from Baumgartner WA et al: *Heart and heart-lung transplantation*, ed 2, Philadelphia, 2002, Saunders.)

ventilation/perfusion (V/Q) mismatch occurs. In the event of elevated pulmonary artery pressures, pharmacologic vasodilation or afterload reduction can be instituted. Patients with pulmonary hypertension potentially may have a greater V/Q mismatch, resulting in larger A-aO_2 gradients.[103,105]

Immunosuppression for lung recipients is essentially the same as that for HLT patients. Initiation of steroids depends on institutional preference and healing of the bronchial anastomosis.

Surveillance of rejection and infection is similar to that in HLT. Pulmonary function testing is not initiated until the second or third week postoperatively to allow for surgical recovery.[107] Decreased lung function because of fluid shifts, microatelectasis, and splinting from incisional pain would interfere with accurate testing. Unlike HLT, in unilateral lung transplantation the transplanted lung functions in parallel with the native lung, which can be expected to retain any pathology.[108] The patient must be measured by a comparison with his or her own baseline and not with normal standards. This concept also can be applied to the immediate postoperative period of intubation during the evaluation of arterial blood gases. Oxygenation and ventilation occur in both the diseased and transplanted lungs, and parameters for evaluation need to be adjusted accordingly.

PATIENT EDUCATION

It is important that patient education is provided to cover all aspects of the immunosuppressive medication regimen, signs and symptoms of infection, role of pulmonary function tests, transbronchial biopsy, and clinical signs of pulmonary failure. In addition, a discussion of lifestyle adjustments, long-term considerations, and follow-up visits is included.

LONG-TERM CONSIDERATIONS

Clinically, SLT recipients function as well as other patients with only one lung. With physical exertion, some patients may complain of shortness of breath. A combination of chest roentgenogram, bronchoscopic examination, and pulmonary function testing is used in the detection and diagnosis of rejection and infection.

One-year survival between 1996 and 2001 was 76% for SLT and 78.3% for DLT.[3] The lack of donors is evident in the fact that there are currently 3915 people on the waiting list even though only 1085 lung transplants were performed in 2003.[3]

LIVER TRANSPLANTATION

Liver transplantation was first attempted in canine models in the 1950s. The outcomes were unsuccessful because of technical complications, infection, and graft failure.[109,110] The effort to improve surgical technique continued, and successful liver transplantation in dogs was achieved several years later by both Moore et al[111,112] and Starzl et al.[113] In 1963 Starzl and colleagues[114] performed the first human liver transplant operation. Although the patient died intraoperatively, this attempt pioneered the possibility of liver transplantation in human beings.

The first successful human liver transplant was performed in 1967, also by Starzl and his colleagues,[115] in a patient with malignant hepatoma. The patient survived 1 year before succumbing to recurrent disease. Patient 1-year survival rates in the late 1960s and throughout the 1970s remained less than 50% despite continued improvements in the surgical techniques. These early attempts were hindered by difficulty of the surgery, poor methods of organ preservation, and inadequate immunosuppression.

Cyclosporine clinical trials began in 1979 and revolutionized liver transplantation. One-year survival rates in the early 1980s increased to 70% and higher.[116,117] This improvement in survival rates prompted the National Institutes of Health (NIH) to declare that liver transplantation was no longer experimental, but rather an accepted therapeutic modality for patients with end-stage liver disease.[118] This position statement by the NIH resulted in an increase in the number of liver transplant centers worldwide and in the number of liver transplants as well. According to UNOS, each year more liver transplants are being performed than in the previous year. Fewer than

Box 41-15

LIVER DISEASES AT END-STAGE, COMMONLY TREATED WITH LIVER TRANSPLANTATION

CHOLESTATIC LIVER DISEASES
Biliary atresia
Primary sclerosing cholangitis
Primary biliary cirrhosis

CHRONIC HEPATOCELLULAR DISEASES
Viral hepatitis (types A, B, C, D, E)
Alcoholic liver disease (Läennec disease)
Autoimmune hepatitis
Cryptogenic cirrhosis
Drug-induced liver disease

VASCULAR DISEASES
Budd-Chiari syndrome
Veno-occlusive disease

FULMINANT AND SUBFULMINANT HEPATIC FAILURE
Viral hepatitis (types A, B, C, D, E)
Drug-induced (acetaminophen, isoniazid overdoses)
Fulminant Wilson's disease

INBORN METABOLIC DISORDERS
Wilson's disease
α_1-Antitrypsin deficiency
Hemochromatosis
Tyrosinemia
Glycogen storage disease, types I and II

PRIMARY HEPATIC MALIGNANCIES
Hepatocellular carcinoma
Hemangioendothelioma
Hepatoblastoma

Box 41-16

LIVER TRANSPLANTATION CONTRAINDICATIONS

ABSOLUTE CONTRAINDICATIONS
Brain death
Metastatic malignancies
Extrahepatic malignancy
Active drug or alcohol abuse
Advanced cardiopulmonary disease
Acquired immunodeficiency syndrome (AIDS)
Extrahepatic sepsis

RELATIVE CONTRAINDICATIONS
Physiologic age
Advanced renal disease
Multiple hepatic malignancies
Moderate cardiopulmonary disease
Peripheral vascular disease
Psychosocial behaviors indicating noncompliance to medical regimens
HIV-positive

200 liver transplants were performed in 1983, more than 3000 in 1993, and over 5600 in 2003.[3] Current patient survival rates for liver transplantation are approximately 85% at 1 year and greater than 70% at 5 years.[119]

INDICATIONS AND SELECTION

Liver transplantation must be considered for any patient who suffers from irreversible acute or chronic liver disease that is progressive and has no therapy of established efficacy. Diseases of the liver may be categorized as chronic, vascular, fulminant or subfulminant, inborn errors of metabolism, and hepatic malignancies. Box 41-15 lists the most common diseases seen in patients who undergo liver transplantation. In the United States, the single most common indication for liver transplantation in adults is chronic viral hepatitis C (see the Clinical Application feature on Transplantation).[120] In the pediatric population biliary atresia and metabolic disorders account for more than 70% of the diseases leading to transplantation.[121]

Candidate selection is an important aspect of transplantation. Given the shortage of available organs, the transplant team must have a reasonable assurance of a successful outcome. Timing of transplantation is of utmost importance. The patient must not be so ill as to be unable to survive the surgery but yet is experiencing deterioration in the quality of life. In general, liver transplantation is not to be offered to persons such as the following:

- Those who would not likely survive major surgery
- Those who would not survive the effects of long-term immunosuppression
- Those who have a disease that is likely to recur quickly and fatally after transplantation
- Those who are not willing to comply with long-term and sometimes difficult and demanding medical regimens

The absolute contraindications in Box 41-16 fall under these four specific considerations. Having one relative contraindication may not rule out transplantation, but having several may predict poor outcome. Chronologic age is less important than physiologic age. Reports of transplantation in the older population conclude with favorable results.[122] Certain diseases can recur after transplantation, such as viral hepatitis,[123-126] sclerosing cholangitis,[125] biliary malignancies,[126] and others. In the case of viral hepatitis, serologic indicators of replication of virus are followed closely. In the presence of aggressively replicating virus and in certain malignancies, it is in the patient's best interest not to proceed to transplantation because it would actually hasten his or her demise. Multicenter protocols are important in evaluating outcomes and efficacies when performing transplantations in patients with diseases that recur. The decision to offer liver transplantation to any patient must be based on evaluation criteria, which vary among institutions

CLINICAL APPLICATION

Transplantation

Mr. A received a liver transplant secondary to chronic hepatitis C. After his surgery, he is admitted to the critical care unit. His blood pressure (BP) is 130/82; temperature (T), 96.8° F; and pulse (P), 86. He has one dressing across his abdomen and two Jackson-Pratt drain lines on his right side. He is intubated, moving all limbs, and opening his eyes when the nurse speaks to him. His laboratory values include white blood cell count (WBC), 6230/mm³; hematocrit (Hct), 26.3%; hemoglobin (Hgb), 9.8 g/dl; aspartate aminotransferase (AST/SGOT), 55 units/L; alanine aminotransferase (ALT/SGPT), 650 units/L; γ-glutamyltransferase (GGT), 730 units/L; total bilirubin, 16.6 mg/dl; prothrombin time (PT), 23.5 sec; international normalized ratio (INR), 2.0; creatinine, 1.8 mg/dl; and albumin, 3.2 g/dl.

1. What are the nurse's immediate goals?
2. What laboratory tests are commonly used to monitor liver functions?

Postoperative 12 hours, Mr. A is alert and is extubated. His vital signs are BP, 100/60; P, 113; T, 98.5° F; and respiratory rate (RR), 20/min with breath sounds absent in the right base and decreased in the left base. His pulse oximetry is 98%. His urine output has been 60 to 75 ml/hr. His laboratory values now are WBC, 7100 units/L; Hct, 23.3%; Hgb, 7.8 g/dl; AST/SGOT, 615 units/L; ALT/SGPT, 730 units/L; GGT, 940 units/L; total bilirubin, 18.5 mg/dl; PT, 23.0 sec; INR, 2.0; and serum creatinine, 1.0 mg/dl.

3. Which of the above values should concern the nurse most at this time?
4. What signs would indicate primary nonfunction of the liver allograft?

Postoperative 5 days, Mr. A complains of insomnia, trembling hands, and diarrhea. He is afebrile with stable vital signs. His medications include tacrolimus 4 mg PO bid; prednisone 20 mg PO daily; mycophenolate mofetil 1000 mg PO bid; acyclovir 200 mg PO tid; sulfamethoxazole and trimethoprim (Bactrim single-strength), 1 PO daily; Nystatin 5 ml, swish and swallow qid.

5. What is the most common reason for Mr. A's complaints?
6. What is the most common complication after liver transplant?

---

evolve   For the discussion of this Clinical Application, see the Evolve website.

---

and which will be modified as advances in technical ability, immunosuppression, and perioperative management continue. Without complications, the average hospital stay following liver transplantation is 7 to 14 days.[119]

Recipient Evaluation. The candidate for liver transplant undergoes a thorough evaluation to determine the etiology and severity of the liver disease, to establish the need for transplantation rather than other interventions, and to identify objective indications and contraindications. Evaluation begins with a carefully elicited patient history (Box 41-17). A comprehensive approach includes laboratory, radiographic, and diagnostic testing and multidisciplinary consultations (Box 41-18). Not every patient undergoes every test and consult. Careful history taking and a good physical examination will direct the initial diagnostic testing. For instance, a patient with a past history of malignancy would undergo extensive testing to rule out metastases, whereas a patient with fulminant hepatic failure may have a more abbreviated work-up that is focused on determining etiology and potential for hepatic recovery.

During the work-up the candidate's support systems are evaluated by the entire transplant team: the surgeon, the hepatologist, the clinical transplant nurse coordinator, the social worker, the dietitian, and the financial

Box 41-17

PRETRANSPLANT HISTORY FOR A PATIENT WITH END-STAGE LIVER DISEASE

- Risk factors for viral hepatitis: transfusions, IV drug abuse, tattoos, other parenteral exposure
- Family history of liver disease
- Associated disorders: hypothyroidism, osteoporosis, infertility, arthritis
- Onset, duration, and description of symptoms/complications: jaundice, lethargy, bleeding disorders, pruritus, confusion, ascites, edema, melenic stools, abdominal pain, bone pain or fractures, chronic diarrhea, gynecomastia (in men), amenorrhea (in women)
- Current and past medical histories: hospitalizations, surgeries
- Social history: exposure to alcohol, drugs, toxins, use of tobacco products
- Status of immunizations

counselor. Other services, such as cardiology, nephrology, psychiatry, gynecology, anesthesia, infectious disease, endocrinology, hematology, rheumatology, and oral surgery or dentistry, may also be included in the evaluation. Ideally, all immunizations are brought up to date in

Box 41-18

SAMPLE OF A PRETRANSPLANT EVALUATION FOR LIVER TRANSPLANTATION

LABORATORY TESTS

Liver function profiles: transaminases (AST, ALT, GGT); alkaline phosphatase; bilirubin; albumin; prothrombin time; partial thromboplastin time; clotting factors; cholesterol; triglycerides

Renal function profile with electrolytes: blood urea nitrogen, creatinine, sodium, potassium, carbon dioxide, chloride

Hematology: CBC, reticulocytes, erythrocyte sedimentation rate

Thyroid function: T_3RIA; T_4RIA; thyroid-stimulating hormone; T_4, T_3 uptake

Serologies for hepatic viruses and other infectious diseases: viral hepatitis (A, B, C, D, E); cytomegalovirus, Epstein-Barr virus, herpes I and II, parvovirus, RPR, HIV

Blood type and antibody screen

Immunologic profiles: antinuclear antibody; antimitochondrial antibody; anti–smooth muscle antibody; immunoglobulins (A, G, M)

Nutritional profiles: vitamin levels (A, D, E, B_{12}, folate); iron studies with ferritin

Tumor markers: α-fetoprotein, CEA, PSA, CA 19-9

Miscellaneous: ceruloplasmin, α_1-antitrypsin level and phenotype

Urine

24-Hour protein and electrolytes, cultures, creatinine clearance, urinalysis, copper

Stool

Ova, cysts, parasites, occult blood, 48-hour fecal fats, cultures

Gastrointestinal Work-Up

Endoscopy, colonoscopy, endoscopic retrograde cholangiopancreatography, liver biopsy

Pulmonary Profile

Arterial blood gases, pulmonary function studies

Radiographic and Diagnostic Tests

Chest x-ray, ultrasound of liver including vascular studies

Other, Optional Tests

Doppler studies; sinus x-ray; computerized tomography (abdomen, chest, head); electrocardiogram; echocardiogram; cardiac stress test; cardiac catheterization; mammogram; peripheral vascular studies; carotid ultrasound; abdominal angiography; percutaneous cholangiogram; bone mineral density

AST, Aspartate transaminase; *ALT,* alanine aminotransferase; *GGT,* γ-glutamyltransferase; *CBC,* complete blood count; *T_3RIA;* serum triiodothyronine (T_3); *T_4RIA,* serum triiodothyronine (T_4); *RPR,* rapid plasma reagin; *HIV,* human immunodeficiency virus; *CEA,* carcinoembryonic agents; *PSA,* prostate-specific antigen; *CA 19-9,* investigational cancer antigen.

an attempt to minimize postoperative infections. The patient and family receive education regarding the evaluation, the transplant waiting list, surgery, postoperative management including immunosuppression, and long-term follow-up. At the conclusion of the evaluation, one of several outcomes is possible: (1) the patient is deemed a transplant candidate, (2) the patient is deemed not a candidate, or (3) the patient may be a candidate some time in the future if certain criteria are met. These criteria may be of a physical nature (e.g., it is too early in the disease process to list now, in which case the patient will be followed at set intervals). The criteria also may be of a psychosocial nature (e.g., the patient must attend a formal rehabilitation program or undergo treatment of depression).

After candidacy has been determined and the patient is ready for transplantation, his or her social security number is entered into the national computer system operated by UNOS. Objective criteria are used to place a patient on the waiting list. This data is used in a formula to determine the patient's score. This score is directly associated with the patient's risk of death within 3 months: the higher the score, the higher the risk. The Model for End-Stage Liver Disease (MELD) formula is used to calculate risk of mortality in patients 12 years and older.[119]

The MELD objective criteria include serum total bilirubin, serum creatinine, and prothrombin time (PT) and international normalized ratio (INR). The Pediatric End-Stage Liver Disease (PELD) formula is used for patients 11 years of age and younger.[119] The PELD objective criteria include date of birth, gender, weight, height, serum albumin, serum total bilirubin, PT, and INR.

Placement on the waiting list is determined by blood type, weight, and patient urgency. Patients with acute fulminant hepatic failure are considered in most urgent need. They are placed at the top of the list. Patients with chronic end-stage liver disease are prioritized on the list by their MELD/PELD score. The higher the score, the higher the patient is on the list. Waiting time is only used as a tie-breaker for patients with equal scores. Each UNOS region has special exception cases that must be voted on by the regional review board (comprised of one member from each transplant center in the region). These exceptions request higher-than-calculated MELD/PELD scores for patients with special problems that are not addressed by only using the objective criteria, such as children with intractable pruritis.

Next, one of the most difficult phases begins—the waiting period. It is not possible to anticipate when an appropriate organ will become available. Thus the patient may feel his or her life is being put "on hold." Because of the shortage of donors, it is not uncommon for the patient in the critical care unit to die awaiting transplantation; this is especially true for pediatric recipients. And knowing that another person must die so that he or she may live can cause feelings of guilt as the patient hopes for a liver to become available. In addition, the patient with end-stage liver disease knows that the only alternative to transplantation is death. By understanding the basic social processes that patients experience while awaiting transplantation, nurses can facilitate health promotion activities.[127] It is therefore important for the patient and family to receive ongoing psychosocial assessment and to attend pretransplant support groups, which are available at most transplant centers.

Pretransplant Phase. The patient with end-stage liver disease awaiting a transplant may be one of the most challenging to care for in the critical care unit. Hepatic encephalopathy, coagulopathies, portal hypertension, severe fluid and electrolyte imbalances, cardiac compromise, and renal deterioration are not uncommon. Frequent mental status assessments of the patient are important in determining continued candidacy for transplant. Hepatic encephalopathy may improve with administration of antibiotics and laxatives or may proceed to stage IV coma. Protection of the airway is especially important in an encephalopathic patient who is not intubated. In these circumstances, if hematemesis or vomiting occurs, intubation and use of paralytic agents may be necessary to protect the patient's airway. Diagnostic studies may be needed to evaluate the possibility of intracranial bleed. Maintain the head of the patient's bed 30 to 45 degrees to avoid even slight increases in intracranial pressure. Patients who have chronic liver disease also have nutritional deficits. They require supplements of the fat-soluble vitamins (A, D, E, and K), may be on protein restrictions to reduce serum ammonia levels, and may experience severe muscle wasting.

Consequences of portal hypertension must be corrected. Gastrointestinal hemorrhage from varices may respond to administration of propranolol or sclerotherapy. Portal hypertension may be reduced by transjugular intrahepatic portosystemic shunting (TIPS) in interventional radiology. Rarely, the patient may need to undergo surgical intervention with a vascular shunt created between the portacaval system and the mesangial, splenic, or renal vascular systems. Patients with massive ascites usually have total body fluid overload but are intravascularly contracted and require sodium restriction and administration of colloidal fluids, such as albumin, along with diuretics. Careful documentation of fluid intake and output, daily weight measurements, and frequent measurement of vital signs are needed to monitor fluid status. Ascites can interfere with lung expansion and can compromise oxygenation. Patients with large, distended abdomens also find adequate oral nutri-

tion difficult. Use of diuretics to control ascites is common, but can compromise kidney function, even worsen hepatorenal syndrome. Paracentesis (removal of ascites) may be required for intractable ascites. However, frequent large-volume paracentesis can also contribute to renal demise.

Spontaneous bacterial peritonitis (SBP) can be manifested in the patient with end-stage liver disease by an acute decline in the hepatic and renal function, accompanied by fever, abdominal pain, and hepatic encephalopathy. Paracentesis fluid will show increased white blood cells with or without a positive culture. Patients are treated aggressively with antibiotics and are temporarily deferred from transplantation during treatment for and recovery from SBP.

Determining Donor Suitability. The two criteria necessary for matching a donor liver to a recipient are blood type and body size. Human lymphocyte antigen (HLA) tissue typing is not used in the matching of donor livers because this has not been shown to significantly affect patient outcomes. Donors are carefully screened for infectious diseases and metastatic carcinomas because these can be transmitted to the recipient. The transplant center is notified by an OPO that a liver is available. If the organ is accepted, the patient is contacted by the transplant team. In very urgent situations the donor blood type may not be compatible with the recipient's; for example, an A-type donor and an O-type recipient. Despite this incompatibility, liver transplantation can be successful. There may be some early postoperative complications, such as mild hemolysis, but long-term follow-up of patients with recipient-donor ABO incompatibility has been favorable.[128]

Once a donor liver becomes available, it is necessary to expedite the preoperative preparation of the recipient. The use of University of Wisconsin (UW) preservation solution has allowed for longer cold ischemia time (the length of time from when an organ is removed from the donor, flushed, and packed in ice for storage until it is transplanted). However, cold ischemia times of longer than 12 hours are correlated with increased recipient morbidity and mortality.[129]

LIVER TRANSPLANT SURGICAL PROCEDURE

Liver transplant surgery is lengthy and technically difficult, often lasting 4 to 12 hours. The procedure involves the combined efforts of surgeons, anesthesiologists, nurse anesthetists, operating room nurses and technicians, perfusionists, and personnel from the blood bank and laboratory and radiology departments, to name a few. The patient is taken to the operating room for anesthesia induction, insertion of large-bore intravenous catheters that allow high-volume fluid infusion, and insertion of a pulmonary artery catheter for hemodynamic monitoring. Other devices such as an arterial line, a nasogastric tube, and a urinary drainage catheter are also inserted. The patient is positioned on the operating room table in such a way as to minimize pressure that may cause ischemia and chronic injury to tissue and peripheral nerves.

The surgery can be divided into three stages: (1) recipient hepatectomy, (2) vascular anastomoses with donor liver, and (3) biliary anastomosis.

Stage 1 is the longest and most difficult part of the surgery since it involves removal of the native liver. It is complicated even more by coagulopathies, adhesions, portal hypertension, and venous collaterals. Before completion of this stage, the patient may be put on venovenous bypass (Fig. 41-10). Not all patients require this procedure. A centrifugal pump cycles the blood out via iliac and portal vein cannulas and returns it to the central circulation via the axillary or subclavian vein. Advances in surgical techniques, anesthesia, and fluid management have shortened the length of surgery enough to warrant not using venovenous bypass on all liver transplants.

Stage 2 comprises the four vascular anastomoses: suprahepatic inferior vena cava, infrahepatic vena cava, hepatic artery, and portal vein. There are many variations and adaptations, such as use of vascular patches, used depending on both donor and recipient anatomy. If venovenous bypass is used, it is removed after the infrahepatic vena cava anastomosis and before the hepatic artery anastomosis.

Stage 3, biliary anastomosis, can be achieved in two ways: choledochojejunostomy (bile duct to jejunum) and choledochocholedochostomy (bile duct to bile duct). Choledochojejunostomy is done in patients with diseased bile ducts such as those with biliary atresia or sclerosing cholangitis. It is also known as a *Roux-en-Y* procedure and is shown in Fig. 41-11. The choledochocholedochostomy is performed when the patient has a healthy and intact common bile duct and is shown in Fig. 41-12. The patient returns from surgery with or without an external stent or T-tube. If an external stent or T-tube is present, it is connected to a bag into which bile drains. Patients who do not have external biliary tubes present may have an internal stent inserted in the bile duct across the biliary anastomosis. Eventually the internal stent moves and is passed with the stool.

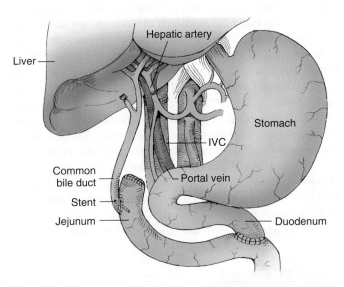

Fig. 41-11 Roux-en-Y procedure (choledochojejunostomy). *IVC,* Inferior vena cava.

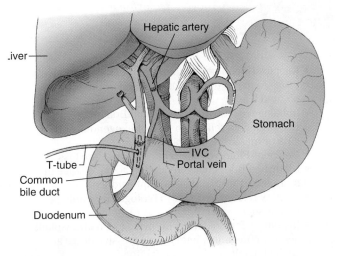

Fig. 41-12 Choledochocholedochostomy procedure. *IVC,* Inferior vena cava.

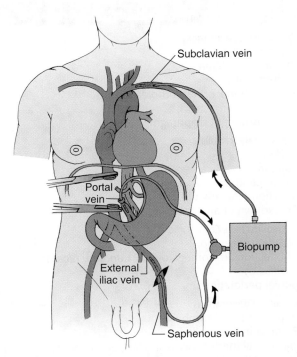

Fig. 41-10 Venovenous bypass during removal of the native liver. The portal and iliac veins are cannulated, and blood is circulated via a centrifugal pump to the subclavian vein.

POSTOPERATIVE MEDICAL AND NURSING MANAGEMENT

The common nursing diagnoses associated with liver transplantation are listed in the Nursing Diagnoses feature on Liver Transplantation. After surgery, some patients may be extubated before arriving in the critical care unit. But most will arrive unreversed from anesthesia. Immediate goals include (1) reestablishment of normal body temperature, (2) hemodynamic stabilization, and (3) maintenance of an effective airway. Postoperative hypothermia is common after an orthotopic liver transplant (OLT). The critical care nurse must achieve rewarming safely by methods such as using warming blankets, heating lamps, and head covers. Hemodynamic stabilization is a particular challenge, because the patient may arrive hypervolemic, euvolemic, or hypovolemic and also be hypertensive or hypotensive. Assessment of total body fluids versus intravascular fluid status is important. Accurate measurements of hemodynamic function such as arterial blood pressure, peripheral blood pressure, central venous pressure (CVP), pulmonary artery pressure (PAP), pulmonary artery occlusion pressure (PAOP) or "wedge" pressure, urinary output, patency of drains, and bile totals are assessed frequently to evaluate true volume status. Choice of replacement fluid and pharmacologic agent for correcting volume and blood pressure abnormalities is transplant center–specific. These protocols vary as to use of albumin or fresh-frozen plasma and use of intravenous renal-dose dopamine or prostaglandin, as well as other agents and solutions. Still, the goals are all the same: optimize tissue perfusion and deliver oxygen to all tissues, especially the newly transplanted graft.

Electrolyte abnormalities can occur after OLT. Disturbances in potassium and magnesium levels are common. High serum levels are usually associated with renal impairment; low levels can be the result of drug side effects, such as diuretic therapy. The patient also may be hypernatremic or hyponatremic, which will complicate correction of volume status and replacement fluids.

Ventilatory support of the patient is maintained until anesthesia has been metabolized and cleared by the new liver and the patient awakens. Frequent measurement of arterial blood gas levels, continuous pulse oximetry, and assessment of breath sounds are needed. The patient may require changes in ventilatory settings, suctioning to remove secretions, or administration of pharmacologic agents to correct acid-base imbalances. Pulmonary complications are common, as listed in Box 41-19. After extubation, patients must be encouraged to perform incentive spirometry exercises and to turn, cough, and deep breathe frequently to help prevent atelectasis and pneumonia. Respiratory treatments with bronchodilators, prophylactic antimicrobials, and chest physiotherapy also may be used.

Management of coagulopathies is important in the early postoperative phase. Characterization and careful measurement of drain lines and drainage from incisions

---

NURSING DIAGNOSES — Liver Transplantation

- Risk for Infection risk factor: immunosuppressive drugs required to prevent rejection of the transplanted liver
- Imbalanced Nutrition: Less Than Body Requirements related to lack of exogenous nutrients or increased metabolic demand
- Deficient Fluid Volume related to absolute loss
- Disturbed Body Image related to actual change in body, structure, function, or appearance
- Anxiety related to threat to biologic, psychologic, and/or social integrity
- Readiness for Enhanced Knowledge: Posttransplant Self-Care Regimen, immunosuppressive drugs and clinical manifestations of infection.

Box 41-19

COMMON COMPLICATIONS AFTER LIVER TRANSPLANT

PULMONARY COMPLICATIONS
Pleural effusion
Pulmonary edema
Pneumonia
Pneumothorax or hemothorax
Atelectasis
Paralysis of right diaphragm

BILIARY COMPLICATIONS
Leaks
Strictures
Obstruction
Infection (cholangitis)
Breakdown of anastomosis

GASTROINTESTINAL COMPLICATIONS
Bleeding/ulceration
GI Infections (cytomegalovirus, *Candida*, *Clostridium difficile*)
Bowel perforations

VASCULAR COMPLICATIONS
Hepatic artery thrombosis
Portal vein thrombosis
Vena caval thrombosis
Peripheral and/or central line sepsis
Hepatic vein thrombosis

are needed along with other nursing assessments of blood loss, such as signs of hypovolemia, tachypnea, tachycardia, or poor peripheral oxygenation. A sudden increase in abdominal girth, sanguineous nasogastric output, and black, tarry stools are hallmarks of bleeding problems and must be reported immediately. Laboratory monitoring to assess blood loss and coagulopathies includes hematocrit, hemoglobin, platelet count, prothrombin time, partial thromboplastin time, fibrinogen, and fibrin split products. Reversal of coagulopathies is done judiciously with consideration for the potential to thrombose newly anastomosed blood vessels in the liver. Blood products such as platelets, fresh-frozen plasma, and specific factors can be given along with pharmacologic agents such as vitamin K.

Neurologic assessment of the patient is important in the early postoperative phase to determine mental status and graft function. Patients who preoperatively were encephalopathic will generally be slower to clear mentally. But with good hepatic function, the patient should be alert and oriented within 1 to 2 days. Neurologic assessment also can be influenced by certain pharmacologic agents, including the immunosuppressants, which can cause both peripheral and central neurologic side effects. The critical care nurse must always be aware of the potential for intracranial bleeds in a patient who has coagulopathies, serum sodium imbalances, and hemodynamic instability. All of these can interfere with pain management, since pharmacologic agents used for pain can mask deterioration in mental status. Medications to relieve pain are administered, but other nonpharmacologic nursing interventions also must be used.

Renal function can be altered after a liver transplant because of acute tubular necrosis, intrinsic kidney disease, or poor liver function. Some studies estimate 21% to 73% of OLT patients develop renal failure.[129] Patients are managed with attention to fluid and electrolyte imbalances; avoidance of nephrotoxic drugs; and occasionally ultrafiltration, continuous renal replacement treatments, or intermittent hemodialysis. With good liver function, kidney function usually improves. But certain immunosuppressive agents and antimicrobials can deleteriously affect renal function. Adjustments in doses or avoidance of use must be balanced with assessment of kidney and liver function.

Immunosuppressive therapy places the transplant patient at an increased risk of infection. Infectious complications continue to be the leading cause of death in the OLT patient,[122,130] and the potential for infection is greatest when patients receive high doses of immunosuppressants. Good hand-washing techniques and Standard Precautions must be practiced by all persons who come into contact with the transplant patient throughout the hospitalization. Infections are treated with appropriate antimicrobials specific to the invading organism. Prophylactic therapies are commonly used as well.[122,130]

Careful attention to any external biliary drain line is important. If the patient has an external biliary drain, the critical care nurse documents color, character, and amount of drainage and reports any changes. Biliary complications can occur after OLT. Posttransplant complications, including biliary ones, are listed in Box 41-19.

Posttransplant Assessment of Liver Function. The standard laboratory measures used to follow graft function are serum aspartate aminotransferase (AST/SGOT), alanine aminotransferase (ALT/SGPT), alkaline phosphatase, and γ-glutamyltransferase (GGT); serum bilirubin; and prothrombin times. In the first few postoperative days, the serum levels may continue to rise before peaking and subsequently falling. These liver function tests (LFTs) are measured frequently in the first few days after surgery. As liver function improves, the frequency of laboratory testing decreases.

The patient with suspected primary nonfunction of the graft will demonstrate (1) hemodynamic instability, (2) progressive renal deterioration, (3) coagulopathies and abnormal serum liver function laboratory tests, (4) hypoglycemia, (5) continued ventilatory dependence, and (6) an inability to awaken from anesthesia.

Continued nonfunction of the graft will necessitate relisting the patient for another donor liver. Early signs of optimal graft function include improving kidney function, mental alertness, a high to normal serum glucose, and early extubation. The serum ALT, AST, GGT, and alkaline phosphatase may peak on the third or fourth day but subsequently will decrease. The serum bilirubin may take 1 week before beginning to fall and may have a mild elevation when the external biliary drainage tube is clamped or following a blood transfusion. Early mobilization and physical therapy are encouraged.

The nasogastric tube is removed when its output is minimal, bowel sounds return, and the patient is extubated. If the patient is expected to be intubated longer than several days, total parenteral nutrition (TPN) may be started. Otherwise, nutrition may begin orally or by feeding tube as soon as bowel function returns. The diet is slowly advanced as tolerated. Central venous catheters and arterial lines are removed. The urinary catheter is removed as soon as the patient is awake enough to be continent. Drain lines are removed as drainage outputs become minimal. As the patient begins to participate in self-care, plans are made to transfer the patient out of the critical care unit to the transplant nursing unit.

On the transplant unit, laboratory data and vital signs continue to be monitored on a routine basis. Self-care protocols are promoted.[131] Increasing levels of physical therapy are encouraged and diet is advanced, and much of the nurse's effort is spent teaching the patient and family.

Rejection Surveillance. Acute rejection in OLT is a cellular-mediated event and is suspected any time the serum liver function laboratory tests (LFTs) become elevated over the previous levels. An elevation of the LFTs usually precedes any other sign of acute rejection of the liver allograft. Sometimes the patient also exhibits fever, a drop in bile output (if a T-tube is still connected to a drainage bag), and a change in the color and viscosity of the bile. At first the patient may not have any other physical symptoms, but eventually malaise may occur and the urine may darken and stools become clay-colored. An acute elevation in LFT's can signal rejection of the liver graft. However, certain infections, such as cytomegalovirus, may also cause LFTs to increase. A liver biopsy may be indicated to determine cause of liver dysfunction. Acute rejection can occur anytime after transplant, but most commonly it occurs in the first few months and even as early as in the first week. The majority of liver transplant patients experience at least one acute rejection episode. Treatment of acute rejection requires increasing immunosuppression (i.e., an increase in tacrolimus or steroid dose, possibly an addition of monoclonal or polyclonal antilymphocyte antibodies, or other newer pharmacologic agents). Immunosuppressant protocols vary from center to center and are usually very successful at reversing acute rejection.

Chronic rejection is a humoral event and is progressive and nonreversible. Chronic rejection in a liver transplant patient usually requires retransplantation if the patient is still considered a candidate.

PATIENT EDUCATION

Considerable attention is focused on patient education and discharge planning. Discharge booklets are helpful in the education process. It is important for the patient to learn how to self-administer medications, monitor vital signs, care for incision and T-tube (if present), prevent infections, and identify problems that must promptly receive medical attention. Because it is not uncommon for patients to be discharged within 2 weeks after an OLT, it is important for discharge instructions to begin as soon as the patient is mentally alert. Patients discharged early may require home health nurse referrals to assist with follow-up of incision care, intravenous therapies, and more. In addition, education must be provided about rejection surveillance, signs and symptoms of infection, lifestyle changes if needed, long-term transplant medication considerations, and the follow-up visit schedule.

LONG-TERM FOLLOW-UP

If the OLT patient does not live in the same city in which the surgery was performed, after discharge from the hospital he or she usually remains in the immediate area of the transplant center before returning home. During this period the patient may be monitored by a home health nurse and also is seen in clinic several times a week by the transplant team. Continued serologic testing is done to monitor graft function, to determine blood levels of certain immunosuppressive agents, and to monitor for postoperative complications. Although many of these complications can be managed successfully in the outpatient setting, readmissions do occur. Because rejections, readmissions, grieving for the donor, and pharmacologic side effects can create anxiety for the family and the patient, they are encouraged to attend transplant support groups if offered by the center. Once patients do return home, they are encouraged to resume a close relationship with their local primary care physician and gastroenterologist. Because of the proliferation in the number of liver transplants being performed, it is not unreasonable for these patients to be admitted to a non–tertiary care hospital for management of some long-term posttransplant complications. Thus even nurses who work for hospitals that do not perform transplants may have the opportunity to care for these patients.

Liver transplant patients need long-term follow-up for hypertension, renal insufficiency, obesity, dyslipidemias, biliary and infectious complications, and malignancies.[122] Early intervention affects both quality and length of life. Behavior modification and therapeutic lifestyle changes should be frequently reinforced to positively affect long-term health. Financial concerns are a major source of stress in this patient population. The largest group of transplant recipients are those who have suffered from some type of chronic liver disease. They often are disabled for some length of time before transplant and already have experienced financial stressors related to illness. As these patients live longer with liver transplants, issues of insurability, continued disability, and even the ability to obtain work have to be addressed.[119,132]

Transplantation offers hope for survival, but at considerable expense. Many insurance providers, including Medicare, provide partial reimbursement for liver transplantation. The costs, however, can be staggering. Liver transplant surgery has been reported to be the single most costly procedure in health care.[133] In this age of managed health care, it becomes a challenge for institutions to provide this labor-intensive, life-saving procedure economically. In attempts to control costs and optimize outcomes, insurance companies are designating "centers of excellence." This will mean more patients will travel some distances to receive transplants. As competition for the health care dollar increases, workloads and the character of the work itself will change. Nurses must remain in the forefront, providing research for cost-effective health care techniques.[127,131,134]

Clinical trials are seeking to identify new drugs and to define improved treatment protocols.[135] With increasing choices of therapies, drugs will be selected for patients in whom other immunosuppressive therapies fail or for patients who develop severe side effects.[136] Studies on tolerance and chimerism also may influence future immunosuppressive protocols.[119] As recipients on the list wait longer, improved methods of medical management of end-stage liver disease and bridges to transplantation become more necessary, such as chemoembolization of hepatomas and transjugular intrahepatic portosystemic shunting.

A limiting factor in liver transplantation today continues to be the shortage of organ donors.[137] Attention also is being focused on ways to increase the number and availability of donor organs. Reduced-size organs are a common occurrence.[138] Split livers, a technique of dividing one liver and transplanting two recipients, is possible.[138] Studies are exploring the roles of xenografts and bioartificial liver devices used to support the patient awaiting a homograft.[138] Expanded criteria for deceased donors has lead to changes in posttransplant recipient therapies.[139] The use of living donors for both pediatric and adult recipients will continue.[119,138,140] Recipient selection criteria also will continue to be redefined for diseases and conditions such as hepatic malignancies[137] and HIV-positivity.[141] As recipients live longer and healthier lives, the issue of reproduction will become more common.[119] These and other factors will influence the future of liver transplantation.

KIDNEY TRANSPLANTATION

The first successful kidney transplant was performed in 1954 in Boston. Today it is the treatment of choice for patients with end-stage kidney disease (ESKD). It allows the recipient to enjoy a much less restricted lifestyle and provides a more cost-effective method of treating ESKD than long-term dialysis.[142] Advances in the study of the immune system and the development of new immunosuppressant medications have allowed for increased graft survival rates for both cadaveric and living, related kidney transplants.

In the early years of transplantation, large doses of oral steroids were the immunosuppressant of choice for preventing graft rejection. Large doses or prolonged use of oral steroids can cause severe osteoporosis, decreased wound healing, and many of the Cushing's syndrome symptoms.[143] In the late 1970s cyclosporine was added to the list of immunosuppressive medications used to prevent rejection. Cyclosporine represented a breakthrough in immunosuppressive agents, and the graft survival rates soared.[144] Today, there are many agents to choose from, and most transplant centers use a combination of agents to prevent rejection. This combining of medications is done in an attempt to lower the doses of each so that the associated side effects can be minimized.

In 2003 13,857 kidney transplants were performed in the United States. However, 56,864 patients were on the UNOS Scientific Registry patient waiting list that year for kidney transplant.[3] Finding new medications and ways to increase the number of donor organs recovered are two of the challenges that the transplant community faces.

SELECTION FOR TRANSPLANTATION

Many disease processes can lead to ESKD. Therefore potential recipients must undergo numerous laboratory tests and some noninvasive physical testing before they can be approved as candidates (Box 41-20). After transplantation, the patient's immune system will be purposely and controllably compromised. Because of this, there are several contraindications to transplant (Box 41-21).

If any or a combination of these risk factors is present, the patient is determined to be at too high a risk for transplantation and the immunosuppressant regimen

---

Box 41-20

KIDNEY TRANSPLANTATION EVALUATION

- Chem 24; human leukocyte antigen tissue typing; prothrombin time; partial thromboplastin time; complete blood count with differential; platelet count; human immunodeficiency virus; hepatitis; cytomegalovirus; Epstein-Barr virus; lipid profile; urine for analysis, culture, and sensitivities; 24-hour urine for creatinine clearance and protein (if patient still produces urine); dialysate fluid for culture and sensitivity (if patient is on continuous ambulatory peritoneal dialysis)
- Kidney ultrasound or spiral computed tomography (CT); chest x-ray posteroanterior and lateral views; electrocardiogram; stress test and cardiac catheterization (if indicated); weight management (if overweight); a colonoscopy (if more than 55 years of age); mammogram (for women over age 35); and a venogram (for patients with diabetes)
- Consultants: psychologist/psychiatrist, urologist, transplant surgeon or transplant nephrologists, social worker, dietitian, chaplain, and financial counselor

---

Box 41-21

CONTRAINDICATIONS TO KIDNEY TRANSPLANTATION

- Malignancy during the past 3 years
- Active infectious process
- Advanced cardiopulmonary disease
- High risk for surgery
- Noncompliance with current medical regimen
- Recreational drug use
- Other serious contributing disease processes

that they must follow. The alternative for such a patient is to decrease or eliminate the risk factors that can be controlled and be reevaluated at a later date. If the candidate is unwilling to eliminate the high-risk behaviors that he or she can control, the only alternative is to remain on dialysis in order to survive.

KIDNEY TRANSPLANT SURGICAL PROCEDURE

When the kidney to be transplanted is procured from the donor, living and related or cadaveric, the ureter, renal vein, and renal artery are dissected, leaving as much length as possible.

Living, Related Donor Surgery. If the donor is living and related, the procurement can take place either as a laparoscopic procedure or as an open procedure. Once the kidney is secured, it is flushed with a cold electrolyte preservative solution until the venous return is clear.[145] This usually requires approximately 500 ml of solution.[146] The kidney is then transported into the recipient's operating room to be transplanted.

Cadaver Donor Surgery. If the donor is a cadaver donor, the kidney is flushed with a cold, electrolyte preservative solution and simultaneously cooled externally as quickly as possible. It can be transported either on a kidney perfusion machine or packed in an iced preservation solution. After it is procured and placed in the hypothermic solution, it can be maintained for 48 to 72 hours before it must be transplanted.[146] However, most transplant centers attempt to transplant the organ as soon after procurement as possible to avoid both cold ischemic injury and acute tubular necrosis (ATN).[147] At the time of procurement, the kidney is visualized in situ to note color, shape, and form. It is palpated to determine firmness, and a biopsy is often taken to rule out undiagnosed renal dysfunction or other disease.

Recipient Surgery. The patient is anesthetized in the usual manner, and a urinary catheter is placed. A curvilinear incision is made 3 to 4 cm above the symphysis pubis that extends to the iliac crest (Fig. 41-13, *A*). The kidney is to be placed in the extraperitoneal space of either the right or left iliac fossa. The muscles and fascia are divided and retracted medially to expose the iliac vessels. The renal artery is anastomosed end-to-side or end-to-end to the external iliac artery, and the vein is sutured end-to-side or end-to-end to the common iliac vein (Fig. 41-13, *B*).[147] During the surgery, a CVP ranging from 8 to 16 mm Hg must be maintained and a systolic blood pressure at or above the patient's baseline should be maintained to ensure adequate perfusion of the transplanted kidney.

After the revascularization procedures are completed, the ureteral anastomosis is done. The most common method used is an ureteroneocystostomy. During this procedure, an incision is made in the dome of the recipient's bladder. The donor ureter is tunneled through the recipient's mucosal layer and is sutured end-to-side to

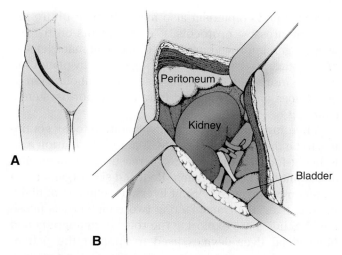

Fig. 41-13   Placement of the renal graft into the iliac fossa. **A,** The incision depicted is for the right side of the abdomen, representing graft implantation in the right iliac fossa. **B,** The iliac vessels are exposed. (Modified from Smith SL: *AACN tissue and organ transplantation: implications for professional nursing practice,* St Louis, 1990, Mosby.)

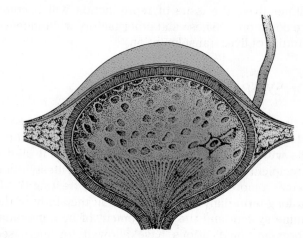

Fig. 41-14   Ureteroneocystostomy reconstruction of the urinary tract. The donor ureter is passed through a posterior bladder wall tunnel and anastomosed to the bladder mucosa. (From Smith SL: *AACN tissue and organ transplantation: implications for professional nursing practice,* St Louis, 1990, Mosby.)

the mucosal opening (Fig, 41-14).[147] If the patient has a history of bladder surgeries, augmentations, or infections, a ureteroureterostomy can be done in which the donor ureter is anastomosed to the recipient's ureter.[146]

POSTTRANSPLANT MEDICAL MANAGEMENT AND NURSING CARE

After the transplant is completed and the patient is stable and ready for discharge from the recovery room, most transplant centers admit the patient directly to the organ transplant unit or to the critical care unit. Serious

NURSING DIAGNOSES — Kidney Transplantation

- Deficient Fluid Volume related to absolute loss
- Ineffective Renal Tissue Perfusion related to decreased renal blood flow
- Risk for Infection risk factor: immunosuppressive drugs to prevent rejection of the transplanted kidney
- Disturbed Body Image related to actual change in body structure, function, or appearance
- Anxiety related to threat to biologic, psychologic, and/or social integrity
- Enhanced Readiness to Learn: Posttransplant Self-Care Regimen, immunosuppressive drugs and clinical manifestation

complications can occur in the immediate postoperative period, and a sound knowledge base of postoperative nursing care, renal function, anatomy, and immunosuppressive medications is imperative for the nurse.

Caring for the Newly Transplanted Patient. Nursing diagnoses used to manage kidney transplant patient care are listed in the Nursing Diagnoses feature on Kidney Transplantation.

If the transplanted organ is working well, fluid status in the patient, monitored by CVP, patient weight, and vital signs observation, must be regulated very closely. Adequate hydration is an absolute necessity for continued graft function in the immediate postoperative period. Hypovolemia can lead to compromised blood flow to the kidney, ATN, and possible graft failure. The new kidney will be producing large amounts of urine, and replacement fluids, usually maintained at a "1 ml : 1 ml" (one-to-one) ratio, must be sustained.

Electrolyte balance is also of grave concern. Because of the large volumes of urine produced, the potential exists for hypokalemia, hypomagnesemia, and hypocalcemia, leading to possible cardiac compromise. These electrolytes must be monitored at least every 4 to 6 hours and replaced as necessary. Assessment of the BUN and creatinine levels is also necessary every 4 to 6 hours to monitor graft function and determine the need for dialysis.

The complete blood count and platelet count should be monitored every 4 to 6 hours. Blood loss during the operation is minimal, generally 500 ml or less. Abrupt decreases or continuously falling counts may indicate hemorrhage at an anastomosis site, requiring a return to the operating room for repair. Despite minimal blood loss during surgery, transfusion of blood products after the surgery is often necessary. Frequent observation and assessment of the surgical incision is needed to evaluate for drainage and swelling.

Urine output volume and color should be monitored at least every 30 minutes. The bladder anastomosis is fragile, and clots occluding the catheter are not uncommon. The bladder must remain decompressed for several days to promote proper healing. If clots occlude the end of the catheter, gentle irrigation/aspiration may be necessary. If the clot cannot be dislodged or aspirated out, it may be necessary to change the catheter. Painful bladder spasms also can occur and require the use of pain medications and opiates to relax the bladder, usually in the form of a belladonna and opium suppository.

If the kidney is not functioning in the immediate postoperative period, the patient's fluid status must be monitored very closely. Hypervolemia in these patients may be so great that respiratory compromise occurs. Electrolyte dilution, because of the fluid overload, is a concern. Output monitoring and bladder decompression still must be maintained. If the kidney function is slow to recover, a dopamine IV drip is often initiated. Low-dose dopamine at 3 mcg/kg/min aids in renal perfusion and may help the kidney function return faster. However, closer observation of blood pressure then becomes necessary to observe for potentially serious hypertension that would require medical management. If significant fluid overload or respiratory compromise occurs, oxygen therapy and dialysis treatments may be necessary for several days.

Initiation of induction immunosuppressant therapy begins at the time of transplant, usually in the form of a polyclonal antithymocyte/antilymphocyte IV compound or IV monoclonal antibody compound. These compounds remove the lymphocytes from the patient's system, preventing rejection and suppressing the immune system until oral agents can be safely administered and blood levels are sufficient to allow the IV agent to be discontinued. Because the patient is now immunocompromised, strict aseptic technique is required to prevent infection. Thorough hand washing, aseptic dressing changes, discontinuation of any unnecessary invasive lines, and limiting the number of visitors are necessary protective mechanisms.

Because of the patient's immunocompromised status, subtle changes in the patient's temperature, white blood cell counts, and wound drainage can signal an active infection. Patients also are susceptible to opportunistic native organisms such as *Candida*, pneumocystis pneumonia, cytomegalovirus (CMV), Epstein-Barr virus (EBV), and *herpes simplex* infections.

PATIENT EDUCATION

The average length of stay in the hospital for an uncomplicated kidney transplant is 5 to 7 days.[142,144] In the first few days after transplant, the patient must learn to care

Box 41-22

Signs and Symptoms of Kidney Rejection

- Increased tenderness over the transplanted kidney site
- Decreased urine output
- Increased serum creatinine levels, above the patient's baseline
- Fever
- Rapid weight gain of 4 to 6 pounds in a 24-hour period
- Swelling, usually in the hands and feet

for him- or herself and the new organ. Medication regimens are very complicated, and most centers initiate a self-medication program at the patient's bedside as a training tool. Patients are taught the signs and symptoms of infection and graft rejection (Box 41-22), transplant clinic protocols, and new dietary limitations. Frequent transplant clinic visits to check the functioning of the organ and to adjust down the doses of immunosuppressant medications are necessary for the first few months after transplantation.[142]

Long-Term Considerations

Rejection of the organ is of ongoing concern for all transplant patients. The graft function is monitored closely, and if rejection is suspected, a biopsy is performed. If the biopsy reveals acute rejection, rescue therapy is initiated. This therapy can be in the form of high-dose IV steroids in the case of mild rejection or IV monoclonal antibody for moderate to severe rejection. If the biopsy reveals chronic rejection, the oral immunosuppressant medications are increased or recycled to the higher doses used immediately after transplant. No two patients' immune systems are exactly alike. The immunosuppressant medication regimen required to prevent rejection must be tailored to each patient individually. The goal is to create a balance among medications which allows the patient to fight off most infections and yet avoid rejection of the transplanted organ.

Patient compliance with the complicated medical regimen required to maintain a transplanted organ is of major concern. Adequate teaching of the importance of taking the medications as instructed is of paramount importance. Patients are reluctant to take the medications appropriately if they are experiencing severe or disfiguring side effects. Decreasing the dose of the medications can often alleviate these side effects but may lead to a rejection episode.

Patients often have financial concerns. A 1-month supply of medications can often cost more than $1000, and paying for the medications long-term can be a bur-

den too great for some patients. The federal government helps to pay for the immunosuppressant medications for 30 months after transplant. After 30 months, the patient is considered to be cured and the government assistance ends. This forces the patient to assume the full financial responsibility for the medications that are required to maintain the transplant.

Kidney transplantation has changed a great deal during the past 40 years. Continuing research with new immunosuppressant medications is the key to continued advances in this dynamic field. Increasing public awareness of the need for donor organs is one strategy to increase the donor pool. Combating rumors and false information with good public education campaigns is important. Considering older patients as potential donors, as well as deceased after cardiac death donors, are additional strategies. Transplanting donor organs into more patients and helping patients keep their organs functioning longer is the primary focus of all the kidney transplant centers around the world.

PANCREAS TRANSPLANTATION

The single most common cause of end-stage kidney disease (ESKD) in Western societies today is insulin-dependent (type 1) diabetes mellitus (DM).[148] Despite meticulous glycemic control, dietary restrictions, healthy exercise programs, and advances in disease-modifying medication regimens, most patients with type 1 DM will develop end-stage kidney disease requiring long-term dialysis treatments.[148] The first pancreas transplants were performed in 1966 with little success. Advances in immunosuppressive medications, diagnosis of rejection, management of the exocrine secretions, and improved surgical techniques have dramatically improved success rates. There were 898 kidney/pancreas transplants and 548 pancreas-only transplants performed in 2003; however, the number of patients awaiting kidney/pancreas or pancreas-only transplants in 2003 was 3619.[3] The advances in immunosuppressant medications and diagnosis of rejection have resulted in 1-year patient and graft survival rates of 92% and 80%, respectively.[149]

Selection for Transplantation

Patients who are selected for pancreas transplantation must undergo a thorough medical examination similar to that for other transplant candidates (Box 41-23). The disease processes involved in diabetes mellitus and their effect on all major body systems require that special care be taken to ensure the candidate is in the best possible condition before transplantation. Severe and often life-threatening complications can occur posttransplantation if the major body systems have not been properly evaluated before transplantation.

Box 41-23

PANCREAS TRANSPLANTATION PRETESTING

- Blood chemistries, tissue typing, and viral studies similar to those for kidney transplant candidates
- Complete cardiovascular work-up, including cardiac catheterization
- Complete vascular studies, particularly of the lower extremities, to ensure proper vascularization of the graft
- Nerve conduction studies to evaluate for neuropathy
- Urologic and bladder-function studies
- Consultations as required for all transplant candidates

PANCREAS TRANSPLANT SURGICAL PROCEDURE

The surgical techniques for pancreas transplantation are diverse, and no standard methodology is used by all programs. The principles are consistent and include the following three concepts:

1. Provide adequate arterial blood flow to the pancreas and duodenal segment.
2. Provide adequate venous outflow of the pancreas via the portal vein.
3. Provide management of the pancreatic exocrine secretions.

The native pancreas is not removed. The majority of transplant centers put the pancreas on the right and the kidney on the left (Fig. 41-15). However, a few transplant centers place both organs on the right side as shown in Fig. 41-16.

Arterial Blood Flow to the Pancreas and Duodenal Segment. Pancreas graft arterial revascularization typically is accomplished using the recipient right common or external iliac artery. The Y graft of the pancreas is anastomosed end-to-side. Positioning of the head of the pancreas graft cephalad or caudad is not relevant with respect to successful arterial revascularization.

Venous Outflow via Portal Vein. The entire iliac vein is dissected from the vena cava to the distal external iliac vein. All the deep internal iliac venous branches are divided. The portal vein is then anastomosed end-to-side to the common iliac vein and the donor iliac Y extension graft is anastomosed end-to-side to the common iliac artery illustrated in Fig. 41-17.

Bowel or Bladder Drainage of Pancreatic Exocrine Secretions. Handling the exocrine drainage of the pancreas is one of the most challenging aspects of the transplantation procedure. Drainage to the bowel offers the most physiologic way of handling the exocrine secretions as illustrated in Fig. 41-18. The graft is usually placed intraperitoneally. The abdomen is entered through a midline incision. The peritoneum is incised over the common iliac artery from the aortic bifurcation to the distal por-

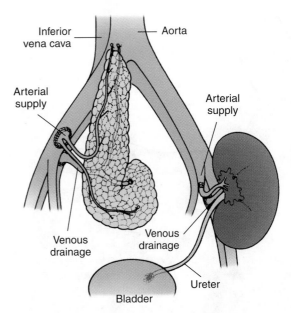

Fig. 41-15 Placement of organs during simultaneous kidney-pancreas transplant. (Modified from Smith SL: *AACN tissue and organ transplantation: implications for professional nursing practice,* St Louis, 1990, Mosby.)

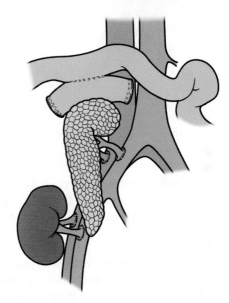

Fig. 41-16 Ipsilateral placement of simultaneous pancreas and kidney allograph. (Copyright Indiana University School of Medicine, Office of Visual Media.)

tion of the external iliac artery. The native ureter is identified and preserved.

The urinary diversion option for pancreatic exocrine drainage is handled by an anastomosis of the duodenal segment to the bladder as seen in Fig. 41-19.

Enteric Drainage Advantages. Approximately 75% of pancreas transplantations are performed with enteric (bowel) drainage, while the remainder are performed with urinary diversion (bladder drainage).

Enteric drainage is the draining of exocrine secretions

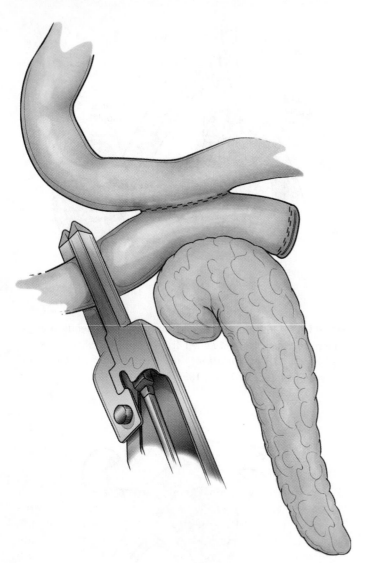

Fig. 41-17 Exocrine management by bowel diversion. Segment of donor bowel remains attached to minimize handling of pancreas. (Copyright Indiana University School of Medicine, Office of Visual Media.)

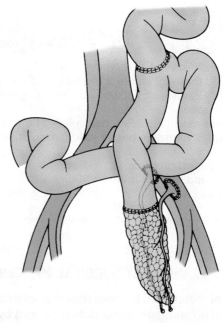

Fig. 41-18 Exocrine management by enteric drainage (Roux-en-Y jejunum). (Modified from Smith SL: *AACN tissue and organ transplantation: implications for professional nursing practice*, St Louis, 1990, Mosby.)

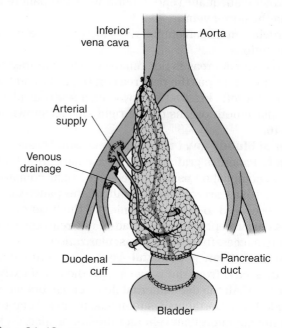

Fig. 41-19 Exocrine management by urinary diversion. (Modified from Smith SL: *AACN tissue and organ transplantation: implications for professional nursing practice*, St Louis, 1990, Mosby.)

into the bowel. The pancreas, with a segment of the donor duodenum, is transplanted onto the recipients' small bowel. All of the enzymes are then drained into the bowel and excreted with the stool. Enteric drainage of pancreas grafts is physiologic with respect to the delivery of pancreatic enzymes and bicarbonate into the intestines for resorption. Enteric drainage has many advantages. Patients experience fewer metabolic, infectious, and dysfunctional bladder complications. It is associated with lower reoperation and leakage rates. However, it does have a major disadvantage in that the bladder drainage allows for monitoring of pancreatic enzymes, as a direct measure of pancreatic function, and the enteric drainage does not. With the successful application of the new immunosuppressant agents and the reduction of the incidences of rejection, enteric drainage of the pancreas transplantations has enjoyed a successful rebirth.

Ischemic Time. The cold ischemia time of the pancreas before implantation should be minimized. Pancreas allografts do not tolerate cold ischemia as well as kidney allografts. Ideally the pancreas should be revascularized within 24 hours from the time of cross-clamping at procurement.

Simultaneous Kidney-Pancreas Transplant. Simultaneous kidney-pancreas transplant has a higher risk of complications; however, it is also associated with better graft outcomes. Simultaneous kidney-pancreas transplant is associated with higher rates of technical complications, lower rejection rates, higher-risk patients, longer time on waiting list, and, with a patient currently undergoing continuous peritoneal ambulatory dialysis, a higher risk of intraabdominal infection and ascites.

Pancreas Transplant After Kidney Transplant. Pancreas transplant after kidney transplant has a lower risk of complications; however, it is associated with poorer graft outcomes. A pancreas transplant after a kidney transplant is associated with lower technical complications, better kidney (possibly living related donor), and lower risk of leakage. However, with different donors for each organ, the possibility for immunologic complications increases.

POSTTRANSPLANT MEDICAL MANAGEMENT AND NURSING CARE

After surgery the patient is taken to the intensive care unit. Even though these patients now have a functioning pancreas, they are at high risk for surgical complications because of the long-term effects of diabetes. Oxygenation, hemodynamics, and cardiac status must be monitored closely. If a simultaneous kidney transplant is performed, fluid and electrolyte management is indicated including intravenous fluid replacement, monitoring intake and output, and monitoring potassium, BUN, and creatinine levels. A nasogastric tube is usually placed and remains for 24 to 48 hours after surgery.

A continuous insulin drip may be placed to rest the graft, maintaining blood glucose levels between 130 and 170 mg/dl. Frequent blood glucose monitoring is essential for patient safety while on the continuous insulin infusion.

The same aseptic techniques used for kidney transplant recipients are used for pancreas transplant recipients. An increased potential for urinary drainage catheter (Foley) occlusion exists for pancreas transplant recipients who undergo the urinary diversion technique. The enzymes make the urine more viscous, and they irritate the anastomosis site on the bladder, causing an increased risk of bleeding. The same gentle aspiration techniques can be used to clear out the clots. Continuous bladder irrigation may be necessary to keep the catheter flowing (see the Nursing Diagnoses feature on Pancreas Transplantation).

PATIENT EDUCATION

Patient education is provided to cover all aspects of the immunosuppressive medication regimen, risk for infection, blood glucose testing, and signs and symptoms of

---

NURSING DIAGNOSES | Pancreas Transplantation

- Risk for Infection risk factor: immunosuppressive drugs required to prevent rejection of pancreas
- Imbalanced Nutrition: Less Than Body Requirements related to lack of exogenous nutrients and increased metabolic demand
- Disturbed Body Image related to actual change in body structure, function, or appearance
- Anxiety related to threat to biologic, psychologic, and/or social integrity
- Activity Intolerance related to prolonged immobility or deconditioning
- Readiness for Enhanced Knowledge: Posttransplant Self-Care Regimen, immunosuppressive drugs and clinical manifestation of infection

---

recurrent diabetes. In addition, long-term considerations and a schedule of follow-up visits are always reviewed.

LONG-TERM CONSIDERATIONS

Rejection in this patient population may be very difficult to detect. Serum amylase levels in pancreas-only transplant are not effective in monitoring graft function, and blood glucose levels become elevated only in the late stages of rejection. Urine amylase levels in patients with the urinary diversion are an effective means of monitoring for rejection. If a kidney transplant is performed simultaneously with the pancreas, an increase in the serum creatinine level is predictive of rejection. Because of the fragility of pancreas tissue, a pancreas biopsy is rarely performed. However, a renal biopsy specimen may be obtained to determine rejection and treatment options. Treatment of pancreas rejection is the same as treatment for all other types of organ rejection.

Compliance with the medication regimen is always a concern. Taking the immunosuppressants as prescribed by the physicians is very important. Patients with functional pancreas grafts continue to need glucose monitoring at home, and often forget to do so since they no longer require insulin. Continued monitoring with frequent clinic visits is required for several months after transplant.

Islet Cell Transplantation. Islet cell transplantation continues to be investigational. Research continues to be conducted in this dynamic field and perhaps one day will allow for a nonsurgical means of transplantation. As with all other organs, donors are in short supply. Finding ways to increase the number of donors, perfecting surgical techniques, and developing advances in immunosuppressant medications will offer an insulin-free treatment option and may one day represent the treatment of choice for insulin-dependent DM.[149]

SUMMARY

The fields of organ donation and solid organ transplantation have made dramatic progress in the last 50 years. There is every reason to believe that this trajectory will continue. As transplantation becomes more widespread, more nurses will encounter a patient who has undergone a solid organ transplant. Even more likely is that a critical care nurse will assist with the care of a potential organ donor. Knowledge of the rationales for care is essential to delivering safe and high-quality patient care.

REFERENCES

1. Beecher HK: A definition of irreversible coma: report of the Harvard Medical School committee to examine the definition of brain death, *JAMA* 205(6):337-340, 1968.
2. Uniform Brain Death Act, 12 Uniform Law Annotated (ULA) 15 (1978) (superseded by Uniform Determination of Death Act, 12 ULA. 236 (Supp. 1982).
3. United Network for Organ Sharing (UNOS): on the Internet at www.unos.org.
4. National Organ Transplant Act of 1984, Pub. L. 98-507, 98 Stat. 2339 (1984).
5. Organ Donation and Recovery Improvement Act of 2004, Pub. L. 108-216 (H.R. 3926).
6. National Transplant Act of 1984, Title 42, US Code (USC), beginning Section 273.
7. Title 42, Public Health. Chapter IV, Part 482, Subpart C, Section 482.45.
8. Ehrle R, Shafer T, Nelson K: Referral, request, and consent for organ donation: best practice—a blueprint for success, *Crit Care Nurse* 19(2):32, 1999.
9. Verble M, Worth J: Adequate consent: its content in the donation discussion, *J Transplant Coordination* 8(2): 101, 1998.
10. Riley L, Coolican M: Needs of families of organ donors: facing death and life, *Crit Care Nurse* 19(2):53, 1999.
11. Verble M, Worth J: Overcoming families' fears and concerns in the donation discussion, *Progress in Transplantation* 10(3):155, 2000.
12. Division of Health Care Services: Non-heart-beating organ transplantation: practice and protocols, *IOM*, 2001.
13. Sullivan J, Seem D, Chabalewski F: Determining brain death, *Crit Care Nurse* 19(2):1999.
14. Wijdicks EFM: Determining brain death in adults, *Neurology* 45:1003, 1995.
15. Powner DJ, Darby JM, Kellum JA: Proposed treatment guidelines for donor care, *Progr Transplantation* 14(1): 16-26, 2004.
16. Department of Health and Human Services: Health Care Financing Administration. Medicare and Medicaid Programs; Hospital Conditions of Participation; Identification of Potential Organ, Tissue, and Eye Donors and Transplant Hospitals. Provision of Transplant-Related Data. Final Rule.63, *Fed Reg* 63(119):33856-33875, 1998.
17. McCoy J, Argue P: The role of critical care nurses in organ donation: a case study, *Crit Care Nurse* 19(2):48-52, 1999.
18. Bartucci MR, Seller MC: The immunology of transplant rejection. In Sigardson-Poor KM, Haggerty LM, editors: *Nursing care of the transplant patient*, Philadelphia, 1990, Saunders.
19. Bierer BE: Immunosuppressive agents targeting T-cell activation pathways. In Sollinger H, Przepiorka D, editors: *Recent developments in transplantation medicine*, vol 1, *New immunosuppressant drugs*, Glenview, Ill, 1994, Physicians & Scientists.
20. Colling EG, Hubbell EA: Immunologic aspects of organ transplantation. In Williams BAH, Grady KL, Sandiford-Guttebiel DM, editors: *Organ transplantation*, New York, 1991, Springer.
21. Young JB: Clinical challenges in thoracic organ transplantation: case studies in immunosuppressive therapy, *J Heart Lung Transplant* 19:718, 2000.
22. Carrier M et al: A 10-year experience with intravenous thymoglobulin in induction of immunosuppression following heart transplantation, *J Heart Lung Transplant* 18: 1218, 1999.
23. Morris RE: Overview of immunosuppressive drugs for transplantation: where are we? How did we get here? And where are we going? *Clin Transplant* 7:138, 1993.
24. Payne JL: Immune modification and complications of immunosuppression, *Crit Care Nurs Clin North Am* 4:43, 1992.
25. Schreiber SL, Crabtree GR: The mechanism of action of cyclosporin A and FK506, *Immunol Today* 13:136, 1992.
26. Crandell B: Immunosuppression. In Sigardson-Poor KM, Haggerty LM, editors: *Nursing care of the transplant recipient*, Philadelphia, 1990, Saunders.
27. White M et al: Pharmacokinetic, hemodynamic, and metabolic effects of cyclosporine Sandimmune versus the microemulsion Neoral in heart transplant recipients, *J Heart Lung Transplant* 16:787, 1997.
28. Meulle EA et al: Pharmacokinetics and tolerability of a microemulsion formulation of cyclosporine in renal allograft recipients—a concentration-controlled comparison with the commercial formulation, *Transplantation* 57:1178, 1994.
29. Eisen HJ et al: Multicenter, double-blind, randomized study of Neoral vs Sandimmune in heart transplantation: one year results, *J Heart Lung Transplant* 18:93, 1999.
30. Steinberg SM et al: Randomized, open label preference study of two cyclosporine capsule formulations (usp modified) in stable solid-organ transplant recipients, *Clin Ther* 25(7):2037, 2003.
31. Staschak SM, Zamberlan K: Recent development: FK506. In Sigardson-Poor KM, Haggerty LM, editors: *Nursing care of the transplant recipient*, Philadelphia, 1990, Saunders.
32. Przepiorka D: Tacrolimus: preclinical and clinical experience. In Sollinger H, Przepiorka D, editors: *Recent developments in transplantation medicine*, vol 1, *New immunosuppressant drugs*, Glenview, Ill, 1994, Physicians & Scientists.
33. Young CJ, Sollinger H: Mycophenolate mofetil (RS-61443). In Sollinger H, Przepiorka D, editors: *Recent developments in transplantation medicine, vol 1, New immunosuppressant drugs*, Glenview, Ill, 1994, Physicians & Scientists.
34. Allison AC, Eugui EM, Sollinger HW: Mycophenolate mofetil (RS-61443): mechanisms of action and effects in transplantation, *Transplant Reviews* 7:129, 1993.

35. White-Williams C: Immunosuppressive therapy following cardiac transplantation, *Crit Care Nurs Q* 16:1, 1993.

36. Morris RE: New immunosuppressive molecules for control of organ transplant rejection. In Williams BAH, Sandiford-Guttenbiel DM, editors: *Trends in organ transplantation,* New York, 1996, Springer.

37. Pethig K et al: Mycophenolate mofetil for secondary prevention of allograft vasculopathy following heart transplantation: a prospective, randomized, intravascular ultrasound controlled trial, *J Heart Lung Transplant* 18:77, 1999.

38. Keogh A et al: Three-year results of the double-blind randomized multicenter trial of mycophenolate mofetil in heart transplant patients, *J Heart Lung Transplant* 18: 53, 1999.

39. Pethig K et al: Mycophenolate mofetil for secondary prevention of cardiac allograft vasculopathy: Influence on inflammation and progression of intimal hyperplasia, *J Heart Lung Transplant* 23:61, 2000.

40. Eisenberg MS et al: Elevated levels of plasma C-reactive protein are associated with decreased graft survival in cardiac transplant recipients, *Circulation* 102:2100, 2000.

41. Meier-Kreische H et al: Mycophenolate mofetil versus azathioprine therapy is associated with a significant protection against long-term renal allograft function deterioration, *Transplantation* 75:1341, 2003.

42. Ingle GT et al: Sirolimus: continuing the evolution of transplant immunosuppression, *Ann Pharmacother* 34:1044, 2000.

43. McAlister VC et al: Sirolimus-tacrolimus combination immunosuppression, *Lancet* 355:376, 2000.

44. Radovancevic B, Vrtovec B: Sirolimus therapy in cardiac transplantation, *Transplant Proc* 35:171S, 2003.

45. Mancini D et al: Use of Rapamycin slows progression of cardiac transplantation vasculopathy, *Circulation* 108:48, 2003.

46. Eisen H et al: Everolimus for the prevention of allograft rejection and vasculopathy in cardiac transplant recipients, *New Engl J Med* 349:847, 2003.

47. Kahan BD et al: Immunosuppressive effects and safety of a sirolimus/cyclosporine combination regime for renal transplantation, *Transplantation* 66:1040, 1998.

48. Watson CJE et al: Sirolimus: a potent new immunosuppressant for liver transplantation, *Transplantation* 67: 505, 1999.

49. Augustine J et al: Experience with everolimus, *Transplant Proc* 36:500S, 2004.

50. Carrier M, Jenicek M, Pelletier LC: Value of monoclonal antibody OKT3 in solid organ transplantation: a meta-analysis, *Transplant Proc* 24:2586, 1992.

51. Van Gelder T et al: A randomized trial comparing safety and efficacy of OKT3 and a monoclonal anti-interleukin-2 receptor antibody (BT563) in the prevention of acute rejection after heart transplantation, *Transplantation* 62: 51, 1996.

52. Pascual J et al: Anti-interleukin-2 receptor antibodies: basiliximab and daclizumab, *Nephrol Dialysis Transplant* 16:1756, 2001.

53. Webster A et al: Interleukin 2 receptor antagonists for renal transplant recipients: a meta-analysis of randomized trials, *Transplantation* 77:166, 2004.

54. Cherikh WS et al: Association of the type of induction immunosuppression with posttransplant lymphoproliferative disorder, graft survival, and patient survival after primary kidney transplantation, *Transplantation* 76:1289, 2003.

55. Reitz B: The history of heart and heart-lung transplantation. In Baumgartner WA, Reitz BA, Achuff SC, editors: *Heart and heart-lung transplantation,* Philadelphia, 1990, Saunders.

56. Losse B: Indications and selection criteria for cardiac transplantation, *Thorac Cardiovasc Surg* 38:276, 1990.

57. Dillon TA et al: Cardiac transplantation in patients with preexisting malignancies, *Transplantation* 52:82, 1991.

58. Edwards BS et al: Cardiac transplantation in patients with preexisting neoplastic diseases, *Am J Cardiol* 65:501, 1990.

59. Badellino NM et al: Cardiac transplantation in diabetic patients, *Transplant Proc* 22:2384, 1990.

60. Ladowski JS et al: Heart transplantation in diabetic recipients, *Transplantation* 49:303, 1990.

61. Rhenman MJ et al: Diabetics and heart transplantation, *J Heart Transplant* 7:356, 1988.

62. Hurst JW et al: *The heart,* ed 7, New York, 1990, McGraw-Hill.

63. Aziz TM et al: Orthotopic cardiac transplantation technique: a survey of current practice, *Ann Thorac Surg* 68: 1242, 1999.

64. Rees AP et al: Valvular regurgitation and right-side cardiac pressures in heart transplant recipients by complete Doppler and color flow evaluation, *Chest* 104:82, 1993.

65. Angerman CE et al: Anatomic characteristics and valvular function of the transplanted heart: thoracic versus transesophageal echocardiographic findings, *J Heart Transplant* 9:331, 1990.

66. Jacquet L et al: Cardiac rhythm disturbance early after orthotopic heart transplantation: prevalence and clinical importance of observed abnormality, *J Am Coll Cardiol* 16:832, 1990.

67. Sievers HH et al: An alternative technique for orthotopic cardiac transplantation with preservation of the normal anatomy of the right atrium, *Thorac Cardiovasc* 39:70, 1991.

68. Miniati DH Robbins RC: Techniques in orthotopic cardiac transplantation: a review, *Cardiol Rev* 9131, 2001.

69. Brandt M: Influence of bicaval anastomoses on late occurrence of atrial arrhythmia after heart transplantation, *Ann Thorac Surg* 64:70, 1997.

70. Dibiase A et al: Frequency and mechanism of bradycardia in cardiac transplant recipients and need for pacemakers, *Am J Cardiol* 67:1385, 1991.

71. Whitman GR, Hicks LE: Major nursing diagnoses following cardiac transplantation, *J Cardiovasc Nurs* vol 2, 1988.

72. Billingham ME et al: A working formulation for the standardization of nomenclature in the diagnosis of heart and lung rejection: heart rejection study group, *J Heart Lung Transplant* 9:587, 1990.

73. Hunt SA et al: Total lymphoid irradiation for treatment of intractable cardiac allograft rejection, *J Heart Lung Transplant* 10:211, 1991.

74. Futterman LG: Cardiac transplantation: a comprehensive nursing perspective, II, *Heart Lung* 17:631-638, 1988.

75. Merigan TC et al: A controlled trial of ganciclovir to prevent cytomegalovirus disease after heart transplantation, *N Engl J Med* 326:1182, 1992.

76. Patel R et al: Cytomegalovirus prophylaxis in solid organ transplant recipients, Transplantation, 61:1279, 1996.

77. Snydman DR et al: Final analysis of primary cytomegalovirus disease prevention in renal transplant recipients with a cytomegalovirus-immune globulin: comparison of the randomized and open label trials, *Transplant Proc* 23:1357, 1991.

78. George MJ et al: Use of ganciclovir plus cytomegalovirus immune globulin to treat CMV pneumonia in orthotopic liver transplant recipients, *Transplant Proc* 25:22-24, 1993.

79. Cytomegalovirus infections in the immunocompromised transplant patient: diagnosis and treatment (special symposium review), San Francisco, 1991, Professional Healthcare Communications.

80. Gao S et al: Accelerated coronary vascular disease in the heart transplant patient: coronary arteriographic findings, *J Am Coll Cardiol* 12:334, 1988.

81. Sharples LD et al: Risk factor analysis for the major hazards following heart transplantation, rejection, infection and coronary occlusive disease, *Transplantation* 52:244, 1991.

82. Stark RP, McGinn AL, Wilson RF: Chest pain in cardiac transplant recipients, *N Engl J Med* 324:1791, 1991.

83. Decampli WM et al: Characteristics of patients surviving more than ten years after cardiac transplantation, *J Thoracic Cardiovasc Surg* 109:1103, 1995.

84. Lough ME et al: Impact of symptom frequency and symptom distress on self-reported quality of life in heart transplant recipients, *Heart Lung* 16:193, 1987.

85. Packa RD: Quality of life of adults after a heart transplant, *J Cardiovasc Nurs* 13:12, 1989.

86. Evans RW et al: *The national heart transplantation study: final report*, Seattle, 1984, Battelle Human Affairs Research Centers.

87. Lough ME: Quality of life issues following heart transplantation, *Prog Cardiovasc Nurs* 1:17, 1986.

88. Marshall SE et al: Selection and evaluation of recipients for heart-lung and lung transplantation, *Chest* 98:1488, 1990.

89. Egan TM, Kaiser LR, Cooper JD: Lung transplantation, *Curr Probl Surg* 10:673, 1989.

90. Hutter JA: Heart-lung transplantation: better use of resources, *Am J Med* 85:4, 1988.

91. Klepetko W et al: Domino transplantation of heart-lung and heart: an approach to overcome the scarcity of donor organs, *J Heart Lung Transplant* 10:129, 1991.

92. Theodore J, Lewiston N: Lung transplantation comes of age, *N Engl J Med* 322:772, 1991.

93. Hakim M et al: Selection and procurement of combined heart and lung grafts for transplantation, *J Thorac Cardiovasc Surg* 95:474, 1988.

94. Starnes V: Heart-lung transplantation: an overview, *Cardiol Clin* 8:159, 1990.

95. Starnes VA et al: Cystic fibrosis: target population for lung transplantation in North America in the 1990s, *J Thorac Cardiovasc Surg* 103(5):1008, 1992.

96. Conte JV, Reitz B: Operative technique of single-lung, bilateral lung, and heart-lung transplantation. In Baumgartner WA, Reitz BA, Achuff SC, editors: *Heart and heart-lung transplantation*, Philadelphia, 1990, Saunders.

97. Valentine VG et al: Clinical diagnosis in heart and lung allograft rejection. In Solez K, Racusen LC, Billingham ME, editors: *Solid organ transplant rejection*, New York, 1996, Marcel Dekker.

98. Yousem SA et al: A working formulation for the standardization of nomenclature in the diagnosis of heart and lung rejection: lung rejection study group, *J Heart Lung Transplant* 9:593, 1990.

99. Theodore J: Pulmonary function in the uncomplicated human transplanted lung, *ACP* 2:301, 1987.

100. Baldwin JC: Comparison of cardiac rejection in heart and heart-lung transplantation, *J Heart Transplant* 6:352, 1987.

101. Theodore J, Starnes VA, Lewiston NJ: Obliterative bronchiolitis, *Clin Chest Med* 11:309, 1998.

102. Glanville AR et al: Obliterative bronchiolitis after heart-lung transplantation: apparent arrest by augmented immunosuppression, *Ann Intern Med* 107:300, 1987.

103. Starnes VA et al: Current trends in lung transplantation: lobar transplantation and expanded use of single lungs, *J Thorac Cardiovasc Surg* 104:1060, 1992.

104. Meyers BF, Patterson A: Lung transplantation: Current status and future prospects, *World J Surg* 23:1156, 1999.

105. Cooper JD et al: Bilateral pneumectomy (volume reduction) for chronic obstructive pulmonary disease, *J Thoracic Cardiovasc Surg* 109:116-119, 1995.

106. Cohen RG, Starnes VA: Living donor lung transplantation, *World J Surg* 25:244, 2001.

107. Marshall SE et al: Prospective analysis of serial pulmonary function studies, transbronchial biopsies in single-lung transplant recipients, *Transplant Proc* 23:1217, 1991.

108. Gaissert HA et al: Comparison of early functional results after volume reduction or lung transplantation for chronic obstructive pulmonary disease, *J Thoracic Cardiovasc Surg* 111:296, 1996.

109. Welch CS: A note on transplantation of the whole liver in dogs, *Transplant Bulletin* 2(2):54, 1955.

110. Cannon GA: Organs, *Transplant Bulletin* 3(1):7, 1956 (communication).

111. Moore FD et al: One-stage homotransplantation of the liver following total hepatectomy in dogs, *Transplant Bulletin* 6:103, 1959.

112. Moore FD et al: Experimental whole organ transplantation of the liver and of the spleen, *Ann Surg* 152(3):374, 1960.

113. Starzl TE et al: Reconstructive problems in canine homotransplantation with special reference to the postoperative role of hepatic vein flow, *Surg Gynecol Obstet* 11:733, 1960.

114. Starzl TE et al: Homotransplantation of the liver in humans, *Surg Gynecol Obstet* 117(6):659, 1963.

115. Starzl TE et al: Orthotopic homotransplantation of the human liver, *Ann Surg* 168(3):392, 1968.

116. Cosimi AB: Update on liver transplantation, *Transplant Proc* 23(4):2083, 1991.

117. Starzl TE et al: Liver transplantation with the use of cyclosporin A and prednisone, *N Engl J Med* 305:266, 1981.

118. National Institutes of Health: National Institutes of Health Consensus Development Conference Statement: liver transplantation—June 20-23, 1983, *Hepatology* 4(1S):107S, 1984.

119. Cupples SA, Ohler L: *Transplantation nursing secrets*, Philadelphia, Pa, 2003, Hanley & Belfus.

120. Terrault NA: Hepatitis C virus and liver transplantation, *Semin Gastrointest Dis 2000*, 11(2):96, 2000.

121. Ginns L, Cosimi A, Morris P: *Transplantation*, Malden, Mass, 1999, Blackwell Science.

122. Cupples, SA and Ohler, L (editors): *Solid organ transplantation: a handbook for primary care providers*, New York, 2002, Springer.

123. Lake JR: Transplantation for chronic viral hepatitis. In Busuttil RW, Klintmalm GB, editors: *Transplantation of the liver*, Philadelphia, 1996, Saunders.

124. Harren P et al: Incidence and treatment of recurrent hepatitis C after liver transplantation, *J Transplant Coordination* 6:24, 1996.

125. Crippen J: Transplantation for sclerosing cholangitis. In Busuttil RW, Klintmalm GB, editors: *Transplantation of the liver*, Philadelphia, 1996, Saunders.

126. Porayko MK, Kondo M, Steers JL: Liver transplantation: late complications of the biliary tract and their management, *Semin Liver Dis* 15:139, 1995.

127. Baker M, McWilliams C: How patients manage life and health while waiting for a liver transplant, *Progress Transplant* 13(1):47, 2003.

128. Farges O et al: Long-term results of ABO-incompatible liver transplantation, *Transplant Proc* 27:1701, 1995.

129. Ojo A et al: Chronic renal failure after transplantation of a non-renal organ, *N Engl J Med* 349(10):931, 2003.

130. Preksaitis J, Green M, Avery R, editors: *American Society of Transplantation Infectious Disease Community of Practice Infectious Disease Guidelines,* Mt Laurel, NJ, 2004, American Society of Transplantation.

131. Randolf S, Sholtz K: Self care guidelines: finding a common ground, *J Transplant Coordination* 9(3):156, 1999.

132. Thomas DJ: The lived experience of people with liver transplants, *J Transplant Coordination* 5:65, 1995.

133. Morrissey M, Rustand L: Financial consideration in liver transplantation. In Busuttil RW, Klintmalm GB, editors: *Transplantation of the liver,* Philadelphia, 1996, Saunders.

134. Whiteman K et al: The effect of continuous lateral rotation therapy on pulmonary complications in liver transplant, *Am J Crit Care* 4(2):133, 1995.

135. Eason J et al: Steroid-free liver transplantation using rabbit antithymocyte globulin and early tacrolimus therapy, *Transplantation* 75(8):1396, 2003.

136. Nair S et al: Sirolimus monotherapy in nephrotoxicity due to calcineurin inhibitors in liver transplant recipients, *Liver Transplant* 9(2):126, 2003.

137. Prince M, Hudson J: Liver transplantation for chronic liver disease: advances and controversies in an era of organ shortage, *Postgrad Med J* 78:135, 2002.

138. Stuart F, Abecassis M, Kaufman, D: *Organ transplantation,* ed 2, Georgetown, Tx, 2003, Landis Bioscience.

139. Loss G et al: Does lamivudine prophylaxis eradicate persistent HBV DNA from allografts derived from anti-HBc positive donors? *Liver Transplant* 9(12):1258, 2003.

140. Brown R et al: A survey of liver transplantation from living adult donors in the U.S., *N Engl J Med* 348(9):818, 2003.

141. Kuo P, Stock P: Transplantation in the HIV⁺ patient, *Am J Transplant* 1:13, 2001.

142. Fisher R et al: Quality of life after renal transplantation, *J Clin Nurs* 7(6):553, 1998.

143. Clayton LH, Dilley KB: Cushing's syndrome, *Am J Nurs* 98(7):40, 1998.

144. Bush WW: Overview of transplantation immunology and pharmacotherapy of adult solid organ transplant recipients: focus on immunosuppression, *AACN Clin Issues Adv Pract Acute Crit Care* 10(2):253, 1999.

145. Cerilli GJ: *Organ transplantation and replacement,* Philadelphia, 1988, Lippincott.

146. Simmons RL et al: *Manual of vascular access, organ donation, and transplantation,* London, 1984, Springer-Verlag.

147. Kumar A et al: Combined kidney and pancreatic transplantation: ideal for patients with uncomplicated type 1 diabetes and chronic renal failure, *Br Med J* 318(7188):886, 1999.

148. Steen DC: Current state of pancreas transplantation, *AACN Clin Issues Adv Pract Acute Crit Care* 10(2):164, 1999.

149. Robertson RP et al: Pancreas and islet transplantation for patients with diabetes, *Diabetes Care* 23(1):112-116, 2000.

*U*nderstanding the pathology of a disease, the areas of assessment on which to focus, and the usual medical management allows the critical care nurse to more accurately anticipate and plan nursing interventions. This chapter focuses on hematologic and oncologic disorders commonly seen in the critical care environment.

OVERVIEW OF COAGULATION AND FIBRINOLYSIS

Hemostasis, the ability of the body to control bleeding and clotting, is an intricate balancing act between the coagulation mechanism and fibrinolysis. There are four major actions involved in achieving hemostasis: (1) local vasoconstriction to reduce blood flow; (2) platelet aggregation at the injury site and formation of a platelet plug; (3) formation of a fibrin mesh to strengthen the plug; and finally (4) dissolution of the clot once tissue repair is complete.[1] Disruption of the normal hemostatic balance can result in devastating hemorrhagic or thrombotic conditions.

COAGULATION MECHANISM

The coagulation mechanism consists of 13 factors that work together through a series of feedback loops to achieve hemostasis (Table 42-1 and Fig. 42-1). Depending on the initial triggering event, either the extrinsic or intrinsic coagulation pathways will be intiated.[1,2] The extrinsic pathway begins when vascular injury occurs, resulting in release of tissue factor and activation of coagulation factor VII. The intrinsic pathway is activated when the damaged subendothelium comes into direct contact with circulating blood. In this contact phase, proteins activate additional coagulation factors (XII, XI, IX, and VIII).[1] It is at this point that the two pathways converge into a common pathway where prothrombin and fibrinogen are converted to their active forms, resulting in clot formation.[3,4]

CLOT FORMATION

Platelets are activated by the arrival of thrombin at the site of injury (Fig. 42-2).[2] Local platelets change shape and become sticky, beginning to aggregate along the vessel wall. Activated platelets undergo degranulation, releasing several factors to assist in clot formation. Serotonin and histamine, two potent vasoconstrictors, help limit blood loss while the clot is forming. The prostaglandin thromboxane A_2 (TxA_2) contributes to vasoconstriction and promotes further platelet degranulation. Adenosine diphosphate (ADP) recruits platelets by increasing adherence and degranulation.[2,3] Thus the process continues.

At the convergence of the intrinsic and extrinsic pathways, factor X is converted into its active form, thereby allowing the conversion of prothrombin to thrombin. Thrombin then converts fibrinogen to fibrin. Strands of fibrin form and radiate around the newly formed clot, essentially creating a net in which platelets, red blood cells, and white blood cells (WBCs) are trapped.[1] Finally, the clot is further secured to the site as platelet actomyosin causes it to contract and consolidate.[2]

REGULATORY MECHANISMS

Under normal conditions, there are feedback systems that prevent the coagulation process from spinning out of control. Prostacyclin-I_2 (PGI_2) is a prostaglandin released from damaged endothelial cells. It functions to counteract the effects of TxA_2, serotonin, and histamine through vasodilation and inhibition of platelet degranulation.[1-3] Another means of regulating clot formation is through inhibition of enzymes necessary for activation of coagulation factors along both the intrinsic and extrinsic pathways, resulting in the inability to convert prothrombin to thrombin. The most important of these is antithrombin III; however, both protein C and protein S play a role in thrombin inhibition.[5]

FIBRINOLYSIS

The process of fibrinolysis promotes dissolution and remolding of the clot to promote repair of the vessel wall

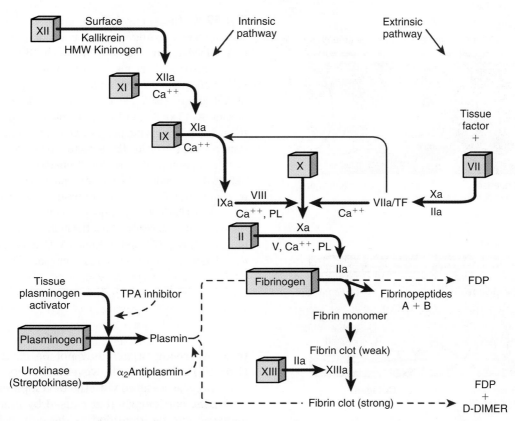

Fig. 42-1 Coagulation cascade. Fibrin clot formation results from the generation of thrombin, which is dependent on the sequential interaction of proenzymes and activated coagulation factors in the intrinsic, extrinsic, and common pathways of coagulation. *HMW,* High–molecular-weight; *PL,* phospholipids; *FDP,* fibrin degradation product; *Ca^{++},* calcium. (From Noble J: *Textbook of primary care medicine,* ed 3, St Louis, 2001, Mosby.)

Table 42-1	Coagulation Factors and Common Names
Factor	**Common Name**
I	Fibrinogen
II	Prothrombin
III	Tissue factor
IV	Calcium
V	Proaccelerin
VI	Accelerin
VII	Proconvertin
VIII	Antihemophilic
IX	Christmas factor
X	Stuart
XI	Plasma thromboplastin antecedent
XII	Hageman factor
XIII	Fibrin stabilizing factor

and maintain flow through the vessel lumen (Fig. 42-2, *D*).[2] Fibrinolysis begins as soon as the fibrin clot is formed. Circulating plasminogen, a precursor to the powerful enzyme plasmin, binds to fibrin and is trapped within the newly formed clot. The injured epithelial wall releases tissue plasminogen activator (tPA) which converts the plasminogen to its active state, plasmin. The plasmin begins to digest the fibrin, rapidly breaking down the clot.[2,4] When fibrin is broken down, fibrin degradation products are released that act as anticoagulants as well.

DISSEMINATED INTRAVASCULAR COAGULATION

DESCRIPTION

Disseminated intravascular coagulation (DIC) is a syndrome that arises as a complication of other serious or life-threatening conditions. Although not likely to be seen often, it can seriously hamper diagnosis and treatment efforts in the critically ill patient. An understanding of the etiology and pathophysiologic mechanisms of DIC can assist in anticipation of the occurrence of the syndrome, recognition of signs and symptoms, and prompt intervention. Also known as consumptive coagulopathy, DIC is characterized by both bleeding and thrombosis, which result from depletion of clotting factors, platelets,

A Vasoconstriction

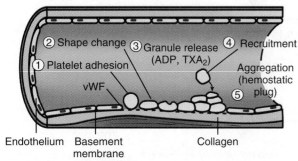

B Primary Hemostasis

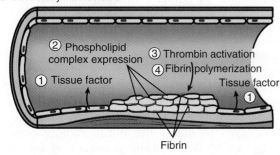

C Secondary Hemostasis

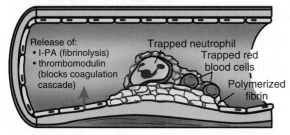

D Thrombus and Antithrombotic Events

Fig. 42-2 Diagrammatic representation of the normal hemostatic process. **A,** After vascular injury, local neurohumoral factors induce a transient vasoconstriction. **B,** Platelets adhere to exposed extracellular matrix (ECM) via von Willebrand factor (vWF) and are activated, undergoing a shape change and granule release; released adenosine diphosphate (ADP) and thromboxane A_2 (TxA_2) lead to further platelet aggregation to form the primary hemostatic plug. **C,** Local activation of the coagulation cascade (involving tissue factor and platelet phospholipids) results in fibrin polymerization, "cementing" the platelets into a definitive secondary hemostatic plug. **D,** Counterregulatory mechanisms, such as release of tissue type plasminogen activator (t-PA) (fibrinolytic) and thrombomodulin (interfering with the coagulation cascade), limit the hemostatic process to the site of injury. (From Cotran RS, Kumar V, Collins T: *Robbins pathologic basis of disease,* ed 6, Philadelphia, 1999, Saunders.)

and red blood cells (RBCs). If not treated quickly, DIC will result in multiple organ failure and death.[6]

ETIOLOGY

There are many clinical events that can prompt the development of DIC in the critically ill patient, although the true underlying trigger may not be clearly identifiable (Box 42-1). There are, however, some commonly known conditions associated with the development of DIC.

Sepsis, particularly that caused by gram-negative organisms, can be identified as the culprit in as many as 20% of cases, making it the most common cause of DIC. In this instance, endotoxins serve as a trigger for activation of tissue factor and the extrinsic coagulation pathway. Metabolic acidosis and hypoperfusion associated with shock syndromes can result in increased formation of free radicals and damage to tissues. Again, tissue factor is activated, resulting in DIC. Massive trauma or burns can also be frequently associated with DIC. Direct tissue damage activates the extrinsic coagulation pathway, while damage to endothelial surfaces activates the intrinsic pathway.[3] Obstetric emergencies such as abruptio placenta, retained placenta, or incomplete abortion are also associated with the development of DIC. Tissue factor is notably concentrated in the placenta, so damage or disruption of this structure can activate coagulation pathways resulting in coagulopathy.[7]

PATHOPHYSIOLOGY

Regardless of etiology, the common thread in the development of DIC is damage to the endothelium that results in activation of the coagulation mechanism (Fig. 42-3). The extrinsic coagulation pathway plays a major role in the development of DIC. Direct damage to the endothelium results in the release of tissue factor and activation of this pathway. However, it is the secondary surge of thrombin formation as a result of activation of the intrinsic coagulation pathway that leads to the massive disruption of the delicate balance that is hemostasis. Excessive thrombin formation results in rapid consumption of coagulation factors and depletion of regulatory substances—protein

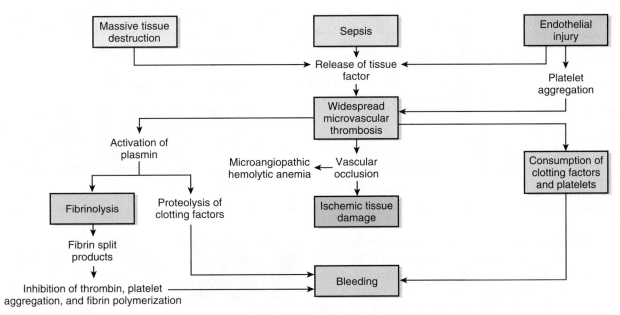

Fig. 42-3 Pathophysiology of disseminated intravascular coagulation. (From Cotran RS, Kumar V, Collins T: *Robbins pathologic basis of disease,* ed 6, Philadelphia, 1999, Saunders.)

Box 42-1

ETIOLOGIES OF DISSEMINATED INTRAVASCULAR COAGULATION

OBSTETRIC COMPLICATIONS
Abruptio placentae
Retained dead fetus
Septic abortion
Amniotic fluid embolism
Toxemia

INFECTIONS
Gram-negative sepsis
Meningococcemia
Rocky Mountain spotted fever
Histoplasmosis
Aspergillosis
Malaria

NEOPLASMS
Carcinomas of pancreas, prostate, lung, and stomach
Acute promyelocytic leukemia

MASSIVE TISSUE INJURY
Traumatic
Burns
Extensive surgery

MISCELLANEOUS
Acute intravascular hemolysis
Snakebite
Giant hemangioma
Shock
Heat stroke
Vasculitis
Aortic aneurysm
Liver disease

From Cotran RS, Kumar V, Collins T: *Robbins pathologic basis of disease,* ed 6, Philadelphia, 1999, Saunders.

C, protein S, and antithrombin.[5] With no checks and balances, thrombi continue to form along damaged epithelial walls, resulting in occlusion of the vessels. As occlusion reaches a critical level, tissue ischemia ensues, leading to further tissue damage and perpetuating the process. Eventually, end-organ function is affected by the ischemia and failure is evident.[8]

In response to the formation of clots, the fibrinolytic system is activated. As plasmin breaks down the fibrin clots, fibrin split products are released and act as anticoagulants as well.[3,7] Coupled with depletion of circulating clotting factors, activation of fibrinolysis results in excessive bleeding. The end result is shock and further tissue ischemia that aggravate end-organ dysfunction and failure. Death is imminent if this destructive cycle is not interrupted.[8]

ASSESSMENT AND DIAGNOSIS

Favorable outcomes in the presence of DIC depend on accurate and timely diagnosis of the condition. Realization of the role underlying pathology plays, recognition of clinical manifestations, and assessment of appropriate laboratory values are key steps in this process.

Clinical Manifestations. Clinical manifestations are related to the two primary pathophysiologic mechanisms present in DIC: the formation of thrombi and bleeding. Thrombi in peripheral capillaries can lead to cyanosis, notably in the fingers, toes, ears, and nose. In severe, untreated cases this peripheral ischemia may progress to gangrene.[3,5,6,9] As the condition progresses, ischemia worsens and end organs are affected. The result of this more central ischemia can be respiratory insufficiency and failure, acute tubular necrosis (ATN), bowel infarct,

Table 42-2	Common Signs and Symptoms of Disseminated Intravascular Coagulation	
System	**Signs Related to Hemorrhage**	**Signs Related to Thrombi**
Integumentary	Bleeding from gums, venipunctures and old surgical sites, epistaxis, ecchymoses	Peripheral cyanosis, gangrene
Cardiopulmonary	Hemoptysis	Dysrhythmias, chest pain, acute myocardial infarction, pulmonary embolus, respiratory failure
Renal	Hematuria	Oliguria, acute tubular necrosis, renal failure
Gastrointestinal	Abdominal distention, hemorrhage	Diarrhea, constipation, bowel infarct
Neurologic	Subarachnoid hemorrhage	Altered level of consciousness, cerebral vascular accident

and cerebral vascular accident (CVA). The tissue damage that results perpetuates the anomalies present in DIC.

As coagulation factors are depleted, bleeding from intravenous (IV) and other puncture sites is noted. Ecchymoses may result from even routine interventions such as the use of a manual blood pressure (BP) cuff, bathing, or turning.[3] Bloody drainage may also be noted from surgical sites, drains, and urinary catheters. With progression of DIC, the patient is at risk for severe gastrointestinal or subarachnoid hemorrhage.[3,6] Table 42-2 lists many of the common signs and symptoms of DIC.

Laboratory Findings. Laboratory tests used to diagnose DIC essentially assess the following four basic characteristics of this syndrome: (1) increased coagulant activity, (2) increased fibrinolytic activity, (3) impaired regulatory function, and (4) the presence of end-organ failure.

Continuous activation of the coagulation pathways results in consumption of coagulation factors. Because of this, the prothrombin time (PT), the activated partial thromboplastin time (aPTT), and the international normalized ratio (INR) will all be elevated. Although the platelet count may fall within normal ranges, serial examination will reveal a declining trend in values. An unexpected drop of at least 50% in the platelet count, particularly in the presence of known contributing factors and associated signs and symptoms, is highly indicative of DIC.[1] In addition, fibrinogen levels drop as more and more clots are formed. Thrombus formation in small vessels narrows the vessel lumen, forcing red blood cells to squeeze through. This results in damage and fragmentation of these cells, which can be seen on microscopic examination of blood samples. Damaged, fragmented red blood cells are called *schistocytes*.[3,6,10]

In response to the excess clotting activity, the fibrinolytic process accelerates and levels of by-products increase. This is reflected in marked elevation of fibrin degradation products (FDP). Another key laboratory test used to evaluate the degree of clot dissolution, and therefore the severity of the coagulopathy, is the D-dimer level.[1] D-dimers are exclusively indicative of clot degradation because, unlike FDPs, which also result from

Table 42-3	Key Laboratory Studies in Disseminated Intravascular Coagulation
Test	**Value**
Prothrombin time (PT)	>12.5 seconds
Platelets	<50,000/mm³, or at least 50% drop from baseline
Activated partial thromboplastin time (aPTT)	>40 seconds
D-dimer	>250 ng/ml
Fibrin degradation products (FDP)	>40 mcg/ml
Fibrinogen	<100 mg/dl

breakdown of free circulating fribrin, D-dimers only result from dissolution of clots.[3] With progression of the coagulopathy, normal regulatory mechanisms are disrupted. This disruption is reflected in decreasing levels of inhibitory factors such as protein C, factor V, and antithrombin III.[3,6]

Finally, unchecked DIC resulting in occlusion of vessels and tissue ischemia leads to end-organ dysfunction. Respiratory failure, indicated by abnormal arterial blood gases (ABGs); liver failure, indicated by increasing liver enzymes; and renal impairment, indicated by rising blood urea nitrogen (BUN) and creatinine (Cr) levels are common findings in advanced DIC.

No single laboratory study can confirm the diagnosis of DIC but there are several key results that are strong indicators the condition is present (Table 42-3). The International Society of Thrombosis and Hemostasis emphasizes early detection of DIC through observation of abnormal trends in laboratory values.[5]

MEDICAL MANAGEMENT

Without question, the primary intervention in DIC is prevention. Being aware of those conditions that commonly contribute to the development of DIC and treating them vigorously and without delay is the best defense against this devastating condition.[3,5,6,9,10] However, once DIC is identified, maintaining organ perfusion and slowing consumption of coagulation factors is paramount to achieving a favorable outcome.[3]

Multiple organ dysfunction syndrome (MODS) is frequently a result of DIC and only serves to exacerbate the underlying pathology. Therefore, it is essential to prevent end-organ ischemia and damage by supporting blood pressure and circulating volume. Administration of IV fluids, inotropic agents, and if overt hemorrhaging is evident, infusion of packed RBCs, would be appropriate to replace blood volume and essential, oxygen-carrying red blood cells.

In the presence of severe platelet depletion (<50,000/mm[3]) and severe hemorrhage, platelet transfusions are often indicated.[5,6] However, caution must be used when administering platelets because antiplatelet antibodies may be formed. These antibodies may then become activated during future platelet transfusions and elicit DIC.[3]

Replacement of clotting factors in the patient with DIC is thought by some to perpetuate the coagulopathy; however, there is little scientific evidence to support this theory.[1] Fibrinogen levels less than 100mg/dl would indicate the appropriateness of administering cryoprecipitate. Prolonged PT would indicate the need for fresh-frozen plasma.[3,5,6]

Slowing consumption of coagulation factors by inhibiting the processes involved in clot formation is also a strategy in treating DIC. The use of heparin, particularly low–molecular-weight heparin, to prevent formation of future clots is controversial. It is contraindicated in those patients with DIC accompanying recent surgery or gastrointestinal (GI) or central nervous system (CNS) bleeding. However, it has been found to be beneficial in obstetrical emergencies such as retained placenta or incomplete abortion, severe arterial occlusions, or MODS caused by microemboli.[3,6] Inhibitors such as aminocaproic acid may be used in conjunction with heparin.[6]

The use of recombinant human protein C is gaining popularity in treating DIC, especially in the presence of sever sepsis. Protein C acts as an anticoagulant and works to restore normal inhibition of coagulation pathways. However, it has been associated with an increased incidence of intracerebral bleeding and must be used with caution in patients with severely decreased platelets.[3,5]

Thrombin production in DIC surpasses that of antithrombins and other regulatory factors that would normally be present to inactivate thrombin and all of its subsequent actions. The use of antithrombin III has just recently been approved in the United States. Ongoing research is yielding very promising results in the treatment of DIC. Another promising avenue of research is occurring around the use of protease inhibitors. Normally, protease molecules inhibit the conversion of fibrinogen to fibrin in the coagulation mechanism. In DIC, this normal inhibitory mechanism is impaired. The introduction of protease inhibitors through IV infusion may therefore be advantageous in arresting DIC.[3]

NURSING MANAGEMENT

Nursing management of the patient with DIC incorporates a variety of nursing diagnoses (see the Nursing Diagnoses feature on Disseminated Intravascular Coagulation). Assessment and monitoring are the primary weapons in the critical care nurse's arsenal where DIC is concerned. Knowing the diseases and conditions that are most often associated with DIC and understanding the pathophysiologic mechanisms involved enables the critical care nurse to anticipate its development and intervene quickly.

Frequent assessments should include parameters for neurologic status, renal function, cardiopulmonary function, and skin integrity that indicate impaired tissue or organ perfusion. Particular parameters to include are mental status, BUN and Cr, urine output, vital signs, hemodynamic values, cardiac rhythm, arterial blood gases and pulse oximetry, skin breakdown, ecchymoses, or hematomas.[6]

The critical care nurse must recognize and support the patient's vital physiologic functions. Administration of IV fluids, blood products, and inotropic agents to provide adequate hemodynamic support and tissue oxygenation is essential in preventing or combating end-organ damage. Close monitoring of vital signs, hemodynamic parameters, intake and output, and appropriate laboratory values will assist the critical care nurse in administering and titrating appropriate agents.

NURSING DIAGNOSES | **Disseminated Intravascular Coagulation**

- Deficient Fluid Volume related to active blood loss
- Decreased Cardiac Output related to alterations in preload
- Risk for Infection
- Anxiety related to threat to biologic, psychologic, and/or social integrity
- Compromised Family Coping related to critically ill family member

NIC   Bleeding Precautions

Definition: Reduction of stimuli that may induce bleeding or hemorrhage in at-risk patients

Activities

Monitor the patient closely for hemorrhage

Note hemoglobin/hematocrit levels before and after blood loss, as indicated

Monitor for signs and symptoms of persistent bleeding (e.g., check all secretions for frank or occult blood)

Monitor coagulation studies, including prothrombin time (PT), partial thromboplastin time (PTT), fibrinogen, fibrin degradation/split products, and platelet counts, as appropriate

Monitor orthostatic vital signs, including blood pressure

Maintain bed rest during active bleeding

Administer blood products (e.g., platelets and fresh-frozen plasma), as appropriate

Protect the patient from trauma, which may cause bleeding

Avoid injections (IV, IM, or SQ), as appropriate

Instruct the ambulating patient to wear shoes

Use soft toothbrush or toothettes for oral care

Use electric razor, instead of straight-edge, for shaving

Tell patient to avoid invasive procedures; if they are necessary, monitor closely for bleeding

Coordinate timing of invasive procedures with platelet or fresh-frozen plasma transfusions, if appropriate

Refrain from inserting objects into a bleeding orifice

Avoid taking rectal temperatures

Tell patient to avoid lifting heavy objects

Administer mediations (e.g., antacids), as appropriate

Instruct patient to avoid aspirin and other anticoagulants

Instruct patient to increase intake of foods rich in vitamin K

Use therapeutic mattress to minimize skin trauma

Prevent constipation (e.g., encourage fluid intake and stool softeners), as appropriate

Instruct the patient and/or family on signs of bleeding and appropriate actions (e.g., notify the nurse), should bleeding occur

From Dochterman JM, Bulechek GM: *Nursing Interventions Classification,* ed 4, St Louis, 2004, Mosby.
IV, Intravenous; *IM,* intramuscular; *SQ,* subcutaneous.

Awareness of the patient's bleeding potential necessitates adjustments to normal nursing interventions (see the Nursing Interventions Classification feature on Bleeding Precautions). Avoid unnecessary venipunctures that may result in bleeding, bruising, or hematomas by drawing blood from and administering medications through existing arterial or venous lines. Avoid the use of manual or automatic blood pressure cuffs whenever possible. If tracheal or oral suctioning is necessary, the use of low-level suction is recommended.[6] Meticulous skin care is advised, keeping the skin moist and using specialty mattresses and beds as appropriate to prevent breakdown. Finally, use gentle care when bathing or turning the patient to prevent bruising or hematoma formation.

The development of DIC in the already critically ill patient can cause a great deal of stress in both the patient and his or her significant others. It is imperative to provide psychosocial support throughout this crisis. Calm reassurance and uncomplicated explanations of the care the patient is receiving can help allay much of the anxiety experienced. Be sure to answer all questions and provide information in the terms best understood by all. The use of an interpreter where English is not the primary language can enhance understanding and help avoid misconceptions. Providing spiritual support as requested may also be of assistance.

Collaborative management of the patient with DIC is outlined in Box 42-2.

Box 42-2

COLLABORATIVE MANAGEMENT

DISSEMINATED INTRAVASCULAR COAGULATION
- Identify and eliminate the underlying cause
- Provide hemodynamic support to prevent end-organ ischemia
  - Intravenous fluids
  - Positive inotropic agents
- Administer blood and blood components
  - Fresh-frozen plasma
  - Platelets
  - Cryoprecipitate
  - Antithrombin III
- Administer medications
  - Heparin
  - Aminocaproic acid
  - Protein C
  - Antithrombin III
- Initiate bleeding precautions
- Maintain surveillance for complications
  - Hypovolemic shock
  - Peripheral ischemia
  - Central ischemia
  - Multiple organ dysfunction syndrome (MODS)
- Provide comfort and emotional support

THROMBOCYTOPENIA

DESCRIPTION

Thrombocytopenia is defined as a platelet count less than 140, 000/mm^3.[11] Similarly to DIC, thrombocytopenia often results from another underlying condition that affects the platelet count. Thrombocytopenia found in adults is more common in women than in men, affecting them most often between the ages of 20 and 50 years.[12]

ETIOLOGY

Onset of thrombocytopenia often follows a viral infection, pregnancy, administration of certain medications (e.g., heparin, thiazide diuretics, chemotherapeutic agents), malignancies, splenomegaly, blood transfusions, or alcoholism.[8,12] Regardless of the precipitating condition, the development of thrombocytopenia occurs in relation to one of four mechanisms: (1) decreased platelet production, (2) increased platelet destruction, (3) splenic sequestration of platelets, and (4) platelet dilution.[11] The most common form of thrombocytopenia seen in the critical care unit is idiopathic thrombocytopenic purpura (ITP).[13]

PATHOPHYSIOLOGY

In ITP, lymphocytes produce antibodies that begin to destroy existing platelets. The cause of this autoimmune response is unknown.[12,14,15] With insufficient platelets available, the normal coagulation pathways are disrupted. Inadequate hemostasis ensues and bleeding results. Although life-threatening GI or intracerebral bleeding can occur, the bleeding seen in ITP does not result in deep visceral hemorrhage and hematoma.[11]

ASSESSMENT AND DIAGNOSIS

Idiopathic thrombocytopenic purpura is characterized by the gradual onset of signs and symptoms.[15] The diagnosis is primarily based on findings in the patient history and physical exam.[16]

Clinical Manifestations. Petechial hemorrhages, small red spots noted primarily on legs and oral mucosa, are most indicative of a platelet disorder, unlike larger hematomas that are most commonly associated with coagulation disorders.[13,14] Bruising unrelated to trauma is another common sign of ITP.[14] Common signs and symptoms of ITP are listed in Table 42-4.

Unusual bleeding is a hallmark of ITP. Excessive bleeding from the gums following dental work, spontaneous epistaxis, blood noted in the urine or stool and, in women, unusually heavy menses are typically seen. More rarely, retinal hemorrhage or intracerebral bleeding may be present.[13-15]

Table 42-4	Common Signs and Symptoms and Laboratory Studies Seen With Idiopathic Thrombocytopenia Purpura
System	**Signs and Symptoms**
Integumentary	Petechial hemorrhage of lower extremities, ecchymoses, gingival bleeding, spontaneous epistaxis
Neurologic	Sudden, severe headache; nausea and/or vomiting; seizures; focal neurologic deficits; decreased level of consciousness
Renal	Hematuria
Gastrointestinal	Hematemesis, melena, hematochezia
Other	Heavy menses in women, retinal hemorrhage
Laboratory	Decreased platelet count, often <30,000 mm^3

Laboratory Findings. A complete blood count will reveal a severely diminished platelet count, often falling below 30,000/mm^3.[13] The number of red and white blood cells and hemoglobin levels will be normal. Coagulation studies and bleeding times likewise will be normal.

MEDICAL MANAGEMENT

In most cases, ITP resolves spontaneously and treatment is not necessary. However, in mild cases where diminished platelets counts result in symptoms, administration of oral corticosteroids is appropriate.[11,13] Platelet counts will rise to normal levels with 2 to 6 weeks and dosages can then be tapered off.

However, in patients exhibiting life-threatening hemorrhage, rapid intervention is necessary. Administration of intravenous immunoglobulin (IV Ig) suppresses the platelet-destroying antibody response. This therapy is extremely expensive and is reserved for the most severe manifestations of ITP.[15] High-dose methylprednisone can be given IV and has been found to be very effective in treating ITP.[16] Platelet transfusion is also recommended following administration of IVIg and/or methylprednisone. When steroid therapy fails to arrest the condition, surgical removal of the spleen is considered.[13,15,16]

NURSING MANAGEMENT

Nursing management of the patient with ITP incorporates a variety of nursing diagnoses (see the Nursing Diagnoses feature on Idiopathic Thrombocytopenia Purpura). Nursing interventions are directed toward bleeding prevention (see the NIC feature on Bleeding Precautions) and supportive measures. Recognizing potential hazards and providing a safe care environment is of utmost concern. For example, padding bed rails can protect the patient from bruising. Substituting sponge-tipped oral care devices for firm-bristled toothbrushes can help minimize mucosal trauma and bleeding. Also instruct the patient to blow the nose gently to avoid instigating epistaxis. When shaving patients, the use of an electric razor is preferred to reduce the risk of laceration associated with a blade. Avoid venipuncture and intramuscular injections.[17] In the event venipuncture is required, prolonged pressure on the site may be necessary to arrest bleeding. Careful administration of prescribed medications and monitoring for adverse effects of platelet transfusions is also required. Finally, monitoring for complicating or contributing factors such as hemorrhage and infection is paramount.

Collaborative management of the patient with ITP is outlined in Box 42-3.

NURSING DIAGNOSES

Idiopathic Thrombocytopenia Purpura

- Deficient Fluid Volume related to active blood loss
- Powerlessness related to lack of control over current situation and/or disease progression
- Disturbed Body Image related to actual change in body structure, function, or appearance

---

Box 42-3

COLLABORATIVE MANAGEMENT

IDIOPATHIC THROMBOCYTOPENIA PURPURA
- Administer medications
  - Glucocorticoids
  - IV Ig immunoglobulin
- Prepare patient for splenectomy if unresponsive to medication therapy
- Administer platelets
- Initiate bleeding precautions
- Maintain surveillance for complications
  - Intracranial or other major hemorrhage
  - Severe blood loss
- Provide comfort and emotional support

HEPARIN-INDUCED THROMBOCYTOPENIA

DESCRIPTION

Another form of thrombocytopenia seen in critical care patients is heparin-induced thrombocytopenia (HIT). There are two distinct types of HIT. The most common form is type 1 HIT. Seen in up to 30% of patients receiving heparin therapy, this nonautoimmune condition manifests within a few days of initiation of therapy. Platelet depletion is moderate, counts are usually less than 100,000/mm^3, and the condition is transient, often resolving spontaneously. Discontinuation of heparin is not required. The second form is type 2 HIT, which is less commonly encountered but has more severe consequences.[18-20] This discussion is limited to type 2 HIT.

ETIOLOGY

Type 2 HIT is an immune-mediated response to the administration of heparin therapy. It has been observed in 3% to 5% of patients treated with unfractionated heparin and has also occurred after exposure to low–molecular-weight heparin (LMWH), though to a lesser degree. The disorder is characterized by severe thrombocytopenia during heparin therapy. Diagnostically it is identified by a platelet count less than 50,000/mm^3 or at least a 50% decrease from the baseline platelet count from the initiation of therapy. Onset is usually 5 to 14 days from the first exposure to heparin, but the onset can be within hours of a reexposure to heparin.[13,19-21] Depending on the source, mortality rates are reported as high as 30%.[19-21]

PATHOPHYSIOLOGY

The thrombocytopenia that occurs with type 2 HIT is related to the formation of heparin-antibody complexes. These complexes release a substance known as platelet factor 4 (PF4). PF4 attracts heparin molecules, forming immunogenic complexes that adhere to platelet and endothelial surfaces (Fig. 42-4). Activation of platelets stimulates the release of thrombin and the subsequent formation of platelet clumps.[18]

Thus patients with type 2 HIT are at a greater risk of developing thrombosis rather than bleeding. Vessel occlusion can result in the need for limb amputation, stroke, acute myocardial infarction, and even death.[11,18-21] The resultant formation of thrombi is the primary characteristic of HIT that distinguishes it from other forms of thrombocytopenia and gives rise to its more descriptive name, "white clot syndrome."[18]

ASSESSMENT AND DIAGNOSIS

HIT can be associated with severe consequences. Rapid recognition of risk factors and subsequent development of signs and symptoms is essential in treating this condition.

Clinical Manifestations. Common signs and symptoms are listed in Table 42-5. The clinical manifestations of HIT are related to the formation of thrombi and subsequent vessel occlusion. Most thrombotic events are venous, although both venous and arterial thrombosis can occur.[21] Thrombotic events typically include deep vein thrombosis, pulmonary embolism, limb ischemia thrombosis, thrombotic stroke, and myocardial infarction.[21] The presence of blanching and the loss of peripheral pulses, sensation, or motor function in a limb is indicative of peripheral vascular thrombi. Neurologic signs and symptoms such as confusion, headache, and impaired speech can signal the onset of cerebral artery occlusion and stroke. Acute myocardial infarction may be heralded by dyspnea, chest pain, pallor, and alterations in blood pressure. Thrombi in the pulmonary vasculature may result as evidenced by pleuritic pain, rales, and dyspnea.[11,13,18]

Laboratory Findings. The key indicator in identifying the development of HIT is the platelet count. General consensus in the literature states that a platelet count of less than 50,000/mm^3 or a sudden drop of 30% to 50% from the patient's baseline following initiation of heparin therapy is highly indicative of HIT.[13,18,21]

More recently, two types of assays have become available to assist in confirming the diagnosis of HIT: (1) functional assays, based on platelet aggregation or the release of granular contents such as serotonin, and (2) assays that identify the HIT antigen. Functional assays are highly sensitive in detecting the presence of HIT. The two most common functional assays are heparin-induced platelet aggregation (HIPA) and serotonin release assay (SRA). The enzyme-linked immunosorbent assay (ELISA) actually identifies the presence of the HIT antigen.[18]

MEDICAL MANAGEMENT

Early identification is critical to managing the effects of type 2 HIT. The College of American Pathologists recommendations include obtaining a baseline platelet count before initiation of therapy and routine monitoring during the highest risk period, 5 to 10 days following initiation.[21] When a decrease in the platelet count is detected, heparin therapy should be discontinued immediately and the patient should be tested for the presence of heparin antibodies.[11,18,20,21]

If the original indication for heparin still exists or new thromboses occur, an alternative form of anticoagulation is usually necessary.[13,18,21]

Direct thrombin inhibitors (DTIs) are being used with increasing frequency to treat HIT. DTIs bind directly to the thrombin molecule, thereby inhibiting its action.[18] The FDA has approved two such drugs for use in the United States: lepirudin and argatroban. Warfarin, although commonly used to treat deep vein thrombosis, is not indicated as a sole agent in treating HIT because of its prolonged onset of action.[18,21] Studies have shown that the use of warfarin without concomitant use of DTIs can significantly increase the incidence of thrombosis in patients with HIT. Comparative information on these medications is provided in the Pharmacologic Management Table on Heparin-Induced Thrombocytopenia.[18,20] The optimal duration of anticoagulation in patients with HIT is not known.[21]

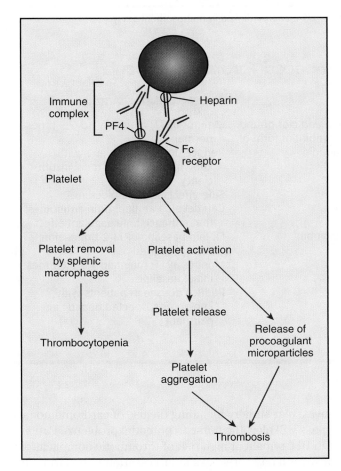

Fig. 42-4 Pathophysiology of heparin-induced thrombocytopenia. First, heparin binds to platelet factor 4 (PF4), forming a highly reactive antigenic complex on the surface of platelets. Susceptible patients then develop an antibody (IgG) to the heparin/PF4 antigenic complex. Once produced, the IgG then activates the platelets via their F$_C$ receptors. Thrombocytopenia develops as the reticuloendothelial system consumes activated platelets, platelet microaggregates, and IgG-coated platelets. (Courtesy GlaxoSmithKline, Philadelphia, Pa.)

Table 42-5	Common Signs and Symptoms and Laboratory Data Seen With Heparin-Induced Thrombocytopenia
System	**Signs and Symptoms**
Cardiac	Chest pain, diaphoresis, pallor, alterations in blood pressure, dysrhythmias
Vascular	Arterial—Pain, pallor, pulselessness, paresthesia, paralysis
	Venous—Pain, tenderness, unilateral leg swelling, warmth, erythema, a palpable cord, pain upon passive dorsiflexion of the foot, and spontaneous maintenance of the relaxed foot in abnormal plantar flexion (Homans' sign)
Pulmonary	Dyspnea, pleuritic pain, rales, chest pain, chest wall tenderness, back pain, shoulder pain, upper abdominal pain, syncope, hemoptysis, shortness of breath, wheezing
Renal	Thirst, decreased urine output, dizziness, orthostatic hypotension.
Gastrointestinal	Abdominal pain, vomiting, bloody diarrhea, abnormal bowel sounds
Neurologic	Confusion, headache, impaired speech patterns, hemiparesis or hemiplegia, vision disturbances, dysarthria, aphasia, ataxia, vertigo, nystagmus, sudden decrease in consciousness
Laboratory	Platelets $< 50,000/mm^3$ or sudden drop of 30%-50% from baseline; positive HIPA, SRA, ELISA

HIPA, Heparin-induced platelet aggregation; *SRA,* serotonin release assay; *ELISA,* enzyme-linked immunosorbent assay.

Pharmacologic Management: Heparin-Induced Thrombocytopenia

DRUG	DOSAGE	ACTIONS	SPECIAL CONSIDERATIONS
Lepirudin (Refludan)	Loading dose: 0.4 mg/kg IV bolus IV infusion: 0.15 mg/kg/hr	Used to inhibit free and clot-bound thrombin; a recombinant form of leech-derived hirudin	Monitor aPTT; maintain 1.5-2.5 times normal Reduce dosage in patients with known or suspected renal insufficiency Side effects include bleeding Can develop antilepirudin antibodies that enhance anticoagulant effect
Argatroban	Loading dose: None IV infusion: 1.5 mcg/kg/min	Used to inhibit thrombin	Obtain baseline aPTT 2 hours after therapy started Monitor aPTT; maintain 1.5-3.0 times initial baseline Reduce dosage in patients with known or suspected hepatic impairment

IV, Intravenous; *aPTT,* activated partial thromboplastin time.

NURSING MANAGEMENT

Nursing management of the patient with HIT incorporates a variety of nursing diagnoses (see the Nursing Diagnoses feature on Heparin-Induced Thrombocytopenia). Nursing interventions include monitoring all patients on heparin for signs and symptoms of HIT, ensuring that all heparin is discontinued, maintaining surveillance for complications, and providing comfort and emotional support. The critical care nurse plays a pivotal role in prevention and detection of heparin-induced thrombocytopenia. Initial assessment is crucial to identifying those patients at risk for developing HIT. Ascertaining past medical history that includes previous heparin therapy, deep vein thrombosis, or cardiovascular surgery including the use of cardiopulmonary bypass will alert the nurse to potential problems. Patients with HIT remain at high risk of thrombotic complications for several days or weeks after cessation of heparin. Vigilant monitoring, early recognition of signs and symptoms, and prompt notification of the physician are key roles of the critical care nurse. Ensuring that all heparin has been removed from the patient's hemodynamic pressure monitoring system and avoiding the use of heparin flushes to maintain the patency of other intravenous lines is also essential.[21]

Patient Education. Finally, prevention of subsequent episodes in patients sensitized to heparin is necessary. Patient and family education is essential (see the Patient

Education feature on Heparin-Induced Thrombocytopenia). The use of medical alert bracelets and listing heparin allergies in the medical record will be necessary to avoid this serious complication in the future.

Collaborative management of the patient with type 2 HIT is outlined in Box 42-4.

TUMOR LYSIS SYNDROME

DESCRIPTION

Tumor lysis syndrome (TLS) refers to a variety of metabolic disturbances that may be seen with the treatment of cancer. A potentially lethal complication of various forms of cancer treatment, TLS occurs when large numbers of neoplastic cells are rapidly killed, resulting in the release of large amounts of potassium, phosphate, and uric acid into the systemic circulation. It is most commonly seen in patients with lymphoma, leukemia, or multiple metastatic conditions.[22-24]

ETIOLOGY

Though most often associated with the use of chemotherapeutic and biologic agents and radiation in the treatment of malignant disorders, TLS can in rare instances occur spontaneously. The development of TLS has been linked to other pathophysiologic conditions such as elevated WBC counts, large tumors or multiple organ involvement, and renal insufficiency.[17,23]

Box 42-4

COLLABORATIVE MANAGEMENT

HEPARIN-INDUCED THROMBOCYTOPENIA
- Stop all heparin exposure
  - Unfractionated and low–molecular-weight heparins by any route
  - Heparin flushes
  - Heparin-coated vascular access devices
- Begin therapy with an alternative anticoagulant
  - Lepirudin
  - Argatroban
- Maintain surveillance for complications
  - Deep vein thrombosis
  - Pulmonary emboli
  - Acute limb ischemia
  - Cerebral vascular accident
  - Acute myocardial infarction
- Administer antifibrinolytic therapy (as indicated) if thrombosis occurs
- Prepare patient for surgical embolectomy (as indicated) if thrombosis occurs
- Provide comfort and emotional support

PATHOPHYSIOLOGY

The primary mechanism involved in the development of TLS is the destruction of massive numbers of malignant cells, either by chemotherapy or radiation. This mass destruction results in the release of large amounts of potassium, phosphorus, and nucleic acids, leading to severe metabolic disturbances such as hyperuricemia, hyperkalemia, hyperphosphatemia, and hypocalcemia (Table 42-6). Death in TLS is most often due to complications of renal failure or cardiac arrest.[22]

Table 42-6	**Characteristic Electrolyte Abnormalities Encountered in Tumor Lysis Syndrome and Their Clinical Consequences**		
Electrolyte	**Pathophysiology**	**Clinical Consequence**	**Treatment Options**
Potassium	Rapid expulsion of intracellular K^+ into the circulation due to cell lysis.	Adverse skeletal and cardiac manifestations (e.g., ventricular dysrhythmia, weakness, paresthesias)	Insulin/glucose, sodium bicarbonate, inhaled beta-agonist, K-binding resins, dialysis, calcium gluconate
Phosphate	Release of intracellular PO_4^- due to cell lysis. May be compounded by renal dysfunction.	Muscle cramps, tetany, dysrhythmias, seizures	Dialysis, phosphate binders
Calcium	Precipitation of the calcium phosphate complex because of the rapid increase in the phosphorous concentration.	Muscle cramps, tetany, dysrhythmias, seizures, renal failure (acute nephrocalcinosis)	Calcium gluconate (treatment should be reserved for those with neuromuscular irritability)
Uric acid	Cell lysis leads to increased levels of purine nucleic acids into the circulation that are metabolized to uric acid.	Renal failure (uric acid nephropathy)	Hydration, dialysis, xanthine oxidase inhibitors, alkalization of urine, urate oxidase

From Davidson MB et al: Pathophysiology, clinical consequences, and treatment of tumor lysis syndrome, *Am J Med* 116:546, 2004.

Hyperuricemia. Tumor cells undergo rapid growth and development, and therefore large amounts of nucleic acids are present within them. When therapy is initiated, tumor cell destruction causes the release of nucleic acids, which are metabolized into uric acid. Metabolic acidosis ensues, resulting in crystallization of the uric acid in the distal tubules of the kidney and leading to obstruction of flow. Glomerular filtration rates drop as the kidneys are unable to clear the increasing amounts of uric acid. Consequently, renal insufficiency and eventually acute renal failure occurs. For further discussion on acute renal failure see Chapter 30.

Hyperuricemia associated with TLS can be potentiated by several other factors including elevated levels before the initiation of therapy. Other causes of increased uric acid production are elevated WBC counts, destruction of WBCs, and enlargement of the lymph nodes, the spleen, or the liver.[22-24]

Hyperkalemia. In addition to release of nucleic acids, destruction of tumor cells also results in the release of potassium. Renal insufficiency related to hyperuricemia prevents adequate excretion of potassium, and levels rise. The resultant hyperkalemia may have a profound effect on intracellular and extracellular fluid levels.[22] Left untreated, hyperkalemia can have devastating consequences including cardiac arrest and death.[22,24]

Hyperphosphatemia and Hypocalcemia. Phosphorus levels also rise as a consequence of tumor cell destruction. Calcium ions then bind with the excess phosphorus, creating calcium phosphate salts and bringing about hypocalcemia. These salts precipitate in the kidney tubules, worsening renal insufficiency. Hypocal-

Table 42-7	**Common Findings in Tumor Lysis Syndrome**
Diagnostic Parameter	**Findings**
Clinical	Weight gain, edema, diarrhea, lethargy, muscle cramps, nausea and vomiting, paresthesia, weakness, oliguria, uremia, seizures
Laboratory	↑ potassium, phosphorus, uric acid, BUN, Cr ↓ calcium, creatinine clearance, pH, bicarbonate, $Paco_2$
Diagnostic	Positive Chvostek's and Trousseau's signs, hyperactive deep tendon reflexes, dysrhythmias, ECG changes

BUN, Blood urea nitrogen; *Cr,* creatinine; *Paco₂,* partial pressure of carbon dioxide; *ECG,* electrocardiogram.

cemia causes tetany and cardiac dysrhythmias, which can result in cardiac arrest and death.[22,24]

ASSESSMENT AND DIAGNOSIS

Detection and recognition of TLS is accomplished through assessment of clinical manifestations, evaluation of laboratory findings, and other diagnostic tests. Table 42-7 provides a summary of common findings in TLS.[22-24]

Clinical Manifestations. Clinical manifestations are related to the metabolic disturbances associated with

TLS. The patient history will reveal an unexplained weight gain following initiation of chemotherapy or radiation treatments. The weight gain is associated with fluid retention due to electrolyte disturbances. Other early signs heralding the onset of TLS include diarrhea, lethargy, muscle cramps, nausea and vomiting, paresthesias, and weakness.

Laboratory Findings. Laboratory findings will demonstrate electrolyte disturbances such as elevated potassium and phosphorus levels and a decreased calcium level. Uric acid levels will also rise. Elevations in BUN and Cr and a decreased creatinine clearance are also indicative of TLS. Metabolic acidosis will be evident by the presence of decreased pH, bicarbonate levels, and partial pressure of carbon dioxide ($Paco_2$) on arterial blood gases.

Other Diagnostic Tests. Physical examination will reveal positive Chvostek's and Trousseau's signs related to hypocalcemia. Hyperactive deep tendon reflexes are indicative of both hyperkalemia and hypocalcemia.[22] Potassium and calcium disturbances also result in changes that can be noted on the electrocardiogram (ECG) such as peaked or inverted T waves, altered QT intervals, widened QRS complexes, and dysrhythmias.[22-24]

MEDICAL MANAGEMENT

Medical interventions are aimed at maintaining adequate hydration, treating metabolic imbalances, and preventing life-threatening complications (see Table 42-6).[17,22,24] Administration of IV fluids may be necessary early on if inadequate hydration exists. The administration of isotonic saline (0.9% normal saline [NS]) reduces serum concentrations of uric acid, phosphate, and potassium.[24] The use of nonthiazide diuretics and/or low-dose dopamine to maintain adequate urine output may also be required.[25] If renal failure is present, hemodialysis should be considered.[24]

Electrolytes and arterial blood gases are closely monitored. Dietary restrictions of potassium and phosphorus may be necessary. Hyperuricemia can be treated with administration of sodium bicarbonate and allopurinol. If potassium levels rise dangerously, kayexalate may be given orally or, if the patient is unable to tolerate oral medications due to nausea and vomiting, rectal instillation may be used. If the patient is oliguric, glucose and insulin infusions may be given to facilitate lowering the potassium levels. Phosphorus-binding antacids can be used when hyperphosphatemia is present. Stool softeners may be necessary to treat the constipation often associated with the administration of these antacids. Finally, calcium gluconate may be required to replace calcium.[22,25]

NURSING MANAGEMENT

Nursing management of the patient with TLS incorporates a variety of nursing diagnoses (see the Nursing Di-

agnoses feature on Tumor Lysis Syndrome). Assessment and continued monitoring of the patient is an important role of the critical care nurse when caring for the patient with TLS. Recognizing critical laboratory changes or development of symptoms and notifying the physician in a timely manner is essential. Insertion of a urinary catheter and maintenance of the IV site is necessary in monitoring and ensuring adequate intake and output. Frequent vital signs and daily weight should also be monitored.

Nursing interventions are also aimed at preventing complications. Instituting seizure precautions will be necessary, especially if calcium levels are disrupted. Insertion of a nasogastric tube is appropriate if nausea or vomiting is present. Dietary adjustments will also be necessary, such as potassium and phosphorus restrictions in the presence of elevated serum levels, and providing additional fiber to combat the constipation associated with the administration of antacids.

Education of the patient and family is also a primary role of the critical care nurse. All treatments and interventions should be explained before carrying them out and questions answered at a level understandable to the patient and family. Before discharge, potential risk factors and identification of early signs and symptoms should be reviewed.

Collaborative management of the patient with TLS is outlined in Box 42-5.

HOSPITAL-ACQUIRED ANEMIA OF THE CRITICALLY ILL

DESCRIPTION AND ETIOLOGY

Hospital-acquired anemia is a common problem seen in critically ill patients and demonstrates many of the same characteristics as those encountered in chronic disease. Much research has been focused on identifying the con-

---

Box 42-5

COLLABORATIVE MANAGEMENT

TUMOR LYSIS SYNDROME
- Facilitate adequate renal function
  - Volume hydration with 0.9% NS
  - Nonthiazide diuretics
  - Low-dose dopamine
- Treat hyperkalemia
  - Kayexalate
  - Glucose and insulin
- Treat hyperuricemia
  - Sodium bicarbonate
  - Allopurinol
- Treat hyperphosphatemia
  - Dietary restrictions
  - Phosphorus-binding antacids
- Treat hypocalcemia
  - Calcium gluconate
- Maintain surveillance for complications
  - Acute renal failure
  - Cardiac dysrhythmias
- Provide comfort and emotional support

NS, Normal saline.

---

tributing factors and interventions related to this issue. Frequent phlebotomy, coagulopathies, and nutritional deficits are just a few reasons for this increasing problem.[26] In addition, demand for human blood products is outstripping current and projected supplies, and public confidence in the safety of our blood supply is deteriorating.[27,28] For these reasons, recent research has been focused on determining ways to minimize iatrogenic blood losses, improve blood salvage techniques, and develop alternatives to traditional blood transfusion therapy.

Risks Associated With Blood Transfusions. Studies have shown that as many as 50% of transfusions administered in the intensive care unit (ICU) are related to nosocomial anemia.[26,27,29] Although the risks associated with transfusions have significantly decreased with the advent of better screening techniques and safer storage mechanisms, it is highly unlikely that the risks will be eradicated completely.

Transmission of Infection. Protecting our blood supply from viral contamination depends on the appropriate selection of donors and meticulous screening of the donated blood for contaminants. Current methods for detecting contaminants in blood are quite sophisticated, but they are not able to detect viruses when the donor is in the seroconversion period.[26] Viruses that can be transmitted through blood transfusion include hepatitis B and C, HIV, and cytomegalovirus.[26,27,29,31]

Less commonly, bacterial contamination may occur. This is most often due to inadequate skin disinfection at the phlebotomy site, an undetected bacteremia in the donor, or minute leaks in the blood storage container itself. Common bacterial contaminants include *Serratia, Yersinia, Pseudomonas,* and *Campylobacter* species.[29,30]

Immunosuppression. Among other studies, Project Impact, sponsored by the Society for Critical Care Medicine, has produced data that link blood transfusions in the critically ill with an increase in nosocomial infections such as pneumonia and surgical site infections.[26,30] This increased nosocomial rate may be linked to immunosupression related to the transfusion itself.[26,27,29] Decreased lymphocytes, changes in T cell ratios, dysfunctional B cells, and activation of immune cells have been attributed to blood transfusions.

Circulatory Overload. The introduction of increased volume during blood transfusions may also be related to fluid volume overload problems. The delicate balance necessary to maintain stability in the critically ill patient can be disrupted by the introduction of blood volume and necessary flush solutions. The inability of compromised renal and cardiovascular systems to handle the additional fluid load may result in pulmonary edema or heart failure.[26,27]

Stored Blood. The average shelf life of a unit of blood is anywhere from 21 to 42 days.[26,28] This period depends on the storage solution, the type of processing used, and the storage system itself.[30] As blood ages during storage, changes take place in the blood itself that contribute to blood-related complications.[27,29] RBCs break down, releasing potassium and bilirubin, which may result in dangerous elevations of these substances in the patient receiving the transfusion. The breakdown of the RBCs also results in depletion of oxygen-carrying capacity of the transfused blood. Citrate is used as a preservative and can bind with calcium released from damaged RBCs, resulting in hypocalcemia.[30]

Clerical Risk Factors. The process of blood transfusion from initial donor to actual recipient requires a tremendous amount of documentation; nonetheless, room is still left for error, which can lead to mismatching of patient and donor blood types. Hemolytic reactions are the unfortunate, and often deadly, consequence of these preventable errors.[26,27]

BLOOD CONSERVATION STRATEGIES

As more and more patients and clinicians opt for the limited use of blood products, strategies for conserving blood and preventing unnecessary loss become an important part of the critical care nurse's standard of care. These strategies include minimizing blood loss, managing oxygen delivery and consumption, stimulating production of RBCs, and understanding transfusion safety and alternative agents.

Minimizing Blood Loss. Frequent laboratory tests have been shown to be a major culprit in the development of nosocomial anemia in critically ill patients.[27,29] Blood losses are due to actual volume of samples and discards when drawing from venous access lines. Critical care nurses can be instrumental in significantly decreasing blood loss in this arena. The use of pediatric collection tubes and point-of-care testing are techniques that yield valid diagnostic results but require smaller blood samples. Closed-loop vascular devices that retain the sterility of the potential discard and allow its return to the patient are also being used. Noninvasive monitoring devices such as pulse oximetry and capnography can reduce the need for arterial blood gas analysis.

The critical care nurse plays a key role in preventing and managing hemorrhagic blood loss in the critical patient. Control of hypertension, which can contribute to significant hemorrhage, can be accomplished through fluid management and the administration of antihypertensive and vasodilatory medications as needed. Blood salvage devices can be employed to collect shed blood and return it to the patient. There are several pharmacologic agents that can also assist in achieving hemostasis and prevent further blood loss. Aprotinin, a serine protease inhibitor, affects both coagulation and fibrinolysis without affecting platelet function. Desmopressin is a potent vasoconstrictor and also affects clotting factor VIII.[31] Aminocaproic acid inhibits activation of plasminogen.[32] All work to control bleeding.

Managing Oxygen Delivery and Consumption. Illness-related stress, blood loss from surgery, infection, pain, and anxiety all contribute to the higher than normal demand for oxygen seen in the critically ill patient.[29] Monitoring pulse oximetry is useful in identifying activities and interventions that can contribute to the imbalance between supply and demand. Supplemental oxygen therapy will assist in maintaining available oxygen supplies. Promoting a restful environment through modulation of nursing care activities and providing pain and sedation control can assist in decreasing the demand for oxygen. It is important to monitor cardiac output and other hemodynamic parameters in order to manage interventions that optimize oxygen delivery. Administration of fluids and inotropic agents optimizes blood pressure and cardiac output, and vasodilators are used to decrease afterload and improve efficiency of cardiovascular function.

Stimulating Production of RBCs. Insufficient erythropoiesis can also contribute to anemia on the critically ill patient. The administration of epoetin alpha has been shown to be helpful in stimulating the production of red blood cells, reducing the need for transfusions.[27,29-32] Iron preparations such as ferrous sulfate, iron sucrose, or iron gluconate may be administered to provide necessary iron stores for the increased erythropoiesis.

Encouraging Safer Transfusions and Alternative Agents. Finding ways to decrease the risks associated with blood transfusions and make the blood supply safer for patients is a high priority. Better, more sensitive screening tests, irradiation, and removal of leukocytes are a few of the current methods in use today. Plasma ex-

pander manufactured from nonhuman sources are also available. Autologous transfusions, where the patient donates his or her own blood before a surgical procedure or other anticipated need, has also been a common practice for many years. More recently, science has been using recombinant DNA technology to develop safe alternatives to blood transfusions. The use of blood from other species is also being researched in the quest to provide safe and effective products for use in severe anemia.[33]

SPECIAL CONSIDERATIONS IN THE SURGICAL PATIENT

The surgical patient who wants to avoid the use of blood transfusions presents special problems. However, there are several strategies that can be used during surgery to minimize the need for transfusions.

Pharmacologic Agents. Antifibrinolytic agents such as aprotinin and aminocaproic acid can be administered to promote hemostasis. Vasopressin or desmopressin (DDAVP) are potent vasoconstrictors that can slow blood leakage from small vessels.[31,32]

Autologous Blood Donation. The patient undergoing surgery who wants to avoid blood transfusions may choose to donate his or her own blood several weeks before surgery. Autologous donation can also be accomplished intraoperatively. This technique provides the patient with fresh, whole blood to be used during surgery. Intraoperative autologous donation is used most often in emergency or traumatic surgery.[32]

Platelet Sequestration. Like intraoperative autologous blood donation, platelet-pheresis may be performed just before beginning surgery. The platelets are then reinfused when necessary.[32] Although controversial, this procedure has been shown to be effective in decreasing chest tube drainage following cardiovascular bypass surgery.

Blood Salvaging. Also called autotransfusion, blood salvage devices collect blood from the operative site, separate and wash the RBCs, and return them to the patient. Similarly to autologous donation, the patient receives his or her own blood and avoids the risks associated with nonautologous blood transfusions.

Anesthesia-Induced Hypotension. The use of induced hypotension is controversial and results have been inconsistent.[28] Hypotension can lead in tissue ischemia and result in cardiac dysrhythmias, acute myocardial infarction, cerebrovascular accidents, and damage to renal or hepatic cells. However, controlled mild hypotension may be useful when a large blood loss is anticipated, such as in the context of orthopedic procedures.[31]

Surgical Techniques and Instruments. Technology has provided many tools that have made it possible to significantly decrease surgical blood loss and the need for blood transfusions. Minimally invasive procedures such as laparoscopic and endoscopic approaches and advances in interventional radiologic techniques have made a significant contribution. The gamma knife, the argon beam coagulator, and the harmonic scalpel are examples of tools that have also been instrumental in decreasing the need for postoperative transfusions.

REFERENCES

1. McCance KL: Structure and function of the hematologic system. In McCance KL, Huether SE, editors: *Pathophysiology: the biologic basis for disease in adults and children,* ed 4, St Louis, 2002, Mosby.
2. Feinstein DI: Hemostasis and coagulation disorders. In Beers MH, Berkow R: *The Merck manual of diagnosis and therapy,* ed 17, Whitehouse Station, NJ, 1999, Merck Research Laboratories.
3. Geiter H: Disseminated intravascular coagulation, *Dimens Crit Care Nurs* 22:108, 2003.
4. Doshi SN, Marmur JD: Evolving role of tissue factor and its pathway inhibitor, *Crit Care Med* 30:S241, 2002.
5. Toh CH, Dennis M: Disseminated intravascular coagulation: old disease, new hope, *Br Med J* 327:974, 2003.
6. Bick RL: Disseminated intravascular coagulation: current concepts of etiology, pathophysiology, diagnosis, and treatment, *Hematol Oncol Clin North Am* 17:149, 2003.
7. Lapointe LA, VonRueden KT: Coagulopathies in trauma patients, *AACN Clin Iss Crit Care Nurs* 13:192, 2002.
8. Wada H: Disseminated intravascular coagulation, *Clin Chim Acta* 344:13, 2004.
9. Slofstra SH, Spek CA, Ten Cate H: Disseminated intravascular coagulation, *Hematol J* 4:295, 2003.
10. Messmore HL, Wehrmacher WH: Disseminated intravascular coagulation: a primer for primary care physicians, *Postgrad Med* 111:2002. Available on the Internet at http://www.postgradmed.com/issues/2002/03_02/messmore.htm.
11. George JN: Platelet disorders. In Beers MH, Berkow R: *The Merck manual of diagnosis and therapy,* ed 17, Whitehouse Station, NJ, 1999, Merck Research Laboratories.
12. McFarland J: Pathophysiology of platelet destruction in immune (idiopathic) thrombocytopenic purpura, *Blood Rev* 16:1, 2002.
13. Horrell CJ, Rothman J: Establishing the etiology of thrombocytopenia, *Nurse Pract* 25:68, 2002.
14. George JN: Idiopathic thrombocytopenic purpura: current issues for pathogenesis, diagnosis, and management in children and adults, *Curr Hematol Rep* 2:381, 2003.
15. Silverman MA: Idiopathic thrombocytopenic purpura, available on the Internet at http://www.emedicine.com/emerg/topic282.htm, 2003.
16. George JN et al: Diagnosis and treatment of idiopathic thrombocytopenic purpura. American Society of Hematology ITP Practice Guideline Panel, *Am Fam Physician* 54: 2437, 1996.
17. Otto SE: *Oncology nursing clinical reference,* St Louis, 2004, Mosby.
18. Housholder-Hughes SD, Bennett J: *The nurses' role in managing HIT: preventing life- and limb-threatening thrombosis,* Aliso Viejo, CA, 2003, American Association of Critical Care Nurses.
19. Walenga JM, Frenkel EP, Bick RL: Heparin-induced thrombocytopenia, paradoxical thromboembolism, and other adverse effects of heparin-type therapy, *Hematol Oncol Clin North Am* 17:259, 2003.
20. Shar MR, Spencer JP: Heparin-induced thrombocytopenia occurring after discontinuation of heparin, *J Am Board Fam Pract* 16:148, 2003.
21. Warkentin TE, Greinacher A, editors: *Heparin-induced thrombocytopenia,* ed 3, New York, 2004, Marcel Dekker.
22. Robison J: Tumor lysis syndrome. In Chernecky CC, Berger BJ, editors, *Advanced and critical care oncology nursing,* Philadelphia, 1998, WB Saunders.
23. Cantril CA, Haylock PJ: Tumor lysis syndrome, *Am J Nurs* 104(4):49, 2004.
24. Davidson MB et al: Pathophysiology, clinical consequences, and treatment of tumor lysis syndrome, *Am J Med* 116:546, 2004.
25. Ezzone SA: Tumor lysis syndrome, *Semin Oncol Nurs* 15:202, 1999.
26. Pearl RG, Pohlman A: Understanding and managing anemia in critically ill patients, *Crit Care Nurse* 22(6):S1, 2002.
27. Pohlman A, Craven JH, Lindsay K: Conserving blood in the intensive care unit, *Crit Care Nurse* 21(6):S1, 2001.
28. Ozawa S, Shander A, Ochani TD: A practical approach to achieving bloodless surgery, *AORN J* 74:32, 2001.
29. Vernon S, Pfeifer GM: Blood management strategies for critical care patients, *Crit Care Nurse* 23(6):34, 2003.
30. Brown M, Whalen PK: Red blood cell transfusion in critically ill patients, *Crit Care Nurse* 20(6):S1, 2000.
31. Physicians and Nurses for Blood Conservation: websites at http://www.pnbc.ca/preop.body.en.html http://www.pnbc.ca/intraop.body.en.html http://www.pnbc.ca/postop.body.en.html
32. Reger TB, Roditski D: Bloodless medicine and surgery for patients having cardiac surgery, *Crit Care Nurse* 21(4):35, 2001.
33. Schaefer J: Advances and dilemmas in recombinant blood products, *J Infusion Nurs* 25:305, 2002.

Nursing Management Plans

NURSING MANAGEMENT PLAN
Activity Intolerance

Definition: Insufficient physiologic or psychologic energy to endure or complete required or desired daily activities

Activity Intolerance Related to Cardiopulmonary Dysfunction

Defining Characteristics
- Chest pain with activity
- Electrocardiographic changes with activity
- Heart rate elevations 15 beats/min above baseline with activity for patients on beta-blockers or calcium channel blockers
- Heart rate elevations above baseline 5 minutes after activity
- Breathlessness with activity
- SpO_2 <92% with activity
- Postural hypotension when moving from supine to upright position
- Patient reports fatigue with activity

Outcome Criteria
- Heart rate elevations are <20 beats/min above baseline with activity and are <10 beats/min above baseline with activity for patients on beta-blockers or calcium channel blockers.
- Heart rate returns to baseline 5 minutes after activity.
- Chest pain with activity is absent
- Patient reports tolerance to activity.

Nursing Interventions and Rationale
1. Encourage active or passive range-of-motion exercises while the patient is in bed *to keep joints flexible and muscles stretched.*
2. Teach patient to refrain from holding breath while performing exercises and *to avoid the Valsalva maneuver.*
3. Encourage performance of muscle-toning exercises at least 3 times daily, *because a toned muscle uses less oxygen when performing work than an untoned muscle.*
4. Progress ambulation *to increase tolerance to activity.*
5. Teach patient to take pulse *to determine activity tolerance:* Take pulse for full minute *before exercise* and then for 10 seconds and multiply by 6 *at exercise peak.*

Activity Intolerance Related to Prolonged Immobility or Deconditioning

Defining Characteristics
- Systolic blood pressure (SBP) drop >20 mm Hg; heart rate increase >20 beats/min with postural change
- Syncope with postural change
- Patient reports lightheadedness with postural change

Outcome Criteria
- SBP drop is <10 mm Hg; heart rate increase is <10 beats/min with postural change.
- Syncope or lightheadedness is absent with postural change.

Nursing Interventions and Rationale
1. Instruct the patient how to perform straight leg raises, dorsiflexion/plantar flexion, and quadriceps-setting and gluteal-setting exercises *to increase muscular and vascular tone.*
2. Consult with physician regarding the administration of fluids to ensure that the patient is hydrated to 24-hour fluid requirements per body surface area (BSA) *to increase preload and thus stroke volume and cardiac output.*
3. Reposition patient incrementally *to avoid syncope:*
   - Head of bed to 45 degrees, and hold until symptom-free.
   - Head of bed to 90 degrees, and hold until symptom-free.
   - Dangle until symptom-free.
   - Stand until symptom-free, and ambulate.
4. Collaborate with physician regarding patient's activity level *to ensure patient's safety.*

NURSING MANAGEMENT PLAN
Acute Confusion

Definition: Abrupt onset of a cluster of global, transient changes and disturbances in attention, cognition, psychomotor activity, level of consciousness, and/or sleep/wake cycle

Acute Confusion Related to Sensory Overload, Sensory Deprivation, and Sleep Pattern Disturbance

Defining Characteristics
Early Symptoms
- Sudden onset of global cognitive function impairment (from hours to days)
- Restlessness, agitation, and combative behavior
- Drowsiness (can lead to loss of consciousness)
- Slurring of speech, inappropriate statements or "word salad," mumbling, or inappropriate gestures
- Short attention span (needs questions repeated); inability to learn new material
- Disordered sleep/wake cycle
- Disorientation to person, time, place, and situation
- Difficulty in separating dreams from reality (may experience bizarre dreams or nightmares)
- Anger at staff for continued questions about his or her orientation

Later Symptoms
- Symptoms that tend to fluctuate throughout the day and night
- Continuations of early symptoms, which may be more frequent or of longer duration
- Illusions
- Hallucinations
- Extreme agitation (e.g., attempts to climb out of bed, pull out catheters, rip off dressings)
- Calling out in loud voice, swearing, or attempting to bite or hit people who approach patient

Nursing Interventions and Rationale
1. Determine and document the patient's dominant spoken language, his or her literacy, and the language(s) in which he or she is literate. *Sometimes people are not literate in their spoken language; or less commonly, they are literate only in their second language.*
2. Determine and document patient's premorbid degree of orientation, cognitive capabilities, and any sensory-perceptual deficits. *Assuming that the patients were or were not fully oriented before critical care admission bases the nurse's assessment on possibly erroneous assumptions.*

For Sensory Overload
1. Initiate each nurse/patient encounter by calling the patient by name and identifying yourself by name. *This fosters reality orientation and assists the patient in filtering irrelevant or impersonal conversation.*
2. Assess the patient's immediate physical environment from his or her viewpoint, and explain equipment, its sounds, and its therapeutic purpose. Demonstrate audible and visual alarms, and explain possible alarm conditions. *This decreases alienation of the patient*

from the technologic environment and reduces the inherent sense of fear and urgency accompanying alarm conditions.
3. For each procedure performed, provide "preparatory sensory information" (i.e., explain procedures in relation to the sensations the patient will experience, including duration of sensations). *Preparatory sensory information enhances learning and lessens anticipatory anxiety.*
4. Limit noise levels. Certainly, audible alarms cannot and must not be silenced, and many critical, albeit noisy, activities must take place in the critical care area. It has been shown, however, that noise levels produced by clinical personnel exceed those levels designated as "acceptable" and are often greater than those generated by technologic devices. Staff conversations must be kept soft enough that they are inaudible to the patient whenever possible. Critical care personnel are to assume that everything said at or around a patient's bedside is intended for that patient's awareness and that it will be interpreted as pertaining to him or her. *As in the discussion that follows, conversations about the patient but not to him or her foster depersonalization and delusions of reference.*
5. Enforce nighttime noise limits.
6. Readjust alarm limits on physiologic monitoring devices as the patient's condition changes (improves or deteriorates) *to lessen unnecessary alarm states.*
7. Consider use of headphones and audiocassette or compact disk player with patient's favorite and/or subliminal or classical music. *This can effectively filter out assaultive noise of the critical care environment and supplant it with familiar, soothing sounds and rhythms.*
8. Modify lighting. Day/night cycles need to be simulated with environmental lighting. At no time should overhead fluorescent lights be turned on abruptly without warning the patient, assisting him or her out of the supine position, and/or shielding his or her eyes with gauze or a face cloth. *Continuous bright lighting sustains anxiety and promotes circadian rhythm desynchronization.*
9. To the extent possible, shield patients from viewing urgent and emergent events in the critical care unit. *Resuscitation efforts, albeit difficult to conceal, engender fear in the patient and a sense of instability and vulnerability (e.g., "I'm next").* When such an event occurs, the nurse needs to elicit the patient's cognitive and emotional reaction; thoughts, impressions, and feeling need to be shared and misconceptions clarified. A useful approach for the nurse in this interchange is that of emphasizing the differences be-

tween the patient at hand and the one resuscitated (e.g., "He was considerably older," "more unstable," "had serious lung disease").

10. Ensure patients' privacy, their modesty, and, at the very least, their dignity. Physical exposure and nudity, although seemingly pale in importance compared with such priorities as physiologic assessment and stabilization, are primal indignities in all individuals. Patients must be kept minimally exposed. When, in the course of assessment and intervention, it becomes necessary to expose the patient, the nurse is to first verbally apologize for this necessity. *To be naked is to feel vulnerable; to be vulnerable is to feel fearful. In this regard, fear is an emotion concomitant to critical care that is preventable through nursing intervention.*

For Sensory Deprivation

1. Provide reality orientation in four spheres (personal, place, time, and situation) at more frequent intervals than when testing. Convey this information in the context of routine conversation. *Sample statements:* "Mr. Clark, this is Tuesday morning and you're in University Hospital. Your heart surgery was yesterday morning, and you're doing well. My name is Joe, and I'm your nurse today." *The patient is made to feel patronized by repetitions such as, "Do you know where you are?"* Given the effects of general anesthesia, narcotic analgesics, sedatives, and sleep, it is expected that some degree of disorientation will exist normally.

2. Ensure the patient's visual access to a calendar. Of interest, the design of most state-of-the-art critical care units now reflects many of the principles of sensory stimulation. One such coronary care unit was designed with a large wall clock facing the patient. A patient who had spent more than 1 week in this unit later reflected that one of the most "distressing, frustrating" aspects of his stay in the coronary care unit was the monotonous, inescapable attention to the clock and its painfully slow documentation of the passing of time.

3. Apprise the patient of daily news events and the weather.

4. Touch patients for the express purpose of communicating caring. Hold their hands, stroke their brows, rub the skin on an aspect of the arms. *Touch is the universal language of caring. In the setting of critical care, in which there is considerable physical body manipulation, it is useful and important to contrast assaultive touch with comforting touch.* Touch can be used as a technique for distraction from painful stimuli when used in conjunction with uncomfortable procedures. (*IMPORTANT:* See discussion of the use of touch in management of the patient experiencing hallucinations.)

5. Foster liberal visitation by family and significant others. Encourage significant others to touch the patient as consistent with their individual comfort level and cultural norms.

6. Structure and identify opportunities for the patient to exercise decision-making skills, however small. *Although not so designated, patients with sensory*

alterations experience a type of "cognitive deprivation" as well.

7. Assist patients to find meaning in their experiences. Explain the therapeutic purpose of all they are asked to do for themselves and all that is done with them and for them. Avoid statements such as "Will you turn to that side for me?" or "I need you to swallow this medication." *These statements implicitly convey that the maneuver has some value for the nurses versus the patients.* Similarly, use "thank you" judiciously. *This simple salutation, when used indiscriminately, suggests something was done to benefit the nurses and not the patients.* Patients need to find meaning and to identify their roles in the experience of critical illness and critical care. The sensations that constitute this experience and those that do not are made bearable and intelligible when attached to a larger picture of their conditions, treatment, and progress.

For Hallucinations

1. Approach the patient with a calm, matter-of-fact demeanor. *The goal of this interaction is for the nurse to demonstrate external control. This helps decrease the anxiety and fear that generally accompany hallucinations and allows the patient to feel safe. Anxiety is transferable.*

2. Address the patient by name. *This is a useful presentation of reality because self-identity is the last sphere of orientation to vanish.*

3. In responding to the patient's description of the hallucination, do not deny, argue, or attempt to disprove the existence of the perceived event. *Statements such as "There are no voices coming from that air vent" or "Look, I'm brushing my hand across the wall, and there are no bugs" confuse the patient further, because the hallucination, although frightening, is his or her perceived reality.*

4. Express to the patient that your experiences are dissimilar, and acknowledge how frightening his or hers must be. sample statements: "I don't hear (see, etc.) what you do, but I know how frightening such an experience must be to you. I'm Joe, your nurse, and I'm going to stay with you until the voices (etc.) go away." Remain with any patient who is experiencing a hallucination. *Feelings of fear and anxiety often accelerate when a patient is left alone. He or she needs someone to represent a nonthreatening reality. In addition, validating the patient's feelings demonstrates acceptance and sensitivity to the experience and promotes trust.*

5. Do not explore the content of the hallucination with the patient by asking about its nature or character. *The nurse is the patient's link with reality. Pursuit of a detailed description of a hallucination may signify to the patient that the nurse accepts his or her sensory distortion as factual. This may further confuse the patient and distance him or her more from reality.* (An exception is the patient who the nurse suspects is experiencing auditory hallucinations [i.e., hearing "voice commands"]. To ascertain that the voices are not telling the patient to harm him- or

herself, it is appropriate for the nurse to ask simply and concretely, "What are the voices saying?") The nurse can help bridge the gap between the patient's misperception and reality by addressing the feelings (e.g., fear, anxiety) and/or meanings (e.g., danger, death) engendered by the hallucination. Determining how the misperception affects the patient emotionally, acknowledging those feelings, and using a calm, controlled, matter-of-fact approach will provide the trust and comfort the patient needs to tolerate this frightening experience. In other words, deal with the intent more than the content of the hallucination. *The resultant decrease in anxiety will enable the patient to focus more accurately on his or her immediate environment.*

6. Talk concretely with the patient about things that are really happening. Sample statements: "How does your chest incision feel this afternoon, Mr. Clark?" "Your sister Kate was here to see you, but you were sleeping. She went down to the cafeteria and will be back." "Your secretions are a little easier for you to cough up today." *Interpretation of reality-based stimuli by the nurse encourages the patient to focus on actual circumstances and discourages a preoccupation with sensory misperceptions.*

7. There may be circumstances in which it is appropriate for the nurse simply to distract the patient by changing the topic. This tactic is useful in situations of escalating anxiety and confusion or when all else fails. Topics need to consist of basic themes that are universally understood and culturally congruent, such as music, food, or weather. They may also be topics of special interest to the patient, such as hobbies, crafts, or sports. Topics that evoke strong emotions, such as politics, religion, or sexuality, are to be avoided with most patients. *This is especially true of the patient with reality distortions; sometimes hallucinations and delusions are expressions of repressed conflicts associated with religious, sexual, or aggressive issues. Pursuit of such subjects could increase confusion and anxiety.*

8. Consider the following regarding the use of touch. *Touch presents a nonthreatening external reality and can therefore be useful in the management of patients with sensory alterations. However, for the patient experiencing hallucinations (as well as delusions and illusions), touch can be readily misinterpreted as, for instance, aggression or pain, or it can actually provide the basis for a tactile illusion.* Therefore avoid the use of touch as an intervention strategy for any patient who demonstrates escalating anxiety or paranoid, suspicious, or mistrustful thoughts.

9. For auditory hallucinations:
   a. *Patient behaviors:* Head cocked as if listening to an unseen presence; lips moving.
   b. *Therapeutic nurse responses:* "Mr. Clark, you appear to be listening to something." If the patient acknowledges voices: "I don't hear any voices, but I know this is troubling you. The voices will go away. Nothing is going to harm you. I'm Joe, your nurse, and I'll be here with you."

   c. *Nontherapeutic nurse responses:* "Tell me about your conversations with these voices." "To whom do these voices belong—anyone you know?"

10. For visual hallucinations:
    a. *Patient behaviors:* Staring into space as if focused on an unseen object; startled movements and anxious facial expression.
    b. *Therapeutic nurse responses:* "Mr. Clark, something seems to be troubling you. Tell me what it is." If patient states he visualizes people, images, or the devil in his environment and implies a sense of danger, respond, "There are only nurses and doctors here, Mr. Clark. I know this must be upsetting, but these images will go away. We're here with you in the hospital. Nothing will happen to you."
    c. *Nontherapeutic nurse responses:* "Describe the people you see. What are they wearing?" "What does the devil mean in your life? What about God?"

For Delusions

1. Explain all unseen noises, voices, and activity simply and clearly. *They readily feed a delusional system. Sample statements:* "That is Dr. Smith. He's come to see you and other patients here in the hospital." "The voices and activity you hear are from the bedside of the patient behind this curtain. He's being helped by one of the nurses."

2. Avoid the "negative challenge" of the patient's delusions (e.g., "Nobody here stole your belongings" or "Doctors and nurses do not harm people"). Similarly, avoid defending the referents of the patient's belief: "Nurses are good" and "Doctors mean well." *Remember, a delusion is a belief, albeit false, that cannot be changed with logic. To attempt this change is to challenge the patient's belief system and thereby escalate his or her anxiety, further blurring the boundaries between reality and the patient's internally-based "logic."*

3. For the patient with persecutory delusions who refuses food, fluids, or medications because of a belief that they have been poisoned or are tainted, permit the refusal unless it is a life-threatening event. Try again in 20 minutes; allow the patient to choose an alternative selection of food or to read the label on the unit's medication. Coercion, show of force, or engagement in complicated, logical justifications will only heighten the patient's suspiciousness and possibly reinforce the delusional belief. *When the patient feels more in control, he or she need not rely on the "paradoxical" quality of the delusion to equip him or her with a false sense of power. His or her power instead is derived from making reality-based decisions.*

4. Staff members should be particularly careful not to engage in unnecessary laughter or whispering within view of the delusional patient. *The delusional patient is hypervigilant, scanning the environment for evidence to corroborate or confirm his or her belief that staff members are colluding against him or her; clearly, laughter and whispers easily suggest this belief, this delusion of reference. This rationale pertains to the patient experiencing hallucinations and/or illusions as well.*

5. Observe the principles detailed in the third intervention of "For Hallucinations."

For Illusions

1. As with the management of delusions, the nurse simply and briefly interprets a reality-based stimulus for the patient in a calm, matter-of-fact manner. ***Seen and unseen noises, voices, activity, and people can provide the stimulus for a sensory misinterpretation, an illusion.***

2. There should be minimal stimulation in the patient's immediate environment. Nursing interventions detailed previously under "Sensory Overload" are especially relevant here.

3. The theme of the nurse's verbal approach to the patient experiencing illusions is similar to that outlined for hallucinations and delusions: address the feeling and meaning associated with the experience, not the content of the sensory misinterpretation.

    a. *Patient behaviors:* Eyes darting, startled movements, frightened facial expression. "I know who you are. You're the devil come to take me to hell."

    b. *Therapeutic nurse responses:* "I'm Joe, your nurse. I know this experience is troubling for you. You're in the hospital, and no one here will harm you."

    c. *Nontherapeutic nurse responses:* "There are no such things as devils and angels." "Do you think the devil would be dressed in white?" ***The first nontherapeutic nurse response carries a parental tone (i.e., "You know better than that."), thus infantilizing the patient and adding to his or her feelings of powerlessness over the environment. The second nontherapeutic response reflects obvious logic, which is not in the patient's sensory domain; therefore it cannot be processed and only adds to his or her confused state.***

4. Observe the principles detailed in the fifth intervention of "For Hallucinations."

NURSING MANAGEMENT PLAN

Acute Pain

Definition: Unpleasant sensory and emotional experience arising from actual or potential tissue damage or described in terms of such damage (International Association for the Study of Pain); sudden or slow onset of any intensity from mild to severe with an anticipated or predictable end and a duration of less than 6 months

Acute Pain Related to Transmission of Perception of Cutaneous, Visceral, Muscular, or Ischemic Impulses

Defining Characteristics

Subjective
- Patient verbalizes presence of pain
- Patient rates pain on scale of 1 to 10 using a visual analog scale

Objective
- Increase in blood pressure (BP), heart rate (HR), and respiratory rate (RR)
- Pupillary dilation
- Diaphoresis, pallor
- Skeletal muscle reactions (grimacing, clenching fists, writhing, pacing, guarding or splinting of affected part)
- Apprehension, fearful appearance
- May not exhibit any physiologic change

Outcome Criteria

(*NOTE:* Outcome is highly variable, depending on individual patient and pain circumstance factors.)
- Patient verbalizes that pain is reduced to a tolerable level or is totally relieved.
- Patient's pain rating is lower on scale of 1 to 10.
- BP, HR, and RR return to baseline 5 minutes after administration of intravenous (IV) narcotic or 20 minutes after administration of intramuscular (IM) narcotic.

Nursing Interventions and Rationale

1. Modify variables that heighten the patient's experience of pain.
   - Explain to the patient that frequent, detailed, and seemingly repetitive assessments will be conducted *to allow the nurse to better understand the patient's pain experience, not because the existence of pain is in question.*
   - Explain the factors responsible for pain production in the individual. Estimate the expected duration of the pain if possible.
   - Explain diagnostic and therapeutic procedures to the patient in relation to sensations the patient should expect to feel.
   - Reduce the patient's fear of addiction by explaining the difference between drug tolerance and drug addiction. Drug tolerance is a physiologic phenomenon in which a drug does begins to lose effectiveness after repeated doses; drug dependence is a psychologic phenomenon in which narcotics are used regularly for emotional, not medical, reasons.
   - Instruct the patient to ask for pain medication when pain is beginning and not to wait until it is intolerable.
   - Explain that the physician will be consulted if pain relief is inadequate with the present medication.
   - Instruct patient in the importance of adequate rest, especially when it reduces pain *to maintain strength and coping abilities and to reduce stress.*
2. Collaborate with physician regarding pharmacologic interventions.
   - For postsurgical or posttraumatic cutaneous, muscular, or visceral pain, perform the following:
     a. Medicate with narcotic maximally to break the pain cycles as long as level of consciousness and vital signs are stable: check patient's previous response to similar dosage and narcotic. *NOTE:* First dose received postoperatively is usually reduced by one half *to evaluate patient's individual response to medication.*
     b. Continuous pain requires continuous analgesia.
        (1) Establish optimal analgesic dose that brings optimal pain relief.
        (2) Offer pain medication at prescribed regular intervals rather than making patient ask for it *to maintain more steady blood levels.*
        (3) Consider waking patient to avoid loss of opiate blood levels during sleep.
     c. If administering medication on as-necessary (PRN) basis, give it when the patient's pain is just beginning, rather than at its peak. Advise patient to intercept pain, not endure it, or several hours and higher doses of narcotics may be necessary to relieve pain, leading to a cycle of undermedication and pain alternating with overmedication and drug toxicity.
     d. Perform rehabilitation exercises (turn, deep breathe, leg exercises, ambulate) shortly before peak of drug effect *because this will be the optimal time for the patient to increase activity with the least risk of increasing pain.*
     e. When making the transition from one drug to another or from IM or IV to oral (PO) medication, the use of an equianalgesic chart is helpful. Equianalgesic means *approximately* the same pain relief. Many consider the IM and IV dose of medications equianalgesic; however, others recommend using one half the IM dose for the IV dose. To effectively use analgesics, each patient requires an individual choice of drug, dose, time interval, and route. The patient's response should be closely monitored to determine if the right analgesic choice was made.
     f. To assess effectiveness of pain medication, do the following:
        (1) Reevaluate pain 5 minutes after IV and 20 minutes after IM medication administration, observe patient's behavior, and ask patient to rate pain on scale of 1 to 10.

(2) Collaborate with physician to add or delete other medications that potentiate the action of analgesics, such as antiemetics, hypnotics, sedatives, or muscle relaxants.

(3) Observe for indicators of undertreatment: report of pain not relieved; observed restlessness, sleeplessness, irritability, and anorexia; decreased activity level.

(4) Observe for indicators of overtreatment: hypotension or bradycardia; respiratory rate <10/min; excessive sedation.

g. If IV patient-controlled analgesia (PCA) is used, perform the following. (*NOTE*: PCA allows patients to administer small doses of their prescribed medication when they feel the need. Constant levels of the drug in the blood stream mean lower doses can be used to obtain analgesia. Pain control is improved because the patient is in control and experiences less fear of unrelieved pain. Reduced net narcotic use is noted, as is less sedation. Critical care patients appropriate for PCA are those who are alert, such as burn patients, trauma patients without head injury, and some postoperative patients.)

(1) Instruct the patient on what the drug is, the dose, and how often it can be self-administered by pushing the button to activate the PCA machine. For example, "When you have pain, instead of asking the nurse to bring medication, push the button that activates the machine and a small dose of the pain medicine will be injected into your IV line. You can keep your pain under control by administering additional medicine as soon as your pain begins to return or increases. Also, push the button before undertaking a painful activity, such as ambulation. Try to balance your pain relief against sleepiness, and don't activate the machine if you start to feel sleepy. If your pain medicine seems to stop working despite pushing the button several times, call the nurse to check your IV. If you are not receiving adequate pain relief, the nurse will call your doctor."

(2) Monitor vital signs, especially BP and RR, every hour for the first 4 hours, and assess postural HR and BP before initial ambulation.

(3) Monitor respirations every 2 hours while patient is on patient-controlled analgesia.

(4) If patient's respirations decrease to <10/min or if patient is overly sedated, anticipate IV administration of naloxone.

h. If epidural narcotic analgesia is used, do the following: (*NOTE:* The delivery of narcotics, such as morphine or fentanyl, by epidural route to specific receptors in the spinal cord selectively blocks pain impulses to the brain for up to 24 hours. Effective analgesia can be obtained without many of the negative side effects or serum narcotic concentrations.)

(1) Keep patient's head elevated 30 to 45 degrees after injection *to prevent respiratory depressant effects.*

(2) Observe closely for respiratory depression up to 24 hours after injection. Monitor respiratory rate every 15 minutes for 1 hour; every 30 minutes for 7 hours; and every hour for the remaining 16 hours.

(3) Assess for adequate cough reflex.

(4) Avoid use of other central nervous system (CNS) depressants, such as sedatives.

(5) Observe for reports of pruritus, nausea, and vomiting.

(6) Anticipate administration of naloxone for respiratory depression (and smaller doses of naloxone for pruritus).

(7) Assess for and treat urinary retention.

(8) Assess epidural catheter site for local infection. Keep catheter taped securely *to prevent catheter migration.*

• For peripheral vascular ischemic pain (hypothetic vascular occlusion of leg), do the following:

a. Correctly identify and differentiate ischemic pain from other types of pain. (*NOTE:* Ischemic pain is usually a burning, aching pain made worse by exercise and lessened or relieved by rest. Eventually the pain occurs at rest. Coldness and pallor of extremity may be noted, especially if the limb is elevated above the heart level. Rubor and mottling of the skin may be evident from prolonged tissue anoxia and inability of damaged vessels to constrict. Eventually cyanosis and gangrenous tissue will be evident. Chronic ischemia leads to visible changes in the limb, such as flaking skin, brittle nails and hair, leg ulcers, and cellulitis).

b. Administer pain medications, and evaluate their effectiveness as previously described. Remember that the pain of ischemia is chronic and continuous and can make the patient irritable and depressed.

c. Treat the cause of the ischemic pain, and institute measures to increase circulation to the affected part.

3. Initiate nonpharmacologic interventions.

• Treat contributing factors; provide explanations (see intervention no. 2 at beginning of this nursing management plan).

• Apply comfort measures.

a. Use relaxation techniques, such as back rubs, massage, warm baths, music, and aroma therapy. Use blankets and pillows *to support the painful part and reduce muscle tension.* Encourage slow, rhythmic breathing.

b. Encourage progressive muscle relaxation techniques.

(1) Instruct patient to inhale and tense (tighten) specific muscle groups and then relax the muscles as exhalation occurs.

(2) Suggest an order for performing the tension/relaxation cycle (e.g., start with facial muscles and move down body, ending with toes).

c. Encourage guided imagery.

(1) Ask patient to recall an experienced image that is very pleasurable and relaxing and involves at least two senses.

(2) Have patient begin with rhythmic breathing and progressive relaxation and then travel mentally to the scene.

(3) Have the patient slowly experience the scene (how it looks, sounds, smells, feels).

(4) Ask patient to practice this imagery in private.

(5) Instruct patient to end the imagery by counting to three and saying, "Now I'm relaxed." If person does not end the imagery and falls asleep, the purpose of the technique is defeated.

NURSING MANAGEMENT PLAN

Anxiety

Definition: Vague uneasy feeling of discomfort or dread accompanied by an autonomic response (the source often nonspecific or unknown to the individual); a feeling of apprehension caused by anticipation of danger. It is an alerting signal that warns of impending danger and enables the individual to take measures to deal with threat

Anxiety Related to Threat to Biologic, Psychologic, and/or Social Integrity

Defining Characteristics

Subjective
- Verbalizes increased muscle tension
- Expresses frequent sensation of tingling in hands and feet
- Relates continuous feeling of apprehension
- Expresses preoccupation with a sense of impending doom
- Reports has difficulty falling asleep
- Repeatedly expresses concerns about changes in health status and outcome of illness

Objective
- Psychomotor agitation (fidgeting, jitteriness, restlessness)
- Tightened, wrinkled brow
- Strained (worried) facial expression
- Hypervigilance (scans environment)
- Startles easily
- Distractibility
- Sweaty palms
- Fragmented sleep patterns
- Tachycardia
- Tachypnea

Outcome Criteria
- Patient effectively uses learned relaxation strategies.
- Patient demonstrates significant decrease in psychomotor agitation.
- Patient verbalizes reduction in tingling sensations in hands and feet.
- Patient is able to focus on the tasks at hand.
- Patient expresses positive, future-based plans to family and staff.
- Patient's heart rate and rhythm remain within limits commensurate with physiologic status.

Nursing Interventions and Rationale
1. Instruct the patient in the following simple, effective relaxation strategies:
   - If not contraindicated for cardiovascular reasons, tense and relax all muscles progressively from toes to head.
   - Perform slow deep-breathing exercises.
   - Focus on a single object or person in the environment.
   - Listen to soothing music or relaxation tapes with eyes closed.

   Progressive toe-to-head relaxation releases the muscular tension that may be a stress-related effect resulting from the threat or change in the patient's health status and outcome of illness. Deep-breathing exercises provide slow, rhythmic, controlled breathing patterns that relax the patient and distract him or her from the effects of his or her illness and hospitalization. Focusing on a single object or person helps the patient dismiss myriad disorienting stimuli from his or her visual-perceptual field, which can have a dizzying, distorted effect. A clear sensorium allows him or her to feel more in control of his or her environment. Music or words expressed in soft, low tones tend to produce soothing, relaxing effects that counteract or inhibit escalating anxiety and provide respites from the patient's situational crisis. Closed eyes eliminate distracting visual stimuli and promote a more restful environment.

2. Actively listen to and accept the patient's concerns regarding the threats from his or her illness, outcome, and hospitalization. *Active listening and unconditional acceptance validate the patient as a worthwhile individual and assure him or her that his or her concerns, no matter how great, will be addressed. Knowledge that he or she has an avenue for ventilation will assuage anxiety.*

3. Help the patient distinguish between realistic concerns and exaggerated fears through clear, simple explanations. *Sample statements:* "Your lab results show that you're doing OK right now." "The shortness of breath you're experiencing is not unusual." "The pain you described is expected, and this medication will relieve it." *A patient who is informed about his or her progress and is reassured about expected symptoms and management of care will be better equipped to maintain a more realistic perspective of his or her illness and its outcome. Thus anxiety emanating from imagined or exaggerated fears will likely be assuaged or averted.*

4. Provide simple clarification of environmental events and stimuli that are not related to the patient's illness and care. *Sample statements:* "That loud noise is coming from a machine that is helping another patient." "The visitor behind the curtain is crying because she's had an upsetting day." "That gurney is here to take another patient to x-ray." *Clarification of events and stimuli that are unrelated to the patient helps to disengage him or her from the extant anxiety-provoking situations surrounding him or her, thus avoiding further anxiety and apprehension.*

5. Assist the patient in focusing on building on prior coping strategies to deal with the effects of his or her illness and care. *Sample statements:* "What methods have helped you get through difficult times in the past?" "How can we help you use those methods now?" (See the nursing management plan for Ineffective Coping, for interventions that assist patients to use coping strategies effectively.)

Use of previously successful coping strategies in conjunction with newly learned techniques arms the patient with an arsenal of weapons against anxiety, providing him or her with greater control over the situational crisis and decreased feelings of doom and despair.

6. Give the patient permission to deny or suppress the effects of his or her illness and hospitalization with which he or she cannot cope or control. *Sample statements:* "It's perfectly okay to ignore things you can't handle right now." "How can we help ease your mind during this time?" "What are some things or tasks that may help distract you?" *Adaptive denial can be helpful in reducing feelings of anxiety in patients with life-threatening illness.*

NURSING MANAGEMENT PLAN
Autonomic Dysreflexia

Definition: Life-threatening, uninhibited sympathetic response of the nervous system to a noxious stimulus after a spinal cord injury at T7 or above

Autonomic Dysreflexia Related to Excessive Autonomic Response to Noxious Stimuli (e.g., Distended Bladder, Distended Bowel, Skin Irritation)

Defining Characteristics

Major
- Paroxysmal hypertension (sudden periodic elevated blood pressure [BP] greater than 20 mm Hg above patient's normal BP); for many spinal cord injury patients, a normal BP may be only 90/60 mm Hg
- Bradycardia (most common; pulse <60 beats/min) or tachycardia (pulse <100 beats/min)
- Diaphoresis (above the injury)
- Facial flushing
- Pallor (below the injury)
- Pounding headache (a diffuse pain in different portions of the head and not confined to any nerve distribution area)

Minor
- Nasal congestion
- Engorgement of temporal and neck vessels
- Conjunctival congestion
- Chills without fever
- Pilomotor erection (goose bumps) below the injury
- Blurred vision
- Chest pain
- Metallic taste in mouth
- Horner syndrome (constriction of the pupil, partial ptosis of the eyelid, enophthalmos, and sometimes loss of sweating over the affected side of the face)

Outcome Criteria
- BP has returned to patient's norm.
- Pulse rate is >60 or <100 beats/min (or within patient's norm).
- Headache is absent.
- Nasal stuffiness, sweating, and flushing above level of injury are absent.
- Chills, goose bumps, and pallor below level of injury are absent.
- Patient verbalizes causes, prevention, symptoms, and treatment of condition.

Nursing Interventions and Rationale
1. Place the patient on cardiac monitor, and assess for bradycardia, tachycardia, or other dysrhythmias. *Disturbances of cardiac rate and rhythm can occur because of autonomic dysfunction associated with dysreflexia.*
2. Do not leave the patient alone. One nurse monitors the BP and patient status every 3 to 5 minutes while another provides treatment.
3. Place the patient's head of bed to upright position *to decrease BP and promote cerebral venous return.*
4. Remove any support stockings or abdominal binder to reduce venous return.
5. Investigate for and remove offending cause of dysreflexia:
   a. Bladder
      - If indwelling catheter not in place, catheterize patient immediately.
      - Lubricate catheter with lidocaine jelly before insertion.
         - Drain 500 ml of urine, and recheck BP.
         - If BP still elevated, drain another 500 ml of urine.
      - If BP declines after the bladder is empty, serial BP must be monitored closely *because the bladder can go into severe contractions causing hypertension to recur.*
      - Collaborate with physician regarding the instillation of 30 ml tetracaine through the catheter *to decrease the flow of impulses from the bladder.*
      - If indwelling catheter is in place, check for kinks or granular sediment that may indicate occlusion.
      - If catheter is plugged, irrigate it gently with no more than 30 ml of sterile normal saline solution. If the bladder is in tetany, fluid will go in but will not drain out. Atropine is sometimes administered *to relieve bladder tetany.*
      - If unable to irrigate catheter, remove it and prepare to reinsert a new catheter; proceed with its lubrication, drainage, and observation as outlined above.
   b. Bowel
      - Using glove lubricated with anesthetic ointment, check rectum for fecal impaction.
      - If impaction is felt, *to decrease flow of impulses from bowel,* insert anesthetic ointment into rectum 10 minutes before manual removal of impaction.
      - A low, hypertonic enema or a suppository may be given to assist bowel evacuation.
   c. Skin
      - Loosen clothing or bed linens as indicated.
      - Inspect skin for pimples, boils, pressure sores, and ingrown toenails, and treat as indicated.
6. If symptoms of dysreflexia do not subside, have available the intravenous (IV) solutions and antihypertensive drugs of the physician's choosing (e.g., hydralazine, nifedipine, phentolamine, diazoxide, sodium nitroprusside). Administer medications, and monitor their effectiveness. Assess BP and pulse.
7. Instruct patient about causes, symptoms, treatment, and prevention of dysreflexia.
8. Encourage patient to carry medical bracelet or informational card to present to medical personnel in the event dysreflexia may be developing.

NURSING MANAGEMENT PLAN
Compromised Family Coping

Definition: Usually supportive primary person (family member or close friend) provides insufficient, ineffective, or compromised support, comfort, assistance, or encouragement that may be needed by the client to manage or master adaptive tasks related to his/her health challenge

Compromised Family Coping Related to Critically Ill Family Member

Defining Characteristics
- Disruption of usual family functions and roles
- Inability to accept or deal with crisis situation; use of defense mechanisms (e.g., denial, anger); unrealistic expectations of patient's outcome and care provided; judgmental toward health care providers
- Nonrecognition that family is in state of crisis
- Inappropriate emotional outbursts; arguments among family and with others; inability to respond to each other's feelings or support each other
- Misinterpretation of information; short attention span with repeated questions about information already provided; members not sharing information with each other
- Inability to make decisions regarding changes in family structure or about course of care for ill member; noncooperation among family members
- Expressions of grief, hopelessness, powerlessness, and isolation; do not seek or respond to support services
- Hesitancy to spend time with ill person in the critical care unit, or inappropriate behavior when visiting (may upset patient)
- Neglect of own personal health; fatigue, apathy; refusal of offers for respite time

Outcome Criteria
- The family will express an understanding of course/prognosis of illness, therapies, and alternative measures.
- The family will diminish or resolve conflicts and cooperate in decision making.
- The family will develop trust and mutual support for each member and form a cohesive unit.
- The family will support ill person in making decisions (if capable) or respect prior wishes regarding provision of health care.
- Family efforts will be directed toward a purpose and readjust to changes in life patterns and role function. Members will accept responsibility for changes.
- The family will identify and use effective coping strategies.
- The family will identify and use available resources as needed to facilitate resolution of the crisis.
- The family will have a sense of control and confidence in meeting personal and collective needs.

Nursing Interventions and Rationale
1. Identify family's perception of the crisis situation. Determine family structure; roles' developmental phase; and ethnic, cultural, and belief factors that may affect communication with family and the plan of care. Identify strengths of the family. *All initial nursing interventions should be directed toward resolving the crisis situation. Understanding and using family* *theory principles will facilitate this process and individualize care.*
2. Provide honest and accurate information in language persons can understand. Give updated information as appropriate. Listen! *This facilitates open communication among family and health care providers, projects a caring attitude and concern for them and patient, and assists family in making decision and being involved with the plan and goals of care.*
3. Encourage liberal visitation with patient. Before the visit, prepare family members for what they will observe in a technical environment. Inform them about patient's appearance, behaviors (etc.) that may be distressing to them. Explain the etiology of patient responses to stimuli (e.g., pain, trauma, surgery, medication), and explain that these behaviors are being monitored and are usually temporary. Encourage them to touch the patient and let the patient know of their presence. *This prevents a strong emotional reaction to an unfamiliar and frightening situation, involves family as support to each other and to the patient, demonstrates the nurse's concern for them as persons, and facilitates satisfaction with care being provided for their loved one.*
4. Identify and support effective coping behaviors. *This aids in the family's sense of control and resolution of helplessness/powerlessness.*
5. Observe for signs of fatigue and the need for emotional/spiritual support and respite from hospital waiting routine. Encourage family to verbalize feelings. Provide information on available resources. Alert interdisciplinary team members (social, psychologic, spiritual) to family needs. Provide pager device (if available), or obtain phone numbers when family leaves the hospital premises. *This provides support and comfort, facilitates hope, resolves sense of isolation, gives sense of security, and diminishes guilt feeling for attending to personal needs.*
6. Instruct family in simple care-giving techniques, and encourage participation in patient's care. *This facilitates giving a sense of "normalcy" to experience, self-confidence, and assurance that good care is being provided.*
7. Serve as advocate for patient and family. Teach family how to negotiate with the health care delivery system, and include them in health care team conferences when appropriate. *This facilitates informed decision making, promotes control and satisfaction, and permits mutual goal-setting.*
8. Consider nonbiologic or nonlegal family relationships. Encourage contact with patient and participation in care.

This facilitates holistic care and support of emotional ties and demonstrates respect for the family unit and relationships.

9. Provide emotional support and compassion when patient's condition worsens or deteriorates. *The use of touch and expression of concern for the patient and family convey comfort and trust in the health care provider and respect and assurance that the family's loved one will receive appropriate care and attention.*

NURSING MANAGEMENT PLAN
Decreased Cardiac Output

Definition: Inadequate blood pumped by the heart to meet the metabolic demands of the body

Decreased Cardiac Output Related to Alterations in Preload

Defining Characteristics
- Cardiac output <4.0 L/min
- Cardiac index <2.5 L/min/m^2
- Heart rate >100 beats/min
- Urine output <30 ml/hr or 0.5 ml/kg/hr
- Decreased mentation, restlessness, agitation, confusion
- Diminished peripheral pulses
- Blue, gray, or dark purple tint to tongue and sublingual area
- Systolic blood pressure <90 mm Hg
- Subjective complaints of fatigue

Reduced Preload:
- Right atrial pressure <2 mm Hg
- Pulmonary artery occlusion pressure <5 mm Hg

Excessive Preload:
- Right atrial pressure >6 mm Hg
- Pulmonary artery occlusion pressure >12 mm Hg

Outcome Criteria
- Cardiac output 4-8 L/min
- Cardiac index 2.5-4 L/min/m^2
- Right atrial pressure 2-8 mm Hg
- Pulmonary artery occlusion pressure 5-12 mg Hg

Nursing Interventions and Rationale
1. Collaborate with physician regarding the administration of oxygen to maintain an SpO$_2$ >92% *to prevent tissue hypoxia.*
2. Maintain surveillance for signs of decreased tissue perfusion and acidosis *to facilitate the early identification and treatment of complications.*
3. Monitor fluid balance and daily weights *to facilitate regulation of the patient's fluid balance.*

For Reduced Preload Secondary to Volume Loss:
1. Collaborate with physician regarding the administration of crystalloids, colloids, blood, and blood products *to increase circulating volume.*
2. Limit blood sampling, observe intravenous lines for accidental disconnection, apply direct pressure to bleeding sites, and maintain normal body temperature *to minimize fluid loss.*
3. Position patient with legs elevated, trunk flat, and head and shoulders above the chest *to enhance venous return.*

4. Encourage oral fluids (as appropriate), administer free water with tube feedings, and replace fluids that are lost through wound or tube drainage *to promote adequate fluid intake.*
5. Maintain surveillance for signs of fluid volume excess and adverse effects of blood and blood product administration *to facilitate the early identification and treatment of complications.*

For Reduced Preload Secondary to Venous Dilation:
1. Collaborate with physician regarding the administration of vasocontrictors *to increase venous return.*
2. Maintain surveillance for adverse effects of vasoconstrictor therapy *to facilitate the early identification and treatment of complications.*
3. If patient is hyperthermic, administer tepid bath, hypothermia blanket, and/or ice bags to axilla and groin *to decrease temperature and promote vasoconstriction.*

For Excessive Preload Secondary to Volume Overload:
1. Collaborate with physician regarding the administration of the following:
   - Diuretics to remove excessive fluid.
   - Vasodilators to decrease venous return.
   - Inotropes to increase myocardial contractility.
2. Restrict fluid intake and double concentrate intravenous drips *to minimize fluid intake.*
3. Position patient in semi-Fowler's or high-Fowler's position *to reduce venous return.*
4. Maintain surveillance for signs of fluid volume deficit and adverse effects of diuretic, vasodilator, and inotropic therapies *to facilitate the early identification and treatment of complications.*

For Excessive Preload Secondary to Venous Constriction:
1. Collaborate with physician regarding the administration of vasodilators *to promote venous dilation.*
2. Maintain surveillance for adverse effects of vasodilator therapy *to facilitate the early identification and treatment of complications.*
3. If patient is hypothermic, wrap patient in warm blankets or administer hyperthermia blanket *to increase temperature and promote vasodilation.*

Decreased Cardiac Output Related to Alterations in Afterload

Defining Characteristics
- Cardiac output <4 L/min
- Cardiac index <2.5 L/min/m^2
- Heart rate >100 beats/min
- Urine output <30 ml/hr
- Decreased mentation, restlessness, agitation, confusion

- Diminished peripheral pulses
- Blue, gray, or dark purple tint to tongue and sublingual area
- Systolic blood pressure <90 mm Hg
- Subjective complaints of fatigue

Reduced Afterload:
- Pulmonary vascular resistance <100 dynes/sec/cm^{-5}
- Systemic vascular resistance <800 dynes/sec/cm^{-5}

Excessive Afterload:
- Pulmonary vascular resistance >250 dynes/sec/cm^{-5}
- Systemic vascular resistance >1200 dynes/sec/cm^{-5}

Outcome Criteria
- Cardiac output 4-8 L/min
- Cardiac index 2.5-4 L/min/m^2
- Pulmonary vascular resistance 80-250 dynes/sec/cm^{-5}
- Systemic vascular resistance 800-1200 dynes/sec/cm^{-5}

Nursing Interventions and Rationale
1. Collaborate with physician regarding the administration of oxygen to maintain an SpO$_2$ $>92\%$ *to prevent tissue hypoxia.*
2. Maintain surveillance for signs of decreased tissue perfusion and acidosis *to facilitate the early identification and treatment of complications.*

For Reduced Afterload:
1. Collaborate with physician regarding the administration of vasocontrictors *to promote arterial vasoconstriction and prevent relative hypovolemia.* If decreased preload is present, implement nursing management plan

of care, Decreased Cardiac Output Related to Alterations in Preload.
2. Maintain surveillance for adverse effects of vasoconstrictor therapy *to facilitate the early identification and treatment of complications.*
3. If patient is hyperthermic, administer tepid bath, hypothermia blanket, and/or ice bags to axilla and groin *to decrease temperature and promote vasoconstriction.*

For Excessive Afterload:
1. Collaborate with physician regarding the administration of vasodilators *to promote arterial vasodilation.*
2. Collaborate with physician regarding initiation of intraaortic balloon pump *to facilitate afterload reduction.*
3. Promote rest and relaxation and decrease environmental stimulation *to minimize sympathetic stimulation.*
4. Maintain surveillance for adverse effects of vasodilator therapy *to facilitate the early identification and treatment of complications.*
5. If patient is hypothermic, wrap patient in warm blankets or administer hyperthermia blanket *to increase temperature and promote vasodilation.*
6. If patient is in pain, treat pain *to reduce sympathetic stimulation.* Implement nursing management plan of care, Acute Pain Related to Transmission and Perception of Cutaneous, Visceral, Muscular, or Ischemic Impulses.

Decreased Cardiac Output Related to Alterations in Contractility

Defining Characteristics
- Cardiac output <4 L/min
- Cardiac index <2.5 L/min/m^2
- Heart rate >100 beats/min
- Urine output <30 ml/hr
- Decreased mentation, restlessness, agitation, confusion
- Diminished peripheral pulses
- Blue, gray, or dark purple tint to tongue and sublingual area
- Systolic blood pressure <90 mm Hg
- Subjective complaints of fatigue
- Right ventricular stroke work index <7 g/m^2/beat
- Left ventricular stroke work index <35 g/m^2/beat

Outcome Criteria
- Cardiac output 4-8 L/min
- Cardiac index 2.5-4 L/min/m^2
- Right ventricular stroke work index 7-12 g/m^2/beat
- Left ventricular stroke work index 35-85 g/m^2/beat

Nursing Interventions and Rationale
1. Collaborate with physician regarding the administration of oxygen to maintain an SpO$_2$ $>92\%$ *to prevent tissue hypoxia.*

2. Maintain surveillance for signs of decreased tissue perfusion and acidosis *to facilitate the early identification and treatment of complications.*
3. Ensure preload is optimized. If preload is reduced or excessive, implement nursing management plan of care, Decreased Cardiac Output Related to Alterations in Preload.
4. Ensure afterload is optimized. If afterload is reduced or excessive, implement nursing management plan of care, Decreased Cardiac Output Related to Alterations in Afterload.
5. Ensure electrolytes are optimized. Collaborate with physician regarding the administration of electrolyte replacement therapy *to enhance cellular ionic environment.*
6. Collaborate with physician regarding the administration of inotropes *to enhance myocardial contractility.*
7. If myocardial ischemia present, implement nursing management plan of care, Altered Cardiopulmonary Tissue Perfusion.

Decreased Cardiac Output Related to Alterations in Heart Rate or Rhythm

Defining Characteristics
- Cardiac output <4 L/min
- Cardiac index <2.5 L/min/m^2
- Heart rate >100 beats/min
- Urine output <30 ml/hr or 0.5 ml/kg/hr
- Decreased mentation, restlessness, agitation, confusion
- Diminished peripheral pulses
- Blue, gray, or dark purple tint to tongue and sublingual area
- Systolic blood pressure <90 mm Hg

- Subjective complaints of fatigue
- Heart rate <60 beats/min
- Dysrhythmias

Outcome Criteria
- Cardiac output 4-8 L/min
- Cardiac index 2.5-4 L/min/m^2
- Absence of dysrhythmias or return to baseline
- Heart rate >60 beats/min

Nursing Interventions and Rationale
1. Collaborate with physician regarding the administration of oxygen to maintain an SpO$_2$ >92% *to prevent tissue hypoxia.*
2. Ensure electrolytes are optimized. Collaborate with physician regarding the administration of electrolyte therapy *to enhance cellular ionic environment and avoid precipitation of dysrhythmias.*
3. Collaborate with physician and pharmacist regarding patient's current medications and their effect on heart rate and rhythm *to identify any prodysrhythmic or bradycardic side effects.*

4. Maintain surveillance for signs of decreased tissue perfusion and acidosis *to facilitate the early identification and treatment of complications.*
5. Monitor ST segment continuously *to determine changes in myocardial tissue perfusion.* If myocardial ischemia is present, implement nursing management plan of care, Altered Cardiopulmonary Tissue Perfusion.

For Lethal Dysrhythmias or Asystole
1. Initiate Advanced Cardiac Life Support interventions and notify physician immediately.

For Nonlethal Dysrhythmias
1. Collaborate with physician regarding administration of antidysrhythmic therapy, synchronized cardioversion, and/or overdrive pacing *to control dysrhythmias.*
2. Maintain surveillance for adverse effects of antidysrhythmic therapy *to facilitate the early identification and treatment of complications.*

For Heart Rate <60 Beats/Min
1. Collaborate with physician regarding the initiation of temporary pacing *to increase heart rate.*

Decreased Cardiac Output Related to Sympathetic Blockade

Defining Characteristics
- Decreased cardiac output (CO) and cardiac index (CI)
- Systolic blood pressure (SBP) <90 mm Hg or below patient's baseline
- Decreased right atrial pressure (RAP) and pulmonary artery occlusion pressure (PAOP)
- Decreased systemic vascular resistance (SVR)
- Bradycardia
- Cardiac dysrhythmias
- Postural hypotension

Outcome Criteria
- CO and CI are within normal limits.
- SBP is >90 mm Hg or returns to baseline.
- RAP and PAOP are within normal limits.
- SVR is within normal limits.
- Sinus rhythm is present.
- Dysrhythmias are absent.
- Fainting or dizziness with position change is absent.

Nursing Interventions and Rationale
1. Implement measures to prevent episodes of postural hypertension:
   - Change patient's position slowly to allow the cardiovascular system time to compensate.

   - Apply antiembolic stockings to promote venous return.
   - Perform range of motion exercises every 2 hours to prevent venous pooling.
   - Collaborate with the physician and physical therapist regarding the use of a tilt table to progress the patient from supine to upright position.
2. Collaborate with the physician regarding the administration of the following:
   - Crystalloids and/or colloids to increase the patient's circulating volume, which increases stroke volume and subsequently cardiac output.
   - Vasopressors if fluids are ineffective to constrict the patient's vascular system, which increases resistance and subsequently blood pressure.
3. Monitor cardiac rhythm for bradycardia and/or dysrhythmias, *which can further decrease cardiac output.*
4. Avoid any activity that can stimulate the vagal response *because bradycardia can result.*
5. Treat symptomatic bradycardia and symptomatic dysrhythmias according to unit's emergency protocol or Advanced Cardiac Life Support (ACLS) guidelines.

NURSING MANAGEMENT PLAN
Decreased Intracranial Adaptive Capacity

Definition: Intracranial fluid dynamic mechanisms that normally compensate for increases in intracranial volumes are compromised, resulting in repeated disproportionate increases in intracranial pressure (ICP) in response to a variety of noxious and non-noxious stimuli

Decreased Intracranial Adaptive Capacity Related to Failure of Normal Intracranial Compensatory Mechanisms

Defining Characteristics
- ICP >15 mm Hg, sustained for 15-30 minutes
- Headache
- Vomiting, with or without nausea
- Seizures
- Decrease in Glasgow Coma Scale score of 2 or more points from baseline
- Alteration in level of consciousness, ranging from restlessness to coma
- Change in orientation: disoriented to time and/or place and/or person
- Difficulty or inability to follow simple commands
- Increasing systolic blood pressure of more than 20 mm Hg with widening pulse pressure
- Bradycardia
- Irregular respiratory pattern (e.g., Cheyne-Stokes, central neurogenic hyperventilation, ataxic, apneustic)
- Change in response to painful stimuli (e.g., purposeful to inappropriate or absent response)
- Signs of impending brain herniation:
  - Hemiparesis or hemiplegia
  - Hemisensory changes
  - Unequal pupil size (1 mm or more difference)
  - Failure of pupil to react to light
  - Dysconjugate gaze and inability to move one eye beyond midline if third, fourth, or sixth cranial nerves involved
  - Loss of oculocephalic or oculovestibular reflexes
  - Possible decorticate or decerebrate posturing

Outcome Criteria
- ICP is ≤15 mm Hg.
- Cerebral perfusion pressure (CPP) is >60 mm Hg.
- Clinical signs of increased ICP as previously described are absent.

Nursing Interventions and Rationale
1. Maintain adequate CPP.
   a. Collaborate with physician regarding the administration of volume expanders, vasopressors, or antihypertensives *to maintain the patient's blood pressure within normal range.*
   b. Implement measures to reduce ICP.
      - Elevate head of bed 30 to 45 degrees *to facilitate venous return.*
      - Maintain head and neck in neutral plan (avoid flexion, extension, or lateral rotation) *to enhance venous drainage from the head.*
      - Avoid extreme hip flexion.
      - Collaborate with the physician regarding the administration of steroids, osmotic agents, and diuretics and need for drainage of cerebrospinal fluid (CSF) if a ventriculostomy is in place.
      - Assist patient to turn and move self in bed (instruct patient to exhale while turning or pushing up in bed) *to avoid isometric contractions and Valsalva maneuver.*
2. Maintain patent airway and adequate ventilation and supply oxygen *to prevent hypoxemia and hypercarbia.*
3. Monitor arterial blood gas (ABG) values and maintain Pao_2 >80 mm Hg, $Paco_2$ at 25-35 mm Hg, and pH at 7.35-7.45 *to prevent cerebral vasodilation.*
4. Avoid suctioning beyond 10 seconds at a time; hyperoxygenate and hyperventilate before and after suctioning.
5. Plan patient care activities and nursing interventions around patient's ICP response. Avoid unnecessary additional disturbances, and allow patient up to 1 hour of rest between activities as frequently as possible. *Studies have shown the direct correlation between nursing care activities and increases in ICP.*
6. Maintain normothermia with external cooling or heating measures as necessary. Wrap hands, feet, and male genitalia in soft towels before cooling measures *to prevent shivering and frostbite.*
7. With physician's collaboration, control seizures with prophylactic and as-necessary (PRN) anticonvulsants. *Seizures can greatly increase the cerebral metabolic rate.*
8. Collaborate with the physician regarding the administration of sedatives, barbiturates, or paralyzing agents *to reduce cerebral metabolic rate.*
9. Counsel family members to maintain calm atmosphere and avoid disturbing topics of conversation (e.g., patient condition, pain, prognosis, family crisis, financial difficulties).
10. If signs of impending brain herniation are present, implement the following:
    a. Notify the physician at once.
    b. Be sure head of bed is elevated 45 degrees and patient's head is in neutral plane.
    c. Administer mainline intravenous (IV) infusion slowly to keep-open rate.
    d. Drain CSF as ordered if a ventriculostomy is in place.
    e. Prepare to administer osmotic agents and/or diuretics.
    f. Prepare patient for emergency computed tomography (CT) head scan and/or emergency surgery.

NURSING MANAGEMENT PLAN

Deficient Fluid Volume

Definition: Decreased intravascular, interstitial, and/or intracellular fluid. This refers to dehydration, water loss alone without change in sodium

Deficient Fluid Volume Related to Absolute Loss

Defining Characteristics
- Cardiac output (CO) <4 L /min
- Cardiac index (CI) <2.2 L /min
- Pulmonary artery occlusion pressure (PAOP), pulmonary artery diastolic (PAD) pressure less than normal or less than baseline, central venous pressure (CVP) less than normal or less than baseline (PAOP <6 mm Hg)
- Tachycardia
- Narrowed pulse pressure
- Systolic blood pressure (SBP) <100 mm Hg
- Urinary output <30 ml/hr
- Pale, cool, moist skin
- Apprehensiveness

Outcome Criteria
- CO is >4 L /min, and CI is >2.2 L /min.
- PAOP, PAD, and CVP are normal or back to baseline level.
- Pulse is normal or back to baseline.
- SBP is >90.
- Urinary output is >30 ml/hr.

Nursing Interventions and Rationale
1. Secure airway, and administer high-flow oxygen.
2. Place patient in supine position with legs elevated *to increase preload.* For patient with head injury, consider using low-Fowler's position with legs elevated.
3. For fluid repletion, use the 3:1 rule, replacing three parts of fluid for every unit of blood lost.
4. Administer crystalloid solutions using the fluid challenge technique: infuse precise aliquots of fluid (usually 5 to 20 ml/min) over 10-minute periods; monitor cardiac loading pressure serially *to determine successful challenging.* If the pulmonary PAOP or PAD elevates more than 7 mm Hg above beginning level, the infusion should be stopped. If the PAOP or PAD rises only to 3 mm Hg above baseline or falls, another fluid challenge should be administered.
5. Replete fluids first before considering use of vasopressors, *since vasopressors increase myocardial oxygen consumption out of proportion to the reestablishment of coronary perfusion in the early phases of treatment.*
6. When blood replacement is indicated, replace it with fresh packed red cells and fresh frozen plasma *to keep clotting factors intact.*
7. Move or reposition patient minimally *to decrease or limit tissue oxygen demands.*
8. Evaluate patient's anxiety level, and intervene through patient education or sedation *to decrease tissue oxygen demands.*
9. Maintain surveillance for signs and symptoms of fluid overload.

Deficient Fluid Volume Related to Decreased Secretion of Antidiuretic Hormone (ADH)

Defining Characteristics
- Confusion and lethargy
- Decreased skin turgor
- Thirst
- Weight loss over short period
- Decreased PAOP
- Decreased CVP
- Urinary output >6 L/day
- Serum sodium >148 mEq/L
- Serum osmolality >295 mOsm/kg
- Urine osmolality <100 mOsm/kg
- Urine specific gravity <1.005

Outcome Criteria
- Weight returns to baseline.
- Urinary output is >30 ml/hr and <200 ml/hr.
- Serum osmolality is 280-295 mOsm/kg.
- Urine specific gravity is 1.010-1.030.

Nursing Interventions and Rationale
1. Record intake and output every hour, noting color and clarity of urine *because color and clarity are an indication of urine concentration.*
2. Monitor ECG rhythm continuously for dysrhythmias *caused by electrolyte imbalance.*
3. Collaborate with physician regarding administration of vasopressin or desmopressin *to replace ADH.*
   a. Monitor patient for adverse effects of medications (i.e., headache, chest pain, abdominal pain) *caused by vasoconstriction.*
   b. Report adverse effects to physician immediately.
4. Collaborate with physician regarding intravenous fluid and electrolyte replacement therapy *to restore fluid balance, correct dehydration, and maintain electrolyte balance.*
   a. Administer hypotonic saline *to replace free water deficit.*
5. Provide oral fluids low in sodium such as water, coffee, tea, or orange juice *to decrease sodium intake.*
6. Weigh patient daily (at same time, in same amount of clothing, and preferably with same scale) *to ensure accuracy of readings.*
7. Reposition patient every 2 hours *to prevent skin integrity issues caused by dehydration.*

8. Provide mouth care every 4 hours *to prevent breakdown of oral mucous membranes.*
9. Collaborate with physician regarding administration of medications to prevent constipation *caused by dehydration.*

10. Maintain surveillance for symptoms of hypernatremia (muscle twitching, irritability, seizures), hypovolemic shock (hypotension, tachycardia, decreased CVP and PAOP), and deep vein thrombosis (calf pain, tenderness, swelling).

Deficient Fluid Volume Related to Relative Loss

Defining Characteristics
- PAOP, PAD pressure, CVP less than normal or less than baseline
- Tachycardia
- Narrowed pulse pressure
- SBP <100 mm Hg
- Urinary output <30 ml/hr
- Increased hematocrit level

Outcome Criteria
- PAOP, PAD, and CVP are normal or back to baseline.
- SBP is >90 mm Hg.

- Urinary output is >30 ml/hr.
- Hematocrit level is normal.

Nursing Interventions and Rationale
1. Collaborate with the physician regarding the administration of intravenous (IV) fluid replacements (usually normal saline solution or lactated Ringer's solution) at a rate sufficient to maintain urinary output >30 ml/hr. Colloid solutions are avoided in the initial phases (but can be used later) because of the possibility of increased edema formation *as a result of the increased capillary permeability.*

NURSING MANAGEMENT PLAN
Deficient Knowledge

Definition: Absence or deficiency of cognitive information related to a specific topic

Deficient Knowledge Related to Cognitive/Perceptual Learning Limitations (e.g., sensory overload, sleep deprivation, medications, anxiety, sensory deficits, language barrier)

Defining Characteristics
- Verbalized statement of inadequate knowledge of skills
- Verbalization of inadequate recall of information
- Verbalization of inadequate understanding of information
- Evidence of inaccurate follow-through of instructions
- Inadequate demonstration of a skill
- Lack of compliance with prescribed behavior

Outcome Criteria
- Patient participates actively in necessary and prescribed health behaviors.
- Patient verbalizes adequate knowledge or demonstrates adequate skills.

Nursing Interventions and Rationale
1. Determine specific cause of patient's cognitive or perceptual limitation.
2. Provide uninterrupted rest period before teaching session *to decrease fatigue and encourage optimal state for learning and retention.*
3. Manipulate environment as much as possible *to provide quiet and uninterrupted learning sessions.*
   - Ensure that lights are bright enough to see teaching aids but not too bright.
   - Schedule care and medications to allow uninterrupted teaching periods.
   - Move patient to quiet, private room for teaching if possible.
4. Adapt teaching sessions and materials to patient's and family's levels of education and ability to understand.
   - Provide printed material appropriate to reading level.
   - Use terminology understood by the patient.
   - Provide printed materials in patient's primary language *if possible.*
   - Use interpreters during teaching sessions *when necessary.*
5. Teach only present-tense focus during periods of sensory overload.
6. Determine potential effects of medications on ability to retain or recall information.
   - Avoid teaching critical content while patient is taking sedatives, analgesics, or other medications that affect memory.
7. Reinforce new skills and information in several teaching sessions. Use several senses when possible in teaching session (e.g., see a film, hear a discussion, read printed information, and demonstrate skills related to self-injection of insulin).
8. Reduce patient's anxiety.
   - Listen attentively, and encourage verbalization of feelings.
   - Answer questions as they arise in a clear and succinct manner.
   - Elicit patient's concerns, and address those issues first.
   - Give only correct and relevant information.
   - Continually assess response to teaching session, and discontinue if anxiety increases or physical condition becomes unstable.
   - Provide nonthreatening information before more anxiety-producing information is presented.
   - Plan for several teaching sessions so information can be divided into small, manageable packages.

Deficient Knowledge Related to Lack of Previous Exposure to Information

Defining Characteristics
- Verbalized statement of inadequate knowledge or skills
- New diagnosis or health problem requiring self-management or care
- Lack of prior formal or informal education about the specific health problem
- Demonstration of inappropriate behaviors related to management of health problem

Outcome Criteria
- Patient verbalizes adequate knowledge about or performs skills related to disease process, its causes, factors related to onset of symptoms, and self-management of disease or health problem.
- Patient actively participates in health behaviors required for performance of a procedure or in those behaviors enhancing recovery from illness and preventing recurrence or complications.

Nursing Interventions and Rationale
1. Determine existing level of knowledge or skill.
2. Assess factors that affect the knowledge deficit
   - Learning needs, including patient's priorities and the necessary knowledge and skills for safety.
   - Learning ability of client, including language skills, level of education, ability to read, preferred learning style.
   - Physical ability to perform prescribed skills or procedures; consider effect of limitations imposed by treatment such as bedrest, restriction of movement by intravenous or other equipment, or effect of sedatives or analgesics.
   - Psychologic effect of stage of adaptation to disease.
   - Activity tolerance and ability to concentrate.
   - Motivation to learn new skills or gain new knowledge.

3. Reduce or limit barriers to learning:
   - Provide consistent nurse/patient contact to encourage development of trusting and therapeutic relationship.
   - Structure environment to enhance learning; control unnecessary noise, interruptions.
   - Individualize teaching plan to fit patient's current physical and psychologic status.
   - Delay teaching until patient is ready to learn.
   - Conduct teaching sessions during period of day when patient is most alert and receptive.
   - Meet patient's immediate learning needs as they arise (e.g., give brief explanation of procedures when they are performed).
4. Promote active participation in the teaching plan by the patient and family:
   - Solicit input during development of plan.
   - Develop mutually acceptable goals and outcomes.
   - Solicit expression of feelings and emotions related to new responsibilities.
   - Encourage questions.
5. Conduct teaching sessions, using the most appropriate teaching methods.
6. Repeat key principles, and provide them in printed form *for reference at a later time.*
7. Give frequent feedback to patient when practicing new skills.
8. Use several teaching sessions when appropriate. *New information and skills should be reinforced several times after initial learning.*
9. Initiate referrals for follow-up if necessary:
   - Health educators.
   - Home health care.
   - Rehabilitation programs.
   - Social services.
10. Evaluate effectiveness of teaching plan, based on patient's ability to meet preset goals and objectives *to determine need for further teaching.*

NURSING MANAGEMENT PLAN
Disturbed Body Image

Definition: Confusion in mental picture of one's physical self

Disturbed Body Image Related to Actual Change in Body Structure, Function, or Appearance

Defining Characteristics
- Actual change in appearance, structure, or function
- Avoidance of looking at body part
- Avoidance of touching body part
- Hiding or overexposing body part (intentional or unintentional)
- Trauma to nonfunctioning part
- Change in ability to estimate spatial relationship of body to environment
- Verbalization of the following:
  —Fear of rejection or reaction by others
  —Negative feeling about body
  —Preoccupation with change or loss
  —Refusal to participate in or to accept responsibility for self-care of altered body part
- Personalization of part or loss with a name
- Depersonalization of part or loss by use of impersonal pronouns
- Refusal to verify actual change

Outcome Criteria
- Patient verbalizes the specific meaning of the change to him or her.
- Patient requests appropriate information about self-care.
- Patient completes personal hygiene and grooming daily with or without help.
- Patient interacts freely with family or other visitors.
- Patient participates in the discussions and conferences related to planning his or her medical and nursing management in the critical care unit and transfer from the unit.
- Patient talks with trained visitors (support-group representatives) at least twice about his or her loss.

Nursing Interventions and Rationale
1. Evaluate patient's mental, physical, and emotional state; recognize assets, strengths, response to illness, coping mechanisms, past experience with stress, and support system.
2. Appraise the response of family and significant others. *Body image is derived from the "reflected appraisals" of family and significant others.*
3. Determine the patient's goals and readiness for learning.
4. Provide the necessary information to help the patient and family adapt to the change. Clarify misconceptions about future limitations.
5. Permit and encourage the patient to express the significance of the loss or change; note nonverbal behavior responses.
6. Allow and encourage the patient's expression of anxiety. *Anxiety is the most predominant emotional response to a body image disturbance.*
7. Recognize and accept the use of denial as an adaptive defense mechanism when used early and temporarily.
8. Recognize maladaptive denial as that which interferes with the patient's progress and/or alienates support systems. Use confrontation.
9. Provide an opportunity for the patient to discuss sexual concerns.
10. Touch the affected body part *to provide the patient with sensory information about altered body structure and/or function.*
11. Encourage and provide movement of altered body part *to establish kinesthetic feedback. This enables the person to know his or her body as it now exists.*
12. Prepare the patient to look at the body part. Call the body part by its anatomic name (e.g., stump, stoma, limb) as opposed to "it" or "she." *The use of impersonal pronouns increases a sense of fantasy and depersonalization of the body part.*
13. Allow the patient to experience excellence in some aspect of physical functioning—walking, turning, deep breathing, healing, self-care—and point out progress and accomplishment. *This helps to balance the patient's sense of dysfunction with function.*
14. Avoid false reassurance. Acknowledge the difficulty of incorporating the altered body part or function into one's body image. *This evidences the nurse's sensitivity and promotes trust.*
15. Talk with the patient about his or her life, generativity, and accomplishments. *Patients with disturbances in body image frequently see themselves in a distortedly "narrow" sense. Encouraging a wider focus of themselves and their life reduces this distortion.*
16. Help the patient explore realistic alternatives.
17. Recognize that incorporating a body change into one's body image takes time. Avoid setting unrealistic expectations and *thereby inadvertently reinforcing a low self-esteem.*
18. Suggest the use of additional resources such as trained visitors who have mastered situations similar to those of the patient. Refer the patient to a psychiatric liaison nurse or psychiatrist if needed.

Disturbed Body Image Related to Functional Dependence on Life-Sustaining Technology (e.g., ventilator, dialysis, IABP, halo traction)

Defining Characteristics
- Actual change in function requiring permanent or temporary replacement
- Refusal to verify actual loss
- Verbalization of the following: feelings of helplessness, hopelessness, powerlessness, fear of failure to wean from technology

Outcome Criteria
- Patient verifies actual change in function.
- Patient does not refuse or fight technologic intervention.
- Patient verbalizes acceptance of expected change in lifestyle.

Nursing Interventions and Rationale
1. Evaluate patient's response to the technologic intervention.
2. Assess responses of family and significant others. **Body image is derived from the "reflected appraisals" of family and significant others.**
3. Provide information needed by patient and family.
4. Promote trust, security, comfort, and privacy.
5. Recognize anxiety. Allow and encourage its expression. **Anxiety is the most predominant emotion accom-** **panying body image alterations.** Implement nursing management plan of care, Anxiety.
6. Assist patient to recognize his or her own functioning and performance in the face of technology. For example, assist patient to distinguish spontaneous breaths from mechanically delivered breaths. **The activity will assist in weaning patient from the ventilator when feasible. To establish realistic, accurate body boundaries, a patient needs help to separate himself or herself from the technology that is supporting his or her functioning. Any participation or function on the part of the patient during periods of dependency is helpful in preventing and/or resolving an alteration in body image.**
7. Plan for discontinuation of the treatment (e.g., weaning from ventilator). Explain procedure that will be followed, and be present during its initiation.
8. Plan for transfer from the critical care environment.
9. Document care, ensuring an up-to-date management plan is available to all involved caregivers.

NURSING MANAGEMENT PLAN
Disturbed Sleep Pattern

Definition: Time-limited disruption of sleep (natural, periodic suspension of consciousness) amount and quality

Disturbed Sleep Pattern Related to Fragmented Sleep

Defining Characteristics
- Decreased sleep during one block of sleep time
- Daytime sleepiness
- Decreased sleep
  —Less than one half of normal total sleep time
  —Decreased slow-wave, or rapid-eye-movement (REM), sleep
- Anxiety
- Fatigue
- Restlessness
- Disorientation and hallucinations
- Combativeness
- Frequent awakenings

Outcome Criteria
- Patient's total sleep time approximates patient's normal.
- Patient can complete sleep cycles of 90 minutes without interruption.
- Patient has no delusions or hallucinations.
- Patient has reality-based thought content.

Nursing Interventions and Rationale
1. Assess normal sleep pattern on admission and any history of sleep disturbance or chronic illness that may affect sleep or sedative/hypnotic use. Promote normal sleep activity while patient is in critical care unit. Assess sleep effectiveness by asking patient how his or her sleep in the hospital compares with sleep at home. *The best treatment for sleep pattern disturbance is prevention.*
2. Promote comfort, relaxation, and a sense of well-being. Treat pain; change, smooth, or refresh bed linens at bedtime; and provide oral hygiene. Eliminate stressful situations before bedtime. Use relaxation techniques, imagery, music, massage, or warm blankets. Other interventions may include having a close family member sit beside the bed and providing the patient with his or her own garments or coverings. Individual patients may prefer quiet or may prefer the background noise of the television or music to best promote sleep. Provide a comfortable room temperature.
3. Minimize noise, particularly that of the staff and noisy equipment. Reduce the level of environmental stimuli. Dim lights at night.
4. Foods containing tryptophan (e.g., milk, turkey) may be appropriate *because these promote sleep.*
5. Plan nap times to assist in approximating the patient's normal 24-hour sleep time.
6. Minimize awakenings *to allow for at least 90-minute sleep cycles.* Continually assess the need to awaken the patient, particularly at night. Distinguish between essential and nonessential nursing tasks. Organize nursing management to allow for maximal amount of uninterrupted sleep while ensuring close monitoring of the patient's condition. Whenever possible, monitor physiologic parameters without waking the patient. Coordinate awakenings with other departments, such as respiratory therapy, laboratory, and x-ray, *to minimize sleep interruptions.*
7. Be aware of the effects of commonly used medications on sleep. *Many sedative and hypnotic medications decrease REM sleep.* Sedative and analgesic medications should not be withheld, but rather, drugs that minimally disrupt sleep are to be used to complement comfort measures, with dosages reduced gradually as the medication is no longer necessary. Do not abruptly withdraw REM-suppressing medications *because this can result in "REM rebound."*
8. Document amount of uninterrupted sleep per shift, especially sleep episodes lasting longer than 2 hours. This can be effectively documented as part of the 24-hour flow sheet and reported routinely, shift to shift. *Sleep pattern disturbance is diagnosed, treated, and resolved more efficiently when formally documented in this manner.*

NURSING MANAGEMENT PLAN
Dysfunctional Ventilatory Weaning Response

Definition: Inability to adjust to lowered levels of mechanical ventilator support that interrupts and prolongs the weaning process

Dysfunctional Ventilatory Weaning Response (DVWR) Related to Physical, Psychologic, or Situational Factors

Defining Characteristics

Mild DVWR
- Responds to lowered levels of mechanical ventilator support with:
  —Restlessness
  —Slightly increased respiratory rate from baseline
  —Expressed feelings of increased need for oxygen; breathing discomfort; fatigue; warmth
  —Queries about possible machine malfunction
  —Increased concentration on breathing

Moderate DVWR
- Responds to lowered levels of mechanical ventilator support with:
  —Slight baseline increase in blood pressure <20 mm Hg
  —Slight baseline increase in heart rate <20 beats per minute (beats/min)
  —Baseline increase in respiratory rate <5 breaths/min
  —Hypervigilance to activities
  —Inability to respond to coaching
  —Inability to cooperate
  —Apprehension
  —Diaphoresis
  —Eye-widening ("wide-eyed look")
  —Decreased air entry on auscultation
  —Color changes: pale, slight cyanosis
  —Slight respiratory accessory muscle use

Severe DVWR
- Responds to lowered levels of mechanical ventilator support with:
  —Agitation
  —Deterioration in arterial blood gases from current baseline
  —Baseline increase in blood pressure >20 mm Hg
  —Baseline increase in heart rate >20 beats/min
  —Respiratory rate increases significantly from baseline
  —Profuse diaphoresis
  —Full respiratory accessory muscle use
  —Shallow, gasping breaths
  —Paradoxic abdominal breathing
  —Discoordinated breathing with the ventilator
  —Decreased level of consciousness
  —Adventitious breath sounds, audible airway secretions
  —Cyanosis

Outcome Criteria
- Airway is clear.
- Underlying disorder is resolving.
- Patient is rested, and pain is controlled.
- Nutritional status is adequate.
- Patient has feelings of perceived control, situational security, and trust in the nurses.
- Patient is able to adapt to selected levels of ventilator support without undue fatigue.

Nursing Interventions and Rationale
1. Communicate interest and concern for the patient's well-being, and demonstrate confidence in ability to manage weaning process *to instill trust in the patient.*
2. Use normalizing strategies (e.g., grooming, dressing, mobilizing, social conversation) *to reinforce the patient's self-esteem and feeling of identity.*
3. Identify parameters of the patient's usual functioning before the weaning process begins *to facilitate early identification of problems.*
4. Identify the patient's strengths and resources that can be mobilized *to enhance the patient's coping and maximize weaning effort.*
5. Note concerns that adversely affect the patient's comfort and confidence, and manage them discretely *to facilitate the patient's ease.*
6. Praise successful activities, encourage a positive outlook, and review the patient's positive progress to date *to increase the patient's perceived self-efficacy.*
7. Inform the patient of his or her situation and weaning progress *to permit the patient as much control as possible.*
8. Teach the patient about the weaning process and how he or she can participate in the process.
9. Negotiate daily weaning goals with the patient *to gain cooperation.*
10. Position the patient with the head of the bed elevated *to optimize respiratory efforts.*
11. Coach the patient in breath control by regular demonstrations of slow, deep, rhythmic patterns of breathing *to assist with dyspnea.*
12. Remain visible in the room and reassure the patient that help is immediately available if needed *to reduce the patient's anxiety and fearfulness.*
13. Encourage the patient to view weaning trials as a form of training, regardless of whether the weaning goal is achieved *to avoid discouragement.*
14. Encourage the patient to maintain emotional calmness by reassuring, being present, comforting, talking down if emotionally aroused, and reinforcing the idea that he or she can and will succeed.
15. Monitor the patient's status frequently *to avoid undue fatigue and anxiety.*
16. Provide regular periods of rest by reducing activities, maintaining or increasing ventilator support, and providing oxygen as needed before fatigue advances.
17. Provide distraction (e.g., visitors, radio, television, conversation) when the patient's concentration starts to create tension and increases anxiety.

18. Ensure adequate nutritional support, sufficient rest and sleep time, and sedation or pain control *to promote the patient's optimal physical and emotional comfort.*
19. Start weaning early in the day *when the patient is most rested.*
20. Restrict unnecessary activities and visitors who do not cooperate with weaning strategies *to minimize energy demands on the patient during the weaning process.*

21. Coordinate necessary activities *to promote adequate time for rest and relaxation.*
22. Monitor the patient's underlying disease process *to ensure it is stabilized and under control.*
23. Advocate for additional resources (e.g., sedation, analgesia, rest) needed by the patient *to maximize comfort status.*
24. Develop and adhere to an individualized plan of care *to promote the patient's feelings of control.*

NURSING MANAGEMENT PLAN
Excess Fluid Volume

Definition: Increased isotonic fluid retention

Excess Fluid Volume Related to Increased Secretion of Antidiuretic Hormone (ADH)

Defining Characteristics
- Headache
- Decreased sensorium
- Weight gain over short period
- Intake greater than output
- Increased pulmonary artery occlusion pressure (PAOP)
- Increased central venous pressure (CVP)
- Urine output <30 ml/hr
- Serum sodium <120 mEq/L
- Serum osmolality <275 mOsm/kg
- Urine osmolality greater than serum osmolality
- Urine sodium >200 mEq/L
- Urine specific gravity >1.03

Outcome Criteria
- Weight returns to baseline.
- Urine output is >30 ml/hr.
- Serum sodium is 135-145 mEq/L.
- Urine specific gravity is 1.005-1030.

Nursing Interventions and Rationale
1. Monitor electrocardiogram (ECG) rhythm continuously for dysrhythmias *caused by electrolyte imbalance.*
2. Restrict patient's fluids to 500 ml less than output per day *to decrease fluid retention.*
3. Provide patient chilled beverages high in sodium content such as tomato juice or broth *to increase sodium intake.*
4. Collaborate with physician regarding administration of demeclocycline, lithium, and/or narcotic agonists *to inhibit renal response to ADH.*
5. Collaborate with physician regarding administration of hypertonic saline and furosemide *for rapid correction of severe sodium deficit and diuresis of free water.*
   a. Administer hypertonic saline at a rate of 1 to 2 ml/kg/hr until the patient's serum sodium is increased no greater than 1 to 2 mEq/L /hr.
6. Weigh patient daily (at same time, in same amount of clothing, and preferably with same scale) *to ensure accuracy of readings.*
7. Provide frequent mouth care *to prevent breakdown of oral mucous membranes.*
8. Initiate seizure precautions *because patient is at high risk as a result of hyponatremia.*
   a. Pad side rails of bed to protect patient from injury.
   b. Remove any objects from immediate environment that could injure patient in the event of a seizure.
   c. Keep appropriate-size oral airway at bedside to assist with airway management postseizure.
9. Collaborate with physician regarding administration of medications to prevent constipation *caused by decreased fluid intake and immobility.*
10. Maintain surveillance for symptoms of hyponatremia (head-ache, abdominal cramps, weakness) and congestive heart failure (dyspnea, rales, increased CVP and PAOP).

Excess Fluid Volume Related to Renal Dysfunction

Defining Characteristics
- Weight gain that occurs during a 24- to 48-hour period
- Dependent pitting edema
- Ascites in severe cases
- Fluid crackles on lung auscultation
- Exertional dyspnea
- Oliguria or anuria
- Hypertension
- Engorged neck veins
- Decrease in urinary osmolality as renal failure progresses
- CVP >15 cm of H_2O
- PAOP 20-25 mm Hg

Outcome Criteria
- Weight returns to baseline.
- Edema or ascites is absent or reduced to baseline.
- Lungs are clear to auscultation.
- Exertional dyspnea is absent.
- Blood pressure returns to baseline.
- Heart rate returns to baseline.
- Neck veins are flat.
- Mucous membranes are moist.

Nursing Interventions and Rationale
1. Promote skin integrity of edematous areas by frequent repositioning and elevation of areas where possible. Avoid massaging pressure points or reddened areas of skin *because this results in further tissue trauma.*
2. Plan patient care to provide rest periods *to not heighten exertional dyspnea.*
3. Weigh patient daily (at same time, in same amount of clothing, and preferably with same scale).
4. Instruct the patient about the correlation between fluid intake and weight gain, using commonly understood fluid measurements; for example, ingesting 4 cups (1000 ml) of fluid results in an approximate 2-pound weight gain in the anuric patient.

NURSING MANAGEMENT PLAN
Hyperthermia

Definition: Body temperature elevated above normal range

Hyperthermia Related to Increased Metabolic Rate

Defining Characteristics
- Increased body temperature above normal range
- Seizures
- Flushed skin
- Increased respiratory rate
- Tachycardia
- Skin warm to touch
- Diaphoresis

Outcome Criteria
- Temperature is within normal range.
- Respiratory rate and heart rate are within patient's baseline range.
- Skin is warm and dry.

Nursing Interventions and Rationale
1. Monitor temperature every 15 minutes to 1 hour until within normal range and stable and then every 4 hours *to maintain close surveillance for temperature fluctuations and evaluate effectiveness of interventions.*
   a. Use temperature taken from pulmonary artery catheter or bladder catheter if available *because these methods closely reflect core body temperature.*
   b. Use tympanic membrane temperature *if core body temperature devices are unavailable.*
   c. Use rectal temperature if none of the methods listed above are available.
2. Collaborate with physician regarding administration of antithyroid medications *to block the synthesis and release of thyroid hormone.*
3. Collaborate with physician regarding the use of cooling blanket *to facilitate heat loss via conduction.*
   a. Wrap hands, feet, and genitalia to protect them from maceration during cooling and decrease chance of shivering.
   b. Avoid rapidly cooling the patient and overcooling the patient because this initiates the heat-conserving response (i.e., shivering).
4. Place ice packs in patient's groin and axilla *to facilitate heat loss via conduction.*
5. Maintain patient on bedrest *to decrease the effects of activity on the patient's metabolic rate.*
6. Provide tepid sponge baths *to facilitate heat loss via evaporation.*
7. Decrease the patient's room temperature *to facilitate radiant heat loss.*
8. Place fan near patient to circulate cool air *to facilitate heat loss via convection.*
9. Provide patient with nonrestrictive gown and lightweight bed coverings *to allow heat to escape from the patient's trunk.*
10. Collaborate with physician and respiratory therapist on the administration of oxygen to maintain SpO_2 >90% *because patient has increased oxygen consumption secondary to increased metabolic rate.*
11. Collaborate with physician regarding use of antipyretic medications *to facilitate patient comfort.*
12. Collaborate with physician regarding use of intravenous and oral fluids *to maintain adequate hydration of the patient.*

Hyperthermia Related to Pharmacogenic Hypermetabolism (Malignant Hyperthermia)

Defining Characteristics
Early Signs
- Blood pressure (BP) >140/90 mm Hg
- Profuse diaphoresis
- Pulse rate >100 beats/min
- Masseter and general skeletal muscle rigidity and fasciculations
- Tachypnea
- Decreased level of consciousness

Late Signs
- Increasing core body temperature up to 42° to 43° C (107.6° to 109.4° F)
- Hot skin
- High-output left ventricular failure
  - Systemic BP <90 mm Hg
  - Pulse rate >100 beats/min and ventricular dysrhythmias
  - Cardiac index (CI) >4.0 L /min/m^2

- Pulmonary artery occlusion pressure (PAOP) and pulmonary artery diastolic (PAD) pressure >15 mm Hg; possible pulmonary edema
- Continued skeletal muscle rigidity and fasciculations
- PaO_2 <80 mm Hg
- Respiratory and metabolic acidosis
- Fixed, dilated pupils
- Seizures/coma/decerebrate posturing
- Urinary output <30 ml/hr; urine color reddish brown (myoglobinuria)
- Prolonged bleeding (disseminated intravascular coagulation [DIC])

Outcome Criteria
- Core body temperature is below 38.3° C (101° F).
- Muscle rigidity and fasciculations are absent.
- Patient is alert and oriented.
- Pupils are normoreactive.

Nursing Interventions and Rationale

1. Obtain the emergency kit for malignant hyperthermia. It is recommended that health care institutions have an emergency malignant hyperthermia kit available that contains the items mentioned in the following plan.
2. Collaborate with the physician to implement measure to rapidly decrease metabolism:
   a. Administer dantrolene (Dantrium), *which relaxes skeletal muscles by reducing the release of calcium from the sarcoplasmic reticulum.*
   b. Observe for infiltration of dantrolene into surrounding tissues. *Dantrolene is very alkaline and irritating to tissues.*
3. Collaborate with the physician to initiate cooling measures:
   a. Administer cold intravenous (IV) solutions (IV bag has been submerged in ice bath before solution is administered).
   b. Provide cool-water sponge bath.
   c. Apply cooling blanket until temperature is within $1°$ to $3°$ F of desired level *to avoid "overshoot," in which excessive cooling lowers the body temperature below the desired range.*
   d. Institute iced saline lavages of stomach, rectum, and bladder.
   e. Monitor core temperature continuously *to avoid overcooling.*
4. Collaborate with physician to implement interventions to reverse metabolic and respiratory acidosis:
   a. Administer sodium bicarbonate as necessary *to treat metabolic acidosis.*
   b. Hyperventilate patient with 100% oxygen; then ventilate with 15-20 ml/kg tidal volume at 15-20 breaths/min.
   c. Assess arterial blood gas (ABG) values frequently, and make ventilatory adjustments as necessary *to remedy hypoxemia and hypercarbia.*
5. Collaborate with physician to provide adequate nutrients to the tissues, and correct electrolyte imbalances:
   a. Administer 50% dextrose and regular insulin *to increase glucose uptake into liver to meet hypermetabolic needs of body and enhance the movement of potassium from extracellular fluid back into the cells.*
   b. Monitor serum electrolytes *to assess efficacy of previously mentioned action.*
   c. Monitor blood urea nitrogen (BUN) and creatinine levels *to evaluate for renal failure.*
   d. Monitor serum enzyme levels, particularly creatine phosphokinase (CPK) elevations *for indication of degree of muscle hyperactivity.*
6. Collaborate with physician to correct cardiovascular instability and dysrhythmias:
   a. Titrate vasoactive and inotropic drips per protocol to desired systemic BP, PAOP, and/or PAD.
   b. Follow critical care emergency standing orders about the administration of antidysrhythmic agents.
7. Collaborate with physician to maintain a high urinary output (>50 ml/hr):
   a. Administer osmotic agents (mannitol) *for excretion of excess fluid load and to increase urinary output to prevent renal failure.*
   b. Administer diuretics (furosemide) *to enhance secretion of myoglobin, potassium, sodium, and magnesium.*
   c. Administer supplemental potassium chloride as indicated by serum potassium levels.
   d. Administer steroids (e.g., Solu-Cortef) *for its mineralocorticoid effect of potassium excretion, to increase glomerular filtration rate, and to reduce cerebral edema.*
8. Maintain surveillance for hematologic abnormalities:
   a. Monitor coagulation studies *for indications of DIC and for efficacy of heparin therapy.*
   b. Assess stool/urinary/nasogastric (NG) drainage for occult blood.
9. Weigh patient daily (at same time, in same amount of clothing, and preferably with same scale) *to assist in assessment of hydration status.*

NURSING MANAGEMENT PLAN

Hypothermia

Definition: Body temperature below normal range

Hypothermia Related to Decreased Metabolic Rate

Defining Characteristics
- Reduction in body temperature below normal range
- Shivering
- Pallor
- Piloerection
- Hypertension
- Skin cool to touch
- Tachycardia
- Decreased capillary refill

Outcome Criteria
- Temperature is within normal range.
- Heart rate is within patient's baseline range.
- Skin is warm and dry.
- Capillary refill is normal.

Nursing Interventions and Rationale
1. Monitor temperature every 15 minutes to 1 hour until within normal range and stable and then every 4 hours *to maintain close surveillance for temperature fluctuations and evaluate effectiveness of interventions.*
   a. Use temperature taken from pulmonary artery catheter or bladder catheter if available *because these methods closely reflect core body temperature.*
   b. Use tympanic membrane temperature *if core body temperature devices are unavailable.*
   c. Use rectal temperature if none of the methods listed above are available.
2. Collaborate with physician regarding administration of thyroid medications *to replace lacking thyroid hormone.*
3. Collaborate with physician regarding the use of fluid-filled heating blanket *to facilitate rewarming via conduction.*
4. Initiate forced air-warming therapy *to facilitate convective heat gain.*
5. Provide patient with warm blankets *to facilitate heat transfer to the patient.*
6. Increase the patient's room temperature *to decrease radiant heat loss.*
7. Replace wet patient gown and bed linen promptly *to decrease evaporative heat loss.*
8. Warm intravenous fluids and blood products *to facilitate rewarming via conduction.*

Hypothermia Related to Exposure to Cold Environment, Trauma, or Damage to the Hypothalamus

Defining Characteristics
- Core body temperature below 35° C (95° F)
- Skin cold to touch
- Slurred speech, incoordination
- At temperature below 33° C (91.4° F):
  —Cardiac dysrhythmias (atrial fibrillation, bradycardia)
  —Cyanosis
  —Respiratory alkalosis
- At temperatures below 32° C (89.6° F):
  —Shivering replaced by muscle rigidity
  —Hypotension
  —Dilated pupils
- At temperatures below 28° to 29° C (82.4° to 84.2° F):
  —Absent deep tendon reflexes
  —(3 to 4 breaths/min to apnea)
  —Ventricular fibrillation possible
- At temperatures below 26° to 27° C (78.8° to 80.6° F):
  —Coma
  —Flaccid muscles
  —Fixed, dilated pupils
  —Ventricular fibrillation to cardiac standstill
  —Apnea

Outcome Criteria
- Core body temperature is greater than 35° C (95° F).
- Patient is alert and oriented.
- Cardiac dysrhythmias are absent.
- Acid-base balance is normal.
- Pupils are normoreactive.

Nursing Interventions and Rationale
1. Monitor core body temperature continuously.
2. Collaborate with the physician regarding the need for intubation and mechanical ventilation.
   a. Heated air or oxygen can be added *to help rewarm the body core.*
   b. Do not hyperventilate the hypothermic patient because carbon dioxide production is low and this action may induce severe alkalosis and precipitate ventricular fibrillation.
3. Maintain cardiopulmonary resuscitation (CPR) and advanced cardiac life support (ACLS) until core body temperature is up to at least 29.5° C (85.1° F) before determining that patients cannot be resuscitated. *Electrical defibrillation is usually successful in terminating ventricular fibrillation if the temperature is greater than 28°C (82.4° F).*
4. Administer cardiac resuscitation drugs sparingly *because as the body warms, peripheral vasodilation occurs. Drugs that remain in the periphery are suddenly released, leading to a "bolus effect" that may cause fatal dysrhythmias.*
5. Monitor arterial blood gas (ABG) values *to direct further therapy,* and ensure that the pH, PaO_2, and $PaCO_2$ are corrected for temperature.

6. Rewarm patient rapidly *because the pathophysiologic changes associated with chronic hypothermia have not had time to evolve.*
   a. Institute rapid, active rewarming by immersion in warm water (38° to 43° C) (100.4° to 109.4° F).
   b. Apply thermal blanket at 36.6° to 37.7° C (97.9° to 99.9° F). Some researchers suggest rewarming only the torso or trunk first, leaving the extremities exposed to room temperature. *This is to prevent early peripheral vasodilation with abrupt redistribution of intravascular volume. This also prevents colder blood trapped in the extremities from returning to the body core before the heart is rewarmed.*
   c. Perform rapid core rewarming with heated (37° to 43° C; 98.6° to 109.4° F) intravenous (IV) infusion, hemodialysis, peritoneal dialysis, and colonic or gastric irrigation fluids.
7. Monitor peripheral circulation because gangrene of the fingers and toes is a common complication of accidental hypothermia.

NURSING MANAGEMENT PLAN
Imbalanced Nutrition: Less Than Body Requirements

Definition: Intake of nutrients insufficient to meet metabolic needs

Imbalanced Nutrition: Less than Body Requirements Related to Lack of Exogenous Nutrients and Increased Metabolic Demand

Defining Characteristics
- Unplanned weight loss of 20% of body weight within the past 6 months
- Serum albumin <3.5 g/dl
- Total lymphocytes <1500/mm³
- Anergy
- Negative nitrogen balance
- Fatigue; lack of energy and endurance
- Nonhealing wounds
- Daily caloric intake less than estimated nutritional requirements
- Presence of factors known to increase nutritional requirements (e.g., sepsis, trauma, multiple organ dysfunction syndrome [MODS])
- Maintenance of nothing by mouth (NPO) status for >7-10 days
- Long-term use of 5% dextrose intravenously
- Documentation of suboptimal calorie counts
- Drug or nutrient interaction that might decrease oral intake (e.g. chronic use of bronchodilators, laxatives, anticonvulsives, diuretics, antacids, narcotics)
- Physical problems with chewing, swallowing, choking, and salivation and presence of altered taste, anorexia, nausea, vomiting, diarrhea, or constipation

Outcome Criteria
- Patient exhibits stabilization of weight loss or weight gain of ½ lb. daily.
- Serum albumin is >3.5 g/dl.
- Total lymphocytes are <1500/mm³.
- Patient has positive response to cutaneous skin antigen testing.
- Patient is in positive nitrogen balance.
- Wound healing is evident.
- Daily caloric intake equals estimated nutritional requirements.
- Increased ambulation and endurance are evident.

Nursing Interventions and Rationale
1. Inquire if patient has any food allergies and food preferences to ensure the food provided to the patient is not contraindicated.
2. Monitor patient's caloric intake and weight daily to ensure adequacy of nutritional interventions.
3. Collaborate with dietitian regarding patient's nutritional and caloric needs to determine the appropriateness of the patient's diet to meet those needs.
4. Monitor patient for signs of nutritional deficiencies to facilitate evaluation of extent of nutritional deficient.
5. Provide patient with oral care prior to eating to ensure optimal consumption of diet.
6. Assist patient to eat as appropriate to ensure optimal consumption of diet.
7. Collaborate with physician regarding the administration of parenteral and enteral nutrition as needed.

NURSING MANAGEMENT PLAN

Impaired Gas Exchange

Definition: Excess or deficit in oxygenation and/or carbon dioxide elimination at the alveolar-capillary membrane

Impaired Gas Exchange Related to Alveolar Hypoventilation

Defining Characteristics
- Abnormal arterial blood gas (ABG) values (decreased PaO_2, increased $PaCO_2$, decreased pH, decreased SaO_2)
- Somnolence
- Neurobehavioral changes (restlessness, irritability, confusion)
- Tachycardia or dysrhythmias
- Central cyanosis

Outcome Criteria
- ABG values are within patient's baseline.
- Central cyanosis is absent.

Nursing Interventions and Rationale
1. Initiate continuous pulse oximetry or monitor SpO_2 every hour.
2. Collaborate with physician on the administration of oxygen to maintain an SpO_2 >90%.
   a. Administer supplemental oxygen via appropriate oxygen-delivery device *to increase driving pressure of oxygen in the alveoli.*
   b. If supplemental oxygen alone is not effective, administer continuous positive airway pressure (CPAP) or mechanical ventilation with positive end-expiratory pressure (PEEP) *to open collapsed alveoli and increase the surface area for gas exchange.*
3. Prevent hypoventilation.
   a. Position patient in high-Fowler's position or semi-Fowler's position *to promote diaphragmatic descent and maximal inhalation.*
   b. Assist with deep-breathing exercises and/or incentive spirometry with sustained maximal inspiration 5 to 10 times/hr *to help reinflate collapsed portions of the lung.* See the nursing management plan for Ineffective Breathing Pattern Related to Decreased Lung Expansion for further instructions.
   c. Treat pain, if present, *to prevent hypoventilation and atelectasis.* Implement the nursing management plan of care, Acute Pain Related to Transmission and Perception of Cutaneous, Visceral, Muscular, or Ischemic Impulses.
4. Assist physician with intubation and initiation of mechanical ventilation as indicated.

Impaired Gas Exchange Related to Ventilation/Perfusion Mismatching or Intrapulmonary Shunting

Defining Characteristics
- Abnormal ABG values (decreased PaO_2, decreased SaO_2)
- Somnolence
- Neurobehavioral changes (restlessness, irritability, confusion)
- Central cyanosis

Outcome Criteria
- ABG values are within patient's baseline.
- Central cyanosis is absent.

Nursing Interventions and Rationale
1. Initiate continuous pulse oximetry, or monitor SpO_2 every hour.
2. Collaborate with physician on the administration of oxygen to maintain an SpO_2 >90%.
   a. Administer supplemental oxygen via appropriate oxygen-delivery device *to increase driving pressure of oxygen in the alveoli.*
   b. If supplemental oxygen alone is not effective, administer CPAP or mechanical ventilation with PEEP *to open collapsed alveoli and increase the surface area for gas exchange.*
3. Position patient to optimize ventilation/perfusion matching.
   a. For patient with unilateral lung disease, position with the good lung down *because gravity will improve perfusion to this area, and this will best match ventilation with perfusion.*
   b. For patient with bilateral lung disease, position with the right lung down *because this lung is larger than the left and affords a greater area for ventilation and perfusion,* or change position every 2 hours, favoring positions that improve oxygenation.
   c. Avoid any position that seriously compromises oxygenation status.
4. Perform procedures only as needed and provide adequate rest and recovery time in between *to prevent desaturation.*
5. Collaborate with the physician regarding the administration of the following:
   a. Sedatives *to decrease ventilator asynchrony and facilitate patient's sense of control.*
   b. Neuromuscular blocking agents *to prevent ventilator asynchrony and decrease oxygen demand.*
   c. Analgesics *to treat pain if present.* Implement the nursing management plan of care, Acute Pain Related to Transmission and Perception of Cutaneous, Visceral, Muscular, or Ischemic Impulses.
6. If secretions are present, implement the nursing management plan of care, Ineffective Airway Clearance Related to Excessive Secretions or Abnormal Viscosity of Mucus.

NURSING MANAGEMENT PLAN
Impaired Spontaneous Ventilation

Definition: Decreased energy reserves results in an individual's inability to maintain breathing adequate to support life

Impaired Spontaneous Ventilation Related to Respiratory Muscle Fatigue or Metabolic Factors

Defining Characteristics
- Dyspnea and apprehension
- Increased metabolic rate
- Increased restlessness
- Increased use of accessory muscles
- Decreased tidal volume
- Increased heart rate
- Abnormal arterial blood gas (ABG) values (decreased Pao_2, increased $Paco_2$, decreased pH, decreased Sao_2)
- Decreased cooperation

Outcome Criteria
- Metabolic rate and heart rate are within patient's baseline.
- Patient experiences eupnea.
- ABG values are within patient's baseline.

Nursing Interventions and Rationale
1. Collaborate with the physician regarding the application of pressure support to the ventilator *to assist patient in overcoming the work of breathing imposed by the ventilator and endotracheal tube.*
2. Carefully snip excess length from the proximal end of the endotracheal *tube to decrease dead space and thereby decrease the work of breathing.*
3. Collaborate with the physician and dietitian to ensure that at least 50% of the diet's nonprotein caloric source is in the form of fat versus carbohydrates *to prevent excess carbon dioxide production.*
4. Collaborate with the physician and respiratory therapist regarding the best method of weaning for individual *patients because each situation is different and a variety of weaning options are available.*
5. Collaborate with the physician and physical therapist regarding a progressive ambulation and conditioning plan *to promote overall muscle conditioning and respiratory muscle functioning.*
6. Determine the most effective means of communication for the patient *to promote independence and reduce anxiety.*
7. Develop a daily schedule and post it in patient's room *to coordinate care and facilitate patient's involvement in the plan.*
8. Treat pain, if present, *to prevent respiratory splinting and hypoventilation.* Implement the nursing management plan of care, Acute Pain Related to Transmission and Perception of Cutaneous, Visceral, Muscular, or Ischemic Impulses.
9. Ensure that patient receives at least 2- to 4-hr intervals of uninterrupted sleep in a quiet, dark room. Collaborate with the physician and respiratory therapist regarding the use of full ventilatory support at night *to provide respiratory muscle rest.*
10. Place patient in semi-Fowler's position or in a chair at the bedside *for best use of ventilatory muscles and to facilitate diaphragmatic descent.*
11. Explain the weaning procedure to the patient before the trial *so that patient will understand what to expect and how to participate.*
12. Monitor patient during the weaning trial for evidence of respiratory muscle fatigue *to avoid overtiring the patient.*
13. Provide diversional activity during the weaning trial *to reduce the patient's anxiety.*
14. Collaborate with physician and respiratory therapist regarding the removal of the ventilator and artificial airway when patient has been successfully weaned.

NURSING MANAGEMENT PLAN
Impaired Swallowing

Definition: Abnormal functioning of the swallowing mechanism associated with deficits in oral, pharyngeal, or esophageal structure or function

Impaired Swallowing Related to Neuromuscular Impairment, Fatigue, and Limited Awareness

Defining Characteristics
- Evidence of difficulty swallowing
  —Drooling
  —Difficulty handling oral secretions
  —Absence of gag, cough, and/or swallow reflex
  —Moist, wet, gurgling voice quality
  —Decreased tongue and mouth movements
  —Presence of dysarthria
  —Difficulty handling solid foods:
  Uncoordinated chewing or swallowing
  Stasis of food in the oral cavity
  Wet-sounding voice or change in voice quality
  Sneezing, coughing, or choking with eating
  Delay in swallowing of more than 5 seconds
  Change in respiratory patterns
  —Difficulty handling liquids:
  Momentary loss of voice or change in voice quality
  Nasal regurgitation of liquids
  Coughing with drinking
- Evidence of aspiration:
  —Hypoxemia
  —Productive cough
  —Frothy sputum
  —Wheezing, crackles, or rhonchi
  —Temperature elevation

Outcome Criteria
- Evidence of swallowing difficulties is absent.
- Evidence of aspiration is absent.

Nursing Interventions and Rationale
1. Collaborate with physician and speech therapist regarding swallowing evaluation and rehabilitation program *to decrease the incidence of aspiration.*
2. Collaborate with physician and dietitian regarding a nutritional assessment and nutritional plan *to ensure that the patient is receiving enough nutrition.*
3. Place the patient in an upright position with the head midline and the chin slightly down *to keep food in the anterior portion of the mouth and to prevent it from falling over the base of the tongue into the open airway.*
4. Provide patient with single-textured soft foods (e.g., cream cereals) that maintain their shape *because these foods require minimal oral manipulation.*
5. Avoid particulate foods (e.g., hamburger) and foods containing more than one texture (e.g., stew) *because these foods require more chewing and oral manipulation.*
6. Avoid dry foods (e.g., popcorn, rice, crackers) and sticky foods (e.g., peanut butter, bananas) *because these foods are difficult to manipulate orally.*
7. Provide patient with thick liquids (e.g., fruit nectar, yogurt) *because thick liquids are more easily controlled in the mouth.*
8. Thicken thin liquids (e.g., water, juice) with a thickening preparation or avoid them *because thin liquids are easily aspirated.*
9. Place foods in the uninvolved side of the mouth *because oral sensitivity and function are greatest in this area.*
10. Avoid the use of straws *because they can deposit the liquid too far back in the mouth for the patient to handle.*
11. Serve foods and liquids at room temperature *because the patient may be overly sensitive to heat or cold.*
12. Offer solids and liquids at different times *to avoid swallowing solids before being properly chewed.*
13. Provide oral hygiene after meals *to clear food particles from the mouth that could be aspirated.*
14. Collaborate with physician and pharmacist regarding oral medication administration *to adjust medication regimen to prevent aspiration and choking and to ensure all prescribed medications are swallowed.*
15. Crush tablets (if appropriate) and mix with food that is easily formed into a bolus, use thickened liquid medications (if available), and/or embed small capsules into food *to facilitate oral medication administration.*
16. Inspect mouth for residue after all medication administration *to ensure medication has been swallowed.*
17. Educate patient and family on the swallowing problem, rehabilitation program, and emergency measures for choking.

NURSING MANAGEMENT PLAN
Impaired Verbal Communication

Definition: Decreased, delayed, or absent ability to receive, process, transmit, and use a system of symbols

Impaired Verbal Communication Related to Cerebral Speech Center Injury

Defining Characteristics
- Inappropriate or absent speech or responses to questions
- Inability to speak spontaneously
- Inability to understand spoken words
- Inability to follow commands appropriately through gestures
- Difficulty or inability to understand written language
- Difficulty or inability to express ideas in writing
- Difficulty or inability to name objects

Outcome Criterion
- Patient is able to make basic needs known.

Nursing Interventions and Rationale
1. Consult with physician and speech pathologist *to determine the extent of the patient's communication deficit (e.g., whether fluent, nonfluent, or global aphasia is involved).*
2. Have the speech therapist post a list of appropriate ways to communicate with the patient in the patient's room *so that all nursing personnel can be consistent in their efforts.*
3. Assess the patient's ability to comprehend, speak, read, and write.
   - Ask questions that can be answered with a "yes" or a "no." If a patient answers "yes" to a question, ask the opposite (e.g., "Are you hot?" "Yes." "Are you cold?" "Yes."). *This may help determine whether in fact the patient understands what is being said.*
   - Ask simple, short questions, and use gestures, pantomime, and facial expressions to give the patient additional clues.
   - Stand in the patient's line of vision, giving a good view of your face and hands.
   - Have the patient try to write with a pad and pencil. Offer pictures and alphabet letters at which to point.
   - Make flash cards with pictures or words depicting frequently used phrases (e.g., glass of water, bedpan).
4. Maintain an uncluttered environment, and decrease external distractions *that could hinder communication.*
5. Maintain a relaxed and calm manner, and explain all diagnostic, therapeutic, and comfort measures before initiating them.
6. Do not shout or speak in a loud voice. *Hearing loss is not a factor in aphasia, and shouting will not help.*
7. Have only one person talk at a time. *It is more difficult for the patient to follow a multisided conversation.*
8. Use direct eye contact, and speak directly to the patient in unhurried, short phrases.
9. Give one-step commands and directions, and provide cues through pictures and gestures.
10. Try to ask questions that can be answered with a "yes" or a "no," and avoid topics that are controversial, emotional, abstract, or lengthy.
11. Listen to the patient in an unhurried manner, and wait for his or her attempt to communicate.
    - Expect a time lag from when you ask the patient something until the patient responds.
    - Accept the patient's statement of essential words without expecting complete sentences.
    - Avoid finishing the sentence for the patient if possible.
    - Wait approximately 30 seconds before providing the word the patient may be attempting to find (except when the patient is very frustrated and needs something quickly, such as a bedpan).
    - Rephrase the patient's message aloud *to validate it.*
    - Do not pretend to understand the patient's message if you do not.
12. Encourage the patient to speak slowly in short phrases and to say each word clearly.
13. Ask the patient to write the message, if able, or draw pictures if only verbal communication is affected.
14. Observe the patient's nonverbal clues for validation (e.g., answers "yes" but shakes head "no").
15. When handing an object to the patient, state what it is *because hearing language spoken is necessary to stimulate language development.*
16. Explain what has happened to the patient, and offer reassurance about the plan of care.
17. Verbally address the problem of frustration over inability to communicate, and explain that both the nurse and the patient need patience.
18. Maintain a calm, positive manner, and offer reassurance (e.g., "I know this is very hard for you, but it will get better if we work on it together").
19. Talk to the patient as an adult. Be respectful, and avoid talking down to the patient.
20. Do not discuss the patient's condition or hold conversations in the patient's presence without including him or her in the discussion. *This may be the reason some aphasic patients develop paranoid thoughts.*
21. Do not exhibit disapproval of emotional utterances or spontaneous use of profanity; instead, offer calm, quiet reassurance.
22. If the patient makes an error in speech, do not reprimand or scold but try to compliment the patient by saying, "That was a good try."

23. Delay conversation if the patient is tired. ***The symptoms of aphasia worsen if the patient is fatigued, anxious, or upset.***

24. Be prepared for emotional outbursts and tears from patients who have more difficulty in expressing themselves than with understanding. The patient may become depressed, refuse treatment and food, ignore relatives, and push objects away. Comfort the patient with statements such as, "I know it's frustrating and you feel sad, but you are not alone. Other people who have had strokes have felt the way you do. We will be here to help you get through this."

NURSING MANAGEMENT PLAN
Ineffective Airway Clearance

Definition: Inability to clear secretions or obstructions from the respiratory tract to maintain a clear airway

Ineffective Airway Clearance Related to Excessive Secretions or Abnormal Viscosity of Mucus

Defining Characteristics
- Abnormal breath sounds (displaced normal sounds, adventitious sounds, diminished or absent sounds)
- Ineffective cough with or without sputum
- Tachypnea, dyspnea
- Verbal reports of inability to clear airway

Outcome Criteria
- Cough produces thin mucus.
- Lungs are clear to auscultation.
- Respiratory rate, depth, and rhythm return to baseline.

Nursing Interventions and Rationale
1. Assess sputum for color, consistency, and amount.
2. Assess for clinical manifestations of pneumonia.
3. Provide for maximal thoracic expansion by repositioning, deep breathing, splinting, and pain management *to avoid hypoventilation and atelectasis.* If hypoventilation is present, implement the nursing management plan of care, Ineffective Breathing Pattern Related to Decreased Lung Expansion.
4. Maintain adequate hydration by administering oral and intravenous fluids (as ordered) *to thin secretions and facilitate airway clearance.*
5. Provide humidification to airways via oxygen-delivery device or artificial airway *to thin secretions and facilitate airway clearance.*
6. Administer bland aerosol every 4 hours *to facilitate expectoration of sputum.*
7. Collaborate with the physician regarding the administration of the following:
   a. Bronchodilators *to treat or prevent bronchospasms and facilitate expectoration of mucus.*
   b. Mucolytics and expectorants *to enhance mobilization and removal of secretions.*
   c. Antibiotics *to treat infection.*
8. Assist with directed coughing exercises *to facilitate expectoration of secretions.* If patient is unable to perform cascade cough, consider using huff cough (patients with hyperactive airways), end-expiratory cough (patient with secretions in distal airway), or augmented cough (patient with weakened abdominal muscle).
   a. Cascade cough—instruct patient to do the following:
      (1) Take a deep breath, and hold it for 1 to 3 seconds.
      (2) Cough out forcefully several times until all air is exhaled.
      (3) Inhale slowly through the nose.
      (4) Repeat once.
      (5) Rest, and then repeat as necessary.
   b. Huff cough—instruct patient to do the following:
      (1) Take a deep breath, and hold it for 1 to 3 seconds
      (2) Say the word "huff" while coughing out several times until air is exhaled
      (3) Inhale slowly through the nose
      (4) Repeat as necessary
   c. End-expiratory cough—instruct patient to do the following:
      (1) Take a deep breath, and hold it for 1 to 3 seconds.
      (2) Exhale slowly.
      (3) At the end of exhalation, cough once.
      (4) Inhale slowly through the nose.
      (5) Repeat as necessary, or follow with cascade cough.
   d. Augmented cough—instruct patient to do the following:
      (1) Take a deep breath, and hold it for 1 to 3 seconds.
      (2) Perform one or more of the following maneuvers to increase intraabdominal pressure:
         (a) Tighten knees and buttocks.
         (b) Bend forward at the waist.
         (c) Place a hand flat on the upper abdomen just under the xiphoid process and press in and up abruptly during coughing.
         (d) Keep hands on the chest wall and press inward with each cough.
      (3) Inhale slowly through the nose.
      (4) Rest and repeat as necessary.
9. Suction nasotracheally or endotracheally as necessary *to assist with secretion removal.*
10. Reposition patient at least every 2 hours or use continuous lateral rotation therapy *to mobilize and prevent stasis of secretions.*
11. Allow rest periods between coughing sessions, suctioning, or any other demanding activities *to promote energy conservation.*

NURSING MANAGEMENT PLAN
Ineffective Breathing Pattern

Definition: Inspiration and/or expiration that does not provide adequate ventilation

Ineffective Breathing Pattern Related to Decreased Lung Expansion

Defining Characteristics
- Abnormal respiratory patterns (hypoventilation, hyperventilation, tachypnea, bradypnea, obstructive breathing)
- Abnormal arterial blood gas (ABG) values (increased $Paco_2$, decreased pH)
- Unequal chest movement
- Shortness of breath, dyspnea

Outcome Criteria
- Respiratory rate, rhythm, and depth return to baseline.
- Minimal or absent use of accessory muscles.
- Chest expands symmetrically.
- ABG values return to baseline.

Nursing Interventions and Rationale
1. Treat pain, if present, **to prevent hypoventilation and atelectasis.** Implement the nursing management plan of care, Acute Pain Related to Transmission and Perception of Cutaneous, Visceral, Muscular, or Ischemic Impulses.
2. Position patient in high-Fowler's or semi-Fowler's position **to promote diaphragmatic descent and maximal inhalation.**
3. Assist with deep-breathing exercises and incentive spirometry with sustained maximal inspiration 5 to 10 times/hr **to help reinflate collapsed portions of the lung.**
   - Deep breathing—instruct patient to:
     a. Sit up straight or lean forward slightly while sitting on edge of bed or chair (if possible).
     b. Take in a slow, deep breath.
     c. Pause slightly, or hold breath for at least 3 seconds.
     d. Exhale slowly.
     e. Rest, and repeat.
   - Incentive spirometry—instruct patient to:
     a. Exhale normally.
     b. Place lips around the mouthpiece, and close mouth tightly around it.
     c. Inhale slowly and as deeply as possible, noting the maximal volume of air inspired.
     d. Hold maximal inhalation for 3 seconds.
     e. Take the mouthpiece out of mouth, and slowly exhale.
     f. Rest, and repeat.
4. Assist physician with intubation and initiation of mechanical ventilation as indicated.

Ineffective Breathing Pattern Related to Musculoskeletal Fatigue or Neuromuscular Impairment

Defining Characteristics
- Unequal chest movement
- Shortness of breath, dyspnea
- Use of accessory muscles
- Tachypnea
- Thoracoabdominal asynchrony
- Abnormal ABG values (increased $Paco_2$, decreased pH)
- Nasal flaring
- Assumption of 3-point position

Outcome Criteria
- Respiratory rate, rhythm, and depth return to baseline.
- Use of accessory muscles is minimal or absent.
- Chest expands symmetrically.
- ABG values return to baseline.

Nursing Interventions and Rationale
1. Prevent unnecessary exertion **to limit drain on patient's ventilatory reserve.**
2. Instruct patient in energy-saving techniques **to conserve patient's ventilatory reserve.**
3. Assist with pursed-lip and diaphragmatic breathing techniques **to facilitate diaphragmatic descent and improved ventilation.**
   - Diaphragmatic breathing—instruct the patient to:
     a. Sit in the upright position.
     b. Place one hand on the abdomen just above the waist and the other on the upper chest.
     c. Breathe in through the nose, and feel the lower hand push out; the upper hand should not move.
     d. Breathe out through pursed lips, and feel the lower hand move in.
4. Position patient in high-Fowler's or semi-Fowler's position **to promote diaphragmatic descent and maximal inhalation.**
5. Assist physician with intubation and initiation of mechanical ventilation as indicated.

NURSING MANAGEMENT PLAN
Ineffective Cardiopulmonary Tissue Perfusion

Definition: Decrease in oxygen resulting in the failure to nourish the tissues at the capillary level

Ineffective Cardiopulmonary Tissue Perfusion Related to Decreased Coronary Blood Flow

Defining Characteristics
- Angina for more than 30 min
- ST-segment elevation on 12-lead electrocardiogram (ECG)
- Elevated troponin I
- Elevated CK-MB enzymes
- Apprehension
- Shortness of breath

Outcome Criteria
- Systolic blood pressure (SBP) is >90 mm Hg.
- Mean arterial pressure (MAP) is >60 mm Hg.
- Heart rate is <100 beats/min.
- Pulmonary artery (PA) pressures are within normal limits or back to baseline.
- Cardiac index (CI) is >2.2 L /min/m^2.
- Urine output is >0.5 ml/kg/hr or >30 ml/hr.
- 12-lead ECG is normalized without new Q waves.
- Angina is absent.
- CK-MB enzymes and troponin I levels are within normal range.

Nursing Interventions and Rationale
1. Collaborate with the physician regarding the administration of thrombolytic therapy or percutaneous transluminal coronary angioplasty (PTCA) *to restore myocardial blood flow.*
2. Collaborate with the physician regarding the administration of aspirin, anti-platelet therapy and heparin *to prevent recurrent thrombosis and inhibit platelet function.*
3. Collaborate with the physician regarding the administration of beta-blockers *to decrease myocardial oxygen demand and prevent recurrent ischemia.*
4. Collaborate with the physician regarding the administration of angiotensin-converting enzyme (ACE) inhibitors *to block the conversion of angiotensin I to angiotensin II, a potent vasoconstrictor.*
5. Collaborate with physician regarding the administration of sublingual nitroglycerin (NTG) and/or intravenous (IV) NTG infusion *to augment coronary blood flow and reduce cardiac work by decreasing preload and afterload.*
6. Collaborate with physician regarding the administration of morphine *to control pain.*
7. Collaborate with physician regarding the administration of oxygen at 2 L/min to achieve SpO$_2$ >90% *to maximize myocardial oxygen supply.*
8. Maintain the patient on bed rest with bedside commode privileges *to minimize myocardial oxygen demand.*
9. Monitor patient's hemodynamic and cardiac rhythm status:
   a. Select electrocardiographic (ECG) monitoring leads based on infarct location and rhythm to obtain the best rhythm for monitoring.
   b. Evaluate cardiac rhythm for presence of dysrhythmias which are common complications of myocardial ischemia.
   c. Collaborate with physician regarding the administration of antidysrhythmic medications.
   d. Assess serum electrolytes (potassium and magnesium) and arterial blood gases (ABGs).
   e. Collaborate with physician regarding the administration of electrolytes to correct any imbalances.
   f. Monitor ST segment continuously to determine changes in myocardial tissue perfusion.
   g. Monitor patient's BP at least every hour as many conditions (drugs, dysrhythmias, myocardial ischemia) may cause hypotension (SBP <90 mm Hg).
   h. Treat symptomatic dysrhythmias according to unit's emergency protocol or Advanced Cardiac Life Support (ACLS) guidelines.
10. Instruct patient to avoid the Valsalva maneuver as forced expiration against a closed glottis causes sudden and intense changes in systolic blood pressure and heart rate.

NURSING MANAGEMENT PLAN
Ineffective Cerebral Tissue Perfusion

Definition: Decrease in oxygen resulting in the failure to nourish the tissues at the capillary level

Ineffective Cerebral Tissue Perfusion Related to Decreased Blood Flow

Defining Characteristics
- Decreased level of consciousness
- Hemiparesis or hemiplegia
- Visual changes
- Aphasia
- Dysphagia
- Facial droop
- Cognitive deficits
- Ataxia

Outcome Criteria
- Absence of neurologic deficits
- Blood pressure within ordered parameters

Nursing Interventions and Rationale
1. Collaborate with physician regarding the administration of thrombolytic therapy *to facilitate lysis of the clot and restoration of blood flow to affected area.*
2. Monitor the patient for alterations in blood pressure, oxygenation, temperature, rhythm and glucose levels.
3. Collaborate with physician regarding the administration vasodilators for hypertension *to maintain the patient's blood pressure within desired range.* Use caution in lowering blood pressure *as hypotension decreases cerebral blood flow.*
   a. Patients receiving thrombolytic therapy—keep systolic blood pressure (SBP) <185 mm Hg and diastolic blood pressure (DPB) <110 mm Hg.
   b. Patients not receiving thrombolytic therapy—keep SBP <220 mm Hg and DBP <140 mm Hg
4. Collaborate with physician regarding the administration of intravenous fluids and vasocontrictors for hypotension *as hypotension decreases cerebral blood flow.*
5. Collaborate with physician regarding the administration of oxygen to maintain SpO$_2$ >95% *to prevent hypoxemia and potential worsening of the neurologic injury.*
6. Collaborate with physician regarding administration of acetaminophen for elevated temperature *as hyperthermia is associated increase morbidity in the stroke patient.*
7. Collaborate with the physician regarding the treatment of dysrhythmias *due to increased sympathetic nervous system stimulation.*
8. Collaborate with the physician regarding the administration of insulin for hyperglycemia *as elevated blood glucose as been linked to an increase the area of infarct.*
9. Collaborate with the speech therapist regarding the patient's ability to swallow before initiating oral feedings *to ensure patient is not at risk for aspirating.*
10. Collaborate with the physical therapist to assess the patient's ability to ambulate safely *to ensure the patient is not at risk for falling* and ability to perform activities of daily living *to facilitate discharge home.*
11. Maintain surveillance for complications such as increased intracranial pressure, seizures, and acute respiratory failure.

Ineffective Cerebral Tissue Perfusion Related to Hemorrhage

Defining Characteristics
Intracerebral Hemorrhage
- Alteration in level of consciousness
- Nausea and vomiting
- Headache
- Seizures
- Hypertension
- Focal neurologic deficits

Subarachnoid Hemorrhage
- Sudden onset of severe headache, nausea, and/or vomiting
- Symptoms of meningeal irritation:
  - Nuchal rigidity and pain
  - Back pain
  - Bilateral leg pain
  - Kernig's sign: resistance to full extension of the leg at the knee when the hip is flexed
  - Brudzinski's sign: flexion of the hip and knee during passive neck flexion
- Photophobia and visual changes
- Sudden loss of consciousness
- Altered level of consciousness
- Seizures
- Focal neurologic deficits

Outcome Criteria
- Patient is oriented to time, place, person, and situation.
- Pupils are equal and normoreactive.
- BP is within patient's norm.
- Motor function is bilaterally equal.
- Headache, nausea, and vomiting are absent.
- Patient verbalizes importance of and displays compliance with reduced activity.

Nursing Interventions and Rationale
1. Assess for indicators of increased intracranial pressure (ICP) and brain herniation (see the nursing management plan Decreased Intracranial Adaptive Capacity Related to Failure of Normal Intracranial Compensatory Mechanism).

2. Collaborate with the physician regarding the administration of anticonvulsant medications *to prevent the onset of seizures or to control seizures.*
3. Collaborate with physician regarding the administration vasodilators for hypertension *to avoid further bleeding.* Use caution in lowering blood pressure *as hypotension decreases cerebral blood flow.*
4. Initiate precautions *to prevent rebleeding.*
   a. Ensure bed rest in a quiet environment *to lessen external stimuli.*
   b. Maintain a darkened room *to lessen symptoms of photophobia.*
   c. Restrict visitors, and instruct them to keep conversation as nonstressful as possible.
   d. Administer prescribed sedatives as prescribed *to reduce anxiety to promote rest.*
   e. Administer analgesics as prescribed *to relieve or lessen headache.*
   f. Provide a soft, high-fiber diet and stool softeners *to prevent constipation, which can lead to straining and increased risk of rebleeding.*
   g. Assist with activities of daily living (feeding, bathing, dressing, toileting).
   h. Avoid any activity that could lead to increased ICP; ensure that patient does not flex hips beyond 90 degrees and avoids neck hyperflexion, hyperextension, or lateral hyperrotation *that could impede jugular venous return.*

NURSING MANAGEMENT PLAN
Ineffective Coping

Definition: Inability to form a valid appraisal of the stressors, inadequate choices of practiced responses, and/or inability to use available resources

Ineffective Coping Related to Situational Crisis and Personal Vulnerability

Defining Characteristics
- Verbalization of inability to cope. *Sample statements:* "I can't take this anymore." "I don't know how to deal with this."
- Ineffective problem solving (problem lumping). *Sample statements:* "I have to eliminate salt from my diet. They tell me I can no longer mow the lawn. This hospitalization is costing a mint. What about my kids' future? Who's going to change the oil in the car? This is an incredible amount of time away from work."
- Ineffective use of coping mechanisms
  —Projection: blames others for illness or pain
  —Displacement: directs anger and/or aggression toward family. *Sample statements:* "Get out of here. Leave me alone." Cursing, shouting, or demanding attention; striking out or throwing objects
  —Denial: of severity of illness and need for treatment
- Noncompliance. *Examples:* activity restriction; refusal to allow treatment or to take medications
- Suicidal thoughts (verbalizes desire to end life)
- Self-directed aggression. *Examples:* disconnects or attempts to disconnect life-sustaining equipment; deliberately tries to harm self
- Failure to progress from dependent to more independent state (refusal or resistance to care for self)

Outcome Criteria
- Patient verbalizes beginning ability to cope with illness, pain, and hospitalization. *Sample statements:* "I'm trying to do the best I can." "I want to help myself get better."
- Patient demonstrates effective problem solving (lists and prioritizes problems from most to least urgent).
- Patient uses effective behavioral strategies to manage the stress of illness and care.
- Patient demonstrates interest or involvement in illness or environment. *Examples:* patient does the following:
  —Requests medications when anticipating pain.
  —Questions course of treatment, progress, and prognosis.
  —Asks for clarification of environmental stimuli and events.
  —Seeks out supportive individuals in his or her environment.
  —Uses coping mechanisms and strategies more effectively to manage situational crisis.
  —Demonstrates significant reduction in impulsive, angry, or aggressive outbursts (projection, shouting, cursing) directed toward family.
  —Verbalizes future-based plans, with cessation of self-directed aggressive acts and suicidal thoughts.
  —Willingly complies with treatment regimen.
  —Begins to participate in self-care.

Nursing Interventions and Rationale
1. Actively listen and respond to patient's verbal and behavioral expressions. ***Active listening signifies unconditional respect and acceptance for the patient as a worthwhile individual. It builds trust and rapport, guides the nurse toward problem areas, encourages the patient to express concerns, and promotes compliance.***
2. Offer effective coping strategies to help the patient better tolerate the stressors related to his or her illness and care. Give permission to vent feelings in a safe setting. *Sample statements:* "I don't blame you for feeling angry or frustrated." "Others who are ill like you have expressed similar feelings." "I will listen to anything you want to share with me." "We don't have to talk; I'd like to sit here with you." "It's perfectly OK to cry." ***Individuals who are provided with opportunities to express their feelings will be better able to release pent-up emotions and derive a greater sense of relief and comfort. Thus they are less likely to resort to overly impulsive, aggressive acts, which may harm self or others.***
3. Inform the family of the patient's need to displace anger occasionally but that you will be working with the patient to help him or her release his or her feelings in a more constructive, effective way. ***Family members who are well-informed are better equipped to cope with their loved one's emotional anguish and outbursts. They are less likely to waste energy on feelings of guilt, fear, anger, or despair and can use their strength to help the patient in more constructive ways. The knowledge that their loved one is being cared for emotionally, as well as physically, will offer family members a greater sense of comfort and understanding. They will feel nurtured and respected by the nurse's attempt to include them in the process.***
4. With the patient, list and number problems from the most to least urgent. Assist him or her in finding immediate solutions for most urgent problems; postpone those that can wait; delegate some to family members; and help him or her to acknowledge problems that are beyond his or her control. ***Listing and numbering problems in an organized fashion help to break them down into more manageable "pieces" so that the patient is better able to identify solutions for those that are solvable and to suppress those that are less relevant or not amenable to interventions.***
5. Identify individuals in the patient's environment who best help him or her to cope, as well as those who do not.

Validate your observations with the patient. *Sample statements*: "I notice you seemed more relaxed during your daughter's visit." "After the clergy left, you were able to sleep a bit longer than usual; would you like to see him more often?" "Your grandson was a bit upset today; I'll be glad to talk to him if you like." ***Supportive persons can invoke a calming effect on the patient's physiologic and psychologic states. Conversely, well-meaning but nonsupportive individuals can have a deleterious effect on the patient's ability to cope and must be carefully screened and counseled by the nurse.***

6. Teach the patient effective cognitive strategies to help him or her better manage the stress of critical illness and care. Help him or her construct pleasant thoughts, situations, or images that can simultaneously inhibit unpleasant realities. *Examples*: a day at the beach, a walk in the park, drinking a glass of wine, or being with a loved one. ***Pleasant thoughts and images constructed during critical illness and care tend to inhibit or reduce the intensity of the unpleasant, stressful effects of the experience.***

7. Assist the patient in using coping mechanisms more effectively so he or she can better manage his or her situational crisis.
   - Suppression of problems beyond his or her control
   - Compensation for illness and its effects; focusing on his or her strengths, interests, family, and spiritual beliefs
   - Adaptive displacement of anger, fear, or frustration through healthy, verbal expressions to staff. ***Effective use of coping mechanisms helps to assuage the patient's painful feelings in a safe setting. Thus the patient is strengthened and need not resort to the use of more ineffective defenses to eliminate anxiety.***

8. Initiate a suicidal assessment if the patient verbalizes the desire to die, states that life is not worth living, or exhibits self-directed aggression. *Sample statement:* "We know that this is a bad time for you. You're saying repeatedly that you want to die. Are you planning to harm yourself?" If the response is "yes," remain with the patient, alert staff members, and provide for psychiatric consultation as soon as possible. Continue to express concern to the patient and protect him or her from harm. ***Suicidal thoughts as a result of ineffective coping or exhaustion of coping devices are not an uncommon occurrence in critically ill patients. If the mood state is distressing enough, a patient may seek relief by attempting a self-destructive act. Although the patient may not imminently have the energy to succeed in his or her attempt, voicing a specific plan signifies a depressed mood state and depletion of coping strategies. Thus immediate intervention is needed, since the attempt may be successful when the patient's energy is restored.***

9. Encourage the patient to participate in self-care activities and treatment regimen in accordance with his or her level of progress. Offer praise for his or her efforts toward self-care. ***Patients who take an active role in their own treatment and progress are less apt to feel like helpless or powerless victims. This greater sense of control over their illness and environment will guide them more swiftly toward becoming as independent as possible.***

NURSING MANAGEMENT PLAN
Ineffective Gastrointestinal Tissue Perfusion

Definition: Decrease in oxygen resulting in the failure to nourish the tissues at the capillary level

Ineffective Gastrointestinal Tissue Perfusion Related to Decreased Gastrointestinal Blood Flow

Defining Characteristics
- Abdominal pain
- Melena
- Abdominal distention
- Hyperactive to absent bowel sounds range from hyperactive to absent
- Guarding
- Fever
- Hypotension
- Tachycardia
- Altered mental status
- Urine output <30 ml/hr

Outcome Criteria
- Normal bowel sounds
- Absence of abdominal pain, distention, and guarding
- Urinary output is >30 ml/hr.
- Vital signs at baseline
- Normal mentation

Nursing Interventions and Rationales
1. Collaborate with physician regarding the administration of crystalloids, colloids, blood, and blood products *to maintain adequate circulating volume.* Implement the nursing management plan, Deficit Fluid Volume Related to Absolute Loss.
2. Collaborate with physician regarding pain management. Implement the nursing management plan, Acute Pain Related to Transmission and Perception of Cutaneous, Visceral, Muscular, or Ischemic Impulses.
3. Collaborate with physician regarding the administration of oxygen to maintain SpO_2 >92% *to prevent hypoxemia and potential worsening of the gastrointestinal injury.*
4. Collaborate with physician regarding the administration of electrolyte replacement therapy *to maintain adequate electrolyte balance.*
5. Collaborate with dietitian regarding administration of nutrition *as patient will be unable to eat.* Implement the nursing management plan, Imbalanced Nutrition: Less Than Body Requirements.
6. Maintain surveillance for complications such as gastrointestinal hemorrhage, hypovolemic shock, and septic shock.
7. Collaborate with physician regarding preparation for surgery *to remove infarcted bowel.*

NURSING MANAGEMENT PLAN
Ineffective Peripheral Tissue Perfusion

Definition: Decrease in oxygen resulting in the failure to nourish the tissues at the capillary level

Ineffective Peripheral Tissue Perfusion Related to Decreased Peripheral Blood Flow

Defining Characteristics
- Weak and/or unequal peripheral pulses
- Delayed capillary refill
- Ischemic pain from extremity
- Cool skin on extremity
- Pale extremity
- Paresthesias from extremity

Outcome Criteria
- Peripheral pulses are full and equal bilaterally.
- Capillary refill is equal bilaterally.
- Ischemic pain is absent.
- Skin temperature is equal in both extremities.
- Skin is pink and warm in both extremities.
- Paresthesias are absent.

Nursing Interventions and Rationale
1. Collaborate with physician regarding the administration of antiplatelet, anticoagulant, and/or thrombolytic therapy.
2. Collaborate with physician regarding pain management. Implement the nursing management plan of care, Acute Pain Related to Transmission and Perception of Cutaneous, Visceral, Muscular, or Ischemic Impulses.
3. Ensure patient is adequately hydrated *to decrease blood viscosity.*
4. Maintain affected extremity in dependent position if possible *to enhance blood flow.*
5. Keep affected extremity warm and protect it from injury. *Do not apply heat directly to the affected extremity as this can result in injury.*
6. Maintain surveillance for pain, pallor, pulselessness, paresthesia, paralysis, and poikilothermia *as indicators of abrupt change in blood flow.*
7. Maintain surveillance for tissue breakdown and arterial ulcers *as indicators of injury.*
8. Prepare patient for possible surgery or interventional procedure to restore blood flow.

NURSING MANAGEMENT PLAN

Ineffective Renal Tissue Perfusion

Definition: Decrease in oxygen resulting in the failure to nourish the tissues at the capillary level

Ineffective Renal Tissue Perfusion Related to Decreased Renal Blood Flow

Defining Characteristics
- Anuria or oliguria
- Decreased urinary creatinine clearance
- Increased serum creatinine
- Increased blood urea nitrogen (BUN)
- Electrolyte abnormalities: potassium, sodium
- Increased MAP, pulmonary artery occlusion pressure (PAOP), pulmonary artery diastolic (PAD) pressure, central venous pressure (CVP) secondary to fluid overload
- Sinus tachycardia
- Metabolic acidosis
- Crackles on lung auscultation
- Engorged neck veins
- Fluid weight gain
- Pitting edema
- Mental status changes
- Anemia

Outcome Criteria
- CO is >4.0 L /min.
- CI is >2.2 L /min/m^2.
- MAP, PAOP, PAD, and CVP are within normal limits for patient.
- Electrolytes are within normal range.
- Serum creatinine and BUN are within normal range.
- Normal acid-base balance.
- Level of consciousness is normal.
- Lungs are clear on auscultation.
- Urinary output is within normal limits, or patient is stable on dialysis.
- Hemoglobin and hematocrit values are stable.

Nursing Interventions and Rationale
1. Monitor intake and output, urine output, and patient weight.
2. Collaborate with physician regarding the administration of crystalloids, colloids, blood, and blood products *to increase circulating volume and maintain MAP >70 mm Hg.*
3. Collaborate with physician regarding the administration of inotropes *to enhance myocardial contractility and increase CI to >2.5 L /min.*
4. Collaborate with physician regarding the administration of diuretics to the oliguric patient *to flush out cellular debris and increase urine output.*
5. Minimize the patient's exposure to nephrotoxic drugs *to decrease damage to kidneys.*
6. Monitor blood levels of drugs cleared by kidneys *to avoid accumulation.*
7. Monitor patient for signs of electrolyte imbalance *due to impaired electrolyte regulation.*
8. Maintain surveillance for signs and symptoms of fluid overload.
9. Monitor patient's clinical status and response to dialysis therapy *to ensure the patient is receiving safe and effective dialytic therapy.*

NURSING MANAGEMENT PLAN
Powerlessness

Definition: Perception that one's own action will not significantly affect an outcome; a perceived lack of control over a current situation or immediate happening

Powerlessness Related to Lack of Control Over Current Situation and/or Disease Progression

Defining Characteristics

Severe
- Verbal expressions of having no control or influence over situation
- Verbal expressions of having no control or influence over outcome
- Verbal expressions of having no control over self-care
- Depression over physical deterioration that occurs despite patient's compliance with regiments
- Apathy

Moderate
- Nonparticipation in care or decision making when opportunities are provided
- Expressions of dissatisfaction and frustration about inability to perform previous tasks and/or activities
- Lack of progress monitoring
- Expressions of doubt about role performance
- Reluctance to express true feelings, fearing alienation from caregivers
- Passivity
- Inability to seek information about care
- Dependence on others that may result in irritability, resentment, anger, and guilt
- No defense of self-care practices when challenged

Low
- Passivity

Outcome Criteria
- Patient verbalizes increased control over situation by wanting to do things his or her way.
- Patient actively participates in planning care.
- Patient requests needed information.
- Patient chooses to participate in self-care activities.
- Patient monitors progress.

Nursing Interventions and Rationale
1. Evaluate the patient's feelings and perception of the reasons for lack of power and sense of helplessness.
2. Determine as far as possible the patient's usual response to limited control situations. Determine through ongoing assessment the patient's usual locus of control (i.e., believes that influence over his or her life is exerted by luck, fate, powerful persons [external locus of control] or that influence is exerted through personal choices, self-effort, self-determination [internal locus of control]).
3. Support patient's physical control of the environment by involving him or her in care activities; knock before entering room if appropriate; ask permission before moving personal belongings. Inform the patient that, although an activity may not be to his or her liking, it is necessary. *This gives the patient permission to express dissatisfaction with the environment and the regimen.*
4. Personalize the patient's care using his or her preferred name. *This supports the patient's psychologic control.*
5. Provide therapeutic rationale for all the patient is asked to do for himself or herself and for all that is being done for and with him or her. Reinforce the physician's explanations; clarify misconceptions about the illness situation and treatment plans. *This supports the patient's cognitive control.*
6. Include the patient in care planning by encouraging participation and allowing choices wherever possible (e.g., timing of personal care activities; deciding when pain medicines are needed). Point out situations in which no choices exist.
7. Provide opportunities for the patient to exert influence over himself or herself and his or her body, thereby affecting an outcome. For example, share with the patient the nurse's assessment of his or her breath sounds and explain that they can be improved by self-initiated deep-breathing exercises. *Feedback that the patient has been successful in helping clear his or her lungs reinforces the influence he or she does retain.*
8. Encourage family to permit patient to do as much independently as possible *to foster perception of personal power.*
9. Assist the patient to establish realistic short-term and long-term goals. *Setting unrealistic or unattainable goals inadvertently reinforces the patient's perception of powerlessness.*
10. Document care to provide for continuity *so that the patient can maintain appropriate control over the environment.*
11. Assist the patient to regain strength and activity tolerance as appropriate, *thus increasing a sense of control and self-reliance.*
12. Increase the sensitivity of the health team members and significant others to the patient's sense of powerlessness. Use power over the patient carefully. Use the words "must," "should," and "have to" with caution *because they communicate coercive powers and imply that the objects of "musts" and "shoulds" are of benefit to the nurse versus the patient.*
13. Plan with the patient for transfer from the critical care unit to the intermediate unit and eventually to home.

NURSING MANAGEMENT PLAN

Risk for Aspiration

Definition: At risk for entry of gastrointestinal secretions, oropharyngeal secretions, solids, or fluids into tracheobronchial passages

Risk Factors
- Impaired laryngeal sensation or reflex
- Reduced level of consciousness
- Extubation
- Impaired pharyngeal peristalsis or tongue function
  - Neuromuscular dysfunction
  - Central nervous system dysfunction
  - Head or neck injury
- Impaired laryngeal closure or elevation
  - Laryngeal nerve dysfunction
  - Artificial airways
  - Gastrointestinal tubes
- Increased gastric volume
  - Delayed gastric emptying
  - Enteral feedings
  - Medication administration
- Increased intragastric pressure
  - Upper abdominal surgery
  - Obesity
  - Pregnancy
  - Ascites
- Decreased lower esophageal sphincter pressure
  - Increased gastric acidity
  - Gastrointestinal tubes
- Decreased antegrade esophageal propulsion
  - Trendelenburg or supine position
  - Esophageal dysmotility
  - Esophageal structural defects or lesions

Outcome Criteria
- Breath sounds are normal, or there is no change in patient's baseline breath sounds.
- Arterial blood gas (ABG) values remain within patient's baseline.
- There is no evidence of gastric contents in lung secretions.

Nursing Interventions and Rationale
1. Assess gastrointestinal function *to rule out hypoactive peristalsis and abdominal distention.*
2. Position patient with head of bed elevated 30 degrees *to prevent gastric reflux through gravity.* If head elevation is contraindicated, position patient in right lateral decubitus position *to facilitate passage of gastric contents across the pylorus.*
3. Maintain patency and functioning of nasogastric suction apparatus *to prevent accumulation of gastric contents.*
4. Provide frequent and scrupulous mouth care *to prevent colonization of the oropharynx with bacteria and inoculation of the lower airways.*
5. Ensure that endotracheal/tracheostomy cuff is properly inflated *to limit aspiration of oropharyngeal secretions.*
6. Treat nausea promptly; collaborate with physician on an order for antiemetic *to prevent vomiting and resultant aspiration.*

Additional Interventions for Patient Receiving Continuous or Intermittent Enteral Tube Feedings
7. Position patient with head of bed elevated 45 degrees *to prevent gastric reflux.* If a head-down position becomes necessary at any time, interrupt the feeding 30 minutes before the position change.
8. Check placement of feeding tube either by auscultation or radiographically at regular intervals (e.g., before administering intermittent feedings and after position changes, suctioning, coughing episodes, or vomiting) *to ensure proper placement of the tube.*
9. Monitor patient for signs of delayed gastric emptying *to decrease potential for vomiting and aspiration.*
   a. For large-bore tubes, check residuals of tube feedings before intermittent feedings and every 4 hours during continuous feedings. Consider withholding feedings for residuals greater than 150% of the hourly rate (continuous feeding) or greater than 50% of the previous feeding (intermittent feeding).
   b. For small-bore tubes, observe abdomen for distention, palpate abdomen for hardness or tautness, and auscultate abdomen for bowel sounds.

NURSING MANAGEMENT PLAN
Risk for Infection

Definition: At increased risk for being invaded by pathogenic organisms

Risk Factors
- Inadequate primary defenses (broken skin, traumatized tissue, decreased ciliary action, stasis of body fluids, change in pH secretions, altered peristalsis)
- Inadequate secondary defenses (decreased hemoglobin, leukopenia, suppressed inflammatory/immune response)
- Immunocompromise
- Inadequate acquired immunity
- Tissue destruction and increased environmental exposure
- Chronic disease
- Invasive procedures
- Malnutrition
- Pharmacologic agents (antibiotics, steroids)

Outcome Criteria
- Total lymphocyte count is >1000/mm^3.
- White blood cell count is within normal limits.
- Temperature is within normal limits.
- Blood, urine, wound, and sputum cultures are negative.

Nursing Interventions and Rationale
1. Perform proper hand hygiene before and after patient care *to reduce the transmission of microorganisms.*
2. Use aseptic technique for insertion and manipulation of invasive monitoring devices, intravenous (IV) lines, and urinary drainage catheters *to maintain sterility of environment.*
3. Stabilize all invasive lines and catheters *to avoid unintentional manipulation and contamination.*
4. Use aseptic technique for dressing changes *to prevent contamination of wounds or insertion sites.*
5. Change any line placed under emergent conditions within 24 hours *because aseptic technique is usually breached during an emergency.*
6. Collaborate with the physician to change any dressing that is saturated with blood or drainage *because these are mediums for microorganism growth.*
7. Minimize use of stopcocks and maintain caps on all stopcock ports *to reduce the ports of entry for microorganisms.*
8. Avoid the use of nasogastric tubes, nasoendotracheal tubes, and nasopharyngeal suctioning in the patient with a suspected cerebrospinal fluid leak *to decrease the incidence of central nervous system infection.*
9. Change ventilator circuits with humidifiers no more often than every 48 hours *to avoid introducing microorganisms into the system.*
10. Provide the patient with a clean manual resuscitation bag *to avoid cross-contamination between patients.*
11. Provide meticulous mouth care at least every 4 hours and suction oropharyngeal subglottic secretions (in patients with artificial airways) *to avoid accumulation.*
12. Cleanse in-line suction catheters with sterile saline according to the manufacturer's instructions *to avoid accumulation of secretions within the catheter.*
13. Maintain the head of the bed elevated at 30 to 45 degrees in patient artificial airways *to decrease the incidence of aspiration.*
14. Use disposable sterile scissors, forceps, and hemostats *to reduce the transmission of microorganisms.*
15. Maintain a closed urinary drainage system *to decrease incidence of urinary infections.*
16. Keep the urinary drainage tubing and bag below the level of the patient's bladder *to prevent the backflow of urine.*
17. Assess the urinary drainage tubing for kinks *to prevent stasis of urine.*
18. Protect all access device sites from potential sources of contamination (nasogastric reflux, draining wounds, ostomies, sputum).
19. Refrigerate parenteral nutrition solutions and opened enteral nutrition formulas *to inhibit bacterial growth.*
20. Maintain daily surveillance of invasive devices for signs and symptoms of infection.
21. Notify physician of elevated temperature or if any signs or symptoms of infection are present.

Additional Interventions for Patient Receiving Immunosuppressive Drugs
22. Obtain blood, urine, and sputum cultures for temperature elevations >38° C (100.4° F) *inasmuch as elevation likely is caused by bacteremia or bladder or pulmonary infection.*
23. Auscultate breath sounds at least every 6 hours. *Pulmonary infection is the most common type of infection, and changes in breath sounds might be an early indication.*
24. Inspect wounds at least every 8 hours for redness, swelling, and/or drainage, *which may indicate infection.*
25. Inspect overall skin integrity and oral mucosa for signs of breakdown, *which place the patient at risk for infection.*
26. Notify physician of new-onset cough. *Even a nonproductive cough may indicate pulmonary infection.*
27. Monitor white blood cell count daily, and report leukocytosis or sudden development of leukopenia, *which may indicate an infectious process.*

28. Protect patient from exposure to any staff or family member with contagious lesion (e.g., herpes simplex) or respiratory infections.

29. Collaborate with dietitian regarding the patient's nutritional status and need for augmentation of nutritional intake as necessary *to prevent debilitation and increased susceptibility to infection.*

30. Collaborate with physician to remove invasive lines and catheters as soon as possible *to decrease potential portals of entry.*

31. Teach patient the clinical manifestations of infection. *A knowledgeable patient will seek medical attention promptly, which will result in earlier treatment and a decreased risk that infection will become life-threatening.*

NURSING MANAGEMENT PLAN

Situational Low Self-Esteem

Definition: Development of a negative perception of self-worth in response to a current situation

Situational Low Self-Esteem Related to Feelings of Guilt About Physical Deterioration

Defining Characteristics
- Inability to accept positive reinforcement
- Lack of follow-through
- Nonparticipation in therapy
- Not taking responsibility for self-care (i.e., self-neglect)
- Self-destructive behavior
- Lack of eye contact

Outcome Criteria
- Patient verbalizes feelings of self-worth.
- Patient maintains positive relationships with significant others.
- Patient manifests active interest in appearance by completing personal grooming daily.

Nursing Interventions and Rationale
1. Evaluate the meaning of health-related situation. How does the patient feel about himself or herself, the diagnosis, and the treatment? How does the present fit into the larger context of his or her life?
2. Assess the patient's emotional level, interpersonal relationships, and feeling about himself or herself. Recognize the patient's uniqueness (how the hair is worn, preference for name used).
3. Help the patient discover and verbalize feelings and understand the crisis by listening and providing information.
4. Assist the patient to identify strengths and positive qualities that increase the sense of self-worth. Focus on past experiences of accomplishment and competency. Help the patient with positive self-reinforcement. Reinforce the obvious love and affection of family and significant others.
5. Assess coping techniques that have been helpful in the past. Help the patient decide how to handle negative or incongruent feedback about the situation.
6. Encourage visits from family and significant others. Facilitate interactions, and ensure privacy. Help family members entering the critical care unit by explaining what they will see. Increase visitors' comfort with equipment; offer chairs and other courtesies.
7. Encourage the patient to pursue interest in individual or social activities, even though difficult in the critical care unit.
8. Reflect caring, concern, empathy, respect, and unconditional acceptance in nurse/patient relationships.
9. Remember that for the patient the nurse is a significant other who provides important appraisals of the patient and who can facilitate the change process.
10. Help the family support the patient's self-esteem.
11. Provide for continuity of nurse assignment to ensure consistent contacts that can *facilitate support of the patient's self-esteem.*

NURSING MANAGEMENT PLAN

Unilateral Neglect

Definition: Lack of awareness and attention to one side of the body

Unilateral Neglect Related to Perceptual Disruption

Defining Characteristics
- Neglect of involved body parts and/or extrapersonal space
- Denial of existence of the affected limb or side of body
- Denial of hemiplegia or other motor and sensory deficits
- Left homonymous hemianopia
- Difficulty with spatial-perceptual tasks
- Left hemiplegia

Outcome Criteria
- Patient is safe and free from injury.
- Patient is able to identify safety hazards in the environment.
- Patient recognizes disability and describes physical deficits present (e.g., paralysis, weakness, numbness).
- Patient demonstrates ability to scan the visual field to compensate for loss of function or sensation in affected limb(s).

Nursing Interventions and Rationale
1. Adapt environment to patient's deficits *to maintain patient safety.*
   - Position the patient's bed with the unaffected side facing the door.
   - Approach and speak to the patient from the unaffected side. If the patient must be approached from the affected side, announce your presence as soon as entering the room *to avoid startling the patient.*
   - Position the call light, bedside stand, and personal items on the patient's unaffected side.
   - If the patient will be assisted out of bed, simplify the environment *to eliminate hazards* by removing unnecessary furniture and equipment.
   - Provide frequent reorientation of the patient to the environment.
   - Observe the patient closely, and anticipate his or her needs. In spite of repeated explanation, the patient may have difficulty retaining information about the deficits.
   - When patient is in bed, elevate his or her affected arm on a pillow *to prevent dependent edema and support the hand in a position of function.*
2. Assist the patient to recognize the perceptual defect.
   - Encourage the patient to wear any prescriptive corrective glasses or hearing aids *to facilitate communication.*
   - Instruct the patient to turn the head past midline *to view the environment on the affected side.*
   - Encourage patient to look at the affected side and to stroke the limbs with the unaffected hand. Encourage handling of the affected limbs *to reinforce awareness of the affected side.*
   - Instruct the patient to look for the affected extremity when performing simple tasks *to know where it is at all times.*
   - After pointing to them, have the patient name the affected parts.
   - Encourage the patient to use self-exercises (e.g., lifting the affected arm with the unaffected hand).
   - If the patient is unable to discriminate between the concepts of "right" and "left," use descriptive adjectives such as "the weak arm," "the affected leg," or "the good arm" to refer to the body. Use gestures, not just words, to indicate right and left.
3. Collaborate with the patient, physician, and rehabilitation team *to design and implement a beginning rehabilitation program for use during the critical care unit stay.*
   - Use adaptive equipment (braces, splints, slings) as appropriate.
   - Teach the patient the individual components of any activity separately, and then proceed to integrate the component parts into a completed activity.
   - Instruct the patient to attend to the affected side, if able, and to assist with the bath or other tasks.
   - Use tactile stimulation *to reintroduce the arm or leg to the patient.* Rub the affected parts with different textured materials *to stimulate sensations (warm, cold, rough, soft).*
   - Encourage activities that require the patient to turn the head toward the affected side, and retrain the patient to scan the affected side and environment visually.
   - If the patient is allowed out of bed, cue him or her with reminders to scan visually when ambulating. Assist and remain in constant attendance *because the patient may have difficulty maintaining correct posture, balance, and locomotion.* There may be vertical-horizontal perceptual problems, with the patient leaning to the affected side to align with the perceived vertical. Provide sitting, standing, and balancing exercises before getting the patient out of bed.
   - Assist patient with oral feedings.
     a. Avoid giving patient any very hot food items that could cause injury.
     b. Place the patient in an upright sitting position if possible.
     c. Encourage the patient to feed himself or herself; if necessary, guide the patient's hand to the mouth.
     d. If the patient is able to feed himself or herself, place one dish at a time in front of the patient. When the patient is finished with the first, add another dish. Tell the patient what he or she is eating.
     e. Initially place food in patient's visual field; then gradually move the food out of the field of vision and teach the patient to scan the entire visual field.
     f. When the patient has learned to visually scan the environment, offer a tray of food with various dishes.

g. Instruct the patient to take small bites of food and to place the food in the unaffected side of the mouth.

h. Teach the patient to sweep out pockets of food with the tongue after every bite *to eliminate retained food in the affected side of the mouth.*

i. After meals or oral medications, check the patient's oral cavity for pockets of retained material.

4. Initiate patient and family health teaching.
   • Assess to ensure that both the patient and the family understand the nature of the neurologic deficits and the purpose of the rehabilitation plan.

• Teach the proper application and use of any adaptive equipment.

• Teach the importance of maintaining a safe environment, and point out potential environmental hazards.

• Instruct family members how to facilitate relearning techniques (e.g., cueing, scanning visual fields).

APPENDIX

Physiologic Formulas for Critical Care

HEMODYNAMIC FORMULAS

MEAN (SYSTEMIC) ARTERIAL PRESSURE (MAP)

$$MAP = \frac{(Diastolic \times 2) + (Systolic \times 1)}{3}$$

SYSTEMIC VASCULAR RESISTANCE (SVR)

$$\frac{MAP - RAP}{CO} = \begin{array}{l} SVR \text{ in units} \\ (Normal \text{ range } 10\text{-}18 \text{ units}) \end{array}$$

$$\frac{MAP - RAP}{CO} \times 80 = \begin{array}{l} SVR \text{ in dynes/sec/cm}^{-5} \\ (Normal \text{ range } 800\text{-}1400 \\ dynes/sec/cm^{-5}) \end{array}$$

SYSTEMIC VASCULAR RESISTANCE INDEX (SVRI)

$$\frac{MAP - RAP}{CI} \times 80 = \begin{array}{l} SVR \text{ in dynes/sec/cm}^{-5}/m^2 \\ (Normal \text{ range } 2000\text{-}2400 \\ dynes/sec/cm^{-5}) \end{array}$$

PULMONARY VASCULAR RESISTANCE (PVR)

$$\frac{PAP \text{ mean} - RAP}{CO} = \begin{array}{l} PVR \text{ in units} \\ (Normal \text{ range } 1.2\text{-}3 \text{ units}) \end{array}$$

$$\frac{PAP \text{ mean} - RAP}{CO} \times 80 = \begin{array}{l} PVR \text{ in dynes/sec/cm}^{-5} \\ (Normal \text{ range } 100\text{-}250 \\ dynes/sec/cm^{-5}) \end{array}$$

PULMONARY VASCULAR RESISTANCE INDEX (PVRI)

$$\frac{PAP \text{ mean} - PAOP}{CI} \times 80 = \begin{array}{l} PVR \text{ in dynes/sec/cm}^{-5}/m^2 \\ (Normal \text{ range } 225\text{-}315 \\ dynes/sec/cm^{-5}/m^2) \end{array}$$

RAP, Right atrial pressure; *CO*, cardiac output; *CI*, cardiac index; *SV*, stroke volume; *HR*, heart rate; *PAP mean*, pulmonary artery mean pressure; *PAOP*, pulmonary artery occlusion pressure; *BSA*, body surface area; *MAP*, mean arterial pressure.

LEFT CARDIAC WORK INDEX (LCWI)

Step 1. $MAP \times CO \times 0.0136 = LCW$

Step 2. $\dfrac{LCW}{BSA} = \begin{array}{l} LCWI \\ (Normal \text{ range } 3.4\text{-}4.2 \text{ kg-m/m}^2) \end{array}$

LEFT VENTRICULAR STROKE WORK INDEX (LVSWI)

Step 1. $MAP \times SV \times 0.0136 = LVSW$

Step 2. $\dfrac{LVSW}{BSA} = \begin{array}{l} LVSWI \\ (Normal \text{ range } 50\text{-}62 \text{ g-m/m}^2) \end{array}$

RIGHT CARDIAC WORK INDEX (RCWI)

Step 1. $PAP \text{ mean} \times CO \times 0.0136 = RCW$

Step 2. $\dfrac{RCW}{BSA} = \begin{array}{l} RCWI \\ (Normal \text{ range } 0.54\text{-}0.66 \text{ kg-m/m}^2) \end{array}$

RIGHT VENTRICULAR STROKE WORK INDEX (RVSWI)

Step 1. $PAP \text{ mean} \times SV \times 0.0136 = RVSW$

Step 2. $\dfrac{RVSW}{BSA} = \begin{array}{l} RVSWI \\ (Normal \text{ range } 7.9\text{-}9.7 \text{ g-m/m}^2) \end{array}$

CORRECTED QT INTERVAL (QTc)

$$\frac{QT}{\sqrt{RR}} = QTc$$

BODY SURFACE AREA

Many hemodynamic formulas can be indexed or adjusted to body size by use of a BSA nomogram (Fig. A-1). To calculate BSA:
1. Obtain height and weight.
2. Mark height on the left scale and weight on the right scale.

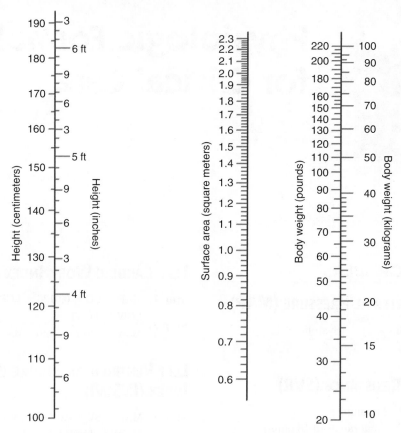

Fig. A-1 Body surface area (BSA) nomogram.

3. Draw a straight line between the two points marked on the nomogram.

The number where the line crosses the middle scale is the BSA value.

PULMONARY FORMULAS

CALCULATION OF THE SHUNT EQUATION (Qs/Qt)

$$\frac{Qs}{Qt} = \frac{Cco_2 - Cao_2}{Cco_2 - Cvo_2}$$

Cco_2 = capillary oxygen content (calculated value)
Cao_2 = arterial oxygen content (calculated value)
Cvo_2 = venous oxygen content (calculated value)

Normal value is less than 5%.

CALCULATION OF THE PULMONARY CAPILLARY OXYGEN CONTENT (Cco₂)

$$Cco_2 = (Hgb \times 1.34 \times Sco_2) + (Pco_2 \times 0.003)$$

Hgb = hemoglobin (measured via laboratory sample or arterial blood gas)
Sco_2 = pulmonary capillary oxygen saturation
Pco_2 = partial pressure of oxygen in capillary blood

Normal value is greater than 19 ml/dl.

CALCULATION OF ARTERIAL OXYGEN CONTENT (Cao₂)

$$Cao_2 = (Hgb \times 1.34 \times Sao_2) + (0.003 \times Pao_2)$$

Hgb = hemoglobin (measured via laboratory sample or arterial blood gas)
Sao_2 = arterial oxygen saturation (measured via arterial blood gas)
Pao_2 = partial pressure of oxygen in arterial blood (measured via arterial blood gas)

Normal range is 17 to 20 ml/dl.

CALCULATION OF VENOUS OXYGEN CONTENT (Cvo₂)

$$Cvo_2 = (Hgb \times 1.34 \times Svo_2) + (0.003 \times Pvo_2)$$

Hgb = hemoglobin (measured via laboratory sample or arterial blood gas)
Svo_2 = mixed venous oxygen saturation (measured via mixed venous blood gas or oximetric pulmonary artery catheter)
Pvo_2 = partial pressure of oxygen in mixed venous blood (measured via mixed venous blood gas)

Normal range is 12 to 15 ml/dl.

CALCULATION OF ALVEOLAR PRESSURE OF OXYGEN (PAO$_2$)

$$PAO_2 = FiO_2 \times (Pb - PH_2O) - PaCO_2/RQ$$

FiO$_2$ = fraction of inspired oxygen (obtained from oxygen settings)

Pb = barometric pressure (assumed to be 760 mm Hg at sea level)

PH$_2$O = water pressure in the lungs (assumed to be 47 mm Hg)

PaCO$_2$ = partial pressure of carbon dioxide in arterial blood (measured via arterial blood gas)

RQ = respiratory quotient (assumed to be 0.8)

Normal range is 60 to 100 mm Hg.

CALCULATION OF PaO$_2$/FiO$_2$ RATIO

$$PaO_2/FiO_2 \text{ Ratio} = \frac{PaO_2}{FiO_2}$$

PaO$_2$ = partial pressure of oxygen in arterial blood (measured via arterial blood gas)

FiO$_2$ = fraction of inspired oxygen (obtained from oxygen settings)

Normal range is greater than 400 mm Hg.

CALCULATION OF ARTERIAL/ALVEOLAR RATIO

$$PaO_2/PAO_2 \text{ Ratio} = \frac{PaO_2}{PAO_2}$$

PaO$_2$ = partial pressure of oxygen in arterial blood (measured via arterial blood gas)

PAO$_2$ = partial pressure of oxygen in alveoli (calculated value)

Normal value is greater than 0.74.

CALCULATION OF ALVEOLAR-ARTERIAL GRADIENT

$$P(A - a)O_2 = PAO_2 - PaO_2$$

PAO$_2$ = partial pressure of oxygen in alveoli (calculated value)

PaO$_2$ = partial pressure of oxygen in arterial blood (measured via arterial blood gas)

Normal range is 25 to 65 mm Hg or 100% O$_2$.

CALCULATION OF THE DEADSPACE EQUATION (VD/VT)

$$\frac{Vd}{Vt} = \frac{PaCO_2 - PetCO_2}{PaCO_2}$$

PaCO$_2$ = partial pressure of carbon dioxide in arterial blood (measured via arterial blood gas)

PetCO$_2$ = partial pressure of carbon dioxide in exhaled gas (measured via end-tidal CO$_2$ monitor)

Normal range 0.2 to 0.4 (20% to 40%).

CALCULATION OF STATIC COMPLIANCE (C$_{ST}$)

This value is calculated on mechanically ventilated patients.

$$C_{ST} = \frac{Vt}{PP - PEEP}$$

Vt = tidal volume (obtained from ventilator)

PP = plateau pressure (measured via ventilator)

PEEP = positive end-expiratory pressure (obtained from ventilator)

Normal range is 60 to 100 ml/cm H$_2$O.

CALCULATION OF DYNAMIC COMPLIANCE (C$_{DY}$)

This value is calculated on mechanically ventilated patients.

$$C_{DY} = \frac{Vt}{PIP - PEEP}$$

Vt = tidal volume (obtained from ventilator)

PIP = peak inspiratory pressure (obtained from ventilator)

PEEP = positive end-expiratory pressure (obtained from ventilator)

Normal range is 40 to 80 ml/cm H$_2$O.

NEUROLOGIC FORMULAS

CALCULATION OF CEREBRAL PERFUSION PRESSURE (CPP)

$$CPP = MAP - ICP$$

MAP = mean arterial pressure (measured via arterial line or blood pressure cuff)

ICP = intracranial pressure (measured via intracranial pressure monitoring device)

Normal range is 60 to 150 mm Hg.

Calculation of Arteriojugular Oxygen Difference (AjDO₂)

$$AjDO_2 = (SaO_2 - SjvO_2) \times 1.34 \times Hgb$$

SaO_2 = arterial oxygen saturation (measured via arterial blood gas)

$SjvO_2$ = jugular venous oxygen saturation (measured jugular blood gas or jugular venous catheter)

Hgb = hemoglobin (measured via laboratory sample or arterial blood gas)

Normal range is 5 to 7.5 ml/dl.

ENDOCRINE FORMULAS

Calculation of Serum Osmolality

$$\text{Serum Osmolality} = 2(Na^+ + K^+) + \frac{Glucose}{18} + \frac{BUN}{2.8}$$

Na^+ = sodium
K^+ = potassium
BUN = blood urea nitrogen

Normal range is 275 to 295 mOsm/kg of water.

Estimation of Fluid Volume Deficit in Liters

$$\text{Fluid Volume Deficit} = \frac{0.6 \text{ (kg/weight)} \times (Na^+ - 140)}{140}$$

Na^+ = sodium

RENAL FORMULA

Clearance

$$\text{Clearance} = U \times \frac{(V)}{(P)}$$

U = concentration of substance in urine
V = time
P = concentration of substance in plasma

Normal range depends on substance measured.

NUTRITIONAL FORMULAS*

Formulas for Estimating Caloric Needs

Step 1. Calculate basal energy expenditure (BEE). This is the energy needed for basic life processes such as respiratory function and maintenance of body temperature.

Women: BEE = 795 + 7.18 × weight (kg)
Men: BEE = 879 + 10.20 × weight (kg)

---

*Deitch EA: *Crit Care Clin* 11:735, 1995; Owen OE et al: *Am J Clin Nutr* 4:1, 1986; Owen OE et al: *Am J Clin Nutr* 46:875, 1987; Garrel DR, Jobin N, de Jonge LH: *Nutr Clin Prac* 11:99, 1996.

Step 2. Multiply by an appropriate stress factor to meet the needs of the ill or injured patient (see the following table). If the patient has more than one stress present (e.g., burn and pneumonia), use only the stress factor for the highest level of stress.

Type of Stress	Multiply the Value Obtained in Step 2 by
Fever	1 + 0.13/°C elevation above normal (or 0.07/°F)
Pneumonia	1.2
Major injury	1.3
Severe sepsis, burn of 15%-30% of body surface area (BSA)	1.5
Burn of 31%-49% BSA content (calculated value)	1.5-2
Burn ≥ 50% BSA	1.8-2.1

Estimating Protein Needs

Protein needs vary with degree of malnutrition and stress.

Condition	Multiply Desirable Body Weight (kg) by
Healthy individual or well-nourished elective surgery patient	0.8-1 g protein
Malnourished or catabolic state (e.g., sepsis, major injury)	1.2-2+ g protein
Burns	
15%-30% BSA	1.5 g protein
31%-49% BSA	1.5-2 g protein
≥50% BSA	2-2.5 g protein

Example of a Calculation of Calorie and Protein Needs

A 28-year-old female patient has a fracture of the left femur and burns to 40% of her BSA after an automobile accident. Her height is 1.65 m (5'5") and her weight is 59.1 kg (130 lb).

Energy Needs
1. BEE + 795 + 7.18 × 59.1 = 1219 calories/day
2. Energy needs for injury = 1219 calories × 1.74 = 2133 calories/day

Protein Needs
Protein needs = 59.1 kg × 1.75 g = 103 g/day

Index

SPECIAL FEATURES

CLINICAL APPLICATIONS

DATA COLLECTION

EVIDENCE-BASED COLLABORATIVE PRACTICE *NEW!*

NURSING DIAGNOSIS